Second edition

Diagnostic Cytopathology

Commissioning Editor: Michael J Houston
Project Development Manager: Sheila Black
Project Manager: Camilla Rockwood
Illustration Manager: Mick Ruddy
Designer: Sarah Russell
Illustrator: Jenni Miller

Second Edition

Diagnostic
Cytopathology

Edited by

Winifred Gray MB BS FRCPath
Consultant Cytopathologist/Histopathologist, John Radcliffe Hospital, Oxford, UK

Grace T McKee BA MB BS
Associate Pathologist, Massachusetts General Hospital,
Associate Professor, Harvard Medical School, Boston, USA

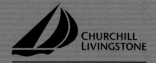
CHURCHILL
LIVINGSTONE

CHURCHILL
LIVINGSTONE

An imprint of Elsevier Science Limited

© 2003, Elsevier Science Limited. All rights reserved.

First edition 1995
Second edition 2003

ISBN 0 443 06473 3

British Library Cataloguing in Publication Data
A catalogue record for this book is available from the British Library

Library of Congress Cataloging in Publication Data
A catalog record for this book is available from the Library of Congress

Note
Medical knowledge is constantly changing. As new information becomes available, changes in treatment, procedures, equipment and the use of drugs become necessary. The editors and the publishers have taken care to ensure that the information given in this text is accurate and up to date. However, readers are strongly advised to confirm that the information, especially with regard to drug usage, complies with the latest legislation and standards of practice.

 ELSEVIER SCIENCE your source for books, journals and multimedia in the health sciences

www.elsevierhealth.com

The
publisher's
policy is to use
**paper manufactured
from sustainable forests**

Typesetting and Colour Separation by RDC Tech Group
Printed in China by RDC Group Limited

Contributors

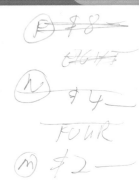

Måns Åkerman MD PhD FIAC
Associate Professor of Pathology,
Senior Cytopathologist, University Hospital, Sweden

Margaret Ashton-Key DM MRCPath
Consultant Histo/Cytopathologist, Department of Cellular
Pathology, Royal Sussex County Hospital, Brighton, UK

Fredrick G Barker MB FRCPath
Consultant Pathologist, Department of Histopathology
Hillingdon Hospital, Middlesex, UK

Christopher Barratt PhD
Professor of Reproductive Medicine, Assisted Conception
Unit, Birmingham Women's Hospital, Birmingham, UK

Mathilde E Boon
Senior Pathologist and Director, Leiden Cytology and
Pathology Laboratory, Leiden, Netherlands

Ian D Buley MA BM BCh FRCPath
Consultant Pathologist, Clinical Director and Senior
Clinical Lecturer, Cellular Pathology, John Radcliffe
Hospital, Oxford, UK

Stuart Coghill BMSc MbChB FRCPath
Consultant Histopathologist, Department of Cellular
Pathology, The General Hospital, Northhampton, UK

Marigold Curling MB BS MRCS LRCP
Consultant Cytopathologist, St Bartholomew's Hospital,
London, UK

W Bastiaan de Boer MBBS BMedSci FRCPA
Consultant Pathologist, Division of Tissue Pathology
Path Centre, QEII Medical Centre, Nedlands, Australia

Alastair R S Deery BSc MB BS FRCPath
Consultant Pathologist and Honorary Senior Lecturer,
Royal Free Hospital and School of Medicine, London, UK

J Denton MSc
Research Fellow, Department of Osteoarticular Pathology,
University of Manchester, Manchester, UK

Vikram Deshpande MD
Fellow in Cytopathology, Harvard Medical School
Department of Pathology, Massachusetts General Hospital,
Boston, MA, USA

Anthony J Freemont MD FRCPath FRCP
Professor of Osteoarticular Pathology, Laboratory Medicine
Academic Group, University of Manchester, Manchester, UK

Felicity Frost MB BS FRCPA FIAC
Consultant Pathologist and Head, Cytology Unit,
The Western Australia Centre for Pathology and Medical
Research, Perth, Australia

Winifred Gray MB BS FRCPath
Consultant Pathologist, Department of Cellular Pathology,
John Radcliffe Hospital, Oxford, UK

Rebecca Harrison BSc MBChB FRCPath
Consultant Pathologist, Departmant of Cytopathology,
School of Medical Science, The University of Birmingham,
Birmingham, UK

C Simon Herrington MA MBBS DPhil MRCP FRCPath
Professor of Pathology, Department of Pathology,
Duncan Building, Royal Liverpool University Hospital,
Liverpool, UK

Alec J Howat MB BS FRCPath MIAC
Consultant Histo/Cytopathologist, Pathology Laboratory,
Royal Preston Hospital, Preston, UK

Jane Johnson BSc(Hons) MB BS FRCPath
Consultant Histopathologist/Cytopathologist, Department
of Histopathology, Nottingham City Hospital NHS Trust,
Nottingham, UK

Thomas Krausz MD FRCPath
Director of Anatomic Pathology, Department of Pathology,
University of Chicago, Chicago, IL, USA

Irmeli Lautenschlager MD PhD
Senior Scientist, Department of Microbiology,
Helsinki University Central Hospital, Finland

Sanjiv Manek BSc MBBS FRCPath Dip RCPath (cyt)
Consultant Gynaecological Pathologist, Department of
Cellular Pathology, John Radcliffe Hospital, Oxford, UK

Euphemia McGoogan MBChB FRCPath MIAC
Senior Lecturer, Pathology Department, University of
Edinburgh and Associate Medical Director,
Lothian University Hospitals Trust, Edinburgh, UK

Grace T McKee BA MB BS
Associate Pathologist, Department of Cytopathology, Massachusetts General Hospital; Associate Professor, Harvard Medical School, Boston, MA, USA

Paul R McKenzie MBBS FRCPA Dip. Cytopath.
Senior Staff Specialist in Anatomical Pathology, Department of Anatomical Pathology, Royal Prince Alfred Hospital, Camperdown, Australia

David Melcher MA (Cantab) MB ChB (Cape Town) FRCPath FIAC
Formerly Consultant Histo/Cytopathologist, Department of Cellular Pathology, Royal Sussex County Hospital, Brighton, UK

Bernard Naylor MD ChB FRCPath FIAC
Professor Emeritus of Pathology, University of Michigan, Ann Arbour, MI, USA

Alan B P Ng MBBS FIAC FRCPA FASCP FASD
Formerly Consultant Pathologist, Head of Department of Anatomic Pathology, Royal Prince Alfred Hospital, Professor of Pathology, University of Sydney, Sydney, Australia

Rachel Oommen MB BS MD MRCPath
Consultant Histopathologist, Department of Cellular Pathology, William Harvey Hospital, Ashford, Kent, UK

Svante R Orell ML(Stockholm) FRCPA FIAC
Consultant Pathologist, Clinpath Laboratories, Kent Town, Australia

Ibrahim Ramzy MD
Professor of Pathology & Obstetrics and Gynaecology, Department of Pathology, Baylor College of Medicine, Houston, TX, USA

Denny Sakkas PhD
Director of Assisted Reproduction Laboratories, Department of Obstetrics and Gynecology, Yale University School of Medicine, New Haven, CT, USA

John B Schofield MB BS FRCPath
Head of Cellular Pathology and Associate Medical Director, Maidstone and Tunbridge Wells NHS Trust and Kent Cancer Centre, Preston Hall, Kent, UK

Keith B Shilkin MBBS FRCPA FRCPath FHKCPath
Consultant Pathologist and Clinical Professor of Pathology, Path Centre, Perth, Australia

Lambert Skoog MD PhD
Professor of Clinical Cytology, Department of Pathology and Cytology, Karolinska Hospital, Stockholm, Sweden

Russell Smith FIBMS
Formerly Clinical Cytologist, Department of Cellular Pathology, Royal Sussex County Hospital, Brighton, UK

Peter A Smith BSc MBBS FRCPath
Consultant Cytopathologist, University Department of Pathology, Royal Liverpool University Hospital, Liverpool, UK

Greg Sterrett MB BS FRCPA FIAC
Consultant Pathologist, Cytology Unit, The Western Australia Centre for Pathology and Medical Research, Clinical Associate Professor, University of Western Australia, Nedlands, Australia

Edneia Tani MD PhD
Associate Professor of Pathology, Division of Clinical Cytology, Department of Pathology and Cytology, Karolinska Hospital, Stockholm, Sweden

Walter R Timperley MA DM FRCPath
Professor of Neuropathology (retired), Department of Neuropathology, Royal Hallamshire Hospital, Sheffield, UK

Mathew Tomlinson PhD
Senior Andrologist and Honorary Research Fellow, Assisted Conception Unit, Birmingham Women's Hospital, Birmingham, UK

Xenia Tyler MB ChB FRCPath
Consultant in Histopathology and Cytopathology, Department of Cellular Pathology, Norfolk and Norwich Hospital, Norwich, UK

Eva Von Willebrand MD PhD
Senior Scientist, Associate Professor in Clinical Immunology, Transplantation Laboratory, University of Helsinki, Helsinki, Finland

Christine Waddell MSc MB ChB DObs RCOG
Consultant Cytopathologist, Honorary Senior Clinical Lecturer, Department of Cytology, Birmingham Women's Hospital, Birmingham, UK

Adrian Warfield MB ChB FRCPath
Consultant Pathologist, Honorary Senior Lecturer in Clinical Pathology, Department of Cellular Pathology, The Medical School, University of Birmingham, Birmingham, UK

Elaine D Waters MB BS FRCPA FIAC
Senior Consultant Cytopathologist, Dalkeith, Australia

Geoffrey Watson
Department of Anatomical Pathology, Royal Prince Alfred Hospital, Camperdown, Australia

Darrel Whitaker FIMLS CFIAC PhD MRCPath
Consultant Clinical Cytologist, Division of Tissue Pathology, Path Centre, Nedlands, Australia

Jennifer A Young MA MD FRCPath FFPath RCPI
Senior Lecturer and Honorary Consultant in Cytopathology, Department of Pathology, University of Birmingham Medical School, Birmingham, UK

Preface to the First Edition

This book aims to provide the reader with an easily accessible, comprehensive account of the diagnostic applications of exfoliative and aspiration cytology in laboratory use at the present time. To this end, a systemic and organ-based approach has been adopted. Descriptive text, plentiful illustrations, summaries of major diagnostic criteria and discussion of the pitfalls and limitations of cytology are included for conditions with well-established findings. The rapidly expanding areas of breast screening, transplantation and investigation of immunosuppressed patients by cytology are addressed in separate chapters to highlight their increasing importance.

The text is primarily concerned with the morphological features seen on routine light microscopy. However, in recent years cytopathology, like histopathology, has extended its diagnostic repertoire and therapeutic applications by incorporating some of the technical developments available and the advances in molecular pathology. Wherever appropriate, therefore, details of the use of ancillary procedures such as immunocytochemistry and electron microscopy have been included. Nevertheless, confident assessment of cell morphology remains the backbone of diagnosis; it is also an essential preliminary to the selection and correct interpretation of special techniques.

The book has been constructed as a benchbook for use by both experienced and trainee pathologists and for the laboratory staff engaged in primary screening work. It is not, however, a technical manual. The emphasis throughout is on how to achieve a diagnosis by microscopy. In general, only a brief overview of specimen preparation has been given, except occasionally to impart a particular piece of technical advice relevant to subsequent interpretation of the findings. There are many excellent accounts of basic laboratory procedures to which the reader may refer for details of preparatory techniques and for staining protocols. Magnification for the illustrations is given according to the objective used: low, medium or high power (LP, MP, HP respectively) or OI for oil immersion.

In contrast to histopathology, the initial assessment of many cytology samples is carried out by staff of varied training and experience. With this in mind, the chapters relating to subjects such as gynaecological screening and the respiratory system, for example, pay great attention to the normal anatomy, histology and normal cytological appearances and to the clinical relevance of findings. Other chapters, notably those concerned with the interpretation of fine needle aspiration biopsies, where evaluation is usually the responsibility of medically qualified staff, concentrate largely on the diagnostic findings.

A textbook of this size could not be written without the help of many people. I am greatly indebted to all of the authors of the chapters and to everyone who gave us encouragement and support during the process of writing the book. Colleagues from around the world have kindly provided some of the illustrations. These are much appreciated. I would like to add my personal thanks to all whose skills in photography, typing, word processing and the provision of sound critical advice were so necessary for completion of the book.

Finally, I would especially thank the publishers, not just for their expertise and seemingly endless patience, but particularly for the generous allowance of colour illustrations they have agreed to grant us. Cytopathology is the most visual of all sciences, requiring accurate colour discrimination as well as pattern recognition and constant vigilance. These ancient survival skills can really only be taught by long apprenticeship. It is hoped, however, that the chapters to follow, and their illustrations, will contribute to the understanding and enjoyment of the subject.

Winifred Gray

Oxford
1995

Preface to the Second Edition

Seven years have elapsed since the first edition of Diagnostic Cytopathology. In that time the whole field of cytology has expanded and developed, new techniques have emerged and the range of diagnostic opportunities in exfoliative and aspiration cytology has continued to grow. The time is right for a new edition.

Readers will note that some chapters have been rewritten, others updated, there are new illustrations for new entities and certain chapters have been adjusted to include new terminology. Several chapters are now merged and a completely new chapter on automation for cervical screening has been introduced. The Editor has been enormously helped in all of this by having an Associate Editor, Dr Grace McKee, who now works as an Associate Professor at Massachusetts General Hospital in Boston. Her influence on the book will span the variations in approaches to cytology on the two sides of the Atlantic.

Many thanks are due to all of the authors for the huge efforts that have gone into each chapter. Thanks are also due for all the assistance we have had from secretaries, colleagues, photographers and, not least, our own families. On a sadder note, the loss of several of the original authors who have since died is deeply regretted. As experts in their field, their contribution to this edition of the book still stands and has been acknowledged by each of the chapter authors.

It is hoped that this second edition of Diagnostic Cytopathology will provide its users with all necessary assistance in cytological diagnosis and will also capture the interest and enthusiasm of newcomers to cellular pathology. For the foreseeable future there will be a need for pathologists who can recognise the faces of the normal and abnormal cells they encounter at the microscope.

Winifred Gray

Oxford
2002

Contents

Introduction

1 Cytopathology: the past, the present, and a glimpse into the new millennium

Bernard Naylor and Ibrahim Ramzy

A simplified version of historical research is that of tracing an idea or observation in a certain field to its earliest proponent or discoverer and then citing, in chronological order, the names of subsequent investigators, as if their work constituted a direct continuance of a single line of thought. Such an approach is apt to give a false linear concept of scientific evolution, by ignoring the fact that ideas and observations may often be multicentric in origin, and their roots may extend beyond the boundaries of any particular field, into related or even unrelated fields. Cytology is a good example of this[1].

The early historical era

The first edition of *Diagnostic Cytopathology* covered the development of the discipline from its meagre beginnings in the nineteenth century, to its full acceptance by pathologists and clinicians by the end of the twentieth century. By then it had become obvious that new techniques and methods were in the stage of being adopted or investigated as to their applicability to cytopathology in the twenty-first century. However, we should not allow ourselves to lose sight of the origins of cytopathology in the nineteenth century.

Observations of normal and abnormal human cells, either exfoliated, or in imprints or scrapes, were steadily and independently recorded throughout the nineteenth century[2–5] and by the first decade of the twentieth, exfoliated cancer cells had been described in all of the types of specimens in which we look for them today[6]. These early reports however, were mostly regarded as scientific curiosities of little or no practical value. One fine example, published in 1861[7], 22 years before the birth of Papanicolaou, featured an exquisite drawing of cancer cells in pharyngeal secretion obtained post-mortem from a man who died with a growth in this throat (Fig. 1.1). To anyone looking at this illustration in 2002, it is obvious that the patient died from keratinizing squamous cell carcinoma.

For those interested in the history of the development of cytopathology, especially of the nineteenth century and up to the fifth decade of the twentieth century, its early historical era, we recommend the articles History of Cytodiagnosis[3] and The Century for Cytopathology[8], and the book: *History of Clinical Cytology: A Selection of Documents*[4]. Essentially, the situation even at the beginning

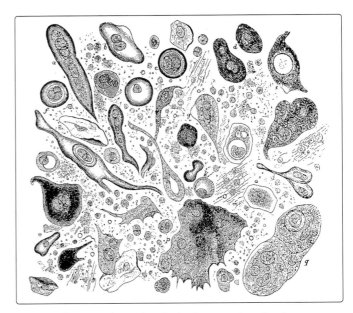

Fig. 1.1 Pharyngeal secretion obtained post-mortem showing keratinizing squamous cell carcinoma. This drawing appeared in the medical literature 22 years before the birth of Papanicolaou.

of the fifth decade of the twentieth century was that cytopathology as a diagnostic discipline hardly existed, that few pathologists had any knowledge of or interest in the subject, and that gynaecologists were unaware of its potential to benefit their patients.

The era of development and expansion

The second and most important era of cytopathology began in 1941, with the publication by Dr George N. Papanicolaou, an anatomist, and Dr Herbert F. Traut, a gynaecologist, of an article in the *American Journal of Obstetrics and Gynecology*: The diagnostic value of vaginal smears in carcinoma of the uterus[9]. Drs Papanicolaou and Traut were members of the faculty of Cornell University Medical School in New York City. Their article was followed in 1943 by their famous monograph *Diagnosis of Uterine Cancer by the Vaginal Smear*[10], with its superbly executed water coloured drawings of exfoliated cells and tissues. Gynaecologists, especially in the United States, were quick to grasp the significance of these two publications, which were succeeded over the next two decades by many more publications by Papanicolaou and his co-workers dealing with the cytological diagnosis of cancer in a variety of other organs.

Despite these seminal publications of 1941 and 1943 on the cytological diagnosis of uterine cancer, cytopathology did not become firmly accepted as part of the practice of anatomic pathology and in the training of anatomic pathologists for the next 15 to 25 years, with its acceptance varying to some extent between different countries and continents. There was a widely prevailing attitude about this situation, well-expressed by Gloyne in 1919, speaking of cancer cells in pleural fluids: 'Most pathologists are now agreed that it is practically impossible to identify these cells in film preparations'[11].

This statement epitomized the attitude that many pathologists felt toward cytopathology: many still remained sceptical or unsure of the validity of the diagnosis of cancer by cytology alone. The notion that cancer, whose unique attribute is its ability to invade tissue and metastasize, could be diagnosed by examining cells that had dropped off from an epithelial surface, seemed to smack of fraud. This is no longer the situation: virtually every major hospital in developed countries now provides a comprehensive service in cytopathology, and very few persons are now being trained in anatomical pathology without having exposure to the discipline.

Before dealing with the series of events that brought about this change, it may be of interest to learn more about the father of cytopathology, Dr George N. Papanicolaou (1883–1962). (A comprehensive and detailed account of the life and character of Dr Papanicolaou can be found in the books: *The Pap Smear: Life of George N. Papanicolaou*[12], by C. Erskine Carmichael and *A Woman Wanders Through Life and Science*[13], by Irena Koprowska. Also of interest are the articles of Koss, Koprowska and Naylor[14–16]).

Dr Papanicolaou was born in 1883 in the coastal town of Kymi on the island of Evia, one of the largest of the Greek Aegean Islands. His father, a general medical practitioner, was at one time mayor of the town. One hundred years later this small town, in collaboration with the Greek Government, the University of Athens and the Greek Society of Cytology, celebrated the 100th anniversary of the birth of its famous son (Figs 1.2–1.4)[16].

George Papanicolaou graduated in medicine from the University of Athens in 1904 and decided early in his professional life not to follow in his father's professional footsteps. He subsequently worked as a physiologist on the oceanographic vessel of Prince Albert I of Monaco, *L'Hirondelle II*. He acquired a doctorate in philosophy in natural sciences from the University of Munich, and served

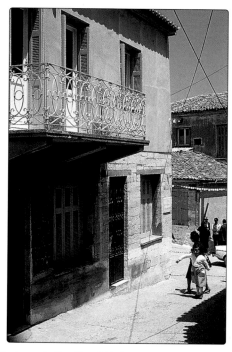

Fig. 1.3 The house in Kymi in which Papanicolaou was born and lived as a young child. It is now a municipal office.

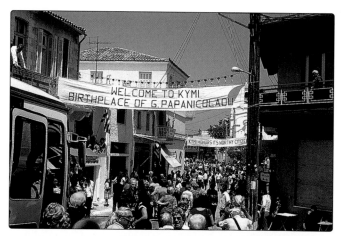

Fig. 1.2 15 May 1983. The town of Kymi on the Greek Aegean Island of Evia celebrates the 100th anniversary of the birth of Papanicolaou. (Figs 1.2–1.5 with permission, *Acta Cytol* 1988; **32**: 613–621.)

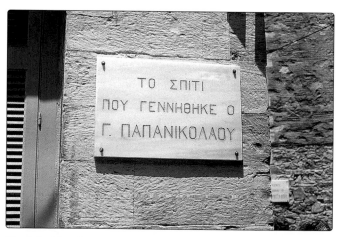

Fig. 1.4 The plaque on the house in which Papanicolaou was born, which reads in translation: 'The house where G. Papanicolaou was born.'

in the Greek Army during the Balkan wars, when he associated with Americans, volunteers to the Greek cause.

Undoubtedly, it was this contact with Americans, coupled with the poor prospects of launching a scientific career in Europe, which influenced Dr Papanicolaou to venture to the United States. The recently married Papanicolaous arrived in New York in 1913, where Dr Papanicolaou obtained a position in the Department of Anatomy at Cornell University. There he pursued his research on the oestrous cycle of mammals, using cellular samples from the vaginas of guinea pigs. Later he extended this work to humans and, inevitably, received vaginal smears from women with cervical cancer. He soon realized that he was able to recognize cancer cells in these smears, not that he was searching for them; he observed and recognized them serendipitously.

Cancer cells in vaginal smears had been recognized and briefly described and illustrated in publications of the nineteenth century[4,5,8]. Dr Papanicolaou's contribution to this field of cytopathology was two-fold: he recognized the importance of wet fixation of cytological specimens and he systematically began to accumulate examples of cancer cells in vaginal smears, culminating in his paper New Cancer Diagnosis[17], presented under the auspices of the Kellogg Foundation at the Third Race Betterment Conference in Battle Creek, Michigan, in January 1928. (Battle Creek, 160 miles east of Chicago, is well known in the United States as the world headquarters of Kellogg's, the cereal company.)

At virtually the same time, Dr Aurel A. Babeş (1885–1961), a distinguished academic pathologist in Romania, also published a major article[18] on the same subject in which he accurately described the appearance of cells of squamous cell carcinoma in scrapings of the uterine cervix. This article was preceded in January and April 1927, by two presentations of the subject by Babeş and his colleague Professor Constantin Daniel at meetings of the Bucharest Gynaecology Society[19,20]. However, these presentations made virtually no impact on the cytological scene. Babeş' technique of preparing, staining and examining vaginal smears was substantially different from that of Papanicolaou and would never have lent itself to mass screening for cervical cancer without modification.

The publications of Papanicolaou and Traut in 1941 and 1943 launched the second era of cytopathology, the era of development and expansion. This era saw the advent of screening for cervical cancer, which has revealed that undetected cervical cancer exists in all populations and that its detection by cytological screening is possible and practical. Concurrently with this development, the cytological method of cancer diagnosis began to be more widely applied to the respiratory, alimentary and urinary tracts as well as to the serous cavities and the central nervous system.

In 1954, Papanicolaou published his *magnum opus*, the comprehensive *Atlas of Exfoliative Cytology*[21]. Though

formally retired from Cornell University in 1951, his activity continued undiminished until his death in 1962, at the age of 77 years. He was buried in the country of his adoption, not too far from the university where he had spent most of his professional life (Fig. 1.5). In 1973, Greece honoured the memory of Dr Papanicolaou by issuing a postage stamp bearing his likeness. His adopted country, the United States, honoured its famous citizen in 1978, and in 1984, Cyprus issued a stamp depicting both Dr and Mrs Papanicolaou (Fig. 1.6); Mrs Papanicolaou was Dr Papanicolaou's long-time assistant in the laboratory.

This emphasis on the development of gynaecological cytology by Papanicolaou and his colleagues should not

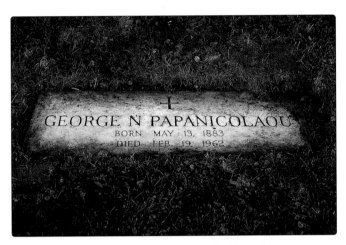

Fig. 1.5   The gravestone of Dr Papanicolaou in Clinton, New Jersey.

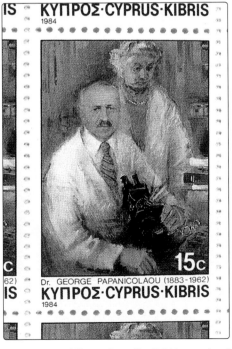

Fig. 1.6   Postage stamp of Cyprus issued in 1984 honouring the memory of Dr and Mrs Papanicolaou. (With permission, Director of Cyprus Postal Services.)

detract from many, carefully executed, earlier or contemporary studies of the cytology of other organs, reviewed in the publications of Grunze and Spriggs[3,4]. But unquestionably the impetus to the development of cytopathology as we know it today resulted from the painstaking research of Papanicolaou in the United States.

Inevitably, societies promoting cytology were founded locally, nationally and internationally. The forerunner of these was the Inter-society Cytology Council, founded in 1951 and later known as the American Society of Cytopathology. Many other societies developed over the next few decades, for example the International Academy of Gynecologic Cytology (1957), later known as International Academy of Cytopathology, the British Society for Clinical Cytology (1961), the Australian Society of Cytology (1969), and the European Federation of Cytology Societies (1969). These societies now have major roles in maintaining high standards in cytopathology by their educational activities, their contribution to the certification of pathologists and technicians in cytopathology, their influence in research, and their contribution to legislation that affects the practice of cytopathology.

The era of consolidation

A third era of cytopathology, an era of consolidation, was heralded by two publications: the first issue of *Acta Cytologica* in 1957, now the oldest journal devoted exclusively to cytopathology, and four years later, in 1961, by the publication of *Diagnostic Cytology and Its Histopathologic Bases* by Leopold G. Koss in association with Grace R. Durfee[22]. The publication of the Koss book in 1961 (Fig. 1.7), now in its fourth edition, brought together under one cover not only a body of theoretical and practical knowledge of cytopathology, but also the correlation between cytology and histopathology, a matter of great importance to anatomical pathologists who have an interest in cytopathology.

As might be expected, the last 50 years has seen an explosion in the literature of cytopathology, with thousands of articles and scores of books written on the subject. In the English language alone, there are now four journals devoted exclusively to cytopathology: *Acta Cytologica, Diagnostic Cytopathology, Cytopathology,* and *Cancer Cytopathology,* begun in 1957, 1985, 1990 and 1997, respectively.

A most important development in this era of consolidation occurred in the mid-1980s, when the technique of fine needle aspiration (FNA) cytology, long accepted and practised in Europe, especially in Sweden[23], became widely adopted throughout the world. Not only was this an outcome of the spread of cytopathological expertise, but it was also fostered by the development in radiology of diagnostic angiography, ultrasound, and computed tomography. These techniques have enabled the performance of fine needle aspiration of virtually any deeply seated organ, giving cytopathologists the opportunity to render valuable diagnostic service to clinicians and their patients. Paradoxically, it was in the United States that the first series of aspirations for neoplasms was published, from Memorial Hospital for Cancer and Allied Diseases in New York City[24-26], yet Memorial Hospital's influence in this field was insignificant; another half century had to pass before aspiration cytology became firmly established in the USA.

This development of aspiration cytology is in keeping with the prediction made to one of us in conversation with Dr Koss in 1978, that one of the biggest advances in anatomic pathology in the forthcoming decade would be the development and application of aspiration cytology. The events in this field confirmed the accuracy of this prediction and have now brought us, we believe, to the end of the third era of cytopathology, the era of consolidation. The ending of this era was summarized succinctly by Dr George L. Wied, Editor of *Acta Cytologica,* when he said 'The cytologic Crusades are over' (1990).

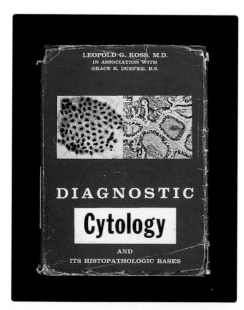

Fig. 1.7 An important landmark in cytopathology: the first edition of *Diagnostic Cytology and Its Histopathologic Bases,* published in 1961. (With permission, Dr Leopold G. Koss.)

The fourth era

A major event in cytopathology, one which straddles the end of the era of consolidation and the forthcoming era, is the attempt to define internationally acceptable terminology for the reporting of cervicovaginal cytology, an aspect of cytopathology that has been bedevilled by a variety of reporting systems that have not been understandable from one institution to another. This confusion was engendered by the reporting system that Dr Papanicolaou devised in the 1940s and which he maintained until his death, a system which employed 'classes' expressed as the roman numerals I to V, with Class I denoting no abnormality and Class V conclusive evidence of malignancy. Over the years, many laboratories adopted a class system of reporting, but unfortunately a certain class report from one laboratory often meant something different from the same class report of another laboratory, thus vitiating any comparison of results between laboratories. Prominent gynaecological cytopathologists in the United States, such as the late Drs James Reagan and Stanley Patten never used the Papanicolaou classes, preferring to replace them with readily understandable diagnostic statements. Their pleas to others to adopt such a method of reporting was often to no avail, since many clinicians believed they knew exactly what a Class III report meant, unlike cytopathologists who never had a consensus on the morphologic criteria for formulating such a report.

In December 1988, a workshop was convened at the National Cancer Institute in Bethesda, Maryland, to hammer out reporting terminology that would be a reflection of the development of cervical cancer and the near impossibility of discriminating with any degree of consistency between certain degrees of squamous intraepithelial neoplasia in cytological preparations. The outcome of this workshop, The Bethesda System for Reporting Cervical/Vaginal Cytology Diagnoses, was promulgated several months later, to be followed by a revision published in 1992[27] with another planned for 2001. Reports according to The Bethesda System provide information as to the quality of the cellular sample, a general categorization of the cellular findings, and a descriptive diagnosis of any abnormality. The system lends itself to computer entry, and its adoption could facilitate quality assurance measures and the international exchange of data.

In the 12 years since its initial publication, The Bethesda System has received general support in the USA from professional societies and has gained widespread acceptance in laboratory practice. Virtually all cervicovaginal cytology reports in the USA are now expressed in the Bethesda terminology. Several reasons may account for the acceptance of The Bethesda System: frustration with terminology of the past, the intrinsic simplicity and adequacy of The Bethesda System, and the need for standardized reporting terminology to deal with the advent of government-mandated proficiency tests in the USA for cervical cytology. However, many European countries, including the United Kingdom, have retained their three-tier system for reporting dyskaryosis (dysplasia) on the ground that, as yet, no firm scientific basis exists for introducing a change that reduces the information conveyed by the present terminology.

Governmental imposed proficiency testing for persons practising gynaecological cytology, is a direct outcome of an exposé published in *The Wall Street Journal* in November, 1987[28]. This dealt with the excessive demands made on their cytology technicians by certain for-profit commercial laboratories in the USA dealing with cervicovaginal cytology. This article caused an outcry in the news media in the USA, resulting in stringent Federal Rules regulating the laboratory practice of gynaecological cytology and the imposition of proficiency testing, which has not yet been implemented. To the reader, this may seem to be only one nation's concern: it should, however, serve as a warning to those practising gynaecological cytopathology in other countries not to demand excessive output from cytology technicians and not to neglect quality assurance practices.

Into the new millennium: innovations in technology

The dawn of the third millennium provides an opportunity to pause and attempt a glimpse at future developments, beyond the Fourth Era of cytopathology. Two major aspects are noteworthy: (1) impact of new technology with its prospects and limitations and (2) challenges facing cytopathology by the expectations of a society that demands perfect outcome, and how to prepare future cytopathologists and technologists to meet these challenges.

Imaging techniques and sampling devices

Perhaps the greatest challenge that faces the next era of cytopathology is to expedite the processing of cervicovaginal specimens while achieving maximum accuracy of interpretation. Accomplishing this goal has been a dream since the 1950s, when Mellors and colleagues in New York[29,30] studied the nucleic acid content of the squamous carcinoma cell using the fluorochrome berberine sulphate and observed measurable differences of fluorescence between benign cells and cancer cells. This was followed by numerous clinical studies of cytological specimens employing the same principle, but the method eventually fell into disuse when it was found that the degree of discrimination required by observers using this technique was essentially similar to that required with the standard Papanicolaou method. Nevertheless, recent technical innovations in several fields have left a clear impact on the discipline, shaping the ability and application of cytopathology in the diagnosis and management of disease. These advances are by no means limited to automated screening of cervicovaginal material; they include significant innovations in imaging modalities, sampling devices, tumour markers, and the emerging field of molecular diagnostics.

The evolution of imaging modalities enhances visualization and sampling of lesions that are not easily localized by older methods. Progress in this arena is expected to result in more refined and sensitive techniques that are more comfortable and carry less risk for the patient, and, as such, will certainly have an impact on the ability to sample areas that are now difficult or too risky to reach. Stereotactic localization and the ability to visualize masses in three dimensions, will continue to be enhanced in the future. Modern breast imaging is playing an important role in combating one of the most common cancers plaguing the human race. Current imaging technology also allows the determination of functional changes in some organs such as the brain, an organ that is still shrouded in a mysterious veil, often frustrating researchers and clinicians. The implication of these improvements in imaging for cytopathology is simple: if an organ or a lesion can be reached, a demand for interpretation of material procured from it will soon be created.

Sampling devices greatly influence the diagnostic accuracy of any test and the ability to establish definitive diagnoses. The use of new brushes and similar devices is now the standard of care, not only for gynaecologists seeking to sample the endocervix, but also for gastroenterologists, urologists and pulmonologists[31,32]. Indeed, the marriage of imaging and sampling techniques undoubtedly opens new fields. The use of flexible endoscopy and ultrasound to guide FNA by gastroenterologists is but one example of such development[33]. Although some of these new techniques enhance the role of cytology, others may actually replace traditional cytology, as in the case of ultrasound-guided core needle biopsy that has all but replaced FNA cytology as the method of choice for sampling the prostate and, in some institutions, the breast. The focus should always be on what is best for patients rather than how to save a specific procedure for a given organ. In this dynamic milieu, the role of cytology continues to evolve; witness the degree to which today's surgeons, chest physicians and endocrinologists are dependent on their cytology laboratory, as compared with the situation only 10 years ago.

Automated screening and processing

Fuelled by miniaturization and an almost logarithmic increase in computing power, automation is playing an increasingly significant role in the practice of cytology. Several companies raced to take advantage of this tremendous computer power to enhance the speed and accuracy of screening, and to relieve technicians of the burden of screening hundreds of normal smears to find the few abnormal ones. Pressures from the manufacturers were being brought to bear on the public and clinicians to demand 'State of the Art' processing and screening. Guidelines for instruments used for primary and for secondary screening were developed by the International Academy of Cytology[34] and by the Intersociety Working Group (ISWG), a group that included representatives from American and other national organizations of pathologists, technologists, and gynaecologists. The group also attempted to quench the thirst of the public and physicians for balanced, truthful and unbiased information about the

new liquid based technology and computerized screening[35–37].

Liquid-based technology offers automated processing to enhance specificity and sensitivity, especially with cervicovaginal cytology[38]. The lack of cellular debris, blood and exudate improves the ability to detect cellular abnormalities and may speed up the time required for screening. Rapid cell transfer from the sampling device to the transporting fluid containing the fixative ensures preservation of cell detail with minimal artifactual changes. Two technically ingenious automated processors, the ThinPrep[39,40] illustrated in Figure 1.8, and the Autocyte[41,42] in Figure 1.9, passed rigorous testing. Both devices are deemed satisfactory for routine screening purposes, by the US Department of Health and Human Services. Not only that, but US governmental rules now allow a cytology technician to screen more specimens prepared by this method rather than the limit of 100 specimens prepared by the conventional Papanicolaou smear technique. Liquid-based technology will certainly evolve with time; further modifications will be dictated by the requirements for automated screening, tumour marker studies, immunocytochemistry, the ability to use the material for *Human papillomavirus* and other molecular testing. After the initial flurry of excitement has subsided, time will bring to light the limitations of such techniques, giving way to more realistic and balanced expectations.

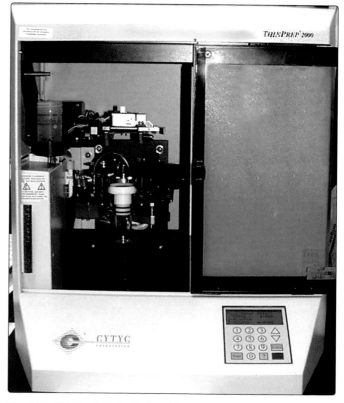

Fig. 1.8   ThinPrep® device for liquid-based smear preparation.

The advent of *automated screening* perhaps will distinguish the new era of cytopathology[43]. The quest for a fully automated screening system, first attempted by Tolles in New York in 1955[44], with a machine called the Cytoanalyzer, continues unabated. Wied surveyed the history of attempts since the 1960s to automate the screening of gynaecological cytology specimens fully and concluded that full automation was an impossible goal within the twentieth century. He stated 'If automation has a place in screening cytological samples, it will be in an interactive mode where the system scans the sample and shows so-called 'alarms' to a human observer for final analysis[5].

Automated screening devices met with mixed success until an increase in computing power permitted the development of several instruments[45]. The Papnet® system was designed for the analysis of conventionally prepared and stained smears, either for pre-screening or for quality assurance of slides found to be negative on prior manual screening. After training a neural network system on a series of normal smears, it will recognize abnormal cells or cells that differ from the normal reference. The abnormal cells are then displayed on a high-resolution television monitor for human assessment (Fig. 1.10). This two-stage system has great promise in that its approach does not use the traditional image analysis techniques that require image segmentation[46]. Unfortunately, for economic reasons, the system has been withdrawn from the market.

The Autopap® system was originally developed by Neopath and is currently part of the Tripath Imaging® system (Fig. 1.11). It uses three separate algorithms addressing single cells, thin cell groups, and thick cell groups and evaluates multiple cellular features to assign a score between 0.0 and 1.0 to each conventional smear. The score reflects the likelihood of having a significant abnormality, and the cut-off point can be adjusted to alter sensitivity and specificity, thus refining the ability to discriminate between significant preneoplastic and other less significant lesions. The system can be used for rescreening negative smears, thus reducing false negatives[47,48]. It can also be used as a primary screener to eliminate the need for manual screening of a percentage of smears, with the lowest score the ones least likely to be abnormal.

Although the new automated technology is available, its adoption as the standard of care is still under debate, particularly in the USA. Despite financial difficulties that led to consolidation of manufacturers and technologies, screening automation will stay in some form and economies of scale will eventually help to lower cost. Marriage of automated screening with automated processing will ensure more standardization of the way cells are spread and stained, thus improving the quality and reliability of automated screening.

Cytotechnologists will continue to have an important role to play, but their job description, and consequently the training requirements, will have to change. They will need to be more computer literate and will have to spend more time examining atypical cases, the cases that the automatic screener has designated as worthy of review[49]. There would be a challenge to seek new skills and to broaden the horizon. These changes are expected to improve patient care and reduce the risk of technologists becoming victims

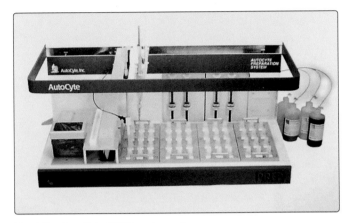

Fig. 1.9   AutoCyte PREP® equipment.

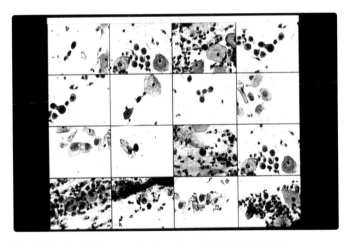

Fig. 1.10   Panel of images displayed from the Papnet® system.

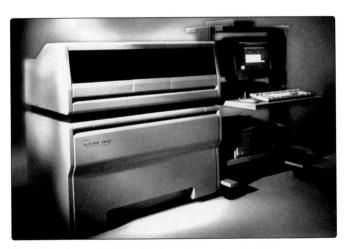

Fig. 1.11   Autopap 300® system for automated screening.

of the deadly 'burn-out' syndrome. On the other hand, looking only at cases the automatic screening machine classifies as abnormal may produce its own kind of tedium.

Tumour markers and molecular techniques

New *tumour and proliferation markers* are being developed for histological sections all the time, but many can be applied to fine needle aspirates by the use of immunocytochemical techniques. The specificity of many markers does not withstand the test of time, while others, such as prostate specific antigen (PSA) and CA 125, continue to hold their ground. It is safe to predict that the armamentarium will be expanded in due time to encompass a wide variety of prognostic markers for different malignancies beyond the few that we have today, such as the HER-2/neu and steroid receptors for breast cancer.

Molecular techniques undoubtedly will play a bigger role in the future[50]. Fluorescence *In Situ* Hybridization (FISH), polymerase chain reaction (PCR), gel-based analysis and Diagnostic Chip technology will leap forward with the advancing knowledge of genetics of disease, derived from mapping of the human genome. The development of sensitive techniques to detect the genomes for HPV, present in almost all cervical squamous and glandular cancers, raises hope that a molecular test capable of identifying patients with increased potential to develop cancer may offer an alternate to the Pap smear as we know it. The cost and availability of such testing may limit its role to the identification of mild changes that are likely to develop significant abnormality, but which are lacking clear morphological characteristics of preneoplasia. Cases cytologically interpreted as atypical squamous cells of undetermined significance (ASCUS), mild dyskaryosis, or low-grade squamous intraepithelial lesion, may be triaged to colposcopy only if the hybrid capture test for high risk HPV serotypes is positive[51,52]. To avoid unacceptable false results, these tests must be able to distinguish a latent or transient viral infection from an active one. Newer tests will undoubtedly be refined to increase their specificity and drop their cost to encourage their use, particularly in developing countries where a simple self-obtained test administered by the patient would be a welcome addition to our diagnostic resources.

Molecular probes for non-random translocations in leukemias, lymphomas, solid soft tissue sarcomas and for other cancer-related abnormalities are available, and the growing list includes p53 tumour suppressor gene, retinoblastoma gene, familial polyposis gene, neurofibromatosis gene and many others. Probe detection by fluorochrome has progressed from a single colour per hybridization to multicolour spectrally distinguishable probes for the 22 somatic chromosomes and the two sex chromosomes simultaneously. Miniaturization of

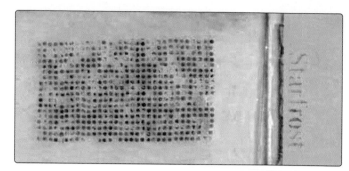

Fig. 1.12 Tissue microarray showing an array of 576 prostatic biopsy specimens on a single glass slide (Courtesy of Dr Gustavo Ayala, Houston, Texas).

computers has also allowed the development of new generations of flow cytometers. Cell cycle analysis can now be easily performed by flow cytometry of needle aspirates or by computerized image analysis. Both techniques, which can be easily adapted to cytology specimens, continue to undergo changes to enhance their sensitivity and specificity.

Microarray technologies, recently developed based on computer chip manufacturing methods, appear to have a great potential application by allowing high-throughput analysis of samples by the use of a large number of biological molecular markers[53–57]. These arrays can be of tissue blocks, oligonucleotides, cDNA or proteins (Fig. 1.12). Each type of array is used for a different reason, and has its own limitation and potential. For example, probes made from tumour RNA can be used to test the expression levels of thousands of genes placed on a single slide to detect mutations. To cytopathologists, these developments present a challenge and an excellent opportunity. At one point, treatment of malignancies may require classification by molecular techniques in addition to those of cytomorphology or histomorphology. This is not unlike the need for immunophenotyping in managing lymphomas, or HER2 expression for breast cancer. New classifications of tumours by criteria that cannot be discernible by morphology alone may arise. It is unlikely that a single biomarker assessed by any technique, be it molecular, immunohistochemical or flow cytometric, is specific for a malignant phenotype; thus the continuous need for morphology. Prostate specific antigen (PSA) is a good example of a specific marker that is elevated in cancer, but which can also be elevated with inflammation.

Molecular testing is not a threat to pathologists, but an opportunity for us to embrace the new technology and develop it. Cytopathologists can play a major role, since they will be asked to do more with smaller and smaller samples. A fine needle aspirate would be morphologically evaluated to ensure the presence of adequate sample and to identify it as being derived from a malignant neoplasm; the remainder of the specimen would then be triaged for molecular or other ancillary studies.

Meeting new professional challenges

Perhaps one of the major challenges that cytopathology increasingly faces is to meet the expectations of a society that demands perfect outcomes and clinical colleagues who are becoming more dependent on cytological methods. Although this is a reflection of success of cytopathology as a discipline, it dictates a need for evolution in the relationship between cytopathologists and other physicians, including surgical pathologists, and society. Unfortunately, the legal profession attempts to portray cytopathology as an exact science with well defined criteria for what is normal and what is abnormal; an unrealistic concept. In the quest to attain perfection we have attempted, as an example, to break down the continuum of slightly, moderately and markedly abnormal cells into clearly, but arbitrarily, defined entities. This blurs the fact that severe dysplasia (dyskaryosis) overlaps with moderate dysplasia on one side, and carcinoma *in situ* on the other side of the spectrum.

Although achieving perfection is a noble goal, the unrealistic expectation carries the risk of portraying one of the most successful cancer screening tools women have as an unreliable test in the eyes of the public. Cytologists should also resist the alternative temptation to report any slight cellular change from the perfect prototype as atypical squamous or glandular cells of undetermined significance (ASCUS or AGUS), thus practising legally 'safe' cytopathology, but resulting in unnecessary colposcopy, distress and expense for many patients.

Integration between surgical pathology and cytopathology, an inevitable outcome of acceptance of cytopathology by surgical pathologists, will gather more momentum in the future. When cytopathology started, 'true' pathologists (i.e. surgical pathologists) did not want to have anything to do with it, and it was left to gynaecologists, who saw the misery of cervical cancer first hand, to embrace the technique in its infancy. Although some surgical pathologists are still sceptical, the success of cytology and the widening of the sphere of influence of both subspecialties have gradually eroded the barrier that separates surgical pathology from cytopathology. More surgical pathologists will come to realize that squash techniques, touch preparations and bench aspirates, will offer them a valuable and different perspective of a resected specimen. These in-between techniques will be the routine standard of care, particularly in intraoperative consultations of thyroid nodules (the best way to see nuclear changes of papillary cancer) and lymph nodes (in lymphomas) and during prostatic or cervical cancer surgery. The methods can also provide useful information about intraoperative liver core biopsies, lung biopsies (granuloma versus cancer) and brain tumours[58]. Minute fragments of valuable material, such as is often the case with pituitary gland, pancreas and orbital needle biopsy specimens, should not be sacrificed at the edge of the frozen section knife, when a touch preparation might yield the diagnosis.

The ever-changing panorama of cytopathology and its scope will dictate the training of practitioners of cytopathology, both in content and methodology, to meet the demands of the future. Pathologists of the twenty-first century, particularly those who run an active FNA service, have to be capable of communicating effectively with patients and clinical colleagues. As the complexity, sophistication and cost of testing increases, wiser selection of tests and laboratory utilization become more critical, thus highlighting the interdependency between the treating physician and the pathologist.

Solid training in general anatomical pathology is critical for the proper training of a broad-based cytopathologist. Medical students should be exposed to the world of cytopathology, including fine needle aspiration and proper utilization of the laboratory early in their formative medical years. Future generations of cytotechnologists will encounter a broader practice, with samples from different organs arriving on their microscope stage. In order to cope with, and be able to detect abnormalities, more in depth knowledge of cytopathology of organs other than those from the female genital tract will be necessary. The increased accessibility to the Internet will continue to shape the future of delivery of new information, not only to physicians and technologists, but also to patients. It should not come as a surprise to us that some patients will show up in the FNA clinic already with many questions about their disease, after spending the previous night surfing the web at home. As the world becomes more interconnected, cytopathology is being offered a wonderful opportunity to enlighten, educate and change the perception of pathology and cytopathology through this medium.

Epilogue

The dawn of the third millennium opens up an opportunity for cytology to grow and have an impact on patient care in many ways. Many new techniques will disappear with the sunset, but others will thrive or evolve in a different format. The demand to get more information from smaller specimens will increase, clearly a golden opportunity to apply new methods to analyse cytological material. The evolution of cytopathology has been 'multicentric' in origin, which confirms the view expressed by Papanicolaou recorded at the beginning of this chapter.

If Dr Papanicolaou were alive today, he would be amazed and gratified by the events and the advances that have taken place in cytology since he gave his paper 'New cancer diagnosis' some 74 years ago (1928): The application of cytology to diagnosis of cancer in all of the systems of the body, the development of successful screening programmes for cervical cancer, the flourishing of aspiration cytology, the surge of interest in automated cytology screening systems, the application of molecular technology, immunocytochemistry and other sophisticated techniques to cytology specimens, the development of education and training in cytopathology for technicians and pathologists, the publication of journals devoted exclusively to cytopathology, and the development of numerous societies of cytology. These constitute an impressive list of achievements since Dr Papanicolaou made the tedious journey from New York to Battle Creek in 1928.

References

1 Papanicolaou G N. Historical landmarks in exfoliative cytology. In: *Trans First International Cancer Congress*. Chicago: 1956; 93–99

2 Hajdu S I. Cytology from antiquity to Papanicolaou. *Acta Cytol* 1977; **21**:668–676

3 Spriggs A I. History of cytodiagnosis. *J Clin Pathol* 1977; **30**: 1091–1102

4 Grunze H, Spriggs A I. *History of Clinical Cytology: A Selection of Documents*. Darmstadt: Ernst Giebler, 1983; 2nd edn

5 Wied G L. Clinical cytology: past, present and future. *Beitr Onkol* 1990; **38**: 1–58

6 Naylor B. The history of exfoliative cancer cytology. *Univ Mich Med Bull* 1960; **26**: 289–296

7 Beale L S. Results of the chemical and microscopic examination of solid organs and secretions: Examination of sputum from a case of cancer of the pharynx and the adjacent parts. *Arch Med* (London) 1861; **2**: 44–46

8 Naylor B. The century for cytopathology. *Acta Cytol* 1999; **44**: 709–725

9 Papanicolaou G N, Traut H F. The diagnostic value of vaginal smears in carcinoma of the uterus. *Am J Obstet Gynecol* 1941; **42**:193–205

10 Papanicolaou G N, Traut H F. *Diagnosis of Uterine Cancer by the Vaginal Smear*. New York: Commonwealth Fund, 1943

11 Gloyne SR. The clinical pathology of thoracic puncture fluids. *Lancet* 1919; **1**: 935–937

12 Carmichael C E. *The pap smear: Life of George N. Papanicolaou*. Springfield: Charles C Thomas, 1973

13 Koprowska I. *A Woman Wanders Through Life and Science*. Albany: State University of New York, 1997

14 Koss L G. George N. Papanicolaou – some reminiscences. *Acta Cytol* 1977; **17**: 1–2

15 Koprowska I. George N. Papanicolaou – as we knew him. *Acta Cytol* 1977; 630–638

16 Naylor B. Perspectives in cytology. From Battle Creek to New Orleans. *Acta Cytol* 1988; **32**: 613–621

17 Papanicolaou G N. *New Cancer Diagnosis*. Proceedings of the 3rd Race Betterment Conference. Battle Creek: Race Betterment Foundation, 1928; 528–534

18 Babeş A. Diagnostic du cancer du col utérin par les frottis. *Presse Méd* 1928; **36**: 451–454

19 Daniel C, Babeş A. *Posibilitatea diagnosticului cancerului cu ajutorul frotiului*. Proceedings of the Bucharest Gynaecology Society, Bucharest, January 1927; 55

20 Daniel C, Babeş A. *Diagnosticul cancerului colului uterin prin frotiu*. Proceedings of the Bucharest Gynaecology Society, Bucharest, April 1927; 23

21 Papanicolaou G N. *Atlas of Exfoliative Cytology*. New York: Commonwealth Fund; 1954

22 Koss L G. *Diagnostic Cytology and its Histopathologic Bases*. Philadelphia: J B Lippincott, 1961; 1st edn

23 Koss L G. Aspiration biopsy – a tool in surgical pathology. *Am J Surg Pathol* 1988; **12**: 43–53

24 Martin H E, Ellis H B. Biopsy by needle puncture and aspiration. *Ann Surg* 1930; **92**:169–181

25 Coley B L, Sharp G S, Ellis E B. Diagnosis of bone tumors by aspiration. *Am J Surg* 1931; **13**: 215–224

26 Stewart F W. The diagnosis of tumors by aspiration. *Am J Pathol* 1933; **9**: 801–812

27 The Bethesda system for reporting cervical/vaginal cytologic diagnoses: Report of the 1991 workshop. Luff R D, Chairman, The Bethesda system editorial committee. *Human Pathol* 1992; **23**: 719–720

28 Bogdanich W. Lax laboratories: Hurried screening of Pap smears elevates error rate of the test for cervical cancer. *The Wall Street Journal* 1987; November 2: 1

29 Mellors R C, Glassman A, Papanicolaou G N. A microfluorometric scanning method for the detection of cancer cells in smears of exfoliated cells. *Cancer* 1952; **5**: 458–468

30 Mellors R C, Keane J F, Papanicolaou G N. Nucleic acid content of the squamous cancer cell. *Science* 1952; **116**: 265–269

31 Kohlberger P D, Stani J, Gitsch G et al. Comparative evaluation of seven cell collection devices for cervical smears. *Acta Cytol* 1999; **43**: 1023–1026

32 Tao L C: *Cytopathology of the Endometrium. Direct Intrauterine Sampling*. Chicago: ASCP Press, 1993; 1–55

33 Gress F, Gottlieb K, Sherman S et al. Endoscopic ultrasonography-guided fine-needle aspiration biopsy of pancreatic cancer. *Ann Intern Med* 2001; **134**: 459–464

34 Specifications for automated systems as submitted by their developers. Editorial Office, International Academy of Cytology. *Analyt Quant Cytol Histol* 1991; **13**: 300–306

35 Intersociety Working Group for Cytology Technologies. Proposed guidelines for primary screening instruments for gynecologic cytology. *Am J Clin Pathol* 1998; **109**: 10–15

36 Intersociety Working Group for Cytology Technologies. Proposed guidelines for secondary screening (rescreening) instruments for gynecologic cytology. *Acta Cytol* 1998; **42**: 273–276

37 McGoogan E, Colgan T J, Ramzy I. Cell preparation methods and criteria for sample adequacy. International Academy of Cytology Task Force summary. *Acta Cytol* 1998; **42**: 25–32

38 Austin R M, Ramzy I. Increased detection of epithelial cell abnormalities by liquid-based gynecologic cytology preparations: A review of accumulated data. *Acta Cytol* 1998; **42**: 178–184

39 Hutchinson M L, Cassin C M, Ball H G. The efficacy of an automated preparation device for cervical cytology. *Am J Clin Pathol* 1991; **96**: 300–305.

40 Linder J, Zahniser D. ThinPrep Papanicolaou testing to reduce false-negative cervical cytology. *Arch Pathol Lab Med* 1998; **122**: 139–144

41 Tench W: Preliminary assessment of the Autocyte PREP: Direct-to-vial performance. *J Reprod Med* 2000; **45**: 912–916

42 Bishop J W, Bigner S H, Colgan T J et al. Multicenter masked evaluation of Autocyte PREP thin layers with matched conventional smears. *Acta Cytol* 1998; **42**: 189–197

43 Linder J. The coming era of cytologic automation. *Am J Clin Pathol* 1991; **96**: 293–294

44 Tolles W E. The cytoanalyzer: An example of physics in medical research. *Trans NY Acad Sci* 1955; **17**: 250–256

45 Data on automated cytology systems as submitted by their developers. Editorial Office, International Academy of Cytology. *Analyt Quant Cytol Histol* 1991; **13**: 300–306

46 Koss L G. Cervical (Pap) smear. New directions. *Cancer* 1993; **71**: 1406–1412 (Suppl)

47 Wilbur D C, Prey M U, Miller W M et al. The Autopap system for primary screening in cervical cytology. *Acta Cytol* 1998; **42**: 214–220

48 Patten S F, Lee J S J, Wilbur D C et al. The AutoPap 300 QC system multicenter clinical trials for use in quality control rescreening of cervical smears: Prospective and archival sensitivity studies. *Cancer Cytopathol* 1997; **81**: 343–347

49 Williams C, Rosenthal D L. Cytopathology in the 21st century. *Am J Clin Pathol* 1993; **99**: S31–33

50 Patterson B, Domanik R, Wernke P. Molecular biomarker-based screening for early detection of cervical cancer. *Acta Cytol* 2001; **45**: 36–47

51 Anton R C, Ramzy I, Schwartz M R et al. Should ASCUS be qualified? An assessment including comparison between conventional and liquid-based technologies. *Cancer (Cancer Cytopathol)* 2001; **93**: 93–99

52   Fait G, Kupferminc M J, Daniel Y *et al.* Contribution of human papillomavirus testing by hybrid capture in the triage of women with repeated abnormal Pap smears before colposcopy referral. *Gynecol Oncol* 2000; **79**: 177–180

53   Rimm D L. Impact of microarray technologies on cytopathology. *Acta Cytol* 2001; **45**: 111–114

54   Rimm D L, Camp R, Charette L *et al.* Tissue microarray: a new technology for amplification of tissue resources. *Cancer J* 2001; **7**:24–31

55   Borrebaeck C A. Antibodies in diagnostics: From immunoassays to protein chips. *Immunol Today* 2000; **21**: 379–382

56   MacBeath G, Schreiber S L. Printing proteins as microarrays for high-throughput function determination. *Science* 2000; **289**: 1760–1763

57   Moch H, Kononen T, Kallioniemi O P *et al.* Tissue microarrays: what will they bring to molecular and anatomic pathology? *Adv Anat Pathol* 2001; **8**: 14–20

58   Goodman J C. Central nervous system, pituitary gland and pineal gland. In: Ramzy I ed: *Clinical Cytopathology And Aspiration Biopsy: Fundamental Principles and Practice*. New York: McGraw-Hill, 2000; 2nd edn.

Section 2

Respiratory system

2 Normal respiratory tract and inflammatory conditions

Winifred Gray

Introduction

The founders of clinical cytology in the nineteenth century were quick to appreciate the value of microscopic examination of material from the respiratory tract[1,2]. At first, clinicians were understandably preoccupied with sputum diagnosis of infective lung diseases, especially tuberculosis, and of other benign conditions. With increasing recognition of bronchogenic carcinoma in the early part of the twentieth century, however, examination of sputum and bronchial secretions for malignant cells became an important investigative procedure[3-7].

Recent developments in sampling techniques have changed the practice of respiratory tract cytology, although new methods have not completely supplanted more traditional ones. Bronchial brushings, fine needle aspiration (FNA) and lavage procedures usually yield better diagnostic material than that obtained by simple exfoliative sampling[8-10]. Bronchoalveolar lavage provides sequential access to well preserved cells to study the natural history of disease processes[11]. Radiological imaging allows FNA sampling of lesions at virtually any site within the thorax and has improved the safety of these procedures[12-15]. Past and present reviews highlight the value and specialized nature of this branch of cytology[16,17]. The Papanicolaou Society of Cytopathology has recently issued guidelines in the United States on the procurement, assessment for adequacy and examination of respiratory tract cytology samples[18].

Chapter 2 here describes briefly some of the methods used in specimen preparation and discusses the cytology of non-neoplastic conditions of the respiratory tract in relation to their clinical context and histology. Recognition of pulmonary and mediastinal neoplasms and the diagnostic accuracy of cytology for tumours form the basis of Chapter 3.

Preparatory techniques and diagnostic applications

Upper respiratory tract

Spontaneous nasal secretions may be collected on a moistened cotton or silk swab[19], or with a gently abrasive rhinobrush[20], or simply by nose blowing. Direct smears should be made promptly before drying out occurs, fixing slides in alcohol for staining by the Papanicolaou method. May-Grünwald-Giemsa (MGG) staining of air-dried preparations is used to assess eosinophil levels in cases of allergic rhinitis, challenging with a series of inhaled allergens to identify the underlying cause[21,22]. Increased exfoliation of epithelial cells has also been noted in cases of nasal hyper-reactivity[23].

Nasopharyngeal sampling by silk swab has been used for rapid diagnosis of nasopharyngeal carcinoma, and has been proposed as an effective screening method in areas with a high incidence of this tumour[19]. Pharyngeal and laryngeal samples are usually collected under direct vision by scraping the lesion with a spatula or swab and preparing the material as described for nasal samples. FNA is appropriate if there is an intact mucosa covering a tumour such as a lymphoma.

Sputum

Sputum is a complex mucoid product resulting from disease or damage within the airways. Microscopic examination of this material may yield information about both benign and malignant conditions[24]. The procedure has certain advantages over other investigations, being non-invasive, cheap and easily repeated. For diagnosis of malignancy, three separate specimens are advised, giving a diagnostic accuracy of up to 70% in some series[25].

Sputum can be processed in a variety of ways. The traditional 'pick and smear' method, whereby the sample is inspected for suspicious material, tissue particles or bloodstained areas, is still in general use. The material is smeared between two microscope slides, fixed in alcohol and stained by the Papanicolaou method. This is the optimal stain for routine sputum examination, displaying nuclear and cytoplasmic features to great advantage[26]. Safety precautions should be maintained during handling and every specimen must be regarded as potentially infective. Thin layer preparation methods, as described in Chapters 1 and 31, yield well preserved clearly displayed cells without background debris, excellent for diagnosis of malignancy, but not for some of the inflammatory conditions where the background detail is of critical importance. These liquid-based samples provide valuable spare material for special stains, including immunocytochemistry.

Although sputum does not deteriorate overnight if refrigerated, longer delays require prefixation of the sample in an equal volume of 70% alcohol. However, cell preservation may be poor, as fixation is impeded by mucus, which tends to become stringy, making handling of these samples difficult[27].

Liquefaction of sputum samples with subsequent concentration of the entire specimen provides a high yield of abnormal cells but at the expense of cell preservation. Liquefaction can be achieved in various ways including enzymatic digestion[28–30]. Techniques for concentrating liquefied samples by centrifugation or filtration have also been described[31,32]. These methods are useful when material is needed for teaching or research[33].

A mechanical procedure for liquefying sputum combining prefixation and concentration, the Saccomanno method[34], is used in many laboratories, especially in the USA. The sample is prefixed in 50% alcohol, then processed in a mechanical blender for 5–10 s. The fluid is filtered or centrifuged and direct smears made from the cell pellet. Cell blocks can also be prepared by this method. One drawback is the tendency for cell groups to fragment, with potential loss of diagnostic information. Direct comparison with the 'pick-and-smear' technique on the same specimens has, however, shown greater diagnostic accuracy and fewer false negative results by the Saccomanno method[35].

A Megafunnel has been used for concentrating sputum on to slides, yielding preparations similar to those produced by the Saccomanno method, but providing better material for immunostaining and requiring a shorter screening time[36].

Induced sputum

Where sputum production is poor, it can be increased artificially by inhalation of an aerosolized irritant solution. Since the introduction of this method in 1958[37] many modifications have emerged[38–41]. Methacholine, hypertonic saline, or a combination with propylene glycol are in common use, inducing sputum production after about 20 min. Physiotherapy may be necessary in some cases. The procedure has proved to be particularly effective for obtaining adequate sputum samples in non-smokers[39], and is useful for investigation of opportunistic infections in immunocompromised hosts, obviating the need for repeated bronchoalveolar lavage or open lung biopsy[42].

Bronchial aspirates and washings

The flexible fibreoptic bronchoscope, developed in Japan in the 1960s, has provided a greatly improved technique for aspirating secretions directly from the lumen of the bronchus or trachea compared with the rigid bronchoscope previously used[43,44].

Bronchial washings are also more easily obtained, instilling normal saline into the bronchus and withdrawing the fluid by suction to collect washings from a large area of mucosa. Direct preparations can be made, or concentration procedures by liquid-based cytology, the Saccomanno method or membrane filtration, may be employed[27].

Bronchial brushings

Using a flexible bronchoscope, the bronchoscopist can obtain a brush sample from the surface of a tumour under direct vision. Material from the brush is then wiped on to microscope slides, fixed in alcohol and stained by the Papanicolaou method. This procedure is frequently combined with bronchial washing[45,46].

Bronchoalveolar lavage

Bronchoalveolar lavage (BAL) sampling of the cellular exudate in the peripheral airways and alveolar spaces is accomplished under local anaesthetic by wedging the tip of the bronchoscope in a subsegmental bronchus, then instilling and aspirating aliquots of normal saline into a trap. The lavage fluid thus obtained is centrifuged and can be processed in a number of different ways depending on the condition under investigation[47–49].

Elucidation of pulmonary infiltrates and identification of opportunistic infections in immunocompromised patients are important applications of this procedure[50,51]. Part of the sample should be submitted for microbiological culture and the remainder prepared as smears after centrifugation or by cytocentrifuge. Papanicolaou staining should be combined with other stains for opportunistic organisms as described in Chapter 22.

BAL was originally developed in the 1920s as a therapeutic procedure in the management of phosgene poisoning and also for treatment of pulmonary alveolar proteinosis and asthma. More recently, differential counts on the inflammatory cell population in lavage fluid have been shown to reflect the histological findings in cases of pulmonary fibrosis and non-infectious granulomatous lung disease. Since the 1990s, serial lavage has found a place in monitoring progress of these conditions[52–54]. The initial lavage material obtained includes upper airways contents and should therefore be discarded.

BAL also has a limited role in diagnosis of peripheral lung cancers[55], as described in Chapter 3.

Fine needle aspiration

Using the method of fine needle aspiration (FNA), material may be obtained either by a transbronchial or transthoracic approach; usually the latter. The procedure has come into increasing prominence in recent years and is of particular value when less invasive tests have failed to achieve a diagnosis or are inappropriate. The introduction of radiological imaging has improved the accuracy of sampling, while use of a fine gauge needle (19–22G) makes the procedure safe and well tolerated[15,56,57].

Since the 1980s, there has been a steady increase in the use of FNA as an initial investigation of localized lung lesions, a position traditionally held by sputum examination. The rapidity and accuracy of diagnosis and its cost effectiveness make FNA the procedure of choice for appropriate cases. The resulting shift in laboratory workload pattern has implications for training of staff and for reporting practices.

Percutaneous transthoracic FNA was developed in the 1930s to examine peripheral lung lesions beyond the reach of the bronchoscope and for investigating patients who were a poor surgical risk[58]. *Transbronchial FNA* was introduced in 1978 to sample lesions extrinsic to the bronchus, or where surface necrosis would prevent accurate direct sampling. Aspiration is performed at bronchoscopy using a flexible metal needle to which suction is applied[15,59].

Whichever method is used, the aspirated sample is smeared on to slides using a blood film technique, or with more pressure if solid particles are present. Some slides should be air-dried for MGG staining and others fixed in alcohol for the Papanicolaou method. Spare material obtained by rinsing the needle in normal saline or tissue culture medium can be processed as a cell block or made into cytospin preparations for other stains and for immunocytochemistry. Alternatively, the entire sample may be processed for thin layer preparations. Electron microscopy, tumour proliferation studies and cytogenetic analysis are among the additional procedures that can be performed on FNA material[60].

Complications are few but include pneumothorax, minor degrees of which were found in up to 40% of cases in one early series, although not often requiring active treatment[58]. Lung haemorrhage is rare with fine needle sampling, but the procedure is obviously contraindicated in patients with a bleeding diathesis.

Structure and function of the respiratory tract

Anatomically, the respiratory system includes the nasal passages, sinuses and nasopharynx, the oropharynx and larynx, trachea, bronchi and bronchioles, and the air spaces beyond. Transportation of gases is the primary function of the upper respiratory tract and airways, but there is also an important role in warming and moistening inspired air, removing particulate material and providing an initial immunological defence against inhaled microorganisms. Gaseous exchange is carried out within the alveoli and other complex activities take place in the lung parenchyma, including further pulmonary defence mechanisms, some endocrine functions and maintenance of homeostasis.

Not surprisingly, there are many variations in cell structure throughout the respiratory system, and their delicate balance is frequently disturbed by disease. A comprehensive knowledge of the normal findings is therefore necessary to understand the pathological changes encountered in cytological specimens[61,62].

Normal histology of the respiratory tract

Two different types of epithelium form the mucosa of the respiratory tract, their exact distribution varying with age. Stratified squamous epithelium covers areas liable to

abrasion, such as the nasal vestibule, nasopharynx, lingual surface of the epiglottis and the vocal cords. Elsewhere a complex layer of glandular cells is found.

The *squamous mucosa* is composed of basal, parabasal, intermediate and superficial cells, and is not keratinized in health. Outside the basement membrane of this epithelium lies a fibrocollagenous stroma containing blood vessels, lymphatics, nerves and seromucinous glands (Fig. 2.1). Inflammatory cells of the immune system, mainly lymphocytes, plasma cells and macrophages are also seen, migrating into the overlying epithelium. In strategic areas lymphoid cells aggregate into organized tissue masses forming the tonsils and adenoids.

The bronchial tree and remainder of the upper airways are lined by specialized *respiratory epithelium* (Fig. 2.2). This consists of a pseudostratified layer of *ciliated tall columnar*

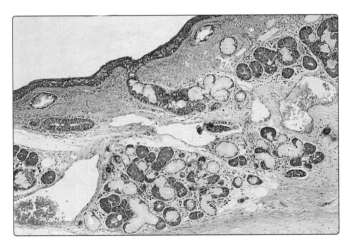

Fig. 2.1   Normal bronchial wall showing the lining mucosa resting on fibrocollagenous submucosa containing seromucinous glands, blood vessels and lymphatic channels. (H&E × LP)

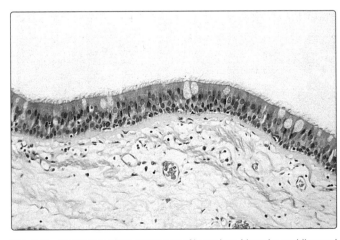

Fig. 2.2   Normal respiratory mucosa of bronchus. Note the multilayered pseudostratified columnar epithelium composed mainly of ciliated cells with occasional goblet cells. A distinct single layer of reserve cells can be seen resting on the basement membrane. Deep to this the submucosa includes a few capillaries, lymphatics and inflammatory cells. (H&E × MP)

cells interspersed with mucin secreting *goblet cells*, which have microvilli on their luminal surfaces. There are approximately five ciliated cells for each goblet cell. Mucin from the goblet cells coats the airways with a sticky layer within which inhaled particles, organisms and cell debris are trapped. The cilia have a metachronous beat which sweeps this material upwards, to be expectorated or swallowed.

Two further cell types are present in respiratory epithelium. Small *reserve cells* rest on the basement membrane, forming an undifferentiated stem cell population from which regeneration of bronchial mucosa takes place after injury (Fig. 2.2). Inconspicuous round cells with neuroendocrine properties are also found situated towards the basement membrane. Known as *Feyrter* or *K (Kultschitzsky) cells*, they are most numerous in the smaller bronchi where they are grouped around capillaries and nerve fibres forming neuroepithelial bodies. They contain neurosecretory granules producing locally active polypeptide hormones, and belong to the APUD (amine precursor uptake and decarboxylation) cell system.

Bronchioles, the first branches of bronchi without cartilaginous support in their walls, are lined by a single layer of non-ciliated columnar cells interspersed with a few goblet cells. In addition there are tall columnar cells, the *Clara cells*, producing surfactant. Terminal bronchioles are lined by low columnar epithelium and are involved solely in air conduction. They are continuous with respiratory bronchioles, which mark the commencement of gaseous exchange. Here the lining becomes cuboidal, merging with flattened epithelial cells in the alveolar ducts. These lead into rotunda-like spaces called alveolar sacs. The periphery of each sac is partitioned into alveoli, the main site of gaseous exchange (Fig. 2.3).

The principal cells lining alveoli are known as *type I* and *type II pneumocytes*. In addition, there are many macrophages of bone marrow derivation, forming an important component of cytology samples from the lower airways. They adhere to the walls of alveoli, ingesting cellular debris and foreign material, which is then transported to the bronchial tree or to lymphatic channels arising at the level of the terminal bronchioles.

It has been estimated that type I pneumocytes cover approximately 90% of the alveolar wall area, but form only about 40% of the lining cell population[62]. Their cytoplasm is thinly spread out to allow maximal exchange of gas between the alveolar space and the underlying capillaries. Type II pneumocytes comprise 60% of the lining cells numerically, but are bulky and rounded, occupying less than 10% of the alveolar surface area. Their cytoplasm is dense, containing spherical laminated osmiophilic bodies when examined by electron microscopy, composed of the precursors of pulmonary surfactant. These cells are also the progenitors of type I pneumocytes.

General cytological findings in respiratory samples

Only a few of the many different cells lining the respiratory tract are seen with any regularity in cytological preparations. The distribution of cells varies considerably with the nature of the sample, but is of importance in assessing specimen adequacy. The appearances to be described for normal and abnormal cells are those seen with Papanicolaou staining unless otherwise specified.

Squamous cells (Fig. 2.4) are numerically the most common cells in sputum, but are less frequent in other specimens and usually absent from FNA samples. Superficial and intermediate cells predominate, staining pinkish orange and green respectively, in Papanicolaou stained smears. They have small central pyknotic or vesicular nuclei, as seen in squames from other sites.

Bronchial epithelial cells (Fig. 2.5) are profuse in brushings, but less common in sputum as they do not exfoliate readily. They are infrequent in FNA material. Columnar or

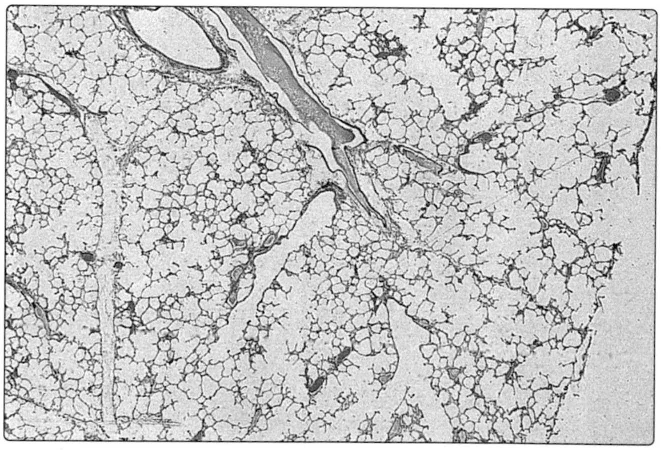

Fig. 2.3   Normal lung parenchyma. This lung lobule shows terminal and respiratory bronchioles, alveolar ducts, sacs and alveoli. (Reticulin stain × LP) (Courtesy of Dr M S Dunnill, Oxford, UK)

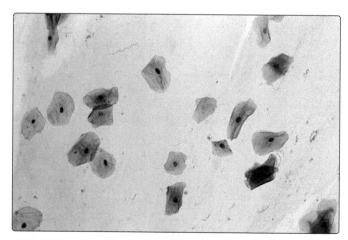

Fig. 2.4   Normal oral squamous cells in a sputum sample consisting mainly of saliva. The cells are of superficial and intermediate type but there is no keratinization. (Papanicolaou × HP)

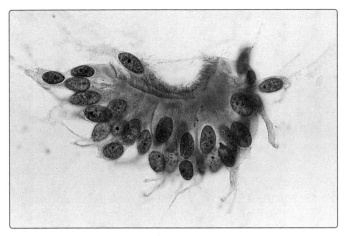

Fig. 2.5   Bronchial epithelial cells in a bronchial brushing sample. These tall columnar cells show the tapering point of anchorage at one end and dark terminal bar, bearing pink cilia at the opposite end of the cell. Nuclei are regular, ovoid in shape and basal in position. Chromatin is finely divided and small nucleoli are visible. (Papanicolaou × HP)

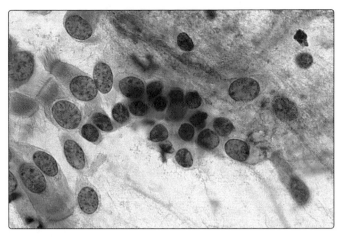

Fig. 2.7   Reserve cells in a crowded group of small cells with dark nuclei and very little cytoplasm, surrounded by columnar epithelial cells. There is a suggestion of nuclear moulding at the right edge of the group. Bronchial brushing. (Papanicolaou × HP)

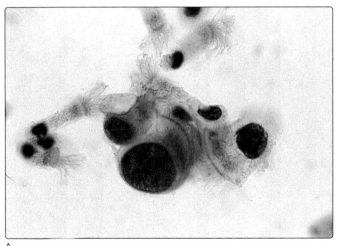

A

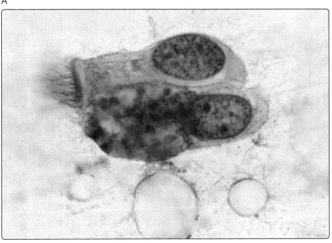

B

Fig. 2.6   (A) Bronchial cells with nuclei of variable size and shape, but still within the normal range. Bronchial brushing (× HP). (B) Single bronchial epithelial cell and goblet cell, the latter showing distension centrally due to the presence of greenish grey mucin. Bronchial brushing. (Papanicolaou × OI)

triangular in shape, the cells lie singly, in short ribbons or in flat sheets which often have a straight 'anatomical' edge. They have delicate cyanophilic cytoplasm, bluish grey with MGG stains, tapering at the point of previous anchorage. Nuclei vary considerably in size and shape but are usually basal and rounded or oval (Fig. 2.6A), with open granular or condensed chromatin and a single small nucleolus. Multinucleation may be seen. Cilia are often still preserved, arising from a dark stained terminal bar at the broader end of the cell.

Goblet cells are inconspicuous in sputum unless hyperplastic, but are quite often seen in brushings and increase in number with chronic bronchial irritation. They are columnar but are distended centrally by globules of mucin, which overlie or displace the nucleus (Fig. 2.6B).

Reserve cells (Fig. 2.7) are rarely present in sputum but are sometimes seen in brushings and lavage specimens, mainly in reactive states. They form sheets of small regular cells slightly larger than lymphocytes, with a high nuclear/cytoplasmic ratio, coarse chromatin and a narrow rim of green cytoplasm.

Macrophages (Figs 2.8, 2.9) are the hallmark of a satisfactory sputum sample and are found in the majority of pulmonary specimens. In sputum, the adequacy of a sample is claimed to be directly proportional to the number of alveolar macrophages it contains[63]. Round or oval dissociated cells, they are usually over 10 μm in diameter but vary greatly in size and shape. Their cytoplasm is poorly defined, cyanophilic and often vacuolated. Phagocytosed material, usually carbon, may be present. They have central or eccentric nuclei, rounded or bean-shaped, with coarse chromatin and visible nucleoli. Binucleation is common and the cells may form giant cells with numerous nuclei.

Inflammatory cells, mainly polymorphonuclear leucocytes and lymphocytes, are invariably present in low numbers and are only of diagnostic significance if markedly

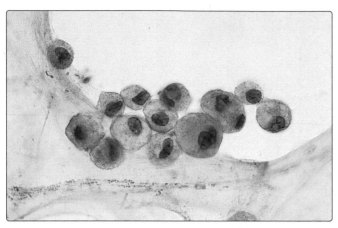

Fig. 2.8   Macrophages forming a streak of dissociated cells in sputum. Note the variation in cell size and finely vacuolated cytoplasm with a few particles of ingested carbon. Most of the nuclei are eccentrically placed, varying in shape and size. Nucleoli are visible and several cells show binucleation. (Papanicolaou × HP)

increased. A preponderance of one inflammatory cell type may however be significant, for example, when eosinophils are conspicuous.

Clara cells, *Feyrter cells* and *types I and II pneumocytes* are prone to rapid degenerative changes and are not recognizable in respiratory samples unless hyperplastic or neoplastic.

Other cytological components of respiratory samples

Non-cellular material and extraneous elements are seen in many specimens, and should be firmly identified to avoid misinterpretation. The possibilities are virtually unlimited.

Mucus is almost invariably present in specimens obtained via the airways unless mucolytic agents have been used. It forms a pale translucent background material staining variably, and may be smooth or stringy in texture, usually with streaks of enmeshed inflammatory cells. Densely stained inspissated mucus (Fig. 2.10A) may obscure cell detail, or give a false impression of cytological abnormality

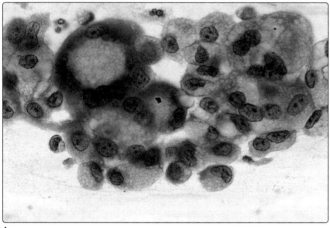

A

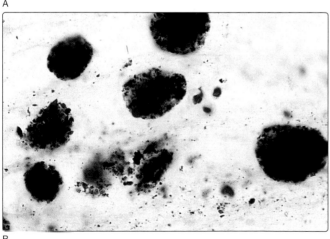

B

Fig. 2.9   (A) Multinucleated macrophages are common, seen here aggregated with mononuclear forms. Their nuclei are randomly arranged at the periphery. (B) Carbon pigment in macrophages varies greatly in amount, but may obscure the nucleus entirely, as in this sputum sample from a coal miner. (Papanicolaou × HP)

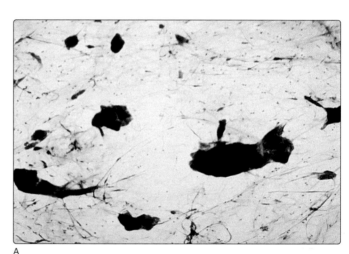

A

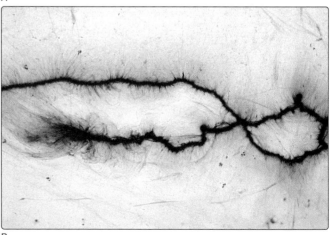

B

Fig. 2.10   (A) Inspissated mucus in sputum or bronchial secretions may stain so darkly that detailed examination is required to exclude the presence of abnormal cells. Sputum. (Papanicolaou × MP). (B) Curschmann's spiral composed of a compressed cast of mucus from a small bronchiole. The form, size and staining of these structures are extremely variable. Sputum. (Papanicolaou × HP)

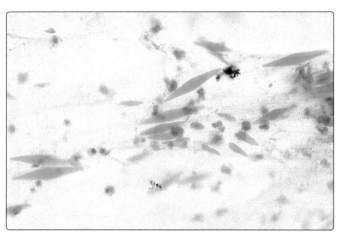

Fig. 2.11   Charcot Leyden crystals are bright orange or yellow and needle shaped. Eosinophils are often present since the crystals form from breakdown products of their granules. Sputum. (Papanicolaou × HP)

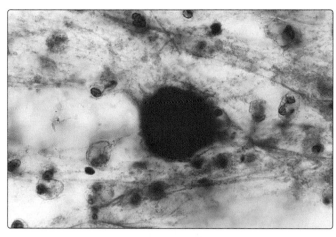

Fig. 2.13   Psammoma body in sputum showing the typical laminated structure. No evidence of malignancy was found in this patient. (Papanicolaou × HP)

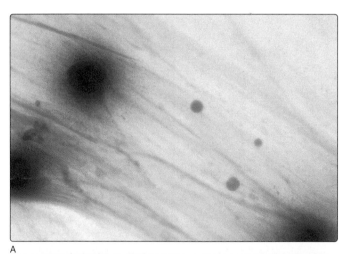

A

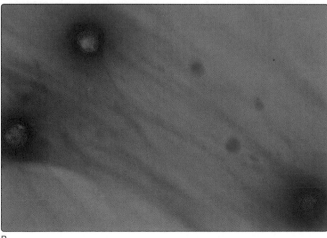

B

Fig. 2.12   Calcified blue bodies are birefringent inorganic concretions seen here on routine light microscopy (A) and by polarized light (B). Sputum. (Papanicolaou × HP)

on low power magnification. Coils of compressed mucus known as *Curschmann's spirals* (Fig. 2.10B) are frequently seen in sputum from smokers or patients with obstructive airways disease, especially asthmatics. The spirals are casts of the small bronchioles and vary considerably in structure[64,65].

Inorganic material of various types may be seen and can have diagnostic significance. The most common of these include:

Charcot-Leyden crystals (Fig. 2.11), derived from the breakdown products of eosinophil granules, appear in conditions evoking pulmonary eosinophilia as orange, yellow or pinkish stained diamond or needle shaped crystals[66].

Calcific blue bodies and *corpora amylacea* are similar in routine preparations. The former consist largely of calcium carbonate and show central birefringence (Fig. 2.12)[67,68]. Corpora amylacea are non-calcified rounded structures composed of glycoproteins including amyloid. They stain pale pink, are Congo red positive and exhibit birefringence. Both of these are seen in various chronic lung diseases[67].

Psammoma bodies (calcospherites) are laminated non-refractile calcified concretions sometimes found in the presence of malignancy, although not necessarily closely associated with tumour cells[67]. Isolated psammoma bodies may be seen in the absence of any tumour formation (Fig. 2.13).

Ferruginous bodies (see Fig. 2.70) are formed when filamentous dust particles such as asbestos become coated with protein and iron in the lung parenchyma[69]. They vary from 5–200 μm in length, are light brown in colour and stain blue with Perl's stain for iron[70].

Contaminants may be added to respiratory samples at any stage from collection to microscopy. Following this time sequence, they include:

Food particles, seen in association with saliva, especially in samples from elderly patients. Meat fibres are elongated and may show cross-striations. Vegetable cells usually have

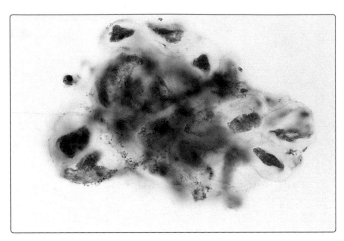

Fig. 2.14 Vegetable matter in sputum may simulate degenerate malignant cells. The salivary nature of the specimen and the thick cellulose walls with lack of nuclear detail are helpful features. Sputum. (Papanicolaou × HP)

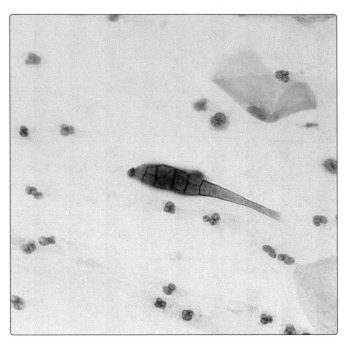

Fig. 2.15 Alternaria sp. organism in sputum, probably an aerial contaminant. (Papanicolaou × HP)

thick straight cellulose walls although of variable appearance. They can be confused with benign or malignant respiratory tract cells[71], but have refractile cell walls and a repetitive structure, lacking the pleomorphism of tumour cells and the true nuclear features of malignancy (Fig. 2.14).

Colonial growth of normal oral flora, including bacteria and yeasts, frequently occurs when there is delay in preparation of samples. The organisms occur mainly in areas of saliva and do not elicit any inflammatory reaction.

Parasitic or saprophytic flora from the mouth, such as non-pathogenic entamoebae, have been described (see Fig. 2.48)[72]. Mites have been found in respiratory specimens and are occasionally significant clinically, since they may be associated with an actual infestation of diseased airways[72].

Aerial contaminants are acquired during specimen collection in transit, or at the time of preparation in the laboratory. Pollen is an obvious external contaminant and must be distinguished from fungal spores. Fungal species may be seen, originating from air, soil or water. The water-borne plant pathogen *Alternaria* is not uncommon, forming light brown conidia 30 μm in length, with an internal segmented structure (Fig. 2.15). Although potentially pathogenic in immunosuppressed patients, they are present only in small numbers as contaminants[73,74].

Carryover of cells from another sample can occur during processing, usually leaving the cells 'out of context', often in a slightly different plane of focus or at one edge of the slide[75]. Cross-contamination by tumour cells is a potential source of false positive diagnosis of malignancy.

Criteria for assessing adequacy of samples

A sample providing enough cells for confident accurate diagnosis can be regarded as adequate. However, misleading reports are sometimes given if the specimen does not include appropriate material confirming the origin of the sample, or if there is insufficient abnormal material to ensure correct interpretation. Hence, it is one of the prime tasks of the cytologist to assess whether a specimen is suitable for diagnosis or whether the test should be repeated. Furthermore, when tumour cells are found, localization of their site of origin may not always be possible. This question mainly arises with sputum samples where cells from upper or lower respiratory tract tumours may exfoliate into the sputum[76].

Sputum specimens are judged adequate when plentiful pulmonary macrophages can be identified[13,63]. The presence of columnar cells is ambiguous since they may be from the nasal passages or upper airways. Macrophage counts have been used to quantify the adequacy of sputum specimens[63,77], and to relate these findings to smoking status[78], but the procedures are too time consuming for routine laboratory work. Samples consisting mainly of saliva should always be screened fully as malignant cells are occasionally found.

Bronchial brushings usually show a profusion of epithelial cells or tumour cells since the material is obtained under direct vision. If the sample is scanty, poor fixation and air-drying of the cells lead to swelling of nuclei and loss of chromatin detail. *Bronchial washings* are generally less cellular than brushings, but are usually well-fixed, since preparation is undertaken in the laboratory. Alveolar macrophages provide unequivocal evidence of appropriate sampling.

Bronchoalveolar lavages contain many macrophages and, provided the first aliquot is discarded, should be virtually free from any cells from the upper airways. In a study of over 1500 lavage samples prepared by filtration and cytocentrifugation, however, Chamberlain *et al.* reported an unsatisfactory rate of 30% as judged by: fewer than 10 alveolar macrophages/high power field; fewer macrophages than cells from the airways; a mucopurulent exudate; cellular changes due to degeneration; or the presence of laboratory artefacts[79]. These criteria are important when inflammatory cells are to be quantified[53,80]. Adequate sampling is also essential in evaluating specimens for opportunistic infections[81,82].

Fine needle aspiration samples from solid lung nodules pose no problem for assessment of quality when the cells obtained are interpretable and in keeping with the site aspirated. It is important to remember, however, that negative findings do not necessarily contribute to diagnosis, since while they may be correct, they may also be misleading[83]. Scanty preparations with a few normal lung parenchymal cells, macrophages and occasional fragments of bronchial epithelium are all that will be seen if the needle misses the lesion. Mesothelial cells in pavemented sheets are sometimes aspirated on traversing the pleural cavity.

Heavily bloodstained aspirates with rather scanty cells are often poorly fixed due to the presence of blood. Even in these smears, however, diagnostic fields may be found. Inadequate sampling can be minimized by immediate assessment of the specimen and repeating the procedure if necessary.

Non-specific reactive changes in cytological preparations

The majority of respiratory specimens from patients with conditions other than tumours show findings reflecting non-specific host responses. These include the effects of damage by environmental agents, as well as changes seen in many of the more common respiratory infections and chronic chest diseases. Appropriate clinical details and judicious use of special stains may enable the cytologist to confirm the diagnosis in some cases.

Reactive squamous cells from the upper respiratory tract are seen particularly in sputum. They have slightly enlarged hyperchromatic nuclei and have come to be known as 'Pap cells' since first described by Dr George Papanicolaou in his own sputum, due to laryngitis[13]. They have little diagnostic significance.

Anucleate keratinized squamous cells are only noteworthy in sputum if present in large numbers, when they suggest an area of hyperkeratosis due to a focus of chronic irritation. The surface cells from keratotic lesions exfoliate readily, whether the underlying process is benign or malignant. The specimen must be assessed carefully to determine whether it is of upper or lower respiratory tract origin, and whether there are any cells with nuclear features suspicious of malignancy. Cells from an area of benign hyperkeratosis are usually mature anucleate squames compared with the bizarre-shaped deep orange cells shed from the keratinized surface of a well-differentiated squamous carcinoma.

Hyperplasia of bronchial epithelial cells can be induced by many different noxious agents. In simple repair processes, sheets of actively regenerating cuboidal to columnar cells are seen, with enlarged nuclei, vesicular chromatin and prominent nucleoli[84] (Fig. 2.16). Multinucleation is a frequent finding and has been described in cells adjacent to malignant neoplasms[85]. Papillary clusters of epithelial cells are sometimes shed, mimicking clumps of adenocarcinoma cells. Their nuclei are difficult to examine when the clusters are dense, but they should retain a normal chromatin pattern (Fig. 2.17). Nevertheless, these cell groups are a classical diagnostic pitfall in respiratory tract cytology[86].

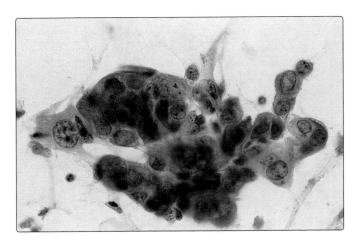

Fig. 2.16 Hyperplasia of bronchial epithelial cells in repair is associated with disorganization of cells, nuclear enlargement and pleomorphism and prominent nucleoli, as seen in this group of cells in BAL fluid from a transplant patient. (Papanicolaou × HP)

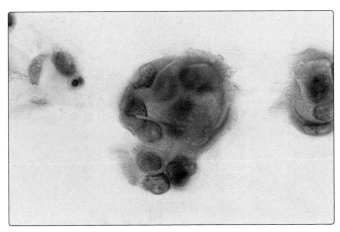

Fig. 2.17 Hyperplastic bronchial epithelial cells forming a papillary cluster, with cilia visible on the surface of the group. The nuclei are enlarged but bland-looking. Their depth of focus requires careful examination at high magnification. Bronchial brushing. (Papanicolaou × OI)

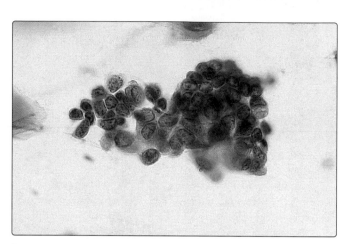

Fig. 2.18 Reserve cell hyperplasia in bronchial brushings from a patient with a squamous carcinoma of bronchus. Note the enlarged active nuclei in this disorganized group of small crowded cells, the high nuclear/cytoplasmic ratio and the narrow rim of cytoplasm. (Papanicolaou ×HP)

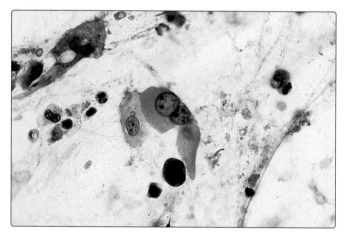

Fig. 2.19 Alveolar cell damage and hyperplasia in BAL from a leukaemic patient receiving cyclosporin treatment. The cells at centre are enlarged and rectangular with dense green cytoplasm, swollen nuclei and prominent nucleoli. Note lack of cilia. A damaged epithelial cell is present at top left. (Papanicolaou ×OI)

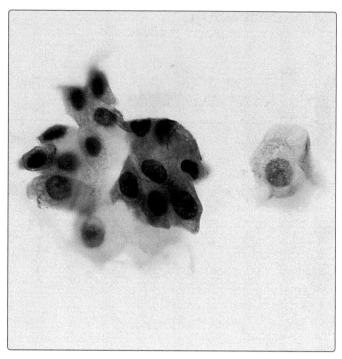

Fig. 2.20 Squamous metaplasia in sputum from a middle-aged smoker. The group is composed of cohesive small polygonal cells with regular darkly stained nuclei. Cytoplasmic staining is variable but there is no keratinization. (Papanicolaou × OI)

Reserve cell hyperplasia (Fig. 2.18) is less easily recognized in cytology specimens. Groups of small cohesive crowded cells with a high nuclear/cytoplasmic ratio and dense chromatin are typical. Nuclear moulding may be seen, hence the cells can be confused with a small cell carcinoma, as described in Chapter 3. Absence of necrosis and cell dissociation, and the uniformity of nuclear size and shape are helpful features[87].

Hyperplasia of type II pneumocytes and bronchiolar cells (Fig. 2.19) usually occurs as a result of specific toxic effects on the lung and the regeneration that follows. The cells are polygonal or rectangular, occurring singly or in twos and threes or sometimes in larger clusters, and they may show cytoplasmic vacuolation. The nuclei are swollen, with prominent nucleoli and pale or dense chromatin. Such cells are not easy to identify with confidence unless an accurate

history is available to alert the cytologist to their origin. They differ from hyperplastic bronchial cells in lacking cilia and in their dissociated cell pattern, with no associated columnar or goblet cells. Distinction from bronchioloalveolar cell carcinoma has sometimes been virtually impossible[88–90]. There is usually less profuse shedding of cells in reactive hyperplasia than in neoplasia and the cells are in flatter groups, without such a striking depth of focus as is required to inspect the nuclei of malignant cells[91].

Squamous metaplasia (Fig. 2.20) is one of the most common responses of bronchial epithelium to persistent injury[92,93]. It is preceded by reserve cell hyperplasia and is a frequent finding in smokers[94–96]. Small fragmented groups of polygonal cells of parabasal size, with regular large bland looking nuclei are found in the early stages. Dissociation increases as the metaplasia progresses to become atypical or dysplastic, and keratinization develops in longstanding atypical metaplasia. A more detailed description of atypical metaplasia is given in Chapter 3.

Ciliocytophthoria (Fig. 2.21) is a degenerative process affecting bronchial epithelium whereby columnar cells fragment into rounded cytoplasmic remnants, some of which still show tufts of cilia, while others contain pyknotic nuclear material. The change was first observed by Papanicolaou in 1956 in association with viral infections[97], but can be seen in a range of acute and chronic pulmonary diseases, and in the presence of bronchial carcinoma[98].

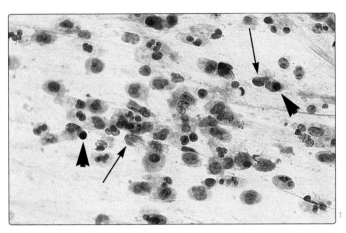

Fig. 2.21   Ciliocytophthoria in sputum from a patient with squamous carcinoma. Scattered fragments of cytoplasmic remnants present, some ciliated (arrows), others with pyknotic nuclei (arrowheads). (Papanicolaou × HP)

Inflammatory and infective diseases of the respiratory tract

Infection by microorganisms is the most common cause of inflammation in the lung. In the majority of such cases, cytology has little to offer in the investigative sequence, since the findings are very often non-specific, the diagnosis depending on firm identification of the organism by culture. This applies particularly to bacterial infections. Certain types of infection, however, can be recognized cytologically: fungal elements may be seen, and some viral infections produce diagnostic cytopathic effects. An important additional role for the cytologist lies in helping to exclude an underlying tumour in cases of unexplained or recurrent chest infection.

Pneumonia

The term pneumonia denotes acute inflammation of lung parenchyma due to invasion by micro-organisms. This is in contradistinction to pneumonitis where physical agents are involved, or alveolitis, which is due to allergic or fibrosing inflammatory reactions within the alveoli[99]. Although the incidence of pneumonia and its mortality have fallen substantially with the advent of antibiotics, the disease remains an important cause of morbidity and death, especially at the extremes of life and in debilitated or immunosuppressed patients.

The usual sequence of events once organisms have lodged in the alveoli or distal airways is an immediate acute inflammatory response, with outpouring of oedema fluid, fibrin, neutrophil polymorphs and red blood cells (Fig. 2.22A). Some organisms produce a rapidly spreading infection, involving the entire lobe in a process of consolidation. Other organisms are subject to host defence mechanisms limiting spread to a more patchy distribution. These two processes are known as lobar pneumonia and bronchopneumonia, respectively. The distinction is by no means absolute, but remains valid in many cases. Certain

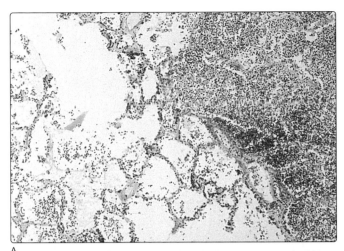

A

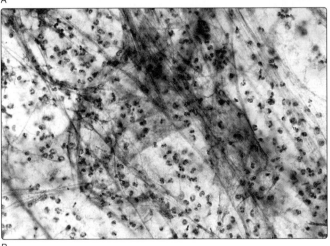

B

Fig. 2.22   (A) Lobar pneumonia in histological section of lung. The alveoli are filled with a dense exudate of neutrophil polymorphs producing consolidation of the parenchyma, most marked on the right. (H&E × LP) (B) Sputum from a patient with bronchopneumonia, showing many polymorphs entangled in the streaks of mucus and absence of macrophages. (Papanicolaou × HP)

viruses and mycoplasma organisms induce interstitial pneumonia involving inflammation of alveolar walls rather than alveolar spaces[100].

Appropriate treatment and adequate host responses lead to complete resolution of inflammation in many cases, but other outcomes such as abscess formation or fibrosis may supervene in adverse circumstances. The nature of the infectious agent influences the type of inflammatory reaction, creating a more indolent chest infection in some cases. In other cases, the immune system may contribute to progression of the disease, as happens in tuberculosis.

There are marked variations in incidence of different types of pulmonary infection throughout the world, but the increasing number of patients with impaired immunity and the comparative ease of international travel have led to changes in traditional epidemiological patterns. It is therefore important to have a full history when assessing cases of respiratory infection.

Bacterial pneumonia

Cytological findings

▶ Grossly purulent or bloodstained sputum
▶ Predominance of neutrophil polymorphs
▶ Cell debris and degenerate epithelial cells
▶ Exfoliation of epithelial cell groups
▶ Causative organisms are sometimes identified

Sputum samples are the most common specimens to be submitted for cytology in cases of pneumonia, often prompted by the need to exclude a bronchial carcinoma rather than to establish the diagnosis of chest infection. Sputum production may be poor, especially in immunosuppressed patients; induced sputum or bronchoalveolar lavage are then more appropriate. FNA is unlikely to be attempted unless an abscess has developed, which may necessitate exclusion of malignancy.

Macroscopically, sputum is often purulent or noted to be rusty due to the presence of blood. Neutrophil polymorphs dominate the microscopic picture (Fig. 2.22B), often at the expense of pulmonary macrophages, obscuring all other cells in some cases. The specimen may be deemed unsatisfactory for cytological assessment if epithelial cells are totally obscured.

Cell debris is prominent in the early stages, whatever sampling method has been used, and degenerative changes such as cytoplasmic vacuolation or ciliocytophthoria may be seen. Clusters of bronchial epithelial cells often show hyperplastic or atypical changes, such as enlarged hyperchromatic nuclei and prominent nucleoli. These features can result from pre-existing lung disease, such as chronic bronchitis or bronchiectasis.

In most cases of pneumonia the causative organisms cannot be identified cytologically. In cases of immunosuppression, special stains including Gram, Ziehl Neelsen, PAS and Grocott should be performed. Gram-positive cocci may be demonstrated but cannot be identified further without microbiological culture.

Higher bacteria, such as Actinomyces organisms (Fig. 2.23) have a more definitive appearance, forming colonies of radiating filamentous Gram-positive bacteria which may be visible in macroscopic samples as 'sulphur granules'[101]. The related organism, Nocardia (Fig. 2.24) stains faintly pink by the Papanicolaou method, exhibits negative staining with MGG and is well demonstrated by Grocott's silver stain[102-104]. Nocardia pneumonia is a recognized cause of infection after cardiac transplantation, often producing a solitary nodule, which may be subjected to FNA[105].

Legionella organisms, the bacteria causing Legionnaires' disease, have been described in sputum, bronchial samples and FNA material[106]. They are tiny Gram-negative bacilli which can be demonstrated by silver stains or by immunofluorescence.

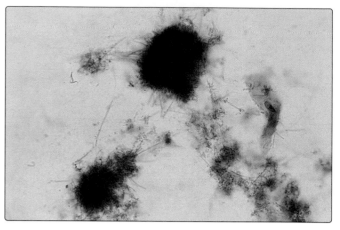

Fig. 2.23   Actinomycotic organisms presenting in colonies of filamentous organisms in sputum with no significant inflammation. The patient was immunosuppressed and had evidence of chest infection but the colonies may represent overgrowth from the oropharynx in this setting. (Papanicolaou ×HP)

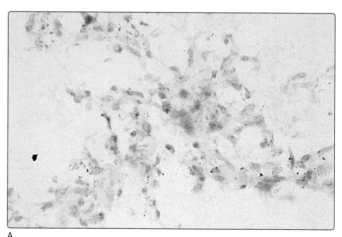

A

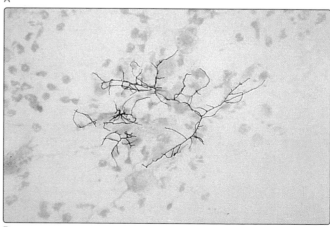

B

Fig. 2.24   (A) FNA of a nodular lung lesion in an immunosuppressed patient showing amorphous inflammatory debris, with no diagnostic features on H&E staining. (× HP). (B) Grocott staining of the same material reveals delicate filamentous organisms characteristic of *Nocardia asteroides*, subsequently confirmed on culture. (× HP) (Courtesy of Dr G Sterrett, Perth, Western Australia)

Diagnostic pitfalls

In some circumstances epithelial atypia may be extreme and difficult to distinguish from malignancy[107]. Close liaison with clinical staff is needed in these cases, with judicious use of other investigations, and where necessary, the adoption of a wait-and-see policy.

Stains for organisms must be interpreted with care so that overgrowth of commensals from the oropharynx is not mistaken for an infection. It is important to note the context of the organisms. They are unlikely to be significant, if mixed in type and found mainly in areas of saliva without accompanying inflammatory cells.

Pulmonary tuberculosis

The incidence of infection by the organism *Mycobacterium tuberculosis* fell dramatically in developed countries during the twentieth century, due to improvements in public health and the advent of effective chemotherapy. Nevertheless, tuberculosis remains one of the major causes of morbidity and mortality throughout the world, and is again occurring more frequently in western countries. This is partly attributable to the increasing numbers of disadvantaged groups within affluent societies. In part, this is due to the emergence of resistant strains of the organism and also because conditions associated with immunosuppression are becoming more common[108]. The latter group of patients are also susceptible to infection with atypical mycobacteria such as *M. avium-intracellulare*, *M. kansasii* and *M. fortuitum*[109].

The natural history and pathogenesis of pulmonary tuberculosis were expounded by Rich, in 1951[110]. The causative organism was isolated in 1852 by Koch, and antibiotic treatment has been available from the 1940s. Awareness of the pathology and cytological findings is important to ensure early diagnosis and treatment.

Primary infection usually occurs in childhood by droplet spread. The organisms are localized in the lung parenchyma and the draining hilar lymph nodes, forming a primary tuberculous complex. Macrophages and lymphocytes mount a defence reaction; however, persistence of organisms and their breakdown products leads to swelling of macrophages, which take on an epithelioid appearance. After about a week some of the epithelioid cells fuse to form Langhans' giant cells, with many nuclei arranged in an arc at one pole of the cell. Lymphocytes accumulate around the periphery of this collection of cells, and the whole circumscribed focus of inflammation is known as a granuloma. Within about 2 weeks, the centre of the granuloma starts to undergo necrosis of a characteristic soft cheesy consistency, a process termed caseation (Fig. 2.25). Epithelioid histiocytes and Langhans' giant cells tend to form palisades around the edge of the caseous material and it is in this area that acid-fast tubercle bacilli are most often found.

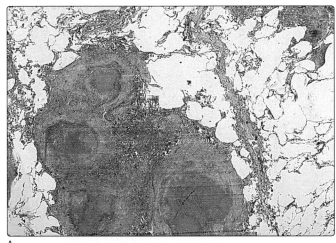

A

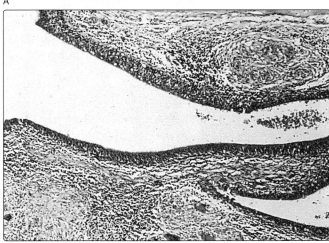

B

Fig. 2.25   (A) Caseating granulomata in lung parenchyma due to pulmonary tuberculosis. The granulomata are well formed and confluent with amorphous eosinophilic caseation necrosis at centre. (H&E × LP) (B) Section of bronchial wall with discrete epithelioid giant cell granulomata in the submucosa, a less common site for these lesions than in the lung parenchyma. Note the intact mucosa over the surface, impeding direct *sampling by cytology. (H&E × MP) (Courtesy of Dr M S Dunnill, Oxford,* UK)

As immunity develops resolution occurs, leaving a peripheral lung scar and calcified draining lymph nodes. If the number of infecting organisms is large, however, or the patient is debilitated, infection may spread elsewhere in the lung or via the bloodstream to other organs. Tuberculous bronchopneumonia and miliary tuberculosis develop in this way. Even when, as usually happens, healing is the early outcome, reinfection may occur at any time, usually by reactivation of a dormant focus of organisms in the lung. This secondary or adult infection takes the form of progressive granulomatous bronchopneumonia with caseation, cavitation and extensive lung destruction.

Recognition of this stage of the disease is important in cytology. The patient has a cough productive of sputum. Bronchoscopy may be undertaken for the collection of washings and brushings to exclude malignancy and to obtain material for culture. Effusions are common.

Localized pulmonary lesions occur, simulating malignancy radiologically and inviting fine needle aspiration sampling. Thus a variety of methods of cytological diagnosis may be employed. The findings are well documented in sputum and bronchial secretions[111-113]. The characteristic features of granuloma formation are best seen in FNA material[102,114-116].

Cytological findings *(Figs 2.26–2.28)*

▶ A mixed inflammatory exudate
▶ Epithelioid histiocytes
▶ Langhans' giant cells are infrequently found
▶ Fragmented granulomas may be seen in FNA material
▶ Caseation is inconspicuous
▶ Organisms may be demonstrated in FNA samples

An analysis undertaken in Brazil by Tani *et al.* in 1987[113] of over 100 tuberculous cytology samples other than FNAs revealed increased numbers of macrophages in 100%, excess neutrophils in 98% and increased lymphocytes in 85% of the specimens. Epithelioid cells were present in 56% and giant cells in only 40% of the samples.

Epithelioid histiocytes are elongated macrophages with pale cytoplasm devoid of any tangible ingested material such as carbon pigment. Their nuclei are drawn out and indented or folded, producing a variety of footprint-like shapes. The chromatin is finely divided and nucleoli are usually inconspicuous. The cells are arranged in loose aggregates in sputum or washings, but may be aspirated in ragged clumps by FNA (Fig. 2.26). Macrophages of more usual type can also be seen.

Langhans' giant cells are characteristic of the disease but are not often seen in cytology samples, apart from FNA material[117]. They are 2 to 10 times the size of mononuclear macrophages and may contain up to 100 or so ovoid nuclei, typically distributed at one pole of the cell (Fig. 2.27). This feature and absence of ingested carbon help to distinguish them from other multinucleated pulmonary macrophages. The cytoplasm is amphophilic with Papanicolaou staining or pale blue with MGG.

Caseation necrosis is suggested by the presence of pale amorphous material, not easily seen in Papanicolaou stained sputum or bronchial secretions, but recognizable in FNA samples as faintly granular light blue stained debris in MGG or H&E preparations (Fig. 2.28), sometimes speckled darker blue if calcification has occurred. It is within the caseous material that tubercle bacilli are most likely to be found.

Lavage fluid from patients with AIDS who have tuberculosis typically contains many lymphocytes and enlarged foamy macrophages, but it is unusual to find a definite granulomatous picture in these samples[118]. A thin purulent background may be seen.

Mycobacterium tuberculosis may be demonstrated, especially in FNA material, with the use of the Ziehl

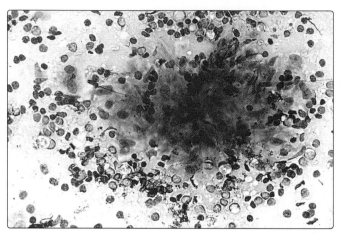

Fig. 2.26 Ragged fragment from an epithelioid granuloma in FNA sample from a patient with pulmonary tuberculosis. Pale histiocytic cells with elongated nuclei can be seen forming the granuloma; lymphocytes and other inflammatory cells are present in the debris at the periphery. (MGG × HP)

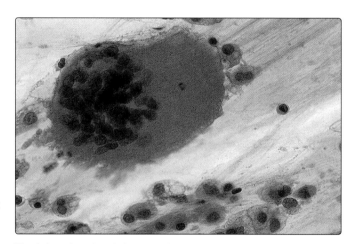

Fig. 2.27 Langhans' giant cell with abundant amphophilic cytoplasm containing many rounded or oval nuclei grouped at one pole. Note absence of any ingested material. Bronchial washing. (Papanicolaou × HP)

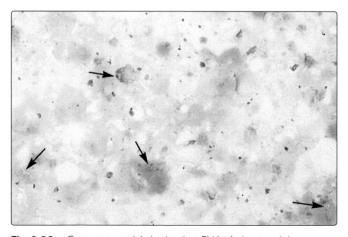

Fig. 2.28 Caseous material obtained on FNA of a lung nodule subsequently confirmed as tuberculous. Within the amorphous debris negative images of the tubercle bacillus can be made out (arrows). (H&E × HP) (Courtesy of Dr G Sterrett, Perth, Western Australia)

Neelsen stain, which reveals a beaded magenta pink straight or slightly curved slender bacillus 1–4 μm in length. Fluorescent methods, such as Rhodamine-auramine staining are quicker to screen if there are large amounts of material. The organisms are sometimes visible as negative staining images within caseous material in FNA preparations stained by MGG (Fig. 2.28). Negative images of the organisms are seen in sputum when there is a high load of acid fast-stained bacilli[119].

Atypical mycobacteria differ slightly in morphology, but cannot be firmly distinguished without culture[120]. When no spare material is available, slides can be decolourized and restained successfully. Nevertheless, culture is essential in all cases, submitting as much material as possible.

Diagnostic pitfalls

The combination of epithelioid histiocytes and Langhans' giant cells is highly suggestive of tuberculosis but is not pathognomonic since either or both cell types can be seen in other conditions with granulomatous inflammation (see Table 2.2).

Caseation necrosis may closely resemble tumour necrosis. A careful search for evidence of granuloma formation or for remnants of malignant nuclei should resolve this problem.

Atypical strains of mycobacteria causing lung infections are morphologically similar to *M. tuberculosis* and can only be distinguished by culture[121].

Viral infections

In contrast to pneumonia due to bacteria, viral infections frequently induce specific cytopathic changes enabling the pathologist to give a firm indication of the causative agent. This is particularly important since other methods of diagnosis may take longer to complete, may not be available, or may not be as accurate. For example, a study by Weiss *et al.*[122] comparing cytology of lavage fluid with immunofluorescence, *in situ* hybridization and viral culture for the diagnosis of cytomegalovirus infection in immunocompromised patients revealed greater sensitivity and specificity for cytology when extensive sampling was used. It is important, however, to obtain confirmation by culture whenever possible if viral respiratory infections are suspected on cytology.

The cytopathic effects are noted mainly in sputum and bronchial secretions[123,124] and can be seen on Papanicolaou staining. Immunostaining will provide firm identification of the virus. Non-specific inflammatory, reactive and degenerative changes are also often present, providing a background to the diagnosis.

Non-specific cytological findings

▶ Necrosis and inflammation

▶ Ciliocytophthoria
▶ Bronchial and alveolar cell hyperplasia

Inflammatory cell exudation and necrotic debris are a frequent finding in the early stages, especially in those infections that cause extensive necrosis of bronchial mucosa such as the influenza and parainfluenza viruses[175]. Ciliocytophthoria, the degenerative change already described, whereby bronchial columnar epithelial cells fragment into ciliated and nucleated remnants with cytoplasmic swelling and nuclear pyknosis, is a variable feature. The phenomenon was first described in adenovirus infections, but is not specific, occurring in other infections and also in association with neoplasia and radiotherapy[97,98].

Bronchial and alveolar cell hyperplasia may be seen, producing clusters of enlarged epithelial cells with swollen hyperchromatic nuclei and prominent nucleoli, as found in a variety of inflammatory states. These changes are easily confused with malignancy but the cohesiveness of the groups in only small numbers and absence of single dissociated abnormal cells favour a reactive process[126].

Specific cytopathic cytological findings

▶ Intranuclear inclusion bodies
▶ Loss of nuclear chromatin pattern
▶ Multinucleation
▶ Cytoplasmic inclusions

The best recognized of these changes are seen in *Herpesvirus hominis* infections[127]. *Herpes simplex* virus[128–130] causes tracheobronchitis initially, but this may progress to necrotizing bronchopneumonia in debilitated or immunodeficient patients[125,128,129]. Varicella-zoster and cytomegalovirus (CMV) also induce cytopathic effects in the respiratory tract, usually as part of a more generalized systemic infection[130–133]. Others less often encountered, although common causes of respiratory disease, include respiratory syncytial virus[134], measles[135] and adenovirus[136].

Herpes simplex virus (Fig. 2.29)

Bronchial epithelial cells and macrophages become multinucleated, with swollen nuclei clustered tightly together, leading to characteristic moulding of nuclear contours. Loss of chromatin pattern follows, due to the presence of viral inclusions. Nuclei take on an empty homogenized or 'ground glass' appearance, with a prominent surrounding nuclear membrane.

As the condition progresses, brightly stained eosinophilic Cowdry type A inclusions develop in the nucleus. These are often triangular or wedge-shaped and may appear refractile. Immunocytochemical methods can be used for definitive identification of herpetic inclusions[137].

The cell changes often occur in a clean background, although if necrotizing pneumonia has supervened acute inflammatory cells and necrotic debris are seen. Herpetic

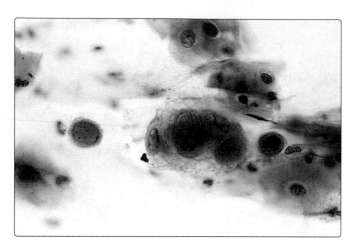

Fig. 2.29   *Herpes simplex* virus cytopathic effects in bronchial columnar epithelium in sputum from a patient on immunosuppressive therapy. The cells are swollen and degenerate with enlarged nuclei, which have a 'ground glass' appearance (see single cell on left). Note the multinucleation and nuclear moulding. (Papanicolaou × OI)

infections may be associated with atypical changes in bronchial epithelium[138]; conversely, patients with treated lung cancer are predisposed to herpetic infections if treatment involves immunosuppression.

Varicella-zoster

Cytologically, the changes in the respiratory tract induced by the Varicella-zoster[130,132] virus are virtually identical to those of herpes simplex infection. The most helpful distinction is the presence of typical skin manifestations. Where necessary, the diagnosis can be confirmed by immunofluorescence or immunocytochemical methods.

Cytomegalovirus *(Fig. 2.30)*

In cytomegalovirus infection[131,132], characteristic large inclusion bodies appear in the nuclei of macrophages and other cells of the respiratory tract. They are surrounded by a halo and the nuclear membrane is thickened giving an 'owl's eye' appearance. The number of inclusions is said to reflect the intensity of the infection[139,140].

Small basophilic cytoplasmic inclusions develop as the disease progresses. These consist of protein-coated viral particles, which impart a finely granular texture to the cytoplasm. The inclusions are difficult to identify in routine preparations[118]. Infected cells swell and undergo degeneration or necrosis, but multinucleation and nuclear moulding are usually not a conspicuous feature.

Combined infections can occur, especially in immunosuppressed patients. *Pneumocystis carinii* may be seen, or there may be evidence of a second virus such as *herpes simplex*, inducing multinucleation and moulding. Bronchoalveolar lavage fluid has been used for rapid detection of CMV by direct *in situ* hybridization[141].

Respiratory syncytial virus

Multinucleated giant cells are the hallmark of respiratory syncytial virus[134] infection, as seen histologically. Basophilic

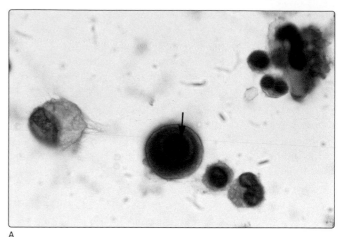

A

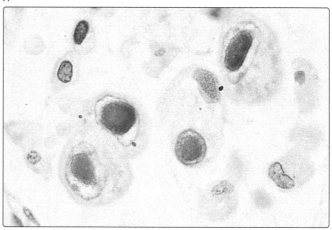

B

Fig. 2.30   Cytomegalovirus inclusion bodies in a bronchoalveolar lavage sample from a transplant patient. (A) (Papanicolaou × OI) (B) (Immunoperoxidase × OI)

inclusions have been described in the cytoplasm of multinucleated and mononuclear cells and in Type II pneumocytes during the course of the illness[142].

Measles virus *(Fig. 2.31)*

Multinucleation of epithelial cells is the characteristic feature of measles pneumonia[135], producing tightly clustered hyperchromatic nuclei at the centre of the cell cytoplasm. Eosinophilic inclusions in both nucleus and cytoplasm may be seen in these multinucleated cells.

Adenovirus infection

In adenovirus infection[136], small eosinophilic inclusions in infected nuclei appear early and these have been described as rosette cells because of the radiating pattern of the chromatin. Some cells have been noted to have a larger basophilic inclusion with loss of the chromatin pattern, being referred to as smudge cells.

Ciliocytophthoria is a striking accompaniment to adenovirus infection, although not specific. Much acute inflammatory exudate will be seen during the stage of active infection.

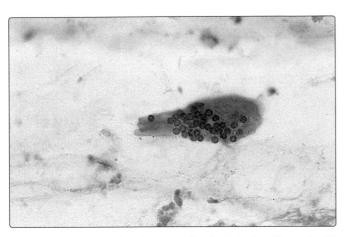

Fig. 2.31   Multinucleation due to measles virus infection. Giant cells with closely packed small dark nuclei in sputum from a child with measles. (Papanicolaou × HP)

Diagnostic pitfalls

In viral infections, clumps of hyperplastic epithelial cells may lead to a false diagnosis of adenocarcinoma, particularly bronchioloalveolar cell carcinoma[126]. A diagnosis of tumour should only be made if individual cells showing the nuclear changes of malignancy are identified and if there is appropriate correlation between the cytological and clinical findings.

The specific changes in different viral infections produce overlapping pictures, hence the need to confirm the identity of the virus by methods such as culture, immunocytochemistry or by serology. Furthermore, several viruses may be present, especially in immunosuppressed patients, and this may not be apparent on routine cytology.

In transplant patients, identification of a virus such as CMV does not necessarily signify active infection unless associated with tissue damage. Lung biopsy may be necessary to establish the presence of viral pneumonia in these patients.

Fungal infections

Fungus cells are generally composed of septate or non-septate hyphae that branch and twine to form a tangled mass known as a mycelium. The hyphae show expansions distally (conidiophores), from which chains of spores (conidia) emerge under aerobic conditions, producing a so-called fruiting head. Some fungi exhibit dimorphism, appearing either as hyphae or as round or oval yeast forms. The yeasts may be arranged in chains resembling hyphae and these are known as pseudohyphae[143].

Infection and allergy are the two most important pathological effects produced in the lung by fungi. Those causing infection are either true pathogens or opportunistic organisms. The latter are saprophytic fungi, only causing disease if the host defences are lowered. They evoke a different range of clinical and pathological responses, compared with infections in immunocompetent people, sometimes with very little inflammatory reaction or granuloma formation.

The presence of fungi in respiratory specimens raises one of three possibilities. First, they may be contaminants from the mouth or atmosphere. Second, there may be saprophytic colonization of an area of pre-existing diseased lung such as a cavity or bronchus, without any invasion of tissues. Third, there could be an active infection (mycosis), with growth of fungi in the lung parenchyma.

Deciding which of these applies to a given cytological sample requires access to clinical details, including any history of immunosuppression, and to the radiological findings. Salivary specimens contaminated by bacterial and fungal overgrowth contrast clearly with the presence of pure fungus in a deep cough sample of sputum or a lavage specimen from a patient with a genuine infection. Inflammatory debris is usually present when there is invasion of tissues by fungi or if a fungal ball (mycetoma) has formed in cavitated lung.

Unlike the bacterial and viral infections already discussed, fungi can often be identified with some precision in respiratory samples, because of their characteristic morphology. Culture of the organism is necessary for confirmation, however.

Aspergillosis

Fungi of the Aspergillus genus are world-wide in distribution and are present in soil and atmosphere. There are about 600 species of Aspergillus organisms, but fewer than 10 are pathogenic to humans. Of these *A. fumigatus* is the most common, *A. niger* and *A. flavus* being much less frequent pathogens. The different species cannot be distinguished by morphology alone[143].

Cytological findings *(Figs 2.32–2.34)*

▶ Septate hyphae 3–4 µm in width
▶ Dichotomous branching at 45° angles
▶ Fruiting heads form in aerobic conditions
▶ Stained by Papanicolaou, PAS and Grocott methods
▶ Potentially a contaminant but should always be reported

Narrow septate hyphae showing dichotomous branching into two equal divisions at a regular angle of 45° are typical of this organism. Unless disrupted by the preparation, the hyphae appear to radiate outwards in a 'sunburst' pattern (Fig. 2.32).

The hyphae stain variably by the Papanicolaou method and are very pale on H&E staining, but are well shown by the periodic acid-Schiff (PAS) stain. Grocott's methenamine silver method (Fig. 2.33) shows the branching structure as stark black hyphae but their septation may not be obvious. They are refractile under polarized light.

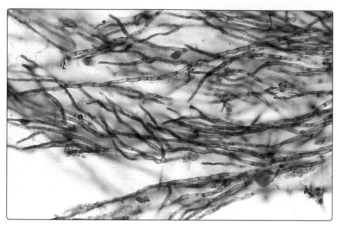

Fig. 2.32 Aspergillus hyphae in a 'sunburst' pattern in lavage fluid from a patient receiving cytotoxic therapy for non-Hodgkin's lymphoma. The hyphae are septate with dichotomous branching. (Papanicolaou × HP)

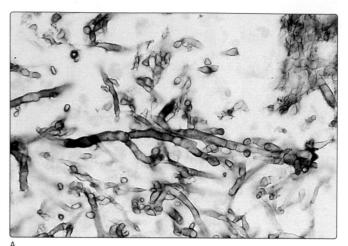

A

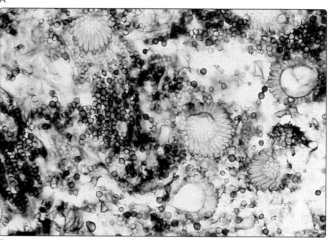

B

Fig. 2.33 (A) Aspergillus hyphae from a pulmonary mycetoma found at post mortem in an elderly man treated for a bronchial carcinoma. (Grocott's methenamine silver × HP) (B) Aspergillus fruiting heads and conidiophores from the same mycetoma. (Grocott stain × HP) (Courtesy of Dr A Padel, Stoke Mandeville, UK)

Fruiting heads develop at the ends of hyphae in aerobic conditions. They consist of pale flask-shaped vesicles from which a projecting crown of stalks bearing chains of conidia can be seen (Fig. 2.33). This structure resembles a brush, hence the name of the genus, derived from the brush known as an aspergillum, used for sprinkling holy water.

Types of pulmonary involvement by Aspergillus[144]

1. Superficial saprophytic colonization of the airways
This is not uncommon in cases of bronchial mucosal damage such as in cystic fibrosis or bronchiectasis, and is usually not associated with any tissue invasion. However hyphae are found in bronchial specimens or sputum from these patients.

2. Allergic bronchopulmonary aspergillosis
In this condition, there is a type III hypersensitivity reaction to the presence of the fungus in the airways, with damage to the bronchial mucosa and lung parenchyma. There may be a long-standing history of asthma, the main cytological features of which are described later in this chapter.

Cases of allergic bronchopulmonary fungal disease develop severe mucoid plugging of the airways, and it is in these plugs with their associated necrotic debris that the hyphae are seen. They may be difficult to identify on Papanicolaou staining but samples can be destained and re-stained by the methenamine silver stain or cell blocks of the mucoid plugs may be helpful (see Fig. 2.57). The diagnosis is an important one and should be borne in mind when sputum or lavage samples include large amounts of eosinophilic debris[145].

3. Pulmonary aspergilloma
Any cavitating lung disease can provide a setting for this form of saprophytic colonization of the lung tissue. Tuberculosis, bronchiectasis, pulmonary infarcts and necrotic carcinomas are among the pre-existing conditions that have been documented. There is no invasion of the lung parenchyma unless cavitation has arisen in lung

destroyed by invasive aspergillosis, as can happen in severely immunocompromised patients.

The cytological findings in sputum, lavage or FNA material include necrotic and inflammatory debris, with fragments of fungal hyphae, some of which may show fruiting heads (Fig. 2.33). Fan-shaped crystals of calcium oxalate are deposited in the fungal ball, especially when *A. niger* is the organism involved (Fig. 2.34)[146]. These refractile crystals may be expectorated or aspirated, or may be found in pleural fluid from an associated effusion, providing a useful clue to the presence of the fungus[147,148].

The fungus goes through phases of growth and death, during which calcification may occur. Haemoptysis is a common presenting symptom in long-standing cases, due to erosion of small vessels in the cavity wall. Atypical hyperplastic or metaplastic epithelial cells are sometimes seen and must be distinguished from malignancy, while remembering that necrotic carcinoma can be the seat of an aspergilloma.

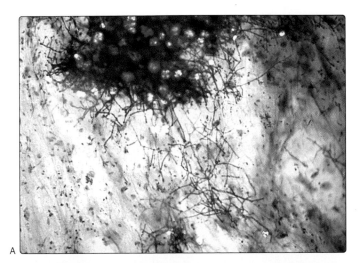

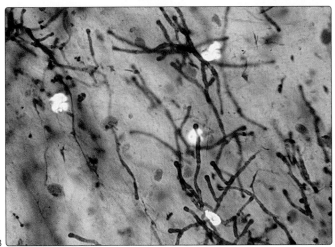

Fig. 2.34 A, B Oxalate crystals are seen on medium and high magnification in this aspiration sample from a patient with a mycetoma of lung. Their presence is confirmed by the use of polarized light and should prompt a thorough search for the accompanying hyphae. (Papanicolaou × MP, HP) (Courtesy of Dr G Sterrett, Perth, Western Australia)

Ultimately the diagnosis rests on a combination of the characteristic radiological appearances of an opacity capped by a meniscus of air, the opacity moving as the patient changes position, together with identification of the organism by morphology, serology and culture.

4. Invasive pulmonary aspergillosis
Invasion of the lung parenchyma is seen only in debilitated patients with immunosuppression, whether iatrogenic or due to a disorder of the immune system. The nature of the immunological deficit determines the pattern of damage to the lung.

Various classifications of the disease have emerged, not distinguishable by cytological methods, and the reader is therefore referred to more detailed accounts for further information[144]. Necrotizing bronchopneumonia, haemorrhagic pulmonary infarction, granulomatous inflammation, abscess formation and lobar pneumonia are among the different pathological reactions found.

The cytological findings relate to the pathological process that has evolved, and are not specific unless the fungus itself is seen. Fungal identification in bronchoalveolar lavage fluid from immunocompromised patients has been reported to have a sensitivity of 64% compared with 40% sensitivity on culture[149], but published results vary considerably[150]. Estimation of aspergillus antigen levels in lavage fluid has also been reported[151]. Oxalic acid levels in lavage fluid are raised, but this finding is not specific as it occurs in CMV infection and also in other conditions[152].

Diagnostic pitfalls

Certain other fungi resemble Aspergillus closely. Candida hyphae are thinner but are prone to swell if degenerate and may then be wrongly identified. Zygomycetes, particularly Mucor species, are also similar although their hyphae are broader with no or very few septa. Culture is necessary for definite identification.

Candidiasis

The ubiquitous Candida fungus is dimorphic, occurring both in budding yeast form and as hyphae. Healthy individuals harbour the organism as a harmless oral mucosal saprophyte, but in the presence of immunosuppression disseminated infection may involve the respiratory tract. Candida is said to be the most frequent of all causes of opportunistic infection and although several potentially pathogenic species exist, *Candida albicans* is by far the most common[142]. Individual species can only be distinguished by culture.

Cytological findings (Fig. 2.35)

► Septate hyphae 3–5 μm in diameter
► Yeast cells 2–4 μm in size
► Chains of yeasts forming pseudohyphae
► Stains with Papanicolaou, PAS and Grocott

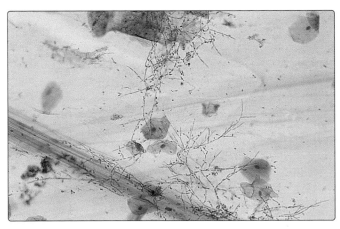

Fig. 2.35 Candida spores and chains of pseudohyphae are abundant in this sputum sample which included many salivary squamous cells and few inflammatory cells. This suggests overgrowth of fungal elements from oral contamination rather than genuine fungal infection. (Papanicolaou × MP)

Yeast forms and hyphae usually occur together in human infections. The hyphae have a delicate branching septate structure. They are found radiating in a disorganized fashion from a mycelial clump or as single hyphal strands separated in the process of preparing the sample. The yeast cells may elongate into budding chains to form pseudohyphae.

Both yeasts and hyphae stain pale pink by the Papanicolaou method but are inconspicuous in MGG stained material. They are well shown by PAS and methenamine silver stains.

Types of pulmonary involvement by Candida species[144]

The patients are virtually always immunosuppressed or have an underlying predisposing condition such as diabetes mellitus, recent surgery or severe burns. Infection follows aspiration of organisms into the lungs or is by haematogenous dissemination. Bronchopneumonia results from the former mode of spread, while the latter causes tiny miliary abscesses in adults. Infants with indwelling venous catheters colonized by the fungus have been found to develop multiple infected pulmonary infarcts. This rarely happens in adults with haematogenous lesions, although other fungi such as Aspergillus do cause haemorrhagic infarction in severely immunocompromised adults.

Significance of Candida in cytological specimens

This may be difficult to ascertain in sputum, washings, brushings and lavages since the organism is such a frequent contaminant[137,153]. When present in acute inflammatory debris in samples from a patient with an appropriate history, it is important to report the finding and ensure that material is sent for culture, although a positive culture may not signify actual lung infection[118].

Raised levels of Candida antigen in bronchoalveolar lavage fluid have been reported by Ness et al. as evidence of significant pulmonary infection. Over 90% of their patients with Candida pneumonia gave positive results by latex agglutination, whereas controls and cases with candidiasis elsewhere were negative, except in those patients in the latter group who had sustained intrapulmonary haemorrhage[154].

FNA specimens, especially transthoracic aspirations, may provide definitive evidence of infection. The yeasts and hyphae are found in a non-specific inflammatory background, which includes neutrophil polymorphs unless the patient has agranulocytosis. Sometimes a picture of granulomatous inflammation is present. As with other samples, culture is essential for confirmation.

Diagnostic pitfalls

These apply to all fungal infections and fall into two categories: the need to identify the fungus accurately with confirmation by culture, and the need to establish whether the presence of the organism is of any clinical significance. The clinical history is important, but so also is the cytological setting, since Candida is part of the normal oral flora and is a frequent coincidental finding in sputum. It is also a common contaminant from water baths, stain solutions and other laboratory sources and may be seen in many different specimens.

A genuine infection is suspected when hyphae and pseudohyphae are intimately related to inflammatory debris in a sample that is clearly of lower respiratory tract origin. Open lung biopsy may be necessary to establish that fungal hyphae are invading tissues. There is less of a problem with FNA material, especially when collected by the transthoracic route.

Candida species must be distinguished from other mycelial fungi such as Aspergillus spp., which branch at 45° and do not form budding yeast cells, and from the fungi with yeast-like forms, for example Cryptococcus, Histoplasma, Torulopsis spp. and others[155]. These organisms do not produce budding pseudohyphae or mycelia. Thus the dimorphism of Candida species can be helpful in identification.

Phycomycosis (mucormycosis)

This group of opportunistic fungal infections, also known as zygomycosis or hyphomycosis, occurs in individuals predisposed by leukaemia, lymphoma and other tumours, in cases of severe burns, renal failure or malnutrition, and as a complication of chemotherapy, diabetes mellitus and drug addiction. The fungi are widespread in nature but only a few, such as Rhizopus, Mucor and Absidia, are likely to be encountered in human infections[143]. The disease runs a fulminant course, with haemorrhagic infarction of the lung due to the ability of the fungal hyphae to invade blood vessel walls, inducing thrombosis[144].

Cytological findings (Fig. 2.36)

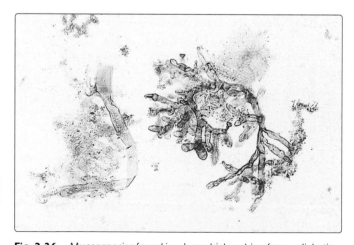

Fig. 2.36 Mucor species found in a bronchial washing from a diabetic patient. Note the broad non-septate hyphae branching at irregularly spaced variable angles. (Toluidine blue × HP) (Courtesy of Professor B Naylor, Michigan, USA)

▶ Non-septate hyphae of variable width (5–50 μm)
▶ Irregular branching at up to 90° angles
▶ Pale staining with most staining methods

All of the fungi of this group appear similar in cytological preparations. The hyphae are thick-walled and non-septate, with a ribbon-like structure averaging 10–15 μm in width. They divide at angles of up to 90°, with irregular spacing between divisions.

Papanicolaou stains show light green or pink hyphae which appear broader than Aspergillus or Candida spp.; they stain less strongly with silver impregnation stains, haematoxylin and eosin, and by PAS. They have been likened to a tangled mass of cellophane ribbons[145].

Diagnostic pitfalls

Problems in diagnosis of mucormycosis are similar to those already described for fungal infections in general. The organisms are common contaminants. They must therefore be seen in the appropriate context, although cellular reaction is sometimes slight in opportunistic infections. The thick-walled hyphae can be taken for plant cells, and when folded they may appear septate, resembling Aspergillus species. Culture is necessary for precise identification.

Cryptococcosis

Cryptococcus neoformans is the causative agent of this world-wide disease, the natural habitat of the fungus being the detritus of birds' nests and pigeon roosts. The birds are not affected but the fungus is pathogenic to humans, colonizing the airways after inhalation or producing outright infection of the lung if the strain is a virulent one. Healthy individuals are able to confine the organism to a single focus, which often resolves but may recur or spread further in the lung parenchyma. If dissemination occurs the fungus exhibits neurotropism, leading to central nervous system involvement and meningitis. Debilitated patients have a rapidly progressive infection with early haematogenous spread in lungs and brain[143].

Early in lung infection, a bronchopneumonic process is seen and the affected area has a slimy surface due to the thick gelatinous capsule, a feature of this organism. At a later stage a more defined focus of firm fibrotic tissue is seen, with very few fungi in the lesion[144]. Extensive lung destruction, cavitation and calcification are rare but the radiological findings can simulate a lung tumour. Because of this, cytology plays a considerable part in diagnosis, and the findings in sputum, lavage fluid, bronchial secretions and FNA material are well documented[156–159].

Cytological findings (Fig. 2.37)

▶ Yeast cells 5–20 μm in size
▶ Thick mucoid capsule

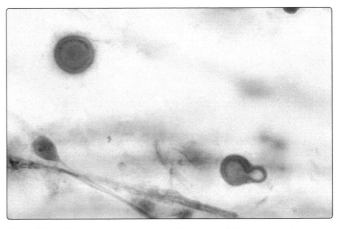

Fig. 2.37 *Cryptococcus neoformans* in sputum stained by mucicarmine to demonstrate the thick mucoid capsule. Note the single budding by a narrow neck, characteristic of this fungus. (× OI)

▶ Single narrow-necked budding
▶ Green cytoplasm with clear capsule on Papanicolaou staining
▶ PAS and mucicarmine stains show the capsule

The fungal cells are rounded yeasts with a thick mucoid capsule of variable width surrounding each organism, holding them apart from one another and any other cytological material present. They reproduce readily by single budding from the parent cell via a thin isthmus, leaving a slight pointed protrusion, which imparts a teardrop shape to the parent organism. Pseudohyphae are rarely seen.

With Papanicolaou staining, the central fungus is dark green or grey and the capsule is clear or only faintly stained. The organisms stain black with Grocott's methenamine silver, but again the capsule is clear. The mucopolysaccharide capsule stains bright pink with Mayer's mucicarmine and PAS stains. Indian ink preparations highlight the dark organism within its clear halo.

Cryptococcal infection may evoke very little inflammation, or there may be an intense acute inflammatory reaction. A granulomatous response with epithelioid histiocytes and giant cells can also occur.

Diagnostic pitfalls

Problems arise from failure to identify the rather inconspicuous smaller forms of the organism unless familiar with their appearance. They may be mistaken for starch granules or artefacts by the unwary[160].

Coccidioidomycosis

The causative agent of this disease is a dimorphic fungus found in desert soils of certain geographical areas, notably in the southern USA, and in Central and Southern America. It produces asymptomatic or indolent granulomatous chest infections by inhalation of airborne arthrospores, which have ruptured from mycelia in the soil. Infection is usually self limiting, but may be chronic and progressive in immunocompromised patients[143].

Productive cough, fever, chest pain, night sweats and weakness are among the presenting symptoms. In persistent disease, miliary granulomas, fibrosis and cavitation occur. The pathology is similar to that of tuberculosis, apart from the presence of endospores lying within large spherules. Radiologically, there may be confusion with carcinoma or tuberculosis[144].

The fungus has been described in sputum and bronchial washings[161], in lavage fluid[162] and in FNA material[163]. Awareness of the disease outside endemic areas is necessary today, with increasing travel and the rise in numbers of immunocompromised patients.

Cytological findings[164]

▶ Intact or collapsed spherules 20–60 μm in diameter
▶ Nucleated endospores 1–5 μm in size
▶ Eosinophilic staining in Papanicolaou preparations
▶ Strongly stained by Grocott method

Intact spherules containing endospores, collapsed spherules and their released endospores are all found. They can be seen in any type of cytological preparation, but are best demonstrated in FNA material. Hyphae are not usually seen. Spherules show a thick cyst wall, eosinophilic or variable by Papanicolaou staining, but which stains strongly with methenamine silver (Fig. 2.38). They may be packed with endospores or empty. Endospores are nucleated and are 1–5 μm in size, but larger yeast cells and deformed degenerate spores may also be seen. A variable amount of inflammatory debris is found, more pronounced if bronchopneumonia or miliary disease is present. Neutrophil polymorphs or evidence of granulomatous inflammation may be seen.

Diagnostic pitfalls

The endospores are easily confused with other small yeasts, particularly Histoplasma and Candida. The endospores of Coccidioides organisms do not bud. Spherules resemble the large cyst-like cells of Rhinosporidium, and when empty they can be mistaken for the large yeast cells of *Blastomyces dermatitidis*, which shows broad-necked budding. These are problems of differential diagnosis, which can be resolved by experience in identification of fungi, and ultimately by culture.

Histoplasmosis

This lung infection is caused by the widely distributed dimorphic fungus *Histoplasma capsulatum var. capsulatum*, but a related fungus *H. capsulatum var. duboisii*, confined to Africa, can on occasion cause similar lung as well as systemic disease.

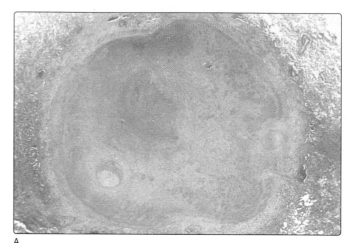

A

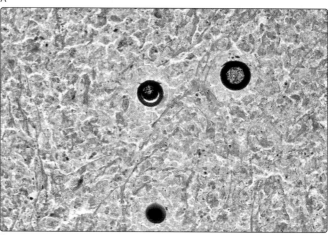

B

Fig. 2.38   *Coccidioides immitis* was found to be the cause of this solitary granulomatous lung lesion in an engineer who had worked briefly in Texas where it is assumed he contracted the infection. The histological section (A) (H&E × LP) shows an indolent caseating granuloma within which fungal spherules are demonstrated by Grocott staining (B). (× HP) (Courtesy of Dr M S Dunnill, Oxford, UK)

The more common condition due to *H. capsulatum var. capsulatum* arises by inhalation of spores from soil contaminated by bird droppings. Although occurring world-wide, it is an endemic infection in some areas of southern USA, Central America and the north of South America[143].

The organism is an obligatory pathogen, but causes only a subclinical or minor illness in most cases. After inhalation, the yeasts are taken up by pulmonary macrophages and are rapidly disseminated to many organs without causing significant pathology. In the lung, a solitary lesion or sometimes multiple localized lesions may develop, producing respiratory symptoms and radiological shadows. Severe systemic disease is only seen in patients with impaired immunity[144].

Histoplasmosis is less frequently recognized than other fungal conditions but the diagnosis has been made in a variety of specimens, including bronchial washings and lavage fluid[165] and in FNA material. The coin lesions seen radiologically are an appropriate target for FNA sampling, but in patients with AIDS diffuse bilateral pulmonary infiltrates are more usually seen, requiring bronchoalveolar lavage for diagnosis[166].

Cytological findings (Figs 2.39, 2.40)

▶ Intracellular yeasts 2–5 μm in size
▶ Poorly visualized on Papanicolaou staining
▶ Strongly stained by the Grocott method

The yeast forms are minute rounded single budding organisms not easily seen in Papanicolaou stained preparations, but shown clearly by the methenamine silver method. Characteristically they are intracellular, having been ingested by macrophages and polymorphs (Fig. 2.39). A small halo can usually be made out surrounding the yeast cells, emphasizing their presence[118].

Their intracellular position is a helpful point of distinction from other small yeasts such as Candida spp.,

which are not usually phagocytosed in this way[167]. This raises the possibility of other intracellular organisms, however, including *Toxoplasma gondii* and Leishmania species. The latter two protozoans do not take up silver stains[165]. Free forms of Histoplasma are inconspicuous in routine preparations and difficult to identify confidently in Grocott stained material (Fig. 2.40).

The standard counterstains used with methenamine silver, such as light green, do not always allow the intracellular position of the fungus to be established with certainty. Counterstaining with haematoxylin and eosin is said to help in identifying the location of the organisms, and not infrequently reveals a mixed infection in immunosuppressed patients[165]. Immunocytochemical staining can be applied to bronchoalveolar lavage specimens for identification of the organisms[168].

Blastomycosis

Infection caused by the dimorphic soil fungus *Blastomyces dermatitidis* occurs mainly in some southern states of North

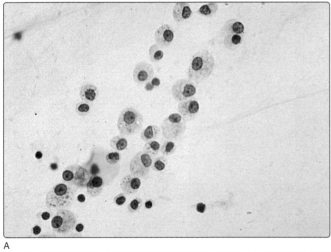

A

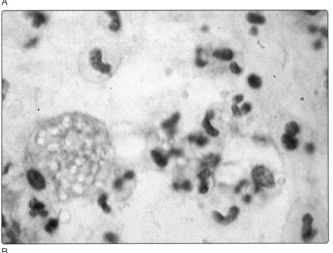

B

Fig. 2.39   (A) *Histoplasma capsulatum* in sputum showing finely vacuolated macrophages which on higher magnification (B), are seen to contain unstained organisms typical of histoplasmosis. (Papanicolaou × MP, OI)

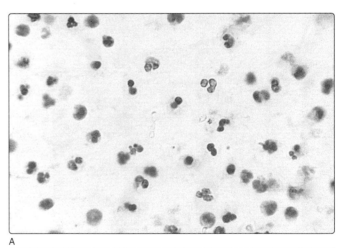

A

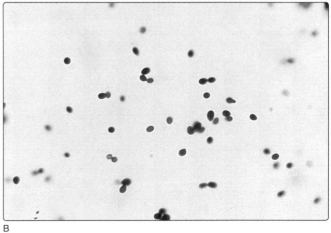

B

Fig. 2.40   (A) Histoplasma organisms shown here in FNA material dispersed in a background of inflammatory cells. They are faintly refractile but difficult to recognize with this stain. (H&E × HP) (B) Grocott staining reveals scattered yeast cells, which have been released from their intracellular position within histiocytes. (× OI)

America and in parts of Central America, although occasional cases have been reported elsewhere. Inhalation of conidia from the soil is followed by an acute or chronic pneumonic process, the latter mimicking tuberculosis or carcinoma in its course. Many other organs may also be involved[143].

Histologically, the lungs show either microabscesses or a granulomatous reaction, followed by fibrosis and cavitation. A striking host response is sometimes seen in this and other fungal infections, producing a dense eosinophilic rim radiating around an individual organism. This material consists of antigen-antibody complexes formed in a hypersensitized individual and is known as the Hoeppli-Splendore phenomenon[144].

A cytological diagnosis can be made from any respiratory tract sample including FNA material. The presence of organisms is evidence of active infection. Confirmation of the diagnosis is obtained by culture or by direct immunofluorescence, which can be performed on smears or histological sections.

Cytological findings[169] *(Fig. 2.41)*

▶ Yeast cells 8–15 μm in diameter
▶ Refractile cell wall, poorly stained in Papanicolaou samples
▶ Strong staining with Grocott's method
▶ Single broad-based budding

The round yeast form shows a dense refractile poorly stained wall, forming a halo around the cell. This may give the impression of a capsule, but the halo is mucicarmine negative and stains strongly with Grocott's technique. The cytoplasm may show a few brown granules with Papanicolaou stain, but most of the cells have shrunken central blue grey cytoplasm. Single budding is seen, the daughter cell remaining closely applied to the parent, creating the appearance of a broad-based attachment. Hyphae are not formed.

Inflammatory cells reflect tissue changes, consisting either of polymorphs or chronic inflammatory cells of granulomatous type. Sometimes organisms are visible in the giant cells as well as lying free. The Hoeppli-Splendore phenomenon has been described in cytological samples[170].

Diagnostic pitfalls

Organisms can be mistaken for host cells in Papanicolaou stained preparations, assuming the core of cytoplasm to be the nucleus[171]. Positive silver staining resolves this problem.

Confusion with other large yeasts can occur, particularly *Histoplasma capsulatum var. duboisii* in cases from Africa. The latter has a different pattern of budding, said to have an hourglass appearance, and is often intracellular. Other organisms such as Cryptococcus or Paracoccidioides have different structure and a different geographical distribution.

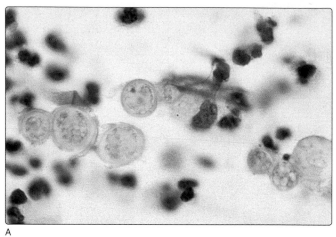

A

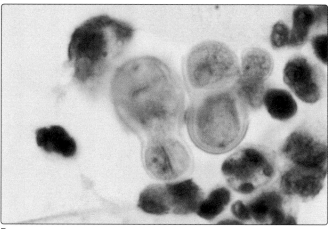

B

Fig. 2.41 *Blastomyces dermatitidis* seen in a bronchoalveolar lavage specimen. The yeast has a thick clear zone peripherally with greyish-blue staining of cytoplasm centrally. Broad-based budding can be seen in B. (Papanicolaou × HP and OI)

Paracoccidioidomycosis

This disease occurs in Central and South America, the habitat of the dimorphic pathogenic soil fungus *Paracoccidioides brasiliensis*. Systemic infection develops after inhalation of hyphae and a bronchopneumonic illness may ensue, progressing to fibrosis, granulomatous inflammation and cavitation[143].

Cytological findings[172]

▶ Variable sized yeasts 6–60 μm in diameter
▶ Stains with Papanicolaou and Grocott methods
▶ Multiple budding

The yeast form is a round organism reproducing by a highly characteristic process of multiple budding. The daughter cells remain attached around the periphery of the parent cell. This appearance, which has been likened to a steering wheel, enables accurate morphological identification of the infection in sputum, bronchial secretions, lavages and FNA samples.

A type of alveolar proteinosis (lipoproteinosis) develops in some patients with paracoccidioidomycosis and may also occur in association with histoplasmosis. Evidence of this may be found in cytological specimens, as described in Chapter 22.

Penicillium species

Several members of this group are known to cause lung infections in healthy or immunosuppressed individuals[173], although they are much less common as a source of opportunistic infection than the fungi already described. *P. marneffei* is a dimorphic member of the group known to cause endemic mycosis in South-east Asia and southern China[174]. It is prone to infect the lungs and has been detected in lavage fluid[175]. The yeast form must be distinguished from Pneumocystis infection, which requires different treatment.

Cytological findings *(Fig. 2.42)*

► Yeast cells 2–6 μm in size
► Poorly visualized on Papanicolaou staining
► Well stained by Grocott's method

The organism is dimorphic, unlike other species of Penicillium. The yeasts are inconspicuous on Papanicolaou staining but Grocott's technique reveals rounded, oval, elongated or cup-shaped cells, some with a thickened dot on the capsule.

Diagnostic pitfalls

The differential diagnosis includes Pneumocystis organisms, which are less variable in shape and do not include elongated forms. They have paired dots on the capsule and are grouped in plaques of alveolar exudate, whereas *P. marneffei* is either intracellular or randomly distributed extracellularly.

Other fungal infections of lung

Many other fungal infections have been detected by cytological methods, notably *Sporothrix schenkii*[176], *Petriellidium boydii*, previously known as *Allescheria boydii*[177] and *Alternaria*[74].

Pneumocystis carinii

This organism, which has become increasingly important as a cause of opportunistic infection, was initially regarded as a protozoan, but is now classified within the order of fungi[178,179]. It is widespread in nature, being present in soil and atmosphere.

Infection occurs by inhalation, causing a treatable form of pneumonia in patients with immunosuppression from any cause, particularly in transplant cases and patients with AIDS.

Patients develop patchy or confluent consolidation of the lungs, producing radiological opacities. The presentation is

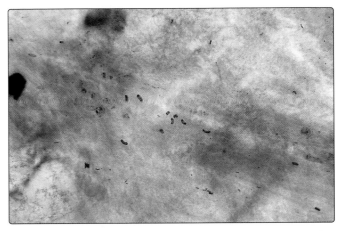

Fig. 2.42   *Penicillium marneffi* in lavage fluid from a patient with AIDS who had recurrent episodes of infection with this organism. The tiny yeast cells vary markedly in shape and size. They are inconspicuous without the use of Grocott or other silver stains. (× HP)

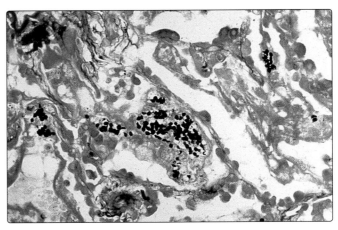

Fig. 2.43   *Pneumocystis carinii* pneumonia in section of lung stained by Grocott's method to demonstrate the silver positive organisms lying in casts of amorphous debris which fill the alveolar spaces. (× MP)

often insidious, with fever, cough and shortness of breath. Histology shows foamy pale pink exudates with haematoxylin and eosin staining, filling alveolar spaces, and it is within these exudates that the cyst wall of the organism can be demonstrated by the methenamine silver method (Fig. 2.43). There is often little inflammatory reaction to the presence of the infection[180].

The organism exists as a nucleated trophozoite 1–5 μm in size, which is capable of amoeboid movement and attaches to type I pneumocytes by means of filopodia. It develops into a cyst 5–8 μm in diameter, the wall of which is focally thickened, giving an appearance of paired inclusions on light microscopy. The cyst contains merozoites, which mature into trophozoites on release from the cyst, thus completing the lifecycle[181].

Cytology has an established role in the diagnosis of Pneumocystis infection, and the findings are well described in sputum, particularly induced sputum[182,183], and in bronchoalveolar lavage fluid[184]. There are also accounts of diagnosis from tracheal aspirates[185], bronchial washings[186] and brushings[187] as well as from percutaneous FNA material[188].

Cytological findings *(Figs 2.44, 2.45)*

▶ Amphophilic proteinaceous alveolar casts
▶ Honeycomb appearance of unstained cysts on Papanicolaou staining
▶ Cysts 5–8 μm outlined within casts by Grocott's method
▶ Trophozoites outside the cysts are not usually visible

Diagnosis is made by recognition of cystic forms of the organism in clusters within proteinaceous alveolar casts[189,190]. The latter are sometimes disrupted by specimen preparation, scattering the cysts widely. Intact alveolar casts are recognizable in Papanicolaou stained material as vaguely rounded amphophilic three-dimensional structures up to 100 μm across. They tend to be

eosinophilic centrally and more cyanophilic at the periphery, with a honeycomb texture due to the presence of the unstained cysts. Finding these casts in Papanicolaou stained samples is strongly predictive of Pneumocystis infection, with a sensitivity of up to 83% and a specificity of 100%[191,192].

Traditionally, definitive cytological diagnosis rests on staining the cysts and this can be achieved in various ways[193,118], listed in Table 2.1. Grocott's modification of the Gomori methenamine silver stain is in common use, revealing cysts with several dot- or comma-shaped internal structures due to areas of thickening of the cyst wall. These cannot be seen in every cyst and are obscured if silver staining is heavy. Collapsed empty cysts are often present, assuming crescent or cup-like shapes. Degenerate cysts stain faintly and may be difficult to recognize with confidence.

Other histochemical stains advocated for demonstrating the cysts have the advantage of a shorter preparation time than the Grocott method. For example, a modified toluidine blue method (Fig. 2.46) has been shown to have equivalent sensitivity to methenamine silver staining, but

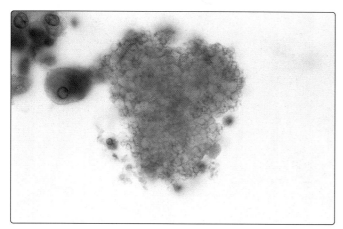

Fig. 2.44 Alveolar cast forming a plaque of amphophilic material with a honeycomb pattern due to the presence of unstained *Pneumocystis carinii* cysts. Bronchoalveolar lavage sample from an HIV positive haemophiliac patient. (Papanicolaou × HP)

Table 2.1	Methods for identification of *Pneumocystis carinii*
Grocott's modification of Gomorri's methenamine silver stain	
Papanicolaou stain	
Toluidine blue stain	
MGG or Diff-Quik stain	
Cresyl violet stain	
Haematoxylin and eosin stain	
Gram and Gram-Wiegert stain	
Acridine orange stain	
Immunofluorescence methods	
Immunocytochemistry	
DNA hybridization	
Polymerase chain reaction	
Electron microscopy	

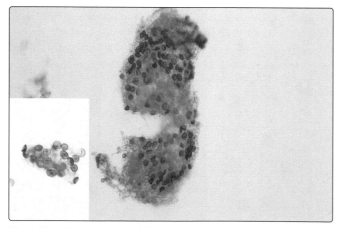

Fig. 2.45 *Pneumocystis carinii* cysts within an alveolar plaque stained by Grocott's methenamine silver method. The inset shows detailed structure of the cysts, several of which contain single or paired darkly stained dots. Trophozoites cannot be seen. Induced sputum. (× HP, OI)

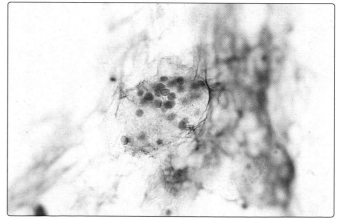

Fig. 2.46 *Pneumocystis carinii* in a plaque stained with modified toluidine blue method, a more rapid technique than the traditional Grocott stain. Bronchoalveolar lavage. (× HP)

is easier and quicker to perform as the reagents do not need fresh preparation for each specimen[194,195]. However the stain involves using concentrated sulphuric acid, making it less acceptable as a laboratory procedure.

Fluorescent microscopy using monoclonal antibodies to cyst wall protein is a sensitive diagnostic technique, although more elaborate than the simpler staining procedures described earlier[196,197]. Pneumocystis detection kits are now available[198]. Immunocytochemical methods can also be used but are relatively expensive and time consuming[199].

Recently, Wakefield and associates have used the polymerase chain reaction to amplify specific segments of DNA from respiratory samples for diagnosis of Pneumocystis infection. They found that amplification of DNA with ethidium bromide enhanced the diagnostic yield in lavage fluid[200] and in induced sputum[201]. The pick-up rate in the latter series was increased from 35% using silver stains to 90% with DNA amplification, including several positive samples that were deemed inadequate on silver staining. The authors suggest it might therefore be possible to use DNA amplification on saliva alone for diagnosis of Pneumocystis.

Trophozoites can be demonstrated by MGG or Diff-Quik stains, but are inconspicuous unless oil immersion magnification is used. Electron microscopy reveals the detailed structure of these organisms[181] but this procedure does not contribute to routine cytological diagnosis.

Diagnostic pitfalls

A reliable rapid method of diagnosis is essential in patient management in order to initiate effective treatment at the earliest possible opportunity. Exclusion of Pneumocystis infection is also important in these immunosuppressed patients to hasten investigation of other treatable conditions.

Despite claims that a definitive diagnosis can be made on Papanicolaou stained preparations alone, recognition can be difficult when only a few casts are present. There are notable variations in the numbers of organisms present in different conditions. Thus patients with AIDS with an extremely heavy load of organisms give a higher diagnostic yield than post transplant cases. The findings on routine stained samples may be tentative without further confirmation by special stains[202].

Studies on the significance of the number of cysts found in cytological specimens are of interest. Pitchenk et al. have pointed out that only very small numbers of silver stained cysts may be found in induced sputum samples from patients who are found to have large numbers on transbronchial lung biopsy[182]. A separate study by Carmichael et al., however, suggested that fewer than five cysts in induced sputum may not represent a significant finding as such cases did not develop evidence of infection on follow-up[203]. Colangelo et al. suggest that the ratio of residual Pneumocystis casts to nucleated cells in lavage fluid taken 21 days after completion of treatment can be used to predict the risk of relapse of pneumonia in AIDS patients over the ensuing six months[204].

Other fungi with budding yeasts such as Histoplasma capsulatum, Candida and Cryptococcus neoformans may be mistaken for Pneumocystis. This risk can be avoided by the use of immunofluorescent staining[205].

Other conditions associated with alveolar casts and amorphous exudate include pulmonary alveolar proteinosis, tracheobronchial amyloidosis and aggregates of degenerate red blood cells adherent to mucus[189]. These structures can usually be distinguished in Papanicolaou stained preparations if appropriate criteria are applied, since there are no cysts within the plaques.

Grocott's or other staining procedures should always be performed with appropriate positive control material. Ideally a cytological preparation should be used as a control since the cysts stain more readily in histological sections than in cytology samples, which may therefore be understained.

Papanicolaou-stained preparations should always accompany the special stains and should be fully screened even if Pneumocystis has already been confirmed. This is necessary to ensure recognition of multiple opportunistic infections or other conditions to which immunocompromised patients are predisposed, such as pulmonary haemorrhage or lymphoma. Cytomegalovirus may be found in association with Pneumocystis pneumonia and other dual infections also occur.

A further reason for screening Papanicolaou stained preparations is to compare the amount of material present with different staining methods so as to detect artefactual loss of deposit from the slide. This can be a problem with Grocott preparations. Further slides should be stained if significant loss has occurred.

In samples from patients with treated Pneumocystis infection, cysts may fail to take up the silver stain, even in the presence of recognizable foamy casts in Papanicolaou stained preparations. Additional Grocott staining may reveal a few empty cysts (Fig. 2.47) but eventually the casts take on a hyalinized appearance and then the cysts can no longer be identified[202]. There is evidence that size of cysts relates to response to treatment, suggesting that smaller forms have a thinner cyst wall[206].

Parasitic infections

Parasitic disease of the lung is much less common than fungal, bacterial or viral infection in developed countries. A few parasites infect human lungs as part of their regular lifecycle, but the majority have a different animal host. Infection may be caused by protozoa, nematodes, trematodes, cestodes, arthropods and leeches. Cytological

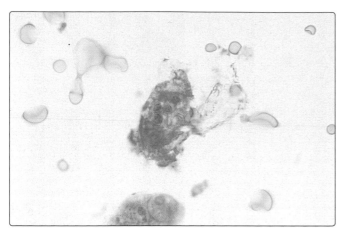

Fig. 2.47 Poorly stained Pneumocystis in Grocott stained induced sputum from an immunosuppressed patient treated with sulphonamide for 5 days prior to the collection of this sample. Only occasional cysts were found, with variable staining of the residual structures and no honeycomb casts were identified in the Papanicolaou stained material. (× HP)

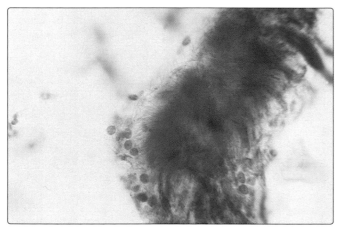

Fig. 2.48 *Entamoeba gingivalis* organisms adherent to actinomyces-like organisms in sputum. Their presence may not signify infection in this setting, as they are saprophytic in the mouth especially if there is poor dental hygiene (Papanicolaou × HP).

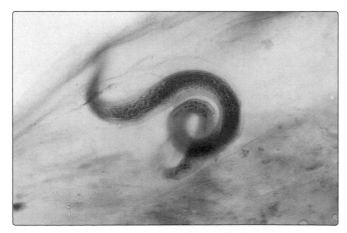

Fig. 2.49 *Strongyloides stercoralis* larva in sputum from an immunosuppressed patient. The coiled shape is a characteristic feature but the indentation at the tail cannot be made out. (Papanicolaou × HP)

findings have only been described for some of these. The reader is referred to more specialized textbooks of parasitology and pulmonary pathology for detailed descriptions of parasites not documented in the cytological literature[207,208].

Other protozoa which have been recognized by cytology in respiratory specimens include *Entamoeba gingivalis*[72,209] (Fig. 2.48) and *Entamoeba histolytica*[209,210], *Giardia lamblia*[211], and Trichomonas organisms[212]. The cytological findings in many of the protozoal infections that are recognized pulmonary pathogens in AIDS have not yet been documented[118,213], but the cytological features of *Toxoplasma gondii* pneumonia in cardiac transplant recipients have recently been described in bronchoalveolar lavage fluid. The trophozoites were best shown by haematoxylin and eosin or MGG stains[214].

Among the nematodes or roundworms found in cytological samples *Strongyloides stercoralis* is important as a cause of haemorrhagic pneumonia in patients receiving high doses of steroids or with impaired immune responses from other causes. Loosely coiled worm-like larvae are expectorated in sputum, measuring 400–500 µm in length (Fig. 2.49)[215,216]. They are thickened at one end and have a notch near the end of the tail, features which are helpful in identification.

Filariasis due to *Wucheria bancrofti* has been diagnosed in pharyngeal and laryngeal smears[217] and also in FNA material[218]. The related worm *Dirofilaria immitis* has also been described in man on FNA[219] although the natural host is the dog. *Schistosoma mansoni* has recently been described in bronchoalveolar lavage fluid[220].

Trematodes identified in sputum and FNA samples include the lung flukes *Paragonimus westermani*[221,222] and *P. kellicotti* which are recognized by finding the golden coloured birefringent ova. They lie in a necrotic inflammatory background with many eosinophils and Charcot Leyden crystals[223].

Of the cestodes that have been described, *Echinococcus granulosus*, the causative agent of hydatid disease, can be identified by finding hooklets and scolices in inflamed necrotic debris in sputum or bronchial secretions[224,225]. FNA is generally regarded as contraindicated in hydatid disease since leakage of cyst contents leads to wide dissemination of the infection. Leakage has been reported in 25% of pulmonary hydatid cysts after FNA in one series[226].

Non-specific inflammatory lung conditions
Chronic obstructive airways disease
Chronic bronchitis and emphysema are linked by having a common aetiological agent, namely inhaled tobacco smoke, and together form a spectrum of lung disease associated with recurrent chest infections. Chronic bronchitis is defined by the presence of hypertrophy of the bronchial mucous glands with increased sputum production. Emphysema results from irreversible destruction of the

respiratory portion of the lung parenchyma, causing breathlessness[227,228]. Clinically, both conditions are frequently present together, although one or other change usually predominates. Sufferers from chronic obstructive airways disease (COAD) are at risk of developing bronchial carcinoma due to the carcinogenic effects of tobacco smoke

Cytological findings *(Fig. 2.50)*

Any or all of the following features may be found in sputum but it should be noted that the overall picture is not specific.

▶ Clusters of hyperplastic bronchial epithelial cells
▶ Goblet cell and reserve cell hyperplasia
▶ Ciliocytophthoria and other degenerative cell changes
▶ Squamous metaplasia, initially regular, becoming atypical
▶ Increased neutrophil polymorphs and macrophages
▶ Curschmann's spirals

Diagnostic pitfalls

These are important because chronic bronchitis is common and the associated changes are not always easy to assess. They have been described in detail in considering non-specific reactive changes in sputum.

Hyperplastic epithelial clusters and goblet cells must be distinguished from adenocarcinoma, bronchoalveolar carcinoma and metastatic carcinoma cells[86,94,229]. The presence of a few cilia around the border of some of the groups is evidence of reactive change. Nuclear features may not be clearly discernible for evaluation of malignancy, but macronucleoli are suspicious of malignancy. Adenocarcinoma cells tend to exfoliate more profusely than benign cells.

Reserve cell hyperplasia may resemble small cell carcinoma on low power magnification, but closer

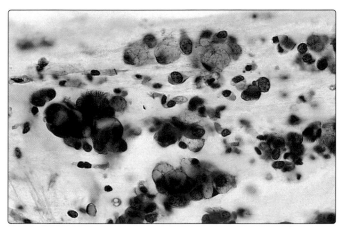

Fig. 2.50 Clusters of hyperplastic bronchial epithelium and goblet cells in a bronchial washing from a patient with severe chronic obstructive airways disease. (Papanicolaou × HP)

inspection reveals more uniform nuclei with regular chromatin and little or no nuclear moulding between the reserve cells. Absence of necrosis is also a helpful feature[88].

Squamous metaplasia in chronic bronchitis mimics squamous carcinoma as the cells become increasingly atypical[230–232]. In early metaplasia nuclear changes do not suggest malignancy, the cells retain their cohesiveness and lack the bizarre shapes and abnormal keratinization of their malignant counterparts. Progressive nuclear and cytoplasmic abnormalities develop, accompanied by loss of cohesion. Differentiation between these cells and invasive or in situ carcinoma is discussed at greater length in Chapter 3.

Bronchiectasis

Irreversible damage by severe respiratory infection may result in permanent dilatation of bronchi associated with production of foul-smelling sputum[233]. Less common than in the past, due to effective use of antibiotics in childhood infections, bronchiectasis is now associated mainly with congenital bronchial abnormalities, cystic fibrosis, asthma, allergic bronchopulmonary aspergillosis and lung tumours. Stagnation of mucus in dilated bronchi predisposes to episodes of infection with further damage to the bronchial tree. Ultimately pulmonary fibrosis and altered vasculature complicate the clinical course of the disease.

Cytological findings

As with chronic obstructive airways disease, the findings represent a combination of various non-specific changes.

▶ Sputum may be purulent, mucoid or blood stained
▶ Neutrophil polymorphs are increased
▶ In follicular bronchiectasis, lymphocytes predominate
▶ Hyperplasia of epithelial cells
▶ Regular or atypical squamous metaplasia

Diagnostic pitfalls

Hyperplastic bronchial epithelial clumps may be confused with adenocarcinoma cells as in chronic bronchitis[86,229]. The same criteria can be used to distinguish benign from malignant clusters, but guarded reporting is necessary[234].

Atypical metaplastic cells (Fig. 2.51) must be distinguished from squamous carcinoma cells, relying on the presence of numerous cells fulfilling the nuclear criteria of malignancy for a diagnosis of carcinoma to be made. Isolated bizarre keratinized cells may be seen in sputum in long-standing bronchiectasis[233–235].

Allergic bronchopulmonary disease

This group of disorders includes extrinsic and intrinsic asthma, allergic bronchopulmonary aspergillosis, eosinophilic pneumonia and extrinsic allergic alveolitis or

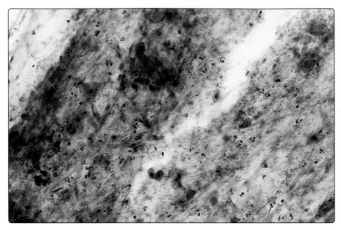

Fig. 2.51   Bronchiectasis showing inflammatory debris with many degenerate keratinized squamous metaplastic cells arising from the wall of a large bronchiectatic cavity. The nuclei are irregular but do not appear frankly malignant. Sputum. (Papanicolaou × MP)

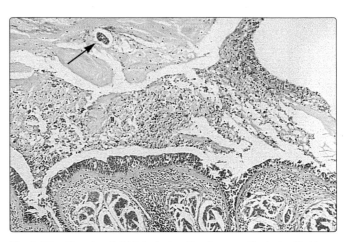

Fig. 2.52   Bronchus in histological section from a patient who died in status asthmaticus. There is a large plug of mucus in the lumen surrounded by a serous exudate containing inflammatory cells, mainly eosinophils. Fragmentation of mucosa is present and an ovoid cluster of epithelial cells can be seen lying at the upper border (arrow). (H&E × MP)

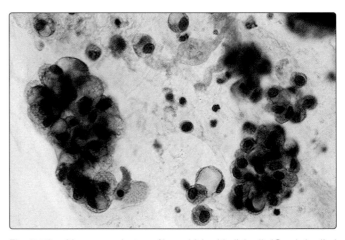

Fig. 2.53   Numerous clusters of bronchial epithelial cells (Creola bodies) in the sputum of a patient during an attack of asthma. A hint of cilia on a few of the cells can be seen at this magnification but the grouping is similar to that of bronchoalveolar cell carcinoma. (Papanicolaou × HP)

hypersensitivity pneumonitis. Cytology plays an important role in assessment of asthmatic patients but is less helpful in diagnosing eosinophilic pneumonia and extrinsic allergic alveolitis. The latter two conditions may in time progress to pulmonary fibrosis. There is an overlap in the pathogenesis of these overtly allergic disorders and some fibrosing or granulomatous lung diseases associated with complicated immunological disturbances.

Bronchial asthma

Although the exact definition is still debated[228], bronchial asthma is characterized by widespread narrowing of airways, fluctuating over short periods of time but largely reversible. The underlying mechanism is a type I allergic response to a variety of external or intrinsic allergens which are not always firmly identifiable.

During an acute attack of asthma there is extensive loss of bronchial epithelium, associated with an outpouring of mucus and serous fluid into the bronchial lumen. Many eosinophils are present in this exudate, which forms viscous obstructive mucoid plugs in the airways (Fig. 2.52). The wall of the bronchus is thickened due to oedema; spasm of the smooth muscle also occurs, increasing bronchial obstruction still further[236].

The changes usually resolve spontaneously or with treatment, although areas of squamous metaplasia may persist, and in some patients collapse and consolidation of the lung parenchyma occurs. Fungal infection may supervene, leading to a type III allergic reaction, with damage to the bronchi and adjacent lung tissue[237]. In Great Britain Aspergillus is the organism most commonly found when this complication occurs.

Characteristic changes in sputum or lavage fluid enable confirmation of asthma to be given in many cases[238]. However, it should be noted that other allergic diseases such as Churg Strauss syndrome and polyarteritis nodosa can be associated with an asthmatic presentation both

clinically and cytologically[239]. Recently it has been suggested that asthmatic changes in the lower airways are reflected in the nasal mucosa, which is more accessible for cytological sampling[21].

Cytological findings (Figs 2.53–2.56)

The findings are well displayed during acute attacks of asthma, but can persist after the attack has subsided.

► Visible mucus plugs may be seen in lavage fluid
► Many bronchial epithelial cell clusters in sputum
► Eosinophils and Charcot Leyden crystals
► Curschmann's spirals
► Inflammatory debris may contain fungal hyphae

Clusters of ciliated bronchial epithelial cells may be papillary or reniform in shape and have well defined

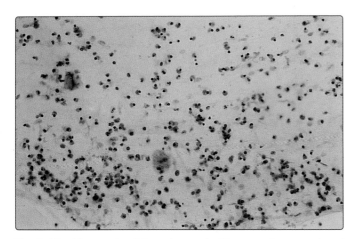

Fig. 2.54 Many eosinophils can be seen in this sputum from an asthmatic child. They have bilobed or, if degenerate, single lobed nuclei and the cytoplasm is filled with eosinophilic granules stained by Papanicolaou. (× HP)

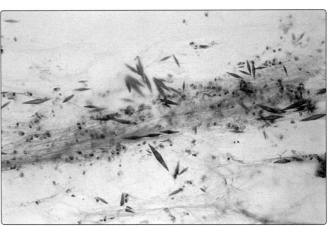

Fig. 2.55 Charcot Leyden crystals in sputum from an asthmatic patient showing the characteristic acicular form and bright orange staining. (Papanicolaou × HP)

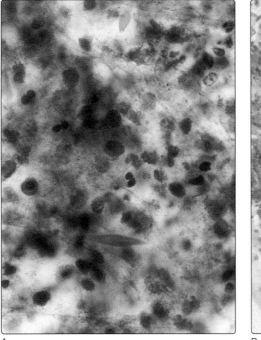

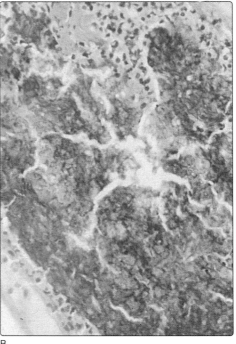

A   B

Fig. 2.56 (A) Sputum from a case of Churg Strauss syndrome, consisting largely of inflammatory debris but fragmented Charcot Leyden crystals can just be made out. (Papanicolaou × HP) (B) Eosinophilic inflammatory debris and inspissated mucus in cell block section of sputum from an asthmatic. (H&E × HP)

borders due to preservation of the terminal plates. They have come to be known as Creola bodies after a young girl in whom they were reported, assuming initially that they were adenocarcinoma cells[240,241].

Eosinophils are usually present. Larger than neutrophil polymorphs, with pink cytoplasmic granules and bilobed nuclei, they are best shown by H&E or MGG stains. Mononuclear or degranulated forms occur, but are not readily identified. Charcot Leyden crystals may be found in all types of cytological material from asthmatic patients. They are formed from breakdown of granules of

eosinophils. Their acicular octahedral form and bright orange colouration with Papanicolaou staining are characteristic and eye-catching[66]. A combination of these findings provides a cytological picture, which is strongly suggestive of bronchial asthma in an appropriate clinical setting.

Amorphous inflammatory debris is sometimes the only finding in the sputum of asthmatics (Fig. 2.56)[145]. Careful searching may reveal fragments of Charcot Leyden crystals in the debris, or fungal elements may occasionally be found (Fig. 2.57). Needle-shaped oxalate

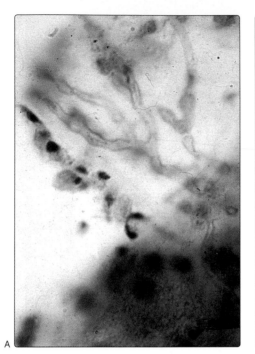 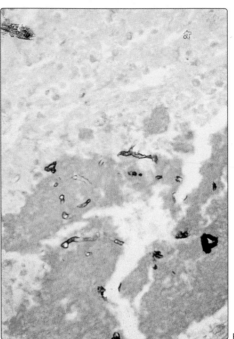

A   B

Fig. 2.57   Aspergillus hyphae seen faintly in the Papanicolaou stained cell block of sputum (A) from a patient with allergic bronchopulmonary aspergillosis, but stained with clarity by Grocott's method (B). (× OI) (Courtesy of Dr G Sterrett, Perth, Western Australia)

crystals arranged in rosettes or wheatsheaf patterns have been noted in sputum and FNA material from cases of aspergillosis associated with asthma. They result from precipitation of oxalic acid, which is produced by the fungus (see Fig. 2.34). They have been regarded as evidence of the presence of Aspergillus even when the fungus itself cannot be identified[148].

Diagnostic pitfalls

Profuse exfoliation of epithelial clusters always raises the possibility of bronchioloalveolar carcinoma[240,126]. The presence of cilia at the borders of groups or the terminal bar are helpful benign features. There is generally more nuclear abnormality in carcinomatous clumps, but the three-dimensional nature of the groups may impair assessment of nuclear detail. As a working principle, it is inadvisable to make a definite diagnosis of this tumour in the presence of a history of asthma. Radiology may help and FNA can provide diagnostic evidence of fungal infection or tumour if a localized lesion is present.

Increased numbers of eosinophils in sputum do not simply equate with a diagnosis of asthma. Increases are also found in conditions such as chronic bronchitis, eosinophilic pneumonia, lung tumours and parasitic infestations[242].

Fungal elements may be overlooked unless anticipated. They can be sparse and degenerate, or hidden beneath inflammatory debris. Destaining a Papanicolaou preparation and restaining with methenamine silver or making use of cell blocks may reveal the hyphae (Fig. 2.57).

Non-infective granulomatous lung disease

Infections such as tuberculosis are responsible for most of the treatable granulomatous diseases of lung but there are numerous other important disorders associated with granuloma formation. The common causes are listed in Table 2.2.

Granulomata can sometimes be firmly identified in FNA material whereas in sputum and bronchial brushings the findings are often non-specific. Open lung biopsy, for so long the traditional method of diagnosis, is still usually employed to elucidate the nature of granulomatous lung disease. However FNA combined with microbiological culture has proved valuable in establishing the aetiology of infective granulomata[243,244]. Bronchoalveolar lavage is useful in the primary diagnosis of granulomatous lung disease and for monitoring disease progress[245,52].

Sarcoidosis

This is one of the most common of non-infective granulomatous disorders, exemplifying the changes seen in many other idiopathic granulomatous lung conditions. It is a systemic disease of unknown aetiology affecting mainly young or middle aged patients, especially women. The respiratory tract is involved in over 90% of cases. Cellular immunity is depressed systemically, but there are increased

Table 2.2   Some conditions associated with pulmonary granulomata

Infections	Occupational exposure
Bacteria	Asbestosis
Mycobacterium tuberculosis and other mycobacteria	Silicosis
	Heavy metals
Nocardia asteroides	Aluminium
Fungi	Beryllium
Aspergillus fumigatus, niger, flavus	Organic dusts (extrinsic allergic alveolitis)
Blastomyces dermatitidis	**Idiopathic lung diseases**
Candida albicans	Sarcoidosis
Coccidioides immitis	Rheumatoid disease
Cryptococcus neoformans	Wegener's granulomatosis
Histoplasma capsulatum, duboisii	Allergic angiitis and granulomatosis
Paracoccidioides immitis	Necrotizing sarcoid granulomatosis
Rhinosporidium seeberi	Lymphomatoid granulomatosis
Sporothrix schenkii	
Torulopsis glabrata	Bronchocentric granulomatosis
Trichosporon capitatum	
Zygomycetes	Granulomatous disease of childhood
Parasites	**Iatrogenic causes**
Arthropods	Drug toxicity
Cestodes	Radiation exposure
Nematodes	Oxygen therapy
Protozoa	**Other conditions**
Trematodes	Foreign body reaction
	Tumour related granulomas

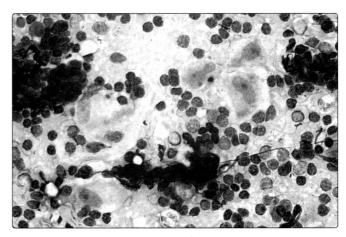

Fig. 2.58   Epithelioid histiocytes and lymphocytes in FNA material from a middle-aged woman with a lung shadowing due to pulmonary and hilar lymph node sarcoidosis. Note the elongated pale footprint-shaped nuclei of the epithelioid cells and their poorly stained cytoplasm. (MGG × HP)

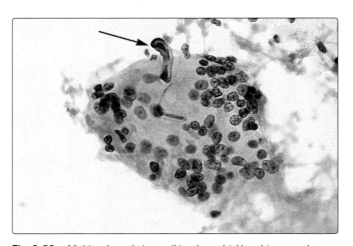

Fig. 2.59   Multinucleated giant cell in a bronchial brushing sample from a patient with sarcoidosis. The cytoplasm contains a partly dislodged Schaumann body, seen at the upper border of the cell (arrow). (Papanicolaou × OI) (Courtesy of Professor B Naylor, Michigan, USA)

numbers of activated T lymphocytes, especially T helper cells, at sites of granuloma formation[246,247]. Cytological findings have been documented in sputum, lavage fluid and FNA samples[247–251].

Cytological findings *(Figs 2.58, 2.59)*

▶ Epithelioid histiocytes
▶ Small and large giant cells, some of Langhans' type
▶ Increased lymphocytes, especially T helper cells

Epithelioid histiocytes are the most characteristic feature, either dissociated or in clusters of spindle shaped cells with pale cytoplasm and elongated footprint-shaped nuclei (Fig. 2.58). Single cells are more often seen in sputum and washings, whereas in FNA smears, ragged fragments of intact granulomata may be found.

Large and small multinucleated giant cells of histiocytic origin accompany the mononuclear cells. They are often of Langhans' type, with nuclei orientated at one pole of the cell, their cytoplasm devoid of any ingested carbon particles. Occasionally crystalline cytoplasmic inclusions are visible, either in the form of large conchoidal structures known as Schaumann bodies (Fig. 2.59), or smaller star-shaped asteroids. Inclusions are more readily seen in cell blocks prepared from FNA material than in

direct spreads[250], but they have also been noted in sputum[248].

Lymphocytes may be found in abundance, especially in lavage fluid, reflecting a profuse lymphocytic exudate into the alveoli while the disease is active. The lymphocytes are predominantly of T cell type, constituting 10–70% of the inflammatory cell population, and are mainly T helper cells. Healthy non-smokers have levels below 7%[252]. The ratio of lymphocytes to neutrophil polymorphs, macrophages and other inflammatory cells is helpful in supporting the diagnosis of sarcoidosis and in monitoring response to treatment or progression of the disease.

Diagnostic pitfalls

A diagnosis of sarcoidosis can only be made in the appropriate clinical setting since other granulomatous disorders may produce an identical picture cytologically. Infective causes of granulomatous lung disease must always be excluded by stains for acid fast bacilli, fungi and other organisms, and culture of the sample is essential. Lavage and FNA specimens may have to be divided to provide material for culture.

Foreign body reactions should be excluded by examination of the material under polarized light. Granuloma formation due to substances such as beryllium or aluminium can be excluded in this way, as can silicosis. Carbon pigment in the giant cells suggests they are not derived from a granulomatous process.

Elongated epithelioid histiocytes have been confused with connective tissue cells in FNA material[102]. Microarchitecture may still be discernible in granulomas, in contrast to the dispersed pattern of connective tissue cells. Moreover, the footprint nuclei of epithelioid cells are unlike the elliptical and spindle shaped nuclei of fibroblasts or smooth muscle cells.

FNA samples containing significant amounts of necrotic debris accompanying granulomatous material are unlikely to have originated from sarcoidosis. Tuberculosis and necrotic tumour tissue are more usual sources. Keratinizing squamous carcinomas frequently evoke a foreign body giant cell response[102].

Other granulomatous diseases

Several other less common granulomatous lung conditions have yielded cytological material enabling the correct diagnosis to be proposed. These include connective tissue diseases such as rheumatoid arthritis, systemic lupus erythematosus and scleroderma, and inflammatory disorders of blood vessels in which vasculitis is the primary lesion.

The connective tissue diseases, thought to be due to autoimmune and immune complex mediated injury to collagen, are associated with a variety of pulmonary manifestations including granulomatous inflammation, pulmonary fibrosis and pleural effusions[244–254]. Cytological findings are variable and are only of use in diagnosis in the light of the clinical features.

Localized granuloma formation in rheumatoid arthritis can be mistaken for malignancy radiologically when there is central necrosis and cavitation. Atypical metaplasia has been found in samples from rheumatoid patients and this, together with background necrosis, may suggest a carcinoma. Strict criteria of malignancy must be sought[255].

Vasculitis may be a component of many different lung disorders including collagen diseases. However there are several conditions in which vasculitis, necrosis and a granulomatous pulmonary infiltrate are the main features. Wegener's granulomatosis is the most common, producing multiple fluctuating lesions in lungs, nasal passages and kidneys. The Churg Strauss syndrome also forms part of this spectrum.

Wegener's granulomatosis has been suggested on FNA findings by the presence of fragmented eosinophilic granular necrotic collagen, aggregates of palisaded histiocytes including some giant cells, and an acute inflammatory cell infiltrate[256]. Specific confirmation of the diagnosis can be made serologically using the ANCA test, based on the recognition of an antineutrophil cytoplasmic antibody. Confirmatory ANCA testing should be prompted by the above cytological findings when the clinical setting is appropriate[256].

Interstitial lung disease in pulmonary fibrosis

This group of inflammatory disorders of lung parenchyma includes a range of pathological fibrosing conditions with clinical and radiological similarities, leading to a variable degree of restrictive ventilatory impairment[257]. As a general principle, persistent inflammation in any organ is accompanied by fibrosis, and in the lung, 25% of which is composed of fibrous tissue, pulmonary fibrosis is the common end result of many different disease processes. The best known of these are listed in Table 2.3. In many cases, however, a causative agent cannot be identified with certainty[258].

Fibrosis of the lung develops either within alveolar spaces following active inflammation, resulting in fibrosing alveolitis (Fig. 2.60), or in the alveolar walls leading to interstitial fibrosis (Fig. 2.61). In many patients both processes occur simultaneously. The onset may be acute and severe as in the Hamman Rich syndrome, or insidious with gradual progression, the common course in idiopathic pulmonary fibrosis. An important subgroup includes patients with bronchiolitis obliterans in whom low-grade

---

Table 2.3 Conditions associated with pulmonary fibrosis

Industrial diseases	**Iatrogenic causes**
Silicosis	Cytotoxic antibiotics
Coal worker's pneumoconiosis (massive pulmonary fibrosis)	Alkylating agents
	Antimetabolites
Asbestosis	Antirheumatic drugs
Heavy metal exposure	Radiation therapy
Organic dusts exposure	Oxygen toxicity
Immune disorders	**Direct lung injury**
Rheumatoid disease	Adult respiratory distress
Systemic sclerosis	syndrome
Dermatomyositis	Paraquat poisoning
Sjögren's syndrome	**Idiopathic conditions**
Coeliac disease	Fibrosing alveolitis
End stage granulomatous disease	Bronchiolitis obliterans
	Organizing pneumonia
Sarcoidosis	Pulmonary haemosiderosis
Fungal infections	Histiocytosis X
Mycobacterial infections	Alveolar proteinosis
Viral infections	
Mycoplasma pneumonia	

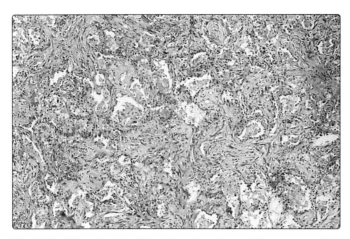

Fig. 2.60   Fibrosing alveolitis and cryptogenic organizing pneumonitis in a section of lung. Most of the alveolar spaces are filled with loose nodular connective tissue, which can be seen extending along alveolar ducts. (H&E × MP)

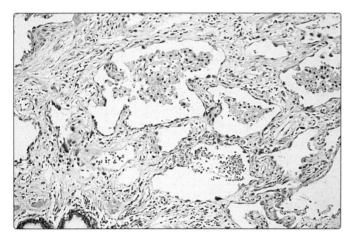

Fig. 2.61   Section of lung with idiopathic interstitial fibrosis. The alveolar walls are thickened by fibrous tissue and alveolar epithelium is prominent. A few inflammatory cells and macrophages can be seen in the distorted alveolar spaces. (H&E × HP)

inflammation and tongues or nodules of loose fibrosis affect the small airways. These cases respond to steroid therapy, as do some of the patients with cryptogenic fibrosing alveolitis, the terminology applied to cases of interstitial fibrosis and inflammation of unknown aetiology[259, 260].

The classification of pulmonary fibrosis has evolved over time as new information about the pathogenesis of the differing patterns of disease has emerged[258,261]. In most cases cytology cannot determine the cause of the disease process but some indication as to prognosis and effectiveness of treatment can be obtained by monitoring inflammatory cell ratios in bronchoalveolar lavage fluid[262]. Accurate quantification of cells requires meticulous attention to detail. The first aliquot of lavage fluid is usually discarded as it includes bronchial content. Cytocentrifugation of subsequent material gives good display of cells but membrane filtration methods have been recommended to ensure full harvesting of the cellular component[47].

Cytological findings

▶ **Inflammatory cell-ratios in lavage fluid**

There is an extensive literature on the analysis of inflammatory cell content following descriptions of techniques in the early 1980s[53,54], relating changes to the two broad groups seen on histology[263-265].

There may be a predominance of neutrophil polymorphs, as exemplified by early idiopathic pulmonary fibrosis[266], occupational dust diseases and collagen-vascular disorders. These patients usually show an associated increase in macrophage and lymphocyte counts as well[267].

In the second group, lymphocytes are the predominant cell, with virtually complete absence of polymorphs. Sarcoidosis and extrinsic allergic alveolitis are examples of this pattern[268]. In sarcoidosis the lymphocytes are mainly of T helper subtype, whereas in extrinsic allergic alveolitis T suppressor cells predominate. There may be marked eosinophilia in eosinophilic pneumonia and to a lesser extent in cryptogenic fibrosing alveolitis.

▶ **Epithelial cell changes** *(Figs 2.62–2.64)*

Long-standing pulmonary fibrosis is frequently associated with abnormalities of bronchial and alveolar epithelial cells regardless of the underlying cause. Type I pneumocytes undergo necrosis at an early stage, to be replaced by type II pneumocytes which enlarge, become cuboidal and eventually atypical. Bronchiolar epithelium also undergoes reactive and hyperplastic changes, and may extend to line the fibrosed alveolar spaces.

These epithelial cells sometimes show striking nuclear changes, with enlargement, hyperchromasia, prominent nucleoli and heavily stained nuclear membranes (Figs 2.62, 2.63). Multinucleation may be seen. Bronchial cells are shed in larger clusters (Fig. 2.64) than alveolar cells, which are generally in twos and threes or present as single cells. The distinction may, however, not always be obvious, especially when cytoplasmic degeneration has occurred.

The appearances may bear a close resemblance to the cytology of malignancy, forming a well-recognized source of false positive diagnosis. To complicate the situation, peripheral lung tumours are prone to develop in long-standing pulmonary fibrosis. The problem of differentiating hyperplasia from malignancy is more likely to arise with sputum and bronchial secretions than in FNA material, where a pure population of tumour cells gives a diagnostic picture.

Safeguards against overdiagnosis of malignancy

A profusion of epithelial cell clusters in respiratory tract samples from patients with diffuse radiological shadowing or a known diagnosis of pulmonary fibrosis should be reported with caution. In general, numerous clusters

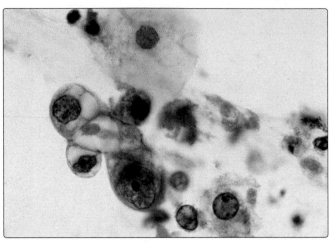

Fig. 2.62 Hyperplasia of type II pneumocytes. These cells are from a BAL specimen in a patient with idiopathic pulmonary fibrosis. There were moderate numbers of single and paired enlarged rectangular, rounded or polygonal cells with nuclear changes regarded at the time of reporting as suspicious of malignancy. Subsequent post mortem examination showed atypical alveolar cell hyperplasia accompanying the fibrosis, but no tumour was found. (Papanicolaou × HP)

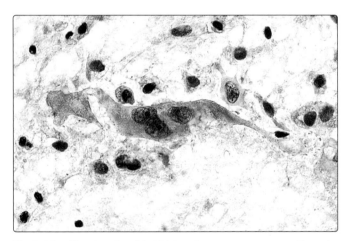

Fig. 2.63 Fibrosing alveolitis. This imprint smear was prepared from the lung section of fibrosing alveolitis shown in Fig. 2.60. Solitary bizarre cells with atypical nuclei such as shown here, reflect the alveolar cell hyperplasia seen on histology. (Toluidine blue × HP)

containing many cells are more suggestive of malignancy, whereas smaller groupings and single cells are more typical of alveolar cell hyperplasia.

The presence of cilia around the periphery of cell clumps indicates a reactive rather than a neoplastic process (Fig. 2.64). Swollen cells with enlarged nuclei found in cases of pulmonary fibrosis usually still maintain a fairly normal nuclear/cytoplasmic ratio compared with adenocarcinoma cells. A marked inflammatory cell component in this setting should raise the possibility of a reactive condition, although the finding by no means excludes tumour.

If only limited material is available it is worth suggesting further sampling. Where the findings are highly suspicious of malignancy but the diagnosis is not confirmed, monitoring the patient over time may reveal a

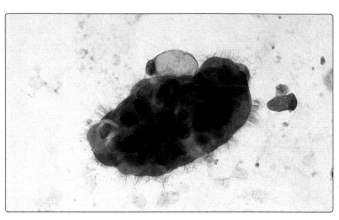

Fig. 2.64 Fibrosing alveolitis. A clump of hyperplastic epithelial cells with a fringe of cilia visible along the outer border. Although the group is too dense for assessment of nuclear detail, the presence of cilia indicates that it is benign. (Papanicolaou × HP)

bronchioloalveolar cell carcinoma in a few cases, an example of a false 'false positive' diagnosis[269].

Specific types of pulmonary fibrosis

Certain types of lung damage eventually leading to pulmonary fibrosis will be described in further detail since the onset of fibrosis is preceded or accompanied by important cytological findings. These conditions include drug-induced toxicity, radiotherapy, other iatrogenic changes and industrial lung disease due to toxic chemicals or dusts.

Drug-induced pulmonary toxicity

Therapeutic agents may injure the lung directly by cytotoxic effects or a hypersensitivity reaction, or they may induce systemic conditions which in turn are associated with damage to the lung[270-272]. An example of the latter type of iatrogenic disease is the systemic lupus erythematosus syndrome induced by drugs such as hydralazine, procainamide or phenytoin.

Direct toxic effects exerted on bronchiolar or alveolar cells by various compounds and hypersensitivity drug reactions causing alveolitis form an important group for cytologists since early recognition of these treatment complications can be lifesaving. Not surprisingly, the most severe lung damage is due to cytotoxic drugs used as chemotherapy for tumours, particularly haematological malignancies. Some of the earliest accounts of these effects related to the use of bleomycin and busulphan in such patients[270]. Many other drugs have also been found to cause diffuse lung damage or pulmonary fibrosis as a side effect of their therapeutic action (Table 2.4).

Assessment of specimens for drug-induced lung disease is often complicated by the use of multiple drug therapy, and also the possibility that the underlying condition may itself have produced lung changes. The mechanisms of pulmonary injury by drugs have been widely reviewed[271-274].

Table 2.4   Some drugs associated with pulmonary toxicity

Non-cytotoxic drugs	Cytotoxic drugs
Antibacterial agents	Cytotoxic antibiotics
Nitrofurantoin	Bleomycin
Sulphasalazine	Mitomycin
Analgesics	Cyclosporin A
Aspirin	Nitrosoureas
Anticonvulsants	Carmustine
Antiarrhythmic agents	Alkylating agents
Amiodarone	Busulphan
Antirheumatic drugs	Cyclophosphamide
Penicillamine	Chlorambucil
Gold salts	Melphalan
Colchicine	Antimetabolites
Diuretics	Methotrexate
Opiates	Azathioprine
Sympathomimetics	Cytosine arabinoside
Tranquillizers	Other cytotoxic drugs
	Procarbazine
	Vinca alkaloids

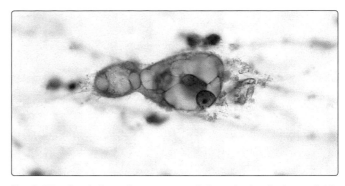

Fig. 2.65   Atypical type II pneumocytes in bronchoalveolar lavage fluid from a young man with acute lymphoblastic leukaemia. He was receiving Cyclosporin therapy and had developed breathlessness with diffuse lung shadowing. Note the degenerative vacuolation of cytoplasm and the enlarged abnormal nuclei with prominent nucleoli. (Papanicolaou × HP)

Cytological findings[266] (Figs 2.65–2.67)

▶ Atypical alveolar and bronchiolar cells
▶ Inflammatory debris
▶ Regenerative epithelium in sheets
▶ Lymphocytes and eosinophils in hypersensitivity pneumonitis

A clear history of drug exposure is necessary for diagnosis. In multiple drug therapy, identification of the responsible agent is not usually possible from the cytological findings alone, but requires accurate clinical correlation. Early descriptions of the findings in sputum were given by Bedrossian and Corey in 1978[275], followed by documentation of similar changes in bronchial secretions[276], and in bronchoalveolar lavage fluid[277–281].

Swollen polygonal or rectangular epithelial cells are present in modest numbers, scattered singly, paired or in small groups (Fig. 2.65). They have dense greenish grey cytoplasm, often showing degenerative vacuolation. The nuclei are enlarged and have prominent nucleoli, with condensation of chromatin on the nuclear membrane. They may be hyperchromatic or depleted of chromatin. Cell groups are flat and often acinar in arrangement. A spectrum of changes has been described, including complete disintegration of the nucleus, leaving anucleate cytoplasmic remnants[282,283].

The origin of these large single and paired cells has been investigated by electron microscopy, revealing type II pneumocytes with degeneration of lamellar bodies and cytoplasmic degranulation[284,273]. Type I pneumocytes undergo necrosis at an early stage of exposure, accompanied by oedema and haemorrhage. Other evidence of damage to the epithelium of the airways is sometimes present in the early stages, consisting of inflammatory and necrotic debris, with ragged sheets of

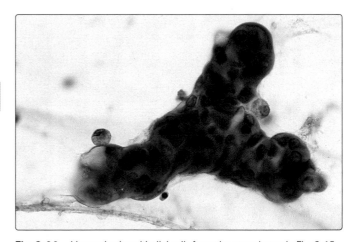

Fig. 2.66   Hyperplastic epithelial cells from the case shown in Fig. 2.65 This is a large three-dimensional group of cells and is therefore likely to be bronchial in origin. Nuclei are difficult to examine but appear enlarged and hyperchromatic. (Papanicolaou × HP)

regenerative inflamed bronchial epithelium composed of swollen cells with enlarged nuclei and prominent nucleoli (Figs 2.66, 2.67).

The inflammatory cell component in lavage fluid is variable, depending on the nature of the damage and the drug. In cases of drug-induced hypersensitivity pneumonitis, there are many lymphocytes and eosinophils[279,285]. Increased neutrophils are seen in lavage fluid in bleomycin induced toxicity[286], and are also a feature of other drug reactions, e.g. to gold therapy[277].

An unusual cytological picture has been documented with the antiarrhythmic drug amiodorone[287–290] which, in addition to causing damage to pneumocytes and pulmonary fibrosis, also produces changes in alveolar macrophages. In lavage fluid the macrophages comprise up to 85% of the cell population and develop pale lacy cytoplasm due to the presence of numerous osmiophilic inclusion bodies, derived from damaged lysosomes. A recent study of multivesiculated macrophages in fine needle aspiration material from lung masses found a case

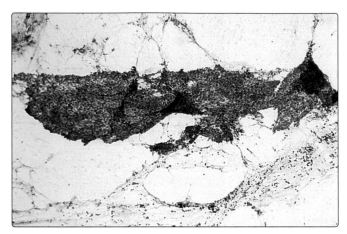

Fig. 2.67   Repair changes in bronchial epithelium. Large ragged sheet of bronchial epithelial cells seen in bronchoalveolar lavage fluid from a patient receiving chlorambucil. The nuclear pleomorphism, prominent nucleoli, and ill-defined cell boundaries are typical of a repair process. (Papanicolaou × MP)

of Amiodorone exposure in which 95% of macrophages showed multivesiculation and this was also present in other cells in the sample[291]. This toxic effect is seen in 6% of patients receiving the drug and may be associated with pleural effusions containing similar macrophages.

Oxygen toxicity

Therapeutic use of oxygen for patients needing artificial ventilation results in alveolar damage proportionate to the concentration of oxygen rather than the duration of exposure. There is initial oedema, haemorrhage and hyaline membrane formation in the alveoli, with necrosis of type I pneumocytes. Pulmonary fibrosis may ensue.

Premature neonates with respiratory distress syndrome treated with oxygen are at special risk of damage to the epithelium of airways and alveoli. The changes have been studied in tracheal aspirates and are liable to progress to pulmonary fibrosis if the infant survives[292–294].

Cytological findings

▶ Atypical type II pneumocytes
▶ Groups of hyperplastic bronchial and bronchiolar cells
▶ Squamous metaplastic cells

Shedding of atypical type II pneumocytes, arranged singly, in pairs and in small groups, is similar to the pattern found in other toxic lung reactions. Hyperplasia of bronchial and bronchiolar cells leads to exfoliation of cell clusters which may be ciliated. These are found in many reactive conditions due to chronic benign lung disease. Squamous metaplasia of bronchial mucosa is seen and samples may include atypical metaplastic cells as the changes progress.

Radiation effects

Despite recent refinements in radiological techniques, the use of radiotherapy in the treatment of intrathoracic

tumours is still associated with the risk of cytotoxic effects on the epithelial cells of airways and alveoli. The changes cause diagnostic problems, particularly when monitoring for tumour recurrence[295]. Radiotherapy for tumours outside the thorax, such as breast or head and neck cancers, is less likely to injure the lungs, but it should be noted that cell damage is not necessarily confined to the area directly irradiated.

Histologically, within a day or two of irradiation the bronchial epithelial cells and type I pneumocytes undergo necrosis; there is an outpouring of haemorrhagic oedema fluid with hyaline membrane formation. Type II pneumocytes undergo hyperplasia and subsequently may transform into type I cells. They may also become increasingly atypical in cases of severe damage, with progression to fibrosis.

Cytological findings[296] (Figs 2.68, 2.69)

▶ All epithelial cell types affected
▶ Swelling of cytoplasm, bizarre shapes, enlarged nuclei
▶ Multinucleation
▶ Cytoplasmic vacuolation and amphophilia
▶ Macronucleoli
▶ Metaplasia and dysplasia in later stages

Squamous, columnar and alveolar epithelial cells are affected and the changes are of a similar nature in each cell type. Cytomegaly and nuclear enlargement go hand in hand, maintaining a nuclear/cytoplasmic ratio that is either normal or only slightly raised. Multinucleation is a frequent finding, with coarse but uniform chromatin and multiple irregular nucleoli or macronucleoli. Cytoplasmic degenerative changes consist of fine or gross vacuolation of cell cytoplasm and variable staining.

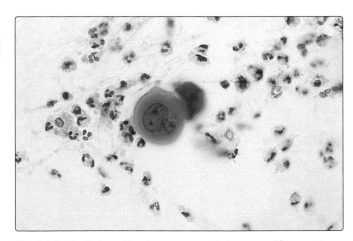

Fig. 2.68   Radiation effects in squamous cells in sputum from a patient with carcinoma of the oesophagus treated by radiotherapy. The cells show nuclear enlargement, binucleation and prominent nucleoli. There was no evidence of pulmonary metastases and the patient remains well. (Papanicolaou × HP)

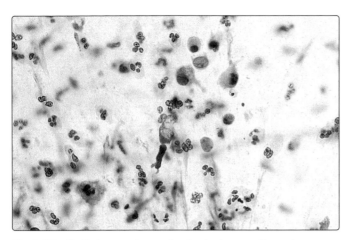

Fig. 2.69 Radiotherapy changes leading to degeneration and fragmentation of epithelial cell cytoplasm with ciliocytophthoria. (Papanicolaou × HP)

Squamous metaplasia is seen in the healing phase and may persist for many years. Atypical features in metaplastic or alveolar cells can regress or become more pronounced with time.

Diagnostic pitfalls

A false positive diagnosis of malignancy may be made. The presence of nuclear and cytoplasmic changes in many different cell types is a pointer to the correct diagnosis, as is the relatively normal nuclear/cytoplasmic ratio. Knowledge of the patient's treatment and of the histology of the tumour treated by radiotherapy are clearly also important.

Radiation changes may camouflage malignant cells from a tumour recurrence. A high nuclear/cytoplasmic ratio and irregular distribution of chromatin are features of malignancy and are not part of the usual spectrum of radiation changes.

Adult respiratory distress syndrome

This serious form of lung damage was first described by Ashbaugh and associates in 1967 at which time it carried a mortality rate of nearly 70%[297]. The mortality remains over 50% despite progress in understanding the underlying mechanisms[298,299]. The syndrome follows conditions such as severe trauma, pancreatitis or septicaemia, developing within 1–3 days of these catastrophic illnesses, with the onset of acute pulmonary oedema and inflammation, accompanied by proliferation of type II pneumocytes and fibroblasts. Local release of highly reactive free oxygen radicals and of enzymes such as proteases from neutrophils are postulated to cause direct damage to the lung parenchyma. Rapidly progressive pulmonary fibrosis may follow.

The cytological findings in adult respiratory distress syndrome have been recorded by Grotte et al.[300] who describe exfoliation of clusters of hyperplastic bronchoalveolar cells as seen in many other types of lung damage. It is important to distinguish such groups from adenocarcinoma cells, given the clinical setting.

Organ transplantation

The lung is the seat of many of the complications arising in patients who have had organ transplantation, regardless of the nature of the transplant. The risks have been reviewed by Ettinger and Trulock[301] and the findings in bronchoalveolar lavage fluid have been documented by Selvaggi[302] (see Chapter 21).

Infectious complications generally relate to the degree of immunosuppression required to prevent rejection of the graft, whereas non-infectious conditions arise either from mechanical problems due to surgery or result from the direct toxic effects of the treatment regime. Graft versus host disease or transplant rejection may supervene.

Opportunistic infections, of which the most common are cytomegalovirus and *Pneumocystis carinii* pneumonia, *herpes simplex* virus infection and aspergillosis, have been considered earlier in this chapter and are also discussed in Chapter 22.

Non-infectious complications such as adult respiratory distress syndrome, cyclosporin A toxicity, bronchiolitis obliterans and, in the longer term, pulmonary fibrosis, may all have cytological manifestations. These are mainly seen in bronchoalveolar lavage fluid and the findings, frequently non-specific, have already been described in this chapter. Accurate clinical details are necessary to interpret the findings correctly.

Industrial exposure to chemicals and dusts

Toxic chemicals such as insecticides have been implicated in the pathogenesis of pulmonary fibrosis. Damage to the alveolar lining cells is followed by changes similar to those seen in oxygen toxicity described above, posing the same diagnostic problems for the cytologist.

Organic dusts can induce pulmonary fibrosis in susceptible individuals. Originally described in 1958 as farmer's lung, the underlying mechanism is a hypersensitivity pneumonitis, also known as extrinsic allergic alveolitis. It is an industrial hazard in a wide range of occupations in which there is exposure to moulds or animal proteins. The condition may resolve on treatment or progress to pulmonary fibrosis. Histologically, lymphocytic alveolitis and chronic interstitial inflammation are seen, with the formation of small non-caseating granulomata[265,303].

The cytological findings vary with the stage of the disease. Lavage specimens show a raised lymphocyte count with an excess of T suppressor cells and sometimes of cytotoxic T cells[266,267]. Specific antibodies, immune complexes and complement components are also detectable in lavage fluid[268]. Later, hyperplastic or atypical type II pneumocytes may appear as pulmonary fibrosis supervenes. The changes are non-specific and a firm diagnosis can only be achieved by clinicopathological correlation.

Mineral pneumoconiosis may result from inhalation of dusts, gases or mineral fibres. This is an important group of occupational lung diseases, not least because there is often a question of industrial compensation. A range of pathological changes are known to occur, including fibrosis, cavitation, granulomatous inflammation, progressive massive fibrosis, asthma, emphysema, alveolar proteinosis and an increased risk of neoplasia. These diverse responses vary with the nature of the exposure, its duration and the interplay with other factors such as cigarette smoking. A comprehensive account of these aspects of occupational lung disease has been given by Churg and Green[304].

Cytology can be used to monitor the inflammatory cell ratios in lavage fluid in pneumoconiosis associated with fibrosis. In addition, refractile particulate material may be apparent in the cytoplasm of macrophages in respiratory specimens. These particles can be identified specifically using electron probes or other procedures[267].

Lavage fluid from cases of *silicosis* and other related pneumoconioses shows raised levels of polymorphs initially and may also have increased numbers of lymphocytes and macrophages. Type II pneumocytes appear in the fluid later in small numbers and may become atypical[305]. Davison and associates have described lavage findings in hard-metal workers; the changes included the presence of many macrophages, with some increase in eosinophils and lymphocytes. Bizarre giant cells were seen, derived from both macrophages and type II pneumocytes, diminishing on treatment and with cessation of exposure[306].

Asbestosis is one of the few mineral related lung diseases in which the fibres may be recognized in routine cytological preparations. Most cases result from industrial exposure but in a few patients it is difficult to establish this link; domestic exposure is known to account for a small proportion of the remainder. All types of asbestos are capable of causing pulmonary fibrosis, but the risk varies, being greater for crocidolite and amosite than for chrysotile, and also related to both duration and extent of exposure. In addition to diffuse fibrosis, asbestos is associated with development of mesothelioma, pleural plaque formation and benign recurrent effusions; there is also an increased incidence of bronchial carcinoma. The cytopathology of mesothelioma is discussed fully in Chapter 6.

Asbestos fibres (Fig. 2.70) are composed of variable proportions of silica, magnesium and iron. They vary in length and shape in their natural state, chrysotile being smaller and curved in contrast to the more solid larger fibres of the amphibole group. Fibres measuring up to 5 μm are usually cleared from the lungs without causing disease, whereas longer ones are phagocytosed by alveolar macrophages. They are then coated with protein and iron to produce inactivated fibres known as ferruginous or asbestos bodies. These structures are up to 200 μm in length and are usually dumbbell, beaded or drumstick in shape, their golden brown coating concentrated on the pointed ends of the fibres. Similar deposits may form around other mineral fibres, hence the more general term ferruginous bodies[70,307–309].

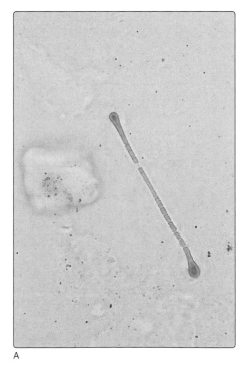
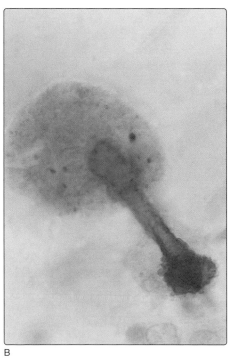

A   B

Fig. 2.70   (A) Asbestos bodies in sputum. Note the golden brown coating with expansions at the two ends. In the second example (B) the asbestos body lies partly within a macrophage. (Papanicolaou × HP, OI)

Identification of large numbers of typical asbestos bodies in respiratory samples from patients with pulmonary fibrosis provides strong evidence of an aetiological association. Asbestos bodies, even in small numbers, should be regarded as an important finding in any cytological preparation, including FNA material[310]. However, a study by Roggli *et al.* of asbestos body counts in lavage fluid from 20 asbestos workers suggested that very low counts are non-specific and only high levels are indicative of significant industrial exposure[311]. Leiman has pointed out that asbestos bodies in FNA material are commonly a marker for conditions other than asbestosis, such as carcinoma, lung abscess or tuberculosis[312].

Other benign pulmonary conditions

Thromboembolism

Thrombotic occlusion of the pulmonary arterial tree is a remarkably common event, usually embolic in origin, arising most often from peripheral venous thrombosis, but sometimes due to thrombus formed locally. Infarction of lung parenchyma follows only if the pulmonary circulation is already compromised.

Cytological changes in thromboembolic disease have been described by Berkheiser[313], and appear to be independent of whether or not actual infarction of the lung parenchyma has occurred. The abnormalities may be seen in sputum, washings or FNA samples and can cause problems in differentiation from malignancy[314–316].

Cytological findings

▶ Bloodstained sputum
▶ Haemosiderin laden macrophages
▶ Hyperplastic epithelial cell groups
▶ Squamous metaplasia

Sputum may be frankly bloodstained in the early stages if infarction occurs. This is followed by the appearance of macrophages laden with brown haemosiderin pigment as the blood is broken down.

Hyperplasia of bronchoalveolar epithelium is a notable feature, although the precise origin of the clusters of atypical cells exfoliated in sputum may not always be certain. The cells are rounded and swollen and show enlarged hyperchromatic nuclei with prominent nucleoli. Clusters vary from three or four grouped cells up to much larger collections in which cell details are difficult to visualize. Squamous metaplasia occurs as organization proceeds and may be atypical.

Diagnostic pitfalls

There is a risk of false positive diagnosis of malignancy if clusters of hyperplastic epithelial cells are not assessed correctly. Attention to nuclear details and the presence of other features such as iron-laden macrophages will reduce the likelihood of this mistake. This is a diagnosis that may be missed for want of consideration.

Congestive cardiac failure

Left ventricular failure from whatever cause subjects the lungs to congestion which if persistent leads to microscopic haemorrhage into alveoli. Degradation of the blood then occurs and is associated with accumulation of haemosiderin-laden macrophages in the alveoli. These cells may be expectorated in large numbers or found in lavage or FNA material. Sputum samples are sometimes submitted specifically requesting detection of such cells for confirmation of heart failure as a cause of wheezing and shortness of breath, so-called cardiac asthma.

Cytological findings *(Fig. 2.71)*

▶ Watery sputum, or tinged with blood
▶ Haemosiderin laden macrophages

Sputum samples are often watery in consistency unless infection has supervened. The specimen may be streaked with blood or rusty, especially if mitral stenosis is the underlying cause or if pulmonary embolism with infarction has occurred.

Macrophages stuffed with coarsely granular dark or golden brown iron pigment are the hallmark of the condition microscopically and these have come to be known as heart failure cells. Although recognizable on Papanicolaou staining, they are best demonstrated by Perl's Prussian blue stain to confirm the iron content.

Diagnostic pitfalls

Other types of pigment must be excluded. Carbon, in black or dark brown granules, is the most common pigment in

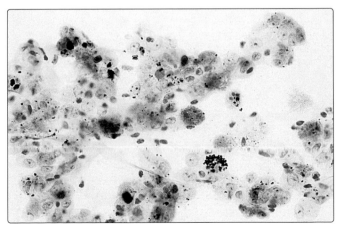

Fig. 2.71   Iron-laden macrophages in sputum stained by Perl's Prussian blue method. The sample is from a patient with congestive cardiac failure. Black carbon pigment is also visible. (Perl's stain × HP)

respiratory samples, obscuring iron if deposition is heavy. Perl's stain is then essential for detection of the iron.

Other sources of haemorrhage into the lung must be considered. Thus iron laden macrophages identical to

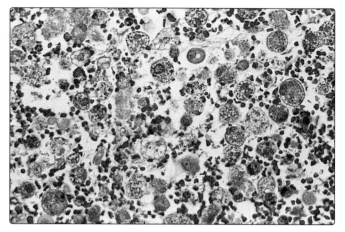

Fig. 2.72 Many iron-laden macrophages in bronchoalveolar lavage fluid from a patient with Goodpasture's syndrome. The iron pigment is coarsely clumped and golden brown in colour. (Papanicolaou × HP) (Courtesy of Professor B Naylor, Michigan, USA)

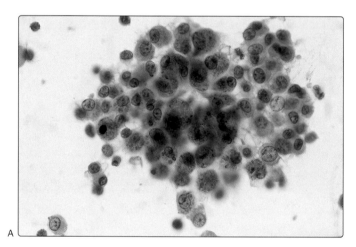

A

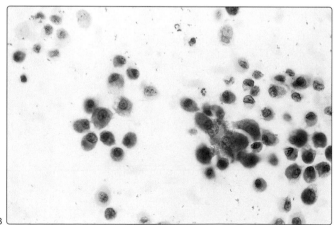

B

Fig. 2.73 (A, B) Bronchoalveolar lavage fluid from a 1-year-old child with idiopathic haemosiderosis. Only the macrophages containing iron take up the Prussian blue stain. (A, Papanicolaou; B, Perl's stain × HP)

heart failure cells can be seen after pulmonary infarcts, in shock lung[317], in idiopathic pulmonary haemosiderosis and Goodpasture's syndrome[318], (Figs. 2.72, 2.73) and in patients with a haemorrhagic diathesis. There is also the possibility of local haemorrhage from a bronchial carcinoma.

Lipoid pneumonitis

Inflammation of lung parenchyma due to the presence of lipid substances is generally the result of either local obstruction to a bronchus with accumulation of lipoidal tissue breakdown products distally, or to inhalation or aspiration of oily material. These are known as endogenous and exogenous lipoid pneumonitis or pneumonia respectively.

Exogenous sources include industrial oil inhalation and the risk of an iatrogenic origin from medications such as nose drops. The most common cause of endogenous lipoid pneumonia is an obstructing bronchial tumour, but there are also iatrogenic endogenous causes, for instance postoperative bronchial obstruction or due to embolization of contrast medium to the lungs. Amiodarone toxicity is associated with accumulation of phospholipids in lung and other tissues.

The hallmark of lipoid pneumonitis, whatever the cause, is the presence of lipid-laden macrophages and pools of free lipid in the alveoli and interstitial tissues (Fig. 2.73). Other inflammatory cells are almost always present, and the inflammation may become granulomatous. Cholesterol clefts from cell breakdown are seen when bronchial obstruction is present.

Cytological findings (Fig. 2.74)

▶ Vacuolated swollen macrophages
▶ Giant cells
▶ A mixed inflammatory background

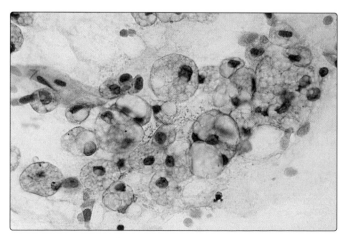

Fig. 2.74 Large lipid-laden macrophages in bronchial washings from the case illustrated in Fig. 2.73. Their cytoplasmic vacuoles show considerable variation in size and shape and some multinucleation can be seen. A few other inflammatory cells are also present. (Papanicolaou × HP) (Courtesy of Professor B Naylor, Michigan, USA)

Sputum findings were originally described by Losner *et al.* in 1950[319]. Lavage fluid findings have also been documented[320]. Characteristically, there are numerous vacuolated fat laden macrophages, including multinucleated forms, which may have bizarre shapes and copious cytoplasm. The presence of fat can be confirmed by oil red O staining. Other inflammatory cells may be present, in varying numbers, and in cases due to an obstructing tumour malignant cells may be seen.

Diagnostic pitfalls

Small droplets of fat in macrophages may be seen in sputum from many patients without signifying lipoid pneumonia. Cigarette smokers are especially prone to show this. The paucity of fat and absence of bizarre multinucleated cells ensure that the conditions are not usually confused. Pneumonia due to aspiration of food may include fatty material but there is usually evidence of mixed aspiration including plant products and bacterial contamination[321].

Bizarre vacuolated cells may be mistaken for malignancy, notably adenocarcinoma or liposarcoma. The former error can be avoided by staining for fat, while the rare occurrence of liposarcoma in lung is associated with only few abnormal tumour cells and the cells show greater nuclear pleomorphism.

Fat laden macrophages can be found transiently in sputum in some conditions without progressing to pneumonitis. An example of this is seen with fat embolism after fractures or orthopaedic surgery, when fat is released into the venous circulation and thence deposited in the lungs. Sputum examination in such patients almost invariably reveals the presence of free lipid or some fat in macrophages, which is of no consequence clinically unless massive enough to induce pulmonary oedema or allow the passage of the fat into the systemic circulation.

Talc granuloma

Foreign material, such as particles of talc, trapped in pulmonary vessels after intravenous injection of substances mixed with talc as a base, evoke a granulomatous inflammatory reaction in the lung parenchyma, leading to diffuse or focal nodular radiological shadowing. These lesions may be investigated by FNA, yielding non-specific inflammation with or without granulomatous elements. The foreign material itself can sometimes be identified in the aspirated material with the help of polarizing light (Fig. 2.75).

Pulmonary amyloidosis

Amyloid is the term used for a group of fibrillary proteins deposited in tissues either as diffuse infiltration of organs or as localized tumorous masses. The protein itself may be derived from the light chains of immunoglobulin molecules (AL), or may be secondary to chronic infections (AA); less common types are the amyloid protein found in old age (AS) and that associated with rare endocrine tumours (AE).

Involvement of the respiratory tract may be tracheobronchial or parenchymal in distribution and at either site deposition can be localized, nodular, multifocal or diffuse. Other organs are affected in the majority of cases.

The cytology of tracheobronchial amyloid deposits has been described by Chen[322] and has been noted in bronchial brushings[323] and in FNA material in a number of reports, as reviewed by Dundore *et al.* who point out that recognition of amyloid in FNA material is important as it may obviate the need for surgery[324]. Michael and Naylor have highlighted the differential diagnosis and pitfalls in the identification of amyloid in a range of cytology specimens[325].

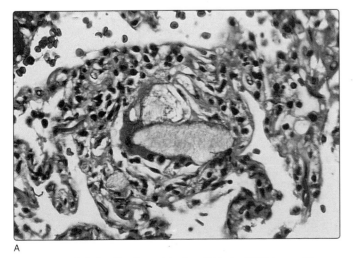
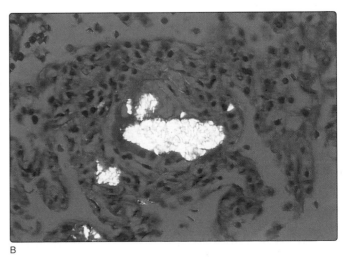

A   B

Fig. 2.75   (A) Refractile talc particles in cell block of FNA lung, with surrounding macrophage reaction. The patient was thought to be an intravenous drug user. Birefringence is apparent with polarized light (B). (H&E × HP) (Courtesy of Professor B Naylor, Michigan, USA)

Cytological findings *(Fig. 2.76)*

▶ Smooth amorphous eosinophilic plaques of amyloid
▶ Congo red stain positive, with apple-green birefringence

Corpora amylacea have similar staining properties but are more rounded in outline and when polarized after Congo red staining show alternating segments of green and yellow birefringence.

Other types of amorphous plaque such as those due to alveolar proteinosis or *Pneumocystis carinii* infection must be considered. In both of these conditions the plaques have a foamy structure. Definitive differentiation can be made with the Congo red stain.

Pulmonary alveolar proteinosis

This rare disease was associated with known exposure to dusts in about half of the cases originally described by Rosen *et al.* in 1958[326], but the condition is probably multifactorial in origin, and there is a strong association with immunosuppression[327]. The characteristic feature is accumulation of lipid-rich proteinaceous material filling alveolar spaces but evoking little or no inflammation. This material has been shown by electron microscopy to contain large amounts of surfactant[328,329]. Hyperplasia of type II pneumocytes may occur and a few cases progress to pulmonary fibrosis if untreated. An underlying defect in the macrophage system of the lung has been postulated[328]. Patients present with severe shortness of breath and copious sputum production. Samples of this sputum or lavage fluid from a therapeutic lavage procedure may be received.

Cytological findings[290] *(Figs 2.77, 2.78)*

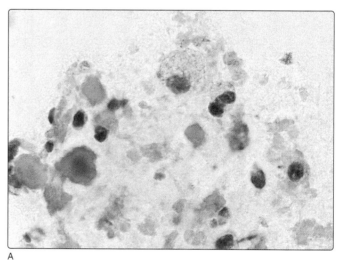

A

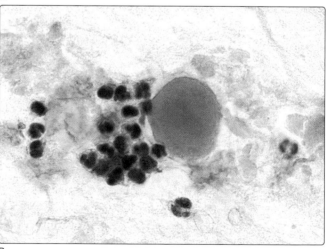

B

Fig. 2.77 (A,B) Pulmonary alveolar proteinosis: plaques of granular eosinophilic and cyanophilic material seen in bronchoalveolar lavage fluid. The patient was a middle-aged man presenting with breathlessness and bilateral pulmonary infiltrates. The plaques differ in distribution, size and texture from those of Pneumocystis infection or amyloidosis, but both of these must be considered in the differential diagnosis. (Papanicolaou and H&E × HP) (Courtesy of Professor B Naylor, Michigan, USA)

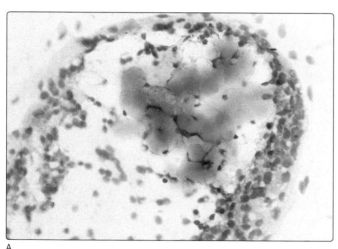

A

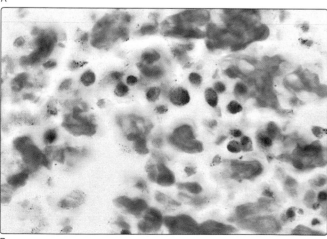

B

Fig. 2.76 (A) Amyloid in a lung aspirate from a patient with a plasmacytoma. There were scattered plaques of amphophilic material of variable size and shape, as shown here, with a few histiocytes and plasma cells. (Papanicolaou × HP) (B) Congo red staining confirms the diagnosis. (× MP) (Courtesy of Professor B Naylor, Michigan, USA)

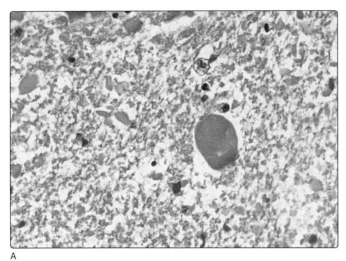

A

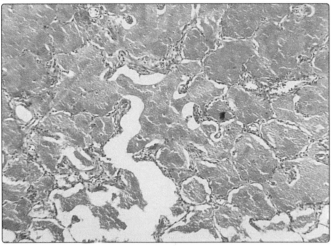

B

Fig. 2.78   Pulmonary alveolar proteinosis plaques in cell block of FNA material (A) and in histological section (B). The proteinaceous precipitate is eosinophilic and fills the alveolar spaces in the lung section. Note the virtual absence of any inflammatory reaction. (H&E × HP, MP) (Courtesy of Professor B Naylor, Michigan, USA)

▶ Lavage specimens are opaque or milky on gross inspection
▶ A background of rounded amphophilic plaques and debris
▶ Osmiophilic laminated structure on electron microscopy

Rounded fragments of amorphous material of variable size, with amphophilic or pale eosinophilic staining properties are seen on light microscopy. Cholesterol crystals may be identified[330]. Few, if any, inflammatory cells are seen. Electron microscopy is necessary for a definitive diagnosis, revealing rounded lamellated structures identical to the osmiophilic bodies of type II pneumocytes and composed of surfactant[290]. In a few cases particulate dusts are identified.

Diagnostic pitfalls

Alveolar casts of *Pneumocystis carinii* infection bear some resemblance to the amorphous material expectorated in alveolar proteinosis. The former have a honeycomb structure on Papanicolaou staining due to cysts within the plaques, as demonstrated by silver stains.

A condition closely simulating alveolar proteinosis has been documented in a few cases of Pneumocystis infection, in which the alveoli contain large amounts of lipid, hence the name given to this finding, lipoproteinosis. Careful searching reveals the Pneumocystis organisms. Other amorphous materials should also be excluded, such as inspissated mucus, which stains deep blue, and amyloid which shows a positive reaction with Congo red staining.

Thermal injury

Detailed studies of the acute and longer-term effects of thermal injury on cells of the airways have been undertaken[331,332]. Severe burns from inhalation of smoke or hot gases results in partial or complete necrosis of bronchial epithelium and the extent of damage may determine the overall prognosis. A neutrophilic response in alveoli and airways is an early event. Healing is accompanied by squamous metaplasia. Reversible atypical squamous metaplasia has been observed in firemen[333].

A study by Clark *et al.*[334] of bronchoalveolar lavage cells in 42 fire victims revealed that respiratory tract damage was greatest when smoke inhalation was accompanied by cutaneous burns. Their findings suggest that there is an excessive release of chemical mediators from neutrophil polymorphs, directly damaging the lung parenchyma, and also depleting the alveolar population of mature macrophages. These combined effects then predispose to overwhelming bacterial infection.

Cytological findings

▶ Thick mucoid sputum or bronchial aspiration samples
▶ Many damaged epithelial cells
▶ Polymorphs and macrophages increased in lavage fluid
▶ Squamous metaplasia occurs early
▶ Secondary infection is common

Thick mucus is recovered by bronchial aspiration in cases of severe burns. Destruction of cilia, the terminal plate or even entire epithelial cell groups may be seen, but in less injured patients these damaged cells are mixed with exfoliated normal cells. Squamous cells may be present in abundance and may be misshapen, with hyperchromatic nuclei and multinucleation.

Secondary infection is a serious risk for the patient. *Herpes simplex* or cytomegalovirus pneumonia, fungal infections such as candidiasis, and bacterial pneumonia, particularly due to Pseudomonas organisms, are the most common.

Plasma cell granuloma/inflammatory myofibroblastoma

This solitary lung nodule of variable size often follows a respiratory infection and usually occurs in young adults,

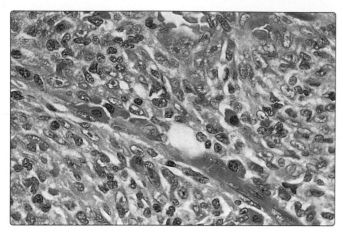

Fig. 2.79   Plasma cell granuloma of lung (inflammatory myofibroblastoma) in histological section. A mixture of inflammatory cells including plasma cells can be seen in a background of spindle cell connective tissue. The patient was a male of 22, presenting with a lung mass two months after an ill-defined respiratory tract infection. (H&E, × HP)

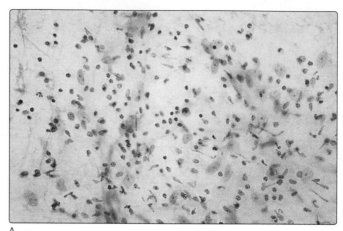

A

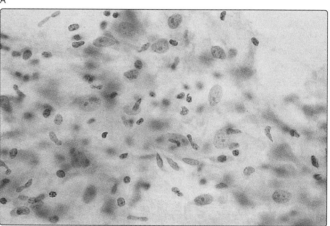

B

Fig. 2.80   (A,B) Plasma cell granuloma (inflammatory myofibroblastoma) of lung in FNA smear showing a mixed population of spindle cells and inflammatory cells. A few plasma cells with eccentric nuclei can be made out, together with histiocytes, lymphocytes and occasional polymorphs. Note the large active nuclei and prominent nucleoli in the spindle cell component. (Papanicolaou × MP, HP) (Courtesy of Dr G Sterrett, Perth, Western Australia)

although no age is exempt[335]. Previously known as 'inflammatory pseudotumour', the lesions may present clinically as a neoplasm and may therefore be investigated by FNA. The histology is diverse (Fig. 2.79), with variable numbers of foamy macrophages (xanthoma cells), lymphocytes, plasma cells, polymorphs and sometimes also a few giant cells. There is a background of collagen with spindle-shaped fibroblastic cells, which often have a storiform pattern of growth. Some of these cells have now been shown by electron microscopy to have the characteristics of myofibroblasts and the lesion in currently classified as an inflammatory myofibroblastoma, a low-grade tumour[336]. Regression may occur with time but most of these lesions are excised, so as to exclude malignancy.

Cytological findings *(Fig. 2.80)*

▶ Mixed inflammatory picture, including plasma cells, polymorphs, eosinophils and mast cells
▶ Foamy histiocytes or giant cells
▶ Fibroblasts and collagen

The cytological findings have been reported by several authors[337-339]. Smears made from FNA material show a mixture of inflammatory cells, including plasma cells, epithelial cells and spindle shaped stromal cells. Xanthoma cells with finely vacuolated cytoplasm may be more numerous than plasma cells. Although the findings are non-specific, it is helpful to make the diagnosis since conservative management may be appropriate in certain cases.

Role of cytology in non-neoplastic pulmonary disease

Such an array of inflammatory processes, reactive changes, hyperplasias, infective diseases and fibrosing conditions provides a great diagnostic challenge. Because the

cytological findings are often non-specific they are at times more a source of frustration than reward. Three main contributions to diagnosis can be claimed on behalf of cytopathology.

The first and most reliable is in confirmation of a diagnosis of infection by recognition of the causative agent or its cytopathic effects. Many of the fungal, viral and parasitic infections fall into this group. They are of increasing importance with the rise in numbers of immunosuppressed patients. Cytology provides a relatively cheap, quick, non-invasive and dependable method of diagnosis for these cases. Culture of the material obtained, whether directly from the airways or by fine needle aspiration, is important in cases showing acute inflammation or necrosis[340].

The next contribution lies in recognition of characteristic changes in respiratory tract samples which, when combined with clinical information, give direction or add weight to the clinical diagnosis. The cytological findings in sputum of asthmatics, in lavage fluids in cases of drug toxicity, or in FNA material that includes granuloma formation are among the many examples of this important diagnostic role.

Thirdly, negative findings in cytology are of value clinically since they contribute to the evidence required to exclude malignancy. A study by Zakowski and associates[341] of the significance of negative findings in FNA specimens in establishing the absence of malignancy found a negative predictive value of 53.3%. Their figures included inadequate samples. The main factor contributing to false negative diagnosis was sampling error. The converse role, namely that of establishing a diagnosis of malignancy, is discussed in Chapter 3.

The diagnostic accuracy of respiratory tract cytology for non-neoplastic disease ranges from the high level of sensitivity and specificity in the recognition of fungal and some viral infections, to the entirely non-specific findings in many of the common chronic inflammatory conditions. No meaningful overall figure for accuracy can be calculated, although estimation for certain diagnoses and particular procedures has been discussed in the course of this chapter.

The accuracy of any cytological diagnosis is dependent on obtaining samples that are both appropriate and adequate. This is apparent from studies contrasting different sampling procedures. Orenstein and associates[190] reported a sensitivity of 94.4% using bronchoalveolar lavage for the diagnosis of *Pneumocystis carinii* pneumonia in AIDS patients. Induced sputum has generally been found to have a much lower sensitivity of 60–70%, but in a direct comparison of induced sputum and lavage for diagnosis in AIDS patients, Leigh *et al.*[342] achieved a sensitivity of 94.7% for induced sputum by adhering to a strict protocol for collection and handling of samples.

The advent of bronchoalveolar lavage and increasing use of fine needle aspiration have undoubtedly provided new diagnostic applications and opportunities for research into benign pulmonary disease[343–345]. The role of cytology in this field seems likely to continue to grow.

References

1 Finlayson R. The vicissitudes of sputum cytology. *Medical History* 1958; **2**: 24

2 Grunze H, Spriggs A I. *History of Clinical Cytology*, 2nd edn. Darmstadt: G-I-T Verlag Ernst Giebeler, 1983; 97–116

3 Dudgeon L S, Wrigley C H. On the demonstration of particles of malignant growth in the sputum by means of the wet-film method. *J Laryngol Otol* 1935; **50**: 752–753

4 Wandall H H. A study on neoplastic cells in sputum as a contribution to the diagnosis of primary lung cancer. *Acta Chir Scand* 1944; **91**: 1–143

5 Herbut P A, Clerf L H. Bronchogenic carcinoma: diagnosis by cytological study of bronchoscopically removed secretions. *JAMA* 1946; **130**: 1006–1012

6 Papanicolaou G N, Cromwell H A. Diagnosis of cancer of the lung by the cytological method. *Dis Chest* 1949; **15**: 412–418

7 Woolner L B, McDonald J R. Bronchogenic carcinoma: diagnosis by microscopic examination of sputum and bronchial secretions; a preliminary report. *Proc Staff Meetings Mayo Clin* 1947; **22**: 369–381

8 Muers M F, Boddington M M, Cole M, Murphy D. Cytological sampling at fibreoptic bronchoscopy: comparison of catheter aspirations and brush biopsies. *Thorax* 1982; **37**: 457–461

9 Bonfiglio T A. Fine needle aspiration biopsy of the lung. *Pathol Ann* 1982; **16**: 159–180

10 Johnston W W. Percutaneous FNAB of the lung. *Acta Cytol* 1984; **28**: 218–224

11 Walters E H, Gardiner P V. Bronchoalveolar lavage as a research tool. *Thorax* 1991; **46**: 613–618

12 House A J S, Thomson K R. Evaluation of a new transthoracic needle for biopsy of benign and malignant lung lesions. *Am J Radiol* 1977; **140**: 215–220

13 Nordenstrom B E W. Technical aspects of obtaining cellular material from lesions deep in the lung. A radiologist's view and description of screw-needle sampling technique. *Acta Cytol* 1984; **28**: 233–242

14 Ell S R. Imaging techniques. In: Bibbo M ed. *Comprehensive Cytopathology*. Philadelphia: W B Saunders Co., 1991; 615–620

15 Siddiqui M T, Saboorian M H, Gokaslan S T et al. The utility of transbronchial (Wang) fine needle aspiration in lung cancer diagnosis. *Cytopathology* 2001; **12**: 7–14

16 Johnston W W, Frable W J. *Diagnostic Respiratory Cytopathology*. Paris: Masson, 1979

17 Koss L G. A quarter of a century of cytology. *Acta Cytol* 1977; **21**: 639–642

18 Papanicolaou Society of Cytopathology Taskforce and Standards of Practice. Guidelines of the Papanicolaou Society of Cytopathology for the examination of cytologic specimens obtained from the respiratory tract. *Diagn Cytopathol* 1999; **21**: 61–69

19 Lau S K, Hsu C S, Sham J S T, Wei W I. The cytological diagnosis of nasopharyngeal carcinoma using a silk swab stick. *Cytopathology* 1991; **2**: 239–246

20 Person C G A, Svensson C, Grieff L et al. The use of the nose to study the inflammatory response of the respiratory tract. *Thorax* 1992; **47**: 993–1000 (Editorial)

21 Pelikan Z. The changes in the nasal secretions of eosinophils during the immediate nasal response to allergen challenge. *J Allerg Clin Immunol* 1983; **72**: 657–682

22 Jean R, Lellouch-Tubiana A, Brunet-Langot D et al. Nasal eosinophilia in children: its use in the nasal allergen provocation test. *Diagn Cytopathol* 1988; **4**: 23–27

23 Rivasi F, Bergamini G. Nasal cytology in allergic processes and other syndromes caused by hyperreactivity. *Diagn Cytopathol* 1988; **4**: 99–105

24 Payne C R, Hadfield J W, Stovin P G et al. Diagnostic accuracy of cytology and biopsy in primary bronchial carcinoma. *J Pathol* 1981; **34**: 773–778

25 Ng A B P, Horak G C. Factors significant in the diagnostic accuracy of lung cytology in bronchial washings and sputum samples. II. Sputum samples. *Acta Cytol* 1983; **27**: 397–402

26 Papanicolaou G N. A new procedure for staining vaginal smears. *Science* 1942; **2469**: 438–439

27 Johnston W W, Frable W J. Cytopreparatory methods. In: Johnston W W and Frable W J eds. *Diagnostic Respiratory Cytopathology*. New York: Masson 1979

28 Haynes E. Trypsin as a digestant of sputum and other broth fluids preliminary to examination for acid-fast bacilli. *J Lab Clin Med* 1942; **27**: 806–809

29 Umiker W, Young L, Waite B. The use of chymotrypsin for the concentration of sputum in the cytologic diagnosis of lung cancer. *Univ Mich Med Bulletin* 1958; **24**: 265

30 McCarty S A. Solving the cytopreparation problem of mucoid specimens with a mucoliquifying agent (Mucolexx) and nucleopore filters. *Acta Cytol* 1972; **16**: 221–223

31 Takahashi M, Urabe M. A new cell concentration method for cancer cytology of sputum. *Cancer* 1963; **16**: 199–204

32 Liu W. Concentration and fractionation of cytologic elements in sputum. *Acta Cytol* 1966; **10**: 368–372

33 Campbell G M, Imrie J E A. The respiratory tract: normal structure, function and methods of investigation. In: Coleman D V,

Chapman P A eds. *Clinical Cytotechnology*. London: Butterworths, 1989

34 Saccomanno G, Saunders R P, Ellis H *et al*. Concentration of carcinoma on atypical cells in sputum. *Acta Cytol* 1963; **7**: 305–310

35 Rizzo T, Schumann G B, Riding J M. Comparison of the pick-and-smear and Saccomanno methods for sputum cytologic analysis. *Acta Cytol* 1990; **34**: 907–908

36 Michel R, Davidson L, Sladon Timm S *et al*. Saccomanno smear slides and Megafunnel slides for sputum specimens: a comparison. *Acta Cytol* 1997; **41**:1774–1780

37 Bickerman H A, Sproul E E, Barach A L. An aerosol method of producing bronchial secretions in human subjects: a clinical technique for detection of lung cancer. *Dis Chest* 1958; **33**: 347–362

38 Olsen R G, Froeb H F, Palmer L A. Sputum cytology after inhalation of heated propylene glycol. *JAMA* 1961; **178**: 668–670

39 Pederson B, Brons M, Holm K *et al*. The value of provoked expectoration in obtaining sputum samples for cytologic investigation: a prospective, consecutive and controlled investigation of 134 patients. *Acta Cytol* 1985; **29**: 750–752

40 Erozan Y S. Cytopathology in the diagnosis of pulmonary disease. In: Seigelman S S, Stitik F P, Summer W R eds. *Multiple Imaging Procedures*, Vol. 1. *Pulmonary System, Practical Approaches to Pulmonary Diagnosis*. New York: Grune & Stratton, 1979

41 Bigby T D, Margolskee D, Curtis J L *et al*. The usefulness of induced sputum in the diagnosis of Pneumocystis carinii pneumonia in patients with the acquired immunodeficiency syndrome. *Amer Rev Respir Dis* 1986; **133**: 515–518

42 Nasr A, Finkle H I. Assessing the adequacy of induced sputum for the evaluation for Pneumocystis carinii pneumonia. *Acta Cytol* 1991; **35**: 251

43 Ikeda S. Flexible bronchofiberscope. *Ann Otol Rhinol Laryngol* 1970; **79**: 916

44 Walloch J. Pulmonary cytopathology in historical perspective. In: Gruhn J G, Rosen S T eds. *Lung Cancer. The Evolution of Concepts*. New York: Field & Wood, 1989

45 Marsh B R, Frost J K, Erozan Y S *et al*. Flexible fiberoptic bronchoscopy. Its place in the search for lung cancer. *Ann Otol Rhinol Laryngol* 1973; **82**: 757–764

46 Zavala D C. Diagnostic fiberoptic bronchoscopy: technique and results of biopsy in 600 patients. *Chest* 1975; **68**: 12–19

47 Hunninghake G W, Gadek J E, Kawanami O *et al*. Inflammatory and immune processes in the human lung in health and disease: evaluation by bronchoalveolar lavage. *Am J Pathol* 1979; **97**: 149–206

48 Saltini C, Hance A J, Ferrans V J *et al*. Accurate quantification of cells recovered by bronchoalveolar lavage. *Am Rev Respir Dis* 1984; **130**: 650–658

49 Lindner J, Rennard S I. *Bronchoalveolar Lavage*. Chicago: American Society of Clinical Pathologists, 1988

50 Young J A, Hopkin J M, Cuthbertson W P. Pulmonary infiltrates in

immunocompromised patients: diagnosis by cytological examination of bronchoalveolar lavage fluid. *J Clin Pathol* 1984; **37**: 390–397

51 Stover D E, Zaman M B, Hajdu S I *et al*. Bronchoalveolar lavage in the diagnosis of diffuse pulmonary infiltrates in the immunosuppressed host. *Ann Intern Med* 1984; **101**: 1–7

52 Gee J B L, Fick R B. Bronchoalveolar lavage. *Thorax* 1980; **35**: 1–8 (Editorial)

53 Crystal R G, Gadek J E, Ferrans V J *et al*. Interstitial lung disease: current concepts of pathogenesis, staging and therapy. *Amer J Med* 1981; **70**: 542–568

54 Zavala D C, Hunninghake G W. Lung lavage. In: Flenley D C, Petty T L eds. *Recent Advances in Respiratory Medicine*, no 3. Edinburgh: Churchill Livingstone, 1983; 21–23

55 Linder J, Radio S J, Robbins R A *et al*. Bronchoalveolar lavage in the cytologic diagnosis of carcinoma of the lung. *Acta Cytol* 1987; **31**: 796–801

56 Bonfiglio T A. Fine needle aspiration biopsy of the lung. *Pathol Ann* 1982; **16**: 159–180

57 Koss L G, Woyke S, Olszewski W. Aspiration biopsy. *Cytologic Interpretation and Histologic Bases*. New York: Igaku-Shoin, 1985

58 Dahlgren S. Lungs. In: Zajicek J ed. *Aspiration Biopsy Cytology*, part 1. *Cytology of Supradiaphragmatic Organs*. Basel: S Karger, 1974; 195–208

59 Wang K P, Brower R, Haponik E F, Siegelman S. Flexible transbronchial needle aspiration for staging of bronchial carcinoma. *Chest* 1983; **84**: 571–576

60 Buley I D. Update on special techniques in routine cytopathology. *J Clin Pathol* 1993; **46**: 881–885 (Editorial)

61 Wang N-S. Anatomy. In: Dail D H, Hammar S P eds. *Pulmonary Pathology*. New York: Springer-Verlag, 1988

62 Stevens A, Lowe J S. Respiratory system. In: Stevens A, Lowe J S eds. *Histology*. London: Gower, 1992

63 Greenberg S D. Recent advances in pulmonary pathology. *Human Pathol* 1993; 14:901–912

64 Walker K R. Anatomy and histochemistry of respiratory spirals. *Acta Cytol* 1982; **26**: 747

65 Antonakopoulos G N, Lambrinaki E, Kyrkou K A. Curschmann's spirals in sputum: histochemical evidence of bronchial gland ductal origin. *Diag Cytopathol* 1987; **3**: 291–294

66 Gleich G. The eosinophils: new aspects of structure and function. *J Allergy & Clin Immunol* 1977; **60**: 73–82

67 Schmitz B, Pfitzer P. Acellular bodies in sputum. *Acta Cytol* 1984; **28**: 136–138

68 Kung I T M, Hsu C, Chan S C W *et al*. Frequency of 'blue bodies' in pulmonary cytology specimens. *Diag Cytopathol* 1987; **3**: 284–286

69 Gross P, de Treville R T P, Cralley L J, Davis J M G. Pulmonary ferruginous bodies; development in response to filamentous dusts and a method of isolation and concentration. *Arch Pathol* 1968; **85**: 539–546

70 Wheeler T M, Johnson E H, Coughlin D, Greenberg S D. The sensitivity of detection of asbestos bodies in sputa and bronchial washings. *Acta Cytol* 1988; **32**: 647–650

71 Weaver K M, Kovak P M, Naylor B. Vegetable cell contaminants in cytologic specimens: their resemblance to cells associated with various normal and pathologic states. *Acta Cytol* 1981; **25**: 210–214

72 Dao A H. Entamoeba gingivalis in sputum smears. *Acta Cytol* 1985; **29**: 632–633

73 Farley M L, Mabry L C. Mites in pulmonary cytology specimens. *Diag Cytopathol* 1989; **5**: 416–426

74 Radio S, Rennard S I, Ghafouri M A, Lindner J A. Cytomorphology of Alternaria in bronchoalveolar lavage specimens. *Acta Cytol* 1987; **31**: 243–248

75 Hussain O A N, Grainger J M, Sims J. Cross contamination of cytological smears with automated staining machines and bulk manual staining procedures. *J Clin Pathol* 1978; **31**: 63–68

76 Johnston W W. Cytopathology of the lung: diagnostic applications of sputum, bronchial brushings and fine needle aspiration biopsy. In: Wied G L, Keebler C M, Koss L G, Reagan J W eds. *Compendium on Diagnostic Cytology*. Chicago: Tutorials of cytology, 1988; 321–322

77 Roby T J, Swan G E, Schumann G B, Enkena L C Jr. Reliability of a quantitative interpretation of sputum cytology slides. *Acta Cytol* 1990; **34**: 140–146

78 Roby T J, Swan G E, Sorensen K W *et al*. Discriminant analysis of lower respiratory components associated with cigarette smoking, based on quantitative sputum cytology. *Acta Cytol* 1990; **34**: 147–154

79 Chamberlain D W, Braude A C, Rebuck A S. A critical evaluation of bronchoalveolar lavage: criteria for identifying unsatisfactory specimens. *Acta Cytol* 1987; **31**: 599–605

80 Davis G, Giancola M, Costanza M, Law R. Analyses of sequential bronchoalveolar lavage samples from healthy human volunteers. *Am Rev Respir Dis* 1982; **126**: 611–616

81 De Fine L, Saleba K, Gibson B *et al*. Cytologic evaluation of bronchoalveolar lavage specimens in immunosuppressed patients with suspected opportunistic infections. *Acta Cytol* 1987; **31**: 235–242

82 Martin W J II, Smith T E, Sanderson D R *et al*. Role of bronchoalveolar lavage in the assessment of opportunistic pulmonary infection: utility and complications. *Mayo Clinic Proc* 1987; **62**: 545–557

83 Deely T J. ed. *Needle Biopsy*. Glasgow: Butterworth, 1974

84 Saito Y, Imai T, Sato M *et al*. Cytologic study of tissue repair in human bronchial epithelium. *Acta Cytol* 1988; **32**: 622–628

85 Chalon J, Tang C-K, Gorstein F *et al*. Diagnostic and prognostic significance of tracheobronchial epithelial multinucleation. *Acta Cytol* 1978; **22**: 316–320

86 Koss L G, Richardson H L. Some pitfalls of cytological diagnosis of lung cancer. *Cancer* 1955; **8**: 937–947

87 Naib Z M. Pitfalls in the cytologic diagnosis of oat cell carcinoma of the lung. *Acta Cytol* 1964; **8**: 34–38

88 Kern W H. Cytology of hyperplastic and neoplastic lesions of terminal bronchioles and alveoli. *Acta Cytol* 1965; **9**: 372–379

89 Berkheiser S W. Bronchiolar proliferation and metaplasia associated with bronchiectasis, pulmonary infarcts and anthracosis. *Cancer* 1959; **12**: 499–508

90 Scoggins W G, Smith R H, Frable W J, O'Donohue W J Jr. False-positive diagnosis of lung carcinoma in patients with pulmonary infarcts. *Ann Thorac Surg* 1977; **24**: 474–480

91 Smith J H, Frable W J. Adenocarcinoma of the lung: cytologic correlation with histologic type. *Acta Cytol* 1974; **18**: 316–320

92 Kierszenbaum A L. Bronchial metaplasia: observations on its histology and cytology. *Acta Cytol* 1965; **9**: 365–371

93 Nasiell M. Metaplasia and atypical metaplasia in the bronchial epithelium: a histopathologic and cytopathologic study. *Acta Cytol* 1966; **10**: 421–427

94 Saccomanno G, Saunders R P, Klein M G et al. Cytology of the lung in reference to irritant, individual sensitivity and healing. *Acta Cytol* 1970; **14**: 377–381

95 Auerbach O, Stout A P, Hammond E C, Garfinkel L. Changes in bronchial epithelium in relation to cigarette smoking and in relation to lung cancer. *N Engl J Med* 1961; **265**: 253–267

96 Neweoehner D E, Kleinerman J, Rice D B. Pathologic changes in peripheral airways of young cigarette smokers. *N Engl J Med* 1974; **291**: 755–758

97 Papanicolaou G N. Degenerative changes in ciliated cells exfoliating from the bronchial epithelium as a cytologic criterion in the diagnosis of diseases of the lung. *New York Med J* 1956; **56**: 2647

98 Papanicolaou G N, Bridges E L, Railey C. Degeneration of the ciliated cells of the bronchial epithelium (ciliocytophthoria) in its relation to pulmonary disease. *Am Rev Resp Dis* 1961; **83**: 641–659

99 Dunnill M S. Bacterial pneumonia. In: Dunnill M S ed. *Pulmonary Pathology*, 2nd edn. Edinburgh: Churchill Livingstone, 1987; 147–170

100 Blackmon J A. Bacterial infections. In: Dail D H, Hammar S P eds. *Pulmonary Pathology*. New York: Springer Verlag, 1988; 157–158

101 Lazzari G, Vineis C, Cugini A. Cytologic diagnosis of primary pulmonary actinomycosis: a report of two cases. *Acta Cytol* 1981; **25**: 299–301

102 Orell S R, Sterrett G F, Walters M N-I, Whitaker D. Lung, mediastinum, chest wall and pleura. In: Orell S R, Sterrett G F, Walters M N-I, Whitaker D eds. *Manual and Atlas of Fine Needle Aspiration Cytology*, 2nd edn. Edinburgh: Churchill Livingstone, 1992; 178–180

103 Pollock P G, Meyers D S, Frable W J et al. Rapid diagnosis of actinomycosis by thin-needle aspiration biopsy. *Am J Clin Pathol* 1978; **70**: 27–30

104 Pollock P G, Valicenti J F Jr, Meyers D S et al. The use of fluorescent and special staining techniques in the aspiration of nocardiosis and actinomycosis. *Acta Cytol* 1978; **22**: 575–579

105 Ettinger N A, Trulock E P. Pulmonary considerations in organ transplantation: state of the art, part 3. *Am Rev Resp Dis* 1991; **144**: 433–451

106 Walker A N, Walker G K, Feldman P S. Diagnosis of Legionella micadei pneumonia from cytologic specimens. *Acta Cytol* 1983; **27**: 252–254

107 Nasiell M. Comparative histological and sputum cytological studies of the bronchial epithelium in inflammatory and neoplastic lung disease. *Acta Pathol Microbiol Scand* 1968; **72**: 501–518

108 Watson J M. Tuberculosis in Britain today. *BMJ* 1993; **306**: 221–222 (Editorial)

109 Auerbach O, Dail D H. Atypical mycobacteria. In: Dail D H, Hammar S P eds. *Pulmonary Pathology*. New York: Springer Verlag, 1988; 184–186

110 Rich A R. *The Pathogenesis of Tuberculosis*, 2nd edn. Oxford: Blackwell, 1951

111 Nasiell M, Roger V, Nasiell K et al. Cytologic findings indicating pulmonary tuberculosis. I. The diagnostic significance of epithelioid cells and Langhans giant cells found in sputum of bronchial secretions. *Acta Cytol* 1972; **16**: 146–151

112 Roger V, Nasiell M, Nasiell K et al. Cytologic findings indicating pulmonary tuberculosis. II. The occurrence in sputum of epithelioid cells and multinucleated giant cells in pulmonary tuberculosis, chronic non-tuberculous inflammatory lung disease and bronchogenic carcinoma. *Acta Cytol* 1972; **16**: 538–542

113 Tani E M, Schmitt F C L, Oliviera M L S et al. Pulmonary cytology in tuberculosis. *Acta Cytol* 1987; **31**: 460–463

114 Dahlgren S E, Lind B. Aspiration cytology in the diagnosis of pulmonary tuberculosis. *Scand J Resp Dis* 1972; **53**: 196–201

115 Linsk J A, Franzen S. FNA diagnosis of benign lung processes. In: Linsk J A, Franzen S eds. *Clinical Aspiration Cytology*. Philadelphia: Lippincott, 1983

116 Rajwanshi A, Bhambbani S, Das D K. Fine needle aspiration cytology diagnosis of tuberculosis. *Diagn Cytopathol* 1987; **3**: 13–16

117 Silverman J F, Marrow H G. Fine needle aspiration cytology of granulomatous diseases of the lung, including nontuberculous Mycobacterial infection. *Acta Cytol* 1985; **29**: 535–541

118 Strigle SM, Gal AA. A review of pulmonary cytopathology in the acquired immunodeficiency syndrome. *Diagn Cytopathol* 1989; **5**: 44–54

119 Singh N, Bahia A, Tickoo SK, Avora VK, Gupta K. Negative-staining refractile mycobacteria in Romanowsky-stained smears. *Acta Cytol* 1995; **39**: 1017

120 Snider D E, Hopewell P C, Mills J et al. Mycobacterioses and the acquired immunodeficiency syndrome. *Am Rev Resp Dis* 1987; **136**: 492–496

121 Wolinsky E. State of the art: non-tuberculous mycobacteria and associated diseases. *Am Rev Resp Dis* 1979; **119**: 107–159

122 Weiss R L, Snow G W, Schumann G B, Hammond M E. Diagnosis of cytomegalovirus pneumonitis on bronchoalveolar lavage fluid: comparison of cytology, immunofluorescence, and in situ hybridization with viral isolation. *Diag Cytopathol* 1991; **7**: 243–247

123 Naib Z M, Stewart J A, Dowdle W R et al. Cytological features of viral respiratory tract infections. *Acta Cytol* 1968; **12**: 167–171

124 Frable W J, Frable M A, Seney F D. Viral infections of the respiratory tract: cytopathologic and clinical analysis. *Acta Cytol* 1977; **21**: 32–36

125 Winn W C Jr, Walker D H. Viral infections. In: Dail D H, Hammar S P eds. *Pulmonary Pathology*. New York: Springer Verlag, 1988

126 Spriggs A I, Cole M, Dunnill M S. Alveolar cell carcinoma: a problem in sputum diagnosis. *J Clin Path* 1982; **35**: 1370–1379

127 Graham B S, Snell J D. Herpes simplex virus infection of the adult lower respiratory tract. *Medicine* 1983; **62**: 384–393

128 Frable W J, Kay S. Herpes virus infection of the respiratory tract: electron microscopic observation of the virus in cells obtained from sputum cytology. *Acta Cytol* 1977; **21**: 391–393

129 Vernon S E. Cytologic features of nonfatal herpesvirus tracheobronchitis. *Acta Cytol* 1982; **26**: 237–242

130 Koprowska I. Intranuclear inclusion bodies in smears of respiratory secretions. *Acta Cytol* 1961; **5**: 219–228

131 Warner N E, McGrew E A, Nonos S. Cytologic study of the sputum in cytomegalic inclusion disease. *Acta Cytol* 1964; **8**: 311–315

132 Jain U, Mani K, Frable W J. Cytomegalic inclusion disease: cytologic diagnosis from bronchial brushing material. *Acta Cytol* 1973; **17**: 467–468

133 Takeda M. Virus identification in cytologic and histologic material by electron microscopy. *Acta Cytol* 1969; **13**: 206–209

134 Naib Z M, Stewart J A, Dowdle W R et al. Cytological features of viral respiratory tract infections. *Acta Cytol* 1968; **12**: 162–171

135 Beale A J, Campbell W. A rapid cytological method for the diagnosis of measles. *J Clin Pathol* 1959; **12**: 335–337

136 Bayon M N, Drut R. Cytologic diagnosis of adenovirus infection. *Acta Cytol* 1991; **35**: 181–182

137 Bedrossian C W, DeArce E A L, Bedrossian U L et al. Herpetic tracheobronchitis detected at bronchoscopic cytology by the immunoperoxidase method. *Diagn Cytopathol* 1985; **1**: 292–295

138 Selvaggi S M, Gerber M. Pulmonary cytology in patients with the acquired immunodeficiency syndrome. *Diagn Cytopathol* 1986; **2**: 187–193

139 An-Foraker S, Haesaert S. Cytomegalic virus inclusion body in bronchial brushing material. *Acta Cytol* 1977; **21**: 181–182

140 Buchanan A J, Gupta R K. Cytomegalovirus infection of the lung: cytomorphologic diagnosis by fine needle aspiration cytology. *Diagn Cytopathol* 1986; **2**: 341–342

141 Hilborne L H, Nieberg R K, Cheng L *et al.* Direct in situ hybridization for rapid detection of cytomegalovirus in bronchoalveolar lavage. *Am J Clin Pathol* 1987; **87**: 766–769

142 Saced Zaman S, Seykara J T, Hodinka R L *et al.* Cytological manifestations of respiratory syncytial virus pneumonia in bronchoalveolar lavage fluid: a case report. *Acta Cytol* 1996; **40**: 546–551

143 Salfelder K. *Atlas of Fungal Pathology.* Dordrecht: Kluwer Academic, 1990

144 Chandler F W, Watts J C. Fungal infections. In: Dail D H, Hammar S P eds. *Pulmonary Pathology.* New York: Springer Verlag, 1988

145 Young J A. ed. *Colour Atlas of Pulmonary Cytopathology.* London: Harvey Miller, 1985

146 Kurrein F, Green G H. Localised deposition of calcium oxalate around a pulmonary Aspergillus niger fungus ball. *Amer J Clin Pathol* 1975; **64**: 556

147 Reyes C V, Kathuria S, MacGlashan A. Diagnostic value of calcium oxalate crystals in respiratory and pleural cytology: a case report. *Acta Cytol* 1979; **23**: 65–68

148 Fabry M L, Mabry L, Munoz L A, Diserens H W. Crystals occurring in pulmonary cytology specimens: association with Aspergillus infection. *Acta Cytol* 1985; **29**: 737–745

149 Levy H, Horak D A, Tegtmeier B R *et al.* The value of bronchoalveolar lavage and bronchial washings in the diagnosis of invasive pulmonary aspergillosis. *Resp Med* 1992; **86**: 243–248

150 Saito H, Anaissie E J, Marice R C *et al.* Bronchoalveolar lavage in the diagnosis of pulmonary infiltrates in patients with acute leukemia. *Chest* 1988; **94**: 745–749

151 Andrews C P, Weiner M H. Aspergillus antigen detection in bronchoalveolar lavage fluid from patients with invasive aspergillosis and aspergillomas. *Am J Med* 1982; **73**: 372–380

152 Benoit G, de Chauvin M F, Cordonnier C *et al.* Oxalic acid levels in bronchoalveolar lavage fluid from patients with invasive pulmonary aspergillosis. *Am Rev Resp Dis* 1985; **132**: 748–751

153 DeFine L A, Saleba K P, Gibson B B *et al.* Cytologic evaluation of bronchoalveolar lavage specimens in immunosuppressed patients with suspected opportunistic infections. *Acta Cytol* 1987; **31**: 235–242

154 Ness M J, Rennard S I, Vaughn W P *et al.* Detection of Candida antigen in bronchoalveolar lavage fluid. *Acta Cytol* 1988; **32**: 347–352

155 Chandler F W. Pathology of the mycoses in patients with the acquired immunodeficiency syndrome (AIDS). *Curr Topics Med Microb* 1986; **1**: 1–23

156 Prolla J C, Rosa U W, Xavier R G. The detection of Cryptococcus neoformans in sputum cytology: report of one case. *Acta Cytol* 1970; **14**: 87–91

157 Gupta R K. Diagnosis of unsuspected pulmonary cryptococcosis with sputum cytology. *Acta Cytol* 1985; **26**: 645–648

158 Rosen S E, Koprowska I. Cytologic diagnosis of a case of pulmonary cryptococcosis. *Acta Cytol* 1982; **26**: 499–502

159 Silverman J F, Johnsrude I S. Fine needle aspiration cytology of granulomatous cryptococcosis of the lung. *Acta Cytol* 1985; **29**: 157–161

160 Johnston W W, Frable W J. Cellular changes associated with nonneoplastic diseases. In: Johnston W W, Frable W J eds. *Diagnostic Respiratory Cytopathology.* New York: Masson, 1979; 93

161 Guglietti L C, Reingold I M. The detection of Coccidioides immitis in pulmonary cytology. *Acta Cytol* 1968; **12**: 332–334

162 Wallace J M, Catanzaro A, Moser K M *et al.* Flexible fiberoptic bronchoscopy for diagnosing pulmonary coccidioidomycosis. *Am Rev Respir Dis* 1981; **123**: 286–290

163 Freedman S I, Ang E P, Haley R S. Identification of coccidioidomycosis of the lung by fine needle aspiration biopsy. *Acta Cytol* 1986; **30**: 420–424

164 Rosenthal D L. Cytopathology of pulmonary disease. In: Wied G L ed. *Monographs in Clinical Cytology*, vol. 11 Basel: S Karger, 1988

165 Blumenfeld W, Gan G L. Diagnosis of histoplasmosis in bronchoalveolar lavage fluid by intracytoplasmic localisation of silver-positive yeast. *Acta Cytol* 1991; **35**: 710–712

166 Wheat L J, Slama T G, Zeckel M L. Histoplasmosis in the acquired immune deficiency syndrome. *Am J Med* 1985; **78**: 203–210

167 Johnston W W. Cytologic correlations. In: Dail D H, Hammar S P eds. *Pulmonary Pathology.* New York: Springer-Verlag, 1988

168 Klatt E C, Cosgrove M, Meyer P R. Rapid diagnosis of disseminated histoplasmosis in tissues. *Ann Int Med* 1985; **103**: 533–538

169 Johnston W W, Amatulli J. The role of cytology in the primary diagnosis of North American blastomycosis. *Acta Cytol* 1970; **14**: 200–204

170 Subramony C, Cason Z, O'Neal R M. Splendore-Hoeppli phenomenon around blastomyces in cytologic preparation. *Acta Cytol* 1984; **28**: 684–686

171 Daniel W C, Nair S V, Bluestein J. Light and electron microscopic observations of Blastomyces dermatitidis in sputum. *Acta Cytol* 1979; **23**: 223–226

172 Tani E M, Franco M. Pulmonary cytology in paracoccidioidomycosis. *Acta Cytol* 1984; **28**: 571–575

173 Remali S, Lofti C, Ismael A *et al.* Penicillium marneffi infection in patients with the human immunodeficiency virus. *Acta Cytol* 1995; **39**: 798–802

174 Tsui W M S, Ma K F, Tsang D N C. Disseminated Penicillium marneffei infection in HIV-infected subject. *Histopathol* 1992; **20**: 287–293

175 Chan J K C, Tsang D N C, Wong D K K. Penicillium marneffei in bronchoalveolar lavage fluid. *Acta Cytol* 1989; **33**: 523–526

176 Farley M L, Fagan M F, Mabry L, Wallace R Jr. Presentation of Sporothrix schenkii in pulmonary cytology specimens. *Acta Cytol* 1991; **35**: 389–395

177 Louria D B, Lieberman P H, Collins H S, Blevins A. Pulmonary mycetoma due to Allescheria boydii. *Arch Intern Med* 1966; **117**: 748–751

178 Miller R F, Mitchell D M. Pneumocystis carinii pneumonia. AIDS and the lung: up date 1992. 1. *Thorax* 1992; **47**: 305–314

179 Pixley F J, Wakefield A E, Banerji S, Hopkin J M. Mitochondrial gene sequences show fungal homology for Pneumocystis carinii. *Molec Microbiol* 1991; **5**: 1347–1351

180 Dunnill M S. Fungal disease of lung. In: Dunnill M S ed. *Pulmonary Pathology*, 2nd edn. Edinburgh: Churchill Livingstone, 209–215

181 Sobonya R E. Pneumocystis infection. In: Dail D H, Hammar S P eds. Pulmonary pathology. New York: Springer-Verlag, 1988; 301–313

182 Pitchenk A E, Gangei P, Torres A *et al.* Sputum examination for Pneumocystis carinii in the acquired immunodeficiency syndrome. *Am Rev Respir Dis* 1986; **133**: 226–229

183 Bigby T D, Margolskee D, Curtis J L *et al.* The usefulness of induced sputum in the diagnosis of Pneumocystis carinii pneumonia in the acquired immunodeficiency syndrome. *Am Rev Respir Dis* 1986; **133**: 515–518

184 Young J A, Stone J W, McGonigle R J, Adu D, Michael D. Diagnosing pneumocystis carinii pneumonia by cytological examination of bronchoalveolar lavage fluid: report of 15 cases. *J Clin Pathol* 1986; **39**: 945–949

185 Karpel J P, Prezant D, Appel D *et al.* Endotracheal lavage for the diagnosis of Pneumocystis carinii pneumonia in intubated patients with acquired immune deficiency syndrome. *Crit Care Med* 1986; **14**: 741

186 Rorat C, Garcia R L, Skolom J. Diagnosis of Pneumocystis carinii pneumonia by cytologic examination of bronchial washings. *JAMA* 1985; **254**: 950–951

187 Hartman B, Koss M, Hui A *et al.* Pneumocystis carinii pneumonia in the acquired immunodeficiency syndrome (AIDS): diagnosis with bronchial brushings, biopsy and bronchoalveolar lavage. *Chest* 1985; **87**: 603–607

188 Wallace J M, Batra P, Gong H *et al.* Percutaneous needle lung aspiration for diagnosing pneumonitis in the patient with the acquired immunodeficiency syndrome (AIDS). *Am Rev Respir Dis* 1985; **131**: 389–392

189 Greaves T S, Strigle S M. The recognition of Pneumocystis carinii in routine Papanicolaou-stained smears. *Acta Cytol* 1985; **29**: 714–720

190 Orenstein M, Webber C A, Heurich A E. Cytologic diagnosis of Pneumocystis carinii infection by bronchoalveolar lavage in acquired immune deficiency syndrome. *Acta Cytol* 1985; **29**: 727–731

191 Dugan J M, Avitable J M, Rossman M D, Ernst C, Atkinson B F. Diagnosis of Pneumocystis carinii pneumonia by cytologic evaluation of Papanicolaou-stained bronchial specimens. *Diagn Cytopathol* 1988; **4**: 106–111

192 Stanley M W, Henry M J, Iber C. Foamy alveolar casts: diagnostic specificity for Pneumocystis pneumonia in bronchoalveolar lavage fluid cytology. *Diagn Cytopathol* 1988; **4**: 113–115

193 Guarner J, Robboy S S, Gupta P K. Cytologic detection of Pneumocystis carinii: a comparison of Papanicolaou and other histochemical stains. *Diagn Cytopathol* 1986; **2**:133–137

194 Regan M C, Ayers L W. A five minute modified toluidine blue O stain for the detection of Pneumocystis carinii (abs). *Amer J Clin Pathol* 1987; **88**: 533–534

195 Paradis I L, Ross C, Dekker A, Dauber J. A comparison of modified methenamine silver and toluidine stains for the detection of Pneumocystis carinii in bronchoalveolar lavage specimens from immunosuppressed patients. *Acta Cytol* 1990; **34**: 511–516

196 Elvin K M, Bjorkman A, Linder E *et al.* Pneumocystis carinii pneumonia: detection of parasites in sputum and bronchoalveolar fluid by monoclonal antibodies. *BMJ* 1988; **297**: 381–384

197 Kovaks J A, Ng V L, Masur H *et al.* Diagnosis of Pneumocystis carinii pneumonia: improved detection in sputum with use of monoclonal antibodies. *N Engl J Med* 1988; **318**: 589–593

198 Wehle K, Blanke M, Koenig G, Pfitzer P. The cytological diagnosis of Pneumocystis carinii by fluorescence microscopy of Papanicolaou stained bronchoalveolar lavage specimens. *Cytopathol* 1991; **2**: 113–120

199 Wazir J F, Macrorie S G, Coleman D V. Evaluation of the sensitivity, specificity and predictive value of monoclonal antibody 3F6 for the detection of Pneumocystis carinii pneumonia in bronchoalveolar lavage specimens and induced sputum. *Cytopathol* 1994; **5**: 82–89

200 Wakefield A E, Pixley F J, Banerji S *et al.* Detection of Pneumocystis carinii with DNA amplification. *Lancet* 1990; **336**: 451–453

201 Wakefield A E, Guiver L, Miller R F, Hopkin J M. DNA amplification of induced sputum samples for diagnosis of Pneumocystis carinii pneumonia. *Lancet* 1991; **337**:1378–1379

202 Naryshkin S, Daniels J, Freno E, Cunningham L. Cytology of treated and minimal Pneumocystis carinii pneumonia and a pitfall of the Grocott methenamine silver stain. *Diagn Cytopathol* 1991; **7**: 41–47

203 Carmichael A, Bateman N, Nayagam M. Examination of induced sputum in the diagnosis of Pneumocystis carinii pneumonia. *Cytopathol* 1991; **2**: 61–66

204 Colangelo G, Baughman R P, Dohn M N, Frame P T. Follow-up bronchoalveolar lavage in AIDS patients with Pneumocystis carinii pneumonia: Pneumocystis carinii burden predicts early relapse. *Am Rev Resp Dis* 1991; **143**: 1067–1071

205 Cregan P, Yamamoto A, Lum A *et al.* Comparison of four methods for rapid detection of Pneumocystis carinii in respiratory specimens. *J Clin Microbiol* 1990; **28**: 2432–2436

206 Wazir J F, Wodsworth J, Coleman D V. Pneumocystis carinii pneumonia: relationship between cyst size and response to treatment. *Cytopathol* 1994; **5**; 90–92

207 Salfelder K. Atlas of parasitic pathology. Dordrecht: Kluwer Academic, 1992

208 Baird J K, Neafie R C, Connor D H. Parasitic infections. In: Dail D H, Hammar S P eds. *Pulmonary Pathology*. New York: Springer-Verlag, 1988

209 Rosenberg M, Rachman R. Entamoeba gingivalis in sputum: its distinction from Entamoeba histolytica. *Acta Cytol* 1970; **14**: 361–362

210 Kenney M, Eveland L K, Yermakov V. Amoebiasis: unusual location in lung. *NY State J Med* 1975; **75**: 1542–1543

211 Stevens W J, Vermiere P A. Giardia lamblia in bronchoalveolar lavage fluid. *Thorax* 1981; **26**: 875

212 Osborne P T, Giltman L I, Ulhman E O. Trichomonads in the respiratory tract: a case report and review of the literature. *Acta Cytol* 1984; **28**: 218–224

213 Kiriazis A P, Kiriazis A A. Incidence and distribution of opportunistic lung infections in AIDS patients related to intravenous drug use: a study of bronchoalveolar lavage cytology by the Diff-Quik stain. *Diagn Cytopathol* 1993; **9**:487–491

214 Gordon S M, Gal A A, Hertzler G L *et al.* Diagnosis of pulmonary toxoplasmosis by bronchoalveolar lavage in cardiac transplant recipients. *Diagn Cytopathol* 1993; **9**: 650–654

215 Wang T, Reyes C V, Kathuria S, Strinden C. Diagnosis of Strongyloides stercoralis in sputum cytology. *Acta Cytol* 1980; **24**: 40–43

216 Chaydhuri B, Nanos S, Soco J N, McGrew F A. Disseminated Strongyloides stercoralis infestation detected by sputum cytology. *Acta Cytol* 1980; **24**: 360–362

217 Munjal S, Gupta J, Munjal K R. Microfilariae in laryngeal and pharyngeal brushing smears from a case of carcinoma of the pharynx. *Acta Cytol* 1985; **29**: 1009–1010

218 Avasthi R, Jain A P, Swaroop K, Samal N. Bancroftian microfilariasis in association with pulmonary tuberculois. *Acta Cytol* 1991; **35**: 717–718

219 Ro J Y, Tsakalalis P J, White V A *et al.* Pulmonary dirofilariasis: the great imitator of primary or metastatic lung tumor. A clinicopathologic analysis of seven cases and a review of the literature. *Hum Pathol* 1989; **20(1)**: 69–76

220 Abdulla M A, Hombre S M, Al-Juwaiser A. Detection of Schistosoma mansoni in bronchoalveolar lavage fluid: a case report. *Acta Cytol* 1999; **43**: 856–858

221 Willie S M, Snyder R N. The identification of Paragonimus westermani in bronchial washings. *Acta Cytol* 1977; **21**: 101–102

222 Rangdaeng S, Alpert L C, Khiyami A *et al.* Pulmonary paragonimiasis: report of a case

with diagnosis by fine needle aspiration cytology. *Acta Cytol* 1992; **36**: 31–36

223 McCallum S M. Ova of the lung fluke Paragonimus kellicotti in fluid from a cyst. *Acta Cytol* 1975; **19**: 279–280

224 Allen A R, Fullmer C D. Primary diagnosis of pulmonary echinococcosis by the cytologic technique. *Acta Cytol* 1972; **16**: 212–216

225 Frydman C P, Raissi S, Watson C W. An unusual pulmonary and renal presentation of echinococcosis: report of a case. *Acta Cytol* 1989; **33**: 655–658

226 Lewall D B, McCorkell S J. Rupture of echinococcal cysts: diagnosis, classification and clinical implications. *Am J Roentgenol* 1986; **146**: 391–394

227 Ciba Guest Symposium. Terminology, definitions and classifications of chronic pulmonary emphysema and its related conditions. *Thorax* 1959; **14**: 286–299

228 Fletcher C M, Pride N B. Definitions of emphysema, chronic bronchitis, asthma and airflow obstruction: 25 years on from Ciba Symposium. *Thorax* 1984; **39**: 81–85 (Editorial)

229 Nasiell M. Abnormal columnar cell findings in bronchial epithelium: a cytologic and histologic study of lung cancer and non-cancer cases. *Acta Cytol* 1967; **11**: 397–402

230 Saccomanno G, Saunders R P, Archer V E *et al.* Cancer of the lung: the cytology of sputum prior to the development of carcinoma. *Acta Cytol* 1965; **9**: 413–423

231 Saccomanno G, Archer V E, Auerbach O *et al.* Development of carcinoma of the lung as reflected in exfoliated cells. *Cancer* 1974; **33**: 256–270

232 Nasiell M, Vogel B. Cytomorphology of benign changes and early carcinoma of the lung. In: Wied G L, Keebler C M, Koss L G, Reagan J W eds. *Compendium on Diagnostic Cytology*, 6th edn. Chicago: Tutorials of Cytology, 1990; 305–313

233 Dunnill M S. Bronchiectasis. In: Dunnill M S ed. *Pulmonary Pathology*, 2nd edn. Edinburgh: Churchill Livingstone, 1987; 81–95

234 Kaweka M. Cytological evaluation of the sputum in patients with bronchiectasis and the possibility of erroneous diagnosis of carcinoma. *Acta Union Intern Cancer* 1959; **15**: 469–473

235 Garrett M. Cellular atypias in sputum and bronchial secretions associated with tuberculosis and bronchiectasis. *Am J Clin Pathol* 1960; **34**: 237–246

236 Dunnill M S. Asthma. In: Dunnill M S ed. *Pulmonary Pathology*, 2nd edn. Edinburgh: Churchill Livingstone, 1987; 61–79

237 Sanerkin N G, Seal R M E, Leopold J G. Plastic bronchitis, mucoid impaction of the bronchi and allergic bronchopulmonary aspergillosis, and their relationship to bronchial asthma. *Ann of Allergy* 1966; **24**: 586–594

238 Sanerkin N G, Evans D M D. The sputum in bronchial asthma: pathognomic patterns. *J Pathol Bacterial* 1965; **89**: 535–541

239 Leavitt R., Fauci A S. State of Art: Pulmonary Vasculitis. *Am Rev Respir Dis* 1986; **134**: 149–166

240 Naylor B. Creola bodies: their 'discovery' and significance. *Cytotechnol Bull* 1985; **22**: 33–34

241 Naylor B, Railey C. A pitfall in the cytodiagnosis of sputum of asthmatics. *J Clin Pathol* 1982; **17**: 84–89

242 Vieira V G, Prolla J C. Clinical evaluation of eosinophils in the sputum. *J Clin Pathol* 1979; **32**: 1054–1057

243 Arroyo J, Gordan V, Postic B. Transthoracic needle aspiration in the management of pulmonary infections. *J Sc Med Assoc* 1981; 427–432

244 Pontifex A H, Roberts F J. Fine needle aspiration biopsy cytology in the diagnosis of inflammatory lesions. *Acta Cytol* 1985; **29**: 979–982

245 Hunninghake G W, Gadek J E, Kawanami O et al. Inflammatory and immune processes in the human lung in health and disease: evaluation by bronchoalveolar lavage. *Am J Pathol* 1979; **97**: 149–206

246 Hunninghake G W, Crystal R G. Pulmonary sarcoidosis: a disorder mediated by excess helper T lymphocyte activity at sites of disease activity. *N Engl J Med* 1981; **305**: 429–434

247 Rossi G A, Sacco O, Cosulich E et al. Pulmonary sarcoidosis: excess of helper T lymphocytes and T cell subset imbalance at sites of disease activity. *Thorax* 1984; **39**: 143–149

248 Aisner S C, Gupta P K, Frost J K. Sputum cytology in pulmonary sarcoidosis. *Acta Cytol* 1977; **21**: 394–398

249 Crystal R G. Pulmonary sarcoidosis: a disease characterised and perpetuated by activated lung T-lymphocytes. *Ann Intern Med* 1981; **94**: 73–94

250 Vernon S E. Nodular pulmonary sarcoidosis: diagnosis with fine needle aspiration biopsy. *Acta Cytol* 1985; **29**: 473–476

251 Pauli G, Pelletier A, Bohner C, Roeslin N, Warter A, Roegel E. Transbronchial needle aspiration in the diagnosis of sarcoidosis. *Chest* 1984; **85**: 482–484

252 Keogh B A, Crystal R G. Alveolitis: the key to interstitial lung disorders. *Thorax* 1982; **37**: 1–10 (Editorial)

253 Walker W C, Wright V. Pulmonary lesions and rheumatoid arthritis. *Medicine* 1968; **47**: 501–520

254 Olsen E G, Lever J V. Pulmonary changes in systemic lupus erythematosus. *Br J Dis Chest* 1972; **66**: 71–77

255 Johnston W W, Frable W J. Epidermoid carcinoma, keratinizing and non-keratinizing. In: Johnston W W, Frable W J eds. *Diagnostic Respiratory Cytopathology*. New York: Masson, 1979; 151–174

256 Pitman M B, Szyfelbein W M, Niles J, Fienberg R. Clinical utility of fine needle aspiration biopsy in the diagnosis of Wegener's granulomatosis: a report of two cases. *Acta Cytol* 1922; **36**: 222–229

257 Corrin B. Diseases characterized by restrictive ventilatory impairment. In: Corrin B ed. *Pathology of the Lungs*. London: Churchill Livingstone, 2000; 239–277

258 Dunnill M S. Pulmonary fibrosis. In: Dunnill M S ed. *Pulmonary Pathology*.

Edinburgh: Churchill Livingstone, 1987; 251–282

259 Geddes D M. BOOP and COP. *Thorax* 1991; **46**: 545–547 (Editorial)

260 Bellomo R, Finlay M, McLaughlin P, Tai E. Clinical spectrum of cryptogenic organizing pneumonitis. *Thorax* 1991; **46**: 554–558

261 Nicholson A. The pathology and terminology of fibrosing alveolitis and the interstitial pneumonias. *Imaging* 1999; **11**: 1–12

262 Morrison H M, Stockley R A. The many uses of bronchoalveolar lavage. *BMJ* 1988; **296**: 1758 (Editorial)

263 Haslam P L, Turton C W G, Heard B et al. Bronchoalveolar lavage in pulmonary fibrosis: comparison of cells obtained with lung biopsy and clinical features. *Thorax* 1980; **35**: 9–18

264 Hunninghake G W, Kawanami O, Ferrans V J et al. Characterization of the inflammatory and immune effector cells in the lung parenchyma of patients with interstitial lung disease. *Am Rev Resp Dis* 1981; **123**: 407–412

265 Salvaggio J E. Hypersensitivity pneumonitis. *J Allergy Clin Immunol* 1987; **79**: 558–571

266 Hunninghake G W, Gadek J E, Lawley T J, Crystal R G. Mechanism of neutrophil accumulation in the lung of patients with idiopathic pulmonary fibrosis. *J Clin Invest* 1981; **68**: 259–269

267 Reynolds H Y. State of art. Bronchoalveolar lavage. *Am Rev Resp Dis* 1987; **135**: 250–263

268 Fink J N, DeShazo R. Immunological aspects of granulomatous and interstitial lung diseases. *JAMA* 1987; **258**: 2938–2944

269 Tao L C, Sanders D E, Weisbrod G L. Value and limitations of transthoracic and transabdominal fine needle aspiration cytology in clinical practice. *Diagn Cytopathol* 1986; **2**: 271–276

270 Akoun G M, Mayoud C M, Milleron B J, Perrot J Y. Drug-induced pneumonitis and drug-induced hypersensitivity pneumonitis. *Lancet* 1984; **i**: 1362

271 Cooper J A D, White D A, Matthay R A. State of art. Drug-induced pulmonary disease. Part 1: Cytotoxic drugs. *Am Rev Resp Dis* 1986; **133**: 321–340

272 Cooper J A D, White D A, Matthay R A. State of art. Drug-induced pulmonary disease. Part 2: Noncytotoxic drugs. *Amer Rev Resp Dis* 1986; **133**: 488–505

273 Bedrossian C W M. Iatrogenic and toxic injury. In: Dail D H, Hammar S P eds. *Pulmonary Pathology*. New York: Springer-Verlag, 1988; 511–534

274 Bedrossian C W M. Pathology of drug-induced lung diseases. *Sem Resp Med* 1982; **4**: 98–106

275 Bedrossian C W M, Corey B J. Abnormal sputum cytopathology during chemotherapy with bleomycin. *Acta Cytol* 1978; **22**: 202–207

276 Koss L G. *Diagnostic Cytology and its Histopathologic Bases*, 4th edn. Philadelphia: Lippincott, 1992

277 Ettensohn D B, Roberts N T, Condemi J J. Bronchoalveolar lavage in gold lung. *Chest* 1984; **85**: 569–570

278 White D A, Gellene R, Rankin J R et al. Methotrexate pneumonitis: bronchoalveolar lavage findings suggest an immune mediated disorder. *Am Rev Resp Dis* 1984; **129**: A64 (Abstract)

279 Munn N J, Baughman R P, Ploysongsang Y et al. Bronchoalveolar lavage in acute drug hypersensitivity pneumonitis probably caused by phenytoin. *South Med J* 1984; **77**: 1594–1596

280 Akoun G M, Mayaud C M, Touboul J L et al. Use of bronchoalveolar lavage if the evaluation of methotrexate lung disease. *Thorax* 1987; **42**: 652–655

281 Huang M S, Colby T V, Goellner J R, Martin W J. Utility of bronchoalveolar lavage in the diagnosis of drug-induced pulmonary toxicity. *Acta Cytol* 1989; **33**: 533–538

282 Koss L G, Melamed M R, Mayer K. The effect of busulphan on human epithelia. *Am J Clin Pathol* 1965; **44**: 385–397

283 Stover D E, Zaman M B, Hajdyu S I et al. Bronchoalveolar lavage in the diagnosis of diffuse pulmonary infiltrates in the immunosuppressed host. *Ann Intern Med* 1984; **101**: 1–7

284 Bedrossian C W M, Luna M A, Mackay B, Lichtiger B. Ultrastructure of pulmonary bleomycin toxicity. *Cancer* 1973; **32**: 44–51

285 Pesci A, Bertorelli G, Marchioni M. T-lymphocytes in bronchoalveolar lavage fluid in hypersensitivity pneumonitis. *Chest* 1985; **87**: 133–134

286 Fathey P J, Utell M J, Mayewski R J et al. Early diagnosis of bleomycin pulmonary toxicity using bronchoalveolar lavage in dogs. *Am Rev Resp Dis* 1982; **126**: 126–130

287 Martin W J II, Williams D E, Dines D E, Sanderson D R. Interstitial lung disease assessment by bronchoalveolar lavage. *Mayo Clin Proc* 1983; **58**: 751–755

288 Israel-Biet D, Venet A, Caubarrere I et al. Bronchoalveolar lavage in amiodorone pneumonitis: cellular abnormalities and their relevance to pathogenesis. *Chest* 1987; **91**: 214–221

289 Stein B, Zaatari G S, Pine J R. Amiodorone pulmonary toxicity: clinical, cytologic and ultrastructural findings. *Acta Cytol* 1987; **31**: 357–361

290 Mermolja M, Rott T, Debeljak A. Cytology of bronchoalveolar lavage in some rare pulmonary disorders: pulmonary alveolar proteinosis and amiodorone pulmonary toxicity. *Cytopathology* 1994; **5**: 9–16

291 Reyes C V, Thompson K S, Jensen J. Multivesiculated macrophages: their implications in fine needle aspiration cytology of lung mass lesions. *Diagn Cytopathol* 1998; **19**: 98–101

292 D'Ablang G III, Bernard B, Zaharov I et al. Neonatal pulmonary cytology and bronchopulmonary dysplasia. *Acta Cytol* 1975; **19**: 21–27

293 Kanbour A, Doshi N, Fujikura T. Neonatal tracheobronchial cytology of bronchopulmonary dysplasia. *Acta Cytol* 1980; **24**: 60

294 Doshi N, Kanbour A, Fujikura T, Klionsky B. Tracheal aspiration cytology in neonates with respiratory distress. *Acta Cytol* 1982; **26**: 15–21

295 Johnston W W, Frable W J. Cellular alterations resulting from irradiation and chemotherapy for cancer. In: Johnston W W, Frable W J eds. *Diagnostic Respiratory Cytopathology*. New York: Masson, 1979; 66–69

296 Koss L G. *Diagnostic Cytology and its Histopathologic Bases*, 4th edn. Philadelphia: Lippincott, 1992; 749–753

297 Ashbaugh D G, Bigelow D B, Petty T L, Levine B E. Acute respiratory distress in adults. *Lancet* 1967; ii: 319–323

298 Rocker G M, Wiseman M S, Pearson D, Shale D J. Diagnostic criteria for adult respiratory distress syndrome: time for reappraisal. *Lancet* 1989; i: 120–123

299 Donnelly S C, Haslett C. Cellular mechanisms of acute lung injury: implications for future treatment in the adult respiratory distress syndrome. *Thorax* 1992; 47: 260–263 (Editorial)

300 Grotte D, Stanley M W, Swanson P E et al. Reactive type II pneumocytes in bronchoalveolar lavage fluid from adult respiratory distress syndrome can be mistaken for cells of adenocarcinoma. *Diagn Cytopathol* 1990; 6: 317–322

301 Ettinger N A, Trulock E P. Pulmonary considerations of organ transplantation: state of the art. Part 1. *Amer Rev Resp Dis* 1991; 143: 1386–1405. Part 2. 1991; 144: 213–223. Part 3. 1991; 144: 433–451

302 Selvaggi S M. Bronchoalveolar lavage in lung transplant patients. *Acta Cytol* 1992; 36: 674–679

303 Hammar S P. Extrinsic allergic alveolitis. In: Dail D H, Hammar S P eds. *Pulmonary Pathology*. New York: Springer-Verlag, 1988; 379–392

304 Churg A, Green F H Y eds. *Pathology of Occupational Lung Disease*. New York: Igaku Shoin, 1988

305 Schuyler M R, Gaumer H R, Stankus R P et al. Bronchoalveolar lavage in silicosis. *Lung* 1980; 157: 95–102

306 Davison A G, Haslam P L, Gorrin B et al. Interstitial lung disease and asthma in hard-metal workers: bronchoalveolar lavage, ultrastructural, and analytical findings and results of bronchial provocation tests. *Thorax* 1983; 38: 119–128

307 Churg A, Warnock M L. Analysis of the cores of ferruginous (asbestos) bodies from the general population I. Patients with and without lung cancer. *Lab Invest* 1977; 37: 280–286

308 Churg A, Warnock M L, Green N. Analysis of the cores of ferruginous (asbestos) bodies from the general population II. True asbestos bodies and pseudoasbestos bodies. *Lab Invest* 1979; 40: 31–38

309 Mazzucchelli L, Radelfinger H, Kraft R. Nonasbestos ferruginous bodies in sputum from a patient with graphite pneumoconiosis. *Acta Cytol* 1996; 40: 552–554

310 Roggli V L, Johnston W W, Kaminsky D B. Asbestos bodies in fine needle aspirates of the lung. *Acta Cytol* 1984; 28: 493–498

311 Roggli V L, Piantadosi C A, Bell D Y. Asbestos bodies in bronchoalveolar lavage fluid: a study of twenty asbestos-exposed individuals and comparison to patients with other interstitial lung disease. *Acta Cytol* 1986; 30: 470–476

312 Leiman G. Asbestos bodies in fine needle aspirates of lung masses: markers of underlying pathology. *Acta Cytol* 1991; 35: 171–174

313 Berkheiser J W. Bronchiolar proliferation and metaplasia associated with thrombolism: a pathological and experimental study. *Cancer* 1963; 16: 205–211

314 Scoggins W G, Smith R H, Frable W J, O'Donahue W J. False positive cytological diagnosis of lung carcinoma in patients with pulmonary infarcts. *Ann Thor Surg* 1977; 24: 474–480

315 Bewtra C, Dewan N, O'Donahue W J. Exfoliative sputum cytology in pulmonary embolism. *Acta Cytol* 1983; 27: 489–499

316 Silverman J F, Weaver M D, Shaw R, Newman W J. Fine needle aspiration cytology of pulmonary infarct. *Acta Cytol* 1985; 29: 162–166

317 Friedman-Mor Z, Chalon J, Katz J S et al. Tracheobronchial and pulmonary cytologic changes in shock. *J Trauma* 1979; 16: 58–62

318 Drew W L, Finley T N, Golde D W. Diagnostic lavage and occult pulmonary haemorrhage in thrombocytopenic immunocompromised patients. *Am Rev Resp Dis* 1977; 116: 215–221

319 Losner S, Volk B W, Slade W R, Nathanson L, Jacobi M. Diagnosis of lipid pneumonia by examination of sputum. *Am J Clin Pathol* 1950; 20: 539–545

320 Silverman J F, Turner R C, West R L, Dillard T A. Bronchoalveolar lavage in the diagnosis of lipoid pneumonia. *Diagn Cytopathol* 1989; 5: 3–8

321 Cowell J L, Feldman P S. Fine needle aspiration diagnosis of aspiration pneumonia (phytopneumonitis). *Acta Cytol* 1984; 28: 77–80

322 Chen K T K. Cytology of tracheobronchial amyloidosis. *Acta Cytol* 1984; 28: 133–135

323 Neifer R A, Amy R W M. Cytology of tracheobronchial amyloidosis. *Acta Cytol* 1985; 29: 187–188

324 Dundore P A, Aisner S C, Templeton P A, Krasna M J et al. Nodular pulmonary amyloidosis: diagnosis by fine-needle aspiration cytology and a review of the literature. *Diagn Cytopathol* 1993; 9: 562–564

325 Michael C W, Naylor B. Amyloid in cytologic specimens: differential diagnosis and pitfalls. *Acta Cytol* 1999; 43: 746–755

326 Rosen S H, Castleman B, Liebow A A. Pulmonary alveolar proteinosis. *N Engl J Med* 1958; 258: 1123–1142

327 Bedrossian C W M, Luna M A, Conklin R H, Miller W C. Alveolar proteinosis as a consequence of immunosuppression: a hypothesis based on clinical and pathologic observations. *Hum Pathol* 1980; 11: 527–535

328 Hook G E R, Bell D Y, Gilmor D B et al. Composition of bronchoalveolar lavage effluents from patients with pulmonary alveolar proteinosis. *Lab Invest* 1978; 39: 342–357

329 Dail D H. Pulmonary alveolar (lipo) proteinosis. In: Dail D H, Hammar S P eds. *Pulmonary Pathology*. New York: Springer-Verlag, 1988; 561–567

330 Pulmonary alveolar proteinosis: a report of two cases with diagnostic features in bronchoalveolar lavage specimens. *Acta Cytol* 1998; 42: 377–383

331 Ambiavagar M, Chalon J, Zargham I. Tracheobronchial cytologic changes following lower airway thermal injury. *J Trauma* 1974; 14: 280–289

332 Cooney W, Dzuira B, Harper R, Nash G. The cytology of sputum from thermally injured patients. *Acta Cytol* 1972; 16: 433–437

333 Koss L G. Respiratory tract cytology in the evaluation of thermal injury. In: Koss L G ed. *Diagnostic Cytology and its Histopathologic Bases*, 4th edn. Philadelphia: J B Lippincott Co, 1992; 747–748

334 Clark C J, Reid W H, Pollock A J et al. Role of pulmonary alveolar macrophage activation in acute lung injury after burns and smoke inhalation. *Lancet* 1988; 872–874

335 Corrin B. Inflammatory myofibroblastic tumour. In: Corrin B ed. *Pathology of the Lungs*. London: Churchill Livingstone, 2000; 587–590

336 Pettinato G, Manival JC, de Rosa N et al. Inflammatory myofibroblastic tumours (plasma cell granuloma) – clinicopathologic study of 20 cases with immunohistochemical and ultrastructural observations. *Am J Clin Pathol* 1990; 94: 538–546

337 Koss L G, Woyke S, Olszewski W. *Aspiration Biopsy. Cytologic Interpretation and Histologic Bases*. New York: Igaku-Shoin, 1984; 327–328

338 Thunnissen F B J M, Arends J W, Buchholtz R T F, ten Velde G. Fine needle aspiration cytology of inflammatory pseudotumor of the lung (plasma cell granuloma): report of four cases. *Acta Cytol* 1989; 33: 917–921

339 Machicao C N, Sorensen K L, Abdul-Karim F W, Somrak T M. Transthoracic fine needle aspiration in inflammatory pseudotumor of the lung. *Diagn Cytopathol* 1989; 5: 400–403

340 Krane J F, Renshaw A A. Relative value and cost effectiveness of culture and special stains in fine needle aspirates of the lung. *Acta Cytol* 1988; 42: 305–311

341 Zakowski M F, Gatscha R M, Zaman M B. Negative predictive value of fine needle aspiration cytology. *Acta Cytol* 1992; 36: 283–286

342 Leigh T R, Hume C, Gazzard B et al. Sputum induction for diagnosis of Pneumocystis carinii pneumonia. *Lancet* 1989; 205 206

343 Morrison H M, Stockley R A. The many uses of bronchoalveolar lavage. *BMJ* 1988; 296: 1758

344 Rohwedder J J. The solitary pulmonary nodule: a new diagnostic agenda. *Chest* 1988; 93: 1124–1125

345 Afify A, Davila RM. Pulmonary fine needle aspiration biopsy: assessing the negative diagnosis. *Acta Cytol* 1999; 43: 601–604

3 Tumours of lung and mediastinum

Greg Sterrett, Felicity Frost and Darrel Whitaker

Pulmonary tumours

Cytological procedures for tumour diagnosis

The various techniques for obtaining pulmonary material for cytological diagnosis of neoplasia are generally selected in order of their degree of invasiveness and complication.

Sputum cytology is non-invasive, relatively inexpensive, and can detect between 60–90% of malignancies if 3–5 specimens are examined[1-3]. It has the disadvantage of not localizing the lesion precisely, is much less sensitive for peripheral than for central lung lesions, and may result in delays in diagnosis for hospital inpatients if multiple samples are needed.

Bronchial brushings and washings by fibreoptic bronchoscopy (FOB) can reach and sample up to 90% of malignant lesions and have a very low rate of complications[1,4,5], although very peripheral lesions, pleural lesions, and submucosal and mediastinal masses cannot be diagnosed.

Transbronchial fine needle aspiration at the time of FOB makes submucosal and paratracheal lesions accessible with little or no extra risk[6-10] and increases the sensitivity of a bronchoscopic diagnosis of malignancy[6,11]. Some authors advocate the routine use of this method together with immediate reporting[12].

Bronchoalveolar lavage (BAL) obtains cells from alveolar regions, is most useful in the study of interstitial lung disease, and for diagnosing alveolar infections such as *Pneumocystis carinii* pneumonia, but may also provide a diagnosis in peripheral malignancies such as bronchioloalveolar carcinoma and metastatic carcinoma[13,14].

Percutaneous fine needle aspiration (FNA) accesses virtually all sites within the thorax, and is particularly useful when FOB has not given a diagnosis[15]. It may be the first choice in lesions of mediastinum[16,17], pleura, chest wall, lung apex and medial upper lobe[18].

Large needle biopsy is generally restricted to pleural-based or chest wall lesions because of the greater risk of complications, particularly haemorrhage, in the lung, though it is used safely in some areas of the mediastinum, particularly with newer techniques of automatic rapid core sampling. There are also recent reports of lung sampling with a low complication rate and a higher rate of specific diagnosis, particularly in benign lesions[19-21].

Mediastinoscopy, open lung biopsy or lobectomy are seldom required for the diagnosis of malignancy, although in some lesions, e.g. lymphomas within the lung and mediastinum and some specific benign or reactive processes, which generally do not yield diagnostic cytological material, these techniques may be necessary for diagnosis and accurate subtyping.

Historical perspective

While respiratory cytodiagnosis had its birth in the late 1800s[22], it was not until the 1930s and 1940s that sputum cytology as a means of detecting or diagnosing lung cancer became a widespread and established clinical practice; the work of Dudgeon[23] and Wandall[24] is singled out for its clarity of description and quality of results.

The next decades brought expanded use of this modality of cytodiagnosis and with it, more precise cytological subtyping of lung cancer and an evaluation of accuracy and clinical value[2,25,26]. Papanicolaou and Koprowska[27] were the first to report the cytological findings from a case of carcinoma *in situ* of the lung. The sputum cytological detection of early lung cancer and its precursors became the subject of attention during the 1960s and 1970s with the introduction and investigation of screening programmes for asymptomatic high risk groups, mainly cigarette smoking older males[28-31]. The effects of industrial exposure to carcinogens, including radon[32] and asbestos[33,34], were also investigated by sputum cytology.

Rigid bronchoscopic biopsy was the standard method of obtaining specimens for definitive diagnosis as a basis for management until the advent of flexible fibreoptic bronchoscopy in the 1960s. Bronchial brushings and washings became more widely accepted as techniques which were as accurate as biopsy diagnoses, and which added to the overall sensitivity of FOB diagnosis. This technique also enabled the sampling of more peripheral and smaller lesions[35,36]. Bronchoalveolar lavage (BAL) was introduced mainly as a tool for investigating nonmalignant interstitial lung disease (see Chapter 2)[37], but has since found some favour in the diagnosis of peripheral diffusely growing malignancies[13,14,38,39].

Fine needle aspiration cytology of the lung in many ways paralleled exfoliative cytology of the respiratory tract, initial reports of detection of lung cancer occurring as early as 1886[40]. However, the modern era of needle aspiration cytology of lung began in the 1960s by Swedish workers[41,42], with the development and refinement of fluoroscopic imaging providing better localization of peripheral thoracic lesions, and the use of finer needles leading to fewer complications. By the 1980s, fine needle aspiration cytology was established as having a pivotal role in the diagnosis and management of intrathoracic lesions[43,44].

The last few decades have seen ample demonstration of the sensitivity and predictive value of cytodiagnosis, an acceptance of all cytological modalities as a basis for management, and gradual extension of the range of diagnoses to virtually all neoplastic processes affecting the lung and mediastinum. Surgical procedures are decreasingly used as a basis for initial diagnosis[45]. Significant recent contributions confirming the accuracy and value of these techniques have come from individual workers[1,43,46–49] and from monographs and textbooks with comprehensive cytological descriptions of intrathoracic lesions[50–60a].

Recent changes in practice

Sputum cytology was the traditional focus for teaching respiratory cytology for many years; however, the emphasis has been altered by the introduction of fibreoptic bronchoscopy (FOB) and fine needle aspiration. In our practice, since around the mid-1980s, there has been a marked reduction in the numbers of sputum samples sent for cytology; these now constitute less than 20% of the numbers sent in 1990.

In an era of financial constraint, a 2–3 day wait for the results of series of sputum cytology samples is often unacceptable for hospital inpatients, although it is an ideal technique for outpatient diagnosis before admission to hospital. Rapid sputum reporting may improve the usefulness of the technique. Bender et al.[61] suggest that pre- or post-bronchoscopy sputum cytology adds little in sensitivity to the detection of carcinoma and proposed reporting on stored sputum only if bronchoscopy is negative, so as to cut costs; this is disputed by others who suggest that pre- and post-bronchoscopy sputum are of some value[62,63]. Goldberg-Kahn et al.[64] suggested that sputum examination had the highest cost per correct diagnosis of any biopsy or cytology method, and was not cost effective except for large unresectable lesions. However in Raab's study[65], sputum cytology as the first diagnostic test was able to lower medical care costs and the mortality risk of management, with large potential cost savings.

Fibreoptic bronchoscopy samples, including biopsy, brushings, washings or aspiration of secretions[66], remain the mainstay of diagnosis for central lung tumours. Adding transbronchial FNA increases the sensitivity of diagnosis although considerable experience is necessary to achieve acceptable results[67]. Combined study of biopsy and cytology material enhances the sensitivity of diagnosis of malignant tumours[68] and their specific subtyping. Washings are sent as part of the procedure and are routinely processed, and, in

our experience, add a small increment to sensitivity, mainly when brush or biopsy cannot reach more peripheral tumours; nevertheless some workers have doubted their value[63].

In company with a fall in sputum samples there has been an increase in the use of percutaneous fine needle aspiration because of its rapidity, ease of performance, confirmation of the site of abnormality and relatively low risk. Only about 10% of patients require treatment for pneumothorax. The emphasis on the use of FNA has shifted from the diagnosis of malignancy in inoperable patients and confirmation of metastatic tumour to its use as a definitive diagnostic procedure[15]. Blumenfeld et al. found that FNA provided 50% of their malignant cytological diagnoses in lung, BAL in 47% and sputum in only 3% of malignancies[69]. Steffee et al., reviewing their results from a decade apart, showed a rapid rise in the use of transbronchial needle aspiration and a corresponding fall in sputum samples. FNA samples gave the highest rate of positive diagnoses (95–97%)[70].

Lesions of all sites including mediastinum and deep hilar lesions are sampled with increasing flexibility and accuracy when accompanied by CT or other imaging techniques. Lung function studies and radiology can be used to predict the risk of pneumothorax, allowing safer selection of patients for outpatient FNA[71,72]. The use of the transbronchial route[73], non-aspiration technique[74,75], endoscopic ultrasound guided FNA[76] and coaxial needle sampling, allows the radiologist and pathologist great flexibility in obtaining material. Having the pathologist at the procedure can reduce the number of needle passes, reduce unsatisfactory samples[77], increase sensitivity of diagnosis[78], allow optimal handling of material for ancillary tests[79] and improves the predictive value of negative results[80]. Intraoperative FNA may be valuable for surgeons confronting lesions hazardous to biopsy[81,82]. Thoracoscopic aspiration may be used where percutaneous aspiration is contraindicated because of the risk of pneumothorax[83]. High rates of cytohistological correlation for common tumours have been demonstrated[43,44], and the value of FNA in the diagnosis of more unusual tumours including those of mediastinum and pleura is accepted, particularly when allied with cell block preparations, immunoperoxidase studies and electron microscopy.

The use of bronchoalveolar lavage has increased rapidly since 1990, particularly in the management of interstitial lung disease and in the diagnosis of opportunistic infection, especially in immunosuppressed patients (see Chapter 2). It has a widening range of clinical applications[84]. Although rarely used as a primary method of diagnosis of malignancy, in patients with diffuse or patchy peripheral lung shadowing which might be due to malignancy or infection, BAL can provide a diagnosis and may be as sensitive as other methods[14,85]; it is particularly useful in conditions such as lymphangitic carcinomatosis[13].

Pulmonary microvascular cytology of blood samples derived from wedged pulmonary artery catheter specimens has been described recently as an aid to the diagnosis of diffusely growing carcinomas or lymphangitic carcinomatosis[86] where other methods have failed.

Complications and contraindications

FOB is avoided in patients with moderate to severe coagulation disorders. Pneumothorax, significant bronchospasm and haemoptysis occur rarely (less than 0.15% of cases) and mortality is extremely low (less than 0.05%)[87]. Concurrent fluoroscopy may reduce the rate of pneumothorax, while supplemental oxygen decreases the rate of hypoxaemia and cardiac complications in pre-disposed patients.

FNA is not performed in unconscious or uncooperative patients or in those with respiratory failure, haemorrhagic diathesis or intractable coughing. Pneumothorax is a common complication although only 4–10% of patients require intercostal catheters[87]. Patients with emphysema are at greater risk[71,72]. Minor degrees of haemoptysis are occasionally seen. Rare cases of air embolism are described and fatalities are exceptionally rare[88]. Needle track implantation by tumour is extremely rare[89,90].

Technical considerations
Types of specimen
Sputum

Technical aspects of sputum collection, transport and laboratory procedures are described in Chapter 2. Although the 'pick and smear' method of preparation is generally used, the Saccomanno method has been adopted by many workers. It has been suggested that this technique may disrupt cell aggregates and make diagnosis more difficult for tumours such as small cell carcinoma and adenocarcinoma[91], but equally good results have been achieved by either method in some authors' hands[92]; a higher sensitivity with the Saccomanno technique is claimed by some[93].

A diagnosis of malignancy is more likely to be made from a deep cough sample with abundant macrophages[94]. Nevertheless, salivary or other unsatisfactory samples should still be screened. Carcinoma cells, in particular small cell cancer, may be detected in sputum samples that appear entirely salivary. Physiotherapy or methacholine-induced deep cough samples are useful in those patients who find it difficult to produce satisfactory samples initially[95].

Bronchial brushings and washings

These samples are generally prepared in the endoscopy theatre by resident staff; air drying artefact is the most common defect in brushing samples, and is particularly so in a teaching institution where there is a continual flow of new operators. It is therefore an advantage to have cytotechnology staff present at the bronchoscopy.

Fine needle aspiration

In most institutions, these samples are taken by the radiologist, who will select sampling devices such as simple thin needles, thin core needles or large core biopsy needles according to the site of the lesion and to minimize the likelihood of complications. Long bevel needles of 23 or 22 gauge give very satisfactory material for smears, cell blocks or electron microscopy. Rapid microscopical assessment of smears in the radiology theatre enables satisfactory sampling to be confirmed and the most useful ancillary test can be selected, including sending material for microbiological assessment. The non-aspiration technique may be particularly valuable for haemorrhagic tumours[74].

Core needle biopsies taken by automated devices are useful for pleural-based lesions and for parenchymal tumours extending to the pleura.

Bronchoalveolar lavage

Details of this technique are given in Chapter 2. Differential washings are an accepted part of the procedure. The first sample removes bronchial lumen content, and the second provides a good alveolar sample[54]. Up to 30% of routinely submitted samples may have a paucity of macrophages, an excess of bronchial epithelial cells, a mucopurulent component or degenerative changes rendering them unsuitable for assessment[96].

Ancillary techniques

Cell blocks on FNA samples are most easily prepared by using powdered thrombin to induce clotting on a slide or watch glass and by fixing and processing the resulting pellet as for biopsy material, so removing washing or centrifugation steps. We regard cell blocks as essential and prepare them in all but the most straightforward cases. They are useful for 'microhistology' to detect architectural features not evident in smears, for cytochemistry using mucin stains, and for immunohistochemistry. Cell blocks prepared from sputum or brushings or washings may also be of value for the diagnosis of carcinoma[97].

Fluid based samples may improve the quality of smears by reducing the amount of blood-staining or inflammation in the background[98–100].

In our laboratory immunoperoxidase studies, including lymphoma studies and hormone receptor assays, are performed on cell blocks, and others have noted their advantages: negative controls and panels of markers can be performed on the same or adjacent cells. Chess and Hajdu[101] have documented the potential for misleading immunocytochemical results in smears. Brown and Gatter[102] suggest that low cellularity and mucus, which prevents antibody access, make preparations of respiratory brushings unsuitable for immunocytochemistry, although others achieve good results with respiratory samples. Recent advances include the use of differential cytokeratin staining (e.g. for CK 7 and 20) and thyroid transcription factor (TTF) in the identification of likely primary sites of origin of carcinomas[103–104] and MART-1 antibodies for the specific recognition of melanoma[105]. Most non-mucinous adenocarcinomas and large cell carcinomas of lung are CK 7 and TTF positive and CK 20 negative, whereas TTF staining is unusual in morphologically similar tumours of other sites. Immunocytochemistry on FNA specimens is a highly effective method of subclassification of tumours[106].

Samples for electron microscopy are gently washed into glutaraldehyde and processed by standard protocols[107–109]. Electron microscopy has particular value in FNA samples from the thorax, because of the variety of lesions encountered[110–115]. Rapid EM processing and reporting enables this technique to be incorporated into day-to-day practice[116]. We find most value in the unequivocal diagnosis of neuroendocrine differentiation, melanoma and mesothelioma, and in subclassification of small round cell tumours, large cell malignancies and pleomorphic spindle cell tumours, particularly when immunocytochemistry has not been helpful.

Other techniques such as evaluating nucleolar organizing regions (AgNORs)[117] or DNA ploidy studies have also been applied to smears and may help in diagnostically difficult cases[118]. Computer assisted screening appears to be highly sensitive in diagnosis[119]. Molecular techniques such as PCR-based enriched single strand conformation polymorphism (E-SSCP) are promising methods of detection which may have an application in screening owing to their ability to detect mutations in small numbers of abnormal cells amongst large populations of non-neoplastic cells[120].

General approach to cytological diagnosis of neoplasia

The cytological appearances of the common lung malignancies vary in different types of specimen. Sputum samples and bronchial washings show similar findings, in particular, the dispersed cell population in keratinizing squamous cell carcinomas, the slightly degenerate shrunken hyperchromatic nuclei of oat cell carcinoma, and the prominence of three-dimensional cell aggregates in adenocarcinoma; washings also contain larger, more disorganized cell groups[121].

Bronchial brushings and FNA samples share similarities and will in general be treated together in the text. Cell aggregation is more often seen. Traumatization of disorganized cell groups may make tumour subtyping more difficult[121]. In brushings, the presence of normal bronchial material provides a useful contrast to neoplastic material, though for small cell carcinoma and carcinoid tumours, traumatized bronchial cells may provide difficulties, rather than help in diagnosis.

Unequivocal cytological diagnosis can occasionally be based on a few cells or cell groups, although as in cytological material in general, diagnosis in respiratory samples is most safely made on abundant well-preserved material. Samples taken by fibreoptic bronchoscopy are best

examined together; we strongly recommend correlation of cytological and histological material before final reports are issued. Such correlation enhances sensitivity of diagnosis, optimizes tumour typing and may prevent confusion if material with different appearances is present in biopsy and cytological samples.

For those approaching fine needle diagnosis for the first time, the full range of possible lesions must be known, as well as the pitfalls. This area is more likely to provide a false positive diagnosis of malignancy because of the wide range of lesions sampled and cell changes observed[122,123]. The 'standard of proof' for histological diagnosis and subtyping of tumours now often includes immunostaining or ultrastructural investigations, and these ancillary techniques must also be available for use on cytological material.

Classification of pulmonary tumours

Table 3.1 is a summary of the most commonly encountered lung neoplasms and tumour-like lesions, and includes an adaptation of the WHO lung tumour classification[124,125]. In the text the common entities are considered in more detail.

Bronchogenic carcinoma
Incidence and importance

In the Western world bronchogenic carcinoma is the leading cause of death from cancer in men and among the leading causes in women[124]. Despite overwhelming evidence accumulated over the last five decades that most cases are caused by tobacco smoking, there has been an increase in incidence of lung cancer throughout the world. Reduced incidence has only been shown in special subgroups such as health workers and in younger age groups accompanying reduced levels of smoking. The effects of smoking in the developing countries have yet to be felt in full.

Although the need for precise cytological and histological diagnosis of lung cancer will be with us for some time, all subtypes of lung cancer continue to have a dismal prognosis. The 5-year survival rate is approximately 6% for squamous cell carcinoma and 2% for small cell carcinoma[124]. Operable tumours constitute only 20% of malignancies and, even in these, survival is only of the order of 20–30% at 5 years. The use of advanced chemotherapy for small cell and non-small cancer has resulted in an increase in survival time with best results in limited stage disease.

Pathogenesis

A current working model for the pathogenesis of lung cancer includes carcinogenic exposure, followed by chromosome deletions and translocations in replicating bronchial epithelial cells, particularly involving chromosome region p3. Clonal abnormalities are presumed to arise by activation of myc and ras family and other oncogenes or deactivation of tumour suppressors such as the retinoblastoma gene (Rb) and p53. These are

Table 3.1 Pulmonary tumours (adapted from WHO Classification[124,125])

Carcinoma of the lung

Squamous cell carcinoma (variants: papillary, clear cell, small cell, basaloid)

Small cell carcinoma (variants: combined with other forms of carcinoma)

Adenocarcinoma
- (a) Acinar adenocarcinoma
- (b) Papillary adenocarcinoma
- (c) Bronchioloalveolar carcinoma (mucinous, non-mucinous or mixed)
- (d) Solid adenocarcinoma with mucin
- (e) Other variants: well-differentiated foetal; mucinous, mucinous cystadenocarcinoma; signet ring cell; clear cell

Large cell carcinoma
- (a) Large cell neuroendocrine carcinoma
- (b) Basaloid
- (c) Lymphoepithelioma-like
- (d) Clear cell
- (e) Rhabdoid phenotype

Carcinomas with pleomorphic, sarcomatoid or sarcomatous elements
- (a) Spindle or giant cell
- (b) Carcinosarcoma
- (c) Pulmonary blastoma

Other primary epithelial neoplasms

Carcinoid tumours
- (a) Typical carcinoid (variants: adenopapillary, clear cell, oncocytic, spindle, melaninogenica)
- (b) Atypical carcinoid

Tumours of seromucinous gland/salivary gland type
- (a) Mucoepidermoid carcinoma
- (b) Adenoid cystic carcinoma
- (c) Acinic cell carcinoma
- (d) Mucous cell adenoma
- (e) Oncocytic adenoma
- (f) Pleomorphic adenoma

Papillary tumours of bronchus/lung
- (a) Juvenile papillomatosis
- (b) Squamous cell papilloma and papillary carcinoma
- (c) Papillary adenoma and adenocarcinoma

Mucinous cystadenoma

Alveolar adenoma

Sclerosing haemangioma/pneumocytoma

Thymoma

Malignant melanoma

Secondary malignancies

Connective tissue neoplasms

Chondroid hamartoma/chondroma

Granular cell tumour

Benign clear cell ('sugar') tumour

Localized fibrous tumour

Inflammatory myofibroblastic tumour

Epithelioid haemangioendothelioma

Primary pulmonary artery sarcoma

Leiomyosarcoma

Malignant fibrous histiocytoma

Neurogenic sarcoma

Rhabdomyosarcoma

Germ cell neoplasms

Teratoma mature/immature

Lymphoproliferative disease

Lymphoid interstitial pneumonia

Nodular lymphoid hyperplasia

Low grade marginal zone B-cell lymphoma of the mucosa-associated lymphoid tissue (MALT)

Lymphomatoid granulomatosis (angiocentric non-Hodgkin's lymphoma)

Other non-Hodgkin's lymphomas

Hodgkin's lymphoma

Plasmacytoma

Histiocytosis X (Langerhan's histiocytosis)

Other localized mass lesions

Amyloid tumour

Hyalinizing granuloma

---

accompanied by the release of autocrine growth factors including abnormal forms of gastrin releasing peptide (GRP; Bombesin), insulin-like growth factor and transferrin-like growth factor, particularly in small cell carcinomas. Acquisition of the invasive or malignant phenotype is associated with a large number of genetic changes including various other oncogene family mutations and chromosome deletions affecting multiple chromosomes[125,126].

Though the sequence of accumulated genetic abnormalities is supported by a large body of molecular biological evidence, the identification of such changes has not yet been profitably applied to diagnosis[126]. Some differences between histological subtypes in terms of the frequency of different molecular abnormalities have been detected[127]. For example squamous cell carcinomas have the highest frequency of p53 mutations, but p53 is also often mutated in small cell and large cell neuroendocrine carcinomas. Rb mutations are seen in only about 15% of

non-small cell carcinomas, but in 80–100% of small cell tumours. The incidence of ras oncogene mutations is very low in small cell cancer, but much higher in non-small cell cancer subtypes, particularly in adenocarcinoma, and mainly in smokers[127]. These differences are insufficiently precise to aid in tumour subtyping. Nevertheless the high frequency of ras and other mutations in non-small cell lung cancer, and the ease of detection in sputum samples using PCR techniques raises the possibility of future screening using molecular techniques[128].

The dysplasia/carcinoma *in situ*/invasive carcinoma sequence for squamous cell carcinoma has been well demonstrated morphologically and epidemiologically, but precursors of large cell carcinoma and small cell carcinoma have not been established. The concept of lung scarring as an aetiopathogenetic factor for adenocarcinoma has come under attack; scars associated with cancers are most likely secondary to the neoplasm[124]. Atypical alveolar hyperplasia is a likely precursor for peripheral adenocarcinomas[124].

Heterogeneity of lung carcinoma

Although subclassification of lung carcinoma follows accepted guidelines[124,125], variable differentiation in different parts of a tumour renders the subtyping of lung lesions by the use of small biopsies or cytological samples prone to some error. Estimates of the proportion of tumours of mixed cell type by light microscopy are up to 40% of all lung carcinomas. In Roggli's series of systematically sectioned resected tumours, 10% of predominantly non-small cell tumours had a component of small cell carcinoma, and 40% of all tumours had a component of some other major subtype[129].

Even further heterogeneity is shown if electron microscopic or immunocytochemical studies are performed. In Dunnill and Gatter's series examined in this way, only 27% of resected tumours were homogeneous in cell type[130]. Adelstein showed a non-small cell component in 10% of small cell tumours in biopsy material[131]. Autopsy studies of patients with small cell carcinoma have shown up to 25% of tumours with large cell, giant cell, squamous cell or carcinoid components, and small numbers showed pure squamous tumours, large cell or adenocarcinoma[132]. Some of this discrepancy may represent the effect of treatment or selective survival of non-small cell elements after therapy; nevertheless, such heterogeneity should be borne in mind when evaluating the accuracy of cytodiagnosis and the degree of concordance of cytological and histological diagnoses based on small amounts of material.

Lung carcinoma subtyping and interobserver agreement

Squamous cell carcinoma has been generally regarded as the most common subtype (30–50%) followed by adenocarcinoma (15–30%), small cell carcinoma (15–30%), and large cell undifferentiated tumours (5–15%) depending on the nature of the series examined[124]. Some changes in prevalence have occurred, e.g. the increase in adenocarcinomas particularly in women smokers in the USA, to the point where adenocarcinoma may now be the most common subtype overall[133], and the increase in squamous and small cell cancer compared to adenocarcinoma in Japan[134]. Changes in types of histological or cytological samples used for diagnosis and in reporting practices for these samples may have been partly responsible.

The main role of the pathologist is to distinguish between small and non-small cell carcinomas, as in general, the former will require chemotherapy, while the latter will be managed surgically or with palliative radiotherapy or different chemotherapy regimes. When adequate material is available for study by experienced pathologists, the consistency of the distinction between small cell and non-small cell types in histological material is in the order of 90%[135]. However, high interobserver agreement for the diagnosis and subclassification of small cell carcinoma has been achieved using current simplified international classifications[136,137]. Interobserver agreement for non-small cell cancers may be less and the variation shown in reported results for cytohistological subtyping should again be assessed against this background.

Staging is the most important prognostic indicator[124]. Subdivision of squamous tumours into well, moderately and poorly differentiated tumours seems to be of prognostic value[138], but there does not appear to be a difference between survival rates for well, moderately or poorly differentiated adenocarcinomas. Among resectable non-small cell tumours, large cell carcinoma may have a worse prognosis.

Subtyping by electron microscopy shows some differences from typing by light microscopy[130,139]; this has no proven biological or clinical significance as a routine practice but allows better subclassification of unusual tumours, and a higher rate of correlation with cytological tumour typing than with histopathology[140,141].

Neuroendocrine differentiation in lung carcinomas

Neuroendocrine lesions of the lung are an area of continuing debate, and the relevance of this differentiation in various histological types of lung carcinoma remains uncertain. The application of new techniques including electron microscopy, immunocytochemistry, cell culture and molecular biology has enhanced our understanding of the interrelationship between these lesions[142–147], but clinical studies of various forms of therapy for them are preliminary. Some have suggested a worse prognosis overall or greater responsiveness to chemotherapy than similar tumours without neuroendocrine features[148] however this issue is controversial[124].

Neuroendocrine differentiation in the form of dense core granules, peptide or amine hormone production and neuroendocrine cytochemical markers such as synaptophysin, chromogranin, gastrin releasing peptide (bombesin) and neural cell adhesion molecules (N-CAM)[149] can be demonstrated in association with a range of lung malignancies. These include small cell carcinoma, atypical carcinoid, carcinoid tumours, large cell neuroendocrine carcinoma and some examples of undifferentiated large cell carcinoma, squamous cell carcinoma and adenocarcinoma[142–147].

A consensus has been reached on the classification of these lesions. The WHO Classification recognizes carcinoid tumours, atypical carcinoids, large cell neuroendocrine carcinoma and small cell carcinoma as separate entities[125]. Studies have shown clear differences in prognosis using criteria easily applied in histological material[150]. However, mitotic rate appears to be the most important criterion and one which is not easily translated to cytological diagnosis. Cytology can usually separate lesions into carcinoid tumours, atypical carcinoids and small cell carcinomas but experience with large cell neuroendocrine tumours is less well documented. There also remains a small group of borderline tumours where a distinction between small cell carcinoma and atypical carcinoid, or small cell carcinoma and large cell neuroendocrine carcinoma is problematical despite adequate material.

Squamous cell carcinoma

This form of lung carcinoma is usually located centrally within the lung in main bronchi or branches and is often associated with bronchial obstruction and secondary pneumonia, or central necrosis and cavitation. Classification depends on the identification of cytoplasmic keratinization or intercellular bridges. Ultrastructurally, bundles of tonofibrils, well-formed desmosomes, concentric layering of tonofibrils around the nucleus and deposition of membrane coated granules are features of squamous differentiation[124].

Cytological findings: sputum and bronchial washings

► Abnormal squamous cells with large or pyknotic hyperchromatic nuclei
► Bizarre cell shapes, abnormal keratinization
► Cell dissociation especially in differentiated tumours
► Tumour diathesis

The cytological diagnosis of squamous cell carcinoma from sputum samples or bronchial washings depends on the identification of abnormal squamous cells with malignant nuclear criteria, including enlargement, dense hyperchromasia, angularity and irregular chromatin distribution or 'black ink' chromatin. Large nucleoli are uncommonly seen, and are not a constant feature within a given group of cells.

Bizarre enlarged cell shapes including spindle and caudate cells, cell engulfment giving rise to 'birds-eye cells', ghost keratinized cell outlines, keratinous debris and a background of necrosis and blood help confirm invasive squamous cell carcinoma (Figs 3.1, 3.2). Intense orange-yellow staining and a refractile appearance of the cytoplasm is a feature of keratinizing tumours (Figs 3.1–3.3); the degree of intensity of staining is characteristic of malignancy and unlike reactive hyperkeratosis.

A dispersed or single cell pattern is usually present in keratinizing tumours, whereas non-keratinizing tumours present in cell groups which are disorganized, often show a spindle morphology and cytoplasmic density with well-defined cell borders. They are less likely to be associated with necrosis.

Cavitating tumours often give rise to purulent sputum containing large amounts of necrotic debris and neutrophils (Fig. 3.4). Malignant cells are 'hyperkeratinised', shrunken, degenerate and include many ghost cells[151]. Diagnostic cells may sometimes be inconspicuous (Fig. 3.4).

In sputum, the diagnosis may occasionally be made on a few cells with sufficiently abnormal nuclei and cytoplasmic

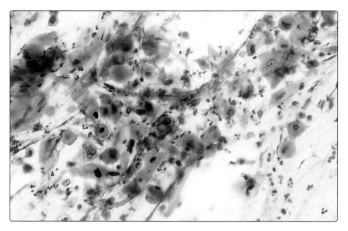

Fig. 3.1 Sputum: keratinizing squamous cell carcinoma. Irregularly shaped keratinizing squamous cells in a background of necrotic debris. (Papanicolaou × HP)

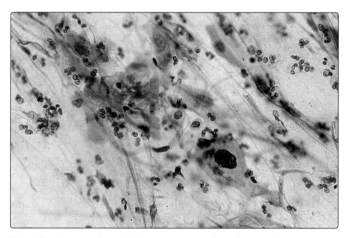

Fig. 3.2 Sputum: keratinizing squamous cell carcinoma. Caudate and fibre cells. (Papanicolaou × HP)

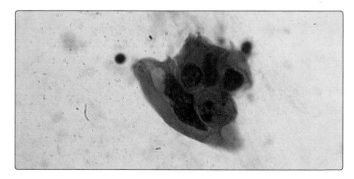

Fig. 3.3 Sputum: keratinizing squamous cell carcinoma. Aggregate of intensely orangeophilic cells with densely hyperchromatic irregular nuclei. Cell engulfment. (Papanicolaou × HP)

shape; however, in this situation we would usually require a consistent clinical background such as a mass on chest X-ray before issuing an unequivocally malignant report. If bizarre cell shapes, ghost cells and keratinous debris are present without intact nuclei, this is also strong evidence of

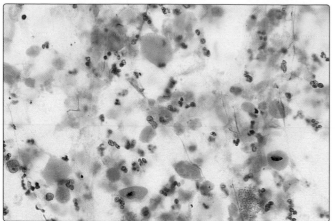

Fig. 3.4   Sputum: Keratinizing squamous cell carcinoma. Abundant necrotic and inflammatory debris and small numbers of keratinized cells, but without definite nuclear criteria of malignancy. (Papanicolaou × MP)

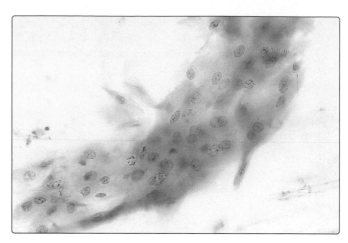

Fig. 3.5   Sputum: upper respiratory tract squamous cells. Cohesive sheet of squamous cells with some nuclear enlargement, but with degenerative features and no significant nuclear irregularity, pleomorphism or hyperchromasia. (Papanicolaou × HP)

carcinoma, although in general it is advisable to recommend that additional samples be taken for identification of malignant nuclear morphology.

Diagnostic pitfalls

Pitfalls in sputum and washings include upper respiratory tract cells with reactive changes, the dysplasia/carcinoma *in situ* sequence, reactive changes due to mycetoma, radiation effect, drug effect, instrumentation or pulmonary embolism and infarction[152], degenerating Herpes virus affected cells, vegetable cells with bizarre morphology and contaminant abnormal cells from oropharyngeal or oesophageal carcinomas. The authors have seen one case of oral pemphigus where some cells in sputum closely mimicked carcinoma.

Upper respiratory tract cells shed from inflammatory lesions or adjacent to ulcers present as small parakeratotic-like aggregates or sheets of eosinophilic or orangeophilic cells with pyknotic nuclei, which show some variation in nuclear size. Cell dispersal may be seen, but a combination of irregular cell shapes and marked nuclear irregularity is not found (Fig. 3.5).

The atypical hyperplasia/dysplasia/carcinoma *in situ* sequence in bronchial epithelium[28–30,153–155] is represented in sputum by a range of cytological appearances. The findings in regular squamous metaplasia are described in Chapter 2. Atypical squamous metaplasia/dysplasia presents as small sheets of squamous cells with nuclear pleomorphism and hyperchromasia, but without the bizarre cell configuration or fully developed nuclear criteria of carcinoma (Fig. 3.6).

Higher grade intraepithelial abnormalities (severe dysplasia) show more advanced nuclear abnormalities and some dispersal. Carcinoma *in situ* tends to present in sputum as single cells, which are rounded, small and with central nuclei showing nuclear atypia including irregular

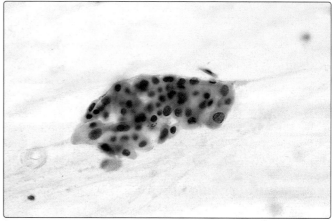

A

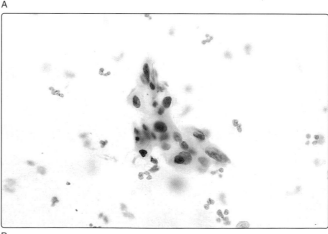

B

Fig. 3.6   (A, B) Sputum: atypical squamous metaplasia. Cohesive aggregates of squamous cells showing nuclear hyperchromasia, enlargement and slight pleomorphism, but without nuclear criteria of malignancy. Clean background. (Papanicolaou × HP)

Subsequent investigation reveals invasive carcinoma in quite a high proportion of patients with cytological changes suggesting severe dysplasia or carcinoma *in situ*[155].

In some centres and as part of screening programmes, clinically and radiologically inapparent *in situ* tumours or early invasive carcinoma have been detected, pursued actively, and localized by sputum cytology, endoscopy and selective brushings, washings and biopsy[158,159]. Extraordinary effort is necessary to detect these lesions in an asymptomatic population and to investigate the bronchial tree exhaustively[158], limiting the value of this approach for screening.

Although 5-year survival may be of the order of 65–90% for small occult carcinomas, the overall survival for screened patients is not significantly better than for non-screened groups[160]. For the authors, the importance of recognizing the morphological features of *in situ* or early cancers has therefore been to separate these cases from obvious invasive carcinoma and not to overdiagnose malignancy. On the few occasions when selective brushings and washings have been performed in our hospital to attempt to localize these lesions detected by sputum, we have been reminded of the need for extreme care in specimen labelling, and the possibilities of cross-contamination of samples.

The changes described above, which suggest premalignancy or *in situ* carcinoma, but occurring in patients without clinical abnormality, may disappear from sputum and may not be followed by the detection or development of carcinoma despite careful bronchoscopic studies over a number of years. This is a further argument in favour of a cautious approach to diagnosis[161]. The natural history of *in situ* bronchogenic carcinoma is uncertain, as is the value of local treatment for these lesions, which are often multifocal. Despite these reservations, regular repeat sputum samples and follow up bronchoscopies have been recommended for patients with cytological findings suggesting severe dysplasia or carcinoma *in situ* in whom initial bronchoscopy reveals no abnormality[156].

Cavities within the lung undergo squamous metaplasia and marked inflammatory changes due to associated infection, including *Aspergillus mycetoma* and tuberculosis[162]. These lesions can on occasions shed spindle-shaped aggregates of atypical metaplastic squamous cells, keratinized cells or reactive cells into sputum, raising the possibility of malignancy. Other infective processes such as blastomycosis and paracoccidioidomycosis[163] have been associated with highly atypical reactive/metaplastic squamous cells.

Chemotherapeutic agents such as bleomycin and busulphan may give rise to cells resembling severe atypical squamous metaplasia or even carcinoma[164,165]. Pulmonary embolism is a recognized cause of atypical reactive squamous cells which may give rise to false positive diagnoses, although few examples are recorded in the

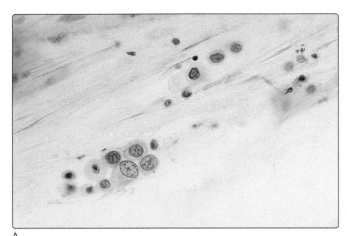

A

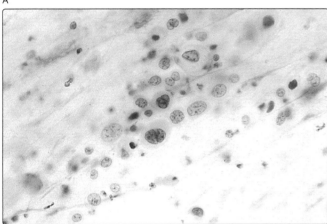

B

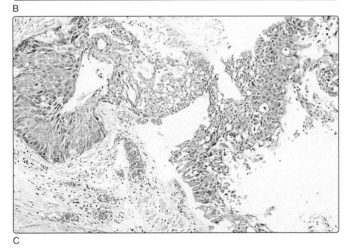

C

Fig. 3.7 Sputum: squamous carcinoma *in situ* pattern. (A, B) Dispersed rounded cells, with some nuclear irregularity and pleomorphism and variable hyperchromasia, but without bizarre cell shapes or a necrotic background. (Papanicolaou × HP) (C) Squamous carcinoma *in situ*; histological section from necropsy. (H&E × LP)

outlines and hyperchromasia, but again without pleomorphic or bizarre cell shapes (Fig. 3.7). This appearance probably also corresponds to early invasive carcinoma and an accurate distinction between these two lesions is not possible[156,157]. Further samples should be collected if this morphological change is encountered.

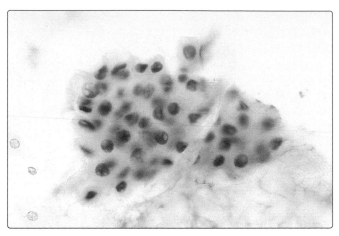

Fig. 3.8 Sputum: vegetable cells resembling abnormal squamous cells. Absence of defined chromatin pattern in nuclei. Cell wall birefringence was observed under polarized light. (Papanicolaou × HP)

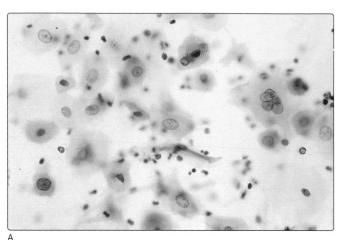

A

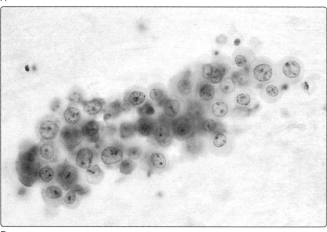

B

Fig. 3.9 Sputum: pemphigus vulgaris. (A) Dispersed orangeophilic cells with some nuclear pleomorphism and hyperchromasia. (B) Loose aggregate of cells of immature type with nuclear enlargement, prominent nucleoli and irregular nuclear membrane, presumably from the base of a regenerating ulcer. (Papanicolaou × HP)

literature; Bewtra *et al.* describe patients with pulmonary embolism in which there were metaplastic squamous cells with marked atypia in sputum and brushings, although the most striking changes were in reactive bronchiolar cells[166]. Instrumentation of the respiratory tract can produce regenerative and degenerative changes resembling squamous cancer[167]. Patients with lung transplants often undergo BAL to detect infectious agents. Opari *et al.* found atypical epithelial cells in nine patients over a 7-year period, associated with diffuse alveolar damage, rejection or infection. There was significant overlap between the cytological findings and those of malignancy.

Vegetable material can usually be recognized by the birefringent structure of the cell wall, but may sometimes provide difficulties (Fig. 3.8)[168]. Radiation effect has similar morphology to that in other sites (see Fig. 3.11).

Cells from oropharyngeal carcinomas or upper oesophageal cancers may shed into sputum. Matsudo *et al.*[169] report a surprisingly high sensitivity (60–70%) of detection of such tumours by sputum cytology; in screening programmes for lung cancer, such lesions may be detected by cytology before being symptomatic. The cells are usually present only in very small numbers and their morphology is usually that of a very well-differentiated tumour. Our experience accords with that of Matsudo, who showed that such cases do not have either the bizarre cell morphology or the abundant cellular material seen in diagnostic sputum samples of bronchogenic carcinoma. Synchronous laryngeal and bronchial tumours also shed cells into sputum[170].

In the single case of oral pemphigus seen by the authors, many abnormal cells were shed into sputum from oral ulcers. The cells presented in loose disorganized aggregates or as single eosinophilic squamous cells, displaying large rounded nuclei, prominent nucleoli, and a high nuclear/cytoplasmic ratio (Fig. 3.9). There was a strong suspicion of carcinoma until the clinical background to the case was realized.

Cytological findings: bronchial brushings and FNA samples

These are similar to sputum findings, although tumour tissue often shows greater aggregation and, in FNA material in particular, tumours often appear less differentiated than in brushings or sputum because of a higher component of deeper non-keratinizing tumour tissue.

Diagnostic pitfalls

In situ carcinoma in bronchial brushings may present as large cohesive aggregates similar to the microbiopsies of cervical intraepithelial neoplasia seen in cervical smears (Fig. 3.10). Where there is monotony of nuclear morphology in large cohesive aggregates, and especially where there may be an anatomical edge to the aggregates, we would add in our reports that an *in situ* lesion could not be excluded and further investigation is necessary for

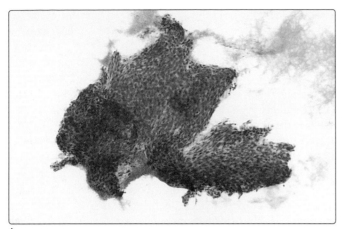

A

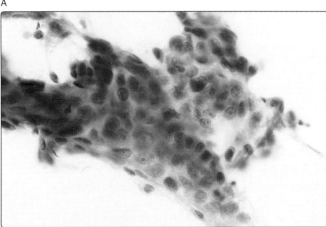

B

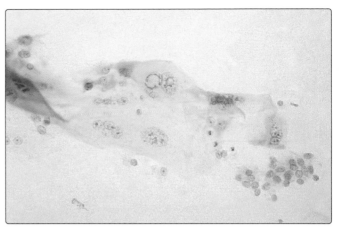

Fig. 3.11 Bronchial brushings: radiotherapy effect. Marked nuclear and cellular enlargement with bizarre multinucleate cells, some showing nuclear vacuoles. (Papanicolaou × MP)

Contamination of transbronchial FNA samples by intraepithelial tumour has been reported; observing lymphocytes in company with tumour cells in mediastinal or transtracheal or transbronchial FNA would help exclude this pitfall[171].

Papillary or polypoid predominantly intraluminal carcinomas may shed squamous cells with malignant morphology into sputum or brushing samples, despite being non-invasive or minimally invasive. These lesions are rarely encountered but may provide particular difficulty in diagnosis in both cytological and small bronchial biopsy samples. They require a combined cytohistological assessment and knowledge of the bronchoscopic and chest radiographic appearances for correct management, which may involve segmental resection rather than pneumonectomy or lobectomy.

In FNA, sources of error include a granulomatous reaction and the acute inflammation and suppuration accompanying central cavitation of tumours. Changes due to radiation (Fig. 3.11) and chemotherapy (Fig. 3.12) in brushings are found particularly in those treated for small cell carcinoma. The cells produced may be large with irregular nuclei, prominent nucleoli and abundant dense cytoplasm. They may not show any degenerative features and may have alarming nuclear morphology; however, the clinical background, prominence of multinucleation, low nuclear/cytoplasmic ratio, lack of hyperchromasia and the scattered nature of the cells amongst normal bronchial cells helps exclude squamous or other large cell carcinoma.

Epithelial repair, having essentially similar morphology to that seen in cervical smears, is occasionally seen in brushings samples, particularly in patients who undergo multiple endoscopic procedures[172]. Large cohesive sheets of cells with enlarged nuclei and prominent nucleoli, absence of dispersed abnormal cells and correlation with biopsy findings have been helpful in diagnosis (Fig. 3.13 and see Fig. 3.30).

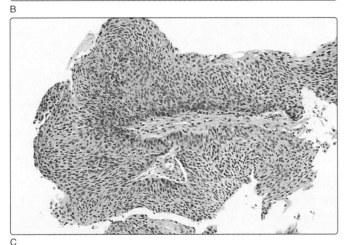

C

Fig. 3.10 Bronchial brushings: squamous cell carcinoma *in situ*. (A) Large cohesive aggregate of hyperchromatic cells. (Papanicolaou × LP) (B) Disorganized but cohesive aggregate of squamous cells with nuclear enlargement, hyperchromasia and cyanophilic cytoplasm. (Papanicolaou × HP) (C) Bronchial biopsy: histological section showing *in situ* carcinoma only. (H&E × MP)

diagnosis. We have also seen a few cases of brushings of *in situ* or early invasive lesions where a population of dispersed rounded squamous cells without marked pleomorphism was present in smears, similar to their presentation in sputum.

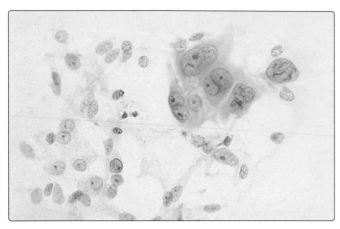

Fig. 3.12 Bronchial brushings: chemotherapy effect. Small sheet of enlarged binucleate cells. Nuclei lack hyperchromasia. Cellular changes following chemotherapy for small cell carcinoma; check bronchoscopy (Papanicolaou × HP)

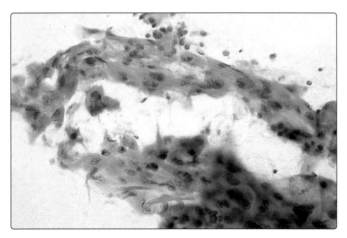

Fig. 3.13 Bronchial brushings: epithelial repair. Cohesive monolayered sheet of cells. Some nuclear enlargement and irregularity but uniform chromatin pattern. No free cells. Changes observed in a repeat bronchoscopy specimen. (Papanicolaou × HP)

Necrosis in other large cell carcinomas simulates keratinization[44,173] particularly in H&E preparations and more often in FNA samples; Papanicolaou staining is better at separating necrosis from the orangeophilia of keratin. In FNA samples there is a tendency to view cytoplasmic density or a sheet-like growth in other large cell carcinomas as an indicator of squamous differentiation, and this is a cause of mistyping. Rare tumours may have a pseudovascular or pseudoglandular growth[174].

Small cell carcinoma

This tumour is usually central or hilar in position, grows rapidly, disseminates widely and has a very poor overall prognosis. Chemotherapy improves survival time and produces some long-term survivors. Small stage I tumours are only rarely detected cytologically[175] or histologically, and the only accepted place for surgery is for small peripheral tumours. Associated paraneoplastic syndromes such as the Eaton-Lambert myasthenic syndrome and syndromes produced by peptide hormone secretion such as ADH and ACTH are well described.

The new WHO classification[125] has abandoned a subdivision into tumours of oat cell type, where tumour cells are shrunken and more poorly preserved, and tumours of intermediate type, with slightly more cytoplasm and larger better preserved nuclei. In well-preserved tissue the oat cell subgroup vanishes suggesting that this subtype is an artefact of poor preservation[176]. Experts fail to separate 'oat cell' from 'intermediate' tumours reliably[177]. The term used for tumours with a mixture of cell types is 'combined' carcinoma including areas of any other non-small cell morphology including large cell neuroendocrine carcinoma. These constitute up to 10% of small cell tumours[131]. All appear to behave in a similar aggressive fashion; the mixed small and large cell group has not been shown to have separate clinical significance[128].

Ultrastructurally, most small cell carcinomas show a few intracytoplasmic dense core neurosecretory granules concentrated in small cytoplasmic processes, but these may be lacking in some tumours of classical appearance and in the small cell/large cell tumours. If neuroendocrine granules are not seen by electron microscopy in a tumour where there is diagnostic difficulty, and there is ultrastructural evidence of glandular or squamous differentiation, this would place a diagnosis of small cell carcinoma in some doubt. However, some small cell tumours, which behave aggressively, may show variable combinations of squamous, glandular or neuroendocrine differentiation ultrastructurally.

Chromogranin A and synaptophysin are neuroendocrine markers, which are demonstrable in the cytoplasm of small cell carcinomas. Paranuclear dot-like positivity for keratin is also commonly seen in tumour cells. Tome *et al.*[178] suggested that antibodies NCC-LU243 and NCC-LU246 against cluster 1 antigen/N-CAM stained virtually all cells of small cell carcinoma in various types of preparations, and with a strong membrane staining pattern; non-small cell tumours showed only focal non-specific cytoplasmic staining.

Some other antibodies, including those to CD44[179], preferentially react with non-small cell tumours[180,181].

Cytological findings: sputum and bronchial washings

► Elongated groupings of small dissociating tumour cells
► Scant cytoplasm, irregular moulded nuclei
► Coarsely stippled chromatin, inconspicuous nucleoli
► Degenerative changes common

In sputum this tumour usually presents in small rounded or elongated aggregates within streaks of mucus. The aggregates are generally loosely arranged with a complement of dissociated cells. The tumour cells are small

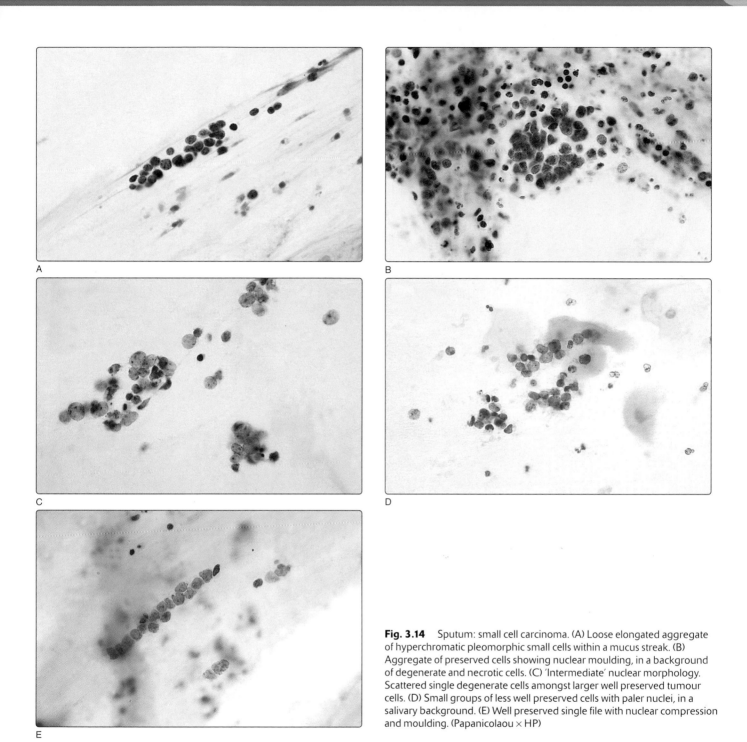

Fig. 3.14   Sputum: small cell carcinoma. (A) Loose elongated aggregate of hyperchromatic pleomorphic small cells within a mucus streak. (B) Aggregate of preserved cells showing nuclear moulding, in a background of degenerate and necrotic cells. (C) 'Intermediate' nuclear morphology. Scattered single degenerate cells amongst larger well preserved tumour cells. (D) Small groups of less well preserved cells with paler nuclei, in a salivary background. (E) Well preserved single file with nuclear compression and moulding. (Papanicolaou × HP)

to medium sized with minimal cytoplasm and demonstrate nuclear pleomorphism within the aggregates, together with nuclear moulding and irregularity of nuclear outline. Nucleoli are inconspicuous. A uniformly hyperchromatic nucleus with a flat or stippled chromatin pattern is most commonly seen; distinct nuclear membranes are not a feature (Figs 3.14, 3.15).

Although cells are only 2–3 times lymphocyte size in most cases, they may be larger if better preserved and may then have a more open chromatin pattern and more easily visible nucleoli; large nucleoli would suggest some other primary or secondary carcinoma. Degenerative change may also contribute to loss of chromatin pattern and often the nuclei are pale-staining with haematoxylin. Nuclear pyknosis may render assessment difficult. Mitotic figures are seldom found in sputum samples; however, single cell necrosis within aggregates and abundant apoptotic cell breakdown all indicate a high mitotic rate and cell turnover.

The close apposition of tumour cells in a rapidly growing tumour with minimal cytoplasm and fragile nuclei leads to

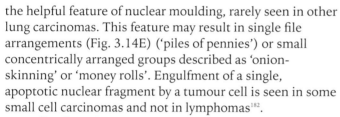

Fig. 3.15   Sputum: small cell carcinoma. Aggregate of tumour cells showing uniform nuclear hyperchromasia, pleomorphism and irregularity of nuclear outline, inconspicuous nucleoli and nuclear moulding. Nuclear membranes are ill-defined. (Papanicolaou × OI)

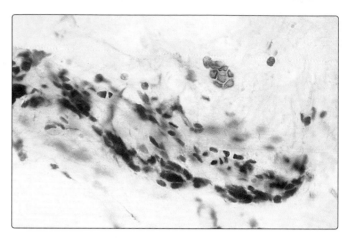

Fig. 3.16   Sputum: degenerate bronchial epithelium. Streaks of traumatized, poorly preserved epithelial cells. One group of cells showing cell moulding but with retained cytoplasm between nuclei. (Papanicolaou × HP)

the helpful feature of nuclear moulding, rarely seen in other lung carcinomas. This feature may result in single file arrangements (Fig. 3.14E) ('piles of pennies') or small concentrically arranged groups described as 'onion-skinning' or 'money rolls'. Engulfment of a single, apoptotic nuclear fragment by a tumour cell is seen in some small cell carcinomas and not in lymphomas[182].

Small cell carcinomas are commonly accompanied by considerable necrosis; however, the background may be entirely clean and we have seen diagnostic material in paucicellular mucoid or salivary samples with no necrosis or accompanying inflammation.

Definitive diagnosis rests on finding a number of well preserved aggregates; a diagnosis should not be made on poorly preserved material or one or two abnormal cells alone.

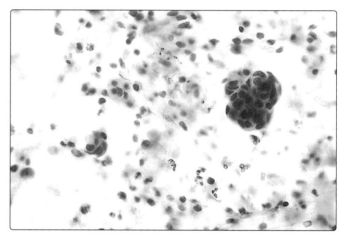

Fig. 3.17   Sputum: post-bronchoscopy changes. Several aggregates of bronchial epithelial cells demonstrating cellular moulding, but with retained cytoplasm between nuclei. (Papanicolaou × HP)

Diagnostic pitfalls

The most common difficulties in diagnosis in sputum arise from degenerate bronchial cells, and in the distinction between small and non-small cell tumours of primary and metastatic origin[183]. Reactive lymphocytes are said to provide diagnostic difficulties but this is rare in our experience; poorly preserved cells from lymphoma may give problems. Inspissated mucus may, on occasion, mimic degenerate aggregates of small cell carcinoma cells.

Degenerate bronchial epithelial cells can generally be easily distinguished from small cell carcinoma (Fig. 3.16). They show a similar degree of degenerative change from nucleus to nucleus within the cluster, with no well-preserved cells among the clusters; a mixture of preserved and degenerate cells within a cluster is more a feature of small cell carcinoma.

Regenerating bronchial cells generally show little pleomorphism, and although they do show moulding, this

usually occurs with a distinct intact rim of cytoplasm rather than the nucleus to nucleus moulding often seen in small cell carcinoma (Fig. 3.17). Observing adjacent, better preserved bronchial cells or a range of degenerative change within an area of the smear is most helpful in diagnosis.

Metastatic breast carcinoma (Fig. 3.18), prostatic carcinoma, and small celled squamous carcinomas may provide difficulties in differential diagnosis. The abundant cytoplasm usually seen in these tumours will generally be the best guide to excluding small cell cancer. More pronounced three-dimensional clustering, cohesion and prominent nucleoli are features unlike small cell carcinoma and more indicative of adenocarcinoma, either primary or secondary.

Malignant lymphoma is occasionally very difficult to distinguish from small cell carcinoma (see Fig. 3.66C); small cell carcinomas may occasionally be very dispersed and lymphomas may show apparent grouping of cells due to

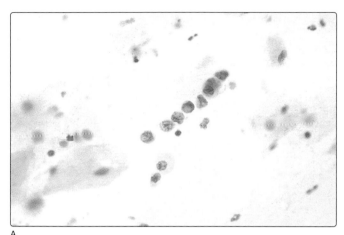

A

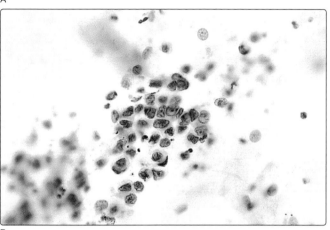

B

Fig. 3.18   Sputum: metastatic breast carcinoma. (A) Single file structure of small cells closely mimicking small cell carcinoma. (B) Loose aggregate of cells showing several engulfed cells. (Papanicolaou × HP)

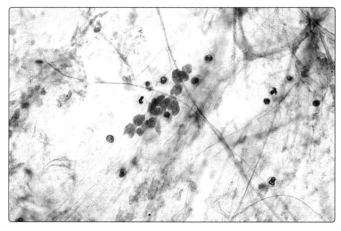

Fig. 3.19   Sputum: aggregate of acellular material, possibly mucus. Resemblance to degenerate nuclei of small cell carcinoma. No chromatin pattern is evident. (Papanicolaou × HP)

artefact. Cell engulfment or engulfment of an apoptotic body and nuclear moulding is not seen in lymphoma[182].

One interesting non-cellular mimic of small cell carcinoma is inspissated mucus or debris (Fig. 3.19) which can collect to form moulded aggregates reminiscent of carcinoma although without any 'nuclear' structure. Limiting diagnosis to well preserved material will prevent error.

We have not seen carcinoid tumours exfoliating into sputum, although others mention this as a problem in differential diagnosis; we have not recognized reserve cells or reserve cell hyperplasia, although these may also, on occasion, resemble small cell carcinoma[52].

Cytological findings: bronchial brushings and FNA samples

► Better preserved larger cells than in sputum
► Some nuclear moulding and cell clustering present
► Open chromatin pattern
► Nucleoli visible
► Artefactually crushed cells and nuclei

In brushings (Fig. 3.20) and FNA samples (Fig. 3.21) the better preservation of cells leads to larger nuclei, sometimes more evident cytoplasm albeit never abundant, a more open chromatin network and more easily visible small nucleoli. Streaks of nuclear material, smeared cells, and tear-drop cells emphasize the fragility of nuclei. The fine strands of haematoxyphilic material extending from nuclei are a characteristic traumatization artefact rarely seen in other types of malignancy[184]. Some cell clustering is usually maintained and moulding may be seen, less commonly than in sputum.

The so-called intermediate variant of small cell carcinoma is an 'artefact of good preservation' and one not seen in sputum samples. Well-preserved material in FNA and brushing samples presents in this form and may show definitely larger nuclei than in sputum (Fig. 3.22). Although subdivisions into oat cell and intermediate categories are neither reproducible nor biologically significant, we retain this category in our teaching. We find this particularly useful for FNA reporting, where there is a tendency to assign some tumours to the non-small cell category unless the considerably larger size of well-preserved small cells is not kept in mind.

Diagnostic pitfalls

In FNA and bronchial brushing samples, a distinction between 'intermediate' small cell carcinoma and other poorly differentiated tumours, particularly large cell carcinoma, small celled or basaloid squamous carcinomas (Fig. 3.23) and secondary tumours, e.g. from breast, are among the most common diagnostic problems.

Critical attention to nuclear morphology is valuable. If there are uniformly hyperchromatic nuclei with granular chromatin, inconspicuous nucleoli and minimal or no cytoplasm, the neoplasm will generally fall into the small cell group histologically; whereas vesicular nuclei and

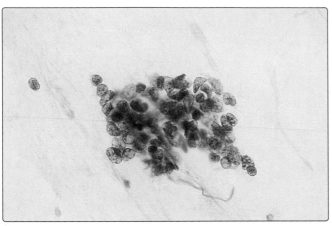

A

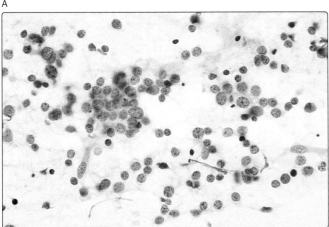

B

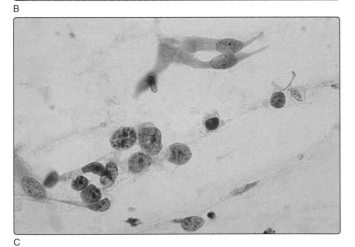

C

Fig. 3.20 Bronchial brushings: small cell carcinoma. (A) Clusters of small cells with granular, stippled nuclear chromatin; nuclear moulding, absent cytoplasm. (Papanicolaou × HP) (B) More dispersed pattern with numerous single bare nuclei, but showing considerable nuclear pleomorphism. (Papanicolaou × HP) (C) Granular stippled chromatin pattern, micronucleoli, nuclear moulding and minimal cytoplasm. Compare with single bronchial cells. (Papanicolaou × OI)

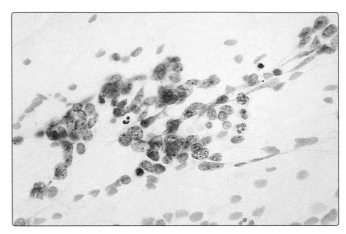

Fig. 3.21 FNA: small cell carcinoma. Traumatized nuclear fragments. Uniform stippled hyperchromatic nuclear chromatin pattern. Minimal cytoplasm. (Papanicolaou × HP)

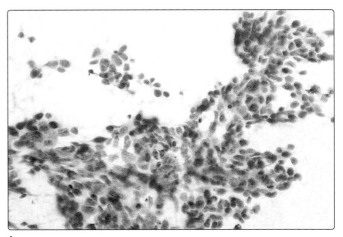

A

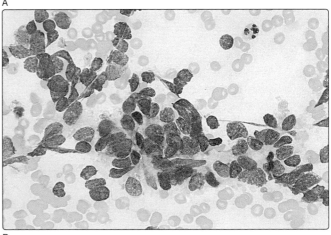

B

Fig. 3.22 FNA: small cell carcinoma, 'intermediate' morphology. Larger, better preserved nuclei than usually seen in sputum and more cohesive aggregates. (A, H&E × MP; B, MGG × HP)

prominent nucleoli, together with well-marked nuclear membranes are generally evidence of non-small cell type. There are exceptions to this, small celled squamous carcinomas providing particular difficulty. Marked cell cohesion is a feature more often seen in squamous cell carcinomas.

Electron microscopy demonstrating neuroendocrine differentiation is helpful in problematic cases. It is

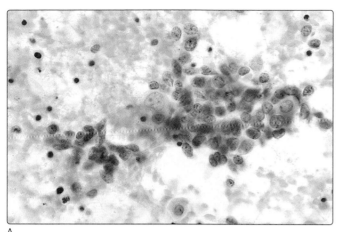

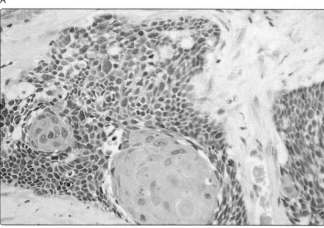

Fig. 3.23   Bronchial brushings: small celled squamous carcinoma.
(A) Loose aggregates of small cells, but including some with cyanophilic
cytoplasm and vesicular nuclei with easily visible nucleoli. Some single cells
with intact cytoplasm. These findings would enable a diagnosis of
carcinoma, but do not permit definite tumour typing. Small cell carcinoma
or a variant is difficult to exclude. (Papanicolaou × HP) (B) Bronchial biopsy:
Squamous cell carcinoma with small celled and larger celled areas.
(H&E × HP)

suggested that nucleolar organizing region (AgNOR)
counts showing few nuclear granules indicate small cell
carcinoma; poorly differentiated non-small cell tumours
have high counts with granules arranged in loose clusters[117].

Combined tumours with components of small cell and
squamous cell or glandular carcinoma are occasionally
diagnosed by cytology[185]; Zaharopoulos et al.[186] discuss the
cytology of small cell variants in detail. This is, however, a
rare finding in routine cytological material; Stuart-Harris et
al.[136] describe less than 2% of such tumours in routine
diagnostic material from small cell cancers. We have seen a
few cases of small cell carcinoma in brushings where an
accompanying component of atypical but not overtly
malignant squamous cells had arisen from overlying
intraepithelial change rather than representing evidence of
a combined tumour.

Mixed small and large cell carcinomas are diagnosed with
less frequency in cytological or endoscopic biopsy samples

than autopsy studies[131,137]. In FNA sampling, a few large cells
are quite commonly seen in association with an otherwise
typical small cell pattern and these do not alter the
diagnosis; however, the presence of aggregates of larger
cells with prominent nucleoli should lead to some caution.
Yang et al. suggested that a mixed morphology could result
from degenerative changes[187].

Cytological material from small celled areas of squamous
carcinoma or basaloid carcinoma (Fig. 3.23) may closely
mimic small cell anaplastic carcinoma[188,189]. If we see
mixtures of cell types we generally request further cytology
for ancillary studies, biopsy or electron microscopic
confirmation of tumour type.

In FNA material the distinction between small cell
carcinoma and atypical carcinoid and large cell
neuroendocrine carcinoma can be difficult (see Fig. 3.50).
A morphological spectrum of neuroendocrine malignancy
from typical carcinoid through to small cell carcinoma is
well recognized, even though on epidemiological grounds
small cell carcinoma constitutes an entirely separate
clinicopathological subgroup. Peripheral growth or small
size and clinical stage I tumours, or those in non-smokers,
should be diagnosed on cytology as small cell carcinoma
with care because at least some of these may be termed
atypical carcinoids at resection or benefit from resection
rather than chemotherapy.

Follicle centre cell lymphomas with pronounced cell
pleomorphism, nuclear irregularity and some cell
aggregation may resemble small cell carcinoma in FNA
samples. Dispersed cells of small cell carcinoma usually do
not maintain cytoplasm whereas lymphoma cells usually
do. Lymphoglandular bodies in the background in MGG
preparations suggest lymphoma and help to exclude
carcinoma.

In brushings samples a mixture with bronchial
epithelium may provide difficulties as small numbers of
tumour cells may be obscured by traumatized bronchial
epithelium. In addition, traumatized bronchial epithelial
cells stripped of cytoplasm may artefactually aggregate and
simulate carcinoma. Such cases require study either to trace
a continuum between benign, well preserved cells and
traumatized cells in benign cases, or to demonstrate an
unequivocal contrast between neoplastic and non-
neoplastic epithelium in malignant cases.

Marchevsky et al. describe cells from a pulmonary
tumorlet in a brushings sample which resembled small cell
carcinoma[190].

Adenocarcinoma – bronchogenic

These tumours, defined histologically by the formation of
acinar or papillary structures, or mucin secretion, tend to
occur more peripherally within the lung than squamous cell
or small cell tumours. Adenocarcinomas are
ultrastructurally very variable. Some contain cells
resembling Clara cells or type II pneumocytes or non-

specific secretory cells; ultrastructural evidence of squamous or neuroendocrine differentiation may also be seen[124].

Secretory products vary in appearance and include intracytoplasmic mucin granules, intracytoplasmic lumina or intracellular lumens containing mucus; surface morphology includes microvilli covered by fibrillar glycocalyx and junctional complexes. There are no specific light microscopic features to prove that a tumour is a primary lesion. A diagnosis of primary lung adenocarcinoma therefore requires clinicopathological correlation and reasonable efforts towards exclusion of tumours at other sites. Immunocytochemistry for thyroid transcription factor, cytokeratin subsets (CK 7 and 20) and other markers can help exclude metastases[103–105]. The demonstration of oncogenic HPV types by PCR or other hybridization technique can help prove a metastasis from cervix.

Cytological findings: sputum and bronchial washings

▶ Cell aggregates are a characteristic feature
▶ Large eccentric pleomorphic nuclei
▶ Prominent nucleoli
▶ Abundant pale or vacuolated cytoplasm

In sputum, the hallmark of the presentation of adenocarcinoma is the cell aggregate. Cells are shed in flattened or three-dimensional clusters with enlarged eccentric nuclei showing moderate nuclear pleomorphism, irregular but well defined nuclear membranes, nuclear hyperchromasia or hypochromasia and abundant pale or lacy cytoplasm which may be vacuolated (Fig. 3.24). Many cells demonstrate prominent rounded central nucleoli.

In poorly differentiated forms, the cell clusters are more irregular and disorganized, and a higher nuclear/cytoplasmic ratio is often seen (Fig. 3.25). Some tumours present with a largely dispersed pattern (Fig. 3.26); cell dispersal may be particularly pronounced in poorly differentiated tumours undergoing necrosis. Distortion of nuclei by large vacuoles may cause indentation of the nucleus, whereas in other cases cytoplasmic vacuolation may be fine. Papillary fragments or true acinar structures with central lumina may be seen.

Hyperchromasia and chromatin abnormalities are less valuable in establishing a diagnosis of malignancy in adenocarcinoma than in other lung carcinomas. Marked nuclear enlargement, anisocytosis within a cluster and nuclear irregularity and folding are the most important malignant nuclear criteria for this neoplasm.

Diagnostic pitfalls

Shed bronchial epithelial aggregates, particularly from asthmatic patients, were historically a pitfall in diagnosis.

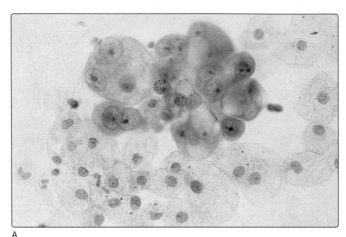

A

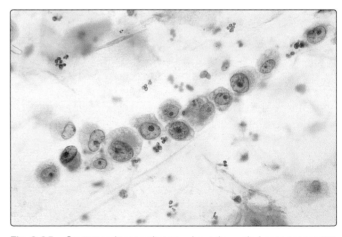

B

Fig. 3.24   Sputum: adenocarcinoma – bronchogenic. (A, B) Aggregate of malignant glandular cells with marked nuclear enlargement, vesicular nuclear chromatin pattern, prominent nucleoli and some nuclear irregularity. Variable cytoplasmic vacuolation. (Papanicolaou × HP)

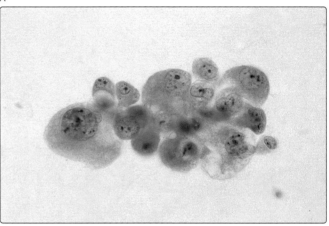

Fig. 3.25   Sputum: adenocarcinoma – bronchogenic. Loose aggregates but showing eccentric nuclei within pale cytoplasm. (Papanicolaou × HP)

Early detailed studies of this problem[191] delineated criteria for distinguishing this material from adenocarcinoma. The ciliated cell surface of larger fragments, as well as the presence of an anatomical or polarized edge with palisaded cells, and a terminal bar are diagnostic features of benign

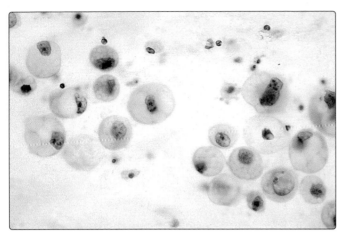

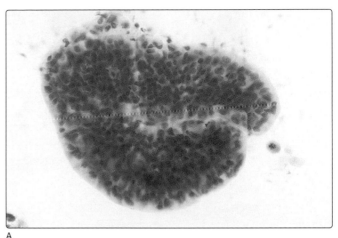

A

Fig. 3.26 Sputum: adenocarcinoma – bronchogenic. Dispersed cell pattern; eccentric nuclei; vacuolated cytoplasm resembling macrophage cytoplasm, but with unequivocal nuclear features of malignancy. (Papanicolaou × HP)

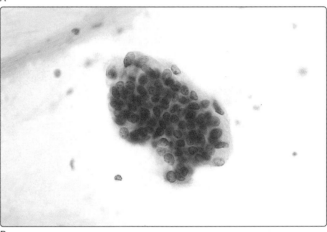

B

Fig. 3.27 Sputum: reactive/shed bronchial epithelium. Post bronchoscopy changes. (A) Large fragment of bronchial epithelium with an 'anatomical edge'. (Papanicolaou × MP) (B) More disorganized fragment of bronchial epithelium with a suggestion of an anatomical border, without obvious cilia but with some apical mucin. (Papanicolaou × HP)

clusters which are generally not seen in adenocarcinoma (Fig. 3.27). A background of eosinophils and eosinophilic debris is a useful warning sign indicating allergic bronchial disease. Fragments or groups of reactive bronchiolar or bronchial epithelium as a result of pneumonitis, bronchiolitis or pulmonary infarction[152,166], may also have markedly atypical nuclear features (Fig. 3.28).

A risk of false positive diagnosis as a result of type II pneumocyte hyperplasia or bronchiolar cell hyperplasia occurs in fibrosing alveolitis[192] and diffuse alveolar damage (adult respiratory distress syndrome, ARDS). Similarly, patients receiving oxygen therapy in association with infection, e.g. in AIDS related infections, may shed abnormal cells resembling adenocarcinoma[193], particularly in BAL samples[194] where the numbers of such cells may be higher due to the sampling process (see Fig.3.37). These groups of atypical cells may also be found in sputum but usually in small numbers. The clinical background, where there is usually no suspicion of lung carcinoma, is often helpful in preventing misdiagnosis.

Cytological findings: bronchial brushings and FNA samples

▶ Sheets, rosettes and acinar groupings, columnar cells and mucin production suggest adenocarcinoma
▶ Rounded nuclei, prominent nucleoli
▶ Clean or mucinous background

In brushings or FNA samples monolayered sheets, columnar cells or evidence of mucin secretion are valuable criteria in confirming glandular differentiation (Fig. 3.29). Rosettes or acinar structures may be seen. Material is, however, more likely to occur in disorganized aggregates, and rounded or three-dimensional cell aggregates are less often a feature. A combination of rounded nuclei with large

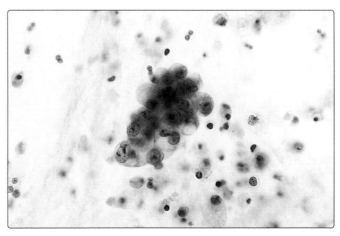

Fig. 3.28 Sputum: reactive bronchiolar cells. Three-dimensional glandular cell clusters with considerable anisokaryosis and prominent nucleoli. Young male with pneumonia. Resolution of all symptoms while in hospital and well on follow-up. (Papanicolaou × HP)

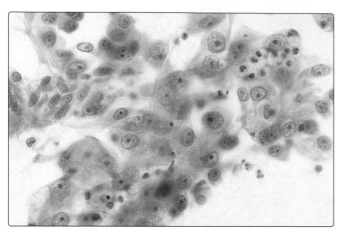

Fig. 3.29   Bronchial brushings: adenocarcinoma. Sheet of adenocarcinoma cells contrasting with adjacent small clusters of bronchial epithelial cells. Uniform nuclear morphology with prominent cell membranes, vesicular nuclei, large nucleoli and abundant pale cytoplasm, together with some columnar cell forms, indicating glandular differentiation. (Papanicolaou × HP)

central nucleoli seen in most cells within a cell aggregate which demonstrates pale, fragile cytoplasm, is most likely to indicate adenocarcinoma though some large cell carcinomas may present in this way. The smear background is generally clean. There may be a macrophage reaction and some cell debris particularly in mucinous tumours, but necrosis is generally not a feature, particularly in the better-differentiated adenocarcinomas.

Diagnostic pitfalls

Reactive or reparative changes in bronchiolar epithelium may resemble adenocarcinoma (Fig. 3.30).

Pseudoglandular growth pattern in squamous carcinomas can mimic adenocarcinoma or vascular tumours[174].

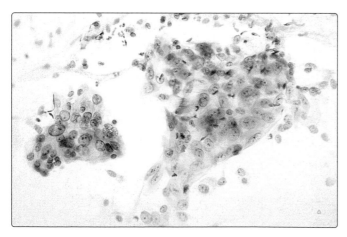

Fig. 3.30   Bronchial brushings: reactive changes, post-bronchoscopy. Monolayered sheet of epithelial repair together with an aggregate of regenerating bronchial cells with some variation in nuclear size. (Papanicolaou × HP)

Rare adenocarcinoma variants such as mucinous cystadenocarcinoma have been studied in FNA samples[195].

Adenocarcinoma – bronchioloalveolar (BAC)

These lesions are peripheral tumours, rare in pure form but common as mixtures with other patterns of histological growth including papillary and more solid forms. Several clinicopathological subtypes exist including localized or solitary lesions, those with a more diffuse spreading growth, and those with multiple foci of tumour possibly indicating either multifocal origin or aerogenous spread.

Histologically, this pattern of growth can be mimicked by metastatic tumour of various sites although this is uncommonly a clinical problem. Tumours of non-secretory, mucinous and pleomorphic type have been identified histologically; ultrastructurally the cells may show features in common with bronchial epithelial cells, mucin secreting cells, Clara cells, type II pneumocytes or combinations of these[124].

Cytological findings: sputum and bronchial washings[196–202]

▶ Numerous small glandular clusters
▶ Regular small cells with ample cytoplasm
▶ Some nuclear hyperchromasia or vesicular nuclei with prominent nucleoli
▶ Clean mucoid background

In sputum this diagnosis is relatively easy if many, small three-dimensional glandular cell clusters of varying size are present throughout a smear, despite the component cells being rather small and regular (Figs 3.31, 3.33). The malignant cells usually have abundant cytoplasm, particularly in the mucinous or secretory type, and even though the nuclei may appear relatively uniform, critical evaluation often shows either hyperchromatic nuclei with some nuclear irregularity or more vesicular nuclei and prominent central nucleoli.

Our approach to this diagnosis in sputum is to identify clusters of glandular cells as of bronchiolar type, then to assess the numbers and size of clusters, and finally, the morphology of individual cells within the clusters. An assessment of the number of clusters is important as the likelihood of carcinoma increases with the amount of material present. The nuclear morphology of these tumours is often bland and an individual cluster indistinguishable from reactive bronchiolar cells. The size of the clusters is also important. A large number of cells within individual clusters is more likely to occur in malignancy than in a reactive bronchiolar proliferation.

We have not found cytoplasmic vacuoles compressing and distorting the nucleus to be a useful malignant criterion; this feature may be seen in benign or malignant bronchiolar clusters. A clean or mucoid background is common. If a prominent inflammatory background is present, caution is

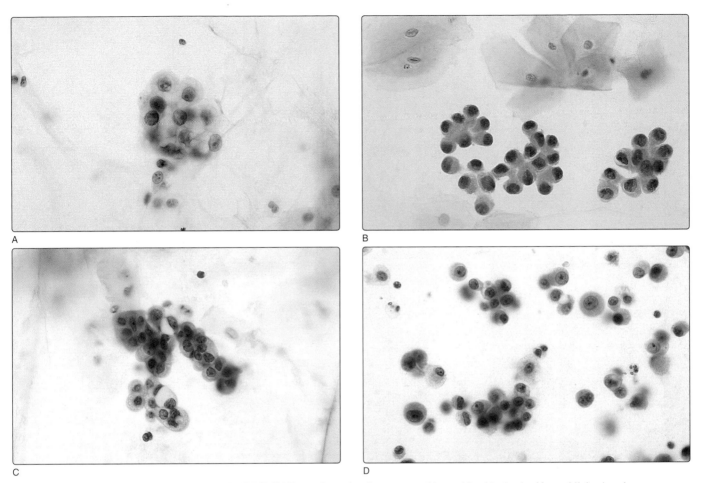

Fig. 3.31   Adenocarcinoma – bronchioloalveolar (BAC). (A) Three-dimensional aggregate with considerable depth of focus. Minimal nuclear pleomorphism or enlargement. Abundant pale vacuolated cytoplasm. This individual cluster is difficult to distinguish from a reactive bronchiolar cell aggregate. (B, C) Multiple aggregates with more variation in cytoplasmic density. (D) Dispersed cell pattern with some cells resembling macrophages. (Papanicolaou × HP)

appropriate although it is worth noting that prominent neutrophil ingestion by tumour cells may occasionally be seen in a clean background, a phenomenon linked to granulocyte stimulating factor production by the tumour cells[203].

Other patterns of cytological presentation are described with this tumour, including a single cell presentation (Fig. 3.31D) closely resembling a macrophage reaction and dispersal associated with degeneration. More pleomorphic forms may shed cells indistinguishable from adenocarcinoma of bronchogenic type or large cell anaplastic carcinoma (see Fig. 3.36). Some tumours are associated with psammoma bodies[200,204].

Diagnostic pitfalls

This neoplasm may be particularly difficult to diagnose if there is minimal material. In sputum, three-dimensional aggregates of reactive bronchiolar cells as a result of pneumonia, tuberculosis, infarction, bronchiolitis,

bronchitis or conditions such as interstitial lung disease are an important differential diagnostic problem, as described in Chapter 2. A few small groups of atypical bronchiolar type epithelial cells should never be used as the basis for a malignant diagnosis. The clinical background to the case may provide important additional information; some of the most atypical reactive bronchiolar cells we have observed were in a very young patient with pneumonia in whom there was no clinical suspicion of malignancy (Fig. 3.32).

In diagnostically difficult cases, multiple sputum samples may eventually allow a diagnosis to be reached although with some cases we cannot be unequivocal in reporting and rely on clinical progression of disease to help establish the diagnosis. This procedure is recommended by other authors[177]. Reactive bronchiolar proliferation will usually resolve within 2–3 weeks and persistence of such abnormal cells for more than a month or so would argue strongly in favour of neoplasia. In the series of atypical bronchiolar cells associated with pulmonary emboli reported by Bewtra et al.[146], the cells were shed in the second and third weeks after infarction but then resolved.

Fig. 3.32 Sputum: markedly atypical reactive bronchiolar cells. (Same case as **Fig. 3.28**.) There would be a risk of false positive diagnosis of malignancy without the clinical information in this case. (Papanicolaou × HP)

Tumours with a single cell presentation may be extremely difficult to recognize and distinguish from, e.g. a macrophage reaction. Degenerating benign cells may show nuclear irregularity, and diagnosis should be based on well-preserved material[201]. Single cell degeneration imparts a somewhat squamous appearance to the cells; though widespread necrosis is not a feature of this tumour and, if present in an adenocarcinoma, would argue for metastatic rather than primary carcinoma.

Metastatic tumours such as breast and prostatic carcinoma shed small aggregates of cells with similar appearance to the ones described; tight cellular moulding in three-dimensional aggregates would be more in favour of secondary breast carcinoma.

In those patients with diffuse alveolar damage (adult respiratory distress syndrome), BAL samples can contain numerous reactive glandular cell aggregates with morphological features suggesting adenocarcinoma. In the study by Grotte *et al.*[194], the cells were shown by electron microscopy to be highly reactive type II pneumocytes; Linder also alludes to the many reactive bronchiolar cells seen in BAL compared with sputum[54].

Cytological findings: bronchial brushings and FNA samples[198,202,205–209]

▶ Best recognized in FNA samples
▶ Cellular aspirate, monotonous cell population
▶ Arrangements in cell balls, sheets and papillae
▶ Intranuclear cytoplasmic inclusions

In bronchial brushings, this diagnosis is not often made but we have seen examples in BAL specimens (Fig. 3.33); this method may be particularly useful for diagnosis of this type of tumour because of its peripheral location. In FNA samples the material is usually diagnostic. Abundant material including monolayered sheets[209], small three-dimensional cell balls resembling those seen in sputum, and papillae

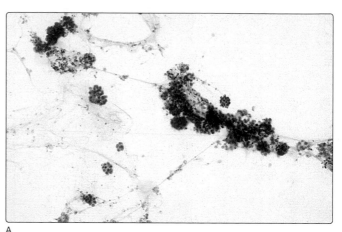

A

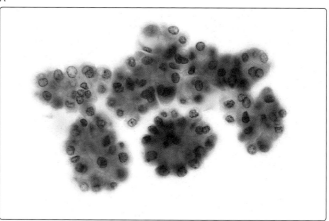

B

Fig. 3.33 Bronchial washings/lavage: bronchioloalveolar carcinoma. (A) Large numbers of bronchiolar type cell aggregates of varying size. (Papanicolaou × LP) (B) Moderate variation in nuclear size with some nuclear irregularity. (Papanicolaou × HP)

composed of monotonous cells with fine granular chromatin, some with intranuclear cytoplasmic inclusions, are characteristic (Fig. 3.34). Psammoma bodies may be seen in a small proportion of tumours (less than 10%)[207].

Mucinous or 'secretory' forms give rise to an appearance like that of sheets of endocervical mucosa (Fig. 3.35). Mixtures of secretory and non-secretory material are commonly seen. Mucinous tumours may show prominent nuclear grooves[209]. Pleomorphic forms with more dispersal are not identifiable as having a bronchioloalveolar growth pattern (Fig. 3.36). In some FNA cases individual cells may show no malignant nuclear criteria (Fig. 3.34) and the architectural features, including cell ball and papillary formation, are most important in recognizing the neoplasm.

Diagnostic pitfalls

Reactive bronchiolar epithelium in BAL samples may give cause for concern (Fig. 3.37). Such epithelium in FNA samples is usually only present in small amounts; abundant

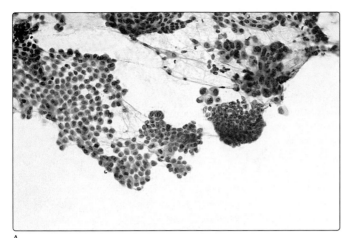

A

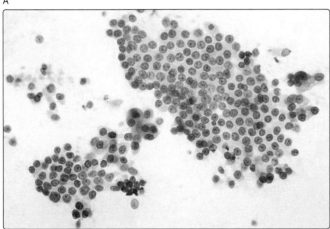

B

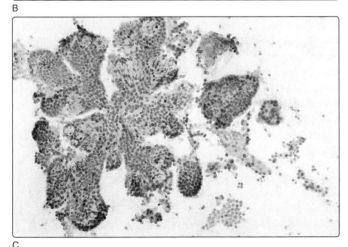

C

Fig. 3.34   FNA: bronchioloalveolar carcinoma. Well-differentiated, non-mucinous type. (A, B) Monolayered sheets of very regular bronchiolar cells, together with scattered three-dimensional aggregates. (C) Papillary structures. (H&E, × MP)

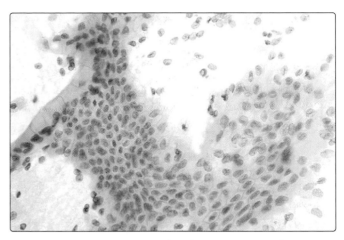

Fig. 3.35   FNA: mucinous bronchioloalveolar carcinoma. Monolayered sheet of regular cells with abundant apical mucin. (H&E × MP)

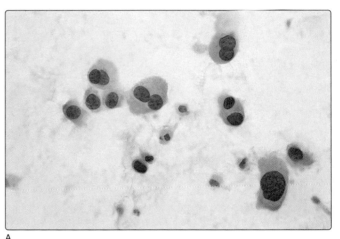

A

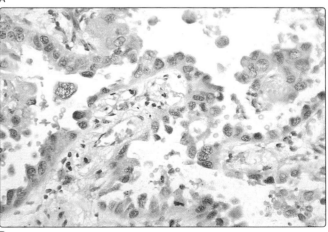

B

Fig. 3.36   FNA: pleomorphic bronchioloalveolar carcinoma. (A) Dispersed pattern of pleomorphic cells showing abundant dense cytoplasm. (H&E ×HP) (B) Resected tumour showing lepidic growth pattern of markedly pleomorphic cells. (H&E × MP)

bronchiolar epithelium of non-ciliated type should raise the possibility of BAC. Reactive sheets are usually smaller; malignant ones show associated architectural three-dimensionality. Irregular nuclear outlines and large nucleolar size are helpful features in distinguishing BAC from reactive bronchiolar proliferations[208], whereas a lack of hyperchromasia, prominence of cell borders, terminal plates, goblet cells and cell or nuclear moulding are more characteristic of benign reactive epithelial proliferations[207].

93

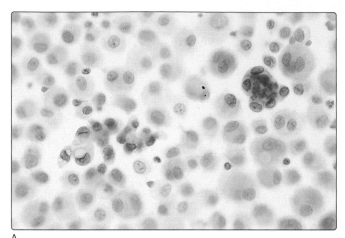

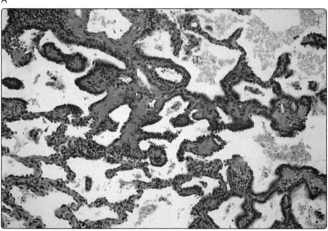

Fig. 3.37 Bronchoalveolar lavage: reactive bronchiolar cell proliferation. (A) Aggregates of glandular cells showing quite marked variation in nuclear size including some irregular nuclear margins and psammoma body formation. Such cases are rare but pose a risk of false positive diagnosis, requiring careful clinical correlation. (Papanicolaou × HP) (B) Open lung biopsy. Interstitial pneumonitis with patchy bronchiolization of alveolar walls. Diagnosed as extrinsic allergic alveolitis. (H&E × LP)

In FNA samples, metastatic tumours (Fig. 3.38) and epithelial mesothelioma[210] are potential differential diagnostic problems, resolved by clinical evaluation or by ancillary testing.

Intranuclear inclusions have been described as a feature of BAC; they may, however, be seen occasionally in reactive bronchiolar epithelium, in the bronchiolar epithelium of hamartomas and in papillary bronchogenic carcinoma[211]. The distinction between this last entity and BAC is arbitrary at times. Psammoma bodies also occur in other types of adenocarcinoma[212] and in mesothelioma.

Well-differentiated BAC may have a prolonged clinical course of up to 6–8 years after diagnosis before spread outside the lung occurs. They are a possible source of a so-called 'false-false-positive' diagnosis of malignancy[213]. A long clinical course does not, therefore, necessarily disprove a cytological diagnosis; small tumours may be difficult to find in lobectomy specimens, may have a similar

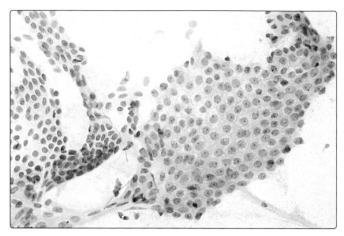

Fig. 3.38 FNA: metastatic prostatic carcinoma. Cell pattern mimicking BAC. (H&E × MP)

consistency to lung tissue and may require careful gross and microscopic examination of excised tissues[213].

Large cell carcinoma

Histologically, this subgroup is defined by exclusion as a non-small cell carcinoma without evidence of squamous or glandular differentiation: the prognosis is similar to or slightly worse than non-small cell cancers in general[214].

Ultrastructural assessment reveals subtle features of differentiation in most cases; such subclassification does not appear to have prognostic importance[188].

The diagnosis cannot be established by small biopsies or cytological preparations, because of an inability to sample lesions widely. Terms such as 'non-small cell carcinoma – further tumour typing not possible' or 'poorly differentiated large cell carcinoma' are generally proffered in cytological material. The WHO Classification recognizes basaloid, lymphoepithelioma-like, clear cell and rhabdoid variants. Pure giant cell carcinoma and spindle or sarcomatoid tumours are now described as carcinomas with pleomorphic, sarcomatoid or sarcomatous elements (Table 3.1).

Cytological findings

▶ Disorganized groups of large clearly malignant cells
▶ Pleomorphic single cell population
▶ Variable cytoplasm, high nuclear/cytoplasmic ratio
▶ Intracytoplasmic neutrophils and necrotic background

In sputum, these neoplasms tend to shed disorganized aggregates of large obviously malignant pleomorphic tumour cells, often with a prominent dispersed element of single cells. They have variable amounts of cytoplasm including some tumours with a high nuclear/cytoplasmic ratio and minimal cytoplasm, others with abundant cell cytoplasm or numerous multinucleated forms (Fig. 3.39). Tumours shedding predominantly spindle-cell forms are also described.

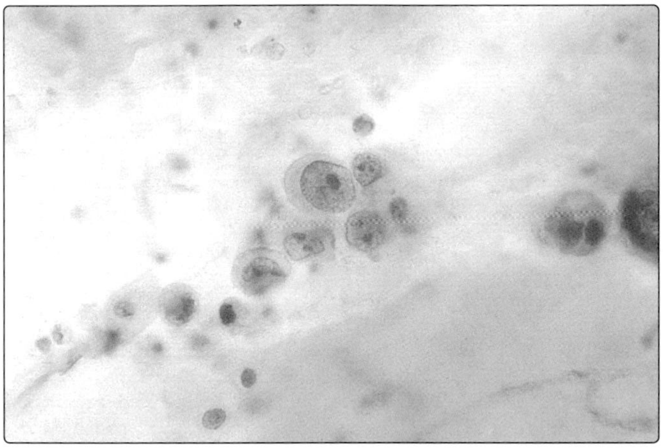

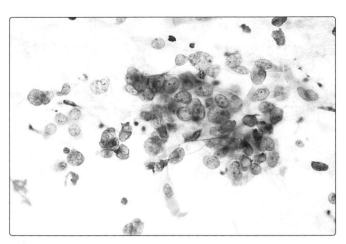

Fig. 3.39 Sputum: poorly differentiated large cell carcinoma. Loose aggregate of malignant cells. No specific features of cell differentiation. The findings here would favour carcinoma but other anaplastic malignancies, including melanoma, could not be excluded. (Papanicolaou × HP)

Fig. 3.41 Bronchial brushings: poorly differentiated carcinoma. The vesicular nuclear chromatin, distinct cell membranes and preserved cytoplasm helps exclude small cell carcinoma, but further specific tumour typing cannot be suggested. (Papanicolaou × HP)

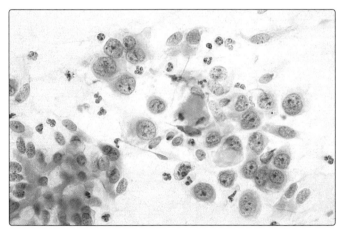

Fig. 3.40 Bronchial brushings: poorly differentiated large cell carcinoma. Loose aggregates of pleomorphic malignant cells without specific features to indicate differentiation. (Papanicolaou × HP)

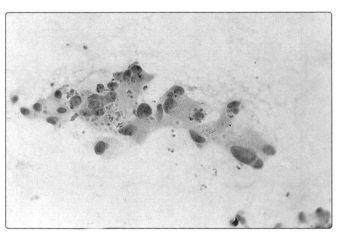

Fig. 3.42 FNA: pleomorphic large cell carcinoma. Prominent giant cell component and neutrophil ingestion. (H&E × MP)

In brushings and FNA samples, similar features are seen including disorganized aggregates or dispersed large pleomorphic cells (Figs 3.40, 3.41). Neutrophil ingestion may be a feature of tumour cells with abundant cytoplasm (Figs 3.42, 3.43). Necrosis is a common accompaniment of large cell carcinomas in any type of cytological sample.

Broderick *et al.*[215] describe the cytological appearances in sputum and washings in pure giant cell tumours, in which a dispersed population of very large pleomorphic malignant cells with few aggregates was observed; phagocytosis of inflammatory cells was common. Naib described similar appearances in sputum[216]. Craig *et al.*[217] presented a case in which brushings and FNA samples showed similar features including phagocytosis of tumour cells, and in which the tumour had probably arisen in a pre-existing bronchioloalveolar cell carcinoma. Figure 3.43 shows an example in FNA material.

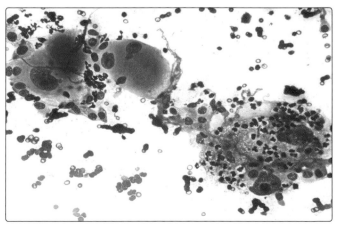

Fig.3.43 FNA: pure giant cell carcinoma. Bizarre malignant giant cells; prominent neutrophil ingestion. (MGG x HP)

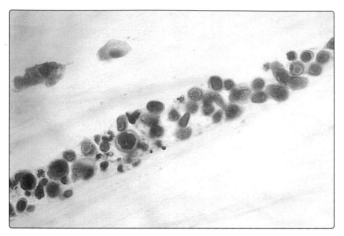

Fig. 3.44   Sputum: herpes virus changes. Low power appearances somewhat resembling carcinoma. (Papanicolaou × MP)

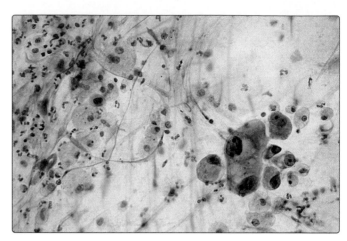

Fig. 3.45   Sputum: adenosquamous carcinoma. Keratinizing malignant cells and an aggregate of adenocarcinoma cells. (Papanicolaou × HP)

Diagnostic pitfalls

In sputum, cell aggregates should not be mistaken for evidence of glandular differentiation when the component cells are totally disorganized. In FNA samples, necrosis causing eosinophilia is commonly mistaken for keratinization[44] although this is a feature more of H&E than Papanicolaou staining, which distinguishes between necrosis and keratinization more easily.

Drug and chemotherapy effect may result in highly atypical large cells, and often with multinucleation (see Fig. 3.12). After treatment for small cell carcinoma we occasionally see this change in bronchial brushings taken as part of patient follow-up and it is not usually a problem in diagnosis because of the clinical background and the few abnormal cells seen.

Radiotherapy effect usually results in cells with a low nuclear/cytoplasmic ratio, multinucleation and degenerative nuclear changes including vacuolation (see Fig. 3.11). These changes are seldom a problem in interpretation, if the clinical background is known[218]. Epithelial 'repair' similar in appearance to that seen in cervical smears (see Fig. 3.13), is also occasionally found, particularly in patients with repeated bronchoscopies for diagnosis of lung cancer[172].

Megakaryocytes[219] occasionally occur in brushings and FNA samples but in small numbers and are unlikely to be mistaken for malignant cells. Viral effect (Fig. 3.44) is seldom a problem.

Other metastatic undifferentiated carcinomas, malignant melanoma and sarcoma may all give cells of similar appearance to primary large cell carcinomas.

Adenosquamous carcinoma

Tumours with an intimate mixture of squamous and glandular growth pattern are uncommon if a significant proportion of both tumour types is required for diagnosis. Smaller foci of glandular or squamous differentiation in tumours of other types are commonly seen. Adenosquamous tumours are said to be more often peripheral in location and to be of poor prognosis. We have rarely made the diagnosis cytologically (Fig. 3.45).

Large cell neuroendocrine tumours

McDowell in 1981[144] described cases which had been reported as large cell or squamous cell carcinoma or adenocarcinoma histologically and which showed cytoplasmic dense core neurosecretory granules, and demonstrated these features in 4% of 150 lung tumours. Others suggested that up to 9% of non-small cell carcinomas of the lung might contain neurosecretory granules[146]. In some studies this has not necessarily been an indicator of poor prognosis: however, others have suggested more aggressive behaviour in these tumours, and responsiveness to chemotherapy[148].

Large cell neuroendocrine carcinoma is now recognized as an entity distinct from atypical carcinoid tumour and small cell carcinoma[127,150]. Histologically, cell nesting with palisading, rosettes or trabeculae; large cells with a low nuclear/cytoplasmic ratio; prominent nucleoli, vesicular chromatin, a high mitotic rate and abundant necrosis are suggested as features helping to identify this tumour by light microscopy[127,150]. Identification of neuroendocrine phenotype by immunocytochemistry or electron microscopy is necessary for diagnosis. A mitotic rate of >10/10 high power fields (HPF) distinguishes these lesions from atypical carcinoid tumours (2–10 mitoses/10 HPF). These lesions have an extremely poor prognosis, similar to small cell carcinoma[150]. Cytological descriptions are few and diagnosis may be difficult. Nicholson and Ryan describe loose cell aggregates in a background of singly dispersed cells, tumour cells clinging to capillaries; rosette formations, delicate, granular cytoplasm, inconspicuous nucleoli, moulding in high grade tumours, and speckled or dusty chromatin patterns as general criteria useful in identifying neuroendocrine differentiation[220].

Carcinoid tumours

These constitute only 1% of lung tumours. They occur predominantly in earlier age groups, in the fourth and fifth decades, in contrast to patients with bronchogenic carcinoma. The tumour has an origin in a main bronchus in 85% of cases, but may be more peripheral particularly in spindle cell forms.

The classic or typical carcinoid tumour consists of uniform cells with small round to oval nuclei, few nucleoli and granular eosinophilic cytoplasm, arranged in nests, trabeculae or a mosaic pattern. Variants include clear cell tumours, papillary and oncocytic tumours and spindle cell forms. Five to ten percent of typical cases with no features of malignancy will metastasize, although superficially invasive tumours, tumours less than 3 cm in diameter and those without lymph node metastases at diagnosis generally behave in a biologically benign fashion.

Cytological findings[220–230]

▶ Best seen in brushings and FNA samples
▶ Uniform small cells, rounded nuclei, stippled chromatin
▶ Marked cell dissociation, some palisades or trabeculae
▶ Bare nuclei are common but necrosis is rare
▶ Plexiform vascular fragments in FNA samples

Typical/classical carcinoid

In typical/classical carcinoids, tumour cells are uncommonly seen in sputum as these neoplasms are usually submucosal, even when they assume an intrabronchial polypoid growth. In brushings or FNA samples, a dispersed cell population with some trabecula or palisading of small cell clusters, a uniform population of small cells with small amounts of intact cytoplasm and monotonous rounded or oval nuclei with a finely granular or stippled nuclear chromatin are diagnostic features (Figs 3.46–3.48).

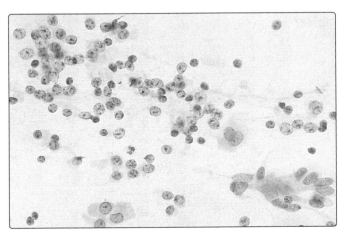

Fig. 3.46 Bronchial brushings: carcinoid tumour. Dispersed cells including many bare nuclei with coarsely clumped 'neuroendocrine' chromatin pattern. Absence of mitotic activity, necrosis or cell traumatization. (Papanicolaou × HP)

The 'neuroendocrine nucleus' with its round or oval shape, regular outline and coarsely stippled nuclear chromatin is a useful diagnostic criterion to keep in mind. Tumour cell nuclei are usually robust, and traumatized cells, cell debris or

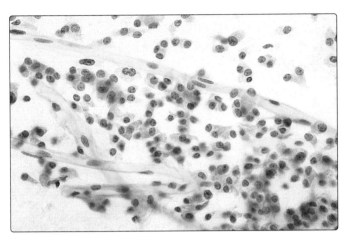

Fig. 3.47 FNA: carcinoid tumour. Dispersed population of regular small neuroendocrine cells. Background of plexiform capillaries. (Papanicolaou × MP)

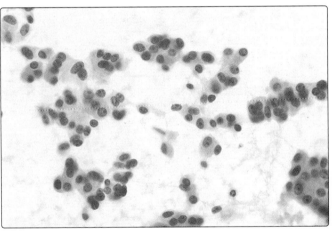

A

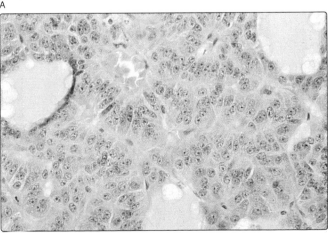

B

Fig. 3.48 FNA: carcinoid tumour. (A) Clumps, cords and trabeculae of tumour cells. (H&E × HP) (B) Histological section showing 'neuroendocrine nuclei'. (H&E × HP)

streaks of nuclear material are not a feature, although bare nuclei are prominent in some cases. Necrosis or inflammatory changes are not usually seen but these lesions are highly vascular and may yield haemorrhagic samples.

In brushings, a contrast with bronchial epithelial cells may be a useful feature although stripped bronchial cell nuclei and carcinoid tumour nuclei may be very similar[223] and small amounts of tumour tissue may be overlooked[221]. Traumatization of cells by the procedure may very rarely lead to an appearance resembling small cell carcinoma[228].

In FNA samples, a plexiform background of small blood vessels and adherence of cells to vascular cores is a striking feature in most cases (Fig. 3.47) and is an important additional diagnostic criterion. Anderson *et al.*[221] found this feature in 21 of 23 cases, including spindle and atypical tumours; Mitchell *et al.*[229] also draw attention to this finding.

Bronchioloalveolar carcinoma cells are usually larger, have more abundant cytoplasm, evidence of sheet-like growth and lack a vascular component. Strong positive staining for synaptophysin or chromogranin would favour carcinoid[221]. Intranuclear cytoplasmic inclusions are seen occasionally in carcinoids[221] as well as in BAC. Sclerosing haemangioma/pneumocytoma can produce similar cytological appearances to carcinoid, but is a very rare neoplasm[221].

Spindle cell carcinoid

Spindle cell carcinoid tumours are usually more peripheral and only seen in FNA material. They may show a closer resemblance to small cell carcinoma, or more rarely mesenchymal tumours (Fig. 3.49), but uniformity of nuclear size, absence of moulding, nuclear smearing and background debris all help to exclude small cell carcinoma[231,232]. A background of capillary blood vessels is unlike small cell carcinoma.

Adenocarcinoid

Adenocarcinoid is a term used in some cytological descriptions for tumours confirmed to be neuroendocrine ultrastructurally and with histological features of carcinoid tumours but showing glandular differentiation with or without mucin secretion. They are not recognized in the WHO classification but may be a useful concept to keep in mind when low grade or columnar cell lesions are encountered. Cytologically, they may show columnar cells with round or oval nuclei in sheets, syncytia or stratified groups[233,234] and may be difficult to diagnose by cytology alone. Pilotti *et al.*[234] advise that carcinoids with glandular features should be considered when FNA material from asymptomatic patients with coin lesions suggests a glandular neoplasm, with an orderly structure of clusters and relatively uniform nuclei.

Atypical carcinoid tumours

This subgroup constitutes about 10% of carcinoid tumours but may provide great diagnostic difficulty. Arrigoni *et al.*[235] suggested that nuclear pleomorphism, mitoses and necrosis

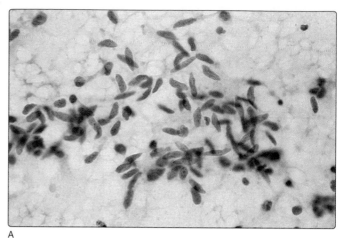

A

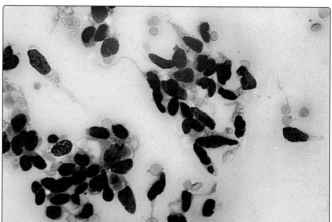

B

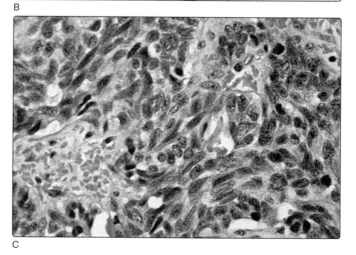

C

Fig. 3.49 Imprint from resected lung specimen: carcinoid tumour, spindle cell type. Unusually elongated cells with a mesenchymal appearance. (A, H&E × HP; B, MGG × HP; C, Histological section H&E × MP)

in tumours of carcinoid architecture predicted more aggressive behaviour. In his series regional or distant metastases were evident in up to 70% of patients and were associated with a death rate of 30%. More recent studies have verified these findings[150] and suggest that a mitotic rate of 2–10/10 HPF or coagulative necrosis defines a subgroup of neuroendocrine tumours with a biological behaviour between typical carcinoid and large cell neuroendocrine carcinoma or small cell carcinoma.

These neoplasms usually possess neuroendocrine cytological characteristics including rounded or oval nuclei, uniform stippled chromatin and some dispersed cells with intact cytoplasm[220,236–238]. In FNA samples, increased pleomorphism and identification of any mitotic activity or necrosis helps distinguish these from typical carcinoids. The absence of widespread moulding, smeared fragile nuclei, abundant single cell necrosis or abundant mitotic activity, and the presence of cohesive acinar, rosette or sheet-like groups with palisading helps exclude small cell carcinoma. Nevertheless it is accepted that there is an overlap in cytological appearances between this lesion and small cell carcinoma or large cell neuroendocrine carcinoma, (Fig. 3.50) and that even on bronchial biopsy such a distinction may be very difficult[220,230,236–238].

Argyrophilia can be seen in some of these tumours in contrast to small cell carcinomas, but this technique is difficult to apply in practice. Markers such as chromogranin, synaptophysin and bombesin may be unequivocally positive in neuroendocrine tumours, but are less valuable in subtyping.

Ultrastructural study allows reliable detection of neuroendocrine differentiation. Evaluation of the number, size and location of neurosecretory granules, cell processes and junctions can be undertaken and nuclear morphology assessed, and it may also help in subtyping these lesions. In atypical carcinoids, neurosecretory granules are less numerous, smaller and more concentrated in cytoplasmic processes than in ordinary carcinoids. Immunohistochemistry or electron microscopy of FNA material or histological material is required for definitive diagnosis[150].

Adenoid cystic carcinoma

These tumours occur as primary lesions, generally of major bronchi[239–242], or as metastatic spread to the lung from other sites[243–245]. If the large acellular basement membrane spheres and fingers so characteristic of this tumour are evident in a background of small cells with uniform nuclei, the diagnosis can be made cytologically (Fig. 3.51). Such spheres are more easily seen in MGG than in Papanicolaou stained preparations. They may not be present in FNA samples from the peripheral infiltrating areas of the tumour (Fig. 3.52), nor in brush samples, and distinction from other small cell neoplasms is then very difficult. Tumour shedding into brushings may not occur until after biopsy[241]. Radhika et al.[243] describe tight branching tubular clusters of malignant cells giving a cylindroid appearance as an additional criterion for diagnosis.

Mucoepidermoid carcinoma

In current practice this term is restricted to low grade tumours of bronchial gland origin. Nguyen[242] describes FNA material from two low-grade bronchial tumours as showing

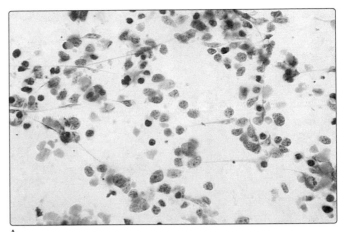

A

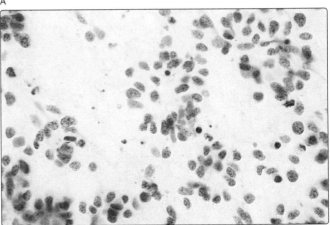

B

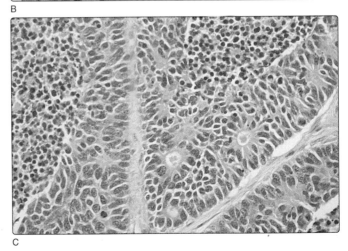

C

Fig. 3.50 FNA: high-grade neuroendocrine carcinoma. (A) Smear appearances closely resembling small cell carcinoma, including necrosis, streaks of nuclear debris and cells with minimal cytoplasm. (Papanicolaou × HP) (B) Prominent rosette formation in some parts of the smear, unlike the pattern seen in small cell carcinoma. (Papanicolaou × HP) (C) Histological section showing rosettes and necrosis. (H&E × IP) There was a high mitotic rate and a pattern consistent with large cell neuroendocrine carcinoma.

features similar to salivary gland lesions, including groups of only moderately pleomorphic squamous cells with intracytoplasmic mucus. Brooks and Baandrup[246] found a mixture of intermediate cells, squamous and mucinous

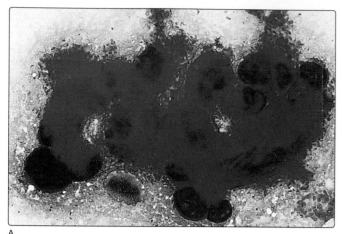

A

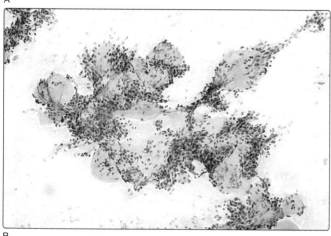

B

Fig. 3.51   FNA: metastatic adenoid-cystic carcinoma. Primary tumour in the oral cavity. (A, B) Numerous hyaline globules of basement membrane material with intervening small hyperchromatic tumour cells. (A, MGG × LP; B, H&E × LP)

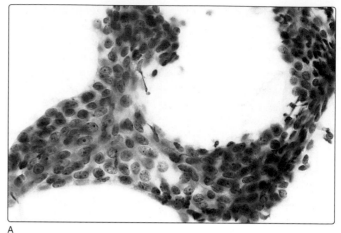

A

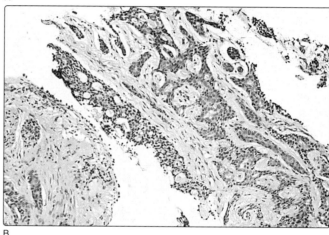

B

Fig. 3.52   Transbronchial FNA: recurrent adenoid-cystic carcinoma. (A) Irregular cord of poorly differentiated carcinoma cells, not diagnosable as adenoid-cystic in type without reference to previous histology. (Papanicolaou × HP) (B) Bronchial biopsy sample at the time of transbronchial FNA showing recurrent adenoid-cystic carcinoma. (H&E × MP)

cells in an FNA sample from a peripheral tumour. Tao[247] describes clusters of uniform squamous cells, mucus secreting cells associated with squamous cells and spindle cells. Segletes *et al.* were able to suggest the diagnosis in three cases based on combinations of mucinous, squamous and intermediate cells[248]. In our single case, the tumour cells were predominantly intermediate squamous cells with a 'transitional' appearance and only focal mucin secretion. The cytomorphology of high-grade tumours is probably indistinguishable from large cell carcinoma of adenosquamous type[247].

Metastatic carcinoma

Metastatic tumours to the thorax constitute up to 15–20% of lesions diagnosed by cytology in some series[43]. The principles of cytological diagnosis of metastatic tumour of lung are the same as those of the surgical pathologist in assessing tissue: detailed knowledge of the clinical history must be available, together with earlier cytological and histological preparations for review and comparison with current material[1,43,249]. Using this approach, a cytological

diagnosis is highly reliable, although metastatic tumour may occasionally be misinterpreted as primary, and primary lung cancer may, on occasions, be misinterpreted as a metastasis or may mimic other unusual tumours, including sarcomas.

Immunohistochemistry is a valuable guide[103,103a,250,251] although a careful clinicopathological approach is still necessary because of an overlap in immunophenotype between primary and metastatic tumours. Mucinous tumours are particularly difficult to characterize.

Attention has been drawn to the common occurrence of new primary tumours when metastases are suspected clinically[252], and double primaries may also be encountered[253]. Metastatic tumour, particularly renal cell and colonic carcinomas[254], may mimic primary tumours clinically either by growing as an endobronchial lesion or because of a bronchioloalveolar growth pattern.

In more recent cytological literature, unusual metastatic lesions such as breast carcinoma with osteoclastic giant cells[255], metaplastic breast carcinoma with prominent squamous cell components[256], or chondroid elements[257], adrenal carcinoma[258], choriocarcinoma[259], meningioma[260,261], mesothelioma[262,263], medullary carcinoma of thyroid[264], adamantinoma of tibia[265], ameloblastoma[266], pleomorphic adenoma of salivary glands[267] and granulosa cell tumour[268] have all been confirmed cytologically. Occasional examples of unusual lesions such as leiomyosarcoma continue to be described in sputum[269].

Cytological findings

▶ Aggregates of tumour cells stand out in clean background
▶ Some metastases recognizable morphologically
▶ Cell blocks, special stains, immunocytochemistry helpful

In sputum the occurrence of very large aggregates of adenocarcinoma cells 'dropped' into a clear background is, to us, suggestive of metastatic tumour and is somewhat different from the pattern in most primary tumours although it will occur with some BACs. This may correspond to alveolar casts of malignant cells, which are shed intact[60]. In addition, a number of carcinomas have such distinctive cytological characteristics as to be readily identifiable. For example, metastatic well-differentiated colonic carcinoma often presents with palisaded, elongated nuclei in aggregates and in a background of confluent necrosis (Fig. 3.53)[270]. The cell aggregates may have a papillary structure.

In FNA or bronchial brushings of samples from colonic carcinoma, the additional criteria of well formed glandular structures showing abundant apical mucin, and well-defined cytoplasmic borders are seen. In any sample a background of necrosis in the presence of a well-differentiated adenocarcinoma is unlike most primary lung carcinoma.

Breast carcinoma in sputum forms small cohesive morules of small cells showing tight cellular apposition and moulding (Fig. 3.54), single files of cells or larger masses of loosely arranged cells (see Fig. 3.18)[271]. A more dispersed pattern is seen in FNA material.

Metastatic renal cell carcinoma with central macronucleoli and abundant clear cytoplasm may be highly

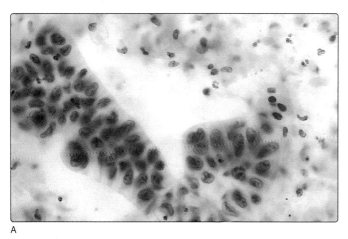

A

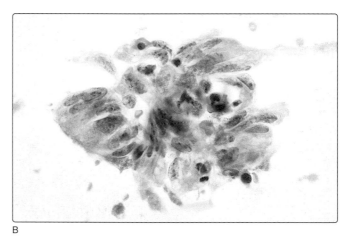

B

Fig. 3.53 Metastatic colonic adenocarcinoma. Columnar morphology of the malignant glandular cells in sputum (A) and brushings (B). (A) Aggregate of malignant glandular cells with a columnar cell form and in a background of necrosis. (Papanicolaou × HP) (B) Columnar cell form of malignant cells with elongated nuclei and abundant apical cytoplasm. (Papanicolaou × HP)

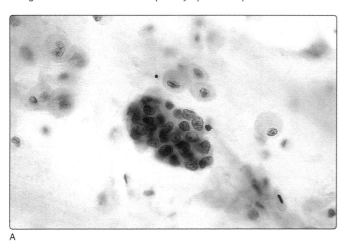

A

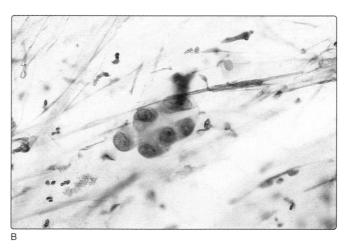

B

Fig. 3.54 Sputum: metastatic breast carcinoma. Cohesive aggregates of small malignant cells. Note the intracytoplasmic lumen in (B). (Papanicolaou × HP)

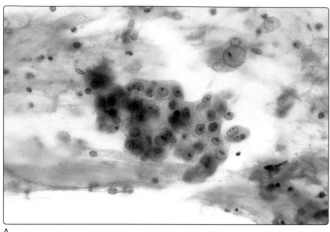

A

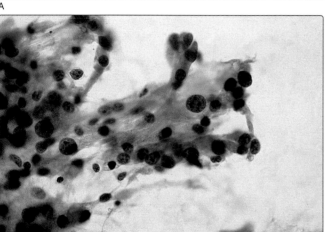

B

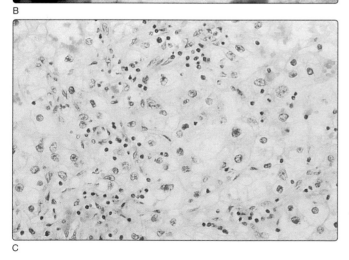

C

Fig. 3.55 Metastatic renal cell carcinoma. (A) Sputum. Disorganized aggregate of glandular cells with rounded nuclei, prominent nucleoli and abundant cytoplasm. (Papanicolaou × HP) (B) FNA. Disorganized aggregates of malignant glandular cells. Cyanophilic cytoplasm without a clear cell appearance. (Papanicolaou × HP) (C) Cell block preparation demonstrating clear cell carcinoma. (H&E × MP)

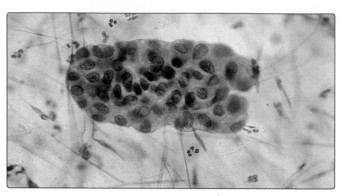

Fig. 3.56 Sputum: metastatic prostatic carcinoma. Cohesive three-dimensional aggregate of small malignant cells. (Papanicolaou × HP)

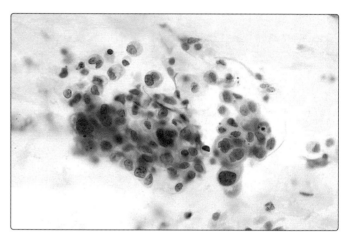

Fig. 3.57 Sputum: metastatic transitional cell carcinoma. Disorganized aggregate of malignant cells showing no particular differentiation. Distinction from poorly differentiated squamous or adenocarcinoma not possible on cytological appearances. (Papanicolaou × HP)

cell morphology[272]. FNA of some concurrent primary tumours with essentially similar cytomorphology allowed confirmation of the diagnosis. As with Linsk and Franzen's series[273], close resemblance to adrenal carcinoma was observed and the value of ultrastructural assessment was emphasized in this differential diagnosis, as well as between renal and hepatocellular carcinoma. In our experience, cytoplasmic clearing may not be a particular feature in smears, although it is prominent in cell-blocks.

Prostatic carcinoma often presents in sputum as aggregates of small cells with round nuclei and prominent nucleoli (Fig. 3.56)[271]. We have seen a case in FNA, with close cytological resemblance to BAC (see Fig. 3.38). Transitional cell carcinoma is of variable appearance (Fig. 3.57, 3.58); clinical features are usually the major determinant of diagnosis in metastatic sites, but a combination of spindle and pyramidal-shaped cells with dense cytoplasm and cytoplasmic vacuoles may help in establishing a cytological diagnosis[274]. Cercariform cells (CCs) were identified by Powers and Elbadawi as diagnostic clues for transitional cell carcinoma[275]. These are cells with a

characteristic (Fig. 3.55). In Nguyen's series of 16 cases of renal cell carcinoma metastatic to various sites including lung, 13 showed mixtures of granular and vacuolated cytoplasm, and three showed either pure granular or clear

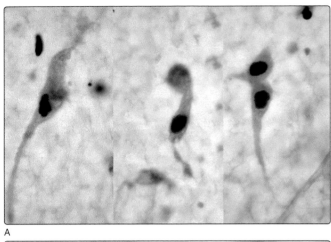

A

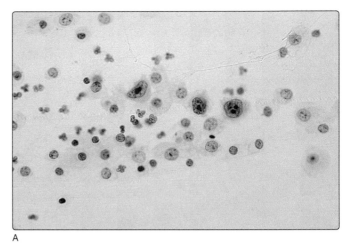

A

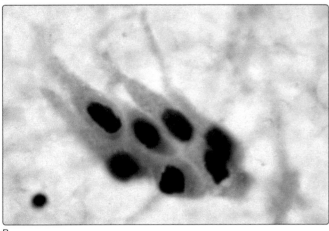

B

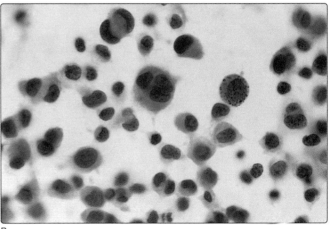

B

Fig. 3.58 FNA: metastatic transitional cell carcinoma. (A) Cercariform cells with bulbous ends and long cytoplasmic processes. (B) Sheet of squamoid cells with long cytoplasmic processes. (Papanicolaou × HP)

Fig. 3.59 Metastatic malignant melanoma. (A) Sputum: Amelanotic tumour. (Papanicolaou × HP) (B) FNA: characteristic dispersal, multinucleation, dense cytoplasm and some intracytoplasmic pigment. (H&E × HP)

nucleated globular body and a unipolar cytoplasmic process with a bulbous end (Fig. 3.58). Hida and Gupta[276] found that other poorly differentiated epithelial tumours may show such cells but usually in small numbers. All TCCs had at least some CCs. Renshaw and Madge[277] found CCs in 57% of TCCs compared to 14% of non-small cell lung cancer. CCs were mainly seen in TCCs without squamous differentiation.

Other tumours, including melanoma[278] (Fig. 3.59B) or metastatic adenoid cystic carcinoma (see Fig. 3.51), may also be easily recognized. Amelanotic melanoma can, of course, provide significant difficulties (Fig. 3.59A). Large cell carcinomas of lung may exhibit very similar cytological features to melanoma, including dispersal, multinucleation and intranuclear cytoplasmic inclusions; spindle cell melanoma may resemble sarcoma, sarcomatoid carcinoma or mesothelioma. We have also seen melanomas which display marked cohesion, cellular engulfment and an onion skinning appearance, and some resembling lymphoma or small cell carcinoma. Blaustein[279] reported melanin pigment in a breast carcinoma metastatic to lung, presumably as a result of transport of epidermal pigment into tumour cells.

Metastatic squamous cell carcinoma is not specifically distinguishable cytologically from primary tumours although it has been our impression that tumour cells are somewhat smaller in secondary cervical cancer than in primary lung cancer. Identification of oncogenic or high risk HPV DNA or positive CK 7 staining[103a] may also be helpful in characterizing them as metastatic female genital tract tumours; most well-differentiated squamous cell carcinomas of lung are CK7 negative, and HPV DNA is uncommonly found in lung carcinomas.

Benign papillary bronchial tumours

Juvenile papillomatosis is most frequently an upper respiratory tract lesion associated with human papilloma virus that may occasionally involve distal bronchi.

Solitary papillomas of bronchi show a range of epithelial types, including some with simple or keratinizing metaplastic epithelium and others with a more transitional appearance; tumours of purely glandular type are also rarely

103

seen. Multifocal lesions are extremely difficult to treat and may extend into lung parenchyma although they are histologically benign. Occasionally, examples of malignant change are described.

In our single case of *squamous papilloma,* bronchial brushings revealed keratinous material and mature

A

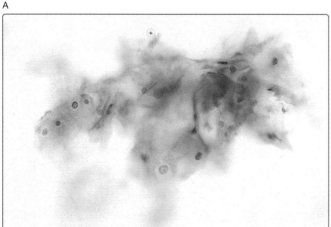

B

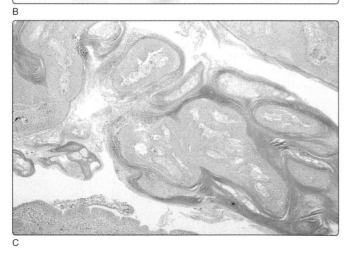

C

Fig. 3.60 Bronchial brushings: squamous papilloma of bronchus. (A) Large masses of keratinous and parakeratotic material. (Papanicolaou × LP) (B) Keratinizing benign squamous cells showing some perinuclear clearing. (Papanicolaou × HP) (C) Histology of resected specimen showing keratinizing squamous cell papilloma. (H&E × LP)

squamous cells, but a diagnosis was not possible without biopsy (Fig. 3.60). Roglic's experience was similar[280]. In a case report by Rubel and Reynolds[281], the brushings and sputum samples of multiple papillomas showed features similar to human papilloma virus effect in other sites; histological appearances also resembled condyloma. In the case reported by Weingarten[282], multifocal tracheobronchial papillomatosis in a 62-year-old man yielded cohesive clusters of overlapping squamous cells together with masses of keratin including keratin plugs, parakeratotic material and small vacuolated squamous cells.

We have seen one case of *papillary adenoma,* in which highly cohesive papillary clusters of small regular glandular cells were present in brushings samples (Fig. 3.61); concomitant biopsy established the diagnosis.

Brightman *et al.*[283] reported a rare case of a combined squamous cell papilloma and mucous gland adenoma in which large squamous cells, smaller polygonal cells and papillary groups of cylindrical cells were present in FNA smears.

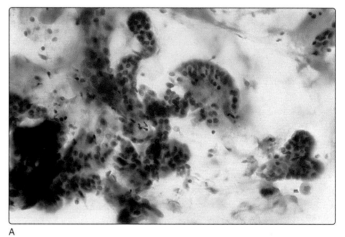

A

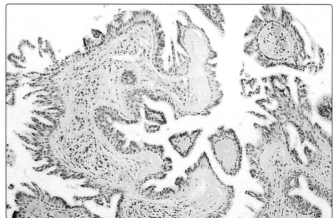

B

Fig. 3.61 Bronchial brushings: papillary adenoma of bronchus. (A) Papillary aggregates of glandular cells without nuclear atypia. The findings were thought unusual but a diagnosis was not suggested on this material. (Papanicolaou × HP) (B) Bronchial biopsy specimen establishing the diagnosis of papillary adenoma. (H&E × MP)

Other rare tumours

FNA samples of a *benign clear cell ('sugar') tumour* of lung were described as showing large irregular clusters of benign polygonal and spindle shaped cells with vacuolated granular PAS positive cytoplasm[284]. A distinction from inflammatory pseudotumour, renal cell carcinoma, clear cell carcinoid or carcinoma was difficult without ultrastructural assessment. The neoplastic cell is thought to be a perivascular cell related to smooth muscle.

Cwierzyk *et al.* describe the appearances of *pulmonary oncocytoma* in bronchial brushings[285]. Syncytial clusters of monotonous epithelial cells with abundant, rather dense, amphophilic cytoplasm were observed within mucus. Granular staining in PAS preparations was seen. Nuclei were round or oval with minimal variation, and had finely stippled chromatin. The tumour was 1.5 cm in diameter, polypoid and projected into the bronchial lumen; the mitochondrion-rich nature of the cytoplasm was observed ultrastructurally. There were no neurosecretory granules, although the cells resembled carcinoid tumour cells. Multicentric oncocytoma has also been diagnosed by FNA

by demonstrating PTAH staining of tumour cell granules and absence of neuroendocrine markers in cell blocks[286].

Benign mesenchymal tumours
Chondroid hamartoma

These lesions constitute 5–10% of small solitary rounded peripheral lung masses and are important because they may be easily recognized cytologically, definitively diagnosed and require no further diagnostic or therapeutic procedures.

Cytological findings

▶ Myxoid connective tissue and cartilage
▶ Sheets of epithelial cells
▶ Fat and macrophages in the background

In FNA samples, the combination of fibrillar myxoid connective tissue, hyaline cartilage (Fig. 3.62), bronchiolar epithelium and fat is diagnostic[287–294]. In some cases, macrophages may be present in abundance in the background. The fibrillar myxoid material is the most

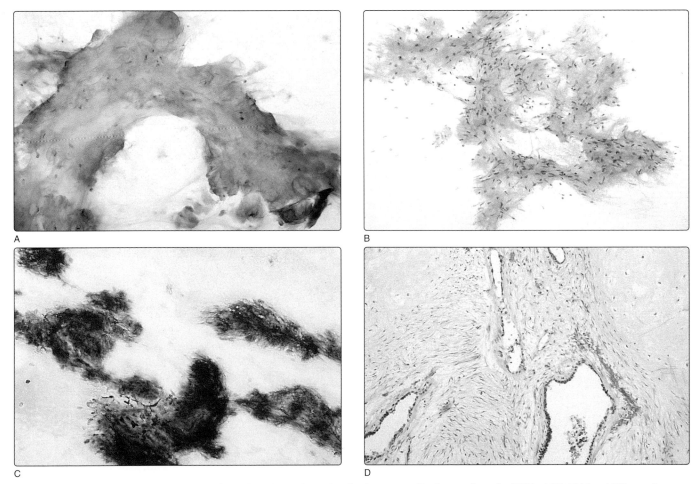

Fig. 3.62 FNA: chondroid hamartoma. (A) Core of hyaline cartilage showing lacunae and background matrix. (H&E × MP) (B) Myxoid fibrous tissue. (H&E × MP) (C) Fibromyxoid tissue showing striking magenta metachromasia. (MGG × LP) (D) A resected specimen showing fibromyxoid tissue, mature cartilage and trapped bronchiolar epithelium. (H&E × MP)

distinctive element of the tumour, and the single most useful diagnostic indicator. It is magenta or purple in MGG preparations and pale orange or grey in Papanicolaou stained material, where it can be more easily overlooked (Fig. 3.62). Positive staining for S 100 helps distinguish this material from collagenous fibrous tissue[294].

Diagnostic pitfalls

Bronchiolar epithelium presents in sheets, may be abundant, and often shows some nuclear enlargement and intranuclear cytoplasmic inclusions (Fig. 3.63), which may lead to an incorrect suspicion of epithelial malignancy. Chondrocytes may also be misinterpreted[288]. For this reason the lesion is a quite common source of false positive diagnosis of malignancy. Mature cartilage has a homogeneous waxy purple/grey appearance in H&E stained material and is sparsely cellular, containing chondrocytes in lacunae. Contamination from chest wall

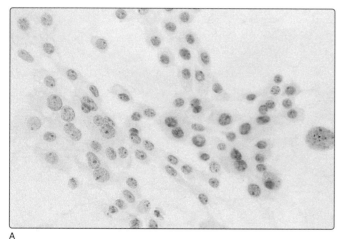

A

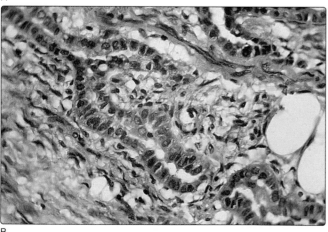

B

Fig. 3.63   FNA: chondroid hamartoma. (A) Bronchiolar epithelium with a moderate degree of variation in nuclear size and shape. (H&E × HP) (B) Resection specimen showing abundant proliferated bronchiolar epithelium. (H&E × HP)

costal cartilage or tracheal or bronchial cartilage might lead to a false diagnosis if reliance is placed on cartilage alone.

Sclerosing haemangioma (pneumocytoma)

This lesion is a rare benign tumour generally presenting as an incidental finding on chest X-ray, and occurring as a solitary rounded mass, mainly in women. Many of the patients are of Asian descent. The range of histological patterns is diverse. It is uncertain which cellular component is neoplastic, although the epithelial cell element is currently favoured[124].

Cytological findings

► Diagnosis possible in FNA material
► Bronchiolar epithelial-type around blood spaces
► Eosinophilic cytoplasm, rounded nuclei, small nucleoli

FNA sampling in one reported case showed aggregates of epithelial-like tumour cells surrounding blood spaces. The neoplastic cells were of medium size with round or oval folded nuclei, finely reticular chromatin, small nucleoli and moderate amounts of eosinophilic cytoplasm[295]. Arrangements of cells along septa probably represented detached larger blood vessel walls. Tao[57] refers to a similar case with a proliferating network of blood vessels and adherent, irritated alveolar cells.

In several case reports, papillary or sheet-like groups of epithelial cells are described[296] having a resemblance to bronchioloalveolar carcinoma[296,297]. Kaw and Nayak[298] reported on a case presenting cytologically with a combination of bland spindle cells and epithelial cells, either bronchiolar or type II pneumocytes. Wojcik *et al.*[299] diagnosed a case in which regular epithelial-like cells were arranged in loose fragments containing sclerotic stromal cores; cell block preparations revealed a papillary pattern together with angiomatous areas. Haemosiderin-laden macrophages were also seen. Intranuclear inclusions were evident in the epithelial-like cells. Our single case was a young Asian male with a long history of haemoptysis and a 10 cm rounded opacity in the lung. Aspiration showed highly cellular smears composed mainly of epithelial-like cells and some macrophages. (Fig. 3.64) The abundance of material and the sheet-like presentation in smears resembled BAC. A definite diagnosis of malignancy was not given because of the unusual clinical findings and absence of nuclear criteria of malignancy. The diagnosis was made on the excised specimen. Carcinoid tumour might also provide differential diagnostic problems[221].

Granular cell tumour

Bronchial tumours constitute only 5–10% of the total incidence of these tumours. They are now accepted as being of Schwann cell derivation. In the lung they usually present as endobronchial nodules, although they may sometimes grossly mimic infiltrative malignancy.

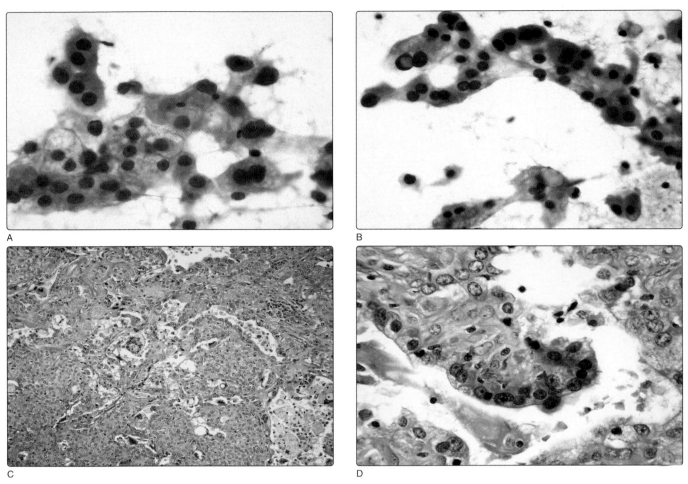

Fig. 3.64 FNA: sclerosing haemangioma/pneumocytoma. (A, B) Sheets of bronchiolar type cells with moderate pleomorphism and prominent intranuclear cytoplasmic inclusions. (H&E × HP) (C, D) Resected specimen. (C, H&E × LP; D, H&E × MP)

Cytological findings

► Single or grouped cells, abundant granular cytoplasm
► Some pleomorphism but low nuclear/cytoplasmic ratio
► Positive staining with S 100

Chen[300] reported a case in which brushings smears showed characteristic abundant eosinophilic granular cytoplasm, a few spindle cell forms and some binucleated cells. Füezesi et al.[301] studied a multicentric lesion diagnosed in cell blocks of bronchial lavage samples. Single cells and groups of tumour cells with abundant, granular cytoplasm were distinguishable from macrophages and epithelial cells. Glant et al.[302], Mermolja et al.[303] and Thomas et al.[304] described similar cytomorphology, including components of strap-like and spindle cell forms. Smith et al. report a mediastinal case diagnosed by FNA[305].

Positive S 100 staining helps confirm the cell type[306]. Occasionally giant or bizarre polygonal cells are described in cytological preparations[302,303], but this appearance is still generally associated with benign biological behaviour. In our limited experience with this tumour in FNA samples of several sites, the very low nuclear/cytoplasmic ratio is distinctive and helps distinguish the cells even from macrophages; the large ill-defined cytoplasmic granules in Papanicolaou stained samples are most helpful (Fig. 3.65). The tumour is rarely diagnosed in exfoliated material[307].

Lymphoma, leukaemia and related disorders

Non-Hodgkin's malignant lymphomas of extrapulmonary origin and of all histological subtypes quite frequently affect the lung during the course of the disease. Primary lymphoproliferative disorders are uncommon and are virtually confined to adults. The majority of primary tumours are low grade B-cell lymphomas of marginal zone (MALT) type, or high-grade large cell lymphomas mainly of B cell type. An angiocentric infiltration is seen in many non-Hodgkin's lymphomas of lung (so-called lymphomatoid granulomatosis pattern). This may occur in low-grade tumours with a pure small cell component as well as high-grade tumours including T cell rich B-cell lymphomas[124]. The clinical background to primary marginal zone (MALT) lung lymphomas includes pre-existing immunopathic disorders such as Sjögren's syndrome and dysproteinaemia.

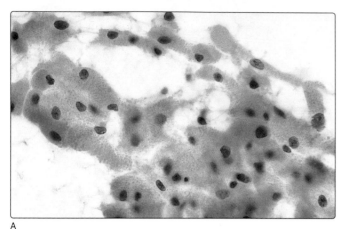

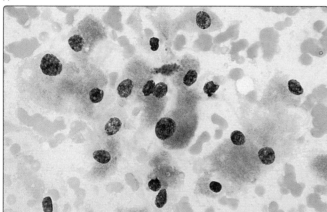

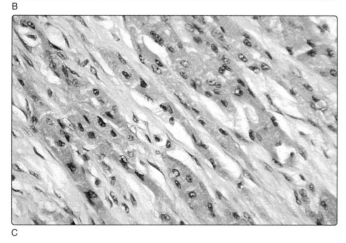

Fig. 3.65 FNA: granular cell tumour. Malignant chest wall lesion, which metastasized to bone. (A, B) Loose aggregates and dispersed cells with abundant granular cytoplasm, rounded nuclei with some variation in shape and size and some strap shaped and spindle cell forms. (A, Papanicolaou × HP; B, MGG × HP) (C) Resected specimen showing cords and clumps of granular cells within a fibrous stroma. (H&E × HP)

AIDS patients can have interstitial lymphoid infiltrates, which progress to frank lymphoma, or present with high-grade large cell or blastic tumours[308]. The lung is not uncommonly involved in post-transplant lymphoproliferative disorders[309]. Gross patterns of lung involvement by lymphoma include masses with or without

cavitation, localized areas of consolidation, multiple nodules or diffuse infiltrates[124].

Reactive lymphoid infiltrations, including prominent germinal centre formation, may be associated with lymphoma, and representative sampling can be difficult to achieve by any cytological method. The existence of widespread benign or reactive lymphoproliferations of the lung, as expressed in the term pseudolymphoma has been disputed, mainly on the basis of frequent subsequent development of frank malignant lymphoma. However lymphoid interstitial pneumonia appears to be a benign process[124] and cases of nodular lymphoid hyperplasia continue to be reported[310].

Hodgkin's lymphoma is rarely seen as a primary lung lesion[311], but the lung is a common site of relapse, particularly for nodular sclerosing disease. Tumour deposits are usually nodular and may cavitate or produce endobronchial lesions.

Extramedullary plasmacytoma is occasionally seen in lung parenchyma but the lung is seldom involved in multiple myeloma.

Leukaemic infiltration of minor degree is commonly seen in the lung at post mortem, although only a small percentage of patients develop clinically significant disease leading to cytodiagnosis. The clinical background is often complex and differential diagnosis of pulmonary infiltrates will include infection and cytotoxic lung damage.

In our experience confirmation of recurrent tumour is often possible cytologically. On the other hand, definitive diagnosis of *primary lymphoma* generally requires open biopsy. Respiratory samples often provide a preliminary cytological diagnosis; however sufficient material for immunophenotyping and/or genotyping is usually considered necessary for definitive diagnosis. BAL samples may be useful for this purpose[312–315] and immunoelectrophoresis of lavage fluid may also prove monoclonality[315]. Flow cytometry in combination with cytology may allow diagnosis without surgical procedures[316]. Cell block preparations are useful for immunocytochemistry[317].

Cytological findings

▶ More readily diagnosed by BAL or FNA than in sputum
▶ Large cell lymphomas easier to diagnose than small/mixed
▶ Loosely aggregated lymphoid cells, intact cytoplasm
▶ Vesicular nuclei, no moulding, nucleoli visible
▶ Subtyping possible in BAL and FNA material

The literature on the cytodiagnosis of pulmonary involvement by non-Hodgkin's lymphomas is not large. Tao[57] gives a thorough discussion of criteria for diagnosis in his monograph. Bonfiglio *et al.* reported on a series of 16 FNA cases[318]. Large cell lymphomas were most easily diagnosed. Small or mixed cell lesions were diagnostically difficult, although an unequivocal diagnosis was given in eight of 14 lymphomas sampled overall, and a strong suggestion of the diagnosis was made in a further five. Bardales *et al.*[317] report on the diagnosis of leukaemias and non-Hodgkin's lymphomas in exfoliated samples from 20 patients including five presenting with pulmonary disease. In 29 of 31 specimens a diagnosis of malignancy was made. The diagnoses of primary lung lymphoma were all confirmed histologically. A monotonous, dispersed cell population was usually seen and necrosis was often evident in washings and brushings. Gattuso *et al.* reported on seven cases of post-transplant lymphoproliferative disease involving lung[309]. They described two patterns, a polymorphous smear pattern with a spectrum of mature and immature lymphocytes and scattered histiocytes and plasma cells, and a monotonous pattern of large lymphoid cells.

Several of our cases of large B-cell lymphoma presented first with groups of loosely arranged medium-sized cells with intact cytoplasm lying within mucus streaks of sputum. Nuclei were vesicular with irregular outlines and had usually prominent, often multiple, nucleoli (Figs 3.66, 3.67). Artefactual aggregation may occur (Fig. 3.66C) and mimic epithelial clusters, but nuclear moulding is not seen nor is engulfment of apoptotic debris by tumour cells, both features of small cell carcinoma.

More abundant material is obtained by FNA and we have made preliminary diagnoses in cases of primary lymphoma later confirmed histologically (Figs 3.67, 3.68). We have seen recurrent lymphoma of various types in sputum, and small-cleaved cell tumours in brushings and FNA samples. Several of our cases of lymphomatoid granulomatosis have not yielded sufficient cells for assessment. FNA samples of several cases of low-grade lymphoplasmacytoid lymphoma yielded a monotonous population of small lymphocytes with plasmacytoid forms, and were provisionally diagnosed cytologically.

Hodgkin's lymphoma usually yields a mixed inflammatory cell background and variable numbers of Hodgkin's mononuclear cells or Reed-Sternberg cells (Figs 3.69, 3.70). Suprun and Koss[319,320] described diagnostic Reed-Sternberg cells lying singly in sputum in a background of inflammatory cells in 10 cases of Hodgkin's lymphoma. Reale *et al.*[321] described six patients in which malignant cells consistent with Hodgkin's lymphoma were seen in sputum. In two cases of nodular sclerosing disease, large cells with vacuolated cytoplasm and multilobated nuclei thought to correspond to lacunar cells were also evident. Flint *et al.*[322] reported on 13 cases of pulmonary involvement by Hodgkin's disease sampled by FNA in which classic Reed-Sternberg cells and/or lacunar cells were identified in most cases and mononuclear Hodgkin's cells in all, generally in a mixed cell background.

Wisecarver *et al.*[323] studied the appearance of Hodgkin's disease in BAL samples. Unequivocal diagnoses of

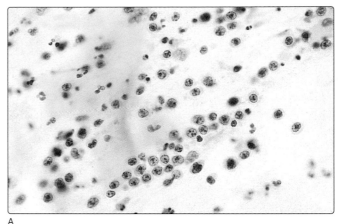

A

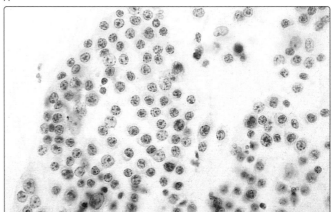

B

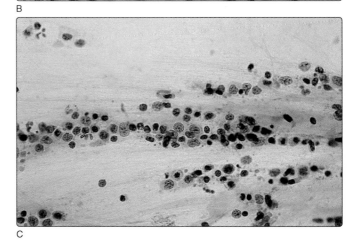

C

Fig. 3.66   Sputum: large cell/immunoblastic lymphoma. (A, B) Dispersed population of cells with vesicular rounded nuclei, multiple nucleoli and small amounts of intact cytoplasm surrounding individual cells. No aggregation. (A and B, Papanicolaou × HP) (C) Dispersal with a few apparent loose aggregates. Single cell degeneration within the abnormal cells. This pattern was not distinguishable from small cell carcinoma. (Papanicolaou × HP)

Hodgkin's lymphoma were made in six cases; the background cell population was often a marked lymphocytosis, the lymphocytes generally being small and monotonous. Reiben *et al.*[324] diagnosed intrapulmonary Hodgkin's disease with bronchial brush cytology and other cases have been reported from sputum[325], washings[317] or

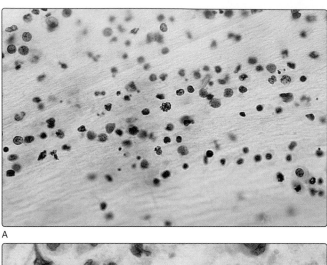

A

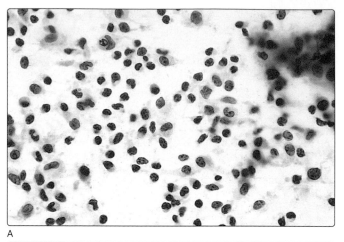

A

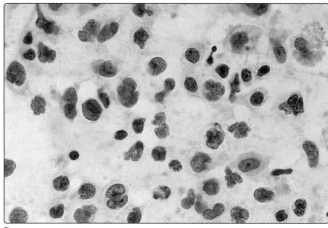

B

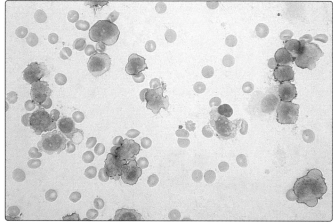

B

Fig. 3.67   Malignant lymphoma with hyperlobated nuclei. (A) Sputum: dispersed population of abnormal cells with irregular convoluted and hyperlobated nuclei. (Papanicolaou HP) (B) FNA lung/mediastinal mass: dispersed cells with unequivocal nuclear features of malignancy and suggesting hyperlobated malignant lymphoma cells. Confirmed by open biopsy. (H&E × HP)

FNA and BAL samples[326,327], including cases in which the diagnosis had not previously been suspected[325,328].

Dissemination of chronic lymphocytic leukaemia is occasionally diagnosed in sputum. Many dispersed cells showing the characteristic blocked nuclear chromatin pattern may allow confirmation of lung involvement in patients with a previous diagnosis and consistent clinical findings. However, large numbers of rather similar cells can be seen as a reactive process, e.g. in follicular bronchitis, and primary diagnosis by sputum is not made.

Single case examples of other lymphoid related lesions are reported. Ludwig and Balachandran[329] described cells with characteristic nuclear grooves or folds in bronchial wash and CSF samples from a patient with a disseminated mycosis fungoides. Rosen et al.[330] and Shaheen and Oertel[331] report similar findings in sputum and aspirates. Vernon[332] describes a signet-ring cell lymphoma, in which bronchial brushings contained lymphoid cells with variable nuclear irregularity and striking cytoplasmic vacuoles, often

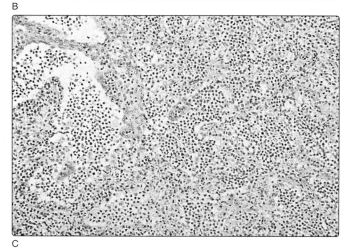

C

Fig. 3.68   FNA: non-Hodgkin's malignant lymphoma. Multiple nodules throughout both lung fields in a young woman. (A) Dispersed population of atypical lymphoid cells suggesting a lymphoproliferative disorder. (Papanicolaou × HP) (B) Cytocentrifuge preparation showing membrane staining for MT1 (Clonab) antigen in tumour cells, suggesting a T-cell lymphoma. (C) Open biopsy specimen showing non-Hodgkin's lymphoma. The tumour was an unusual T-cell neoplasm with NK cell phenotype and large granular lymphocyte morphology on electron microscopy. (H&E × MP)

compressing the nucleus; he warns of the possibility of confusion with epithelial malignancy, particularly adenocarcinoma.

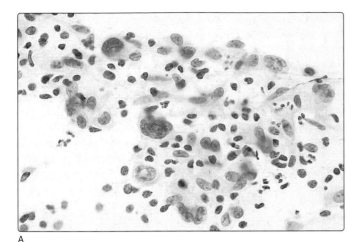

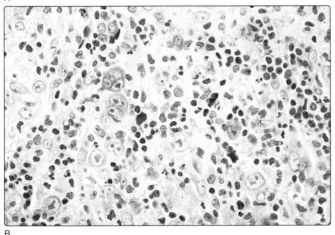

Fig. 3.69 FNA lung: Hodgkin's lymphoma. (A) Recurrent tumour within lung tissue. Syncytial masses of abnormal lymphoreticular cells including Reed-Sternberg cells. (H&E × HP) (B) Histology of previous lymph node biopsy. (H&E × MP)

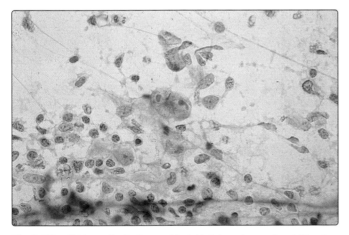

Fig. 3.70 FNA mediastinal mass: Hodgkin's lymphoma. Reed-Sternberg cell in a background of lymphoid cells and atypical mononuclear cells. Cytological findings suggesting Hodgkin's lymphoma, confirmed on formal biopsy. (Papanicolaou × HP)

Goldstein et al.[333] suggested that lung involvement by immunoblastic lymphadenopathy might be diagnosed by identifying large numbers of immunoblasts in sputum in a patient with a previous diagnosis on lymph node biopsy. Williams et al.[334] demonstrated the angioinvasive nature of the lymphoid infiltrate in cell blocks of an FNA specimen from lymphomatoid granulomatosis.

Multiple myeloma within brushings samples was documented by Riazmontazer et al.[335]; bronchial washings contained aggregates and dispersed cells in which the degree of clustering initially suggested an epithelial tumour. Chollet et al.[336] and Auerswald et al.[337] used immunostaining to quantitate Langerhans cells in BAL samples and suggested that >5% of Langerhan's cells strongly supported the diagnosis of Langerhan's histiocytosis. However an increase in these cells in lung is found in smokers and in localized reactive processes and open biopsy is still often undertaken.

Bardales et al.[317] point out several pitfalls in diagnosis including the need for immunocytochemistry to distinguish Hodgkin's lymphoma from anaplastic large cell lymphoma and other malignancies, the resemblance of megakaryocytes to malignant cells and the need to report only on blood free samples in leukaemic patients with lung infiltrates.

Sarcoma in the lung

There are reports of the diagnosis of sarcoma being made in sputum[338] and several FNA series of primary or metastatic sarcomas have been published[339,340]. They suggest that many single cells and spindle shaped cells, poorly cohesive or in flat aggregates, with fragile cytoplasm and finely granular nuclear chromatin, small nucleoli and bizarre multinucleation were general indicators of mesenchymal malignancy. A distinction between high-grade sarcoma, primary or secondary, melanoma and sarcomatoid carcinoma is usually not possible without comparison with histological material, cell block immunocytochemistry or electron microscopy. Attention has been drawn to the nuclear atypia, which may mimic malignancy in benign neural tumours.

FNA of primary and secondary malignant fibrous histiocytomas (MFH) of lung yields variable mixtures of fibroblast-like and histiocyte-like cells, including isolated large malignant cells with elongated or comet-shaped configuration, together with multinucleate forms and some loose aggregates (Fig. 3.71)[339–345]. Similar findings are reported in material from bronchial brushings[346]. Nguyen[344] documents a myxoid variant with similar appearances, but includes a pink, myxoid background. Distinction from anaplastic or spindle cell (sarcomatoid) carcinoma or melanoma is difficult[347], although the finely granular nuclear chromatin of MFH is said to contrast with the coarse granularity of carcinoma. Lipoblast-like cells may resemble a liposarcoma[343].

Kim describes similar appearances in fibrosarcomas, leiomyosarcoma and several undifferentiated sarcomas, although leiomyosarcomatous nuclei were more truncated and their cytoplasmic tails shorter[340]. Logrono et al.[348]

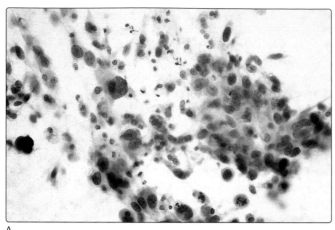

A

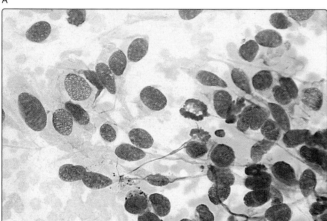

B

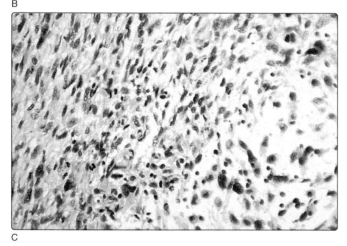

C

Fig. 3.71 FNA: metastatic malignant fibrous histiocytoma. (A) Varied population of malignant cells including some epithelial-like aggregates, spindle and giant cell forms and abundant haemosiderin pigment. (Papanicolaou × IP) (B) Predominantly spindle cell forms including mitotic figures. Fragile spindle shaped cytoplasmic processes. Diagnosis made by reference to the previous resection specimen. (MGG × HP) (C) Previous resection specimen from thigh tumour. (H&E × MP)

diagnosed primary fibrosarcoma by FNA and core biopsy with relevant immunocytochemistry including non-reactivity for keratin, S 100, desmin, alpha smooth muscle actin and CD 34. Krumerman[349] and Sawada et al.[350] describe

the cytology of several cases of primary leiomyosarcoma in which the diagnosis was made preoperatively. Other reactive processes such as inflammatory pseudotumour[351] or traumatized elements of bronchial wall enter the differential diagnosis[352].

Nguyen[353] described an example of pulmonary angiosarcoma in which bronchial brushings show clusters and sheets of round or oval nuclei with focal gland-like and cleft-like arrangements, and with pale ill-defined cytoplasm. The findings were suggestive of an epithelial tumour such as adenocarcinoma or carcinoid, and the final diagnosis required lobectomy and histological examination. Epithelioid haemangioendothelioma has been described in sputum samples[354] and presented as isolated cells or in small sheets of cells with convoluted nuclei and prominent nucleoli resembling adenocarcinoma cells.

Dermatofibrosarcoma protruberans was diagnosed by Perry et al.[355] on the basis of a storiform arrangement of slender spindle cells demonstrated in FNA smears. Nickels and Koivuniemi[356] studied five cases of malignant haemangiopericytoma in FNA samples, including three lung lesions. Knob-like formations of neoplastic cells with round or oval irregular hyperchromatic nuclei and pale indistinct cytoplasm were characteristic. Adherence of tumour cells to capillary vessels was a feature resembling carcinoid tumour. The overall findings were not considered sufficiently distinctive to be diagnostic on smears alone, although immunocytochemistry[357], ultrastructure or cell block preparations may be diagnostic. Silverman et al.[358] and Saleh et al.[359] describe cases of metastatic malignant schwannoma in FNA samples. Examples of metastatic endometrial stromal sarcoma[360], giant cell tumour of bone[361,362], chondrosarcoma of nasal sinuses[363], osteosarcoma[364], synovial sarcoma[365,366], angiosarcoma[367], pleuropulmonary blastoma of childhood[368,369], alveolar soft part sarcoma presenting as lung metastases[370], and a primary chondrosarcoma[371] are also reported. Primitive neuroectodermal tumour (PNET) is most commonly encountered as a chest wall lesion, or a metastasis but may occasionally be seen as a primary tumour of lung. Figure 3.72 shows material from a lung FNA in a 35-year-old woman. The tumour cells were positive for synaptophysin and CD 99 and negative for epithelial, lymphoid and melanocytic markers in cell block preparations. A diagnosis of PNET was made and treatment given on this basis.

Pulmonary blastoma

These tumours are rare aggressive malignant neoplasms usually situated peripherally in lung and composed of epithelial and mesenchymal elements[124]. They occur at any age, but often in younger adult males. The histological appearances resemble fetal lung. The epithelial elements consist of tubules lined by glycogen-rich columnar cells, and the mesenchymal elements are composed of small, loosely arranged spindle cells. Cartilage and smooth or

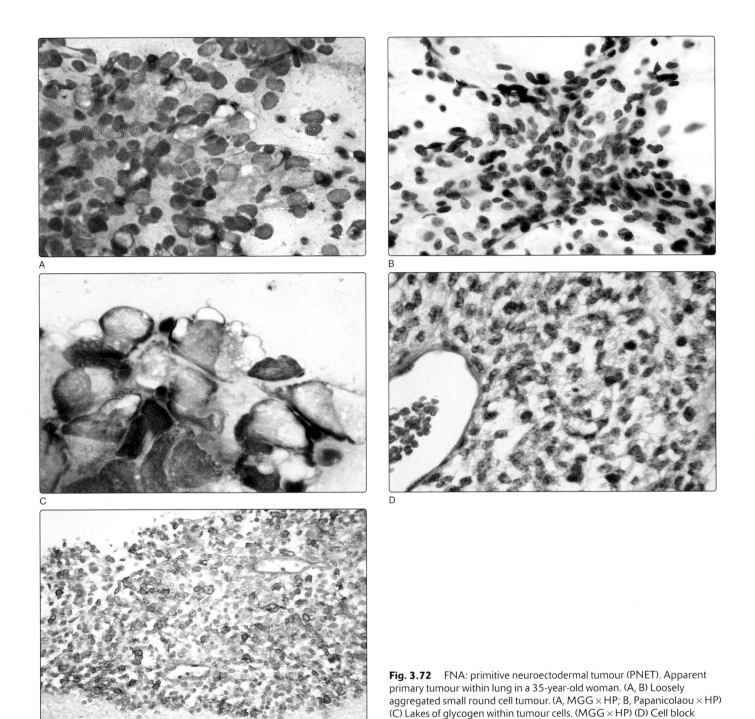

A

B

C

D

E

Fig. 3.72 FNA: primitive neuroectodermal tumour (PNET). Apparent primary tumour within lung in a 35-year-old woman. (A, B) Loosely aggregated small round cell tumour. (A, MGG × HP; B, Papanicolaou × HP) (C) Lakes of glycogen within tumour cells. (MGG × HP) (D) Cell block preparation. (H&E × HP) (E) CD 99 staining in tumour cells. (IPOX × MP)

striated muscles are sometimes seen. Immunocytochemistry suggests a true mixed epithelial-mesenchymal tumour. The early age at which many tumours occur supports a difference from carcinosarcoma or sarcomatoid carcinoma.

Cosgrove *et al.*[372] diagnosed a tumour in cell blocks of an FNA sample by observing a biphasic pattern of branching glands lined by multilayered columnar epithelium with subnuclear vacuoles and surrounded by a primitive stroma.

We have been shown a similar case (Fig. 3.73) where the diagnosis was made on FNA material. In other descriptions the epithelial component was usually evident but the mesenchymal element was more difficult to appreciate, generally leading to diagnoses of carcinoma[372–376]. In our single case, in brushings of recurrent tumour, small malignant cells with a rather close resemblance to small cell carcinoma were seen (Fig. 3.74). The epithelial and mesenchymal elements may merge.

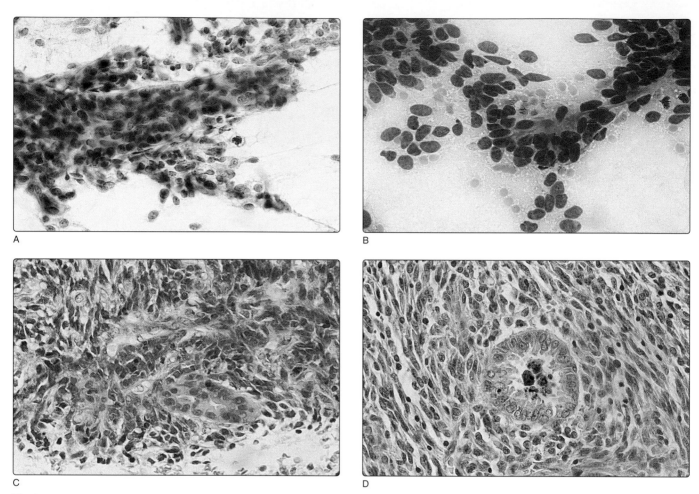

Fig. 3.73 FNA: pulmonary blastoma. (A) Aspirated material from lung lesion showing a biphasic pattern including epithelial-like and mesenchymal-like cells. (Papanicolaou × HP) (B) Predominantly spindle cell morphology. (MGG × HP) (C) Cell block from metastasis within abdomen showing biphasic glandular and primitive mesenchymal pattern. (H&E × MP) (D) Lung resection specimen showing biphasic glandular and primitive stromal pattern. (H&E × MP) The diagnosis in this case was made following the aspiration of the abdominal metastasis.

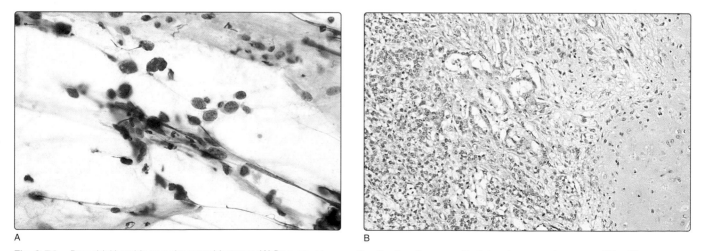

Fig. 3.74 Bronchial brushings: pulmonary blastoma. (A) Recurrent tumour. Small cell malignancy of indeterminate type but compatible with recurrent blastoma. (Papanicolaou × HP) (B) Resected specimen showing biphasic glandular and primitive stromal pattern, together with cartilage. (H&E × LP)

In Non's case[374], tumour cell aggregates resembled the clusters of endometrial stromal cells seen in so-called exodus in cervical smears, and endometriosis might also be a consideration. Malignant teratoma, Wilm's tumour or other biphasic lesions such as synovial sarcoma are difficult to exclude without detailed clinical information or evaluation of serum markers or histological material. Lee and Cho[377] report on the cytological findings in a case of adenocarcinoma of foetal type which may have some relationship to blastoma.

Pulmonary carcinosarcoma

This rare neoplasm, composed of malignant epithelial and bizarre sarcomatous components, often presents with a pedunculated mass affecting a major bronchus. It is likely that the lesion represents a form of sarcomatoid carcinoma and there is a similar prognosis to other poorly differentiated lung cell carcinomas. Cabarcos et al.[378] reported polygonal squamous cells and fusiform fibrosarcomatous cells in an FNA sample. In the case of Finley et al.[379], FNA cytodiagnosis depended on identifying squamous epithelial and mesenchymal smear patterns and dual staining for keratins and vimentin. Ishizuka et al.[380] describe a case in which sputum samples showed a combination of malignant squamous and rhabdomyosarcomatous cells with cross striations allowing the diagnosis to be suggested.

Mediastinal tumours

A broad range of neoplasms is encountered in this site (Table 3.2). Approximately 40% of mediastinal masses are malignant. Tumours in children are more likely to be neurogenic neoplasms, enterogenous cysts, teratomatous or vascular lesions. In adults, the most common lesions are metastases, cysts of thymic, pericardial or enteric origin, followed by thymomas, neurogenic tumours and lymphomas, with lesser numbers of germ cell tumours. All lesions are accessible to fine needle sampling by transthoracic, transbronchial or transtracheal routes[16,17,381–385]. Powers et al.[386], in a multi-institutional analysis, report metastatic carcinoma in 60% of lesions sampled by FNA; malignant lymphoma and thymoma were the most frequent primary tumours. Shabb et al.[387] gave a correct diagnosis in 86% of lesions sampled. A total of 57% of their cases were primary neoplasms, 24% were metastases and 12% were other benign conditions.

FNA of this site has a low rate of complication and can be performed safely even when superior vena caval obstruction is present[388]. FNA by the transbronchial or transcranial routes is particularly useful for the diagnosis and staging of metastatic lung carcinoma. Mediastinal cystography is useful in the diagnosis of cysts or in cyst drainage. Fluoroscopy and CT are generally necessary for needle guidance and the latter has the advantage of localizing the needle tip to within millimetres, thus avoiding such rare

---

Table 3.2   Mediastinal tumours (adapted from WHO Classification[390])

Thymoma
Spindle/medullary (A); lymphocyte rich/predominantly cortical (B1); cortical (B2); mixed (AB); epithelial/atypical (B3)
Encapsulated; minimally invasive; widely invasive

Thymic carcinoma
Squamous cell carcinoma (keratinizing; non-keratinizing)
Lymphoepithelioma-like
Sarcomatoid
Clear cell
Basaloid
Mucoepidermoid
Papillary
Undifferentiated

Neuroendocrine neoplasms
Carcinoid tumour (typical, atypical; spindle, pigmented)
Small cell carcinoma and variants
Large cell neuroendocrine carcinoma

Lymphoproliferative disease
Castleman's disease (angiofollicular lymphoid hyperplasia)
Non-Hodgkin's lymphoma
Large cell lymphoma, B-cell, with sclerosis
Lymphoblastic
Marginal zone lymphoma of mucosa associated lymphoid tissue (MALT)
Hodgkin's lymphoma

Neural neoplasms
Schwannoma

Neurofibroma
Ganglioneuroma/ganglioneuroblastoma
Neuroblastoma
Paraganglioma
Neurogenic sarcoma

Germ cell neoplasms
Seminoma (germinoma)
Non-seminomatous germ cell tumours
  Teratoma: mature; immature
  Embryonal carcinoma
  Endodermal sinus/yolk sac tumour
  Choriocarcinoma
  Mixed tumours

Non-neoplastic cystic lesions
Bronchogenic cyst
Oesophageal and gastroenteric cyst
Thymic cyst unilocular/multilocular (associated with Hodgkin's lymphoma, germinoma; AIDS)
Pericardial cyst
Lymphangioma

Other mediastinal mass lesions
Thymic hyperplasia
Thyroid enlargement: retrosternal or ectopic
  Multinodular goitre
  Thyroid neoplasms
Parathyroid adenoma

complications as cardiac puncture. CT scanning also can exclude aneurysm and delineate relationships with adjacent structures, including large vessels.

The authors' approach to diagnosis relies particularly on cell block preparations and electron microscopy because of the extraordinary variability of neoplasms of this site. Dabbs and Silverman[110] and Taccagni et al.[114] emphasized the value of ultrastructural diagnosis particularly for thymoma, germ cell tumours, carcinoid tumours and small cell carcinoma. Geisinger summarizes differential diagnostic problems and potential pitfalls in this site[389].

Thymoma

Thymic epithelial neoplasms are a common primary neoplasm of the anterior mediastinum. Most cases are biologically benign encapsulated lesions, although in up to 20% of cases, invasion of adjacent tissues including pleura, pericardium and/or lung may occur. This pattern of invasive growth may be seen in lesions of quite benign cytological appearance, without significant nuclear pleomorphism or mitotic activity. Epithelial thymomas show a range of cell size and morphology lymphocyte content; in some neoplasms the epithelial cells may be completely obscured by accompanying lymphocytes showing various degrees of activation.

The WHO classification of thymic epithelial tumours (see Table 3.2) is histogenetically based, and may not be easily applicable to cytological or small biopsy samples[390]. Other classifications recognize a spectrum of differentiation from thymoma through atypical thymoma to thymic carcinoma[391]. Tao et al.[392] subdivided their cases of thymic neoplasms cytologically into small, intermediate and large epithelial cell types with or without an accompanying lymphocytic component, large pleomorphic epithelial cell type (cytologically malignant and presumably corresponding to thymic carcinoma), and spindle cell tumours.

Cytological findings[383,392–400]

► Cohesive aggregates of epithelial cells
► Variable lymphocytic infiltration; may obscure fragments
► Epithelial cells have pale cytoplasm, regular nuclei
► Spindle cell types show granular chromatin

In our experience benign thymomas give rise to cohesive fragments with virtually no free epithelial cells (Fig. 3.75). Lymphocytic infiltration may almost completely obscure epithelial cells and it requires close scrutiny to detect epithelial cells within aggregates (Fig. 3.75). The component epithelial cells usually have oval or rounded pale vesicular nuclei with small nucleoli and minimal mitotic activity (Figs 3.75, 3.76). Cytoplasm is moderate in amount, pale and with indistinct borders. Spindle cell tumours show a more homogeneous granular chromatin and less conspicuous nucleoli (Fig. 3.77). Lymphoepithelial

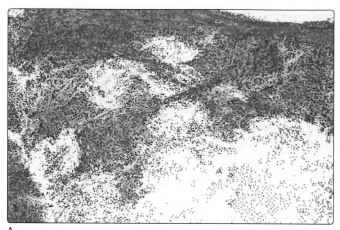

A

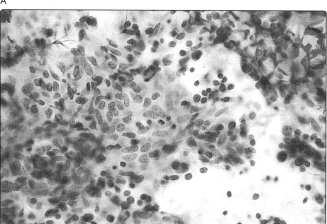

B

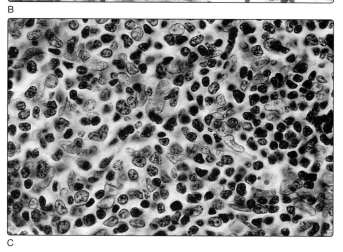

C

Fig. 3.75 FNA: lymphoepithelial thymoma. (A) Cohesive tissue fragments with a background of dispersed lymphoid cells. (Papanicolaou × LP) (B) Biphasic pattern of cohesive oval or spindle cells and a background of smaller lymphoid cells. (Papanicolaou × HP) (C) Resected tumour with biphasic epithelial/spindle cell pattern. (H&E × HP)

tumours may be diagnosed on cytological findings alone, but confirmation of the epithelial nature of the tumour cells by immunohistochemistry is now routine and is essential for spindle cell tumours without a lymphoid component, when mesenchymal tumours enter the differential diagnosis.

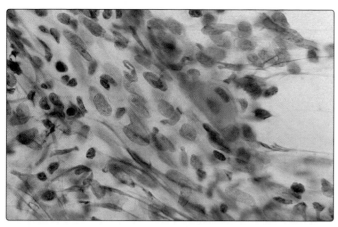

Fig. 3.76   FNA: lymphoepithelial thymoma. Metastatic tumour within lung tissue. Hassall's corpuscles with surrounding oval epithelial cells and a smaller component of lymphoid cells. (Papanicolaou × HP)

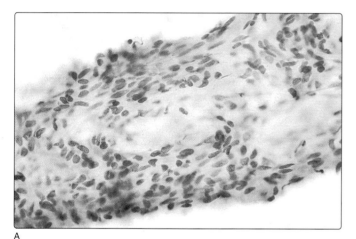

A

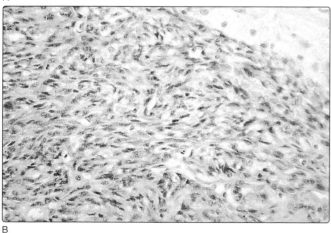

B

Fig. 3.77   FNA: spindle cell thymoma. (A) Cohesive fragment of spindle cells. (H&E × MP) (B) Resection specimen. (H&E × MP)

Diagnostic pitfalls

In tumours with a high lymphoid content, Hodgkin's or non-Hodgkin's lymphoma and angiofollicular lymphoid hyperplasia are all considerations. The degree of cohesiveness of the tissue in thymoma is generally unlike that in Hodgkin's or non-Hodgkin's lymphoma. However, attention has been drawn to sclerosing large cell non-Hodgkin's lymphoma as a source of error in this regard[401]. These tumours present with large fragments of cohesive cells consisting of a mixture of lymphoid cells and a background of connective tissue. The light microscopic pattern may mimic epithelial thymoma or carcinoma. Cell block sections demonstrating keratin or EMA staining in thymomas[393], and lymphoid markers in large cell lymphomas, are the most useful ancillary tests (see Fig. 3.80)

Spindle cell tumours, including connective tissue neoplasms of various types, mesothelioma, or submesothelial fibromas may all be difficult to distinguish from spindle cell thymoma without ancillary investigations. Electron microscopy often proves valuable. Slagel *et al.* describe a range of lesions presenting with spindle cells in FNA samples. Eleven percent of their series of mediastinal lesions had a significant component of spindle cells, including examples of inflammatory lesions, lymphomas of Hodgkin's and non-Hodgkin's type, connective tissue neoplasms, melanoma, squamous carcinoma and thymoma[402].

Some tumours may be predominantly cystic and misinterpreted as non-neoplastic unless care is taken to sample the wall of the lesion[403].

Malignant thymoma

Two distinct subgroups are recognized. The first is a group of tumours without cytological evidence of malignancy, with aggressive local behaviour. Such tumours may occasionally metastasize (Fig. 3.76). The diagnosis usually requires a combination of clinical/surgical assessment and open biopsy for accurate assessment.

Spahr and Frable[404] describe a case of invasive thymoma that exfoliated tumour cells into bronchial brushings and washings samples. Clusters of epithelial cells and a background of lymphocytes were evident, and these were closely intermixed in some of the material. The epithelial cells showed benign morphology.

The second group of cytologically malignant tumours (thymic carcinoma) are uncommon[405,406]. There is a wide range of histological subtypes, including keratinizing squamous cell, large cell non-keratinizing, lymphoepithelioma-like, sarcomatoid, basaloid, mucoepidermoid, clear cell and small cell types. In several of our cases a cytological diagnosis of carcinoma could be made, and origin from thymus suggested, although a specific origin from thymus can only be accepted after clinical and biopsy evidence excludes other primary sites (Fig. 3.78). Some biologically aggressive cases with less obvious malignant cytological features may also be encountered (Fig. 3.79)[407].

Neuroendocrine tumours

The full range of neuroendocrine epithelial tumours is found here although carcinoid tumours tend to be atypical

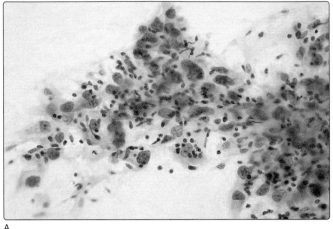

A

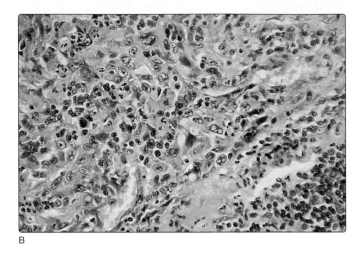

B

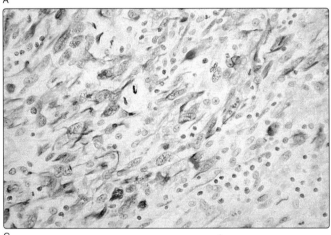

C

Fig. 3.78   FNA: malignant thymoma (thymic carcinoma) (A) Disorganized aggregate of large malignant cells. The degree of cohesion suggests an epithelial origin. Background of lymphocytes. Thymic carcinoma was suggested when clinical evaluation revealed no other primary lesion (H&E × HP) (B, C) Resected specimen. Anaplastic malignancy with epithelial features confirmed on staining for cytokeratins. (B, H&E × HP; C, Cytokeratin stain AE1-AE3 × HP)

in morphology and biologically aggressive. Diagnosis by FNA, cell block immunocytochemistry and electron microscopy is well described[408–410]. A spindle cell tumour has been reported in FNA material[411].

Lymphoma

The primary diagnosis of non-Hodgkin's lymphoma in this site and a distinction from Hodgkin's lymphoma or other anaplastic malignancies requires immunophenotyping and sometimes genotyping. Cytological diagnosis may be used for management for recurrent tumours and when sufficient material for ancillary testing by flow cytometry, or cell block or thin core biopsy material is also available. Figure 3.80 shows FNA material from a mediastinal mass in a 60 year-old man. A diagnosis of malignancy was made on smears, but definitive tumour typing as a B-cell non-Hodgkin's lymphoma was made on a thin core sample. Tumour cells were negative for epithelial and melanocytic markers and negative for Hodgkin's disease markers.

Germ cell tumours

Seminoma (germinoma) is most commonly seen in young adult males. Predominantly cystic forms are described and tumour deposits may undergo massive necrosis[412]. Lung and mediastinum are also sites of metastasis from testicular tumours (Fig. 3.81). Primary benign cystic teratomas occur here (Fig. 3.82), as well as teratocarcinomas (Fig. 3.83), embryonal carcinoma, endodermal sinus tumours (Fig. 3.84) and choriocarcinoma, or combinations of these.

A combination of cytological findings and serum estimations of markers such as β-HCG or αFP may allow unequivocal diagnosis and management without recourse to open biopsy (Figs 3.83, 3.84)[413,414]. Motoyama found that among the germ cell tumours only germinomas could be specifically diagnosed in smears but that thymomas were easily distinguished from germ cell tumours.[414] Placental alkaline phosphatase, CD 30, keratins, alpha-fetoprotein and hCG were useful in differential diagnosis. Further cytological descriptions are found in Chapter 19.

Neural tumours

These lesions are discussed in more detail in Chapter 40. Dahlgren and Ovenfors describe the findings in a series of schwannian tumours[415]. Palombini and Vetrani[416,417] outline the FNA pattern in mediastinal ganglioneuroblastoma and ganglioneuroma; in one case there was a mixture of polyhedral cells including binucleate forms with abundant

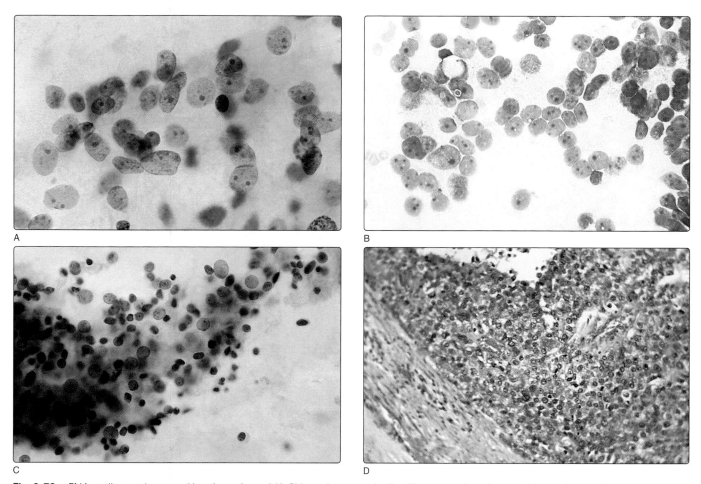

Fig. 3.79   FNA: malignant thymoma (thymic carcinoma) (A, B) Loosely arranged cells with some nuclear pleomorphism and rosette formation. Borderline cytological criteria of malignancy. (Papanicolaou × HP; MGG × HP) (C) Sputum cytology: loose aggregates of neoplastic cells with a background of lymphocytes. (Papanicolaou × HP) (D) Tumour tissue within inferior vena cava at necropsy. (H&E × MP)

eosinophilic cytoplasm and smaller cells with an oval or spindle shape. Some of the larger cells closely resembled neurons, with axonal projections. The findings suggested ganglioneuroblastoma and were confirmed by elevated VMA and HVA estimations. In other cases, the fibrillar material between tumour cells, especially evident in MGG preparations and thought to correspond to collections of neurites emanating from tumour cells, was an important diagnostic feature.

Other mediastinal tumours

Heimann *et al.*[418] describe a case of thymolipoma where lymphoid cells, mature adipose tissue and groups of epithelial cells were found in FNA samples and included a few Hassall's corpuscles. Immunostaining of lymphocytes for pan-T and antithymocyte markers was positive and cytokeratin was demonstrated in the epithelial cells. The large size of the lesion and fat density on CT scanning were features in support of the diagnosis. Mishriki *et al.*[419] diagnosed a Hurthle cell neoplasm arising in mediastinal ectopic thyroid in a FNA sample in conjunction with electron microscopy, and De Las Casas *et al.* report a similar

case diagnosed on intraoperative cytology[420]. Attal *et al.* diagnosed myxoid liposarcoma based on the distinctive arborizing vascular pattern and myxoid background[421]. Cytological findings in mediastinal melanotic schwannomas were described by Marco *et al.*[422] and Prieto-Rodriguez *et al.*[423].

Accuracy of diagnosis

Sensitivity of diagnosis of malignancy

For sputum cytology, sensitivity ranges from around 50–60% for peripheral lesions and metastases, to 70–85% for central lesions when five or six specimens can be examined[1–3,46,48,49,61–63]. Sensitivity may be as low as 40% in routine practice[424]. Blood stained specimens and larger tumours are associated with a higher yield[94]. A tabular literature review by Bocking[97] gives a useful summary of the range of results. Bronchoscopic brushings and washings achieve 90% sensitivity for central lesions and 70% for peripheral lesions[4,5,48,61,63,68,354,425,426]. By adding transbronchial FNA, this accuracy can be extended[6–11]. Bronchoalveolar lavage gives similar sensitivity in some authors'

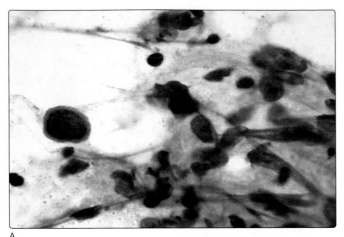

A

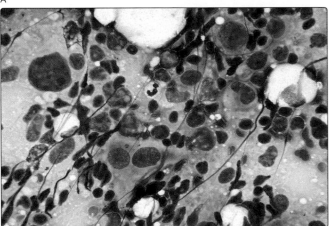

B

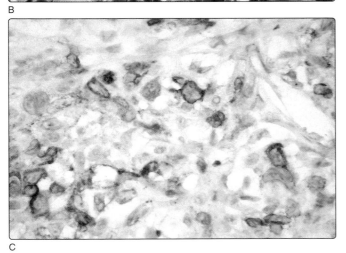

C

Fig. 3.80   FNA: large B-cell non-Hodgkin's lymphoma. (A, B) Mixed cell population of large malignant cells, some small lymphoid cells, and connective tissue elements. (A, H&E × HP; B, MGG × HP) (C) Thin core sample showing positive immunostaining for B cell marker (CD 20). (IPOX × HP)

hands[13,14,38,39]. The sensitivity of fibreoptic bronchoscopic biopsy (for histology) is similar, around 90% for central and up to 70–80% for more peripheral lesions; brushings and biopsy are complementary. Multiple sampling often increases the yield[427].

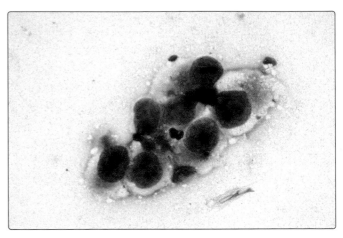

Fig. 3.81   FNA lung: metastatic testicular seminoma. Aggregate of tumour cells with abundant pale cytoplasm, large nuclei and macronucleoli. The tumour was more cohesive than the usual seminoma. (MGG × HP)

Fine needle aspiration sensitivity is usually over 80% and up to 95% in selected series[15,42–44,58], varying according to the size and depth of the lesion and the experience of the radiologist[428]. A negative result by any single diagnostic method cannot exclude malignancy; however, using a selection or combination of these diagnostic methods up to 98% of central lesions and 94% of peripheral lung tumours may be diagnosed pretherapeutically[55]. In special sites such as the mediastinum a cytological diagnosis may be reached in 80% of cases[16,17,386].

Comparisons of the accuracy of the various techniques used to obtain cytological material suggest that these are complementary and that the physician can select which may be most effective based on the clinical features of the lesion for individual patients. Considerations such as the economics of hospital stay may also enter into such assessment.

Predictive value of malignant diagnosis

A 100% predictive value of malignant diagnosis is the aim, because cytological diagnosis is to be used for definitive management decisions[429,430]. The positive predictive value of malignancy has been near this level for experienced workers for many years.

In our own practice, we have had rare false positive diagnoses of malignancy over the last 15 years. For example, a case of highly atypical reactive bronchial epithelial proliferation in sputum was interpreted as metastatic adenocarcinoma in a patient with a previous history of colonic carcinoma. In FNA material we have misdiagnosed malignancy in an atypical mesothelial cell reaction, the epithelial proliferation in chondroid hamartoma, pleomorphic fibroblastic cells in benign pleural fibroma, and a mediastinal ectopic multinodular thyroid tissue. However, the false positive rate overall has been less than 0.1% of malignant diagnoses and this is of a similar order to most recent reports for sputum, brushings and FNA diagnoses.

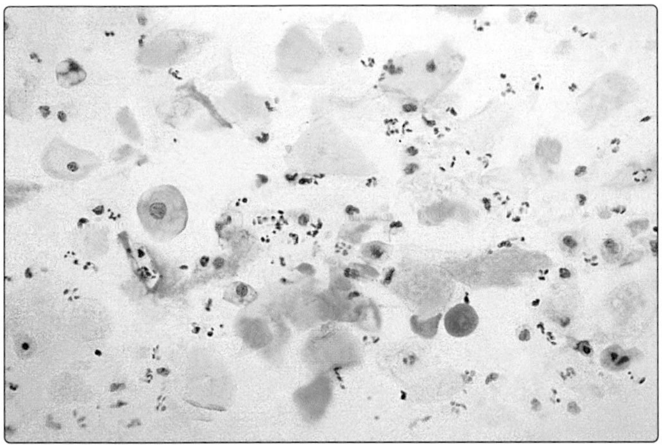

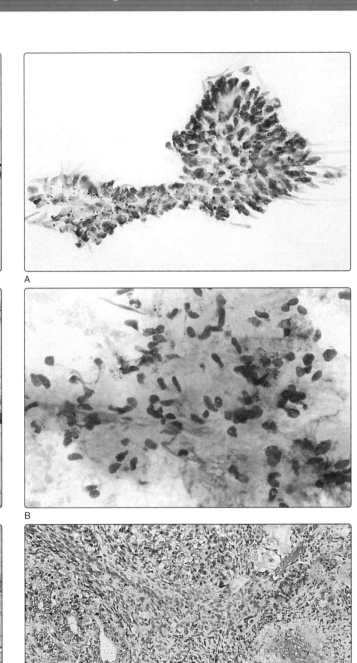

Fig. 3.82 FNA: cystic mature teratoma of mediastinum. (A) Anucleate squamous cells, keratinous debris and mature squamous cells together with an inflammatory cell component. (Papanicolaou × HP) (B) Ciliated columnar epithelium in a background of mucoid debris. (MGG × HP) (C) Resected tumour showing mature endodermal and ectodermal elements. (H&E × LP)

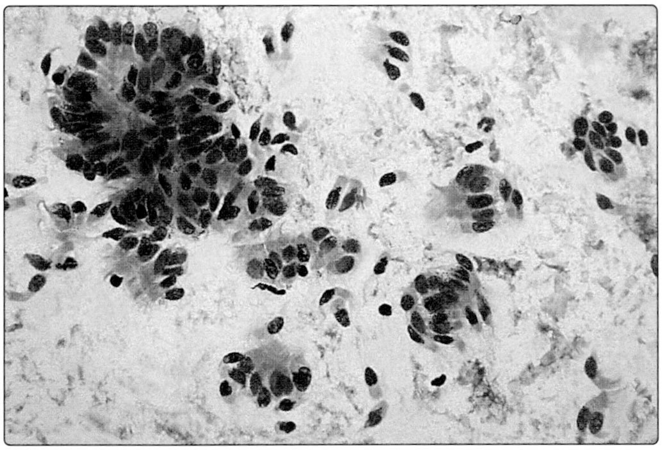

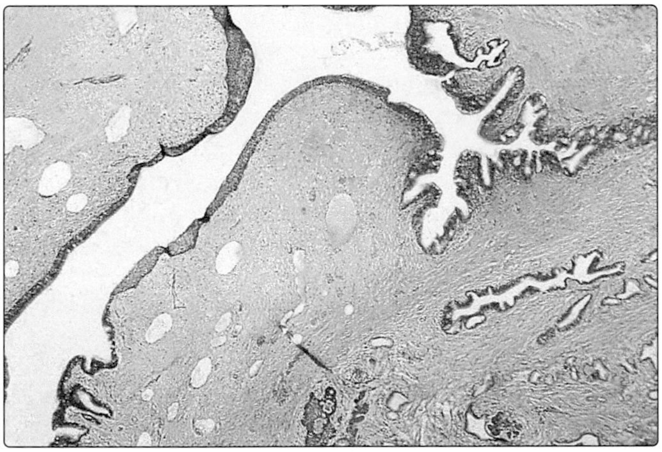

Fig. 3.83 FNA: primary malignant teratoma involving lung and mediastinum. (A) Cohesive epithelial elements with malignant nuclear features and abundant apoptotic debris. (Papanicolaou × HP) (B) Fibromyxoid mesenchymal tissue. (MGG × HP) (C) Resected tumour showing glandular and mesenchymal elements together with areas of cartilage formation. (H&E × MP) On the FNA findings, consideration was given to diagnoses of pulmonary blastoma or metastatic Wilm's tumour as well as teratoma. The patient was treated as teratoma on the basis of the cytological findings and markedly elevated serum markers prior to resection of the mass.

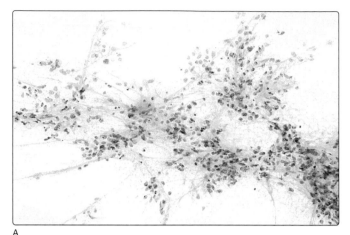

A

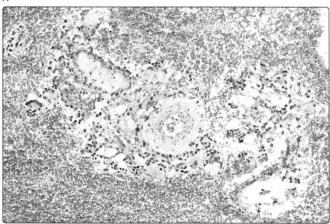

B

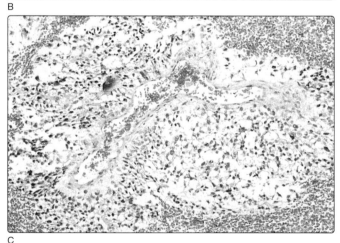

C

Fig. 3.84   FNA: metastatic endodermal sinus tumour within lung and mediastinum. (A) Loosely arranged neoplastic tissue but without specific diagnostic features. (H&E × MP) (B, C) Cell block preparations with histological pattern in keeping with metastatic endodermal sinus tumour. (H&E × MP)

A diagnosis of 'markedly atypical' cells may even be associated with over 99.9% specificity for malignancy[431]. Recent reviews highlight the most likely non-neoplastic cytological mimics of malignancy[432–434]. Kern[435,436] and Cagle[437] allude to the difficulty of obtaining cytohistological correlation after a marked decline in autopsy rates, pointing

out that there is a tendency to overestimate false positive rates if cytohistological correlation is based on subsequent biopsy, particularly endoscopic, without adequate clinical followup. Caya et al.[438] suggest that only open lung biopsy, autopsy or the results of long term clinical follow-up should be used in evaluating accuracy.

Tumour typing

Sputum cytology provides extremely accurate tumour subtyping; for typing small cell carcinoma; sputum may be the most accurate modality[46]. Definitive typing of squamous cell and adenocarcinoma is also extremely accurate in sputum[2,3,46]. The accuracy of tumour typing for FNA and brushings is high, with over 90% sensitivity and predictive value[43,44].

For small cell carcinoma FNA gives over 90% sensitivity of diagnosis and most workers show a very high predictive value/specificity[43,44,79,439]. However in some workers experience only 90% of diagnoses are confirmed[440], and there is thus room for conservatism and a cautious approach to small cell carcinoma diagnosis by FNA. In problematic cases, repeat cytology or biopsy specimens are of most value.

In brushings and FNA samples subtyping of large cell carcinomas is more difficult than in sputum although approximately 80% of large cell tumours may be typed accurately and up to 80–90% of predictions of type are correct[43,44].

Hess et al.[140] reviewed cytological criteria for tumour typing and suggested that revised data based on objective cytoplasmic features of functional differentiation allowed a more reliable diagnosis. Their categories had more in common with ultrastructural characterization of lung tumours than conventional histological diagnosis and led to a high proportion of diagnosis of combined squamous and glandular tumours and few cases of large cell anaplastic carcinoma. Similar views were expressed by Mennemeyer[141]. Such studies have further emphasized the heterogeneity of lung cancer and the high frequency of ultrastructural evidence of both glandular and squamous differentiation in tumours from non-small cell categories.

Diagnosis of benign neoplasms

Dahlgren et al.[394] diagnosed eight of 13 thymomas by FNA; schwannoma, lymphoma and carcinoid tumours provided some diagnostic difficulty. Tao et al.[392] were able to diagnose all of the 37 FNA cases they encountered and, in most of our cases, FNA material with or without ancillary testing allowed diagnosis. Dahlgren et al.[415] diagnosed most benign neurogenic tumours although 18 gauge needles were used; in our experience, diagnostic material is difficult to obtain with 23 or 22 gauge needles in deep neural neoplasms and thin core sampling is of value if clinically feasible. Over 90% of chondroid hamartomas can be recognized by FNA[289–291]. Reports of most other benign neoplasms involve only small numbers of cases.

References

1   Johnston W W, Bossen E H. Ten years of respiratory cytopathology at Duke University Medical Centre. I. The cytopathologic diagnosis of lung cancer during the years 1970 to 1974, noting the significance of specimen number and type. *Acta Cytol* 1981; **25**: 103–107

2   Koss L G, Melamed M R, Goodner J T. Pulmonary cytology – a brief survey of diagnostic results from 1 July 1952 until 31 December 1960. *Acta Cytol* 1964; **8**: 104–113

3   Ng A B P, Horak G C. Factors significant in the diagnostic accuracy of lung cytology in bronchial washing and sputum samples. II. Sputum samples. *Acta Cytol* 1983; **27**: 397–402

4   Bibbo M, Fennessy J J, Lu C-T et al. Bronchial brushing technique for the cytologic diagnosis of peripheral lung lesions. A review of 693 cases. *Acta Cytol* 1973; **17**: 245–251

5   Ng A B P, Horak G C. Factors significant in the diagnostic accuracy of lung cytology in bronchial washing and sputum samples. I. Bronchial washings. *Acta Cytol* 1983; **27**: 391–396

6   Bhat N, Bhagat P, Pearlman E et al. Transbronchial needle aspiration biopsy in the diagnosis of pulmonary neoplasms. *Diagn Cytopathol* 1990; **6**: 14–17

7   Horsley J R, Miller R E, Amy R W M, King E G. Bronchial submucosal needle aspiration performed through the fiberoptic bronchoscope. *Acta Cytol* 1984; **28**: 211–217

8   Rosenthal D L, Wallace J M. Fine needle aspiration of pulmonary lesions via fiberoptic bronchoscopy. *Acta Cytol* 1984; **28**: 203–210

9   Schenk D A, Bower J H, Bryan C L et al. Transbronchial needle aspiration staging of bronchogenic carcinoma. *Am Rev Respir Dis* 1986; **134**: 246–248

10 Wang K P. Flexible transbronchial needle aspiration biopsy for histologic specimens. *Chest* 1985; **88**: 860–863

11 Reichenberger F, Weber J, Tamm M et al. The value of transbronchial needle aspiration in the diagnosis of peripheral pulmonary lesions. *Chest* 1999; **116**: 704–708

12 Govert J A, Dodd L G, Kussin P S, Samuelson W M. A prospective comparison of fiberoptic transbronchial needle aspiration and bronchial biopsy for bronchoscopically visible lung carcinoma. *Cancer* 1999; **87**: 129–134

13 Levy H, Horak D A, Lewis M I. The value of bronchial washings and bronchoalveolar lavage in the diagnosis of lymphangitic carcinomatosis. *Chest* 1988; **94**: 1028–1030

14 Linder J, Radio S J, Robbins R A et al. Bronchoalveolar lavage in the cytologic diagnosis of carcinoma of the lung. *Acta Cytol* 1987; **31**: 796–801

15 Levine M S, Weiss J M, Harrell J H et al. Transthoracic needle aspiration biopsy following negative fiberoptic bronchoscopy in solitary pulmonary nodules. *Chest* 1988; **93**: 1152–1155

16 Adler O B, Rosenberger A, Peleg H. Fine needle aspiration biopsy of mediastinal masses: evaluation of 136 experiences. *AJR* 1983; **140**: 893–896

17 Bartholdy N J, Anderson M J, Thommesen P. Clinical value of percutaneous fine needle aspiration biopsy of mediastinal masses. Analysis of 132 cases. *Scand J Thor Cardiovasc Surg* 1984; **18**: 81–83

18 Rohwedder J J. The solitary pulmonary nodule. A new diagnostic agenda. *Chest* 1988; **93**: 1124–1125

19 Arakawa H, Nakajima Y, Kurihara Y et al. CT-guided transthoracic needle biopsy: a comparison between automated biopsy gun and fine needle aspiration. *Clin Radiol* 1996; **51**: 503–506.

20 Bocking A, Klose K C, Kyll H J, Hauptmann S. Cytologic versus histologic evaluation of needle biopsy of the lung, hilum and mediastinum. Sensitivity, specificity and typing accuracy. *Acta Cytol* 1995; **39**: 463–471.

21 Greif J, Marmor S, Schwarz Y, Staroselsky A N. Percutaneous core needle biopsy vs. fine needle aspiration in diagnosing benign lung lesions. *Acta Cytol* 1999; **43**: 756–760.

22 Grunze H, Spriggs A. *History of Clinical Cytology*. A selection of documents. Darmstadt: G-I-T Verlag Ernst Giebeler, 1980

23 Dudgeon L S, Wrigley C H. On the demonstration of particles of malignant growth in the sputum by smears of the wet film method. *J Laryngol Otol* 1935; **50**: 752–763

24 Wandall H H. A study on neoplastic cells in sputum as a contribution to the diagnosis of primary lung cancer. *Acta Chir Scand* 1944; **91**(suppl 93): 1–143

25 Foot N C. Identification of types of pulmonary cancer in cytologic smears. *Am J Pathol* 1952; **28**: 963–977

26 Woolner L B, McDonald J R. Diagnosis of carcinoma of the lung; value of cytologic study of sputum and bronchial secretions. *JAMA* 1949; **139**: 497–502

27 Papanicolaou G N, Koprowska I. Carcinoma-in-situ of the right lower bronchus; case report. *Cancer* 1951; **4**: 141–146

28 Auerbach O, Stout A P, Hammond E C, Garfinkel L. Changes in bronchial epithelium in relation to cigarette smoking and in relation to lung cancer. *N Engl J Med* 1961; **265**: 253–267

29 Nasiell M. Metaplasia and atypical metaplasia in the bronchial epithelium: a histopathologic and cytopathologic study. *Acta Cytol* 1966; **10**: 421–427

30 Saccomanno G, Archer V E, Auerbach O et al. Development of carcinoma of the lung as reflected in exfoliated cells. *Cancer* 1974; **33**: 256–270

31 Woolner L B, Fontana R S, Cortese D A et al. Roentgenographically occult lung cancer: pathologic findings and frequency of multicentricity during a 10 year period. *Mayo Clinic Proc* 1984; **59**: 453–466

32 Saccomanno G, Huth G C, Auerbach O, Kuschner M. Relationship of radioactive radon daughters and cigarette smoking in the genesis of lung cancer in uranium miners. *Cancer* 1988; **62**: 1402–1408

33 Greenberg S D, Hurst G A, Christianson S C et al. Pulmonary cytopathology of former asbestos workers. Report of the first year. *Am J Clin Pathol* 1976; **66**: 815–822

34 Whitaker D. Asbestos bodies in sputum. *Acta Cytol* 1978; **22**: 443–444

35 Hattori S, Matsuda M, Sugiyama T, Matsuda H. Cytologic diagnosis of early lung cancer: brushing method under X-ray television fluoroscopy. *Dis Chest* 1964; **45**: 129–142

36 Hattori S, Matsuda M, Nishihara H, Horai T. Early diagnosis of small peripheral lung cancer — cytologic diagnosis of very fresh cancer cells obtained by the TV-brushing technique. *Acta Cytol* 1971; **15**: 460–467

37 Hunninghake G W, Gadek J E, Kawanami O et al. Inflammatory and immune processes in the human lung in health and disease: evaluation by bronchoalveolar lavage. *Am J Pathol* 1979; **97**: 149–206

38 Sestini P, Rottoli L, Gotti C et al. Bronchoalveolar lavage diagnosis of bronchioloalveolar carcinoma. *Eur J Resp Dis* 1985; **66**: 55–58

39 Springmeyer S C, Hackman R, Carlson J J, McClellan J E. Bronchioloalveolar cell carcinoma diagnosed by bronchoalveolar lavage. *Chest* 1983; **83**: 278–279

40 Menetrier P. Cancer primitif du poumon. *Bull Soc Anat* 1886; **61**: 643–647

41 Dahlgren S E, Nordenstrom B. *Transthoracic Needle Biopsy*. Stockholm: Almquist and Wiksell, 1966

42 Dahlgren S E. Aspiration biopsy of intrathoracic tumours. *Acta Pathol Microbiol Scand (B)* 1967; **70**: 566–576

43 Johnston W W. Percutaneous fine needle aspiration biopsy of the lung. A study of 1015 patients. *Acta Cytol* 1984; **28**: 218–224

44 Mitchell M L, King D E, Bonfiglio T A, Patten S F Jr. Pulmonary fine needle aspiration cytopathology. A five year correlation study. *Acta Cytol* 1984; **28**: 72–76

45 Fraire A E, McLarty J W, Greenberg S D. Changing utilization of cytopathology versus histopathology in the diagnosis of lung cancer. *Diagn Cytopathol* 1991; **7**: 359–362

46 Johnston W W, Bossen E H. Ten years of respiratory cytopathology at Duke University Medical Center. II. A comparison between cytopathology and histopathology in typing of lung cancer between the years 1970–1974. *Acta Cytol* 1981; **25**: 499–505

47 Johnston W W. Ten years of respiratory cytopathology at Duke University Medical Centre. III. The significance of inconclusive cytopathologic diagnosis during the years 1970 to 1974. *Acta Cytol* 1982; **26**: 759–766

48 Johnston W W. Fine needle aspiration biopsy versus sputum and bronchial material in the diagnosis of lung cancer. A comparative study of 168 patients. *Acta Cytol* 1988; **32**: 641–646

49 Johnston W W. Histologic and cytologic patterns of lung cancer in 2580 men and women over a 15 year period. *Acta Cytol* 1988; **32**: 163–168

50 Bonfiglio T A. *Cytopathologic Interpretation of Transthoracic Fine Needle Biopsies*. New York: Masson, 1983

51 Canti G. *A Colour Atlas of Sputum Cytology*. The early diagnosis of lung cancer. Ipswich: Wolfe Publishers, 1992

52 Johnston W W, Frable W J. *Diagnostic Respiratory Cytopathology*. New York: Masson, 1979

53 Kato H, Konaka C, Ono J et al. *Cytology of the Lung*. Techniques and interpretation. Tokyo: Igaku-Shoin, 1983

54 Linder J, Rennard S. *Bronchoalveolar Lavage*. Chicago: American Society of Clinical Pathologists Press, 1988

55 Rosenthal D L. Cytopathology of pulmonary disease, vol. 11. In: Wied G L ed. *Monographs in Clinical Cytology*. Basel: Karger, 1988

56 Saccomanno G. *Diagnostic Pulmonary Cytology*, 2nd edn. Chicago: American Society of Clinical Pathologists Press, 1986

57 Tao L C. *Guides to Clinical Aspiration Biopsy*. Lung, pleura and mediastinum. Tokyo: Igaku-Shoin, 1988

58 Young J A. *Colour Atlas of Pulmonary Cytopathology*. Oxford: Harvey Miller Press, 1985

59 Koss L G. *Diagnostic Cytology and its Histopathologic Bases*, 4th edn. Philadelphia: Lippincott, 1992

60 Johnston W W, Elson C E. Respiratory tract. In: Bibbo M ed. *Comprehensive Cytopathology*. Philadelphia: WB Saunders, 1991; 320–398

60a De May R. *The Art and Science of Cytopathology*. Chicago: ASCP Press, 1996

61 Bender B L, Cherock M, Sotos S N. Effective use of bronchoscopy and sputa in the diagnosis of lung cancer. *Diagn Cytopathol* 1985; **1**: 183–187

62 Castella J, de la Heras P, Puzo C et al. Cytology of postbronchoscopically collected sputum samples and its diagnostic value. *Respiration* 1981; **42**: 116–121

63 Chopra S K, Genovesi M G, Simmons D H, Gothe B. Fiberoptic bronchoscopy in the diagnosis of lung cancer. Comparison of pre- and post-bronchoscopy sputa, washings, brushings and biopsies. *Acta Cytol* 1977; **21**: 524–527

64 Goldberg-Kahn B, Healy J C, Bishop J W. The cost of diagnosis: a comparison of four different strategies in the workup of solitary radiographic lung lesions. *Chest* 1997; **111**: 870–876

65 Raab S S, Hornberger J, Raffin T. The importance of sputum cytology in the diagnosis of lung cancer: a cost-effectiveness analysis. *Chest* 1997; **112**: 937–945

66 Piaton E, Grillet-Ravigneaux M H, Saugier B, Pellet H. Prospective study of combined use of bronchial aspirates and biopsy specimens in diagnosis and typing of centrally located lung tumours. *BMJ* 1995; **310**: 624–627

67 Rodriguez de Castro F, Diaz Lopez F, Serda G J et al. Relevance of training in transbronchial fine-needle aspiration technique. *Chest* 1997; **111**: 103–105

68 Naryshkin S, Daniels J, Young N A. Diagnostic correlation of fiberoptic bronchoscopic biopsy and bronchoscopic cytology performed simultaneously. *Diagn Cytopathol* 1992; **8**: 119–123

69 Blumenfeld W, Singer M, Glanz S, Hon M. Fine-needle aspiration as the initial diagnostic modality in malignant lung disease. *Diagn Cytopathol* 1996; **14**: 268–272

70 Steffee C H, Segletes L A, Geisinger K R. Changing cytologic and histologic utilization patterns in the diagnosis of 515 primary lung malignancies. *Cancer* 1997; **81**: 105–115

71 Fish G D, Stanley J H, Miller K S et al. Post biopsy pneumothorax: estimating the risk by chest radiography and pulmonary function tests. *AJR* 1988; **150**: 71–74

72 Poe R H, Kallay M C, Wicks C M, Odoroff C L. Predicting risk of pneumothorax in needle biopsy of the lung. *Chest* 1984; **85**: 232–235

73 Dasgupta A, Mehta A C. Transbronchial needle aspiration. An underused diagnostic technique. *Clin Chest Med* 1999; **20**: 39–51

74 Akhtar M, Ali M A, Huq M, Faulkner C. Fine needle biopsy: comparison of cellular yield with and without aspiration. *Diagn Cytopathol* 1989; **5**: 162–165

75 Yue X-H, Zheng S-F. Cytologic diagnosis by transthoracic fine needle sampling without aspiration. *Acta Cytol* 1989; **33**: 805–808

76 Fritscher-Ravens A, Petrasch S, Reinacher-Schick A et al. Diagnostic value of endoscopic ultrasonography-guided fine-needle aspiration cytology of mediastinal masses in patients with intrapulmonary lesions and nondiagnostic bronchoscopy. *Respiration* 1999; **66**: 150–155

77 Santambrogio L, Nosotti M, Bellaviti N et al. CT-guided fine-needle aspiration cytology of solitary pulmonary nodules: a prospective, randomized study of immediate cytologic evaluation. *Chest* 1997; **112**: 423–425

78 Johnsrude I S, Silverman J F, Weaver M D, McConnell R W. Rapid cytology to decrease pneumothorax incidence after percutaneous biopsy. *AJR* 1985; **144**: 793–794

79 Stewart C J, Stewart I S. Immediate assessment of fine needle aspiration cytology of lung. *J Clin Pathol* 1996; **49**: 839–843

80 Conces D J Jr, Schwenk G R, Doering P R, Glant M D. Thoracic needle biopsy. Improved results utilizing a team approach. *Chest* 1987; **91**: 813–816

81 Christ M L, Fry W A. Intraoperative fine needle aspiration and rapid diagnosis of thoracic lesions. *Appl Pathol* 1986; **4**: 125–131

82 De Caro L F, Pak H Y, Yokota S et al. Intraoperative cytodiagnosis of lung tumours by needle aspiration. *J Thorac Cardiovasc Surg* 1983; **85**: 404–408

83 Bousamra M 2nd, Clowry L Jr. Thoracoscopic fine-needle aspiration of solitary pulmonary nodules. *Ann Thorac Surg* 1997; **64**: 1191–1193

84 Goldstein R A, Rohatgi P K, Bergofsky E H et al. Clinical role of bronchoalveolar lavage in adults with pulmonary disease. *Am Rev Respir Dis* 1990; **142**: 481–486

85 Radio S J, Rennard S I, Kessinger A et al. Breast carcinoma in bronchoalveolar lavage. *Arch Pathol Lab Med* 1989; **113**: 333–336

86 Masson R G, Krikorian J, Lukl P et al. Pulmonary microvascular cytology in the diagnosis of lymphangitic carcinomatosis. *N Engl J Med* 1989; **321**: 71–76

87 Sterrett G F, Whitaker D, Glancy J. Fine needle aspiration of lung, mediastinum and chest wall. *Pathol Annu* 1982; **17** (part 2): 197–228

88 Pereira P. A fatal case of cerebral artery gas embolism following fine needle biopsy of the lung. *Med J Aust* 1993; **159**: 755–757

89 Moloo Z, Finley R J, Lefcoe M S et al. Possible spread of bronchogenic carcinoma to the chest wall after a transthoracic fine needle aspiration biopsy. A case report. *Acta Cytol* 1985; **29**: 167–169

90 Muller N L, Bergin C J, Miller R R, Ostrow D N. Seeding of malignant cells into the needle track after lung and pleural biopsy. *J Can Assoc Radiol* 1986; **37**: 192–194

91 Perlman E J, Erozan Y S, Howdon A. The role of the Saccomanno technique in sputum cytopathologic diagnosis of lung cancer. *Am J Clin Pathol* 1989; **91**: 57–60

92 Risse E K J, van't Hof M A, Laurini R N, Vooijs P G. Sputum cytology by the Saccomanno method in diagnosing lung malignancy. *Diagn Cytopathol* 1985; **1**: 286–291

93 Rizzo T, Schumann G B, Riding J M. Comparison of the pick-and-smear and Saccomanno methods for sputum cytologic analysis. *Acta Cytol* 1990; **34**: 875–880

94 Risse E K J, Vooijs G P, van't Hof M A. Relationship between the cellular composition of sputum and the cytologic diagnosis of lung cancer. *Acta Cytol* 1987; **31**: 170–176

95 Pederson B, Brons M, Holm K et al. The value of provoked expectoration in obtaining sputum samples for cytologic investigation. A prospective, consecutive and controlled investigation of 134 patients. *Acta Cytol* 1985; **29**: 750–752

96 Chamberlain D W, Braude A C, Rebuck A S. A critical evaluation of bronchoalveolar lavage. Criteria for identifying unsatisfactory specimens. *Acta Cytol* 1987; **31**: 599–605

97 Bocking A, Biesterfeld S, Chatelain R et al. Diagnosis of bronchial carcinoma on sections of paraffin-embedded sputum. Sensitivity and specificity of an alternative to routine cytology. *Acta Cytol* 1992; **36**: 37–47

98 Fischler DF, Toddy SM. Nongynecologic cytology utilizing the ThinPrep Processor. *Acta Cytol* 1996; **40**: 669–675

99 Motherby H, Nicklaus S, Berg A et al. Semiautomated monolayer preparation of bronchial secretions using AutoCyte PREP. *Acta Cytol* 1999; **43**: 47–57

100 Wang H H, Sovie S, Trawinski G et al. ThinPrep processing of endoscopic brushing specimens. *Am J Clin Pathol* 1996; **105**: 163–167

101 Chess Q, Hajdu S I. The role of immunoperoxidase staining in diagnostic cytology. *Acta Cytol* 1986; **30**: 1–7

102 Brown D C, Gatter K C. Use of bronchial brushings in the immunocytochemical assessment of human lung tumours. *Acta Cytol* 1988; **32**: 432

103 Blumenfeld W, Turi G K, Harrison G et al. Utility of cytokeratin 7 and 20 subset analysis as an aid in the identification of primary site of origin of malignancy in cytologic specimens. *Diagn Cytopathol* 1999; **20**: 63–66

103a Chu P, Wu E, Weiss L M. Cytokeratin 7 and cytokeratin 20 expression in epithelial neoplasms: a survey of 435 cases. *Mod Pathol* 2000; **13**: 962–972

104 Kaufmann O, Dietel M. Expression of thyroid transcription factor-1 in pulmonary and extrapulmonary small cell carcinomas and other neuroendocrine carcinomas of various primary sites. *Histopathology* 2000; **36**: 415–420

105 Fetsch P A, Marincola F M, Filie A et al. Melanoma-associated antigen recognized by T cells (MART-1): the advent of a preferred immunocytochemical antibody for the diagnosis of metastatic malignant melanoma with fine-needle aspiration. *Cancer* 1999; **87**: 37–42

106 Raab S S, Slagel D D, Hughes J H et al. Sensitivity and cost-effectiveness of fine-needle aspiration with immunocytochemistry in the evaluation of patients with a pulmonary malignancy and a history of cancer. *Arch Pathol Lab Med* 1997; **121**: 695–700

107 Akhtar M, Ali M A, Owen E W. Application of electron microscopy in the interpretation of fine needle aspiration biopsies. *Cancer* 1981; **48**: 2458–2463

108 Akhtar M, Bakry M, Al-Jeaid A S, McClintock J A. Electron microscopy of fine-needle aspiration biopsy specimens: a brief review. *Diagn Cytopathol* 1992; **8**: 278–282

109 Lazzaro A V. Technical note: improved preparation of fine needle aspiration biopsies for transmission electron microscopy. *Pathol* 1983; **15**: 399–402

110 Dabbs D J, Silverman J F. Selective use of electron microscopy in fine needle aspiration cytology. *Acta Cytol* 1988; **32**: 880–884

111 Davies D C, Russell A J, Tayar R et al. Transmission electron microscopy of percutaneous fine needle aspirates from lung: a study of 70 cases. *Thorax* 1987; **42**: 296–301

112 Neill J S A, Silverman J F. Electron microscopy of fine-needle aspiration biopsies of the mediastinum. *Diagn Cytopathol* 1992; **8**: 272–277

113 Sehested M, Francis D, Hainau B. Electron microscopy of transthoracic fine needle aspiration biopsies. *Acta Pathol Microbiol Immunol Scand (A)* 1983; **91**: 457–461

114 Taccagni G, Cantaboni A, Dell'Antonio G et al. Electron microscopy of fine needle aspiration biopsies of mediastinal and paramediastinal lesions. *Acta Cytol* 1988; **32**: 868–879

115 Wills E J, Carr S, Philips J. Electron microscopy in the diagnosis of percutaneous fine needle aspiration specimens. *Ultrastruct Pathol* 1987; **11**: 361–387

116 Kurtz S M. Rapid ultrastructural examination of FNAs in the diagnosis of intrathoracic tumours. *Diagn Cytopathol* 1992; **8**: 289–292

117 Ascoli V, Barsotti P, Facciolo F et al. Nucleolar organizer regions in the fine needle aspirates of lung tumours. *Cytopathol* 1990; **1**: 277–286

118 Chern J H, Lee Y C, Yang M H et al. Usefulness of argyrophilic nucleolar organizer regions score to differentiate suspicious malignancy in pulmonary cytology. *Chest* 1997; **111**: 1591–1596

119 Hoda RS, Saccomanno G, Schreiber K et al. Automated sputum screening with PAPNET system: a study of 122 cases. *Hum Pathol* 1996 ;**27**: 656–659

120 Marchetti A, Buttitta F, Carnicelli V et al. Enriched SSCP: a highly sensitive method for the detection of unknown mutations. Application to the molecular diagnosis of lung cancer in sputum samples. *Diagn Mol Pathol* 1997; **6**: 185–191

121 Bedrossian C W M, Rybka D L. Bronchial brushing during fiberoptic bronchoscopy for the cytodiagnosis of lung cancer: comparison with sputum and bronchial washings. *Acta Cytol* 1976; **20**: 446–453

122 Tao L C, Sanders D E, Weisbrod G L et al. Value and limitations of transthoracic and transabdominal fine-needle aspiration cytology in clinical practice. *Diagn Cytopathol* 1986; **2**: 271–276

123 Cagle P T, Kovach M, Ramzy I. Causes of false results in transthoracic fine needle aspirates. *Acta Cytol* 1993; **37**: 16–20

124 Corrin B. *Pathology of the Lungs*. Edinburgh: Churchill Livingstone, 2000

125 WHO. Histological typing of lung and pleural tumours. *World Health Organization International Classification of Tumours*. Berlin: Springer, 1999

126 Minna J D, Sekido Y, Fong K M, Gazdar A F. Molecular biology of lung cancer. In: de Vita V T, Hellman S, Rosenberg S A eds. *Cancer: Principles and Practice of Oncology*, 5th edn., Lipincott-Raven, Philadelphia: 1997; 849–857

127 Slebos R J C, Wagenaar S S, Meijer C J L M et al. Frequency and significance of ras oncogene alterations in human lung tumours. *Proc Am Assoc Cancer Res* 1990; **31**: 310–315

128 Ronai Z, Yabubovskaya MS, Zhang E, Belitsky G A. K-ras mutation in sputum of patients with or without lung cancer. *J Cell Biochem Suppl* 1996; **25**: 172–176

129 Roggli V L, Vollmer R T, Greenberg S D et al. Lung cancer heterogeneity: a blinded and randomized study of 100 consecutive cases. *Hum Pathol* 1985; **16**: 569–579

130 Dunnill M S, Gatter K C. Cellular heterogeneity in lung cancer. *Histopathol* 1986; **10**: 461–475

131 Adelstein D J, Tomashefski J F, Snow N J et al. Mixed small cell and non-small cell lung cancer. *Chest* 1986; **89**: 699–704

132 Matthews M J. Effects of therapy on the morphology and behaviour of small cell carcinoma of the lung – a clinicopathologic study. *Prog Cancer Res Ther* 1979; **11**: 155–165

133 Auerbach O, Garfinkel L. The changing pattern of lung carcinoma. *Cancer* 1991; **68**: 1973–1977

134 Tanaka I, Matsubara O, Kasuga T et al. Increasing incidence and changing histopathology of primary lung cancer in Japan. A review of 282 autopsied cases. *Cancer* 1988; **62**: 1035–1039

135 Rilke F, Carbone A, Clemente L et al. Surgical pathology of resectable lung cancer. *Prog Cancer Res Ther* 1979; **11**: 129–142

136 Hirsch F R, Matthews M J, Aisner S et al. Histopathologic classification of small cell lung cancer. Changing concepts and terminology. *Cancer* 1988; **62**: 973–977

137 Stuart-Harris R, Boyer M, Greenberg M et al. The histopathological classification of small cell lung cancer: application of the IASLC classification in 124 cases. *Lung Cancer* 1992; **8**: 63–70

138 Katlic M, Carter D. Prognostic implications of histology; size and location of primary tumours. *Prog Cancer Res Ther* 1979; **11**: 143–150

139 Leong AS-Y. The relevance of ultrastructural examination in the classification of primary lung tumours. *Pathol* 1982; **14**: 37–46

140 Hess F G, McDowell E M, Trump B F. Pulmonary cytology. Current status of cytologic typing of respiratory tract tumours. *Am J Pathol* 1981; **103**: 323–333

141 Mennemeyer R, Hammar S P, Bauermeister D E et al. Cytologic, histologic and electron microscopic correlations in poorly differentiated primary lung carcinoma. A study of 43 cases. *Acta Cytol* 1979; **23**: 297–302

142 Gould V E, Linnoila R I, Memoli V A, Warren W H. Neuro-endocrine cells and neuro-endocrine neoplasms of the lung. *Pathol Annu* (part I), 1983; **18**: 287–330

143 Hammond M E, Sause W T. Large cell neuro-endocrine tumours of the lung. Clinical significance and histopathologic definition. *Cancer* 1985; **56**: 1624–1629

144 McDowell E M, Wilson T S, Trump B F. Atypical endocrine tumours of the lung. *Arch Pathol Lab Med* 1981; **105**: 20–28

145 Mooi W T, Dewar A, Springall D R et al. Non small cell lung carcinomas with neuro-endocrine features. A light microscopic, immunohistochemical and ultrastructural study of 11 cases. *Histopathol* 1988; **13**: 329–337

146 Neal M H, Kosinski R, Cohen P, Orenstein J M. Atypical endocrine tumours of the lung. A histologic, ultrastructural and clinical study of 19 cases. *Hum Pathol* 1986; **17**: 1264–1277

147 Warren W H, Penfield Faber L, Gould V E. Neuro-endocrine neoplasms of the lung. A clinicopathologic update. *J Thorac Cardiovasc Surg* 1989; **98**: 321–323

148 Graziano S L, Tatum A H, Newman N B *et al*. The prognostic significance of neuroendocrine markers and carcinoembryonic antigen in patients with resected stage I and II non-small cell lung cancer. *Cancer Res* 1994; **54**: 2908–2913

149 Souhami R L. The antigens of lung cancer. *Thorax* 1992; **47**: 53–56

150 Travis W D, Rush W, Flieder D B *et al*. Survival analysis of 200 pulmonary neuroendocrine tumors with clarification of criteria for atypical carcinoid and its separation from typical carcinoid. *Am J Surg Pathol* 1998; **22**: 934–944

151 Lavoie R R, McDonald J R, Kling G A. Cavitation in squamous carcinoma of the lung. *Acta Cytol* 1977; **21**: 210–214

152 Kern W H. Cytology of hyperplastic and neoplastic lesions of terminal bronchioles and alveoli. *Acta Cytol* 1965; **9**: 372–379

153 Koprovska I, An S H, Corsey D *et al*. Cytologic patterns of developing bronchogenic carcinoma. *Acta Cytol* 1965; **9**: 424–430

154 Saccomanno G, Saunders R P, Archer V E *et al*. Cancer of the lung: the cytology of sputum prior to the development of carcinoma. *Acta Cytol* 1965; **9**: 413–423

155 Saccomanno G, Archer V E, Auerbach O *et al*. Development of carcinoma of the lung as reflected in exfoliated cells. *Cancer* 1974; **33**: 256–270

156 Risse E K J, Vooijs G P, van't Hof M A. Diagnostic significance of 'severe dysplasia' in sputum cytology. *Acta Cytol* 1988; **32**: 629–634

157 Saito Y, Imai T, Nagamoto N *et al*. A quantitative cytologic study of sputum in early squamous cell bronchogenic carcinoma. *Analyt Quant Cytol Histol* 1988; **10**: 365–370

158 Sato M, Saito Y, Nagamoto N *et al*. Diagnostic value of differential brushing of all branches of the bronchi in patients with sputum positive or suspected positive for lung cancer. *Acta Cytol* 1993; **37**: 879–883

159 Woolner L B. Recent advances in pulmonary cytology: early detection and localization of occult lung cancer in symptomless males. In: Koss L G, Coleman D V eds. *Advances in Clinical Cytology*, vol. 1. London: Butterworths, 1981

160 Fontana R S. Screening for lung cancer: recent experience in the United States. *Cancer Treat Res* 1986; **28**: 91–111

161 Band P R, Feldstein M, Saccomanno G. Reversibility of bronchial marked atypia: implication for chemoprevention. *Cancer Detect Prevent* 1986; **9**: 157–160

162 Garret M. Cellular atypias in sputum and bronchial secretions associated with tuberculosis and bronchiectasis. *Am J Clin Pathol* 1960; **34**: 237–246

163 deMattos M C F I, de Oliveira M L S. Pseudoepitheliomatous proliferation, a pitfall in sputum cytology. *Diagn Cytopathol* 1991; **7**: 656–657

164 Bedrossian C W M, Corey B J. Abnormal sputum cytopathology during chemotherapy with bleomycin. *Acta Cytol* 1978; **22**: 202–207

165 Koss L G, Melamed M R, Mayer K. The effect of busulphan on human epithelia. *Am J Clin Pathol* 1965; **44**: 385–397

166 Bewtra C, Dewan N, O'Donahue W J Jr. Exfoliative sputum cytology in pulmonary embolism. *Acta Cytol* 1983; **27**: 489–496

167 Berman J J, Murray R J, Lopez-Plaza I M. Widespread posttracheostomy atypia simulating squamous cell carcinoma. *Acta Cytol* 1991; **35**: 713–716

168 Weaver K M, Novak P M, Naylor B. Vegetable cell contaminants in cytologic specimens. Their resemblance to cells associated with various normal and pathologic states. *Acta Cytol* 1981; **25**: 210–214

169 Matsuda M, Nagumo S, Horai T, Yoshino K. Cytologic diagnosis of laryngeal and hypopharyngeal squamous cell carcinoma in sputum. *Acta Cytol* 1988; **32**: 655–657

170 Willet G D, Schumann G B, Genack L. Primary cytodiagnosis of synchronous small-cell cancer and squamous-cell carcinoma of the respiratory tract. *Acta Cytol* 1984; **28**: 610–613

171 Baker J J, Solanki P H, Schenk D A *et al*. Transbronchial fine needle aspiration of the mediastinum. Importance of lymphocytes as an indicator of specimen adequacy. *Acta Cytol* 1990; **34**: 517–523

172 Saito Y, Imai T, Sato M *et al*. Cytologic study of tissue repair in human bronchial epithelium. *Acta Cytol* 1988; **32**: 622–628

173 Suprun H, Pedio G, Ruttner J R. The diagnostic reliability of cytologic typing in primary lung cancer with a review of the literature. *Acta Cytol* 1980; **24**: 494–500

174 Smith A R, Raab S S, Landreneau R J, Silverman J F. Fine-needle aspiration cytologic features of pseudovascular adenoid squamous-cell carcinoma of the lung. *Diagn Cytopathol* 1999; **21**: 265–270

175 Bell W R Jr, Johnston W W, Bigner S H. The cytologic diagnosis of occult small-cell undifferentiated carcinoma of the lung. *Acta Cytol* 1982; **26**: 73–77

176 Lee T-K, Esinhart J D, Blackburn L D, Silverman J F. The size of small cell lung carcinoma cells: ratio to lymphocytes and correlation with specimen size and crush artifact. *Acta Cytol* 1992; **36**: 265

177 Hirsch F R, Matthews M J, Aisner S *et al*. Histopathologic classification of small cell lung cancer: changing concepts and terminology. *Cancer* 1988; **62**: 973–977

178 Tome Y, Hirohashi S, Noguchi M *et al*. Immunocytologic diagnosis of small-cell lung cancer in imprint smears. *Acta Cytol* 1991; **35**: 485–490

179 Ariza A, Mate J L, Isamat M *et al*. Standard and variant CD44 isoforms are commonly expressed in lung cancer of the non-small cell type but not of the small cell type. *J Pathol* 1995; **177**: 363–368

180 Koprowska I, Zipfel S A. The potential usefulness of monoclonal antibodies in the determination of histologic types of lung cancer in cytologic preparations. *Acta Cytol* 1988; **32**: 675–679

181 Tabatowski K, Vollmer R T, Tello J W *et al*. The use of a panel of monoclonal antibodies in ultrastructurally characterised small cell carcinomas of the lung. *Acta Cytol* 1988; **32**: 667–674

182 Walker W P, Wittchow R J, Bottles K *et al*. Paranuclear blue inclusions in small cell undifferentiated carcinoma: a diagnostically useful finding demonstrated in fine-needle aspiration biopsy smears. *Diagn Cytopathol* 1994; **10**:212–215

183 Naib Z M. Pitfalls in the cytologic diagnosis of oat cell carcinoma of the lung. *Acta Cytol* 1964; **8**: 34–38

184 Davenport R D. Diagnostic value of crush artefact in cytologic specimens. Occurrence in small cell carcinoma of the lung. *Acta Cytol* 1990; **34**: 502–504

185 Rollins S D, Genack L J, Schumann G B. Primary cytodiagnosis of dually differentiated lung cancer by transthoracic fine needle aspiration. *Acta Cytol* 1988; **32**: 231–234

186 Zaharopoulos P, Wong J Y, Stewart G D. Cytomorphology of the variants of small cell carcinoma of the lung. *Acta Cytol* 1982; **26**: 800–808

187 Yang G C. Mixed small cell/large cell carcinoma of the lung. Report of a case with cytologic features and ultrastructural correlation. *Acta Cytol.* 1995; **39**: 1175–1181

188 Dugan J M. Cytologic diagnosis of basal cell (basaloid) carcinoma of the lung. A report of two cases. *Acta Cytol.* 1995; **39**: 539–542

189 Vesoulis Z. Metastatic laryngeal basaloid squamous cell carcinoma simulating primary small cell carcinoma of the lung on fine needle aspiration lung biopsy. A case report. *Acta Cytol.* 1998; **42**: 783–787

190 Marchevsky A, Nieburgs H E, Olenko E *et al*. Pulmonary tumourlets in cases of 'tuberculoma' of the lung with malignant cells in brush biopsy. *Acta Cytol* 1982; **26**: 491–494

191 Naylor B, Bailey C. A pitfall in the cytodiagnosis of sputum of asthmatics. *J Clin Pathol* 1964; **17**: 87–89

192 McKee G, Parums D V. False-positive cytodiagnosis in fibrosing alveolitis. *Acta Cytol* 1990; **34**: 105–107

193 Selvaggi S M, Rerber M. Pulmonary cytology in patients with the acquired immunodeficiency syndrome (AIDS). *Diagn Cytopathol* 1986; **2**: 187–193

194 Grotte D, Stanley M W, Swanson P E *et al*. Reactive type II pneumocytes in bronchoalveolar lavage fluid from adult respiratory distress syndrome can be mistaken for cells of adenocarcinoma. *Diagn Cytopathol* 1990; **6**: 317–322

195 Cohen J-M, Kreitzer R, Dicpinigaitis P. Mucinous cystadenocarcinoma of the lung; correlation of intraoperative cytology with histology. *Acta Cytol* 1991; **35**: 626

196 Elson C E, Moore S P, Johnston W W. Morphologic and immunocytochemical

studies of bronchiolo-alveolar carcinoma at Duke University Medical Centre 1968–1986. *Analyt Quant Cytol Histol* 1989; **11**: 261–274

197 Gupta R K. Value of sputum cytology in the differential diagnosis of alveolar cell carcinoma from bronchogenic carcinoma. *Acta Cytol* 1981; **25**: 255–258

198 Lozowski W, Hajdu S I. Cytology and immunocytochemistry of bronchioloalveolar carcinoma. *Acta Cytol* 1987; **31**: 717–725

199 Roger V, Nasiell M, Linden M, Enstad I. Cytologic differential diagnosis of bronchioloalveolar carcinoma and bronchogenic adenocarcinoma. *Acta Cytol* 1976; **20**: 303–307

200 Smith J H, Frable W J. Adenocarcinoma of the lung. Cytologic correlation with histologic types. *Acta Cytol* 1974; **18**: 316–320

201 Spriggs A I, Cole M, Dunnill M S. Alveolar-cell carcinoma: a problem in sputum cytodiagnosis. *J Clin Pathol* 1982; **35**: 1370–1379

202 Tao L C, Delarue N C, Sanders D, Weisbrod G. Bronchioloalveolar carcinoma: a correlative clinical and cytologic study. *Cancer* 1978; **42**: 2759–2767

203 Kimura M, Hiruma S, Hara S, Hashimoto S. Cytopathology of granulocyte colony-stimulating factor-producing lung adenocarcinoma. *Acta Cytol* 1997; **41**: 952–953

204 Gupta P K, Verma K. Calcified (psammoma) bodies in alveolar cell carcinoma of the lung. *Acta Cytol* 1972; **16**: 59–61

205 Tao L-C, Weisbrod G L, Pearson F G et al. Cytologic diagnosis of bronchioloalveolar carcinoma by fine needle aspiration biopsy. *Cancer* 1986; **57**: 1565–1570

206 Silverman J F, Finley J L, Park H K et al. Fine needle aspiration cytology of bronchioloalveolar-cell carcinoma of the lung. *Acta Cytol* 1985; **29**: 887–894

207 Silverman J F, Finley J L, Park H K et al. Psammoma bodies and optically clear nuclei in bronchiolo-alveolar cell carcinoma. Diagnosis by fine needle aspiration biopsy with histologic and ultrastructural confirmation. *Diagn Cytopathol* 1985; **1**: 205–215

208 Jarrett D D, Betsill W L. A problem-orientated approach regarding the fine needle aspiration cytologic diagnosis of bronchioloalveolar carcinoma of the lung: a comparison of diagnostic criteria with benign lesions mimicking carcinoma. *Acta Cytol* 1987; **31**: 684–685

209 Auger M, Katz R L, Johnston D A. Differentiating cytological features of bronchioloalveolar carcinoma of the lung in fine-needle aspirations: a statistical analysis of 27 cases. *Diagn Cytopathol* 1997; **16**: 253–257

210 Broghamer W L, Collins W M, Mojsejenko I K. The cytohistopathology of a pseudomesotheliomatous carcinoma of the lung. *Acta Cytol* 1978; **22**: 239–242

211 Tsumuraya M, Kodama T, Kameya T et al. Light and electron microscopic analysis of intranuclear inclusions in papillary adenocarcinoma of the lung. *Acta Cytol* 1981; **25**: 523–532

212 Chen K T K. Psammoma bodies in fine needle aspiration cytology of papillary adenocarcinoma of the lung. *Diagn Cytopathol* 1990; **6**: 271–274

213 Tao L-C, Weisbrod G, Ritcey E L, Ilves R. False 'false positive' results in diagnostic cytology. *Acta Cytol* 1984; **28**: 450–455

214 Albain K S, True L D, Golomb H M et al. Large cell carcinoma of the lung. Ultrastructural differentiation and clinical pathologic correlations. *Cancer* 1985; **56**: 1618–1623

215 Broderick P A, Corvese N L, Lachance T, Allard J. Giant cell carcinoma of the lung: a cytologic evaluation. *Acta Cytol* 1975; **19**: 225–230

216 Naib Z M. Giant cell carcinoma of the lung: cytologic study of the exfoliated cells in sputa and bronchial washings. *Chest* 1961; **40**: 69–73

217 Craig I D, Desrosiers P, Lefcoe M S. Giant cell carcinoma of the lung. A cytologic study. *Acta Cytol* 1983; **27**: 293–298

218 Albright C D, Hafiz M A. Cytomorphologic changes in split course radiation treated bronchogenic carcinomas. *Diagn Cytopathol* 1988; **4**: 9–13

219 Chess Q. Megakaryocytes in bronchial brushings. *Acta Cytol* 1988; **23**: 130

220 Nicholson S A, Ryan M R. A review of cytologic findings in neuroendocrine carcinomas including carcinoid tumors with histologic correlation. *Cancer* 2000; **90**: 148–161

221 Anderson C, Ludwig M E, O'Donnell M, Garcia N. Fine needle aspiration cytology of pulmonary carcinoid tumours. *Acta Cytol* 1990; **34**: 505–510

222 Collins B T, Cramer H M. Fine needle aspiration cytology of carcinoid tumors. *Acta Cytol.* 1996; **40**: 695–707

223 Gephardt G N, Belovich D M. Cytology of pulmonary carcinoid tumours. *Acta Cytol* 1982; **26**: 434–438

224 Givens C D Jr, Marini J J. Transbronchial needle aspiration of a bronchial carcinoid tumour. *Chest* 1985; **88**: 152–153

225 Horan D C, Bonfiglio T A, Patten S F Jr. The needle aspiration cytopathology of bronchial carcinoid tumours. An analytical study of the cells. *Analyt Quant Cytol* 1982; **4**: 105–109

226 Kim K, Mah C, Dominquez J. Carcinoid tumours of the lung: cytologic differential diagnosis in fine-needle aspirates. *Diagn Cytopathol* 1986; **2**: 343–346

227 Lozowski W, Hajdu S I, Melamed M R. Cytomorphology of carcinoid tumours. *Acta Cytol* 1979; **23**: 360–365

228 Kyriakos M, Rockoff S D. Brush biopsy of bronchial carcinoid – a source of cytologic error. *Acta Cytol* 1972; **16**: 261–268

229 Mitchell M L, Parker F P. Capillaries. A cytologic feature of pulmonary carcinoid tumours. *Acta Cytol* 1991; **35**: 183–185

230 Nguyen G K. Cytopathology of pulmonary carcinoid tumors in sputum and bronchial brushings. *Acta Cytol* 1995; **39**: 1152–1160

231 Craig J D, Finley R J. Spindle cell carcinoid of lung. Cytologic, histopathologic and ultrastructural features. *Acta Cytol* 1982; **26**: 495–498

232 Fekete P S, Cohen C, DeRose P B. Pulmonary spindle cell carcinoid. Needle aspiration biopsy, histologic and immunohistochemical findings. *Acta Cytol* 1990; **34**: 50–56

233 Nguyen G-K, Shnitka T K. Aspiration biopsy cytology of adenocarcinoid tumour of the bronchial tree. *Acta Cytol* 1987; **31**: 726–730

234 Pilotti S, Rilke F, Lombardi L. Pulmonary carcinoid with glandular features. Report of 2 cases with positive fine needle aspiration cytology. *Acta Cytol* 1983; **27**: 511–514

235 Arrigoni M G, Woolner L B, Bernatz P E. Atypical carcinoid tumour of lung. *J Thorac Cardiovasc Surg* 1972; **64**: 413–421

236 Szyfelbein W M, Ross J S. Carcinoids, atypical carcinoids and small cell carcinoma of the lung: differential diagnosis of fine needle aspiration biopsy specimens. *Diagn Cytopathol* 1988; **4**: 1–8

237 Frierson H F Jr, Covell J L, Mills S E. Fine needle aspiration cytology of atypical carcinoid of the lung. *Acta Cytol* 1987; **31**: 471–475

238 Jordan A G, Predmore L, Sullivan M M, Memoli V A. The cytodiagnosis of well differentiated neuro-endocrine carcinoma. A distinct clinicopathologic entity. *Acta Cytol* 1987; **31**: 464–470

239 Buchanan A T, Fauck R, Gupta R K. Cytologic diagnosis of adenoid cystic carcinoma in tracheal wash specimens. *Diagn Cytopathol* 1988; **4**: 130–132

240 Gupta R K, McHutchison A G R. Cytologic findings of adenoid cystic carcinoma in a tracheal wash specimen. *Diagn Cytopathol* 1992; **8**: 196–197

241 Lozowski M S, Mishriki Y, Solitaire G B. Cytopathologic features of adenoid cystic carcinoma. Case report and literature review. *Acta Cytol* 1983; **27**: 317–322

242 Nguyen G-K. Cytology of bronchial gland carcinoma. *Acta Cytol* 1988; **32**: 235–239

243 Radhika S, Dey P, Rajwanshi A et al. Adenoid cystic carcinoma in a bronchial washing. A case report. *Acta Cytol* 1993; **37**: 97–99

244 Anderson R J, Johnston W W, Szpak C A. Fine needle aspiration of adenoid cystic carcinoma metastatic to the lung. Cytologic features and differential diagnosis. *Acta Cytol* 1985; **29**: 527–532

245 Smith R C, Amy R W. Adenoid cystic carcinoma metastatic to the lung. Report of a case diagnosed by fine needle aspiration biopsy cytology. *Acta Cytol* 1985; **29**: 535–536

246 Brooks B, Baandrup U. Peripheral low grade mucoepidermoid carcinoma of the lung – needle aspiration cytodiagnosis and histology. *Cytopathol* 1992; **3**: 259–265

247 Tao L C, Robertson D I. Cytologic diagnosis of bronchial mucoepidermoid carcinoma by fine needle aspiration biopsy. *Acta Cytol* 1978; **22**: 221–224

248 Segletes L A, Steffee C H, Geisinger K R. Cytology of primary pulmonary mucoepidermoid and adenoid cystic

carcinoma. A report of four cases. *Acta Cytol* 1999; **43**: 1091–1097

249 Burke M D, Melamed M R. Exfoliative cytology of metastatic cancer in lung. *Acta Cytol* 1968; **12**: 61–74

250 Saleh H, Masood S. Value of ancillary studies in fine-needle aspiration biopsy. *Diagn Cytopathol* 1995; **13**: 310–315

251 O'Reilly P E, Brueckner J, Silverman J F. Value of ancillary studies in fine needle aspiration cytology of the lung. *Acta Cytol* 1994; **38**: 144–150

252 Korfhage L, Broghamer W L, Richardson M E et al. Pulmonary cytology in the post-therapeutic monitoring of patients with bronchogenic carcinoma. *Acta Cytol* 1986; **30**: 351–355

253 Ebihara Y, Fukushima N, Asakuma Y. Double primary lung cancers; with special reference to their exfoliative cytology and to the rare malignant 'mixed' tumour of the salivary-gland type. *Acta Cytol* 1980; **24**: 212–223

254 Braman S S, Whitcomb M E. Endobronchial metastasis. *Arch Intern Med* 1975; **135**: 543–547

255 Ludwig R A, Gero M. Bronchoscopic cytology of metastatic breast carcinoma with osteoclast like giant cells. *Acta Cytol* 1987; **31**: 365–368

256 Selvaggi S, Kissner D, Qureshi F. Metastatic metaplastic carcinoma of the breast. Diagnosis by bronchial brush cytology. *Diagn Cytopathol* 1989; **3**: 396–399

257 Chell S E, Nayar R, De Frias D V, Bedrossian C W. Metaplastic breast carcinoma metastatic to the lung mimicking a primary chondroid lesion: report of a case with cytohistologic correlation. *Ann Diagn Pathol* 1998; **2**: 173–180

258 Varma S, Amy R W. Adrenal cortical carcinoma metastatic to the lung. Report of a case diagnosed by fine needle aspiration biopsy. *Acta Cytol* 1990; **34**: 104–105

259 Craig I D, Shum D T, Desrosiers P et al. Choriocarcinoma metastatic to the lung: a cytologic study with identification of human choriogonadotrophin with an immunoperoxidase technique. *Acta Cytol* 1983; **27**: 647–650

260 Tao L C. Pulmonary metastases from intracranial meningioma diagnosed by aspiration biopsy cytology. *Acta Cytol* 1991; **35**: 524–528

261 Baisden B L, Hamper U M, Ali S Z. Metastatic meningioma in fine-needle aspiration (FNA) of the lung: cytomorphologic finding. *Diagn Cytopathol* 1999; **20**: 291–294.

262 Ehya H. Cytology of mesothelioma of the tunica vaginalis metastatic to the lung. *Acta Cytol* 1985; **29**: 79–84

263 Whitaker D, Sterrett G F, Shilkin K B, Walters M N-I. Malignant mesothelioma cells in sputum. *Diagn Cytopathol* 1986; **2**: 21–24

264 Hamilton C, Bigner S H, Wells S, Johnston W W. Metastatic medullary carcinoma of the thyroid in sputum – a light and electron microscopic study. *Acta Cytol* 1983; **27**: 49–53

265 Tabei S Z, Abdollahi B, Nili F. Diagnosis of metastatic adamantinoma of the tibia by pulmonary brushing cytology. *Acta Cytol* 1988; **32**: 579–581

266 Levine S E, Mossler J A, Johnston W W. The cytopathology of metastatic ameloblastoma. *Acta Cytol* 1981; **25**: 295–298

267 Landolt U. Pleomorphic adenoma of the salivary glands metastatic to the lung: diagnosis by FNA cytology. *Acta Cytol* 1990; **34**: 101–102

268 Liu K, Layfield L J, Coogan A C. Cytologic features of pulmonary metastasis from a granulosa cell tumor diagnosed by fine-needle aspiration: a case report. *Diagn Cytopathol* 1997; **16**: 341–344.

269 Ali S Z, Kronz J D, Plowden K M, Erozan Y S. Metastatic pulmonary leiomyosarcoma: cytopathologic diagnosis on sputum examination. *Diagn Cytopathol* 1998; **18**: 280–283

270 Flint A, Lloyd R. Colon carcinoma metastatic to the lung. Cytologic manifestations and distinction from primary pulmonary adenocarcinoma. *Acta Cytol* 1992; **36**: 230–235

271 Kern W H, Schweizer C. Sputum cytology of metastatic carcinoma of the lung. *Acta Cytol* 1976; **20**: 514–520

272 Nguyen G-K. Fine needle aspiration biopsy cytology of metastatic renal cell carcinoma. *Acta Cytol* 1988; **32**: 409–414

273 Linsk J A, Franzen S. Aspiration cytology of metastatic hypernephroma. *Acta Cytol* 1984; **28**: 250–260

274 Johnson T L, Kini S R. Cytologic features of transitional cell carcoma. *Diagn Cytopathol* 1993; **9**: 270–278

275 Powers C N, Elbadawi A. "Cercariform" cells: a clue to the cytodiagnosis of transitional cell origin of metastatic neoplasms? *Diagn Cytopathol* 1995; **13**: 15–21

276 Hida C A, Gupta P K. Cercariform cells: are they specific for transitional cell carcinoma? *Cancer* 1999; **87**: 69–74

277 Renshaw A A, Madge R. Cercariform cells for helping distinguish transitional cell carcinoma from non-small cell lung carcinoma in fine needle aspirates. *Acta Cytol* 1997; **41**: 999–1007

278 Friedman M, Forgioni H, Shanbhag V. Needle aspiration of metastatic melanoma. *Acta Cytol* 1980; **24**: 7–15

279 Blaustein R L. Fine needle aspiration of a metastatic breast carcinoma of the lung with melanin pigmentation. A case report. *Diagn Cytopathol* 1990; **6**: 364–365

280 Roglic M, Jukic S, Damjanov I. Cytology of the solitary papilloma of the bronchus. *Acta Cytol* 1975; **19**: 11–13

281 Rubel L R, Reynolds R E. Cytologic description of squamous cell papilloma of the respiratory tract. *Acta Cytol* 1979; **23**: 227–230

282 Weingarten J. Cytologic and histologic findings in a case of tracheobronchial papillomatosis. *Acta Cytol* 1981; **25**: 167–170

283 Brightman I, Morgan J A, Zwehl D, Sheppard M N. Cytological appearances of a solitary squamous cell papilloma with associated mucous cell adenoma in the lung. *Cytopathol* 1992; **3**: 253–257

284 Nguyen G-K. Aspiration biopsy cytology of benign clear cell ('sugar') tumour of the lung. *Acta Cytol* 1989; **33**: 511–515

285 Cwierzyk T A, Glasberg S S, Virshup M A, Cranmer J C. Pulmonary oncocytoma: report of a case with cytologic, histologic and electron microscopic study. *Acta Cytol* 1985; **29**: 620–623

286 Laforga J B, Aranda F I. Multicentric oncocytoma of the lung diagnosed by fine-needle aspiration. *Diagn Cytopathol* 1999; **21**: 51–54

287 Hamper U M, Khouri N F, Stitik F P, Siegelman S S. Pulmonary hamartoma: diagnosis by transthoracic needle-aspiration biopsy. *Radiol* 1985; **155**: 15–18

288 Curtin C T, Proux J, Davis E. Cartilaginous hamartoma of the lung: a potential pitfall in pulmonary fine needle aspiration. *Acta Cytol* 1988; **32**: 764

289 Dahlgren S E. Needle biopsy of intrapulmonary hamartoma. *Scand J Respir Dis* 1966; **47**: 187–194

290 de Rooij P D, Meijer S, Calame J et al. Solitary hamartoma of the lung; is thoracotomy still mandatory? *Neth J Surg* 1988; **40**: 145–148

291 Dunbar F, Leiman G. The aspiration cytology of pulmonary hamartomas. *Diagn Cytopathol* 1989; **5**: 174–180

292 Ramzy I. Pulmonary hamartomas: cytologic appearances of fine needle aspiration biopsy. *Acta Cytol* 1976; **20**: 15–19

293 Sinner W N. Fine needle biopsy of hamartomas of the lung. *AJR* 1982; **138**: 65–69

294 Wiatrowska B A, Yazdi H M, Matzinger F R, MacDonald L L. Fine needle aspiration biopsy of pulmonary hamartomas. Radiologic, cytologic and immunocytochemical study of 15 cases. *Acta Cytol* 1995; **39**: 1167–1174

295 Chow L T-C, Chan S-K, Chow W-H, Tsui M-S. Pulmonary sclerosing haemangioma. Report of a case with diagnosis by FNA. *Acta Cytol* 1992; **36**: 287–292

296 Wang S E, Nieberk R K. Fine needle aspiration cytology of sclerosing haemangioma of the lung, a mimicker of bronchioloalveolar carcinoma. *Acta Cytol* 1985; **30**: 51–54

297 Gottschalk-Sabag S, Hadas-Halpern I, Glick T. Sclerosing haemangioma of lung mimicking carcinoma diagnosed by fine needle aspiration (FNA) cytology. *Cytopathology* 1995; **6**: 115–120

298 Kaw Y T, Nayak R N. Fine needle biopsy cytology of sclerosing haemangioma of the lung. A case report. *Acta Cytol* 1993; **37**: 933–937

299 Wojcik E M, Sneige N, Lawrence D D, Ordonez N G. Fine needle aspiration cytology of sclerosing haemangioma of the lung: case report with immunohistochemical study. *Diagn Cytopathol* 1993; **9**: 304–309

300 Chen K. Cytology of bronchial benign granular cell tumour. *Acta Cytol* 1991; **35**: 381–384

301 Füezesi L, Höer P-W, Schmidt W. Exfoliative cytology of multiple endobronchial granular cell tumour. *Acta Cytol* 1989; **33**: 516–518

302 Glant M D, Wall R W, Ransburg G. Endobronchial granular cell tumour: cytology of a new case and review of the literature. *Acta Cytol* 1979; **23**: 477–482

303 Mermolja M, Rott T. Cytology of endobronchial granular cell tumour. *Diagn Cytopathol* 1991; **7**: 524–526

304 Thomas L, Risbud M, Gabriel J B *et al*. Cytomorphology of granular cell tumour of the bronchus. A case report. *Acta Cytol* 1984; **28**: 129–132

305 Smith A R, Gilbert C F, Strausbauch P, Silverman J F. Fine needle aspiration cytology of a mediastinal granular cell tumor with histologic confirmation and ancillary studies. A case report. *Acta Cytol.* 1998; **42**: 1011–1016

306 Guillou L, Gloor E, Anani P, Kaelin R. Bronchial granular cell tumour – report of a case with preoperative cytologic diagnosis on bronchial brushings and immunohistochemical studies. *Acta Cytol* 1991; **35**: 375–380

307 Naib Z M, Goldstein H G. Exfoliative cytology of a case of bronchial granular cell myoblastoma. *Dis Chest* 1962; **42**: 645–647

308 Strigle S M, Gal A A. A review of pulmonary cytopathology in the acquired immunodeficiency syndrome. *Diagn Cytopathol* 1989; **5**: 44–54

309 Gattuso P, Castelli M J, Peng Y, Reddy V B. Posttransplant lymphoproliferative disorders: a fine-needle aspiration biopsy study. *Diagn Cytopathol* 1997; **16**: 392–395

310 Abbondanzo S L, Rush W, Bijwaard K E, Koss M N. Nodular lymphoid hyperplasia of the lung: a clinicopathologic study of 14 cases. *Am J Surg Pathol* 2000; **24**: 587–597

311 Yousem S A, Weiss L M, Colby T V. Primary pulmonary Hodgkin's disease. A clinicopathologic study of 15 cases. *Cancer* 1986; **57**: 1217–1224

312 Davis W B, Gadek J E. Detection of pulmonary lymphoma by bronchoalveolar lavage. *Chest* 1987; **91**: 787–789

313 Gouldesbrough D R, McGoogan E. Primary pulmonary lymphoma: a case diagnosed by bronchial cytology and immunocytochemistry. *Histopathol* 1988; **13**: 465–467

314 Myers J L, Fulmer J D. Bronchoalveolar lavage in the diagnosis of pulmonary lymphomas. *Chest* 1989; **91**: 642–643

315 Oka M, Kawano K, Kanda T, Hara K. Bronchoalveolar lavage in primary pulmonary lymphoma with monoclonal gammopathy. *Am Rev Resp Dis* 1988; **137**: 957–959

316 Zaer F S, Braylan R C, Zander D S *et al*. Multiparametric flow cytometry in the diagnosis and characterization of low-grade pulmonary mucosa-associated lymphoid tissue lymphomas. *Mod Pathol* 1998; **11**: 525–532

317 Bardales R H, Powers C N, Frierson H F Jr *et al*. Exfoliative respiratory cytology in the diagnosis of leukemias and lymphomas in the lung. *Diagn Cytopathol* 1996; **14**: 108–118.

318 Bonfiglio T A, Dvoretsky P M, Piscioli F *et al*. Fine needle aspiration biopsy in the evaluation of lymphoreticular tumours of the thorax. *Acta Cytol* 1985; **29**: 548–553

319 Suprun H, Koss L G. The cytological study of sputum and bronchial washings in Hodgkin's disease with pulmonary involvement. *Cancer* 1964; **17**: 674–680

320 Suprun H Z. Cytodiagnosis of Hodgkin's disease in sputum specimens. *Acta Cytol* 1984; **28**: 190–191

321 Reale F R, Variakojis D, Compton J, Bibbo M. Cytodiagnosis of Hodgkin's disease in sputum specimens. *Acta Cytol* 1983; **27**: 258–261

322 Flint A, Kumar N B, Naylor B. Pulmonary Hodgkin's disease. Diagnosis by fine needle aspiration. *Acta Cytol* 1989; **32**: 221–225

323 Wisecarver J, Ness M, Rennard S *et al*. Bronchoalveolar lavage in the assessment of pulmonary Hodgkin's disease. *Acta Cytol* 1988; **32**: 766–767

324 Reiben A E, Ben-Shachar M, Malberger E. Cytologic diagnosis of pulmonary Hodgkin's disease via endobronchial brush preparation. *Chest* 1989; **96**: 948–949

325 Fullmer C D, Morris R P. Primary cytodiagnosis of unsuspected mediastinal Hodgkin's disease. Report of a case. *Acta Cytol* 1972; **16**: 77–81

326 Levij I S. A case of primary cavitary Hodgkin's disease of the lungs, diagnosed cytologically. *Acta Cytol* 1972; **16**: 546–549

327 Morales F M, Matthews J I. Diagnosis of parenchymal Hodgkin's disease using bronchoalveolar lavage. *Chest* 91; **5**: 785–786

328 Eisenberg R S, Dunton B L. Hodgkin's disease first suggested by sputum cytology. *Chest* 1974; **65**: 218–219

329 Ludwig R A, Balachandran I. Mycosis fungoides: the importance of pulmonary cytology in the diagnosis of a case with systemic involvement. *Acta Cytol* 1983; **27**: 198–201

330 Rosen S E, Vonderheid E C, Koprowski I. Mycosis fungoides with pulmonary involvement: cytopathologic findings. *Acta Cytol* 1984; **28**: 51–57

331 Shaheen K, Oertel Y C. Mycosis fungoides cells in sputum. A case report. *Acta Cytol* 1984; **28**: 483–486

332 Vernon S E. Cytodiagnosis of 'signet-ring'-cell lymphoma. *Acta Cytol* 1981; **25**: 291–294

333 Goldstein J, Leslie H. Immunoblastic lymphadenopathy with pulmonary lesions and positive sputum cytology. *Acta Cytol* 1978; **22**: 165–167

334 Williams W L. Clark D A, Saiers J H. Fine needle aspiration diagnosis of lymphomatoid granulomatosis. A case report. *Acta Cytol* 1992; **36**: 91–94

335 Riazmontazer N, Bedayat G. Cytology of plasma cell myeloma in bronchial washing. *Acta Cytol* 1989; **33**: 519–522

336 Chollet S, Soler P, Dournovo P *et al*. Diagnosis of pulmonary histiocytosis X by immunodetection of Langerhans' cells in bronchoalveolar lavage fluid. *Am J Pathol* 1984; **115**: 225–232

337 Auerswald U, Barth J, Magnussen H. Value of CD-1 positive cells in bronchiolar lavage fluid for the diagnosis of pulmonary histiocytosis X. *Lung* 1991; **169**: 305–309

338 Fleming W H, Jove D F. Primary leiomyosarcoma of the lung with positive sputum cytology. *Acta Cytol* 1975; **19**: 14–20

339 Crosby J H, Hoeg K, Hager B. Transthoracic fine needle aspiration of primary and metastatic sarcoma. *Chest* 1984; **85**: 696–697

340 Kim G, Naylor B, Han I H. Fine needle aspiration cytology of sarcomas metastatic to the lung. *Acta Cytol* 1986; **30**: 688–694

341 Hsiu J-G, Kreuger J K, D'Amato N A, Moris J R. Primary malignant fibrous histiocytoma of the lung. *Acta Cytol* 1987; **31**: 345–350

342 Kawahara E I, Nakanishi I, Kuroda Y, Morishita T. Fine needle aspiration biopsy of primary malignant fibrous histiocytoma of the lung. *Acta Cytol* 1988; **32**: 226–230

343 Lozowski M S, Mishriki Y Y, Epstein H. Metastatic malignant fibrous histiocytoma in lung examined by fine needle aspiration: case report and literature review. *Acta Cytol* 1980; **24**: 350–354

344 Nguyen G-K, Jennot A. Cytopathologic aspects of pulmonary metastasis of malignant fibrous histiocytoma, myxoid variant: fine needle aspiration biopsy of a case. *Acta Cytol* 1982; **26**: 349–353

345 Yang H-L, Weaver L L, Fot P R. Primary malignant fibrous histiocytoma of the pleura. A case report. *Acta Cytol* 1983; **27**: 683–687

346 Fujita Y, Shimizu T, Yamazaki K *et al*. Bronchial brushing cytology features of primary malignant fibrous histiocytoma of the lung. A case report. *Acta Cytol.* 2000; **44**: 227–231

347 Schantz H D, Ramzy I, Tio F O, Buhaug J. Metastatic spindle cell carcinoma. Cytologic features and differential diagnosis. *Acta Cytol* 1985; **29**: 435–441

348 Logrono R, Filipowicz E A, Eyzaguirre E J, Sawh R N. Diagnosis of primary fibrosarcoma of the lung by fine-needle aspiration and core biopsy. *Arch Pathol Lab Med* 1999; **123**: 731–735

349 Krumerman M S. Leiomyosarcoma of the lung: primary cytodiagnosis in two consecutive cases. *Acta Cytol* 1977; **21**: 103–108

350 Sawada K, Fukuma S, Seki Y *et al*. Cytological features of primary leiomyosarcoma of the lung: report of a case diagnosed by bronchial brushing procedure. *Acta Cytol* 1977; **21**: 770–773

351 Michacao C N, Sorensen K, Abdul-Karim F W, Somrak T M. Transthoracic needle aspiration in inflammatory pseudotumours of the lung. *Diagn Cytopathol* 1989; **5**: 400–403

352 Takeda M, Burechailo F A. Smooth muscle cells in sputum. *Acta Cytol* 1969; **13**: 696–699

353 Nguyen G-K. Exfoliative cytology of angiosarcoma of the pulmonary artery. *Acta Cytol* 1985; **29**: 624–627

354 Nowels K W, Burford-Foggs A et al. Epithelioid haemangioendothelioma. Cytomorphology and histological features of a case. Diagn Cytopathol 1989; 5: 75–78

355 Perry M D, Furlong J W, Johnston W W. Fine needle aspiration cytology of metastatic dermatofibrosarcoma protuberans. A case report. Acta Cytol 1986; 30: 507–512

356 Nickels J, Koivuniemi A. Cytology of malignant haemangiopericytoma. Acta Cytol 1979; 23: 119–125

357 Saleh H A, Haapaniemi J. Aspiration biopsy cytology of malignant hemangiopericytoma metastatic to the lungs. Cytomorphologic and immunocytochemical study of a case. Acta Cytol 1997; 41: 1265–1268

358 Silverman J F, Weaver M D, Gardner N et al. Aspiration biopsy cytology of malignant schwannoma metastatic to the lung. Acta Cytol 1985; 29: 15–18

359 Saleh H, Beydoun R, Masood S. Cytology of malignant schwannoma metastatic to the lung. Report of a case with diagnosis by fine needle aspiration biopsy. Acta Cytol 1993; 37: 409–412

360 Zaharopoulos P, Wong J Y, Lamke C R. Endometrial stromal sarcoma. Cytology of pulmonary metastasis including ultrastructural study. Acta Cytol 1982; 26: 49–54

361 Eisenstein R, Battifora H A. Malignant giant cell tumour of bone: exfoliation of tumour cells from pulmonary metastases. Acta Cytol 1966; 10: 130–133

362 Szyfelbein W M, Schiller A L. Cytologic diagnosis of giant cell tumour of bone metastatic to lung: a case report. Acta Cytol 1979; 23: 460–464

363 Gattuso P, Reddy V B, Castelli M J. Fine needle aspiration biopsy of paranasal chondrosarcoma metastatic to lung. Acta Cytol 1990; 34: 102–104

364 Dodd L G, Chai C, McAdams H P, Layfield L J. Fine needle aspiration of osteogenic sarcoma metastatic to the lung. A report of four cases. Acta Cytol 1998; 42: 754–758

365 Costa I, Lerma E, Esteve E et al. Aspiration cytology of lung metastasis of monophasic synovial sarcoma. Report of a case. Acta Cytol 1997; 41: 1289–1292

366 Kilpatrick S E, Teot L A, Stanley M W et al. Fine-needle aspiration biopsy of synovial sarcoma. A cytomorphologic analysis of primary, recurrent, and metastatic tumors. Am J Clin Pathol 1996; 106: 769–775

367 Mullick S S, Mody D R, Schwartz M R. Angiosarcoma at unusual sites. A report of two cases with aspiration cytology and diagnostic pitfalls. Acta Cytol 1997; 41: 839–844

368 Drut R, Pollono D. Pleuropulmonary blastoma: diagnosis by fine-needle aspiration cytology: a case report. Diagn Cytopathol 1998; 19: 303–305

369 Gelven P L, Hopkins M A, Green C A et al. Fine-needle aspiration cytology of pleuropulmonary blastoma: case report and review of the literature. Diagn Cytopathol 1997; 16: 336–340

370 Logrono R, Wojtowycz M M, Wunderlich D W et al. Fine needle aspiration cytology and core biopsy in the diagnosis of alveolar soft part sarcoma presenting with lung metastases. A case report. Acta Cytol 1999; 43: 464–470

371 Stanfield B, Powers C N, Desch C E et al. Fine needle aspiration cytology of an unusual primary lung tumour, chondrosarcoma: a case report. Diagn Cytopathol 1991; 7: 423–426

372 Cosgrove M, Chandrasoma P T, Martin S E. Diagnosis of pulmonary blastoma by fine needle aspiration biopsy: cytologic and immunocytochemical findings. Diagn Cytopathol 1991; 7: 83–87

373 Francis D, Jacobsen M. Pulmonary blastoma: preoperative cytologic and histologic findings. Acta Cytol 1979; 23: 437–442

374 Non D P Jr, Lang W R, Patchefsky A, Takeda M. Pulmonary blastoma. Cytopathologic and histopathologic findings. Acta Cytol 1976; 20: 381–386

375 Spahr J, Draffin R, Johnston W W. Cytopathologic findings in pulmonary blastoma. Acta Cytol 1979; 23: 454–459

376 Yokoyama S, Hayashida Y, Nagahama J et al. Pulmonary blastoma: a case report. Acta Cytol 1992; 36: 293–297

377 Lee K G, Cho N H. Fine needle aspiration cytology of pulmonary adenocarcinoma of fetal type. Report of a case with immunohistochemical and ultrastructural studies. Diagn Cytopathol 1991; 7: 408–414

378 Cabarcos A, Dorronsoro M G, Beristain J. Pulmonary carcinosarcoma: a case study and review of the literature. Br J Dis Chest 1985; 79: 83–94

379 Finley J L, Silverman J F, Dabbs D J. Fine needle aspiration cytology of pulmonary carcinosarcoma with immunocytochemical and ultrastructural observations. Diagn Cytopathol 1988; 4: 239–243

380 Ishizuka T, Yoshitake J, Yamada T et al. Diagnosis of a case of pulmonary carcinosarcoma by detection of rhabdomyosarcoma cells in sputum. Acta Cytol 1988; 32: 658–662

381 Das D K, Pant C S, Rath B et al. Fine needle aspiration diagnosis of intrathoracic and intra-abdominal lesions: review of experience in the paediatric age group. Diagn Cytopathol 1993; 9: 383–393

382 Linder J, Olsen G A, Johnston W W. Fine needle aspiration biopsy of the mediastinum. Am J Med 1986; 81: 1005–1008

383 Sterrett G F, Whitaker D, Shilkin K B, Walters M N-I. Fine needle aspiration cytology of mediastinal lesions. Cancer 1983; 51: 127–135

384 Weisbrod G L. Percutaneous fine needle aspiration biopsy of the mediastinum. Clin Chest Med 1987; 8: 27–41

385 Weisbrod G L, Lyons D J, Tao L-C, Chamberlain D W. Percutaneous fine needle aspiration biopsy of mediastinal lesions. AJR 1984; 143: 525–529

386 Powers C N, Silverman J F, Geisinger K R, Frable W J. Fine-needle aspiration biopsy of the mediastinum. A multi-institutional analysis. Am J Clin Pathol 1996; 105: 168–173

387 Shabb N S, Fahl M, Shabb B et al. Fine-needle aspiration of the mediastinum: a clinical, radiologic, cytologic, and histologic study of 42 cases. Diagn Cytopathol 1998; 19: 428–436

388 Reyes C V, Thompson K S, Massarani-Wafai R, Jensen J. Utilization of fine-needle aspiration cytology in the diagnosis of neoplastic superior vena caval syndrome. Diagn Cytopathol 1998; 19: 84–88

389 Geisinger K R. Differential diagnostic considerations and potential pitfalls in fine-needle aspiration biopsies of the mediastinum. Diagn Cytopathol 1995; 13: 436–442

390 WHO. Histological typing of tumours of the thymus. World Health Organization International Classification of Tumours. Berlin: Springer, 1999

391 Suster S, Moran C A. Primary thymic epithelial neoplasms: spectrum of differentiation and histological features. Semin Diagn Pathol 1999; 16: 2–17

392 Tao L C, Griffith Pearson F, Coper J D et al. Cytopathology of thymoma. Acta Cytol 1984; 28: 165–170

393 Ali S Z, Erozan Y S. Thymoma. Cytopathologic features and differential diagnosis on fine needle aspiration. Acta Cytol 1998; 42: 845–854

394 Dahlgren S E, Sandstedt B, Sunstrom C. Fine needle aspiration cytology of thymic tumours. Acta Cytol 1983; 27: 1–6

395 Miller J, Allen R, Wakefield J S L. Diagnosis of thymoma by fine needle aspiration cytology: light and electron microscopic study of a case. Diagn Cytopathol 1987; 3: 166–169

396 Pak H Y, Yokota S B, Friedberg H A. Thymoma diagnosed by transthoracic fine needle aspiration. Acta Cytol 1982; 26: 210–216

397 Sajjad S M, Lukeman J M, Llamas L, Fernandez T. Needle biopsy diagnosis of thymoma. Acta Cytol 1982; 26: 503–506

398 Shin H J, Katz R L. Thymic neoplasia as represented by fine needle aspiration biopsy of anterior mediastinal masses. A practical approach to the differential diagnosis. Acta Cytol 1998; 42: 855–864

399 Sherman M E, Black-Schaffer S. Diagnosis of thymoma by needle biopsy. Acta Cytol 1990; 34: 63–68

400 Suen K, Quenville N. Fine needle aspiration cytology of uncommon thoracic lesions. Am J Clin Pathol 1981; 75: 803–809

401 Silverman J F, Raab S S, Park H K. Fine needle aspiration cytology of primary large cell lymphoma of the mediastinum. Cytomorphological features with potential pitfalls in diagnosis. Diagn Cytopathol 1993; 9: 209–215

402 Slagel D D, Powers C N, Melaragno M J et al. Spindle-cell lesions of the mediastinum: diagnosis by fine-needle aspiration biopsy. Diagn Cytopathol 1997; 17: 167–176

403 Pinto M M, Dovgan D, Kaye A D, Chinniah A. Fine needle aspiration for diagnosing a thymoma producing CA-125. A case report. Acta Cytol 1993; 37: 929–932

404 Spahr J, Frable W J. Pulmonary cytopathology of an invasive thymoma. *Acta Cytol* 1981; **25**: 163–166

405 Finley J L, Silverman J F, Strausbach P et al. Malignant thymic neoplasms. Diagnosis by fine needle aspiration biopsy with histologic, immunocytochemical and ultrastructural confirmation. *Diagn Cytopathol* 1986; **2**: 118–125

406 Kaw Y T, Esparza A R. Fine needle aspiration cytology of primary squamous carcinoma of the thymus. A case report. *Acta Cytol* 1993; **37**: 735–739

407 Riazmontazer N, Bedayat G, Izadi B. Epithelial cytologic atypia in a fine needle aspirate of an invasive thymoma. A case report. *Acta Cytol* 1992; **36**: 387–390

408 Gherardi G, Marveggio C, Placidi A. Neuroendocrine carcinoma of the thymus: aspiration biopsy, immunocytochemistry, and clinicopathologic correlates. *Diagn Cytopathol* 1995; **12**: 158–164

409 Nichols G L Jr, Hopkins M B 3rd, Geisinger K R. Thymic carcinoid. Report of a case with diagnosis by fine needle aspiration biopsy. *Acta Cytol* 1997; **41**: 1839–1844

410 Wang D Y, Kuo S H, Chang D B et al. Fine needle aspiration cytology of thymic carcinoid tumor. *Acta Cytol* 1995; **39**: 423–427

411 Dusenbery D. Spindle-cell thymic carcinoid occurring in multiple endocrine neoplasia I: fine-needle aspiration findings in a case. *Diagn Cytopathol* 1996; **15**: 439–441

412 Dunsmore N, Sherman M E, Erozan Y S. Massive necrosis: a pitfall in the cytopathologic diagnosis of primary mediastinal seminoma. *Diagn Cytopathol* 1991; **7**: 323–324

413 Sangalli G, Livirghi T, Girordano F et al. Primary mediastinal embryonal carcinoma and choriocarcinoma. A case report. *Acta Cytol* 1986; **30**: 543–546

414 Motoyama T, Yamamoto O, Iwamoto H, Watanabe H. Fine needle aspiration cytology of primary mediastinal germ cell tumors. *Acta Cytol* 1995; **39**: 725–732

415 Dahlgren S E, Ovenfors C-O. Aspiration biopsy diagnosis of neurogenous mediastinal tumours. *Acta Radiol Diagn (Stockh)* 1970; **10**: 289–298

416 Palombini L, Vetrani A. Cytologic diagnosis of ganglioneuroblastoma. *Acta Cytol* 1976; **20**: 286–287

417 Palombini L, Vetrani A, Veccione R et al. The cytology of ganglioneuroma on fine needle aspiration smear. *Acta Cytol* 1982; **26**: 259–260

418 Heimann A, Sneige N, Shirkhoda A, De Caro L F. Fine needle aspiration cytology of thymolipoma. A case report. *Acta Cytol* 1987; **31**: 335–359

419 Mishriki Y Y, Lane B P, Lozowski M S, Epstein H. Hürthle cell tumour arising in the mediastinal ectopic thyroid and diagnosed by fine needle aspiration. Light microscopic and ultrastructural features. *Acta Cytol* 1983; **27**: 188–192

420 De Las Casas L E, Williams H J, Strausbauch P H, Silverman J F. Hurthle cell adenoma of the mediastinum: intraoperative cytology and differential diagnosis with correlative gross, histology, and ancillary studies. *Diagn Cytopathol* 2000; **22**: 16–20

421 Attal H, Jensen J, Reyes CV. Myxoid liposarcoma of the anterior mediastinum. Diagnosis by fine needle aspiration biopsy. *Acta Cytol* 1995; **39**: 511–513

422 Marco V, Sirvent J, Alvarez Moro J et al. Malignant melanotic schwannoma fine-needle aspiration biopsy findings. *Diagn Cytopathol* 1998; **18**: 284–286

423 Prieto-Rodriguez M, Camanas-Sanz A, Bas T et al. Psammomatous melanotic schwannoma localized in the mediastinum: diagnosis by fine-needle aspiration cytology. *Diagn Cytopathol* 1998; **19**: 298–302

424 Gledhill A, Bates C, Henderson D et al. Sputum cytology: a limited role. *J Clin Pathol* 1997; **50**: 566–568

425 Hsu C. Cytologic diagnosis of lung tumours from bronchial brushings of Chinese patients in Hong Kong. *Acta Cytol* 1983; **27**: 641–696

426 Lachman M F, Schofield K, Cellura K. Bronchoscopic diagnosis of malignancy in the lower airway. A cytologic review. *Acta Cytol* 1995; **39**: 1148–1151

427 Popp W, Merkle M, Schreiber B et al. How much brushing is enough for the diagnosis of lung tumours? *Cancer* 1992; **70**: 2278–2280

428 Layfield L J, Coogan A, Johnston W W, Patz E F. Transthoracic fine needle aspiration biopsy. Sensitivity in relation to guidance technique and lesion size and location. *Acta Cytol* 1996; **40**: 687–690

429 Caya J G, Gilles L, Tieu T M et al. Lung cancer treated on the basis of cytologic findings: an analysis of 112 patients. *Diagn Cytopathol* 1990; **6**: 313–316

430 Caya J G, Wollenberg N J, Clowry L J, Tieu T M. The diagnosis of pulmonary small cell anaplastic carcinoma by cytologic smears: a 13 year experience. *Diagn Cytopathol* 1988; **4**: 202–205

431 Benbasset J, Regev A, Slater P. Predictive value of sputum cytology. *Thorax* 1987; **42**: 165–172

432 Naryshkin S, Young N A. Respiratory cytology: a review of non-neoplastic mimics of malignancy. *Diagn Cytopathol* 1993; **9**: 89–97

433 Ritter J H, Wick M R, Reyes A et al. False-positive interpretations of carcinoma in exfoliative respiratory cytology. Report of two cases and a review of underlying disorders. *Am J Clin Pathol* 1995; **104**: 133–140

434 Silverman J F. Inflammatory and neoplastic processes of the lung: differential diagnosis and pitfalls in FNA biopsies. *Diagn Cytopathol* 1995; **13**: 448–462

435 Kern W H. The diagnostic accuracy of sputum and urine cytology. *Acta Cytol* 1988; **32**: 651–654

436 Kern W H. The elusive 'false positive' sputum and urine cytology. *Acta Cytol* 1990; **34**: 587–588

437 Cagle P T, Kovach M, Ramzy I. Causes of false results in transthoracic fine needle lung aspirates. *Acta Cytol* 1993; **37**: 16–20

438 Caya J G, Clowry L T, Wollenberg N J, Tieu T M. Transthoracic fine needle aspiration cytology. Analysis of 82 patients with detailed verification criteria and evaluation of false negative cases. *Am J Clin Pathol* 1984; **82**: 100–103

439 Delgado P I, Jorda M, Ganjei-Azar P. Small cell carcinoma versus other lung malignancies. Diagnosis by fine-needle aspiration cytology. *Cancer (Cancer Cytopathology)* 2000; **90**: 279–285

440 Weisbrod G L, Cunningham I, Tao L C, Chamberlain D W. Small cell anaplastic carcinoma: cytological histological correlations from percutaneous fine needle aspiration biopsy. *J Can Assoc Radiol* 1987; **38**: 204–208

Serous cavities

4 Reactive effusions

Thomas Krausz and Frederick Barker

The normal serous cavities

The pleural cavities, pericardial cavity and peritoneal cavity are the serous cavities. Each is a potential cavity but is normally collapsed, containing only a small volume of lubricant fluid. The visceral and parietal surfaces of each cavity are lined by a membrane, the mesothelium, which is continuous where the surfaces meet; hence the viscera are actually external to the serous cavities and invaginate the visceral mesothelium. The serous fluid lubricates the movement of the lungs relative to the chest wall, and of the heart relative to the pericardium. It also lubricates movement of the digestive tract.

The visceral and parietal surfaces of the serous cavities are lined by a single layer of mesothelial cells which is supported by vascular connective tissue. The mesothelial cells have long microvilli on their free surface, while pinocytotic vesicles are present in their cytoplasm, generally close to the luminal and abluminal surfaces. The cytoplasm contains numerous intermediate filaments; these can be detected by immunochemistry and electron microscopy, which show them to be most numerous around the nucleus. Tight junctions are present between cells. The connective tissue contains collagen fibres in a polysaccharide matrix, which is also permeated by capillaries and lymphatics. The pleura of humans has been studied most; in some respects the visceral and parietal pleurae differ, for the visceral pleura is thicker, while stomata are present between the parietal mesothelial cells, and measure 2–12 μm across.

The volume of fluid present in each serous cavity is known to be small but is difficult to measure accurately in humans. It has been estimated to be about 1 ml in the pericardial sac, a little more in the pleural spaces, and rather more, perhaps as much as 50 ml, in the peritoneal cavity[1]. In the pleural cavity in mammals, the volume has been found to be 0.1–0.2 ml/kg body weight[2].

Formation of the fluid involves the passage of fluid out of the capillaries in the serous membranes into the connective tissue, which it must then pass through to reach the mesothelial layer. The rate of formation of fluid will increase if the capillary pressure rises, if the capillary oncotic pressure falls, or if inflammation increases capillary permeability. Resistance to the flow of fluid through the connective tissue depends in part upon the degree of hydration of the tissue. In dehydrated subjects, the collagen fibres and polysaccharide molecules are closely packed and offer considerable resistance to the passage of fluid, but as hydration increases, the separation of the molecules widens to the point at which channels open up through the connective tissue. In this situation, the resistance to the flow of fluid becomes low[3,4].

To reach the serous cavity, the fluid has finally to cross the mesothelial cell. Two routes appear to be possible: between cells and through the cytoplasm in pinocytotic vesicles. The mesothelial cell layer is known to offer little resistance to the flow of water and solutes; even molecules as large as albumin cross the layer with ease[5].

The mechanisms of resorption of fluid are less certain. The older view concerning the pleural cavity assumed that the visceral pleura was perfused by the pulmonary circulation, and hence that the mean capillary pressure in the visceral pleural circulation (8 mmHg) was lower than that in the parietal pleural circulation (22 mmHg), as the latter is part of the systemic circulation. It followed that, due to hydrostatic and oncotic forces, there was a net movement of fluid across the pleural space from the parietal to the visceral pleura, where the fluid was resorbed by the visceral capillaries. It was also assumed that some resorption by lymphatics took place[6].

The more recent view differs in several respects. It is now thought that in humans the visceral pleural arterial supply is derived from the bronchial circulation and hence is systemic[2]; moreover, the thicker visceral pleura may impede flow of fluid in either direction, so that the greater part of the flow of fluid is probably across the parietal pleura. Pleural fluid probably re-enters the parietal pleura via the stomata between the mesothelial cells, and is resorbed mainly by the lymphatics. The formation of a transudate (see later) could then be most readily explained by impaired lymphatic drainage. In the common setting of congestive heart failure, the rise in the mean right atrial pressure would be transmitted via the large veins to the lymphatics compromising lymphatic flow.

The fluid dynamics of the pericardial and peritoneal cavities have been less studied, and it is not certain whether similar mechanisms operate. It is notable that in circulatory disturbances such as right ventricular failure, effusions accumulate most readily in the peritoneum; this appears to be because of the ease with which fluid can leave the congested sinusoids of the liver and reach the peritoneal space.

Injury to the mesothelial cell layer occurs in various situations including inflammation, infection, neoplasia and trauma. The mechanisms of regeneration have not been extensively investigated; the historical view was that dividing mesothelial cells spread over the injured area from the periphery[7] but this view was challenged when it was found that the rate of healing was the same regardless of the size of the injured area[8]. Various mechanisms of regeneration were proposed subsequently including the postulated existence of a submesothelial cell layer which would proliferate and differentiate in response to mesothelial injury[9]. Recently, experimenters following mesothelial regeneration with quantitative methods using tritiated thymidine have argued strongly against the hypothesis of a submesothelial cell layer and in favour of regeneration by mesothelial cells[10].

The molecular interactions between the mesothelial cell and other cells have been studied. CD44, which exists in several forms, is the principal receptor for hyaluronic acid, which is secreted by mesothelial cells. Certain tumour cells, particularly those of adenocarcinomas of the ovary, produce CD44 which some investigators consider to be implicated in the adhesion of the tumour cells to the peritoneal surface via hyaluronic acid[11,12], while others think that hyaluronic acid is actually a barrier to adhesion[13].

Transudates and exudates

Two mechanisms underlie the development of serous effusions. Transudates form as a result of physical disturbance of the circulation, usually a rise in venous pressure or a decrease in oncotic pressure, while exudates form as a result of increased capillary permeability, which is usually due to inflammation. The distinction between the two types of effusion is not clear-cut because transudates may be complicated by secondary inflammation.

Transudates

The cellular content and protein content of a pure transudate are low and are similar to those of normal serous fluid. The cells present are usually macrophages, mesothelial cells and lymphocytes. It may be difficult to distinguish the first two types of cell by morphology and more so if the mesothelial cells are dissociated. It is common to see degenerate mesothelial cells or macrophages in which the cytoplasm has several vacuoles or a large vacuole compressing the nucleus, producing a signet ring appearance, which can be confused with adenocarcinoma. This is discussed further below. Small numbers of mast cells may be seen in transudates from the peritoneum.

The concentration of protein in a pure transudate is usually not more than about 30 g/l. Pure transudates occur most commonly in the peritoneal cavity; conditions with

which they are associated include cardiac, liver and renal failure. In the pleural cavity transudates are usually associated with cardiac or renal failure.

Exudates

Exudates form as a result of increased permeability of the capillaries in the serosal wall and protein and cells pass through the capillary walls much more readily than is the case with transudates. In consequence, in a typical exudate the cellular content is much greater than that of a transudate and a greater variety of cells is usually present. These cells may be inflammatory or neoplastic, depending on the cause of the exudate. The concentration of protein is often greater than that found in a transudate, but not invariably so as there is considerable overlap between the ranges. The protein usually contains fibrin, and the higher the concentration of protein, the more likely is the fluid to clot.

When exudates form in a case of infection, micro-organisms may be present, while in cases of trauma or fistula, foreign material may be found in the exudate.

Molecular studies have shown that the mesothelium is not a passive bystander in inflammatory conditions. Stimulated mesothelial cells release numerous substances including nitric oxide, enzymes, platelet-derived growth factor, monocyte chemotactic peptide and interleukins[14].

Cells in normal serous fluid

Normal ranges of types and concentrations of cells in serous fluids have not been established with confidence since the volumes of fluid in the normal serous cavities are small and are spread thinly over large areas, making sampling without significant trauma practically impossible. In 1933 a study was reported in which pleural fluid was aspirated from healthy men; the concentration of cells was in the range 1700–6200 cells/ml, most cells being large mononuclear cells and the remainder being lymphocytes and mesothelial cells[15]. In the pleural cavity in animals, the types of cell present are similar[2], and number about 1500 cells/µl.

Laparoscopy allows sampling of peritoneal fluid without much disruption of the serous membrane, and fluid may sometimes be obtained by culdocentesis. Such samples have contained a preponderance of macrophages with relatively few lymphocytes and mesothelial cells, but clusters of mesothelial cells have been found, even with psammoma bodies. If endosalpingiosis is present in the peritoneum, clusters of epithelial cells with psammoma bodies may be found in the peritoneal fluid. The presence of cilia on the epithelial cells will distinguish them from mesothelial cells. However, if there is nuclear atypia, the possibility of a serous carcinoma should be considered. Obtaining samples of pericardial fluid is difficult, and most commonly used to be done at thoracotomy[16]. The introduction of radiologically guided fine needle aspiration has made sampling feasible without surgery.

Mesothelial cells

The mesothelial cell is the only cell specific to the serous membranes. When the serosa is injured, e.g. by inflammation, or stimulated, e.g. by ascites, the mesothelial cells undergo proliferation. In histological sections from proliferated mesothelium the cells may be multilayered or form papillae, and in this state the cells are more likely to be shed into the serous fluid. Single mesothelial cells are round and often have an indistinct cytoplasmic membrane. The cytoplasm is a dense green when stained by the Papanicolaou method, and blue or deep blue when stained by the May-Grunwald-Giemsa (MGG) method. The nucleus is large, round or elliptical and often has a single nucleolus. In addition to single cells, clusters are often found; these may consist of clumps of many cells, or of only a few cells. When there are only two or three cells together, they often display a feature called 'windows', in which a lozenge-shaped, empty space separates adjacent cells, the cytoplasm of which only touches at either end of the lozenge (Fig. 4.1). This phenomenon may sometimes be seen, however, in adenocarcinoma[17].

The diameter of the mesothelial cell is quite variable. The smallest cells are little larger than a red cell, but the range extends to several tens of microns. The largest cells are usually multinucleated (Fig. 4.2). Mesothelial cells in mitosis may be seen (Fig. 4.3).

Examination by electron microscopy reveals that the surface of the mesothelial cell bears microvilli which differ from those of epithelial cells by being longer and thinner (Fig. 4.4). Thick, blunt, cytoplasmic protrusions have also been described[18]. These two features may be responsible for the fluffy 'brush' border which mesothelial cells often display, particularly when the MGG stain is used.

Glycogen is often present in mesothelial cells. It is not stained by the Papanicolaou or MGG techniques and so appears as a peripheral ring of tiny spaces in the cytoplasm. The granules are revealed by staining with PAS and are diastase-labile. It may also be present as fine granules distributed throughout the cytoplasm, or as very coarse granules arranged in a large crescent; in this last form, it is more often found in the cells of malignant mesothelioma than in benign mesothelial cells (Fig. 4.5). Mesothelial cells also synthesize hyaluronic acid; this can be demonstrated rarely in some cytoplasmic vacuoles and more regularly on the cell surface by staining with Alcian blue. Prior treatment with hyaluronidase should abolish or greatly reduce the staining, but the technique is a difficult one and requires stringent controls.

Lipids may be present in mesothelial cells, usually in small amounts in the form of microvacuoles around the nucleus (Fig. 4.6A). These microvacuoles can be seen in wet or MGG preparations as unstained droplets, but confirmation of their nature is provided by a fat stain, such as oil red-O. Lipid droplets may be more prominent and more extensively distributed in the cytoplasm in some cases of mesothelioma.

Occasionally, mesothelial cells contain small amounts of pigment, usually haemosiderin or lipofuscin, which are brown in the Papanicolaou stain or greenish-blue with MGG. These pigmented mesothelial cells can be confused with macrophages, and the distinction between the two types of cell must be made with other morphological criteria. Pigmented mesothelial cells also have to be distinguished from cells of metastatic melanoma.

A further source of confusion is the presence in some mesothelial cells of large vacuoles in the mesothelial cytoplasm. These may be round, or, if very large, they may extend partially around the nucleus and nearly fill the cytoplasm (Fig. 4.6C). These vacuoles are considered to be a degenerative feature; neither glycogen, mucin nor lipid can be demonstrated in them, which helps in distinction from adenocarcinoma.

The various types of vacuolation just described cause resemblance between mesothelial cells and macrophages but, in general, mesothelial cytoplasm is more dense and lacks the diffuse microvacuolation often found in

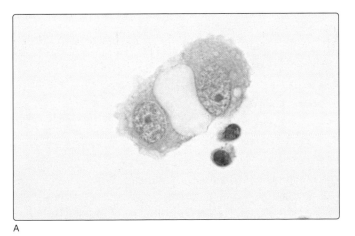

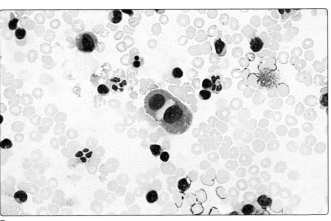

A   B

Fig. 4.1   Mesothelial cells with intercellular spaces. Pleural effusion. (A, Papanicolaou × OI; B, MGG × HP)

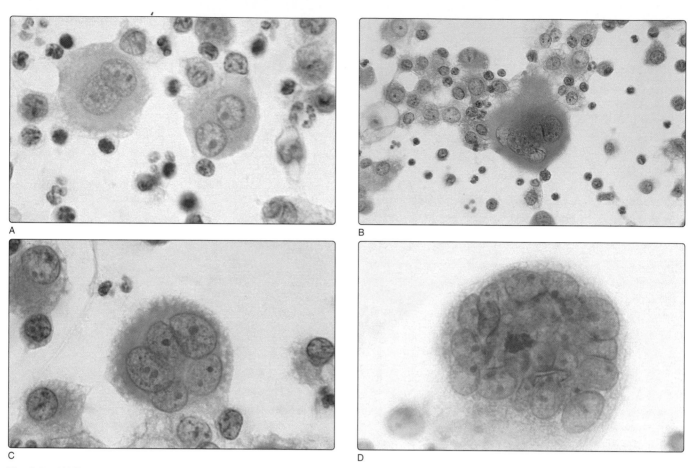

Fig. 4.2   (A) Binucleate mesothelial cells. Ascites. (Papanicolaou) (B) A multinucleate mesothelial cell. Bi- and multinucleation do not indicate malignancy, though they are more common in mesothelioma. Pleural fluid. (Papanicolaou) (C) Multinucleate mesothelial cell. Pleural fluid. (Papanicolaou) (D) A giant, multinucleate mesothelial cell with one nucleus in mitosis. Pleural fluid. (Papanicolaou × OI)

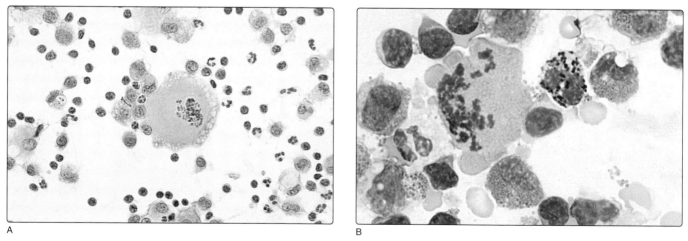

Fig. 4.3   Mesothelial cells in mitosis. Peritoneal fluid. Mitosis by itself does not denote malignancy. (A, Papanicolaou × HP; B, MGG × OI)

macrophages. The mesothelial nucleus is more deeply staining and has a smoother contour and in multinucleated cells, mesothelial nuclei are not usually distorted (Fig. 4.7). The morphological distinction between mesothelial cells and adenocarcinoma showing

little pleomorphism can be very difficult, but immunochemistry using a panel of antibodies[19] will usually help (Fig. 4.8). Many antibodies have been tested in the hope of finding markers that will distinguish between mesothelial cells and adenocarcinoma and there

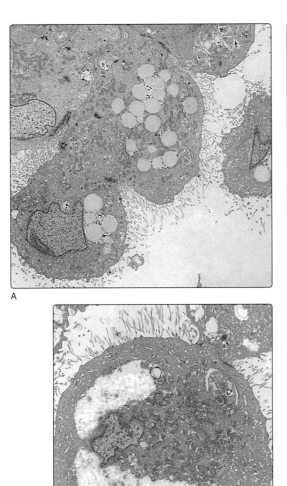

A

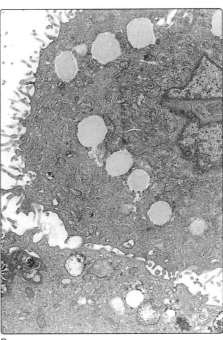

B

C

Fig. 4.4 Ultrastructure of mesothelial cells. Lipid vacuoles and long microvilli are shown in (A) and (B), and long microvilli in C. (EM) (With permission from Oxford University Press 1992)

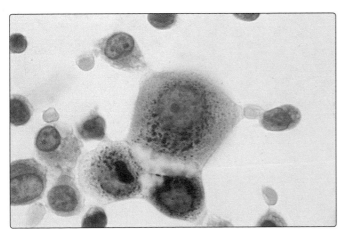

Fig. 4.5 Glycogen in the cytoplasm of mesothelial cells can occur in dispersed granules or large lakes. Pleural fluid. (PAS × OI)

are now some promising candidates. Calretinin[20,21], fibronectin[22], thrombomodulin[23] and CA125[24,25] favour mesothelial cells, while GLUT1[26], CA19-9[27] and Ber EP4[28] are among the newer antibodies which favour adenocarcinoma. Integrin[29] and lectin[30] profiles also show promise. This topic is covered further in Chapter 5.

Mesothelial cells may appear in another form if they are present in fluid obtained by peritoneal washing during laparotomy or laparoscopy. The procedure dislodges large, flat sheets of cells which, when examined with the microscope, can be seen to consist of a monolayer of uniform cells in a mosaic pattern (Fig. 4.9); there is seldom any risk of mistaking this appearance for carcinoma.

True papillary fragments of mesothelium have a core of connective tissue, which is invested with mesothelial cells. Microscopic examination reveals that these papillae have

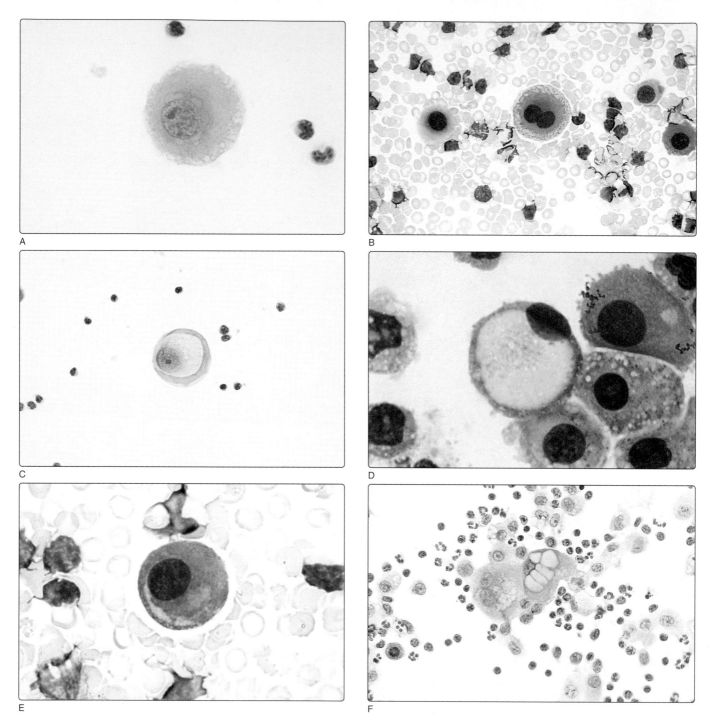

Fig. 4.6 Vacuolated mesothelial cells. In (A) (Papanicolaou × OI) and (B) (MGG × OI), there is peripheral microvacuolation, while in (C) (Papanicolaou × HP) and (D) (MGG × HP) a large vacuole nearly fills the cytoplasm. Crescentic vacuolation is present in (E) (MGG × OI), and in (F) (Papanicolaou × HP) several vacuoles are moulded together. Pleural effusion.

depth, and the lack of cells in the core of connective tissue will be apparent. The core will be stained green or brown with the Papanicolaou stain.

The possibility of confusion with adenocarcinoma is real, and the distinction depends on the absence of malignant features in the nuclei. The nuclear detail may be obscured in these papillae, in which case examination of smaller fragments and single cells, if any, may help to make the distinction. Rarely, mesothelial papillae may calcify, and hence the presence of psammoma bodies does not distinguish adenocarcinoma from benign mesothelial papillae[31]. Endosalpingiosis, which was mentioned earlier, can be distinguished from mesothelial papillae by its ciliated epithelium.

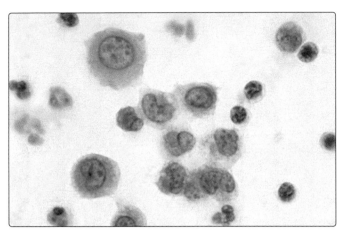

Fig. 4.7 A mesothelial cell (top left of centre) with macrophages. The nuclear characteristics of the macrophages distinguish them from the mesothelial cell. Ascites. (Papanicolaou × OI)

Macrophages

Like the mesothelial cell, the macrophage is found in almost every sample of serous fluid. It is a large cell with a mean diameter of about 30 µm but the variation in size is great. The outline of the cell is round, and the cytoplasm is microvacuolated or lace-like. With the Papanicolaou stain, it is a lighter green than the cytoplasm of the mesothelial cell. When viewed along an appropriate axis, the nucleus is indented and located off-centre; its chromatin is granular but nucleoli, if present at all, are small. Macrophages are less often found in clusters than mesothelial cells, but they sometimes occur in loosely cohesive sheets, which lack the mosaic uniformity of sheets of mesothelial cells.

As a result of degeneration or phagocytic activity, the cytoplasm of a macrophage may contain a single large vacuole or a few large vacuoles (Fig. 4.10); such vacuolation may also be seen in mesothelial cells and in adenocarcinoma. In extreme cases the vacuole may so distend the cytoplasm that the nucleus is compressed, producing an appearance similar to that of signet ring carcinoma. The true nature of the cells will be apparent if a range of forms can be found, but in other cases immunocytochemistry may be necessary. The phagocytic activity of macrophages may be apparent from the presence of other foreign matter in the cytoplasm, such as engulfed leucocytes or red cells, or cellular debris ('tingible body macrophages') (Fig. 4.11). In biliary peritonitis bile pigment has been found in macrophages and free bile in peritoneal fluid[32].

Although multinucleated macrophages are common in histological specimens, they are unusual in serous effusions, with the exception of effusions occurring in rheumatoid disease. In most other instances, multinucleated cells can be shown to be mesothelial cells.

Lymphocytes

Lymphocytes, like macrophages and mesothelial cells, are present in almost every sample of serous fluid. The small

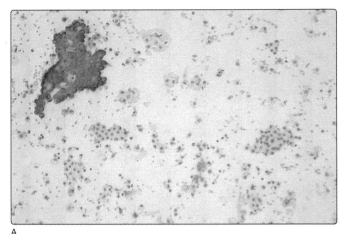

A

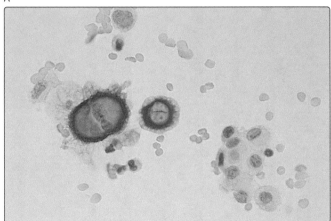

B

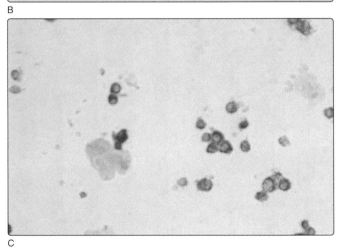

C

Fig. 4.8 Immunocytochemistry is helpful in certain cases to distinguish between mesothelial cells and macrophages. (A) Cytokeratin highlights mesothelial cells in a group while macrophages are unstained. (B) The perinuclear ring-like arrangement of cytokeratin filaments is typical of mesothelial cells. (C) CD68 stains macrophages but not mesothelial cells. Pericardial effusion.

lymphocyte is the type most commonly found and is little larger than a red cell. The cell is practically all nucleus, with only a rim of basophilic cytoplasm. The chromatin of the round nucleus is uniformly granular and is stained intensely; examination under oil may reveal a slight

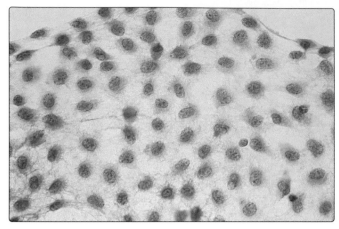

Fig. 4.9 Mesothelial cells in a cohesive sheet one layer thick. Peritoneal fluid. (Papanicolaou × HP)

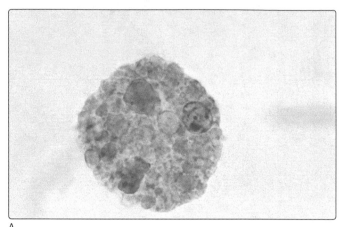

A

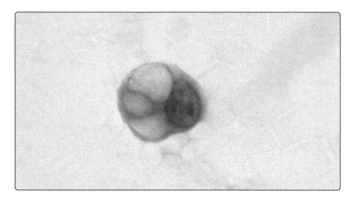

Fig. 4.10 A vacuolated macrophage. This should not be confused with adenocarcinoma. Peritoneal fluid. (Papanicolaou × OI)

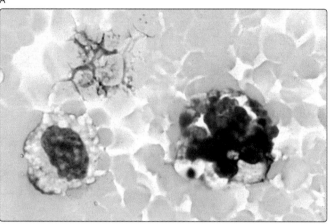

B

Fig. 4.11 Pigmented macrophages. In this case the pigment was haemosiderin but lipofuscin is also found. Peritoneal fluid. (A, Papanicolaou × OI; B, MGG × OI)

indentation of the nucleus (Fig. 4.12). Immunocytochemical staining has shown that the majority of small lymphocytes in serous fluids are T cells[33,34].

It may sometimes be necessary, particularly in pleural effusions, to distinguish small lymphocytes from the cells of oat cell carcinoma (small cell carcinoma). Oat cells often aggregate and exhibit moulding, which means that the surface of one cell may be concave where it abuts on an adjacent convex surface of another cell; lymphocytes have less tendency to aggregate and when they do make contact they do not deform. In other morphological respects the two types of cell are rather similar, although they can be distinguished by immunocytochemistry.

Very infrequently, an occasional lymphocyte may be seen in which hyaline droplets of immunoglobulin are present in the cytoplasm; these Mott cells are several times the diameter of a small lymphocyte, and have been described in both benign effusions and in effusions containing cells of lymphoplasmacytoid lymphoma[35].

Immature lymphoid cells constitute a small proportion of the cells found in benign effusions; these cells have a larger volume of easily visible cytoplasm than small lymphocytes,

and larger, less densely stained nuclei with one or more nucleoli.

Neutrophils

Neutrophils are also present in virtually every specimen of serous fluid. Their concentration varies enormously, from the occasional cell, which might be seen in a sample of serous fluid from a case of heart failure, to the large numbers of cells, which are found in purulent effusions. The typical neutrophil is a little larger than a red cell; its cytoplasm stains weakly green with the Papanicolaou method, but the granules in the cytoplasm are difficult to see. In an MGG preparation the pale pink granules are more easily discerned. The lobated nucleus, which is the most characteristic feature of the cell, is clearly demonstrated by either method: three is the commonest number of lobes, but smaller and larger numbers occur. A strand of chromatin links adjacent lobes (Fig. 4.13A). Neutrophils are often seen in states of degeneration; the nucleus fragments into small, discrete basophilic globules, which are said to resemble drops of mercury, and as the plasma membrane loses its integrity the cytoplasm expands.

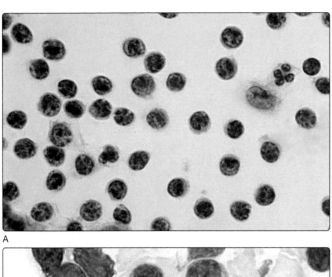

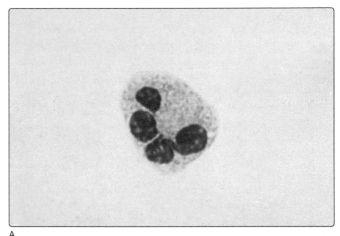

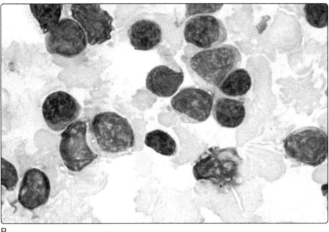

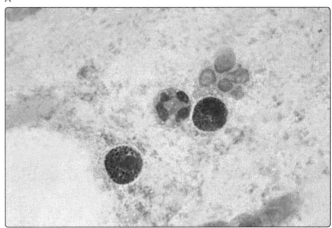

Fig. 4.12 A lymphocyte predominant effusion. In such cases the possibility of small lymphocytic lymphoma or chronic lymphocytic leukaemia cannot be excluded. Pleural effusion. (A, Papanicolaou ×OI; B, MGG × OI)

Eventually disintegration reaches a point at which the cell becomes unrecognizable.

Eosinophils

An occasional eosinophil is present in most serous effusions, but in some circumstances the eosinophil is numerous. In preparations stained by the Papanicolaou technique, the most conspicuous feature is the bilobed nucleus. The lobes are larger and rounder than those of the neutrophil; only a small proportion of eosinophils has a greater number of lobes than two. The cytoplasm stains green but it is seldom possible to discern granules. By contrast, when the MGG method is used, the orange-red granules in the cytoplasm are obvious. Another stain sometimes used is chromotrope 2R, which colours the granules a dull red (Fig. 4.13B). If an eosinophil has discharged its granules, it can still be recognized by its nuclear morphology.

'Eosinophilic' effusions have long been considered to be a distinct class of effusion. The concentration or percentage of eosinophils in a fluid which is required in order for an

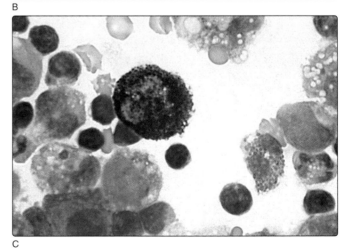

Fig. 4.13 Granulocytes. (A) A neutrophil. (MGG × OI) (B) Eosinophils stained with chromotrope 2R × HP. The granules of the neutrophil are unstained. (C) A basophil with metachromatic purple granules. (MGG × OI)

effusion to be described as eosinophilic cannot be determined logically, and the definitions which have appeared in the literature are arbitrary: most definitions have fallen in the range 5–50%. The clinical associations are varied, including mechanical factors such as trauma and pneumothorax[36], infectious conditions such as tuberculosis, fungal and parasitic infections and pneumonia, and conditions such as allergy, malignancy and pulmonary infarction[37]. As one might expect, most of these associations are with pleural eosinophilic effusions and, in fact, eosinophilic effusions in the other serous cavities are very seldom found. A correlation between the duration of a pneumothorax, the percentage of eosinophils in the pleural fluid and the concentration of interleukin 5 has been reported[38]. In about one-third of all eosinophilic effusions, no precipitating factor is found. Notwithstanding the disparate situations in which eosinophilic effusions develop, one feature which unites them is their generally good prognosis; most do eventually resolve, although in a few cases it may take a year or two[39-41].

Peritoneal eosinophilic effusions have been described in association with similar conditions to the above but also with peritoneal dialysis[42,43]. This procedure introduces plastic into the peritoneum and is a source of small quantities of materials such as starch. It is presumed that some subjects experience a hypersensitivity reaction, which provokes the effusion[44].

Pericardial eosinophilic effusions are extremely rare but have been described in eosinophilic conditions involving the lung[45].

Plasma cells

These are occasionally found in effusions associated with chronic inflammation, and also in some cases of lymphoreticular neoplasia. In the Papanicolaou stain, they may be difficult to distinguish from lymphocytes, but the MGG stain reveals the aggregated chromatin of the eccentric nucleus, and the strongly amphophilic cytoplasm. The pale halo next to the nucleus corresponds to the Golgi complex.

Mast cells and basophils

Mast cells and basophils are infrequently found in serous fluids. They are hardly ever present in appreciable numbers, except in mast cell proliferative diseases and some types of myeloid leukaemia respectively. Their granules are normally seen in MGG preparations (Fig. 4.13C), in which they are stained deep red or blue[46], but not in Papanicolaou preparations.

Distinction between the two types of cell in effusions is not particularly easy as they have many features in common, but the nucleus of the basophil is less likely to be obscured by the granules than is the nucleus of the mast cell. The granules of the mast cell are AS-D chloroacetate esterase positive, while those of the basophil show little activity. The basophil granules are relatively soluble in water and are easily lost in the staining baths if immersion is prolonged. Histamine is present in the granules of both types of cell, as are mucopolysaccharides; the latter confer the property of metachromasia on the granules. Receptors for IgE can be detected on the surface of mast cells and basophils.

Investigations in humans[47] and animals[48] have shown that mast cells and basophils are derived from precursor cells in the marrow, and possibly even from the same precursor. A circulatory cell without granules migrates into the tissues and there matures into a granulated mast cell.

Red cells

A few red cells can be found even in clear samples of serous fluid (Fig. 4.14), while in blood-stained fluid, the cells will be numerous. Lysis of red cells produces a xanthochromia when the haemoglobin becomes degenerate. Intact red cells, when seen in serous fluid stained by the Papanicolaou technique, are light green or orange discs about 7 µm across and have the usual biconcave shape (Fig. 4.15). However, the fixation step usually causes lysis of the red cells, which then appear as ghosts with a green rim, while the released haemoglobin forms an amorphous pale green background. If the morphology of the red cells is of concern, it is necessary to use some other stain such as MGG, which renders them orange red and does not cause lysis. The various abnormal forms of red cell which occur in some haemoglobinopathies,

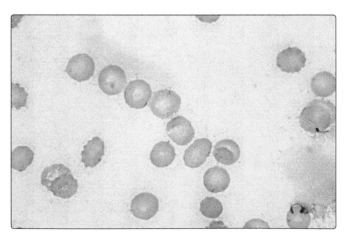

Fig. 4.14   Red cells. The biconcave shape is responsible for the paler staining at the centre of each cell. Peritoneal fluid. (MGG × OI)

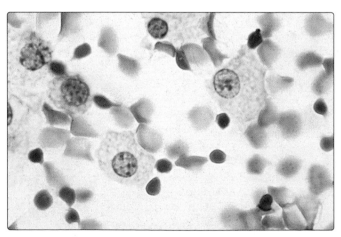

Fig. 4.15   Red cells. These are stained orange-red. Pleural fluid. (Papanicolaou × OI)

anaemias and myeloproliferative disorders may also be seen in serous fluids as well as in the blood.

Red cells in fluids are sometimes engulfed by macrophages without lysis and can be seen distending the cytoplasm of the macrophage. This is seldom of pathological significance.

Megakaryocytes

Megakaryocytes are seldom found in effusions. When they are present, it is usually in association with some abnormality of haemopoiesis such as a myeloproliferative disorder or in association with secondary involvement of the bone marrow by carcinoma or lymphoma[49,50].

One case has been described in which megakaryocytes were found in a haemorrhagic pleural effusion, which developed in a patient who was taking an anticoagulant[51].

The morphology of megakaryocytes in effusions is best demonstrated by the MGG stain; the mature cells are large and have multiple nuclei, each with a nucleolus. Recognition of atypical or immature forms is less easy, and there may be a possibility of confusion with neoplastic cells; immunostaining for factor VIII related antigen will often help as megakaryocytes are usually positive[52,53].

Types of effusions

Effusions associated with malignancy, which are discussed in Chapter 5 are excluded here. As mentioned earlier, transudates usually result from hydrostatic disturbances while exudates are generally associated with inflammation; this may be either specific or non-specific.

Non-specific effusions

Non-specific inflammatory effusions are much more common than specific effusions. Non-specific in this context refers to the content of the effusion, not to the underlying cause, which may well be specific (e.g. a bacterial pneumonia causing a pleuritis). The effusion usually contains a mixture of inflammatory cells such as neutrophils and lymphocytes, and often macrophages and mesothelial cells, in variable proportions. Red cells are also usually present, sometimes in sufficient numbers to colour the fluid. It is a commonly held clinical belief that a blood-stained effusion is likely to be malignant, but this is often not the case. In addition to cells, the effusion may contain fibrin, which may be seen with the microscope as weakly basophilic trails. If the fibrin content is great enough, the fluid may clot. Chylous effusions, in which the fluid has a milky appearance, are uncommon. Malignant lymphoma accounts for the largest group; other causes of lymphatic obstruction such as carcinoma, notably bronchial carcinoma, can produce similar effusions. They can also result from accidental or surgical trauma to the cisterna chyli or lymphatic duct. Chylous ascites may complicate lymphangioleiomyomatosis[54].

In general, it is not possible by examination of a non-specific effusion to deduce the underlying cause, although there are two relatively uncommon special cases that suggest possible causes. One case is that in which most or all of the inflammatory cells are neutrophils, which constitutes a purulent effusion; in the pleural cavities, this is often called an empyema. Some of the neutrophils are likely to be degenerate, and the DNA released from these cells into the fluid makes it sticky. The majority of cases of empyema occur in association with bacterial pneumonia; it may or may not be possible to detect micro-organisms in the fluid. Other associations are with pulmonary malignancy or infarction, and some cases develop through secondary bacterial infection of a serous effusion. Purulent effusions in the other two serous cavities are rare, and when they occur it is usually in association with malignancy or infarction of a viscus.

The other special case is that in which the inflammatory cells in the effusion are predominantly lymphocytes, usually small and mature. The most common associations are with pulmonary malignancy and with tuberculosis[55] and, as was noted above in connection with purulent effusions, most lymphocytic effusions occur in the pleural cavities. As would be expected, a few lymphocytic effusions arise through direct involvement of the serous membranes by malignant lymphoma of small lymphocytic type or by chronic lymphocytic leukaemia. The distinction of these conditions from inflammatory effusions poses difficulties, which are discussed in Chapter 5. A primary effusion lymphoma has been described. This occurs mainly in patients with HIV infection and takes the form of a proliferation of large, atypical lymphoid cells in the serous cavities. The cells are of B lineage and may contain sequences from herpesvirus 8 (Kaposi's sarcoma-associated virus) and from Epstein-Barr virus[56–60].

Specific effusions

Specific inflammatory effusions occur in association with two connective tissue diseases, namely rheumatoid arthritis and systemic lupus erythematosus.

Rheumatoid disease

Rheumatoid disease, when it involves extra-articular sites, is one of the conditions that produces palisaded granulomas. These comprise a central area of necrosis surrounded by radially directed elongated histiocytes. Multinucleated macrophages may also be present but are not usually prominent. If such granulomas develop in serous membranes, an effusion may form but, in addition, macrophages and necrotic debris may be released into the fluid.

Cytological findings

► Elongated histiocytes
► Granular necrotic debris
► Multinucleated histiocytes

The multinucleated histiocytes, when they are present in an effusion, do not differ from such cells found in effusions in other circumstances (Fig. 4.16). The elongated histiocytes have round or elongated nuclei, and quite often more than one nucleus, while the cytoplasm is moderately dense (Fig. 4.17). The necrotic debris is often present in large amounts relative to the cells, is of variable tinctorial quality and occurs in granules many times larger than the diameter of a leucocyte (Fig. 4.18). These granules characteristically have fuzzy borders.

The combination of two types of histiocyte and necrotic debris in an effusion is considered to be pathognomonic of rheumatoid disease[61,62]. In practice, rheumatoid effusions also contain a mixture of inflammatory cells such as are found in many other types of effusion; mesothelial cells are infrequent. If wet films, stained or unstained, are prepared from rheumatoid effusions, droplets of lipid are sometimes visible in the cytoplasm of neutrophils. Similar cells may be seen in joint fluid from patients with arthritis, in which situation they are called ragocytes (see Chapter 42). Even in joint fluid ragocytes are not specific to rheumatoid arthritis, and similar cells have been found in serous effusions in conditions unrelated to arthropathy. The cells are hence of only limited value in diagnosing a rheumatoid effusion[63].

Degenerative changes often complicate a rheumatoid effusion. Inflammatory cells may undergo karyorrhexis, and decomposition of cell membranes releases cholesterol, which may crystallize in the form of flat, rhomboidal plates which are unstained in MGG preparations (Fig. 4.19) and can also be seen by phase contrast[46].

Most rheumatoid effusions occur in the pleural space, while a few develop in the pericardium. In a rheumatoid effusion

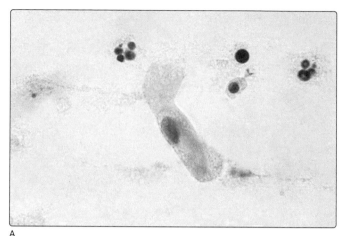

A

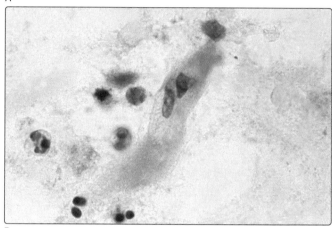

B

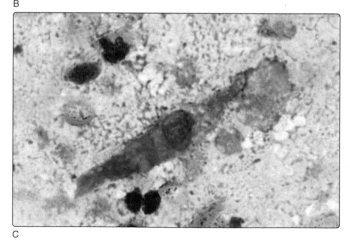

C

Fig. 4.17 Elongated histiocytes in rheumatoid disease. Pleural effusion. (A, B, Papanicolaou × OI; C, MGG × OI)

A

B

Fig. 4.16 Multinucleated histiocytes in rheumatoid disease. Pleural effusion. (A, Papanicolaou × HP; B, MGG × HP)

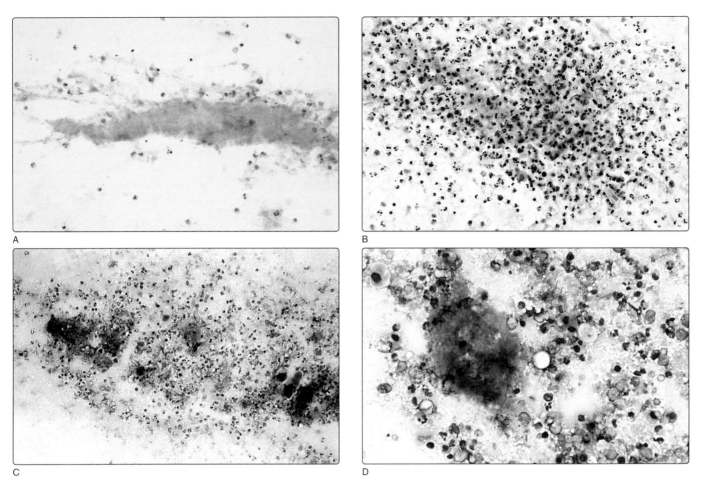

Fig. 4.18   Necrotic debris in rheumatoid disease. Pleural effusion. (A, B, Papanicolaou × HP; C, D, MGG × HP)

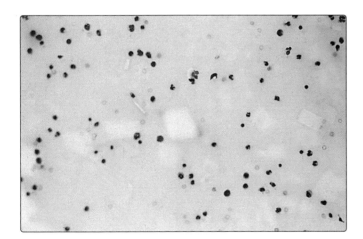

Fig. 4.19   Cholesterol crystal outlines in rheumatoid disease. Pleural effusion. (MGG × HP)

the complement cascade is activitated through the classical and alternate pathways, and the distinction between rheumatoid disease, malignancy and tuberculosis by measuring the concentrations of complement components has been described[64]. Hyaluronan concentrations are elevated in rheumatoid effusions but less so than in effusions associated with malignant mesothelioma[65].

Systemic lupus erythematosus

Serous effusions may develop in patients with systemic lupus erythematosus (SLE); any serous cavity may be involved, but the peritoneum is the least common site. Occasionally, an effusion is the presenting sign of the illness.

Cytological findings

► LE cells with ingested nuclear material
► Degenerating cells
► Nuclear debris

The fluid contains the inflammatory cells and mesothelial cells found in many other conditions, but there may also be LE cells, which are almost pathognomonic. These cells are similar to the LE cells which can be found in the blood and bone marrow in this illness, and consist of a phagocyte (usually a neutrophil), which has ingested homogenized nuclear material from another cell. The nuclear material, the staining reaction of which varies from acidophilic to basophilic, assumes a rounded shape and fills most of the cytoplasm of the neutrophil, displacing the nucleus to the side (Fig. 4.20). Sometimes the displaced nucleus loses its lobation. There may be a background of degenerating cells

147

and nuclear debris. It was formerly thought that LE cells only developed in specimens after they had been taken from the patient, but while it is true that the concentration of these cells increases if the specimen is left to stand for some time, there is no doubt that the cells can be found in freshly drawn specimens. It should be noted that there have been occasional reports of typical LE cells having been found in effusions from subjects whose illnesses were not wholly typical of SLE; therefore, the LE cell should not be considered absolutely diagnostic of the condition[66,67]. It is important to distinguish LE cells from so-called 'Tart' cells (named after a patient). Tart cells are phagocytes that have ingested an unaltered nucleus; being found in many conditions, they are not specific to SLE[68]. An eosinophilic pleural effusion has been described in SLE[69].

Other conditions associated with benign effusions

Congestive heart failure

Congestive heart failure, if severe, may be associated with serous effusions. The mechanism is hydrostatic, producing a transudate, and although any cavity may be involved, pleural effusions are the most common. There are no specific features. The concentration of cells is usually low, and neutrophils are not numerous, except in the occasional case where infection supervenes and stimulates exudation. Red cells and phagocytosed haemosiderin may be present.

Pneumonia

Pulmonary infections may cause pleural effusions if the inflammation of the lung involves the pleura. An exudate accumulates in the pleural space; the cellular composition of the exudate is variable, and although the types of inflammatory cells present are not specific for any particular infecting organism, it is true that a predominance of lymphocytes in the exudate at an early stage is more commonly associated with tuberculosis, legionella or a viral pneumonia than with other types of pneumonia. If, in these pneumonias, a secondary bacterial infection should develop, the concentration of neutrophils in the pleural fluid is likely to increase, rendering the composition of the effusion entirely non-specific. A curious feature of tuberculous pleural effusions is that they seldom contain

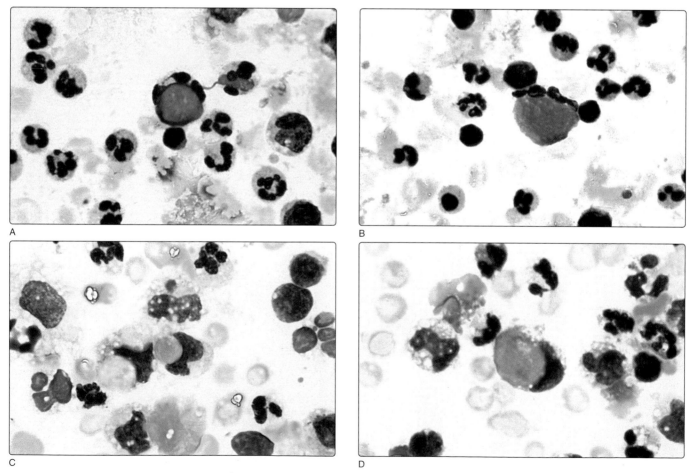

A   B   C   D

Fig. 4.20   LE cells in systemic lupus erythematosus. In (A) and (B) a neutrophil is distended by homogeneous violet material. In (C) and (D) a macrophage contains similar material. Pleural effusion. (MGG × OI)

many mesothelial cells. The reason is obscure but it may be that the inflammatory exudate or a layer of fibrin traps the mesothelial cells and prevents their exfoliation[70].

In a small proportion of cases of effusion associated with pneumonia, it may be possible to detect the infecting organism in the fluid by microscopy or culture; this is more likely when there is empyema. Viral inclusions in mesothelial cells in cases of herpes virus and cytomegalovirus infection have been reported, and it is sometimes possible to confirm the presence of cytomegalovirus by immunocytochemistry when the morphological features are absent[71].

Now that immunosuppressive therapy for malignancy, autoimmune disease and transplantation is in common use, fungal infections have become of considerable importance. HIV infection and the use of antibiotics also facilitate infection by fungi. The lungs are much the most common site of fungal infection, and diagnosis is usually made by examination of sputum or of specimens obtained by bronchoscopy. When serous effusions occur, their composition is usually non-specific, and it is uncommon to find fungi in the fluids; there have been occasional reports of Candida, Aspergillus, Coccidioides and Blastomyces. A case of pleural effusion in which *Pneumocystis carinii* was found has been reported[72]. The circumstance in which fungi are most likely to be found in an effusion is that of overwhelming infection, which is often a terminal development.

Bacteria and fungi, when present, are often rendered visible if Papanicolaou and MGG stains are used in conjunction. The former stain colours some fungi (e.g. Candida) brick red, while MGG stains bacteria dark blue and fungal walls pale blue. Where there is a clinical suspicion of infection, however, it is better to use appropriate stains such as Gram, PAS and methenamine-silver. A specific stain such as the last of these is essential if Pneumocystis is to be detected.

Endometriosis

Endometriosis is the presence of endometrial glands and stroma at sites outside the endometrial cavity. The ovary is the commonest site outside the uterus, followed by the pelvic peritoneum. It is very rare for endometriosis to occur in the pleura[73–75]. Effusions in the serous cavities, due to endometriosis, are also very rare but have been reported. Diagnosis of the effusion as being due to endometriosis is exceedingly difficult and it has been assumed depends on finding recognizable endometrial tissue. Unfortunately, endometrial cells, whether single or in groups, notoriously resemble mesothelial cells or macrophages in fluids, and are often degenerate[76]. Differences in the expression of cytokeratins by endometrium and mesothelium have been used to identify endometrial cells in effusions[77]. A recent report, however, suggests that the presence of haemosiderin-laden macrophages in peritoneal fluid is a more recognizable and specific indicator of endometriosis[78]. In practice, a diagnosis is not commonly made without a biopsy. Specimens of peritoneal washings taken from patients with endometriosis may contain fragments that can be identified as endometrial glands and stroma after embedding as a paraffin block. Cytokines such as vascular endothelial growth factor, interleukins 6 and 8, and tumour necrosis factor alpha are found in elevated concentrations and are secreted by activated macrophages[79–81].

The related condition of endosalpingiosis occurs in the pelvic organs and peritoneum. Exfoliated cells and clusters of cells may be more easily recognized than endometrial cells, as mentioned earlier. Psammoma bodies may be found in these conditions and lead to an erroneous diagnosis of malignancy[82].

Cirrhosis

In the majority of cases of cirrhosis associated with ascites, the fluid contains benign looking macrophages and mesothelial cells. In a small proportion of patients, however, necrosis of the liver stimulates the mesothelial cells, which may be found in the fluid in clusters and papillae, and may have atypical nuclei. The benign nature of the cells can still be recognized in most of these cases as the nuclei are still of uniform size and appearance. If hepatocellular carcinoma with ascites complicates cirrhosis it is sometimes possible to recognize malignant hepatocytes in the ascitic fluid[83].

Peritoneal dialysis

This technique, commonly used in the treatment of renal failure, involves the instillation of several litres of dialysing solution into the peritoneal cavity for a few hours at a time.

Cytological findings

▶ Increased nuclear:cytoplasmic ratio in mesothelial cells
▶ Nuclear hyperchromasia and clumped chromatin
▶ Mitoses
▶ Spectrum of changes from atypical to normal

Cytological examinations of the used fluid have been made, although the procedure is not routine. The most notable features described are an increased nuclear/cytoplasmic ratio of the mesothelial cells accompanied by nuclear hyperchromasia, clumping of chromatin and increased numbers of mesothelial cells in mitosis. The mitotic figures may even appear atypical. It is important to realize that these changes are reactive or degenerative, clues to which are that the proportion of atypical cells in the sample is small and that a spectrum of cells varying from typical to atypical may be present[84–86].

The peritoneum may undergo a form of squamous metaplasia, cells exfoliated from which may be observed in the peritoneal fluid[87]. Inflammatory cells may be in the fluid in variable concentrations; neutrophils and lymphocytes have been reported. Eosinophils are found in almost all patients at some time (see earlier).

The nature of the stimuli causing these changes is a matter of speculation. The solutes or glucose in the dialysing fluid[86], air and extraneous material introduced by the catheter have been suggested.

Photodynamic therapy may induce atypical changes in mesothelial cells[88].

Mucus

Curschmann's spirals are commonly observed in cytological specimens prepared from sputum, and are believed to consist of a string of mucus, usually assuming a helical form. They have occasionally been described in cervical smears, in which mucus is normally present. However, there are a few reports of their presence in serous effusions, in which their occurrence is harder to explain, although in some of these examples there was a mucinous adenocarcinoma or pseudomyxoma peritonei, either of which could be a source of extracellular mucus. Curschmann's spirals in serous effusions are not known to have any practical implication[89,90]. Pseudomyxoma may also produce a diffuse mucinous background[91].

Asbestos bodies

Asbestos bodies in pleural effusions are very rarely observed. They are similar to those seen in sputum or in the tissue of the lung, being fibres several tens of microns long and encrusted with clumps of ferruginous material. The route by which they reach the pleural cavity from the lung is uncertain; it has been suggested that trauma or a fistula involving the visceral pleura may be involved, or that the thoracocentesis needle may puncture the lung. Benign effusions related to exposure to asbestos are uncommon and asbestos fibres have rarely been demonstrated in them[92].

Many inhaled asbestos fibres are trapped in the bronchial mucus, which is ultimately swallowed. This gives the fibres access to the lumen of the gastrointestinal tract; nevertheless, the fibres appear not to have been reported in the peritoneal cavity, nor in the pericardial sac.

Types of specimens and preservation

Most specimens of serous fluid are obtained by passing a wide-bore needle through the skin and into the serous cavity. This allows the fluid to be aspirated from any of the cavities. Samples of fluid may also be obtained during surgical procedures. An additional technique, which is used to obtain so-called peritoneal 'washings' involves the instillation of small volumes of physiological saline into selected areas of the peritoneal cavity, followed by aspiration of the fluid. Cells exfoliate from the serous membranes during this procedure and the fluid can be examined in the same way as an effusion.

Sterile universal containers are suitable for transport; if it is considered necessary to eliminate the possibility of

clotting, citrate, heparin or EDTA can be added. 2 ml of 3.8% sodium citrate, 1 unit of heparin or 13 mg of EDTA in a 20 ml bottle are suitable amounts. Cellular detail is at its best when the specimen is fresh but if a delay in slide preparation is unavoidable, cells will survive quite well at 4°C.

Technical methods

Several methods of preparation are available, each having its own advantages. All begin, however, with removal of clotted material, if any has formed. This may contain entrapped, diagnostic cells, so it is usual to fix it in buffered formalin and process it for paraffin sections.

The fluid is then shaken to produce a uniform suspension of cells and a sample is centrifuged at 2000 rpm for 5 minutes. The supernatant is discarded. A small drop of the deposit is placed on a glass slide with a pipette and spread evenly and quickly. Smears for Papanicolaou staining are placed immediately in 95% ethanol or other suitable fixative and left to fix; the time between spreading and immersion should be as short as possible (not more than a few seconds) to prevent drying artefact. Smears for MGG staining are spread thinly and air dried as quickly as possible and fixed in methanol. These are the routine methods of staining used most often. A mucin stain may be helpful in the examination of fluid in cases of suspected adenocarcinoma; PAS with and without diastase digestion is suitable for demonstrating the presence of mucin, and is performed on alcohol-fixed slides. Similarly, immunocytochemistry may help to differentiate mesothelial cells from adenocarcinoma, and can be performed on air-dried acetone fixed or ethyl alcohol fixed slides. Fixation gives better preservation of cytological detail. Heavy contamination with blood can make smears difficult to assess. Most of the red cells can be removed after the first centrifugation by applying the deposit to a sucrose solution with a density gradient and centrifuging again. This separates cells according to their densities, and the method can be extended to allow various cell types to be isolated. Suitable solutions are available commercially.

If a very rapid report is required, it is possible to examine a wet film, which is prepared by placing one drop each of sediment and of a stain such as toluidine blue on a slide, mixing them and putting on a cover slip. Specimens containing numerous obviously malignant cells can be diagnosed by this technique. It is also good for the identification of crystals, such as cholesterol, haematoidin and Charcot-Leyden, which may not survive processing to permanent slides. A further advantage is that samples containing numerous malignant cells can be processed separately from other specimens, reducing the risk of contamination of staining baths. The disadvantages are that the preparation is not permanent, cytological detail is not assessed as easily as in permanent smears, so that specimens containing small numbers of malignant cells may not be diagnosed as positive, and the method has no step in which there is microbicidal action, so that the samples from patients infected with dangerous pathogens are not rendered harmless.

References

1 Hessen I. Roentgen examination of pleural fluid: a study of the localisation of free effusions, the potentialities of diagnosing minimal quantities of fluid and its existence under physiological conditions. *Acta Radiol (suppl) (Stockholm)* 1951; **86**: 1–80

2 Sahn S A. State of the Art. The pleura. *Am Rev Resp Dis* 1988; **138**: 184–234

3 Granger H J. 1981. Physicochemical properties of the extracellular matrix. In: Hargens A R ed. *Tissue Fluid Pressure And Composition*. Baltimore: Williams and Wilkins, 43–61

4 Granger H J. Role of the interstitial matrix and lymphatic pump in regulation of transcapillary fluid balance. *Microvascular Res* 1979; **18**: 209–216

5 Rasio E. 1987. The physiology of fluid exchange between the circulation and the body cavities. In: Jones J S P ed. *Pathology of the Mesothelium*. London: Springer-Verlag, 15–32

6 Pistolesi M. State of the Art. Pleural liquid and solute exchange. *Am Rev Resp Dis* 1989; **140**: 825–847

7 Cunningham R S. The physiology of the serous membranes. *Physiol Rev* 1926; **6**: 242–280

8 Ellis H, Harrison T W, Tugh T B. The healing of peritoneum under normal and pathological conditions. *Br J Surg* 1965; **52**: 471–476

9 Whitaker D, Papadimitriou J M, Walters M N-I. The mesothelium and its reactions. A review. *CRC Crit Rev Toxicol* 1982; **10**: 81–144

10 Mutsaers S E, Whitaker D, Papadimitriou J M. Mesothelial regeneration is not dependent on subserosal cells. *J Pathol* 2000; **190**: 86–92

11 Kayastha S, Freedman A N, Piver M S *et al.* Expression of hyaluronan receptor, CD44S, in epithelial ovarian cancer is an independent predictor of survival. *Clin Cancer Res* 1999; **5**(5): 1073–1076

12 Cannistra S A, DeFranzo B, Niloff J, Ottensmeir C. Functional heterogeneity of CD44 molecules in ovarian cancer lines. *Clin Cancer Res* 1995; **1**(3): 333–342

13 Jones L M, Gardner M J, Catterall J B, Turner G A. Hyaluronic acid secreted by mesothelial cells: a natural barrier to ovarian cancer cell adhesion. *Clin Exp Metastasis* 1995; **13**(5): 373–380

14 Kroegel C, Antony V B. Immunobiology of pleural inflammation: potential implications for pathogenesis, diagnosis and therapy. *Eur Respir J* 1997; **10**(10): 2411–2418

15 Yamada S. Uber die serose flussigkeit in der pleurahohle der gesunden menschen. *Z Gesamte Exp Med* 1933; **90**: 342–348

16 Ramsey S J, Tweeddale D N, Bryant L R, Braunstein H. Cytologic features of pericardial mesothelium. *Acta Cytol* 1970; **14**: 283–290

17 Yu G H, Sack M J, Baloch Z W *et al.* Occurrence of intercellular spaces (windows) in metastatic adenocarcinoma in serous fluids: a cytomorphologic, histochemical and ultrastructural study. *Diagn Cytopathol* 1999; **20**(3): 115–119

18 Domagala W, Woyke S. Transmission and scanning electron microscopic studies of cells in effusions. *Acta Cytol* 1975; **19**: 214–224

19 Shield P W, Perkins G, Wright R G. Immunocytochemical staining of cytologic specimens. How helpful is it? [See comments]. *Am J Clin Pathol* 1996; **105**(2): 139–162

20 Barberis M C, Faleri M, Veronese S *et al.* A selective marker of normal and neoplastic mesothelial cells in serous effusions. *Acta Cytol* 1997; **41**(6): 1757–1761

21 Oates J, Edwards C. HBME-1, MOC-31, WT1 and calretinin: an assessment of recently described markers for mesothelioma and adenocarcinoma. *Histopathology* 2000; **36**(4): 341–347

22 Lee J S, Nam J H, Lee M C *et al.* Immunohistochemical panel for distinguishing between carcinoma and reactive mesothelial cells in serous effusions. *Acta Cytol* 1996; **40**(4): 631–636

23 Kennedy A G, King G, Kerr K M. HBME-1 and antithrombomodulin in the differential diagnosis of malignant mesothelioma of the pleura. *J Clin Pathol* 1997; **50**(10): 859–862

24 Carpenter P M, Gamboa G P, Dorion G E *et al.* Radiation-induced CA 125 production by mesothelial cells. *Gynecol-Oncol* 1996; **63**(3): 328–332

25 Pabst T, Ludwig C. [CA 125–a tumor marker?]. *Schweiz Med Wochenschr* 1995; **125**(24): 1195–1200

26 Burstein D E, Reder I, Weiser K *et al.* GLUT1 glucose transporter: a highly sensitive marker of malignancy in body cavity effusions. *Mod Pathol* 1998; **11**(4): 392–396

27 Fetsch P A, Abati A, Hijazi Y M. Utility of the antibodies CA 19–9, HBME-1, and thrombomodulin in the diagnosis of malignant mesothelioma and adenocarcinoma in cytology. *Cancer* 1998; **84**(2): 101–108

28 Bailey M E, Brown R W, Mody D R *et al.* Ber-EP4 for differentiating adenocarcinoma from reactive and neoplastic mesothelial cells in serous effusions. Comparison with carcinoembryonic antigen, B72.3 and Leu-M1. *Acta Cytol* 1996; **40**(6): 1212–1216

29 Koukoulis G K, Shen J, Monson R *et al.* Pleural mesotheliomas have an integrin profile distinct from visceral carcinomas. *Hum Pathol* 1997; **28**(1): 84–90

30 Kortsik C S, Freudenberg N, Riede U *et al.* Lectin binding sites and immunocytochemical characterization of normal pleural mesothelium. *Gen Diagn Pathol* 1995; **141**(2): 141–146

31 Kern W H. Benign papillary structures with psammoma bodies in culdocentesis fluid. *Acta Cytol* 1969; **13**: 178–180

32 Elsheikh T M, Silverman J F, Sturgis T M, Geisinger K R. Cytologic diagnosis of bile peritonitis. *Diagn Cytopathol* 1996; **14**(1): 56–59

33 Guzmann J, Bross K J, Wurtemburger G *et al.* Tuberculous pleural effusions: Lymphocyte phenotypes in comparison with other lymphocyte-rich effusions. *Diagn Cytopathol* 1989; **5**: 139

34 Domagala W, Emeson E E, Koss L G. T and B lymphocyte enumeration in the diagnosis of lymphocyte-rich pleural fluids. *Acta Cytol* 1981; **25**: 108–110

35 Mott F W. The cerebro-spinal fluid in relation to disease of the nervous system. *BMJ* 1904; **2**: 1954–1960

36 Spriggs A I. Pleural eosinophilia due to pneumothorax. *Acta Cytol* 1979; **23**: 425

37 Bower G. Eosinophilic pleural effusion. A condition with multiple causes. *Am Rev Resp Dis* 1967; **95**: 746–751

38 Smit H J, van den Heuvel M M, Barbierato S B *et al.* Analysis of pleural fluid in idiopathic spontaneous pneumothorax; correlation of eosinophil percentage with the duration of air in the pleural space. *Respir Med* 1999; **93**(4): 262–267

39 Jarvinen K A J, Kahampaa A. Prognosis in cases with eosinophilic pleural effusion. 17 cases followed for 5–12 years. *Acta Med Scand* 1959; **164**: 245–251

40 Veress J F, Koss L G, Schreiber K. Eosinophilic pleural effusions. *Acta Cytol* 1979; **23**: 40–44

41 Koss L G. *Diagnostic Cytology and its Histological Bases*, 4th edn. Philadelphia: Lippincott, 1992; 1099–1101

42 Wachter B, Jager-Arand E, Engers R *et al.* Eosinophilic gastroenteritis with serosa involvement. A rare differential diagnosis of ascites. *Z Gastroenterol* 1992; **30**(7): 469–472

43 Vandewiele I A, Maeyaert B M, Van-Cutsem E J *et al.* Massive eosinophilic ascites: differential diagnosis between idiopathic hypereosinophilic syndrome and eosinophilic gastroenteritis. *Acta Clin Belg* 1991; **46**(1): 37–41

44 Lee S, Schoen I. Eosinophilia of peritoneal fluid and peripheral blood associated with chronic peritoneal dialysis. *Am J Clin Pathol* 1967; **47**: 638–640

45 Jolobe O M P, Melnick S C. Asthma, pulmonary eosinophilia and eosinophilic pericarditis. *Thorax* 1983; **38**: 690–691

46 Spriggs A I, Boddington M M. 1989. *Atlas of Serous Fluid Cytopathology*. Dordrecht: Kluwer Academic

47 Denburg J A, Richardson M, Telizyn S, Bienenstock J. Basophil/mast cell precursors in human peripheral blood. *Blood* 1983; **61**: 775–780

48 Zucker-Franklin D, Grusky G, Hirayama N, Schnipper E. The presence of mast cell precursors in rat peripheral blood. *Blood* 1981; **58**: 544–551

49 Stephenson R W, Britt D A, Schumann G B. Primary cytodiagnosis of peritoneal extramedullary haematopoiesis. *Diagn Cytopathol* 1986; **2**: 241–243

50 Yazdi H M. Cytopathology of extramedullary haemopoiesis in effusions and peritoneal washings: a report of three cases with immunohistochemical study. *Diagn Cytopathol* 1986; **2**: 326–329

51 Bartziota E V, Naylor B. Megakaryocytes in a hemorrhagic pleural effusion caused by anticoagulant overdose. *Acta Cytol* 1986; **30**: 163–165

52 Kumar N B, Naylor B. Megakaryocytes in pleural and peritoneal fluids: prevalence, significance, morphology and cytohistological correlation. *J Clin Pathol* 1980; **33**: 1153–1159

53 Vilaseca J, Arnau J M, Tallada N, Salas A. Megakaryocytes in serous effusions. *J Clin Pathol* 1981; **34**: 939

54 Joliat G, Stalder H, Kapanci Y. Lymphangiomyomatosis: a clinicoanatomical entity. *Cancer* 1973; **31**: 455–461

55 Ellison E, Lapuerta P, Martin S E. Cytologic features of mycobacterial pleuritis: logistic regression and statistical analysis of a blinded, case-controlled study. *Diagn Cytopathol* 1998; **19**(3): 173–176

56 Vadmal M S, Smilari T F, Brody J P et al. Cytodiagnosis of a primary effusion lymphoma. A case report. *Acta Cytol* 1998; **42**(2): 374–376

57 Mansour G, Charlotte F, Calvez V et al. AIDS-related primary lymphoma of the pleural cavity. A case report. *Acta Cytol* 1998; **42**(2): 371–373

58 Ansari M Q, Dawson D B, Nador R et al. Primary body cavity-based AIDS-related lymphomas (see comments). Comment in: *Am J Clin Pathol* 1996; **105**(2): 221–229

59 Drexler H G, Uphoff C C, Gaidano G, Carbone A. Lymphoma cell lines: in vitro models for the study of HHV-8 + primary effusion lymphomas (body cavity-based lymphomas). *Leukemia* 1998; **12**(10): 1507–1517

60 Hasserjian R P, Krausz T. 1999. Diagnosis of primary and secondary lymphomatous effusions. In: Lowe D G, Underwood J C E eds. *Recent Advances in Histopathology* 18, New York: Churchill Livingstone, 118–123

61 Naylor B. The pathognomonic cytologic picture of rheumatoid pleuritis. *Acta Cytol* 1990; **34**: 465–473

62 Boddington M M, Spriggs A I, Morton J A, Mowat A G. Cytodiagnosis of rheumatoid pleural effusions. *J Clin Pathol* 1971; **24**: 95–106

63 Delbarre F, Kahan A, Amor B, Krassinine G. Le ragocyte synovial. Son interet pour le diagnostic des maladies rheumatismales. *Presse Med* 1964; **72**: 2129–2132

64 Salomaa E R, Viander M, Saaresranta T, Terho E O. Complement components and their activation products in pleural fluid. *Chest* 1998; **114**(3): 723–730

65 Soderblom T, Petterson T, Nyberg P et al. High pleural fluid hyaluronan concentrations in rheumatoid arthritis. *Eur Respir J* 1999; **13**(3): 519–522

66 Schett G, Steiner G, Smolen J S. Nuclear antigen histone H1 is primarily involved in lupus erythematosus cell formation. *Arthritis-Rheum* 1998; **41**(8): 1446–1455

67 Hidalgo C, Vladutio A O. Lupus erythematosus cells in serum and pleural fluid of a patient with negative fluorescent antinuclear antibody test. *Am J Clin Pathol* 1987; **87**: 660–662

68 Hargraves M M, Richmond H, Morton R. Presentation of two bone marrow elements: the 'tart' cell and the 'LE' cell. *Proc Staff Meet Mayo Clin* 1948; **23**: 25–28

69 Kojima T, Umeno M, Takaki K et al. A case of SLE with the onset of pleuritis showing eosinophilia and elevation of serum IgE. *Fukuoka Igaku Zasshi* 1996; **87**(4): 97–101

70 Spriggs A I, Boddington M M. Absence of mesothelial cells from tuberculous pleural effusions. *Thorax* 1960; **15**: 169–171

71 Goodman Z D, Gupta P K, Frost J K, Erozan Y S. Cytodiagnosis of viral infections in body cavity fluids. *Acta Cytol* 1979; **23**: 204–208

72 Balachandran I, Jones D B, Humphrey D M. A case of Pneumocystis carinii in pleural fluid, with cytologic, histologic and ultrastructural documentation. *Acta Cytol* 1990; **34**: 486–490

73 Zaatari G S, Gupta P K, Bhagavan B S, Jarboe R R. Cytopathology of pleural endometriosis. *Acta Cytol* 1982; **26**: 227–232

74 Flanagan K L, Barnes N C. Pleural fluid accumulation due to intra-abdominal endometriosis: a case report and review of the literature [see comments]. *Thorax* 1996; **51**(10): 1064

75 Shek Y, De Lia J E, Pattillo R A. Endometriosis with a pleural effusion and ascites. Report of a case treated with nafarelin acetate. *J Reprod Med* 1995; **40**(7): 540–542

76 Gaulier A, Jouret-Mourin A, Marsan C. Peritoneal endometriosis. Report of a case with cytologic, cytochemical and histopathologic study. *Acta Cytol* 1983; **27**: 446–449

77 Van der Linden P J, Dunselman G A, de Goeij A F et al. Epithelial cells in peritoneal fluid—of endometrial origin? *Am J Obstet Gynecol* 1995; **173**(2): 566–570

78 Stowell S B, Wiley C M, Perez-Reyes N, Powers C N. Cytologic diagnosis of peritoneal fluids. Applicability to the laparoscopic diagnosis of endometriosis. *Acta Cytol* 1997; **31**(3): 817–822

79 Harada T, Enatsu A, Mitsunari M et al. Role of cytokines in progression of endometriosis. *Gynecol Obstet Invest* 1999; **47**(suppl 1): 34–39; discussion 39–40

80 Shifren J L, Tseng J F, Zaloudek C J et al. Ovarian steroid regulation of vascular endothelial growth factor in the human endometrium: implications for angiogenesis during the menstrual cycle and in the pathogenesis of endometriosis. *J Clin Endocrinol Metab* 1996; **81**(8): 3112–3118

81 McLaren J, Prentice A, Charnock-Jones D S et al. Vascular endothelial growth factor is produced by peritoneal fluid macrophages in endometriosis and is regulated by ovarian steroids. *J Clin Invest* 1996; **98**(2): 482–489

82 Fanning J, Markuly S N, Hindman T L et al. False positive malignant peritoneal cytology and psammoma bodies in benign gynecologic disease. *J Reprod Med* 1996; **41**(7): 504–508

83 Falconieri G, Zanconati F, Colautti I et al. Effusion cytology of hepatocellular carcinoma. *Acta Cytol* 1995; **39**(5): 893–897

84 Carlon G, Della Giustina D. Atypical mesothelial cells in peritoneal dialysis fluid. *Acta Cytol* 1983; **27**: 706–708

85 Hoeltermann W, Schlotmann-Hoeler E, Winkelmann M, Pfitzer P. Lavage fluid from continuous ambulatory peritoneal dialysis: a model for mesothelial cell changes. *Acta Cytol* 1989; **33**: 591–594

86 Fok F K, Bewtra C, Hammeke M D. Cytology of peritoneal fluid from patients on continuous ambulatory peritoneal dialysis. *Acta Cytol* 1989; **33**: 595–598

87 Selgas R, Fernandez de Castro M, Viguer J M et al. Transformed mesothelial cells in patients on CAPD for medium- to long-term periods. *Perit Dial Int* 1995; **15**(8): 305–311

88 Garza O T, Abati A, Sindelar W F et al. Cytologic effects of photodynamic therapy in body fluids. *Diagn Cytopathol* 1996; **14**(4): 356–361

89 Wahl R W. Curschmann's spirals in pleural and peritoneal fluids. Report of 12 cases. *Acta Cytol* 1986; **30**: 147–151

90 Naylor B. Curschmann's spirals in pleural and peritoneal fluids. *Acta Cytol* 1990; **34**: 474–478

91 Pisharodi L R, Bedrossian C W. Cytologic diagnosis of pseudomyxoma peritonei: common and uncommon causes. *Diagn Cytopathol* 1996; **14**(1): 10–13

92 Ferrer J, Balcells E, Orriols R et al. Benign asbestos pleural effusion. Report of a first series in Spain. *Med Clin Barc* 1996; **107**(14): 535–538

5 Metastatic disease and lymphomas

John Schofield and Thomas Krausz

Introduction

Aspiration of the serous cavities is a simple and relatively non-invasive technique to achieve a diagnosis. In malignant conditions, accumulation of serous fluid is more commonly due to secondary involvement of the serous membranes than primary malignant tumour of the mesothelium (malignant mesothelioma). Such involvement may be either by direct extension or by metastasis. Even in cases where there is a known tumour this may not directly account for the effusion, e.g. when there is remote lymphatic obstruction, infection, hypoalbuminaemia or pulmonary embolism.

The range of malignant neoplasms that may affect the mesothelial surfaces and result in serous effusions, is wide. However, there are some tumours with a particular propensity for serous membrane involvement, and these will be discussed in order of incidence. Mesothelioma is covered in the following chapter. As correct identification of tumours is crucial for therapeutic purposes, it is of great importance to assess the cause of serous effusions accurately. In a number of cases, the effusion may be the presenting feature of malignant disease[1], and it is advisable that diagnosis is not delayed as this may increase morbidity and mortality. Involvement of the serous cavities generally implies a very poor prognosis and, as always in cytopathology, caution should be taken not to 'overdiagnose'. If a definitive diagnosis cannot be made despite careful analysis and the application of special techniques, a 'suggestive' report may be issued, with the recommendation of examination of further cytological or histological material in an attempt to reach a definite diagnosis. Correlation between clinical history, radiographic and pathological findings is important for ensuring correct diagnosis.

The relative frequency of involvement by metastatic tumours differs according to age, sex and cavity involved (Table 5.1)[2]. In children, leukaemia and lymphoma are the most frequent tumours to involve the serous cavities, followed by nephroblastoma, neuroblastoma, embryonal rhabdomyosarcoma and Ewing's tumour. In adult males, peritoneal involvement is most often seen in association with tumours of the gastrointestinal tract or malignant lymphoma whereas pleural involvement is commoner in lung carcinoma, followed by tumours of the gastrointestinal

Table 5.1 Relative incidence of serous membrane involvement by metastatic tumours and lymphoma according to age and sex (modified from reference no 17)

	Pleural	**Peritoneal**
Adult female	Breast	Ovary
	Ovary	Breast
	GI tract (stomach, oesophagus, colon)	GI tract (stomach, pancreas, colon)
	Lung	Lymphoma
	Lymphoma	Others
	Others	
Adult male	Lung	GI tract (stomach, pancreas, colon)
	GI tract (oesophagus, stomach, colon)	Lymphoma
	Lymphoma	Others
	Others	
Child	Leukaemia/lymphoma	Leukaemia/lymphoma
	Small round cell tumour (including neuroblastoma, nephroblastoma and rhabdomyosarcoma)	Small round cell tumour (including neuroblastoma, nephroblastoma and rhabdomyosarcoma)
	Others	Others

tract and malignant lymphoma. In adult females, peritoneal involvement is most often seen with ovarian carcinoma followed by breast carcinoma, gastrointestinal carcinomas and malignant lymphoma, whereas pleural involvement is commonest in breast carcinoma followed by ovarian carcinoma, gastrointestinal carcinomas, lung carcinoma and malignant lymphoma. Involvement of the pericardium in adults of both sexes is seen principally in lung and breast carcinomas and lymphoma.

In many cases, a primary tumour is already known and the onus is to identify the presence of metastatic tumour cells and to confirm that these are consistent with the known primary. If the primary site is not already established, morphological, immunocytochemical and other studies may be used to help provide a definitive diagnosis of primary site or a narrow differential. These techniques are discussed in a later section.

The number of malignant cells present in an effusion varies greatly, and in some cases only small numbers may be present. These are easily masked by the benign constituents of the fluid, especially if there is an associated inflammatory cell infiltrate or haemorrhage, leading to a false negative result. However, it is even more important to recognize the full range of morphological appearances of normal and reactive cells in effusions to avoid a false positive result. Cells in effusions are no longer subject to the anatomical constraints imposed by their normal 'host' tissues, and this often leads to a different morphological appearance. For example, many cells, benign or malignant, become more rounded. Reactive mesothelial cells show a range of morphology, which may overlap with that of neoplastic mesothelial cells and metastatic carcinoma, particularly adenocarcinoma. In addition, macrophages may occasionally show degenerative features simulating adenocarcinoma. Ancillary techniques, such as immunohistochemistry or electron microscopy may be required to differentiate between these cell types in some cases.

A number of benign conditions are particularly well known for their propensity to simulate malignancy. Paramount amongst these are causes of chronic effusions with marked mesothelial hyperplasia, in particular chronic renal failure, congestive heart failure and cirrhosis of the liver. Markedly atypical mesothelial cell clusters occur in patients receiving peritoneal dialysis, possibly representing reaction to the dialysate[3]. Acute pleural effusions, sometimes with marked mesothelial cellularity and atypia, are seen in pulmonary embolism, in some cases with associated eosinophilia[4,5]. However, in only about 10% of cases of pleural effusion due to pulmonary embolism does the degree of cellularity and atypia raise the possibility of a malignant tumour[5]. Endometriosis[6] and endosalpingiosis[7] can rarely be confused with malignancy (see Chapter 4) and it is important to remember that psammoma bodies are not diagnostic of carcinoma[7,8]. Mullerian inclusions can occasionally be identified[9]. Megakaryocytes may be rarely present in effusions, causing confusion because of their size and resemblance to multinucleated tumour cells; they are commonest in patients with myelofibrosis[10] but have been reported in the absence of extramedullary haemopoiesis in a patient with anticoagulant overdosage[11]. Other multinucleated giant cells may be of mesothelial or macrophage origin and are seen in some reactive conditions (see Chapter 4). Ciliated cells or detached ciliated cell tufts may occasionally be present in fluids[12]. They are seen most frequently following surgery to the gynaecological tract or in peritoneal lavage specimens, and have no clinical relevance[13]. Although the presence of cilia strongly suggests that cells are benign, in exceptional cases adenocarcinoma cells (usually from a serous ovarian carcinoma) may possess cilia[14,15]. Peritoneal washings produce a different spectrum of appearances from those seen in effusions and can cause diagnostic difficulties[16].

Various techniques are available to refine diagnosis in this field; immunocytochemistry is most widely used but electron microscopy, flow cytometry, cytogenetics, morphometry, confocal microscopy, fluorescent *in situ* hybridization (FISH), reverse transcriptase polymerase chain reaction (RT-PCR) and biochemical analysis of the fluid may also be valuable. These techniques are covered in subsequent sections.

Specimen collection, general treatment of fluids and routine staining techniques have been discussed in preceding chapters and are reviewed elsewhere[17,18]. However, diagnosis of malignant disease in serous fluids can be enhanced by special techniques in the preparation of fluids; a short synopsis of these can be found at the end of this chapter. Papanicolaou, May-Grünwald-Giemsa (MGG) and mucin stains are routinely performed on direct smears or cytospin preparations. Cytospin preparations are extremely valuable to concentrate the cell population. The cell block technique can be helpful, in a few cases being the only way to make a definite diagnosis. Removal of cellular fragments using a celloidin bag has been advocated[19]. Histological processing of any clot present in the specimen, which is likely particularly if a specimen has not been collected into a citrated container, should be performed; often malignant cells may be present in high concentration. These techniques also have the advantage of enabling serial sections to be cut for immunocytochemical or other analysis, either to confirm a diagnosis or for retrospective study[20].

General characteristics of malignant cells in serous effusions

Crucial to the diagnosis of metastatic tumour involving the pleura is the identification of the foreign cells, allowing the recognition of a dual population of benign and malignant cells. Serous fluid containing malignant cells may have a wide range of appearances: the effusion may be sparsely cellular but contain scattered tumour cells, or it may be highly cellular; in the latter case, mesothelial cells, inflammatory cells or tumour cells may predominate.

Detection of the dual population may be easy but in some cases it is hampered, usually by one of three situations: when there is a relative paucity of malignant cells in a background rich in either mesothelial cells or inflammatory cells; when there is an excess of malignant cells and not enough mesothelial cells to allow easy comparison; and when malignant cell morphology shows a particularly striking similarity to mesothelial cells making distinction difficult. Of these, the two most frequently encountered problems are the identification of malignancy when the tumour cells are scanty and the recognition of tumours showing strong resemblance to reactive mesothelium. Careful analysis of both the morphological appearances of individual cells and the way the cells are arranged is required for accurate diagnosis.

Arrangement of benign and malignant cells in fluids

The way cells are arranged in effusions gives us particular insight into their nature. Essentially, cells either lie singly or form groups, which may originate by a number of different mechanisms. The serous fluid can be regarded as a culture medium in which exfoliated cells are suspended. If they divide, the architecture of the arrangements they form is dependent purely on the specialization of the cells, particularly on properties of the cell membranes, and not on the usual constraints of the tissues. However, some groups seen in serous fluid are not due to division of the cells; preformed groups may separate from the serous membrane, or single cells may join together in the fluid to form aggregates.

Cells which possess junctional complexes, such as epithelial and mesothelial cells, tend to be seen as tight clumps, from which they may dissociate. Cells lacking junctional complexes tend not to form tight clumps, but lie separately; if they are apposed, they may form small loose aggregates. Unfortunately, the morphology of clumps and aggregates often overlaps. Confocal microscopy with three-dimensional reconstruction of cell clusters has been advocated but this technique is not widely available[21].

Mesothelial cells usually lose adhesion from their neighbours and exfoliate into the fluid as single cells, although whole sheets may become detached. These flat sheets have regularly arranged nuclei and are especially seen in washings of the pelvic cavity[22,23] where they may cause diagnostic problems[16]. The formation of three-dimensional clumps is not a feature of this cell type. Thus, benign mesothelial cells in effusions are either separated (although clustering of T lymphocytes may occur around them) or form small groups, generally of less than 10 cells; these groups have a scalloped border and true acinus formation does not occur. Spaces may be seen between the cells, so called mesothelial windows, into which microvilli,

found all over the surface of the cells, project. However, these 'windows' are not entirely specific for mesothelial cells and can be occasionally encountered in metastatic adenocarcinoma[24]. If there is papillary hyperplasia of the serous membrane and the papillae become detached, they may appear in the fluid. These papillary formations have a fibrovascular core and rarely may contain a psammoma body; it is important not to confuse them with the papillary formations of a borderline tumour or well-differentiated serous carcinoma of the ovary or peritoneum. Cytological features, particularly nuclear/cytoplasmic ratio (see later), are important in this distinction.

Macrophages usually lie separately, but may form loose aggregates or, in some cases, small sheets making distinction from mesothelial cells difficult. Generally they have bland nuclear morphology and are not easily confused with malignant cells. Conversely, in some cases of gastric carcinoma the tumour cells can be very bland, simulating macrophages or mesothelial cells, and thus easily overlooked.

Large clumps of cells are characteristic of carcinomas, especially adenocarcinoma. Features aiding in the distinction between adenocarcinoma and mesothelial cell groups are summarized in Table 5.2. The characteristics of particular note in the recognition of adenocarcinoma are the formation of large, very cohesive clumps of cells with a smooth, 'hard' outline. The cells are usually densely packed and the nuclei often appear to overlap. The groups may be of several types, but all indicate differentiation of tumour cells to form glandular structures. They include papillary formations, acinar formations, proliferation spheres and solid cell clusters[25].

Table 5.2 Morphological and histochemical features distinguishing reactive mesothelial cells, mesothelioma cells and adenocarcinoma cells

Feature	Reactive mesothelium	Mesothelioma	Adenocarcinoma
Cellularity	Variable	Usually high	Variable
Edges of groups	Often berry-like clumps with scalloped contour	Often berry-like clumps with scalloped contour	Often smooth contoured clumps with 'hard' edges
Papillary structures	Rare	May be seen	May be seen
Acinar structures	Not seen	May be seen	Common
Cell sheets	May be seen, especially in washings	Rare	Not seen
Multinucleated cells	Sparse	Frequent	May be seen
Nuclei	Round with smooth contours	Enlarged, round, generally smooth contour	Variably-sized, often irregular in contour
Nucleoli	May be prominent	Often macronucleoli	Often prominent
N:C ratio	Tends to be low with little cell-to-cell variability	Tends to be low with little cell-to-cell variability	Tends to be high with cell-to-cell variability
Cytoplasm	Usually abundant and dense with peripheral 'fuzziness'	Usually abundant and dense with peripheral 'fuzziness'	Variable, not dense; sharp cell border
Cytoplasmic vacuolation	May be seen	May be seen	Often seen
Cytoplasmic glycogen	Often seen	Often abundant	May be seen
Cytoplasmic neutral mucin	Not seen	Not seen	Often seen
Cytoplasmic acidic mucin (hyaluronidase resistant)	Not seen	Not seen	Often seen
Cytoplasmic lipid	Frequent, small perinuclear vacuoles	Frequent, small perinuclear vacuoles	Often extensive in renal cell carcinomas; sometimes seen in others

Papillary formations have a central fibrovascular core covered by tumour cells and are only seen in adenocarcinomas with a true papillary nature such as papillary serous ovarian carcinoma and papillary carcinoma of thyroid. In such tumours, psammoma bodies may also be identified in the fluid. Papillary formations are also seen in some cases of mesothelioma. The presence of 'collagen balls' in clot or cell block specimens is a useful marker for mesothelial rather than epithelial origin[26,27].

Acinar formations are diagnostic of adenocarcinoma, and are composed of cells arranged around a central glandular lumen. The nuclei are polarized away from the centre; in cell block preparations, basal lamina may be seen around the acinus. Intracytoplasmic or luminal mucin may be apparent. These structures are most frequently encountered in ovarian, endometrial and gastrointestinal adenocarcinomas.

Proliferation spheres are well-circumscribed, rounded, three-dimensional cell groups, generally composed of non-vacuolated cells. The groups may be solid or may be hollow with an 'empty' centre, a feature most easily appreciated in histological sections of cell blocks. These are not true acini, because the cells are orientated with their basal aspect innermost and often have microvilli on the external aspect. Although characteristic of breast carcinoma, they can sometimes be seen in other types of adenocarcinoma. Mesothelial cells may also form similar spheres, but careful scrutiny of the cytological features, often most easily appreciated at the edge of the sphere, usually reveals typical mesothelial cell morphology; mesothelial clusters are more commonly solid or may occasionally have a fibrovascular core, and generally have a soft outline with a prominent or exaggerated 'berry-like' configuration.

Solid cell clusters are more irregular in shape than well-formed clumps, but are probably the most common grouping pattern encountered. The cells are arranged in a haphazard fashion without any evidence of orientation, but retain a definite three-dimensional structure. This structure may be large (more than 15 cells) and generally has a 'hard' outline. Distinction from mesothelial cell aggregates may be difficult, but in carcinoma the nuclei are packed more closely together as well as showing nuclear abnormalities. It should be emphasized that a careful examination of the cell clusters is important for accurate diagnosis. Using the fine focus allows the observer to analyse each individual cell and to appreciate the overall architecture of the group. Because the cytological details may be more difficult to identify than in single, loose-lying cells, this process is sometimes overlooked by the inexperienced cytologist. A characteristic cell grouping, the so-called 'raspberry body' has been identified in some cases of clear cell carcinoma of the ovary[28]. Features of particular value in the distinction between mesothelial cell clusters and adenocarcinoma clumps are shown in Table 5.2.

It is important to remember that not all cohesive groups of glandular cells in serous fluid are malignant.

Endometriosis can involve either the peritoneum or rarely the pleura and can easily be confused with metastatic carcinoma[6]. Furthermore, endosalpingiosis can strongly resemble well-differentiated serous ovarian adenocarcinoma and must be considered before making this diagnosis[7].

Non-cohesive tumour cells are characteristically seen in certain tumour types, principally non-epithelial tumours such as lymphoma; cells from such tumours do *not* form tight clumps, e.g. if such cells adhere to each other they form loose aggregates. Similar diffuse patterns can be seen in sarcoma, melanoma and very poorly differentiated carcinomas.

Features of individual malignant cells

It is important to realize that no single feature allows the accurate recognition of malignant cells in every case; a synthesis of various observations gleaned by careful analysis of the cells is required for this purpose. These characteristics will be discussed in turn, but are further elaborated in the section dealing with the appearances of specific tumours. One of the most challenging problems is distinction of mesothelial cells from tumour cells, so their morphology is briefly reviewed.

The mesothelial cell has a central or eccentric round nucleus with one or more small nucleoli; the chromatin is pale and well dispersed, and the nuclear membrane is smooth without chromatin condensation. The cytoplasm, which is often copious and dense in the perinuclear area due to numerous cytoskeletal filaments, fades to the edge of the cell. The cytoplasmic membrane appears slightly blurred and sometimes 'ruffled'; this appearance is partly due to artefactual swelling of surface microvilli. A ring of minute lipid vacuoles is sometimes present, usually adjacent to the nucleus. Reactive change is signalled by enlargement of the cell and the nucleus with retention of the nuclear/cytoplasmic ratio; both nucleus and cytoplasm become more densely stained and may form binucleate or rarely multinucleate cells. Occasional mitotic figures are often present and do not indicate malignancy, but the presence of numerous mitoses is suspicious, particularly in a highly cellular effusion. A marked increase in numbers of mitoses may be seen during treatment with cytotoxic drugs causing metaphase arrest. Degenerative vacuolation is common and can sometimes be extreme causing confusion with signet ring cell adenocarcinoma. Conversely, in some cases adenocarcinoma cells may have a very bland nuclear appearance and a striking resemblance to mesothelial cells; ancillary techniques may be required to make this distinction.

The following parameters are of particular value in the recognition of malignant cells in serous fluids:

1. *Nuclear size and nuclear/cytoplasmic ratio (N:C ratio)* are very valuable in the detection of malignancy. Malignant cells typically show marked nuclear enlargement and

increased N:C ratio. However, exceptions occur; in some cases the adenocarcinoma cells may be distended with mucin leading to a decreased N:C ratio; mesotheliomas also tend to have a relatively low N:C ratio. Both reactive and malignant mesothelial cells can reach quite large sizes, retaining a near normal N:C ratio. The cells of small cell carcinoma and lymphoma have a markedly abnormal N:C ratio; they are usually smaller than macrophages or mesothelial cells. The large numbers of such cells in the fluid with a monomorphic pattern is a useful indicator of clonal expansion.

2. *Nuclear hyperchromatism* is a valuable feature in the diagnosis of malignancy. Most malignant cells have an increased DNA content, leading to a marked increase in nuclear staining intensity in Papanicolaou and H&E stained preparations; this is less easily appreciated with MGG staining. However, some tumour cells do not show this feature; often adenocarcinoma may have rather pale nuclei with condensation of the nuclear chromatin around the nuclear membrane. A clumped chromatin pattern may occasionally be seen, but often the nucleus is vesicular, a feature best seen in histologically processed cell blocks.

3. *Nuclear contour*. In general, benign cells have a smooth nuclear contour. Malignant cells may show marked convolution of the nucleus with irregularities of the nuclear membrane, which often appears more prominent due to the chromatin condensation. The presence of irregular nuclear outlines is strongly suggestive of malignancy; this feature is particularly prominent in squamous cell carcinoma but is not present in all malignant cells. Nuclear grooves or 'creases' are more common in malignant cells, and are often prominent is gastric carcinoma cells.

4. *Nucleoli* are often conspicuous in malignant cells. However, small nucleoli are commonly present in macrophages and mesothelial cells. Enlarged nucleoli are sometimes encountered in reactive mesothelial cells, although more common in mesothelioma. Some malignant cells, such as those of small cell carcinoma and Merkel cell tumour, characteristically have minute or absent nucleoli, which can be a useful diagnostic sign.

5. *Intranuclear inclusions* can be useful when present, as they do not appear to occur in benign epithelial or mesothelial cells. Melanoma cells may have dense sharply circumscribed spherical nuclear inclusions, sometimes with a central area of pallor[29]; paler intranuclear cytoplasmic invaginations can be seen in the nucleus of cells of lymphoplasmacytoid lymphoma (Dutcher bodies)[30], and similar features can be seen in papillary thyroid carcinoma[31] and some adenocarcinomas, especially from lung.

6. *Mitoses*, if present in large numbers, are a valuable indicator of malignancy. Although an occasional mitotic figure is often observed among reactive mesothelial cells, the presence of several normal, or any abnormal, mitotic figures, is strongly suggestive of malignancy. Rarely, abnormal mitoses can be seen in mesothelial cells and an immunoblastic response may result in many mitotic figures[32]. Increased numbers of mitoses may also be the result of cytotoxic chemotherapy with drugs that induce metaphase arrest.

7. *Cell shape* is also a useful consideration. In general, the majority of cells seen in serous fluids are rounded, even if this may not be their normal configuration when seen in tissues. Irregularly angulated cells are characteristic of squamous cell carcinoma; this appearance is due to the organization of intracytoplasmic cytoskeletal filaments. The presence of bizarre or spindle-shaped cells is suggestive of malignancy, but occasionally fragments of granulation tissue may present in this way. Abnormal mesothelial cells may also be seen following cytotoxic chemotherapy and/or irradiation but in our experience in such cases the nuclear features usually resemble marked reactive change. Occasionally, multinucleation, nuclear hyperchromasia and homogenization occur, often in association with nuclear enlargement. If available, comparison with cells from previous material is helpful.

8. *Cell size*. In practical terms, cell size alone is a poor discriminator between benign and malignant cells in serous fluids. There is a large overlap between the cell size of mesothelial cells and tumour cells, and cell size appears different in air-dried and alcohol fixed material. Malignant cells in general are larger than their benign counterparts, and cell size may be useful in the recognition of a dual population when the malignant cells are substantially different in size from mesothelial cells. Although tumour cells are frequently larger than most mesothelial cells, it is important to note that they may be of similar or smaller size, making them considerably more difficult to identify. In reactive fluids, intermediate sized forms between the resting and activated mesothelial cell will normally be apparent resulting in a range of cells with different sizes (in contrast to the dual population). Unfortunately, mesothelial cells in normal and reactive serous fluid can vary in size from 10–30 µm, and the majority of malignant cells will also fall into this range, limiting the value of cell size in diagnosis. In passing, it should be clear that quoting cell sizes relative to mesothelial cells is not particularly useful.

In general, large cells are seen in many adenocarcinomas, squamous cell carcinomas, melanomas, sarcomas and large cell lymphomas. In most cases, these cells are easily identified and are clearly malignant on morphological grounds. Here the challenge is not the diagnosis of malignancy, but the accurate subclassification of the tumour (see later). Intermediate-sized cells are seen in adenocarcinomas of breast, stomach, pancreas and occasionally lung. These tumours can be particularly difficult to identify in some cases because the dual population of tumour cells and mesothelial cells is not easily appreciated. However, other features in the effusion can help, particularly the arrangement of the cells, their nuclear structure and the nuclear/cytoplasmic ratio. Small cells are seen in some malignant lymphomas, small cell carcinoma and small dark round cell tumours, usually but not exclusively seen in infancy.

9. *Cytoplasmic vacuolation*. Cytoplasmic vacuoles may contain various substances produced or stored by the cell including mucins, lipid, glycogen, or may be due to swelling of intracytoplasmic structures (usually endoplasmic reticulum) as a degenerative phenomenon.

The presence of intracytoplasmic neutral mucin equates with the diagnosis of adenocarcinoma and therefore its demonstration is of vital importance. We recommend *routine* staining for mucin on all serous fluids to avoid overlooking a cytologically bland mucin secreting adenocarcinoma. Lobular carcinoma of breast and carcinoma of stomach, which often manifest as relatively small cells in a dispersed pattern, are particularly easy to miss. However, not all adenocarcinomas contain mucin and a negative result does not exclude this diagnosis.

Various mucins may be elaborated by cells seen in serous fluids. They are generally grouped into neutral and acidic mucins. Neutral mucins are produced by many epithelia, especially those of the gastrointestinal tract, lung and breast. Histochemically they show positivity with PAS before *and* after diastase digestion, and with mucicarmine; the latter stain is more specific for neutral mucin, but less sensitive than PAS. PAS stains vicinal glycol groups present in neutral mucins, glycogen and the carbohydrate portion of glycoproteins and glycolipids. Staining for glycogen is abolished by pre-digestion with diastase. Acidic mucins are present in mesenchymal tissues (including mesothelium) and their tumours, but are also commonly elaborated by metaplastic, dysplastic and neoplastic epithelia. Acidic mucins are subdivided into sialated, weakly sulphated and highly sulphated types. These can be demonstrated using Alcian blue, a basic phthalocyanine dye with the ability to discriminate between sialated and sulphated glycosaminoglycans and glycoproteins. Further distinction can be made by altering the pH and the concentration of magnesium chloride in the technique (critical electrolyte concentration method)[33]. Pretreatment with hyaluronidase or sialidase allows identification of specific acidic mucins, and the former is of particular value in the identification of mesothelioma; this tumour is characterized by the production of acidic mucin rich in hyaluronic acid, therefore demonstrating hyaluronidase sensitive Alcian blue staining at pH 2.5. The high iron diamine technique is specific for highly sulphated mucins, which are often present in gastrointestinal and prostatic adenocarcinomas. The various histochemical methods for detection of mucin in serous fluid samples have been recently reviewed[34].

As mentioned above, not all adenocarcinomas produce mucin and a negative result cannot exclude malignancy. In contrast, PAS staining has been reported in some epithelial mesotheliomas[35,36,37], although this is rare and PAS staining following diastase digestion remains one of the most useful discriminants in distinguishing adenocarcinoma from mesothelioma. Even in adenocarcinomas, not all of the vacuolated cells contain mucin; identification of mucin-negative vacuoles should not deter the observer from further study of the preparation. Of even greater importance, not all large vacuoles contain mucin; a common pitfall is the presence of vacuolation in mesothelial cells undergoing degenerative changes which can closely simulate signet ring cells. Some vacuoles contain glycogen (see later) or lipid, as is often seen in renal cell carcinoma.

10. *Intracytoplasmic pigments* may be valuable in distinguishing benign from malignant cells, and in subtyping malignant cells. It is important to note that a large cell containing pigment is not necessarily a melanoma cell; conversely, an intermediate sized cell containing pigment is not necessarily a macrophage but could be a melanoma cell or a mesothelial cell. If pigment is seen it is wise to elucidate its character precisely; stains for melanin, iron, lipofuscin, bile pigments and others may reveal the true nature of the cells. Haemosiderin may be found in mesothelial cells as well as macrophages. Lipofuscin similarly, can be identified in either mesothelial cells or macrophages. The presence of melanin is diagnostic of melanoma; in most cases the melanin will be seen in tumour cells, but rarely in cases with excessive melanin production it can be phagocytosed by macrophages. Carbon pigment in macrophages is only normally seen following lung trauma or in cases of bronchopleural fistula. Intracellular bile production in malignant cells is only seen in hepatocellular carcinoma. However, rarely, normal hepatocytes may be present in pleural fluid if the right lobe of the liver has been accidentally penetrated during aspiration[17].

11. *Other cell products* including glycogen, myofilaments and keratin can be diagnostic. Mesothelial cells contain diffuse or clumped cytoplasmic glycogen, and this is often markedly increased in the cells of mesothelioma, in which it may completely obscure the nucleus on the PAS preparation. Other glycogen rich tumours include clear cell carcinoma of ovary, seminoma, dysgerminoma, hepatocellular carcinoma, Ewing's sarcoma and rhabdomyosarcoma; generally, the morphology of the tumour cells will allow distinction between these entities. In addition, a small amount is often present in many other tumour types.

Myofilaments imply muscle differentiation, e.g. in smooth muscle tumours and rhabdomyosarcoma. Intracytoplasmic keratinization may be identified in well-differentiated squamous cell carcinoma, resulting in a malignant cell with an angulated rather than round contour, a dense nucleus and hard, glassy cytoplasm. Mesothelial cells have cytoplasm rich in cytokeratin filaments, but these have a striking perinuclear distribution. Squamous metaplasia of the peritoneum occurs rarely.

Psammoma bodies, which are laminated calcified bodies or calcospherules, may be free-lying or associated with papillary clusters of epithelial cells. If present in large numbers they are usually indicative of serous carcinoma or serous borderline tumour; these tumours are usually ovarian, but may rarely originate as a primary tumour of the peritoneum. Careful analysis of the cells in any papillary structure and those lying free in the fluid is mandatory, as psammoma bodies may occur in other papillary tumours, including mesothelioma, and are occasionally seen in reactive mesothelial proliferations and endosalpingiosis. In benign situations, it is rare to see more than an occasional psammoma body in a smear. Any associated cells are usually small and do not show nuclear hyperchromatism or mitotic activity; in papillae there should not be significant multilayering or disorganization. Clearly, while suspicious, the presence of psammoma bodies is *not* diagnostic of malignancy, and the fluid must be judged on the cytological appearances.

Cytoplasmic inclusions of various types can be helpful. Sharply circumscribed, dense, glassy (hyaline) inclusions may be seen in yolk sac tumour and mixed Mullerian tumour. In hepatocellular carcinoma, especially of the fibrolamellar variant, they are 'softer' and less well circumscribed. Characteristic crystalline cytoplasmic inclusions known as Reinke crystalloids are the hallmark of Leydig cell tumour. Similar structures are seen in alveolar soft part sarcoma; the crystals in this condition are strongly PAS positive.

12. *Multiple sex chromatin bodies* in female patients can be used for diagnosis of malignancy. In our experience, in difficult cases they are rarely convincingly seen. The only situation where these may be seen in benign cells is in patients with an abnormal karyotype (47 XXX)[17].

Morphology of specific tumour types
Carcinoma

Cytological findings

▶ Carcinoma cells in serous fluid are usually cohesive and form groups or clumps. However, some carcinomas have a predominantly single cell pattern, which may hamper recognition
▶ The major differential diagnoses of adenocarcinoma in serous fluid are mesothelial cell hyperplasia and mesothelioma. Cytoplasmic vacuolation can occur in any of these conditions; the presence of neutral mucin is diagnostic of adenocarcinoma but is not seen in all cases
▶ The cells of metastatic signet ring cell carcinoma of gastrointestinal tract and lobular carcinoma of the breast are easily missed because their cells are often small and arranged in predominantly single cell pattern; cells from small cell carcinoma can be confused with lymphocytes
▶ Immunocytochemistry may be helpful in identifying or subtyping malignant cells

Adenocarcinoma

Adenocarcinoma is the commonest tumour to show involvement of the serous membranes. Tumours of the breast, lung and ovary are most frequently encountered, followed by tumours of the gastrointestinal tract and the rest of the genitourinary tract. The cells of adenocarcinoma (e.g. Fig. 5.1–5.8) may be closely mimicked by reactive mesothelial cells (Fig. 5.9) and the cells of malignant mesothelioma (Fig. 5.10). Separation of these entities may be possible on routinely stained preparations but in the difficult case mucin stains and immunocytochemistry can be of value. To determine the primary source of adenocarcinoma cells in effusions may be impossible. With knowledge of the clinical data, especially sex and age of the patient, and taking into account the cavity involved and the morphological appearances, the site of origin may be inferred by the experienced cytopathologist in many cases. This skill may be enhanced by judicious use of immunocytochemistry.

Morphological features of adenocarcinoma include the presence of solid cell nests, as well as cells lying singly and

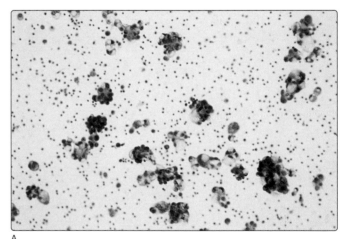

A

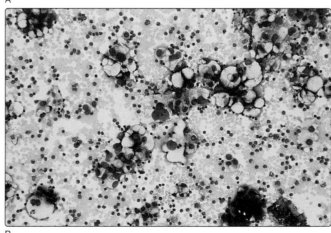

B

Fig. 5.1 Pleural fluid. Adenocarcinoma forming cell clumps, lung primary. Clumps of malignant cells of variable size can be seen; this is the most easily recognized pattern of carcinomatous involvement of serous membranes. (A, Papanicolaou × MP; B, MGG × MP)

in small clusters. In general terms, three different architectural patterns of adenocarcinomatous cells are seen in effusions: a clumped cell pattern (Fig. 5.1), a diffuse cell pattern (Fig. 5.7) and a mixed pattern (see Fig. 5.18). The presence of large cell clumps, recognizable papillae, acini or proliferation spheres makes the diagnosis considerably easier, as reactive mesothelial cells (Fig. 5.9) and many non-carcinomatous tumours (e.g. mesothelioma, Fig. 5.10) tend to form only small aggregates or single cell suspensions. Features aiding in the distinction between adenocarcinoma and mesothelial cell groups are summarized in Table 5.2. Although the cells of adenocarcinoma have a range of appearances, the typical adenocarcinoma cell is large with an eccentrically positioned hyperchromatic nucleus, often with condensation of nuclear chromatin on the nuclear membrane (Figs 5.2–5.4). There may be relative pallor of

the central area of the nucleus, and multinucleation may be seen (Fig. 5.5). The nucleolus is sometimes prominent, single and central or slightly eccentric, but multiple nucleoli can occur or the nucleolus may be indistinct, as in signet ring cell carcinoma. The cytoplasm often contains epithelial mucin, which is present in one or more vacuoles (Fig. 5.6). However, vacuolated cytoplasm does not necessarily signal adenocarcinoma and not all vacuoles are mucin; mesothelial cells typically contain a ring of tiny lipid vacuoles around the nucleus, but may contain larger glycogen or degenerative vacuoles. These vacuoles may even displace the nucleus, simulating a signet ring adenocarcinoma cell. The typical 'windows' between mesothelial cells can be mistaken for epithelial mucin vacuoles by the less experienced. Some cases of adenocarcinoma produce 'windows' identical to those seen

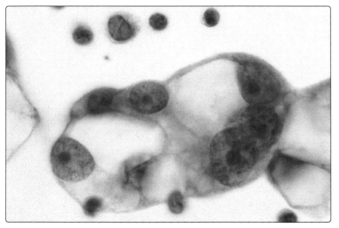

Fig. 5.2 Pleural fluid. Adenocarcinoma, lung primary. Cells within the groups are closely packed and unevenly distributed; the nuclei appear to overlap and prominent nucleoli are seen. Several large vacuoles with sharp edges and pale staining contents are present; special stains are frequently required to identify this material. (Papanicolaou × OI)

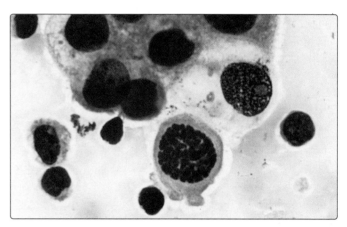

Fig. 5.4 Pleural fluid. Adenocarcinoma, lung primary. The cells show a high nuclear/cytoplasmic ratio. A mitotic figure is present; however, mitoses are not diagnostic of malignancy, and can rarely be seen in benign fluids (see **Fig. 5.9**). (MGG × HP)

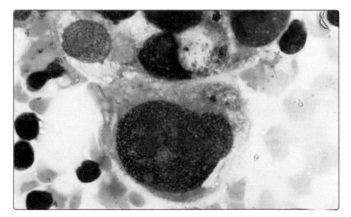

Fig. 5.3 Pleural fluid. Adenocarcinoma, lung primary. Nuclear pleomorphism is more apparent in MGG stained preparations. Several nucleoli can be identified in some nuclei, and one nucleus is indented by a cytoplasmic vacuole. (MGG × OI)

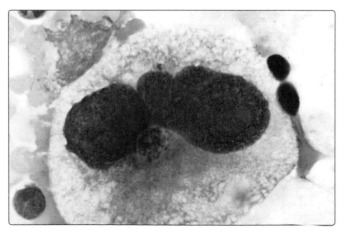

Fig. 5.5 Pleural fluid. Adenocarcinoma, lung primary. Multinucleated adenocarcinoma cells are not uncommon; nuclear size helps to distinguish them from multinucleated macrophages. When numerous they may cause confusion with mesothelioma, in which multinucleation is often particularly prominent. (MGG ×OI)

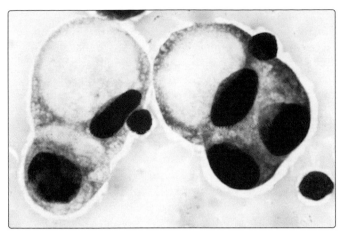

Fig. 5.6 Pleural fluid. Adenocarcinoma, lung primary. Vacuolated cells are often present in serous effusions. In this case, the adenocarcinoma cells contain mucin but similar appearances can be seen in mesothelial cells. A mucin stain is mandatory in such cases. (MGG × OI)

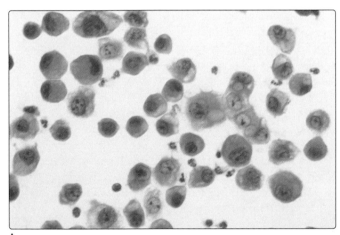

A

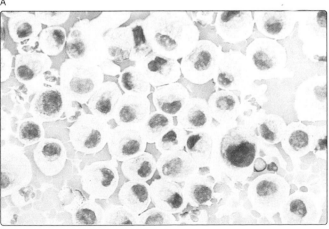

B

Fig. 5.7 Pleural fluid. Adenocarcinoma, dissociated cell pattern, stomach primary. This pattern of involvement is more easily overlooked than the clumped pattern (see **Fig. 5.1**), especially as in some cases (such as this) there is almost a pure tumour cell population and the cells are of similar size to mesothelial cells. However, careful examination of the tumour cells reveals nuclear irregularity and indentation. In addition, an occasional sharp edged vacuole is seen. (A, Papanicolaou × HP; B, MGG ×HP)

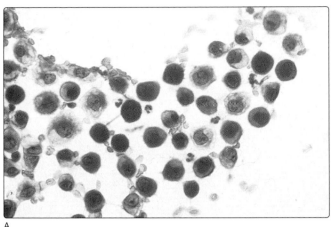

A

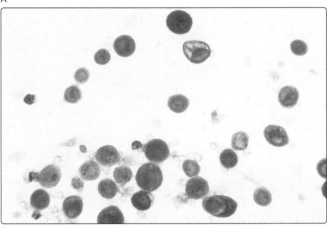

B

Fig. 5.8 Pleural fluid. Adenocarcinoma, stomach primary. Mucin stains are helpful in revealing the true nature of the dispersed cells in this malignant effusion. Almost every cell contains cytoplasmic mucin, some clearly within vacuoles. If mucin is present, the diagnosis is obvious. However, if mucin is scanty or absent, immunocytochemistry (in this case for CEA) is useful to confirm the non-mesothelial nature of the tumour cells. (A, PASD × HP; B, CEA × HP)

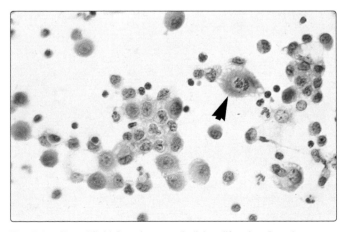

Fig. 5.9 Pleural fluid. Reactive mesothelial proliferation. Reactive mesothelial cells lie singly or in small, fairly regular clusters. Although they may show dramatic nuclear enlargement on occasion, they generally retain a normal nuclear/cytoplasmic ratio. One cell (arrowed) is in mitosis; this may occur in reactive mesothelial proliferation. (Papanicolaou × HP)

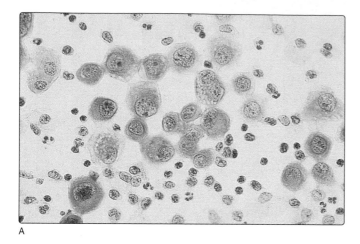

A

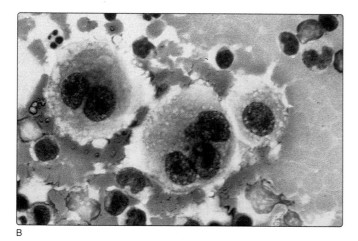

B

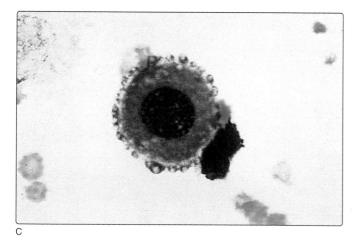

C

Fig. 5.10   Pleural fluid. Mesothelioma. (A) Mesotheliomas generally show a diffuse cell pattern similar to that seen in reactive mesothelial hyperplasia (see **Fig. 5.9**), melanoma (see **Fig. 5.50**) and some adenocarcinomas (see **Fig. 5.8**), including renal cell carcinoma (see **Fig. 5.33**). (B) The mesothelioma cell cytoplasm is dense and glassy due to the abundant cytoskeletal filaments, and there is often a striking resemblance to reactive mesothelial cells, but nuclear enlargement, macronucleolation and multinucleation are often prominent. (C) The surface of mesothelioma cells often shows a ruffled appearance, whereas adenocarcinoma cells tend to have a smoother cytoplasmic boundary (see **Fig. 5.4**). (A, Papanicolaou × HP; B, C, MGG × HP)

between mesothelial cells[24]. Even in adenocarcinoma cells, many of the vacuoles are either degenerative or contain glycogen, and some adenocarcinomas (e.g. renal cell carcinoma) do not produce mucin. Although mucin stains are recommended in this setting, they may be misleading if not studied with care; remnants of large pools of glycogen following inadequate diastase digestion on PAS preparations should not be misinterpreted as mucin.

Lung carcinoma is responsible for about 40% of positive pleural effusions[17]. Morphological appearances vary, and some lung tumours show evidence of divergent differentiation with the coexistence of adenocarcinoma, squamous cell carcinoma, large cell undifferentiated or small cell carcinoma. A range of differentiation can be seen with a few tumours being highly pleomorphic bordering on undifferentiated, and others, notably bronchoalveolar carcinoma, showing a very well-differentiated pattern. Cell clusters are usual (Fig. 5.1), but acinar formations are uncommon; papillary structures and rarely even psammoma bodies may be present. The cells are of variable size, and their nuclei appear to overlap; nuclear pleomorphism is often evident, with prominent nucleoli (Figs 5.2, 5.3). Nuclear/cytoplasmic ratio is increased and mitotic figures are generally present (Fig. 5.4); multinucleated forms are not uncommon, causing confusion with mesothelioma if numerous (Fig. 5.5). The malignant cells generally show evidence of mucin production with intracytoplasmic mucin vacuoles (Fig. 5.6). In well-differentiated bronchoalveolar carcinoma the cells may be exceptionally bland and do not always contain mucin; their cytological features resemble the normal Clara cell or type II pneumocyte towards which these tumours appear to differentiate, even to the recapitulation of the characteristic lamellar bodies seen ultrastructurally. In poorly differentiated lung tumours, mucin may be difficult to identify despite special stains; immunocytochemistry may be of use).

Breast carcinoma is the next most common tumour, and the most common in women, to affect the serous cavities, especially the pleurae. Involvement is chiefly by metastasis, which may occur many years after initial diagnosis. Pleural effusions may rarely be due to aggressive local disease eroding through the chest wall. The cytological appearances are variable depending on the type of tumour, but it is important to realize that this is a tumour which can be overlooked because of the monotonous size and nuclear morphology of the cells (Figs 5.11–5.17). Lobular carcinoma has a particular propensity to disseminate widely and to involve the peritoneal cavity; it may even present with ascites. In contrast, ductal carcinomas more frequently result in pleural effusions. The cells of ductal carcinoma are usually present in serous fluid in large numbers; they often form proliferation spheres (Figs 5.11, 5.12) or may lie singly, and although the cells may contain mucin[38], this is often scanty[39]. While the cells are often quite monotonous,

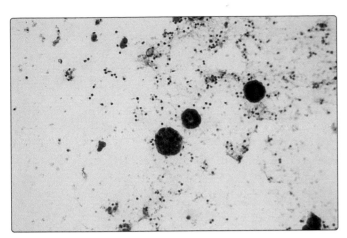

Fig. 5.11 Pleural fluid. Adenocarcinoma, breast primary, ductal type. This case demonstrates the 'proliferation sphere' which is a ball of large tumour cells, often with a hollow centre forming an acinar structure with a smooth external outline. (Papanicolaou × MP)

nuclear pleomorphism is more marked in some examples (Fig. 5.13). The cells of lobular carcinoma are smaller, tend to lie singly and are usually evenly dispersed in the fluid, a pattern rather similar to that seen in lymphoma. In most cases, however, there are at least a few groups revealing the carcinomatous nature of the lesion. The cells tend to form short chains reminiscent of the 'Indian file' pattern seen histologically (Fig. 5.14); this may cause confusion with small cell (oat cell) carcinoma but the typical hyperchromatic, moulded and angulated nuclei of that condition are not seen, and there is generally more cytoplasm. A characteristic feature of lobular carcinoma is the presence of intracytoplasmic lumina (Fig. 5.15), in the classical form composed of a targetoid lesion with a central dot-like core of neutral mucin surrounded by an acidic mucin halo[38] with 'thick' edges[40], best demonstrated by a combined Alcian blue/periodic acid Schiff preparation[41]. The lumina are lined by microvilli and also show strong immunocytochemical staining for epithelial membrane antigen[42]; cytokeratin staining may be of value to identify the tumour cells by their diffuse cytoplasmic staining, in contrast to the perinuclear ring pattern of mesothelial cells (Fig. 5.16). Occasionally, intracytoplasmic lumina grow to such a size that they deform the nucleus, resulting in a signet ring appearance, similar to that seen in signet ring cell carcinoma of the gastrointestinal tract (Fig. 5.17). However, while the intracytoplasmic lumen of breast carcinoma is usually single (occasionally multiple), in gastric signet ring cell carcinoma the pale area corresponds to numerous tiny mucin vacuoles within the endoplasmic reticulum; this multivacuolated appearance can be appreciated using light microscopy at high magnification.

Gastric and oesophageal adenocarcinomas frequently show serous cavity involvement and may be difficult to diagnose as the cells can be very bland, resembling macrophages (see Fig. 5.7). In some cases, the diagnosis is made easier

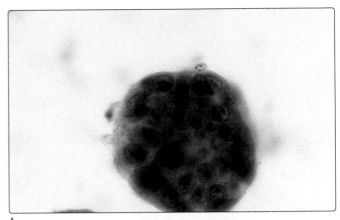

A

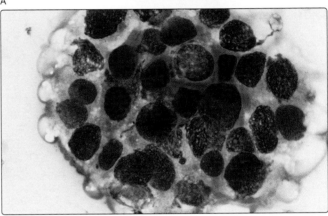

B

Fig. 5.12 Pleural fluid. Adenocarcinoma, breast primary, ductal type. Because of the three-dimensional nature of the proliferation sphere, focussing in various planes is required to extract cytological details. Out of the general plane, the features of individual cells are more easily appreciated; as is often the case in breast carcinoma, the cells have a remarkably monotonous appearance, but they are crowded and possess little cytoplasm. (A, Papanicolaou × HP; B, MGG ×HP)

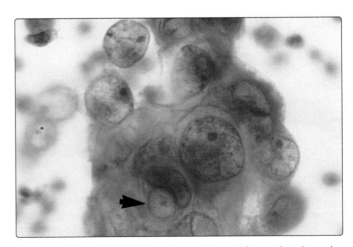

Fig. 5.13 Pleural fluid. Adenocarcinoma, breast primary, ductal type. In this example, in contrast to many breast carcinomas, nuclear pleomorphism is more marked; such pleomorphic ductal carcinomas are difficult to distinguish from adenocarcinomas from other sites. Mucin filled vacuoles, so called intracytoplasmic lumina (arrowed), are often seen in ductal carcinomas, although they are more characteristic of lobular carcinoma of breast. (Papanicolaou × OI)

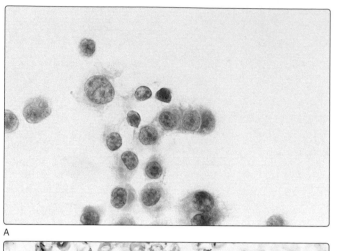

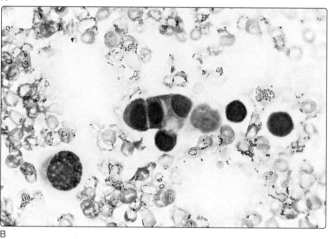

A

B

Fig. 5.14   Ascitic fluid. Adenocarcinoma, breast primary, lobular type. The cells are smaller than those of ductal carcinoma and lie singly or in small groups; because of their size, they are easily overlooked. The cells often form short chains, similar to those seen in small cell carcinoma. (A, Papanicolaou × HP; B, MGG ×HP)

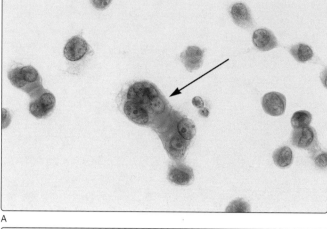

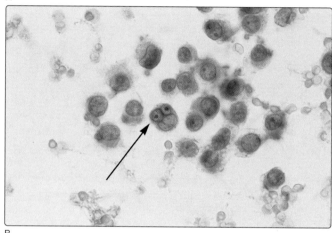

A

B

Fig. 5.15   Ascitic fluid. Adenocarcinoma, breast primary, lobular type. Intracytoplasmic lumina (one arrowed) are generally easily found in lobular carcinoma. They are accentuated by mucin stains; in (B), a tumour cell contains two lumina (arrowed). (A, Papanicolaou × HP; B, PASD × HP)

by the presence of cell clumps (Fig. 5.18). The typical cell type seen in diffuse gastric carcinoma is the signet ring cell, so called due to the displacement of the nucleus to the periphery of the cell by a large mucin vacuole. These cells are often small and round, and may lie dispersed in fluid, as they do in the gastric wall. The nucleus is often not particularly hyperchromatic, but usually contains a prominent central nucleolus. Nuclear grooves or creases may be present. However, similar but often even smaller cells, can be seen in metastatic breast carcinoma. Mesothelial cells with degenerative vacuolation may simulate these cells, and confirmation that vacuoles contain mucin is required (Figs 5.8, 5.19). Often, gastric carcinoma cells contain more acidic mucin (hyaluronidase resistant, Alcian blue positive) than neutral mucin (PAS positive). Interestingly, some vacuoles in undoubtedly malignant cells do not contain mucin. These are presumably degenerative and careful scrutiny of the mucin stains is recommended. In difficult cases,

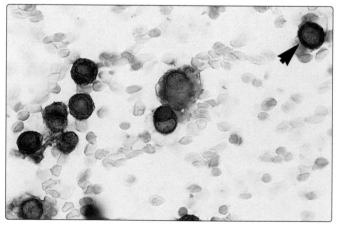

Fig. 5.16   Ascitic fluid. Adenocarcinoma, breast primary, lobular type. When these small uniform cells are dispersed, they may be difficult to differentiate from mesothelial cells. Cytokeratin staining allows this distinction, highlighting the tumour cells that show strong diffuse cytoplasmic reactivity. In contrast, a mesothelial cell (arrowed) shows the typical perinuclear stain in contrast. (Cytokeratin × HP)

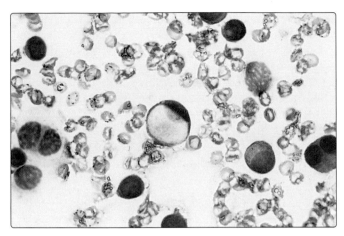

Fig. 5.17 Ascitic fluid. Adenocarcinoma, breast primary, lobular type. Occasionally, intracytoplasmic lumina may grow to such a size as to deform the nucleus producing a signet ring cell, similar to those seen in some intestinal tumours (centre). (MGG × HP)

immunocytochemistry for carcinoembryonic antigen (CEA) may be of value (see Fig. 5.8).

Ovarian tumours, which have breached their capsules typically disseminate by transcoelomic spread, and the cells of such tumours are frequently identified in ascitic fluid. Metastatic involvement of pleura or pericardium is rare. In involvement of the serous cavity, usually large numbers of neoplastic cells are present. They may be arranged in large clusters, acini or papillary structures interspersed by single tumour cells, often showing pronounced cytoplasmic vacuolation. The morphological appearances of these cells are variable but are in keeping with the main histological groups (serous, mucinous and endometrioid carcinomas).

Serous ovarian tumours in effusions are generally composed either of large pleomorphic cells if poorly differentiated, or rather bland small cells if well differentiated, arranged in papillary groups sometimes associated with psammoma (derived from the Greek 'grain

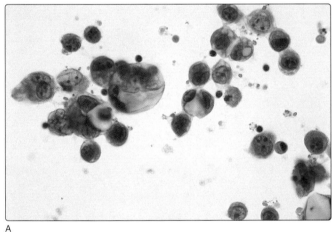

A

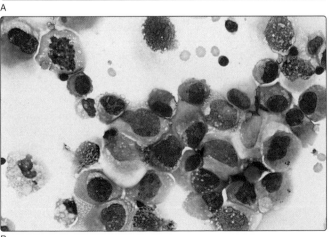

B

Fig. 5.18 Pleural fluid. Adenocarcinoma, oesophageal primary. This case demonstrates the combination of diffuse and clumped cell patterns. The cells contain small vacuoles, more apparent in the MGG stained preparation. In contrast to mesothelial cell vacuoles, they are distributed throughout the cell and are not mainly perinuclear in location. (A, Papanicolaou × HP; B, MGG × HP)

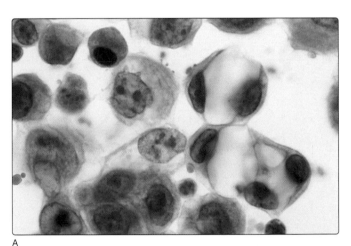

A

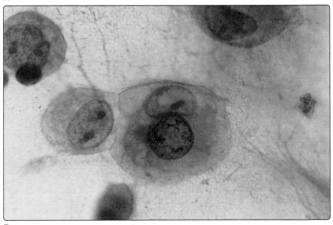

B

Fig. 5.19 Pleural fluid. Adenocarcinoma, oesophageal primary. The cells show marked nuclear irregularity and prominent nucleoli are present. Large cytoplasmic mucin vacuoles compress the nucleus resulting in a signet ring appearance. While this pattern is particularly associated with upper gastrointestinal tumours, it can be seen in other mucin secreting adenocarcinomas. (A, Papanicolaou × OI; B, PASD × OI)

of sand') body formation (Figs 5.20, 5.21). The psammoma body is easily overlooked in MGG preparations where it can simulate a vacuole (Fig. 5.22). The distinction between carcinoma and 'borderline tumour', or adenocarcinoma of low malignant potential, is important for prognosis; conventionally, it is based on the presence or absence of destructive stromal invasion in histological sections of the ovarian tumour. However, both carcinoma and 'borderline tumour' may demonstrate peritoneal involvement, the latter type typically showing implants of 'non-invasive' type histologically. Generally, cells shed from borderline tumours or their implants are small and fairly uniform,

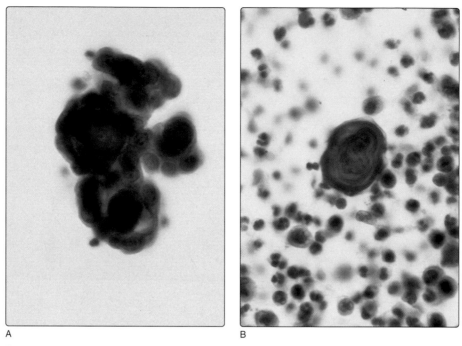

A   B

Fig. 5.20   Ascitic fluid. Psammoma bodies. Psammoma bodies may either be seen in the papillary cores (A) or may lie free in the fluid (B). On Papanicolaou staining, they often take on a brownish yellow hue. (Papanicolaou × HP)

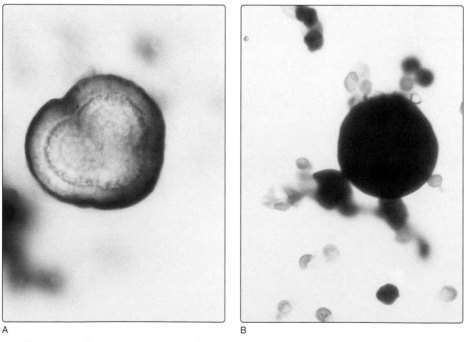

A   B

Fig. 5.21   Ascitic fluid. Psammoma bodies. The laminated nature of the psammoma body can clearly be seen. Staining with alizarin red (B) confirms the presence of calcium. (A, MGG × OI; B, alizarin red × OI)

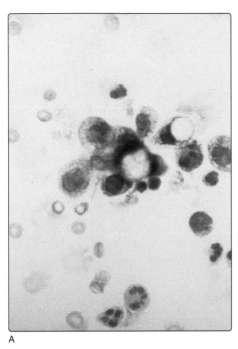
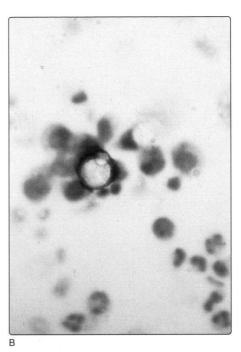

A   B

Fig. 5.22   Ascitic fluid. Adenocarcinoma, ovarian primary, serous type. in MGG stained preparations, psammoma bodies are easily overlooked as they have a clear centre, resembling a vacuole (A). However, careful examination reveals that the structure is refractile. Focusing in several planes may be required to identify the densely stained calcified outer layer (B). (MGG ×HP)

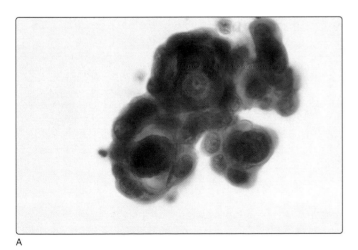
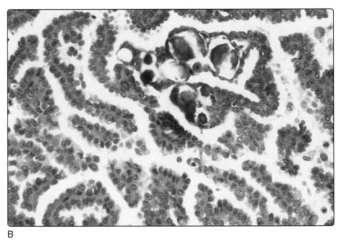

A   B

Fig. 5.23   (A) Ascitic fluid. Ovarian serous borderline tumour. Psammoma bodies are not diagnostic of serous carcinoma; careful study of the associated cells is needed to reach an accurate diagnosis. Distinction between borderline tumour and carcinoma may not be possible on cytological material. In this case there is only mild pleomorphism and the nuclei are relatively pale staining, favouring the diagnosis of borderline tumour. (B) Peritoneal tumour deposit, serous borderline tumour. This shows the typical papillary architecture of a serous ovarian tumour, and the presence of several psammoma bodies. The diagnosis of borderline tumour depends on the exclusion of stromal invasion and requires extensive sampling. (A, Papanicolaou × HP; B, H&E × MP)

with only rare mitotic figures (Fig. 5.23). When present, papillary fragments tend to be larger and more complex than in serous carcinoma (Fig. 5.24). In contrast, in invasive adenocarcinoma, the cells show greater pleomorphism, mitoses are more easily found and the papillary groups tend to be smaller (Fig. 5.25). Cell block preparations of peritoneal washings may be helpful in the distinction between borderline and malignant serous tumours[43]. Rarely, papillary groups may be absent and the

neoplastic population may be composed of dispersed small carcinoma cells similar in morphology to mesothelial cells. Similar tumours may arise from the peritoneum without ovarian involvement.

Mucinous ovarian tumours generally cause turbid serous effusions; free mucin may be visible in the preparations. However, the presence of mucin is not diagnostic of mucinous carcinoma, as it may be due to rupture of a benign mucinous cystadenoma or a borderline mucinous

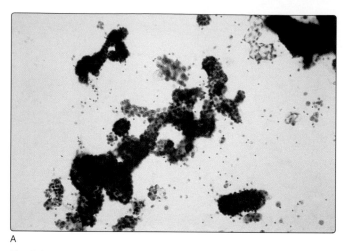

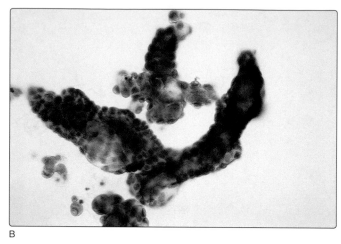

A   B

Fig. 5.24   Ascitic fluid. Ovarian serous borderline tumour. Borderline serous tumours typically give rise to complex branching papillary epithelial structures rather than the smaller clumps seen in serous carcinoma (see **Fig. 5.25**). (A, Papanicolaou × LP; B, Papanicolaou × HP)

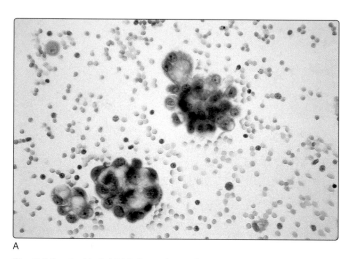

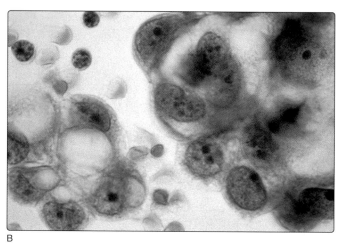

A   B

Fig. 5.25   Ascitic fluid. High-grade ovarian serous carcinoma. (A) In contrast to borderline serous tumours, serous carcinomas generally form small papillary groups and clumps. (B) There is also usually more pronounced cytological atypia, but it should be emphasized that the distinction is made on histological grounds depending on the presence or absence of stromal invasion. (A, Papanicolaou × LP; B, Papanicolaou × LP)

tumour. In mucinous adenocarcinoma, the tumour cells are columnar with often copious intracytoplasmic neutral mucin in better differentiated tumours, but there is nuclear hyperchromasia, pleomorphism and mitotic figures may be seen (Figs 5.26, 5.27). It is important to confirm the mucinous content of the cells, as vacuolation can be seen in serous and endometrioid carcinomas; the former may contain degenerative vacuoles and the latter may contain glycogen granules in the pattern of secretory endometrium.

Pseudomyxoma peritonei is widespread peritoneal involvement by mucin secreting tumour, usually associated with a mucinous borderline tumour or a well-differentiated mucinous adenocarcinoma of ovary or appendix (Figs 5.28–5.30)[44]. It is thought to arise from rupture of a cystic tumour and generalized seeding of tumour cells throughout the abdominal cavity, and results in the accumulation of large amounts of mucin, which can be very difficult to

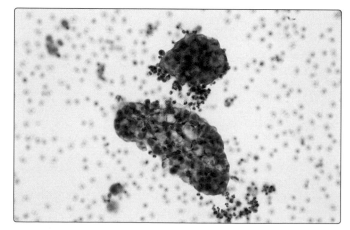

Fig. 5.26   Ascitic fluid. Ovarian mucinous adenocarcinoma. Peritoneal involvement usually results in large strongly cohesive groups of clearly malignant cells containing copious intracytoplasmic mucin. (Papanicolaou × MP)

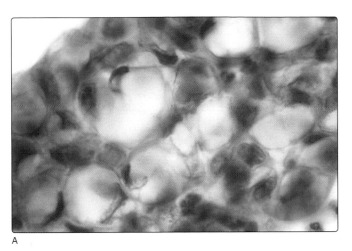

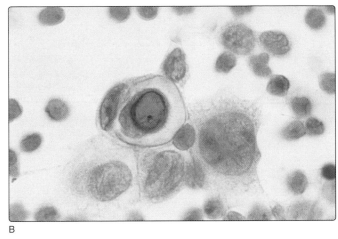

A   B

Fig. 5.27   Ascitic fluid. Ovarian mucinous adenocarcinoma. The cells are large, closely packed and haphazardly arranged; many contain hard-edged vacuoles. The nuclei are hyperchromatic and irregular. The presence of neutral mucin is confirmed using PASD staining. (A, Papanicolaou × OI; B, PASD × OI)

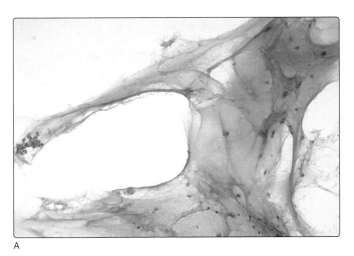

A   B

Fig. 5.28   Ascitic fluid. Ruptured mucocoele resulting in free mucin in the peritoneal cavity. Epithelial mucin appears as a dense homogeneous material, similar to fibrin but lacking its fibrillary appearance. It is an important finding and must not be disregarded. However, it is not diagnostic of malignancy and may result from a ruptured benign mucinous tumour of ovary or, as in this example, appendix. Careful examination for malignant cells must be made, as cases due to adenocarcinoma often contain only few malignant cells (similar to those shown in **Fig. 5.27**). In MGG preparations, epithelial mucin stains a delicate shade of blue. (A, Papanicolaou × MP; B, MGG × MP)

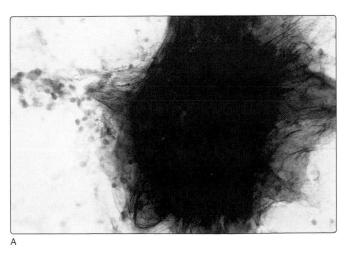

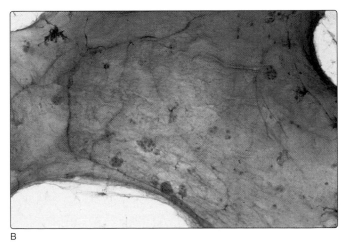

A   B

Fig. 5.29   Ascitic fluid. Free mucin in the peritoneal cavity. Mucin is confirmed as epithelial and not connective tissue mucin (as seen in mesothelioma) by PASD or alcian blue following hyaluronidase digestion. (A, PASD × MP; B, PASD/alcian blue following hyaluronidase digestion × MP)

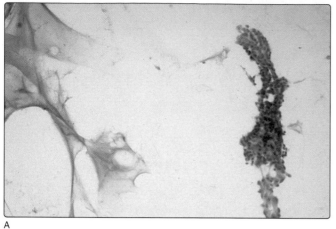

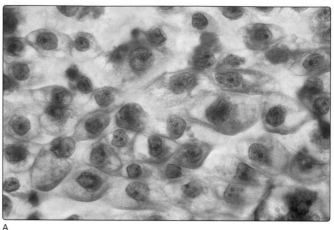

A

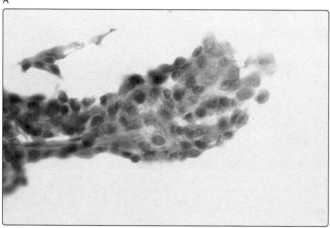

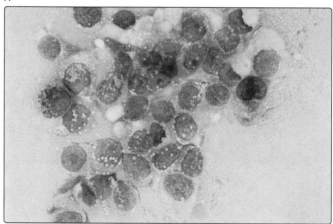

B

B

Fig. 5.30   Ascitic fluid. Free mucin in the peritoneal cavity. The association of neutral mucin with groups of cells does not always indicate malignancy. The cells here are mesothelial cells, not adenocarcinoma; note the organization and lack of crowding. In this case, following a ruptured mucocoele of the appendix, the patient was alive and well 2 years later. The type of primary lesion determines the outcome in these cases; malignant tumours presenting in this manner have a progressive clinical course but this is often protracted, especially in the case of a borderline tumour. (A, B, Papanicolaou × LP, MP)

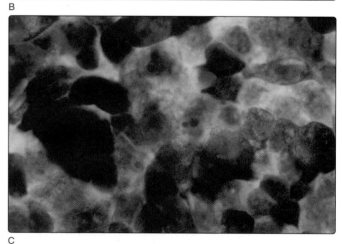

C

Fig. 5.31   Ascitic fluid. Adenocarcinoma, ovarian primary, clear cell type. The large tumour cells show slightly irregular nuclear contour and prominent nucleoli. The cytoplasm is condensed around the cell membrane resulting in a 'vegetable material-like' appearance. In the MGG stained preparation, small vacuoles are apparent in the copious pale cytoplasm. The cells contain numerous PAS positive granules corresponding to cytoplasmic glycogen. (A, Papanicolaou × HP; B, MGG × HP; C, PAS × HP)

aspirate due to its high viscosity. Smears from such a case contain copious PAS positive and hyaluronidase resistant mucin and may be almost or entirely acellular (Figs 5.28, 5.29). Tumour cells are often very scanty or absent and it may be necessary to examine numerous preparations, or even further aspirates, before a definitive diagnosis can also be reached. A malignant diagnosis cannot be based purely on the presence of epithelial mucin since this can also be present as the result of rupture of an appendiceal mucocele or benign mucinous cystadenoma of the ovary. Care must be taken not to overdiagnose malignancy, especially when mucin from a benign tumour is associated with groups of reactive mesothelial cells as is sometimes seen (Fig. 5.30). In these instances, in contrast to the relentless though often protracted course seen in pseudomyxoma peritonei, complete resolution is the norm. Diagnosis requires careful analysis of the mucin secreting cells for abnormal

cytological features. Cell blocks can be particularly helpful in making the diagnosis of pseudomyxoma peritonei, as the viscid fluid is difficult to handle in conventional ways and the cells are often very scanty.

Endometrioid ovarian carcinomas show features similar to adenocarcinoma of the lung or colon. Squamous differentiation is common in this tumour but is not generally apparent in serous fluid[17].

Clear cell ovarian carcinomas in serous fluid typically show the presence of small groups and individual cells with a very well defined, sharp cytoplasmic border and a centrally situated round to oval nucleus, resulting in a 'vegetable material-like' appearance; the cells contain large amounts of cytoplasmic glycogen (Fig. 5.31)[18]. The tumour cells may be cohesive or may dissociate simulating mesothelial cells. In the latter case, immunocytochemistry for HMFG2 and calretinin is useful in identifying the neoplastic cells (Fig. 5.32). Malignant Brenner tumour is rarely encountered in serous fluid[17]. The cells show features similar to those seen in transitional cell carcinoma.

Ovarian malignant mixed Mullerian tumour, in which sarcomatous and adenocarcinomatous differentiation is seen, usually presents with numerous bizarre tumour cells[45,46]. Both components may be apparent or one may predominate. The sarcomatous component may show skeletal muscle differentiation with the production of rhabdomyoblasts. Characteristic cross striations may be present, but immunocytochemical reactivity for desmin and myoglobin is specific and more sensitive. Similar tumours arise from the endometrium and, exceptionally, the fallopian tube.

Renal cell carcinoma, often of clear cell type, is particularly important because it is often difficult to identify in fluids as the tumour cell morphology may be very similar to that of mesothelial cells (Fig. 5.33). Abundant glycogen is present in both cell types, but intracytoplasmic lipid globules, if present in large numbers, are suggestive of renal cell carcinoma; immunocytochemistry may be helpful as many renal cell carcinomas express CD15 (LeuM1)[47]. In some cases of renal cell carcinoma, there is a more cohesive appearance (Fig. 5.34). Numerous tiny lipid and glycogen vacuoles, best seen in MGG preparations, are typical. However, this feature may occasionally be seen in mesothelioma (Fig. 5.35). Papillary renal cell carcinoma

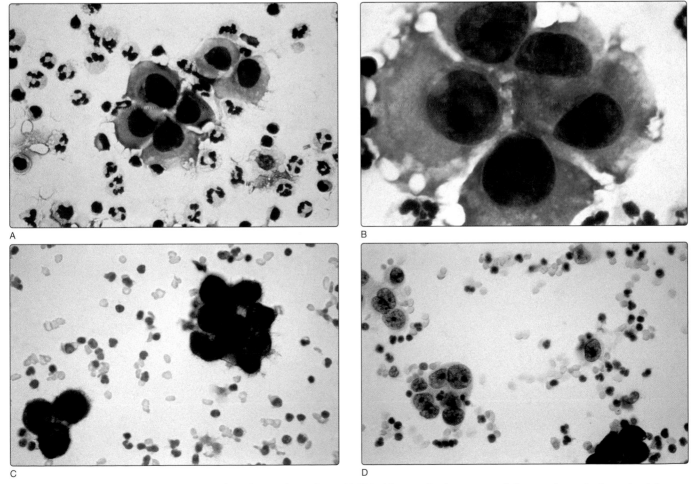

Fig. 5.32 Ascitic fluid. Adenocarcinoma, ovarian primary, clear cell type. (A, B) In this example, the tumour cells have copious cytoplasm, simulating mesothelial cells. (C) Immunocytochemistry for HMFG2 shows strong cytoplasmic staining. (D) Calretinin staining highlights adjacent mesothelial cells; the tumour cells are unstained. (A, Papanicolaou × LP; B, Papanicolaou × HP; C, HMFG2 × MP; D, calretinin × MP)

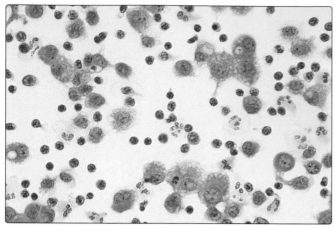

Fig. 5.33 Ascitic fluid. Renal cell carcinoma. Renal cell carcinoma can also simulate mesothelial cells or mesothelioma. Here the malignant cells have a dispersed cell pattern and preserved N:C ratio. Note similarity to **Figs 5.7A** and **5.9** (Papanicolaou × HP)

may also involve the serous membranes although diagnosis may be difficult, as papillae are not invariably present[48].

Colonic carcinoma is one of the most common tumours seen in histological practice, but curiously it is rare to see involvement of the peritoneum resulting in ascites. The tumour cells are normally large, and in well-differentiated tumours the columnar nature may be apparent. Occasionally, cells similar to those seen in gastric carcinoma may be present. Electron microscopic demonstration of microvilli with 'cytoplasmic rootlets' is reported to be characteristic of colonic carcinoma[49].

Endometrial carcinoma may be present in serous fluid, usually ascitic, in advanced disease. The features are identical to those seen in endometrioid carcinoma of the ovary, and tend to lack specificity; the presence of squamous metaplasia may be helpful but is difficult to recognize. Serous carcinoma of endometrium has also been

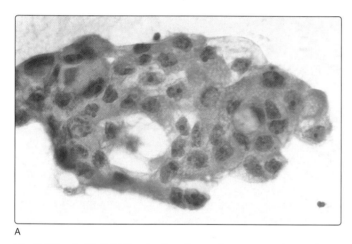

A

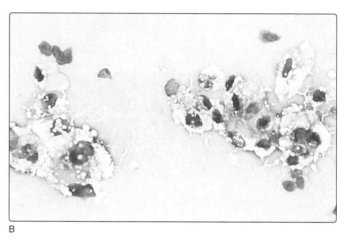

B

Fig. 5.34 Ascitic fluid. Renal cell carcinoma. In contrast to the previous case, the cells form large poorly cohesive clumps. The nuclei are well spaced due to the relatively normal nuclear/cytoplasmic ratio, but there is irregularity of the nuclear membrane. Numerous small cytoplasmic vacuoles can be seen in the MGG preparation; they are almost invisible in the Papanicolaou preparation. Note the similarity to the ovarian clear cell carcinoma (**Fig. 5.31**). The vacuoles contain abundant fat and glycogen. However, lipid microvacuoles are not diagnostic for renal cell carcinoma (see **Fig. 5.35**). (A, Papanicolaou × HP; B, MGG × HP)

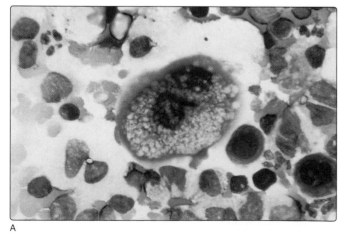

A

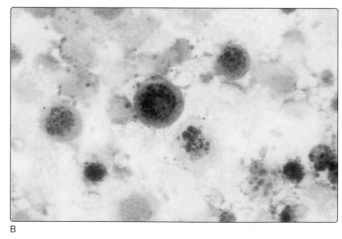

B

Fig. 5.35 Pleural fluid. Mesothelioma. Small dispersed vacuoles can be seen in mesothelioma cells in a pattern almost indistinguishable from that seen in renal cell carcinoma. A lipid stain confirms the nature of the intracytoplasmic vacuoles, as in renal cell carcinoma. However, this extent of lipid accumulation is uncommon in mesothelioma. (A, MGG × HP; B, oil red-O × HP)

reported in ascitic fluid but is essentially indistinguishable from its ovarian counterpart[50].

Many other adenocarcinomas may rarely involve serous cavities, including embryonal carcinoma (see also 'Germ cell tumours'), hepatocellular carcinoma, thyroid, pancreatic and prostatic carcinoma. In many of these cases distinctive cytological features are not present, and the diagnosis relies heavily on adequate clinical information. However, serous membrane involvement by papillary carcinoma of the thyroid, although rare, results in a characteristic appearance: the cells are fairly small, generally arranged in papillary clusters and often contain intranuclear cytoplasmic invaginations and nuclear grooves; psammoma bodies are usually present, except when the tumour assumes a follicular pattern. Immunocytochemistry may be used to confirm the site of origin using antibodies to thyroglobulin. A similar approach can be used to confirm origin of prostatic carcinomas using prostate specific antigen and prostatic acid phosphatase, and hepatocellular carcinoma using polyclonal CEA to reveal a canalicular staining pattern with CD34 positive sinusoidal lining cells[51].

Curschmann's spirals indistinguishable from those seen in the respiratory tract are rarely present in serous fluid. They are thought to be related to altered mucin, and in some cases they are associated with a mucin secreting adenocarcinoma. However, this is not invariable, and it has been postulated that they may be caused by myxoid degeneration of the submesothelial tissues[18].

Squamous cell carcinoma

Involvement of serous cavities by squamous cell carcinoma (SCC) is uncommon. Pleural involvement by SCC of lung is most frequently encountered (Fig. 5.36) but as the majority of these tumours occur centrally, pleural and/or pericardial involvement is seen only occasionally in late stage disease, sometimes associated with pericardial tamponade[52]. SCC of the female genital tract (predominantly cervix) may lead to ascites by peritoneal involvement in advanced local disease, or may involve pleura or pericardium by metastasis, although this is less frequent. Metastasis from any site of SCC may occur, but in practice the majority of the remainder originate from laryngeal primaries. The morphological appearance of metastatic SCC cells is variable and several specific cell types are recognized, reflecting the degree of differentiation shown[53]. Unfortunately, the commonest cell seen in effusions from known squamous cell carcinomas of lung is the undifferentiated/poorly-differentiated type. However, to make a definitive diagnosis of SCC, tumour cells showing convincing squamous differentiation must be present, and this is another reason for the relative rarity of the diagnosis despite the common occurrence of the tumour.

Fibre cells and tadpole cells are relatively infrequent; diagnosis is usually based on the presence of cells showing cytoplasmic keratinization of variable degree, and/or

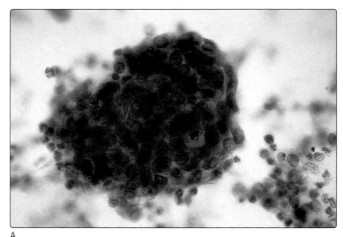

A

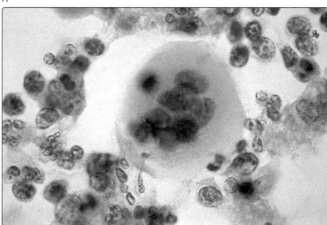

B

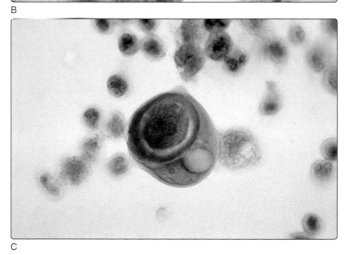

C

Fig. 5.36 Pleural fluid. Squamous cell carcinoma, lung primary. (A) Squamous cell carcinoma usually forms large irregular clumps of malignant cells. Cytoplasmic keratinization, if present, results in cytoplasmic orangeophilia, sometimes with a hard or glassy quality. Squamous carcinoma cells may be multinucleate (B) or show emperipolesis (C). (A, Papanicolaou × LP; B, C, Papanicolaou × HP)

irregular angulated cytoplasmic boundaries due to the large amounts of intracytoplasmic cytokeratin filaments (Fig. 5.36). Cytoplasmic vacuolation may be seen in a few cells in over a quarter of cases, simulating adenocarcinoma

(Fig. 5.37), but this is only rarely present extensively and is unlikely to cause serious diagnostic difficulties. Mucin stains are negative in such cases. Keratin pearls, if present, aid diagnosis but these only occur in well-differentiated tumours and are therefore infrequently seen. However, not all orangeophilic cells in Papanicolaou stained preparations are squamous, mesothelial cells sometimes showing similar changes. Differentiation in a few squamous carcinomas leads to the production of cells with relatively mature cytoplasm with a pyknotic dyskaryotic nucleus or even an anucleate cell. However, the presence of anucleate squamous cells, while strongly suggestive if present in large numbers, is not strictly adequate for the diagnosis of SCC in the absence of cytologically malignant cells. Quite apart from contamination of the specimen or slides by cells shed by operator or technician, there are several other potential sources of anucleate squamous cells including ruptured teratoma[54], squamous metaplasia of the peritoneum and, in the pleural cavity, fistulous communication between the oesophagus or tracheobronchial tree and pleural cavity. In

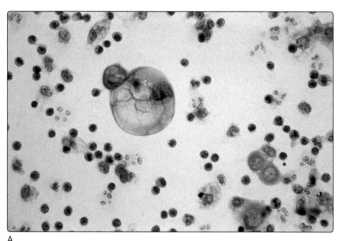

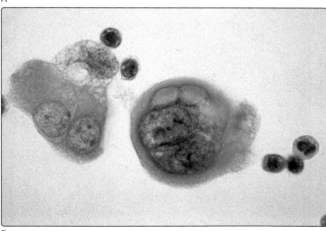

Fig. 5.37 Pleural fluid. Squamous cell carcinoma, lung primary. (A) Metastatic squamous cell carcinoma may be difficult to distinguish from adenocarcinoma if keratinization is scanty. (B) Degenerative nuclear vacuolation may simulate intracellular mucin. (A, Papanicolaou × LP; B, Papanicolaou × HP)

addition, the presence of squamous cells with malignant cells may be seen in endometrioid ovarian adenocarcinoma (see above) or endometrial adenocarcinoma showing squamous differentiation (adenoacanthoma). Cellular fragments of squamous cell carcinoma are present in 40% of fluids positive for SCC[18]. These are less three-dimensional than the clusters seen in adenocarcinoma, being composed of cells with easily seen cell boundaries and centrally positioned hyperchromatic round to oval nuclei (Figs 5.36, 5.37). The cytoplasm may appear orange or pale green in Papanicolaou stained preparations, and intercellular bridges may be apparent.

Transitional cell carcinoma

Transitional cell carcinoma is rarely seen in serous effusions, and then usually in patients with advanced and clinically apparent bladder carcinoma[18]. The tumour cells do not possess particularly characteristic features in fluids, and can resemble mesothelial cells or undifferentiated carcinoma cells. The tumour cells may be vacuolated as a degenerative phenomenon, although glandular differentiation is not uncommon in urothelial malignancies. The specific diagnosis is extremely difficult to make in the absence of an appropriate clinical history.

Undifferentiated carcinoma

This is a diagnosis of exclusion, implying that despite extensive investigation, no features of differentiation other than carcinomatous can be identified. It should not be made without negative mucin stains to exclude glandular differentiation. If studied immunohistochemically and ultrastructurally, the number of genuinely undifferentiated tumours decreases substantially. However, it can be argued that differentiation so discovered may be of little value in biological terms. Involvement of the pleura by the variant of lung carcinoma known as large cell undifferentiated carcinoma may also occur.

Small cell (oat cell) carcinoma

This tumour usually arises in the lung, but may involve a number of other sites including prostate, oesophagus and ovary. It is highly malignant and metastasizes widely, at autopsy over 50% of patients having adrenal metastases. Although pleural and pericardial involvement are most common, peritoneal spread does occur. The cells of small cell (oat cell) carcinoma have a distinctive appearance but because of their relatively small size and inconspicuous cytoplasm they may be confused with lymphocytes or other small celled tumours (Figs 5.38–5.40)[55]. The distinction is chiefly made by the cohesive nature of the carcinoma cells in contrast to lymphoid cells that tend to lie dispersed in fluids. The arrangement of nuclear chromatin is also useful (see later). Typically, the cells of small cell (oat cell) carcinoma are about twice the size of unstimulated lymphocytes and are arranged singly and in small groups and chains with 'moulding' of adjacent nuclei (Figs 5.38,

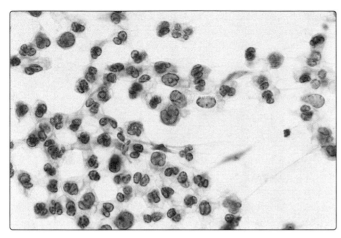

Fig. 5.38 Pleural fluid. Small cell carcinoma, lung primary. The nuclei of small cell carcinoma are two to three times the diameter of a small lymphocyte and have little cytoplasm, resulting in a very high nuclear/cytoplasmic ratio; because of their morphological similarity to lymphocytes, they are easily overlooked. (Papanicolaou × HP)

5.39). In the most extreme example, they resemble stacks of coins, or a silhouette of the vertebral column. When two or more cells touch, one may form a 'cap' on the other, occasionally leading to production of an onion skin-like appearance. The cells are fragile and this can lead to a distorted or crushed appearance. The nuclei are round when the cells lie singly, but when in groups, tend to be more angulated; they are hyperchromatic but rather featureless, nucleoli being usually absent or at least inconspicuous. The presence of prominent nucleoli should prompt reconsideration of the diagnosis. The cytoplasm is scanty, even in the larger cell subtypes of small cell carcinoma, which apart from cell size, show similar features to classical small cell (oat cell) carcinoma. In some cases, larger aggregates or sheets with a pavement-like appearance may be seen; exceptionally, rosette-like structures may be seen in fluid specimens (Fig. 5.40). Distinction from lymphoma has been discussed above; other rare tumours,

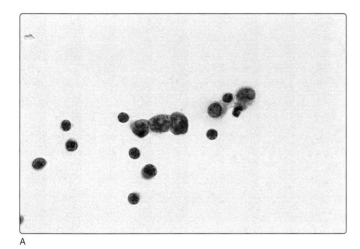

A

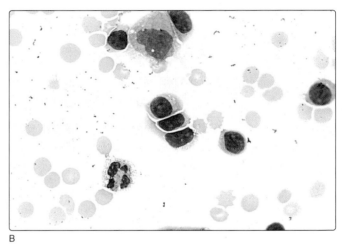

B

Fig. 5.39 Pleural fluid. Small cell carcinoma, lung primary. The malignant nature of the cells is more apparent when they form characteristic short chains; these chains are similar to those seen in lobular breast carcinoma, but where the cells touch they mould around each other giving a 'stack of coins' or 'vertebral column' appearance. Nucleoli are small or absent, a useful differential diagnostic feature (A, Papanicolaou × HP; B, MGG × HP)

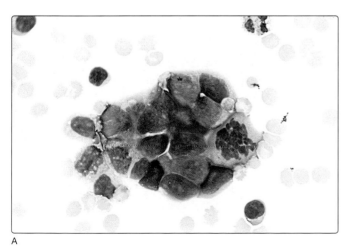

A

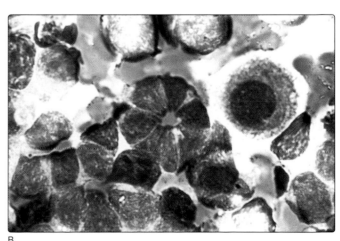

B

Fig. 5.40 Pleural fluid. Small cell carcinoma, lung primary. (A) Larger aggregates of tumour cells may show a pavement-like appearance. (B) Exceptionally, a rosette-like structure may be seen (A, B, MGG × HP)

which show similar appearances, include neuroepithelioma, Ewing's sarcoma and neuroblastoma. Immunocytochemistry may be useful to confirm the diagnosis and in problem cases (see Fig. 5.58). The cells of small cell (oat cell) carcinoma often show a distinctive perinuclear punctate or dot-like accentuation of cytokeratin staining; this finding corresponds to aggregation of intermediate filaments confirmed ultrastructurally and appears restricted to tumours showing neuroendocrine differentiation, the prime example of which is Merkel cell tumour. Immunoreactivity for neurone specific enolase is the rule[56], and many tumours show positivity for the neurosecretory granule related peptide chromogranin. Staining for CD56 (neural cell adhesion molecule, NCAM)[57], Leu 7[58], bombesin, bombesin receptor[59] and many other markers of neuroendocrine differentiation has been reported[60,61].

Lymphoma and leukaemia

Cytological findings

▶ The cells of lymphomas and leukaemias are usually present in large numbers in serous fluids and typically do not form clumps, but aggregation of tumour cells may occur

▶ Well-differentiated lymphocytic lymphoma may be difficult to distinguish from a lymphocyte rich reactive condition; immunocytochemistry is often needed for definite diagnosis

▶ Large cell lymphomas and acute myeloid leukaemias may be confused with other high-grade malignancies such as poorly differentiated carcinoma and melanoma; cytochemistry including immunocytochemistry may be valuable.

▶ Large cell lymphoma may present exclusively involving serous cavities (primary effusion lymphoma, PEL)

Non-Hodgkin's Lymphoma (NHL)

Serous effusions are a common feature of advanced disease, but very occasionally may be the presenting condition. In such instances a careful clinical examination will usually reveal widespread disease. Primary pulmonary or gastrointestinal lymphomas (lymphomas of mucosal associated lymphoid tissue, MALT lymphoma) do not generally give rise to serous effusions unless there is advanced local or widespread disease.

Lymphomas presenting with pleural effusion as their initial manifestation are rare and almost all cases are B-cell lymphomas, mostly diffuse large cell lymphoma, follicular lymphoma and small lymphocytic lymphoma. Many of these cases have mediastinal lymphadenopathy and classification as primary pleural lymphoma is difficult. However, two primary effusion-based lymphomas appear to represent distinct clinicopathological entities[62].

Primary effusion lymphoma (PEL) is a rare body cavity-based NHL, that occurs almost exclusively in HIV positive patients, usually in homosexual men[63,64]. It may involve pleural, pericardial or peritoneal surfaces and usually remains confined to body cavities. A characteristic feature is the presence of human herpes virus 8 (HHV8, Kaposi's

sarcoma-associated herpes virus), as well as clonal Epstein Barr virus sequences; C-myc gene is germ line configuration. Many patients who develop PEL have pre-existing Kaposi's sarcoma. The lymphoma is usually of a large cell type (immunoblastic/anaplastic) and often expresses CD30.

Pyothorax-associated lymphoma (PAL) was initially observed in Asian patients, but is now also recognized in Western patients; seen in the setting of long standing pleural inflammation caused by tuberculosis[65]. It occurs solely in the pleura, often associated with a thoracic mass presenting at least 20 years after initial pleural infection. While morphologically resembling PEL and associated with EBV viral sequences in most cases, HHV8 positive cases have not been described and the tumour cells are CD30 negative. Prognosis for PEL and PAL is poor with death within months of diagnosis[66].

In general, lymphomatous involvement of the serous membranes leads to the production of a serous effusion, which appears typically white and turbid (chylous) but may be clear or blood stained.

The fluid is highly cellular and contains a monotonous population of lymphoid cells. The morphological features of the cells depend on the type of lymphoma (Figs 5.41–5.47)[67]. In general, lymphoid cells have little cytoplasm. The nuclear features vary widely depending on the type of lymphoid cell or malignancy, but the chromatin is usually diffusely dispersed in the nucleus with some condensation around the nuclear membrane in contrast to leukaemia in which this feature is not usually seen. The presence of nucleoli is variable. The nucleus is often deeply indented or 'cleaved' and this is seen in an extreme form in some variants of T cell lymphoma, in which the cells may assume a cerebriform appearance due to the complexity of the numerous nuclear invaginations.

Involvement by *low-grade B-cell lymphoma* may result in a monomorphic population of small lymphoid cells, which may be difficult or impossible to differentiate from those seen in benign lymphocyte rich conditions (Figs 5.41, 5.42). This pattern is seen in well-differentiated lymphocytic lymphoma/chronic lymphocytic leukaemia. The monomorphic nature of the lymphoid cells is a useful feature as in reactive lymphocyte rich effusions there is usually more variation in cell size. A distinctive feature is the nuclear chromatin clumping of the cells of chronic lymphocytic leukaemia; these cells have been referred to as 'cellules grumelées'[68]. The presence of lymphoplasmacytoid cells (Fig. 5.43), often with intranuclear cytoplasmic invaginations (Dutcher bodies), is virtually diagnostic of lymphoplasmacytoid lymphoma[30]. Serous cavity involvement by hairy cell leukaemia with typical morphological and immunocytochemical features has also been reported[69].

In the *high-grade B-cell lymphomas*, the cell size is invariably larger but the characteristic lack of cohesion is

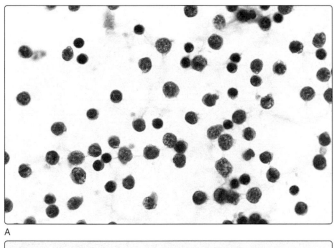

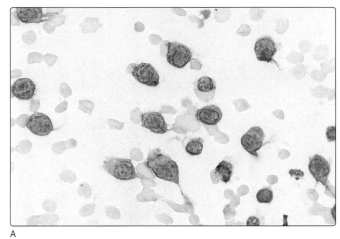

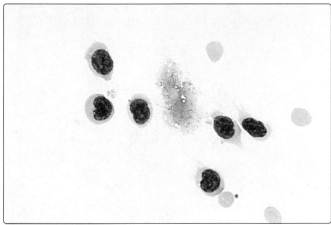

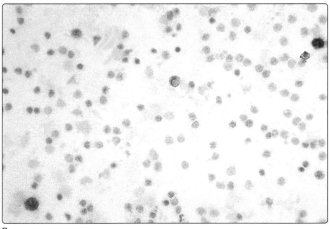

A

B

Fig. 5.41 Pleural fluid. Low-grade B cell non-Hodgkin's lymphoma. The small to medium-sized lymphoid cells are monotonous and the nuclei are indented, not round; the nuclear chromatin is evenly dispersed. A few small T lymphocytes are also present. (A, Papanicolaou × HP; B, MGG × HP)

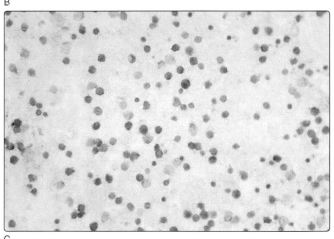

C

Fig. 5.42 Pleural fluid. Low-grade B cell non-Hodgkin's lymphoma. Immunocytochemistry is valuable in such cases to confirm the B cell nature of the cells. Clonality can be demonstrated by staining for immunoglobulin light chains. In this example the tumour cells are lambda light chain restricted. (A, CD20; B, κ-light chain; C, λ-light chain, all × HP)

still apparent; the cells remain individuals and refuse to form tightly packed clumps (Figs 5.44, 5.45). This is probably the most useful diagnostic feature, along with the typical lymphoid nuclear morphology. The chromatin is often rather coarsely clumped and there may be small nucleoli. The cytoplasm is usually inconspicuous; what little cytoplasm can be seen stains intensely blue with MGG. Mitotic figures, including abnormal forms, may be present. Other characteristic features are the presence of individual cell necrosis in high-grade tumours, exemplified by Burkitt's lymphoma; this particular tumour has an unusual and distinctive morphological appearance, the nuclear chromatin being diffuse and finely granular and the cytoplasm containing numerous small vacuoles.

High-grade T-cell lymphomas may involve the serous surfaces as pulmonary involvement is common. Again, these result in a lymphocyte rich effusion, often containing many large highly pleomorphic and often polylobated T lymphoid cells. Eosinophils may be present. This group includes some cases formerly classified as histiocytic lymphoma. Unfortunately, similar morphological features can be seen in a small number of high-grade B-cell lymphomas; immunocytochemistry is essential for this distinction.

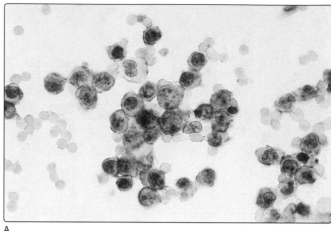

A

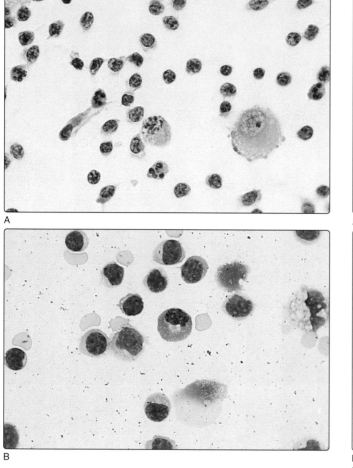

A

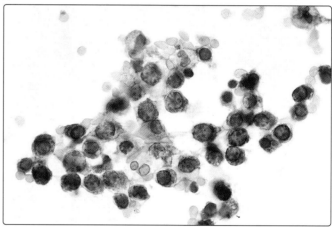

B

Fig. 5.43 Pleural fluid. Low-grade B cell non-Hodgkin's lymphoma (lymphoplasmacytoid). Many of the small lymphoid cells have a clockface distribution of chromatin clumps on the nuclear membrane. Some cells have eccentric nuclei and a pale perinuclear hof indicating plasmacytoid differentiation. (A, Papanicolaou × HP; B, MGG × HP)

B

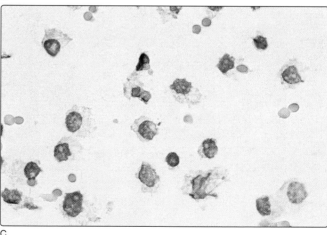

C

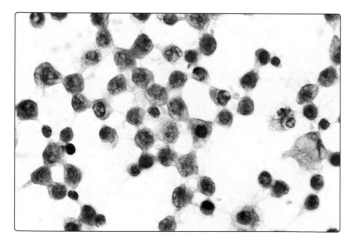

Fig. 5.44 Pleural fluid. High-grade B cell non-Hodgkin's lymphoma (diffuse large B cell). The neoplastic lymphoid cells are large (compare with **Fig. 5.41**). Centroblasts have pale nuclei with chromatin clumped on the nuclear membrane. Occasional cells have central nucleoli. (Papanicolaou × HP)

Fig. 5.45 Pleural fluid. High-grade B cell non-Hodgkin's lymphoma. Immunocytochemistry is valuable in such cases to confirm the B cell nature of the cells. Clonality can be demonstrated by staining for immunoglobulin light chains. In this example the tumour cells are kappa light chain restricted. (A, CD20; B, κ-light chain; C, λ-light chain, all × HP)

Anaplastic large cell lymphoma (Ki-1 lymphoma) may involve the pleura. The cells are large, with highly atypical nuclei and prominent nucleoli (Fig. 5.46); there is immunocytochemical expression of CD30 and often EMA and CD45 Ro; the tumour cells may be negative for LCA

(Fig. 5.47). Epithelioid morphology and expression of epithelial markers such as EMA and rarely cytokeratin can cause confusion with metastatic adenocarcinoma[70].

Low-grade T cell lymphoma rarely involves the serous surfaces but the diagnosis is particularly difficult as the cells are morphologically and immunophenotypically

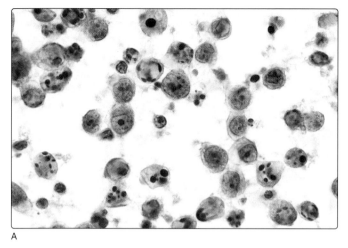 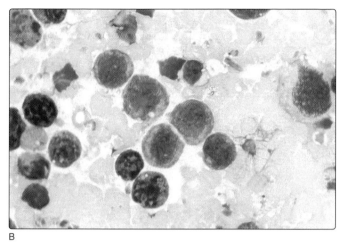

A B

Fig. 5.46   Pleural fluid. Anaplastic large cell lymphoma (Ki 1 lymphoma). The tumour cells are large (compare with **Fig. 5.41** and **5.44**) with prominent nucleoli and there is extensive necrosis. The lymphoid nature of the cells is not easily recognizable, but the diffuse pattern, blue staining cytoplasm (MGG) and peripheral chromatin concentration outlining the nuclear membrane are subtle clues. (A, Papanicolaou × HP; B, MGG × HP)

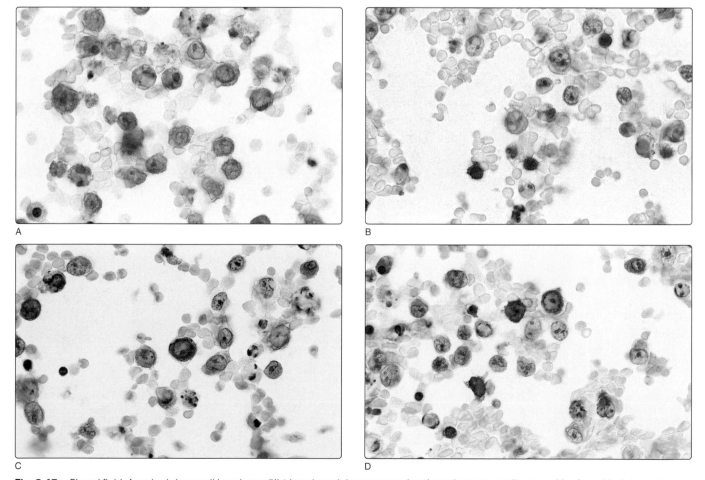

A B

C D

Fig. 5.47   Pleural fluid. Anaplastic large cell lymphoma (Ki 1 lymphoma). Immunocytochemistry: the tumour cells are positive for epithelial membrane antigen (EMA) and negative for leucocyte common antigen (LCA, CD45), causing potential confusion with epithelial malignancy. However, the tumour cells are positive for CD30 (Ber-H2, Ki 1 antigen) and the T-cell marker CD3. This immunophenotype suggests anaplastic large cell lymphoma, although some high-grade T-cell lymphomas may have a similar immunoprofile. (A, EMA; B, LCA; C, CD30; D, CD3, all × HP)

similar to lymphocytes in reactive conditions. Demonstration of aberrant immunophenotype may be of value[71].

Immunocytochemistry is particularly valuable in the diagnosis of lymphocyte rich effusions (Fig. 5.42, 5.45, 5.47)[72-76]. In most reactive conditions, the cells have a T cell phenotype (CD3 and CD45Ro positive). Preponderance of B cells should alert the cytopathologist to the possibility of a B-cell lymphoma. It may be possible to confirm this suspicion by the demonstration of light chain restriction by staining for kappa and lambda light chains. The presence of convincing light chain restriction is evidence of clonal expansion of B cells and is generally regarded to be diagnostic of malignancy (Figs 5.42, 5.45). Gene rearrangement studies are valuable to confirm clonality[77] and the use of flow cytometric evaluation of cell markers may also be helpful[78].

Myeloma

This condition is a rare cause of serous effusion. Involvement is generally seen in the more aggressive (plasmablastic) variants in which the resemblance of the tumour cells to normal plasma cells may be minimal[79,80], although occasionally the cells may be well differentiated, simulating a reactive condition. Generally the diagnosis of myeloma will be known, but initial presentation with serous effusion is occasionally seen. In most cases, numerous neoplastic cells are present. The cells may have very large nuclei and multinucleation is frequent; the nucleus usually retains its eccentric situation in the cell, and the perinuclear Golgi 'hof' may be present in the better-differentiated cells. Peripherally placed clumped chromatin resulting in the typical clock face, or cartwheel appearance, is often less striking than in mature plasma cells, and in many cases a prominent nucleolus is present. The cytoplasm contains large quantities of RNA stainable by pyronin. Immunocytochemical demonstration of light chain restriction is advised to confirm the diagnosis.

Hodgkin's lymphoma

Serous effusions, especially pleural effusions, are not uncommon in Hodgkin's lymphoma[17]. However, the appearances are generally non-specific and the diagnosis is almost always already known; in our experience, definitive diagnosis of Hodgkin's lymphoma involving the serous membranes, which can only be made with certainty if Reed Sternberg (RS) or typical mononuclear Hodgkin's cells can be identified, is an extreme rarity[81]. The RS cell is a large binucleate cell with very prominent eosinophilic nucleoli. These cells have been descriptively termed 'mirror-image', 'owl's eye' and 'butterfly' cells. In histological tissue sections a clear halo is seen around the nuclei; this is a constant artefact of processing and is not seen in cytological material. Mononuclear Hodgkin's cells have a similar nuclear morphology; the advent of immunocytochemistry

has simplified the recognition of this cell type which, like the RS cell, is immunoreactive for CD15 (LeuM1) and CD30 (Ber H2, Ki 1) in most cases[82,83]. The involved serous fluid contains a mixed population of mainly small lymphocytes and plasma cells with an admixture of macrophages and mesothelial cells. Surprisingly, eosinophils are often *not* a major component[17].

Leukaemia

Serous effusions in leukaemic patients are common and many of them are not primarily due to leukaemic infiltration. Because of the immunosuppressive nature of both the disease and its treatment, the patient is prey to a wide range of infective conditions, some of which result in serous effusions. Thus, the presence of a few leukaemic cells in an effusion from a known case of leukaemia (which may of course be contaminants from the blood) should not deter the pathologist from looking further for a cause. Nonetheless, solid leukaemic deposits may occur on or adjacent to serous cavities and may therefore result in effusions (Figs 5.48, 5.49). While it is uncommon for this

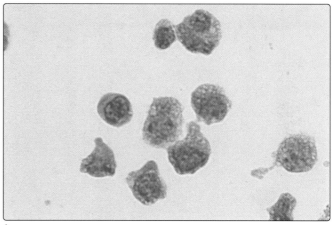

A

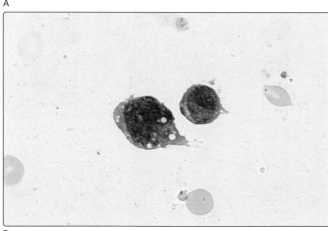

B

Fig. 5.48 Pleural fluid. Acute myeloid leukaemia. Large numbers of myeloid blasts are present. Confirmation can be obtained using chloroacetate esterase staining or immunocytochemistry for myeloperoxidase. (A, Papanicolaou × HP; B, MGG × HP)

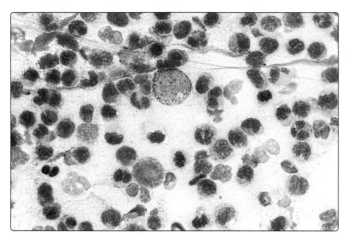

Fig. 5.49 Synovial fluid. Chronic granulocytic leukaemia. Heavily granulated, immature myeloid precursors are present in this knee effusion of a patient with CGL. (MGG × HP)

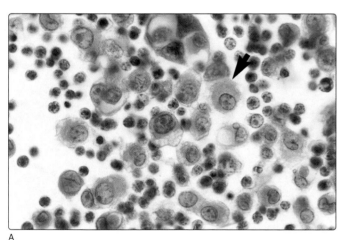

A

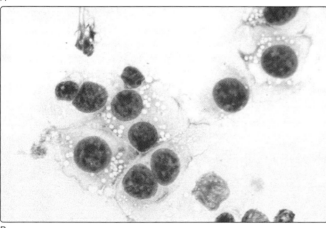

B

Fig. 5.50 Pleural fluid. Melanoma. (A) Malignant melanoma involving the serous cavities results in a diffuse cell population, which is easily missed, as amelanotic melanoma cells may show a striking similarity to mesothelial cells. However, as seen here, melanoma cells have a higher nuclear/cytoplasmic ratio and more prominent nucleoli (centre) than mesothelial cells. A pigmented cell is present (arrowed). (B) Melanoma cells often contain small intracytoplasmic vacuoles similar to those observed in renal cell carcinoma, best shown in MGG stained preparations. (A, Papanicolaou × HP; B, MGG × HP)

to be the presenting condition of leukaemia, monocytic or granulocytic sarcoma (chloroma) may primarily involve lung, abdominal organs or pleura. In involvement of serous membranes by this type of tumour, the serous fluid usually contains large numbers of dispersed neoplastic cells (Fig. 5.48). The cells may form loose aggregates, but the presence of clumps of tightly cohesive cells should prompt reconsideration of this diagnosis. The cells have a variable appearance depending on the type of leukaemia, but most have primitive haematological blast-like morphology, often with some degree of maturation along either monocytic or granulocytic lines (Fig. 5.49). In the former, and in tumours with little maturation, cytoplasmic granulation may be absent and Auer rods cannot usually be seen; stains for myeloid granules, e.g. chloroacetate esterase, may be unhelpful. Immunocytochemical demonstration of lysozyme or CD68 (KP 1) in clearly malignant cells may be diagnostically helpful. However, these markers are also positive in macrophages and care must be taken in interpretation. Hairy cell leukaemia has also been reported in serous cavities[69].

Malignant melanoma

Cytological findings

▶ Melanoma cells tend to lie singly in serous fluids, and can simulate reactive mesothelial cells or mesothelioma. The nucleoli are often prominent and the cytoplasm may be vacuolated, causing confusion with adenocarcinoma

▶ The presence of melanin pigment in tumour cells in serous fluid is one of the most important findings in the diagnosis of melanoma. Other pigments may simulate melanin, thus its nature should be confirmed by cytochemical staining

▶ Amelanotic melanoma has to be distinguished from other malignant tumours, especially mesothelioma and renal cell carcinoma

▶ Immunocytochemistry may be helpful, especially in amelanotic cases, but it must be interpreted with caution; remember that mesothelial cells and adenocarcinoma cells may express S 100 protein

Malignant melanoma involves the serous surfaces by metastatic spread, which may occur many years after the original diagnosis. Indeed, in some cases a pigmented lesion has been removed and thought to be innocuous, only to be shown to be melanoma on later review. In addition, rarely, melanoma may present with a serous effusion from a clinically insignificant or even regressed cutaneous lesion.

The cytological appearances of melanoma in serous fluids are varied (Figs 5.50–5.54)[84]. The cells are almost invariably dispersed due to lack of cohesion, although they may form small loose aggregates. Marked anisocytosis is the norm, with cell sizes in alcohol fixed material largely ranging between 10–20 μm, but with some smaller and some larger cells (Fig. 5.50). Giant melanoma cells up to

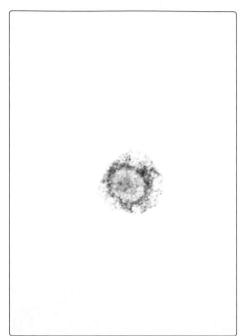

A(i)

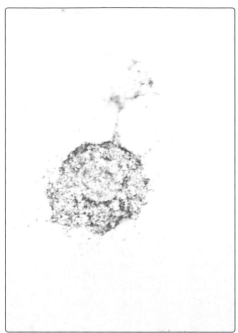

A(ii)

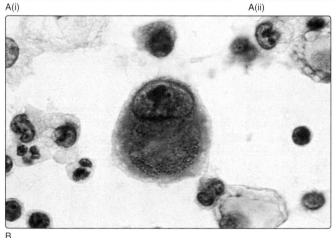

B

Fig. 5.51   Pleural fluid. (A) Melanoma; (B) Mesothelioma. (A) Where cytoplasmic pigment can be identified as melanin, either in melanoma cells or in macrophages (melanophages), a definite diagnosis of melanoma can be made. (B) Not all pigmented tumour cells represent melanoma; the pigment in this mesothelioma cell is pale brown and represents lipofuscin rather than melanin. Lipofuscin can be present in macrophages or benign or malignant mesothelial cells; iron within macrophages can also occasionally cause confusion. Distinction between pigments can be difficult to make reliably without appropriate special stains. (A, Masson-Fontana for melanin × HP; B, Papanicolaou × OI)

300 μm in diameter may be present. In such cases, the cells are easily recognizable as melanoma cells; these large cells usually have abundant cytoplasm containing variable amounts of melanin pigment which is usually finely dispersed or 'dust like'[85]. The pigment is yellowish brown to black in colour in Papanicolaou stained preparations but blue/green in MGG stained smears and can be confirmed as melanin by Masson-Fontana staining (Fig. 5.51); it is prudent also to stain for iron using Perl's Prussian blue reaction and lipofuscin using PAS. In some cases pigmentation may be so heavy as to obscure cytological detail and bleaching may be required to appreciate the morphological features, which incidentally confirms that the pigment is melanin. Note that not all of the pigmented cells will be tumour cells, as macrophages (melanophages) can contain phagocytosed pigment; in the macrophage the pigment is generally clumped and irregular as opposed to the finely dispersed pigment of the melanoma cell, but this

is not invariable. Lipofuscin pigment can occasionally be seen in mesothelioma cells (Fig. 5.51). In up to 60% of cases of melanoma, the cells contain little or no pigment, causing diagnostic confusion, as they frequently resemble reactive mesothelial cells.

The nuclei are large, round to oval, and often eccentrically situated giving a plasmacytoid appearance[86]. Often there is a large well-formed, round or irregular, eosinophilic nucleolus. Intranuclear inclusions, which are in reality cytoplasmic invaginations, are a useful indicator if present. Mitotic figures are often seen and multinucleated cells are not uncommon. Aggregates of cytoplasmic filaments may be present resulting in rhabdoid appearance. Sometimes cytoplasmic vacuolation is a prominent feature, seen in its most extreme form in balloon cell melanoma[84].

In a few cases, the cells will not be of the typical epithelioid cell type described above, but will be spindle cells or small cells with hyperchromatic nuclei. In these cases, and indeed in all amelanotic cases, immunohistochemical confirmation of the diagnosis is helpful (Fig. 5.52). Almost all cases contain large numbers

of cytoplasmic vimentin filaments, and show strong nuclear and often cytoplasmic staining for S 100 protein[87,88]. Most cases also stain with HMB 45, melanoma specific antigen, or Melan A[89–91]. HMB 45, which is more specific but less sensitive than S 100 protein, may occasionally be found in breast carcinoma[92], peripheral nerve sheath tumour, neuroectodermal tumour of infancy[93] and other tumours[94,95]. S 100 protein negative melanoma is an extreme rarity; however, S 100 protein is not infrequently expressed in carcinomas and mesenchymal tumours and can be identified in mesothelial cells[84] and mesothelioma[96]. It is important to note that melanoma cells may occasionally contain cytokeratin[90,97] as well as vimentin.

Ultrastructural analysis can be performed on fresh fluids or on material retrieved from slides or cell blocks and may be useful to demonstrate melanosomes in difficult cases. Finally, in a few difficult cases of melanoma, marked cytoplasmic vacuolation may be present (so-called balloon cell or signet ring cell melanoma) simulating adenocarcinoma; these vacuoles contain glycogen rather than mucin (Fig. 5.53). Very rarely, a mesothelioma may show identical features with both pigmentation and vacuolation (Fig. 5.54), and could show S 100 protein positivity; such cases are a considerable diagnostic challenge.

Sarcoma

Cytological findings

► Sarcomas are only rarely seen in serous fluids, and often present a diagnostic challenge; they are most commonly encountered in children. In practice, the diagnosis is often already known
► The number of malignant cells tends to be low. Their appearance depends on the type of sarcoma, and may be of small round cell, epithelioid cell or spindle cell morphology
► Immunocytochemistry is often required to subtype the tumour cell population

Sarcomas are rare causes of serous effusion[98,99] but may occasionally produce it by direct involvement of the serous cavity (either primary or metastatic) or by obstruction of lymphatic channels. However, it is more common to encounter the morphologically similar sarcomatoid mesothelioma, spindle cell (sarcomatoid, metaplastic) carcinoma and spindle cell melanoma. Nevertheless, almost every known sarcoma type has been described in association with serous effusions and diagnosis may be possible on examination of the fluid. Unfortunately, most sarcomas do not exfoliate readily into serous fluid and the malignant cells are usually scanty; often they do not show specific morphological features of differentiation, and in practice the diagnosis is almost always already known.

The cytological findings are extremely variable[99] but there are four main morphological appearances: pleomorphic large epithelioid cells, pleomorphic spindle cells,

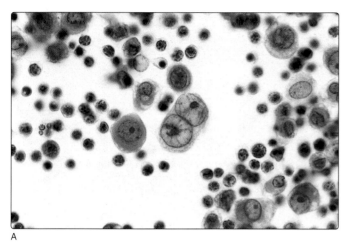
A

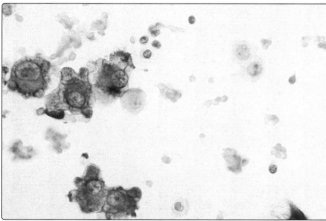
B

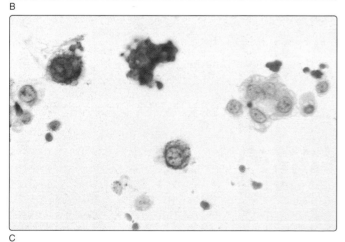
C

Fig. 5.52 Pleural fluid. Melanoma. In cases of amelanotic melanoma, confirmation of the diagnosis can be made by immunocytochemistry. In this case, the differential diagnosis included melanoma, mesothelioma and renal cell carcinoma. Immunocytochemistry showed strong positivity for S 100 protein and also for HMB 45 (melanoma specific antigen). The latter is particularly important as both renal cell carcinoma and mesothelioma may express S 100 protein, albeit usually weakly. (A, Papanicolaou; B, S 100 protein; C, HMB 45 all × HP)

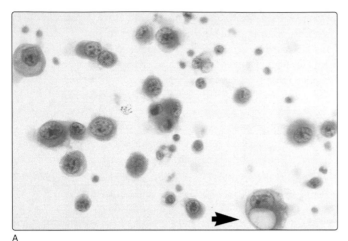

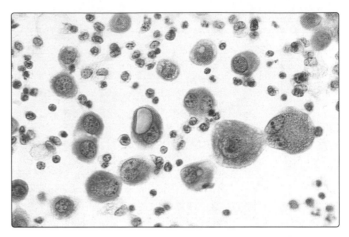

Fig. 5.54   Pleural fluid. Mesothelioma. This case of mesothelioma exemplifies the differential diagnostic problems with melanoma. Tumour cells contain pigment and occasional large sharp edged vacuoles, identical to those seen in melanoma. Pigment stains (see **Fig. 5.51**) and immunocytochemistry (see **Fig. 5.52**) are helpful in such cases. (Papanicolaou × HP)

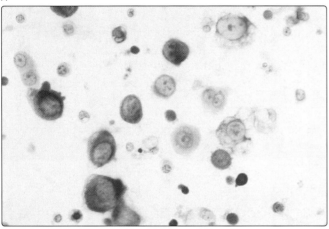

Fig. 5.53   Pleural fluid. Melanoma. Vacuoles are often present in melanoma cells (arrowed), and in extreme cases the so-called balloon cell or signet ring cell melanoma can simulate adenocarcinoma. The vacuoles contain glycogen rather than mucin, so it is important to ensure adequacy of diastase digestion to avoid misinterpretation of PASD stains. Mesothelioma cells also contain large quantities of glycogen, often forming large irregular aggregates. (A, MGG × HP; B, PAS × HP)

monomorphic spindle cells and small blue cells[98]. Each of these categories can be confused with non-sarcomatous tumours, the first two principally with carcinoma, mesothelioma and melanoma, the third with granulation tissue and mesothelioma and the fourth with small cell carcinoma and lymphoma. A full clinical history is essential before making such a diagnosis and immunocytochemistry is particularly helpful in most of these differential diagnoses[29]. The panel should be tailored to address the specific problem (see section on 'Immunocytochemistry'). Mention should be made of the neuroectodermal tumour group[100], including peripheral neuroectodermal tumour, Ewing's sarcoma and the primary small cell tumour of the chest wall in children (Askin's tumour), which may result in a pleural effusion rich in small hyperchromatic cells with little cytoplasm[101]. Malignant fibrous histiocytoma may present with ascites[102] or pleural effusion[103]. Kaposi's sarcoma is a rare cause of

pleural effusions which may be heavily bloodstained and contain occasional monotonous spindle cells; the patient is almost invariably known to have AIDS and there is usually extensive cutaneous involvement. Rhabdomyoblastic differentiation is seen in rhabdomyosarcoma (usually in infants)[104] but similar sarcomatous components may be present in mixed Mullerian tumour of ovary or uterus; these tumours often show extremely bizarre tumour cell morphology. Clear cell sarcoma has also been described in pleural fluid[105].

Although gastrointestinal stromal tumour (GIST) is one of the commonest intra-abdominal spindle cell tumours, exfoliation is unusual and diagnosis by ascitic fluid rarely reported[106]. Immunohistochemistry for c-kit (CD117) is helpful as it is demonstrable in most specimens from GISTs. However, care must be taken as this marker is expressed in other tumour types including synovial sarcoma; cytokeratin positivity helps to support the latter diagnosis.

Germ cell tumours

Germ cell malignancies, including seminoma and its ovarian homologue dysgerminoma[45], yolk sac tumour[107,108], embryonal carcinoma[18], choriocarcinoma[4] and pineal germinoma[109], have been described. The cytological features are similar to the cells in their primary site. The cells of seminoma have a very characteristic appearance[45]; they occur singly and in small clusters, and have large rather bland pale staining nuclei, little vacuolated (glycogen rich) cytoplasm and an associated T lymphocytic population in some cases. The N:C ratio is different from mesothelial cells and immunocytochemistry for cytokeratin is usually negative, whereas that for placental alkaline phosphatase is positive. The cells of embryonal carcinoma are large and pleomorphic with a primitive, vesicular nucleus usually containing one or more prominent nucleoli. Yolk sac tumour may have a range of cytological appearances, from clear cells resembling renal cell carcinoma to regular cells with granular eosinophilic cytoplasm (the hepatoid variant); the typical Schiller-Duval body is not seen in cytological material unless microbiopsies are present[108]. Eosinophilic cytoplasmic inclusions may be present and are a useful diagnostic aid[110]. Often the tumour closely resembles adenocarcinoma and misdiagnosis is possible; the diagnosis should always be considered in very young patients or those with a past history of teratoma, and relevant further study undertaken. Immunocytochemistry for AFP may be positive in the cells and globules but is often very focal and weakly expressed; measurement of AFP in the serous fluid is a more reliable indicator. Choriocarcinoma is only rarely seen in serous fluids[4]. In some cases it is morphologically indistinguishable from adenocarcinoma, but it may be possible to identify both cytotrophoblast and syncytiotrophoblast cells, the latter strongly immunoreactive for βHCG.

Other tumours

Other less common tumours include the small cell tumours of infancy including neuroblastoma[111] and nephroblastoma[112] which are composed of cells with small hyperchromatic nuclei and little cytoplasm; immunocytochemistry may be useful to identify and subclassify this group of tumours[113,114]. Neuroendocrine tumours, e.g. carcinoid tumour[18] and Merkel cell tumour[115], may involve the serous cavities. The former are usually composed of small groups and trabeculae of relatively monomorphic cells with moderate amounts of granular (Grimelius positive) cytoplasm; the latter closely simulate small cell (oat cell) carcinoma in both morphological and immunocytochemical features. Malignant thymoma may present with involvement of either pleural or pericardial cavities[116]. Malignant histiocytosis has been reported in ascitic fluid[117] but this entity has been extensively reclassified and the reported case could represent another lymphoid malignancy. Ascites is not uncommon in hepatocellular carcinoma, but malignant cells can only rarely be demonstrated[51]; occasionally bile can be identified in tumour cells, confirming this diagnosis[118]. Papillary carcinoma of thyroid very rarely involves serous membranes but may be recognizable by the presence of psammoma bodies or the characteristic grooving of the nucleus[31]. Intranuclear cytoplasmic invaginations may also be present but are more common in histologically processed tissue.

Other rare tumours described include Sertoli-Leydig tumour[45], granulosa cell tumour[119], olfactory neuroblastoma[120], choroid plexus carcinoma[121], endometrial stromal sarcoma[122], metastatic meningioma[123] desmoplastic small round cell tumour of the pleura[124] and intra-abdominal desmoplastic small round cell tumour[125].

Finally, most tumours have been encountered at one time or another in serous fluid; those not discussed here are regarded as extreme rarities.

Techniques in diagnosis
Routine techniques

In our practice, routine stains performed on all serous fluids include Papanicolaou, MGG, PAS and PASD. The examination of both Papanicolaou and MGG stains leads to a more accurate identification of most cells in the fluid. Stains for neutral mucin will help to differentiate between adenocarcinoma and reactive mesothelial proliferations, one of the commonest diagnostic dilemmas. However, these stains are not infallible: inadequately digested preparations can lead to false positive diagnosis and therefore it is wise to ensure that the PASD positive material morphologically resembles mucin. Furthermore, some adenocarcinomas do not elaborate mucin. Positive controls should always be performed in parallel on cytological material; neutrophils in the test section are a useful internal positive control. Rare cases of 'mucin-positive' mesothelioma have been reported[37]. On selected cases, staining for acidic mucins with Alcian blue is necessary. In the differentiation between adenocarcinoma and mesothelioma, Alcian blue staining with and without predigestion with hyaluronidase is performed as mesothelioma elaborates hyaluronidase sensitive mucin. Appropriate positive controls must be included to ensure adequate digestion has occurred. Other mucin stains such as high iron diamine and mucicarmine may be of value. Pigment stains should be employed whenever pigment is visible or suspected; Masson-Fontana for melanin, PAS for lipofuscin, Perl's Prussian blue reaction for iron and occasionally, Fouchet's technique for bile are generally used. Other staining techniques should be employed as appropriate.

Ancillary techniques
Immunocytochemistry

The use of immunocytochemistry (ICC) in cytological practice is now widespread and this technique is of great importance in a few otherwise insoluble cases[29,126]. It is of particular value in serous fluid cytodiagnosis (see Figs 5.55–5.60)[127–132]. ICC can be performed on cell suspensions using a flow cytometer[133–138] but in most laboratories direct preparations, cell block sections (Fig. 5.55) or cytospin preparations (Fig. 5.56) are used; we find that cell block sections and cytospins give particularly good results. In most cases, unlike fine needle aspirates, quite large numbers of tumour cells are present and special techniques to optimize the amount of diagnostic material are not usually necessary. Fixation can be tailored to optimum preservation of specific antigens but for routine use, the balance between antigenicity and morphology is best preserved by using alcohol fixation. As always in ICC, a

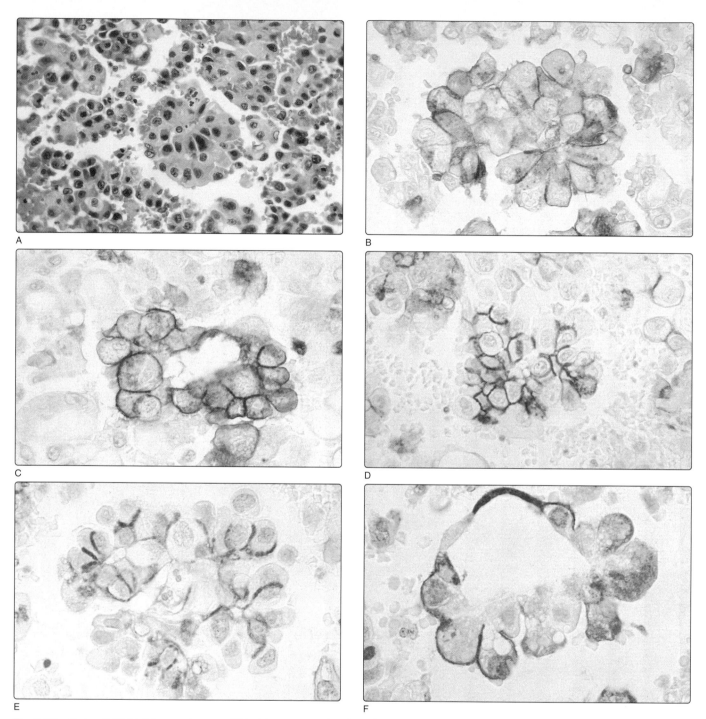

Fig. 5.55 Pericardial fluid. Adenocarcinoma, cell block immunocytochemistry. Cell blocks are particularly valuable for immunocytochemistry as they allow numerous serial sections to be prepared. In addition, exact cellular localization of staining is far easier than in the three-dimensional direct or cytospin preparations. This adenocarcinoma shows a typical immunophenotype; note that Ber-EP4 and AUA 1 stain only where the cells touch, being located on basolateral cell membranes in normal epithelia. HMFG2, CEA and LeuM1 show strong generalized membrane staining and weaker cytoplasmic staining. (A, H&E × HP; B, CEA; C, LeuM1; D, Ber-EP4; E, AUA 1; F, HMFG2; B–F × OI)

panel of markers is required to ensure correct diagnosis. Introduction of heat induced epitope retrieval (HIER, also known as heat-mediated antigen retrieval or HMAR) has enabled a much expanded range of diagnostic antibodies but these techniques must be carefully controlled and

evaluated as increased sensitivity can lead to apparently aberrant results[139].

ICC is principally of value in a few well-defined settings, which will be discussed. The differential diagnoses where ICC is helpful are:

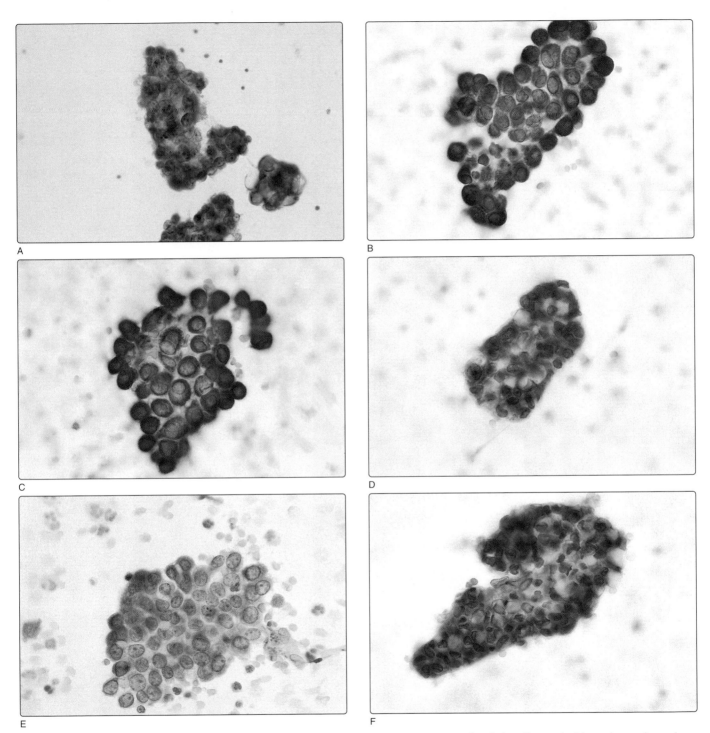

Fig. 5.56 Ascitic fluid. Adenocarcinoma, cytospin preparation immunocytochemistry. Immunocytochemical profile seen in this ovarian carcinoma is similar to that shown in **Fig. 5.55**. Precise localization of staining is more difficult than in cell block sections. (A, Papanicolaou; B, CEA; C, LeuM1; D, Ber-EP4; E, AUA 1; F, HMFG2, all × HP)

1 Adenocarcinoma *vs* reactive mesothelial proliferation
2 Mesothelioma *vs* reactive mesothelial proliferation
3 Adenocarcinoma *vs* mesothelioma
4 Lymphocyte predominant effusion (reactive) *vs* lymphoma
5 Poorly differentiated large cell malignancy: carcinoma *vs* melanoma *vs* lymphoma
6 Small cell malignancy: oat cell *vs* lymphoma *vs* neuroepithelioma *vs* neuroblastoma/nephroblastoma
7 Rarely, spindle cell tumour: carcinoma *vs* sarcoma *vs* sarcomatoid mesothelioma.

ICC may also be helpful to:

1 Increase reliability of prediction of primary site in metastatic carcinoma
2 Supply additional prognostic information

Adenocarcinoma *vs* reactive mesothelial proliferation

Up until the late twentieth century, immunohistochemical distinction between mesothelial cells, mesothelioma cells and metastatic carcinoma cells rested on certain markers in epithelial cells and their absence in mesothelial cells. In the last few years, several antibodies immunoreactive with

benign and malignant mesothelial cells but rarely carcinoma cells have been described. 'Positive' mesothelial markers include calretinin[140–147], thrombomodulin[148], cytokeratin 5/6[148,149], and HMBE-1[150,151], allowing supplementation of the previously available 'carcinoma-specific' panel with 'mesothelial-specific' antibodies[152–154].

In this case, the suggested panel includes: CEA, CD15 (LeuM1), Ber-EP4 (or AUA-1), HMFG2 (or EMA), Cam 5.2, MOC-31, calretinin and cytokeratin 5/6 (Figs 5.55, 5.56, 5.59). B72–3, thrombomodulin, TTF-1, and BG8 may also be of value depending on the clinical setting.

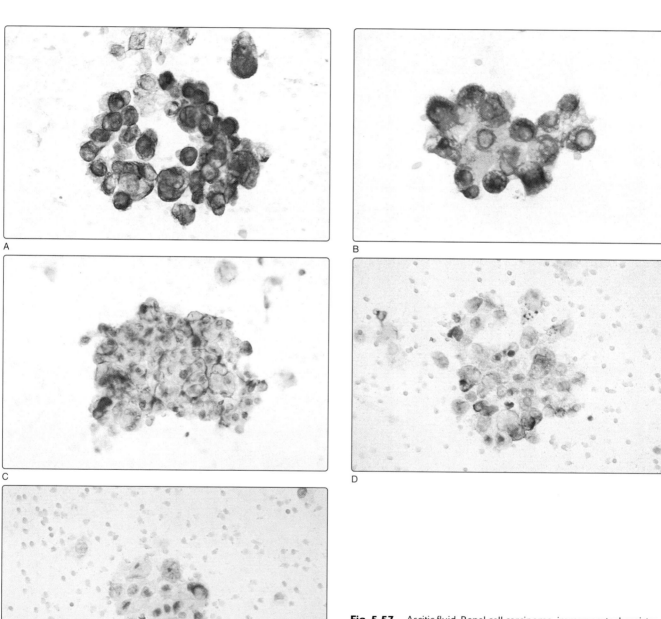

Fig. 5.57   Ascitic fluid. Renal cell carcinoma, immunocytochemistry. Immunocytochemistry shows coexpression of cytokeratin and vimentin, a typical feature of this tumour. There is staining for AUA 1 but that for LeuM1 is weak and for CEA is negative, emphasizing the value of a panel of markers. The frequent occurrence of S 100 protein in this tumour is a potential cause of confusion. (A, cytokeratin; B, vimentin; C, AUA 1; D, LeuM1; E, CEA, all × HP)

Calretinin is a 28 kDa intracellular calcium binding protein originally isolated from chick retinal cells and present in many human neuronal cells. It can also be identified in steroid producing cells of ovary and testis, eccrine glands, renal tubular cells, thymic epithelial cells and mesothelial cells[140] It has been identified in 42–100% of epithelial mesotheliomas (usually strong cytoplasmic and nuclear positivity) and 4–23% of adenocarcinomas (usually weak focal staining). Some of this variation is probably related to the use of different commercially available antibodies. In one study, the Zymed antibody gave a higher rate of positivity with mesothelioma (100% vs Chemicon 74%); fewer than 10% of adenocarcinomas gave focal weak staining with this antibody[142].

Cytokeratin 5/6 (using commercially available monoclonal antibodies D5/16B4) is a marker with high sensitivity for mesothelioma (approaching 100%) and is usually negative or very weakly expressed in pulmonary adenocarcinoma. Positivity is also seen in squamous carcinomas and (focally or weakly) in up to 20% of non-pulmonary adenocarcinomas[143].

Thrombomodulin is a cell surface glycoprotein involved in the regulation of intravascular coagulation and normally expressed on a range of cell types including endothelial, squamous, transitional and mesothelial cells[155,156]. It has been identified in 49–100% of mesotheliomas and 6–42% of pulmonary adenocarcinomas. As the same commercial source was used in these studies, it seems likely that methodological and interpretative factors are responsible for these differences[157]. It is also frequently seen in transitional cell carcinoma and squamous cell carcinoma[155].

HBME-1 is a commercially available monoclonal antibody, which characteristically reacts with mesothelial cells and epithelial mesothelioma, producing a thick membranous staining pattern in contrast to pulmonary adenocarcinoma, which usually manifests diffuse cytoplasmic staining. Several groups have noted a considerable overlap in staining patterns rendering this antibody less useful in routine diagnostic practice[150,151], but some claim excellent results with this antibody[158].

Carcinoembryonic antigen (CEA) is an oncofetal protein, which is particularly valuable, as it is not expressed by reactive mesothelial cells. Originally described in colonic cancer, this antigen is widespread in malignant cells and by no means specific. Although the majority of gastrointestinal adenocarcinomas are positive, this is not the case for some other tumours; in particular, breast carcinomas are often negative[159]. There are occasional reports of CEA positive mesothelial cells[160] and a few CEA positive mesotheliomas have been reported, possibly due to hyaluronic acid staining[161]. False positives may also occur due to the presence of non-specific cross reacting antigen in inflammatory cells[162]. The cells of renal cell carcinoma which are cytologically bland and may show a striking similarity to mesothelial cells are often CEA negative and may be S 100 protein positive, causing confusion with melanoma (Fig. 5.52). Studies using monoclonal rather than polyclonal CEA antibodies have shown CEA positivity in 85–95% of pulmonary adenocarcinomas but not in mesotheliomas[139]. It should be noted that serous carcinoma tends not to express CEA (0–35% cases positive). CEA is unhelpful in distinguishing between serous carcinoma of ovary/peritoneum and papillary mesothelioma[143].

LeuM1 is a differentiation marker present on myelomonocytic cells and most Reed Sternberg cells, and which is also expressed in some adenocarcinomas[47]. It is not present in mesothelial cells but excess hyaluronic acid may result in a false positive result in mesothelioma[161]. This monoclonal antibody reacts with the Lewis[x] antigen designated CD15. In an up-to-date study, Riera reported LeuM1 positivity in 75% of adenocarcinomas of various origins including pulmonary (84% CEA positive). Only two of 57 (3%) of epithelial mesotheliomas showed focal staining. Although LeuM1 is highly specific for distinguishing mesothelioma from adenocarcinoma, it is slightly less sensitive than other markers such as CEA, BG8 and MOC-31[139], and the staining pattern is often focal.

Ber-EP4 is a monoclonal antibody reactive with a 39 kDa basolateral (non-luminal) membrane glycoprotein[163]; while expressed in many adenocarcinomas[146,164,165], focal staining can also be seen in mesotheliomas[166]. While many authors conclude that this marker is useful there remains some controversy concerning the number of positive mesothelioma cases which ranges from 0–87.5%. It seems likely that differences in interpretation are responsible. Using the criterion of a basolateral membrane reaction, Riera reported no staining in 57 mesotheliomas and positivity in 64% of adenocarcinomas of various types[139]. However, Ordoñez has noted staining confined to a few cells only in 18/70 (26%) mesotheliomas whereas 101/110 (92%) of adenocarcinomas were judged to be positive. In this study, all pulmonary adenocarcinomas showed widespread Ber-EP4 positivity but non-pulmonary adenocarcinomas showed a more variable pattern from strong diffuse to focal or (in a few cases) negative. Ordoñez concludes that Ber-EP4 may be valuable to differentiate pulmonary adenocarcinoma from epithelial mesothelioma but it is of less value in distinguishing between non-pulmonary adenocarcinoma and mesothelioma[167].

AUA-1 is a monoclonal antibody directed against a 35 kDa antigen on the basolateral cell membrane; it is reactive with many carcinomas but not mesothelial cells[168,169]. It has a similar reactivity pattern and diagnostic sensitivity profile as Ber-EP4.

HMFG2 (human milk fat globule glycoprotein type 2), a member of the epithelial membrane antigen (EMA) group, is found in many epithelia[42], and is strongly expressed by many carcinomas[42,170]; 54%[171] to 100%[172] of adenocarcinomas have been shown to be positive. The staining pattern is characteristic in adenocarcinoma; there is extensive strong cytoplasmic staining focally with peripheral accentuation due to membrane staining. Distinction between cytoplasmic and membrane staining is less easily appreciated in cytological preparations than in cell blocks; this is due to the three-dimensional nature of the cell membrane in the former. Mesothelial cells show relatively weak cytoplasmic EMA staining, most marked at the periphery of the cell[172]. In mesothelioma, in some cells there is strong peripheral and weak cytoplasmic staining.

Cytokeratin staining patterns can also be helpful; small cell carcinomas characteristically have a perinuclear dot of cytokeratin positivity (Fig. 5.58), in contrast to mesothelial cells which usually have a dense perinuclear ring of cytokeratin filaments (Fig. 5.59); adenocarcinoma cells tend to have less well organized filaments in their cytoplasm[173,174]. Cytokeratin profiles may also be useful in diagnosis, particularly in identification of the unknown primary (see below).

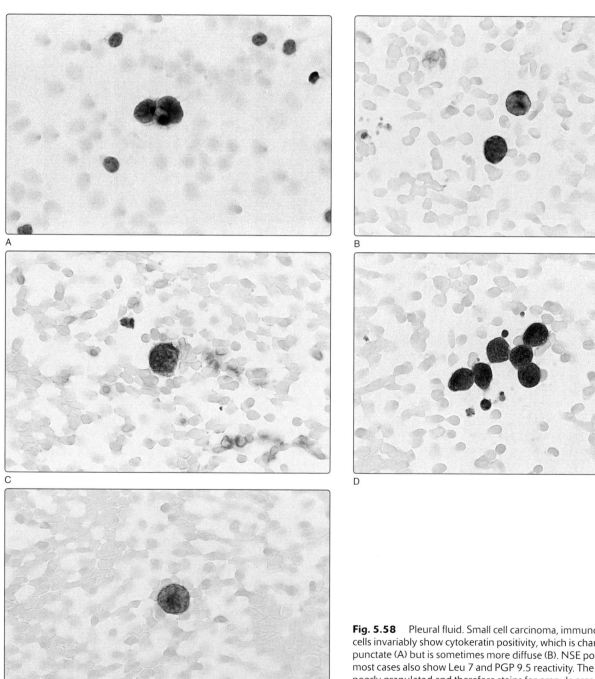

Fig. 5.58 Pleural fluid. Small cell carcinoma, immunocytochemistry. The cells invariably show cytokeratin positivity, which is characteristically punctate (A) but is sometimes more diffuse (B). NSE positivity is the rule; most cases also show Leu 7 and PGP 9.5 reactivity. The cells are usually poorly granulated and therefore stains for granule associated proteins (e.g. chromogranin) are often weak or negative. (A, B, low molecular weight cytokeratin (CAM 5.2); C, NSE; D, PGP 9.5; E, Leu 7, all × HP)

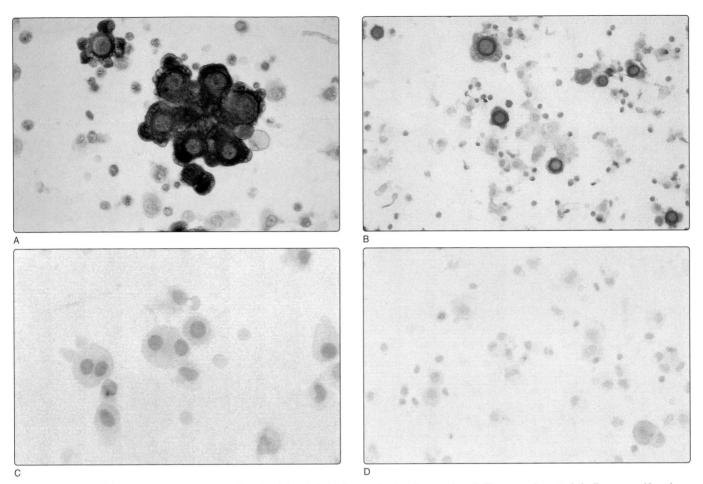

Fig. 5.59 Pleural fluid. Reactive mesothelial proliferation. Mesothelial cells contain abundant cytokeratin filaments, characteristically arranged in a dense perinuclear ring. This contrasts with the strong diffuse cytoplasmic staining seen in carcinoma (see **Fig. 5.57**). No immunostaining is seen for CEA. Use of cytokeratin 5/6 and calretinin usually enables reliable distinction between strongly stained mesothelial cells and (negative) adenocarcinoma cells, but squamous and transitional cell carcinomas may also express these markers. Reactive mesothelial cells may show a weak diffuse cytoplasmic staining for HMFG2 or EMA, but this should be contrasted with the strong membrane and cytoplasmic staining seen in most adenocarcinomas (see **Fig. 5.55**) and the peripheral cytoplasmic staining sometimes seen in mesothelioma (see **Fig. 5.60**). (A, calretinin; B, low molecular weight cytokeratin (CAM 5.2); C, CEA; D, HMFG2, all × HP)

B72.3, which recognizes the tumour associated antigen TAG-72, has been identified in up to 95% of adenocarcinomas in paraffin embedded material[175,176]. Initially it was stated to be absent in reactive mesothelial cells and in a range of benign serous fluids, but further study has shown that this marker is less specific than first thought; it has been seen in reactive mesothelial cells[177] and in occasional mesotheliomas[178], limiting its value. Whereas in some studies, all mesotheliomas were negative for B72.3, others have shown focal positivity in 2–48% of cases. In most authors' experience, 2–5% of epithelial mesotheliomas and about 80% of pulmonary adenocarcinomas show B72.3 positivity[157]. In contrast to CEA, B72.3 is usually positive in serous carcinoma (87% of cases in a recent series) and may be helpful to distinguish these from peritoneal mesotheliomas[143].

BG8 is a monoclonal antibody that reacts with the Lewis[y] antigen first noted in 1989 to be of use in distinguishing between pulmonary adenocarcinoma (18/18 strong

positive) and epithelial mesothelioma (7/30 (23%) weak positive)[179]. This finding was confirmed in a study showing 14/123 (92.7%) pulmonary adenocarcinomas positive and 5/57 (8.8%) of mesotheliomas showing weak reactivity[139]. The authors concluded that BG8 is one of the best markers available in this context and this is supported by a recent review[180].

MOC-31 is a recently recognized monoclonal antibody, which is reactive with a 38 kDa epithelial surface glycoprotein. Strong MOC-31 reactivity has been reported in 89% of adenocarcinomas in contrast to weak focal staining in 5% of epithelial mesotheliomas. In one study, 40/40 pulmonary adenocarcinomas and 20/21 non-mucinous ovarian carcinomas showed MOC-31 reactivity[181]. The sensitivity of MOC-31 has been supported[151] and this appears to be one of the most promising new antibodies but experience is still somewhat limited.

TTF-1 is a homeodomain containing transcription protein expressed in thyroid and lung epithelial cells (type II pneumocytes and Clara cells). It appears to be expressed only in pulmonary adenocarcinomas and some thyroid carcinomas but not in adenocarcinomas of breast, colon, prostate or kidney. As well as distinguishing between pulmonary and non-pulmonary (excluding thyroid) adenocarcinomas, TTF-1 appears to be valuable in differentiating between pulmonary adenocarcinoma and epithelial mesothelioma, being expressed in 18/21 (86%) of pulmonary adenocarcinomas and 0/37 mesotheliomas in one study[182]. This has recently been supported by further studies[180,183,184].

The cytological and immunocytochemical features of mesothelioma are covered in Chapter 6. In distinction between mesothelioma and adenocarcinoma, the suggested panel includes: CEA, HMFG2 (or EMA), CD15 (LeuM1), Ber-EP4 (or AUA-1), Cam 5.2, MOC-31, TTF-1, calretinin and cytokeratin 5/6 (Figs 5.55, 5.56, 5.60). In our experience, no single marker will invariably allow differentiation between mesothelioma and adenocarcinoma. While CEA is a useful marker favouring carcinoma[185], occasional CEA positive mesotheliomas have been reported, and false positives occur due to non-specific cross reacting antigen and hyaluronic acid staining; some carcinomas are CEA negative (see above). Strong extensive positive CD15 (LeuM1), MOC-31, Ber-EP4 or AUA-1 staining virtually excludes mesothelioma. However, there have been reports of weak focal staining of each of these markers in mesothelioma as discussed above[164,178], and results must be interpreted with caution.

As mentioned above, TTF-1, calretinin, HBME-1, thrombomodulin, and CK5/6 have all been suggested as powerful discriminants for this differential; in our hands, CK5/6 and calretinin have proved the most useful positive markers for mesothelial differentiation.

Other markers recently suggested to be useful in the differential diagnosis of carcinoma and mesothelioma include N-cadherin[144], E-cadherin[147,180], WT1 gene product[151,180], Mesothelin (KI)[186], telomerase[187], p53[188–190], Ca125[191], hyaluronate binding probe[192], CD44[148,192], NCAM[193], LeuM5 (CD11a)[194], secretory component[195], and surfactant proteins[183,184]. The value of these markers has yet to be fully evaluated in routine diagnostic practice. A full analysis of mesothelioma immunohistochemistry is covered in Chapter 6 and in recent reviews[155,157,196–198].

Mesothelioma *vs* mesothelial proliferation

This distinction may be particularly difficult in cases of well-differentiated epithelial mesothelioma. In our experience, HMFG2 reactivity is of use in differentiating mesothelioma from mesothelial hyperplasia (Fig. 5.59). Mesothelioma shows focal strong membrane staining whereas mesothelial hyperplasia shows weak or negative cytoplasmic staining. In contrast, adenocarcinoma usually shows extensive strong cytoplasmic and membrane staining[199]. p53 expression and proliferation markers such

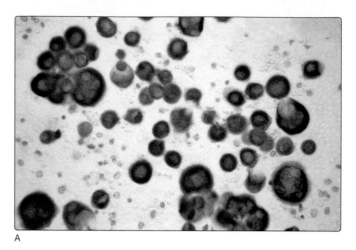

A

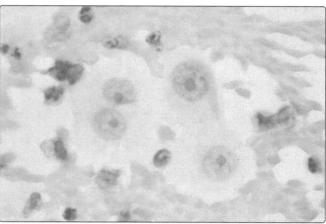

B

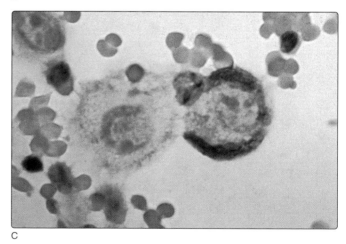

C

Fig. 5.60 Pleural fluid. Mesothelioma. The use of 'mesothelial-specific' antibodies has simplified distinction from adenocarcinoma. Mesothelioma is usually strongly immunoreactive for calretinin and cytokeratin 5/6. In contrast to many adenocarcinomas, mesothelioma cells are negative on immunostaining for CEA (note the non-specific cross reacting staining in neutrophils which acts as a useful internal control). Mesothelioma is also almost invariably negative for Ber H2, AUA 1, Leu MI and secretory component. Compared with reactive mesothelial cells, which are also negative for all the above mentioned markers, mesothelioma cells often show stronger staining for HMFG2, seen as a thick peripheral band without accentuation of the cytoplasmic membrane; adenocarcinoma typically shows mainly membrane and some diffuse cytoplasmic staining (see **Figs 5.55, 5.56**). (A, CK 5/6; B, CEA; C, HMFG2, all × HP)

as Ki67 have also been suggested in this context[188–190,200] but do not appear to be helpful in individual cases[198].

Lymphocyte predominant effusion (reactive) vs lymphoma

In this case, the suggested panel includes: two B-cell markers (CD20, and CD79a), two T-cell markers (CD3 and CD45Ro) and kappa and lambda immunoglobulin light chains (see Figs 5.42, 5.45–5.47). The cells of lymphocyte-rich reactive effusions are T cells, therefore the demonstration of a large population of B cells is almost diagnostic of a B-cell lymphoma; this can be confirmed by the demonstration of immunoglobulin light chain restriction. Distinction between lymphocyte-rich *reactive* effusion and T-cell lymphoma can be difficult and is dependent on morphology. Fortunately, most T-cell lymphomas involving serous cavities are pleomorphic high-grade tumours. Nevertheless, involvement by low-grade peripheral T-cell lymphoma may occur and this may be almost indistinguishable from a lymphocyte-rich reactive effusion. The cells may show nuclear atypia, and loss of T-cell epitopes may be useful in this setting; this is most easily demonstrated by flow cytometry. Molecular techniques may also be helpful.

Serous effusions, particularly pleural effusions, are not uncommon in Hodgkin's disease[4]. However, the diagnosis is usually known and the fluid is generally not examined; when it is, it is often non-diagnostic[81]. The effusion usually contains large numbers of T lymphocytes, with only occasional larger neoplastic cells. Classical Reed Sternberg cells are not easily found; the use of antibodies to CD15 (LeuM1) and CD30 (Ber H2) will identify mononuclear Hodgkin's cells as well as classical Reed Sternberg cells which may be present in very small numbers. It is important to remember that CD15 (LeuM1) is also positive in some adenocarcinomas[47], which may cause confusion, particularly as adenocarcinoma also may be associated with a T lymphocyte rich effusion.

Poorly differentiated large cell malignancy: carcinoma vs melanoma vs lymphoma

The suggested panel of markers in this setting includes cytokeratin (low molecular weight and broad spectrum), vimentin, EMA, LCA, S 100 protein, HMB 45, T and B-cell markers and Ber H2 (CD30). Carcinomas, even poorly differentiated tumours, usually express cytokeratins. However, many other tumours also show this feature, including mesothelioma, synovial sarcoma, epithelioid sarcoma, plasmacytoma, anaplastic large cell lymphoma, leiomyosarcoma, epithelioid angiosarcoma and occasionally rhabdomyosarcoma, chondrosarcoma and melanoma[29,126]. In carcinoma, strong expression of EMA is often seen, especially in tumours of the breast, lung and gastrointestinal tract. A few carcinomas (notably renal cell carcinoma) express S 100 protein, but melanoma is almost invariably S 100 protein positive, even when

amelanotic. Mesothelial cells can also show cytoplasmic S 100 protein staining. Although most melanomas contain vimentin filaments, as mentioned above, a few confusingly contain cytokeratin[90]. Melanoma specific markers, e.g. HMB 45 are also present in most cases[89], but we have occasionally seen HMB 45 positivity in mesothelial cells, and is reported in a number of tumours other than melanoma[92–95]. The majority of lymphomas will express the common leucocyte antigen LCA (CD45), and usually either a B or T-cell marker such as CD20 and CD3 respectively. An occasional example is LCA negative; this usually occurs in the large cell anaplastic variant, which is EMA positive (see Fig. 5.42).

Small cell malignancy: oat cell vs squamous carcinoma vs lymphoma vs neuroblastoma/nephroblastoma vs sarcoma

The panel of markers suggested in this case includes cytokeratin, desmin, LCA, CD20, CD3, CD45Ro, NSE, chromogranin, neurofilament, S 100 protein and Mic-2 (CD99) (see Fig. 5.58). Clearly, the clinical setting is of particular importance here; neuroblastoma is not likely in an 80-year-old person and similarly small cell carcinoma is unlikely in a 3-year-old child. Small cell (oat cell) carcinoma shows cytokeratin positivity, sometimes with punctate paranuclear accentuation as seen in other neuroendocrine neoplasms, exemplified by Merkel cell tumour[115]. In addition, there is usually positivity for neurone specific enolase (NSE)[56], and variable focal staining for chromogranin[59]. Lymphomas are generally positive for LCA (see section on 'Lymphocyte rich effusions'); false positives for this marker are extremely rare[201,202]. Neuroblastomas generally contain neurofilaments; they may also stain for NSE, PGP 9.5 and chromogranin but these may be absent in poorly differentiated examples. Nephroblastoma (Wilms' tumour) can show a bewildering immunocytochemical profile corresponding to the various primitive components present (blastema, mesenchyme including neural and rhabdomyoblastic tissues, and epithelial). Cytokeratin and EMA are found in the epithelial component but blastoma cells contain vimentin only; variable staining is seen for desmin, GFAP and S 100 protein depending on the degree of neural or muscle differentiation. Sarcomas, particularly embryonal rhabdomyosarcoma (desmin, vimentin and myoglobin positive) and Ewing's sarcoma (vimentin and glycogen positive) cannot always be clearly diagnosed on morphological grounds. More recently described markers for Ewing's sarcoma include MIC2 gene product[114,203]. Rarely, melanoma (S 100 protein positive) or a pyknotic or basaloid poorly differentiated squamous cell carcinoma may manifest as a small cell tumour. The latter is distinguished from small cell carcinoma by a more diffuse cytoplasmic cytokeratin staining pattern and negativity for neuroendocrine markers.

Spindle cell tumours: sarcoma *vs* carcinoma *vs* sarcomatoid mesothelioma

Most spindle cell tumours exfoliate much less readily than their epithelioid counterparts or epithelial tumours, and the cells are generally scanty. The suggested panel includes cytokeratin, vimentin, desmin, HMFG2, S 100 protein and smooth muscle actin. Myogenin and Myo D-1 are added if appropriate. Cytokeratin and HMFG2 are present in most carcinomas, although often expressed more weakly in spindle cells than in epithelioid cells. Sarcomatoid mesothelioma invariably coexpresses cytokeratin and vimentin but is generally negative for HMFG2 (except when coexisting with epithelioid mesothelioma in dimorphic pattern). Coexpression of vimentin is common in carcinomas, and occasionally S 100 protein may be present (especially renal cell carcinoma). Sarcomas generally express vimentin and some notable subtypes, synovial sarcoma and the rare epithelioid sarcoma, also express cytokeratin and HMFG2, mimicking carcinoma[204]. Desmin with myogenin indicates rhabdomyoblastic (skeletal muscle) differentiation, whereas desmin with smooth muscle actin positivity generally indicates smooth muscle differentiation (usually leiomyosarcoma, which may also be positive for HMFG2). Malignant nerve sheath tumours may be difficult to diagnose as they express S 100 protein in only 50% of cases. Angiosarcoma expresses endothelial antigens such as factor VIII related antigen, CD31 and CD34, and generally stains with *Ulex europaeus* lectin, but may contain cytokeratin in the epithelioid variant[205]. Spindle cell melanoma is not uncommon but exfoliated cells in serous fluid seldom retain this configuration. However, strong positivity for S 100 protein and vimentin raises the possibility of this diagnosis; here, HMB 45 can be useful but we have seen weak staining in reactive mesothelial cells. Although cytokeratin is usually absent, we and others[90,97] have occasionally seen positive cases. C kit (CD117) is a useful marker for GIST[106], but has reported in other spindle cell tumours including synovial sarcoma.

Increasing reliability of prediction of primary site in metastatic carcinoma

Prediction of site of origin on morphological features alone is in part dependent on the experience of the cytopathologist. However, when clinical information is supplied a much higher rate of prediction can be achieved[17]. In order to refine diagnosis in cases where the primary site is not apparent clinically, some authors have advocated a combined morphological and immunocytochemical approach[51,174,206-208]. Several immunocytochemical approaches can be used including cytokeratin profiles (either individual cytokeratins or cytokeratin clusters)[209,210], intermediate filament coexpression, e.g. vimentin and cytokeratin, detection of antigens such as CEA, CA125[191] which are expressed in a range of tumours, detection of hormone receptors e.g. ER and PR, and finally detection of 'organ specific' markers which point to a unique primary site (see Table 5.3)[206].

Particular problems faced frequently by the cytologist include:

1　Pleural effusion: pulmonary or non-pulmonary adenocarcinoma. Expression of surfactant proteins A and B and thyroid transcription factor 1 (TTF-1) are common in lung cancers, but rare in others (with the obvious exception of thyroid in the case of TTF-1). These markers have been usefully employed to discriminate pulmonary carcinoma from an extrapulmonary primary.

2　Ascitic fluid: ovarian *vs* gastrointestinal *vs* other adenocarcinoma. Differential expression of cytokeratins 7 and 20, CEA and CA125 have been used as a panel to distinguish between these conditions. Colorectal cancer is usually cytokeratin 20 positive but cytokeratin 7 negative in

Table 5.3　Site specific markers

Antibody	Site	Cross reactivity
Prostate specific antigen (PSA)	Prostate	
Prostatic acid phosphatase (PAP)	Prostate	Neuroendocrine carcinomas
Thyroid transcription factor 1 (TTF-1)	Thyroid Lung	Rare
Thyroglobulin	Thyroid	
Uroplakin	Transitional epithelium	
Gross cystic disease fluid 15	Breast	Salivary and sweat gland carcinomas
Surfactant proteins A, B, C	Lung	

Table 5.4　Expression of cytokeratin 7 and cytokeratin 20 in various tumour types* (Modified from Gown[51])

	Cytokeratin 7 positive	Cytokeratin 7 negative
Cytokeratin 20 positive	Transitional cell carcinoma Pancreatic carcinoma Mucinous ovarian carcinoma	Colorectal adenocarcinoma
Cytokeratin 20 negative	Breast adenocarcinoma Pulmonary adenocarcinoma Serous ovarian carcinoma Endometrioid ovarian carcinoma Endometrial adenocarcinoma Thymoma Mesothelioma	Hepatocellular carcinoma Renal cell carcinoma Prostatic adenocarcinoma Squamous cell carcinoma Neuroendocrine carcinoma Gastric adenocarcinoma (less reliable)

*A minority of tumours may express alternative cytokeratin 7/cytokeratin 20 phenotypes

contrast to mucinous carcinoma (cytokeratin 20 positive, cytokeratin 7 positive) and serous and endometrioid ovarian adenocarcinoma (cytokeratin 20 negative, cytokeratin 7 positive). Gastric, renal, prostatic and hepatocellular carcinoma are usually cytokeratin 20 negative, cytokeratin 7 negative[51,206]. Addition of cytokeratin 5/6 can give further information, but this marker is expressed by some breast and transitional cell tumours as well as mesothelioma and squamous cell carcinoma. CA125 is expressed in most serous and endometrioid ovarian tumours, but is not usually expressed by mucinous ovarian tumours or colorectal, prostatic or renal carcinomas. Endometrial carcinomas and carcinomas of the pancreas and biliary tree are often also positive. CEA is often expressed by colorectal cancer, but is common in other carcinomas (e.g. lung). Conversely, a minority of colorectal carcinomas do not express CEA.

Supportive evidence of metastatic breast carcinoma can be obtained by nuclear staining for oestrogen receptor (ER) or progesterone receptor (PR). Not all cases will be positive and some other tumours may express ER/PR but staining is usually weak. A strongly positive result favours breast carcinoma over other primary sites. Those carcinomas that may express ER/PR include neuroendocrine tumours, and carcinomas of thyroid, sweat gland, ovary, endometrium and uterine cervix. Some tumours are almost invariably negative for ER/PR including pulmonary, colorectal and hepatocellular carcinomas.

Other 'site-specific' markers, such as prostate specific antigen, prostatic acid phosphatase, placental alkaline phosphatase, thyroglobulin, calcitonin, alpha-fetoprotein, beta human chorionic gonadotrophin, gross cystic disease fluid protein (as well as the previously mentioned surfactant proteins, WT-1 and TTF-1) may be useful in specific instances to confirm a morphological diagnosis.

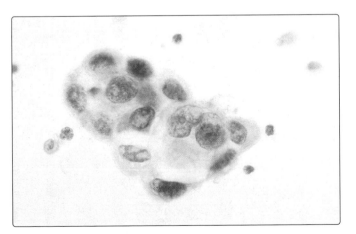

Fig. 5.61 Ascitic fluid. Adenocarcinoma. Immunocytochemistry for tumour associated gene products (in this case p53 protein) may be of value but is not discriminant between adenocarcinoma and mesothelioma. In addition, expression can be seen in some reactive mesothelial cells. (p53 × HP)

However, care should be taken not to over interpret such results as aberrant expression may be seen in some cases.

Despite successes in individual cases, discriminant analysis has shown that cytokeratin 7/cytokeratin 20 immunostaining has a predictive error rate of about 40%. While useful to guide the clinician as a 'first guess', clinical features if available, may be more reliable for deducing the origin of adenocarcinoma cells in effusions[210].

Molecular techniques may also be of value in determining primary site, particularly the use of cytogenetic analysis by FISH[211] (see 'Molecular techniques').

Prognostic markers applied to cytological material

Once a diagnosis has been reached there is increasing evidence that expression of certain markers is associated with superior response to therapy or may indicate a better or worse overall prognosis. This group includes ER, PR, c-erbB-2, p53 and Ki67[212,213]. (Fig. 5.61).

Diagnostic pitfalls in the evaluation of immunocytochemistry

Pitfalls in diagnosis using ICC can only be mentioned briefly here, but are extensively covered elsewhere[29]. A full knowledge of the many problems, which must be taken into account when analysing immunocytochemical preparations, is essential to avoid potentially serious errors. It is crucially important, when interpreting, that background or non-specific staining is not regarded as a positive result (negative controls should always be run) and that positively stained cells can be definitely identified as the 'target' (tumour cell) population and not benign bystanders (polymorphs, macrophages, etc.). This of particular importance in the interpretation of CEA and CD15 (LeuM1) stains. There are several well described confusing staining reactions; they include EMA and cytokeratin positivity in some cases of lymphoma, especially large cell anaplastic lymphoma which may be LCA (CD45) negative (see Fig. 5.47), myeloma, in normal plasma cells and also in certain sarcomas, notably synovial sarcoma, epithelioid sarcoma and leiomyosarcoma. As mentioned earlier, cytokeratin may also rarely be seen in melanoma[97]. Very occasionally, non-lymphoid tumours have been reported to express LCA[201,202]. S 100 protein is expressed in a number of carcinomas, notably renal cell, and does not unequivocally imply neural or melanocytic differentiation; it may also be seen in mesothelial cells[84]. The reader is directed to other texts for a more comprehensive account[29,126].

Electron microscopy

Scanning and transmission electron microscopy may be useful in precise subtyping of cells from serous fluids by their ultrastructural features[214–216]. Both modalities are of some value in distinguishing adenocarcinoma from mesothelioma by the differing morphology of microvillous processes. Scanning electron microscopy, allowing recognition of the characteristics of the cell surface, demonstrates the long and delicate microvilli of mesothelial and mesothelioma cells (see Chapter 4); those of adenocarcinoma are generally shorter and thicker[214]. However, we have encountered occasional metastatic adenocarcinomas, which contain cells with 'pseudomesotheliomatous' microvilli, and therefore several cells should be examined for diagnostic features. Reduplication of the basal lamina has recently been noted in mesothelioma but is not identified in pulmonary adenocarcinoma[217]. Transmission electron microscopy allows the examination of both intracellular and extracellular components. The microvillous morphology is still clearly apparent and allows distinction between adenocarcinoma and mesothelioma in most cases; also of use is the presence of glycogen and the perinuclear arrangement of cytoskeletal filaments in cells of mesothelial origin[218,219].

A further use of electron microscopy is to detect ultrastructural evidence of differentiation in tumours, which appear undifferentiated at light microscopic level. Tight junctions, tonofilaments, basal lamina, mucin, glycogen, myofilaments, melanosomes and dense core neurosecretory granules can be particularly useful if identified in an otherwise anaplastic tumour[218]. The presence of dense core neurosecretory granules indicates neuroendocrine differentiation, but this encompasses a range of tumours with differing biological behaviour: small cell carcinoma and neuroendocrine carcinomas are usually poorly granulated, whereas carcinoid tumours generally contain large numbers of granules. In distinguishing bronchioloalveolar cell carcinoma from other well-differentiated carcinomas, lamellar bodies as seen in normal type II pneumocytes may be helpful[220,221]. The presence of adenocarcinoma cells with cytoplasmic rootlets is strongly suggestive of colonic origin[49]. It is important to realize that, as always in ultrastructural studies, careful identification of the target cell is required to ensure that observations relate to the tumour cells and not unrelated 'bystander' cells.

Flow cytometry

Flow cytometry can be used for DNA analysis[134,222,223] or for immunophenotyping of cells in suspension[133,137]; both of these applications may have value in the analysis of serous fluids. Detection of aneuploidy is a useful pointer towards malignancy, as many malignant tumours are aneuploid; this can be useful when the tumour cells have bland cytological details. However, diagnostic utility is hampered by several problems. Interpretation of DNA histograms is not always easy and may be subject to inter-observer variability; not all malignant tumours are aneuploid, some being diploid or near diploid, and an 'inappropriate' diploid result may be recorded in over 40% of malignant cases[222]. Lack of

sensitivity is also a problem if very small numbers of aneuploid cells (less than 5%) are present, in that they may be masked by the large diploid population[224]. More seriously, occasional false positive results occur as benign tumours may exhibit chromosomal abnormalities[22]; a positive result should prompt a careful reassessment of the cytological appearances, preferably augmented by appropriate immunocytochemistry, but cannot be relied upon by itself for definitive diagnosis. In some cases, examination of a further sample or biopsy for histology may be advised. Recent studies have suggested that the low sensitivity of this technique precludes its use in screening and its potential role is restricted to clarifying cytologically equivocal cases[138,225] A more cogent use of the technique is in the analysis of fluids involved by haematological and lymphoid malignancies; cell surface marker studies may be helpful in distinction from benign causes of lymphocyte rich effusions[71].

Cytogenetics

Cytogenetic study can give additional information in cytological material[226]. There are well documented specific chromosomal abnormalities described in a number of tumours, particularly well documented in sarcomas, including t(x;18) in synovial sarcoma and t(11; 22) in the Ewing's sarcoma/peripheral neuroectodermal tumour group. These abnormalities are reviewed in detail by Heim and Mitelman[227]. Techniques for their demonstration are becoming easier, and specific abnormalities may be useful to support morphological diagnosis. The development of fluorescent *in situ* hybridization has simplified cytogenetic evaluation of tumour cells in fluid specimens[228,229] and it is likely that they will be of increasing use in the future[230].

Morphometry

Morphometry has been used by several groups to distinguish between benign and malignant cells in serous effusions. Various features have been assessed including nuclear and cytoplasmic area[231–233], nuclear and cytoplasmic diameter[234], cumulative area and distribution of cytoplasmic vacuoles[235] and nucleolar number and diameter[233]. These are summarized by van Diest and Baak[236]. Such measurements appear to be valuable in diagnosis, but computer assisted systems are required for optimal measurement; sample sizes of about 300 cells may be required to obtain reproducible results[233] and this is likely to be time consuming. Nucleolar organizer regions visualized using a silver impregnation technique (known as AgNORs) are seen in many malignant cells[237] and are easily demonstrated in cytological material[168]. However, as reactive mesothelial cells may contain increased numbers of AgNORs, overlap between benign and malignant ranges limits the use of this technique in serous fluids and its use is not recommended for diagnostic purposes[168,238]. The role of static DNA cytometry as a diagnostic aid in cytological preparations has recently been reviewed[239,240]. Such techniques are probably best reserved for analysis of problematic cases in specialist centres.

Molecular techniques

Until recently, the main use of *in situ* hybridization (ISH) and polymerase chain reaction (PCR) in cytology has been the identification of viral nuclear material (e.g. human papilloma virus) in infected cells. However, there has been increasing interest in the molecular detection of low level malignant disease in various cytological specimens, such as bone marrow[241], bronchoalveolar lavage fluid[242], and cerebrospinal fluid (CSF)[243,244]. While the role of this technique in routine diagnostic work has yet to be fully evaluated[245], reverse transcriptase PCR (RT-PCR) appears to be a highly sensitive method for detecting malignant epithelial cells in serous effusions[246] as well as lymphoma cells in CSF[243,244]. Point mutations (e.g. p53 and K-ras gene) may also be detected by PCR; some studies suggest that this could be a valuable adjunct to cytological diagnosis in effusion cytology[247].

Fluorescent *in situ* hybridization (FISH) has also shown promise in detecting low level disease[248,249] and subtyping tumours by karyotyping[226]. It has also been shown to be of value in detecting non-Hodgkin's lymphomas in serous effusions[243]. These molecular techniques hold great promise for the future in view of their high sensitivity but are not yet in routine use in most diagnostic cytology laboratories.

Biochemical analysis

Measurement of specific proteins and other substances in serous fluid has been shown to have diagnostic value[250-256]. High total protein and LDH concentrations indicate an exudate rather than a transudate and are usually seen in malignancy, although this is clearly not diagnostic. The most useful markers of metastatic adenocarcinoma are CEA[250] and fibronectin[251]. Ca125 is also of value in detection of Mullerian tumours but may be raised in other tumour types and occasionally is mildly elevated in non-malignant effusions[250]. AFP concentration is usually dramatically elevated in hepatocellular carcinoma and yolk sac tumour, but may reflect very high serum values; while it confirms the presence of an AFP secreting tumour, if does not necessarily imply tumour involvement of the serous membranes. Hyaluronic acid concentration is mildly raised in adenocarcinoma[252] but markedly raised in mesothelioma[252-254]. Measurement of other substances including tumour associated trypsin inhibitor[255] and sialic acid[256] has been advocated but these appear to lack specificity for malignancy.

Technical appendix

Preparation of fluids for routine staining

On receipt, the fluid is described and measured, and any clot is removed and processed for histology. Cellular fragments, if present, can be removed using the celloidin bag technique[19]. Several direct smears are made, some of which are air dried and some ethanol fixed. The fluid is divided and part is diluted with saline and several cytospin preparations are made. The remainder (or another aliquot) is centrifuged and the pellet wrapped in tissue paper and submitted for histological processing[257]. MGG (air-dried) and Papanicolaou (alcohol fixed) stains are performed on direct smears and cytospin preparations; glycogen and mucin stains are routinely performed on alcohol fixed material. Depending on clinical context, further stains are performed generally on alcohol fixed material as cellular detail is considerably better than in air dried smears.

Preparation of fluids for immunocytochemistry

Fluids can be stored at 4°C for 1 to 2 days and still give satisfactory immunostaining, but it is prudent to prepare slides as soon as possible following receipt of the specimen to avoid degeneration and loss of antigenicity[29]. Adhesives such as poly-l-lysine[258] are valuable to promote cellular adhesion and minimize cell loss. ICC can be performed on direct smears, cytospin preparations or sections from cell blocks. For general usage, cytocentrifuge preparations (which concentrate the population of target cells) are preferable to direct smears in most cases. In addition, cytospin preparations have the advantage of requiring less reagent to cover the cell 'buttons' than direct smears. Optimal fixation for ICC depends on the nature of the antigens to be identified; for general use, 95% ethanol gives good cellular morphology and adequate antigen preservation. Air dried smears (which require post fixation in cold acetone) are less easily interpreted, often having a 'smudgy' ICC staining pattern. For preservation of certain markers, some have advocated B5 fixation[5] and other techniques for lymphoid[259] or neuroendocrine[56] markers. Air-dried acetone fixed smears give acceptable preservation of lymphoid markers in our experience.

Preparation of fluids for *in situ* hybridization

Gelatin or poly-l-lysine coated slides are recommended to minimize loss of cells during processing. Rapid fixation is essential for optimal results; for direct smear and cytospin preparations, ethanol gives satisfactory results. Cell blocks should be fixed in buffered formol saline for RNA analysis[260]; Carnoy's fixative is superior for DNA analysis[261]. Bouin's fixative degrades DNA and RNA and is not suitable[262].

Preparation of fluids for electron microscopy

Several techniques are available. The aspirate can be diluted with saline, centrifuged at 2000 rpm for 5 minutes and the pellet fixed in glutaraldehyde for one hour before being processed. Alternatively, the diluted aspirate can be passed through a nucleopore filter, fixed with glutaraldehyde before being post fixed with osmium tetroxide[215]. Cells can also be retrieved from routinely ethanol fixed Papanicolaou stained slides, although the staining process leaches lipid from cell membranes, resulting in some artefactual change[219].

Preparation of fluids for polymerase chain reaction

PCR can be performed on a wide range of sample types. DNA can be successfully extracted from cell deposits frozen in buffer, cell blocks, cytospin preparations, fixed smears and even stained and mounted cytological slides[263]. Prompt preparation is required to prevent action of DNAses.

Fixation should be avoided if possible as DNA denaturation may occur[264], and unfixed specimens can be stored at –70°C for considerable periods[265].

Cell preparation should be protected by wrapping in tin foil prior to freezing. In our hands, cell deposits suspended in buffer and frozen at –70°C give excellent results. In order to extract DNA from stored frozen slides, these should be allowed to return to room temperature before removal of cells using a pipette tip and sterile water. Standard DNA extraction kits can then be employed using 'cell culture' protocols.

References

1 Monte S A, Ehya H, Lang W R. Positive effusion cytology as the initial presentation of malignancy. *Acta Cytol* 1987; **31**: 448–451

2 Hsu C. Cytologic detection of malignancy in pleural effusion. A review of 5255 samples from 3811 patients. *Diagn Cytopathol* 1987; **3**: 8–12

3 Selvaggi S M, Migdal S. Cytological features of atypical mesothelial cells in peritoneal dialysis fluid. *Diagn Cytopathol* 1990; **6**: 22–26

4 Spriggs A I, Boddington M M. *Atlas of Pleural Fluid Cytopathology. A Guide to the Cells of Pleural, Pericardial, Peritoneal and Hydrocele Fluids*. Dordrecht: Kluwer Academic, 1989

5 Nance K V, Silverman J F. The cytology of serous effusions. In: eds. *Cytopathology Annual*. Baltimore: Williams and Williams, 1993

6 Zaatari G S, Gupta P K, Bhagavan B S, Jorboe B R. Cytopathology of pleural endometriosis. *Acta Cytol* 1982; **26**: 227–232

7 Carlson G J, Samuelson J J, Dehner L P. Cytologic diagnosis of florid peritoneal endosalpingosis. *Acta Cytol* 1986; **30**: 494–496

8 Kern W H. Benign papillary structures with psammoma bodies in culdocentesis fluid. *Acta Cytol* 1969; **13**: 178–180

9 Sneige N, Fernandez T, Copeland L J, Katz R L. Mullerian inclusions in peritoneal washings. Potential source of error in cytological diagnosis. *Acta Cytol* 1986; **30**: 271–276

10 Kumar N B, Naylor B. Megakaryocytes in pleural and peritoneal fluids: prevalence, significance, morphology and cytohistological correlation. *J Clin Pathol* 1980; **33**: 1153–1159

11 Bartziota E V, Naylor B. Megakaryocytes in a haemorrhagic pleural effusion caused by anticoagulant overdose. *Acta Cytol* 1986; **30**: 163–165

12 Coleman D V. Ciliated organisms in dialysis fluid. *Lancet* 1986; **i**: 1030

13 Sidawy M K, Chandra P, Oertel Y C. Detached ciliated tufts in female peritoneal washings. A common finding. *Acta Cytol* 1987; **31**: 841–844

14 Kobayashi T K, Teraoka S, Tsujioka T, Yoshida Y. Ciliated ovarian adenocarcinoma cells in ascitic fluid cytology: report of a case with immunocytochemical features. *Diagn Cytopathol* 1988; **4**: 234–238

15 Gupta P K, Albritton N, Erozan Y S, Frost J K. Occurrence of cilia in exfoliated ovarian adenocarcinoma cells. *Diagn Cytopathol* 1985; **1**: 228–231

16 Sneige N, Fanning C V. Peritoneal washing cytology in women: diagnostic pitfalls and clues for correct diagnosis. *Diagn Cytopathol* 1992; **8**(6): 632–640 (discussion 640–642)

17 Koss L G. *Diagnostic Cytopathology and Its Histopathologic Basis*, 4th edn. Philadelphia: Lippincott, 1992

18 Naylor B. Pleural, peritoneal and pericardial fluids. In: Bibbo M ed. *Comprehensive Cytopathology*. Philadelphia: WB Saunders, 1991

19 Bussolati G. A celloidin bag for the histological preparation of cytological material. *J Clin Pathol* 1982; **35**: 574–576

20 Cibas E S, Corson J M, Pinkus G S. The distinction of adenocarcinoma from mesothelioma in cell blocks of effusions: the role of routine mucin histochemistry and immunohistochemical assessment of carcinoembryonic antigen, keratin proteins, epithelial membrane antigen, and human milk fat globule-derived antigen. *Hum Pathol* 1987; **18**: 67–74

21 Michael C W, King J A C, Hester R B. Confocal laser scanning microscopy and three dimensional reconstruction of cell clusters in serous fluids. *Diagn Cytopathol* 1997; **17**:272–279

22 Cibas E S. Effusions (pleural, pericardial, and peritoneal) and peritoneal washings. In: Atkinson B F ed. *Atlas of Diagnostic Cytopathology*. Philadelphia: WB Saunders, 1992

23 Ravinsky E. Cytology of peritoneal washings in gynecologic patients: diagnostic criteria and pitfalls. *Acta Cytol* 1986; **30**: 8–16

24 Yu G H, Sack M J, Baloch Z W et al. Occurrence of intercellular spaces (windows) in metastatic adenocarcinoma in serous fluids. A cytomorphological, histochemical and ultrastructural study. *Diagn Cytopathol* 1999; **20**(3): 115–119

25 Spriggs A I. The architecture of tumour cell clusters in serous effusions. In: Koss L G, Coleman D V eds. *Advances in Clinical Cytology*, vol. 2. New York: Masson, 1984

26 Wojcik E M, Naylor B. 'Collagen balls' in peritoneal washings. Prevalence, morphology origin and significance. *Acta Cytol* 1992; **36**: 466–470

27 Delahaye M, de Jong A A, Versnel M A et al. Cytopathology of malignant mesothelioma. Reappraisal of the diagnostic value of collagen cores. *Cytopathology* 1990; **1**: 137–145

28 Ito H, Hirasawa T, Yasuda M et al. Excessive formation of basement membrane substance in clear-cell carcinoma of the ovary: diagnostic value of the 'raspberry body' in ascites cytology. *Diagn Cytopathol* 1997; **16**(6): 500–504

29 Krausz T, Schofield J B, van Noorden S et al. Application of immunocytochemistry to fine needle aspirates. In: Young J ed. *Fine Needle Aspiration Cytopathology*. Oxford: Blackwell Scientific Publications, 1993

30 Young J A, Crocker J. Pleural fluid cytology in lymphoplasmacytoid lymphoma with numerous intracytoplasmic immunoglobulin inclusions. A case report with immunocytochemistry. *Acta Cytol* 1984; **28**: 419–422

31 Söderström N, Biorklund A. Intranuclear cytoplasmic inclusions in some types of thyroid *Cancer*. *Acta Cytol* 1973; **17**: 191–197

32 Spriggs A I, Boddington M M. *The Cytology of Effusions, Pleural, Pericardial and Peritoneal, and of Cerebrospinal Fluid*, 2nd edn. London: William Heinemann, 1968

33 Scott J E, Dorking J. Differential staining of acid glycosaminoglycan (mucopolysaccharide) by Alcian blue in salt solutions. *Histochem* 1965; **5**: 221–233

34 Yu G H, De Frias D V S, Horcher A M. Evaluation of histochemical methods for the detection of intracytoplasmic mucin in serous effusions. *Cytopathology* 1999; **10**: 298–302

35 Walz R, Koch H K. Malignant pleural mesothelioma: some aspects of epidemiology, differential diagnosis and prognosis. Histological and immunohistochemical evaluation and follow up of mesotheliomas diagnosed from 1964 to January 1985. *Pathol Res Pract* 1990; **186**: 124–134

36 Henderson D W, Shilkin K B, Whittaker D. Reactive mesothelial hyperplasia *vs* mesothelioma, including mesothelioma *in*

situ. A brief review. *Am J Clin Pathol* 1998; **110**: 397–404

37 Cook D S, Attanoos R L, Jalloh S, Gibbs A R. 'Mucin-positive' mesothelioma of the peritoneum: an unusual diagnostic pitfall. *Histopathology* 2000; **37**: 33–36

38 Spriggs A I, Jerrome D W. Intracellular mucin inclusions. A feature of malignant cells in effusions in the serous cavities, particularly due to carcinoma of the breast. *J Clin Pathol* 1975; **28**: 929–936

39 Ashton P R, Hollingsworth A S, Johnson W W. The cytopathology of metastatic breast cancer. *Acta Cytol* 1975; **19**: 1–6

40 Battifora H. Intracytoplasmic lumina in breast carcinoma. A helpful histologic feature. *Arch Pathol* 1975; **99**: 614–617

41 Gad A, Azzopardi J G. Lobular carcinoma of the breast: a special variant of mucin-secreting carcinoma. *J Clin Pathol* 1975; **28**: 711–716

42 Burchell J, Gendler S, Taylor-Papadimitriou J et al. Development and characterisation of breast cancer reactive monoclonal antibodies directed to the core protein of the human milk mucin. *Cancer Res* 1987; **47**: 5476–5482

43 Gammon R, Hameed A, Keyhani-Rofagha S. Peritoneal washing in borderline epithelial tumours in women under 25: The use of cell block preparations. *Diagn Cytopathol* 1998; **18**(3): 212–214

44 Rammou-Kinia R, Sirmakechian-Karra T. Pseudomyxoma peritonei and malignant mucocele of the appendix. *Acta Cytol* 1986; **30**: 169–172

45 Valente P T, Schantz H D, Edmonds P R, Hanjani P. Peritoneal cytology of uncommon ovarian tumors. *Diagn Cytopathol* 1992; **8**: 98–106

46 Modzelewski J R, Silverman J F, Berns L A et al. Serous effusion cytology in gynecologic malignant mixed mullerian tumors. *Diagn Cytopathol* 1995; **12**(4): 309–312

47 Sheibani K, Battifora H, Burke J S, Rappaport H. LeuM1 in human neoplasms: an immunohistological study of 400 cases. *Am J Surg Pathol* 1986; **10**: 227–236

48 Renshaw A A, Comiter C V, Nappi D, Granter S R. Effusion cytology of renal cell carcinoma. *Cancer Cytopathol* 1998; **84**: 148–152

49 Pozalaky Z, McGinley D, Pozalaky I P. Electron microscopic identification of the colorectal origins of tumour cells in pleural fluid. *Acta Cytol* 1983; **27**: 45–48

50 Mesia A F, Tarafder D, Shanerman, A I, Cohen J-M. Peritoneal cytology in uterine papillary serous carcinoma. *Acta Cytol* 1999; **43**(4) 605–609

51 Gown A M, Yaziji H. Immunohistochemical analysis of carcinomas of unknown primary site. *Pathol Case Rev* 1999; **4**(6): 250–259

52 Hoda R S, Cangiarella J, Koss L G. Metastatic squamous cell carcinoma in pericardial effusion: Report of four cases, two with cardiac tamponade. *Diagn Cytopathol* 1998; **18**: 422–424

53 Smith-Purslow M J, Kini S R, Naylor B. Cells of squamous cell carcinoma in pleural, peritoneal and pericardial fluids. Origin and morphology. *Acta Cytol* 1989; **33**: 245–253

54 Cobb C J, Wynn J, Cobb S R, Duane G B. Cytologic findings in an effusion caused by rupture of a benign cystic teratoma of the mediastinum into a serous cavity. *Acta Cytol* 1985; **29**: 1015–1020

55 Spriggs A I, Boddington M M. Oat-cell bronchial carcinoma. Identification of cells in pleural fluid. *Acta Cytol* 1976; **20**: 525–529

56 Springall D R, Lackie P, Levene M M et al. Immunostaining of neurone-specific enolase is a valuable aid to the cytological diagnosis of neuro-endocrine tumours of the lung. *J Pathol* 1984; **143**: 259–265

57 Shipley W R, Hammer R D, Lennington W J, Macon W R. Paraffin immunohistochemical detection of CD56, a useful marker for neural cell adhesion molecule (NCAM), in normal and neoplastic fixed tissues. *Appl Immunohistochem* 1997; **5**: 87–93

58 Michels S, Swanson P E, Robb J A, Wick M A. Leu 7 in small cell neoplasms. *Cancer* 1987; **60**: 2958–2964

59 Said J W, Vimadalal S, Nash G et al. Immunoreactive neuron-specific enolase, bombesin and chromogranin as markers for neuroendocrine lung tumours. *Hum Pathol* 1985; **16**: 237–240

60 Guzman J, Bross K J, Costabel U. Malignant pleural effusions due to small cell carcinoma of the lung. An immunocytochemical cell surface analysis of lymphocytes and tumour cells. *Acta Cytol* 1990; **34**: 497–501

61 Nance K V, Silverman J F. Immunocytochemical panel for the identification of malignant cells in serous effusions. *Am J Clin Pathol* 1991; **95**: 867–874

62 Hasserjian R P, Krausz T. Diagnosis of primary and secondary lymphomatous effusions. In: Lowe D G, Underwood J C E eds. *Recent Advances in Histopathology* 18, London: Churchill Livingstone, 2000; 118–122

63 Jones D, Weinberg D S, Pinkus G S et al. Cytologic diagnosis of primary serous lymphoma. *Am J Clin Pathol* 1996; **106**: 359–364

64 Nador R G, Cesarman E, Chadburn A et al. Primary effusion lymphoma: a distinct clinicopathological entity associated with the Kaposi's sarcoma-associated herpesvirus. *Blood* 1996; **88**: 645–656

65 Aozasa K. Pyothorax-associated lymphoma. *Int J Hematol* 1996; **65**: 9–16

66 Gaidano G, Carbone A. Primary effusion lymphoma: a liquid phase lymphoma of fluid-filled body cavities. *Adv Cancer Res* 2001; **80**: 115–146

67 Spriggs A I, Vanhegan R I. Cytological diagnosis of lymphoma in serous effusions. *J Clin Pathol* 1981; **34**: 1311–1325

68 Seidel T A, Garbes A D. Cellules grumelées: old terminology revisited: regarding the cytologic diagnosis of chronic lymphocytic leukaemia and well differentiated lymphocytic lymphoma in pleural effusions. *Acta Cytol* 1985; **29**: 775–780

69 Krause J R, Dekker A. Hairy cell leukemia (leukemic reticuloendotheliosis) in serous effusions. *Acta Cytol* 1978; **22**: 80–82

70 Dunphy C H, Collins B, Ramos R, Grusso L E. Secondary pleural involvement by an AIDS-related anaplastic large cell (CD30+) lymphoma simulating metastatic adenocarcinoma. *Diagn Cytopathol* 1998; **18**(2): 113–117

71 Picker L J, Weiss L M, Medeiros L J et al. Immunophenotyping criteria for the differential diagnosis of non-Hodgkin's lymphoma. *Am J Pathol* 1987; **128**: 181–201

72 Domagala W, Emerson E E, Koss L G. T and B lymphocyte enumeration in the diagnosis of lymphocyte-rich pleural fluids. *Acta Cytol* 1981; **25**: 108–110

73 Yam L T, Lin D G, Janckila A J, Li C-Y. Immunocytochemical diagnosis of lymphoma in serous effusions. *Acta Cytol* 1985; **29**: 833–841

74 Martin S E, Zhang H-Z, Magyarosy E et al. Immunologic methods in cytology: definite diagnosis of non-Hodgkin's lymphomas using immunologic markers for T and B cells. *Am J Clin Pathol* 1984; **82**: 666–673

75 Robey S S, Cafferty L L, Beschorner W E, Gupta P K. Value of lymphocyte marker studies in diagnostic cytopathology. *Acta Cytol* 1987; **31**: 453–459

76 Guzman J, Bross K J, Costabel U. Malignant lymphoma in pleural effusions: an immunocytochemical and cell surface analysis. *Diagn Cytopathol* 1991; **7**: 113–118

77 Walts A E, Shintaku I P, Said J W. Diagnosis of malignant lymphoma in effusions from patients with AIDS by gene rearrangement. *Am J Clin Pathol* 1990; **94**: 170–175

78 Foucar K, Chen I-M, Crago S. Organisation and operation of a flow cytometric immunophenotyping laboratory. *Semin Diagn Pathol* 1989; **6**: 13–36

79 Sasser R L, Yam L T, Li C Y. Myeloma with involvement of the serous cavities. Cytologic and immunohistochemical diagnosis and literature review. *Acta Cytol* 1990; **34**: 479–485

80 Khoddami M, Esphehani F N, Aslani F S. Ascites as a presenting feature of relapsed multiple myeloma. Report of a case diagnosed by aspiration cytology. *Acta Cytol* 1992; **36**: 325–328

81 Debray C, Hardouin J P, Charlier G, Martin E. La maladie de Hodgkin gastro-duodenale. Son diagnostic valeur du cytodiagnostic du liquide d'ascite. *Sem Hôp* 1961; **37**: 408

82 Hall P A, D'Ardenne A J, Stansfeld A G. Paraffin section immunohistochemistry. II. Hodgkin's disease and anaplastic large cell (Ki-1) lymphoma. *Histopathology* 1988; **13**: 161–169

83 Olson P R, Silverman J F, Powers C N. Pleural fluid cytology of Hodgkin's disease: cytomorphologic features and the value of immunohistochemical studies. *Diagn Cytopathol* 1999; **22**: 21–24

84 Mooi W J, Krausz T. *Biopsy Pathology of Melanocytic Disorders*. London: Chapman & Hall, 1992

85 Hajdu S I, Savino A. Cytologic diagnosis of malignant melanoma. *Acta Cytol* 1973; **17**: 320–327

86 Woyke S, Domagala W, Czerniak B, Strokowska M. Fine needle aspiration cytology of malignant melanoma of the skin. *Acta Cytol* 1978; **24**: 529–538

87 Pinto M M. An immunoperoxidase study of S-100 protein in neoplastic cells in serous effusions. Use as a marker for melanoma. *Acta Cytol* 1986; **30**: 240–244

88 Angeli S, Koelma I A, Fleuren G J, Van Steenis G J. Malignant melanoma in fine needle aspirates and effusions. An immunocytochemical study using monoclonal antibodies. *Acta Cytol* 1988; **32**: 707–712

89 Ordoñez N G, Sneige N, Hickey R C, Brooks T E. Use of monoclonal antibody HMB-45 in the cytologic diagnosis of melanoma. *Acta Cytol* 1988; **32**: 684–688

90 Bishop P W, Menasce L P, Yates A J, Win N A, Banerjee S S. An immunophenotypic survey of malignant melanomas. *Histopathology* 1993; **23**: 159–166

91 Banerjee S S, Harris M. Morphological and immunophenotypic variations in malignant melanoma. *Histopath* 2000; **36**: 387–402

92 Bonetti F, Colombari E, Zamboni G et al. Breast carcinoma positive for melanoma marker (HMB 45). *Am J Clin Pathol* 1989; **22**: 491–495

93 Pelosi G, Bonetti F, Colombari R et al. Use of monoclonal antibody HMB-45 for detecting melanoma cells in fine needle aspiration biopsy samples. *Acta Cytol* 1990; **34**: 460–462

94 Yates A J, Banerjee S S, Bishop P W, Graham K E. HMB-45 in non-melanocytic tumours. *Histopathology* 1993; **23**: 477–478

95 Weeks D A, Chase D R, Malott R L et al. HMB-45 staining in angiolipoma, cardiac rhabdomyoma, other mesenchymal processes, and tuberous sclerosis-associated brain lesions. *Int J Surg Pathol* 1994; **1**: 191–198

96 Rasmussen O O, Larsen K E. S-100 protein in malignant mesotheliomas. *Acta Pathol Microbiol Scand (A)* 1985; **93**: 199–201

97 Zarbo R J, Gown A M, Visscher D W, Crissman J D. Anomolous cytokeratin expression in malignant melanoma: one- and two-dimensional Western blot analysis and immunohistochemical survey of 100 melanomas. *Modern Pathol* 1990; **3**: 494–501

98 Hajdu S I, Hajdu E O. *Cytopathology of Sarcomas and Other Non-Epithelial Tumours.* Philadelphia: Saunders, 1976

99 Abadi M A, Zakowski M F. Cytologic features of sarcomas in fluids. *Cancer Cytopathol* 1998; **84**(2): 71–76

100 Malone M. Soft tissue tumours in childhood. *Histopathology* 1993; **23**: 203–216

101 Askin F B, Rosai D, Sibley R K et al. Malignant small cell tumour of the thoracopulmonary region in childhood. *Cancer* 1979; **43**: 2438–2451

102 Satake T, Matsuyama M. Cytologic features of ascites in malignant fibrous histiocytoma of the colon. *Acta Pathol Japn* 1988; **38**: 921–928

103 Yang H-Y, Weaver L L, Foti P R. Primary malignant fibrous histiocytoma of the pleura. A case report. *Acta Cytol* 1983; **27**: 683–687

104 Hajdu S I, Koss L G. Cytologic diagnosis of metastatic myosarcomas. *Acta Cytol* 1969; **13**: 545–551

105 Nguyen G-K, Schnitka T K, Jewell L D, Wroblewski J A. Exfoliative cytology of clear cell sarcoma metastases in pleural fluid. *Diagn Cytopathol* 1986; **2**: 144–149

106 Kashimura M, Tsukamoto N, Matsuyama T et al. Cytologic findings of ascites from patients with ovarian dysgerminoma. *Acta Cytol* 1983; **27**: 59–62

107 Roncalli M, Gribaudi G, Simoncelli D, Servida E. Cytology of yolk-sac tumour of the ovary in ascitic fluid. *Acta Cytol* 1988; **32**: 113–116

108 Cho K J, Myong N H, Jang J J. Effusion cytology of endodermal sinus tumor of the colon. Report of a case. *Acta Cytol* 1991; **35**: 207–209

109 Kim K, Koo B C, Delaflor R R, Shaikh B S. Pineal germinoma with widespread extracranial metastases. *Diagn Cytopathol* 1985; **1**: 118–122

110 Morimoto N, Ozawa M, Amano S. Diagnostic value of hyaline globules in endodermal sinus tumour. *Acta Cytol* 1971; **25**: 417–420

111 Farr G H, Hajdu S I. Exfoliative cytology of metastatic neuroblastoma. *Acta Cytol* 1971; **16**: 203–206

112 Hajdu S I. Exfoliative cytology of primary and metastatic Wilms' tumors. *Acta Cytol* 1971; **15**: 339–342

113 Sears D, Hadju S I. The cytological diagnosis of malignant neoplasms in pleural and peritoneal effusions. *Acta Cytol* 1987; **31**: 85–97

114 Halliday B E, Slagel D D, Elsheikh T E, Silverman J F. Diagnostic utility of MIC-2 immunocytochemical staining in the differential diagnosis of small blue cell tumours. *Diagn Cytopathol* 1998; **19**(6): 410–416

115 Watson C W, Freidman K J. Cytology of neuroendocrine carcinoma (Merkel-cell) carcinoma in pleural fluid. A case report. *Acta Cytol* 1985; **29**: 397–402

116 Zirkin H J. Pleural fluid cytology of invasive thymoma. *Acta Cytol* 1985; **29**: 1011–1014

117 Aozasa K, Kurokawa K, Kabori Y et al. Malignant histiocytosis showing ascites and recurrent meningeal infiltration. *Acta Cytol* 1980; **24**: 228–231

118 Woyke S, Domagala W, Olszewski W. Ultrastructure of hepatoma cells detected in peritoneal fluid. *Acta Cytol* 1972; **16**: 63

119 Ehya H, Lang W R. Cytology of granulosa cell tumour of the ovary. *Am J Clin Pathol* 1986; **85**: 402

120 Jobst S B, Ljung B-M, Gilkey F N, Rosenthal D L. Cytologic diagnosis of olfactory neuroblastoma. Report of a case with multiple diagnostic parameters. *Acta Cytol* 1983; **27**: 299–305

121 McCallum S, Copper K, Franks D N. Choroid plexus carcinoma: cytologic identification of malignant cells in ascitic fluid. *Acta Cytol* 1984; **32**: 263–266

122 Hong I S. The exfoliative cytology of endometrial stromal sarcoma in peritoneal fluid. *Acta Cytol* 1981; **25**: 277–281

123 Safnaeck J R, Halliday W C, Quinonez G. Metastatic meningioma detected in pleural fluid. *Diagn Cytopathol* 1998; **18**: 453–457

124 Bian Y, Jordan A G, Rupp M et al. Effusion cytology of desmoplastic small round cell tumor of the pleura. *Acta Cytol* 1993; **37**: 77–82

125 Gerald W L, Miller H K, Battifora H et al. Intra-abdominal desmoplastic small round cell tumor. *Am J Surg Pathol* 1991; **15**: 499–513

126 Osborn M, Domagala W. Immunocytochemistry. In: Bibbo M ed. *Comprehensive Cytopathology*. Philadelphia: W B Saunders, 1991

127 Al Nafussi A, Carder P J. Monoclonal antibodies in the cytodiagnosis of serous effusions. *Cytopathology* 1990; **1**: 119–128

128 Flens M J, van der Valk P, Tadema T M et al. The contribution of immunocytochemistry in diagnostic cytology. Comparison and evaluation with immunohistology. *Cancer* 1990; **65**: 2704–2711

129 Li C-Y, Lazcano-Villareal O, Pierre R V, Yam L T. Immunocytochemical identification of cells in serous fluid. *Am J Clin Pathol* 1987; **88**: 696–705

130 Cuijpers V M, Boerman O C, Salet van de Pol M R et al. Immunocytochemical detection of ovarian carcinoma cells in serous effusions. *Acta Cytol* 1993; **37**: 272–279

131 Shield P W, Perkins G, Wright R G. Immunocytochemical staining of cytologic specimens. How helpful is it? *Am J Clin Pathol* 1996; **105**(2): 139–162

132 Bedrossian C W. Diagnostic problems in serous effusions. *Diagn Cytopathol* 1998; **19**(2): 131–137

133 Czerniak B, Papenhausen P R, Herz F, Koss L G. Flow cytometric identification of cancer cells in effusions using Cal monoclonal antibody. *Cancer* 1985; **55**: 2783–2788

134 Croonen A M, van de Valk H C J, Lindeman J. Cytology, immunology and flow cytometry in the diagnosis of pleural and peritoneal effusions. *Lab Invest* 1988; **58**: 725–731

135 Davidson B, Risberg B, Berner A et al. Evaluation of lymphoid cell populations in cytology specimens using flow cytometry and polymerase chain reaction. *Diagn Mol Pathol* 1999; **8**: 183–188

136 Motherby H, Freidrichs N, Kube M et al. Immunocytochemistry and DNA-image cytometry in diagnostic effusion cytology II. Diagnostic accuracy in equivocal smears. *Anal Cell Pathol* 1999; **19**(2): 18–21

137 Risberg B, Davidson B, Dong H P et al. Flow cytometric immunophenotyping of serous effusions and peritoneal washings: comparison with immunocytochemistry and morphological findings. *J Clin Pathol* 2000; **53**: 513–517

138 Laucirica R, Schwartz M R. Clinical utility of flow cytometry in body fluid cytology: To flow or not to flow? That is the question. *Diagn Cytopathol* 2001; **24**: 305–306

139 Riera J R, Astengo-Osuna C, Longmate J A, Battifora H. The immunohistochemical diagnostic panel for epithelial mesothelioma. A reevaluation after heat-induced epitope retrieval. *Am J Surg Pathol* 1997; **21**(12): 1409–1419

140 Doglioni C, Dei-Tos A P, Laurins L et al. Calretinin: A novel immunocytochemical marker for mesothelioma. *Am J Surg Pathol* 1996; **20**: 1037–1046

141 Nagel H, Hammerlein B, Ruschenburg I et al. The value of anti-calretinin antibody in the differential diagnosis of normal and reactive mesothelial vs metastatic tumours in effusion cytology. *Pathol Res Pract* 1998; **194**: 759–764

142 Ordoñez N G. Value of calretinin immunostaining in differentiating epithelial mesothelioma from lung adenocarcinoma. *Mod Pathol* 1998; **20**: 929–933

143 Ordoñez N G. Role of immunohistochemistry in distinguishing epithelial peritoneal mesotheliomas from peritoneal and ovarian serous carcinomas. *Am J Surg Pathol* 1998; **22**: 1203–1214

144 Simsir A, Fetsch P, Mehta D et al. E-cadherin, N-cadherin and calretinin in pleural effusions: the good, the bad, the worthless. *Diagn Cytopathol* 1999; **20**(3): 125–130

145 Chieng D C, Yee H, Cangiarella J F et al. Calretinin staining pattern aids in the differentiation of mesothelioma from adenocarcinoma in serous fluids. *Cancer* 2000; **90**(3): 194–200

146 Sato S, Okamoto S, Ito K, Konno R, Yajima A. Differential diagnosis of mesothelial and ovarian Cancer cell lines in ascites by immunohistochemistry using Ber-EP4 and calretinin. *Acta Cytol* 2000; **44**(3): 485–488

147 Kitazume H, Kitamura K, Mukai K et al. Cytological differential diagnosis among reactive mesothelial cells, malignant mesothelioma and adenocarcinoma: utility of combined E-cadherin and calretinin immunostaining. *Cancer* 2000; **90**(1): 55–60

148 Cury P M, Butcher D N, Fisher C et al. Value of the mesothelium-associated antibodies thrombomodulin, cytokeratin 5/6, calretinin and CD44H in distinguishing epithelioid pleural mesothelioma from adenocarcinoma metastatic to the pleura. *Mod Pathol* 2000; **13**(2): 107–112

149 Ordoñez N G. Value of cytokeratin 5/6 immunostaining in distinguishing epithelial mesothelioma of the pleura from lung adenocarcinoma. *Am J Surg Pathol* 1998; **22**: 1215–1221

150 Ascoli V, Carnovale-Scalzo C, Taccogna S, Nardi F. Utility of HMBE-1 immunostaining in serous effusions. *Diagn Cytopathol* 1995; **12**(4): 303–308

151 Oates J, Edwards C. HMBE-1, MOC-31, WT1 and calretinin: an assessment of recently described markers for mesothelioma and adenocarcinoma. *Histopathology* 2000; **36**(4): 341–347

152 Ordoñez N G. In search of a positive immunohistochemical marker for mesothelioma: an update. *Adv Anat Pathol* 1998; 5;53–60

153 Ordoñez N G. Role of immunohistochemistry in differentiating epithelial mesothelioma from adenocarcinoma. Review and update. *Am J Clin Pathol* 1999; **112**(1): 75–89

154 Chenard-Neu M P, Kabou A, Mechine A et al. Immunohistochemistry in the differential diagnosis of mesothelioma and adenocarcinoma. Evaluation of 5 new antibodies and 6 traditional antibodies. *Ann Pathol* 1998; **18**(6): 460–465

155 Ordoñez N G. The immunohistochemical diagnosis of epithelial mesothelioma. *Hum Pathol* 1999; **30**(3): 313–323

156 Attanoos R L, Goddard H, Gibbs A R. Mesothelioma-binding antibodies: thrombomodulin OV632 and HBME-1 and their use in the diagnosis of malignant mesothelioma. *Histopathol* 1996; **29**: 209–215

157 Ordoñez N G. The immunohistochemical diagnosis of epithelial pleural mesothelioma. *Pathol Case Rev* 1999; **4**(6): 234–241

158 Gonzáles-Lois C, Ballestín C, Sotelo M T et al. Combined use of novel epithelial (MOC-31) and mesothelial (HBME-1) immunohistochemical markers for optimal first line diagnostic distinction between mesothelioma and metastatic carcinoma in pleura. *Histopathol* 2001; **38**: 528–534

159 Orell S R, Dowling K D. Oncofetal antigens as tumour markers in the cytological diagnosis of effusions. *Acta Cytol* 1983; **27**: 625–629

160 Miettinen M, Lehto V-P, Virtanen I. Antibodies to intermediate filament proteins in the diagnosis and classification of human tumours. *Ultrastr Pathol* 1984; **7**: 83–107

161 Robb J A. Mesothelioma vs adenocarcinoma. False positive CEA and LeuM1 staining due to hyaluronic acid. *Hum Pathol* 1989; **20**: 400

162 Schröder S, Klöppel G. Carcinoembryonic antigen and non-specific cross reacting antigen in thyroid Cancer. *Am J Surg Pathol* 1987; **11**: 100–108

163 Latza U, Niedobitek G, Schwarting R et al. Ber-EP4: new monoclonal antibody which distinguishes epithelia from mesothelia. *J Clin Pathol* 1990; **43**: 213–219

164 Gaffey M J, Mills S E, Swanson P E et al. Immunoreactivity for BER-EP4 in adenomatoid tumors and malignant mesotheliomas. *Am J Surg Pathol* 1992; **16**: 593–599

165 Bailey M E, Brown R W, Mody D R et al. Ber EP-4 for differentiating adenocarcinoma from reactive and neoplastic mesothelial cells in serous effusions. Comparison with Carcinoembrionic antigen, B72.3 and LeuM1. *Acta Cytol* 1996; **40**: 1212–1216

166 De Angelis M, Buley I D, Herget A, Gray W. Immunocytochemical staining of serous effusions with the monoclonal antibody BER-EP4. *Cytopathology* 1992; **3**: 111–117

167 Ordoñez N G. Value of the Ber-EP4 antibody in differentiating epithelial pleural mesothelioma from adenocarcinoma. The MD Anderson experience and review of the literature. *Am J Clin Pathol* 1998; **109**: 85–89

168 Soosay G N, Griffiths M, Papadaki L et al. The differential diagnosis of epithelial type mesothelioma from adenocarcinoma and mesothelial proliferation. *J Pathol* 1991; **163**: 299–305

169 Kocjan G, Sweeney E, Miller K D, Bobrow L. AUA 1: new immunocytochemical marker for detecting epithelial cells in body cavity fluids. *J Clin Pathol* 1992; **45**: 358–359

170 Singer S, Boddington M M, Hudson E A. Immunocytochemical reaction of Ca1 and HMFG2 monoclonal antibodies with cells from serous effusions. *J Clin Pathol* 1985; **38**: 180–184

171 To A, Dearnaley D P, Ormerod G et al. Epithelial membrane antigen: its use in the cytodiagnosis of malignancy in effusions. *Am J Clin Pathol* 1981; **77**: 214–219

172 Walts A E, Said J W, Shintaku I P. Epithelial membrane antigen in the cytodiagnosis of effusions and aspirates: immunocytochemical and ultrastructural localisation in benign and malignant cells. *Diagn Cytopathol* 1987; **3**: 41–49

173 Otis C N, Carte D, Cole S, Battifora H. Immunohistochemical evaluation of pleural mesothelioma and pulmonary adenocarcinoma: a bi-institutional study of 47 cases. *Am J Surg Pathol* 1987; **11**: 445–456

174 Kahn H J, Thorner P S, Yeger H et al. Distinct keratin patterns demonstrated by immunoperoxidase staining of adenocarcinomas, carcinoids and mesotheliomas using polyclonal and monoclonal anti-keratin antibodies. *Am J Clin Pathol* 1986; **86**: 566–574

175 Johnston W W, Szpak C A, Thor A, Schlom J. Use of a monoclonal antibody as an immunochemical adjunct to the diagnosis of adenocarcinoma in human effusions. *Cancer* 1985; **45**: 1894–1900

176 Szpak C A, Soper J T, Thor A, Schol J, Johnson W W. Detection of adenocarcinoma in peritoneal washings by staining with monoclonal antibody B-72.3. *Acta Cytol* 1989; **33**: 205–214

177 Esteban J M, Yokota S, Husain S, Battifora H. Immunocytochemical profile of benign and carcinomatous effusions. *Am J Clin Pathol* 1990; **94**: 698–705

178 Ordoñez N G. The immunohistochemical diagnosis of mesothelioma: differentiation from mesothelioma and lung carcinoma. *Am J Surg Pathol* 1989; **13**: 276–291

179 Jordon D, Jagirdar J, Keneko M. Blood group antigens Lewisx and Lewisy in the diagnostic discrimination of malignant mesothelioma vs adenocarcinoma. *Am J Pathol* 1989; **135**: 931–937

180 Ordoñez N G. Value of thyroid transcription factor-1, E-cadherin, BG8, WT1, and CD44S immunostaining in distinguishing epithelial pleural mesothelioma from pulmonary and nonpulmonary adenocarcinoma. *Am J Surg Pathol* 2000; **24**(4): 598–606

181 Ordoñez N G. Value of the MOC-31 monoclonal antibody in differentiating epithelial mesothelioma of the pleura from lung adenocarcinoma. *Hum Pathol* 1998; **29**: 166–169

182 Anwar F, Schmidt R A. Thyroid transcription factor-1 (TTF-1) distinguishes mesothelioma from pulmonary adenocarcinoma. *Lab Invest* 1999; **79**: 181A

183 Khoor A, Whitsett JA, Stahlman MT *et al.* Utility of surfactant protein B precursor and thyroid transcription factor 1 in differentiating adenocarcinoma of the lung from malignant mesothelioma. *Hum Pathol* 1999; **30**(6): 695–700

184 Kaufmann O, Dietel M. Thyroid transcription factor-1 is the superior immunohistochemical marker for pulmonary adenocarcinomas and large cell carcinomas compared to surfactant proteins A and B. *Histopathology* 2000; **36**: 8–16

185 Duggan M A, Masters C B, Alexander F. Immunohistochemical differentiation of malignant mesothelioma, mesothelial hyperplasia, and metastatic adenocarcinoma in serous effusions, utilising staining for carcinoembryonic antigen, keratin and vimentin. *Acta Cytol* 1987; **31**: 807–814

186 Arai T, Yasuda Y, Takaya T *et al.* Application of telomerase activity for screening of primary lung Cancer in broncholalveolar lavage fluid. *Oncol Rep* 1998; **5**(2): 405–408

187 Cunningham V J, Markham N, Shroyer A L, Shroyer K R. Detection of telomerase expression in fine needle aspirations and fluids. *Diagn Cytopathol* 1998; **18**(6): 431–436

188 Mayall F, Hervet A, Manga D, Kriegeskotten A. p53 immunostaining is a highly specific and moderately sensitive marker of malignancy in serous fluid cytology. *Cytopathology* 1997; **8**(1): 9–12

189 Saleh H A, Bober P, Tabaczka P. Improved detection of adenocarcinoma in serous fluids with p53 immunocytochemistry. *Acta Cytol* 1998; **42**(6): 1330–1335

190 Pindzola J A, Kovatich A J, Bibbo M. p53 immunohistochemistry for distinguishing reactive mesothelium from low-grade ovarian adenocarcinoma. *Acta Cytol* 2000; **44**(1): 31–36

191 Carico E, Chicchirichi R, Atlante M *et al.* CA 125 in ovarian cysts, serous effusions and peritoneal washings: immunocytochemical expression. *AntiCancer Res* 1995; **15**(2): 631–634

192 Filie A C, Abati A, Fetsch P, Azumi N. Hyaluronate binding probe and CD44 in the differential diagnosis of malignant effusions: disappointing results in cytology material. *Diagn Cytopathol* 1998; **18**(6): 473–474

193 Lantuejoul S, Laverrierre M H, Sturm N *et al.* NCAM (neural cell adhesion molecule) expression in malignant mesotheliomas. *Hum Pathol* 2000; **31**:415–421

194 Berena J, Sun N C. Application of Leu M5 (CD11c) antibody in the cytodiagnosis of body fluids: preliminary results. *J Clin Lab Anal* 1993; 7: 19–25

195 Kondi-Paphitis A, Addis B J. Secretory component in pulmonary adenocarcinoma and mesothelioma. *Histopathology* 1986; **10**: 1279–1287

196 Whitaker D. The cytology of malignant mesothelioma. *Cytopathology* 2000; **11**: 139–151

197 Yu G, Soma L, Hahn S, Friedberg J S. Changing clinical course of patients with malignant mesothelioma: implications for FNA cytology and utility of immunocytochemical staining. *Diagn Cytopathol* 2001; **24**: 322–327

198 Churg A, Colby T V, Cagle P *et al.* The separation of benign and malignant mesothelial proliferations. *Am J Surg Pathol* 2000; **24**: 1183–1200

199 Battifora H. The pleura. In: Sternberg S S ed. *Diagnostic Surgical Pathology*, 2nd edn. New York: Raven, 1994

200 Saleh H, Bober P, Tabaczka M T. Value of Ki67 immunostain in identification of malignancy in serous effusions. *Diagn Cytopathol* 1999; **20**(1): 24–28

201 Warnke R A, Rouse R V. Limitations encountered in the application of tissue section diagnosis to the study of lymphomas and related disorders. *Hum Pathol* 1985; **16**: 326–331

202 McDonnell J M, Beschorner W E, Kuhajda F P, deMent S H. Common leukocyte antigen staining of a primitive sarcoma. *Cancer* 1987; **59**: 1438–1441

203 Ambros I M, Ambros P F, Strehl S *et al.* MIC 2 is a specific marker for Ewing's sarcoma and peripheral primitive neuroectodermal tumour. *Cancer* 1991; **67**: 1886–1893

204 Fisher C. Synovial sarcoma: ultrastructural and immunohistochemical features of epithelial differentiation in monophasic and biphasic tumours. *Hum Pathol* 1986; **17**: 996–1008

205 Fletcher C D M, Beham A, Bekir S *et al.* Epithelioid angiosarcoma of soft tissue: a distinctive tumor readily mistaken for an epithelial neoplasm. *Am J Surg Pathol* 1991; **15**: 915–924

206 Williams G. Unravelling the unknown primary. *CPD Bulletin* 1999; **1**(4): 140–143

207 Lagendijk J H, Mullink H, Van Diest P J *et al.* Immunohistochemical differentiation between primary adenocarcinomas of the ovary and ovarian metastases of colonic and breast origin. Comparison between a statistical and an intuitive approach. *J Clin Pathol* 1999; **52**(4): 283–290

208 Lagendijk J A, Mullink H, Van Diest P J *et al.* Tracing the unknown primary using immunohistochemistry: differential diagnosis between colonic and ovarian carcinomas as primary sites. *Hum Pathol* 1998; **29**: 491–497

209 Ascoli V, Taccogna S, Scalzo CC, Nardi F. Utility of cytokeratin 20 in identifying the origin of metastatic carcinomas in effusions. *Diagn Cytopathol* 1995; **12**(4): 303–308

210 Filho A L, Bisi H, Alves V A F *et al.* Adenocarcinoma in females detected in serous effusions. Cytomorphological aspects and immunocytochemical reactivity to cytokeratins 7 and 20. *Acta Cytol* 1997; **41**(4): 961–971

211 Eisenberger C F, Wu L, Nichol T *et al.* Comparative microsatellite analysis in discerning origin of disseminated tumour: the case of a patient with malignant ascites and a history of multiple tumours. *Hum Pathol* 1999; **30**: 1111–1113

212 Tawfik M S, Coleman D V. C-myc expression in exfoliated cells in serous effusions. *Cytopathology* 1991; **2**: 83–92

213 Geradts J. Immunohistochemical prognostic and predictive markers in common tumours. *CPD Bulletin Cell Pathol* 1999; **1**(4): 144–147

214 Gondos B, McIntosh K M, Renston R H, King E B. Application of electron microscopy in the definitive diagnosis of effusions. *Acta Cytol* 1978; **22**: 297–304

215 Beals T F. Scanning electron microscopy of body fluids. *Diagn Cytopathol* 1992; **8**: 266–271

216 Sakuma N, Kamei T, Ishihara T. Ultrastructure of pleural mesothelioma and pulmonary adenocarcinoma in malignant effusions as compared with reactive mesothelial cells. *Acta Cytol* 1999; **43**(5): 777–785

217 Di Muzio M, Spoletini L, Strizzi L *et al.* Basal lamina reduplication in malignant epithelioid pleural mesothelioma. *Ultrastruct Pathol* 1998; **22**: 467–475

218 Kobzik L, Antman K H, Warhol M J. The distinction of mesothelioma from adenocarcinoma in malignant effusions by electron microscopy. *Acta Cytol* 1985; **29**: 219–225

219 Beals T F. Cytology and electron microscopy. In: Trump B F, Jones R T eds. *Diagnostic Electron Microscopy*. Chichester: John Wiley, 1980

220 Woyke S, Domagala W, Olszewski W. Alveolar cell carcinoma of the lung: an ultrastructural study of the cancer cells detected in pleural fluid. *Acta Cytol* 1972; **16**: 63

221 Benning T L, Finlay J L, Silverman J F. Alveolar cell carcinoma presenting as malignant pericardial effusion: diagnosis by electron microscopy. *Ultrastructural Pathology* 1992; **16**: 303–306

222 Zarbo R J. Flow cytometric DNA analysis of effusions. A new test seeking validation. *Am J Clin Pathol* 1991; **95**: 2–4

223 Sinton E B, Carver R K, Morgan D L *et al.* Prospective study of concurrent ploidy analysis and routine cytopathology in body cavity fluids. *Arch Pathol Lab Med* 1990; **114**: 188–194

224 Rijken A, Dekker A, Taylor S *et al.* Diagnostic value of DNA analysis in effusions by flow cytometry and image analysis. A prospective study on 102 patients as compared with cytologic examination. *Am J Clin Pathol* 1991; **95**: 6–12

225 Saha I, Dey P, Vhora H, Nijhawan R. Role of DNA flow cytometry and image analysis on effusion cytology. *Diagn Cytopathol* 2000; **22**: 81–85

226 Bousfield L R, Greenberg M L, Pacey F. Cytogenetic diagnosis of cancer from body fluids. *Acta Cytol* 1985; **29**: 768–774

227 Heim S, Mitelman F. Cytogenetics of solid tumours. In: Antony P P, MacSween R N M eds. *Recent Advances in Histopathology*. Edinburgh: Churchill Livingstone, 1992

228 Fiegl M, Kaufmann H, Zojer N *et al.* Malignant cell detection by fluorescence *in*

situ hybridization (FISH) in effusions from patients with carcinoma. *Hum Pathol* 2000; **31**: 448–455

229 Xiao S, Renshaw A, Cibas E S *et al*. Novel fluorescence *in situ* hybridization approaches in solid tumours. *Am J Pathol* 1995; **147**: 896–904

230 Fletcher J A. DNA *in situ* hybridization as an adjunct to tumour diagnosis. *Am J Clin Pathol* 1999; **112**: S11–S18

231 Kwee W S, Veldhuizen R W, Alons C L *et al*. Quantitative differences between benign and malignant mesothelial cells in pleural fluid. *Acta Cytol* 1982; **26**: 401–406

232 Marchevsky A M, Hauptman E, Gil J, Watson C. Computerised interactive morphometry as an aid in the diagnosis of pleural effusions. *Acta Cytol* 1987; **31**: 131–136

233 Scott N, Sutton J, Gray C. Morphometric diagnosis of serous effusions: refinements of differences between benign and malignant cases by use of outlying values and larger sample size. *J Clin Pathol* 1989; **42**: 607–612

234 van Molengraft F J J M, van't Hot M A, Herman C J, Vooijs P G. Quantitative light microscopy of atypical mesothelial cells and malignant cells in ascitic fluid. *Analyt Quant Cytol Histol* 1982; **4**: 217–220

235 Boon M E, Veldhuizen R W, Ruinaard C *et al*. Qualitative distinctive differences between the vacuoles of mesothelioma cells and cells from metastatic carcinoma exfoliated in pleural fluid. *Acta Cytol* 1984; **28**: 443–449

236 van Diest P J, Baak J P A. Morphometry. In: Bibbo M ed. *Comprehensive Cytopathology*. Philadelphia: Saunders, 1991

237 Underwood J C E, Giri D D. Nucleolar organiser regions as diagnostic discriminants for malignancy. *J Pathol* 1988; **155**: 95–96

238 Ribotta M, Donna A, Betta P G *et al*. Quantitative analysis of nucleoli and nucleolar organizer regions in cultured primary human normal, reactive and malignant mesothelial cells. *Pathol Res Pract* 1992; **188**: 536–540

239 Motherby H, Nadjari B, Remmerbach T *et al*. Static DNA cytometry as a diagnostic aid in effusion cytology: II. DNA aneuploidy for identification of neoplastic cells in equivocal effusions. *Anal Quant Cytol Histol* 1998; **20**(3): 162–168

240 Thunnissen F B J M, Buchholtz R T F, Woutersen D P *et al*. Clinical value of DNA image cytometry in effusions with atypia. *Diagn Cytopathol* 1999; **21**(2): 112–116

241 Berois N, Varangot M, Aizen B *et al*. Molecular detection of cancer cells in bone marrow and peripheral blood of patients with operable breast cancer. *Eur J Cancer* 2000; **36**(6): 717–723

242 Ahrendt S A, Chow J T, Xu L H *et al*. Molecular detection of tumour cells in bronchoalveolar lavage fluid from patients with early stage lung cancer. *J Natl Cancer Inst* 1999; **91**(4): 332–339

243 Rhodes C H, Glantz M J, Glantz L *et al*. A comparison of polymerase chain reaction examination of cerebrospinal fluid and conventional cytology in the diagnosis of lymphomatous meningitis. *Cancer* 1996; **77**(3): 543–548

244 Galoin S, Daste G, Apoil P A *et al*. Polymerase chain reaction on cerebrospinal fluid cells in the detection of leptomeningeal involvement by B cell lymphoma and leukaemia: a novel strategy and its implications. *Br J Haematol* 1997; **99**(1): 122–130

245 Burchill S A, Selby P J. Molecular detection of low-level disease in patients with Cancer. *J Pathol* 2000; **190**: 6–14

246 Sakaguchi M, Virmani A K, Ashfaq *et al*. Development of a sensitive, specific reverse transcriptase polymerase chain reaction based assay for epithelial tumour cells in effusions. *Br J Cancer* 1999; **79**(3–4) 416–422

247 Yamashita K, Kuba T, Shinoda H *et al*. Detection of K-ras point mutations in the supernatants of peritoneal and pleural effusions for diagnosis complementary to cytological examination. *Am J Clin Pathol* 1998; **109**(6) 704–711

248 Zojer N, Fiegl M, Angerler J *et al*. Interphase fluorescence *in situ* hybridization improves the detection of malignant cells in effusions from breast Cancer patients. *Br J Cancer* 1997; **75**(3): 403–407

249 Murphy M, Signoretti S, Nasser I *et al*. Detection of concurrent/recurrent non-Hodgkin's lymphoma in effusions by PCR. *Hum Pathol* 1999; **30**: 1361–1366

250 Pinto M M, Bernstein L H, Rudolph R A *et al*. Diagnostic efficiency of carcinoembryonic antigen and CA125 in the cytological evaluation of effusions. *Arch Pathol Lab Med* 1992; **116**: 626–631

251 Siddiqui R A, Kochhar R, Singh V *et al*. Evaluation of fibronectin as a marker of malignant ascites. *J Gastroenterol Hepatol* 1992; **7**: 161–164

252 Hjerpe A. Liquid-chromatographic determination of hyaluronic acid in pleural and ascitic fluids. *Clin Chem* 1986; **32**: 952–956

253 Castor W C, Naylor B. Acid mucopolysaccharide composition of serous effusions. Study of 100 patients with neoplastic and non-neoplastic conditions. *Cancer* 1967; **20**: 462–466

254 Harington J S, Wagner J C, Smith M. The detection of hyaluronic acid in pleural fluids of cases with diffuse pleural mesotheliomas. *Br J Exp Pathol* 1963; **44**: 81–83

255 Rapellino M, Pecchio F, Baldi S *et al*. Tumor-associated trypsin inhibitor (TATI) in pleural effusions. *Scand J Clin Lab Invest* 1991; **207**(suppl): 47–49

256 Chondros K, Dapolla V, Stringou E *et al*. Correlation of total (TSA) and lipid and bound (LSA) sialic acid levels with cytology of cyst or body fluids in Cancer patients. *AntiCancer Res* 1991; **11**: 2103–2106

257 Krogerus L A, Andersson L C. A simple method for the preparation of paraffin-embedded cell blocks from fine needle aspirates, effusions and brushings. *Acta Cytol* 1988; **32**: 585–587

258 Hussain O A N, Millet J A, Grainger J M. Use of poly-l-lysine coated slides in the preparation of cell samples for diagnostic cytology with special reference to urine samples. *J Clin Pathol* 1980; **33**: 309–311

259 Aratake Y, Tamura K, Kotani T, Ohtaki S. Application of the avidin-biotin complex method for the light microscopical analysis of lymphocyte subsets with monoclonal antibodies on air dried smears. *Acta Cytol* 1988; **32**: 117–122

260 Nuovo G J, Silverstein S J. Methods of laboratory investigation. Comparison of formalin, buffered formalin and Bouin's fixative on the detection of human papilloma virus deoxyribonucleic acid from genital lesions. *Lab Invest* 1988; **59**: 720–724

261 Croissant O, Breitburd F, Orth G. Specificity of cytopathic effects of cutaneous papillomaviruses. In: Jablonska S ed. *Clinical Dermatology*. Philadelphia: Lippincott, 1985; 43–55

262 Nuovo G J, Richart R M. Buffered formalin is the superior fixative for the detection of HPV DNA by *in situ* hybridization analysis. *Am J Pathol* 1989; **134**: 837–842

263 Gall K, Pavicic D, Audy-Jurkovic S, Pavellic J. PCR amplification of DNA from stained cytological smears. *J Clin Pathol* 1993; **46**: 378–379

264 Mayall F, Cursons R, Jacobson G, Chang B. Single-strand conformational polymorphism (SSCP)-detected p53 gene mutations are a less sensitive marker of malignancy in pleural fluids than p53 immunostaining. *Cytopathology* 1999; **10**: 259–262

265 Howes G P, Stephenson J, Humphreys S. Sensitive and reliable PCR and sequencing used to detect p53 point mutations in fine needle aspirates of the breast. *J Clin Pathol* 1996; **49**: 570–573

6 Mesotheliomas

Darrel Whitaker, Greg Sterrett and Keith B. Shilkin

Introduction

Although mesotheliomas are relatively uncommon neoplasms, they have attracted considerable interest, out of proportion to their frequency. This appears to be due to a number of factors, including difficulty in establishing a pre-mortem diagnosis, the medicolegal issues centring around compensation for asbestos exposed patients, and also the controversy over the histogenesis of mesothelioma. The incidence of disease has also been rising in many areas, however a trends analysis suggests that at least in some countries the incidence for mesothelioma will peak in the next 30 years (2030)[1].

While the mesothelial lining of the serosal cavities has been recognized since the early days of histology[2], the recognition and acceptance of mesothelioma as a primary neoplasm of the mesothelium has been more recent. Only after the link between asbestos exposure and the subsequent development of malignant mesothelioma was demonstrated by Wagner et al. in 1960[3] was malignant mesothelioma widely accepted as a distinct entity.

Establishing a diagnosis of mesothelioma can be a significant challenge, especially with limited material or away from centres of high prevalence where there is expertise. The diagnostic difficulty stems in part from the marked diversity of histological differentiation, with epithelial, spindle, biphasic and sometimes anaplastic or unusual growth patterns; and partly from the histological similarity in some cases to metastatic adenocarcinoma or other malignancy.

Given the lack of any effective treatment for mesothelioma, the short life expectancy following diagnosis and the need for unequivocal diagnosis in order to support claims for compensation, the clinician's expectation and the responsibility of the pathologist are onerous. Furthermore, the laboratory's role in helping establish the presence, type and degree of any asbestos exposure places the pathologist and laboratory scientist in a rather unique position in the complex medicolegal field.

Controversies over histogenesis have resolved into two main points of view: some argue that the diversity of histological differentiation indicates a multipotential subserosal stem cell[4] as the source of these tumours; others who have studied 'early' mesothelioma believe that surface mesothelial cells are the target of neoplastic change. The latter concept includes the idea of *in situ* mesothelioma[5] and the potential for treatment of this early stage.

Most malignant mesotheliomas initially present as a serous effusion, less often as a pleural mass without effusion. The role of cytology, either of effusions or fine needle aspiration (FNA) samples, in the diagnostic work-up is therefore always important. A detailed knowledge of the cytology of malignant mesothelioma is thus now essential for all who practise diagnostic cytopathology.

Histological classification

Table 6.1 shows a working histopathological classification of mesothelioma and of those mesothelial related neoplasms likely to be encountered in diagnostic cytopathology, either in fluids or FNA samples.

Malignant mesothelioma refers to the histologically aggressive diffusely growing tumours, often associated with asbestos exposure, occurring in the pleura, peritoneum and occasionally the pericardium or tunica vaginalis of the testis. They present as epithelial, biphasic, sarcomatous (spindle cell or desmoplastic) or anaplastic neoplasms (Figs 6.1–6.4). The main features used in diagnosis are the presence of tubuloglandular or papillary structures, biphasic growth pattern, cuboidal nature of tumour cells, eosinophilic dense cytoplasm, immunocytochemical profile including the absence of adenocarcinoma markers and electron microscopic

Table 6.1	Working classification of mesothelial related neoplasms
Malignant mesothelioma	Epithelial
	Biphasic
	Sarcomatous
Unusual or rare variants	
Other neoplasms of mesothelial origin or differentiation	Well-differentiated papillary mesothelioma of peritoneum
	Cystic mesothelioma
	Adenomatoid tumour of male and female genital tract
Neoplasms likely to be of subserosal origin	Benign fibrous tumour of pleura (so-called localized fibrous mesothelioma, benign pleural fibroma)
	Localized malignant fibrous tumours of pleura

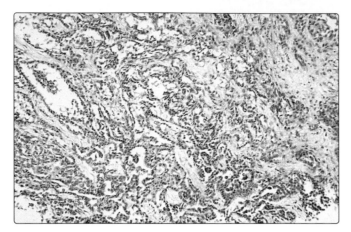

Fig. 6.1 Histological section: mesothelioma, tubulopapillary type. (H&E × LP)

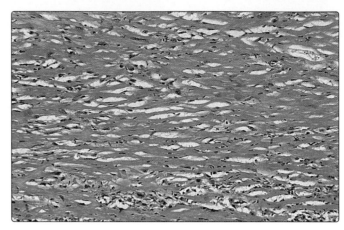

Fig. 6.3 Histological section: desmoplastic mesothelioma. (H&E × LP)

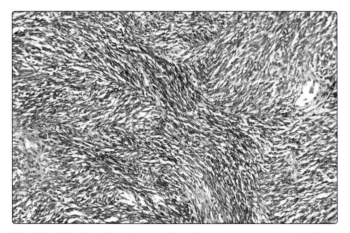

Fig. 6.2 Histological section: spindle cell or sarcomatous mesothelioma. (H&E × LP)

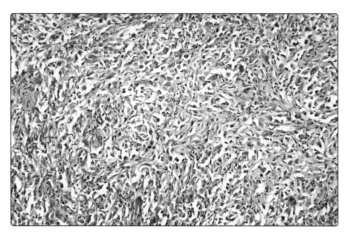

Fig. 6.4 Histological section: anaplastic mesothelioma. (H&E × LP)

evidence of long, thin surface microvilli without a radiating glycocalyx.

Well-differentiated papillary mesotheliomas are uncommon benign neoplasms unrelated to asbestos exposure. They usually present as a pedunculated peritoneal mass often found incidentally at operation. Histologically they appear benign, consisting of a conglomerate of regular cuboidal cells with a simple papillary configuration. Their histological, immunocytochemical and ultrastructural characteristics are indicative of mesothelial derivation.

Cystic mesotheliomas are uncommon cystic tumours unrelated to asbestos exposure and are mainly found in the peritoneal cavity of females. They have a variable behaviour, some benign but prone to recur, while others are more aggressive and may be lethal. Histologically, the tumour is composed of masses of cystic spaces lined by flat or cuboidal cells that immunocytochemically and ultrastructurally demonstrate mesothelial characteristics.

Benign pleural fibroma (localized benign tumour, solitary fibrous tumour, so-called localized fibrous mesothelioma) are tumours of fibrous tissue with or without entrapped

bronchial or mesothelial cells. They grow in an expansive fashion, are generally benign, and rarely cause a serous effusion. They are unrelated to asbestos exposure and are not mesotheliomas despite the frequent use of this term as a synonym.

Malignant fibrous tumours of the pleura comprise a rare group of malignant spindle cell tumours that are usually localized to the pleural cavity. Some are of mesothelial cell origin and others encompass malignant fibrous histiocytoma and other pleural sarcomas. They are not linked with asbestos exposure nor do they usually present with a serous effusion. Many may be chest wall tumours that come to occupy a predominantly pleural location.

For detailed discussion of the classification of mesotheliomas, the reader is referred to the work of Henderson et al.[6].

Aetiology and pathogenesis

Asbestos and malignant mesothelioma

The relationship between asbestos exposure and mesothelioma is now established beyond doubt. The epidemiological and experimental evidence for the oncogenic effect of asbestos on mesothelial tissue is overwhelming[6]. Epidemiological evidence is based on the recognition of high incidence levels of malignant mesothelioma in persons exposed to asbestos. The background incidence of mesothelioma in the unexposed population is 1–2 per million persons per year.

Crocidolite or blue asbestos has been found to be particularly oncogenic and our major experience with mesothelioma has resulted from the operation of a blue asbestos mine and mill at Wittenoom in the north of Western Australia from 1939–66[7]. At the time of writing, the incidence of mesothelioma in Western Australian men is 45 per million per year, the world's highest. Incidence rates of up to 9000 per million per year can occur in people who have been involved in the mining, milling or manufacture of asbestos or asbestos products[8].

The frequency with which malignant mesotheliomas can be directly associated with asbestos exposure varies from series to series, and may be as high as 80%[8]. Another rare cause of mesothelioma in both humans and animals is radiation exposure[9–11] and a small number of so-called spontaneous mesotheliomas seem to exist.

Experimental evidence comes from laboratory animal and tissue culture studies. Various laboratory animals develop mesothelioma following serosal implantation of asbestos. Animal models and, more recently, cell lines have provided a focus for the investigation of the nature and possible mechanisms of the pathogenesis of mesothelioma. Asbestos induced animal mesotheliomas have a similar histomorphology and ultrastructure to the human form and likewise the cytology of mesothelioma in domestic and laboratory animals is similar to that of human mesothelioma[12–16].

From the original work of Stanton and Wrench[17] it seems that long thin fibres (greater than 8 μm in length and less than 0.15 μm wide) are the most oncogenic for mesothelial tissues regardless of chemical composition of the fibre. The exact sequence of events leading to the development of mesothelioma is unknown but recent studies have shown that asbestos fibres cause genetic damage in target cells, either directly by causing chromosomal breaks or indirectly through cytoskeletal filament alteration[18]. This genetic damage may result in aneuploidy, translocation, deletion or other chromosomal damage. Mesothelial cells have proved extremely susceptible to the clastogenic effects of asbestos, though no unique pattern of chromosomal damage has emerged.

Molecular biological studies of the effects of genetic changes are still in their infancy. Lechner[19] found that this asbestos induced chromosomal damage conferred a growth advantage on the affected cells. Some mesothelioma cell lines have expressed C-SIS oncogene and because this codes for part of the platelet derived growth factor (PDGF) which is mitogenic for normal mesothelial cells, an autocrine growth mechanism has been claimed for the interaction between asbestos fibre and mesothelial cell in its transformation[20,21].

Mesothelioma *in situ*

Several studies of human and animal mesotheliomas have made reference to the existence of a preinvasive stage of mesothelioma or mesothelioma *in situ*[5]. This concept has implications for the pathogenesis of mesothelioma and also for the diagnostic histopathologist and cytopathologist. We have seen several cases of 'early mesothelioma' characterized by a gross pleuroscopic appearance of miniscule 'grains of sand' on the pleural surface or very small nodules. Biopsies from these sites show a histological pattern of non-invasive mesothelial growth, occurring either as a monolayer of atypical surface mesothelial cells or as tubular and papillary surface extensions of atypical mesothelial cells (Fig. 6.5). These lesions have stained strongly with the proliferation marker epithelial membrane antigen (EMA, Fig. 6.6) and have also contained levels of

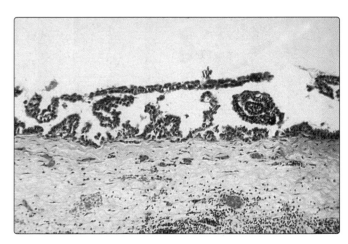

Fig. 6.5 Histological section: mesothelioma *in situ*. Superficial papillary non-invasive growth. (H&E × LP)

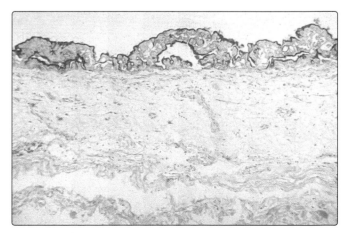

Fig. 6.6 Histological section: mesothelioma *in situ*. Surface non-invasive growth showing strong cellular membrane staining with epithelial membrane antigen (EMA). (IPOX, EMA × LP)

silver-rich nucleolar organizer regions (AgNORs) thought to be consistent with malignancy (see p. 215). In our hands, prominent papillary formation of EMA positive, AgNOR-rich mesothelial cells is characteristic of these early lesions.

The acceptance of *in situ* mesothelioma may have considerable implications for diagnosis. From the histopathologist's point of view the presence or absence of invasion may not then be the sole criterion used in the distinction between benign mesothelial reaction and mesothelioma. The presence of prominent surface growth should prompt further investigation using such ancillary tests as EMA staining and AgNOR counts. In our hands such testing has enhanced the sensitivity of diagnosis of invasive mesothelioma[22] as well as *in-situ* lesions[23].

For the cytopathologist, the importance lies in recognizing that while the cytological picture is unlike a benign reactive proliferation it can be identical to invasive mesothelioma and hence could lead to a 'false positive' cytological interpretation. In either situation, whether histopathological or cytological, if doubt exists and gross tumour is not evident then investigation should proceed by way of pleuroscopy.

Technical aspects

The place of cytology in the diagnosis of mesothelioma is now established[24,25]. Up to 90% of malignant mesotheliomas initially present with serous effusion and because effusion cytology is a safe, quick, inexpensive and reliable test for serosal malignancy, cytodiagnosis should be considered as the first and foremost laboratory investigation in the diagnostic work-up. Furthermore, in the absence of effusions, pleural-based peripheral or, more rarely, pulmonary fissural lesions and metastatic sites such as lymph nodes are readily accessible to FNA sampling[26], which is similarly a reliable, quick and virtually complication-free investigation.

Our approach[27] to the tissue diagnosis of malignant mesothelioma is depicted in Figure 6.7. The pathway chosen depends on whether effusion is present or not. In either situation, we prefer to receive, additionally if possible, a small tissue biopsy sample for histopathological assessment. This combined sampling approach by biopsy and cytology has resulted in maximum sensitivity in the diagnosis of malignant mesothelioma[28]. In this respect our results for this combined approach in the diagnosis of mesothelioma are similar to those obtained with metastatic serosal malignancy[29].

The importance of technique

Without doubt, the single most important consideration in determining whether a cytological diagnosis of malignant mesothelioma can be made with confidence is the degree of technical dedication and skill used in preparing the samples and making the smears. With serous effusion samples we prefer to receive all the fluid which is collected in bottles containing anticoagulant/preservative solution to prevent the formation of fibrin clots and to facilitate blood separation and cell concentration[30]. A note should be made as to the physical appearance of the specimen, especially whether the fluid is viscous as this may indicate an elevated level of hyaluronic acid, which is sometimes present in malignant mesothelioma.

Adequate attention must be given to cell concentration and the removal of blood. With heavily bloodstained samples, the use of density gradients such as Ficoll hypaque is of great advantage in facilitating cellular concentration and the separation of red blood cells. We use both cytocentrifuge preparations and direct smears prepared by the blood film method, and find them complementary. The cytocentrifuge preparations are better for poorly cellular fluids whereas the direct smears provide a better cell distribution in cellular samples, especially those with many cell aggregates. We routinely employ MGG as well as Papanicolaou stained smears as both provide useful information on the nature of the cell cytoplasm (see later).

One crucial step in preparation is the cell concentration procedure, when it is important to remove all traces of

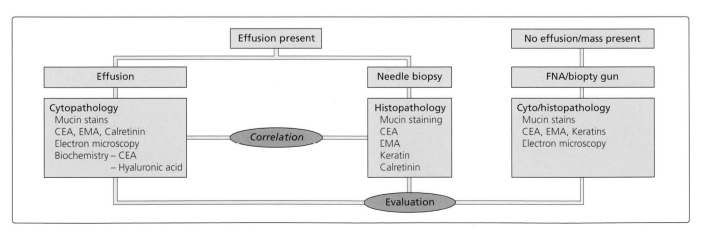

Fig. 6.7   The investigation of suspected mesothelioma.

supernatant from the cell pellet before the direct smears are made. In this way, maximum cell concentration is obtained and the cellular material adheres to the slide and is less likely to float off when placed in fixative solution. Furthermore, this step helps make a thin, transparent smear consisting of a cell monolayer.

Some of the same cell deposit is fixed in formol sublimate for processing into cell blocks. Sections from these are used for all special stains and immunoperoxidase testing. While the value of cell block preparation in effusion cytology in general has been questioned[31], we have no doubt that cell blocks are invaluable for the accurate cytological diagnosis of mesothelioma.

As a further step, some of the cell deposit is fixed in 25% glutaraldehyde for ultrastructural evaluation. Finally, the supernatant can be stored at −20°C for possible future evaluation of hyaluronic acid and carcinoembryonic antigen levels (CEA) (see later). Our serous effusion protocol for the diagnosis of mesothelioma is depicted in Figure 6.8. On reviewing the cytological diagnosis of mesothelioma it was clear that dedication to technical excellence played a vital role in quality of results[1] and that poor samples were the cause of poor results[32].

The multidisciplinary approach

In some instances the cytomorphology may be characteristic and permit a definite diagnosis of malignant mesothelioma on light microscopy alone. However, cytodiagnosis of this site is challenging and is best practised in conjunction with other supporting tests.

Ancillary testing can include cytochemistry, immunocytochemistry, electron microscopy, biochemistry of supernatant fluid, or quantitative studies including AgNOR counting. Information gathered from these various tests not only helps raise the confidence of a cytological diagnosis but also improves the accuracy of diagnosis[25,33,34] and reduces the chance of a false positive diagnosis of malignancy or error in tumour typing.

Malignant mesothelioma

Effusions

Following the excellent early reports[35,36] there have been an ever increasing number of descriptions of the cytological appearances of malignant mesothelioma as seen in serous effusions[31,25,34,51] and in FNA material[26,51–57], reflecting a wealth of experience, albeit somewhat concentrated in regions linked with past industrial exposure to asbestos[25,35,43]. In our view the cytological diagnosis of malignant mesothelioma can be a relatively straightforward exercise though it is often a challenge and occasionally, especially in desmoplastic cases, impossible.

There is general agreement that diagnosis of malignant mesothelioma by effusion cytology involves a two-stage process: first, the distinction of malignant mesothelioma from some form of reactive mesothelial proliferation and, second, its distinction from metastatic malignancy involving the serosa. Because the cytological diagnosis of malignancy is often the greater challenge, we have chosen to pay particular attention to this area.

Cytological criteria for malignancy: mesothelioma effusions

▶ Abundant cell aggregates
▶ Nuclear atypia
▶ Cell enlargement
▶ Macronucleoli

When dealing with epithelial or biphasic mesotheliomas, the single most valuable diagnostic criterion of malignancy is a very cellular effusion with many cell aggregates (Figs 6.9, 6.10). Aggregates range in size from small groups of 20–30 cells to those consisting of 100–200 cells. They may be round, elongated, papilloid or of variable shape. Regardless of size or shape, aggregates in mesothelioma are usually three-dimensional tissue fragments as opposed to

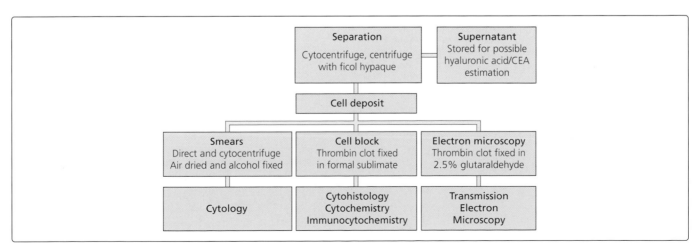

Fig. 6.8 Extended effusion cytology protocol.

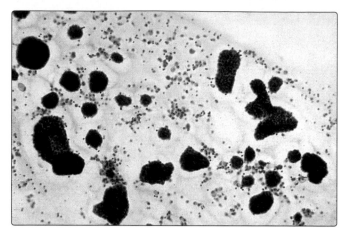

Fig. 6.9   Pleural fluid: cell aggregates. Mesothelioma; many large papillary aggregates. (Papanicolaou × MP)

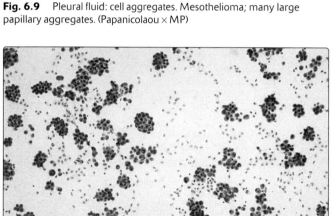

Fig. 6.10   Pleural fluid: cell aggregates. Mesothelioma; many small cell clusters of malignant mesothelial cells. (Papanicolaou × MP)

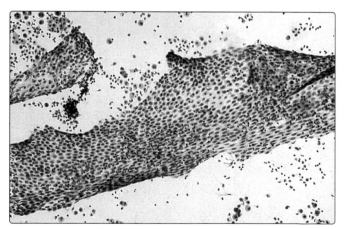

Fig. 6.11   Pleural fluid: benign mesothelium. Flat monolayered sheets of mesothelial cells. (Papanicolaou × LP)

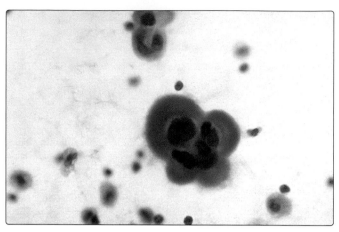

Fig. 6.12   Pleural fluid: nuclear atypia. Cells with mesothelial characteristics; enlarged irregular hyperchromatic nuclei; multinucleation. (Papanicolaou × HP)

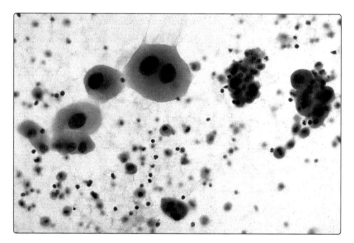

Fig. 6.13   Pleural fluid: enlarged cells. Population of very enlarged malignant mesothelial cells up to 10 times normal size. (Papanicolaou × MP)

flat sheets, the latter being more typical of a benign process (Fig. 6.11).

Nuclear atypia is neither common nor pronounced in mesothelioma[43] and only in about 50–75% of cases does the degree of nuclear abnormality contribute to a diagnosis of malignancy[34]. Nuclear hyperchromasia is usually mild, and irregular nuclear contours are only seen in a small proportion of cases. It should be stressed that generally, as a criterion of malignancy in effusions, nuclear atypia is best and more reliably assessed in small clusters of cells rather than in single cells.

Cell and nuclear enlargement is more pronounced in mesothelioma (Figs 6.12, 6.13) than in reactive proliferation (see Fig. 6.18). This was first described by Naylor[36] who referred to these enlarged cells as 'gigantic forms' of mesothelial cells. Its diagnostic value was subsequently confirmed by other workers[40,46,58]. This feature is variable and in any given case only a few cells may be greatly enlarged. Cytomegaly is usually accompanied by nuclear enlargement without disturbance of the nucleocytoplasmic ratio.

Macronucleoli cannot be used as a sole criterion of malignancy; however, if present in many mesothelial cells they should prompt concern and careful evaluation as they are seen particularly in well-differentiated mesothelioma (Figs 6.14, 6.15)[25,48].

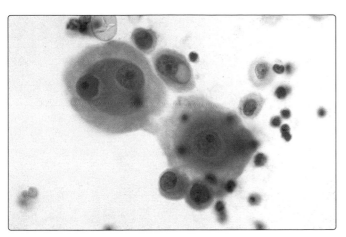

Fig. 6.14 Pleural fluid: prominent nucleoli. Enlarged malignant mesothelioma cells with macronucleoli. (Papanicolaou × HP)

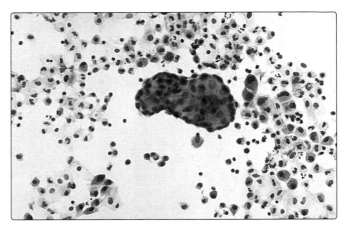

Fig. 6.16 Pleural fluid: benign cell cluster. A well-defined cluster of mesothelial cells in a benign pericardial effusion. (Papanicolaou × HP)

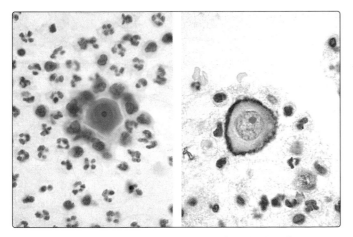

Fig. 6.15 Pleural fluid: prominent nucleoli. Left: isolated malignant mesothelial cell with a solitary central nucleolus and a cuff of inflammatory cells (Papanicolaou × HP). Right: single malignant mesothelial cell with macronucleolus and EMA positive cell border. (EMA)

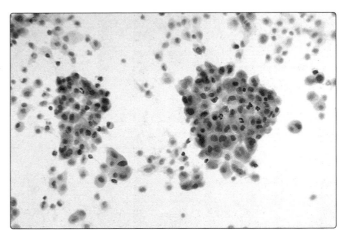

Fig. 6.17 Pleural fluid: benign cell aggregates. Loose aggregates of mesothelial cells in pleural fluid; case of pulmonary embolism. (Papanicolaou × HP)

In summary, we agree with Spriggs and Boddington[45] that 'there is no known criterion nor constellation of criteria which are universally diagnostic of malignancy', however the constellation of criteria described here are very useful in establishing malignancy in suspected cases of mesothelioma; their judicious use has been associated with no false positive diagnoses of malignancy in our hands.

Diagnostic pitfalls

Several diagnostic difficulties can arise. Three main differential diagnostic problems demand attention:

► Cell aggregates in a benign process as a result of a reactive mesothelial proliferation
► Nuclear atypia in reactive mesothelial cells
► Well-differentiated malignant mesothelioma

Because the presence of many cell aggregates is such a key feature for the diagnosis of malignancy there is a need to be

aware of pitfalls when using this criterion. There is general agreement that *within the pleural cavity* the presence of many large cell aggregates signifies malignancy. In the pericardium, and to a lesser degree in the peritoneum, this criterion is of less diagnostic value because there are a few well documented cases of prominent reactive papillary aggregates shedding into a benign pericardial effusion[59,60]. We have seen somewhat similar cases following chest trauma (Fig. 6.16) and in a pericardial effusion subsequent to heart surgery. Such large aggregates of mesothelial cells have also been described in peritoneal effusions[49,61]. Loose aggregates of benign mesothelial cells are a common finding in an effusion subsequent to pulmonary infarction (Fig. 6.17).

One must also make some distinction between effusions and specimens obtained by washing. Many large aggregates of benign mesothelial cells, some surrounding a mass of collagen, 'collagen balls', with or without psammoma bodies (see Fig. 6.52), are well documented in peritoneal washings[2,62]. In female patients, they are believed to originate from the ovarian surface[62].

Reactive mesothelial proliferation is common at the serosal surface covering the tunica vaginalis; hydrocoele fluids often contain many small well formed papillary aggregates identical to the 'collagen balls' described by Wojcik and Naylor[62]. Malignant mesothelioma can occur in this site[62], and give rise to malignant effusions[63]. We agree with Spriggs and Boddington[45], who stress the need for extreme caution when interpreting the significance of papillary aggregates in hydrocoele fluids; almost all such cases will be benign.

Experience suggests that nuclear atypia in single cells or small clusters of reactive mesothelial cells is of lesser concern in the cytological diagnosis of mesothelioma. Nuclear atypia has been described after radiation or chemotherapy[41,49], in dialysis fluids[64] and as a consequence of pancreatitis[65]. It is our policy to be cautious in diagnosing malignancy solely on the basis of a dispersed population of atypical cells. Small numbers of hyperchromatic cells or cells with irregular nuclei are sometimes seen in benign effusions where cells show degenerative effects (Fig. 6.18). Likewise, multinucleate mesothelial cells with hyperchromatic nuclei should generally be disregarded when assessing a difficult case.

Most cytologists now seem to be well aware of the potential pitfall of such mesothelial atypia in the diagnosis of malignancy, and we are not aware of any literature report in the last 20 years of a false positive diagnosis of malignancy based on misinterpretation of reactive mesothelial cells. If in an individual case doubt exists, then immunocytochemical testing with EMA and CEA to confirm malignancy is strongly advised (see later).

Well-differentiated epithelial mesotheliomas can sometimes shed abundant single cells and small cell clusters that lack cellular pleomorphism and nuclear atypia (Fig. 6.19). In these situations, it may be difficult to establish malignancy on cytology alone yet very cellular effusions that are composed entirely of mesothelial cells should be viewed with concern and ancillary testing performed in these cases. Lack of nuclear atypia in well-differentiated malignant mesothelioma can partly be explained by the fact that many mesotheliomas have a diploid nuclear DNA profile when ploidy studies are carried out.

Criteria for mesothelial differentiation

A critical microscopic evaluation of the cellular material of serous effusions includes an assessment of the number, distribution and form of individual cells, an assessment of the size, shape and structure of cell aggregates and an assessment of the cellular background. The following criteria have been found useful in the distinction of malignant mesothelioma from metastatic serosal malignancy (usually adenocarcinoma).

▶ Lack of a 'foreign' population
▶ Structure of cell aggregates
▶ Cytoplasmic characteristics
▶ Cell-to-cell relationships
▶ Vacuoles
▶ Collagen-basement membrane
▶ Glycogen
▶ Squamous-like cells
▶ Hyaluronic acid background network

Cell population

Most observers[38,40,43,44] have noted that in mesothelioma, as opposed to metastatic malignancy, a second or 'foreign' cell population is absent. The cellular picture in mesothelioma usually appears to be uniform, with most if not all cells showing typical dense staining mesothelial cytoplasm. On

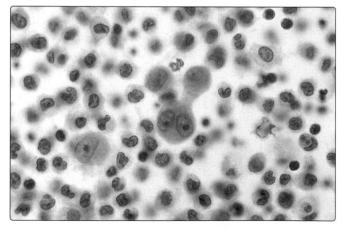

Fig. 6.18 Pleural fluid: reactive mesothelial cells. A population of slightly enlarged mesothelial cells with prominent nucleoli in a background of inflammatory cells. (Papanicolaou × HP)

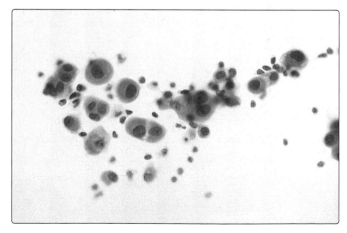

Fig. 6.19 Pleural fluid: well-differentiated mesothelioma. A population of malignant mesothelioma cells lacking nuclear features of malignancy. (Papanicolaou × HP)

closer inspection in some cases this population does include a mixture of cells that are regular and look benign, together with cells showing malignant nuclear criteria. The explanation for this presumably lies in partial involvement of the serosal membrane by tumour and cellular exfoliation from involved and uninvolved areas into the fluid. While not all metastatic effusions have a 'two cell' population, the individual cells usually lack the cytoplasmic density that is characteristic of mesothelial cells.

Structure of cell aggregates

The cell aggregates seen in mesothelioma often have a characteristic structure. Several authors have made reference to the appearance of rounded berry-like external contours of mesothelioma aggregates seen in smears, a feature that is said to contrast with the normally smooth external contours of aggregates from metastatic adenocarcinoma. While this feature is often present, its discriminant value is limited, as many cell aggregates in mesothelioma have a smooth outer surface or an elongate or frond-like form. A better appreciation of cell aggregate architecture can be gained on examination of cell block sections where some of the points described here may be more readily recognized.

Cell aggregate structure can be variable in mesothelioma, even within any one sample, with papillary, hollow, solid or complex forms. The constituent cells of the aggregates are usually cuboidal as opposed to columnar as is common in adenocarcinoma (Fig. 6.20). Larger aggregates are frequently papillary with a stromal core[39,43,47,66], a valuable differential diagnostic feature[43] as such structures are uncommon in adenocarcinoma. Hollow aggregates are common in mesothelioma although in section they are usually small. These need to be distinguished from the true acini of adenocarcinoma. Spriggs[67] has pointed out that the latter are characterized by microvilli lined lumens and noted that microvilli are lacking on their external contours. The identification of the microvillous border is more readily appreciated on PAS, Alcian blue or EMA stained sections. Solid aggregates are usually small and composed only of like cells. Rarely, complex structures more like those described by Spriggs[67] as 'tubulopapillary' are seen in mesothelioma with a 'back-to-back' cell arrangement and with microvilli present at both the luminal and external surfaces.

Characteristic cytoplasm (see Figs 6.21–6.26)

As commented earlier, the size of cells or amount of cytoplasm is often greatly increased in malignancy. Mesothelial cell cytoplasm is usually abundant, dense and basophilic. Its density is similar to that of metaplastic squamous cells as seen in cervical smears. Furthermore, this optical density is maintained in MGG stained smears, a feature that is often of crucial differential diagnostic value (see 'Differential diagnosis from breast carcinoma'). In

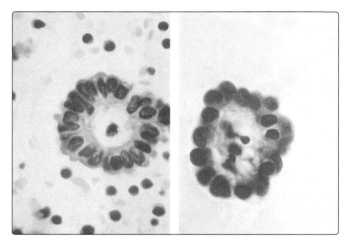

Fig. 6.20 Pleural fluid: cell block sections comparing cell aggregates in mesothelioma and adenocarcinoma. Left: adenocarcinoma; columnar cells with elongated nuclei. Right: mesothelioma; cuboidal cells with rounded nuclei. (H&E × HP)

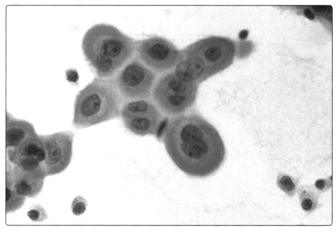

Fig. 6.21 Pleural fluid: cytoplasmic features. Cuboidal cells with dense cytoplasm showing a tinctorial change towards the nucleus and intercellular 'windows'. (Papanicolaou × HP)

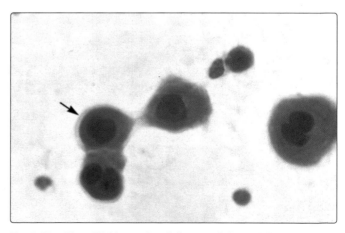

Fig. 6.22 Pleural fluid: cytoplasmic features. Polygonal dense staining malignant mesothelioma cells with 'windows' and a microvillous border (arrow). (Papanicolaou × HP)

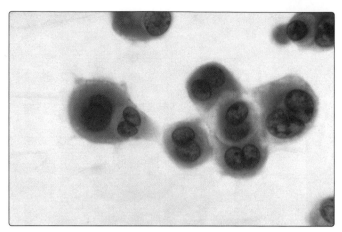

Fig. 6.23 Pleural fluid: cytoplasmic features. Densely staining cuboidal cells showing prominent binucleation, close opposition and 'windows'. (Papanicolaou)

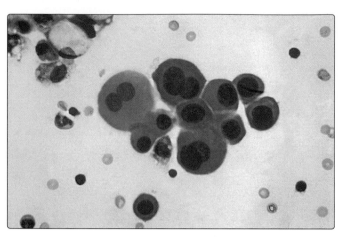

Fig. 6.25 Pleural fluid: cytoplasmic features. Densely staining cytoplasm. (MGG × MP)

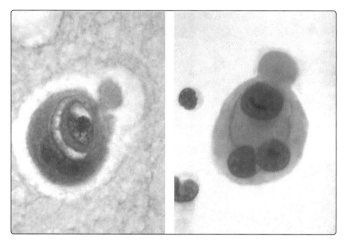

Fig. 6.24 Pleural fluid: cell engulfment in malignant mesothelioma. Left: cell block (H&E). Right: smear. (Papanicolaou × HP)

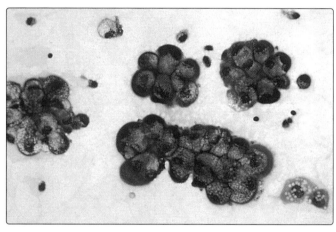

Fig. 6.26 Pleural fluid: cytoplasmic features. Prominent small cytoplasmic vacuoles. (MGG × MP)

Papanicolaou stained smears, mesothelial cytoplasm often shows a characteristic tinctorial gradation from green at the periphery of the cell to reddish orange in the perinuclear zone. The cytoplasmic density of mesothelioma cells can also be seen in H&E stained sections of cell block preparations where, as in biopsy material, the mesothelial cell cytoplasm is dense with a deep dull red hue. This constant cytoplasmic density is most uncommon in metastatic adenocarcinomas.

Cell-to-cell relationships

In good quality preparations at high power magnification individual cells and small cell clusters often reveal a characteristic brush-like border of microvilli. This feature is, of course, the ultrastructural hallmark of mesothelioma. In Papanicolaou stained smears this microvillous border appears as a thin, faint zone at the periphery of the dense cytoplasm or at the intersection of adjacent cells, and is probably responsible, at least in part, for producing the so

called 'window' effect occurring between adjacent cells (Figs 6.21–6.23).

This is a well recognized characteristic of mesothelioma and has important discriminatory value in the distinction between mesothelioma and adenocarcinoma[48]. Electron micrographs of these regions confirm the profuse microvillous formation and reveal that the points of cell-to-cell contact are cell junctions. In degenerate cells these microvillous projections may coalesce producing marked cytoplasmic peripheral blebbing, a feature more readily seen in air-dried MGG stained smears.

Cell engulfment, where one cell is partially or wholly wrapped around another, is common in mesothelioma and such terms as 'embracement' or 'pincer-like grip' have been used to describe this phenomenon (Fig. 6.24). Although cell engulfment can be seen in reactive mesothelial cells it is more common and complex in mesothelioma[48]. Multinucleate malignant cells are often seen in mesothelioma. Sherman and Mark[46] reported finding 1–3 malignant giant cells per high power field in 26 out of 39 cases.

Vacuoles

Vacuolar prominence is normally associated with adenocarcinomas but cytoplasmic vacuoles are not uncommon in mesothelioma (see Figs 6.26, 6.29, 6.33). Two distinct patterns may occur: multiple small vacuoles or solitary large 'hard edged' vacuoles. The small vacuoles are frequently seen localized to the periphery of the cell cytoplasm[35,36] or occasionally at the perinuclear zones. These small vacuoles may represent lipid[68] or glycogen[69,70]. Occasionally, this form of vacuolation is so dominant that the mesothelioma cells assume a macrophage-like appearance[41,42,71,72], yet when tested they maintain the immunocytochemical and ultrastructural phenotypic expression of mesothelial differentiation. It has been suggested that excessive vacuolation is a special feature of peritoneal rather than pleural mesothelioma[42] but in our material we have not been able to confirm this observation.

Larger, often solitary, even signet ring-like vacuoles, while less common, have also been well described and illustrated by many observers[35-37,41,44,46,72,73]. Although some[41,44,73,74] have postulated that these large vacuoles represent a degenerative phenomenon, this seems an unlikely explanation for at least three reasons. First, on Papanicolaou stained smears some of these large vacuoles contain dark grey material, which has a crinkled appearance (see Fig. 6.33). Second, when using alcohol fixed smears it is possible to demonstrate the presence of hyaluronic acid within these vacuoles by Alcian blue stain with and without prior digestion with hyaluronidase. Third, the ultrastructural appearances show many large vacuoles to be microvillous lined neolumens filled with flocculent or granular material consistent with hyaluronic acid[6].

It is therefore likely that many of these larger vacuoles are secretory rather than degenerative in nature. It should be stressed here that in mesothelioma, as opposed to adenocarcinoma, the number of cells with a large vacuole are usually few and may comprise only 1–2% of the cell population.

Collagen-basement membrane

Pathologists have long recognized that the epithelial form of malignant mesothelioma is characterized by papillary growth. It is also some 40 years since Takagi[75] first noted that papillary formation was 'the most significant finding' in an effusion sample from a single case of mesothelioma. That this feature could be of differential diagnostic value in effusions was first suggested by us after studying the nature of mesothelioma and adenocarcinoma cell aggregates in cell block sections (Fig. 6.27)[39]. Since then others[43,47,63,66,76,77] have confirmed this finding, and furthermore, Delahaye et al.[47] have shown that such connective tissue elements can readily be recognized in Romanovsky stained smears.

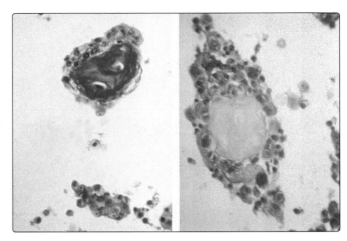

Fig. 6.27   Pleural fluid: collagen cores in mesothelioma cell aggregates; cell block. Left: Weigert van Gieson × HP. Right: H&E × HP

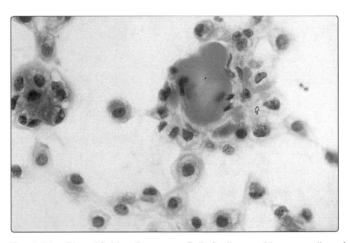

Fig. 6.28   Pleural fluid: collagen core. Ball of collagen with surrounding of mesothelioma cells. (Papanicolaou × MP)

Certainly in some cases of malignant mesothelioma, collagen and/or basement membrane-like material can be a prominent feature and can even be recognized in Papanicolaou stained smears as collections of light green amorphous material (Figs 6.28, 6.29). Moreover, cell block sections stained with PAS also highlight basement membrane-like substance beneath the mesothelial cell (Fig. 6.30). Ultrastructural studies on effusion cells have also documented this link between malignant mesothelioma and the presence of collagen fibres.

There is some experimental evidence to show that malignant mesothelioma cells produce this collagen[18]. It should be stressed that such basement membrane and collagen can occasionally be found in benign mesothelial proliferation[60,76], and that these are commonly found in benign peritoneal washings[62] and benign hydrocoele fluids[45].

Glycogen

Mesothelioma cells may be glycogen rich. This may take the form of small peripheral collections or larger lakes of yellow

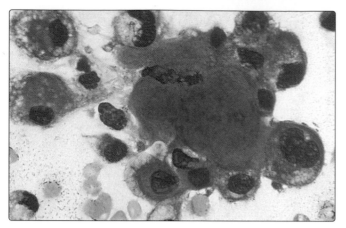

Fig. 6.29 Pleural fluid: collagen core. Ball of collagen and surrounding vacuolated mesothelioma cells. (MGG × HP)

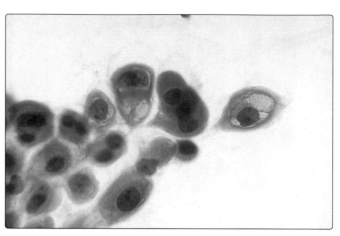

Fig. 6.31 Pleural fluid: glycogen. Abundant refractile yellow staining glycogen. (Papanicolaou × HP)

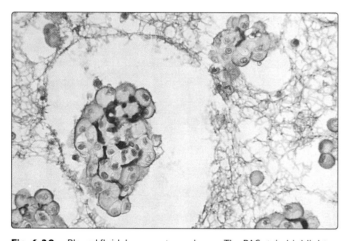

Fig. 6.30 Pleural fluid: basement membrane. The PAS stain highlights the abundant intercellular basement membrane substance and the microvillous borders on the cell surface. (PAS/D × HP)

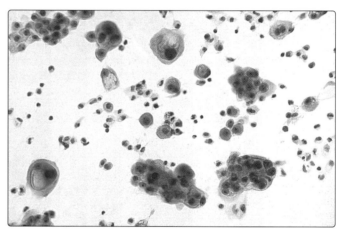

Fig. 6.32 Pleural fluid: squamous-like cell in a background of malignant mesothelial cells. (Papanicolaou × MP)

refractile substance (Fig. 6.31) in Papanicolaou stained smears, an appearance similar to the glycogenated navicular cells seen in some cervical smears. Such glycogen containing cells were found in 59% of our cases and the content was confirmed on cell block sections when stained with PAS with and without diastase digestion. Again, these glycogenated cells may be few or many. Furthermore, electron micrographs of mesothelioma cells also confirm the occurrence of these large lakes of glycogen. This amount and distribution of glycogen is not often seen in metastatic adenocarcinomas.

Squamous-like cells

In Papanicolaou stained smears, in marked contrast to the main population of green staining cells, a few very small, degenerate orange staining cells with pyknotic nuclei are occasionally found (Fig. 6.32). They closely resemble degenerate squamous epithelial cells. These particular cells are exceedingly rare in other types of malignant serous effusion, with the obvious exception of squamous cell

carcinoma, and while they are not common, they are a reasonably good marker of mesothelioma. This appearance may be due to the large amount of keratin filaments present in mesothelioma cell cytoplasm.

Hyaluronic acid network

Occasionally, mesotheliomas produce a very large amount of hyaluronic acid. This may be seen in smears as a peculiar network (Figs 6.33 and 6.34) of fine material or as a granular substance in the background in the thick parts of smears[24,78]. High levels of hyaluronic acid detected in the supernatant biochemically can be sufficient to predict mesothelioma and hence help establish malignancy.

Differential diagnosis of mesothelioma: effusions

There are two important considerations here: benign reactive proliferation and metastatic malignancy.

In an interesting study, Stevens *et al.*[48] used the approach of stepwise logistic regression analysis in an attempt to rank the differential diagnostic features between

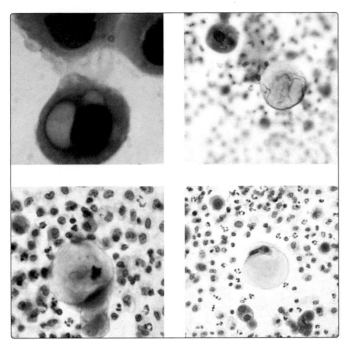

Fig. 6.33   Pleural fluid: hyaluronic acid. Large hard-edged vacuole (top left) and three large solitary vacuoles containing mauve crinkled hyaluronic acid secretion. (Papanicolaou × HP)

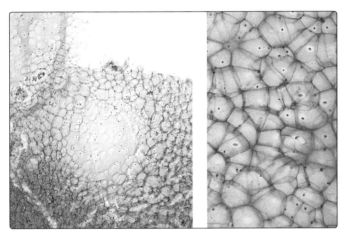

Fig. 6.34   Pleural fluid: hyaluronic acid. Network of bubbles in a smear from an effusion containing abundant hyaluronic acid. (Papanicolaou × LP)

mesothelioma, adenocarcinoma and benign mesothelial proliferation. While this does highlight those discriminants of greatest statistical significance, it does not necessarily follow that the conclusions drawn in the context of the mathematical model can be transferred into routine cytology practice. The approach needs to be verified by prospective studies applied to individual cases.

Reactive proliferation

The cytological distinction of mesothelioma from reactive proliferation has largely been dealt with earlier. While mesothelial proliferation associated with prominent papillary formation has given rise to the suspicion of

malignancy[60,79], in routine clinical practice this problem is rarely encountered. We, like Spriggs[67], are unaware of any false positive diagnosis of malignant mesothelioma or adenocarcinoma being made on the basis of the presence of cell aggregates. However, if aggregates are absent[51], or the degree of nuclear atypia is minimal or there is an inappropriate clinical setting, there is a greater chance for a false negative diagnosis. For these reasons, we routinely employ immunocytochemical testing with EMA, as it serves as a most valuable guide to distinguish the benign from the malignant nature of the cell population (see later).

Metastatic malignancy

The differential diagnosis of mesothelioma from metastatic adenocarcinoma in effusions is important and occasionally this causes great difficulty. The distinction of malignant mesothelioma from metastatic malignancy may present a special challenge in either of two differing cell presentations: first, when the cytological picture is one solely of cell aggregates, and second, when the smears contain only single malignant cells. The exercise involves a critical evaluation of the cellular pattern, including an assessment of aggregate form[28,43,67], the presence or absence of a double cell population[24,45,49], and of cell shape[28,45].

The external contours of cell aggregates seen in adenocarcinoma are generally smooth when compared with the knobbly or berry-contours seen in mesothelioma[25,36-38,46]. While many adenocarcinoma cell aggregates appear semitranslucent on smears and are hollow on section, most mesothelioma aggregates are solid. On cell block section, the cells which form aggregates in adenocarcinoma may be flat or columnar with basally situated nuclei[28,67], whereas mesotheliomatous aggregates are usually composed of cuboidal cells with central nuclei (see Fig. 6.20). Furthermore, the presence of many papillary aggregates with or without loose stroma or stromal tissue/basement membrane in the smear background favours the diagnosis of mesothelioma[39,43,47].

Alternatively, when the cytological picture is without cell aggregates and composed mainly of single cells, distinction of mesothelioma from metastatic malignancy is best carried out with the help of ancillary testing including special stains for epithelial and non-epithelial mucins, immunocytochemical phenotyping and electron microscopy.

Because the cytological picture of metastatic carcinoma of the breast and ovary most closely mimic mesothelioma, particular attention is given to the differential diagnosis of these two conditions.

Metastatic breast carcinoma is noteworthy because of its variable presentation in serous effusions and the close resemblance of the tumour cell cytoplasm to that of mesothelial cells in some cases. Furthermore, the cytological picture may be predominantly cell aggregates, single cells or a mixed cell pattern[80], presumably dependent upon the type of the primary tumour. Large rounded cell aggregates seen in ductal carcinoma of the breast may mimic mesothelioma; however the external contours of the breast carcinoma aggregates are usually smooth and the aggregates have an appearance of a hollow or collapsed sphere[24,67]. Furthermore, on section, these structures are rarely papillary and are mainly hollow with a blastula-like form[67,80].

Mesotheliomas presenting as a single cell pattern or with a single cell pattern and a few small clusters may mimic breast carcinoma as both, especially on Papanicolaou stained smears, may present a single cell with a rather dense cytoplasm. In breast carcinoma the nuclei are usually eccentric and the high cytoplasmic density sometimes seen on Papanicolaou stained smears is often not apparent on MGG staining.

Like breast carcinoma, metastatic ovarian carcinoma may present with a pure population of large cell aggregates. Occasionally these may be papillary as in a serous carcinoma but frequently they are hollow. The value of immunocytochemistry in the differential diagnosis of ovarian serous tumours from mesothelioma is limited, as most are CEA negative, as is mesothelioma. The differential diagnosis of papillary malignancy in serous effusions from females remains difficult and further ancillary testing including ultrastructural assessment is advisable[81].

Unusual patterns

Kho-Duffin et al.[51] have reported on the single cell pattern of malignant mesothelioma where the finding of cell aggregates is either absent or very uncommon. We too have seen such cases, however in our experience this pattern is quite rare (4/400).

As the authors point out, this form of cytological presentation brings a greater challenge into differential diagnosis of mesothelioma from a benign reactive process. We have found that cell enlargement and the extent of exfoliation are the most useful morphological discriminants in this regard. Furthermore EMA testing is invariably positive in these cases thus reinforcing the value of routine EMA testing of all florid mesothelial populations.

Sarcomatous mesothelioma: effusions

Unlike epithelial or biphasic mesotheliomas, the sarcomatous variant usually presents without a serous effusion and these lesions are more effectively sampled by the FNA approach. On the occasion when effusions are present, because of the non-epithelial nature of the tumour cells, exfoliation into the fluid rarely occurs[40,44,49,82]. However, several authors[35,40,41,44,63,82] have reported cases with poorly cellular fluids containing a few malignant spindle cells with large hyperchromatic elongated nuclei and cytoplasmic 'tails'. More voluminous cells with ill-defined wispy cytoplasm, large nuclei and macronucleoli can be seen, especially in the less differentiated tumours (Fig. 6.35). A less common presentation of sarcomatous mesothelioma,

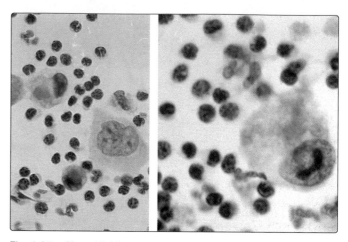

Fig. 6.35 Pleural fluid: sarcomatous mesothelioma. Single pleomorphic malignant cells with large irregular nuclei and, in one, a prominent nucleolus with abundant ill-defined cytoplasm. (Papanicolaou × HP)

either in direct smears or in cell block preparations, is the presence of small tissue fragments of spindle cell growth[40,44,49,55].

On morphology alone, the cytological presentation described above is of a spindle cell malignancy and not distinguishable from other spindle cell malignancies such as malignant fibrous histiocytoma, other soft tissue sarcomas, sarcomatoid lung or renal cell carcinoma or melanomas. However, given adequate cellular material, immunocytochemistry of cell block material and/or ultrastructural examination may enable the distinction between these tumours to be made.

Fine needle aspiration diagnosis of mesothelioma

It is now well recognized that in the absence of serous effusion, FNA sampling of solid lesions is valuable and can permit a sufficiently confident diagnosis of malignant mesothelioma to serve as a basis for clinical management[28,44,53,55]. Not only has the FNA approach been successfully employed in the diagnosis of primary pleural tumours[26,41,53,83-85], it has also been used for lesions in the peritoneum[52,53,55] and in the tunica vaginalis. In addition, it has been of value in assessing lymph node, surgical drain sites and distant subcutaneous involvement by mesothelioma[53,86-88].

Unlike effusion cytology, fine needle sampling can reflect the full range of histological patterns seen in malignant mesothelioma whether epithelial, biphasic, sarcomatous or anaplastic, though the spindle cell component is usually under-represented or absent[53,55]. Sarcomatous or anaplastic tumours may present a diagnostic difficulty on FNA material. Desmoplastic tumours may result in sparsely cellular or inadequate smears for diagnosis, whereas aspirates from anaplastic tumours may produce a high yield of cells that lack any sign of differentiation. In both of these situations additional sampling is necessary and we have found small tissue core biopsy sampling with the 'Biopty Gun' or FNA material collected for ultrastructural examination and immunocytochemical testing to be of assistance.

Cytological findings

Criteria for FNA diagnosis of epithelial/biphasic variants

▶ Flat loosely associated sheets of cells with dense cytoplasm
▶ Cohesive three-dimensional round, elongate or frond-like aggregates of regular cells
▶ Polygonal cells with dense cytoplasm and intercellular 'windows'
▶ Elongate cells with dense cytoplasm and central nuclei
▶ Hyaluronic acid-containing vacuoles in epithelial cells
▶ Isolated spindle cells with ill-defined cytoplasm

The most common FNA presentation of epithelial or biphasic mesotheliomas is of a cellular aspirate with both flat sheets and three-dimensional clusters of epithelial-like cuboidal cells with a variable number of more dispersed polygonal cells. Less common patterns include a picture mainly composed of cohesive aggregates of differing size, and one with a single population of isolated cytoplasmically dense polygonal cells with short cytoplasmic extensions resulting in an appearance resembling metaplastic squamous cells (Figs 6.36–6.38)[83,86,88]. The flat sheets seen in FNA samples of mesothelioma resemble desquamated sheets of normal mesothelium and when a degree of dissociation is evident, the intercellular gaps may be prominent, giving rise to a mosaic or 'spongiotic' appearance[53,54].

Hard-edged hyaluronic acid-containing vacuoles are seen within small numbers of tumour cells (Fig. 6.37); rarely these may be a very pronounced feature, giving rise to a signet ring appearance. In MGG stained smears these vacuoles contain magenta granules; in Papanicolaou stained smears they appear as an amorphous, often crinkled, grey substance. With adequate material it is possible to stain smears with Alcian blue with and without prior digestion by the specific enzyme hyaluronidase in order to confirm the presence of hyaluronic acid.

Criteria for diagnosis of sarcomatous mesothelioma

▶ Cohesive spindle cell tissue fragments
▶ Poorly cellular smears containing spindle cells with oval nuclei

Most authors[26,44,49,53–56] agree that FNA smears from sarcomatous mesotheliomas may present in two patterns, one with ill-defined tissue fragments of variable cohesiveness, and the other of sparsely cellular smears with randomly distributed spindle cells and some background connective tissue. Less well-differentiated lesions are characterized by increased cellular and nuclear pleomorphism, mitotic activity and necrosis.

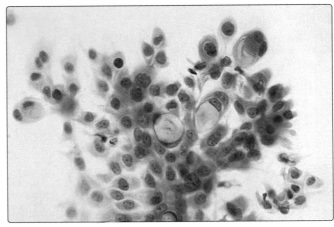

Fig. 6.37 FNA sample: loose sheets of epithelial-like cells with a few mauve staining hyaluronic acid vacuoles. (Papanicolaou × MP)

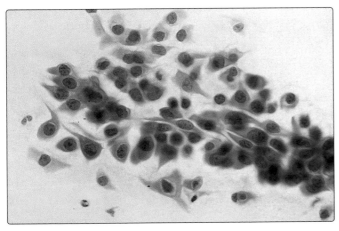

Fig. 6.36 FNA sample: loose clusters of polygonal (metaplastic-like) epithelial cells with dense cytoplasm and cytoplasmic processes. (Papanicolaou × MP)

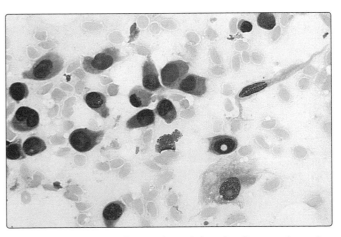

Fig. 6.38 FNA sample: dispersed population of malignant polygonal epithelial cells and a single fibroblastic (spindle) cell. (MGG × MP)

Differential diagnosis

Because of the range of cytological patterns seen in the same material, the differential diagnosis is wide, yet given the appropriate clinical setting and considering the radiographic evidence together with the fine needle findings, a diagnosis may be possible. Clearly, when mesothelioma presents in unusual sites[87,88] or with an unusual radiographic presentation[53,87], the diagnosis is more difficult. It is important to stress the value of setting aside some FNA material for cell block preparation for immunocytochemistry and for electron microscopy in support of the cytological findings.

Benign reactive mesothelium

The finding of a few flat sheets of mesothelium is not uncommon in FNA samples that traverse thoracic or peritoneal serous cavities. Tao noted that the identification of inflammatory cells in between the mesothelial cells supports a reactive rather than neoplastic origin. Benign lesions with a component of hyperplastic mesothelial cells may, on the rare occasion, give rise to a false positive diagnosis of malignancy[26]. If a cell block has been made EMA testing is of great diagnostic value in difficult cases.

Epithelial/biphasic lesions

The differential diagnosis includes a wide range of adenocarcinomas, both primary and secondary, especially those presenting with a combination of flat sheets and papillary clusters of fairly regular cells, e.g. bronchiolar alveolar carcinoma. With biphasic mesothelioma, melanoma and carcinomas with a spindle cell component need to be considered. Once again, cell block preparations are essential for immunocytochemistry testing, and EM is desirable.

Diagnostic pitfalls

▶ Of particular note is the difficulty encountered with some renal cell carcinomas[25,54]. These can present with serosal spread when the primary remains occult. The FNA pattern can be biphasic with loose epithelial sheets and spindle or elongate cells, and furthermore, the immunocytochemical profile of renal cell carcinoma is similar to that of mesothelioma showing positivity to low molecular weight keratins (CAM 5.2), EMA and vimentin but CEA negative

▶ A careful review of the cytomorphological features of one of our cases which was initially thought to represent mesothelioma but which at autopsy subsequently proved to be renal cell carcinoma, showed that many of the elongated epithelial cells had eccentrically placed nuclei, a feature more in keeping with an adenocarcinoma and unlike mesothelioma (see Figs 6.39, 6.40)

Ancillary testing

It has already been stressed that because of the difficulty in establishing a definite diagnosis of malignant mesothelioma on cytomorphology alone, ancillary testing is advocated whenever possible. The range of ancillary tests that can be used in support of cytological findings is wide. It is now commonplace to use a battery of such tests including cytochemistry (special stains), immunocytochemistry, electron microscopy, biochemical assay of supernatant fluid, cytogenetics and quantitative studies.

Immunocytochemistry

Most immunocytochemical studies on mesothelioma and its differential diagnosis from metastatic malignancy have been performed on tissue sections[6,89]. However, cytological material is equally suitable either in direct smears[90,91] or in cell block sections[25,34,92–95]. The latter have found particular favour in effusion and FNA work because they provide morphological information as well as permitting

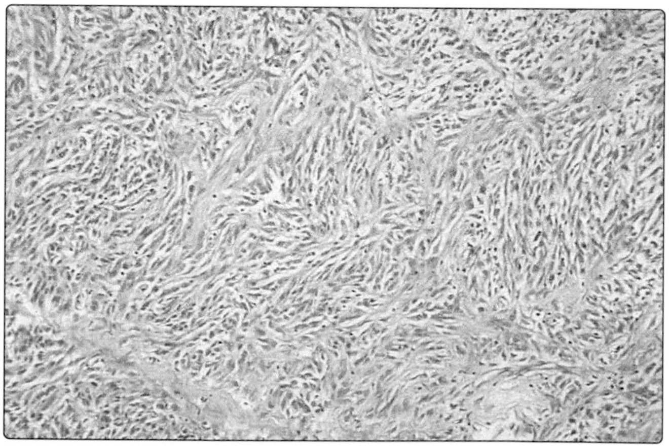

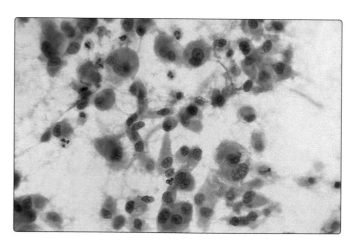

Fig. 6.39 Histological section: renal cell carcinoma. A spindle pattern in metastatic tumour within the pleura. (H&E × LP)

Fig. 6.40 FNA sample: renal cell carcinoma. A population of elongate and more polygonal cells with moderately dense cytoplasm. (Papanicolaou × MP)

consecutive sections that can be tested in an immunochemical profile.

Most immunocytochemical tests are used as phenotypic markers in tumour typing; a few also provide valuable support for the cytological diagnosis of malignancy. By far the most important recent advance is the development of commercially available positive phenotypic markers specific for mesothelioma including calretinin and CK 5/6 (see later). Until this introduction, the main value in immunocytochemical testing lay in the positive identification of metastatic malignancy, i.e. diagnosis by exclusion. There are several antisera that have been used as 'metastatic markers' in the differential diagnosis of mesothelioma in serous effusions. Some were developed as glandular markers and others as myelomonocytic markers, which have found use in this field, they include CEA, LeuM1, B72.3, and Ber EP4.

Carcinoembryonic antigen

CEA was the first immunological marker shown to be of value in the differential diagnosis of mesothelioma[96,97]. There has now been much written about the value of CEA testing in the differential diagnosis of mesothelioma. Mezger et al.[98] reviewed 40 studies and concluded that CEA testing was a most valuable aid in the differential diagnosis of mesothelioma from adenocarcinoma. In cytology specimens almost all mesotheliomas are CEA negative and only in a few cases do occasional tumour cells stain weakly positive[25,92,95,99,100]. A strong positive reaction with CEA would rule out a mesothelioma (Fig. 6.41).

Caution has been advocated in reading too much into a CEA negative result[101], as up to 40% of metastatic malignancies can be CEA negative[98]. However, from a practical point of view as adenocarcinomas usually constitute the main differential diagnostic problem in serous effusions and as most of these (in one series, 51 out of 54) are CEA positive[95], the role of CEA testing remains highly important. As Pinto et al.[81] have pointed out, a negative CEA result in a malignant effusion from males is highly suspicious of malignant mesothelioma; however, renal cell carcinoma continues to be one exception to the rule as it also is usually CEA negative, as are serous ovarian carcinomas in females.

From a practical point of view, we routinely perform CEA testing on serous effusions and continue to find the information of value.

LeuM1

Based on immunohistochemical studies of biopsy material, LeuM1 is identified as a valuable discriminant between mesothelioma and adenocarcinoma. LeuM1 is virtually never expressed in mesothelioma[95,102,103] whereas adenocarcinomas are frequently positive (76–94%) and often most cells are marked[95,102,103]. In our laboratory[95] we have tested LeuM1 against a series of malignant effusions using cell block material and found that 41 of 54 (76%) adenocarcinomas were positive but no case (0/36) of mesothelioma showed any positive staining. Wick et al.[103] found a minute focus of 5–10 cells stained positively in 3/43 cases.

B72.3

B72.3 is a murine monoclonal antibody raised against a high molecular weight glycoprotein (TAG.72) originally found in breast adenocarcinoma[104]. This antibody has been applied to the differential diagnosis of cytology specimens, including serous effusion[105]. Because reactive mesothelial cells are consistently negative and most metastatic malignancies, especially adenocarcinoma, are strongly positive, it has a valuable role in supporting a cytological diagnosis of metastatic malignancy[99,105,106].

However, its role in the diagnosis of mesothelioma is less clear. In biopsy material there appears to be a major quantitative difference between B72.3 expression in adenocarcinomas that show a high proportion of intensely stained positive cells (86%) and in mesothelioma demonstrating few weakly staining cells[107]. Few reports are available on cytology material. Johnson[106] records a negative result in a single case, whereas Linare[94] found two of 10 cases of epithelial mesothelioma gave a strong positive reaction but no comment was given as to the proportion of positive cells.

Of practical importance in the differential diagnosis of malignant effusions is the observation that ovarian adenocarcinomas react positively with B72.3. In this respect B72.3 is a better discriminant than CEA, as many serous tumours are CEA negative. Finally, Szpak et al.[107] have pointed out that B72.3 has no role in the differential diagnosis between reactive mesothelial cells and malignant mesothelioma since both are B72.3 negative.

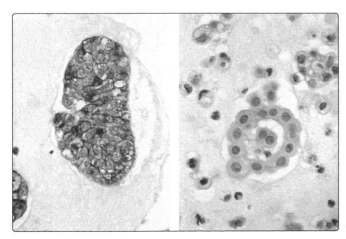

Fig. 6.41   Pleural fluid: cell block sections immunostained for CEA. Left: adenocarcinoma; strong positive cytoplasmic staining. Right: mesothelioma; negative reaction. (IPOX, CEA × HP)

Ber-EP4

Latza et al.[108] first investigated the use of the monoclonal antibody Ber-EP4 in the differential diagnosis of malignant tumours. They noted that benign mesothelial cells were consistently negative in effusions (0/25), and that in histological sections no case of mesothelioma (0/12) stained positive. Subsequently, a few authors have found some reactive mesothelial cells to be positively stained[109,110]. Sheibani et al.[111] found one positive case of mesothelioma in 115 cases tested whereas 87% of adenocarcinomas stained positively. We have also investigated the value of Ber-EP4 monoclonal in the differential diagnosis of mesothelioma from adenocarcinoma in cell block material[112]. All reactive mesothelial cells were negative and most malignant mesotheliomas were negative (42/43). Once again, this monoclonal antibody seems to have comparable value to other glandular markers and thus can be used as part of the immunocytochemical profile as a means of excluding mesothelioma.

Immune markers that aid the cytological diagnosis of malignancy

While as yet there is no absolutely reliable immune 'cancer marker', some antisera, including CEA and epithelial membrane antigen (EMA), have been employed in diagnostic cytology as a means of helping screen for malignant cells or to support a suspected diagnosis of malignancy (usually metastatic malignancy).

Epithelial membrane antigen

To et al.[113] originally reported that EMA was expressed on malignant but not on benign mesothelial cells. Since 1984, we have routinely used EMA (Fig. 6.42) as an adjunct immunocytochemical marker in serous effusion cytology and our experience runs to several hundreds of cases[93]. Based on the testing of mercuric chloride fixed cell block sections our results indicate that strong positive membrane staining with EMA is never seen in a high proportion of cells in reactive effusions; a few weakly positive cells may however be found. This latter finding has led to an opinion by some authors that EMA does not discriminate reliably between reactive and neoplastic mesothelium[101], but we have found that EMA is of practical value for this purpose; other workers are of like view[34,47,94,103,114–116]. On the two occasions in our material when a false positive was thought possible, both patients subsequently proved to have a mesothelioma.

In mesothelioma a strong membrane reaction has been noted[116], and while strong membrane staining is usual, the reaction can be patchy with variability in staining between one cluster and the next cluster and even from cell to cell within the same cluster (Fig. 6.43). Furthermore, we have been unable to confirm the suggestion that the pattern of EMA staining is a reliable discriminant between mesothelioma and adenocarcinoma. However, this does not negate the practical usefulness of EMA in the differential diagnosis of mesothelioma from reactive mesothelial cells. Singh et al.[117] have singled out EMA as the most useful antigen for dealing with 'atypical cells in serous effusion'. In summary, routine EMA staining has proved useful in our hands in supporting a suspected diagnosis of malignancy mesothelioma.

Positive immune markers for mesothelioma

There have been a few reports over the last decade of the production of antimesothelial antibodies and their application to the diagnosis of mesothelioma[118–121]. However, none of these were commercially available. However, recently we have seen the introduction of two antisera (calretinin and CK 5/6) that selectively mark mesothelioma cells with a high specificity and sensitivity. Studies on biopsy material first indicated that commercially available calretinin and cytokeratin 5/6 had a valuable discriminating

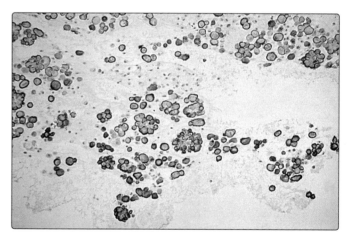

Fig. 6.42   Pleural fluid: cell block sections of mesothelioma, immunostained for EMA. Strong positive staining of cell aggregates for epithelial membrane antigen. (IPOX, EMA × LP)

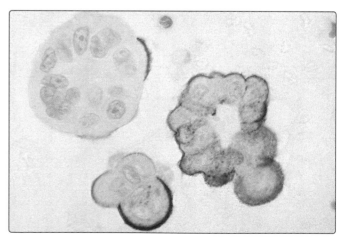

Fig. 6.43   Pleural fluid: cell block sectioned mesothelioma. Three mesothelioma cell clusters showing variable staining for EMA; most reaction product is located on a microvillous border. (IPOX, EMA × HP)

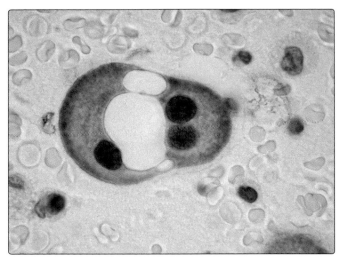

Fig. 6.44 Pleural fluid: cell block section mesothelioma. Cluster of mesothelioma cells showing cytoplasmic and nuclear staining for Calretinin. (IPOX, calretinin × HP)

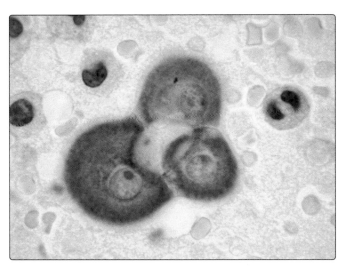

Fig. 6.45 Pleural fluid: Cell block section mesothelioma. Three mesothelioma cells showing diffuse cytoplasmic staining for CK 5/6. (IPOX, CK 5/6 × HP)

role between mesothelioma (positively stained) and adenocarcinoma (negative)[122–126]. It should be noted that as benign mesothelial cells also stain with these two antisera, therefore they cannot be used to discriminate between benign and malignant mesothelial processes. While our experience with these two antisera is still being acquired, results so far suggest their impact on the differential diagnosis of mesothelioma to be the most significant developments at the end of the twentieth century, and we suggest that calretinin at least, will become a critical component of any immunocytochemical panel used. We have now studied both these antibodies on pleural biopsy material and effusion (cell block) samples. Following an initial period of rather poor results the eventual selection of Zymed antisera (for calretinin) and the development of appropriate antigen retrieval and incubation times[127], all 42 cases of mesothelioma studied were positive with a high proportion of cells staining with both nuclear and cytoplasmic diffuse pattern (Fig. 6.44). Similarly, all cases of mesothelioma were positive with cytokeratin 5/6 with a diffuse cytoplasmic picture (Fig. 6.45). Only one case of adenocarcinoma (1 out of 39) gave a positive result with calretinin, and a single (different) case of adenocarcinoma stained moderately positively with cytokeratin 5/6[1]. Clearly, these two positive markers of mesothelioma will bring much greater confidence to the diagnosis of malignant mesothelioma.

Electron microscopy

Ultrastructural examination of tissue or cell concentrates has been widely used as an ancillary tool in the differential diagnosis of mesothelioma. Because mesotheliomas, especially epithelial or biphasic tumours, demonstrate phenotypic structural characteristics that differ in several aspects from adenocarcinoma, many advocate ultrastructural

examination for confirmation of a histological/cytological diagnosis of malignant mesothelioma[6,34,39,40,70,128–131].

While availability and cost may limit electron microscopy to particular centres and EM may be less often used than previously, we disagree with Naylor[24] that EM is of little practical value in the assessment of effusions from cases of suspected mesothelioma. Many cases of malignant mesothelioma can be diagnosed on cytology alone, some more confidently with supportive immunocytochemical staining, but in some situations, either when the clinical or cytological picture is not entirely typical, or when the patient has a previous history of carcinoma, then we believe all possible discriminating tests, including EM, should be performed to establish the diagnosis beyond doubt.

Of practical importance is the fact that cell concentrates from FNA and effusion samples both provide ideal material for electron microscopy; cell preservation is generally much better than that in small tissue biopsies[25,26,34]. We stress here that electron microscopy has little or no role in the differential diagnosis between benign and malignant mesothelial cells[129].

The ultrastructural features of mesothelioma and its differential diagnosis are well documented and are summarized by Henderson[6], Bedrosian[33] and Coleman[131]. In effusion cell samples containing free floating malignant cells, the most important discriminants for mesothelioma are the number, form and distribution of the surface microvilli. A profuse microvillous border composed of long, thin, occasionally branching microvilli lacking basal rootlets or terminal webs or radiating glycocalyx, is characteristic and virtually pathognomonic of malignant mesothelioma. Other features, including the number and distribution of intermediate filaments and the presence and nature of secretory products, also help distinguish mesothelioma from adenocarcinoma (Figs 6.46, 6.47).

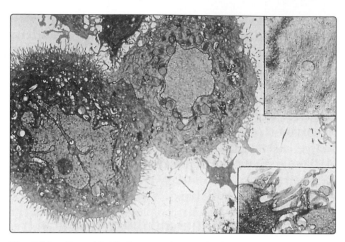

Fig. 6.46 Pleural fluid: electron micrograph of mesothelioma. Two mesothelioma cells with abundant long thin microvilli and abundant intermediate filaments but lacking glycocalyx. (EM × 3750)

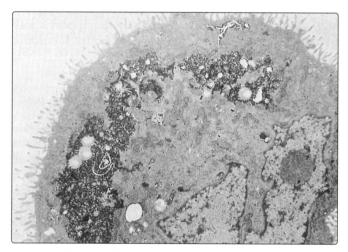

Fig. 6.47 Pleural fluid: electron micrograph of mesothelioma. Long thin microvilli and a crescent shaped lake of glycogen. (EM × 5000)

Quantitative studies

Ancillary tests based on measurement of various elements of the cell have been applied to the distinction of benign from malignant mesothelial tissue. These include DNA ploidy (both flow and static), morphometry and the demonstration of silver staining nucleolar organizer regions (AgNORs).

Ploidy studies

While most material studied has been from tissue samples, neither flow[132,133] nor static[134] DNA ploidy results have proved to be of discriminant value in distinguishing between benign and malignant mesothelial cells. A high proportion of mesotheliomas (range 39–65%) have a diploid profile[132,133,135] and this feature may well, at least in part, explain why many well-differentiated mesotheliomas are difficult to distinguish from reactive mesothelial proliferation by nuclear characteristics alone.

Morphometry

Measurements of such parameters as mean nuclear area, nucleocytoplasmic ratio or a multiparameter approach, have shown that malignant mesothelioma cells can be distinguished from reactive cells in both mesothelial tissue[136,137] and effusion samples[138,139]. Further investigation of this approach should be of value.

AgNORs

The demonstration of AgNORs as a diagnostic tool in pathology is of much greater interest. Greater experience will be necessary to establish whether this test is a reliable marker of malignancy. However, the technique has been applied to the distinction of mesothelioma from reactive mesothelial hyperplasia in tissue biopsy samples with some success[140]. We have used the assay in evaluating several cases of mesothelioma[22]. Soosay et al.[141] have cast some doubt on the absolute discrimination between benign and malignant lesions using this technique; they found overlap between the benign and malignant reference ranges. We found it to be a reliable, if laborious, tool in the discrimination of benign from malignant mesothelial lesions in biopsy material[22,23].

Few reports yet exist on the application of AgNORs in the diagnosis of effusions. Derenzini et al.[142] studied 10 cases of mesothelioma and reactive mesothelial conditions and found clear cut distinction in the distribution and variability of size of AgNORs. More recently Lim et al.[143] applied a modification of the technique using back scatter electron microscopy coupled with image analysis to effusion diagnosis. While noting the cost and time restrictions of this method, they found that the mean AgNOR area was a good discriminant between benign and malignant mesothelial cells.

Biochemistry of serous effusion

While in the past these options have been explored, the advent of positive mesothelial immune markers have probably made these investigations almost redundant.

Hyaluronic acid

Several workers have found quantification of hyaluronic acid to be of differential diagnostic value in the assessment of mesothelioma[144–149]. Depending on the sensitivity of the test system used, it is possible in a proportion of cases to distinguish between mesothelioma and other effusions by variability in levels, with high concentrations of hyaluronic acid in mesotheliomatous effusions.

Carcinoembryonic antigen (CEA)

Faravelli[150] and Whitaker[151] have investigated the usefulness of assessing CEA levels in serous effusion in the differential diagnosis of mesothelioma from adenocarcinoma, as reviewed by Mezger[98]. This relatively simple test is of value, especially when other tests, such as immunocytochemistry and electron microscopy are equivocal, unavailable or unhelpful. In our series, CEA was present in 67% of adenocarcinomas at a concentration above 15 ng/ml, whereas no case of mesothelioma contained more than 2.9 ng/ml.

Cytogenetics

There have been sporadic reports on the potential of cytogenetic analysis as a means of establishing a diagnosis of malignancy in serous effusions and in particular in the diagnosis of mesothelioma[152–155]. Hagmeijer et al.[156] recently examined effusions from 40 cases of mesothelioma by cytogenetic analysis and 30 were found to have abnormal karyotypes.

When the facility is readily available, this form of investigation has value, especially for well-differentiated epithelial mesotheliomas where the demonstration of an abnormal karyotype would add support to a cytological diagnosis.

Cytology of other mesothelial lesions

Other than malignant mesothelioma described above, there are several mesothelial tumours and related lesions[6], which may be sampled for cytodiagnosis (see 'Histological classification', above).

Well-differentiated papillary mesothelioma

Truly benign epithelial mesotheliomas are uncommon and are unrelated to asbestos exposure. They occur mainly in the peritoneum and are usually incidental findings at laparotomy[157,158]. Histologically, they are composed of a conglomerate of papillary-like structures bounded by a single layer of regular, cuboidal mesothelial cells. On examination of limited material the distinction of this entity from reactive mesothelial proliferation can be difficult.

Well-differentiated papillary mesotheliomas rarely cause serous effusions[75,158,159]. However, Burrig[160] briefly mentions the cytological findings of atypical cells in a viscous ascitic fluid from a patient with papillary mesothelioma and Tao[85] illustrates a case with prominent papillary formations in effusion cytology. We have seen a single case of this entity involving both the pleural and peritoneal cavity. The cytologic presentation was of many small rounded clusters and had a similar cytologic picture to some cases of well-differentiated malignant mesothelioma.

There is a single report of FNA findings of such a mesothelioma by Jayaram[161] in a patient with multifocal disease. The FNA smear showed dissociated syncytial and papillary clusters of round tumour cells with a high N/C ratio. The findings were considered to be unlike those usually seen in reactive mesothelial cells, although the difficulty in distinguishing between tumour and reaction was stressed by the author.

Pleural fibroma (synonyms: submesothelial fibrous tumour, solitary fibrous tumour, 'localized fibrous mesothelioma')

In the past there was much debate as to the origin of these pleural tumours; they are now generally regarded as tumours of fibroblasts with or without bronchial epithelial or mesothelial entrapment (Fig. 6.48), rather than being true mesotheliomas. These lesions are pleurally based, well circumscribed, often encapsulated and grow to a considerable size. They are generally unrelated to asbestos exposure. While most are benign some are histologically malignant, or eventually have a malignant clinical course[6,162,163]. These tumours have now been described in a wide range of tissues.

They rarely present with a serous effusion (5/60)[160] and on the few occasions where an effusion is present, cytology is unhelpful[85,160]. They are more likely to be sampled by the FNA approach[26,54,55,161–165]. We have seen aspirates from four cases of localized fibrous lesions of the pleura: two benign and two having a malignant course. All were surprisingly cellular, a feature also noted by Frazer[166], having many spindle fibroblastoid-like cells with oval nuclei (Fig. 6.49), associated with some background collagenous material; occasionally epithelial-like cells were also present. One benign case demonstrated a degree of nuclear atypia that caused a suspicion of malignancy on the FNA material.

The presence of many bare oval nuclei and collagen in the background of the smear was also observed by Dusenbery et al.[167]. They also stressed the value of cell block material in making a precise diagnosis. Immunocytochemical testing for keratin is of value in the differential diagnosis of these tumours; unlike sarcomatoid malignant mesothelioma, the spindle cells of pleural fibroma do not stain with antikeratin antibodies, and most stain positively for CD34 in tumour cells.

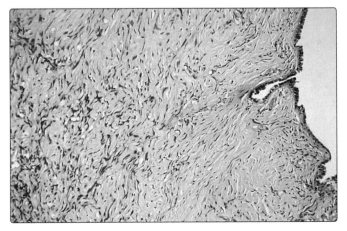

Fig. 6.48 Histological section: benign pleural fibroma. A single layer of benign epithelial (bronchiolar) cells cover dense fibrous tumour tissue. (H&E × LP)

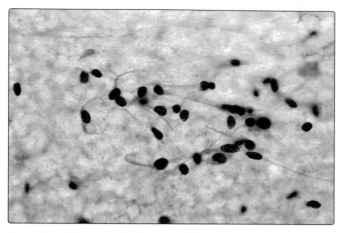

Fig. 6.49 FNA sample: benign pleural fibroma. Several spindle shaped cells. (H&E × HP)

Given the correct clinical setting and adequate cellular material, it is possible to suggest the diagnosis of localized pleural fibrous tumour by the FNA approach though prediction of their ultimate biological behaviour as judged solely on the cytological assessment is not possible.

Cystic mesothelioma of the peritoneum

These are rare and unusual lesions unrelated to asbestos exposure and are mainly found in women[6,168,169]. They are composed of multiple translucent mesothelial lined cysts (Fig. 6.50). There has been debate as to whether these lesions are true tumours or represent a reactive process[168,169]. While most cystic mesotheliomas are benign, they often have a protracted clinical course, tend to recur, and occasionally they can undergo transition to malignancy[6].

We have seen FNA cytology from one case of cystic mesothelioma and effusion cytology from another. The FNA sample (courtesy of Dr V. Caruso) was from a benign tumour; smears were poorly cellular with only a few flat sheets of regular mesothelial cells. This case was similar in appearance to those illustrated by Baddoura[170] and Devaney[171], who also found the predominant cytological picture was of flat sheets of regular mesothelial cells with bland nuclei. Our second patient first presented in 1962 complaining of abdominal discomfort. In 1985 a typical low-grade cystic mesothelial lesion was removed from the surface of the liver (Fig. 6.51). In 1988, the authors received 470 ml of so-called peritoneal fluid; this fluid was very cellular with many papillary-like aggregates. The immunoperoxidase reactions for these aggregates was CEA and EMA negative and, in view of the history and the immunocytochemical results, a somewhat guarded report was issued. Some 2 months later invasive disease was confirmed at laparotomy and the patient died in 1990. In retrospect, within the fluid samples there were clusters of cells with increased nucleocytoplasmic ratio and a marked degree of cell engulfment (Fig. 6.52).

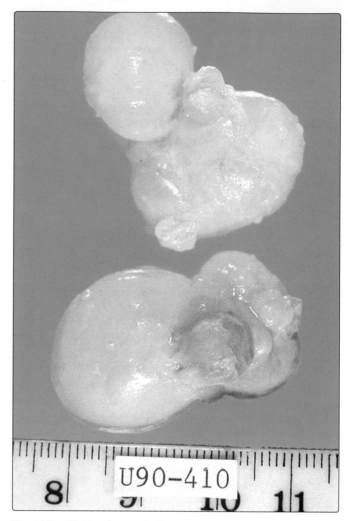

Fig. 6.50 Multicystic mesothelioma. Excised multiloculated cystic peritoneal tumour.

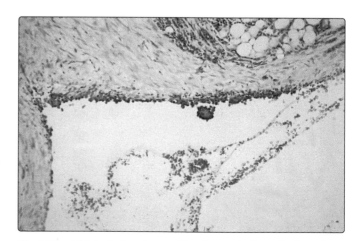

Fig. 6.51 Histological section: multicystic mesothelioma. Surface of one of the cystic spaces lined by proliferating mesothelial cells covering a more solid stromal region. (H&E × LP)

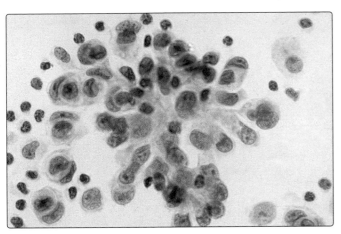

Fig. 6.52 Peritoneal fluid: multicystic mesothelioma. A loose cluster of atypical mesothelial cells with prominent cell engulfment, from a peritoneal fluid sample. (Papanicolaou × HP)

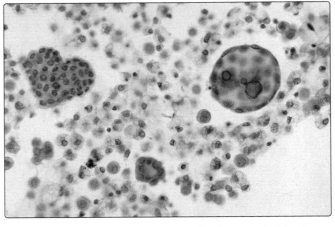

Fig. 6.53 Hydrocoele fluid: aggregates of benign mesothelial cells, one aggregate containing psammoma bodies. (Papanicolaou × MP)

Mesothelioma of the tunica vaginalis testis

(see also Chap. 26)

Both mesothelioma and mesothelial hyperplasia can occur in this site and because hydrocoele usually develops, there are implications for cytodiagnosis. This type of malignant mesothelioma is often associated with asbestos exposure[6,172].

Spriggs and Boddington[45] also describe a case they thought possibly represented mesothelioma. The smears were very cellular with many hollow and papillary mesothelial aggregates. Extreme caution should be used in making such a diagnosis by cytology alone. We have seen several benign hydrocoele fluids containing large numbers of papillary aggregates of regular mesothelial cells, some with psammoma bodies (Figs 6.53, 6.54), and therefore our approach to these findings is to regard them as likely to be benign. Noteworthy is the observation of Grove *et al.*[173] who found that all malignant mesotheliomas in this site presented with heavily blood-stained fluids; hence such samples would warrant a higher degree of clinical suspicion.

Serous papillary tumours of serosal surfaces

There are two lesions that can arise from the mesothelial surface of the peritoneum that have implications for cytodiagnosis: borderline serous tumours[174,175] and serous carcinomas[176,177] as seen in ovarian epithelial neoplasms of this type (see Chaps. 5 and 36).

Accuracy and value of cytological diagnosis

While some[32,178,179] still maintain that the diagnosis of malignant mesothelioma by cytological methods is extremely difficult or of questionable value, good results are usually obtained, especially from areas with a high local incidence of the disease[24,25,34,43,48]. Di Bonito *et al.*[180] reported a

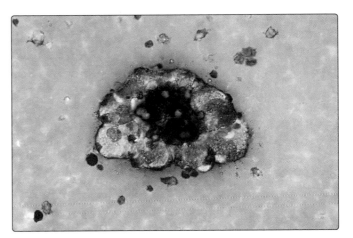

Fig. 6.54 Pelvic washings: a benign aggregate of mesothelial cells with psammoma bodies. (MGG × MP)

sensitivity of 76% on a series of 51 cases, a figure similar to our own (see below).

In our hospital the clinician's view of the relative value of cytology and needle biopsy in establishing a pathological diagnosis of malignant mesothelioma has been analysed by Musk and Christmas[181]. They reported on a consecutive series of 45 cases of mesothelioma in which 41 (91%) had a definite diagnosis on cytology, 37 being serous effusions and 4 FNAs, whereas only 25 out of 45 (55%) of closed needle biopsies gave a definite result.

We have analysed in some detail the mechanism by which the best possible result may be obtained[25,93]. Appropriate sampling[1,32], technical dedication[25,30], better definition of diagnostic criteria[26,47,48], the use of ancillary tests[25,46] and experience are all important[24,25,30,38,46]. Table 6.2 records the diagnostic accuracy reported in a number of series in the literature. Our current sensitivity for effusion diagnosis in malignant mesothelioma is 85%. In our hands the predictive value of an unequivocal diagnosis of malignant mesothelioma on effusion cytology has been 100%.

Table 6.2   Diagnosis in serous effusions.

Year	Authors	Origin of series	Total no. of cytology cases	Malignant diagnosis	Meso.	Meso. adeno.	?Meso.	Neg.	Sensitivity Meso.	Sensitivity Malig.
1962	Klempman[35]	South African asbestos mines	27	24	24	–	–	3	89	89
1963	Naylor[36]	Univ. of Michigan, Ann Arbor	7	6	4	2	–	1	57	86
1971	Oels[182]	Mayo Clinic I	25	15	(15)		1	9	60	60
1972	Roberts[37]	Shipyards (Glasgow)	14	10	8	2	2	2	57	71
1973	Butler[38]	Many referrals	27	25	25	–	1	0	93	93
1976	Sherrin[183]	General hospital	15	1	(1)		(14)		7	7
1976	Elmes[184]	Collected referred series	127	26	7	19			5	20
1977	Jara[185]	Hospital	20	8	1	7	2	11	5	40
1978	Whitaker[40]	Asbestos mine (Western Australia)	12	10	8	2	1	1	60	83
1978	Edge[186]	Shipyards (Barrow)	26	20	20	–	–	6	77	77
1979	Tao[85]	General hospital	22	17	17	–	–	5	77	77
1980	Antman[187]	Shipyards	28	8	1	7	(20)		4	28
1981	Lewis[188]	Local asbestos industry	46	3	3	?	?	?	6	6
1982	Nauta[189]	Hospital	26	9	4	3	(38)		15	35
1984	Law[190]	London chest hospitals	80	20	–	20	21 (17)	39	0	25
1984	Triol[43]	Asbestos factory	75	50	42	8	23	4	56	67
1984	Martensson[191]	Mainly shipyards (Sweden)	31	11	1	10			3	35
1985	Matzel[192]	Chest hospital (Bulgaria)	51	39	21	18	– (14)	12	41	76
1986	Adams[193]	Mayo Clinic II	69	22	18	4	9	38	26	32
1987	Whitaker[93]	Asbestos mine (Western Australia) II	103	83	74	8	10	9	72	81
1987	Strankinga[194]	Hospital (Amsterdam)	25	0	0	–			0	0
1988	Riback[195]	Asbestos insulation workers	182	50			51 (25)	81	31	31
1990	Sherman[46]	Massachusetts hospital	36	26	21	5	6	4	58	72
1992	Whitaker[25]	Author's update to 1 Nov, 1992	83	76	67	9	4	3	80	95

Malig., definite diagnosis of malignancy; Meso., mesothelioma; Meso./adeno, definitely malignant, either mesothelioma or adenocarcinoma; ?Meso., atypical cells, either mesothelioma or reactive proliferation; Neg., negative; (), distinction not made between categories; Sensitivity (number of cases diagnosed/total number of cases) × %.
Modified from ref. 93 and reproduced by permission.

FNA diagnosis

Between 1976–92, the literature reports a total of 72 cases of malignant mesothelioma where FNA sampling was studied. These included one series of 30[55], another of 19[53] and a number of small series or isolated case reports. Recent case reports[57,87,88] demonstrate that FNA diagnosis, especially when coupled with ancillary testing, permits a definite diagnosis on which clinical management can be based.

An analysis of our last 22 cases of malignant mesothelioma seen over the last 6 years and sampled by FNA are as shown in Table 6.3. Of the cases with a definite diagnosis, 12 had a known history of asbestos exposure and a further two were thought clinically to be malignant mesothelioma. All cases were epithelial or biphasic tumours, 11 having contributory special stains/immunoperoxidase staining and six with supportive electron microscopy. In four cases where malignancy was established but not the tumour type, two gave a history of asbestos exposure and the other two had pleural lesions thought clinically to be possible mesothelioma. Two cases

Table 6.3   FNA diagnosis of mesothelioma

Diagnosis	No.	(%)
Malignant mesothelioma	16	73
Malignant possible mesothelioma	4	19
Suspicious of malignancy	2	9

were anaplastic spindle cell malignancies on histopathology and two were well-differentiated spindle cell tumours. Electron microscopy and immunocytochemistry were also unhelpful in these four cases. In two cases with atypical cells only, one had a history of asbestos exposure, and the other had a pleural mass. In both instances, the FNA material was scant with only a few plump atypical spindle cells. Both proved to be sarcomatous mesotheliomas on subsequent 'Biopty Gun' samples.

Sensitivity, specificity/predictive value

Nguyen et al.[57] have reported a series of nine cases diagnosed on FNA with a sensitivity of diagnosis being

78%. Over the same 6-year period, we saw FNA samples from a further three cases where malignant mesothelioma was considered in the differential diagnosis. These included a pleural sarcoma, malignant fibrous histiocytoma of chest wall and a pleural based metastatic deposit from a renal cell carcinoma (see Figs 6.39, 6.40). There were no false positive diagnoses of mesothelioma made on FNA samples.

References

1   Whitaker D. The cytology of malignant mesothelioma. *Cytopathology* 2000, **11**: 139–151

2   Whitaker D, Papadimitriou J M, Walters M N-I. The mesothelium and its reactions: a review. *CRC Crit Rev Toxicol* 1982; **10**: 81–144

3   Wagner J C, Sleggs C A, Marchand P. Diffuse pleural mesothelioma and asbestos exposure in the Northwestern Cape Province. *Br J Ind Med* 1960; **17**: 260–271

4   Bolen J W, Hammar S P, McNutt M A. Reactive and neoplastic serosal tissue. A light microscopic, ultrastructural and immunohistochemical study. *Am J Surg Pathol* 1986; **10**: 34–47

5   Whitaker D, Henderson D W, Shilkin K B. The concept of mesothelioma *in situ*: implications for diagnosis and histogenesis. *Semin Diagn Pathol* 1992; **9**: 151–161

6   Henderson D W, Shilkin K B, Whitaker D *et al*. The pathology of malignant mesothelioma, including immunohistology and ultrastructure. In: Henderson D W, Shilkin K B, Langlois S Le P, Whitaker D eds. *Malignant Mesothelioma*. New York: Hemisphere, 1992; 69–139

7   Layman L. The blue asbestos industry at Wittenoom in Western Australia: A short history. In: Henderson D W, Shilkin K B, Langlois S Le P, Whitaker D eds. *Malignant Mesothelioma*. New York: Hemisphere, 1992

8   de Klerk N H, Armstrong B K. The epidemiology of asbestos and mesothelioma. In: Henderson D W, Shilkin K B, Langlois S Le P, Whitaker D eds. *Malignant Mesothelioma*. New York: Hemisphere, 1992; 223–250

9   Kawashima A, Libshitz H I, Lukeman J M. Radiation-induced malignant pleural mesothelioma. *Can Assoc Radiol J* 1990; **41**: 384–386

10 Pelnar P V. Further evidence of nonasbestos-related mesothelioma. A review of the literature. *Scand J Work Environ Health* 1988; **14**: 141–144

11 Craighead J E. Current pathogenetic concepts of diffuse malignant mesothelioma. *Hum Pathol* 1987; **18**: 544–557

12 Whitaker D, Shilkin K B, Walters M N-I. Cytologic and tissue culture characteristics of asbestos induced mesothelioma in rats. *Acta Cytol* 1984; **28**: 185–189

13 Topov J, Kolev K. Cytology of experimental mesotheliomas induced with crocidolite asbestos. *Acta Cytol* 1987; **31**: 369–373

14 Kramer J W, Nickels F A, Bell T. Cytology of diffuse mesothelioma in the thorax of a horse. *Equine Vet J* 1976; **8**: 81–83

15 Colbourne C M, Boulton J R, Mills J M, Whitaker D. Mesothelioma in two horses. *Aust Vet J* 1992; **69**: 275–278

16 Ricketts S W, Peace C K. A case of peritoneal mesothelioma in a thoroughbred mare. *Equine Vet J* 1976; **8**: 78–80

17 Stanton M R, Wrench C. Mechanisms of mesothelioma induction with asbestos and fibrous glass. *J Nat Cancer Inst* 1972; **48**: 797–821

18 Whitaker D, Manning L S, Robinson B W S, Shilkin K B. The pathobiology of the mesothelium. In: Henderson D W, Shilkin K B, Langlois S Le P, Whitaker D eds. *Malignant Mesothelioma*. New York: Hemisphere, 1992; 25–68

19 Lechner J F, Tokiwa T, LaVeck M A *et al*. Asbestos-associated chromosomal changes in human mesothelial cells. *Proc Natl Acad Sci USA* 1985; **82**: 3884–3888

20 Gerwin B I, Lechner J F, Reddel R R *et al*. Comparison of production of transforming growth factor-b and platelet-derived growth factor by normal human mesothelial cells and mesothelioma cell lines. *Cancer Res* 1987; **47**: 6180–6184

21 Versnel M A, Hagemeijer A, Bouts M J *et al*. Expression of c-sis (PDGF B-chain) and PDGF A-chain genes in ten human malignant mesothelioma cell lines derived from primary and metastatic tumors. *Oncogene* 1988; **2**: 601–605

22 Wolanski K, Whitaker D, Shilkin K B, Henderson D W. The use of EMA and AgNOR testing in the differential diagnosis of mesothelioma from benign reactive mesothelioses. *Cancer* 1998; **82**: 583–590

23 Whitaker D, Shilkin K, Henderson D. Mesothelioma *in situ*. *Cytopathology* 1998; **9**(supp 1): 3–4

24 Naylor B. Pleural, peritoneal and pericardial fluids. In: Bibbo M ed. *Comprehensive Cytopathology*. Philadelphia: Saunders, 1991; 590–610

25 Whitaker D, Sterrett G F, Shilkin K B. Cytological appearances of malignant mesothelioma. In: Henderson D W, Shilkin K B, Langlois S Le P, Whitaker D eds. *Malignant Mesothelioma*. New York: Hemisphere, 1992

26 Orell S R, Sterrett G F, Walters M N-I, Whitaker D. *Manual and Atlas of Fine Needle Aspiration Cytology*, 2nd edn. Edinburgh: Churchill Livingstone, 1992

27 Henderson D W, Whitaker D, Shilkin K B. The differential diagnosis of malignant mesothelioma: A practical approach to diagnosis during life. In: Henderson D W, Shilkin K B, Langlois S Le P, Whitaker D eds. *Malignant Mesothelioma*. New York: Hemisphere, 1992; 183–197

28 Whitaker D, Shilkin K. Diagnosis of pleural malignant mesothelioma in life – a practical approach. *J Pathol* 1984; **143**: 147–175

29 Nance K V, Shermer R W, Askin F B. Diagnostic efficacy of pleural biopsy as compared with that of pleural fluid examination. *Mod Pathol* 1991; **4**: 320–324

30 Whitaker D. Serous effusion diagnosis of malignant mesothelioma. *Australian Institute of Medical Laboratory Scientists Broadsheet* No. 13, 1989

31 Jonasson J G, Ducatman B S. Wang H H. The cell block for body cavity fluids: do the results justify the cost? *Mod Pathol* 1990; **3**: 667–670

32 Renshaw A A, Dean B R, Animan K H *et al*. The role of cytologic evaluation of pleural fluid in the diagnosis of malignant mesothelioma. *Chest* 1997, **111**: 106–109

33 Bedrossian C W M, Bonsib S, Moran C. Differential diagnosis between mesothelioma and adenocarcinoma; a multimodal approach based on ultrastructure and immunocytochemistry. *Semin Diag Pathol* 1992; **2**: 124–140

34 Leong A S Y, Stevens M W, Mukherjee T M. Malignant mesothelioma: cytologic diagnosis with histologic, immunohistochemical and ultrastructural correlation. *Semin Diag Pathol* 1992; **9**: 141–150

35 Klempman S. The exfoliate cytology of diffuse pleural mesothelioma. *Cancer* 1962; **15**: 691–704

36 Naylor B. The exfoliative cytology of diffuse malignant mesothelioma. *J Pathol Bacteriol* 1963; **86**: 293–298

37 Roberts G H, Campbell G M. Exfoliative cytology of diffuse mesothelioma. *J Clin Pathol* 1972; **25**: 577–582

38 Butler E B, Berry A V. Diffuse mesotheliomas. Diagnostic criteria using exfoliative cytology. In: Bogovski P, Gilson J C, Timbrell V, Wagner J C eds. Biological effects of asbestos. *IARC Sci Publ* 1973; No. 8

39 Whitaker D. Cell aggregates in malignant mesothelioma. *Acta Cytol* 1977; **21**: 236–239

40 Whitaker D, Shilkin K B. The cytology of malignant mesothelioma in Western Australia. *Acta Cytol* 1978; **22**: 67–70

41 Lopes-Cardozo P L. *Atlas of Clinical Cytology*. Hertogenbosch: Targa, 1979

42 Boon M E, Kwee W S, Alons C L *et al*. Discrimination between primary pleural and primary peritoneal mesotheliomas by morphometry and analysis of vacuolization pattern of the exfoliated mesothelial cells. *Acta Cytol* 1982; **26**: 103–108

43 Triol J H, Conston A S, Chandler S V. Malignant mesothelioma. Cytopathology of 75 cases seen in a New Jersey community hospital. *Acta Cytol* 1984; **28**: 37–45

44 Ehya H. The cytologic diagnosis of mesothelioma. *Semin Diagn Pathol* 1986; **3**: 196–203

45 Spriggs A I, Boddington M M. Atlas of serous fluid cytopathology. A guide to the cells of pleural, pericardial, peritoneal and hydrocele fluids. In: Gresham G A ed. *Current Histopathology*, vol. 14. Dordrecht: Kluwer Academic Publishers, 1989

46 Sherman M E, Mark E J. Effusion cytology in the diagnosis of malignant epithelioid and biphasic mesothelioma. *Arch Pathol Lab Med* 1990; **114**: 845–851

47 Delahaye M, de Jong A A W, Versnel M A *et al*. Cytopathology of malignant mesothelioma. Reappraisal of the diagnostic value of collagen cores. *Cytopathology* 1990; **1**: 137–145

48 Stevens M W, Leong A S-Y, Fazzalari N L *et al*. Cytopathology of malignant mesothelioma. A step-wide logistic regression analysis. *Diagn Cytopathol* 1992; **8**: 333–341

49 Koss L G, *Diagnostic Cytology and Its Histopathologic Bases*, 4th edn. Philadelphia: Lippincott, 1992

50 Di Bonito L, Falconieri G, Colautti I *et al*. Cytopathology of malignant mesothelioma: a study of its patterns and histological bases. *Diagn Cytopathol* 1993; **9**: 25–31

51 Kho-Duffin J, Tao L-C, Cramer H *et al*. Cytological diagnosis of malignant mesothelioma, with particular emphasis on the epithelial noncohesive cell type. *Diagn Cytopathol* 1999; **20**: 57–62

52 Reuter K, Raptopoulos V, Reale F *et al*. Diagnosis of peritoneal mesothelioma: computed tomography, sonography and fine-needle aspiration biopsy. *Am J Radiol* 1983; **140**: 1189–1194

53 Sterrett G F, Whitaker D, Shilkin K B, Walters M N-I. Fine needle aspiration cytology of malignant mesothelioma. *Acta Cytol* 1987; **31**: 185–193

54 Obers V J, Leiman G, Girdwood R W, Spiro F I. Primary Chest wall and pleura, malignant pleural tumors (mesotheliomas) presenting as localised masses. Fine needle aspiration cytologic findings, clinical and radiologic features and review of the literature. *Acta Cytol* 1988; **32**: 567–575

55 Tao L C. Aspiration biopsy cytology of mesothelioma. *Diagn Cytopathol* 1989; **5**: 14–21

56 Koss L G, Woyke S, Olszewski W. *Aspiration Biopsy: Cytologic Interpretation and Histologic Bases*. New York: Igaku-Shoin, 1984

57 Nguyen G-K, Akin M-R, Villanueva R R, Slatnik J. Cytopathology of malignant mesothelioma of the pleura in fine needle aspiration biopsy. *Diagn Cytopathol* 1999; **21**: 253–259

58 McCaughey W T E, Kannerstein M, Churg J. Tumors and pseudotumors of the serous membranes. In: Hartman W H, Sobin L H eds. *Atlas of Tumor Pathology*, 2nd series, fascicle 20. Washington DC: Armed Forces Institute of Pathology, 1985

59 Becker S N, Pepin D W, Rosenthal D L. Mesothelial papilloma: a case of mistaken identity in pericardial effusion. *Acta Cytol* 1976; **20**: 266–268

60 Spriggs A L, Jerome D W. Benign mesothelial proliferation with collagen

formation in pericardial fluid. *Acta Cytol* 1979; **23**: 428–430

61 Ashton P R. Diagnostic cytology seminar. *Acta Cytol* 1982; **26**: 851–882

62 Wojcik E M, Naylor B. 'Collagen Balls' in peritoneal washings. Prevalence, morphology, origin and significance. *Acta Cytol* 1992; **36**: 466–470

63 Kobayashi Y, Takeda S, Yamamoto T, Goi S. Cytologic detection of malignant mesothelioma of the pericardium. *Acta Cytol* 1978; **22**: 344–349

64 Selvaggi S M, Migdal S. Cytologic features of atypical mesothelial cells in peritoneal dialysis fluid. *Diagn Cytopathol* 1990; **6**: 22–26

65 Kutty C P, Remeniuk E, Varkey B. Malignant-appearing cells in pleural effusion due to pancreatitis. Case report and literature review. *Acta Cytol* 1981; **25**: 412–416

66 Triol J H, Conston A S, Chandler S V D. Distinguishing adenocarcinoma from mesothelioma in effusions (letter). *Hum Pathol* 1987; **18**: 969

67 Spriggs A I. The architecture of tumor cell clusters in serous effusions. In: Koss L G, Coleman D V eds. *Advances in Clinical Cytology*, vol. 2. New York: Masson, 1984

68 Boon M E, Veldhuizen R W, Ruinaard C *et al*. Qualitative distinctive differences between the vacuoles of mesothelioma cells and of cells from metastatic carcinoma exfoliated in pleural fluid. *Acta Cytol* 1984; **28**: 443–449

69 Castelain C G, Pretet S, Kreis, B P. Cytodiagnostic des mesotheliomes pleuraux. *La Presse Medicale* 1969; **77**: 197–199

70 Legrand M. Ultrastructural study of pleural fluid in mesothelioma. *Thorax* 1974; **29**: 164–171

71 Spriggs A I, Grunze H. An unusual cytologic presentation of mesothelioma in serous effusions. *Acta Cytol* 1983; **27**: 288–292

72 Guffani C M, Faleri M L. Benign-appearing mesothelioma cells in a serous effusion. *Acta Cytol* 1985; **29**: 90–92

73 Jones J S P, Lund C, Planteydt H T, Butler E B. *Colour Atlas of Mesothelioma*. Lancaster: MTP Press, 1985; 20–23

74 Takahashi M. *Color Atlas of Cancer Cytology*, 2nd edn. Tokyo: Igaku-Shoin, 1981

75 Takagi F. Studies on tumor cells in serous effusion. *Am J Clin Pathol* 1954; **24**: 663–675

76 Young J A. *Colour Atlas of Pulmonary Cytopathology*. Oxford: Oxford University Press, 1985

77 Barsotti P, Muda A O, Ascoli V *et al*. Ultrastructural histochemistry of mesotheliomas and adenocarcinomas in malignant effusions. *Diagn Cytopathol* 1989; **5**: 154–161

78 Whitaker D. Hyaluronic acid in serous effusion smears. *Acta Cytol* 1986; **30**: 90–91

79 Rosai J, Dehner L P. Nodular mesothelial hyperplasis in hernia sacs. A benign reactive condition simulating a neoplastic process. *Cancer* 1975; **35**: 165–175

80 Danner D E, Gmelich J T. A comparative study of tumor cells from metastatic carcinoma of the breast in effusions. *Acta Cytol* 1975; **19**: 509–516

81 Pinto M M, Bernstein L H, Brogan D A, Criscuolo E M. Carcinoembryonic antigen in effusions. A diagnostic adjunct to cytology. *Acta Cytol* 1987; **31**: 113–118

82 Hajdu S I, Hajdu E O. *Cytopathology of Sarcomas and Other Nonepithelial Malignant Tumours*. Philadelphia: Saunders, 1976

83 Frable W J. *Thin-needle Aspiration Biopsy*. Philadephia: Saunders, 1983

84 Kline T S. *Handbook of Fine Needle Aspiration Biopsy Cytology*, 2nd edn. New York: Churchill Livingstone, 1988

85 Tao L C. The cytopathology of mesothelioma. *Acta Cytol* 1979; **23**: 209–213

86 Linsk J A, Franzen S. *Clinical Aspiration Cytology*. Philadelphia: Lippincott, 1983

87 Musk A W, Dewar J, Shilkin K B, Whitaker D. Miliary spread of malignant pleural mesothelioma without a clinically identifiable pleural tumour. *Aust NZ J Med* 1991; **21**: 460–462

88 Craig F E, Fishback N F, Schwartz J G, Powers C N. Occult metastatic mesothelioma – diagnosis by fine-needle aspiration. A case report. *Am J Clin Pathol* 1992; **97**: 493–497

89 Sheibani K, Esteban J M, Bailey A *et al*. Immunopathologic and molecular studies as an aid to the diagnosis of malignant mesothelioma. *Hum Pathol* 1992; **23**: 107–116

90 Tickman R J, Cohen C, Varma V A *et al*. Distinction between carcinoma cells and mesothelial cells in serous effusions. Usefulness of immunohistochemistry. *Acta Cytol* 1990; **34**: 491–496

91 Wazir J F, Martin Bates E, Woodward G, Coleman D V. Evaluation of immunocytochemical staining as a method of improving diagnostic accuracy in a routine cytopathology laboratory. *Cytopathology* 1991; **2**: 75–82

92 Cibas E S, Corson J M, Pinkus G S. The distinction of adenocarcinoma from malignant mesothelioma in cell blocks of effusions: the role of routine mucin histochemistry and immunohistochemical assessment of carcinoembryonic antigen, keratin proteins, epithelial membrane antigen, and milk fat globule-derived antigen. *Hum Pathol* 1987; **74**: 67–74

93 Whitaker D, Sterrett G, Shilkin K. Early diagnosis of malignant mesothelioma: the contribution of effusion and fine needle aspiration cytology and ancillary techniques. In: Peters G A, Peters B J eds. *Sourcebook on Asbestos Diseases: Medical, Legal and Engineering Aspects*, vol. 4. New York: Garland Law Publishing, 1989; 71–115

94 Linari A, Bussolati G. Evaluation of impact of immunocytochemical techniques in cytological diagnosis of neoplastic effusions. *J Clin Pathol* 1989; **42**: 1184–1189

95 Spagnolo D V, Whitaker D, Carrello S, Radosevich J A, Rosen S T, Gould V E. The use of monoclonal antibody 44–3A6 in cell blocks in the diagnosis of lung carcinoma,

carcinomas metastatic to lung and pleura, and pleural malignant mesothelioma. *Am J Clin Pathol* 1991; **95**: 322–329

96 Wang N S, Huang S N, Gold P. Absence of carcinoembryonic antigen-like material in mesothelioma: an immunohistochemical differentiation from other lung cancers. *Cancer* 1979; **44**: 937–943

97 Whitaker D, Sterrett G F, Shilkin K B. Detection of tissue CEA-like substance as an aid in the differential diagnosis of malignant mesothelioma. *Pathology* 1982; **14**: 255–258

98 Mezger J, Lamerz R, Permanetter W. Diagnostic significance of carcinoembryonic antigen in the differential diagnosis of malignant mesothelioma. *J Thorac Cardiovasc Surg* 1990; **100**: 860–866

99 Duggan M A, Masters C B, Alexander F. Immunohistochemical differentiation of malignant mesothelioma, mesothelial hyperplasia and metastatic adenocarcinoma in serous effusions using staining for carcinoembryonic antigen, keratin and vimentin. *Acta Cytol* 1987; **31**: 807–814

100 Silverman J F, Nance K, Phillips B, Norris H T. The use of immunoperoxidase panels for the cytologic diagnosis of malignancy in serous effusions. *Diagn Cytopathol* 1987; **3**: 134–140

101 Heyderman E, Ridley P D. Malignant mesothelioma. *J R Soc Med* 1989; **82**: 571–572

102 Sheibani K, Battifora H, Burke J S. Antigenic phenotype of malignant mesotheliomas and pulmonary adenocarcinomas. An immunohistologic analysis demonstrating the value of Leu M1 antigen. *Am J Pathol* 1986; **123**: 212–219

103 Wick M R, Mills S W, Swanson P E. Expression of 'myelomonocytic' antigens in mesotheliomas and adenocarcinomas involving the serosal surfaces. *Am J Clin Pathol* 1990; **94**: 18–26

104 Szpak C A, Johnston W W, Lottich S C *et al.* Patterns of reactivity of four novel monoclonal antibodies (B72.3, DF3, B1.1 and B6.2) with cells in human malignant and benign effusions. *Acta Cytol* 1984; **28**: 356–367

105 Johnston W W, Szpak C A, Thor A, Simpson J, Schlom J. Antibodies to tumor-associated antigens: applications in clinical cytology. In: Wied G L, Keebler C M, Koss L G, Reagan J W eds. Compendium on Diagnostic Cytology, 6th edn., *Tutorials of Cytology* 1988; 567–578

106 Johnston W W, Szpak C A, Lottich S C *et al.* Use of a monoclonal antibody (B72.3) as an immunocytochemical adjunct to diagnosis of adenocarcinoma in human effusions. *Can Res* 1985; **45**: 1894–1900

107 Szpak C A, Johnston W W, Roggli V *et al.* The diagnostic distinction between malignant mesothelioma of the pleura and adenocarcinoma of the lung as defined by a monoclonal antibody (B72.3). *Am J Pathol* 1986; **122**: 252–260

108 Latza U, Niedobitek G, Schwarting R *et al.* Ber-EP4: new monoclonal antibody which distinguishes epithelia from mesothelia. *J Clin Pathol* 1990; **43**: 213–219

109 Diaz-Arias A, Loy T, Chapman R, Bickel J. Utility of monoclonal antibody BER-EP4 in the cytologic diagnosis of adenocarcinoma in body fluids. *Mod Pathol* 1991; **4**: Abstract 134

110 Frisman D M, Buckner S H, Nocito J D *et al.* Use of monoclonal antibody BER-EP4 in the diagnosis of effusions. *Mod Pathol* 1991; **4**: Abstract 137

111 Shelbani K, Shin S S, Kezirian J, Weiss L. Ber-EP4 antibody as a discriminant in the differential diagnosis of malignant mesothelioma versus adenocarcinoma. *Am J Surg Pathol* 1991; **15**: 779–784

112 Maguire B, Whitaker D, Carrello S, Spagnolo D. The use of monoclonal antibody Ber-EP4 in cell blocks in the differential diagnosis of malignant mesothelioma and carcinoma in malignant effusions and FNA specimens. *Surg Pathol* 1992; Abstract

113 To A, Coleman D V, Dearnaley D P *et al.* Use of antisera to epithelial membrane antigen for the cytodiagnosis of malignancy in serous effusions. *J Clin Pathol* 1981; **34**: 1326–1332

114 Walts A E, Said J W, Shintaku I P. Epithelial membrane antigen in the cytodiagnosis of effusions and aspirates: immunocytochemical and ultrastructural localization in benign and malignant cells. *Diagn Cytopathol* 1987; **3**: 41–49

115 van der Kwast T H, Versnel M A, Delahaye M *et al.* Expression of epithelial membrane antigen on malignant mesothelioma cells. An immunocytochemical and immunoelectron microscopic study. *Acta Cytol* 1988; **32**: 169–174

116 Leong A S Y, Parkinson R, Milios J. 'Thick' cell membranes revealed by immunocytochemical staining: a clue to the diagnosis of mesothelioma. *Diagn Cytopathol* 1990; **6**: 9–13

117 Singh H K, Silverman J F, Berns L *et al.* Significance of epithelial membrane antigen in the work-up of problematic serous effusions. *Diagn Cytopathol* 1995; **13**: 3–7

118 Singh G, Whiteside T L, Dekker A. Immunodiagnosis of mesothelioma. Use of antimesothelial cell serum in an indirect immunofluorescence assay. *Cancer* 1979; **43**: 2288–2296

119 Donna A, Betta P G, Bellinger D, Marchisini A. New marker for mesothelioma: an immunoperoxidase study. *J Clin Pathol* 1986; **39**: 961–968

120 Hsu S-M, Hsu P-L, Zhao X *et al.* Establishment of human mesothelioma cell lines (MS-1, -2) and production of a monoclonal antibody (anti-MS) with diagnostic and therapeutic potential. *Cancer Res* 1988; **48**: 5228–5236

121 O'Hara C J, Corson J M, Pinkus G S, Stahel R A. A monoclonal antibody that distinguishes epithelial-type malignant mesothelioma from pulmonary adenocarcinoma and extrapulmonary malignancies. *Am J Pathol* 1990; **136**: 421–428

122 Clover J, Oates J, Edwards C. Anti-cytokeratin 5/6: a positive marker for epithelioid mesothelioma. *Histopathology* 1997; **31**: 140–143

123 Doglioni C, Dei Tos A P, Laurino L Iussolino P *et al.* Calretinin: A novel immunocytochemical marker for mesothelioma. *Am J Surg Pathol* 1996; **20**: 1037–1046

124 Gotzos V, Vogl P, Celio M R. The calcium binding protein calretinin is a selective marker for malignant pleural mesotheliomas of the epithelial type. *Pathol Res Pract* 1996; **192**: 137–147

125 Ordonez N G. Value of cytokeratin 5/6 immunostaining in distinguishing epithelial mesothelioma of the pleura from lung adenocarcinoma. *Am J Surg Pathol* 1998; **22**: 1215–1221

126 Ordonez N G. Value of calretinin immunostaining in differentiating epithelial mesothelioma from lung adenocarcinoma. *Mod Pathol* 1998; **11**: 929–933

127 Lam M H, Whitaker D. The value of calretinin and cytokeratin 5/6 in the diagnosis of malignant mesothelioma in cell blocks and pleural biopsies. *Int J Surg Path* 2000; 50: A3

128 Wang N S. Electron microscopy in the diagnosis of pleural mesotheliomas. *Cancer* 1973; **31**: 1046–1054

129 Warhol M J, Hickey W F, Corson J M. Malignant mesothelioma. Ultrastructural distinction from adenocarcinoma. *Am J Surg Pathol* 1982; **6**: 307–314

130 Butler E B, Johnson J F. The use of electron microscopy in the diagnosis of diffuse mesotheliomas using human pleural effusions. In: Wagner J C ed. Biological effects of mineral fibres. *IARC Sci Publ* 1980, No. 30

131 Coleman M, Henderson D W, Mukherjee T M. The ultrastructural pathology of malignant pleural mesothelioma. *Path Annu* 1989; **24**: 303–353

132 Burmer G C, Rabinovitch P S, Kulander B G *et al.* Flow cytometric analysis of malignant pleural mesotheliomas. *Hum Pathol* 1989; **20**: 777–783

133 Dazzi H, Thatcher N, Hasleton P S *et al.* DNA analysis by flow cytometry in malignant pleural mesothelioma: relationship to histology and survival. *J Pathol* 1990; **162**: 51–55

134 Tierney G, Wilkinson M J, Jones J S P. The malignancy grading method is not a reliable assessment of malignancy in mesothelioma. *J Pathol* 1990; **160**: 209–211

135 Dejmek A, Stromberg C, Wikstrom B, Hjerpe A. Prognostic importance of the DNA ploidy pattern in malignant mesothelioma of the pleura. *Analyt Quant Cytol Histol* 1992; **14**: 217–221

136 Marchevsky A M, Gil J G, Caccamo D. Computerized interactive morphometry. *Arch Pathol Lab Med* 1985; **109**: 1102–1105

137 Robutti F, Betta P G, Donna A, Pavesi M. A morphometrically based classification rule for the diagnosis of primary mesothelial lesions. *J Pathol* 1990; **162**: 57–60

138 Christen H, Oberholzer M, Buser M *et al.* Digital image analysis in cytological diagnosis: a morphometric analysis on pleural mesotheliomas. *Anal Cell Pathol* 1989; **1**: 105–122

139 Alons C L, Veldhuizen R W, Boon M E. Learning from quantitation. *Anal Quant Cytol* 1981; **3**: 178–181

140 Ayres J G, Crocker J G, Skilbeck N Q. Differentiation of malignant from normal and reactive mesothelial cells by the argyrophil technique for nucleolar organiser region associated proteins. *Thorax* 1988; **43**: 366–370

141 Soosay G N, Griffiths M, Papakadi L et al. The differential diagnosis of epithelial-type mesothelioma from adenocarcinoma and reactive mesothelial proliferation. *J Pathol* 1991; **163**: 299–305

142 Derenzini M, Nardi F, Farabegoli F et al. Distribution of silver-stained interphase nucleolar organizer regions as a parameter to distinguish neoplastic from nonneoplastic reactive regions as a parameter to distinguish neoplastic from nonneoplastic reactive cells in human effusions. *Acta Cytol* 1989; **33**: 491–498

143 Lim S M, Duggan M A, Ruff M et al. Morphometric analysis of nucleolar organizer regions in benign and malignant peritoneal effusions using backscattered electron microscopy. *J Pathol* 1992; **166**: 53–60

144 Matzel W, Schubert G. Hyaluronic acid in pleural fluids: an additional parameter for clinical diagnosis on diffuse mesothelioma. *Arch Geschwulstforsch* 1979; **49**: 146–154

145 Castor C W, Naylor B. Acid mucopolysaccharide composition of serous effusions. *Cancer* 1967; **20**: 462–466

146 Rasmussen K N, Faber V. Hyaluronic acid in 247 pleural fluids. *Scand J Respir Dis* 1967; **48**: 366–371

147 Roboz J, Greaves J, Silides D et al. Hyaluronic acid content of effusions as a diagnostic aid for malignant mesothelioma. *Cancer Res* 1985; **445**: 1850–1854

148 Hjerpe A. Liquid-chromatographic determination of hyaluronic acid in pleural and ascitic fluids. *Clin Chem* 1986; **32**: 952–956

149 Azumi N, Underhill C B, Kagan E, Sheibani K. A novel biotinylated probe specific for hyaluronate. *Am J Surg Pathol* 1992; **16**: 116–121

150 Faravelli B, Diamore E, Nosenzo M et al. Carcinoembryonic antigen in pleural effusions. Diagnostic value in malignant mesothelioma. *Cancer* 1984; **53**: 1194–1197

151 Whitaker D, Shilkin K B, Stuckey M, Nieuwhof W N. Pleural fluid CEA levels in the diagnosis of malignant mesothelioma. *Pathology* 1986; **18**: 328–329

152 Watts K C, Boyo-Ekwueme H, To A et al. Chromosome studies on cells cultured from serous effusions; use in routine cytologic practice. *Acta Cytol* 1983; **27**: 38–44

153 Mark J. Three chromosomal abnormalities observed in cells of two malignant mesotheliomas studied by banding technique. *Acta Cytol* 1978; **22**: 398–401

154 Bousfield L R, Greenberg M L, Pacey F. Cytogenetic diagnosis of *Cancer* from body fluids. *Acta Cytol* 1985; **29**: 768–774

155 Granados R, Cibas E S, Fletcher J. Cytogenetic analysis is useful in the evaluation of cytologically inconclusive pleural effusions in patients with malignant mesothelioma. *Mod Pathol* 1991; **4**: Abstract 138

156 Hagemeijer A, Versnel M A, van Drunen E et al. Cytogenetic analysis of malignant mesothelioma. *Can Genet Cytogenet* 1990; **47**: 1–28

157 Goepel J R. Benign papillary mesothelioma of peritoneum; a histological, histochemical and ultrastructural study of six cases. *Histopathology* 1981; **5**: 21–30

158 Raju U, Fine G, Greenawald K A, Ohorodnik J M. Primary papillary serous neoplasia of the peritoneum: a clinicopathologic and ultrastructural study of eight cases. *Hum Pathol* 1989; **20**: 426–436

159 Daya D, McCaughey W T E. Well-differentiated papillary mesothelioma of the peritoneum. *Cancer* 1990; **65**: 292–296

160 Burrig K F, Pfitzer P, Hort W. Well differentiated papillary mesothelioma of the peritoneum: a borderline mesothelioma. Report of two cases and a review of the literature. *Virchow Arch (A)* 1990; **417**: 443–447

161 Jayaram G, Ashok S. Fine needle aspiration cytology of well-differentiated papillary peritoneal mesothelioma: report of a case. *Acta Cytol* 1988; **32**: 563–566

162 Okike N, Bernatz P E, Woolner L B. Localized mesothelioma of the pleura. Benign and malignant variants. *J Thorac Cardiovasc Surg* 1978; **75**: 363–372

163 England D M, Hochholzer L, McCarthy M J. Localized benign and malignant fibrous tumors of the pleura. *Am J Surg Pathol* 1989; **13**: 640–658

164 Bonfiglio T. Cytopathologic interpretation of transthoracic fine-needle biopsies. In: Johnston W W ed. *Masson Monographs in Diagnostic Cytopathology*, vol. 4. New York: Masson, 1983

165 Conces D J, Schwenk G R, Doering P R, Glant M D. Thoracic needle biopsy: improved results utilizing a team approach. *Chest* 1987; **91**: 813–816

166 Fraser R S. Transthoracic needle aspiration—the benign diagnosis. *Arch Pathol Lab Med* 1991; **115**: 751–761

167 Dusenbery D, Grimes M M, Frable W J. Fine needle aspiration cytology of localized fibrous tumor of pleura. *Diagn Cytopathol* 1992; **8**: 444–450

168 Weiss S W, Tavassoli F A. Multicystic mesothelioma. An analysis of pathologic findings and biologic behaviour in 37 cases. *Am J Surg Pathol* 1988; **12**: 737–746

169 Ross M J, Welch W R, Scully R E. Multilocular peritoneal inclusion cysts (so called cystic mesotheliomas). *Cancer* 1989; **64**: 1336–1346

170 Baddoura F K, Varma V A. Cytologic findings in multicystic peritoneal mesothelioma. *Acta Cytol* 1990; **34**: 524–528

171 Devaney K, Kragel P J, Devaney E J. Fine-needle aspiration cytology of multicystic mesothelioma. *Diagn Cytopathol* 1992; **8**: 68–72

172 Antman K, Cohen S, Dimitrov N V et al. Malignant mesothelioma of the tunica vaginalis testis. *J Clin Oncol* 1984; **2**: 447–451

173 Grove A, Jensen M, Donna A. Mesotheliomas of the tunica vaginalis testis and hernial sacs. *Virchows Archiv (A) Pathol Anat* 1989; **415**: 283–292

174 McCaughey W T E. Papillary peritoneal neoplasms in females. *Pathol Annu* 1985; **20**: 387–404

175 Bell D A, Scully R E. Serous borderline tumors of the peritoneum. *Am J Surg Pathol* 1990; **14**: 230–239

176 Dalrymple J C, Bannatyne P, Russell P et al. Extraovarian peritoneal serous papillary carcinoma. A clinicopathologic study of 31 cases. *Cancer* 1989; **64**: 110–115

177 Truong L D, Maccato M L, Awalt H et al. Serous surface carcinoma of the peritoneum: a clinicopathologic study of 22 cases. *Hum Pathol* 1990; **21**: 99–110

178 Martensson G. Diagnosing malignant pleural mesothelioma. *Eur Respir J* 1990; **3**: 985–986

179 Scamurra D O. Effusion cytology in the diagnosis of malignant epithelioid and biphasic pleural mesothelioma. *Arch Pathol Lab Med* 1991; **115**: 210

180 DiBonito L, Falconiere G, Colautti I et al. The positive pleural effusion. A retrospective study of cytopathologic diagnoses with autopsy confirmation. *Acta Cytol* 1992; **36**: 329–332

181 Musk A W, Christmas T I. The clinical diagnosis of malignant mesothelioma. In: Henderson D W, Shilkin K B, Langlois S Le P, Whitaker D eds. *Malignant Mesothelioma*. New York: Hemisphere, 1992; 253–258

182 Oels H C, Harrison E G, Carr B T, Bernatz P E. Diffuse malignant mesothelioma of the pleura: a review of 37 cases. *Chest* 1971; **60**: 564–570

183 Sherrin J C, Jackson P. Malignant pleural mesothelioma. *J Thorac Cardiovasc Surg* 1976; **71**: 621–627

184 Elmes P C, Simpson M J C. The clinical aspects of mesothelioma. *Quart Med* 1976; **45**: 427–429

185 Jara F, Hiroshi T, Uma N M R. Malignant mesothelioma of pleura. *NY State J Med* 1977; **77**: 1885–1888

186 Edge J R, Choudhury S L. Malignant mesothelioma of the pleura in Barrow-in-Furness. *Thorax* 1978; **33**: 26–30

187 Antman K H. Malignant mesothelioma. *N Engl J Med* 1980; **303**: 200–202

188 Lewis R J, Sisler G E, MacKenzie J W. Diffuse, mixed malignant pleural mesothelioma. *Ann Thorac Surg* 1981; **31**: 53–60

189 Nauta R J, Osteen R T, Antman K H, Koster J K. Clinical staging and the tendency of malignant pleural mesotheliomas to remain localized. *Ann Thorac Surg* 1982; **34**: 66–70

190 Law M R, Hodson M E, Turner-Warwick M. Malignant mesothelioma of the pleura. Clinical aspects and symptomatic

treatment. *Eur J Respir Dis* 1984; **65**: 162–168

191 Martensson G, Hagmar B, Zettergren L. Diagnosis and prognosis in malignant pleural mesothelioma: a prospective study. *Eur J Respir Dis* 1984; **65**: 169–178

192 Matzel W. Biochemical and cytological features of diffuse mesotheliomas of the pleura. *Arch Geschwulstforsch* 1985; **55**: 259–264

193 Adams V I, Unni K K, Huhm J R *et al*. Diffuse malignant mesothelioma of pleura: diagnosis and survival in 92 cases. *Cancer* 1986; **58**: 1540–1551

194 Strankinga W F, Sperber M, Kaiser M C, Stam J. Accuracy of diagnostic procedures in the initial evaluation and follow-up of mesothelioma patients. *Respiration* 1987; **51**: 179–187

195 Ribak J, Lilis R, Suzuki Y *et al*. Malignant mesothelioma in a cohort of asbestos insulation workers: clinical presentation, diagnosis, and causes of death. *Br J Ind Med* 1988; **45**: 182–187

7 Normal breast cytology and breast screening

Alec Howat and Stuart Coghill

Introduction

To ease the taking and interpretation of cytology specimens of breast and to advise surgical colleagues on prognosis and management, it is important to have a good understanding of relevant anatomy, pathology and clinical practice. An attempt is made in these chapters to make available the core information necessary for the student of breast cytology to integrate the cytological perspective into a clinical and histopathological context. As it is assumed that most readers will already have a good understanding of the histopathology of the breast, the text and illustrations will build on this by correlating cytological appearances with those of histopathology.

In the past, the procedure of obtaining a sample of tissue with a small bore needle and the preparation and interpretation of smears or spun preparations has been variously referred to as 'FNA cytology' or 'FNA biopsy'. It has been recommended[1] that care be taken to avoid any laxity in terminology now that methods are in use for the preparation of histological sections from aspirated specimens. The convention of referring only to the latter method as 'FNA biopsy' will be observed in this section.

Fine needle aspiration (FNA) cytology is a new but now well-established method of obtaining a diagnosis from lesions in superficial and deep locations[2-6]. In the practice of most cytopathologists the vast majority of FNA samples will be from breast.

In the assessment of breast lesions, the most important role of diagnostic cytology is in making the binary decision between benign and malignant. The difference between a benign and malignant lesion is usually dramatic, clinically. It is often surprising to clinical colleagues that there can be any difficulty when the pathologist has been presented with something that can be scrutinized under the microscope. However, these difficulties can be particularly acute for the breast cytologist because of certain characteristic, but not unique, qualities of pathological lesions of the breast.

These qualities include the remarkable ability of the breast to undergo benign hyperplasia and the tendency for many carcinomas of the breast to be bland cytologically. Malignant breast epithelium exhibits the nuclear enlargement, anisonucleosis and chromatin derangements that are the hallmarks of malignancy in a way that is often more subtle than in malignancies at other sites. There is also the tendency of breast carcinomas to provoke a marked stromal reaction. This ensures that, despite ease of access, it can be difficult to extract a diagnostic cytological sample from what may be a clinically obvious carcinoma. The final major difficulty is the imperceptible gradation between the lesions that all histopathologists would regard as benign and those that are obviously malignant. This has not been such a problem in symptomatic patients, but is becoming increasingly important with the developing interest in obtaining cytological samples from very early impalpable lesions.

Further difficulties may arise because the adjacent soft tissues and overlying skin and adnexae may be the host to lesions that are mistaken clinically and cytologically for breast disease. The deep surface of the breast is closely apposed to the underlying skeletal muscle and is only a few millimetres away from the ribs and pleura. These facts explain the contents of some aspirates and the occurrence of some rare complications of FNA such as pneumothorax.

Development and hormonal responsiveness of the breast

It is generally agreed, but not proven, that the development of mature resting functional units of the breast occurs throughout reproductive life, with accentuation in pregnancy, rather than being completed at the time of puberty[7]. Under the influence of oestrogen and then, following menarche, progestogens, and in a complex hormonal milieu of growth hormone, thyroxine and insulin, the breast parenchyma grows by a process of duct elongation and branching. There is also a formation of buds destined to become the lobular structures.

Before puberty, the progenitors of the adult breast are concentrated in a small volume of tissue and so damage to the vestigial organ can result in postpubertal disfigurement. Fortunately the occurrence of masses in the prepubertal breast is rare, but when this does occur FNA offers a means of obtaining a diagnosis without the risk of unnecessary surgery. Pubertal hyperplasia occurs in both males and females and can be temporarily unbalanced or unilateral, but should not be mistaken for a pathological process when seen in the appropriate stage of development of the child. It subsides with progressing sexual maturation.

The physiology of the human breast is in some respects unique among mammals. Even casual observation of other species reminds us that their breasts are diminutive organs in the resting state, becoming prominent only in response to pregnancy, or in some species, as a reaction to copulation in anticipation of pregnancy. The parenchyma of human breast, by contrast, becomes fully developed at puberty and is then subjected to the waxing and waning stimuli of the menstrual cycle, interrupted only by the additional effects of pregnancy until the menopause. Observation of the hormonal responses in the normal breast is difficult and the changes are therefore controversial. However, we have some understanding of events from the study of surgical specimens and medicolegal autopsies in premenstrual women[7].

Following ovulation, rising levels of progesterone cause hyperplasia and dilation of terminal ductules. Mitotic activity appears in the lobular epithelium as does vacuolation, the morphological expression of a low level of secretion. In the secretory phase of the cycle the stroma becomes oedematous, sometimes giving the woman a sensation of fullness of the breasts. Late in the secretory and menstrual phase apoptotic activity occurs with some shedding of epithelial cell debris into the ductal lumina. Secretory products of non-lactating breast are slight and are presumably largely resorbed, only becoming obvious when part of the duct lobular system becomes obstructed by an inflammatory or neoplastic process.

The effects of ageing on breast tissue have been the focus of subjective as well as more objective morphometric scrutiny[8]. Generalized involution of stroma and epithelial elements is the usual morphological finding in normal postmenopausal women but this is predominantly a pre- rather than postmenopausal phenomenon. There is an increase in the incidence of breast carcinoma in postmenopausal women. This is associated with a rise in the incidence of premalignant changes. These are rare and difficult to detect and so the current approach to breast screening is aimed at the detection of early cancer rather than premalignant lesions.

Clinical and technical methods

Aspiration method for palpable breast lumps

Evidence from the literature indicates that optimal results are obtained when a dedicated single aspirator, ideally the pathologist, obtains and interprets the sample using direct smears[9–12]. Many pathologists are wary of re-exposing themselves to the rigours of a clinical role but, if properly defined and understood by both pathologist and clinician responsible for the patient, no problems need be anticipated.

If manning levels or attitudes do not allow the cytopathologist to adopt a clinical role, it is important that aspirations are obtained by a senior clinician with a particular interest in breast disease. The stereotactic sampling of mammographic abnormalities is the province of a diagnostic radiologist with special training in the technique.

However, there are many units where the FNA is taken by a variable number of clinicians, including trainees. Flushing the FNA into a transport medium is then often preferable to the array of poorly prepared direct smears that are usually submitted from such an eclectic collection of aspirators. This procedure is known as 'liquid based cytology (LBC)' and includes the 'Cytospin', the 'ThinPrep' and 'Tripath (Autocyte)' procedures. All LBC techniques involve preparation of interpretive slides in the laboratory[13].

Recently core biopsy has undergone a renaissance in popularity for the primary diagnosis of breast disease, especially in cases considered clinically and/or radiologically malignant or suspicious.

Direct smears aspirated and prepared by a pathologist

It is intended that this section will provide the novice aspirator with the basic information required of the practical aspects of clinical aspiration cytology. There can, however, be no substitute for attending a clinic with a pathologist who has already gained the necessary experience.

The first stage of the procedure is for the cytologist to examine the lesion clinically. As the clinician will have already fully examined both breasts and axillae, the cytologist may safely concentrate on the presenting lesion and most often the patient will provide the best guide as to its location. Occasionally, the patient will deny accurate knowledge of the lesion, saying that her family doctor found it during a routine examination. Similarly the initial assessment by the clinician may locate a further lesion of which the patient was not aware. In these circumstances it is very helpful to have the clinician outline the lesion on the skin using a pen.

In examining the lesion, the cytologist should confirm the presence or absence of tethering to skin or chest wall or in-drawing of the nipple. It is important for training and audit that the cytologist records his description of the lesion including size, location, tissue plane, and whether it is well or poorly defined, hard or soft. These details can be collected efficiently using a proforma including a diagram of a female thorax.

It is also helpful to record the sensation obtained when the needle enters the lesion and include details in the report for subsequent audit. These may be described and correlated in the following way, modified from the United Kingdom National Health Service Breast Screening Programme (NHSBSP) guidelines[14]:

Soft – fibroadenoma, mucoid carcinoma, medullary carcinoma
Rubbery – fibrocystic change, lobular carcinoma, fibroadenoma
Variable resistance with popping sensation – fibrocystic change
Leathery – dense fibrous change, ancient fibroadenoma

Gritty – carcinoma, partial calcification, a few fibroadenomas

Solid – completely calcified ancient fibroadenomas

No resistance – fatty tissue

There has been debate as to the most appropriate gauge of needle to use for breast aspiration[15]. Clearly there is likely to be a compromise as a very large needle will produce too much pain and haemorrhage whereas a needle that is too small will not permit an adequate sample to be taken. The sensitivity of cytodiagnosis was evaluated in two groups of women with symptomatic breast lumps randomly allocated to aspiration with 21 and 23 gauge needles[15]. There was no statistical difference in the sensitivity or specificity achieved with the two needles. In an earlier *in vitro* study[16] it was shown that the amount of epithelium obtained may be greater with the larger needle. It would appear that this is not translated into a major improvement in sensitivity, presumably because an *in vitro* study cannot assess the effects of the presence of blood in the sample. This is a problem more commonly experienced with the larger needle. From observing the patient's reactions it is clear that the 23-gauge needle causes less discomfort.

The use of a multihole needle for obtaining both histological and cytological samples has been described[17] and may bring an increase in diagnostic accuracy but its use has not yet become widespread.

When the aspirate is taken and interpreted by different individuals, it has been shown that sensitivity can be optimized within the limitations of practicality by taking three or four aspirations routinely from each lesion[18]. Cytopathologists who perform the aspirations are able to examine each sample in turn, minimizing the imposition on the patient.

Another modification of the technique that has been recently suggested is the use of a needle without a syringe or the application of suction[19–21]. A syringe is then used to express the sample. Theoretically the sample is obtained by the cutting action of the tip of the needle, suction serving only to increase tissue damage and contamination of the specimen with blood.

Obtaining the aspirate

Apart from interpretive skills, the most important element in accurate breast cytodiagnosis is the technique of aspiration. Each aspirator cytopathologist will develop his or her own technique; the following is intended as a guide.

► The patient should lie on a couch with the head raised.
► Right-handed aspirators should approach from the patient's right, even for aspiration of a lesion in the left breast. If necessary the patient is asked to roll towards the aspirator.
► Not infrequently a patient will report that she can only find the lump when sitting up and leaning forward. It is clearly necessary for the aspirator to find the lesion with the patient in this position. It is generally more comfortable for both the patient and the aspirator if the patient lies down again for the aspirate to be taken.
► A 10 ml syringe should be inserted in the pistol grip if one is available. It is important that the syringe holder is tailored to fit syringes from a specific manufacturer. Some aspirators prefer not to use a syringe holder but novices should begin with one. A needle, 21G (green) or 23G (blue), should be used.
► The syringe is primed with 1–2 ml of air to aid the expulsion of the sample[22].
► The assembled syringe is laid within reach or handed to an assistant along with an opened antiseptic swab.
► An ethylene chloride spray is placed within reach. The pocket of the aspirator's white coat is a convenient location.
► The lump is identified and grasped between the thumb and forefinger of the left hand (right-handed aspirators). It is worth spending some time manipulating the lump so that it is gripped firmly. This is particularly important for deep breast lumps in obese patients.
► It is better not to fix breast lumps against the chest wall but to manipulate them forward between the finger and thumb to reduce the risk of pneumothorax. The gripping of the lump should also put tension on the skin to aid needle penetration.
► When the lump is securely gripped the alcohol swab is used to wipe the area.
► Ethyl chloride spray is then trained on the area until a white frost appears. The use of ethyl chloride is optional but a kindness when two or three attempts are required.
► The needle tip is then pushed into the centre of the lump and negative pressure applied to the syringe. Then the tip of the needle is gently moved backwards and forwards in the same direction, taking care not to rock the needle sideways through the lesion as this is likely to cause bleeding.
► Three or four passes are adequate on a first attempt.
► *It is important not to wait until a 'sample' appears in the hub of the needle. The ideal aspirate is invisible and resides within the shaft of the needle.* When a sample appears in the hub it is generally impaired by heavy contamination with blood.
► The negative pressure is then fully released *before* the tip of the needle is withdrawn from the lesion.
► Without delay, the contents of the needle are expelled on to a single slide to form a spot a few millimetres from the frosted end. The needle should be carefully removed from the syringe, which is then fully recharged with air, allowing the expulsion of any remaining material within the needle. Repeat this twice.
► Place the needle and syringe in a safe disposal container.
► Immediately spread the aspirate with a second slide held at right angles with a gentle, even pressure.
► Allow the sample to dry and immediately label with the patient's name in *pencil*.
► One smear should be fixed in alcohol for those cytopathologists who prefer to report wet-fixed, Papanicolaou-stained smears.
► If the aspirate appears very scanty it may be worth performing an immediate repeat.
► On repeating the aspirate it can be helpful to aim for the periphery of the lesion as some carcinomas have a scirrhous centre, but are more cellular at the growing margins.

▶ To minimize the risk of haematoma formation, a cotton wool ball or gauze pad should be firmly applied to the site by an assistant or the patient. The longer and the greater this pressure, within the limits of comfort, the better.

▶ If the aspirate is not to be stained immediately, it should be placed in a protective slide box *once fully dried* and stained and examined or dispatched to the pathologist.

▶ When the pathologist has not taken the aspirate, it is important to be fully appraised of clinical details. Previous biopsy or cytology report numbers should be quoted.

Liquid based cytology

Cytospin method

This method, which involves collecting FNA in Cytospin collection fluid (CCF), and then making preparations in the laboratory to be stained with Papanicolaou and H&E, is utilized by some laboratories for the following reasons:

▶ An unacceptably high proportion of poorly prepared direct smears by a variety of clinicians

▶ Health and Safety anxiety in making air-dried smears

▶ Lack of research material with direct smears

CCF is an aqueous mixture of denatured ethanol, ispropanol and polyethylene glycol giving a final alcohol concentration of approximately 40%. Methylene blue and tartrazine are also added to give a bright green colour, preventing confusion with other fluids, e.g. formalin, saline etc[23]. The FNA is obtained in the usual way by the aspirator as described previously; the needle and syringe are then flushed into 10 ml of CCF and the specimen taken to the laboratory[24]. The specimen is centrifuged at 3000 rpm (approximately 1500 x *g*) for 5 min. A total of 4 ml of fluid including floating material are aspirated and retained in a 3 x 3/8 inch tube, the rest of the supernatant being carefully discarded. The deposit is then re-suspended in 2 ml of well-mixed reserved supernatant. 0.5 ml is then applied to each of 4 Cytospin cups, prepared with APES-treated slides and 4 drops of cervical smear fixative, and centrifuged using the Cytospin III (Shandon (UK) Ltd) at 1250 rpm for 5 min. Any fluid remaining in the specimen container is aspirated and retained in the 3 x 3/8 inch tube for further investigations, if required. The preparations are dried for 20 min at room temperature or 10 min at 37°C in a fan-assisted slide-dryer. The cytopreparations are then stained with Papanicolaou and/or H&E.

Heavy deposits can be solved using a variety of methods[25], one of the simplest being to gently squeeze two slides together with the buttons longitudinally offset; the buttons must not be allowed to dry before squeezing. Solid fragments of tissue are removed after centrifugation, fixed in Dubosq-Brazil, paper-wrapped and processed to paraffin. Alternatively, the Cytoblock technique may be used[26]. Cytopreparations can be ready in 1–1.5 h. This method may be used in rapid breast clinics that permit more time for diagnosis, as opposed to requiring an immediate result.

The Cytospin method is an acceptable alternative to direct smears for FNAs[24,27-29]; comparing favourably with direct smears[10,30-31], the positive predictive value for malignancy being almost 100%[9,10,24,27-31].

There are a number of merits to the Cytospin method:

1 Relatively low inadequate rate when multiple aspirators perform FNAB

2 Reproducible uniform high quality preparations with excellent morphology

3 Safety, without potentially dangerous air-drying

4 Faster reporting with a small area on the slide; all cytopathologists will know that daunting feeling of having to examine many poorly cellular direct smears

5 Additional material for further diagnostic, prognostic and research methods

There are two main disadvantages to the Cytospin method:

1 Inability to make air-dried MGG stained specimens

2 Relatively higher inadequate rate than that reported with direct smears made by single aspirators where further aspirates can be performed if the first is inadequate

ThinPrep method

This LBC method is similar to the Cytospin method in that the FNAs are flushed into a transport medium, CytoLyt Solution (Cytyc Corporation). The transport solution is centrifuged and resuspended in a preservative solution, PreservCyt, (Cytyc Corporation)[32]. ThinPrep slides are made using the ThinPrep processor (Cytyc Corporation) and routinely stained with the Papanicolaou stain.

In a large study comparing 21 193 conventional breast FNA smears with 7903 ThinPreps, there was no significant difference in diagnostic accuracy[33], the unsatisfactory rate being marginally better for ThinPrep (27.7% *vs* 29.5%). The advantages and disadvantages of ThinPrep compared with direct smears are the same as for the Cytospin method, although reports have stressed the need for a learning period with ThinPrep as the preparations display artefacts not seen in conventional smears[32,33].

Tripath (Autocyte) method

This LBC method (TriPath Imaging Inc.) involves the FNA being sent to the lab in a transport medium and prepared using the Tripath Preparation technique. Studies are limited as the technology is new for non-gynaecological cytology[34].

Core biopsy

The use of core biopsy (CB) has increased predominantly in breast screening programmes; the primary investigation for analysis of a palpable breast mass remains FNA. About two-thirds of cancers detected through the United Kingdom National Health Service Breast Screening Programme (UK NHSBSP) are diagnosed preoperatively by either CB and/or FNA[35], with a decrease in centres solely using FNA from 46% in 1995/6 to 11% in 1996/7. Large calibre stereotactic biopsy systems are in the process of being evaluated[36,37].

CB can be especially useful in specific circumstances: for example when the FNA is inadequate, or when the mammogram shows microcalcification, and for low-grade cancers that are difficult to accurately diagnose as malignant on cytology, hence are reported as suspicious[38]. Although CB has a higher absolute sensitivity and specificity than FNA for impalpable lesions, it has a higher false negative rate[35]. Other disadvantages of CB include the need for histopathological processing thereby precluding 'rapid diagnosis', difficulty in technique and tissue damage and displacement, this being partially related to the size of the cutting needle[39,40]. Pitfalls include granulation tissue, haemorrhage as a direct result of trauma, and displacement of benign epithelium into vessels and stroma. Care must be taken to recognize these potential false positives by observing the lack of tumour stroma and the bland cytology.

Preparative methods

The method for producing reliable evenly spread smears has already been described. There are three staining methods that are routinely used in cytodiagnosis. Each pathologist will tend to favour the method that was used in his or her training department and will not easily be persuaded of the benefits of the alternatives. Those pathologists introduced to cytodiagnosis early in their careers who became accustomed to May-Grunwald-Giemsa (MGG) preparations of serous fluids will feel comfortable with this method in breast cytodiagnosis. Histopathologists will adapt more easily to wet fixed preparations stained with haematoxylin and eosin (H&E) or with the more frequently used Papanicolaou stain favoured by many cytopathologists[41].

There are several advantages that make the MGG method preferable to some pathologists, the most important being the time taken to make and stain the smears. The rapid MGG methods (Diff-Quik, HaemaGurr) take less than 2 min from removal of the needle from the patient to the slide reaching the microscope stage. Other advantages include:

1 Avoidance of air drying artefact
2 Avoidance of cell loss when wet smears are placed in alcohol
3 Fewer steps required, ensuring good quality preparations without the assistance of a cytotechnologist
4 The cells appear much larger in the air dried preparations
5 Extracellular material such as mucin, connective tissue ground substance and intracytoplasmic granules are more easily seen
6 Smears may be examined without a coverslip

The disadvantages are:

1 Thick smears do not stain adequately, which is not a problem when the cytopathologist performs the aspirate

2 Squamous cells may be difficult to identify, but this not a major problem in breast cytodiagnosis

Papanicolaou-stained smears are more useful for detecting subtle nuclear and chromatin changes that may be seen in low-grade carcinomas. With this stain the cells at the bottom of a cluster can be visualized by careful focusing, as cytoplasm retains its translucency.

Artefacts in breast aspirates

Stain precipitate

This is seen most commonly when the second staining reagent of the MGG method is used for many cases, particularly when these are not fully defatted by the first two reagents. The presence of a small amount of precipitate seldom impairs the specimen for diagnostic purposes, but mars photomicrographs. Its appearance should prompt a change of staining solutions.

Starch granules

These refractile spheroids originate from glove starch and are familiar to histopathologists. They are frequently found in breast aspirates when the aspirator sensibly wears gloves to avoid cross infection.

Exploded nuclei

This is the most serious artefact besetting MGG air-dried smears. If widespread, it may render a specimen useless. Furthermore the novice may try to interpret the less affected cells that appear artificially large. The appearance, sometimes called the osmotic effect, is that of a cell whose nucleus has expanded and ruptured with spillage of chromatin at the cell border, forming a flare. This artefact has been attributed to the effects of saline, local anaesthetic fluid and autolysis from slow drying, as when the smear is placed directly into an airtight box. Over-heating when an electric hairdryer is used to ensure rapid drying and the use of excessive pressure when making the smear are also possible culprits.

Crushed nuclei *(Fig. 7.1)*

This is distinct from the phenomenon of exploded nuclei described above as the spilled chromatin is spread in the direction of the smear. It is due to the use of excessive pressure but some types of malignant tumours are particularly prone to this problem, so this finding can be used as a diagnostic pointer.

Air drying of Papanicolaou preparations

In contrast to the more mucin-rich cervical smear, many breast aspirates are scanty, not only in terms of the cellular content but also for the fluid present. These aspirates may dry almost immediately when they are spread on the slide, particularly if humidity is low, and even quite rapid application of fixative may not prevent this artefact. The resulting blurring of nuclear detail demands that

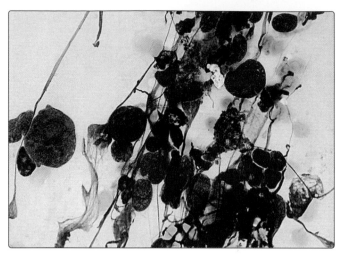

Fig. 7.1 Crushing artefact. These breast carcinoma cells show typical crushing and spreading of the chromatin. The tendency for this artefact to develop is a function of the fragility of the cells and the pressure used to make the smear. (MGG)

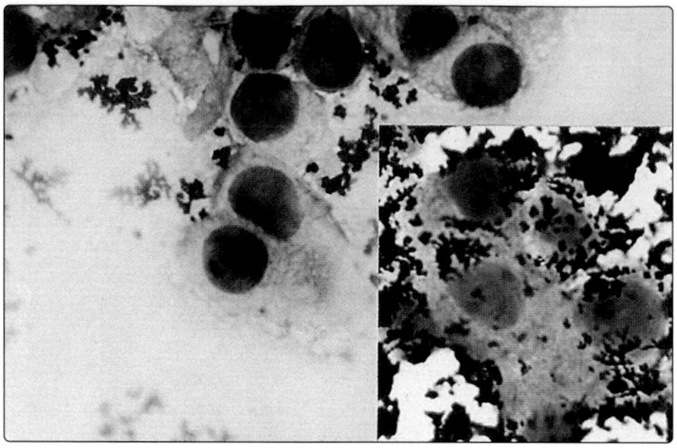

Fig. 7.2 Ultrasound jelly artefact. These breast carcinoma cells show an intermediate degree of damage as a result of the presence of ultrasound jelly. The nuclei show loss of the chromatin detail and the constituent of the jelly is seen as a purple granular precipitate. The inset shows the cells at a slightly more advanced stage of dissolution resulting from a greater concentration of the jelly. (MGG)

interpretation is made with great caution if it is to be undertaken at all.

MGG staining of wet-fixed smears

This problem can arise because of poor clinical liaison. A smear that is incorrectly labelled as air-dried or that is unlabelled and assumed to be air-dried will give a misleading appearance when stained with an MGG method. The cells are more compact and therefore appear smaller and more bland than if they had been air-dried. The staining characteristics are however normal, making it difficult to recognize that the artefact is present. Cytopathologists may be tricked into missing what would otherwise have been an easy malignant diagnosis. The education of clinical colleagues as to the important difference between air-dried and wet-fixed preparations is necessary, for avoidance of the problem with aspiration by the cytopathologist.

Heavily blood-stained aspirates

A few red blood cells provide a scale for comparison with the size of the nucleated cells. The commonest cause of impairment of the quality of aspirates is the presence of a large amount of blood. Epithelial cells are partially obscured and in air-dried aspirates, the stains often do not penetrate the thick film of blood. Fortunately, the film is often thinner at the edge, and in the more cellular aspirates there will be sufficient material to allow a diagnosis. The aspirator cytopathologist has the option of prolonging staining times for thicker aspirates and of repeating the aspirate when all else fails.

Cell lysis by contamination by ultrasound transmission jelly

As ultrasound localization of breast lumps is adopted more widely, this phenomenon poses a threat to cytological

diagnosis[42]. The effect of the jelly on cell morphology is dramatic and, in *in vitro* experiments, varies with the length of exposure before fixation. The phenomenon is seen even in rapidly air-dried samples, presumably from the mixing of the jelly with the sample within the needle rather than on the slide.

Initially, there is some swelling of the cell cytoplasm and nucleus (Fig. 7.2). This can make benign cells more worrying when compared with uncontaminated controls. Cell swelling is closely followed by leakage of nuclear chromatin, then complete dissolution of cell structure to form granular basophilic material and then eventually, a basophilic soup.

Radiologists regard ultrasound jelly as a bland substance. If made aware of its detrimental effects on aspirated cells, they can modify their technique to lessen the risk of contamination.

Complications of FNA of the breast

Complications are few and seldom serious. The only common problem encountered clinically is the formation of a haematoma. This is unpredictable and can be minimized by prolonged pressure following aspiration, but frequently the bleeding occurs very rapidly, even before the needle is withdrawn. This can obscure the lesion, making a second attempt difficult or impossible and can make mammograms difficult to interpret for the following 2 to 3 weeks.

Pneumothorax has been reported as a very rare complication[43-44]. Strict adherence to the method outlined earlier in this chapter should minimize this risk.

Some clinicians have persistent fears that 'needling' a malignancy will help it to disseminate, despite a lack of any evidence that this occurs in breast lesions. The fear may be

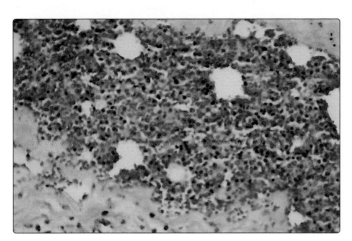

Fig. 7.3   Tumour cells in the tract of a core-biopsy. This is virtually unknown following fine needle aspiration. (H&E)

more justified when large bore biopsy needles are used, than when fine needle sampling is performed. There is evidence that needle tract seeding can occur with various tumours[45–54] but this has not been reported with breast cancer and appears to be a very small risk. In view of the trend towards more conservative surgery for breast cancer, the very small risk from this theoretical problem may be increased but it is unlikely that it will be detectable among the relatively large number of spontaneous chest wall and surgical scar recurrences.

Histological sections of excision biopsy specimens following core biopsy occasionally show epithelial displacement (Fig. 7.3), but this has not been seen following FNA, by the authors.

The interpretation of histopathology specimens taken after a prior fine needle aspiration is usually straightforward, but problems have been reported both with breast and other tissues[55–56]. Mammographic changes induced by haemorrhage following FNA appear to be more of a problem[57–59]. This is a good reason for performing mammography before aspiration. If the radiographs are then made available to the pathologist, the targeting and interpretation even of palpable lesions will be enhanced.

Special methods for cytological diagnosis and determination of the prognosis in breast carcinoma

For the foreseeable future, the mainstay of cytological diagnosis in breast disease will be subjective analysis of the morphology of cells stained using May-Grunwald-Giemsa, Papanicolaou or haematoxylin and eosin methods. Current skills and methodology do not permit cytology alone to reach 100% sensitivity and specificity. However, this is achievable when cytology and mammography are used together[10] but there must be a continuing effort to optimize the application of this powerful technique. With breast screening and an ever improving mammographic

technology there is the expectation that cytological methods will keep pace with the need to diagnose breast carcinomas at an ever earlier stage. As methods of treatment are refined and developed there will be an increasing demand to predict the behaviour of breast neoplasms as early as possible during the disease.

Cytological prognostication

There has been some progress in the prediction of tumour behaviour from cytological assessment. However, while the primary therapeutic manoeuvre in the treatment of breast cancer remains excision of the lesion, there is little to be gained from engaging in assessments of the cytology aimed at deciding the ultimate prognosis. These goals are better achieved with histopathological methodology, and histopathology is likely to remain the gold standard for the future.

Prognostic factors in breast cancer have been the subject of much recent research, mainly using fixed histological material but also cytology preparations. Despite the numerous publications purporting to describe a 'new prognostic marker', multivariate analyses have consistently shown correlation of these new markers with the well-known prognostic factors of tumour size, nodal status, tumour histological type, vascular invasion and tumour grade[60–62]. The ability to predict tumour grade on breast aspirates is of value, especially if neo-adjuvant chemotherapy is being considered. A number of studies have shown some success[63–70], and it has been recommended that cytological grading should be included in breast FNA reports[12]. Demonstration of cells in proliferation using the monoclonal antibody MIB-1, which recognizes parts of the Ki-67 antigen, may be of some help in grading[71].

Investigation of factors that might affect treatment regimes has been undertaken; oestrogen and progesterone receptors (ER and PR) are demonstrable on aspirates[72–76] with decisions regarding tamoxifen or chemotherapy sometimes resting on this information pre-operatively or for inoperable cases. However, for routine cases, most pathologists like to use histology where there is usually some normal breast that can act as an internal positive control. Drugs are being developed that target antigens on cancer cells; for example, trastuzumab (Herceptin) is an agent directed against HER-2/neu (c-erbB-2) oncoprotein which is expressed by a number of high-grade breast cancers containing the HER-2/neu oncogene, and associated with a relatively dismal prognosis[77]. In addition, tumours that are HER-2/neu positive and hormone receptor negative might be those best suited to treatment with adjuvant chemotherapy[78].

Many studies on histological sections, as well as on aspirates, have reported demonstration of other putative prognostic factors including oncogenes, cathepsin-D expression, cell adhesion molecules such as CD44, proteases, metalloproteinases, growth factors, laminin receptors, multidrug resistance-associated protein, tumour suppression genes including p53 and p21, ploidy studies, AgNOR expression and ultrastuctural and morphometric analyses, some with limited clinical value[61-62,79-101]. Computer-based expert systems have been developed to aid cytological assessment of breast lesions and may prove to be of use[102], while ultrastructural analysis has little practical value[103]. In-situ hybridization techniques are also being applied to cytology[104]. It is apparent that, despite all these ingenious attempts to extract the maximum amount of information from aspiration specimens, full histopathological assessment and clinical staging have to be undertaken before rational decisions can be made with respect to therapy and assessment of prognosis[61-62].

The role of FNA in the management of breast disease

Uses of FNA cytology: clinical considerations

Although the very first approaches to microscopic diagnosis of breast neoplasms were cytological, the traditional method of deciding the nature of a palpable breast lump has been excision biopsy and histopathological assessment with or without intraoperative frozen section diagnosis. However, it was generally accepted that it was cruel to subject the patient to a general anaesthetic with the uncertainty of whether a breast would have been removed on recovery. The development of the wide bore biopsy needle was a considerable advance, but is painful for most patients and fails to provide a diagnosis in some carcinomas[105]. The need for histological processing precludes the provision of a diagnosis in the clinic, although the provision of an immediate diagnosis by frozen section[106] or imprint cytology of the needle core[107] in the outpatient clinic has been described.

There have been many studies of series of patients with breast lumps assessed by aspiration cytology[9-13,108-155]. It is now established that by employing the 'triple diagnosis' of clinical assessment, mammography and cytology, a sensitivity and specificity that is effectively 100% can be achieved. If the aspirates are obtained by the clinician and, more particularly, when there are multiple aspirators, this level of accuracy will not be achieved. When the sensitivity or specificity falls significantly below 100% the method rapidly loses value[115,116].

The influence of the skill of the aspirator on the general utility of breast cytodiagnosis has been stressed. Even more important however, is the marked increase in sensitivity when the aspirator receives immediate feedback on individual samples, because of staining and reading the smears in the clinic. Comparison of the results achieved by a pathologist aspirator with that of an experienced surgeon reveals that the advantage gained by the pathologist's clinical participation is an increase of 11% in the complete

sensitivity[9,10]. When it is not possible for the pathologist to obtain the aspirates, it is vitally important that there is close liaison between clinician, pathologist and radiologist at the triple assessment clinic.

Early in the use of FNA cytology, both surgeons and pathologists may become discouraged if the initial results are poorer than expected. Less than optimal results are to be anticipated when any technique is newly adopted. In centres where its introduction is not carefully planned, or where the clinicians or pathologists are less than enthusiastic about the method, there is a risk that the technique will lose credibility before it is properly established. This is particularly likely to happen when multiple aspirators with no formal training in the technique submit samples to a remote laboratory and therefore do not receive immediate feedback on the adequacy of the aspirate. Regular audit of FNA performance is essential.

It has been recommended that implementation should be in three phases with a sequence of in vitro, in vivo and finally in vivo for clinical use[123]. In this way clinicians and pathologists can gain confidence without any risk to patients. It is extremely helpful to pathologists wishing to provide this service for the first time to visit a centre where clinics are already established.

It is also vital to review as many cytological preparations and follow-up histology slides as possible. By this means, a service as good as that in established centres can be provided within a few months. The influence of training on breast cytodiagnostic accuracy has been assessed using a method known as 'receiver operating curve analysis'[124]. Whether or not this method is used to monitor progress, it is essential once routine cytodiagnosis is established, that there is continuing audit. This should include the correlation of cytology and histology, or clinical follow-up in those patients not proceeding to surgery. These data are most efficiently obtained from an integrated cytology/histology computer system, supplemented with follow-up data from the breast clinic.

In making comparisons with other series, it is important to include all those samples that were regarded as inadequate when considering the sensitivity of the method. For some series in which the clinician has obtained the aspirates and in which the sensitivity is relatively high, scrutiny of the methodology suggests that sensitivity has been calculated only on those samples deemed to contain sufficiently large amounts of epithelium. The true sensitivity of the technique must take account of those women (up to 10-20% in some series) for whom a diagnosis could not be made.

Much has been written about the best method of obtaining and handling breast aspirates[9,10,12-14,24,27,29,33]. Of all the factors influencing the utility of the technique, none is more important than the training and experience of the aspirator. It is very important that the sampling of tissue lesions is not regarded as a procedure of similar complexity to the taking of blood samples that may be delegated to inexperienced trainees. This can be a particular problem in a busy institution that has a high ratio of trainees to trained clinicians. There is no doubt that the best results are obtained when the experience is concentrated in the hands of as few individuals as possible.

Furthermore, the best results and the most efficient service are obtained when the aspirate is taken and immediately stained and reported by the same individual. The history, clinical examination, taking and interpreting of the sample then become part of the same diagnostic process. Apart from achieving concentration of expertise in a few individuals, adoption of this policy makes major contributions to diagnostic accuracy. The most important of these is the facility to repeat the aspirate if the initial microscopic findings are inadequate for diagnosis or are inconsistent with the clinical picture. It can be argued that this may be achieved by merely having the cytopathologist 'on hand' for an immediate opinion. While this policy is certainly a major improvement over a remote laboratory service, it is still not ideal. This is because it is never possible to convey verbally or otherwise, the degree to which the taking of the aspirate 'felt' representative. Conversely the degree of confidence that the microscopic appearances are likely to be adequate for diagnosis, and representative of the palpated lump, cannot be adequately assessed in this way. In the Scandinavian countries where FNA was initially developed and is now most widely used, the pathologist aspirator is the most frequent provider of this service.

The provision of a reliable diagnosis in symptomatic breast disease results in delivery of a better quality and more efficient service to the patient. Women attending an outpatient clinic with a palpable lump want to be told immediately that the lesion is benign, rather than experience the anxiety of waiting several days for the diagnosis[156–158]. As most of the patients in a symptomatic breast clinic do not have a malignancy, the provision of an immediate diagnosis is worthwhile. There is however more ambivalence concerning the impact of receiving a malignant diagnosis 'rapidly'[157–159]. It has been demonstrated that breast cancer patients who were provided with an immediate diagnosis had higher levels of depression at 8 weeks compared with those given the diagnosis in the two-stop system[157]. Clearly, whenever news of malignancy is broken to a patient there is likely to be severe distress. It may be argued that women given a malignant diagnosis at the first attendance will have longer to come to terms with the news, to consult with friends and relatives and reach a more rational decision on the appropriate management in discussion with the surgeon[160]; counselling by a trained member of staff can begin immediately. Even if the bad news is not broken to the patient straight away, its availability will allow rapid planning of further

investigations and treatment and will result in a more authoritative and helpful communication with the family doctor.

Close attention is being paid to the costs of different diagnostic and therapeutic methods[160–165]. FNA is a relatively inexpensive investigation and frequently obviates the need for other more costly investigations or admission to hospital for open biopsy. It is possible to demonstrate cost effectiveness even when the sensitivity is only 37% and the specificity 80%[161]. The improved results obtained by an aspirator cytopathologist lead to substantial savings even if it is necessary to employ additional staff[163–164]. Core biopsies prevent open surgery and save considerable healthcare costs, ultrasound-guided biopsies unsurprisingly saving more than those taken stereotactically[165].

In centres where it not possible to establish formal aspiration cytology clinics, the provision of an examination room within the pathology department will allow aspirates to be taken on an *ad hoc* basis. A less time efficient approach is the attendance of the pathologist on the ward or in the clinic when requested. This activity is made more effective if aspirates can be assessed for adequacy by the bedside. The weight and fragility of bench microscopes make them unsuitable for this purpose but there is a pocket microscope of considerable help in this regard[166]. In many centres, a FNA trolley complete with microscope and staining kit is always kept available for the cytopathologist to take to the ward or clinic.

Breast cytology is generally considered to be part of the initial assessment of breast lesions. It has, however, also been used as an adjunct to frozen section and paraffin section histology to assist in reaching a diagnosis[167] and assessing excision margins[168]. There are also reports of its use in the assessment of nipple discharge specimens in symptomatic cases and for screening purposes[169,170].

Benefits of FNA in management of symptomatic breast lesions

► Rapid diagnosis of neoplastic, hyperplastic and inflammatory masses
► Simplification of assessment of the need for further diagnostic tests
► Permits diagnosis of some benign conditions for which there is no need for surgery
► Allows cases to be prioritized when there is a waiting time for surgery
► Provides preoperative diagnosis to allow planning of the operation, fuller preoperative counselling, avoidance of delays for frozen section diagnosis
► Renders unnecessary the need for excisional biopsy in advanced disease, elderly patients, or in cases where the treatment is non-surgical, e.g. neoadjuvant chemotherapy
► It is a rapid means of confirmation of recurrence of previously treated malignancy without recourse to surgery
► Allows reassurance of the patient (and clinician) where a lesion is benign clinically

Limitations of FNA cytology

▶ All FNA diagnoses must be viewed in the light of the clinical picture and other investigations to minimize the risks of a false negative report (usually due to sampling error)
▶ A few false negatives are inevitable

Characteristics of the optimal FNA cytology service for symptomatic breast patients (Fig. 7.4)

1　All symptomatic and screening breast cases are cared for by an integrated breast care team. This team will inevitably and properly be led by a surgeon or team of surgeons

2　The symptomatic breast cases should be seen in a specialist clinic that is exclusively devoted to that purpose. If more than one senior surgeon in an institution participates in breast work, joint clinics are highly desirable

3　Mammographic and cytological diagnoses are available within the breast clinic so that a complete assessment is made on the patient's first visit

4　Mammograms are either taken routinely on the patient's arrival, having been requested by the surgeon on booking the patient to the clinic, or are taken following the clinical assessment, ideally, but not necessarily, before aspiration cytology is obtained

5　The cytologist obtains his/her own aspirates and is prepared to repeat the aspirate when necessary. If a variety of aspirators take the aspirates, use of LBC methods may be preferable

6　A cytology report is issued within the clinic

7　The patient is seen by the surgeon following discussion of the cytology and mammography reports

8　There is a trained breast care nurse available to provide immediate counselling for those patients to whom a malignant diagnosis has been intimated

9　The cytology preparations are reviewed after the clinic, ideally by a second cytologist, before the typed definitive report is issued. Hopefully, amendment of a report will be a rarity

10　The cytologist also participates in the assessment of the subsequent breast histopathology

11　The diagnostic accuracy of cytology and mammography is consistently correlated with the histopathology and clinical outcome by ongoing medical audit

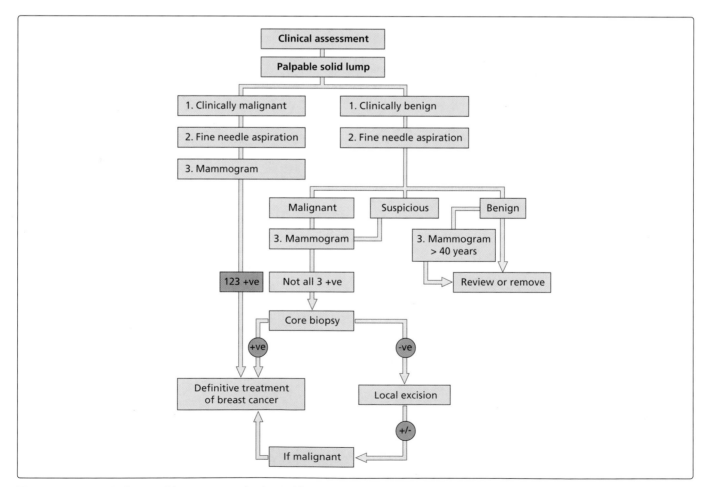

Fig. 7.4　A schematic diagram of the assessment of patients with a palpable breast lump by means of the 'triple test' approach. (Courtesy of Mr S J A Lewis, Northampton, UK)

12 There are regular meetings between the surgeon, radiologist and pathologist to consider individual cases and areas of difficulty

Role of FNA in screening for breast cancer

The UK National Health Service Breast Screening Programme (NHS BSP) invites women between the ages of 50 and 70 years to attend for screening by mammography. With initial setting up of this comprehensive breast screening campaign, scant attention was paid to the possible role of FNA cytology. Cytological diagnosis is the primary tissue investigation in the management of lesions identified by screening in the UK NHS BSP[171], although there has been a swing back to the use of core biopsy with the introduction of new biopsy guns[172]. There has been concern expressed over the value of breast screening[173,174], but the general view is that the programme does indeed reduce death from breast cancer[175]. The experience reported from other countries has been equally encouraging; results obtained for the diagnosis of non-palpable, mammography detected lesions in the breast centres are similar to those obtained for palpable masses. In a large Swedish series[176] of 2594 cases of non-palpable lesions, only one of 429 carcinomas was not detected with the combined assessment by mammography and cytology. In an Australian study involving 404 cases, mammography detected non-palpable breast lesions in 389 women, no case subsequently shown to have carcinoma was diagnosed as benign by radiography and cytology[177]. This study also showed that the sensitivity of stereotactic FNA cytology in detecting ductal carcinoma *in situ* (DCIS) was similar to that for invasive carcinomas. However, the cases of DCIS were more likely to be given a suspicious or atypical diagnosis rather than a definite diagnosis of malignancy.

The effectiveness of breast cytodiagnosis in reducing the need for excision biopsy is reflected in the objectives recommended in the quality assurance guidelines for radiologists in the UK NHS BSP.

▶ When FNA is available, the number of benign biopsies should be less than 20 per 10 000 screened women. The benign:malignant ratio in the prevalence screen should be less than 1:2. The benign:malignant ratio in the incidence screen should be less than 1:4
▶ When FNA is not available, the number of benign biopsies should be less than 40 per 10 000 screened women and the benign:malignant ratio should be less than 3:1 in the prevalence screen. The benign:malignant ratio in the incidence screen should be less than 1:1

Targeting mammographic lesions is most accurately performed with a digitally-controlled stereotaxis apparatus by radiologists and radiographers experienced in its use[178,179]. The sampling of lesions under ultrasound control is a further supplementary method. When ultrasound control is used, care must be taken not to contaminate the specimen with ultrasound contact medium as this can severely damage the specimen.

It is particularly important not to rely solely on the cytological assessment of impalpable lesions when the diagnostic team is still on the learning curve. The duration of this curve depends on the numbers of patients and the previous training of aspirator/cytopathologist but in most centres a reliable service should be available within 6 months.

In contrast to the situation in sampling palpable lumps, experience of imaging methodology is paramount and few cytopathologists would find it possible to extend their role into this field. It is however of considerable value, time permitting, for the cytopathologist to be present when the samples are taken. He or she can ensure that good quality smears are made, provide immediate feedback on the accuracy of the sample, allow correlation of the mammographic and cytological features and, where appropriate, provide an immediate diagnosis.

In manually guided sampling of a palpable lesion it is possible to alter the angle of the needle with each pass thus sampling different parts of the lesion. This is not possible with impalpable lesions and so multiple sampling is recommended with up to five separate attempts, reducing to two or three as experience is gained[180]. Clear instructions as to the preferred methods for obtaining samples from impalpable lesions are available in the UK NHS BSP guidelines[179].

The usual findings in breast aspirates and those found in response to hormonal stimuli

The normal breast, pregnancy and lactation

Histologically, the breast is composed of regularly arranged, radially disposed, independent glandular units forming a bush-like structure, with ducts as branches and lobules as berries. These 15–25 separate units end at the collecting ducts. The collecting ducts lead to lactiferous sinuses, distensible structures that act as a temporary reservoir for milk, which then form the lactiferous ducts that open on to the nipple. The glandular units contain the terminal duct-lobular units (TDLU). The TDLU is the most hormone sensitive part of the breast, is the main functional component, and therefore not surprisingly is the major site of origin for most of the pathological processes. There are tens of thousands of lobules in each breast. Subgross stereomicroscopy of cleared breast tissue reveals that the lobules overlap and mingle with those of adjacent segments.

All these glandular elements are surrounded by connective tissue. The undistinguished interlobular connective tissue contains a very variable amount of adipose tissue. It is this component that accounts for the variable size of the resting breast, a feature relevant to the aspirator as lesions can be difficult to sample in large breasts.

Normal clinical variants: accessory and ectopic breast tissue and intramammary lymph nodes

The breast is not a well demarcated or encapsulated organ and so mammary lobules may be found beyond the normal anatomical boundaries. Most commonly, this is proved by the presentation of ectopic axillary breast tissue as a lump either in pregnancy or because of increased 'breast awareness'. Aspiration of such a lump reveals normal breast tissue components only.

Conversely, lymph nodes from the lower axillary group may be found in the upper outer quadrant or even the lower outer quadrant of the breast where they may present as a lump[181]. The combination of the clinical features and an aspirate of normal or reactive lymphoid tissue permits diagnosis and reassurance.

It is more appropriate to describe the 'usual' contents of a breast aspirate because it is not generally intended to obtain aspirates of 'normal' breast tissue. It is common, however, to see components of normal breast tissue and adjacent structures in aspirates that are taken of palpable and non-palpable lesions.

Cytological findings in breast aspirates

Normal epithelial and myoepithelial cells *(Figs 7.5, 7.6)*

These typically are seen in small cohesive groups or regular monolayers when the orientation is appropriate. Quite frequently the lobular origin of a group is apparent from the acinar shape. Usually however it is not possible to distinguish acinar from duct cells. Normal resting breast epithelial cells have a round to oval nucleus 8–10 μm in diameter with a very small nucleolus or no visible nucleolus. The cytoplasm is scanty and in crowded groups may not be visible. Intimately mixed within the epithelial cell groups, are myoepithelial cells, which are generally recognized by their more compact, denser and more ovoid nuclei. The mixture of epithelial and myoepithelial cell nuclei can give a spurious appearance of anisonucleosis that may trouble the novice, particularly in the more cellular aspirates from hyperplastic lesions.

The responsiveness of the breast epithelium to cyclic hormonal influences has been very elegantly shown in FNA specimens[182]. Post-ovulatory (endometrial secretory phase) aspirates are characterized by an increase in the number of acinar cells. Peripheral orientation of the nuclear chromatin with clearing around a relatively prominent nucleolus is seen. The cytoplasm is lacy and fragile and the epithelial fragments show a multilayered arrangement.

In preovulatory (endometrial proliferative phase) aspirates, the cell borders are more prominent with the cytoplasm appearing more even in consistency and better delineated. The nucleus is smaller and more compact with

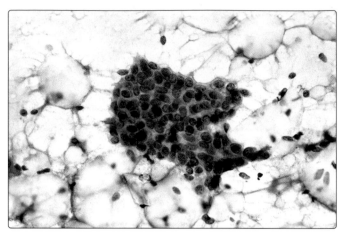

Fig. 7.5 Normal breast. A group of benign ductal cells surrounded by single bipolar nuclei in the background. (Papanicoloau) (Courtesy of Dr G McKee, Boston).

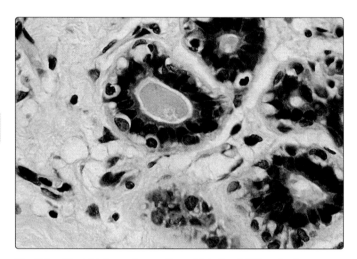

Fig. 7.6 The histology of normal breast lobules. (H&E section)

evenly distributed chromatin. Epithelial fragments appear compact and tend to be arranged in single layered sheets.

Morphometric analyses resulting in grey-level density reliefs and isophote profiles of individual cells reinforce the impression of cyclical changes in breast epithelial cell morphology. Discriminate analysis based on extracted nuclear features was shown to identify correctly the menstrual phase in all cases when applied to 20 cells from each case[182].

Bipolar cell nuclei (stripped, bare, naked or stromal nuclei) *(Fig. 7.5)*

The small ovoid or elongated naked nuclei seen in the background of benign breast aspirates are almost certainly nuclei of fibroblasts from specialized intralobular stroma, although some believe them to be a mixture of myoepithelial cells and connective tissue nuclei. In aspirates, their number correlates well with the amount of specialized stroma seen histologically, being scant in 'normal breast' and abundant in fibroadenomas with cellular stroma, and particularly prominent in phyllodes tumours.

Adipose tissue

This is frequently the sole component of breast aspirates and is a common finding with both benign and malignant aspirates. It is remarkable that the abundant adipose tissue in an aspirate does not prevent the parenchymal elements from adhering to the slide more often. Fatty aspirates contain balloon-like fat cells in clusters of variable sizes, sometimes associated with strands of fibrocollagenous tissue or occasional capillaries. There is invariably some traumatic release of liquid lipid material but this is generally dissolved during the alcohol fixation step in preparation and is not apparent microscopically.

Red blood cells

These can be useful to the cytologist when present in small numbers as a ubiquitous measure of scale, to gauge the size of the nuclei of the epithelial cells in the aspirate. When an aspirate is heavily contaminated with blood the epithelial cell groups are not clearly visible and often show some degree of air-drying. The penetration of Romanowsky stains also is adversely affected by the presence of abundant blood.

Platelets

These appear as small granular amphophilic aggregates.

Skeletal muscle fibres

These are rarely seen if the correct aspiration technique is used. They appear as distinctive elongated cylinders with basophilic cytoplasm, on air-dried smears, orange on Papanicolaou-stained aspirates, with cross striations and peripherally-located nuclei.

Lymphoid cells

If present exclusively and in large numbers in an aspirate, the presence of an intramammary lymph node may be suspected. These nodes are often seen as well-defined, impalpable masses on mammograms.

Reporting protocols

The UK NHS BSP recommends a 5-tier reporting scheme[183,184], summarized as follows:

C1: inadequate/non-diagnostic

This category may be used for any of the following reasons: acellularity, the presence of only blood, fat, bipolar nuclei and macrophages (unless the lesion is a cyst) or too few epithelial groups. However, if the clinical diagnosis is a lipoma then aspiration merely of fat is adequate for diagnosis, placing the report in the benign (C2) category.

C2: Benign (Fig. 7.7)

This category includes normal breast and benign lesions ranging from mastitis to fibroadenoma. The typical pattern here is of benign epithelial cells in cohesive epithelial

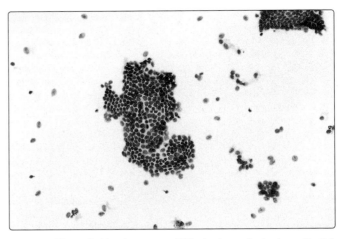

Fig. 7.7   The typical benign pattern (C2) of a sheet of cohesive epithelial cells with bipolar nuclei in the background. (H&E)

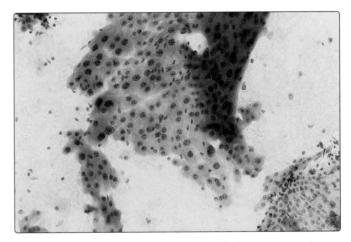

Fig. 7.8   This sheet of apocrine metaplastic cells shows some atypia, eliciting a diagnosis of 'atypical, probably benign' (C3). Histology showed benign fibrocystic change with some atypia in apocrine glandular epithelium. (Papanicolaou)

groups, with a background of bare, bipolar nuclei. A cystic component shows apocrine metaplasia with macrophages and cyst debris. The cellularity of benign lesions is variable, normal tissue being poorly cellular and fibroadenoma highly cellular.

C3: Atypical, probably benign (Fig. 7.8)

This category is usually characterized by a predominantly benign pattern with some atypical features; either nuclear enlargement or pleomorphism. Some fibroadenomas, hyperplastic benign disease and phyllodes tumours can result in a C3 diagnosis.

C4: Suspicious, probably malignant (Fig. 7.9)

Here the pattern is suggestive, but not diagnostic of malignancy. There may be only limited cell discohesion and minimal nuclear pleomorphism. Bipolar nuclei in the background, especially accompanying epithelial cells that are not frankly malignant, indicate that caution should be exercised and the lesion reported as suspicious, rather than

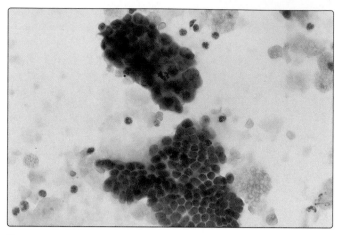

Fig. 7.9   One of these cell groups is benign, the other shows crowding, nuclear pleomorphism and a mitosis. This was reported as 'suspicious, probably malignant' (C4). Histology showed a focus of low-grade DCIS with fibrocystic change. (H&E)

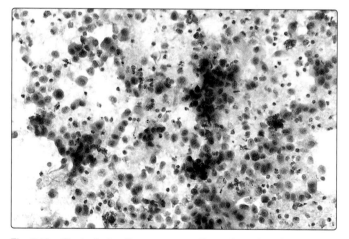

Fig. 7.10   The typical malignant pattern of loose, irregular, highly pleomorphic cells with cell death and many mitoses. (Papanicolaou)

malignant. Low-grade and lobular carcinomas frequently are given a C4 diagnosis.

C5: Malignant *(Fig. 7.10)*

The cytological features are unequivocally malignant. This category includes epithelial, non-epithelial and metastatic tumours to breast. The typical features of malignancy include discohesion of epithelial cells, nuclear pleomorphism, irregularity of the nuclear margin and abnormal nucleoli. Low-grade tumours display mild to moderate pleomorphism while high-grade neoplastic cells show marked nuclear pleomorphism and many mitoses, often bizarre.

A more detailed description of the cytological characteristics of specific entities is provided in Chapters 8 and 9.

Statistical analysis

The UK NHS BSP has published guidelines and statistical data for quality assurance audit of cytology[171,183,184]:

Absolute sensitivity: the number of carcinomas diagnosed as C5 expressed as a percentage of the total number of carcinomas; *recommended target >60%*

Complete sensitivity: the number of carcinomas that were not definitely benign or inadequate on FNA expressed as a percentage of the total number of carcinomas; *recommended target >80%*

Specificity: the number of correctly identified benign lesions (the number of C2 results minus the number of false negatives) expressed as a percentage of the total number of benign lesions; *recommended target >60%*

Positive predictive value of a C5 diagnosis: the number of correctly identified cancers (C5 minus the number of false positives) expressed as a percentage of the total number of C5; *recommended target >95%*

Positive predictive value of a C4 diagnosis: the number of cancers reported as suspicious (C4 minus the number of false suspicious cases) expressed as a percentage of the total number of C4

Positive predictive value of a C3 diagnosis: the number of cancers reported as atypical (C3 minus the number of cases that were benign), expressed as a percentage of the total number of C3

False negative case: a case reported as C2 that subsequently (over the next 3 years) is diagnosed as carcinoma. This will inevitably include 'interval' cancers (cancers that have grown and presented since the previous correctly reported C2)

False negative rate: the number of false negatives expressed as a percentage of the total number of carcinomas; *recommended target <5%*

False positive case: a case reported as C5 that is benign on excision

False positive rate: the number of false positives expressed as a percentage of the total number of carcinomas; *recommended target <1%*

Inadequate rate: the number of C1 cases expressed as a percentage of the total number of cases; *recommended target <25%*

Inadequate rate from cancers: the number of C1 cases that subsequently turn out to be carcinoma, expressed as a percentage of the total number of carcinomas; *recommended target <10%*

Suspicious rate: the number of C3 and C4 expressed as a percentage of the total number of cases; *recommended target <20%.*

Statistics must include all inadequates (C1) as part of the denominator, because removing them will distort comparative studies[24].

Pitfalls in breast cytodiagnosis: an overview

In the diagnosis of breast lesions, difficulties can arise in clinical, mammographic and frozen or paraffin histological assessment[185,186] as well as in cytology. Specific areas of difficulty in cytodiagnosis are highlighted systematically in the Chapters 8 and 9, under the diagnostic headings. In this section, factors that may predispose to mistakes are identified.

Systematic audit of diagnostic performance is the best means of ensuring the maintenance or improvement of standards. When establishing a FNA clinic service, it is advisable to set limitations on the number of cases to be seen per session. The number of cases can be increased gradually, as experience is gained. Where resources are inadequate, it is better not to introduce innovations that cannot be sustained. It is important that the pathologist is never rushed or pressurized into giving a diagnosis against his or her better judgement. Problems may also arise from attempting to provide a diagnosis on a technically inferior or inadequate preparation. This raises a difficult question: 'What is an adequate sample?' For the aspirator cytopathologist, it may be defined as 'a sample or series of samples that contain material consistent with the clinical appearance of the lesion'. When a sample is assessed remotely, this definition cannot be applied unless the clinician aspirator provides a clinical diagnosis such as lipoma or mastitis.

It is generally accepted that any sample that lacks epithelial cells should be deemed inadequate, with certain exceptions, clinical lipomas or lymph nodes for example. Whether a sample containing scanty or distorted epithelial groups is deemed suitable for diagnosis, is highly subjective. On occasion, it is possible to make a confident diagnosis of breast carcinoma on two or three cells, while other cases provide abundant aspirates on which a definite diagnosis cannot be made. Only experience, preferably gained in the clinic, can allow this decision to be made reliably.

A further factor that can impede accurate diagnosis is failure of communication from the clinician, such as omission of clinical information about pregnancy, the patient's age, previous malignancy or radiotherapy. Again, the most reliable solution to this problem is attendance at the clinic. If necessary it may be thought permissible to state on the report that the clinical data were insufficient.

What follows is a summary of common pitfalls arranged in a reasonable descending order of importance.

Diagnostic pitfalls

- Lobular carcinoma cells are relatively small and their malignant nature may be overlooked
- Low-grade ductal carcinoma (e.g. tubular carcinoma) can be mistaken for a benign hyperplasia
- Fibroadenomas can present a very worrying appearance, leading to a risk of a false positive diagnosis, particularly in pregnancy or when they occur in an elderly woman
- A small carcinoma can be overshadowed by a more dominant benign lesion
- Pregnancy or lactation can be associated with 'atypical' epithelial changes and are open to misinterpretation
- Previous radiotherapy can produce cytological abnormalities in patients where the index of suspicion is already high
- Complex proliferative, papillary and atypical hyperplastic lesions may be overdiagnosed as malignant. These can be accompanied by a mammographic appearance that may raise the index of suspicion
- Apocrine cells can give a spurious appearance of atypia, particularly when they become degenerate
- Necrotic debris is seen in necrotic tumours as well as in inflammatory conditions
- Inflammatory conditions such as simple abscess can be associated with marked reactive atypia of epithelial cells

Rare problems

- Fat necrosis can be associated with large reactive macrophages that can mimic carcinoma cells. Conversely some tumours have associated fat necrosis
- Skin adnexal tumours, soft tissue tumours of the chest wall and secondary carcinomas can all present in a way that mimics a primary breast lesion
- Organizing haematoma may contain degenerate material, large spindle cells, large cells containing pigment and prominent nucleoli giving a potential for misdiagnosis as metastatic melanoma
- Granular cell tumour and the macrophages of the commoner duct ectasia can present a similar appearance
- Herpetic infection and eczema of the nipple may be mistaken for Paget's disease of the nipple

References

1 Slater D N. Terminology: fine needle aspiration cytology and biopsy. *Cytopathol* 1991; **2**: 51–54

2 Frable W J. Fine needle aspiration biopsy: a review. *Hum Pathol* 1983; **14**: 9–28

3 Lever J V, Trott P A, Webb A J. Fine needle aspiration cytology. *J Clin Pathol* 1985; **38**: 1–11

4 Bottles K, Miller T R, Cohen M B, Ljung B. Fine needle aspiration biopsy. Has its time come? *Am J Med* 1986; **81**: 525–530

5 Frable W J. Needle aspiration biopsy: past, present and future. *Hum Pathol* 1989; **20**: 504–517

6 McManus D T, Anderson N H. Fine needle aspiration cytology of the breast. A review. *Curr Diagn Pathol* 2001; **7**: 262–271

7 Anderson T J. Genesis and source of breast cancer. *Br Med Bull* 1991; **47**: 305–318

8 Hutson S W, Cowen P N, Bird C C. Morphometric studies of age related changes in normal human breast and their significance for evolution of

mammary cancer. *J Clin Pathol* 1985; **38**: 281–287

9 Padel A F, Coghill S B, Powis S J A. Evidence that the sensitivity is increased and the inadequacy rate decreased when pathologists take aspirates for cytodiagnosis. *Cytopathol* 1993; **4**: 161–165

10 Brown L A, Coghill S B, Powis S J A. Audit of diagnostic accuracy of FNA cytology specimens taken by the histopathologist in a symptomatic breast clinic. *Cytopathol* 1991; **2**: 1–6

11 Snead D R J, Vryenhoef P, Pinder S E et al. Routine audit of breast FNA cytology specimens and aspirator inadequacy rates. *Cytopathol* 1997; **8**: 236–247

12 The uniform approach to breast FNA biopsy. A synopsis. *Acta Cytol* 1996; **40**: 1120–1126

13 Howat A J, Briggs W A. Fine needle aspiration cytology of the breast using the Cytospin method. *Cytopathol* 1999; **10**: 50–53

14 UK Department of Health. *National Health Service Breast Screening Pathology – Guidelines for Cytology*. London: NHS BSP Publication, September 1993; no. 22

15 Brown L, Jagger C, Coghill S B. Which needle? Does it matter? *Cytopathol* 1993; **4**(1): 11

16 Hartley M N, Tuffnell D J, Hutton J L et al. Fine needle aspiration cytology: an *in vitro* study of cell yield. *Br J Surg* 1988, **75**: 380–381

17 Vorherr H. Breast aspiration biopsy with multihole needles for histologic and cytologic examination. *Am J Obstet Gynecol* 1985; **151**: 70–76

18 Pennes D R, Naylor B, Rebner M. Fine needle aspiration biopsy of the breast. Influence of the number of passes and the sample size on the diagnostic yield. *Acta Cytol* 1990; **34**: 673–676

19 Zajdela A, Zillhardt P, Voillemot N. Cytological diagnosis by fine needle sampling without aspiration. *Cancer* 1987; **59**: 1201–1205

20 Mair S, Dunbar F, Becker P J, Du Plessis W. Fine needle cytology – is aspiration suction necessary? A study of 100 masses in various sites. *Acta Cytol* 1989; **33**: 809–813

21 Rajasekhar A, Sundaram C, Chowdhary T et al. Diagnostic utility of fine needle sampling without aspiration – a prospective study. *Diagn Cytopathol* 1991; **7**: 473–476

22 Robinson C R. A new technique for fine needle aspiration biopsy. *Hum Pathol* 1984; **15**: 197

23 Harris S C, Currie A, Anderson G, Howat A J. Transport media for FNA cytology. *J Clin Pathol* 1987; **40**: 1263

24 Howat A J, Stringfellow H F, Briggs W A, Nicholson C M. FNA cytology of the breast: A review of 1,868 cases using the Cytospin method. *Acta Cytol* 1994; **38**: 939–944

25 Briggs W A. Avoiding unreadably thick Cytospin preparations. *Acta Cytol* 1992; **36**: 652–653

26 Cobb N, Slater D N, Beck S. A new filter technique permitting traditional histopathological assessment of FNAs. *Med Lab Sci* 1990; **47**: 172–181

27 Dundas S A C, Mansour P, Zeiderman M et al. Audit of 6 years' experience of breast FNA using the Cytospin method: improvement through multidisciplinary clinical audit. *Cytopathol* 1997; **8**: 230–235

28 Ross D A, Cunningham S C, Vincenti A C, Rainsbury R M. Cytodiagnosis of breast disease using a liquid suspension medium. *Br J Surg* 1993; **80**: 866–867

29 Sirkin W, Auger M, Donat E, Lipa M. Cytospins – an alternative method for FNAC of the breast: a study of 148 cases. *Diagn Cytopathol* 1995; **13**: 266–269

30 Hammond S, Keyhani-Rofagha S, O'Toole R V. Statistical analysis of FNAC of the breast – a review of 678 cases plus 4265 cases from the literature. *Acta Cytol* 1987; **31**: 276–280

31 Zuk J A, Maudsley G, Zakhour H D F. Rapid reporting on FNA of breast lumps in outpatients. *J Clin Pathol* 1989; **42**: 906–911

32 Dey P, Luthra U K, George J et al. Comparison of ThinPrep and conventional preparations on FNA cytology material. *Acta Cytol* 2000; **44**: 46–50

33 Bedard Y C, Pollett A F. Breast FNA. A comparison of ThinPrep and conventional smears. *Am J Clin Pathol* 1999; **111**: 523–527

34 Nicol T L, Kelly D, Reynolds L, Rosenthal D L. Comparison of TriPath thin-layer technology with conventional methods on nongynecologic specimens. *Acta Cytol* 2000; **44**: 567–575

35 Britton P D, McCann J. Needle biopsy in the NHS BSP 1996/7: how much and how accurate? *Breast* 1999; **8**: 5–11

36 Deschryver K, Radford D M, Schuh M E et al. Pathology of large-caliber stereotactic biopsies in nonpalpable breast lesions. *Sem Diagn Pathol* 1999; **16**: 224–234

37 Meyer J E, Smith D N, Lester S C et al. Large-core needle biopsy of nonpalpable breast lesions. *JAMA* 1999; **281**: 1638–1641

38 Pinder S E, Elston C W, Ellis I O. The role of pre-operative diagnosis in breast cancer. *Histopathol* 1996; **28**: 563–566

39 Diaz L K, Porter G A, Venta L A, Wiley E L. *Tumor Displacement in Large Gauge Needle Core Biopsies: Presence in Excision Specimens*. San Francisco: USCAP, March 1999; abstract 93, p. 19A

40 Liberman L, Vuolo M, Dershaw D D et al. Epithelial displacement after stereotactic 11–guage directional vacuum-assisted breast biopsy. *Am J Roentgenol* 1999: **172**: 677–681

41 Vincenti A C. Fine needle aspiration biopsies. *Bull Roy Coll Pathol* 1989; **65**: 17

42 Molyneux A M, Coghill S B. Ultrasound contact jelly causes an artefact in breast aspirates. *Cytopathol* 1993; **5**: 41–45

43 Catania S, Boccato P, Bono A et al. Pneumothorax: a rare complication of fine needle aspiration of the breast. *Acta Cytol* 1989; **33**: 140

44 Stevenson J, James A S, Johnston M A, Anderson I W. Pneumothorax after fine needle aspiration of the breast. *BMJ* 1991; **303**: 924

45 Hales M S, Hsu F S F. Needle tract implantation of papillary carcinoma of the thyroid following aspiration biopsy. *Acta Cytol* 1990; **34**(6): 801–804

46 Fornari F, Civardi G, Cavanna L et al. Complications of ultrasonically guided fine-needle abdominal biopsy: results of a multicenter Italian study and review of the literature. *Scand J Gastroenterol* 1989; **24**(8): 949–955

47 Seyfer A E, Walsh D S, Graeber G M et al. Chest wall implantation of lung cancer after thin-needle aspiration biopsy. *Ann Thorac Surg* 1989; **48**(2): 284–286

48 Kansara G, Hussain M, DiMauro J. A case of plasmacytoma in muscle as a complication of needle tract seeding after percutaneous bone marrow biopsy. *Am J Clin Pathol* 1989; **91**(5): 604–606

49 Moloo Z, Finley R J, Lefcoe M S et al. Possible spread of bronchogenic carcinoma to the chest wall after a transthoracic fine needle aspiration biopsy: a case report. *Acta Cytol* 1985; **29**(2): 167–169

50 Sakurai M, Seki K, Okamura J, Kuroda C. Needle tract implantation of hepatocellular carcinoma after percutaneous liver biopsy. *Am J Surg Pathol* 1983; **7**(2): 191–195

51 Flynn M S, Wolfson S E, Thomas S, Kuhns J G. Fine needle aspiration biopsy in clinical management of head and neck tumors. *J Surg Oncol* 1990; **4**(4): 214–217

52 Augsburger J J, Shields J A, Folberg R et al. Fine needle aspiration biopsy in the diagnosis of intraocular cancer. Cytologic-histologic correlations. *Ophthalmol* 1985; **92**(1): 39–49

53 Tatsuda M, Ikegami H, Horai T, Nakamura S. Diagnosis of lung cancer by percutaneous aspiration biopsy. *Lung Cancer* 1982; **22**(2): 165–173

54 Fortunato R P, Smith E. Ultrasound-guided percutaneous needle biopsy procedures. *Postgrad Radiol* 1981; **1**(3): 237–245

55 Tsang W Y W, Chan J K C. Spectrum of morphologic changes in lymph nodes attributable to fine needle aspiration. *Hum Pathol* 1992; **23**(5): 562–565

56 Tabbara S O, Frierson H F, Fechner R E. Diagnostic problems in tissues previously sampled by fine-needle aspiration. *Am J Clin Pathol* 1991; **96**(1): 76–80

57 Stigers K B, King J G, Davey D D, Stelling C B. Abnormalities of the breast caused by biopsy: spectrum of mammographic findings. *Am J Roent* 1991; **156**: 287–291

58 Klein D L, Sickles E A. Effects of needle aspiration on the mammographic appearance of the breast: a guide to the proper timing of the mammography examination. *Radiology* 1982; **145**: 44

59 Sickles E A, Klein D L, Goodson W H, Hunt T K. Mammography after needle aspiration of palpable breast masses. *Am J Surg* 1983; **145**: 395–397

60 Miller W R, Ellis I O, Sainsbury J R C, Dixon M J. ABC of breast diseases. Prognostic factors. *BMJ* 1994; **309**: 1573–1576

61 Ferno M. Prognostic factors in breast cancer: a brief review. *AntiCancer Res* 1998; **18**: 2167–2171

62 Elston C W, Ellis I O, Pinder S E. Prognostic factors in breast cancer. *Clin Oncol* 1998; **10**: 14–17

63 Robinson I A, McKee G, Nicholson A et al. Prognostic value of cytological grading of fine-needle aspirates from breast carcinomas. *Lancet* 1994; **343**: 947–949

64 Hunt C M, Ellis I O, Elston C W et al. Cytological grading of breast carcinoma – a feasible proposition? *Cytopathol* 1990; **1**: 287–295

65 De-Maublanc M A, Briffod M, Pallud C et al. Fine needle aspiration and prognostic factors in breast cancer. *Bull Cancer* 1990; **77**(suppl 1): 91S–94S

66 Mouriquand J, Pasquier D. Fine needle aspiration of breast carcinoma. A preliminary cytoprognostic study. *Acta Cytol* 1980; **24**(2): 153–159

67 Layfield L J, Robert M E, Cramer H, Giuliano A. Aspiration biopsy smear pattern as a predictor of biologic behaviour in adenocarcinoma of the breast. *Acta Cytol* 1992; **36**: 208–214

68 Mouriquand J, Gozlan-Fior M, Villemain D et al. Value of cytoprognostic classification in breast carcinomas. *J Clin Pathol* 1986; **39**: 489–496

69 Dabbs D. Role of nuclear grading of breast carcinomas in FNA specimens. *Acta Cytol* 1993; **37**: 361–366

70 New N E, Howat A J. Grading of breast carcinoma on FNA specimens (letter). *Acta Cytol* 1994; **38**: 969–970

71 Dalquen P, Baschiera B, Chaffard R et al. MIB-1 (Ki-67) immunostaining of breast cancer cells in cytologic smears. *Acta Cytol* 1997; **41**: 229–237

72 Suthipintawong C, Leong AS-Y, Chan KW et al. Immunostaining of estrogen receptor, progesterone receptor, MIB1 antigen, and c-erbB2 oncoprotein in cytologic specimens: a simplified method with formalin fixation. *Cytopathol* 1997; **17**: 127–133

73 Skoog L, Rutqvist L E, Wilking N. Analysis of hormone receptors and proliferation fraction in fine needle aspirates from primary breast carcinomas during chemotherapy or tamoxifen therapy. *Acta Oncol* 1992; **31**: 139–141

74 Yates A J, Howat A J. Immunocytochemistry on Cytospin FNAs (letter). *Cytopathol* 1993; **4**: 251–252

75 Leung S W, Bedard Y C. Estrogen and progesterone receptor contents in ThinPrep-processed fine needle aspirates of breast. *Am J Clin Pathol* 1999; **112**: 50–56

76 Hudock J A, Hanau C A, Christen R, Bibbo M. Expression of estrogen and progesterone receptor in cytologic specimens using various fixatives. *Diagn Cytopathol* 1996; **15**: 78–83

77 Slamon D, Leyland-Jones B, Shak S et al. Use of chemotherapy plus a monoclonal antibody against Her 2 for metastatic breast cancer that overexpresses Her 2. *NEJM* 2001; **344**: 783–792

78 Willsher P C, Pinder S E, Chan S Y et al. C-erbB2 expression predicts response to preoperative chemotherapy for locally advanced breast cancer. *AntiCancer Res* 1998; **18**: 3695–3698

79 Walker R A, Cowl J. The expression of C-Fos protein in human breast. *J Pathol* 1991; **163**: 323–327

80 Walker R A, Senior P V, Jones J L et al. An immunohistochemical and in situ hybridization study of c-myc and c-erbB2 expression in primary human breast carcinomas. *J Pathol* 1989; **158**: 97–105

81 Foekens J A, Look M P, Bolt de-V et al. Cathepsin-D in primary breast cancer: prognostic evaluation involving 2810 patients. *Br J Cancer* 1999; **79**: 300–307

82 Foekens J A, Dall P, Klijn J G et al. Prognostic value of CD44 expression in primary breast cancer. *Int J Cancer* 1999; **84**: 209–215

83 Giri D D, Dundas S A C, Sanderson P R, Howat A J. Silver binding nucleoli and NORs in breast FNA cytology. *Acta Cytol* 1989; **33**: 173–175

84 Stephenson T J, Royds J A, Silcocks P B et al. Diagnostic associations of p53 immunostaining in FNAC of the breast. *Cytopathol* 1994; **5**: 146–153

85 Rudolph P, Olssen H, Bonatz G et al. Correlation between p53, c-erbB2, and topoisomerase II alpha expression, DNA ploidy, hormonal receptor status and proliferation in 356 node-negative breast carcinomas: prognostic implications. *J Pathol* 1999; **187**: 207–216

86 Nooter K, Brutel de la R, Look M P et al. The prognostic significance of the multidrug resistance-associated protein (MRP) in primary breast cancer. *Br J Cancer* 1997; **76**: 486–493

87 Castronovo V, Colin C, Claysmith A P et al. Immunodetection of the metastasis associated laminin receptor in human breast cancer cells obtained by FNA biopsy. *Am J Pathol* 1990; **137**: 1373–1381

88 Reed W, Hannisdal E, Boehler P J et al. The prognostic value of p53 and c-erbB2 immunostaining is overrated for patients with lymph node negative breast carcinoma. *Cancer* 2000; **88**: 804–813

89 Wu J, Shao Z-M, Shen Z-Z et al. Significance of apoptosis and apoptotic-related proteins, bcl-2 and bax in primary breast cancer. *Breast J* 2000; **6**: 44–52

90 Candlish W, Kerr I B, Simpson H W. Immunocytochemical demonstration and significance of p21 ras family oncogene product in benign and malignant breast disease. *J Pathol* 1986; **150**: 163–167

91 Fromowitz F B, Viola M V, Chao S et al. ras p21 expression in the progression of breast cancer. *Hum Pathol* 1987; **18**: 1268–1275

92 Walker R A, Wilkinson N. p21 ras protein expression in benign and malignant human breast. *J Pathol* 1988; **156**: 147–153

93 Bhattacharjee D K, Harris M, Faragher E B. Nuclear morphometry of epitheliosis and intraduct carcinoma of the breast. *Histopathol* 1985; **9**: 511–516

94 Baak J P A. The relative prognostic significance of nucleolar morphometry in invasive ductal breast cancer. *Histopathol* 1985; **9**: 437–444

95 Parham D M, Robertson A J, Brown R A. Morphometric analysis of breast carcinoma: association with survival. *J Clin Pathol* 1988; **41**: 173–177

96 van Diest P J, Mouriquand J, Schipper N W, Baak J P A. Prognostic value of nucleolar morphometric variables in cytological breast cancer specimens. *J Clin Pathol* 1990; **43**: 157–159

97 Mapstone N P, Zakhour H D. Morphometric analysis of fine needle aspirates from breast lesions. *Cytopathol* 1990; **1**: 349–355

98 St J Thomas J, Mallon E A, George W D. Semiquantitative analyses of fine needle aspirates from benign and malignant breast lesions. *J Clin Pathol* 1989; **42**: 28–34

99 Beerman J, Veldhuizen R W, Blok R A P et al. Cytomorphometry as quality control for fine needle aspiration: a study in 321 breast lesions. *Anal Quant Cytol Histol* 1991; **13**(2): 143–148

100 Walker R A, Camplejohn R S. DNA flow cytometry of human breast carcinomas and its relationship to transferrin and epidermal growth factor receptors. *J Pathol* 1986; **150**: 37–42

101 Williams R A, Charlton I G, Rode J. Comparative ploidy studies using cytological and paraffin section preparations. *Cytopathol* 1991; **2**: 29–37

102 Heathfield H A, Kirkham N, Ellis I O, Winstanley G. Computer assisted diagnosis of fine needle aspirate of the breast. *J Clin Pathol* 1990; **43**: 168–170

103 Akhtar M, Ali M A, Owen E, Bakry M. A simple method for processing fine needle aspiration biopsy specimens for electron microscopy. *J Clin Pathol* 1981; 1214–1216

104 Jackson D P, Payne J, Bell S et al. Extraction of DNA from exfoliative cytology specimens and its suitability for analysis by the polymerase chain reaction. *Cytopathol* 1990; **1**: 87–96

105 Minkowitz S, Moskowitz R, Khafif R A, Alderete M N. Tru-cut needle biopsy of the breast: an analysis of its specificity and sensitivity. *Cancer* 1986; **52**: 320–323

106 Gonzalez E, Grafton W D, Morris D M, Barr L H. Diagnosing breast cancer using frozen sections from Tru-cut registered needle biopsies. Six year experience with 162 biopsies, with emphasis on outpatient diagnosis of breast carcinoma. *Ann Surg* 1985; **202**: 696–701

107 Albert U-S, Duda V, Hadji P et al. Imprint cytology of core needle biopsy specimens of breast lesions. *Acta Cytol* 2000; **44**: 57–62

108 Dixon J M. Immediate reporting of fine needle aspiration of breast lesions. *BMJ* 1991; **302**: 428–429

109 Galea M, Blamey R W. Diagnosis by team work: an approach to conservatism. *Br Med Bull* 1991; **47**: 295–304

110 Franzén S, Zajicek J. Aspiration biopsy in diagnosis of palpable lesions of the breast. Critical review of 3479 consecutive biopsies. *Acta Radiol Ther Phy Biol* 1968; **7**: 241–262

111 Dehn T C B, Clarke J, Dixon J M et al. Fine needle aspiration cytology, with immediate reporting, in the outpatient diagnosis of breast disease. *Ann R Coll Surg Eng* 1987; **69**: 280–282

112 Salter D R, Bassett A A. Role of needle aspiration in reducing the number of unnecessary breast biopsies. *Can J Surg* 1981; **24**: 311–313

113 Dixon J M, Clarke P J, Crucioli V et al. Reduction of the surgical excision rate in benign breast disease using fine needle aspiration cytology with immediate reporting. *Br J Surg* 1987; **74**: 1014–1016

114 Zuk J A, Maudsley G, Zakhour H D. Rapid reporting on fine needle aspiration of breast lumps in outpatients. *J Clin Pathol* 1989; **42**: 906–911

115 Shabot M M, Goldberg I M, Schick P et al. Aspiration cytology is superior to Tru-cut registered needle biopsy in establishing the diagnosis of clinically suspicious breast masses. *Ann Surg* 1982; **196**: 122–126

116 Lee K R, Foster R S, Papillo J L. Fine needle aspiration of the breast. Importance of the aspirator. *Acta Cytol* 1987; **31**: 281–284

117 Palombini L, Fulciniti F, Vetrani A et al. Fine needle aspiration biopsies of breast masses. A critical analysis of 1956 cases in 8 years (1976–1984). *Cancer* 1988; **61**: 2273–2277

118 Fine needle aspiration: editorial. *Cytopathol* 1990; **1**: 57–58

119 Silverman J F, Lannin D R, O'Brien K, Norris H T. The triage role of fine needle aspiration biopsy of palpable breast masses: diagnostic accuracy and cost-effectiveness. *Acta Cytol* 1987; **31**: 731–736

120 Cheung P S Y, Yan K W, Alagaratnam T T. The complementary role of fine needle aspiration cytology and Tru-cut needle biopsy in the management of breast masses. *Aus & NZ J Surg* 1987; **57**: 615–620

121 Shabot M M, Goldberg I M, Schick P et al. Aspiration cytology is superior to Tru-cut needle biopsy in establishing the diagnosis of clinically suspicious breast masses. *Ann Surg* 1982; **196**(2): 122–128

122 Robinson C R. Clinical approach to fine needle biopsy: a note of caution. *Cytopathol* 1990; **1**: 257–258

123 Abele J S, Miller T R, Goodson W H et al. Fine needle aspiration of palpable breast masses. A program for staged implementation. *Arch Surg* 1983; **118**: 859–863

124 Cohen M B, Channing Rogers R P, Hales M S et al. Influence of training and experience in fine needle aspiration biopsy of breast. *Arch Pathol Lab Med* 1987; **111**: 518–520

125 Lamb J, Anderson T J. Influence of cancer histology on the success of fine needle aspiration of the breast. *J Clin Pathol* 1989; **42**: 733–735

126 Brown L A, Coghill S B. Fine needle aspiration cytology of the breast: factors affecting sensitivity. *Cytopathol* 1991; **2**: 67–74

127 Barrows G H, Anderson T J, Lamb J L, Dixon J M. Fine needle aspiration of breast cancer: relationship of clinical factors to cytology results in 689 primary malignancies. *Cancer* 1986; **58**: 1493–1498

128 Gupta R K, Dowle C S, Simpson J S. The value of needle aspiration cytology of the breast, with an emphasis on the diagnosis of breast disease in young women below the age of 30. *Acta Cytol* 1990; **34**: 165–168

129 Sheikh F A, Tinkoff G H, Kline T S, Neal H S. Final diagnosis by fine needle aspiration biopsy for definitive operation in breast cancer. *Am J Surg* 1987; **154**: 470–474

130 Powles T J, Trott P A, Cherryman G et al. Fine needle aspiration cytodiagnosis as a prerequisite for primary medical treatment of breast cancer. *Cytopathol* 1991; **2**: 7–12

131 Hitchcock A, Hunt C M, Locker A et al. A one year audit of fine needle aspiration cytology for the preoperative diagnosis of breast disease. *Cytopathol* 1991; **2**: 167–176

132 Wanebo H J, Feldman P S, Wilhelm M C et al. Fine needle aspiration cytology in lieu of open biopsy in management of primary breast cancer. *Ann of Surg* 1984; **199**(S): 569–572

133 Wolberg W H, Tanner M A, Loh W Y, Vanichsetakul N. Statistical approach to fine needle aspiration diagnosis of breast masses. *Acta Cytol* 1987; **31**: 737–741

134 Wolberg W H, Tanner M A, Loh W Y. Fine needle aspiration for breast mass diagnosis. *Arch Surg* 1989; **124**: 814–818

135 Zarbo R J, Howanitz P J, Bachner P. Interinstitutional comparison of performance in breast fine needle aspiration cytology: a Q-probe quality indicator study. *Arch Pathol Lab Med* 1991; **115**: 743–750

136 Lioe T F, Elliott H, Allen D C, Spence R A. A 3-year audit of fine needle aspirates from a symptomatic breast clinic. *Ulster Med J* 1997; **66**: 24–27

137 Langumuir V K, Cramer S F, Hood M E. Fine needle aspiration cytology in the management of palpable benign and malignant breast disease. *Acta Cytol* 1989; **33**: 93–96

138 Goodson W H, Mailman R, Miller T R. Three year follow up of benign fine-needle aspiration biopsies of the breast. *Am J Surg* 1987; **154**: 58–61

139 Norton L W, Davis J R, Wiens J L, Trego D C, Dunnington G L. Accuracy of aspiration cytology in detecting breast cancer. *Surgery* 1984; **96**: 806–811

140 Strawbridge H T G, Bassett A A, Foldes I. Role of cytology in management of lesions of the breast. *Surg Gynaecol Obstet* 1981; **152**: 1–7

141 Ingram D M, Sterrett G F, Sheiner H J, Shilkin K B. Fine needle aspiration cytology in the management of breast disease. *Med J Aust* 1983; **2**: 170–173

142 Kaufman M, Bider D, Weissberg D. Diagnosis of breast lesions by fine needle aspiration biopsy. *Am Surg* 1983; **49**: 558–559

143 Grant C S, Goellner J R, Welch J S, Martin J K. Fine needle aspiration of the breast. *Mayo Clin Proc* 1986; **61**: 377–381

144 Smallwood J, Herbert A, Guyer P, Taylor I. Accuracy of aspiration cytology in the diagnosis of breast disease. *Br J Surg* 1985; **72**: 841–843

145 Wilkinson E J, Schuettke C M, Ferrier C M et al. Fine needle aspiration of breast masses. An analysis of 276 aspirates. *Acta Cytol* 1989; **33**: 613–619

146 Ciatto S, Cecchini S, Grazzini G et al. Positive predictive value of fine needle aspiration cytology of breast lesions. *Acta Cytol* 1989; **33**: 894–898

147 Nicastri G R, Reed W P, Dzuira BR. The accuracy of malignant diagnoses established by fine needle aspiration cytologic procedures of mammary masses. *Surg Gynecol Obstet* 1991; **172**: 457–460

148 Halevy A, Reif R, Bogokovsky H, Orda R. Diagnosis of carcinoma of the breast by fine needle aspiration cytology. *Surg Gynecol Obstet* 1987; **164**: 506–508

149 Learmonth G M, Hayes M M M, Hacking A et al. Fine needle aspiration biopsy cytology of the breast. A review of the Groote Schuur Hospital experience. *S Afr Med J* 1987; **72**: 525–527

150 Hammond S, Keyhani-Rofagha S, O'Toole R V. Statistical analysis of fine needle aspiration cytology of the breast. A review of 678 cases plus 4265 cases from the literature. *Acta Cytol* 1987; **31**: 276–280

151 Painter R W, Clark W E, Deckers P J. Negative findings on fine-needle aspiration biopsy of solid breast masses: patient management. *Am J Surg* 1988; **155**: 387–390

152 Giard R W M, Hermans J. The value of aspiration cytologic examination of the breast: a statistical review of the medical literature. *Cancer* 1992; **69**: 2104–2110

153 Vetrani A, Fulciniti F, Di-Benedetto G et al. Fine needle aspiration biopsies of breast masses: an additional experience with 1153 cases (1985–1988) and a meta-analysis. *Cancer* 1992; **69**: 736–740

154 Smeets H J, Saltzstein S L, Meurer W T, Pilch Y H. Needle biopsies in breast cancer diagnosis: techniques in search of an audience. *J Surg Oncol* 1986; **32**: 11–15

155 Baildam A D, Turnbull L, Howell A et al. Extended role for needle biopsy in the management of carcinoma of the breast. *Br J Surg* 1989; **76**: 553–558

156 Seckel M, Birney M. Social support, stress and age in women undergoing breast biopsies. *Clin Nurse Spec* 1996; **10**: 137–142

157 Harcourt D, Ambler N, Rumsey N, Cawthorn SJ. Evaluation of a one-stop breast lump clinic: a randomised control trial. *Breast* 1998; **7**: 314–319

158 Poole K, Hood K, Davis B D et al. Psychological stress associated with waiting for results of diagnostic investigations for breast disease. *Breast* 1999; **8**: 334–338

159 Ubhi S, Wright S, Clarke L et al. Anxiety in patients with symptomatic breast disease: effects of immediate versus delayed communication of results. *Ann R Coll Surg Engl* 1996; **78**: 466–469

160 Gui G, Allum W, Perry N et al. One-stop diagnosis for symptomatic breast disease. *Ann R Coll Surg Engl* 1995; **77**: 24–27

161 Lannin D R, Silverman J F, Pories W J, Walker C. Cost-effectiveness of fine needle biopsy of the breast. *Ann Surg* 1986; 474–480

162 Smith T J, Safaii H, Foster E A, Reinhold R B. Accuracy and cost-effectiveness of fine needle aspiration biopsy. *Am J Surg* 1985; **149**: 540 544

163 Kocjan G. Evaluation of the cost effectiveness of establishing a fine needle aspiration cytology clinic in a hospital out-patient department. *Cytopathol* 1991; **2**: 13–18

164 Brown L A, Coghill S B. Cost effectiveness of a fine needle aspiration clinic. *Cytopathol* 1992; **3**: 275–280

165 Liberman L, Feng T L, Dershaw D D *et al.* US-guided core breast biopsy: use and cost-effectiveness. *Radiology* 1998; **208**: 717–723

166 Coghill S B. New techniques, the Lensman microscope: tool or toy? *Cytopathol* 1992; **3**: 317–320

167 Howat A J, Williams R A. Combined scrape cytology and frozen section histology for rapid diagnosis and assessment in breast pathology. *Histopathol* 1990; **17**: 85–96

168 Ku N N K, Cox C E, Reintgen D S *et al.* Cytology of lumpectomy specimens. *Acta Cytol* 1991; **35**: 417–421

169 Petrakis N L, Wrensch M R, Ernster V *et al.* Prognostic significance of atypical epithelial hyperplasia in nipple aspirates of breast fluid. *Lancet* 1987; **29**: 505

170 Takeda T, Matsui A *et al.* Nipple discharge cytology in mass screening for breast cancer. *Acta Cytol* 1990; **34**: 161–164

171 Wells CA, Perera R, White FE, Domizio P. FNA cytology in the UK breast screening programme: a national audit of results. *Breast* 1999; **8**: 261–266

172 Ernst M F, Roukema J A. Diagnosis of non-palpable breast cancer: a review. *Breast* 2002; **11**: 13–22

173 Gotsche P C, Olsen O. Is screening for breast cancer with mammography justifiable? *Lancet* 2000; **355**: 129–134

174 Bunker J P, Houghton J, Baum M. Putting the risk of breast cancer in perspective. *BMJ* 1998; **317**: 1307–1309

175 de Koning H J. Assessment of nationwide cancer-screening programmes. *Lancet* 2000; **355**: 80–81

176 Azavedo E, Svane G, Auer G. Stereotactic fine needle biopsy in 2594 mammographically detected non-palpable lesions. *Lancet* 1989; **1**: 1033–1036

177 Sterrett G, Oliver D, Frayne J *et al.* Stereotactic fine needle aspiration biopsy (SFNB) of breast: preliminary results in Perth with the TRC mammotest machine. Cytological aspects. *Pathol* 1991; **23**: 302–310

178 Svane G, Silfverswärd C. Stereotaxic needle biopsy of non-palpable breast lesions. *Acta Radiol Diag* 1983; **4**: 283–288

179 Yeoman L J, Michel M J, Humphreys S *et al.* Radiographically guided FNA cytology and core biopsy in the assessment of impalpable breast lesions. *Breast* 1996; **5**: 41–47

180 Ciatto S, Bulgaresi P. Multiple sampling to reduce inadequacy rates in stereotaxic

aspiration cytology of the breast. *Acta Cytol* 1991; **35**: 842

181 Jadusingh I H. Intramammary lymph nodes. *J Clin Pathol* 1992; **45**: 1023–1026

182 Malberger E, Gutterman E, Bartfeld E, Zajicek G. Cellular changes in the mammary gland epithelium during the menstrual cycle. A computer image analysis study. *Acta Cytol* 1987; **31**: 305–308

183 Guidelines for non-operative diagnostic procedures and reporting in breast cancer screening. *NHS BSP Publication* 2001; **50**

184 Wells C A, Ellis I O, Zakhour H D *et al.* Guidelines for cytology procedures and reporting on FNAs of breast. *Cytopathol* 1994; **5**: 316–334

185 Keen M E, Murad T M, Cohen M I, Matthies H J. Benign breast lesions with malignant clinical and mammographic presentations. *Hum Pathol* 1985; **16**: 1147–1152

186 Underwood J C E, Parsons M A, Harris S C, Dundas S A C. Frozen section appearances simulating invasive lobular carcinoma in breast tissue adjacent to inflammatory lesions and biopsy sites. *Histopathol* 1988; **13**: 232–234

8 Inflammatory conditions and benign breast lesions

Alec Howat and Stuart Coghill

Introduction

Cytological findings in the great majority of benign lesions of the breast display the classical benign pattern, as described in Chapter 7. What follows is an account of benign breast diseases that may indeed show solely the basic benign pattern or may display specific cytological characteristics.

Inflammatory conditions

The breast is susceptible to a limited range of inflammatory conditions, a few of which have a recognized infective aetiology. Trauma and extravasation of duct contents account for a proportion, but in some conditions, no obvious tissue insult is recognized. Inflammation is characteristically manifest by the presence of dolour, calor, tumour and loss of function. It is the formation of a mass in the breast with or without pain that results in the patient with an inflammatory condition seeking medical assistance. Inflammatory lumps may frequently mimic malignancy both to the patient and on initial clinical assessment. Fine needle aspiration (FNA) can usually provide a reliable generic diagnosis of inflammation and frequently a highly specific one when an organism is cultured from aspirated material. Thus, although these cases represent only a small proportion of patients at a symptomatic breast clinic, they are of considerable interest to the cytologist.

Fat necrosis of the breast (Fig. 8.1)

Fat necrosis of the breast may be associated with mammary duct ectasia and fibrocystic disease when there is rupture of a duct or cyst causing extravasation of contents with secondary necrosis of adjacent fat. It may also follow surgery and radiotherapy[1-6]. Traumatic fat necrosis tends to be more superficial, often occurring in the subcutaneous fat, rather than within the breast itself. There is usually a history of injury 1 or 2 weeks (sometimes longer) before the lump is noted and there may or may not be bruising. Clinically, the lump may be suspicious, even with a hint of skin tethering in healing cases. Aspirates tend to be thick, granular and fatty when spread and contain many foamy macrophages and variable numbers of multinucleate giant cells. Other inflammatory cells may be present, but there is usually a paucity of epithelial elements. The background contains fatty globules and fragments of adipose tissue, some showing degeneration.

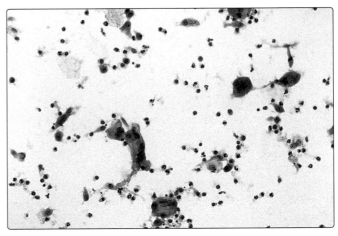

Fig. 8.1   Fat necrosis. Foamy macrophages and foamy multinucleate cells typical of those seen in fat necrosis of the breast. (MGG × HP)

Clinical and cytological findings

▶ History of trauma with or without bruising in the skin
▶ Frequently tender on palpation
▶ Foamy macrophages and multinucleate giant cells with foamy cytoplasm
▶ Fragments of normal as well as degenerate adipose tissue
▶ Variable numbers of other inflammatory cells but usually sparse
▶ Few if any epithelial cells
▶ Free lipid droplets, seen as spaces surrounded by blood
▶ Granular background

Diagnostic pitfalls

▶ Treatable conditions such as tuberculosis or other causes of panniculitides may be mistaken for fat necrosis. Clinically, fat necrosis can imitate carcinoma closely. Failure to examine the active macrophages in a cellular aspirate from fat necrosis closely at high power can reinforce a wrong assumption by the inexperienced

Mammary duct ectasia, plasma cell mastitis, comedo mastitis[7]

Although some authors distinguish between plasma cell mastitis and mammary duct ectasia (also referred to as comedo mastitis), they will be considered as one lesion here. Clinically, this common lesion may mimic carcinoma, as there can be retraction of the nipple associated with a well-defined lesion, usually centrally located. In a fifth of cases there is nipple discharge. Mammography may reveal tubular, annular or linear calcifications. The aetiology is not clear but the basic abnormality is stagnation of secretion, possibly due to loss of elastin support in duct walls, leading to ectasia.

As the many names given to this condition suggest, there is a spectrum of histological appearances reflecting the different stages of the disease process. The most obvious feature is dilatation of large or intermediate ducts that are filled with secretion, foamy macrophages, siderophages and cholesterol crystals that form the inspissated, pasty material seen on gross examination. Epithelial proliferation is not a feature, but reparative changes in epithelium next to areas of inflammation may give rise to a spurious impression of atypia both histologically and cytologically. Stroma surrounding the duct shows scarring and fibrosis or chronic inflammation, frequently with many plasma cells.

The pathologist frequently receives early clues to the diagnosis from the clinical features and the appearance of the aspirate when it is spread on the slide. It is unusually thick, creamy and homogenous. Much of the material appears to dissolve in methanol fixative. The specimen that remains is amorphous debris with variable numbers of foamy macrophages and other inflammatory cells (Fig. 8.2). Occasionally small numbers of atypical epithelial cells are seen. Close examination usually reassures that these show reactive or reparative changes, rather than dysplasia.

Clinical and cytological findings

▶ Discrete lesion often adjacent to the nipple
▶ Abundant, thick spreading pasty aspirate
▶ Loss of much of the material on smears because of dissolution in the methanol fixative
▶ Abundant amorphous debris in smears
▶ Foamy macrophages, occasional giant cells and plasma cells
▶ Scant epithelium which may show reactive atypia

Diagnostic pitfalls

▶ As with fat necrosis, the clinical features can falsely raise the index of suspicion
▶ If epithelium is included, it can appear atypical because of the inflammation
▶ Necrotic carcinomas can be mistaken for duct ectasia; when in doubt reaspirate

Granulomatous mastitis (Figs 8.3–8.4)

Various systemic and local conditions can give rise to the formation of a granulomatous response in the breast[8–14]. Some cases of granulomatous mastitis are part of the spectrum of duct ectasia, but it may occur without duct

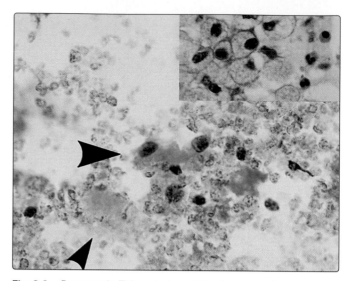

Fig. 8.2   Duct ectasia. This aspirate contained numerous foamy macrophages (upper arrowhead) and amorphous debris (lower arrowhead). There was little if any epithelium. The appearances are typical of those seen in duct ectasia. The inset shows the histological appearances of the same case. (Papanicolaou)

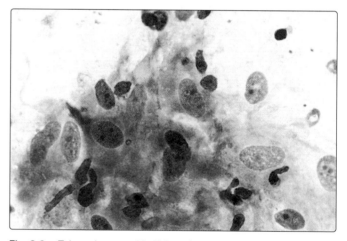

Fig. 8.3   Tuberculous mastitis. This aspirate contained numerous groups of epithelioid histiocytes and occasional giant cells. Cultures and histology confirmed a diagnosis of tuberculous mastitis. (MGG)

dilatation. There is a distinct group in which the granulomatous inflammation is lobulocentric and associated with either recent pregnancy or another cause of high serum prolactin levels, such as phenothiazine therapy[9,10]. Sarcoidosis of the breast is rare, but recognized and can be the presenting sign, compounding diagnostic difficulties[11,12]. Tuberculosis of the breast is more common in developing countries, but does occur in Western society[13].

Other entities that display granulomatous features on aspirates include granulomatous panniculitis (Langerhans cell granulomatosis), granulomatous angiopanniculitis of the breast, Wegener's granulomatosis, rheumatoid nodule, giant cell arteritis, actinomycosis, coccidioidomycosis, foreign body reaction to implanted silicone and tumours[15–19].

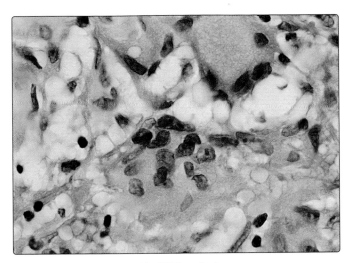

Fig. 8.4   Tuberculous mastitis. (H&E section)

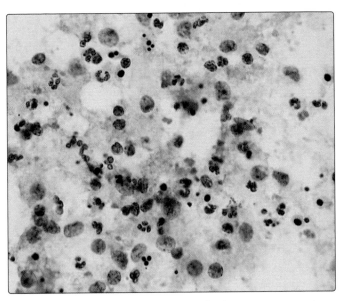

Fig. 8.5   Breast abscess. This aspirate contained numerous macrophages and neutrophil polymorphs with little if any epithelium. (Papanicolaou)

Although clues to the most probable aetiology of the granulomatous infiltration may be had from the gestational history, previous medical history, ethnic origins or other clinical findings, the cytological features will rarely allow a specific diagnosis. The aspirator cytopathologist who recognizes a granulomatous picture is in an ideal position to repeat the aspirate for microbiological examination[13]. Occasionally, the specific diagnosis may be apparent in the cytological preparations. The recognition of the 'sulphur granules' of actinomycosis is an example[15].

As few, if any, of these diseases benefit from surgical intervention, the provision of a specific diagnosis on aspirated material is particularly gratifying. In several series, identification of *Mycobacterium tuberculosis* has been more successful in smears containing inflammatory debris from a cold abscess or necrotic material (47–74%) than in FNA samples containing epithelioid cells alone (26–34%)[20].

Clinical and cytological findings

▶ Sheets or clusters of epithelioid cells with copious cytoplasm and elongated nuclei. The nuclei may have a characteristic slipper-shaped profile
▶ Multinucleate giant cells associated with epithelioid cells. The giant cells often have epithelioid cell characteristics. Langhans type giant cells may be identified
▶ In tuberculosis and fungal infections, a mixture of eosinophilic necrotic debris and inflammatory cells may also be present. If other features of granulomatous disease are absent, special stains and culture for micro-organisms may often be positive

Diagnostic pitfalls

▶ Tuberculosis of the breast may be so similar to carcinoma clinically, that the surgeon may be reluctant to accept a benign diagnosis. It is important to obtain material for

culture, not only to add credibility to the diagnosis but also to ascertain the sensitivity of the organism. Care must be taken with slide preparation including use of a liquid-based method or wet-fixed smears, if the disease is suspected before aspiration is performed
▶ Rarely, carcinomas or lymphomas elicit a granulomatous response. Carcinoma with osteoclast-type giant cells must also be considered. A largely necrotic carcinoma can occasionally give the misleading appearance of a granulomatous condition. Usually however, there will be large numbers of degenerate or not fully necrotic epithelial cells with malignant features. In cases of doubt, a repeat aspirate from the periphery of the lesion will usually provide a more viable sample and confirm the diagnosis

Abscess and acute mastitis *(Fig. 8.5)*

Breast abscesses and acute mastitis occur most commonly, but not invariably, in the puerperium. The diagnosis is usually made clinically and effective antibiotic treatment is given without need for a cytological or tissue diagnosis. Occasionally however, resolution does not occur or is slow and surgical drainage is planned. The possibility of an inflammatory carcinoma may then be considered and an FNA diagnosis sought.

As might be predicted, aspirates contain neutrophil polymorphs and macrophages in considerable numbers as well as abundant cell debris[21]. Occasionally active-looking epithelial cells, derived from adjacent inflamed and possibly lactating breast tissue, are included. These can cause concern but reassurance can be found when the epithelial cell fragments are seen to be infiltrated by inflammatory cells and show no features of malignancy. Usually, the clinical information reinforced by a second aspirate allows an accurate assessment to be made.

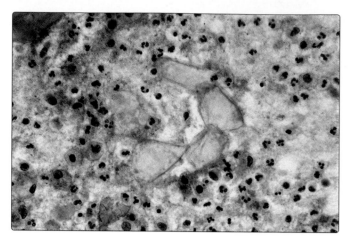

Fig. 8.6 Subareolar abscess. Inflammatory cells, histiocytes and anucleate squames are present. The presence of anucleate squames distinguishes this lesion from mastitis. (MGG) (Courtesy of Dr G McKee, Boston)

Subareolar abscess/mammary duct fistula/Zuska's disease[22,23] *(Fig. 8.6)*

This condition is thought to have some affinity with mammary duct ectasia. It is probably better recognized by surgeons than by pathologists. There is often a history of the recurrent formation of a tender mass in the subareolar region, sinus tract formation and discharge with partial healing. Histologically, excised lesions are seen to consist of an inflammatory sinus tract lined by granulation tissue but often partially by squamous epithelium. Aspirates appear to consist primarily of inflammatory exudate but additionally there may be anucleate squames, multinucleate giant cells and epithelium showing reactive atypia. The cytological appearance is not dissimilar to that of an infected epidermal cyst except that these do not contain ductal cells.

Clinical and cytological findings

▶ Typical history of recurrent inflammatory lesions associated with the nipple
▶ Smears containing anucleate squames, multinucleate giant cells, macrophages and epithelium showing reactive atypia

Diagnostic pitfalls

▶ Other inflammatory conditions including tuberculosis should be considered but the history should be helpful in identifying a mammary duct fistula. Sometimes the reactive atypia in the epithelial component of the aspirate is such that it may be confused with a more significant lesion

Sclerosing lymphocytic lobulitis of the breast[24-26]

This lesion, also referred to as lymphocytic or diabetic mastopathy, has well-documented histopathological features. There is an association with insulin-dependent diabetes mellitus, thyroiditis and arthropathy, although most cases are sporadic without other underlying disease. An overlap with fibrous disease is apparent. It can present as a lump and it might be expected to be the target of a FNA. The cytological features are not specific, merely showing a paucicellular benign pattern with lymphocytes[27].

Amyloid 'tumour'[28]

FNA cytology of subcutaneous fat followed by Congo red staining has been advocated for confirming the diagnosis of systemic amyloidosis. Localized collections of amyloid can occur in a variety of sites including the breast. These deposits have been termed amyloid tumour and present as a solitary localized mass, rarely bilateral. It occurs in older women and can be firm or hard and discrete. It can imitate carcinoma clinically and mammographically.

Cytological preparations show amorphous translucent material similar to thick thyroid colloid. This material stains violet with May-Grünwald-Giemsa and pale pink with the Papanicolaou method. Scanty bland spindle cells are seen, and more rarely, reactive giant cells are a feature. Faced with this picture, the pathologist can take further aspirates for Congo red staining to confirm the diagnosis.

Rare inflammatory conditions

Parasitic lesions in the breast are rare. The cytological appearance of cysticercosis of the breast[29] has been described, however. Myospherulosis[30,31] is a pseudomycotic condition that can occur following the subcutaneous injection of penicillin and presents an intriguing histological appearance. Altered erythrocytes coated with lipid are deposited in the tissues within spherules. In smears they stain brown with MGG staining, but are red in Papanicolaou preparations and are negative with PAS and silver stains.

Silicone implants may leak, giving rise to a local mass and to axillary lymphadenopathy[32]. Aspirates contain numerous macrophages containing large cytoplasmic vacuoles as well as giant cells of foreign body type. Cytopathologists should be aware of the risks of sampling breast lesions adjacent to mammary prostheses. The patient is not always aware of the need to disclose the presence of such devices and the scars can be almost invisible.

Benign breast lesions

Breast cysts

It has now been convincingly established that the cytological examination of cyst fluid that is not blood-stained has little utility[33]. If cyst fluid is blood-stained, it should be examined cytologically, but with the caveat that a negative result will not necessarily exclude the presence of an intracystic carcinoma.

It is also important to re-aspirate any residual mass following the drainage of a cyst whatever the nature of the cyst contents, as a cyst may mask an adjacent carcinoma. It has been suggested that cysts providing haemorrhagic

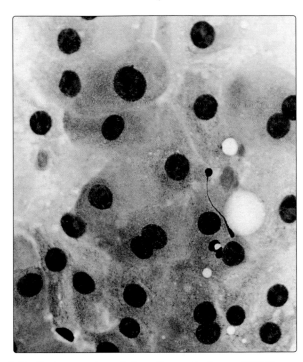

Fig. 8.7   Benign apocrine cells from fibrocystic disease. (MGG)

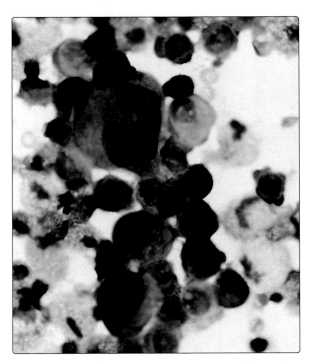

Fig. 8.8   Cyst fluid containing atypical apocrine cells which were deemed suspicious. (MGG)

fluid should be investigated by pneumocystography[34]. When in doubt, however, many surgeons prefer to excise the lesion.

A lesion that provides more than 1 ml of fluid has been defined as a cyst. Not infrequently, however, aspiration of a breast lump will provide a watery sample with a volume sufficiently small to allow it to be spread over one or two slides. Microscopical examination usually reveals a moderate number of benign apocrine cells, providing reassurance that the lesion is a focus of fibrocystic change (Fig. 8.7). Occasionally, a cyst contains apocrine epithelium that shows degenerative changes easily mistaken for atypia (Figs 8.8, 8.9).

Any pathologist who believes that cyst fluids should always be examined should be aware that many general practitioners aspirate cysts in their surgeries and discard the fluid.

Fibrocystic change[35–38] *(Figs 8.10–8.14)*

Clinically, the appearance of this, the most common cause of a palpable breast lump, has certain characteristic findings. The typical patient is between 30 and 50 years old, but an age range of 25 to 70 has been quoted. Often, there is a convincing history of change of the breast lump with the menstrual cycle and fibrocystic lesions are more commonly tender or painful than malignant ones. The palpable lesion is not always well-defined and may range in size from a few millimetres to a change occupying the whole breast.

The condition may be synchronously bilateral, but often the first presentation is as a solitary lesion. Patients are prone to developing multiple sequential lumps and thus

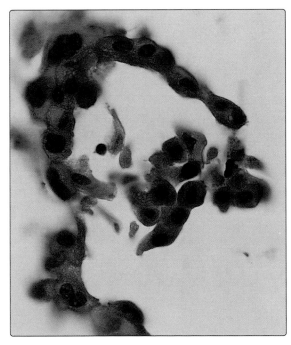

Fig. 8.9   Apocrine cyst lining from the same case as Fig. 8.8. This section showed that the atypical apocrine epithelium showed only degenerate change with no evidence of premalignancy. (H&E section)

may be less anxious about the appearance of further masses than women presenting with the first breast lump. Each lesion must be assessed on its own merits. Some fibrocystic lumps can present appearances that are worrying clinically, mammographically and indeed, histologically.

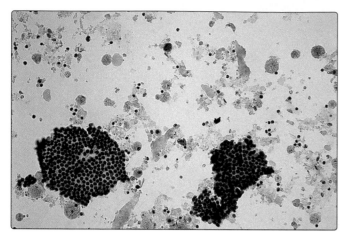

Fig. 8.10 Fibrocystic change with a benign pattern (C2) of ductal cell sheets, bipolar nuclei, cyst debris and macrophages in the background. (H&E)

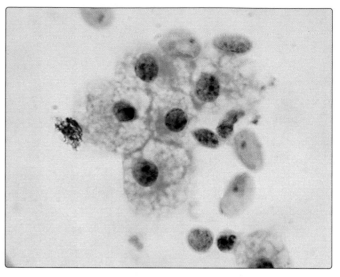

Fig. 8.12 Foamy macrophages in benign fibrocystic disease. (Papanicolaou)

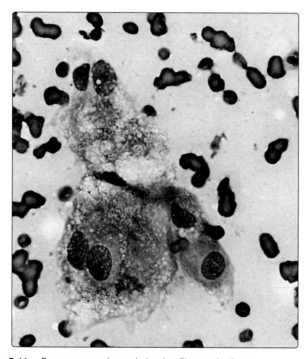

Fig. 8.11 Foamy macrophages in benign fibrocystic disease. (Papanicolaou)

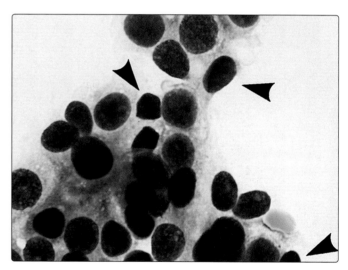

Fig. 8.13 Benign breast epithelium. This field illustrates the typical appearance of benign breast epithelium. The apparent anisonucleosis is spurious and due to the presence of a number of interspersed myoepithelial cells (arrowheads). (MGG)

The spectrum of histological appearances generally included under the heading of 'fibrocystic change' is very wide. The basic histological elements are:

1 The formation of cysts
2 Apocrine metaplasia of cyst lining cells and of duct and lobular epithelium
3 Rupture of the cyst lining with extravasation of contents and associated inflammation
4 Fibrosis of the stroma
5 Chronic inflammation of non-specific type
6 Epithelial hyperplasia of various types
7 Fibroadenomatoid change

Following examination, the aspirator gains a further important diagnostic clue when the needle enters the lump. The fibrous elements frequently present in this condition will often have a distinctly rubbery or leathery feel to the needle. The cellularity of the sample usually bears a relation to the ease with which the specimen is obtained. The distant cytopathologist will be deprived of this component of the diagnostic information. When the needle is gripped by leathery fibrous tissue, a poorly cellular aspirate may be anticipated and a little more vigour can be applied in the movement of the needle. In other cases, the aspirate will often appear watery allowing it to be spread over the whole of one or two slides with ease.

The amount of microscopical material varies considerably, depending on whether the lesion is from the

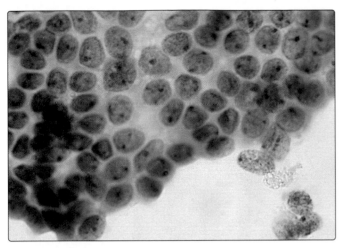

Fig. 8.14 Hyperplasia. The typical appearances of benign hyperplastic breast epithelium. Occasional bipolar nuclei are seen, bottom right. (Papanicolaou)

fibrous or the proliferative ends of the spectrum seen in this condition. The basic pattern is benign, but there may be several cell types present. The most reassuring component is the presence of obviously benign apocrine cells. These may be in large cohesive sheets or dispersed singly or in small groups. The nuclei are large, round and relatively hyperchromatic. The nucleoli are large and prominent, unusually so for a benign epithelial cell. The cytoplasm is abundant and usually granular. Cell borders should be well-defined in contrast to the cells of a low grade apocrine carcinoma that have wispy poorly defined cytoplasmic margins. Further reassurance is obtained from the presence of bipolar nuclei, myoepithelial and stromal.

Clinical and cytological findings

▶ Poorly defined lumpiness on palpation sometimes with a 'shotty' feeling
▶ Either easy needle penetration with variable resistance or marked resistance with a leathery or rubbery feel
▶ Scanty, watery or fatty smear
▶ Benign or uncertain mammogram
▶ Low or moderate cellularity
▶ Apocrine cells either dominating the cellular picture or in variable numbers
▶ Foam cells (of macrophage or epithelial origin)
▶ Sheets or fragments of ductal epithelium with bland nuclei arranged in a honeycomb pattern with admixed myoepithelial cells and dispersed bipolar nuclei
▶ Fat or fibrous stroma in variable quantities

Diagnostic pitfalls

▶ Benign fibrocystic disease may mask an adjacent carcinoma
▶ Apocrine carcinoma can occasionally be interpreted as benign if low-grade

▶ Benign apocrine metaplasia may appear atypical when degenerate

Fibrous disease of the breast (focal fibrosis of the breast, fibrous 'tumour')

For some histopathologists the very existence of this entity is controversial[39]. The features overlap with those of lymphocytic lobulitis[24-27] (p 260). As discussed under lymphocytic lobulitis, there is an increased incidence in diabetic patients[26,40-42]. Clinically obvious palpable lumps that are excised may show what cannot be classified as any other type of benign breast disease.

Some argue that many cases presenting with an indurated mass show stromal changes and parenchymal atrophy that fall within the normal range histologically. Many more cases present to the surgeon than are biopsied. Aspiration is frequently difficult, with dense fibrous tissue gripping the needle, making the routine of several passes hard to accomplish. FNA usually reveals a paucicellular aspirate, perhaps with increased lymphocytes. Often no sample can be expressed from the needle or a trace of acellular fluid is obtained[43]. If the same result is obtained on further aspiration of a lump showing the appropriate clinical features, a presumptive diagnosis of fibrous disease of the breast may be inferred. Follow-up histology confirms that the tissue is composed of virtually acellular collagen.

Clinical and cytological findings

▶ Variable clinical features from a vague thickening to a craggy lump
▶ Penetration of the needle usually difficult and restricted
▶ Acellular or very scanty aspirate containing only bipolar nuclei, resulting in an inadequate diagnosis (C1)

Diagnostic pitfalls

▶ Very scirrhous ductal, or more especially lobular, carcinomas can yield very scanty or acellular aspirates. Confusion of these lesions with benign fibrous change accounts for some false negative cytology reports

Epithelial hyperplasia (proliferative breast disease)

Histologically, the basic appearances described as fibrocystic changes are frequently accompanied by epithelial proliferative changes of various types. Cytologically, this may be suspected when an aspirate, otherwise typical of 'simple' fibrocystic change, is cellular with the additional cells being non-apocrine in type[44,45]. These proliferative changes also commonly occur without detectable fibrocystic change. The histological changes include adenosis (sclerosing, microglandular, 'blunt duct'), hyperplasias (duct hyperplasia, duct papillomatosis), atypical ductal hyperplasia (atypical lobular hyperplasia now being included with lobular carcinoma-*in-situ* under the general heading of lobular neoplasia), adenomyoepithelial hyperplasia, adenosis tumour, apocrine adenosis with and without sclerosis, radial scar and complex sclerosing lesions.

Histopathologists routinely spend much time and effort in classifying and subclassifying these entities. It should be said at the outset that such precision is neither possible nor necessarily desirable on cytological assessment. Thus, at initial evaluation the cytopathologist is forced to become a diagnostic 'lumper' and report the FNA as benign (C2). However, attempts have been made to refine the diagnosis using semiquantative methods[46]. Unfortunately the predictive value is not high[47] and it may therefore be prudent to give a benign diagnosis with further discussion of the case at the triple assessment clinic. The mammographic appearance of some of these lesions, notably the radial scar is, however, distinctive. Pooling of cytological and mammographic information may allow a more specific diagnosis. However, not all radial scars can be diagnosed with confidence on mammograms as some spiculated lesions represent carcinomas. At the present time all stellate lesions are excised even if cytologically benign, in case of missed sampling. Histopathologists are keen to separate ductal and lobular hyperplasia but this is not possible with certainty in cytological assessment.

One rare variant of benign epithelial hyperplasia that does have a distinctive cytological appearance is collagenous spherulosis[48,49] (Figs 8.15, 8.16). In May-Grünwald-Giemsa stained preparations the collagenous spherules are very conspicuous and appear magenta in colour. This lesion should be excluded when a diagnosis of adenoid cystic carcinoma is being considered.

Microcalcifications can be recognized in cytological preparations when present (Fig. 8.17). Their radiological characteristics are diagnostic but they are of little assistance in microscopic diagnosis as they look morphologically similar in both benign and malignant lesions. However, they are useful in confirming that a mammographic lesion containing microcalcifications has been correctly sampled.

Clinical and cytological findings

▶ The clinical picture is usually benign, but can be highly suspicious

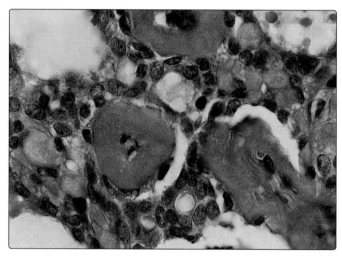

Fig. 8.16   The histology of collagenous spherulosis. (H&E section)

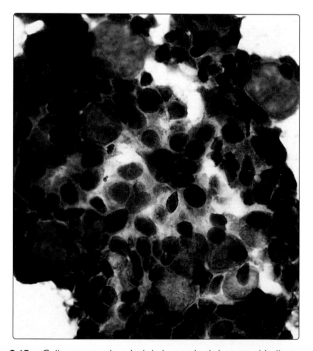

Fig. 8.15   Collagenous spherulosis in hyperplastic breast epithelium. The epithelium is interspersed with pink staining globules resulting in an appearance that is difficult to distinguish from adenoid cystic carcinoma cytologically. (MGG)

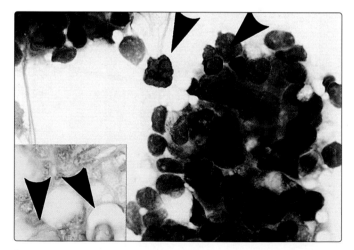

Fig. 8.17   Microcalcifications. The arrowheads indicate the presence of two microcalcifications associated with hyperplastic and atypical breast epithelium. (MGG) The inset shows similar laminated microcalcifications in the histology. (H&E section)

- The mammographic appearance of sclerosing lesions is usually suspicious
- Low or moderate cellularity with small epithelial groups or high cellularity with large flat or folded sheets of cohesive regular cells
- Adenosis lesions may show a microacinar appearance in smears
- Nuclei may be enlarged, but the chromatin pattern is fine and nucleoli inconspicuous
- The epithelial groups contain the smaller darker ovoid nuclei of myoepithelial cells
- Variable numbers of bipolar nuclei between the groups
- Any separate epithelial cells present also have a fine chromatin pattern and small nucleoli
- The nuclear membrane, often difficult to see in compact groups, has a smooth profile
- Macrophages and apocrine cells may be present
- An absence of nuclear atypia, widespread loss of cell cohesion or necrotic debris

Hyperplasia with atypia

By extrapolation from other body sites where premalignancy can be observed *in situ*, and from study of the long-term outcome of many cases of breast disease, it is now widely accepted that there is correlation between the degree of hyperplasia, whether usual type or atypical, and the risk of subsequent development of invasive ductal carcinoma[50–62]. Recent evidence suggests that atypical ductal hyperplasia (ADH) and low-grade DCIS represent low-grade ductal neoplasia even sharing identical chromosomal abnormalities[60]. Much the same is true for atypical lobular hyperplasia and LCIS with some authors favouring the all-encompassing term of lobular neoplasia[60–62]. Risk of the future development of invasive carcinoma is related to the size of the abnormal area of lobular neoplasia, while ADH has been defined as being less than 3 mm in maximum diameter with low-grade cytology. Any atypical ductal proliferation with high-grade cytology must be called DCIS whatever the size[63–65]. The risk of future invasive breast cancer in women showing such abnormalities is shown in Table 8.1.

If aspiration cytology is to reach its full potential, some attempt must be made to identify benign lesions from those

carrying increased risk of carcinoma[44–46,63–66]. These risk-bearing lesions must be viewed in the light of the high total life-time risk for breast cancer. This is 1 in 12 for women in the UK[67,68]. A factor worth noting is that there are problems in categorizing hyperplastic, atypical and premalignant lesions of the breast, with poor interobserver agreement, even in histological assessment of atypical lesions[69].

The main role for cytological assessment of symptomatic benign breast disease together with mammography is in selecting those cases where excision biopsy and detailed histological assessment are indicated. This should then allow an acceptably low benign to malignant biopsy ratio. Close liaison between surgeon, pathologist and radiologist is as important here as in the assessment of breast screening cases. In the past, communication may have been hampered by incompatible radiological and pathological terminologies, which made decisions unnecessarily difficult for the surgeons. A simple cytological reporting classification should be adhered to (see Chapter 7), so that the surgeon understands precisely what is being conveyed by the report. In cases where there is hyperplasia without obvious atypia, the FNA should be reported as benign (C2). When a lesion is clearly atypical but not obviously malignant the diagnosis 'atypical, probably benign' (C3) may be appropriate. Certain features that may lead to a diagnosis of atypia include the following.

Cytological findings

- Increased crowding and overlapping of cells within the groups
- Obvious papillary groups
- Decreased cohesion of epithelial cells
- More variation in nuclear size
- More prominence of nucleoli
- Less evidence of cells of apocrine type

It becomes obvious that the features used to differentiate atypical cases cytologically are very much a matter of degree and are therefore highly subjective. Where there is any doubt as to the presence of atypia, the triple assessment findings should be considered and excision biopsy or follow-up undertaken, as appropriate.

Diagnostic pitfalls

- ALH and LCIS cannot be differentiated cytologically or chromosomally
- ADH and low-grade DCIS cannot be differentiated cytologically or chromosomally
- Fibroepithelial neoplasms may appear atypical when the clinical and mammographic features are not available and the cytology is viewed under a high-power lens
- Low-grade and lobular carcinomas may be mistaken for a hyperplastic process
- Inflammatory lesions may cause quite marked reactive atypia
- Previous radiotherapy may cause atypia

Table 8.1 The relative risk of future breast carcinoma associated with various forms of benign breast disease and *in situ* lesions

Fibrocystic change with no hyperplasia, duct ectasia, sclerosing adenosis	× 1.00
Fibrocystic change with hyperplasia but no atypia, increased risk	× 1.5–2.0
Atypical ductal (ADH) or atypical lobular hyperplasia (ALH), increased risk	× 4–5
Lobular carcinoma in-situ increased risk	× 7–12
DCIS (low-grade) increased risk	× 8–10
DCIS (high-grade) increased risk	× 15–20

Benign fibroepithelial tumours

Fibroadenoma *(Figs 8.18–8.23)*

Despite its name, some authorities believe this lesion almost certainly represents a focal hyperplasia rather than a benign neoplasm. Cytological features[70,71] closely mimic the histological features. When the cytopathologist has the opportunity to obtain the aspirate, the clinical features and cytological appearances allow an accurate diagnosis to be made with ease in most cases.

Fibroadenoma most commonly presents in women between the ages of 20 and 35 years, but can come to the attention of the patient for the first time in later life, sometimes after unrelated weight loss. Increasing use of mammography has increased the diagnosis of longstanding fibroadenomas in older women. These lesions are often of the poorly cellular 'ancient' type.

Histological variants that may lead to special cytological features include the occurrence of apocrine metaplasia in up to 32%[71], haemorrhagic infarction, especially during pregnancy, squamous metaplasia[72] (although this is more common in phyllodes tumour) and stromal metaplasias including the formation of smooth muscle, cartilage, bone or dystrophic calcification. The formation of bone and calcification is commoner in older women and is likely to become apparent on taking the aspirate as the needle may refuse to enter the mass or may give a very gritty sensation.

Particularly in younger women, marked cellularity can be a frequent feature, but the youth of the patient reduces the likelihood of a false positive diagnosis. Rarely (<1 in 1000), carcinoma arises within or infiltrates into a fibroadenoma[73–75]. Some 50% of these are LCIS, 15% DCIS and the remaining 35% show either invasive ductal or invasive lobular carcinoma.

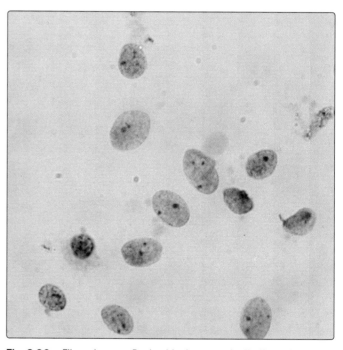

Fig. 8.20 Fibroadenoma. Benign bipolar stromal cells. (Papanicolaou)

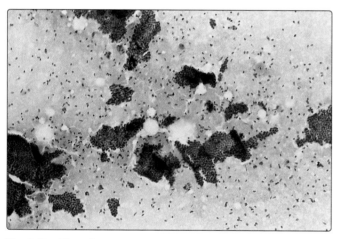

Fig. 8.18 Fibroadenoma. The complex three-dimensional structure of the epithelial component of a typical fibroadenoma is illustrated in this smear. There is a background of bipolar cells. (Papanicolaou)

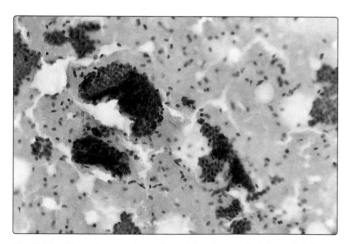

Fig. 8.19 Fibroadenoma. Large branching sheets of benign epithelium are a typical finding in fibroadenoma. (Papanicolaou)

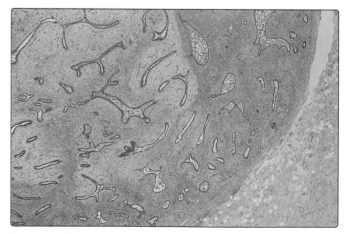

Fig. 8.21 Fibroadenoma. Histology. (H&E)

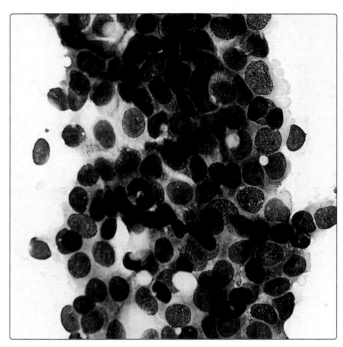

Fig. 8.22 Fibroadenoma. The typical appearances of cohesive benign epithelial cells with admixed myoepithelial cells showing as darker bipolar nuclei. (MGG)

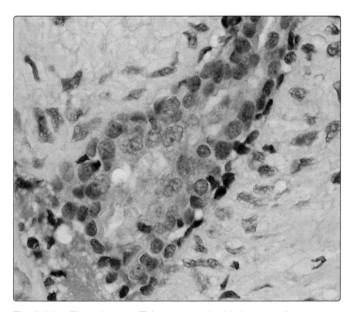

Fig. 8.23 Fibroadenoma. This corresponds with the preceding cytological appearances and the peripheral myoepithelial cells can be seen particularly to the right of the epithelial structure. (H&E section)

An early clue to the diagnosis of fibroadenoma is a firm, discrete and highly mobile lump ('breast mouse') in a young woman. The clinical features of a classical fibroadenoma almost render aspiration cytology superfluous. Surprises can occur, however. In cases showing highly cellular stromal fragments, very large numbers of plump, naked bipolar nuclei with hyperplastic duct cells, giant cells and an absence of apocrine cells, a diagnosis of

phyllodes tumour should be considered[76] but this is more likely in older women.

Good technique is important in securing a diagnostic aspirate from a small, mobile fibroadenoma. It is tempting to prevent the lesion from escaping the needle by fixing it against the chest wall but this increases the risk of pneumothorax in thin subjects. It is advisable to spend a little time fixing the lump between the forefinger and thumb before aspirating. It can also be drawn forward through the soft tissue and supported from behind by the aspirator's thumb and finger. This technique also provides the aspirator with stereotactic and tactile sensations to detect when the needle tip has entered the lesion. The needle usually penetrates easily, but older and more fibrous lesions may be pushed away by the tip of the needle. Very occasionally a lesion that on excision turns out to be a fibroadenoma will give a suspicious gritty sensation on the needle.

To the naked eye the aspirate is usually satisfyingly fat free, and particulate when it is spread, but may appear scanty until it is stained, whereupon large epithelial fragments become apparent.

Microscopically, the diagnosis is often obvious at low power with characteristic large frond-like epithelial groups with peripheral finger-like projections. These are sometimes likened to the antlers of stags. At high power this epithelium is composed of closely packed, uniform cells with an irregular honeycomb appearance, best visualized on the Papanicolaou-stained smear. In air-dried preparations it is only at the edge of the epithelial groups that the cells will be sufficiently flattened to allow satisfactory close examination. The nuclei are approximately the size of one or two erythrocytes and are round or slightly ovoid, having one or two small nucleoli and finely granular chromatin. Myoepithelial cells are seen scattered over the surface of the sheets of ductal epithelial cells.

The other essential feature is the presence of an often generous population of naked bipolar cell nuclei. As the number of these nuclei usually correlates well with the cellularity of the stroma in the subsequent histology it is suggested that these are more likely to be stromal cells than myoepithelial cells. The bipolar cells have condensed chromatin packed into a small elongate nucleus. Although some of the nuclei are truly naked, probably representing myoepithelial cells, many are stromal cells displaying more spindly nuclei and a strand of pale blue cytoplasm at each pole, seen best under high power. In some fibroadenomas a scattering of foamy macrophages or apocrine cells is seen.

Clinical and cytological findings

▶ Typical 5–30 mm diameter well circumscribed mobile lump clinically
▶ Benign mammographic appearances of a round well-defined lesion

► Moderate or high cellularity
► Cohesive sheets with an antler-like appearance and many naked bipolar cell nuclei
► If apocrine or foam cells are present they are few

Diagnostic pitfalls

► More than the occasional fibroadenoma shows features such as reduced cellular cohesion and nuclear enlargement with anisonucleosis and prominent nucleoli that may cause anxiety and give a risk of a false positive diagnosis. It is important that the general low power pattern is fully appreciated before looking at the aspirate at higher power when the spuriously worrying features may be apparent. The recognition of bipolar cells is also particularly important in these cases
► Misdiagnosis of fibroadenoma is the commonest cause of false positive diagnoses, although these are rare

Benign phyllodes tumour (formerly cystosarcoma phyllodes, benign) (Figs 8.24–8.27)

This fibroepithelial neoplasm is seen in women on average 20 years older than those with fibroadenoma[66]. There is however considerable overlap and, while phyllodes tumours tend to be larger on presentation, they may present at any stage of development. Conversely, fibroadenomas may reach 100 mm or more in diameter before the patient seeks help. The differentiation between giant fibroadenoma and benign phyllodes tumour depends entirely on the histological appearance of the stroma[66,77] and the distinction is frequently impossible cytologically[76,78–80].

Late presentation, particularly in a large breast, has resulted in some very large specimens of phyllodes tumour.

On examination, these tumours are softer, less mobile and less well-defined than fibroadenomas. There is usually little resistance to the needle, unless the rare occurrence of metaplastic bone or cartilage is encountered. The aspirate is generally blood free and appears glairy when spread.

The smears are usually very cellular and the differentiation from a cellular fibroadenoma can be impossible. The above clinical features are of assistance in balancing the probabilities. Additionally, the cellularity of the stromal fragments and the size and possible atypia of the many dispersed stromal cells is important, often leading to an atypical, probably benign (C3) diagnosis. MGG

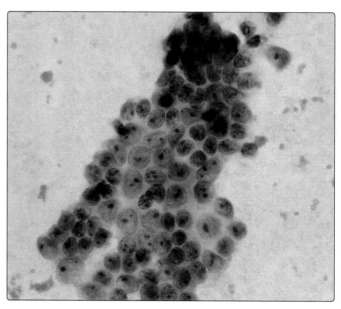

Fig. 8.25 Benign phyllodes tumour. The plump active-looking but essentially benign epithelial nuclei contain quite prominent nucleoli in this aspirate of a benign phyllodes tumour. (Papanicolaou)

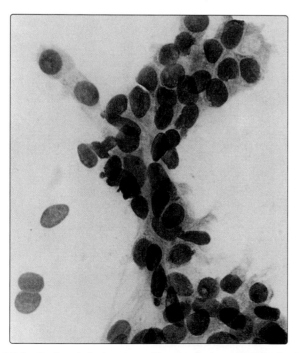

Fig. 8.24 Benign phyllodes tumour. Plump cohesive epithelial cells with numerous naked bipolar cells in the typical clinical setting characterize benign phyllodes tumour. (MGG)

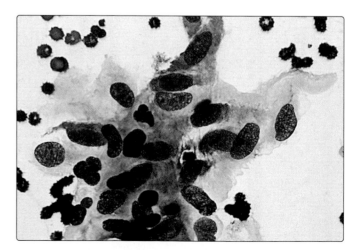

Fig. 8.26 Benign phyllodes tumour stroma. This field illustrates the appearance of the plump stromal cells from a benign phyllodes tumour. (MGG)

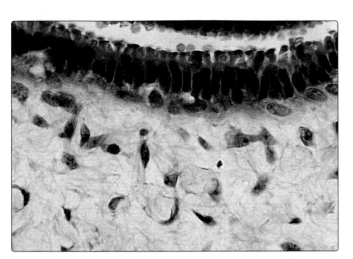

Fig. 8.27   Benign phyllodes tumour. This field was selected for correlation with the preceding aspirates and illustrates the somewhat hyperplastic epithelium and plump stromal cells. (H&E section)

stained preparations may reveal pink or purple staining ground substance within the stromal fragments. The most critical cytological feature in deciding whether the lesion is benign, borderline or malignant, is the degree of atypia of the stromal cells. They may occasionally be frankly malignant cytologically; more commonly the atypia is of a lesser degree suggesting a borderline lesion, which may result in a C3 or C4 diagnosis. Even histological assessment is subjective in this regard and the degree of infiltration that is important in histological assessment is obviously not apparent on cytological preparations. There is a distinct risk of making a false positive diagnosis when assessing a benign phyllodes tumour[78]. Occasional phyllodes tumours contain keratin cysts leading to further diagnostic problems[81].

There is considerable value in making a correct preoperative diagnosis of phyllodes tumour as the enucleation that would be adequate for a fibroadenoma may result in a local recurrence if applied to a phyllodes tumour.

Clinical and cytological findings

▶ Clinically, phyllodes tumours are usually larger than fibroadenomas and present in an older age group
▶ Very cellular smears with occasional large sheets of benign epithelium and many plump stromal cells. The prominence and number of bipolar cells are usually greater than in fibroadenomas
▶ Fragments composed entirely of bipolar cells containing pink or purple ground substance in MGG preparations

Diagnostic pitfalls

▶ Frequently impossible to distinguish from a fibroadenoma
▶ Borderline lesions are difficult to recognize cytologically

Other benign tumours and focal hyperplasias

Microglandular adenosis

Some attention has been drawn to cytological appearances of this rare condition[82], which has been recognized as a potential histopathological diagnostic pitfall[83] since it was described by McDivitt in 1968[84]. The clinical presentation is of a palpable mass that can vary from 3 to 30 mm in diameter.

Findings are of an abundantly cellular aspirate with many cells in small clumps and elongated cohesive three-dimensional tubular arrays. The cells have scant cytoplasm but have round and uniform nuclei. The chromatin pattern is reassuringly fine and evenly dispersed and each nucleus has a single nucleolus. No bipolar cells or other features are seen and an atypical or suspicious diagnosis (C3/C4) may result. There is clearly a risk of making a false diagnosis of tubular carcinoma on the aspirate. This is understandable as even good quality histological sections may present a problem in making this differential diagnosis.

Histologically, the differentiation of this lesion from tubular carcinoma depends on the recognition of a lobular structure in the former. Microglandular adenosis displays very round glandular profiles, complete absence of cellular pleomorphism and each gland is shown on staining to be invested by a complete layer of peritubular reticulin, with no myoepithelial cells. The presence of eosinophilic, PAS positive secretion in the tubular lumina is an important finding in indicating a benign lesion. Tubular carcinoma by contrast shows slight irregularity or angulation of the tubular profiles and should show at least mild cellular pleomorphism. Finding foci of intraduct carcinoma is obviously helpful but cannot be relied upon. Cytological differentiation is therefore even more problematic. The regular honeycomb pattern within the epithelial groups of microglandular adenosis is not found in tubular carcinoma and so the actual arrangement of the nuclei within epithelial groups is very important.

Clinical and cytological findings

▶ Presents clinically as a palpable mass up to 30 mm in diameter
▶ Abundant cellularity
▶ Epithelial cells in small groups and cohesive three-dimensional elongated tubular arrays
▶ The cells have scant cytoplasm, but round uniform nuclei with fine evenly dispersed chromatin and single nucleoli
▶ No bipolar cells

Diagnostic pitfalls

▶ Possible confusion with tubular carcinoma

Complex sclerosing lesion[66,85], radial scar[86–90], sclerosing papilloma[66,85]

These lesions are presented together not to suggest that there is complete histological homology, but because they provide similar cytological features. Their frequently small size and sclerotic nature make the aspiration of sufficient cells for a specific diagnosis difficult. When a sample is obtained, it is generally scanty and shows a mixture of small groups and some dissociated epithelial cells and a few bipolar cells. A provisional preoperative diagnosis may be made on mammography with a poorly cellular cytological sample. As a false negative diagnosis may be feared, particularly in older women, full reassurance will not be obtained without excision biopsy and histopathological assessment. There is, at present, some debate as to whether radial scars convey an increased risk of subsequent breast cancer[89].

Clinical and cytological findings

- ► May present with suspicious mammographic features in screened cases
- ► The sample is poorly cellular but cellular areas may also be represented in the aspirate
- ► Small groups of uniform epithelial cells and dispersed bipolar cells
- ► Apocrine cells may be present, usually in small numbers

Diagnostic pitfalls

- ► The main difficulty is in reaching a diagnosis on a scanty sample

Tubular adenoma[66,85]

The clinical features of this lesion are indistinguishable from fibroadenoma and occasional examples show areas resembling classical fibroadenoma. This suggests some homology between these conditions. Tubular adenomas tend to be easy to aspirate, being softer than the average fibroadenoma.

The cytological features are similar to those of a fibroadenoma but there are fewer bipolar cells and the larger complex epithelial sheets are not a feature. This is reflected in the histology in which there are closely packed tubular structures showing a single epithelial cell layer surrounded by a thinned layer of myoepithelial cells. The relative rarity of these lesions makes it unlikely that a specific diagnosis will be made by FNA cytology and a preoperative diagnosis of fibroadenoma or fibroadenosis is likely.

Clinical and cytological findings

- ► Clinical presentation similar to fibroadenoma
- ► Moderate to highly cellular aspirate with a basic benign pattern

- ► No large antler-like groups are seen
- ► The epithelial cells are cytologically benign and in small groups, some displaying a microacinar arrangement
- ► Bipolar cells are fewer than that in fibroadenomas

Diagnostic pitfalls

- ► These are as for fibroadenoma

Nipple adenoma[66,85,91], papilloma of the nipple ducts, erosive adenosis of the nipple, subareolar papillomatosis

The cytologist will benefit greatly from the opportunity to appraise this lesion clinically. The condition occurs in late middle age and the appearance is that of an eroded and weeping nipple with no mass on either clinical examination or mammography. There is therefore a chance of an erroneous clinical diagnosis of Paget's disease of the nipple with the risk of over treatment. Cytology is of assistance here. Before aspiration it is useful to take contact specimens from any moist eroded area directly on to a slide. Aspiration of the nipple and areola can be acutely painful and so some skill is required to obtain an adequate sample without undue discomfort for the patient. It is important to avoid the areola and to pass the needle through normal skin sampling the nipple lesion obliquely.

The histological pattern of these lesions can be variable with both papillomatous and adenomatous forms. The interpretation may be complicated by the presence of adenosquamous nests that occur where the ductal epithelium interacts with that of the epidermis.

Cytologically, the described appearance is that of considerable cellularity with a profusion of epithelial cells presenting singly and in clusters. Uniform nuclei contain finely distributed chromatin and inconspicuous nucleoli. Some variation in nuclear size and occasional hyperchromatic nuclei should not exclude the diagnosis but clearly there should be no overtly suspicious feature. Small amounts of cellular debris, inflammatory cells and siderophages are also possible. The differentiation from Paget's disease of the nipple with an underlying carcinoma in or associated with the lactiferous ducts should not be a problem.

Clinical and cytological findings

- ► The location is clearly important
- ► Moderate or high cellularity with a basic benign pattern
- ► Dispersed epithelial cells and small groups
- ► Little anisonucleosis, the uniform nuclei showing finely distributed chromatin and small nucleoli
- ► Occasional hyperchromatic nuclei possible
- ► Adenosquamous nests may be apparent
- ► Small amount of debris, inflammatory cells and siderophages may be a feature

Diagnostic pitfalls

▶ Clinically, may be mistaken for Paget's disease of the nipple
▶ Low-grade carcinoma may be difficult to exclude except by local excision, which is in any case appropriate

Adenosis tumour[92] and duct adenoma[93,94]

Adenosis tumour is the term applied to a clinically palpable mass, which histologically is composed of confluent areas of sclerosing adenosis. These lesions are quite uncommon but occur over a wide age range (22–68 with a mean of 40 years). The histology of this lesion has been described by Nielsson[92]. There is hyperplasia of both epithelial and myoepithelial cells with distortion of the lobular structure. The average diameter of the adenosis tumour in this study was 13 mm with a range of 6–23 mm.

Clinically and histologically, there is a risk of misdiagnosis of carcinoma. Cytology therefore has a useful role in preventing such an error at an early stage in the assessment, but cannot be expected to provide a specific diagnosis as the appearances closely resemble benign hyperplastic breast disease of other types. It has been suggested however that cytology is less likely than frozen section to provide a false positive diagnosis[95]. Aspirates show a biphasic pattern of groups of uniform epithelial cells and many elongated bipolar cell nuclei (Figs 8.28, 8.29).

Clinical and cytological findings

▶ Mainly presents in premenopausal women
▶ Moderate to high cellularity
▶ Small groups of uniform epithelial cells and myoepithelial cells
▶ The relationship of sclerosing stroma and microacinar epithelium may be preserved

Diagnostic pitfalls

▶ Clinically may resemble carcinoma

Duct papilloma[66,85] (Figs 8.30, 8.31)

The clinical presentation of duct papilloma of the breast is variable, nipple discharge sometimes being the main symptom, and a palpable mass in other cases. The mean age of presentation is 48, but the lesion can present commonly in the 6th and 7th decades. Smaller lesions may be impalpable but can still produce a bloody discharge appearing from one duct on the nipple. This may direct examination to a particular breast segment where careful palpation may reveal a target for FNA cytology. Benign papillomatous lesions rarely exceed 30 mm in diameter and are usually soft and friable which explains their tendency not to present as a mass. Firmer examples usually transpire to be sclerotic or are intracystic, a feature that becomes rapidly apparent on aspiration. Even where not obviously intracystic, the aspirate is frequently watery and blood-stained.

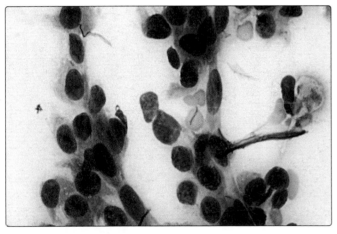

Fig. 8.28 Adenosis tumour. This field illustrates the intimate blend of elongate bipolar ells and epithelial cells that typified this lesion. (MGG)

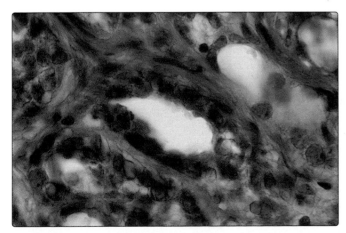

Fig. 8.29 Adenosis tumour. This field illustrates the histological concomitant of the stromal and epithelial cells seen in **Fig. 8.28**. (H&E section)

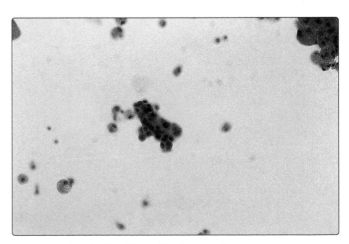

Fig. 8.30 Intraduct papilloma. Nipple smear showing foamy macrophages with a papillary group of epithelial cells. (H&E)

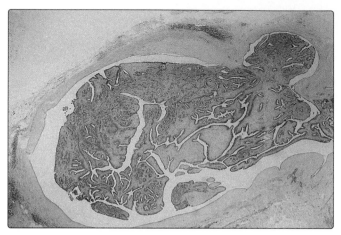

Fig. 8.31   Histology of intraduct papilloma. (H&E)

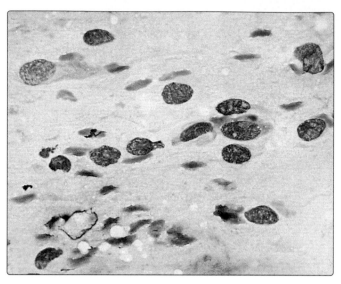

Fig. 8.32   Nodular fasciitis. Moderate numbers of plump spindle cells with scant basophilic cytoplasm but rather plump nuclei were set in a background of amorphous amphophilic material seen at the lower border. (MGG)

The initial cytological assessment may engender anxiety because of variable cellularity, poor cohesion of the epithelial cells and small cell groups. The fact that the aspirate is likely to have come from a woman in the peak age range for carcinoma may heighten suspicion.

Attention to the larger groups may give an impression of a papillary structure and occasional bipolar cells may be found in the background. Apocrine cells are a frequent feature and macrophages are commonly seen. The histological differentiation of a benign papilloma and a well-differentiated papillary carcinoma can be extremely difficult and so not surprisingly the differentiation may be impossible cytologically. With a typical clinical presentation and the above cytological findings, a report suggesting a papillary lesion of uncertain nature requiring excision and histopathological examination is entirely appropriate. Examination of the nipple discharge by gently dabbing it on to a slide, fixing and staining it, is usually helpful. The smear shows blood, abundant foamy macrophages, haemosiderin-laden macrophages and papillary clusters of ductal cells, sometimes accompanied by apocrine cells.

Clinical and cytological findings

▶ Often presents with nipple discharge and the mass identified only after careful palpation
▶ Usually soft on palpation
▶ Variable cellularity with a basic benign pattern
▶ The epithelial cells are often dispersed or in small groups but papillary clusters may be preserved leading to an atypical (C3) result
▶ Small numbers of bipolar cells
▶ Apocrine cells may be present
▶ A small amount of debris and macrophages may be present

Diagnostic pitfalls

▶ Differentiation from a well-differentiated papillary carcinoma may be impossible

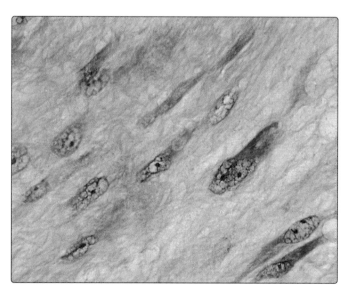

Fig. 8.33   Nodular fasciitis, histology. (H&E)

Benign connective tissue lesions

Benign neoplastic connective tissue lesions also make rare appearances in FNA of breast.

Lipoma[66,85]

The diagnosis of lipoma on FNA cytology depends on the clinical correlation with a soft (usually subcutaneous) lump and an aspirate of mature adipose tissue. Without relevant clinical information the aspirate will be reported as inadequate (C1), rather than benign (C2).

Nodular fasciitis[95,96] (Figs 8.32, 8.33)

This usually occurs in young subjects and is more likely to occupy the subcutaneous plane rather than presenting as a deep mass within the breast. The lesion usually comes to the patient's attention because of localized pain but may present as a mass of up to 20–30 mm. Cytologically, the presence of moderately large numbers of active looking spindle cells may cause anxiety. Knowledge of this possibility is the best protection against overdiagnosis of this entirely benign and probably reactive process.

Clinical and cytological findings

► The clinical presentation is helpful. The patient tends to be young and reports a suddenly appearing tender lump that on examination may appear to be in the deep subcutis rather than the breast tissue itself
► A moderately cellular aspirate may be obtained
► The cells are dispersed in a finely granular amphophilic background. Most are single but occasional small groups of two or three cells are seen
► All the cells have a pronounced spindle shaped-nucleus. Some have no cytoplasm but many are obvious spindle cells with moderately abundant basophilic cytoplasm
► The nuclei are large but uniform with no bizarre forms. Each nucleus has one fairly or very prominent nucleolus and the chromatin has a coarse texture, although is evenly distributed

Diagnostic pitfalls

► As with histological assessment, the main danger is misdiagnosis of a sarcomatous condition. Familiarity with the clinical features of the case minimizes this risk.

Granular cell tumour[97,98] *(Fig. 8.34)*

Granular cell tumours can occur in the breast but are rare, presenting as a firm, painless mass. The abundant cytoplasm of the tumour cells retains its granular quality in cytological preparations. The nuclei are fairly small and round and so, a false positive diagnosis should not be made. However the cytopathologist's threshold may be erroneously raised, as these lesions can mimic scirrhous carcinoma of breast on clinical examination. Malignant granular cell tumours are even more rare but do occur.

Mammary hamartoma or choristoma[99–102]

The histological features of these uncommon lesions are well described, consisting of varying amounts of breast parenchyma and adipose tissue. Cytologically this lesion cannot be reliably distinguished from normal breast tissue or a fibroadenoma.

Gynaecomastia and other benign conditions of the male breast[66,85]

Gynaecomastia is the enlargement of the male breast due to hypertrophy and hyperplasia of both the glandular and stromal components. When arising before the age of 25 it is almost invariably due to pubertal hormonal changes and commonly reverses spontaneously. In later life, the possibility of drug therapy (cimetidine, spironolactone,

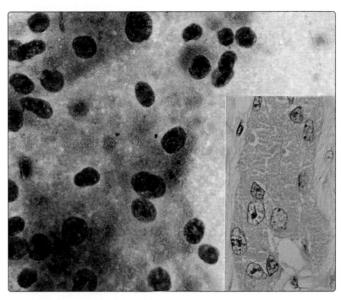

Fig. 8.34   Granular cell tumour. This smear was obtained from a woman presenting with a mass deep within the breast, simulating carcinoma. The appearance was of a cellular smear comprised of cells with poorly defined cytoplasm with a distinctly granular texture. The nuclei showed a fairly marked degree of variation in size and the nucleoli were very prominent. Histologically, this proved to be a malignant granular cell tumour. The appearances of a benign lesion are similar but with rather less nuclear pleomorphism. The inset illustrates the H&E histological appearances of this case. (MGG)

stilboestrol, digitalis, etc.) should be excluded. Other causes include hormone producing tumours (germ cell tumours, interstitial cell tumours of the testis, bronchogenic carcinoma, etc.) and cirrhosis of the liver with resulting failure to metabolize endogenous oestrogen.

Although gynaecomastia may be unilateral, clinical differentiation from carcinoma can occasionally be made with some confidence, as the mass is usually symmetrical and deep to the nipple, whereas carcinoma is more commonly eccentrically placed. Nonetheless, there is a definite role for FNA cytology. The superficial nature of the mass in gynaecomastia generally makes sampling easy but it should be noted that the procedure is particularly painful in the male breast and so good technique is important. Usually the cytological features are obviously benign resembling closely those of benign fibrocystic change or fibroadenoma.

When the condition is florid or in the cellular phase, worrying cytological features may be present and in one series of 24 aspirates of male breast there were several false positive diagnoses[103]. An immunohistochemical approach has been suggested to differentiate gynaecomastia from carcinoma in difficult cases[104].

Clinical and cytological findings

► Usually bilateral but may be unilateral and symmetrically placed in relation to the nipple

► Moderately cellular smears
► Bimodal benign appearance with small to medium sized epithelial fragments and small to moderate numbers of bipolar cells

Diagnostic pitfalls

► The epithelium may appear spuriously atypical
► Low-grade carcinomas of the male breast do occur and may trap the unwary

Fibrocystic change may rarely occur in the male breast[105] as can mammary duct ectasia, sclerosing adenosis, nipple adenoma, intraduct papilloma, neurofibroma and haemangiopericytoma. Myofibroblastoma of the male breast has also been documented[106]. The cytological features described included monomorphic spindle cells with ovoid grooved nuclei, isolated or in clusters with an ill-defined short fascicular pattern. The background contained abundant acellular myxoid appearing material.

Aspiration cytology of the breast in pregnancy

Cytology has an important role in the care of pregnant or nursing women with breast lumps[107]. These lesions are usually benign. In a series of 1612 fine needle aspirates of breast, 25 were identified to be from pregnancy-related masses[108]. Only two cases proved to be malignant. However, carcinomas occurring in pregnancy display notoriously aggressive behaviour with relatively late presentation[109]. Carcinoma of the breast is second only to carcinoma of the cervix as the commonest newly presenting malignancy in pregnancy[110].

The development of a mass during pregnancy may be due to uneven response to hormonal stimulation or enlargement of a pre-existing lesion such as a fibroadenoma. Other masses, such as lactating adenoma and galactocele arise *de novo* in pregnancy. Most galactoceles are so characteristic clinically that no further investigation is undertaken and the majority resolve spontaneously. The commonest cause of a mass during lactation is the development of an abscess. The accompanying pain and erythema usually make the diagnosis obvious but anxiety over the possibility of an inflammatory carcinoma may lead to a request for a FNA cytology diagnosis.

During the 6th to 20th weeks of pregnancy the breast undergoes intensive growth[111]. At the cellular level there is enlargement of both the nuclei and the cytoplasm of duct and lobular epithelial cells. This growth slows dramatically in the third trimester when secretory changes become more prominent. During lactation the secretory cells become smaller and flattened with vacuolation of their cytoplasm. Following the cessation of lactation the breast undergoes an involutionary process over several months, until the terminal duct lobular units return to their resting state.

Changes in steroid receptors, detected by immunohistochemistry have also been noted over the same interval. These changes have been interpreted as representing a prolonged refractory interval to hormonal stimuli and have been cited to help explain the protective effects of early pregnancy against the subsequent development of breast cancer[111]. The potential for prolonged and irregular involution of the breast tissue following pregnancy is of practical diagnostic importance to the cytopathologist.

It is important for the cytopathologist to be informed about pregnancy or lactation when the aspirate is performed by others, to lessen the likelihood of interpretive errors.

Pregnancy related changes

Aspirates taken from fibroadenomas in pregnant or lactating breasts are frequently very cellular and appear quite different from those from resting breasts (Figs 8.35, 8.36).

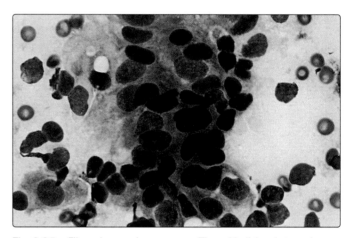

Fig. 8.35 Fibroadenoma in pregnancy. The epithelial and stromal component of a fibroadenoma can appear quite atypical during pregnancy. Recognition of the biphasic cellular components will avoid this error. (MGG)

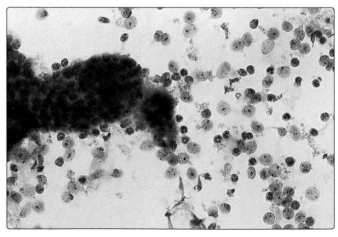

Fig. 8.36 Fibroadenoma in pregnancy. Note the abundant 'active-looking' bipolar nuclei with prominent nucleoli. (Papanicolaou)

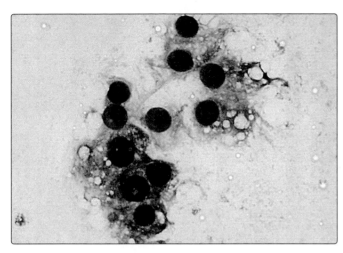

Fig. 8.37 Lactating breast. The typical appearances of lactating breast epithelium. Note the marked vacuolation of the cytoplasm, the active nuclei with prominent nucleoli and the rather 'dirty' background. (MGG)

Acinar cells have abundant granular or vacuolated cytoplasm that is unusually fragile, frequently stripping away, leaving naked nuclei in a granular 'dirty' background (Fig. 8.37). The nuclei are large and round with active vesicular chromatin and a distinct but small nucleolus. As bipolar cells are infrequent and the active epithelial cells poorly cohesive, a spuriously malignant appearance may be noted. However, the presence of lipid-laden secretory material in the background is a helpful feature.

Clinical and cytological findings

▶ An awareness that the patient is pregnant or a nursing mother is obviously important
▶ Clinical data on whether the lump arose in pregnancy or because of enlargement of a pre-existing abnormality may be helpful
▶ The aspirate may be moderately or markedly cellular
▶ The cells are single and well dispersed in a lipid rich foamy or granular background
▶ The cells are large with abundant cytoplasm that is vacuolated or wispy. Bare nuclei are common
▶ The nuclei are noticeably round and uniform with active granular or vesicular, but evenly distributed chromatin. Single prominent nucleoli are noted

Diagnostic pitfalls

▶ The main risk is that the low-power impression of a cellular aspirate of single, large cells is taken as evidence of malignancy when the pathologist is not aware of the pregnant or lactational state of the patient
▶ The distinctive granular background and critical assessment of the nuclear features should prevent this error

Lactating adenoma[112–114]
Lactating adenoma, contrary to what the name might suggest, more commonly occurs during rather than after pregnancy. Its origin is controversial, but most authorities regard it as a fibroadenoma or tubular adenoma modified by the hormonal influences of pregnancy. Aspirates show moderate numbers of cells singly or in groups, including intact lobules and acini. Most cells however are dispersed. There is a characteristic granular or foamy background. The cells show obvious cytoplasmic vacuolation and have large round or ovoid nuclei with a smooth nuclear membrane and fine chromatin with a prominent nucleolus. The appearances are thus similar to those of the pregnancy-related changes. Cytometric analysis reveals no statistically significant difference between the mean nuclear areas of lactating adenoma cells and those of well-differentiated ductal or lobular carcinoma. There is therefore the risk that these lesions will result in a false positive diagnosis.

Clinical and cytological findings

▶ Present in pregnancy rather than puerperium
▶ Moderately cellular aspirates composed of dispersed cells singly or in small groups in a foamy background
▶ The cytoplasm is vacuolated or wispy and stripped epithelial nuclei may be present
▶ The nuclei are uniform and show fine, stippled chromatin and a prominent nucleolus

Diagnositc pitfalls

▶ As for pregnancy related changes

Galactocele[115]
Galactoceles are often easily diagnosed clinically without need for further investigation. However occasionally a galactocele can accumulate abundant inspissated milk to form a large mass, even up to 80 mm in diameter, and this can be clinically worrying. It generally arises shortly after pregnancy, during lactation. The diagnosis may be readily made from the history, confirmed by the aspiration of milk, a procedure both diagnostic and therapeutic. The smears show abundant secretory material with scattered foamy macrophages. Epithelial cells are rarely seen. In the light of the clinical details the diagnosis should be benign, not inadequate.

Clinical and cytological findings

▶ Often occurs during lactation
▶ The aspirated material is composed of milk
▶ The smear shows secretory material and foamy macrophages

Diagnostic pitfalls

▶ The diagnosis should seldom cause a problem

Milk granuloma[116]

Milk granuloma is thought to arise when milk leaks into the mammary stroma. The histological appearance has been only recently (2000) reported and aspirates are likely to have an inflammatory appearance.

Carcinoma in pregnancy

Carcinoma arising in pregnancy is not cytologically distinct, but often tends to be of a high grade[109].

References

1   El Beed N A. Fat necrosis of the breast: an unusual complication of lumpectomy and radiotherapy in breast cancer. Review of literature and report of four new cases. *Eur J Surg Oncol* 1990; **16**(3): 248–250

2   Boyages J, Bilous M, Barraclough B, Langlands A O. Fat necrosis of the breast following lumpectomy and radiation therapy for early breast cancer. *Radiother Oncol* 1988; **13**(1): 69–74

3   Serin D, Martin P, Reboul F *et al*. Localized spontaneous fat necrosis of the breast. *J Gynecol Obstet Biol Reprod* 1985; **14**(2): 205–207

4   Clarke D, Curtis J L, Martinez A *et al*. Fat necrosis of the breast simulating recurrent carcinoma after primary radiotherapy in the management of early stage breast carcinoma. *Cancer* 1983; **52**(3): 442–445

5   Stefanik D E, Brereton H D, Lee T C *et al*. Fat necrosis following breast irradiation for carcinoma: clinical presentation and diagnosis. *Breast* 1982; **8**(4): 4–6

6   Sonobe H, Sato Y, Suzuki Y *et al*. Bilateral fat necrosis of the breast: report of a case. *Acta Med Okahama* 1980; **34**(5): 345–347

7   Dixon J M, Anderson T J, Lumsden A B *et al*. Mammary duct ectasia. *Br J Surg* 1983; **70**(10): 601–603

8   Fletcher A, Magrath I M, Riddell R H, Talbot I C. Granulomatous mastitis: a report of seven cases. *J Clin Pathol* 1982; **35**: 941–945

9   Going J J, Anderson T J, Wilkinson S, Chetty U. Granulomatous lobular mastitis. *J Clin Pathol* 1987; **40**: 535–540

10   Macansh S, Greenberg M, Barraclough B, Pacey F. Fine needle aspiration cytology of granulomatous mastitis. *Acta Cytol* 1990; **34**: 49–42

11   Banik S, Bishop P W, Ormerod L P, O'Brien T E B. Sarcoidosis of the breast. *J Clin Pathol* 1986; **39**: 446–448

12   Gansler T S, Wheeler J E. Mammary sarcoidosis. *Arch Pathol Lab Med* 1984; **108**: 673–675

13   Brown L A, Coghill S B. Fine needle aspiration for the diagnosis and management of granulomatous disease. *Cytopathol* 1992; **3**: 9–15

14   Arnaout A H, Shousha S, Metaxas N, Husain O A N. Intramammary tuberculous lymphadenitis. *Histopathol* 1990; 91–93

15   Pinto M M, Longstreth G, Khoury G. Fine needle aspiration of Actinomyces infection of the breast. *Acta Cytol* 1991; **35**: 409–411

16   Cooper N E. Rheumatoid nodule in the breast. *Histopathol* 1991; **19**: 193 194

17   Wargotz E S, Lefowitz M. Granulomatous angiopanniculitis of the breast. *Hum Pathol* 1989; **20**: 1084–1088

18   Coyne J, Haboubi N Y. Microinvasive breast carcinoma with granulomatous stromal response. *Histopathol* 1992; **20**: 184–185

19   Oberman H A. Invasive carcinoma of the breast with granulomatous response. *Am J Clin Pathol* 1987; **88**: 718–721

20   Rajwananshi A, Bhamhani S, Das D K. Fine needle aspiration cytology diagnosis of tuberculosis. *Diagn Cytopathol* 1987; **3**: 13–16

21   Das D K, Sodhani P, Kashyap V *et al*. Inflammatory lesions of the breast: diagnosis by fine needle aspiration. *Cytopathol* 1992; **3**: 281–289

22   Galblum L I, Oertel Y C. Subareolar abscess of the breast: diagnosis by fine needle aspiration. *Am J Clin Pathol* 1983: **80**(4): 496–499

23   Silverman J F, Lannin D R, Unverferth M, Norris H T. Fine needle aspiration cytology of subareolar abscess of the breast: spectrum of cytomorphologic findings and potential diagnostic pitfalls. *Acta Cytol* 1986; **30**(4): 413–419

24   Lammie G A, Bobrow L G, Staunton M D M *et al*. Sclerosing lymphocytic lobulitis of the breast – evidence for an autoimmune pathogenesis. *Histopathol* 1991; **19**: 13–20

25   Mills S E. Lymphocytic mastopathy: a 'new' autoimmune disease? *Am J Clin Pathol* 1990; **93**: 834–835

26   Morgan M C, Weaver M G, Ceowe J P, Abdul-Karin FW. Diabetic mastopathy: a clinicopathologic study in palpable and nonpalpable breast lesions. *Mod Pathol* 1995; **8**: 349–354

27   Miralles T G, Gosalbez F, Menendez P *et al*. FNA of sclerosing lymphocytic lobulitis. *Acta Cytol* 1998; **42**: 1447–1450

28   Silverman J F *et al*. Localized primary (AL) amyloid tumour of the breast. *Am J Surg Pathol* 1986; **10**(8): 539–545

29   Vuong P. Fine needle aspiration cytology of subcutaneous cysticercosis of the breast. *Acta Cytol* 1989; **33**: 659–662

30   Shabb N, Sneige N, Dekmezian R H. Myospherulosis. Fine needle aspiration cytologic findings in 19 cases. *Acta Cytol* 1991; **35**: 225–228

31   Ferrell L D. Myospherulosis of the breast. Diagnosis by fine needle aspiration. *Acta Cytol* 1984; **28**(6): 726–728

32   Tabatowski K, Elson C E, Johnston W W. Silicone lymphadenopathy in a patient with a mammary prosthesis. *Acta Cytol* 1990; **34**: 10–14

33   Ciatto S, Cariaggi P, Bulgaresi P. The value of routine cytologic examination of breast cyst fluids. *Acta Cytol* 1987; **31**: 301–304

34   Ciatto S, Bravetti P, Cariaggi P. Significance of nipple discharge clinical patterns in the selection of cases for cytologic examination. *Acta Cytol* 1986; **30**: 17–20

35   Love S M, Gelman R S, Silen W. Fibrocystic 'disease' of the breast – a non disease? *N Engl J Med* 1982; **307**(16): 1010–1014

36   Vorherr H. Fibrocystic breast disease: pathophysiology, pathomorphology, clinical picture, and management. *Am J Obstet Gynaecol* 1986; **154**(1): 161–179

37   Berkowitz G S, Kelsey J L, LiVolsi V A *et al*. Risk factors for fibrocystic breast disease and its histopathologic components. *J Natl Cancer Inst* 1985; **75**(1): 43–50

38   Pastides H, Kelsey J L, Holford T R, LiVolsi V A. An epidemiologic study of fibrocystic breast disease with reference to ductal epithelial atypia. *Am J Epidemiol* 1985; **121**(3): 440–447

39   Rivera Pomar J M, Vilanova J R, Burgos Bretones J J. Arocena-G. Focal fibrous disease of breast. A common entity in young women. *Virchows Arch* 1980; **386**(1): 59–64

40   Gump F E, McDermott J. Fibrous disease of the breast in juvenile diabetes. *NY J Med* 1990; **90**(7): 356–357

41   Westinghouse Logan W, Hoffman N Y. Diabetic fibrous breast disease. *Radiol* 1989; **172**(3): 667–670

42   Garstin W I, Kaufman Z, Michell M J, Baum M. Fibrous mastopathy in insulin dependent diabetics. *Clin Radiol* 1991; **44**: 89–91

43   Rollins S D. FNA cytology of diabetic fibrous mastopathy. *Diagn Cytopathol* 1993; **9**: 687–690

44   Khan S A, Masood S, Miller L, Numann P J. Random FNA of the breast of women at increased breast cancer risk and standard risk controls. *Breast J* 1998; **4**: 420–425

45   Ellis I O, Pinder S E. FNA cytology of the breast: refining the diagnosis (editorial). *Cytopathol* 1998; **9**: 289–290

46   Masood S, Frykberg E R, McCellan G L *et al*. Cytologic differentiation between proliferative and nonproliferative breast disease in mammographically guided FNAs. *Diagn Cytopathol* 1991; **7**: 581–590

47   Stanley M W, Henry-Stanley M J, Zera R. Atypia in breast FNA smears correlates poorly with the presence of a prognostically significant proliferative lesion of ductal epithelium. *Hum Pathol* 1993; **24**: 630–635

48   Wells C A, Wells C W, Yeomans P *et al*. Spherical connective tissue inclusions in

epithelial hyperplasia of the breast ('collagenous spherulosis'). *J Clin Pathol* 1990; **43**: 905–908

49 Tyler X, Coghill S B. Fine needle aspiration cytology of collagenous spherulosis of the breast. *Cytopathol* 1991; **2**: 159–162

50 Eliasen C A, Cranor M L, Rosen P P. Atypical duct hyperplasia of the breast in young females. *Am J Surg Pathol* 1992; **16**(3): 246–251

51 Tavassoli F A, Norris H J. A comparison of the results of long-term follow-up for atypical intraductal hyperplasia and intraductal hyperplasia of the breast. *Cancer* 1990; **65**(3): 518–529

52 London S J, Connolly J L, Schnitt S J, Colditz G A. A prospective study of benign breast disease and the risk of breast cancer. *JAMA* 1992; **267**: 941–947

53 Bodian C A, Perzin K H, Lattes R *et al*. Prognostic significance of benign proliferative breast disease. *Cancer* 1993; **71**: 3896–3907

54 Schnitt S J, Connolly J L, Tavassoli F A *et al*. Interobserver reproducibility in the diagnosis of ductal proliferative lesions using standardized criteria. *Am J Surg Pathol* 1992; **16**: 1133–1139

55 Dupont W D, Page D L. Relative risk of breast cancer varies with time since diagnosis of atypical hyperplasia. *Hum Pathol* 1989; **20**(8): 723–725

56 Norris H J, Bahr G F, Mikel U V A. Comparative morphometric and cytophotometric study of intraductal hyperplasia and intraductal carcinoma of the breast. *Anal Quant Cytol Histol* 1988; **10**(1): 1–9

57 Page D L, Dupont W D, Rogers L W. Ductal involvement by cells of atypical lobular hyperplasia in the breast: a long-term follow-up study of cancer risk. *Hum Pathol* 1988; **19**(2): 201–207

58 Page D L, Dupont W D, Rogers L W, Rados M S. Atypical hyperplastic lesions of the female breast. A longterm follow up study. *Cancer* 1985; **55**: 2698–2708

59 Peterse J L, Koolman-Schellekens M A. Atypia in fine needle aspiration cytology of the breast: a histologic follow-up study of 301 cases. *Semin Diagn Pathol* 1989; **6**: 126–134

60 Moinfar F, Denk H. Mammary intraepithelial neoplasia: a logical concept? *Breast J* 1998; **4**: 287–288

61 Barsky S H, Bose S. Should LCIS be regarded as a heterogenous disease? *Breast J* 1999; **5**: 407–412

62 Marshall L M, Hunter D J, Connolly J L *et al*. Risk of breast cancer associated with atypical hyperplasia of lobular and ductal types. *Cancer Epidemiol Biomarkers Prev* 1997; **6**: 297–301

63 Page D L, Steel C M, Dixon J M. ABC of breast diseases: management of carcinoma in-situ and patients at high risk of subsequent breast cancer. *BMJ* 1995; **310**: 39–42

64 Dixon J M, Page D L. Ductal carcinoma in-situ of the breast. *Breast* 1998; **7**: 239–242

65 Abendroth C S, Wang H H, Ducatman B S. Comparative features of carcinoma *in situ* and atypical ductal hyperplasia of the breast on fine needle aspiration biopsy specimens. *Am J Clin Pathol* 1991; **96**: 654–659

66 Jensen R, Page D L. Epithelial hyperplasia. In: Elston CW, Ellis IO eds. 'The Breast' *Systemic Pathology*, 3rd edn, vol. 13, Edinburgh: Churchill Livingstone 1998; 65–90

67 Bunker J P, Houghton J, Baum M. Putting the risk of breast cancer in perspective. *BMJ* 1998; **317**: 1307–1309

68 Haybittle J. Women's risk of dying of heart disease is always greater than their risk of dying of breast cancer (letter). *BMJ* 1999; **318**: 539

69 Rosai J. Borderline epithelial lesions of the breast. *Am J Surg Pathol* 1991; **15**: 209–221

70 Bottles K, Chan J S, Holly E A *et al*. Cytologic criteria for fibroadenoma. *Am J Clin Pathol* 1988; **89**: 707–713

71 Walters T K, Zuckerman J, Nisbet-Smith A *et al*. Fine needle aspiration biopsy in the diagnosis and management of fibroadenoma of the breast. *Br J Surg* 1990; **77**: 1215–1217

72 Sousha S. Squamous metaplasia in fibroadenomas of the breast. *Histopathol* 1986; **10**: 1001–1002

73 Gupta R K, Dowle C. Fine needle aspiration of breast carcinoma in a fibroadenoma. *Cytopathol* 1992; **3**: 49–53

74 Diaz N M, Palmer J O, McDivitt R W. Carcinoma arising within fibroadenomas of the breast; a clinicopathologic study of 105 cases. *Am J Clin Pathol* 1991; **95**: 614–622

75 Buzanowski-Konarky K, Harrison E G Jr, Payne W S. Lobular carcinoma arising in fibroadenoma of the breast. *Cancer* 1975; **35**: 450–456

76 Simi U, Moretti D, Iacconi P *et al*. Fine needle aspiration cytopathology of phyllodes tumour. Differential diagnosis with fibroadenoma. *Acta Cytol* 1988; **31**(1): 63–66

77 Grimes M M. Cystosarcoma phyllodes of the breast: histologic features, flow cytometric analyses and clinical considerations. *Mod Pathol* 1992; **5**: 232–238

78 Dusenbery D, Frable W J. Fine needle aspiration cytology of phyllodes tumor: potential diagnostic pitfalls. *Acta Cytol* 1992; **36**(2): 215–221

79 Rama-Rao C, Narasimhamurthy N K, Jaganathan K *et al*. Cystosarcoma phyllodes: Diagnosis by fine needle aspiration cytology. *Acta Cytol* 1992; **36**(2): 203–207

80 Deen S A, McKee G T, Kissin M W. Differential cytologic features of fibroepithelial lesions of the breast. *Diagn Cytopathol* 1999; **20**: 53–56

81 Agarwal J, Kapila K, Verma K. Phyllodes tumor with keratin cysts: a diagnostic problem in fine needle aspiration of the breast. *Acta Cytol* 1991; **35**(2): 255–256

82 Evans A T, Hussein A H. A microglandular adenosis-like lesion simulating tubular adenocarcinoma of the breast. A case report with cytological and histological appearances. *Cytopathol* 1990; **1**: 311–316

83 Clement P B, Azzopardi J G. Microglandular adenosis of the breast – a lesion simulating tubular carcinoma. *Histopathol* 1983; **7**: 169–180

84 McDivitt R, Bell D A, Greco M A. Tumours of the breast. In: *Atlas of Tumour Pathology*, Washington DC: Armed Forces Institute of Pathology, 2nd series, Fasicle 2, 1968

85 Page D L, Anderson T J. *Diagnostic Histopathology of the Breast*. Edinburgh: Churchill Livingstone, 1987

86 Nielsen M, Jensen J, Anderson J A. An autopsy study of radial scar in the female breast. *Histopathol* 1985; **9**: 287–295

87 Wellings S R, Alpers C E. Subgross pathologic features and incidence of radial scars in the breast. *Hum Pathol* 1984; **15**: 475–479

88 Battersby S, Anderson T J. Myofibroblast activity of radial scars. *J Pathol* 1985; **147**: 33–40

89 Anderson T J, Battersby S. Radial scars of benign and malignant breasts: comparative features and significance. *J Pathol* 1985; **147**: 23–32

90 Jacobs T W, Byrne C, Colditz G *et al*. Radial scars in benign breast biopsy specimens and the risk of breast cancer. *N Engl J Med* 1999; **340**: 430–436

91 Rosen P P, Caicco J A. Florid papillomatosis of the nipple. A study of 51 patients, including nine with mammary carcinoma. *Am J Surg Path* 1986; **10**: 87–101

92 Nielsen B B. Adenosis tumour of the breast – a clinicopathological investigation of 27 cases. *Histopathol* 1987; **11**: 1259–1275

93 Azzopardi J G, Salm R. Ductal adenoma of the breast: a lesion which can mimic carcinoma. *J Pathol* 1984; **144**: 15–23

94 Gusterson B A, Sloane J P, Middwood C *et al*. Ductal adenoma of the breast – a lesion exhibiting a myoepithelial/epithelial phenotype. *Histopathol* 1987; **11**: 103–110

95 Silverman J F, Dabbs D J, Gilbert C F. Fine needle aspiration cytology of adenosis tumour of the breast. *Acta Cytol* 1989; **33**: 181–187

96 Dahl I, Akerman M. Nodular fasciitis. A correlative, cytologic and histologic study of 13 cases. *Acta Cytol* 1981; **25**: 215–222

97 Lowhagen T, Rubio C A. The cytology of the granular cell myoblastoma of the breast. *Acta Cytol* 1977; **21**: 314–315

98 Gibbons D, Leitch M, Coscia J *et al*. FNA cytology and histologic findings of granular cell tumor of the breast: review of 19 cases with clinical/radiologic correlation. *Breast J* 2000; **6**: 27–30

99 Fisher C J, Hanby A M, Robinson L, Millis R R. Mammary hamartoma – a review of 35 cases. *Histopathol* 1992; **20**: 99–106

100 Norris M W, Jones H J, Wargotz E S. Hamartomas of the breast. *Surg Gynecol Obstet* 1991; **173**: 54–62

101 Daroca P J, Reed R J, Love G L, Kraus S D. Myoid hamartomas of the breast. *Hum Pathol* 1985; **16**: 212–219

102 Metcalfe J S, Ellis B. Choristoma of the breast. *Hum Pathol* 1985; **16**: 739–740

103 Russin V L, Lachowicz C, Kline T S. Male breast lesions: gynaecomastia and its distinction from carcinoma by aspiration biopsy cytology. *Diagn Cytopathol* 1989; **5**: 243–247

104 Mottolese M, Bigotti G, Coli A *et al*. Potential use of monoclonal antibodies in the diagnostic distinction of gynaecomastia from breast carcinoma in men. *Am J Clin Pathol* 1991; **96**(2): 233–237

105 Joshi A. FNA cytology in the management of male breast masses: nineteen years of experience. *Acta Cytol* 1999; **43**: 334–338

106 Ordi J, Riverola A, Sole M *et al*. Fine needle aspiration of myofibroblastoma of the breast in a man: a report of two cases. *Acta Cytol* 1992; **36**: 194–198

107 Bottles K, Taylor R N. Diagnosis of breast masses in pregnant and lactating women by aspiration cytology. *Obstet Gynaecol* 1985; **66**S: 76–78

108 Novotny D B, Maygarden S J, Shermer R W, Frable W J. Fine needle aspiration of benign and malignant breast masses associated with pregnancy. *Acta Cytol* 1991; **35**: 676–686

109 Gemignani M L, Petrek J A. Pregnancy-associated breast cancer: diagnosis and treatment. *Breast J* 2000; **6**: 68–73

110 Haas J F. Pregnancy in association with newly diagnosed cancer: a population based epidemiological assessment. *Int J Cancer* 1984; **34**: 229–235

111 Anderson T J. Genesis and source of breast cancer. *Brit Med Bull* 1991; **47**(2): 305–318

112 O'Hara M F, Page D L. Adenomas of the breast and ectopic breast under lactational influences. *Hum Pathol* 1985; **16**: 707–712

113 James K, Bridger J, Anthony P P. Breast tumour of pregnancy ('lactating' adenoma). *J Pathol* 1988; **156**: 37–44

114 Grenko R T, Lee K P, Lee K R. Fine needle aspiration cytology of lactating adenoma of the breast. A comparative light microscopic and morphometric study. *Acta Cytol* 1990; **34**: 21–26

115 Raso D S, Greene W B, Silverman J F. Crystallizing galactocele. A case report. *Acta Cytol* 1997; **41**: 863–870

116 Rytina E R C, Coady A T, Millis R R. Milk granuloma: an unusual appearance in lactational breast tissue. *Histopathol* 1991; 466–467

Malignant breast tumours

Alec Howat and Stuart Coghill

General criteria for malignancy

Before proceeding to discuss the cytological features that lead to a diagnosis of the various forms of breast cancer it may be helpful to review the general cytological features of malignancy in breast tissue, previously mentioned in Chapter 7. It is axiomatic that no single morphological feature can be relied upon to distinguish benign from malignant cells at any site and nowhere is this more true than in the breast. It is the complete picture, considered in the light of what is known about the clinical features of the case that leads to an accurate diagnosis.

Differentiation of benign and malignant lesions

The classical appearances of malignant breast epithelial cells are illustrated in Figures 9.1–9.3. When a case presents with these features, it is a spot diagnosis requiring little deductive thought. Those new to breast cytodiagnosis, and each of us faced with a difficult case, must approach the diagnosis by considering the following features.

Cellularity of the specimen

This is an extremely useful criterion but it must be used with caution. Many benign lesions found in younger women may provide intensely cellular aspirates and conversely, even with vigorous re-aspiration, some more scirrhous carcinomas are reluctant to give up even a few cells.

Dispersal of cells

Lack of cell-to-cell cohesion is a characteristic malignant feature. However the pressure with which the aspirate is spread has an influence on this, providing a further reason

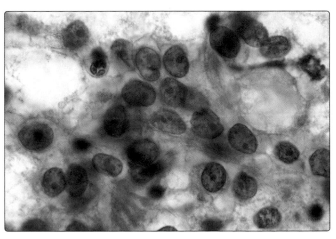

Fig. 9.2 High-grade ductal carcinoma. Notice the poor cell cohesion, pleomorphism, and prominent nucleoli. (Papanicolaou). (Courtesy of Dr G. McKee, Boston)

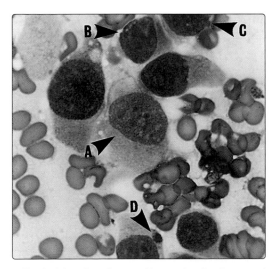

Fig. 9.1 Classical ductal carcinoma of breast showing features of malignancy. (A) coarse chromatin pattern and multiple nucleoli of variable size, with nuclear holes; (B) irregular nuclear membrane; (C) extrusion of chromatin from the surface of the nucleus; (D) extranuclear chromatin. There is also noticeable anisonucleosis and poor cell cohesion. Red cells serve as an index of size. (MGG)

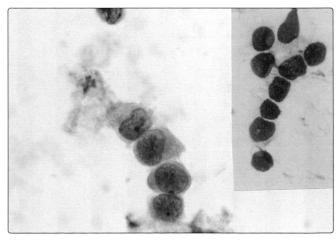

Fig. 9.3 The classical appearance of lobular carcinoma of the breast. The inset shows the corresponding MGG appearance at a lower power. (Papanicolaou)

279

to obtain one's own aspirates. Cellular discohesion is preserved in liquid based cytology (LBC) preparations.

Biphasic pattern with bipolar cells

This is the nearest criterion to an absolute indication of benignancy as shown in Chapters 7 and 8. Unfortunately there are exceptions. Some benign conditions provide few or no bipolar cells. In most of these the aspirates will be poorly cellular. Difficulties therefore arise in assessing scanty aspirates. Some carcinomatous aspirates contain a population of naked epithelial cell nuclei, some of which may be ovoid and therefore mistaken for bipolar cells. Careful attention to the quality of the chromatin and the appearance of the nucleoli should avoid this pitfall. Some malignant aspirates will be 'contaminated' with hyperplastic but benign tissue resulting in a population of bipolar cells that distract attention from the population of malignant cells.

Nuclear size and pleomorphism

A considerable proportion of breast carcinomas is low-grade when assessed histologically. These are categorized as such by the relative lack of nuclear enlargement or pleomorphism. Pathologists experienced in exfoliative cytology will recognize that when a metastatic breast carcinoma is detected in a pleural fluid, a mammary origin will be suggested when the malignant cells have relatively small and bland nuclei. Even when the nuclei in a malignant FNA of breast appear remarkably regular, a diligent search will usually reveal one or two significantly larger nuclei, and a diagnosis of carcinoma can be made.

Lobular carcinoma is even more problematic in this regard than the low-grade ductal carcinoma. The difficulties created by nuclear uniformity and the relatively small nuclear diameters are compounded by characteristically scanty aspirates.

Nucleolar size and pleomorphism

For histopathologists accustomed to haematoxylin and eosin, nucleolar size and characteristics are usually more easily observed in Papanicolaou stained cytological preparation, but May-Grünwald-Giemsa (MGG) stained smears provide just as much detail to an experienced eye. Except for apocrine metaplastic cells, it is unusual for benign epithelial cells to have prominent nucleoli. The presence of multiple large and variable nucleoli within a nucleus is particularly suspicious.

Nuclear membrane irregularity and extranuclear chromatin

These features can be very helpful in difficult cases. Malignant nuclei almost invariably show nuclear profiles in which there are small indentations or projections. Box-shaped and angular nuclei are also suspicious. Extranuclear chromatin is very much a malignant feature but tends to be seen more commonly in higher-grade carcinomas where diagnosis is not a problem.

Nuclear/cytoplasmic ratio and cytoplasmic features

This is of less help than at any other site in the body as normal breast epithelial cells can have scanty cytoplasm and carcinoma cells showing apocrine differentiation may have a great abundance. Intracytoplasmic lumina are an occasional feature of both lobular and ductal carcinoma cells but are only very rarely seen in benign breast epithelium.

Chromatin texture

This is extremely important in difficult cases. In Papanicolaou stained preparations, the appearance of a coarsely and unevenly stippled nucleus with variable but prominent chromocentres suggests malignancy. MGG stained preparations give a more subtle, but no less characteristic appearance of a coarse 'rope-like' texture that, when marked, can give the impression of small nuclear holes.

Nuclear fragility

Malignant nuclei show a greater tendency to rupture under the physical pressure of being smeared. This tendency is variable and is seldom marked in breast aspirates unless excessive pressure is used.

The relationship of nuclei to each other

Marked nuclear moulding is a feature of some breast carcinomas but in others, where there is little cell cohesion, it may be completely absent. Crowded nuclei may show moulding and overlapping but this can also be a feature of benign epithelial groups. Where robust, regular, relatively small cells with virtually no cytoplasm are seen linked in short, straight or slightly curved chains the diagnosis of lobular carcinoma should be entertained.

Mitotic figures

These are rarely seen in breast aspirates except those of high-grade ductal carcinomas. They can be a feature of benign lesions such as fibroepithelial neoplasms. Unless frequent and atypical, they should not be given a heavy diagnostic bias.

Contents of the background

Abundant necrotic material in an otherwise cellular smear is usually attributable to tumour necrosis. Comedocarcinoma and poorly differentiated papillary intracystic carcinomas aspirates can yield much necrotic debris. The presence of blood or fatty tissue should not influence the interpretation, as there is no difference in their incidence in benign and malignant aspirates.

Ductal carcinoma and variants

Different series quote varying proportions of breast carcinomas that fall into the different histological subtypes, reflecting less rigidity in the application of the criteria by some authors[1-3]. Table 9.1 shows the ranges for different subtypes.

Table 9.1   Histological subtypes of invasive breast carcinomas

Ductal of no special type	65–80%
Lobular carcinoma	5–14%
Medullary carcinoma	5–7%
Tubular carcinoma	2–8%
Mucinous carcinoma	2–4%
Papillary carcinoma	1–2%
Apocrine carcinoma	1–4%
Other rare types	<1%

Infiltrating ductal carcinoma of no special type (IDC of NST) or not otherwise specified (NOS)
(Figs 9.4–9.12)

Of all epithelial malignancies of the breast, up to 80% of breast carcinomas fall into this category[1–4]. The general features of malignancy pertain to these all too common tumours. The cellularity of the aspirate will depend on the interplay between the skill of the aspirator, the size of the lesion and the degree of desmoplasia within the lesion. Scirrhous ductal carcinomas provide the lowest cell yield of all breast lesions while high grade, poorly collagenous ductal carcinoma can provide even the novice with a very thick spread of aspirated cells. Similarly, the cellular pattern can be very variable. There can be large three-dimensional arrays of folded epithelium interspersed with smaller groups and occasional single cells. Others show a lack of cohesion that results in a virtual monolayer resembling the low power pattern of a high-grade lymphoma. Occasionally, recognizable acini are apparent but more often there is no hint of an organized relationship between the cells. Within the groups there is loss of polarity, the nuclei can appear

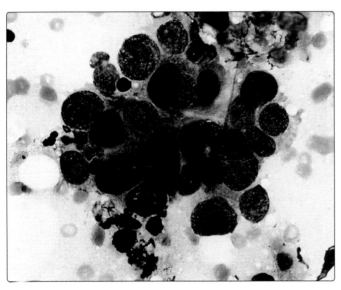

Fig. 9.4   High-grade ductal carcinoma of the breast. (MGG)

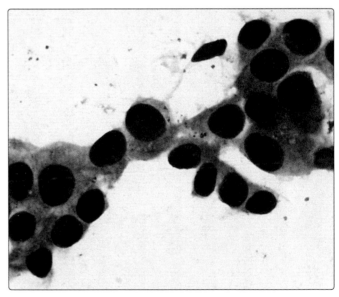

Fig. 9.6   Ductal carcinoma of breast. A typical Grade 2 carcinoma showing moderate anisonucleosis and poor cell cohesion. (MGG)

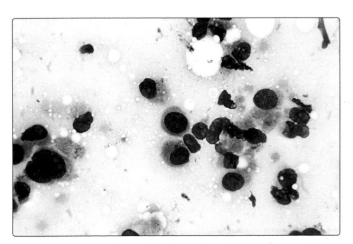

Fig. 9.5   Ductal carcinoma of the breast. Loss of cell cohesion and pleomorphism are apparent. (MGG) (Courtesy of Dr G McKee, Boston)

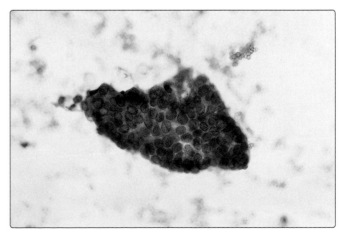

Fig. 9.7   Grade 1 ductal carcinoma with well-preserved cell cohesion but showing nuclear margin irregularities. (Papanicolaou) (Courtesy of Dr G McKee, Boston)

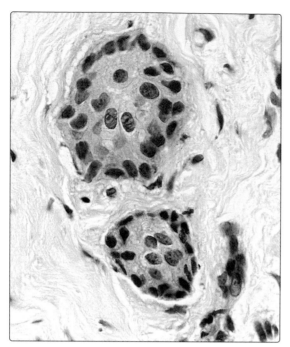

Fig. 9.8   Grade 1 ductal carcinoma. (H&E section)

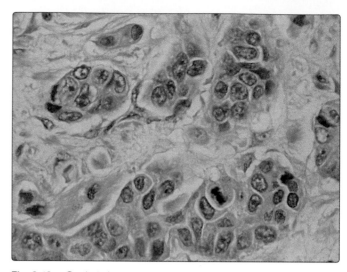

Fig. 9.10   Grade 2 ductal carcinoma. (H&E section)

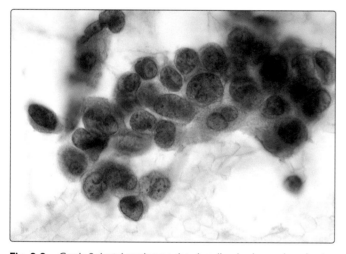

Fig. 9.9   Grade 2 ductal carcinoma showing discohesion and moderate nuclear pleomorphism. (Papanicolaou) (Courtesy of Dr G McKee, Boston)

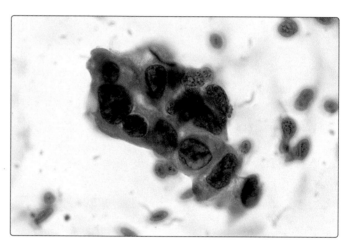

Fig. 9.11   Grade 3 ductal carcinoma. This cluster of cells shows abnormal chromatin, pleomorphism and nuclear margin irregularities but no loss of cohesion. (Papanicolaou) (Courtesy of Dr G McKee, Boston)

crowded and moulded and the general appearance may resemble a syncytium.

The prognosis for women with infiltrating breast cancer is dependent on many factors; those that confer a poorer than average prognosis include an age at presentation of less than 50 years, pregnancy, invasion of skin or nipple, lymph node spread, late diagnosis, large size, high histological grade, infiltrative margins, tumour necrosis, the presence of stromal reaction and angioinvasion[5,6]. A factor most useful in predicting a favourable prognosis is the type of carcinoma, certain types being less aggressive than others[7]. Histological grade is also important with Grade 1 tumours having a significantly better prognosis

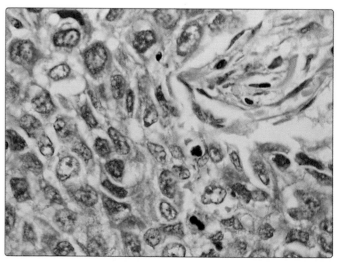

Fig. 9.12   Grade 3 ductal carcinoma. (H&E section)

than Grades 2 and 3[8]. Tumour grade, size and lymph node stage are the criteria used to calculate the 'Nottingham Prognostic Index' (NPI); this has proven robust after many years of audit and is an excellent method of predicting the prognosis for any individual case[2,9,10]. The formula used to calculate the NPI is: 0.2 × size of tumour (cm) + lymph node stage (1–3) + Grade (1–3). The prognostic categories are as follows:

2.1–3.4	Good prognosis with a 79% 15-year survival rate
>3.4–5.0	Intermediate prognosis with a 50% 15-year survival rate
>5.0	Poor prognosis with a 18% 15-year survival rate

It goes without saying that the correct treatment is one of the most important prognostic factors[11]. Large clinical trials are studying the results of chemotherapy for breast cancer[12]. Therapy can be modified depending on pathological factors such as grade[13] or the HER-2/neu (c-erbB-2) expression of the tumour[14]. Radiotherapy and surgery however remain the primary treatment modalities[11].

Non-invasive ductal carcinoma/ductal carcinoma *in situ* (DCIS) and minimally invasive carcinoma

Pure intraduct carcinoma may not produce a palpable lesion[15–17], especially with the availability of mammography for the detection of small lesions, but most pathologists have seen at least one example of a palpable lesion, sometimes quite large, that is composed purely of DCIS. Particularly since the arrival of population screening for carcinoma of the breast, the diagnosis of very early carcinomas has become a major challenge for cytologists. A 1982 report of a large series of breast lesions, initially assessed by cytology, and subsequently found to have only *in situ*, microinvasive and minimally invasive carcinoma, showed that a mere 17.4% were detected cytologically[18]. Since then, experience in sampling very small and impalpable lesions, the quality of stereotactic apparatus[19] and cytological expertise have improved considerably.

FNA cannot be relied upon to distinguish DCIS from IDC. However, recent studies have highlighted certain discriminating features: cohesive groups of epithelial cells and single malignant cells, necrosis, cribriform tissue fragments, stromal fragments with tumour cells, tubules composed of neoplastic cells, cytoplasmic lumina, fibroblast proliferation and elastoid stroma[20–22]. Some invasive tumours have a prominent intraduct component that is an adverse prognostic factor as it predisposes to local recurrence[23].

Low-grade DCIS (cribriform/micropapillary)

This, on its own, carries a good prognosis[24]. The cytological profile of such lesions is one of tumour cells that are mainly clustered in three-dimensional ductal structures in which

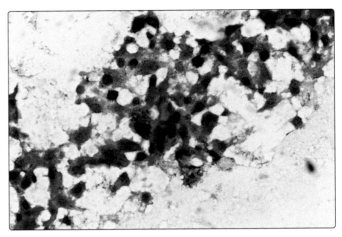

Fig. 9.13 High-grade DCIS. The mixture of obvious malignant cells intimately associated with necrotic debris is characteristic. (MGG) (Courtesy of Dr G McKee, Boston)

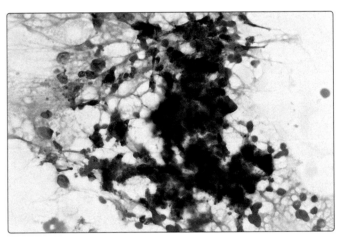

Fig. 9.14 High-grade DCIS. Note the necrotic background material and scattered, obviously malignant ductal epithelial cells. (Papanicolaou)

occasional tumour cells border on central lumina[25]. This reflects the histological cribriform architecture. A few single epithelial cells, but no myoepithelial cells, may be present. The background should be clear or haemorrhagic and without necrosis. The tumour cells are uniform and have a cylindroid shape, with round or oval nuclei showing a mean largest nuclear diameter 1.5–1.6 times that of erythrocytes. The chromatin is finely granular with some condensation along the nuclear membrane and one very small nucleolus.

High-grade DCIS (comedo/solid)

The cells are not distinguishable from those of high-grade IDC. The intimate association of malignant epithelium and necrotic debris is however characteristic (Figs 9.13–9.15). Fragments of dystrophic calcification may be seen.

Mucinous (colloid) carcinoma[26–33] *(Figs 9.16–9.18)*

Depending on the rigidity with which the diagnostic criteria are applied histologically, the incidence of colloid carcinoma

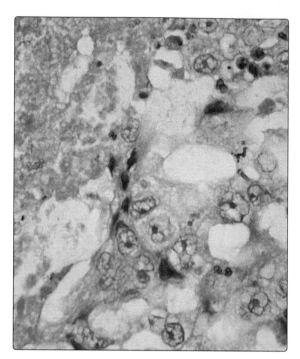

Fig. 9.15   High-grade DCIS with necrosis. (H&E section)

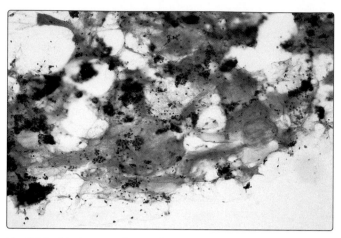

Fig. 9.17   Mucinous carcinoma. Small and fairly bland but malignant ductal epithelial cells, single and in clusters, with abundant orange background mucin. This is often less obvious than in MGG preparations. (Papanicolaou) (Courtesy of Dr G McKee, Boston)

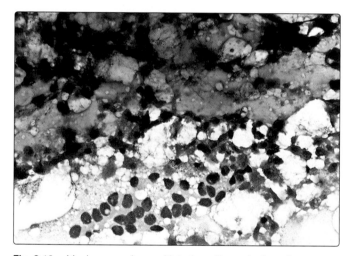

Fig. 9.16   Mucinous carcinoma. Note the uniform, single malignant epithelial cells and the abundant violet-coloured mucin. (MGG) (Courtesy of Dr G McKee, Boston)

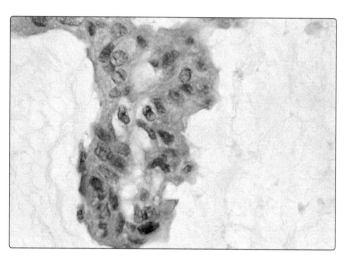

Fig. 9.18   Mucinous carcinoma. (H&E section)

is quoted to be between 1–5% of all breast carcinomas[1–3]. This is typically a tumour of older post-menopausal women occurring at an age of 60 years or more. It tends to be slow growing and has a favourable prognosis with a 5-year survival of up to 86%[2].

On examination these lesions tend to be well defined, hard and mobile. Because of the smooth outline they may be mistaken clinically and mammographically for a fibroadenoma or cyst but awareness of the typical age of presentation for each of these lesions reduces this error. Aspiration is generally easy, giving a sensation on the needle similar to or softer than that of a cellular fibroadenoma. On spreading, the aspirate is often very mucinous.

The cells tend to be in loose aggregates and small cohesive groups bathed in a mucinous background[31–33]. The single cells show eccentricity of the nucleus and little variation of nuclear size or shape when compared with IDC of NST. The chromatin tends to be bland but there may be recognizable hyperchromatism and coarsening. Nucleoli are not prominent. The mucinous nature of the background is usually more immediately obvious in MGG stained smears where the mucin is a bright crimson, than in Papanicolaou stained smears where it is usually wispy and pale grey/green in colour. With either preparation, however, a specific diagnosis is nearly always possible. The favourable prognosis of colloid carcinoma is only maintained in pure forms of the tumour. As otherwise unremarkable ductal carcinomas of any grade can occasionally contain foci of mucin-producing carcinoma, there is the potential for overdiagnosis of this entity on cytological assessment, dependent on the area sampled.

Some colloid carcinomas may be shown to contain endocrine cells histochemically but these are not apparent cytologically[34]. In otherwise typical colloid carcinomas the occasional signet ring cell can be seen. This should not be taken as evidence of a signet ring cell carcinoma, which has a much worse prognosis.

Clinical and cytological findings

- ► Usually well circumscribed on palpation and mammography
- ► The tumour is, on average, larger than IDC of NST at presentation
- ► The tumour is easily penetrated by the needle
- ► On spreading, the aspirate is quite glairy, hinting at a high mucin content
- ► The smear is usually cellular
- ► The epithelial cells present as single cells, loose aggregates and cohesive groups often three-dimensional in appearance
- ► The cells are small, with small, uniform, round nuclei, smooth nuclear outlines, bland, possibly granular, chromatin and inconspicuous nucleoli
- ► The cells are bathed in mucin of variable density. This is more obvious in MGG preparations, where it stains violet
- ► Cells may be vacuolated and occasional signet ring cells are seen
- ► Some cases contain microcalcification

Diagnostic pitfalls

- ► These tumours are so bland cytologically that they may be misdiagnosed as benign, particularly when they occur in younger women. Although biologically these are low-grade tumours, once local spread occurs, eradication can be difficult
- ► It is important to distinguish mucoid carcinoma from primary signet ring carcinoma of breast and the even rarer metastatic signet ring carcinoma of gastrointestinal origin
- ► Some ductal carcinomas of no special type can contain large foci of mucinous carcinoma

Signet ring cell carcinoma[34–37]

These rare lesions occur in a younger age group than colloid carcinomas. In contrast to colloid carcinomas they are invariably aggressive lesions attended by a high risk of metastatic spread. Although both lobular and ductal carcinomas may show cytoplasmic vacuoles in both cytological and histological preparations, lesions showing a sufficient degree to warrant a diagnosis of signet ring cell carcinoma are rare.

With cytological assessment there is a risk of misdiagnosis of mucinous (colloid) carcinoma with an underestimate of the aggressiveness of the lesion. A mistaken diagnosis of metastatic signet ring carcinoma of gastrointestinal origin leads to the assumption of an unduly gloomy prognosis. Awareness of the existence of this lesion should prevent these mishaps.

The cells are usually abundant and poorly cohesive with only small stringy groups. The cells are large with large eccentric, crescentic-shaped nuclei displaced to a marginal position by cytoplasmic mucin. There is quite marked anisonucleosis and moderate to marked hyperchromasia.

Clinical and cytological findings

- ► The clinically malignant nature is usually suspected and this aggressive tumour may present because of metastatic spread
- ► On smearing, the thick, mucinous nature of these lesions may be apparent
- ► Smears are cellular containing poorly cohesive, large malignant cells with moderate to marked anisonucleosis and hyperchromatism
- ► The cytoplasm is abundant and vacuolated
- ► The nucleus is typically crescentic and displaced to the edge of the cell

Diagnostic pitfalls

- ► The distinction from colloid carcinoma must be made
- ► The possibility of metastatic spread from a visceral signet ring carcinoma should be considered

Argyrophil carcinoma of the breast/carcinoma with endocrine features[38–42]

The existence of this entity is controversial as several types of breast carcinoma may contain argyrophil cells and their presence does not provide a discriminator in terms of behaviour. A case diagnosed by FNA in which there were bilateral lesions has been described[41]. The application of the term 'carcinoid tumour' is best avoided, as carcinoid syndrome with its hormonal manifestations has not been described with breast lesions. Clinically, these tumours present like a ductal carcinoma. Cytologically, eccentric nuclei with stippled chromatin may be noted. The cells are said to resemble plasma cells or lymphoid cells[41,42].

Cytological features

- ► Not distinctive clinically but often well circumscribed
- ► Cellular aspirates contain dispersed single cells that appear in small groups
- ► The cells are remarkably uniform with an eccentrically placed nucleus resembling plasma cells
- ► The chromatin is stippled and thickening of the nuclear border may be noted

Diagnostic pitfalls

- ► Lymphoplasmacytoid lymphoma or plasmacytoma can form deposits in soft tissue and breast. This lesion usually displays complete absence of cell cohesion

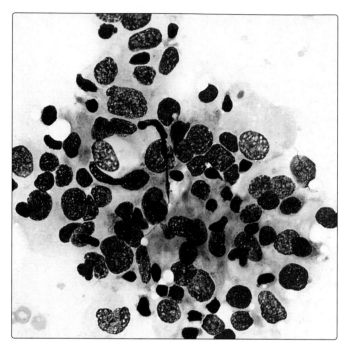

Fig. 9.19   Medullary carcinoma with lymphoid stroma. The characteristic features of large obvious malignant epithelial cells admixed with small lymphoid cells are apparent here. (MGG)

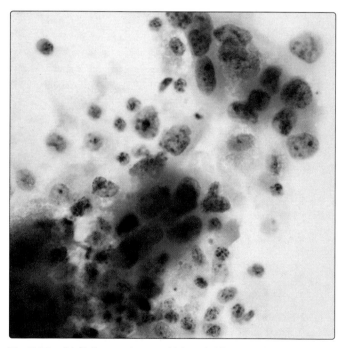

Fig. 9.20   Medullary carcinoma with lymphoid stroma. (Papanicolaou)

Medullary carcinoma with lymphoid stroma[43–47]
(Figs 9.19–9.21)

This is attended by a better than average prognosis, with a 10-year survival of 84% compared with 63% for ductal carcinoma of no special type[46,47]. The quoted incidence is 2–15% of the total number of breast carcinomas, but in series where the incidence is greater than 7% it is likely that

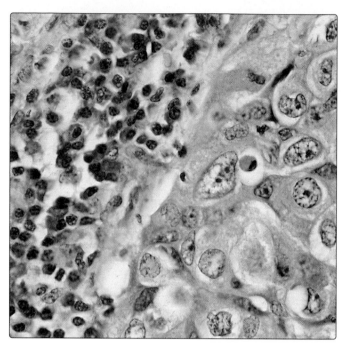

Fig. 9.21   Medullary carcinoma with lymphoid stroma. (H&E section)

the criteria have been too loosely applied. Only those conforming to strict histological criteria display the improved survival[46].

It presents in a younger age group and typically in women under 50. As it is a well-defined, mobile lesion there is a risk of a clinical misdiagnosis of fibroadenoma. Even the macroscopic assessment of a histological specimen may give a similar impression. Aspiration of these lesions is very easy as they are very cellular and contain little stroma. On smearing, the sample is frequently opaque, spreading evenly like a lymphomatous aspirate of a lymph node but usually appearing more granular. Microscopically, the appearance is that of a poorly cohesive, high-grade carcinoma. Syncytial fragments of carcinoma cells are likely to survive intact and these are infiltrated by lymphoid cells and surrounded by a background of small lymphocytes and occasional plasma cells.

Clinical and cytological findings

- A well defined lesion clinically and mammographically
- The lesion is very soft to the needle
- Very cellular smears are easily obtained
- Poorly cohesive large malignant cells with abundant pale staining cytoplasm, some forming syncytial aggregates
- Large angular nuclei with coarse chromatin and prominent nucleoli. Mitotic figures are not unusual
- The background of small lymphocytes and plasma cells is a vital feature but their number is very variable and can be so few that they are overlooked. These cells may be entirely separate from the epithelial cells or intimately mixed with the syncytial groups
- Tumour giant cells are sometimes a feature

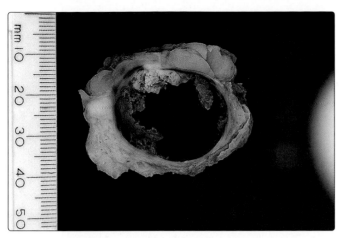

Fig. 9.22 Gross photograph of an intracystic papillary carcinoma.

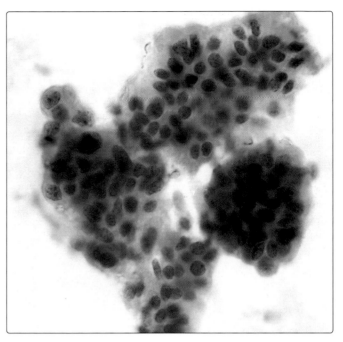

Fig. 9.24 Papillary carcinoma. Note the papillary outline of this epithelial fragment which is composed of cells showing some columnar features. (Papanicolaou)

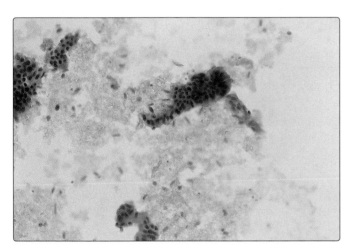

Fig. 9.23 Papillary carcinoma. Low-power view showing papillary structures in a background of elongated spindle cells and necrotic debris. (Papanicolaou)

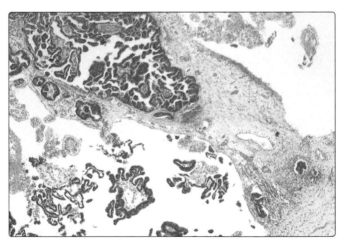

Fig. 9.25 Papillary carcinoma illustrating invasion of the stroma. (H&E section)

Diagnostic pitfalls

▶ If the number of lymphoid cells is low, an erroneous diagnosis of a high grade, poor prognosis carcinoma may be made

Papillary and intracystic carcinoma[48–50] (Figs 9.22–9.27)

Pure papillary carcinoma is a rare lesion although a focal papillary component is seen in up to 4% of all carcinomas[34]. The prognosis is better than that of IDC of NST, with an 80% 5-year survival rate. There can be difficulty in distinguishing histologically between a low-grade papillary carcinoma and a papilloma that has undergone infarction, fibrosis or squamous metaplasia. In addition, benign papillomas can be found in association with intraduct carcinoma of cribriform type, further compounding the difficulties. Non-invasive papillary carcinoma may occur on its own, or represent the predominant component of a lesion that also contains infiltrative carcinoma.

Clinically, these tumours vary in presentation but they may be small, coming to the patient's attention because of associated fibrocystic change or because of the development of a mass due to the cyst around a papillary intracystic carcinoma. They may also present mammographically.

Cytologically, these lesions can be problematic as the nuclear pleomorphism is not always great and bare nuclei may be present[50]. This picture can cause confusion with fibroadenoma or benign papilloma. The smears tend to be cellular with three-dimensional papillary structures that include a fibrovascular core. This appearance may be lost if undue shearing forces have been used in preparing the

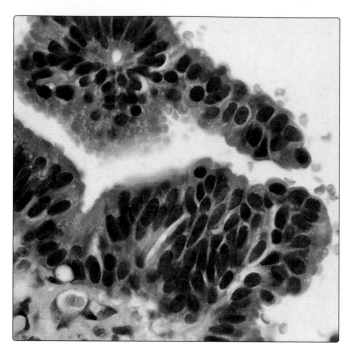

Fig. 9.26 Papillary carcinoma showing papillary fronds. (H&E section)

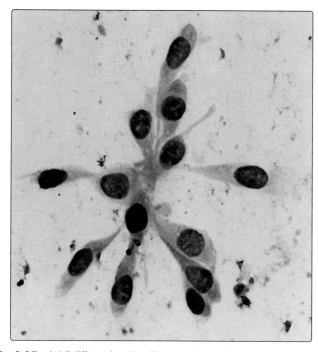

Fig. 9.27 Well-differentiated papillary carcinoma. The cells show a striking elongated appearance. (MGG)

smear. Then, denuded fibrovascular cores may be apparent. The cells often have a definite columnar appearance and may appear in small rows or palisades. Naked nuclei in the background have the same size, shape and chromatin pattern as the epithelial cells and therefore should not be confused with benign bipolar stromal cells. There is frequently a population of haemosiderin laden macrophages in the background.

Clinical and cytological findings

▶ Often small and soft clinically
▶ May be cystic on aspiration
▶ Large cell clusters forming arborizing arrays bearing overlapping, palisaded cells on a fibrovascular core
▶ Cells may be dispersed and the fibrovascular cores denuded
▶ The cells are often distinctly columnar in appearance
▶ Anisonucleosis, hyperchromasia, coarse chromatin, and prominent nucleoli are uncommon
▶ Benign bipolar cells are absent from the background and myoepithelial cells are not seen within the groups

Diagnostic pitfalls

▶ These lesions are usually low-grade and lack obvious cytological features of malignancy often resulting in a suspicious (C4) diagnosis
▶ The diagnosis may be missed if blood stained cyst fluid is discarded rather than sent for cytological examination, although in some cases the cyst fluid is not diagnostic. If there is any residual mass after drainage of cyst fluid, re-aspiration should be undertaken

Invasive cribriform carcinoma[51,52]

When present in its pure histological form, this entity confers a very good prognosis. We have been unable to discern any feature that allows a cytological differentiation of invasive cribriform carcinoma from low-grade IDC of NST.

Tubular carcinoma[53–55] *(Figs 9.28–9.30)*

This low-grade variant of breast carcinoma also has a very good prognosis and adequate primary treatment of a

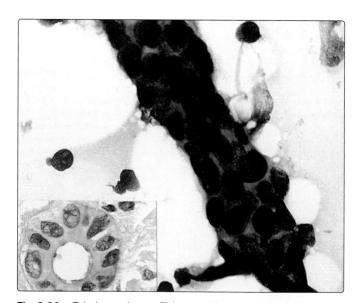

Fig. 9.28 Tubular carcinoma. This smear illustrates the fairly bland appearance of the epithelium in tubular carcinoma. In this fragment the tubule is orientated longitudinally. The inset reveals a tubule sectioned transversely in H&E stained histology. (MGG)

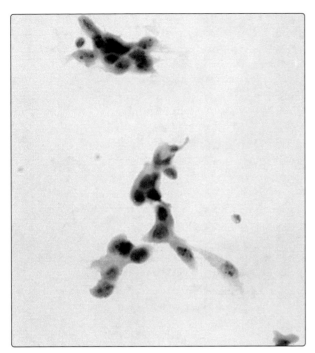

Fig. 9.29 Tubular carcinoma. This is a different case from the one illustrated in **Fig. 9.28** in which the tubular nature of the lesion is difficult to discern in the smear. The presentation is that of a low-grade carcinoma. (Papanicolaou)

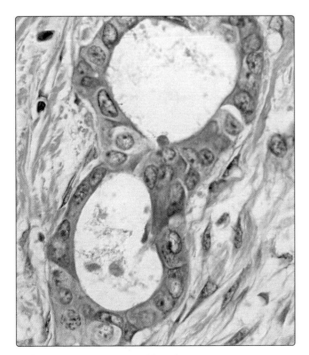

Fig. 9.30 Tubular carcinoma. (H&E section)

classical example should be rewarded by a cure. Being very slow growing lesions and having a significantly collagenous stroma, these tumours commonly present when small or on a routine screening mammogram. Clinically, they are firm and discrete. On aspiration it can be quite difficult to obtain smears that reach even moderate cellularity. Coupled with

the tendency for the cells to exhibit bland nuclear features and their failure to dissociate, the difficulty with sampling these lesions makes the risk of a false negative diagnosis quite high. The cells may have a cuboidal or even columnar appearance but the apical snouts seen on histology are not readily recognized on cytological preparations.

Clinical and cytological findings

► Usually presents when small, but usually clinically and mammographically suspicious
► Fibrous sensation on needle
► Aspirates often poorly cellular with no aspirate more than moderately cellular
► Epithelial cells in cohesive clusters and sheets that have a recognizable acinar structure, but abnormal rigid finger-like groups and cell balls also may be seen
► There is only slight anisonucleosis and mild hyperchromasia. The chromatin is granular with some prominent chromo-centres in wet fixed preparations but the usually single nucleoli are small
► Bipolar nuclei are present in only very occasional cases
► 'Messy' background of cell fragments and stromal elements
► No apocrine or foam cells present

Diagnostic pitfalls

► This type of carcinoma accounts for some false negative cytological diagnoses as the malignant characteristics are very subtle. Frequently the cytological category is suspicious (C4) rather a confident malignant (C5). It is important to take the clinical and mammographic features into account
► There is an overlap in appearance with complex sclerosing lesions and radial scars (p 270), mammographically and cytologically

Squamous cell carcinoma[56–60] *(Figs 9.31, 9.32)*

As its histogenesis is a subject of debate, this is a lesion of considerable interest to the histopathologist. Clinically, it appears to behave similarly to IDC of NST. These lesions, in their pure form, are rare and tend to occur in elderly women. More commonly areas of squamous differentiation occur in otherwise unremarkable ductal carcinomas.

On clinical presentation squamous carcinomas are similar to ductal carcinoma though somewhat larger. An initial clue to the unusual nature of the lesion is obtained when the needle enters a central cystic cavity and thick yellow fluid is withdrawn. This phenomenon occurs most commonly in those tumours showing marked keratinization and will be familiar to those used to taking aspirates from neck nodes involved by secondary squamous carcinoma.

When this type of sample is obtained from breasts, the possibility of fibrocystic change is quickly dispelled by the microscopic appearance of squamous cells of varying degrees of maturity. Advice that straw-coloured fluid from a breast cyst may safely be discarded should not lead to a

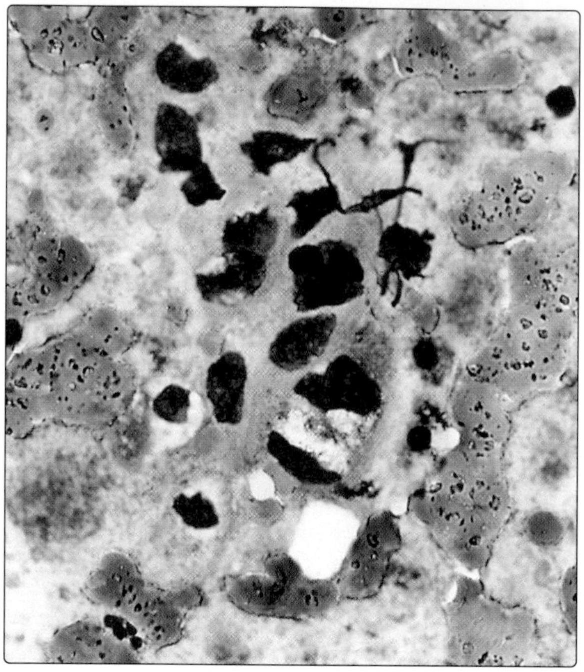

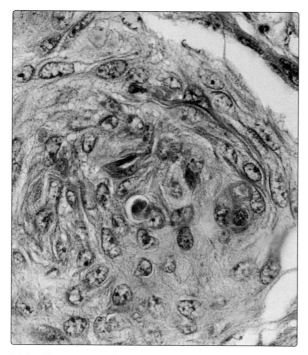

Fig. 9.31 Squamous carcinoma of the breast. These malignant cells have rather condensed chromatin and an angular nuclear outline with fairly abundant, somewhat hyaline basophilic but pale staining cytoplasm. (MGG)

Fig. 9.32 Squamous carcinoma of the breast. (H&E section)

missed diagnosis with this lesion as there is always likely to be a residual mass that will prompt immediate re-aspiration. A further possible source of cytological confusion is with an epidermal cyst. Epidermal cysts are generally very superficial lesions and therefore clinically distinct; however when an epidermal cyst occurs adjacent to the inframammary fold its

true depth may be difficult to assess. More importantly, the squamous cells in epidermal cysts do not display malignant features. Squamous cells may also be seen in aspirates from fibroadenomas and phyllodes tumours with squamous metaplasia and they are also seen in infarcted fibroadenomas[61].

Cytologically, the squamous nature of the less well-differentiated squamous carcinoma is more readily apparent in Papanicolaou stained smears than in air dried ones. Although mature and anucleate squames may be present, there are usually obviously malignant epithelial cells to be found. The cells tend to be single or in small groups, usually with fairly abundant cytoplasm that is keratinized. The intracytoplasmic keratin is well demonstrated as an orange, refractile hue on Papanicolaou-stained smears but stains a more subtle blue with the May-Grünwald-Giemsa stain. There tends to be a dirty background because of necrotic cellular and keratinous debris. An additional feature is the presence of multinucleate giant cells as a reaction to tumour keratin.

Clinical and cytological features

▶ No distinctive clinical features unless there has been central cystic degeneration
▶ Pure squamous carcinomas cannot be confidently diagnosed cytologically as the needle may have sampled only the area of squamous differentiation, missing the main ductal carcinoma component
▶ The cells are usually poorly cohesive with dense angular nuclei. The squamous nature of the cells is more obvious in Papanicolaou stained preparations but in MGG stained smears the dense blue grey cytoplasm is quite distinctive
▶ Necrotic debris is common
▶ Anucleate cells may be present

Diagnostic pitfalls

▶ A squamous carcinoma with a cystic centre may be mistaken clinically for fibrocystic change

Adenoid cystic carcinoma[62–64] (Figs 9.33,9.34)

This uncommon tumour has a very good prognosis but strict histological criteria need to be applied. Ductal carcinoma without special features can have cribriform and papillary areas that may be misdiagnosed as adenoid cystic carcinoma. True adenoid cystic carcinoma accounts for no more than 1 in 1000 breast carcinomas so putative cases must be viewed with a critical eye.

The cytological features are distinctive and are similar to those seen in salivary gland tumours of this type. The cells do not always show obviously malignant features. The presence of globules that stain magenta with MGG was formerly said to be pathognomonic of this entity but collagenous spherulosis of the breast can be identical in this respect[65]. Diagnostic caution is therefore required.

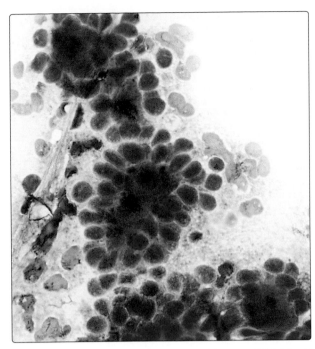

Fig. 9.33 Adenoid cystic carcinoma. The combination of fairly bland but nonetheless malignant epithelial cells and the bright violet globules can be confused with collagenous spherulosis. (MGG)

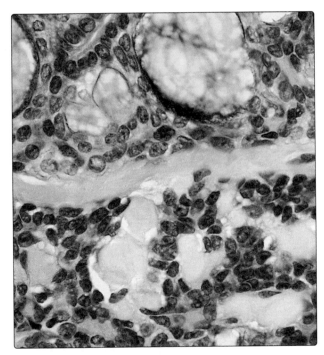

Fig. 9.34 Adenoid cystic carcinoma. (H&E section)

Clinical and cytological findings

► This low-grade lesion tends to be small at presentation, usually in older women
► The aspirate is likely to be moderately cellular with cohesive cell groups

► In MGG-stained preparations the cell groups contain very distinctive magenta coloured bodies which are round or cylindrical, measuring between 0.01–0.08 mm in diameter and up to 0.04 mm in length; they are less apparent in Papanicolaou stained slides being pale blue
► Most cells are three-dimensional groups, many incorporating metachromatic basement membrane bodies. Smaller numbers of single cells and cells in small groups are present
► In the groups the nuclei are crowded and overlapping but where the details are more easily seen they are round or oval with slight but definite anisonucleosis and slight coarsening of the chromatin. Nucleoli are small and generally single
► No bipolar cells are present but 'myoepithelium-like', vimentin-positive cells have been reported[66]

Diagnostic pitfalls

► Some IDC of NST contain areas indistinguishable from adenoid cystic carcinoma
► The very distinctive basement membrane bodies are also seen in aspirates of benign breast disease with collagenous spherulosis. Adenoid cystic carcinoma aspirates do not contain a benign component while collagenous spherulosis aspirates include benign epithelial and many myoepithelial cells

Mucoepidermoid carcinoma[67–70]

Focal squamous and mucinous differentiation may be found independently in ductal carcinomas of breast. When they occur together in a moderate or high-grade lesion there seems little merit in including such a tumour in a special category. When present in a low-grade lesion the term mucoepidermoid tumour may be invoked implying a better than average outcome. The cytological features are similar to those described in the salivary gland.

Apocrine carcinoma[71–74] *(Figs 9.35–9.38)*

Although pure apocrine carcinoma is unusual (1–4% of all breast carcinomas), both ductal carcinoma and a variant of lobular carcinoma can show apocrine features. The prognosis is no different from that of a ductal carcinoma without special features. The importance of this lesion is the potential for confusion with benign apocrine metaplasia. The diagnostic problems that can follow are likely to be most acute when a low-grade, pure apocrine carcinoma presents in a younger woman. Clearly there is a risk of making a diagnosis of fibrocystic change, as benign apocrine cells have a notoriously active appearing nucleus with a large nucleolus. Furthermore low-grade apocrine carcinomas may have very bland cytological features.

Apocrine carcinoma is diagnosed on an aspirate when the cells have malignant nuclei and abundant eosinophilic or amphophilic cytoplasm that may be granular or finely vacuolated. The cell outline tends to be polygonal. Features helpful in the differentiation of benign from malignant apocrine cells are pleomorphic nuclei, poorly defined cell borders and cellular discohesion in the latter.

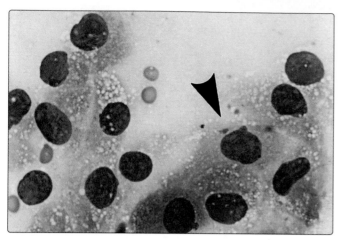

Fig. 9.35   Well-differentiated apocrine carcinoma. Note the irregular nuclear outline with occasional protrusions of chromatin as well as occasional fragments of extranuclear chromatin (arrowhead). Another suspicious feature is the rather poorly defined cellular borders. Compare with the illustrations of benign apocrine epithelium. (MGG)

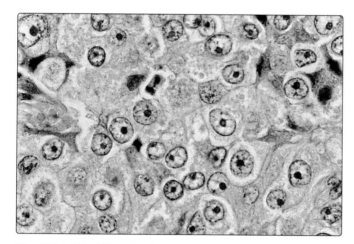

Fig. 9.36   Well-differentiated apocrine carcinoma. (H&E section)

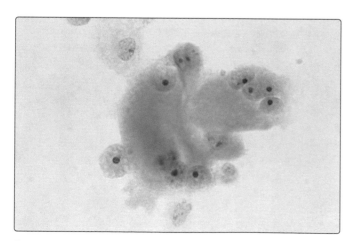

Fig. 9.37   Less well-differentiated apocrine carcinoma. Notice the abundant slightly granular cytoplasm and the very prominent nucleoli. (Papanicolaou)

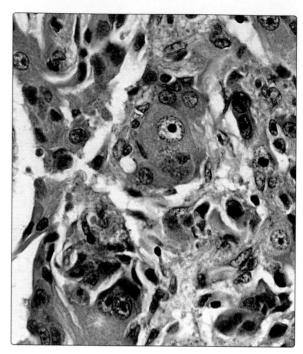

Fig. 9.38   Less well-differentiated apocrine carcinoma. (H&E section)

Clinical and cytological findings

▶ These lesions are not distinct from other types of carcinomas clinically
▶ Aspirates tend to be cellular and the cells dispersed
▶ The cells are large with abundant acidophilic cytoplasm that may be granular but this is less marked than in benign apocrine epithelium
▶ The cell borders tend to be indistinct or ragged in contrast to the well-defined borders of benign apocrine cells. This is an important feature if low-grade apocrine carcinoma is suspected
▶ The nucleus is also large and the chromatin coarse and unevenly distributed
▶ The single nucleolus is very large, sometimes spectacularly so. Multiple nucleoli are also seen in the higher-grade tumours

Diagnostic pitfalls

▶ The main danger is in dismissing a low-grade apocrine carcinoma as apocrine metaplasia
▶ Benign apocrine epithelium can look quite atypical, particularly when the lining of a cyst has become degenerate or inflamed

Secretory carcinoma (formerly juvenile carcinoma)[75–77]

These lesions appear to have an excellent prognosis in women under the age of 20 years. The behaviour in older women is less favourable with late recurrence the rule, occurring up to 20 years after surgery. Although initially described in children, adult cases have been described, including a 73-year-old patient[75]. Clinically, these lesions are well circumscribed and most are less than 20 mm at presentation.

FNA smears tend to be poorly cellular but show abundant material resembling thyroid colloid, which is bubbly or fractured to give a mosaic appearance[77]. This material does not show streaming around embedded epithelial cells as does mucin in a colloid carcinoma. The epithelial cells are single or in small groups. The occasional sheets show a regular arrangement of nuclei. Some of these cells have a bland appearance but others show a more convincingly malignant appearance. They have basophilic granular cytoplasm and large nuclei with one or two distinct nucleoli. Some cases show prominent cytoplasmic vacuolation and signet ring forms.

Clinical and cytological findings

▶ Colloid-like background material imitating a thyroid aspirate
▶ Dispersed cells but some small sheets in which there is regular spacing of the nuclei
▶ Often prominent cytoplasmic vacuolation and signet ring cells
▶ The non-vacuolated cytoplasm appears granular
▶ Malignant nuclear features apparent in only some of the cells which have enlarged nuclei with one or two distinct nucleoli

Diagnostic pitfalls

▶ These are well circumscribed lesions with bland cytological features, which commonly occur in an age group where carcinoma is not expected. There is therefore a risk of false negative diagnosis on cytology
▶ The features closely resemble colloid carcinoma of breast but the background material does not stream around the cells like mucin. Cases with prominent signet ring cells may be mistaken for signet ring cell carcinoma

Glycogen rich (clear cell) carcinoma[78,79]

This lesion carries a significantly worse prognosis than IDC of NST. It may resemble signet ring carcinoma in sections but special stains will readily reveal the cytoplasm to be filled with glycogen and not mucin. In aspirates, the differentiation is made by the central location of the nucleus and the fragility of the abundant pale cytoplasm.

Clinical and cytological findings

▶ An aggressive lesion but otherwise not clinically distinct
▶ Abundantly cellular aspirate
▶ Large dispersed cells with plentiful clear cytoplasm and centrally placed nuclei
▶ Obvious malignant nuclear features, occasionally the chromatin may be condensed and hyperchromatic

Diagnostic pitfalls

▶ The cytological appearance may resemble signet ring carcinoma but the prognosis is in any case similar
▶ Occasionally, clear cell carcinoma of the kidney metastasizes to breast or skin and may present a similar appearance

Carcinoma with osteoclast-like stromal giant cells[80–85]

These rare lesions are of academic interest to histopathologists but the diagnosis appears not to have any practical implications. In tumours with reactive stromal giant cells there is no evidence of phagocytosis but the giant cells show the ultrastructural appearances and immunohistochemical profile of histiocytes. These tumours should be graded as though the giant cells were not present. An important distinction has to be made from carcinomas with bizarre neoplastic giant cells, which are high-grade in their behaviour[86,87].

As might be expected, the cytological appearances of carcinomas with osteoclast like giant cells are characteristic.

Clinical and cytological features

▶ These lesions are usually soft but well circumscribed, mimicking medullary carcinoma clinically
▶ Aspirates are cellular, containing malignant ductal epithelial cells of any grade
▶ The giant cells have abundant basophilic cytoplasm and variable numbers of nuclei but are not cytologically malignant

Diagnostic pitfalls

▶ It is important to differentiate carcinoma with stromal giant cells, which may be low-grade, from carcinoma with tumour giant cells, which is high grade
▶ In cases with a prominent fibroblastic component, as well as stromal giant cells, an erroneous diagnosis of fat necrosis is possible

Invasive lobular carcinoma (Figs 9.39–9.41)

Most histopathologists recognize this entity as a distinctive variety of invasive carcinoma of the breast[88,89]. The criteria for histological diagnosis are subjective, however, and the incidence in different series varies from 3–14% of breast carcinomas[1–3]. The prognosis for classical cases is midway between that of tubular carcinoma and IDC of NST but there is an increased risk of synchronous or asynchronous bilaterality. Overall, however, the outlook is similar for each grade of lobular carcinoma to that of ductal carcinoma of no special type.

Histologically, the most important features of classical invasive lobular carcinoma are the relatively small size of

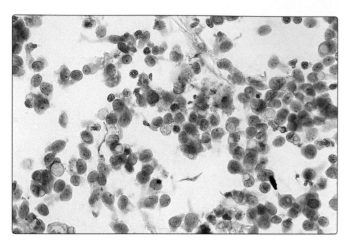

Fig. 9.39   Lobular carcinoma. Dispersed single cells, many containing intracytoplasmic lumina. (Papanicolaou)

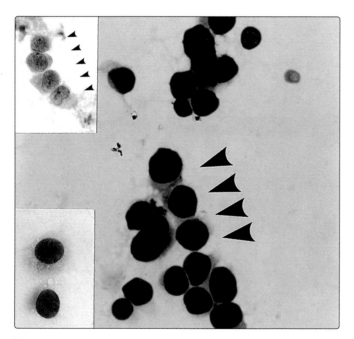

Fig. 9.40   Lobular carcinoma. Notice the tendency for the cells to form short 'Indian file' chains (arrowheads). This phenomenon is also illustrated in a different case stained by the Papanicolaou method (upper inset). The lower inset shows a third case in which the cells were diffusely scattered. Note the double nucleoli and the fairly finely granular chromatin. The cytoplasm is scant and vacuolated. (MGG)

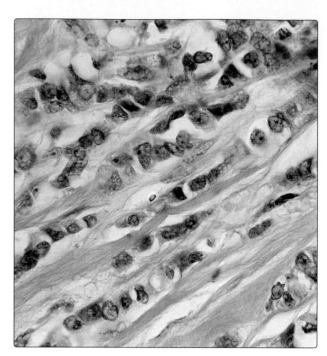

Fig. 9.41   Histological section of invasive lobular carcinoma. (H&E section)

the cells and a tendency not to form acini or cell groups but rather to infiltrate in an 'Indian file'. The presence of *in situ* lobular carcinoma (LCIS) in sections supports the diagnosis. However, as this can also be found in association with otherwise typically ductal varieties of invasive carcinoma, it cannot be regarded as conclusive proof for a lobular origin of the invasive component. Ductal carcinomas frequently 'cancerize' lobules and when the ductal carcinoma cells are small they can closely mimic LCIS[90]. Intracytoplasmic lumina are a feature of many classical invasive lobular carcinomas but are also seen in

some ductal carcinomas. It is also necessary to distinguish mucinous signet ring carcinoma, which is of ductal type[88].

Correct categorization of lobular carcinomas is important because of the characteristic pattern of metastatic spread to retroperitoneum, peritoneum and viscera and to the central nervous system. Awareness of the tumour type allows early diagnosis of what may otherwise be rather unusual symptoms of recurrence.

Lobular carcinomas are important to the cytopathologist because, with the more scirrhous ductal carcinomas, they are responsible for many false negative cytological diagnoses in palpable breast lesions[91,92]. This is because lobular carcinomas, particularly the classical type, tend to yield poorly cellular aspirates composed of small uniform cells with small and relatively bland nuclei. One study cites a malignant diagnosis obtained in only 27% of cases of lobular carcinoma with 30% reported as atypical or suspicious and a false negative rate of 28%[93].

The clinical presentation is not significantly different from that of ductal carcinoma, with a higher incidence of bilaterality. Aspirates, especially when blood-stained, may appear inadequate as the tumour nuclei are sufficiently small to blend into the background of red cells and leucocytes.

A most valuable clue to the presence of lobular carcinoma is the tendency to form 'Indian files' in the aspirate. Seldom do more than three or four cells in one or two groups form a chain in any one aspirate but this is generally sufficient to secure the diagnosis. Although the nuclear/cytoplasmic ratio is high, the nuclear characteristics are not classically those of malignant cells. In Papanicolaou-stained preparations there is a fine stippling of the chromatin but marked hyperchromasia is not a feature and the nucleolus is characteristically very small, except in the histiocytoid or pleomorphic variant in which the nuclei are pleomorphic, the nucleoli prominent and the cytoplasm abundant. MGG-stained preparations show a small, dense and compact nucleus and usually no nucleolus is visible. The nuclear membrane is generally smooth in contour and the variation in nuclear size is slight but detectable. Occasional intracytoplasmic lumina with a target-like appearance may be seen[94]. Signet-ring cells may also be seen.

In short, the presence of sparse, small but bold and robust appearing nuclei with an absence of bipolar stromal cells from a clinically suspicious lump should alert the cytologist to the possibility of an invasive lobular carcinoma. It is not always possible to distinguish lobular carcinoma from the smaller celled varieties of ductal carcinoma but the following features may help.

Clinical and cytological findings

▶ May be clinically bilateral or multifocal at presentation
▶ Scanty aspirates are common. Frequently the first aspirate from a clinically suspicious lump is acellular. The more cellular alveolar variant is easier to sample
▶ Tumour cells are well dispersed and mainly single
▶ Cells are small and easily mistaken for benign epithelium but nuclei have an abnormal appearance that should raise suspicion
▶ Occasional Indian file groupings, usually containing only three or four cells, may be seen
▶ Cytoplasm is scanty, with the nucleus eccentrically placed and some cells may contain an intracytoplasmic lumen with a signet-ring appearance
▶ Nuclei show slight but definite variation in size but tend to be round in shape. The chromatin is stippled but not coarse and the nucleolus inconspicuous in the classic type

Diagnostic pitfalls

▶ Lobular carcinomas account for many of the false negative cases in most series. There are also problems in categorizing the tumour cytologically
▶ It is not always possible to distinguish lobular carcinomas from ductal carcinomas. Cases with prominent intracytoplasmic lumina may be mistaken for signet ring carcinoma
▶ Apocrine differentiation is possible[95,96]. This variant is also known as pleomorphic or histiocytoid lobular carcinoma. Their lobular growth pattern cannot be discerned on cytology, so may be typed as high-grade ductal carcinoma

Other malignant tumours

Metaplastic carcinoma/carcinosarcoma
(Figs 9.42–9.45)

These are high-grade carcinomas in which much of the tumour undergoes metaplastic change producing a

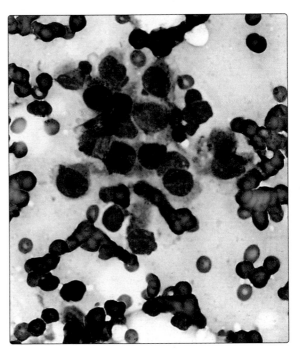

Fig. 9.42 Carcinosarcoma. The appearances in this smear were thought to indicate ductal carcinoma and even in retrospect the more precise diagnosis of carcinosarcoma could not be elicited from the cytology; see **Fig. 9.43**. (MGG)

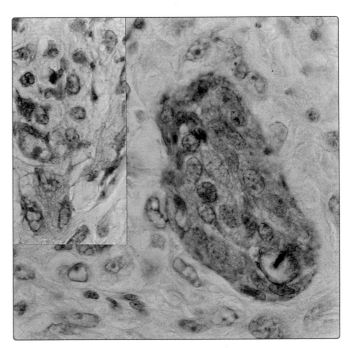

Fig. 9.43 Carcinosarcoma. Main figure: cytokeratin CAM 5.2; inset, vimentin. The dual differentiation was only apparent on histological examination of the case. (Immunochem)

pseudosarcomatous pattern[97]. The sarcomatous element can resemble fibrosarcoma, chondrosarcoma, osteosarcoma, rhabdomyosarcoma, or anaplastic sarcoma with giant cells. These rare tumours represent no more than 0.2% of breast cancers[93,98]. Even more rarely, a pure spindle cell variant is

295

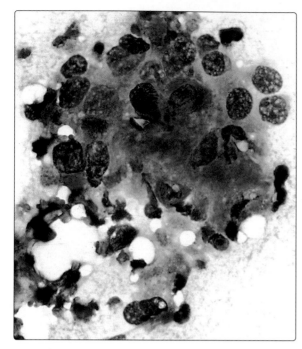

Fig. 9.44 Carcinosarcoma with cartilage formation. The typical malignant cells were associated with abundant crimson material with a somewhat amorphous appearance raising the suspicion of cartilaginous differentiation. (MGG)

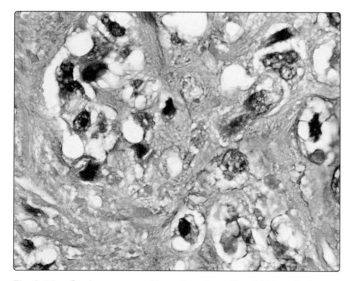

Fig. 9.45 Carcinosarcoma with cartilage formation. (H&E section)

encountered[99–103]. The diagnosis suggests a worse prognosis than that for IDC of NST. The greater the sarcomatous component, the worse the prognosis.

The clinical presentation is not significantly different from that of ductal carcinoma and the average age is the same. Cytologically, there is seldom any difficulty in recognizing the presence of malignancy and occasionally both the epithelial and heterologous elements are recognized in aspirates. If however, as often happens, either the carcinomatous or sarcomatous element predominates there is a possibility that the lesser component will not be apparent or will be overlooked[103].

The epithelial cell component is indistinguishable from a high-grade ductal carcinoma but there may be transitional forms providing a spectrum through to obviously spindle shaped cells. When cartilaginous differentiation is present, magenta-coloured ground substance may be noted. Osteosarcomatous metaplasia does occur. The presence of well-mineralized malignant osteoid can provide a definite clue that a clinically obvious carcinoma has unusual features and the aspirator's needle encounters areas that are very gritty and virtually impenetrable. If osteoclast-like giant cells and malignant spindle cells are present in the aspirate the picture is complete.

Clinical and cytological findings

▶ Clinically, these appear as rapidly growing lesions
▶ The aspirates are usually cellular
▶ The cells may be indistinguishable from those of a high-grade ductal carcinoma of breast depending on the area aspirated
▶ Additional features depending on the extent and type of the metaplastic malignancy may include:
  ▶ Large, malignant multinucleated giant cells
  ▶ Malignant cells associated with fragments of amorphous metachromatic material
  ▶ Large malignant spindle cells singly or in syncytial clusters

Diagnostic pitfalls

▶ The extent and degree of metaplasia are variable and so some cases may be diagnosed as ductal carcinoma without special features on cytological assessment
▶ The aspirate may contain only spindle cells and may be diagnosed as a sarcoma

Borderline and malignant phyllodes tumour[100–108]

The differentiation of benign, borderline and malignant phyllodes tumours can be very difficult histologically. Distinction is based on the degree of atypia and mitotic activity of the stromal cells and the appearance of the margin of the tumour. Cases in which there is a lesser degree of atypia may be classified as borderline lesions.

In frankly malignant cases, pleomorphic, high-grade spindle cells are seen, with a fibrosarcoma-type pattern. Rarely, heterologous sarcomatous elements are present in the form of lipoblasts or malignant cartilage with abundant ground substance. It has to be said, however, that the aspirate does not contain features that predict the 12% of malignant phyllodes tumours that will metastasize. Even histological assessment is subjective in this regard and the extent of infiltration that is important in histological assessment is obviously not apparent to a cytologist. As lymph node spread is not a problem with malignant phyllodes tumours, the treatment of a suspicious example as though it were a carcinoma is clearly inappropriate.

Clinical and cytological findings

▶ Malignant lesions tend to be larger
▶ Properly taken aspirates are always abundantly cellular
▶ Large atypical stromal cells, often in cohesive groups, are always a feature
▶ The epithelial content is variable but tends to be particularly sparse in frankly malignant phyllodes tumours. It is recognizably benign

Diagnostic pitfalls

▶ It is frequently difficult and often impossible to decide whether a phyllodes tumour is benign or low-grade malignant (borderline)

Adenomyoepithelioma

This is a rare tumour of the breast, which usually presents as a solitary mass. This neoplasm has well-documented histological features, with spindle-shaped or polygonal myoepithelial cells surrounding glandular cells[109–112]. The cytological appearances are described in some reports as overlapping with phyllodes tumour[113,114], while another mentions epithelial cells with prominent nuclei[115].

Fibromatosis (desmoid tumour)

Breast is an uncommon location for desmoid tumours but cases have been reported[116]. The patient usually presents with a palpable breast lump, suspicious of carcinoma on clinical and mammographic assessment. However, the aspirate is usually scanty, yielding bland, isolated spindle cells, and small groups of benign ductal cells[117].

Sarcomas

Non-epithelial malignancies, other than malignant phyllodes tumours, occurring as primary lesions in the breast include stromal sarcoma[118], angiosarcoma[119,120], malignant fibrous histiocytoma[121,122] (Figs 9.46, 9.47), liposarcoma[123], lymphoma[124–128], leiomyosarcoma[129], rhabdomyosarcoma[130], chondrosarcoma[131,132] and osteosarcoma[133,134]. The cytological features are identical to those of such lesions presenting at their more usual sites (see Chapters 40, 41).

Metastatic malignancy[135–145]

The incidence of metastatic tumours in the breast is 1 for every 370 new breast carcinomas. Clearly any tumour capable of metastasis will appear in aspirates of breast lesions from time to time. As this event is rare and breast carcinoma is common, a mass developing in the breast of a patient with a known extramammary primary is more likely to be a second primary than a metastasis.

Bronchogenic carcinomas and lymphomas are most likely to create a mass in the breast. Both may present initially in

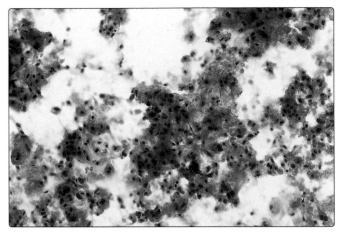

Fig. 9.46 Sarcoma of the breast. This field illustrates poorly cohesive, plump spindle cells with nuclear pleomorphism. (H&E).

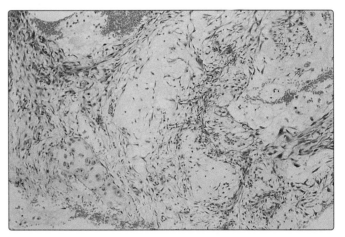

Fig. 9.47 Low-grade myxoid malignant fibrous histiocytoma. (H&E)

this way and the former may be confused with a high-grade ductal carcinoma cytologically (Fig 9.48) and the latter with a low-grade ductal carcinoma or lobular carcinoma. Secondary lymphomas usually involve the breast as a late event. The aspirates are very cellular and the cells poorly cohesive, and so diagnostic difficulties should be avoidable (Fig. 9.49). Amelanotic melanomas with no known primary create a risk of wrong diagnosis.

It is most important that metastatic malignancy is at least considered in all cases that are not completely typical of any of the recognized varieties of breast carcinoma so as to prevent an unnecessary mastectomy.

Cytological findings

▶ Often there will be a history of a recognized extramammary primary tumour
▶ Helpful features are those that are not typical of a primary breast carcinoma such as oat cell appearance, melanin pigment, clear cell differentiation

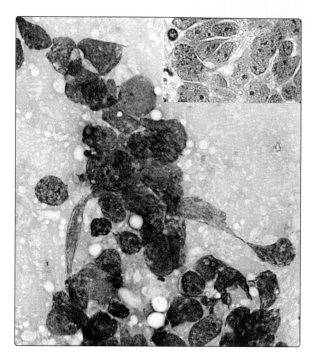

Fig. 9.48 Metastatic anaplastic carcinoma of lung presenting in a fine needle aspirate of breast. The inset shows the histological appearances of this secondary lesion. (MGG)

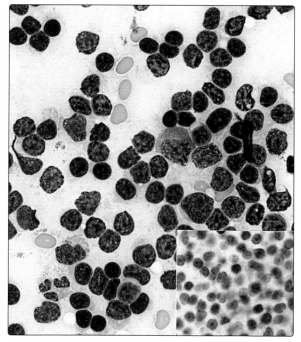

Fig. 9.49 Lymphoplasmacytoid lymphoma recurring as a breast lump. The inset shows the histological appearance for size comparison. (MGG)

Diagnostic pitfalls

▶ Metastatic small cell (non-oat cell) carcinomas and lymphomas can imitate small celled ductal and lobular carcinoma, and amelanotic melanoma may mimic high-grade ductal carcinoma

▶ Renal clear cell carcinoma can imitate clear cell carcinoma of the breast, as can signet ring carcinomas of the gastrointestinal tract

Recurrent breast lesions[146,147]

The major role of aspiration cytology is in the primary diagnosis of malignancy. There is however, an important subsidiary role in the follow-up assessment of patients after treatment is complete. Here too, there is considerable scope for reducing the need for surgery and speeding therapeutic and prognostic evaluation.

This issue has been addressed and the usefulness of FNA in this situation has been confirmed[147]. Interestingly, the problem of inexperienced aspirators obtaining non-representative aspirates may be increased here, possibly reflecting the smaller size of the lesions or the effect of local scar tissue. The cytopathologist had an inadequacy rate of only 6.2% while 45% of the aspirates obtained by the others were not suitable for diagnosis. The sensitivity, specificity, positive and negative predicative values for the cytological findings were 97%, 100%, 100% and 94.7% respectively (excluding inadequates).

Metastasis of breast malignancy to remote sites is commonly detected by exfoliative and aspiration cytology. It is usually possible to indicate that breast is the likely source of the metastatic cells. If the previous history is available, there is seldom any doubt but occasional cases present with distant metastasis before the breast primary is clinically apparent.

Lobular carcinoma exhibits a different pattern of metastatic spread from that of ductal carcinoma. It may therefore present in specimens from unusual sites in cases where the primary tumour has not been detected or in which it has apparently been forgotten by the referring clinician. Diagnostic difficulties may arise when specimens of peritoneum, retroperitoneum, stomach wall, ovaries or uterus are submitted without adequate clinical information and show diffuse infiltration by small tumour cells on histology.

Radiation-induced changes in breast[148–152]

In common with other tissue, breast shows characteristic histological changes following therapeutic irradiation. These changes vary in extent and severity among patients and within individual patients. This variation is not related to the presence of residual carcinoma, radiation dose, patient age, adjuvant chemotherapy or time to post-irradiation sampling.

The most characteristic effect is the presence of atypical epithelial cells in the terminal duct lobular unit, with associated lobular sclerosis and atrophy. This atypia of the epithelium is accompanied by vascular changes and abnormal fibroblasts.

The epithelial atypia can be reflected in the aspiration cytology of lesions in patients where the index of suspicion is already very high.

Clinical and cytological findings

▶ Clearly, it is important to know that the patient has had previous radiotherapy. Not all clinicians are aware of its significance to the cytopathologist and there is always the possibility of a clerical omission on the request form. The aspirator cytopathologist will usually be aware of the possibility from the skin changes or from the history obtained from the patient

▶ The aspirates are usually scanty unless there is a recurrence of the neoplasm

▶ The cells are in small groups and do not exhibit the loss of cohesion seen in carcinoma

▶ Some nuclei may be very large and there is characteristically quite marked anisonucleosis

▶ The nuclear/cytoplasmic ratio is normal, however, and there is usually a scattering of bipolar cells

▶ The appearances of fat necrosis may also be present

Diagnostic pitfalls

▶ Differentiation from recurrent carcinoma can be difficult but attention to the above usually leads to a correct assessment. The main danger is overdiagnosis due to lack of information that the patient has had radiotherapy

References

1 Page D L, Anderson T J. *Diagnostic Histopathology of the Breast*. Edinburgh: Churchill Livingstone, 1987

2 Elston CW, Ellis IO eds. The Breast. *Systemic Pathology*, 3rd edn, vol. 13, Edinburgh: Churchill Livingstone, 1998

3 Rosen P P. The pathological classification of human mammary carcinoma: past present and future. *Ann Clin Lab Sci* 1979; **9**: 144–156

4 Nemoto T, Vana J, Bedwani R N et al. Management and survival of female breast cancer. *Cancer* 1980; **45**: 2917–2924

5 Armstrong K, Eisen A, Weber B. Assessing the risk of breast cancer. *N Engl J Med* 2000; **342**: 564–571

6 Ferno M. Prognostic factors in breast cancer: a brief review. *AntiCancer Res* 1998; **18**: 2167–2171

7 Ellis I O, Galea M, Broughton N et al. Pathological prognostic factors in breast cancer. II. Histological type. Relationship with survival in a large study with long-term follow-up. *Histopathol* 1992; **20**: 479–489

8 Elston C W, Ellis I O. Pathological prognostic factors in breast cancer. I. The value of histological grade in breast cancer: experience from a large study with long-term follow-up. *Histopathol* 1991; **19**: 403–410

9 Haybittle J L, Blamey R W, Elston C W et al. A prognostic index in primary breast cancer. *Br J Cancer* 1982; **45**: 361–366

10 Todd J H, Dowle C, Williams M R et al. Confirmation of a prognostic index in primary breast cancer. *Br J Cancer* 1987; **56**: 489–492

11 Soran A, Vogel V G. Optimal management of primary breast cancer. *Breast J* 1999; **5**: 81–93

12 Early Breast Cancer Trialists' Collaborative Group. Polychemotherapy for early breast cancer: an overview of the randomised trials. *Lancet* 1998; **352**: 930–941

13 Pinder S E, Murray S, Ellis I O et al. The importance of histologic grade of invasive breast carcinoma and response to chemotherapy. *Cancer* 1998; **83**: 1529–1539

14 Willsher P C, Pinder S E, Chan S Y et al. C-erbB2 expression predicts response to preoperative chemotherapy for locally advanced breast cancer. *AntiCancer Res* 1998; **18**: 3695–3698

15 Intraduct carcinoma of the breast (Editorial). *Lancet* 1984; **2**(8393): 24–25

16 Alpers C E, Wellings S R. The prevalence of carcinoma *in situ* in normal and cancer-associated breasts. *Hum Pathol* 1985; **16**: 796–807

17 Page D L, Simpson J F. Ductal carcinoma in-situ – the focus for prevention, screening, and breast conservation in breast cancer. *N Engl J Med* 1999; **340**: 1499–1500

18 Arisio R, Fessia L, Aimone V. Diagnostic possibilities of needle aspiration cytology in minimal breast carcinoma. *G Ital Senologia* 1982; **3**(2): 201–206

19 Romanelli J R, Smith T J. Management of nonpalpable breast lesions: techniques in breast biopsy. *Cancer Invest* 1999; **17**: 624–630

20 Saver T, Young K, Thoresen S O. Fine needle aspiration cytology in the work-up of mammographic and ultrasonographic findings in breast cancer screening: an attempt at differentiating *in situ* and invasive carcinoma. *Cytopathol* 2002; **13**: 101–110

21 Shin H J C, Sneige N. Is a diagnosis of infiltrating versus *in situ* ductal carcinoma of the breast possible in fine-needle aspiration specimens? *Cancer* 1998; **84**: 186–191

22 Bondeson L, Lindholm K. Prediction of invasiveness by aspiration cytology applied to nonpalpable breast carcinoma and tested in 300 cases. *Diagn Cytopathol* 1997; **17**: 315–320

23 Schnitt S J, Connolly J L, Silver B et al. Updated results of the influence of pathologic features on treatment outcome in stage I and II breast cancer. *Int J Radiat Oncol Biol Phys* 1985; **II**(suppl 1): 104

24 Page D L, Dupont W D, Rogers L W, Landenberger M. Intraduct carcinoma of the breast: follow up after biopsy only. *Cancer* 1982; **49**: 751–758

25 Lilleng R, Hagmar B M, Fannants G. Low grade cribriform ductal carcinoma *in situ* of the breast: fine needle aspiration cytology in three cases. *Acta Cytol* 1992; **36**: 48–54

26 Silverberg S G, Kay S, Chitale A R, Levitt S H. Colloid carcinoma of the breast. *J Clin Pathol* 1971; **55**: 355–363

27 Clayton F. Pure mucinous carcinomas of breast. *Hum Pathol* 1986; **17**: 34–38

28 Ferguson D J P, Anderson T J, Wells C A, Battersby S. An ultrastructural study of mucoid carcinoma of the breast: variability of cytoplasmic features. *Histopathol* 1986; **10**: 1219–1230

29 Toikkanen S, Eerola E, Ekfors T O. Pure and mixed mucinous breast carcinomas: DNA stemline and prognosis. *J Clin Pathol* 1988; **41**: 300–303

30 Coady A T, Shousha S, Dawson P M et al. Mucinous carcinoma of the breast: further characterization of its three subtypes. *Histopathol* 1989; **15**: 617–626

31 Palombini L, Fulciniti F, Vetrani A. Mucoid carcinoma of the breast on fine needle aspiration biopsy sample: cytology and ultrastructure. *Appl Pathol* 1984; **2**(2): 70–75

32 Gupta R K, McHutchinson A G R, Simpson J S, Dowle C S. Value of fine needle aspiration cytology of the breast, with an emphasis on the cytodiagnosis of colloid carcinoma. *Acta Cytol* 1991; **35**: 703–709

33 Duane G B, Kanter M H, Branigan T, Chang C. A morphologic and morphometric study of cells from colloid carcinoma of the breast obtained by fine needle aspiration. *Acta Cytol* 1987; **31**: 742–750

34 Rasmussen B B, Rose C, Thorpe S M et al. Argyrophilic cells in 202 human mucinous breast carcinomas. *Am J Clin Pathol* 1985; **84**: 737–740

35 Merino M J, Livolsi V A. Signet ring carcinoma of the female breast: a clinicopathologic analysis of 24 cases. *Cancer* 1981; **48**(8): 1830–1837

36 Hull M T, Seo I S, Battersby J S, Csicsko J F. Signet ring cell carcinoma of the breast. A clinicopathologic study of 24 cases. *Am J Clin Pathol* 1980; **73**(1): 31–35

37 Misonou J, Kanda M, Miyake T et al. An autopsy case of triple cancers including signet-ring cell carcinoma of the breast – report of a rare case with reference to a review of the literature. *Jpn J Surg* 1990; **20**(6): 720–725

38 Battersby S, Dely C J, Hopkinson H E, Anderson T J. The nature of breast dense core granules: chromogranin reactivity. *Histopathol* 1992; **20**: 107–114

39 Ashworth M T, Haqqani M T. Endocrine variant of ductal carcinoma *in situ* of breast: ultrastructural and light microscopical study. *J Clin Pathol* 1986; **39**: 1355–1359

40 Cross A S, Azzopardi J G, Krausz T et al. A morphological and immunocytochemical study of a distinctive variant of ductal carcinoma *in situ* of the breast. *Histopathol* 1985; **9**: 21–37

41 Wee A, Nilsson B, Siew-Meng-Chong, Raju G C. Bilateral carcinoid tumour of the breast: report of a case with diagnosis by fine needle aspiration cytology. *Acta Cytol* 1992; **36**: 55–59

42 Schmitt F C, Brandao M. Carcinoid tumour of male breast diagnosed by fine needle aspiration. *Cytopathol* 1990; **1**: 251–255

43 Wargotz E S, Silverberg S G. Medullary carcinoma of the breast. *Hum Pathol* 1988; **19**: 1340–1346

44 Harris M, Lessells A M. The ultrastructure of medullary, atypical medullary and non-medullary carcinomas of the breast. *Histopathol* 1986; **10**: 405–414

45 Burt A D, Seywright M M, George W D. Mixed apocrine/medullary carcinoma of the breast. Report of a case with fine needle aspiration cytology. *Acta Cytol* 1987; **31**: 322–324

46 Ridolfi R W, Rosen P P, Post A et al. Medullary carcinoma of the breast. A clinical pathological study with 10 year follow up. *Cancer* 1977; **40**: 1365–1385

47 Pedersen L, Holck S, Mouridsen H T et al. Prognostic comparison of three classifications for medullary carcinoma of the breast. *Histopathol* 1999; **34**: 175–178

48 Kline S, Kannan V. Papillary carcinoma of the breast. *Arch Pathol Lab Med* 1986; **110**: 189–191

49 Corkhill M E, Sneige N, Fanning T, El-Naggar A. Fine needle aspiration cytology and flow cytometry of intracystic papillary carcinoma of breast. *Am J Clin Pathol* 1990; **94**: 673–680

50 Papotti M, Gugliotta P, Ghiringhello B, Bussolati G. Association of breast carcinoma and multiple intraductal papillomas: an histological and immunohistochemical investigation. *Histopathol* 1984; **8**: 963–975

51 Page D L, Dixon J M, Anderson T J et al. Invasive cribriform carcinoma of the breast. *Histopathol* 1983; **7**: 525–536

52 Wells C A, Ferguson D J P. Ultrastructural and immunocytochemical study of a case of invasive cribriform breast carcinoma. *J Clin Pathol* 1988; **41**: 17–20

53 Parl F F, Richardson L D. The histologic and biologic spectrum of tubular carcinoma of the breast. *Hum Pathol* 1983; **14**: 694–698

54 Lamb J, McGoogan E. Fine needle aspiration of breast in invasive carcinoma of tubular type and in radial scar/complex sclerosing lesions. *Cytopathol* 1994; **5**: 17–26

55 Bondeson L, Lindholm K. Aspiration cytology of tubular breast carcinoma. *Acta Cytol* 1990; 34(1): 15–20

56 Raju G C. The histological and immunohistochemical evidence of squamous metaplasia from the myoepithelial cells in the breast. *Histopathol* 1991; **17**: 272–275

57 Eggars J W, Chesney T McC. Squamous cell carcinoma of the breast. *Hum Pathol* 1984; **15**: 526–531

58 Lazarevic B, Katatikarn V, Marks R A. Primary squamous cell carcinoma of the breast: diagnosis by fine needle aspiration cytology. *Acta Cytol* 1984; **28**: 321–324

59 Macia M, Ces J A, Becerra E, Novo A. Pure squamous carcinoma of the breast. *Acta Cytol* 1989; **33**: 201–204

60 Chen K T K. Fine needle aspiration cytology of squamous cell carcinoma of the breast. *Acta Cytol* 1990; **34**: 665–667

61 Flint A, Oberman H A. Infarction and squamous metaplasia of intraductal papilloma. *Hum Pathol* 1984; **15**: 764–767

62 Ro J Y, Silva E G, Gallagher H S. Adenoid cystic carcinoma of the breast. *Hum Pathol* 1987; **18**: 1276–1281

63 Düe W, Herbst H, Loy V, Stein H. Characterisation of adenoid cystic carcinoma of the breast by immunohistology. *J Clin Pathol* 1989; **42**: 470–476

64 Wells C A, Nicoll S, Ferguson D J P. Adenoid cystic carcinoma of the breast: a case with axillary lymph node metastasis. *Histopathol* 1986; **10**: 415–424

65 Tyler X, Coghill S B. Fine needle aspiration cytology of collagenous spherulosis of the breast. *Cytopathol* 1991; **2**: 159–162

66 Düe W, Herbst H, Loy V, Stein H. Characterization of adenoid cystic carcinoma of the breast by immunohistology. *J Clin Pathol* 1989; **42**: 470–476

67 Hastrup N, Sehested M. High-grade mucoepidermoid carcinoma of the breast. *Histopathol* 1985; **9**: 887–892

68 Hanna E, Kahn H J. Ultrastructural and immunohistochemical characteristics of mucoepidermoid carcinoma of the breast. *Hum Pathol* 1985; **16**: 941–946

69 Cohen M B, Fisher P E, Holly E A et al. Fine needle aspiration biopsy diagnosis of mucoepidermoid carcinoma of salivary gland. *Acta Cytol* 1990; **34**: 43–49

70 Pettinato G, Insabato G, De Chiara A et al. High-grade mucoepidermoid carcinoma of the breast. *Acta Cytol* 1989; **33**: 195–200

71 Mossler J A, Barton T K, Brinkhous A D et al. Apocrine differentiation in human mammary carcinoma. *Cancer* 1980; **46**: 2463–2471

72 Shousha S, Bull T B, Southall P J, Mazoujian G. Apocrine carcinoma of the breast containing foam cells. An electron microscopic and immunohistological study. *Histopathol* 1987; **11**: 611–620

73 Yates A J, Ahmed A. Apocrine carcinoma and apocrine metaplasia. *Histopathol* 1988; **13**: 228–231

74 Gupta R K, Wakefield S, Naran S, Dowle C C. Immunocytochemical and ultrastructural diagnosis of a rare mixed apocrine medullary carcinoma of the breast in a fine needle aspirate. *Acta Cytol* 1989; **33**: 105–108

75 Krausz T, Jenkins D, Grontoft O et al. Secretory carcinoma of the breast in adults: emphasis on late recurrence and metastasis. *Histopathol* 1989; **14**: 25–36

76 Colandrea J M, Shmookler B M, O'Dowd H J, Cohen M H. Cystic hypersecretory duct carcinoma of the breast. *Arch Pathol Lab Med* 1988; **112**: 560–563

77 D'Amore E S G, Maisto L, Gatteschi M B et al. Secretory carcinoma of the breast: report of a case with fine needle aspiration biopsy. *Acta Cytol* 1986; **30**: 309–312

78 Sorensen F B, Paulsen S M. Glycogen-rich clear cell carcinoma of the breast: a solid variant with mucus. A light microscopic immunohistochemical and ultrastructural study of a case. *Histopathol* 1987; **11**: 857–869

79 Fisher E R, Tavares J, Bulatao I S et al. Glycogen-rich clear cell breast cancer. *Hum Pathol* 1985; **16**: 1085–1090

80 Nielsen B B, Kiaer H W. Carcinoma of the breast with stromal multinucleated giant cells. *Histopathol* 1985; **9**: 183–193

81 McMahon R F T, Ahmed A, Connolly C E. Breast carcinoma with stromal multinucleated giant cells – a light microscopic, histochemical and ultrastructural study. *J Pathol* 1986; **150**: 175–179

82 Stewart C J R, Mutch A F. Breast carcinoma with osteoclast-like giant cells. *Cytopathol* 1991; **2**: 215–219

83 Pettinato G, Petrella G, Manco A et al. Carcinoma of the breast with osteoclast-like giant cells. Fine needle aspiration cytology, histology and electron microscopy of 5 cases. *Appl Pathol* 1984; **2**: 168–178

84 Sugano I, Nagao K, Kondo Y et al. Cytologic and ultrastructural studies of a rare breast carcinoma with osteoclast-like giant cells. *Cancer* 1983; **52**: 74–78

85 Boccato P, Briani G, D'Atri C et al. Spindle cell and cartilaginous metaplasia in a breast carcinoma with osteoclast like stromal cells. A difficult fine needle aspiration diagnosis. *Acta Cytol* 1988; **32**: 75–78

86 Douglas-Jones A G, Barr W T. Breast carcinoma with tumour giant cells. *Acta Cytol* 1989; **33**: 109–114

87 Gupta R K, Holloway L J, Wakefield S, Fauck R J. Fine needle aspiration cytology, immunocytochemistry and electron microscopy in a rare case of carcinoma of the breast with malignant epithelial giant cells. *Acta Cytol* 1991; **35**: 413–416

88 Howell A, Harris M. Infiltrating lobular carcinoma of the breast. *BMJ* 1985; **291**: 1371–1372

89 Nesland J M, Holm R, Johannessen J V. Ultrastructural and immunohistochemical features of lobular carcinoma of the breast. *J Pathol* 1985; **145**: 39–52

90 Kerner H, Lichtig C. Lobular cancerisation: incidence and differential diagnosis with lobular carcinoma *in situ* of breast. *Histopathol* 1986; **10**: 621–629

91 Lamb J, Anderson T J. Influence of cancer histology on the success of fine needle aspiration of the breast. *J Clin Pathol* 1989; **42**: 733–735

92   Brown L A, Coghill S B. Fine needle aspiration of the breast: factors affecting sensitivity. *Cytopathol* 1991; **2**: 67–74

93   Mitnick J S, Gianutsos R, Pollack A H et al. Comparative value of mammography, FNA biopsy, and core biopsy in the diagnosis of invasive lobular carcinoma. *Breast J* 1998; **4**: 75–83

94   Robinson I A, McKee G, Jackson P A et al. Cytological features supporting the diagnosis of lobular cancer. *Diagn Cytopathol* 1995; **13**: 196–201

95   Eusebi V, Betts C, Haagensen D E et al. Apocrine differentiation in lobular carcinoma of the breast. *Hum Pathol* 1984; **15**: 134–140

96   Walford N, Ten Velden J. Histiocytoid breast carcinoma: an apocrine variant of lobular carcinoma. *Histopathol* 1989; **14**: 515–522

97   Kaufman M W, Maerti J R, Gallager H S, Hoehn J I. Carcinoma of the breast with pseudosarcomatous metaplasia. *Cancer* 1984; **53**: 1908–1917

98   Huvos A G, Lucas J C, Foote F W. Metaplastic breast carcinoma. *NY J Med* 1973; May: 1078–1082

99   Gersell D J, Katzenstein A A. Spindle cell carcinoma of the breast. *Hum Pathol* 1981; **12**: 550–561

100 Bauer T W, Rostock R A, Eggleston J C, Baral E. Spindle cell carcinoma of the breast. *Hum Pathol* 1984; **15**: 147–152

101 Raju G C, Wee A. Spindle cell carcinoma of the breast. *Histopathol* 1990; **16**: 497–499

102 Ellis I O, Bell J, Ronan J E, Elston C W, Blamey R W. Immunocytochemical investigation of intermediate filament proteins and epithelial membrane antigen in spindle cell tumours of the breast. *J Pathol* 1988; **154**: 157–165

103 Jebsen P W, Hagmar B M, Nesland J M. Metaplastic breast carcinoma: a diagnostic problem in fine needle aspiration biopsy. *Acta Cytol* 1991; **35**: 396–402

104 Norris H J, Taylor H B. Relationship of histologic features to behaviour of cystosarcoma phyllodes. *Cancer* 1967; **20**: 2090–2099

105 Pietruszka M, Barnes L. Cystosarcoma phyllodes: a clinicopathologic analysis of 42 cases. *Cancer* 1978; **41**: 1974–1983

106 Grimes M M. Cystosarcoma phyllodes of the breast: histologic features, flow cytometric analysis and clinical considerations. *Mod Pathol* 1992; **5**: 232–238

107 Reddick R L, Shin T K, Sawhney D, Siegal G P. Stromal proliferations of the breast. *Hum Pathol* 1987; **18**: 45–49

108 Mentzel T, Kosmehl H, Katenkamp D. Metastasizing phyllodes tumour with malignant fibrous histiocytoma-like areas. *Histopathol* 1991; **19**: 557–560

109 Loose J H, Patchefsky A S, Hollander I et al. Adenomyoepithelioma of the breast: a spectrum of biologic behavior. *Am J Surg Pathol* 1992; 16(9): 868–876

110 Tavassoli F A. Myoepithelial lesions of the breast: myoepitheliosis, adenomyoepithelioma, and myoepithelial

111 Eusebi V, Casadei G P, Bussolati G, Azzopardi J G. Adenomyoepithelioma of the breast with a distinctive type of apocrine adenosis. *Histopathol* 1987; **11**: 305–315

112 Rosen P P. Adenomyoepithelioma of the breast. *Hum Pathol* 1987; **18**: 1232–1237

113 Birdsong G G, Bisharo H M, Costa M J. Adenomyoepithelioma of the breast: report of a case initially examined by fine-needle aspiration. *Diagn Cytopathol* 1993; **9**: 547–550

114 Lee W-Y. Fine needle aspiration cytology of adenomyoepithelioma of the breast: a case indistinguishable from phyllodes tumor in cytologic findings and clinical behavior. *Acta Cytol* 2000; **44**: 488–489

115 Hock Y-L, Chan S-Y. Adenomyoepithelioma of the breast. A case report correlating cytologic and histologic features. *Acta Cytol* 1994; **38**: 953–956

116 Bogomoletz V, Boulenger E, Simatos A. Infiltrating fibromatosis of the breast. *J Clin Pathol* 1981; **34**: 30–34

117 Pettinato G, Manivel J C, Petrella G, Jassim A D. Fine needle aspiration cytology, immunocytochemistry and electron microscopy of fibromatosis of the breast. *Acta Cytol* 1991; **35**: 402–407

118 Rupp M, Hafiz M A, Khalluf E, Sutula M. Fine needle aspiration in stromal sarcoma of the breast. Light and electron microscopic findings with histologic correlation. *Acta Cytol* 1988; **32**: 72–74

119 Liberman L, Dershaw D D, Kaufman R J, Rosen P P. Angiosarcoma of the breast. *Radiology* 1992; 183(3): 649–654

120 Parsi B, Dilhuydy M H, Leger F et al. Cytologic diagnosis of angiosarcoma of the breast. *Arch Anat Cytol Pathol* 1989; 37(5–6): 231–234

121 Langham M R, Mills A S, DeMay R M et al. Malignant fibrous histiocytoma of the breast. *Cancer* 1984; **54**: 558–563

122 Luzzatto R, Grossmann S, Scholl J G, Recktenvald M. Post radiation pleomorphic malignant fibrous histiocytoma of the breast. *Acta Cytol* 1986; **30**: 48–50

123 Austin R M, Dupree W B. Liposarcoma of the breast. *Hum Pathol* 1986; **17**: 906–913

124 Mambo N C, Burke J S, Butler J J. Primary malignant lymphomas of the breast. *Cancer* 1977; **39**: 2033–2040

125 Telesinghe P U, Anthony P P. Primary lymphoma of the breast. *Histopathol* 1985; **9**: 297–307

126 Aozasa K, Ohsawa M, Saeki K et al. Malignant lymphoma of the breast: immunologic type and association with lymphocytic mastopathy. *Am J Clin Pathol* 1992; 97(5): 699–704

127 Pettinato G, Manivel J C, Petrella G, De Chiara A. Primary multilobated T-cell lymphoma of the breast diagnosed by fine needle aspiration cytology and immunocytochemistry. *Acta Cytol* 1991; 35(3): 294–299

128 Hugh J C, Jackson F I, Hanson J, Poppema S. Primary breast lymphoma. An

immunohistologic study of 20 new cases. *Cancer* 1990; 66(12): 2602–2611

129 Arista Nasr J, Gonzalez Gomez I, Angeles A et al. Primary recurrent leiomyosarcoma of the breast. Case report with ultrastructural and immunohistochemical study and review of the literature. *Am J Clin Pathol* 1989; 92(4): 500–505

130 Torres V, Ferrer R. Cytology of fine needle aspiration biopsy of primary breast rhabdomyosarcoma in an adolescent girl. *Acta Cytol* 1985; **29**: 430–434

131 Steiner E, Barrabes M H, Lequang M L et al. A case of a chondrosarcoma of the soft tissues in the wall of the thorax after operation and irradiation of adenocarcinoma of the breast. *J Gynecol Obstet Biol Reprod* 1989; 18(4): 496–499

132 Ladefoged Chr, Nielsen B B. Primary chondrosarcoma of the breast: a case report and review of the literature. *Breast* 1984; 10(4): 26–28

133 Savage A P, Sagor G R, Dovey P. Osteosarcoma of the breast: a case report with an unusual diagnostic feature. *Clin Onco London* 1984; 10(3): 295–298

134 Going J J, Lumsden A B, Anderson T J. A classical osteogenic sarcoma of the breast: histology, immunohistochemistry and ultrastructure. *Histopathol* 1986; **10**: 631–641

135 Hajdu S I, Urban J A. Cancers metastatic to the breast. *Cancer* 1972; **29**: 1691–1696

136 Kelly C, Henderson D, Corris P. Breast lumps: rare presentation of oat cell carcinoma of lung. *J Clin Pathol* 1988; **41**: 171–172

137 Kumar P V, Esfahani F N, Salimi A. Choriocarcinoma metastatic to the breast diagnosed by fine needle aspiration. *Acta Cytol* 1991; **35**: 239–242

138 Matsuda M, Sone H, Ishiguro S et al. Fine needle aspiration cytology of malignant schwannoma metastatic to the breast. *Acta Cytol* 1989; **33**: 373–376

139 Lozowski M S, Faegenburg D, Mishriki Y, Lundy J. Carcinoid tumour metastatic to breast diagnosed by fine needle aspiration. *Acta Cytol* 1989; **2**: 191–194

140 Pettinato G, De-Chiara A, Insabato L, De-Renzo A. Fine needle aspiration biopsy of a granulocytic sarcoma (chloroma) of the breast. *Acta Cytol* 1988; **32**: 67–71

141 Corrigan C, Sewell C, Martin A. Recurrent Hodgkin's disease in the breast. *Acta Cytol* 1990; **34**: 669–672

142 Schwartz J G, Clark E G I. Fine needle aspiration biopsy of mycosis fungoides presenting as an ulcerating breast mass. *Arch Dermatol* 1988; **124**: 409–413

143 Yazdi H M. Cytopathology of endometrial adenocarcinoma metastases to the breast examined by fine needle aspiration. *Am J Clin Pathol* 1982; **78**: 559–563

144 Silverman J F, Feldman P S, Covell J L, Frable W J. Fine needle aspiration cytology of neoplasms metastatic to the breast. *Acta Cytol* 1987; **31**: 291–300

145 Sneige N, Zachariah S, Fanning T V et al. Fine needle aspiration cytology of metastatic neoplasms in the breast. *Am J Clin Pathol* 1989; **92**: 27–35

146 Ciatto S, Bravetti P, Cecchini S *et al*. The role of fine needle aspiration cytology in the differential diagnosis of suspected breast cancer local recurrences. *Tumori* 1990; **76**: 225–226

147 Malberger E, Edoute Y, Toledano O, Sapir D. Fine needle aspiration and cytologic findings of surgical scar lesions in women with breast cancer. *Cancer* 1992; **69**: 148–152

148 Dornfield J M, Thompson S K, Shurbaji M S. Radiation induced changes in the breast: a potential diagnostic pitfall on fine needle aspiration. *Diagn Cytopathol* 1992; **8**: 79–81

149 Peterse J L, Thunnissen F B J M, Van-Heerde P. Fine needle aspiration cytology of radiation-induced changes in nonneoplastic breast lesions. Possible pitfalls in cytodiagnosis. *Acta Cytol* 1989; **33**: 176–180

150 Girling A C, Hanby A M, Millis R R. Radiation and other pathological changes in breast tissue after conservation treatment for carcinoma. *J Clin Pathol* 1990; **43**: 152–156

151 Schnitt S J, Connolly J L, Harris J R, Cohen R B. Radiation-induced changes in the breast. *Hum Pathol* 1984; **15**: 545–550

152 Zbieranowski I, Le-riche J C, Jackson S M, Olivotto I. The use of sequential fine needle aspiration biopsy with flow cytometry to monitor radiation induced changes in breast carcinoma. *Anal Cell Pathol* 1992; **4**: 13–24

Alimentary system

10 The salivary glands

Jennifer A. Young and Adrian T. Warfield

Introduction

As early as 1933, Stewart, writing of his experience at the Memorial Hospital, New York, commented that 'parotid tumours are particularly suited to aspiration' and that he had examined 66 examples[1]. The foundations of current practice were established by the Karolinska group[2] who between 1964–76 published a series of six studies on FNA of the salivary glands[3-8]. By 1987, Layfield et al.[9] in a review of published work identified 36 papers which together contained reports on aspirates from 3000 lesions and many further papers containing detailed descriptions have appeared since then.

There is perhaps no tissue anywhere in the body that is subject to such a diverse and heterogeneous range of tumours and tumour-like conditions (see Table 10.1). While this results in fascinating cytopathology it also produces diagnostic limitations, which must be appreciated by both pathologist and clinician if the extensive benefits of the technique are to be fully and safely utilized in patient management.

Clinical applications

Clinical acumen allied to modern imaging techniques contributes much to the assessment of salivary gland disease, but findings are not uncommonly equivocal. In many instances, and particularly in cases of suspected neoplastic disease, microscopic examination is required for diagnosis. However, preoperative histological biopsy is hazardous as the use of a Vim-Silverman or Trucut needle may damage the facial nerve or lead to fistula formation, and is also associated with tumour seeding in the needle track. Intraoperative frozen section can give rise to inconvenient organizational problems and precludes prior planning of the surgical approach and informed discussion with the patient. Fine needle aspiration (FNA) is, however, virtually risk free[9,10]. Malignant cells have been identified microscopically in the needle track shortly after FNA[11] but reported clinical examples are exceptional.

Par excellence, cytology provides confirmation of benign disease in patients not undergoing surgery and confirmation of malignancy in those unsuitable for attempted curative surgery or with recurrent disease prior to palliative treatment. Overall, surgery can be avoided in between one third and one half of cases[12,13]. In patients undergoing radical surgery preoperative FNA enables the clinician to estimate the degree of urgency and to plan the surgical approach including, in the case of the parotid, the decision to preserve or sacrifice the facial nerve. A preoperative diagnosis also allows counselling of the patient prior to surgery.

With experience, FNA can substantially replace intraoperative frozen section although this is still required to assess the margins of excision. However, it cannot be considered an alternative in every case, as in some instances cytological diagnosis is imprecise, either because of the similarity which exists between the cytomorphology of certain disparate conditions, or because the material obtained by a fine needle is insufficient to adequately sample a large and possibly heterogeneous mass.

Technique

Standard FNA technique is suitable and is applicable not only to the parotid and submandibular glands, but also to the sublingual and minor salivary glands. Aspiration is facilitated by the use of a Cameco or similar syringe holder. The needle-only technique, as described by Zajdela et al.[14], can be employed for lesions that appear likely to be highly vascular. Immunosuppressed patients are prone to salivary gland disease and great care should be taken to avoid needlestick injuries. In high risk cases, the lump should be stabilized by the patient.

Caution is necessary if cystic fluid is aspirated, as this may be from either a simple non-neoplastic cyst or a cystic neoplasm such as Warthin's tumour or mucoepidermoid carcinoma. If at all possible, the wall of the 'cyst' should be re-aspirated in an effort to obtain representative cellular material from a solid area of the lesion. If microbiological culture is required, repeat aspiration for this purpose is advised, as division of a single aspirate is seldom satisfactory.

Diagnosis

The cytological interpretation of an aspirate from what is clinically suspected to be an enlarged salivary gland must be undertaken in two stages. It is first necessary to confirm that the mass is indeed of salivary gland origin and not one of the various other lesions that can mimic salivary gland disease. Once the anatomical site has been established, the cytopathologist can then proceed to consider specific salivary gland disorders and arrive at either a definitive or a differential diagnosis according to the nature of the cellular material.

Lesions which mimic salivary gland disease

The most frequently encountered problem is the distinction between enlarged lymph nodes and sialomegaly. Due to late encapsulation in foetal life, small lymph nodes are not uncommonly enclosed within the parotid. It is not possible to reliably distinguish between intraparotid lymphadenopathy and true salivary gland enlargement by palpation or imaging. FNA of a hyperplastic lymph node yields a mixed population of lymphocytes, follicle centre cells and 'tingible body' macrophages. If perinodal ductal or acinar tissue is traversed by the needle the resulting cell mixture is difficult to separate from salivary gland disease associated with lymphocytosis.

Similarly, metastatic malignancy within an intraparotid lymph node can mimic a primary salivary gland carcinoma. The origin is most commonly squamous cell carcinoma of the face or ear, or malignant melanoma. When a local primary source is clinically apparent it will aid the diagnosis, but the origin may be distant or occult. If the node is substantially replaced by squamous cell or anaplastic carcinoma, the distinction from a primary salivary gland neoplasm cannot be made on FNA preparations. Other entities which can mimic sialomegaly include branchial cleft cyst, nerve sheath tumours, carotid body tumours, parathyroid lesions, pilomatrixoma or other skin adnexal tumours, and soft tissue lesions such as nodular fasciitis and Kimura's disease[15–21].

Normal findings

Acinar cells are large, with abundant cytoplasm and small round uniform nuclei. The cytoplasm is finely granular in serous glands and clear or lightly vacuolated in mucous glands. Either type is fragile and easily disrupted by smearing, so that bare dispersed nuclei may be present in the background. When complete acini are aspirated the cells occur in lobulated groups.

The larger ducts are lined by columnar epithelium and the smaller ones by cuboidal cells. Normal epithelial cells are usually found in flat sheets displaying good cohesion and uniform morphology. Small pointed nuclei arising from myoepithelial cells may occasionally be identified between the epithelium and the basement membrane. Oncocytosis of both ductal and acinar tissue occurs with age and groups of polygonal oncocytes with granular cytoplasm are not uncommon in aspirates from the elderly (see also under 'Developmental disorders').

Non-neoplastic disease

A considerable number of non-neoplastic disorders of known and unknown aetiology occur. Some of these are uncommon but they are important in differential diagnosis and as possible causes of interpretive errors. Many are included under the heading of tumour-like lesions in the current WHO classification (see Table 10.1).

Developmental disorders

Ectopic salivary glands

Salivary gland tissue at other than normal anatomical locations is termed ectopic (heterotopic). The most common sites are periparotid lymph nodes, the middle ear and the lower neck, but it can also occur in more remote regions. Ectopic salivary gland tissue may be the explanation for an otherwise puzzling aspirate. Either normal acinar cells or material indicating benign or malignant disease can be encountered, as any of the salivary gland disorders found in normally placed salivary gland tissue can develop.

Adenomatoid hyperplasia

This is a rare condition of the mucous glands, which occurs almost exclusively in the palate. Its nature is not fully understood but is probably hamartomatous. Clinically, it is generally misdiagnosed as a neoplasm. Aufdemorte *et al.*[22] reported FNA from a case. It is a potential source of a false positive diagnosis of mucoepidermoid carcinoma.

Polycystic disease

Polycystic (dysgenetic) disease of the parotid glands is a rare malformation of the ductal system. It must be included in the differential diagnosis of cystic lesions.

Obstructive disorders

Mucus retention cyst (mucocele)

This is a true cyst lined by epithelium and is probably caused by partial obstruction to the ductal system. When tense and deep seated, mucus retention cysts may lead to clinical suspicion of neoplasia and are therefore not infrequently targets for FNA. Rupture may lead to so-called mucus extravasation phenomenon with muciphages and often a foreign body type giant cell reaction.

Cytological findings

▶ Watery or viscous fluid
▶ Scanty cellularity
▶ Leucocytes and macrophages in variable numbers
▶ Few columnar cell sheets
▶ Many leucocytes and epithelial atypia if secondarily infected

The fluid is watery or viscous depending upon whether the epithelium is predominantly serous or mucinous. It is relatively hypocellular, containing only a few leucocytes and macrophages and perhaps occasional sheets of columnar cells. Secondary infection, however, is not uncommon and then leucocytosis is pronounced and the epithelial cells display reactive and inflammatory changes that can result in marked morphological alterations.

Many tumours contain cystic areas. Small quantities of fluid may be aspirated from both Warthin's tumour and pleomorphic adenoma. Mucinous material may be obtained from a mucoepidermoid carcinoma, acinic cell carcinoma may be cystic and extensive necrosis and liquefaction in high-grade carcinomas can also result in a fluid aspirate. Branchial cysts also occur in the anterior area of the parotid. As indicated under 'Technique', it is most important to re-needle the palpable wall of any 'cyst' so that evidence of a malignant tumour is not overlooked.

Sialolithiasis and sialadenitis *(Fig. 10.1, 10.2)*

Calculi (sialoliths) form in the salivary ducts as the result of mineralization of debris. The submandibular gland is the most common site. Clinically, calculi are associated with pain and swelling and retrograde infection results in *acute* or *chronic sialadenitis*. Changes in the duct wall include squamous, oncocytic and mucous cell metaplasia, and if obstruction is longstanding atrophy and fibrosis of acinar tissue will ensue. Cystic change with a variety of crystalloids may occasionally be encountered[23].

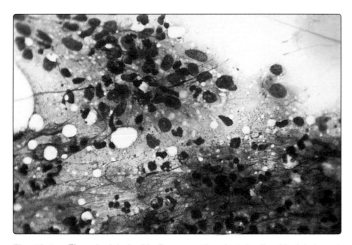

Fig. 10.1 Chronic sialadenitis. Degenerative ductal cells with debris and inflammatory cells. (MGG × MP)

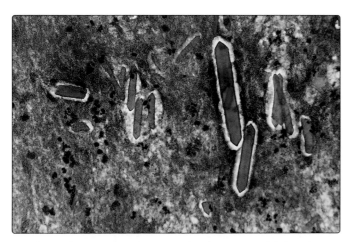

Fig. 10.2 Cystic change with crystalloids. Polymorphs, debris and rhomboid crystals aspirated from a cystic swelling associated with acute sialadenitis. (MGG × MP)

Cytological findings

▶ Scanty aspirate
▶ Ductal cells with possible metaplasia or atypia
▶ Paucity of acinar cells
▶ Inflammatory cells in background debris
▶ Possible cystic change and crystalloids

Aspirates are generally hypocellular and acinar cells are unusual due to the atrophic changes. Severe morphological alterations of the ductal cells are possible, including anisonucleosis and hyperchromasia, and evidence of squamous metaplasia is not uncommon. Polymorphs or lymphocytes and debris are present in the background. The overall cytological appearance can be quite worrying. In particular, *chronic sclerosing sialadenitis* (Küttner tumour) of the submandibular gland, which presents as a firm mass, is associated with marked morphological atypia.

Infections and systemic diseases

Acute sialadenitis

Acute sialadenitis is due to specific bacterial or viral infection such as mumps parotitis. It is usually clinically obvious and FNA is not indicated.

Acquired immunodeficiency syndrome (AIDS)

One of the manifestations of HIV infection is *cystic lymphoid hyperplasia of the salivary glands* in which there is proliferation of the epithelium, cyst formation and lymphocytosis. The resulting lesion is somewhat similar to the changes seen in Sjögren's syndrome. The clinical, histological and cytological features have been described by Finfer *et al.*[24,25] and Chhieng *et al.*[26] *Cytomegalovirus* (CMV) can also cause parotitis in AIDS patients but is generally only one manifestation of systemic infection.

Granulomatous sialadenitis

Granulomatous disease has many causes. Evidence of salivary gland involvement is present in about 6% of cases of *sarcoidosis*[27]. Multinucleated giant cells and clusters of epithelioid cells against a background of lymphocytes are seen in aspirates[28,29]. Tuberculosis, fungal infection, cat scratch disease, brucellosis and toxoplasmosis are included in the differential diagnosis of granulomatous sialadenitis and lymphadenitis, but all are infectious lesions and primary investigation by FNA is unlikely.

Tumour-like lesions

Sialadenosis *(Fig. 10.3)*

This is a non-inflammatory, often bilateral, swelling of the salivary glands, particularly of the parotid. It is due to hypertrophy of the acinar cells. It is associated with systemic diseases such as diabetes. Characteristically, numerous acinar cells are present, the reverse of the findings of chronic sialadenitis, and ductal cells are sparse. Care must be taken not to confuse this entity with well-differentiated acinic cell carcinoma[30].

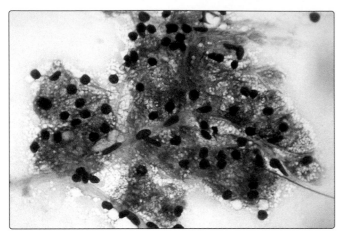

Fig. 10.3 Sialadenosis. One of numerous large groups of plump acinar cells from a case of bilateral sialadenosis of the parotid glands. (MGG × MP)

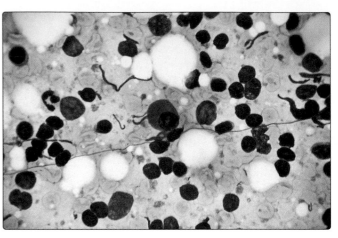

Fig. 10.4 Lymphoepithelial disease. Cells of the lymphoid series with a plasma cell in the centre of the field. (MGG × OI)

Lipomatosis

The salivary glands are invested by fibrofatty connective tissue. The parotid gland and, to a lesser extent, the submandibular gland normally contain fat cells and their fat content generally rises with advancing age. Lipomatosis refers to a diffuse excess of interstitial fat, which may occur in obesity and diabetes and occasionally presents as a swelling. Fatty replacement of parenchyma may also be a consequence of glandular atrophy. Intraparotid and periparotid lipomata and sialolipomata occur and pleomorphic adenoma may show varying degrees of adipocytic differentiation[31]. The interpretation of the significance of fat cells in an aspirate, therefore, depends very much upon their context, the presence of other components and the adequacy of sampling.

Oncocytosis

Foci of oncocytic change in salivary glands and ductal epithelium become more common with increasing age. More diffuse oncocytosis (oncocytic hyperplasia) may occur and it can be difficult, on occasion even impossible, to discriminate between this and oncocytoma or paucilymphocytic Warthin's tumour. Areas of oncocytic differentiation can also occur in pleomorphic adenoma. The interpretation of oncocytic cells in an aspirate depends therefore upon the other elements present and the context of the examination[32].

Lymphoepithelial disease *(Fig. 10.4)*

A spectrum of diseases, ranging from benign lymphoepithelial lesion (*localized myoepithelial sialadenitis or MESA*) to systemic *Sjögren's syndrome* are included in this benign sialadenopathy, believed to be of autoimmune origin[33,34]. The condition is commonest in middle-aged or elderly women and is usually bilateral and symmetrical although sometimes initially unilateral. In cases of Sjögren's syndrome, other manifestations such as dryness of eyes and mouth, rheumatoid arthritis and hypergammaglobulinaemia

are present. Benign lymphoepithelial lesion is the presentation likely to be encountered by cytopathologists.

Cytological findings

▶ Many reactive lymphoid cells, plasma cells and histiocytes
▶ Clusters of myoepithelial cells sometimes present

FNA preparations contain numerous lymphocytes mixed with follicle centre cells, plasma cells and histiocytes. Clusters of myoepithelial cells, if present, are a helpful pointer to the disease but they are not always evident in aspirates. A florid lymphocytosis may be produced by many other conditions including chronic sialadenitis, Warthin's tumour, mucoepidermoid carcinoma and acinic cell carcinoma[35]. Aspiration of perisalivary lymph nodes is another source of lymphoid tissue. The diagnosis of benign lymphoepithelial lesion is best established by correlating the clinical and the cytopathological findings. Benign lymphoepithelial lesion can progress to malignant lymphoma and rarely, myoepithelial or squamous cell carcinoma develops[36].

Necrotizing sialometaplasia

This is a rare condition, which causes ulceration of the palate and is probably of ischaemic aetiology. It very occasionally occurs in other sites following surgery or irradiation. Necrosis of acinar cells is associated with pseudoepitheliomatous hyperplasia and bizarre squamous metaplasia[37,38]. Such material can give rise to a false suspicion of squamous cell or mucoepidermoid carcinoma on histological examination and although FNA material has not personally been examined there is no reason to suppose that the same difficulty would not be present.

Tumours of the salivary gland

Salivary gland tumours are very uncommon. Auclair *et al.*[39] quote the annual incidence around the world as between 0.4 and 13.5 cases per 100,000 population. The percentage of malignant tumours varies from 21.8% to 36.8%. Although the total number of neoplasms arising in the minor glands is much less than in the major glands, the relative incidence of malignancy is very much higher in the former.

Classification

Because of the diverse and heterogeneous nature of salivary gland neoplasms, numerous classifications have evolved over the years[40–43]. The revised World Health Organization (WHO)[42] classification includes an extensive review of adenomas and the introduction of a number of uncommon carcinomas. The essential details of this classification are shown on Table 10.1. Tumour-like lesions (section 7, in Table 10.1), are entities which may be mistaken for true tumours. Descriptions of the majority of these have been given earlier in this chapter.

Table 10.1 WHO histological classification of salivary gland tumours

1. Adenomas
Pleomorphic adenoma
Myoepithelioma
Basal cell adenoma
Warthin's tumour
  (adenolymphoma)
Oncocytoma
Canalicular adenoma
Sebaceous adenoma
Ductal papilloma
Cystadenoma
 	
2. Carcinomas
Acinic cell carcinoma
Mucoepidermoid
  carcinoma
  Low-grade/well
  differentiated
  High-grade/poorly
  differentiated
Adenoid cystic carcinoma
  Glandular/tubular
  Solid
Polymorphous low-grade
  carcinoma
Epithelial-myoepithelial
  carcinoma
Salivary duct carcinoma
Basal cell adenocarcinoma
Sebaceous carcinoma
Oncocytic carcinoma
Papillary
  cystadenocarcinoma
Mucinous
  adenocarcinoma
Adenocarcinoma NOS
Squamous cell carcinoma
Carcinoma in pleomorphic
  adenoma
Myoepithelial carcinoma
	Small cell carcinoma
	Undifferentiated
	  carcinoma
	Other carcinomas
	
	3. Non-epithelial tumours
	Angiomas
	Lipomas
	Neural tumours
	Other benign
	  mesenchymal tumours
	Sarcomas
	
	4. Malignant lymphomas
	Extranodal lymphoma of
	  salivary gland
	Lymphoma of salivary
	  gland nodes
	
	5. Secondary tumours
	6. Unclassified tumours
	7. Tumour-like lesions
	Sialadenosis
	Oncocytosis
	Necrotizing
	  sialometaplasia (salivary
	  gland infarction)
	Benign lymphoepithelial
	  lesion
	Salivary gland cysts
	  Mucocoeles
	  Salivary duct cysts
	  Lymphoepithelial cysts
	  Dysgenetic (polycystic)
	  disease
	Chronic sclerosing
	  sialadenitis of
	  submandibular gland
	  (Küttner tumour)
	Cystic lymphoid
	  hyperplasia in AIDS

Benign salivary gland neoplasms

According to the WHO classification of 1972[40] all benign adenomas not corresponding to pleomorphic adenoma (benign mixed tumour) were included under the rubric of 'monomorphic adenoma' and often little effort was expended to further subclassify them. The revised WHO classification of 1991[42] attempts to refine this group of heterogeneous tumours by separation into morphologically or clinicopathologically distinct entities. It must, however, be acknowledged that, when dealing with such a potentially diverse group of lesions, the morphological variation acceptable within each category and a degree of overlap between each tumour subtype often makes precise classification a challenge for histopathologists, and even more so for the cytopathologist.

Pleomorphic adenoma *(Figs 10.5–10.7)*

Pleomorphic adenoma, the so-called benign mixed tumour, is by far the most common of all salivary gland neoplasms and, particularly in specimens from the parotid, is the

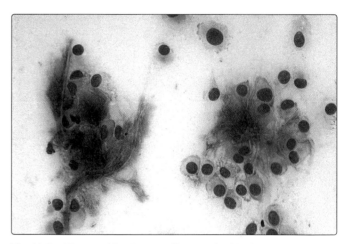

Fig. 10.5 Pleomorphic adenoma. Clusters of epithelial cells intermingled with fibrillary mesenchymal material. (MGG × MP)

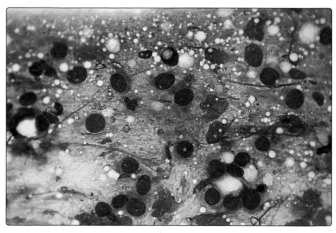

Fig. 10.6 Pleomorphic adenoma. Large dispersed abnormal epithelial cells from a tumour that contained an area of non-invasive carcinoma. (MGG × HP)

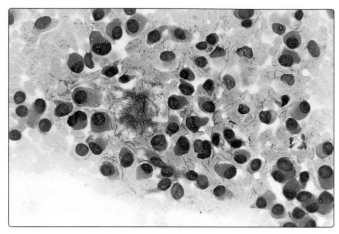

Fig. 10.7 Pleomorphic adenoma. Dispersed plasmacytoid cells and central fragment of mesenchymal material from a myoepithelial cell rich pleomorphic adenoma. (MGG × MP)

lesion most likely to be encountered in FNA practice. The tumour occurs most often in patients aged 30–50 years and is slightly more common in females. It presents as a painless mass, initially mobile, sometimes multinodular, and is occasionally associated with tumours of different types in other salivary glands. Histologically, the typical tumour consists of glandular structures composed of a double layer of epithelial and myoepithelial cells embedded in a mucoid myxomatous stroma. Squamous metaplasia, oncocytosis, mucus production or sebaceous or adipocytic differentiation[31] may occur and the mesenchymal component can undergo chondroid change or even ossification. Cystic areas form in some tumours. In the WHO classification[42] tumours with a high percentage of myoepithelial cells are classified as myoepitheliomas (see later) rather than myoepithelial-rich pleomorphic adenomas.

Cytological findings

▶ Cellular aspirates with large amount of myxoid background matrix
▶ Epithelial cells singly or in sheets
▶ Cell nuclei vary in size but have uniform chromatin
▶ Spindle-shaped mesenchymal cells
▶ Chondroid or other metaplastic changes sometimes seen

The cytological diagnosis of the great majority of pleomorphic adenomas is quite straightforward. Aspirates contain plentiful epithelial cells, which are closely intermingled with loose clusters of mesenchymal cells and fibrillary mucomyxomatous background substance. The epithelial cells lie singly or in sheets and have nuclei of uniform chromasia, although they may vary a little in size. The mesenchymal cells are rounded or spindly with elongated nuclei. The background substance is closely tangled with cells and stains pinkish-grey with Papanicolaou and bright magenta with MGG. Chondroid

change is indicated by a blue reaction with the latter technique. Published studies based on these criteria confirm a high level of accuracy for FNA diagnosis of pleomorphic adenoma[5,9,12,13,44–48].

The paper by Klijanienko and Viehl[48] reviews 412 pleomorphic adenomas, correlating the cytological and histological findings.

Diagnostic pitfalls

Problems in interpretation occur for two reasons: the predominance of one element leading to the apparent absence of the other components, or the presence of atypical cytomorphological features. If the epithelial cells are very numerous and the mesenchymal material is not readily apparent the tumour may be misdiagnosed as some other type of adenoma. Clinically, however, this is of little significance. If the mucomyxomatous component is very abundant it may overwhelm the few epithelial cells present and the lesion may be mistaken for a retention cyst. This is more likely to happen if only MGG stained slides are examined, as the strong magenta reaction may mask other cellular components.

More serious is false suspicion of malignancy[5,9,44,48]. Very occasional examples of pleomorphic adenoma are densely cellular and display marked cytological atypia. This is reflected in FNA specimens in which the epithelial cells can show loss of cohesion and nuclear enlargement and hyperchromasia to a worrying degree. It is important not to over diagnose these changes. On close histological examination many so-called 'atypical' pleomorphic adenomas contain areas of intracapsular malignant change (non-invasive carcinoma, carcinoma *in situ*). This is a very much less serious entity than invasive carcinoma ex-pleomorphic adenoma (see under 'Carcinomas') and while an atypical pleomorphic adenoma necessitates excision with a wide margin, it carries the same excellent prognosis as an 'usual-type' tumour and does not require management as a clinical carcinoma. True carcinoma ex-pleomorphic adenoma is a high-grade invasive neoplasm, which requires much more aggressive treatment and carries a poor prognosis.

A few pleomorphic adenomas contain areas with adenoid cystic-like characteristics[48]. Globules of basement membrane material may be seen in these aspirates. Great caution must be exercised not to confuse this appearance with true adenoid cystic carcinoma. The distinction can be difficult even on histological specimens. If the globules are few and other cellular features of pleomorphic adenoma are present, false suspicion of malignancy should not be raised. Mucin production by pleomorphic adenomas[49] is another difficulty and the differential diagnosis then includes Warthin's tumour and low-grade mucoepidermoid carcinoma. Extensive squamous metaplasia may also raise

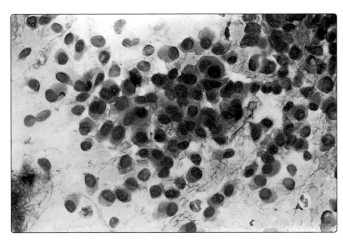

Fig. 10.8 Myoepithelioma. Clusters of small plasmacytoid cells devoid of any mesenchymal material from a tumour in the palate. (MGG × MP)

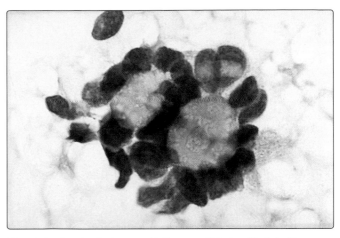

Fig. 10.9 Basal cell adenoma. Uniform small dark epithelial cells arranged around basement membrane material. Note the similarity to adenoid cystic carcinoma. (MGG × OI)

the possibility of mucoepidermoid carcinoma but careful examination of the characteristics of the squamous cells will resolve this problem.

Myoepithelioma *(Fig. 10.8)*

Myoepithelioma (myoepithelial adenoma) in its pure form is a rare, benign tumour composed exclusively of myoepithelial cells, devoid of any stromal component[50]. Many authorities however, would accept a minor epithelial subpopulation, usually less than 5% tumour volume, within this definition. There is a convincing argument for regarding myoepithelioma as one extreme manifestation within the spectrum of appearances of pleomorphic adenoma and absolute discrimination between myoepithelial cell-rich pleomorphic adenoma and myoepithelioma is of little biological consequence. The potential mimicry of other benign or malignant spindle cell or clear cell neoplasms, on the other hand, is of much greater clinical importance. The malignant counterpart of myoepithelioma is myoepithelial carcinoma. With experience the cytomorphological features of myoepithelioma are recognizable in FNA material[51].

Cytological findings

- ▶ Loosely cohesive fusiform or dendritic cells
- ▶ Epithelioid, clear cell or hyaline (plasmacytoid) cells may be a component or predominate
- ▶ Ovoid nuclei with finely dispersed chromatin
- ▶ Little or no epithelial cell population
- ▶ No stromal component

Basal cell adenoma *(Fig. 10.9)*

Basal cell adenomas are a group of benign ductal tumours, further subclassification of which is sometimes problematical[50]. In general, they comprise well-polarized basaloid cells, often with peripheral palisading and accompanying hyaline stroma. A variety of histological growth patterns such as solid, tubular, trabecular and membranous may be encountered and this diversity is recapitulated in FNA material. The membranous variant ('dermal analogue tumour') resembles an eccrine cylindroma of the skin and may occur either in isolation or in association with a variety of cutaneous adnexal neoplasms. The malignant counterpart of these adenomas is basal cell adenocarcinoma.

The hyaline stroma is not uncommonly seen in FNA as metachromatic globules or droplets mantled by epithelial cells, a pattern akin to that in adenoid cystic carcinoma. Such a 'pseudo-adenoid cystic' appearance may also occur in pleomorphic adenoma, basal cell adenocarcinoma and epithelial-myoepithelial carcinoma. With experience, critical examination of the shape and intensity of staining of the stroma, the cytonuclear morphology and any background content of a smear will often facilitate a correct diagnosis, but the differences are at best subtle and, on occasion, definitive interpretation may not be feasible[52,53].

The potential pitfall of mistaking basal cell adenoma for adenoid cystic carcinoma is one that must be kept in mind by all who report FNA of the salivary glands. The consequences of unnecessary sacrifice of the facial nerve are considerable.

Canalicular adenoma is an uncommon related tumour composed of duct-like epithelial structures without a myoepithelial cell layer. It shows a predilection for the upper lip and often undergoes cystic degeneration.

Warthin's tumour (adenolymphoma) *(Fig. 10.10)*

The great majority of these adenomas occur in the parotid[50]. They are much more common in males than in females and most occur in middle-aged or elderly patients. They grow slowly, are often fluctuant and can be bilateral or unilaterally multicentric. Histologically, Warthin's tumour is composed of glandular, often cystic, papillary structures

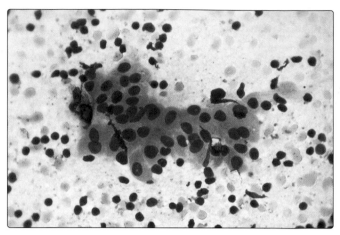

Fig. 10.10   Warthin's tumour. A flat sheet of oncocytic cells surrounded by lymphocytes. (MGG × MP)

with a stroma, which contains lymphoid tissue. The epithelium is double-layered and predominantly oncocytic but mucous or goblet cells and areas of squamous metaplasia may be present. Oncocytic cells are particularly susceptible to trauma and Warthin's tumours may show total or subtotal infarction, either spontaneously or following FNA.

Cytological findings

▶ Watery or mucoid aspirate
▶ Sheets of large pale columnar oncocytes
▶ Admixture of lymphocytes
▶ Background debris

It is usual on aspiration to obtain a small quantity of watery or mucoid fluid, a helpful diagnostic pointer. On microscopy, sheets of flat polyhedral oncocytes are scattered among amorphous debris mixed with lymphocytes[4,54]. Mast cells are common[55,56]. If the epithelial cells are few, the tumour can be mistaken for a non-neoplastic cyst. Laurica et al.[57] and Ballo et al.[58] have highlighted possible sources of diagnostic error.

Oncocytoma

Oncocytoma (oncocytic adenoma) is a rare, benign tumour composed of oncocytes (oxyphil cells)[50]. It differs from Warthin's tumour in that it is more usually unicentric, rarely cystic and contains no significant lymphocytic cell population. Its malignant counterpart is oncocytic carcinoma.

It is well recognized that benign oncocytic cells may exhibit a worrisome degree of nuclear atypia. Conversely, malignant oncocytes may appear deceptively monomorphic with bland nuclear features and, therefore, sometimes the best that can be attained is a diagnosis of 'oncocytic neoplasm', relaying the differential diagnosis with the caveat that malignancy cannot be excluded. Other pitfalls include degenerate oncocytes (pyknocytes) which possess

'pseudokeratinized' orangeophilic cytoplasm masquerading as squamous cells and the problem of clear cell change. Metastatic renal, thyroid and apocrine mammary carcinoma should never be forgotten.

Sebaceous adenoma, other adenomas and ductal papilloma

These are all rare benign tumours, uncommonly aspirated[50]. *Sebaceous adenoma* and *lymphadenoma* are comparable to Warthin's tumour, albeit with sebaceous rather than oncocytic epithelium. Their malignant counterpart is sebaceous carcinoma.

Evidence of sebaceous differentiation may infrequently be seen in normal salivary parenchyma, pleomorphic adenoma, Warthin's tumour proper and mucoepidermoid carcinoma. Voluminous, clear and microvacuolated cytoplasm with round, isomorphic nuclei are the hallmarks of benign sebaceous cells.

Several histological subtypes of ductal papilloma are recognized and usually show a cystic architecture[59]. Papillary and mucinous cystadenomas should also be included in the differential diagnosis of FNA from a cystic lesion.

The existence of *clear cell adenoma* is a contentious issue[60]. Most clear cell tumours in the salivary glands represent malignancy of one sort or another and the temptation to make this benign diagnosis must be approached with extreme caution.

Malignant salivary gland neoplasms

The earlier classifications of salivary gland tumours established the histopathology of the more common types of salivary gland carcinoma and the cytological features of these are now well described. Recent classifications and monographs[42,61] include a number of new or very uncommon malignant tumours, the cytopathology of which is not yet fully explored.

Acinic cell carcinoma *(Fig. 10.11)*

World-wide, acinic cell carcinoma accounts for about 10% of malignant salivary gland tumours. Over 80% occur in the parotid[61]. They are slightly more common in females and can occur at any age, with a mean age of 44 years. They display a spectrum of growth patterns described as solid, microcystic, papillary cystic and follicular[42]. However, the acinar cell is the basis of the terminology and the cytological recognition of well-differentiated acinic cell carcinoma. The more poorly differentiated examples and the less common subtypes are more difficult to recognize.

Cytological findings

▶ Large loosely cohesive cells with fragile granular cytoplasm and small dark nuclei
▶ Bland monomorphic picture
▶ Clean background with bare nuclei but no necrosis

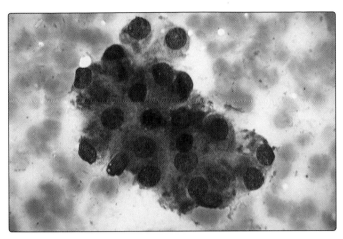

Fig. 10.11 Acinic cell carcinoma. Clusters of large acinic cells containing numerous intracytoplasmic granules. (MGG × OI)

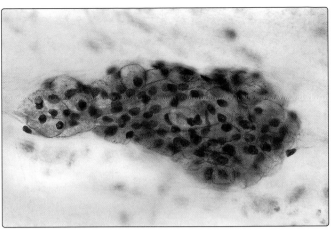

Fig. 10.12 Mucoepidermoid carcinoma. Mucus secreting cells from low-grade carcinoma. (Papanicolaou × MP)

▶ Possible lymphocytosis
▶ Possible evidence of cystic change

The cytological appearance is usually deceptively bland with numerous large delicate cells, granular cytoplasm and uniform nuclei. The granules are purple with Papanicolaou staining red with MGG, and can be highlighted with periodic acid-Schiff. A marked lymphocytosis is seen in about 10% of tumours and evidence of cystic change can be present. The more poorly differentiated carcinomas are difficult to type and are likely to be classified as adenocarcinoma NOS.

The differential diagnosis of well-differentiated acinic cell carcinoma includes, in particular, sialadenosis and, in cases where there is marked lymphocytosis, Warthin's tumour. Mucoepidermoid carcinoma is the most likely primary malignant differential diagnosis but the possibility of metastatic renal cell carcinoma must also be considered. Good descriptions are given by Palmo et al.[62] and Nagel et al[63]. In the latter paper 68% of 58 acinic cell carcinomas were correctly typed by FNA.

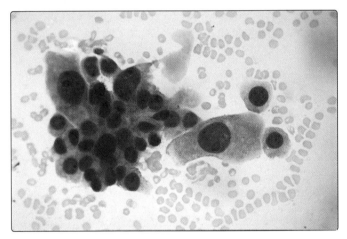

Fig. 10.13 Mucoepidermoid carcinoma. Polygonal malignant squamous epithelial cells and smaller intermediate type cells. (MGG × HP)

Mucoepidermoid carcinoma (Figs 10.12–10.14)

In the files of the Armed Forces Institute of Pathology (AFIP) mucoepidermoid carcinoma is the most common malignant tumour, accounting for 20% of all carcinomas arising in both the major and minor glands[61]. However, there is quite a marked geographic distribution and the incidence in the United Kingdom is very much less (2%)[61].

As the name implies, the tumour has a bimorphic glandular and squamous structure. However, three cell types are identifiable: mucus producing cells, squamous cells and cells intermediate between the two. The *low-grade subtype* contains cystic spaces lined with vacuolated mucus-secreting cells. Intermediate type cells and squamous epithelium are also present. The *high-grade subtype* is a solid, invasive tumour and the abnormal squamous cell component predominates. Prognosis is directly related to the tumour grade.

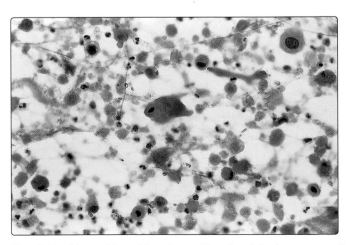

Fig. 10.14 Mucoepidermoid carcinoma. Hyperkeratinized squamous cell debris from a high-grade carcinoma. (Papanicolaou × LP)

Cytological findings

Low-grade tumours:

▶ Extracellular mucoid material
▶ Large vacuolated glandular tumour cells
▶ Intermediate cells with sparse cytoplasm
▶ Inconspicuous malignant squamous type cells

High-grade tumours:

▶ Numerous malignant squamous type cells
▶ Intermediate cells not prominent
▶ Absence of mucus and glandular type cells
▶ Necrosis

The appearance of mucoepidermoid carcinoma in FNA was described by Zajicek et al.[8] and a statistical analysis of the cytomorphological features published by Cohen et al. in 1990[64]. Klijanienko and Viehl[65] have reviewed 50 cases and provide excellent details. Specimens from low-grade tumours contain abundant mucoid material aspirated from the cystic areas coexisting with large pale cells with vacuolated cytoplasm. Intermediate type cells, which have sparse cytoplasm and dark nuclei, are also present but squamous cells may be inconspicuous and display little abnormality. Aspirates from high-grade subtypes show plentiful squamous cells with some intermediate cells but the mucus-producing component of the tumour is seldom evident. The squamous cells show the characteristic cytological stigmata of malignancy including pleomorphic or pyknotic, hyperchromatic nuclei. If well-keratinized forms are present, the classical bright orangeophilic cytoplasm will be seen with Papanicolaou stain.

Diagnostic pitfalls

Problems of diagnosis may be encountered with both the low-grade and high-grade subtype of mucoepidermoid carcinoma. If there are large cystic areas only acellular mucin may be obtained and the tumour mistaken for a non-neoplastic cyst, hence the importance of re-aspirating the wall of cystic lesions, as previously emphasized. Chronic sialadenitis with squamous metaplasia, necrotizing sialometaplasia and adenomatoid hyperplasia are other non-neoplastic conditions, which might be considered in differential diagnosis. Mucus-producing cells, however, are not a feature of sialadenitis and the other two conditions are rare and occur mainly in the palate, a highly unusual site for mucoepidermoid carcinoma. While diagnosis of the high-grade subtype as a malignant tumour is quite straightforward if the aspirate consists solely of squamous cells, precise typing may be impossible. Malignant squamous cells from mucoepidermoid carcinoma, primary squamous cell carcinoma and secondary squamous carcinoma metastatic to intraparotid lymph nodes appear identical in smears and the three entities cannot be distinguished. Very poorly differentiated mucoepidermoid carcinoma will appear similar to undifferentiated primary or metastatic carcinoma.

Adenoid cystic carcinoma (Figs 10.15–10.17)

According to the AFIP, adenoid cystic carcinoma accounts for about 4% of all benign and malignant salivary gland tumours[61]. Since the incorporation of polymorphous low-grade adenocarcinoma into the classification of salivary gland neoplasms[42], the perceived incidence of adenoid cystic carcinoma has fallen, especially in the minor salivary glands[61].

Clinically, the tumour presents as a slowly enlarging mass except in the more aggressive histological subtypes, growth of which can be rapid. Pain due to perineural infiltration is an almost constant symptom. The incidence increases from middle age, with an equal distribution in both sexes.

Like many other salivary gland neoplasms, adenoid cystic carcinoma has a varied histological pattern. Three main

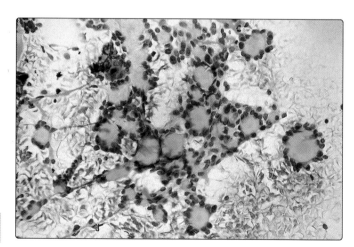

Fig. 10.15 Adenoid cystic carcinoma. Groups of small monomorphic malignant cells arranged around circular 'holes' filled with pale, translucent basement membrane substance. (Papanicolaou × LP)

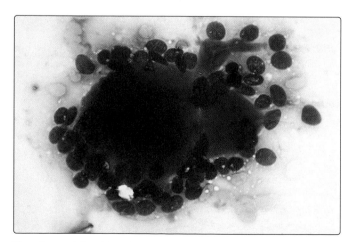

Fig. 10.16 Adenoid cystic carcinoma. Bright magenta globules of basement membrane material surrounded by small malignant cells. (MGG × HP)

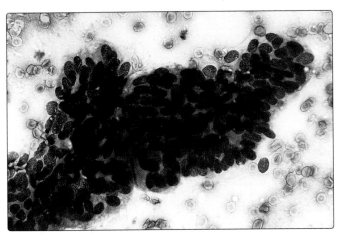

Fig. 10.17   Adenoid cystic carcinoma. Small overlapping malignant cells from a solid pattern carcinoma. (MGG × MP)

types are described: *cribiform, tubular* and *solid*. The cribiform variety is the most common and classically has a 'Swiss cheese' pattern with nests and cords of relatively monomorphic cells arranged concentrically around circular spaces (pseudocysts) filled with mucinous-type material believed to be of basal lamina origin. In the tubular variety the neoplastic cells are similar in appearance but are arranged in ductal structures, which appear tubular when viewed in longitudinal section. The solid variety, which carries the worst prognosis, contains no obvious circular spaces or tubules, displays greater nuclear pleomorphism and may contain areas of necrosis.

Cytological findings

▶ Cellular aspirate
▶ Clusters of monomorphic tumour cells with hyperchromatic nuclei
▶ Globules of mucoid material surrounded by tumour cells in cribriform type
▶ Similar material in elongated processes especially in tubular type
▶ Small anaplastic malignant cells in solid type

The original description of the cytopathology of adenoid cystic carcinoma was provided by Eneroth and Zajicek *et al.*[6] and the main features are substantiated by later studies including major series by Klijanienko and Viehl[66] and Nagel *et al.*[67]. Despite the nomenclature, there is no true cystic component to the tumour and it is most exceptional to obtain fluid on aspiration.

FNA specimens are hypercellular and composed of clusters of small, relatively monomorphic epithelial cells with hyperchromatic nuclei. Characteristically, these are arranged around apparent 'holes' which correspond to the circular spaces (pseudocysts) seen in the cribriform histological pattern. The 'holes' are filled with homogenous globules of mucoid substance. These are translucent, pale

blue and inconspicuous with Papanicolaou stain but are a prominent bright magenta with MGG (Fig. 10.16). Finger-like processes of similar material running between groups of cells can also sometimes be seen. These correspond to areas of tubular differentiation. The solid variety of adenoid cystic carcinoma seldom displays the above distinguishing basement membrane material and resembles a small celled anaplastic carcinoma on FNA.

Diagnostic pitfalls

The globules of amorphous material surrounded by haloes of cells are the clue to establishing a cytological diagnosis of cribriform adenoid cystic carcinoma. When they are numerous, and the clinical features are in keeping, in particular, evidence of involvement of the facial nerve, then the diagnosis is secure. However, as previously indicated, small numbers of similar globules may very occasionally be seen in pleomorphic adenomas. The resemblance between FNA from basal cell adenoma and adenoid cystic carcinoma has also been stressed. As the surgical management of adenoma and carcinoma is quite different accurate distinction is therefore vital. The subtle variation in the character of the matrix of the globules may be helpful in distinguishing the benign tumours[66,67]. In the latter the globules are fewer, less dense and less intensely staining with MGG. However, it is an advisable and safe working rule for cytopathologists that a definitive diagnosis of adenoid cystic carcinoma should not be rendered in the absence of corroborative clinical evidence of pain due to perineural infiltration. This is particularly important with parotid lesions as pleomorphic adenoma is so common in comparison to adenoid cystic carcinoma at this site. Radical surgery for adenoid cystic carcinoma should not be based solely on FNA. Other carcinomas including basal cell carcinoma, epithelial-myoepithelial carcinoma, and low-grade polymorphous adenocarcinoma may all contain globules of basement membrane-like material, but here the distinction is clinically much less important as the surgical treatment is the same as that for adenoid cystic carcinoma. The solid variety of adenoid cystic carcinoma is likely to be called anaplastic carcinoma on cytological diagnosis, but this is of minimal importance in patient management.

Carcinoma ex-pleomorphic adenoma *(Fig. 10.18)*

The entity of malignancy ex-pleomorphic adenoma (malignant mixed tumour) is conventionally taken to encompass the categories of carcinoma ex-pleomorphic adenoma, carcinosarcoma ex-pleomorphic adenoma, and benign, metastasing pleomorphic adenoma. Non-invasive carcinoma (intracapsular carcinoma, carcinoma *in situ*) is also included in this category in the WHO classification[42] (see under 'Pleomorphic adenoma').

Carcinoma ex-pleomorphic adenoma is one of the most common types of carcinoma of the parotid and sublingual

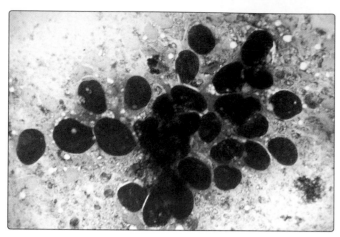

Fig. 10.18 Carcinoma ex-pleomorphic adenoma. Anaplastic malignant cells from a carcinoma in the parotid gland of a patient with a long history of recurrent pleomorphic adenoma. (MGG × OI)

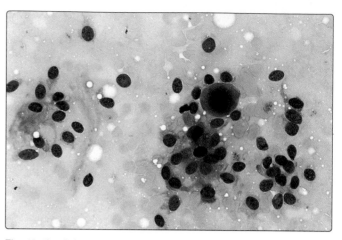

Fig. 10.19 Polymorphous low-grade carcinoma. Uniform sized malignant cells with micropapillary architecture and a solitary globule of basement membrane substance. (MGG × MP) (By kind permission of Dr Ivan Robinson)

glands in the United Kingdom. It accounts for approximately 5% of all epithelial neoplasms and about 20% of all carcinomas of the salivary glands[68]. The risk of malignant transformation of pleomorphic adenoma increases with time and also with recurrences following surgery. A period of accelerated growth and/or the onset of pain engrafted upon a longstanding static or slowly enlarging lump are pointers to malignant transformation. Virtually any pattern or combination of patterns of carcinoma may supervene[61], the commonest being a mixed histological pattern high-grade carcinoma, sometimes not further classifiable. Rarer examples of pure histological subtypes and even low-grade carcinomas are, however, recorded[42,61].

The histological diagnosis of carcinoma ex-pleomorphic adenoma hinges on the recognition of elements of a benign pleomorphic adenoma being admixed with a carcinomatous cell population. Reliable separation of non-invasive (intracapsular, *in situ*) and true invasive carcinoma ex-pleomorphic adenoma is difficult and not always achievable on FNA material. The cellularity, degree of nuclear atypia and presence of necrosis may be helpful features in discriminating between the two, but it is prudent to resist making a definitive diagnosis of carcinoma ex-pleomorphic adenoma (i.e. invasive carcinoma requiring radical surgery) if obvious elements of benign pleomorphic adenoma can be still identified in the aspirate. This reduces the possibility of 'overcall' of non-invasive malignant transformation. Most high-grade invasive carcinomas are diagnosable on FNA, but false negative results are not uncommon with low-grade carcinoma ex-pleomorphic adenoma[69].

Carcinosarcoma ex-pleomorphic adenoma is a less common variation on this theme. The FNA diagnosis rests upon the recognition of a biphasic pattern and classification of the malignant components from first principles.

The exceptionally rare benign metastasizing pleomorphic adenoma is defined by its anomalous biological behaviour, rather than any perceived subtle, histological and cytological differences from its non-metastasizing counterpart.

Polymorphous low-grade (terminal duct) adenocarcinoma *(Fig. 10.19)*

Polymorphous low-grade adenocarcinoma (PLGAC) is predominantly a tumour of minor salivary glandular tissue, commonly arising in the palate. It is characterized by its architectural diversity and cytological uniformity. Solid (lobular), cribriform, tubuloductal, fascicular, papillary and papillocystic growth patterns are recognized and there may be a hyaline stromal component[42]. Any or all of these may be represented in FNA material and although experience is limited, several examples of good descriptions are available in published literature[70–72]. It should be noted in particular that PLGAC may exhibit hyaline globules similar to those seen in adenoid cystic carcinoma or epithelial-myoepithelial carcinoma and, importantly, basal cell and pleomorphic adenomas[70,71,73,74].

Epithelial-myoepithelial (intercalated duct) carcinoma *(Fig. 10.20)*

This very uncommon low-grade carcinoma is most often of parotid origin. It is typified by an organoid growth pattern and a dimorphic cell population[42]. Central epithelial ductal structures are mantled by abluminal myoepithelial cells, which often show clear cell change. FNA material classically shows this bimorphic population, the myoepithelial component occasionally manifesting as fusiform (bipolar), naked nuclei. Hyaline stroma may be encountered[73–75].

Diagnostic pitfalls

Epithelial-myoepithelial carcinoma-like growth may be seen focally in pleomorphic adenoma, in intercalated duct

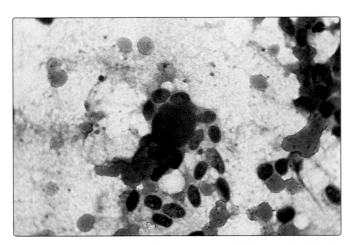

Fig. 10.20 Epithelial-myoepithelial carcinoma. Malignant epithelial cells clustered around a basement membrane globule. (MGG × HP)

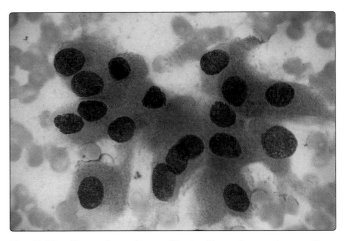

Fig. 10.22 Oncocytic carcinoma. Sheets of large abnormal oncocytic cells from a well-differentiated carcinoma of the parotid. (MGG × OI)

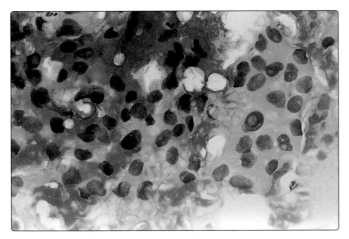

Fig. 10.21 Salivary duct carcinoma. Pleomorphic malignant epithelial cells with plentiful cytoplasm and conspicuous intranuclear vacuoles. (Papanicolaou × HP)

hyperplasia[76] and as part of so-called composite or hybrid tumours. Caution must also be exercised to distinguish epithelial-myoepithelial carcinoma from other salivary tumours of biphasic cellular composition, e.g. adenoid cystic carcinoma and from those with a clear cell component, e.g. mucoepidermoid carcinoma and acinic cell carcinoma[73–75].

Salivary duct (excretory or large duct) carcinoma (Fig. 10.21)

Salivary duct carcinoma is a high-grade, biologically aggressive carcinoma usually of major salivary gland origin. Papillary, solid, cribriform and comedo patterns of growth are recognized[42], the latter resembling ductal carcinoma of the breast. The typical FNA preparation shows plentiful, large, polygonal cells with pleomorphic nuclei. Areas of necrosis are not uncommon. Difficulty may be experienced in separating salivary duct carcinoma from other poorly differentiated carcinomas of the salivary glands, most notably oncocytic carcinoma. Good descriptions and discussion of the differential diagnosis are available from several authors[77–79].

Basal cell adenocarcinoma

This is the malignant counterpart of benign basal cell adenoma and its variants characterized by permeating growth, often with neurotropism and/or angioinvasion[42]. Again, solid, trabecular, tubular and membranous subtypes are described and there may be hyaline stroma and focal squamoid differentiation. The major differential diagnosis lies between adenoid cystic carcinoma and basal cell carcinoma of the skin. The cytological problems are well discussed by Klijanienko[53].

Squamous cell carcinoma

Primary squamous cell carcinoma of the salivary glands is a diagnosis reached largely by exclusion of metastatic disease (either directly into the gland or within intraparotid and periparotid lymph nodes), high-grade mucoepidermoid carcinoma and carcinoma ex-pleomorphic adenoma amongst others. Confounding variables include non-keratinizing pattern, acantholytic or cystic growth pattern and a spindle cell ('pseudosarcomatoid') variant. Benign metaplasia of native gland especially after irradiation or within pleomorphic adenoma or Warthin's tumour must also be considered[80].

Oncocytic carcinoma (adenocarcinoma) (Fig. 10.22)

Oncocytic carcinoma is rare and is the malignant counterpart of benign oncocytoma (oncocytic adenoma). It is a high-grade carcinoma, almost invariably showing clear-cut evidence of malignancy on histology[42]. Caution must, however, be advised in reaching such a diagnosis from FNA material, as oncocytic carcinoma can appear quite bland[81], while benign oncocytic neoplasms and metaplastic/hyperplastic oncocytic proliferations may display a disturbing degree of atypia. Oncocytic carcinoma may exhibit more than a passing resemblance to salivary duct carcinoma, although both are aggressive tumours and absolute discrimination between them on FNA is unlikely to be of prime clinical importance.

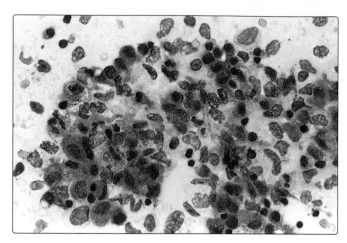

Fig. 10.23   Myoepithelial carcinoma. Small, dark, focally elongated malignant cells. (MGG × MP)

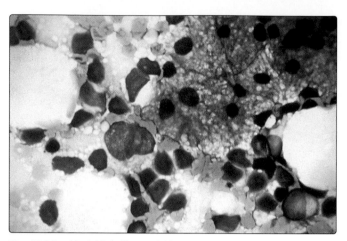

Fig. 10.24   Hodgkin's disease. A binucleate Reed-Sternberg cell with scattered lymphocytes adjacent to a group of acinar cells. (MGG × OI)

Myoepithelial carcinoma (malignant myoepithelioma)
(Fig. 10.23)

The malignant counterpart of benign myoepithelioma is myoepithelial carcinoma and as such, merges with the concept of carcinoma ex-pleomorphic adenoma[82]. It is rare and usually presents as clusters of small cells with hyperchromatic nuclei or many small spindle-shaped cells ('pseudosarcomatoid' pattern). The potential for clear cell, giant cell or plasmacytoid differentiation must be borne in mind, as otherwise these may cause difficulty in interpretation of FNA material.

Undifferentiated and neuroendocrine carcinomas

These include both large cell and small cell variants, the latter comparable to small cell anaplastic ('oat cell') carcinoma of bronchopulmonary origin. Difficulty may be experienced in separating these from other high-grade carcinomas and lymphomas. If there is a conspicuous reactive lymphoid component, the possibility of undifferentiated carcinoma with lymphoid stroma ('malignant lymphoepithelioma'), similar to that more usually encountered in the nasopharynx, must be considered. If sufficient material is received by FNA, a limited panel of immunocytochemical staining may prove invaluable in further sub-classifying this group of tumours[83].

Other primary carcinomas

A heterogeneous variety of uncommon primary salivary gland carcinomas such as sebaceous carcinoma, adenosquamous carcinoma, hyalinizing clear cell carcinoma and adenocarcinoma not otherwise specified, among others, also occur[42,43] and may be aspirated. The correct diagnosis and resolution of differential diagnosis of these, and especially clear cell tumours[60], is best reached from cytomorphological first principles coupled with a thorough knowledge of the classification system, backed by experience of the range of appearances that may be encountered in FNA material. Layfield and Glasgow discuss

the diagnostic dilemma of clear cell lesions of the parotid in their 1993 paper[84] and hyalinizing clear cell carcinoma is described by Milchgrub *et al.*[85].

Non-epithelial tumours

These include angiomas, lipomas, neural tumours and other benign mesenchymal tumours as well as sarcomas[42]. Layfield *et al.*[86] have drawn attention to lipomatous lesions of the parotid gland as a potential source of 'non-diagnostic' FNA reports as the material may be misinterpreted as subcutaneous fat. Otherwise, benign soft tissue neoplasms and sarcomas display the same cytomorphological features as similar tumours in other anatomical sites (see Chapter 40). Chhieng *et al.*[87] reviewed a series of spindle cell lesions of the salivary gland, showing that few were primary non-epithelial tumours on histological follow-up.

Malignant lymphomas *(Fig. 10.24)*

Two separate entities are included here: *extranodal lymphoma of the salivary gland (MALT lymphoma)* and *lymphoma arising in intrasalivary lymph nodes*. It is not possible to separate these two conditions by FNA as the source of the lymphomatous cells cannot be identified. The first type may develop from pre-existing benign lymphoepithelial disease or arise *de novo*. The few cases of the latter personally examined have arisen mainly in transplant recipients. Lymphomas are usually of non-Hodgkin's type (see Chapter 19), but Hodgkin's disease does also occur. When considering the diagnosis of lymphoma the wide range of lesions with a high lymphoid component must be excluded[88]. Allen *et al.* have demonstrated the value of flow cytometry for cell surface marker analysis and/or immunophenotyping[89].

Secondary tumours *(Fig. 10.25)*

Squamous cell carcinoma and malignant melanoma metastatic to the intraparotid/periparotid lymph nodes are the most common secondary tumours[90]. The primary site of squamous cell carcinoma is generally in the head and neck, but may be distant, e.g. in the lung. The cytology is identical

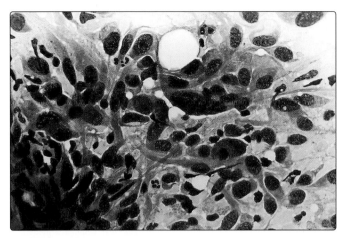

Fig. 10.25 Metastatic sarcoma. Bizarre large malignant cells with frequent spindle forms. (MGG × MP)

to primary squamous cell carcinoma or the squamoid component of mucoepidermoid carcinoma. Metastatic carcinoma of kidney or thyroid must be considered in the differential diagnosis of acinic cell carcinoma and oncocytic tumours. Carcinoma of the breast also spreads to intraparotid lymph nodes as may many other primary tumours. Metastatic sarcoma is occasionally found.

Diagnostic accuracy of fine needle aspiration

As will be appreciated by reading this text, FNA of the salivary glands presents many problems for the cytopathologist (see Table 10.2 for differential diagnosis based on cellular morphology), but with experience and good clinical liaison sensitivity and specificity are high. FNA series with good clinical and histological correlation indicate specificity as high as 94–100% and sensitivity of 81–100%[12–14,44,47,91–95]. When considered from the viewpoint of type-specific diagnostic accuracy of tumours the figure is approximately 80%[42] and is better for benign than

malignant neoplasms. Diagnosis of pleomorphic adenoma is invariably high[48] but mucoepidermoid carcinoma[65] and carcinoma ex-pleomorphic adenocarcinoma[69] can pose problems for even the most experienced, as will the unexpected encounter of a rare tumour.

The overall results of FNA compare favourably with those of frozen section but without the risks and inconvenience. Auclair *et al.* (1991)[96] reviewed published data on frozen sections from the salivary glands. The overall accuracy calculated from 21 series was 96.2% excluding deferred diagnosis. However, as the authors point out that, while the sensitivity for benign lesions which account for 78% of all frozen sections, is excellent, the rates for malignant lesions, with and without deferred diagnoses, are only 77.1% and 85.7%, respectively. Three further studies comparing FNA and frozen sections from the same lesions have shown that the overall accuracy of FNA was higher[9,97,98]. However, frozen section complements cytodiagnosis. FNA examines only a very limited sample of material and neither architectural features nor presence or absence of invasion can be assessed. There remain some occasions when frozen section is advisable, in particular for the confirmation of adenoid cystic carcinoma.

Causes of false negative and false positive errors and diagnostic problems have been reviewed in several papers[94,99–102]. False negative results are generally due to unrepresentative sampling, especially from cystic tumours, and false positive reports from failure to appreciate the difficulties associated with pleomorphic adenoma and basal cell adenoma. Diagnostic problems in general are discussed by Young[102] and MacLeod and Frable[103].

The conclusion reached in 1993 that successful FNA of the salivary glands depends on the recognition of the problem lesions is still valid[104]. Therefore, there are cases where a differential diagnosis is more appropriate than a definitive one. Despite this cautionary note fine needle aspiration of the salivary glands is an accurate, safe and clinically helpful technique.

Table 10.2 Differential diagnosis based on cellular morphology

Morphological feature	Extrinsic lesion	Intrinsic salivary gland lesion
Fat cells	Subcutaneous fat	Fatty replacement with age
	Lipoma	Lipomatosis
		Lipoma/sialolipoma
Cystic change	Branchial cleft cyst	Obstructive sialopathy
		Salivary duct cyst
		Lymphoepithelial cyst
		Polycystic disease
		Warthin's tumour
		Pleomorphic adenoma
		Papillary adenoma
		Mucinous cystadenoma
	Colliquative necrosis in lymph node associated with metastatic carcinoma	Mucoepidermal carcinoma (low-grade)
		Acinic cell carcinoma
		Cystadenocarcinoma

(Continued)

Table 10.2 *(Cont'd)*

Morphological feature	Extrinsic lesion	Intrinsic salivary gland lesion
Lymphoid cells	Benign lymphadenopathy	Chronic sialadenitis
		Granulomatous sialadenitis
		Lymphoepithelial lesion (MESA, Sjögren's, AIDS)
		Warthin's tumour
		Mucoepidermoid carcinoma
		Acinic cell carcinoma
	Malignant lymphoma of nodal origin	Extranodal malignant lymphoma (MALToma)
Squamous epithelial cells	Branchial cleft cyst	Chronic sialadenitis
		Post radiation change
		Necrotizing sialometaplasia
		Pleomorphic adenoma
		Warthin's tumour
	Metastatic squamous cell carcinoma in lymph node	Primary squamous cell carcinoma
		Mucoepidermoid carcinoma (high-grade)
		Adenosquamous carcinoma
Basement membrane type globules	Eccrine cylindroma of sweat gland	Basal cell adenoma
		Pleomorphic adenoma
		Canalicular adenoma
		Adenoid cystic carcinoma
		Basal cell carcinoma
		Epithelial-myoepithelial carcinoma
		Polymorphous low-grade carcinoma
		Focal/diffuse oncocytosis
		Nodular oncocytic hyperplasia
		Oncocytoma
		Warthin's tumour
		Tumour metaplasia in other adenomas
Oncocytic type cells	Metastatic thyroid or renal cell carcinoma in lymph node	Oncocytic carcinoma
		Mucoepidermoid carcinoma
Cohesive groups of small cells with dark, sometimes elongated, nuclei	Nerve sheath tumours	Myoepithelioma
	Basaloid skin appendage tumours	
	Merkel cell carcinoma of skin	Solid form of adenoid cystic carcinoma
	Metastatic small cell carcinoma in lymph node	Myoepithelial carcinoma
		Primary small cell carcinoma
Acinic-type cells	Lymph nodal inclusions	Normal salivary gland
	Heterotopic salivary tissue	Sialadenosis
		Acinic cell carcinoma
		Pleomorphic adenoma
		Clear cell oncocytoma
		Sebaceous adenoma
Clear cells	Metastatic clear cell carcinoma in lymph node e.g. renal, thyroid	Acinic cell carcinoma
		Epithelial: myoepithelial carcinoma
		Mucoepidermoid carcinoma
		Sebaceous carcinoma
Giant cells	Granulomatous lymphadenitis	Granulomatous sialadenitis
		Pleomorphic adenoma
	Metastatic carcinoma	Carcinoma or carcinosarcoma
	Soft tissue sarcoma	ex-pleomorphic adenoma
		Primary sarcoma
Spindle cells	Reactive/proliferative soft tissue lesions	
	Benign mesenchymal neoplasms	Myoepithelioma
		Pleomorphic adenoma
	Sarcoma	Carcinoma/sarcoma
		ex-pleomorphic adenoma
Intranuclear inclusions	Metastatic papillary thyroid carcinoma	Mucoepidermoid carcinoma
		Salivary duct carcinoma

References

1 Stewart F W. The diagnosis of tumours by aspiration. *Am J Pathol* 1933; **9**: 801–813

2 Linsk J A. Aspiration cytology in Sweden: the Karolinska Group. *Diagn Cytopathol* 1985; **1**: 332–335

3 Mavec P, Eneroth C-M, Franzen S *et al.* Aspiration biopsy of salivary gland tumours 1. Correlation of cytologic reports from 652 aspiration biopsies with clinical and histological findings. *Acta Otolaryngol Stockh* 1964; **58**: 472–484

4 Eneroth C-M, Zajicek J. Aspiration biopsy of salivary gland tumours II. Morphologic studies on smears and histologic sections from oncocytic tumours (45 cases of papillary cystadenoma lymphomatosum and 4 cases of oncocytoma) *Acta Cytol* 1965; **9**: 355–561

5 Eneroth C-M, Zajicek J. Aspiration biopsy of salivary gland tumours III. Morphologic smears and histologic sections from 368 mixed tumours. *Acta Cytol* 1966; **10**: 440–454

6 Eneroth C-M, Zajicek J. Aspiration biopsy of salivary gland tumours IV. Morphologic studies on smears and histologic sections from 45 cases of adenoid cystic carcinoma. *Acta Cytol* 1969; **13**: 59–63

7 Eneroth C-M, Zajicek J. Aspiration biopsy of salivary gland tumours V. Morphologic investigations on smears and histologic sections of acinic cell carcinoma. *Acta Radiol Stockh* 1971; 310(Suppl): 85–93

8 Zajicek J, Eneroth C-M, Jakobsson P. Aspiration biopsy of salivary gland tumours VI. Morphologic investigation on smears and histologic sections of 24 cases of mucoepidermoid carcinoma. *Acta Cytol* 1979; **20**: 35–41

9 Layfield L J, Tan P, Glasgow B J. Fine needle aspiration of salivary gland lesions: comparison with frozen sections and histological findings. *Arch Pathol Lab Med* 1987; **111**: 346–353

10 Frable W J. Thin needle aspiration biopsy. *Am J Clin Pathol* 1976; **65**: 168–182

11 Mighell A J, High A S. Histological identification of carcinoma in 21 gauge needle tracks after fine needle biopsy of head and neck carcinoma. *J Clin Pathol* 1997; **51**: 241–243

12 Qizilbash A H, Sianhos J, Young J E N, Archibald S D. Fine needle aspiration biopsy of the major salivary glands. *Acta Cytol* 1985; **29**: 503–512

13 Nettle W J, Orell S R. Fine needle aspiration in the diagnosis of salivary gland lesions. *Aust & NZ J Surg* 1989; **59**: 47–51

14 Zajdela A, Zillhardt P, Voillemot N. Cytological diagnosis by fine needle sampling without aspiration. *Cancer* 1987; **59**: 1201–1205

15 Lowhagen T, Tani E M, Skoog L. Salivary glands and rare head and neck lesions. In: Bibbo M ed. *Comprehensive Cytopathology*. Philadelphia: W B Saunders, 1991; 621–648

16 Engzell B, Franzen S, Zajicek J. Aspiration biopsy of tumours of the neck. II. Cytologic findings in 13 cases of carotid body tumour. *Acta Cytol* 1971; **15**: 25–30

17 Viero R M, Tani E, Skoog L. Fine needle aspiration (FNA) cytology of pilomatrixoma: report on 14 cases and review of the literature. *Cytopathol* 1999; **10**: 263–269

18 Chan M K M, McGuire L J. Fine needle aspiration of an unusual parotid mass. *Acta Cytol* 1989; **33**: 274–276

19 Skoog L, Schmitt F, Tani E. Neuroendocrine (Merkel cell) carcinoma of the skin: immunocytochemical and cytomorphologic analysis on fine needle aspirations. *Diagn Cytopathol* 1990; **6**: 53–57

20 Batsakis J G. Littler E R, Leahy M S. Sebaceous gland lesions of the head and neck. *Arch Otolaryngol* 1972; **95**: 151–157

21 Chan M K M, McGuire L J. Cytodiagnosis of lesions presenting as salivary gland swellings. *Diagn Cytopathol* 1992; 439–443

22 Aufdemorte T B, Ramzy I, Holt G R *et al.* Focal adenomatoid hyperplasia of the salivary glands. A different diagnostic problem in fine needle aspiration biopsy. *Acta Cytol* 1985; **29**: 23–27

23 Gupta R K, Green C, Fauck R *et al.* Fine needle aspiration cytodiagnosis of sialadenitis with crystalloids. *Acta Cytol* 1999; **43**: 390–392

24 Finfer M D, Schniella R A, Rothstein S G, Perky M S. Cystic parotid lesions in patients at risk of the acquired immune deficiency syndrome. *Arch Otolaryngol Head Neck Surg* 1988; **112**: 1290–1294

25 Finfer M D, Gallo L, Perchick A *et al.* Fine needle aspiration biopsy of cystic benign lymphoepithelial lesion of the parotid gland in patients at risk of the acquired immune deficiency syndrome. *Acta Cytol* 1990; **34**: 821–826

26 Chhieng D C, Argosino R, McKenna B J *et al.* Utility of fine needle aspiration in the diagnosis of salivary gland lesions in patients infected with human immunodeficiency virus. *Diagn Cytopathol* 1999; **21**: 260–264

27 Van der Walt J D, Leake J. Granulomatous sialadenitis of the major salivary glands. A clinicopathological study of 57 cases. *Histopathol* 1987; **11**: 131–144

28 Agarwal A P, Jayaram G, Mandal A K. Sarcoidosis diagnosed on fine needle aspiration of salivary glands: a report of three cases. *Diagn Cytopathol* 1989; **5**: 289–292

29 Mair S, Leiman G, Levinsohn D. Fine needle aspiration of parotid sarcoidosis. *Acta Cytol* 1989; **33**: 169–172

30 Gupta S, Sodhani P. Sialadenosis of parotid gland: a cytomorphic and morphometric study of four cases. *Anal Quart Cytol Histol* 1998; **20**: 225–228

31 Seifert G, Donath K, Schäfer R. Lipomatous pleomorphic adenoma of the parotid gland. Classification of lipomatous tissue in salivary glands. *Pathol Res Tract* 1999; **4**: 247–252

32 Sanmann F, Putzke H P. Focal oncocytosis of the salivary glands and etiopathogenetic relations. *Mund Kiefer Gestichtschir* 1997; **2**: 86–89

33 Batsakis J G. The pathology of head and neck tumours: the lymphoepithelial lesion and Sjogren's syndrome, part 16. *Head Neck Surg* 1982; **5**: 150–163

34 Kondratowicz G M, Smallman L A, Morgan D A. A clinicopathological study of myoepithelial sialadenitis and chronic sialadenitis/sialolithiasis. *J Clin Pathol* 1988; **41**: 403–409

35 Chiling C, Dodd L G, Glasgow B. Layfield L T. Salivary gland lesions with a prominent lymphoid component: cytologic findings and differential diagnosis by fine needle aspiration biopsy. *Diagn Cytopathol* 1997; **17**: 183–190

36 Batsakis J G, Bernacki E G, Rice D H, Steibler M E. Malignancy and the benign lymphoepithelial lesion. *The Laryngoscope* 1975; **85**: 389–399

37 Abrams A M, Melrose R J, Howell F V. Necrotising sialometaplasia: a disease simulating malignancy. *Cancer* 1973; **32**: 130–135

38 Fechner R E. Necrotising sialometaplasia. A source of confusion with carcinoma of the palate. *Am J Clin Pathol* 1977; **67**: 315–317

39 Auclair P L, Ellis G L, Gnepp D R *et al.* Salivary gland neoplasms: General considerations. In: Ellis G L, Auclair P L, Gnepp D R eds. *Surgical Pathology of the Salivary Glands*. Philadelphia: W B Saunders, 1991; 135–164

40 Thackray A C, Sobin L H. *Histological Typing of Salivary Gland Tumours*. Geneva: World Health Organisation, 1972

41 Ellis G L, Auclair P L. Classification of salivary gland neoplasms: In: Ellis G L, Auclair P L, Gnepp D R eds. *Surgical Pathology of the Salivary Glands*. Philadelphia: W B Saunders, 1991; 129–134

42 Seifert G, ed. *Histological Typing of Salivary Gland Tumours*. World Health Organisation, Berlin: Springer-Verlag, 1991

43 Ellis G L, Auclair P L. *Tumors of the Salivary Glands*. Washington: Armed Forces Institute of Pathology, 1996

44 Young J A, Smallman L A, Thompson H *et al.* Fine needle aspiration of salivary gland lesions. *Cytopathol* 1990; **1**: 25–33

45 Sismanis A, Merriam J M, Kline T S *et al.* Diagnosis of salivary gland tumours by fine needle aspiration biopsy. *Head Neck Surg* 1981; **3**: 482–489

46 O'Dwyer P, Farrar W B, James A G *et al.* Needle aspiration of major salivary glands. *Cancer* 1986; **57**: 554–557

47 Jayaram N, Ashim D, Rajwandshi A *et al.* The value of fine needle aspiration biopsy in the cytodiagnosis of salivary gland lesions. *Diagn Cytopathol* 1989; **5**: 349–354

48 Klijanienko J, Viehl P. Fine needle sampling of salivary glands lesions 1. Cytology and histology correlation of 412 cases of pleomorphic adenoma. *Diagn Cytopathol* 1996; **14**: 195–200

49 Stanley M W, Lowhagen T. Mucin production by pleomorphic adenomas of the parotid gland: a cytologic spectrum. *Diagn Cytopathol* 1990; **6**: 49–52

50 Ellis G L, Auclair P L, eds. Benign salivary gland neoplasms. In: *Tumors of the Salivary Glands*. Washington: Armed Forces Institute of Pathology, 1996; 39–153

51 Dedd L G, Caraway H P, Luna M A et al. Myoepithelioma of the parotid: report of a case initially examined by fine needle aspiration biopsy. *Acta Cytol* 1994; **38**: 417–421

52 Tawgik O, Tsue T, Pnatazis C et al. Salivary gland neoplasms with basaloid cell features: report of two cases diagnosed by fine needle aspiration cytology. *Diagn Cytopathol* 1999; **21**: 46–50

53 Klijanienko J, El-Nagger A K, Viehl P. Comparative cytological and histologic study of fifteen salivary basal-cell tumors: differential diagnostic considerations. *Diagn Cytol* 1999; **21**: 30–34

54 Klijanienko J, Viehl P. Fine needle aspiration of salivary gland lesions II. Cytology and histology correlation of 71 cases of Warthin's tumor (adenolymphoma). *Diagn Cytopathol*. 1997; **16**: 221–225

55 Bottles K, Lowhagen T, Miller T R. Mast cells in the aspiration cytology differential diagnosis of adenolymphoma. *Acta Cytol* 1984; **29**: 513–515

56 Kobagashi T K, Veda M, Hishino T et al. Association of mast cells with Warthin's tumour in fine needle aspirations of the salivary gland. *Acta Cytol* 1999; **43**: 1052–1058

57 Laurica R, Farum J B, Leopold S K et al. False-positive diagnosis in fine needle aspiration of an atypical Warthin's tumour: histochemical differential stains for cytodiagnosis. *Diagn Cytopathol* 1989; **5**: 412–415

58 Ballo M S, Shin H J C, Sneige N. Sources of diagnostic error in fine needle aspiration diagnosis of Warthin's tumor and clues to a correct diagnosis. *Diagn Cytopathol* 1997; **17**: 230–234

59 Soofer S B, Tabbara S. Intraductal papilloma of the salivary gland. A report of two cases with diagnosis by fine needle aspiration biopsy. *Acta Cytol* 1999; **43**: 1142–1146

60 Eveson J W. Troublesome tumours **2**: borderline tumour of salivary glands. *J Clin Pathol* 1992; **45**: 369–377

61 Ellis G L, Auclair P L, eds. Malignant epithelial tumours. In: *Tumors of the Salivary Glands*. Washington: Armed Forces Institute of Pathology, 1996; 155–371

62 Palmo O, Terri A M, Cristofaro J A, Fiaccavanto S. Fine needle aspiration cytology in two cases of acinic-cell carcinoma of the parotid gland: discussion of diagnostic criteria. *Acta Cytol* 1985; **29**: 516–521

63 Nagel H, Laskawi R, Büter J J et al. Cytologic diagnosis of acinic cell carcinoma of salivary glands. *Diagn Cytopathol* 1997; **16**: 402–412

64 Cohen M B, Fisher P E, Holly E A et al. Fine needle aspiration biopsy of mucoepidermoid carcinoma: statistical analysis. *Acta Cytol* 1990; **34**: 43–49

65 Klijanienko J, Viehl P. Fine needle sampling of salivary gland lesion IV. Review of 50 cases of mucoepidermoid carcinoma with histologic correlation. *Diagn Cytopathol* 1997; **17**: 93–98

66 Klijanienko J, Viehl P. Fine needle sampling of salivary gland lesions III. Cytologic and histologic correlation of 75 cases of adenoid cystic carcinoma: review and experience at the Institute Curie with emphasis on cytologic pitfalls. *Diagn Cytopathol* 1997; **17**: 36–41

67 Nagel H, Hotze H J, Laskawi R et al. Cytologic diagnosis of adenoid cystic carcinoma of salivary glands. *Diagn Cytopathol* 1999; **20**: 358–366

68 Cawson R A, Gleason M J, Eveson J W. Carcinoma of salivary glands. In: *Pathology and Surgery of the Salivary Glands*. Oxford: ISIS Medical Media, 1997; 117–169

69 Klijanienko J, El-Nagger A K, Viehl P. Fine needle sampling in 25 carcinoma ex-pleomorphic adenomas: diagnostic pitfalls and clinical considerations. *Diagn Cytopathol* 1999; **21**: 163–166

70 Klijanienko J, Viehl P. Salivary carcinoma with papillae: cytology and histology analysis of polymorphous low-grade adenocarcinoma and papillary cystadenoma. *Diagn Cytopathol* 1998; **19**: 244–249

71 Gibbons D, Saboorian M H, Vuitch F et al. Fine needle aspiration findings in patients with polymorphous low-grade adenocarcinoma of the salivary glands. *Cancer* 1999; **87**: 31–36

72 Watanabe K, Ono N, Saito A, Suzuki T. Fine needle aspiration cytology of polymorphous low-grade adenocarcinoma of the tongue. *Diagn Cytopathol* 1999; **20**: 167–169

73 Klijanienko J, Viehl P. Fine needle sampling of salivary gland lesions VII. Cytology and histology correlation of five cases of epithelial-myoepithelial carcinoma. *Diagn Cytopathol* 1998; **19**: 405–409

74 Ng W-k, Chou C, Ip P et al. Fine needle aspiration cytology of epithelial-myoepithelial carcinoma of salivary glands : a report of three cases. *Acta Cytol* 1999; **43**: 675–680

75 Yang G C H, Soslaw R A. Epithelial-myoepithelial carcinoma of the parotid. A case of ductal-prominent presentation with cytologic, histologic and ultrastructural correlations. *Acta Cytol* 1999; **43**: 1113–1118

76 Chetty R. Intercalated duct hyperplasia : possible relationship to epithelial-myoepithelial carcinoma and hybrid tumours of salivary gland. *Histopathol* 2000; **37**: 260–263

77 Fyrat P, Cramer H, Feczko J D et al. Fine needle aspiration biopsy of salivary duct carcinoma : report of five cases. *Diagn Cytopathol* 1997; **16**: 526–530

78 Klijanienko J. Viehl P. Cytologic characteristics and histomorphologic correlations of 21 salivary duct carcinomas. *Diagn Cytopathol* 1998; **19**: 333–337

79 Anand A, Brockle E S. Cytomorphological features of salivary duct carcinoma ex pleomorphic adenoma : diagnosis by fine needle aspiration biopsy with histologic correlation. *Diagn Cytopathol* 1999; **20**: 375–378

80 Klijanienko J, Viehl P. Fine needle sampling of salivary gland lesions VI. Cytological review of 44 cases of primary salivary gland squamous-cell carcinoma with histological correlation. *Diagn Cytopathol* 1998; **18**: 174–178

81 Harrison R F, Smallman L A, Watkinson J C, Young J A. Fine needle aspiration of oncocytic carcinoma of the parotid gland. *Cytopathol* 1995; **6**: 54–58

82 Savers A T, Sloman A, Huros A G, Klimstra D S. Myoepithelial carcinoma of the salivary glands: a clinicopathologic study of 25 patients. *Am J Surg Pathol* 2000; **24**: 761–774

83 Mair S, Phillips J I, Cohen R. Small cell undifferentiated carcinoma of the parotid gland: cytologic, histologic, immunohistochemical and ultrastructural features of a neuroendocrine variant. *Acta Cytol* 1988; **33**: 164–169

84 Layfield L J, Glasgow B J. Aspiration cytology of clear-cell lesions of the parotid gland: morphologic features and differential diagnosis. *Diagn Cytopathol* 1993; **9**: 705–712

85 Milchgrub S, Vuitch F, Saboorian M H et al. Hyalinising clear-cell carcinoma of salivary glands in fine needle aspiration. *Diagn Cytopathol* 2000; **23**: 333–337

86 Layfield L J, Glasgow B J, Goldstein N, Lufkin R. Lipomatous lesions of the parotid gland: potential pitfalls in fine needle aspiration diagnosis. *Acta Cytol* 1973; **17**: 351–354

87 Chhieng D C, Cohen J-M, Cangiarella J F. Fine needle aspiration of spindle cell and mesenchymal lesions of the salivary glands. *Diagn Cytopathol* 2000; **23**: 253–259

88 Chiling C, Dodd L G, Glasgow B J, Layfield L. Salivary gland lesions with a prominent lymphoid component: cytologic findings and differential diagnosis by fine needle aspiration biopsy. *Diagn Cytopathol* 1997; **17**: 183–190

89 Allen E A, Ali S Z, Mathew S. Lymphoid lesions of the parotid. *Diagn Cytopathol* 1999; **21**: 170–173

90 Zhang C, Cohen J M, Cangiarella J F et al. Fine needle aspiration of secondary neoplasms involving the salivary glands. *Am J Clin Pathol* 2000; **113**: 21–28

91 Persson P S, Zettergren L. Cytologic diagnosis of salivary gland tumours by aspiration biopsy. *Acta Cytol* 1973; **17**: 351–354

92 Webb A J. Cytologic diagnosis of salivary gland lesions in adult and paediatric surgical patients. *Acta Cytol* 1973; **17**: 51–58

93 Kline T S, Merriam J M, Shapsay S M. Aspiration biopsy cytology of the salivary gland. *Am J Clin Pathol* 1981; **76**: 263–269

94 Cajulus R S, Gokaslan S T, Yu G H, Frias-Hidvegi D. Fine needle aspiration biopsy of the salivary glands: a five year experience with emphasis on diagnostic pitfalls. *Acta Cytol* 1997; **41**: 1412 – 1420

95 Cristallini E G, Ascani S, Farabi R et al. Fine needle aspiration biopsy of salivary glands, 1985–1995. *Acta Cytol* 1997; **41**: 1421–1425

96 Auclair P L, Ellis G L, Gnepp D R *et al*. Salivary gland neoplasms: general considerations. In: Ellis G L, Auclair P L, Gnepp D R eds. *Surgical Pathology of the Salivary Glands. Major Problems in Pathology*, vol. 25, Philadelphia: W B Saunders, 1991; 135–164

97 Cohen M B, Lyung B M E, Boles R. Salivary gland tumours: fine needle aspiration vs. frozen section diagnosis. *Arch Otolaryngeal Head Neck Surg* 1986; **112**: 867–869

98 Chan M K M, McGuire L J, King W *et al*. Cytodiagnosis of 112 salivary gland lesions: correlation with histologic and frozen section diagnosis. *Acta Cytol* 1992; **36**: 353–363

99 Orell S R, Nettle W J S. Fine needle aspiration biopsy of salivary glands: problems and pitfalls. *Pathology* 1988; **20**: 332–337

100 Kocjan G, Nayagam M, Harris M. Fine needle aspiration cytology of salivary gland lesions: advantages and pitfalls. *Cytopathol* 1990; **1**: 267–275

101 Layfield L J, Glasgow B J. Diagnosis of salivary gland tumours by fine needle aspiration cytology. *Diagn Cytopathol* 1991; **7**: 267–272

102 Young J A. Diagnostic problems in fine needle aspiration Cytopathology of the salivary glands. *J Clin Pathol* 1994; **47**: 193–198

103 MacLeod C, Frable W J. Fine needle aspiration biopsy of the salivary gland : problem cases. *Diagn Cytopathol* 1993; **9**: 216–225

104 Young J A, ed. Salivary glands. *Fine Needle Aspiration*. Oxford: Blackwell Scientific, 1993: 48–67

11 Oral cavity

Alastair Deery

Introduction

Within the ordinary experience of the average clinical cytopathologist are benign viral or infective ulcers, abscesses or ulcer cancers of the tongue, lips and buccal surfaces. Frequently, clinical suspicion of lymphoma surrounds tonsillar masses. Uncommonly, fungal plaque-like infections may occur in the intra-nasal spaces and on sinusoidal and buccal mucosae. Rarely apparent soft tissue swelling or nodularity of the palate or cheek walls raises possibilities of accessory salivary gland malignancy or an adenoma. Very rarely visiting leukaemic or lymphomatous infiltrates bulge or distend the gums or cheek. In specialized practice, lesions of Kaposi's disease which may thicken and distort the palate or 'dysplasias' of the lips or tongue may be screened for.

Normal anatomy and histology

The lips, tongue, labial mucosal surfaces of the cheeks, gums, sublingual surfaces of the floor of the mouth, palate, tonsils and pharynx are covered by stratified squamous epithelium. This is cornified over the dorsal aspect of the tongue, over the gums and hard palate. Minor salivary glands composed of ducts and acinar secretory structures are present beneath the squamous mucosae of the lips, buccal or labial surfaces, palate and tongue. The nasopharynx and paranasal sinuses are lined by ciliated columnar epithelium salivary glands. Organized lymphoid tissue, forming Waldeyer's ring, is present in the nasopharyngeal tonsil, adenoids, faucial tonsil and the lingual tonsil. Lesser lymphoid aggregates are present throughout the oral and nasal cavities within the subepithelial tissues. Odontogenic tissues include the tooth root, epithelial remnants of the tooth follicle, enamel organ-type tissue, associated mesodermal soft tissues and bone.

Cytological sampling

From the range of tissues present it can be imagined that any intra- or peri-oral presentation of a mass invites a wide differential diagnosis. The application of wash or scrape cytology and directed aspiration cytology to oral and paranasal sinus lesions needs to take account of the full range of pathologies that visit this site. This emphasizes the critical importance of adapted cytological sampling and processing techniques to permit any given fixation or staining schedule to allow accurate and specific diagnosis. Direct smear techniques are unlikely to afford anything beyond the identification of the commoner epithelial or non-epithelial tumours; with insufficient negative assurance or precision to allow a significant role for cytological diagnosis. Liquid-based collection media have allowed greater possibilities. In very recent times this potential has been commercially 'hi-jacked' and seems threatened with curtailment by the 'old fashioned' convenience use of alcohol-based preservatives, added to the collection media. These unscientific adjustments are made to achieve 'rapid fixation' to allow specimen transport.

So long as the cells remain 'wet' and are osmotically protected however, alcohol preservation and coagulation shrinkage is actually undesirable, prior to making the final preparations on glass slides. Better preservation of cellular morphology is actually achieved on the 'flatter' thinly spread areas of conventional direct smears just by chance! Moreover alcohol pre-fixation excludes the use of Romanowsky stains, severely limiting non-epithelial morphological characteristics and seriously restricting the 'flattening' of the cells seen in subsequent thin-layer preparations. Finally, the addition of alcohol, less importantly perhaps, obliges the use of 'antigen recovery' techniques such as microwaves/pressurized steam 'cooking' to allow immunocytochemical analysis. Alcohol-free, pre-citrated culture media and physiologically adjusted saline solutions offer a scientifically sounder, economic and more flexible alternative. Most importantly, Romanowsky stains are accommodated. Informative acellular constituent proteinaceous materials, e.g. colloid, are not all but lost to alcohol immersion. Coupled with low-acceleration centrifugation, 'flat', thin layer preparations are achieved, without pre-immunocytochemical procedures. Simple room-temperature acetone immersion is all that is required for most antigen-antibody systems.

These fixative-free fluid collection techniques remain 'state of the art' for diagnostic cytopathology when the requirements go beyond simple haematoxylin nuclear staining. The medical and technical ability to extend the use of a very limited cellularity sample, from a nearly painless capillary-action aspirate, taken with a very thin needle, is the justification for use of aspiration cytology. Many alternative handling techniques are described by others who claim success with approaches that actually can only even begin to achieve results at the cost of many repetitions.

Aspiration cytology can be carried out with or without the assistance of an investigative imaging modality. Such procedures are not neutral in their effect. The size, consistency (solid low/high density/cystic) and eventual nature of the lesions aspirated are changed substantially by the decision whether or not to apply ultrasound or computerized tomographic assistance. The aspirators change too often; the decision locally pivots on the relative availability or will, or possibly aptitude, of the specialists involved. For these and all the considerations above it is unfortunately rarely possible to compare the performance of aspiration cytology meaningfully.

The diagnostic criteria for tumours in this area are as described for those same tumours with similar differentiation found in other sites. Some descriptions offered are therefore deliberately brief and more detail is included where there are site specific features.

Inflammatory conditions

Non-specific inflammation

Regenerative and/or degenerative cellular changes in squamous and columnar respiratory-type epithelial cells with associated acute and/or chronic inflammatory cell infiltrates may be found in a wide range of indistinguishable inflammations and focal ulcerations of the mucosae. Allergic conditions of the nasal and paranasal spaces may release an exudate into washes and swabs rich in eosinophils, mast cells and plasma cells in addition (Fig. 11.1).

Candida infection

Candida albicans pseudohyphae and spores are best seen in scrape smears from reddened whitish areas on the oral mucosa. The infection and organism load is commonly very intense in patients with profound immunosuppression, e.g. HIV positive patients' and AIDS patients' (Fig. 11.2) swabs for culture are more sensitive, but possibly less specific.

Herpes viral infection

Primary or recurrent herpes virus infection of the lips or intraoral mucosa presents as painful single or multiple small ulcers, sometimes with associated lymphadenopathy. The infection by *Herpes simplex* viruses (type I or II), usually occurs sporadically in those without chronic immunosuppression. The bizarre syncytial type giant cells with moulded nuclei, beaded degenerate nuclear membranes and basophilic or eosinophilic intranuclear inclusions or clear 'ground glass' nuclei can be easily identified in Papanicolaou stained smears (Fig. 11.3).

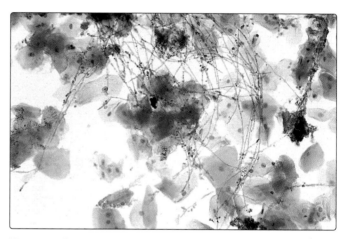

Fig. 11.2 Spatula scrape smear from the buccal mucosa in an AIDS patient. Note numerous interrupted pseudohyphae of candida (1–3 μm) and spores admixed with squamous cell sheets showing amphophilic cytoplasm and nuclear enlargement. (Papanicolaou × HP)

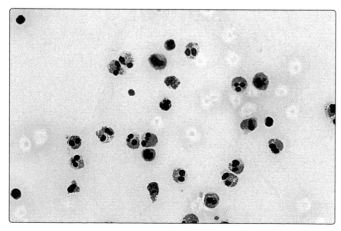

Fig. 11.1 Cytocentrifuge preparation from a maxillary sinus wash in a patient with allergic rhinitis, asthma and nasal polyps. Note the mucus, eosinophils, basophils and plasma cells. (MGG × HP)

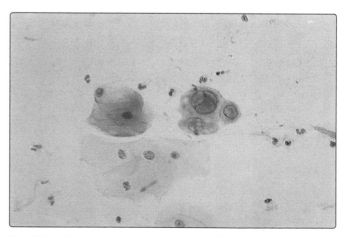

Fig. 11.3 Spatula scrape smear from a painful lip ulcer indicating herpes viral infection. Note the moulded nuclei of the multinucleate giant squamous cells, beaded nuclear membranes, 'ground glass' nuclei and intranuclear inclusions. (Papanicolaou × HP)

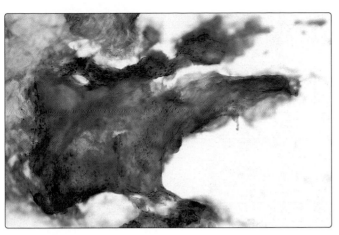

Fig. 11.4   Scalpel scrape smear from an area of grey-white leukoplakia on the buccal mucosa including parakeratotic 'spikes' and 'pearls' and orthokeratotic 'rafts', but not nuclear atypia. (Papanicolaou × MP)

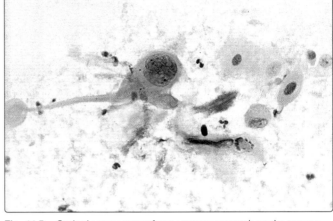

Fig. 11.5   Scalpel scrape smear from a verrucous patch on the tongue edge including atypical keratinized and parabasal type squamous cells. The lesion proved to be Bowenoid *in situ* squamous carcinoma. (Papanicolaou × MP)

Epithelial lesions

Leukoplakia

Clinical leukoplakia or a fixed white mucosal plaque or patch is a relatively common conundrum and will usually reveal bland orthokeratotic cytological appearances (anucleate 'keratinized' squamous cell sheets) and parakeratotic or dyskeratotic artefacts[1], with or without nuclear atypia in cytological smears (Fig. 11.4). In any individual case the smear appearances may not reflect existing underlying *in situ* neoplasia or invasive disease. Leukoplakia requires biopsy and/or careful clinical follow-up[2].

Nasopharyngeal tumours

Paranasal sinus washes will occasionally reveal atypical squamous, transitional or glandular cells indicating underlying malignancy in this site. The appearances are similar to such malignancies in other sites. Squamous tumours are most common and may be very poorly differentiated.

Squamous carcinoma

The existing literature[3–6] almost exclusively directs itself towards the adjunctive cytological diagnosis or 'suspicion' of oral squamous carcinoma, admittedly the most common malignancy arising in the oral cavity. It restricts cytology largely to swab and scrape smear samples. Modern scrape samples on scalpel blades can advantageously be taken directly into liquid collection fluid and shaken to produce a dispersed sample for subsequent centrifugation. The sample may then be treated as for any fluid sample.

Primary clinical suspicion of oral squamous carcinoma may result in incisional or excisional surgical biopsy. Prior scrape or aspiration cytology of an indurated, raised or ulcerated intra-oral lesion in the outpatient clinic, combined with aspiration of any associated cervical lymphadenopathy will establish the diagnosis in the majority of cases and can direct further surgery and/or adjuvant radiotherapy/chemotherapy without the need for further biopsy.

Apparent lymphadenopathy need not of course be related to the visible, presumed primary squamous cancer. In my experience, systematic aspiration of clinically, supposedly involved nodes, has occasionally revealed quite independent benign salivary gland tumours, e.g. an adenolymphoma synchronously discovered alongside squamous carcinoma of the oral cavity in an elderly male. Such outcomes highlight the value of effective investigative aspiration techniques, in contradistinction to conventional delayed histological dissections, which are not sparing upon the patient and sometimes have unjustifiable outcomes.

Follow-up of patients after earlier oral surgery with an assortment of potential recurrences or benign new lumps becomes part of the routine material of the head and neck aspiration clinic. Early 'recurrences' may prove to be 'seromas' or lymphatic cysts. Late recurrences may be second or entirely unrelated tumours. Intermediate 'lumps' at 3 to 6 months are usually metastatic carcinoma and encourage the belief that regional lymph node dissection should possibly be more systematically part of surgical protocols. There is a potential use of aspiration for 'sentinel' lymph node sampling.

In the absence of metastatic disease, scrape cytology of even ulcerated oral lesions cannot reliably and consistently separate *in situ* and invasive squamous tumour (Figs 11.5, 11.6). In this instance, a 'positive' result indicates the need for an adequate, i.e. complete excision, or multiple biopsies of the clinically visible lesional area. Attempts to screen for oral cancer have led some to suggest more innovative approaches to detection, coupling scrape cytology with p^{53} protein immunocytochemistry[7].

Basal cell carcinoma

There are no reports of this tumour occurring in the oral cavity, but occasionally at the lip margin and commonly at

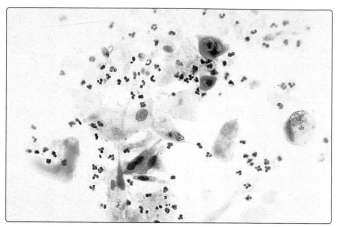

Fig. 11.6   Scalpel scrape smear from a sublingual ulcer revealing atypical keratinized and less differentiated parabasal-type squamous cells. The appearances are similar to those in **Fig. 11.5**, but the lesion proved to be invasive squamous carcinoma. (Papanicolaou × MP)

the nares. The features in scrape cytology; characteristically composed of microbiopsies of hyperchromatic crowded oval cells and similar partly stripped oval pale nuclei, with even chromatin and no visible nucleoli, are pathognomonic; they are elsewhere described under skin tumours (see Chapter 38).

Salivary gland lesions

Tumours of the minor (accessory) salivary glands most commonly occur as nodular or ulcerative lesions in the tongue, hard palate or buccal mucosa and should be clinically distinguishable from tumours, usually pleomorphic salivary adenomas presenting as an intraoral mass arising in the deep part of the parotid gland and pushing into the soft palate from the region of the pharyngeal faucial tonsil. Fine needle aspiration cytology is the procedure of choice under direct peroral visual guidance. A butterfly needle with a small flexible plastic tube to attach to a syringe used perhaps, in conjunction with a pistol grip is a valuable adjunct for 'difficult customers' located posteriorly.

Minor salivary tumours are most commonly malignant, though sometimes low-grade and early stage. A well-differentiated muco-epidermoid tumour may test even an experienced cytopathologist (Fig. 11.7). Palatal tumours often prove to be more easily identified adenoid cystic carcinomas, which carry a poor prognosis (Fig. 11.7B). The criteria for these diagnoses are discussed in Chapter 10, in salivary gland lesions.

Non-epithelial tumours

Orofacial lymphomas

Primary local incidence of nodal and extranodal lymphoma in and around the oral cavity forms a considerable proportion of all lymphomatous presentations[8]. As with all intraoral masses, the initial investigative biopsy should be fine needle aspiration. The diagnosis of lymphoma requires

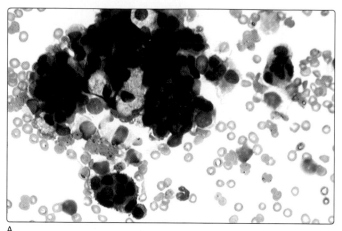

A

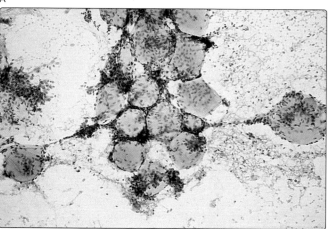

B

Fig. 11.7   (A) Cytocentrifuge preparation from a capillary aspirate of a metastatic low-grade mucoepidermoid carcinoma in a presenting palpable left neck node. No primary major salivary site seemed palpable and a 20 mm lesion was located on both sides of the back of the tongue. Note free mucin background, sheets of bland ductal cells, included goblet cells and outlying aggregates of 'intermediate' type cells. (MGG × MP)
(B) Cytocentrifuge preparation from an aspirate of a small nodular palatal mass revealing an adenoid cystic carcinoma. These lesions are relatively common. Note the cribriform microarchitecture created by the small bland epithelial cells and enclosed or encircled balls of stromal type (fibrillary) mucin linked by fine stromal strands. (Papanicolaou × MP)

a morphological recognition of cell type or types and the appropriate application of immunostaining to define the immunophenotype. This can only be achieved by fastidious technique. All the material should be collected into citrated, buffered physiological saline solution, or cell culture fluid. By means of cell density separation media and cytocentrifuge techniques, it is possible to apply both conventional and special immunocytochemical staining procedures to the characterization of the particular lymphoma in question (Figs 11.8, 11.9).

The separation of lymphoma from poorly differentiated squamous carcinoma and melanoma is not problematic in adequate cytological aspirates appropriately processed. This contrasts with the sometimes insurmountable difficulties experienced in small traumatized histological biopsies,

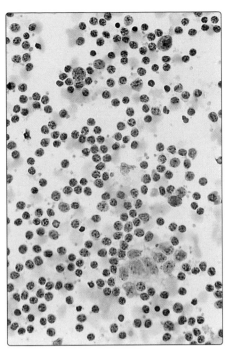

Fig. 11.8   Cytocentrifuge preparation from a capillary aspirate of an isolated 20 mm diameter, sublingual submucosal mass revealing a low-grade non-Hodgkin's B-cell lymphoma, centroblastic-centrocytic subtype. Background small lymphocytes can be seen; a majority population of cleaved centrocyte-like cells with micronucleoli (12 μm) and rare centroblast-like cells (25 μm) with dispersed micronucleoli (<3% of cells). Small cytoplasmic fragments (apoptotic cytoplasmic remnants) can also be seen between tumour cells (so called 'lymphoglandular bodies'); these demonstrated the same IgM kappa immunoglobulin restriction pattern after appropriate immunostains. (Papanicolaou × HP)

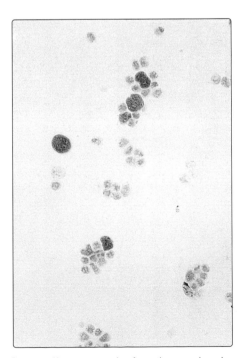

Fig. 11.9   Cytocentrifuge preparation from the same lymphoma as in **Fig. 11.8** stained with an antibody for Ki-67 (nuclear cell cycle related antigen) revealing brown nucleoplasmic and/or nucleolar staining of only 4% of tumour cells, mainly blast cells in cycle. (Ki-67 immunostain (DAKO) × HP)

directing re-biopsy. Most lymphomas are quickly identified cytologically, even without resort to immunocytochemistry, which is nonetheless essential for full characterization. These findings are in contrast to the commonly propounded clinicopathological myth that lymphomas, particularly low-grade lymphomas, are 'difficult' or even 'impossible' to cyto-diagnose. Adequate technique, moreover, permits immunoglobulin heavy and light chain restriction to be demonstrated in virtually all relevant B-cell lymphomas in fresh aspirates, much as in frozen tissue section; a further advantage by comparison with the difficulties experienced in paraffin embedded tissue. Systematic immunocytochemistry applied to all lymphoid cytological infiltrates is the best assurance the populations are as 'reactive' or innocent as they appear on morphological grounds. 'Best guessing' from limited direct preparations means a great many unnecessary anaesthetics, lymph node resections and scars to achieve even an equivalent level of clinical assurance.

Most lymphomas in this territory present as tonsillar, sublingual, buccal or palatal masses, and prove to be mainly non-Hodgkin's B-cell lymphomas (see Chapter 20).

Kaposi's disease

In AIDS patients, Kaposi's sarcoma commonly presents with nodular orofacial masses without ulceration and is particularly often present in the palate. There may or may not be accompanying lymphadenopathy.

Cytological findings

- ▶ Rafts or tangles of thin spindle cells with long parallel cytoplasmic process
- ▶ Discohesive individual plump spindle or epithelioid cells with polar processes and oval nuclei
- ▶ Mild variation in nuclear size and shape, no hyperchromatism
- ▶ Longitudinal nuclear grooves or chromatin lines caused by nuclear infolding (a prominent, but not unique feature of endothelial cells)
- ▶ Micronucleoli
- ▶ Intracytoplasmic bodies
- ▶ Few mitoses
- ▶ Accompanying macrophages with included haemosiderin granules

Diagnosis by aspiration cytology is possible, but usually with difficulty, as a consequence of the paucity of cellular material. The lesions aspirate easily only when within lymph nodes, where the minimal architecture is effaced. If cellular, the aspirate may reveal composite rafts or tangles and singly dispersed individual cells. The cells are spindle or polygonal cells with bland, plump nuclei without hyperchromatism; sometimes with characteristic longitudinal nuclear grooves or infoldings of the nuclear membrane. Diagnostic intracytoplasmic bodies that represent altered ingested red cells might be identified.

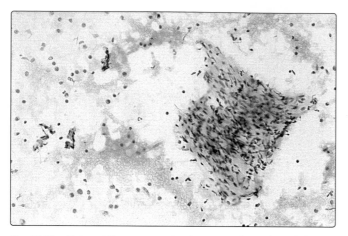

Fig. 11.10 Cytocentrifuge preparation from an aspirate of a nodular palatal mass in an AIDS patient revealing proliferated monotypic endothelial cells consistent with Kaposi's disease. Note the rafted endothelial cells with bland oval nuclei. (Papanicolaou × HP)

These are not specific and may be seen in angiosarcoma. Mitoses are few. Haemosiderin granules may be found in accompanying macrophages. If found, these spindle cells indicate proliferated endothelial cells which can be confirmed by immunocytochemistry, e.g. for factor VIII or CD34 (QB End 10). In the right clinical context they then clearly enough identify Kaposi's sarcoma. The nuclear features however, do not indicate neoplasia on purely cytomorphological grounds (Fig. 11.10).

On fresh aspiration material collected into cell culture fluid, washed, cytospun, air dried and acetone fixed, the spindle cells are usually positively immunostained for factor VIII related antigen, CD34 (QB End 10) and vimentin. They are negative for S100, α smooth muscle actin and desmin. MiB$_1$ or Ki67 immunostaining (reacting with a nuclear cell cycle related antigen) reveals positive nuclear staining in perhaps 1% of the cell population. Occasional spindle cells within the aspirated material will be positive for α actin and possibly are included smooth muscle cells from small vessel walls.

Melanoma

Primary melanoma of the oral cavity is a rare occurrence, mainly in negroid or oriental peoples. The criteria for diagnosis are as found with this tumour in skin (see Chapter 38).

Lipoma

Slow growing pedunculated or sessile lipomas and fibrolipomas may be encountered arising in the tonsillar areas, revealing sheets of mature adipose fibroadipose tissue in aspirates.

Fibroma

Pure fibromas are rare and cannot give a specific aspiration diagnosis even in context, since similar appearances will be seen with post-inflammatory pseudotumours.

Granular cell tumour

Granular cell tumours not uncommonly arise as nodules on the tip or edges of the tongue, in the palate or rarely in the posterior pharyngeal wall. The cytodiagnosis relies, as will this tumour in other sites, on the recognition of aggregated and discohesive, large, bland polygonal cells with granular acidophilic cytoplasm, polar pale nuclei and prominent single nucleoli. Mitoses are not seen. The cytologist may be struck by their similarity to apocrine cells from breast aspirates.

Neurofibroma

Occasionally this growth occurs in the tongue and may be diagnosed by aspiration. Correct identification of microbiopsies of thin spindle cells with sinewy nuclei and processes is necessary, with occasional admixed plump spindle or polygonal cells and often intermingled mast cells, best seen in May-Grünwald-Giemsa (MGG) stained preparations. Sometimes there are characteristic pseudoglandular or pseudocystic spaces present within the otherwise obvious spindle cell, soft tissue fragments, or myxoid areas with dendritic or stellate cells embedded in fibrillary mucin.

Chordoma

The author has seen this tumour which arises from notochordal remnants, presenting as a palatal nodule, having presumably arisen in the nasopharynx.

Sarcoma

Chondrosarcoma, osteosarcoma, rhabdomyosarcoma, fibrosarcoma, leiomyosarcoma and angiosarcoma may all present as primary tumours in the soft tissues and bone of the palate and jaws very rarely and aspiration might be predicted to reveal malignant spindle cells with or without reliable differentiating features, as with soft tissue tumours at other sites (see Chapter 40).

References

1   Silverman S Jr, Bilimoria K F, Bhargava K *et al.* Cytologic, histologic and clinical correlations of precancerous and cancerous oral lesions in 57 518 industrial workers of Gujarat, India. *Acta Cytol* 1977; **21**: 1896–198

2   Silverman S Jr, Gorsky M, Lozada F. Oral leukoplakia and malignant transformation. A follow-up study of 257 patients. *Cancer* 1984; **53**: 563–568

3   Allegra S R, Broderick P A, Corvese N. Oral cytology. Seven year oral cytology screening program in the State of Rhode Island. Analysis of 6448 cases. *Acta Cytol* 1973; **17**: 42–48

4   Folsom T C, White C P , Bromer L *et al.* Oral exfoliative cytology. Review of the literature and report of a three year study. *Oral Surg, Oral Med, Oral Pathol* 1972; **33**: 61–74

5   Hayes R L, Berg G W, Ross W L. Oral cytology: its value and its limitations. *J Am Dent Assoc* 1969; **79**: 649–657

6   Silverman S Jr. Early diagnosis of oral cancer. *Cancer* 1988; **63**: 1796–1799

7   Ogden G R, Cowpe J G, Chisholm D M, Lane D P. p53 immunostaining as a marker for oral cancer in diagnostic cytopathology – preliminary report. *Cytopathol* 1994; **5**: 47–53

8   Bruke J S. Lymphomas. In: Gnepp D R ed. *Pathology of the Head and Neck*. Edinburgh: Churchill Livingstone, 1988; p 335

12 Oesophagus and stomach

Alastair Deery

Introduction

Cytopathology of the gastrointestinal tract languishes in many parts of the world, mainly as a direct consequence of the traditional systematic specialization among anatomical pathologists. If gastrointestinal pathologists have no formative cytopathological training, then the application of cytological techniques often seems not to progress in that centre. Many published cytology texts and atlases have only the barest mention of this territory, with its rich, varied and sometimes difficult pathology. By applying the best sampling techniques (i.e. disposable endoscopic brushes cut off into alcohol free collection fluid, with tissue particles subsequently teased and vortexed from the brush bristles), and considering carefully the appropriate clinical questions to be answered for each segment of the intestine; clinical enthusiasm can be generated and sometimes answered more completely than with other available techniques alone, including biopsy. Ultrasound guided fine needle aspiration cytology has become a preferred method for diagnosis of intra-abdominal tumours in a few centres world-wide, employing trans-abdominal ultrasound[1] or endoscopic ultrasound[2]. This approach has been applied to oesophageal, gastric, pancreatic, hepatic and biliary lesions[1-5]. By taking the transducer close to the area of interest, with endoscopic ultrasound, Wiersema et al.[2] have recently demonstrated a very high accuracy in diagnosis in the oesophagus, stomach, duodenum and rectum. More recently trans-abdominal ultrasound has been demonstrated to have similar efficacy in the diagnosis of colonic neoplasia by Heriot et al.[6] (see Chapter 13).

Throughout the upper and lower intestinal tract, there are infectious and neoplastic processes that may be separately indicated by careful morphology. Dual conventional staining (Papanicolaou and MGG) is necessary to assist with infectious agents, e.g. *Helicobacter pylori*. Any collection and processing techniques need to allow for such considerations systematically. Immunocytochemical staining on parallel preparations will only be possible by adopting liquid collection media. Such staining is particularly important for confirmation of lymphoma or viral agents. Again preparedness requires a systematic or universal approach for all samples.

Normal anatomy and histology

The inner surface of the hollow muscular oesophagus is lined by non-cornified stratified squamous epithelium. Measured from the incisor teeth, the oesophagus extends to 150 mm at the hypopharynx and is approximately 400 mm in length at the junction with the gastric cardia. The sub-diaphragmatic transition zone of 10 to 20 mm is lined variably by off-white squamous epithelium and longitudinal folds of pink columnar, glandular cardiac gastric mucosa.

The cardia of the stomach extends to meet the gastric body a few centimetres from the gastro-oesophageal junction and is lined by very tall columnar, neutral mucinous epithelial cells arranged in tubules. The body, or fundal mucosa, is more complex. The inner quarter of the mucosa is composed of crypts lined by shorter columnar mucinous epithelial cells. The larger, deeper zone is composed of straight or coiled tubules incorporating mucous cells, spherical, parietal acid-secreting eosinophilic cells, cuboidal chief pepsinogen-secreting neutrophilic cells and a variety of pyramidal endocrine cells. The distal third of the stomach, or pyloric antrum, has a mucosa organized much in the same fashion as the body, but with increased mucous cells in the deep zone, fewer pepsinogen-secreting cells and a marked prevalence of gastrin-secreting G cells amongst the endocrine cell population.

The oesophageal and gastric walls are further subdivided: the muscularis mucosae lies beneath the lamina propria: the submucosa is in continuity through both viscera, although within the oesophagus it contains mucous glands and lymphoid aggregates in addition to the blood vessels, lymphatics and ganglion cells found throughout. Beneath the submucosa lie the layers of the muscularis propria. A thin serosa is present only over the stomach.

Cytology sampling methods

The advent of the flexible fibreoptic endoscope in the late 1960s relegated a plethora of washing and irrigation techniques to history[7]. The oblique view endoscope is now the instrument in common use for most oesophageal and gastric investigations and where cost implications are not the only measure of quality; allow the taking of both brush samples for cytopathology and small biopsies for histopathology. A recent five-year audit of gastro-oesophageal malignancy detection within this laboratory where combined samples were taken, revealed an 88% cytological sensitivity, a 73% histological sensitivity (1–3 simultaneous biopsy fragments) and a 96% combined detection rate at a single endoscopic evaluation. This must be compared with histological biopsy study detection rates of oesophageal cancer of 95% after six biopsies and 1200% after seven biopsies where there was endoscopic visualization of cancer[8].

Directional reusable brush samples may be collected and rolled directly on to the surface of glass slides for immediate fixation in alcohol, or less commonly air drying and post-fixation in methanol. Disposable brush samples tips are clipped off advantageously, into buffered saline or cell culture fluid to allow later laboratory processing and a wider range of better quality, identical preparations to be made. The brush sample should, in either case be taken prior to the biopsies, since there is then less blood contamination. This consideration is less critical with disposable brushes, due to the availability of density separation media for the subsequent separation of red cells from fluid wash samples.

The endoscopic brush should be employed like a needle rather than as a swab and jabbed through the surface mucosa or ulcer slough. Brush samples nonetheless benefit over usual small biopsies by including surface mucus or exudate from wider, sometimes unrelated mucosal surfaces and inevitably include an exfoliative sample. This is perhaps best explained by considering the identification of *Helicobacter pylori* in disposable brush wash preparations; the organisms are usually best seen in free wisps or trails of mucus rather than in close association with an epithelial surface (as in section). They are commonplace within oesophageal and duodenal brushes as a result of the wide inclusion of a sometimes cellular exudative gastric mucus sample within these otherwise directed brush samples. This of course considerably improves the yield from such samples by direct comparison with biopsy.

In general and by similar consideration, brush samples are superior to biopsy for the detection of usual epithelial malignancy in the oesophagus and stomach, and certainly in ulcerative epithelial malignancy. Biopsy is, however, superior in the detection of submucosal spreading 'signet-ring' cell carcinoma of the stomach, rare submucosal glandular malignancy of the oesophagus, primary gastric lymphomas or 'maltomas' and non-epithelial stromal tumours.

Normal components of cytological brush smears

Oesophageal brush smears are usually paucicellular in the absence of disease and are composed of superficial and intermediate squamous cells with small pyknotic or vesicular nuclei and variably eosinophilic or basophilic cytoplasm, in Papanicolaou stained preparations. In the absence of any other detectable abnormality, granular layer cells may appear and very occasionally may be accompanied by orthokeratotic or even parakeratotic artefacts. Buccal squamous cells may contaminate the specimen incidentally, contributing to these appearances, and swallowed sputum may be identified as mucus including ciliated respiratory-type cells and perhaps anthracotic pigment-laden alveolar macrophages. Ciliated columnar epithelial cells may rarely be native to this site as a result of remnant mucosa from an early embryonic stage of development[9]. Mixed bacteria, actinomyces and *Candida* spores are all commonly represented. In brush specimens from the lower oesophagus, it is common to observe amounts of gastric mucus and gastric epithelial cells as a reflection of the variable lining mucosa resulting from heterotopia[10], or due to the presence of acquired metaplastic gastric epithelium (Barrett's oesophagus)[11], or because of intrusion of the brush into the stomach.

Gastric brushes are much more cellular than oesophageal brushes in the absence of disease in the normal stomach. Invariably they include some detectable oesophageal or buccal degenerate elements: mucus and inflammatory cells: bare or stripped. Sometime degenerate pale folded gastric epithelial cell nuclei and variable small aggregates, twisted overlapped sheets, and microbiopsies with 'trunk-like' inverted crypts of mucus-type gastric epithelial cells (Fig. 12.1). Dependent on the site of the brushing and the depth of use of the brush, there may be loose aggregates of plump, granular, eosinophilic, spherical acid-secreting parietal cells and more rarely recognizable pale cuboidal pepsinogen-secreting or chief cells (Fig. 12.2).

Food debris is a frequent finding in both oesophageal and gastric specimens. After the ravages of heat coagulation (cooking), mastication (chewing) and enzymatic digestion (chemical catalysis), the morphological details of striated animal muscle fragments and different root vegetable or

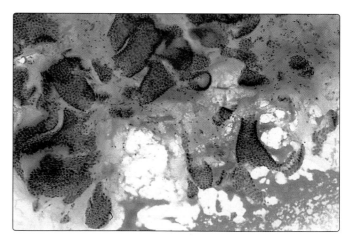

Fig. 12.1   Normal gastric brush smear with blood, mucus and complex sheets of tall columnar mucinous epithelial cells including inverted crypts or tubules ('elephant trunks'). (Papanicolaou × MP)

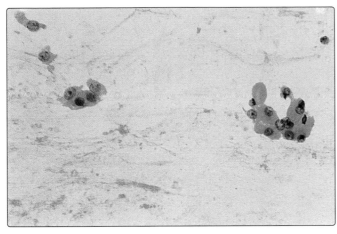

Fig. 12.2   Normal gastric body (fundus) brush including aggregators of granular spherical parietal cells from the deeper mucosal zone. (Papanicolaou × HP)

leafy plant materials may resist zoo-botanical identification. Fine or clumped refractile non-birefringent particles may be present as a consequence of the pre-endoscopic radiographic use of *Gastrograffin*.

Oesophagus

Inflammatory conditions

Reflux or peptic oesophagitis

An incompetent sphincter mechanism either transiently or chronically may lead to reflux of acid gastric contents into the lower oesophagus. A variety of conditions including sliding hiatus hernia, excessive alcohol consumption, pyloric stenosis, diabetic autonomic neuropathy, scleroderma and previous surgery may result in persistence of the reflux. The non-keratinized stratified squamous mucosa appears less resistant to acid or bile than the mucus and alkali-protected specialized columnar gastric glandular mucosa (as with the unprotected endocervical mucinous columnar epithelium and subsequent novel metaplastic squamous epithelium upon exposure to the lower pH vaginal micro-environment within the cervical ectopy). This results in acute inflammation, regenerative squamous hyperplasia, keratosis and subsequent healing, gastric/intestinal type metaplasia or chronic ulceration.

Cytological findings

Typical brush appearances in reflux oesophagitis will include some or all of these features dependent on some combination of the intensity or extensiveness of the changes:

► Increased squamous cellularity and discohesiveness (squamous hyperplasia)
► Clumps of irregular parabasal type squames with enlarged reactive hyperchromatic nuclei and multiple nucleoli (squamous hyperplasia)
► Increased polymorphs and mucus admixed with squamous sheets and perhaps lymphocytes; plasma cells; macrophages and cell debris (active inflammation)
► Eosinophils, which are otherwise unusual (associated with acid reflux chemical inflammation)
► Ulcer slough consisting of clumps of mixed inflammatory cell populations, macrophages; degenerate epithelial cells; fibroblasts; smooth muscle rafts; fibrin; red cells and small capillary or vein walls (ulcer evidence)

If superinfecting organisms such as *Candida* are present, this may destroy the associated appearances preventing the correct interpretation.

Barrett's oesophagus

This is not a congenital condition, but one of change in response to reflux oesophagitis resulting in small intestinal type or gastric type metaplasia in the normally squamous lined oesophagus[12]. In brush smears from the lower oesophagus, gastric epithelial cells are common whatever the putative measured endoscopic travel from the teeth and the condition may not be inferred from this information alone. The presence of small intestinal type epithelial sheets with a brush border on shorter columnar cells or cuboidal cells with goblet cells interspersed among them; will allow the inference; provided it is known the specimen is oesophageal; short of 350 mm and that there is no history of previous intestinal surgical repair.

The condition is pre-neoplastic and may be associated with adenomatous/papillary 'dysplasia' (*in situ* glandular neoplasia) but the risk of progression (particularly that associated with intestinal type metaplasia) has not been determined[13]. In brush smears, in the absence of neoplastic changes, recognition depends on the identification of intestinal type epithelium coupled with inflammatory reflux oesophagitis type changes. A considerable amount of sheeted or rafted epithelium is needed to allow recognition of the 'portholes' or 'flasks' (mucus cells seen from above/below or on edge respectively). The villous border is more difficult to see in cytology preparations than in section.

Radiation changes

Oesophagitis coupled with typical radiation changes in squamous, or included gastric type epithelial cells, is a relatively common finding in brush smears from, e.g. bone marrow transplant patients who receive pre-transplant 'mantle' irradiation to the chest. The changes usually regress, but may go on to cause stricture.

In squamous or gastric epithelial cells, radiation changes may occasionally be present in conjunction with tumour where irradiation is the instituted therapy (uncommon), or with accompanying ulcerative changes with or without additional *Candida* or viral co-infection due to *Cytomegalovirus* (CMV) or *Herpes simplex*. The clinical question is often directed 'unreasonably' towards a single cause of the ulceration and symptoms. The cellular morphology usually includes some combination of ulcer slough; degenerative and regenerative epithelial changes; infective agents; viral cytopathic effects; radiation induced focal cellular gigantism; multinucleation and atypia. Separate evaluation of lymphoid cells, which may be part of the inflammatory reaction, is necessary, to attempt to consider graft-versus-host disease or infiltration by any pre-existing or novel lymphoma or leukaemia. The correct interpretation among these processes might be likened to the quest for the 'Holy Grail'.

It is possible to separate mucopus from ulcer slough, to characterize and identify fungal organisms and specific viral effects and to set out separating irradiation atypia from ordinary regenerative changes. The further separation of possible chemotherapeutic cytotoxic effects from radiation changes, or the separate identification of graft-versus-host disease from common inflammatory alterations is not usually possible in brush smears. The observation of a common 'daughter' population of tumour cells may be unrelated to these changes and is not usually the area of difficulty, though such cells may well also suffer alteration by irradiation induced damage.

Cytological findings

The following is a summary of irradiation induced changes in brush smears:

► Increased epithelial cellularity composed of ragged sheets and aggregates of superficial, intermediate and basal squamous cells, isolated cells and trails of discohesive cells (hyperplasia)
► Dense amphophilia or azurophilia (green) of squamous cell cytoplasm regardless of maturity (metachromatic stain response to cytoplasmic metabolic changes)
► Multinucleation of epithelial cells (disordered cell division and impending cell death)
► Cellular gigantism of both mononuclear and multinucleated cells (disruption of cell division)
► Hydropic nuclear and cytoplasmic swelling with decreasing tincture and cytoplasmic vacuolation (simple common degenerative cellular changes; cytoplasmic changes usually in advance of nuclear alterations)
► Hypo- or hyperchromatism (nuclear stoichiometry of haematoxylin staining adjusts in response to differential fixation within direct smears in addition to condensed chromatin variations in regenerating/degenerating cell nuclei)
► Dispersed prominent macronucleolation (single or multiple in relation to metabolic adjustments)
► Normal nuclear/cytoplasmic ratios despite increased nuclear and cytoplasmic diameters (unlike neoplasia)
► Focal very variable or patchy occurrence of these changes within epithelial cells (heterogeneous cellular pleomorphism unlike the monotonous or homogeneous alterations within neoplasia)
► Degenerate dispersed-type mitoses (failed mitoses in irradiated dying cells)

► Accompanying polymorphonuclear leucocyte infiltration with or without true ulcer slough (active inflammation)
► Plump spindle or bizarre fibroblasts, macrophages and endothelial cells when ulceration is present (evidence of ulcer base material within preparations)

Candida infection

Candida pseudohyphae and spores are relatively common findings in conventional Papanicolaou stained brush smears in the presence of oesophagitis associated with reflux or gastric juice. Superinfection with *Candida* is sometimes seen in acute peptic ulceration, not uncommonly in malignant ulcerations and rarely combined with other infectious ulceration such as herpes[14,15]. In AIDS patients an intense oesophageal candidiasis is common; indeed, the author has correctly inferred the underlying diagnosis as a result of a pattern of intense *Candida* infection alone.

Cytological findings

Brushings of the off-white plaques from the middle or lower oesophagus include acute inflammatory exudates, 'knotted' sheets of squamous epithelial cells with admixed pseudohyphae and budded spores.

Inflammatory squamous cell changes in *Candida* infections include:

► 'Knotted' sheets of amphophilic squamous cells
► Granular layer squames increased
► Parakeratotic 'rafts' or 'whirls'
► Increased superficial and intermediate squamous nuclear diameters
► Vesicular multiple micronucleolated nuclei
► Entrapped 'cytoplasmic' polymorphs and apoptotic polymorph debris within squames

Other fungal or bacterial infections

Very rarely, infections are seen with organisms such as *Mucor*, *Histoplasma* and *Actinomyces*.

A bacterium, *Lactobacillus acidophilus*, may cause intense infection in AIDS and appears as grey-white membranous exudates and slough endoscopically. The organism is then clinically mistaken for *Candida*. In cytological circles it has had a confused nomenclature, often historically being referred to as Leptothrix. Lactobacillus appears as short, straight and long curved thin filaments (under 1 μm diameter). The organisms adopt long linked colony forms in opportunistic infections. These filaments may group in radiate balls or bezoars in brush smears in overwhelming infection or overgrowth and then can appear very similar to *Actinomyces* or *Nocardia*. The latter do not share the background of separate short bacillary and isolated curved and S-shaped filaments, and the balls of organisms are more coarsely filamentous and accompanied by particular interfilamentous fragmented bacteria.

Lactobacillus is most commonly seen in *in-vivo* culture conditions as short and long filamentous forms in cervical or vaginal smears. The long forms are then usually referred to as the mythical Leptothrix, which is unknown in microbiological taxonomy.

Viral infection

Herpes simplex ulceration is not uncommon in the oesophagus[16] and is seen in otherwise healthy, as well as immunosuppressed patients[17]. Clinically, the plaque-like ulcerative slough is usually mistaken for *Candida*. Herpes is rarely seen in this site in AIDS patients, whereas *Cytomegalovirus* is frequently seen in the gastro-oesophageal junction and elsewhere within the gastrointestinal tract[18,19].

Cytological findings

The characteristic features of *Cytomegalovirus* (CMV) seen elsewhere are rarely represented in oesophageal brush smears in AIDS. The plump endothelial cells are delivered by the brush from adjacent gastric margin ulcers, alongside intact squamous mucosa. The endothelial cells bearing the inclusions are degenerate or necrotic and are scattered as rare single mononuclear, or binucleate orangeophilic cells between the squamous sheets. The nuclei are polar and hydropic (swollen) with often shrunken eosinophilic or azurophilic inclusions. The cytoplasmic inclusions are not well seen separately, but form an orange granular haze (Fig. 12.3)

Rarely, the virus is seen in occasional plump proliferating endothelial cells as a 'passenger' within cells in brush smears, otherwise diagnostic of Kaposi's disease (Fig.12.4). The often very degenerate appearances of *Herpes simplex* virus infected squamous cells brushed from vesicles or ulcers in the middle or lower oesophagus may lead inexperienced observers to diagnose cancer of either squamous or glandular type (Figs 12.5–12.7).

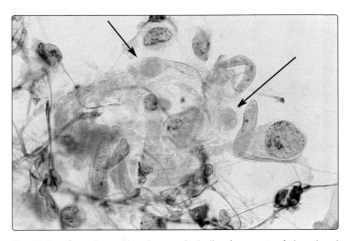

Fig. 12.4 Oesophageal brush smear including fragments of ulcer slough, which on close inspection are composed of tangled rafts of plump spindle and polygonal (histiocytoid) blandly nucleated cells, indicating Kaposi's disease. Cytoplasmic inclusions or bodies, which are probably ingested erythrocytes, are present in some spindle cells (arrows). (Papanicolaou × HP)

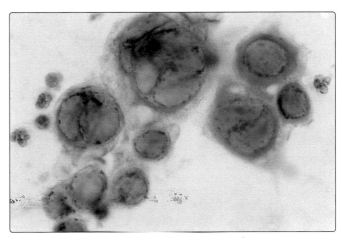

Fig. 12.5 Oesophageal brush smear revealing squamous cytopathic changes with the more typical ground glass inclusions, moulded syncytial giant cells and beaded nuclear membranes so characteristic of *Herpes simplex* infection. (Papanicolaou × HP)

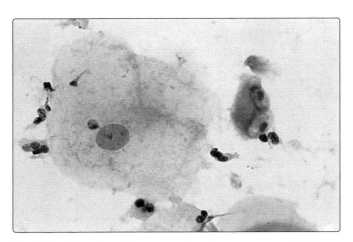

Fig. 12.3 Oesophageal brush smear including squamous epithelial sheets, background mucopus and cytoplasmic debris and an isolated plump degenerate orangeophilic endothelial cell with atypical CMV intranuclear and cytoplasmic inclusions. (Papanicolaou × HP)

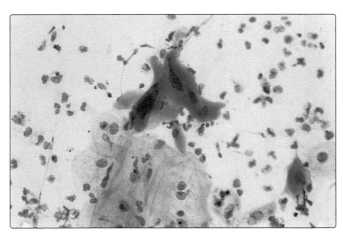

Fig. 12.6 Oesophageal brush smear including orangeophilic multinucleate *Herpes simplex* virus infected cells, mimicking squamous atypia. (Papanicolaou × HP)

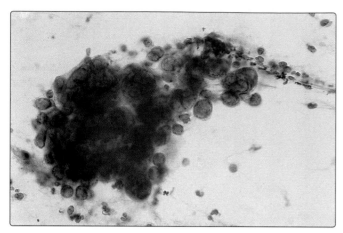

Fig. 12.7   Oesophageal brush smear including clusters of basophilic *Herpes simplex* virus infected giant cells, mimicking adenocarcinoma. (Papanicolaou × MP)

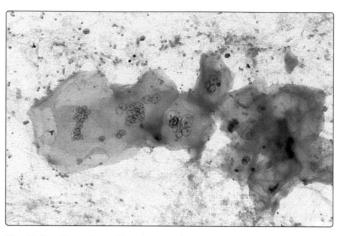

Fig. 12.8   Oesophageal brush smear from a post-bone marrow transplant patient, revealing sheets of squamous cells exhibiting multinucleation, dyskeratosis and dyskaryosis, indicating Human papillomavirus infection/latent reactivation and oesophageal intraepithelial neoplasia. (Papanicolaou × HP)

Table 12.1   Comparative cytological features of *Herpes simplex* and *Cytomegalovirus*

Herpes simplex
Separate mononuclear or bizarre syncytial-type giant, multinucleate squamous cells with moulded nuclei
Eosinophilic or basophilic intranuclear inclusions or 'ground glass' nuclei
Beaded nuclear membranes with alternating marginated chromatin and nuclear holes or gaps

Cytomegalovirus
Single, isolated, amphophilic, often very degenerate endothelial cells or, rarely, gastric epithelial cells
Sometimes binucleate or trinucleate giant cells with inclusions
Large azurophilic 'owl's eye' nuclear inclusions, peri-inclusional clear nuclear halo, marginated nucleolus, intact nuclear envelope
Cloud of smaller eosinophilic intracytoplasmic inclusions

Comparative cytological features of *Herpes simplex* and *Cytomegalovirus* are shown in Table 12.1.

Human papillomavirus (HPV) infection

The author has frequently seen koilocytosis, parakeratosis, dyskeratosis, multinucleation and dyskaryosis in oesophageal squamous cells in AIDS patients and in renal, liver and bone marrow transplant patients (Fig. 12.8), and HPV antigen has been demonstrated in such infections in the oesophagus[20]. Such changes may be seen in occasional cases of squamous carcinoma *in situ* in other patients, though such cases appear rare outside China and Iran.

Clear cell acanthosis (glycogenic acanthosis)

Discrete white plaques occur rarely in the lower oesophagus, which have been said to be squamous hyperplasia without atypia histologically. In the author's experience of two such cases brushed and biopsied, the cytological features were those of HPV infection. A single report has confirmed the presence of HPV DNA in three of six cases (50%) biopsied[21].

Epithelial tumours

Benign papillomas and adenomas

There is no good evidence that benign tumours of these types exist in man. The described 'growths' usually correspond either to inflammatory polyps, HPV associated condylomas or Barrett's associated polypoid hyperplasia or neoplasia.

Malignant epithelial tumours
Squamous carcinoma

There are marked variations in the incidence of this most common malignancy of the oesophagus with striking evidence of local pockets of high incidence in all parts of the world. China accounts for over half of all the world cases; there are high rates of occurrence in Iran and South Africa and, within Europe, in Normandy and Brittany in France. Male to female ratios vary considerably in different localities. Precancerous dysplasia and *in situ* oesophageal intraepithelial neoplasia are closely associated with the high incidence areas. Mass cytological screening with the use of an inflatable abrasive balloon has revealed a continuous range of changes of developing neoplasia akin to those in the cervix within high risk populations[22].

Aetiological factors include smoking in all its forms, tobacco chewing, eating of opiate-pipe tar residues, excessive alcohol consumption, trace element and vitamin deficiencies; but few hereditary factors to date.

Most tumours occur in the middle and lower thirds of the oesophagus, the postcricoid upper third carcinomas associated with the Plummer-Vinson syndrome now being rare. There is synchronous and asynchronous association with tumours in the oropharynx, larynx and respiratory tract, with similar aetiological risk factors.

Macroscopically, the tumours have a variably ulcerating, exophytic or stricturing appearance.

Cytological findings

▶ Ragged solid microbiopsies and syncytial sheets
▶ Dissociated pleomorphic abnormal epithelial cells
▶ Cell debris and/or slough
▶ Variable cytoplasmic differentiation or evidence of keratinization

The microscopic appearance of squamous tumours in brush smears are much as in other sites. Irregular compact microbiopsies with irregularly orientated ragged cellular margins, loose syncytial sheets, trails of discohesive scattered single large cells, pale or dark stripped nuclei and cytoplasmic debris are low power features that prompt the diagnosis at a glance (Figs 12.9, 12.10). Ulcer slough may or may not be present. As with most squamous cancer, the degree of cellular anaplasia is considerable, regardless of any apparent differentiation (defined mainly by the abnormal intracellular accumulation of high molecular weight cytokeratins or keratinization). When little

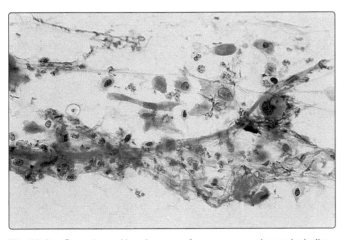

Fig. 12.9 Oesophageal brush smear of squamous carcinoma including scattered discohesive trials of pleomorphic, occasionally keratinized, squamous cells. (Papanicolaou × MP)

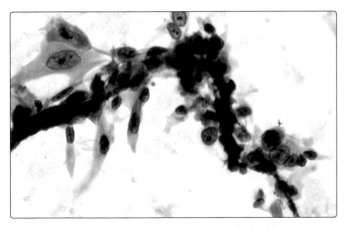

Fig. 12.10 Oesophageal brush smear of a ragged microbiopsy of squamous carcinoma including pleomorphic nuclear detail, coarse chromatin structure, multinucleation and multiple macronucleolation. (Papanicolaou × HP)

keratinization is apparent, it may be difficult to recognize the tumour type, though the degree of cellular anaplasia is unchanged. Discohesive, pleomorphic, multinucleated, often multiple micronucleolated, large epithelial cells, are characteristic. It can be difficult to recognize intercellular bridges cytologically and these assume less importance than in thin tissue sections where they are artefactually highlighted. The condensed nuclear chromatin in malignant squamous cells is usually much increased and very coarse. Pyknotic or karyorrhectic (apoptotic) and pale karyolytic, degenerate ghost cells seem more common in squamous tumours by comparison with glandular malignancies, but are nonetheless non-specific associations and may mislead. Plump spindle cells in rafts and clumped or single 'fibre' cells with or without keratinized cytoplasm are pathognomonic of squamous carcinoma cytologically even when the corresponding histology is said not to be obviously spindle celled. Rare 'smaller celled' monotonous basaloid or transition-celled squamous tumours may occur.

Adenocarcinoma

Unusual adenoid cystic and mucoepidermoid carcinomas are described arising from submucosal mucous glands usually in the middle third of the oesophagus[24,25]. Since they are usually still covered by sometimes hyperplastic squamous epithelium, it seems unlikely that these would present in a brush sample. The author is unaware of any cytological reports of such tumours in this site. Their features would be as with common similar salivary gland and uncommon bronchial gland tumours.

The remaining tumours are typical gastric-type adenocarcinomas and the cytological findings are described later. There may be adjacent dysplasia or *in situ* carcinoma arising in Barrett's oesophagus, where the squamous mucosa has been replaced by columnar epithelium. The malignant potential of this condition has probably been greatly exaggerated by intensive histological studies of simultaneously diagnosed disease.

In all, adenocarcinoma represents less than 5% of primary tumours of the oesophagus and the gastric-type tumours are often not distinguished from gastric carcinoma extending into the gastro-oesophageal junction.

The changes of adenocarcinoma *in situ* in oesophageal brushings are similar to those described for endocervical adenocarcinoma *in situ* or colonic adenomatous *in situ* neoplastic changes. The histological descriptions are similar, although high-grade *in situ* changes are usually synchronous with adjacent invasive tumour at this site[26]. Metastatic adenocarcinoma may rarely metastasize to this site and then can be seen within brush specimens (Figs 12.11, 12.12).

Small cell carcinoma

Perhaps 2–3% of oesophageal carcinomas are said to be of this type[27] although, in the author's experience, this is too high a figure. Endocrine cells have been identified in the

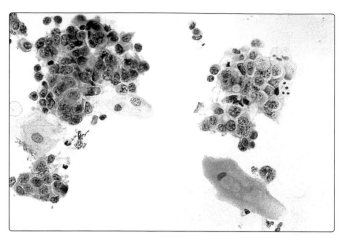

Fig. 12.11 Oesophageal disposable brush smear from an elderly female with a previous history of breast carcinoma, showing clusters of hyperchromatic small glandular epithelial cells with occasional intracytoplasmic mucin vacuolation. The small cell size and ductal mucin pattern suggest a breast rather than oesophageal primary tumour. (Papanicolaou × MP)

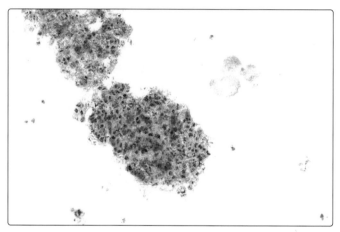

Fig. 12.12 Oesophageal brush of the same tumour (as in **Fig. 12.11**), exhibiting diffusely positive oestrogen receptor immunoperoxidase staining in the tumour cell nuclei. (Oestrogen receptor immunostain × MP)

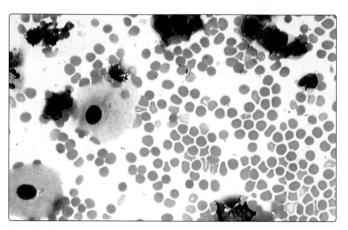

Fig. 12.13 Oesophageal brush smear revealing squamous sheets and files of moulded small hyperchromatic cells characteristic of an uncommon primary small cell carcinoma. (MGG × HP)

Granular cell tumours, neurofibromas, lipomas and angiomas all occur in the oesophagus, although none has been described in cytological samples. These tumours are all submucosal and would be less likely to appear in conventional brush cytology.

Advance in the use of endoscopic ultrasound-guided fine needle aspiration will produce cytological diagnoses of some of these lesions in the near future.

Malignant stromal tumours

There are few reports in the literature of cytological diagnosis of leiomyosarcoma or any of the more unusual sarcomas occurring in this site.

Melanoma

Melanocytes are present in the oesophageal mucosa, but melanoma in the oesophagus is more often secondary than primary. The author has seen a single oesophageal brush sample with metastatic melanoma. The presence of junctional changes in the squamous epithelium is said to distinguish primary from secondary tumours. This feature would only be available in biopsy material.

Leukaemia and lymphoma

Rare primary lymphomas have been described in the oesophagus as histological case reports. Secondary lymphomatous and leukaemic infiltration is more common and Hodgkin's disease has been described. Antemortem cytological diagnosis of acute myeloblastic leukaemic infiltration of the oesophagus has been reported and said to be present in just over 7% of cases at postmortem[30].

Stomach

Inflammatory conditions

Acute gastritis, chronic gastritis, superficial gastritis, atrophic gastritis, peptic ulceration

Brush cytology may reveal several distinctive patterns of inflammation, which variably correspond to underlying

basal layer of the normal oesophageal mucosa. The tumours arise in the middle and lower thirds and are no different cytologically or histologically from 'oat cell' carcinoma of other sites, although they are commoner in females (Fig. 12.13).

A lung primary eroding or metastatic to the oesophagus needs to be excluded before accepting the tumour as a primary oesophageal malignancy. Occasionally tumours are combined with a squamous or glandular tumour[28], or associated *in situ* squamous carcinoma[29].

Non-epithelial tumours

Benign stromal tumours

Polypoid leiomyomas, which may occasionally be ulcerated, arise here as elsewhere in the bowel, within the muscularis propria. There are only rare cytological reports in this site, although this is the commonest benign tumour.

histopathological diagnosis and clinical patterns of symptoms. Cytology has a minor role in the findings in such inflammation.

Acute erosive gastritis

This may be related to excessive consumption of alcohol, the ingestion of drugs such as aspirin, salicylates, corrosive chemicals, uraemia, bacterial toxins, reflux of bile, or to endotoxic shock.

Cytological findings

► Increased cellularity
► Fibrinous mucopurulent material
► Epithelial fragments and dissociated groupings
► Absence of frank ulcer slough

The cytological feature of erosion consists of an altered pattern of large amounts of fibrinous mucopus, with islands of degenerative and regenerative epithelial cells. The smears include fresh blood and fibrin. The fibrin meshes that form combine mucus, polymorphs, stripped gastric epithelial cells and histiocytes. Intact, discohesive, hydropic epithelial cells appear in small loose aggregates with degenerative nuclear and cytoplasmic vacuolation or partial dissolution. Larger sheets or microbiopsies composed of reactive gastric epithelial cells may be seen with pleomorphic vesicular nuclei, prominent nucleoli (nucleolar dispersion), coarsely aggregated nuclear chromatin and amphophilic cytoplasm, with loss of pale mucin. Mitoses may be present. Polymorphs and polymorph debris are seen entrapped or encircled apparently within the cytoplasm of enlarged epithelial cells. These are all degenerative exfoliative appearances in a regenerating epithelial surface and must be sensibly differentiated from neoplasia (Fig. 12.14). There is no

evidence of deeper ulceration signalled by the appearance of ulcer slough.

Chronic continuing gastritis

The relationship of this cytological pattern to chronic gastritis, atrophic gastritis and gastric atrophy is only approximate and often unclear.

Cytological findings

► Microbiopsies of epithelial cells with chronic inflammatory cell infiltration
► Discohesive epithelial cells mingling with lymphocytes and plasma cells
► Acute inflammatory exudate still also present
► Intestinal metaplasia may be seen
► *Helicobacter pylori* identifiable in air-dried preparations

Brush smears may include some acute features, including increased mucopus and fibrin meshes related to acute erosion and reactive (regenerative) epithelial sheets with admixed polymorphs in which the epithelial cells are commonly shortened and cuboidal in appearance, with enlarged nuclei and possess conspicuous, often multiple nucleoli. The key features, however, include microbiopsies of epithelial cells including lamina propria with a prominent lymphocyte and plasma cell population and sometimes follicle centre cells. In addition, there are trails of discohesive epithelial cells with admixed lymphocytes, plasma cells, histiocytes, polymorphs and sometimes eosinophils (Fig. 12.15).

Intestinal metaplasia may be seen in such smears. This is recognized in flat sheets by the identification of an eosinophilic cuboidal or short columnar cell margin, a tenuous fused 'terminal bar' line and short brush or pale ciliated border. Goblet cells are seen every six or seven nuclei within the 'honeycomb' with the mucus above or behind the nucleus, depending on whether the sheet faces out of or into the slide (see Figs 13.2, 13.3). With care and

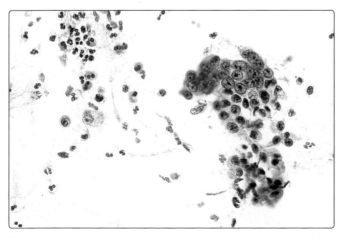

Fig. 12.14 Gastric brush smear including sheets of benign markedly reactive (regenerative) gastric epithelial cells with loss of pale apical mucin, amphophilic cytoplasm, degenerative cytoplasmic vacuolation, pale nucleoplasm, smooth nuclear envelopes and prominent nucleoli. Acute erosive gastritis. (Papanicolaou × MP)

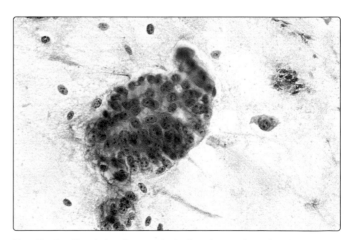

Fig. 12.15 Gastric brush smear including sheets of gastric epithelial cells with inflammatory regenerative and degenerative features. No ulcer slough is present. Chronic gastritis. (Papanicolaou × HP)

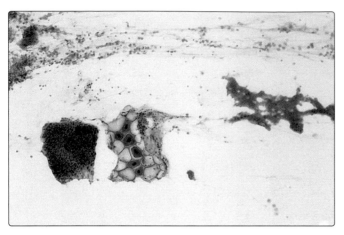

Fig. 12.16 Gastro-oesophageal brush smear revealing ulcer slough, food debris and a large sheet of epithelial cells with surface and included goblet cells (vacuoles over nuclei within sheet). Intestinal metaplasia. (Papanicolaou × MP)

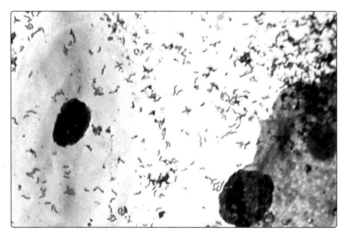

Fig. 12.17 Disposable gastric brush cytospin smear from pylorus including trails of bird's wing-like spiral organisms characteristic of *Helicobacter pylori*. (Romanowsky (MGG) × HP)

practice, 'incomplete' forms of intestinal metaplasia can be recognized. Paneth cells are rare in such examples (Fig. 12.16).

The presence of the spiral bacterium *Helicobacter pylori* has been studied in gastric brush specimens, using modified Romanowsky methods, with considerable success in rapid recognition (Fig. 12.17)[31]. The organism is common in loose association with gastric mucus or epithelial cells in smears. A dry preparation is necessary for processing. Culture testing is a superior, less subjective and more specific technique, however[32].

Ulcerative gastritis

Cytological findings

▶ Ulcer slough as described above
▶ Erosive type exudate
▶ Increased epithelial fragments with marked reactive cellular changes
▶ Possible *Candida* superinfection

All the features of acute erosive gastritis may be present in brush smears from benign chronic ulceration. The determination of the presence of a chronic ulcer requires the recognition of ulcer slough. This appears as compact microbiopsies composed of fibrin mesh, polymorphs, mucus, histiocytes, epithelial cells and then stromal material including small vessels, fibroblasts and lymphoid aggregates (i.e. granulation tissue). The appearance of the deeper layers of the ulcer base is the critical element. In addition, there may be striated animal muscle debris, plant debris, foreign crystalline debris from oral medications and sometimes haemosiderin-laden macrophages as evidence of old haemorrhage. *Candida* pseudohyphae may be present within the slough, representing secondary superinfection.

The epithelial cells within the brush may be from the ulcer edge or base and appear as microbiopsies or small looser sheets of often markedly reactive, or regenerative enlarged glandular cells. There may be marked focal irregular pleomorphism and anisocytosis, hyperchromatic coarse clumped nucleoplasm, prominent multiple nucleation and dark or pale hydropic cytoplasm. Mitoses may be numerous. Polymorphs and lymphocytes are commonly closely admixed amongst the cells of the epithelial groups. The experienced observer will nonetheless rapidly distinguish this chaos from the rather monotonous regular irregularity of clonal neoplasia.

Granulomatous gastritis

Cytological findings

Within brush smears, giant multinucleate histiocytes and histiocytic aggregates are most commonly seen in association with food debris, presumably intruded into an ulcer base. Granulomas related to other specific causes such as Crohn's disease, *Mycobacteria*, bile reflux, *Helicobacter*; or worm infestation are all less likely occurrences.

Viral gastritis

Herpetic ulceration with *Herpes simplex* virus and *Cytomegalovirus* infection may occur in gastric mucosa as in the oesophagus. In AIDS patients, *Cytomegalovirus* ulceration is pre-eminent.

Fungal gastritis

In immunosuppressed patients, fungal infection may be seen in brush smears, most typically due to *Mucor* and *Candida* and sometimes in association with *Cytomegalovirus* ulceration.

Summary of cytological features of gastritis

▶ Purulent brush smears with fresh blood and fibrinomucoid meshes
▶ Mucopus and/or ulcer slough, the latter including small vessels, fibroblasts, lymphocytes and sometimes plasma cells

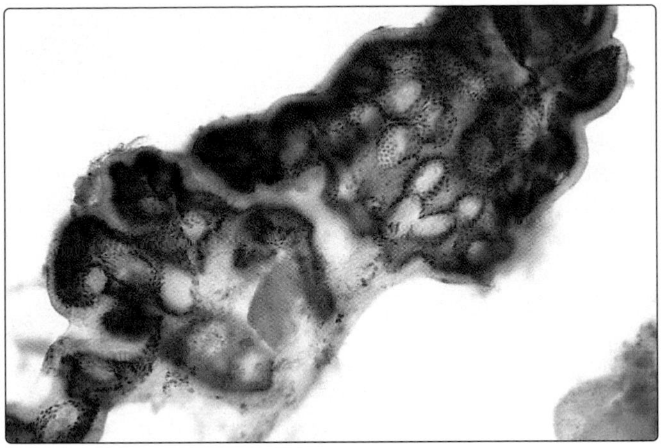

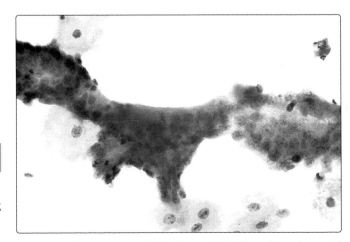

Fig. 12.18 Gastric brush from polypoid lesion in gastric cardia revealing mucoid lakes with an unusually complex microbiopsy of tall mucinous epithelium with racemose pattern and dilated crypts. In context the appearances indicated a 'regenerative' polyp. (Papanicolaou × MP)

▶ Microbiopsies, 'honeycombed' flat sheets, loose aggregates and discohesive trails of variably reactive regenerative and degenerative epithelial cells. Admixed or entrapped polymorphs, lymphocytes and perhaps plasma cells
▶ Epithelial cells show cytoplasmic condensation and loss of pale mucin. Orientation may be lost and some eddying of cells seen within sheets with nuclear overlap
▶ Epithelial cells in regenerative hyperplasia within erosions, ulcers or incipient ulceration are irregularly enlarged with increased nuclear diameters, irregular coarsely clumped chromatin, smooth nuclear envelopes and variable conspicuous nucleation
▶ Mitoses may be few or frequent

Benign epithelial tumours
Benign polyps
Hyperplastic, or regenerative polyps are the commonest type and consist of complex folded epithelium and sometimes mucin-filled cystically dilated crypts. They may be single or multiple. Rarely, they may present characteristic microarchitectural features in brush smears in context with the endoscopic features (Fig. 12.18). The diagnosis rests, however, with the histopathological biopsy.

Adenomatous polyps
These represent a minority of gastric polyps and within histopathological classifications include some types of early gastric cancer.

Cytological findings

Brush smears of such polyps may show complex villous or unusual crypt microarchitecture in microbiopsies, crowding of hyperchromatic columnar nuclei including mitoses or obvious neoplastic cellular atypia in addition. In the latter case, the appearances resemble the features seen in brush smears from colonic adenomas with 'dysplasia' (see Chapter 13). Intestinal metaplasia is common.

The endoscopic features represent vital information, which must cautiously guide the observer against the over-diagnosis of malignancy.

Hamartomatous polyps
There are no cytological reports of distinguishable types of hamartomatous polyps as found in association with Peutz-Jeghers syndrome, Cronkhite-Canada syndrome, or fundic cysts and it seems unlikely that separable microarchitectural features might be identified.

Malignant epithelial tumours
Gastric *in situ* neoplasia
Atypia amounting to *in situ* neoplasia occurs in association with adenomas most commonly and in association with Barrett's oesophagus. Few early gastric carcinomas can be demonstrated to arise on the basis of pre-existing 'dysplasia'. The cytological features are similar to the appearances seen in the colon and indeed, endocervix. That such cases are possessed of neoplastic character is clear and the histological preference for the term 'dysplasia' need not be adopted.

In this laboratory we have seen two patterns of smear appearances emerging: one of hyperplastic epithelial sheets with crowding of polarized nuclei and mild nuclear hyperchromasia; the other of papillary or ciriform tubular configurations with cell size increase, definite nuclear membrane irregularities, nucleolation and 'peppered' chromatin. The first pattern is correlated with mild gastric 'dysplasia'; the second with high grade adenomatous 'dysplasia'; or indeed early gastric carcinoma, histologically. The second pattern requires a cytological report of 'at least *in situ* glandular neoplasia' (Figs 12.19, 12.20).

Early gastric adenocarcinoma
Carcinomas that are histologically confined to the mucosa and submucosa in either case with or without lymph node metastases may be surgically curable[33]. Most such cases

Fig. 12.19 Oesophagogastric brush smear including a sheet of crowded hyperchromatic epithelial cells with enlarged nuclei, peppered chromatin and mitotic figures. High grade adenomatous dysplasia in Barrett's oesophagus. (Papanicolaou, × MP)

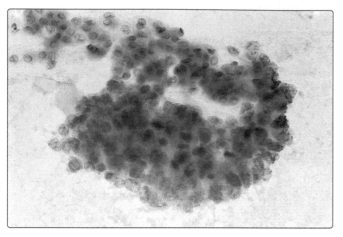

Fig. 12.20   Oesophagogastric brush smear of a papilliform microbiopsy in Barrett's associated high grade dysplasia, alongside degenerate benign epithelium. (Papanicolaou, × HP)

into well, moderately or poorly differentiated groupings of each type (WHO classification).

Lauren more practically divided tumours into a common intestinal type, with papillary and solid patterns and variably well-formed glandular lumina lined by large polar cells, and a less frequent diffuse type characterized by an infiltrative more sclerosing pattern with few gland lumina, a smaller celled population and often abundant intra- and extracellular mucus. The sex ratio for diffuse type carcinomas is equal and intestinal type growths predominate still more in high incidence areas.

There are inconsistencies and difficulties in applying both these and other lesser known classifications to given tumours by different pathologists and the structural criteria of the WHO classification is most popular. There has been no systematic study or correlation of cytological appearances with either histological pattern or clinical outcome.

Cytological findings in gastric adenocarcinoma

► Ulcer slough containing single malignant cells
► Papillary or glandular formations frequently seen
► Signet ring carcinomas show few cells, dissociated, with a prominent mucous vacuole, open chromatin and macronucleolus
► Poorly differentiated tumours may have squamoid features

Brush smears reveal 'signet-ring' type carcinomas with difficulty. Commonly, the tumour cells are few in number in the smears and present as small loose groups or trails of discohesive large pleomorphic cells. This probably reflects the pattern of diffuse mucosal and submucosal spread, but little surface tumour. The clear vacuole compressing a thin marginated nucleus seen in formalin fixed histological material appears different in brushings with alcohol fixation. In smears, the large cells have a marginated, but usually more open nucleus with a prominent commonly single macronucleolus. The intra-cytoplasmic mucin is finely textured and lightly basophilic. A thin rim to the textured mucin may be identified close to, but separate from the cytoplasmic rim (Fig. 12.21). The anaplasia of the cells is evidenced by their lack of any cellular cohesion, their large size, anisonucleosis and anisonucleolinosis.

Other patterns of adenocarcinoma seen cytologically fit variably well with the underlying histology. Papillary and glandular patterns are easily recognized in smears (Fig. 12.22)[38]. Ulcerated solid carcinomas give rise to ragged biopsies with an inflammatory cell infiltrate. Careful inspection may reveal microtubular arrangements or pseudocystic patterns within such fragments of tumour, the latter representing disrupted glandular lumina. Within ulcer slough, it is usually simple to identify degenerate discohesive groups and trails of tumour cells.

Very poorly differentiated tumours may be difficult to categorize as adenocarcinoma. The cells may have high

have occurred and have been studied in Japan. Classification is complicated and divides lesions into a number of subtypes of elevated or depressed cancers from the gross or endoscopic appearances. Most tumours occur in the pyloric antrum following the pattern of more advanced cancer. The majority are tubular (well differentiated), or else 'signet-ring type' (poorly differentiated) cancers.

Cytologically, brush smears from such tiny cancers (3–90 mm in diameter)[34], are no different from more usual advanced tumours.

Adenocarcinoma

Gastric carcinoma is one of the most common malignancies world-wide, with a male predominance and an especially high incidence in Japan, South America, Eastern Europe and Portugal. Since the 1950s, falls in the incidence rates have been recorded in virtually all countries. The causes of this turnaround are largely still obscure, the reasons for declining incidence remaining circumstantial and speculative. Dietary studies reveal some associations with high carbohydrate, low fat and low vitamin C intake. Pathological studies reveal that precancerous conditions include atrophic gastritis and intestinal metaplasia. These conditions, along with non-premalignant conditions such as peptic duodenal ulceration, are all being convincingly linked to exposure to and colonization by *Helicobacter pylori*[35,36]. Early life exposure to this organism has been proposed as critical in determining later susceptibility to the disease[37]. Genetic factors appear to have little influence, but may prove to have a role in pre-selection of those with particular responses to colonization or infection by *Helicobacter*.

Gross appearances of gastric cancer include polypoid, nodular, ulcerative and infiltrative plaque-like, or sclerosing growths. Combinations of these basic patterns occur.

Histological classification of the microscopic pattern divides tumours into papillary, tubular, mucinous and 'signet-ring' cell types, which may be variously combined

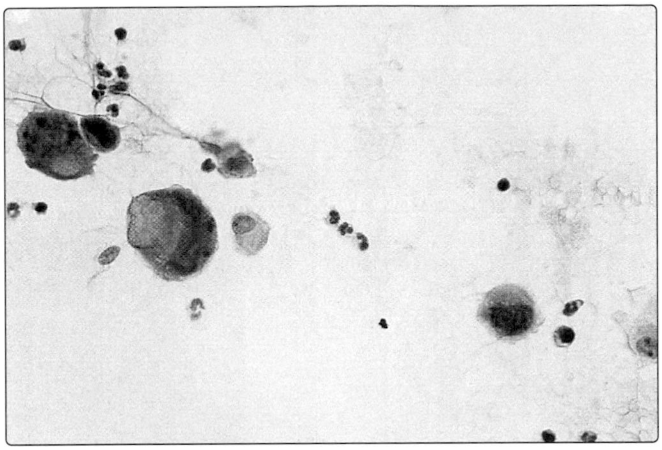

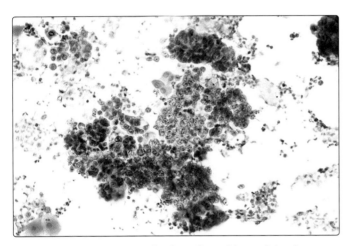

Fig. 12.21 Gastric brush showing one of several scarce trails of dispersed mainly dyshesive 'signet-ring' type large carcinoma cells with marginated nucleolated nuclei and textured cytoplasmic mucin. (Papanicolaou, × HP)

Fig. 12.22 Cytospin preparation from disposable gastric brush incorporating papilliform and solid microbiopsies and clusters of malignant large glandular epithelial cells with prominent, usually single, nucleoli and finely irregular nuclear envelopes. Gastric adenocarcinoma. (Papanicolaou, × MP)

nuclear/cytoplasmic ratios, little evidence of mucin and sometimes a surprisingly small celled or intermediate sized cell pattern, and yet are evidently carcinoma. If present in smears from the gastro-oesophageal junction, patient searching needs to be carried out to separate any squamous or glandular features. One may not depend on associative cytological features of necrosis, such as pyknotic necrotic cells, to type squamous neoplasia. Orangeophilic cytoplasm and even 'tadpole cells' may occasionally appear in adenocarcinoma without later histologically recognizable features of squamous differentiation.

In such poorly differentiated tumours it is identification of specific features of squamous differentiation that usually identify the tumour type i.e. 'fibre' or spindle cells and 'pearls' with or without dyskeratotic central cells. Multiple nucleation and multiple macronucleolation, if present, are on balance features of squamous tumour. Single nucleoli do

not push the likelihood in favour of adenocarcinoma when other features fail. It may occasionally not be possible to place the features in one of the two camps and, more rarely still, a combined tumour is identified in the presence of good features of both differentiations. When only fixed brush smears are received, it is nonetheless possible to lift a coverslip and perform a mucin stain, which may well resolve the issue. The receipt of disposable brushes in fluid makes it practicable to perform such stains consistently as required.

Endocrine cell tumours

Carcinoid tumours of the stomach form a small percentage of such tumours occurring in the gastrointestinal tract. They usually form polypoid or nodular grey masses without or with ulceration in the body or pyloric antrum.

Cytological reports in gastric brushings are non-existent, but the features would be similar to carcinoids in other sites (see Chapter 3).

Non-epithelial tumours
Lymphoma

The majority of primary gastric lymphomas are B-cell lymphomas with a fairly even breakdown of high-grade versus low-grade tumours (REAL classification). Most gastric lymphomas are a result of secondary involvement. Primary gastric lymphomas usually present as single or multiple ulcerated nodular or polypoid masses in the gastric body or polyic antrum. They may also take the form of incipiently ulcerating thickened rugae where the tumour is diffusely infiltrating.

Cytological appearances of gastric lymphomas in smears have been described in the past[39] and have predicted the eventual histological classification in many cases. However, the last decade of the twentieth century has seen the characterization of lymphomas of mucosa-associated lymphoid tissue (MALT) affecting the stomach and intestine and further the introduction of the idea that such lymphomas account for the majority of primary gastric lymphomas[40,41]. It has been proposed that most low-grade tumours and possibly high-grade tumours are derived from a centrocyte-like marginal zone B cell that differentiates either to immunoblast-like, centroblastic or lymphoplasmacytoid and plasmacytic cell types[42].

Most recently[43], it is suggested that the acquisition of MALT in the stomach is dependent on infection by *Helicobacter pylori*. Continued infection is suggested to lead to strain specific T cell drive, B cell proliferation and chronic active gastritis. Continued B cell proliferation is then proposed to result in clonal selection and expansion while apparently still under specific antigen-drive (*Helicobacter* strain specific) via T-cell cytokines. Whether this stage of 'clonal' expansion should be considered reversible lymphoproliferative disease, remains controversial (as with such disease in transplant recipients receiving immunosuppressive therapy) or meets the possible more demanding criteria of autonomous neoplasia. The invariably good prognosis, the localized extent of disease and claims for its cure or reversibility by antibiotic treatment directed against *Helicobacter* infection, might support the former interpretation.

Nonetheless, the elucidation of a mechanism of T-cell dependent B-cell proliferation may prove to have much wider application in understanding T-cell rich B-cell lymphoproliferative disease.

Cytological findings

The identification of lymphoma in brush smears requires the recognition first of an unusual lymphoid population and then the separate analysis of whether that lymphoid population is reactive, derived from lymphocytic gastritis, or neoplastic, that is from a lymphoma of one or another of several cell types.

A certain amount may be achieved by experienced cytomorphological observation and correct assignment of the observed lymphoid populations to the correct lymphoma subcategory. This situation, however, is now clearly theoretically increasingly complex in gastric and intestinal lymphoma. Brush smears and biopsies may not be sufficient to determine the most appropriate treatment and surgery may be curative. Careful immunophenotyping is required to support the morphological assessment. This requirement would seem to preclude the use of brush cytology, except perhaps for the introduction of disposable brushes. In the author's laboratory, after audit of eight biopsy established cases of low-grade maltoma where conventional brushings were also received, a suggestive diagnosis was only offered in three cases cytologically and, after retrospective review, in only one further case, arguably (Figs 12.23–12.25). This compares unfavourably with the majority of cases of leukaemic or high-grade lymphomatous gastric involvement over the same period (Fig. 12.26)

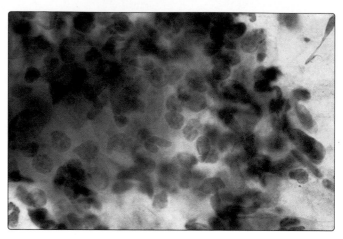

Fig. 12.24   Gastric brush of low grade lymphoproliferative disease of MALT (maltoma) revealing a sheet of epithelial cells (pale elongated nuclei and syncytium of orangeophilic cytoplasm) with intimately infiltrating centrocyte-like cells (a 'lymphoepithelial lesion'). (Papanicolaou, × HP)

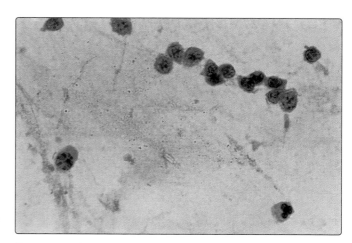

Fig. 12.25   Gastric brush maltoma showing a trail of centrocyte-like cells and an occasional plasma cell. (Papanicolaou, × HP)

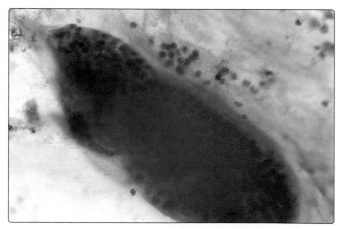

Fig. 12.23   Gastric brush smear including a microbiopsy composed of tall columnar mucinous cells with an admixture of centrocyte-like cells of maltoma (a 'lymphoepithelial lesion'). (Papanicolaou, × MP)

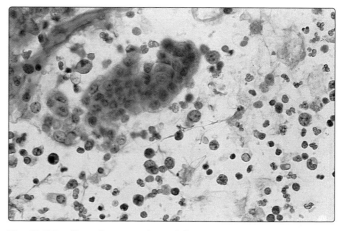

Fig. 12.26   Cytospin preparations of disposable gastric brush specimen featuring a high-grade diffuse large B-cell lymphoma (centroblastic, polymorphic subtype). (Papanicolaou × MP)

Within direct smears, the characteristic 'lymphoepithelial lesions' are hard to see and perhaps because of the wide numbers of differentiated cell types, may be harder still to separate from reactive populations. Intraepithelial lymphocytes are common in lymphocytic gastritis within brushes. The demonstration heavy and light chain restriction is not practicable within a few submitted prefixed, direct brush smears and requires a cell suspension only possible from a disposable brush. In addition, it would perhaps be desirable to identify such lymphoproliferative disease by the application of molecular genetic analysis to distinguish it from morphologically and immunophenotypically similar follicle centre-cell tumours. It is clear that many of these limitations also apply to small biopsies and a more exhaustive approach may be required.

Stromal tumours

The stomach is the most common site in the gastrointestinal tract for stromal tumours of smooth muscle or neural origin. Their submucosal location, characteristically with a central ulcer-crater, might seem to reduce the application of brush cytology. Nonetheless, occasional cytological diagnoses of cases of leiomyosarcoma have been reported[44]. In the presence of a typical endoscopic appearance and with the aid of endoscopic ultrasonography, fine needle aspiration has reportedly provided the reliable differential diagnosis of leiomyomas and leiomyosarcoma in stomach and other sites[45]. It is not clear however, to what extent the clinical or endoscopic details urged the correct diagnosis. These gastric tumours may show scant evidence of smooth muscle differentiation immunocytochemically (desmin) and their often 'epithelioid' cell make-up might be expected to prompt a diagnosis of carcinoma where there are cellular features of neoplasia. The author has indeed reviewed such an instance in gastric brush smears and even 'retrospectroscopically' found the distinction tasking. A malignant stromal tumour in small intestine is presented in Chapter 13, with both usual spindle and epithelioid features.

References

1   Holm H H, Skjolbye B. Interventional ultrasound. *Ultrasound Med Biol* 1996; **22**: 773–789

2   Wiersema M J, Vilmann P, Giovannini M *et al.* Endosonography guided fine needle aspiration biopsy: diagnostic accuracy and complication assessment. *Gastroenterology* 1997; **112**: 1087–1095

3   Vilmann P, Hancke S, Henriksen F W, Jacobsen G K. Endoscopic ultrasonograph guided fine needle aspiration biopsy of lesions in the upper gastrointestinal tract. *Gastrointest Endosc* 1995; **41**: 230–235

4   Chang K J, Katz K D, Durbin T E *et al.* Endoscopic ultrasound guided fine needle aspriation. *Gastrointest Endosc* 1994; **40**: 694–699

5   Giovanni M, Seitz J F, Monges G *et al.* Fine needle aspiration cytology guided by endoscopic ultrasonography: results in 141 patients. *Endoscopy* 1995; **27**: 171–177

6   Heriot A G, Kumar D, Thomas V *et al.* Ultrasonographically guided fine needle aspiration cytology in the diagnosis of colonic lesions. *Br J Surg* 1998; **85**: 1713–1715

7   Husain O A N. Alimentary tract (oesophagus, stomach, colon, rectum). In: Bibbo M ed. *Comprehensive Cytopathology*. London: W B Saunders, 1991; 409–432

8   Graham D Y, Schwarts J T, Cain G D, Gyarkey F. Prospective evaluation of biopsy number in the diagnosis of oesophageal and gastric carcinoma. *Gastroenterol* 1982; **82**: 228

9   Raeburn C. Columnar ciliated epithelium in the adult oesophagus. *J Path Bact* 1951; **63**: 157

10 Hague A K, Merkel M. Total columnar lined oesophagus: a case for congenital origin? *Arch Pathol Lab Med* 1981; **105**: 546

11 Barrett N R. The oesophagus lined with gastric mucous membrane. *Surgery* 1967; **41**: 881

12 Mossberg S M. The columnar lined oesophagus (Barrett's syndrome) – an acquired condition? *Gastroenterol* 1966; **50**: 671

13 Sarr M G, Hamilton S R, Marrone G C, Cameron J L. Barrett's oesophagus: its prevalence and association with adenocarcinoma in patients with symptoms of gastro-oesophageal reflux. *Am J Surg* 1985; **149**: 187

14 Rosen P, Hajdn S I. Visceral herpes virus infection in patients with cancer. *Am J Clin Pathol* 1971; **56**: 459–465

15 Concomitant herpes-monilial oesophagitis: case report with ultrastructure study. *Hum Pathol* 1982; **8**: 760–763

16 Nash G, Ross J S. Herpetic oesophagitis: a common cause of oesophageal ulceration. *Hum Pathol* 1983; **5**: 339

17 Dushmukh M, Shah R, McCallum R W. Experience with herpes oesophagitis in otherwise healthy patients. *Am J Gastroenterol* 1984; **79**: 176

18 Freedman P G, Weiner B C, Balthazar E J. Cytomegalovirus oesophagogastritis in a patient with acquired immunodeficiency syndrome. *Am J Gastroenterol* 1985; **80**: 434

19 Teot L A, Ducatman B S, Geisinger K R. Cytologic diagnosis of cytomegaloviral oesophagitis. A report of three acquired immunodeficiency syndrome-related cases. *Acta Cytol* 1993; **37**(1): 93–96

20 Winkler B, Capo V, Reumann W. Human papillomavirus infection of the oesophagus. A clinicopathologic study with demonstration of papillomavirus antigen by the immunoperoxidase technique. *Cancer* 1985; **55**: 149

21 Williamson A L, Jaskiesicz K, Gunning A. The detection of human papillomavirus in oesophageal lesions. *AntiCancer Res* 1991; **11**(1): 263–265

22 Shu Y J. Cytopathology of the oesophagus. An overview of oesophageal cytopathology in China. *Acta Cytol* 1982; **27**: 7–16

23 Goodner J T, Watson W L. Cancer of the oesophagus: its association with other primary cancers. *Cancer* 1965; **9**: 1248

24 Epstien J I, Sears D L, Tucker R S, Eagan J U S Jr. Carcinoma of the oesophagus with adenoid cystic differentiation. *Cancer* 1984; **53**: 1131

25 Kay S. Mucoepidermoid carcinoma of the oesophagus. Report of two cases. *Cancer* 1968; **22**: 1053

26 Reid B J, Weinstein W M, Lewin K J. Endoscopic biopsy can detect high grade dysplasia or early adenocarcinoma in Barrett's oesophagus without grossly recognizable neoplastic lesions. *Gastroenterol* 1988; **94**: 81

27 Briggs J C, Ibrahim N B N. Oat cell carcinoma of the oesophagus: a clinico-pathological study of 23 cases. *Histopathol* 1993; **7**: 261

28 Ho K-J, Herrera G A, Jones J M, Alexander C B. Small cell carcinoma of the oesophagus: evidence for an unified histogenesis. *Hum Pathol* 1984; **15**: 460

29 Wilson P O G, Crow J, Dhillon A P *et al.* The epithelial origin of a primary oat cell carcinoma of the oesophagus. *J Pathol* 1988; **154**: 93A

30 Fulp S R, Nestok B R, Powell B L *et al.* Leukaemic infiltration of the oesophagus. *Cancer* 1993; **71**(1): 112–116

31 Mendoza M L, Marin-Rabadan P, Carrion I *et al.* Helicobacter pylori infections: rapid diagnosis with brush cytology. *Acta Cytol* 1993; **37**: 181–185

32 Schnell G A, Schubert T. Usefulness of culture, histology and urease testing in the detection of Campylobacter pylori. *Am J Gastroenterol* 1989; **84**: 133–137

33 Hayashida T, Kidocora T. End results of early gastric cancer collected from 22 institutions. *Stom Int* 1969; **4**: 1077

34 Johansen A. Early gastric cancer: a contribution to the pathology and to gastric cancer histogenesis. Copenhagen: Poul Petri, 1981

35 Scott N, Lansdown M, Daiment R. Helicobacter gastritis and intestinal metaplasia in a gastric cancer family. *Lancet* 1990; **I**(335): 728

36 Dixon M. Acid, ulcers and H. pylori. (Commentary) *Lancet* 1993; **342**: 384–385

37 Crooea P. Is gastric carcinoma an infectious disease? (Editorial) *N Engl J Med* 1991; **325**: 1170–1171

38 Lauren P. The two histological main types of gastric carcinoma: diffuse and so called intestinal-type carcinoma. An attempt at a histo-clinical classification. *Acta Pathol Microbiol Immunol Scand* 1972; **64**: 31–49

39 Rubin C E, Massey B W. The preoperative diagnosis of duodenal malignant lymphoma by exfoliative cytology. *Cancer* 1954; **7**: 271

40 Isaacson P G, Spencer J, Finn T. Primary B-Cell gastric lymphoma. *Hum Pathol* 1986; **17**: 72

41 Isaacson P G, Wright D H. Malignant lymphoma of mucosa associated lymphoid tissue. A distinctive type of B-Cell lymphoma. *Cancer* 1983; **52**: 1410

42 Myhre M J, Isaacson P G. Primary B-cell gastric lymphoma – a reassessment of its histogenesis. *J Pathol* 1987; **152**: 1

43 Wotherspoon A C, Orrthiz-Hidalgo C, Falzon M R, Isaacson P G. *Helicobacter pylori*-associated gastritis and primary B cell gastritis lymphoma. *Lancet* 1991; **335**: 175–176

44 Cabre-Fiol V, Villardell F, Sala-Cladera E, Percy Mota A. Preoperative cytological diagnosis of gastric leiomyosarcoma. *Gastroenterol* 1975; **68**: 563

45 Tao L, Davidson D D. Aspiration biopsy cytology of smooth muscle tumours. A cytologic approach to the differentiation between leiomyosarcoma and leiomyoma. *Acta Cytol* 1993; **37**(3): 300–308

13 Small and large intestine

Alastair Deery

Small intestine

Normal anatomy and histology

The small bowel is a mucosa-lined tube of continuously variable diameter, having an endoscopically-measured total length of 3 m in life; measured at death, the relaxed length averages 6 m. It comprises the duodenum (from Latin: *duodeni*, 12 each), measuring 12 fingers' breadths or 20 cm in length, beginning at the pyloric sphincter and describing a right handed C-shaped arc encircling the head of the pancreas; it continues as the jejunum (from Latin: *jejunus*, hungry) and then the ileum (from Latin: *ileum*, groin or flank), where it ends in the ileocaecal sphincter. The normal mucosa is villous throughout, the villi varying in shape, with approximately three times as many crypts between. There are eight times as many columnar enterocytes with a thin microvillous 'brush' border as there are mucus-laden goblet cells lining the villi; both are derived from the more cuboidal crypt stem cells. The crypt bases include a complex variety of endocrine cells and Paneth cells, while the villi incorporate intraepithelial T lymphocytes with a frequency of one to every ten epithelial cells. A myoid cell layer is present beneath the epithelial cells and the lamina propria is composed of lymphocytes, plasma cells, eosinophils and mast cells. The villus cores are composed of small vessels, lymphatics and smooth muscle cells. A muscularis mucosa is continuous throughout and confines specialized, localized Brunner's, antral type mucous glands, into submucosal collections in the duodenum. Within the mucosa there are lymphoid aggregates underlying specialized M cells, or antigen processing epithelial cells, which become more organized into Peyer's patches and extend increasingly into the submucosa as the ileum is reached. The submucosa, in addition to these lymphoid projections, includes blood vessels, lymphatics and nerves (Meissner's plexus) and overlies a muscularis composed of inner circular and outer longitudinal layers, divided by a myenteric nerve plexus (Auerbach's plexus). Beneath these layers is a small bowel serosa composed of fibroadipose tissue invested by blood vessels and lymphatics, and bounded by a mesothelial cell layer.

The pancreatic and common bile ducts open into the second part of the duodenum, usually through a single fused opening in the ampulla of Vater (Chapter 15).

Cytological sampling methods and applications

Most cytological sampling of the small intestine that has been written about has been directed at the collection of duodenal, biliary and pancreatic secretions or washings in order to ascertain the presence of malignancy in the pancreas or biliary tract. The value of cytology for these diagnoses, including more modern methods of sampling, has previously been reviewed[1] and is further dealt with in Chapters 15 and 16.

In the author's own institution, cytology has been employed in the identification of opportunistic infectious agents in duodenal, jejunal and pancreatico-biliary inflammations, detection of tumours in these areas and more routinely in the investigation of ampullary masses. Disposable brush specimens are received ensheathed in their cut-off plastic catheter tips, within 10 ml of balanced salt solution, or cell culture fluid. They are then subsequently vortexed in the laboratory, adjusted for optimal dilution and cytocentrifuged and stained for examination. Six cytospins are made in the first instance (five Papanicolaou, one MGG) with additional preparations for mucin (PASD/Alcian blue), mycobacteria (PAS, ZN) or special histochemical (e.g. Grimelius) or immunocytochemical investigations as required. With this approach, cytological analysis has yielded invaluable novel and additional data in this portion of the intestine, as in any other. This accords with recent publications concerning brush cytology and percutaneous and endoscopic aspiration cytology[2-9].

Normal components of small intestinal brushes

Where no inflammation or tumour is apparent, brush specimens will include: mucus tracts, small numbers of polymorphs, mixed coccal and bacillary bacteria, vegetable and animal striated muscle debris and stripped oval, pale, intestinal epithelial nuclei. There are usually numerous small intestinal type epithelial cells in variably presented finger-like (villous) microbiopsies of usual epithelial orientation, unlike the inverted 'pyjama legs' or 'trunks' seen in gastric brushes. In addition, there may also be inverted or torn cryptal epithelial arrangements, with reversed polarity. The villous epithelial cells usually have recognizable goblet cells interspersed among them, either seen flask like and on edge, or else port-hole like, every seven or eight cells within flat sheets. In the latter instance,

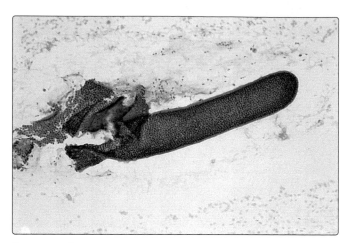

Fig. 13.1 Cytospin preparation of disposable duodenal brush including a villus microbiopsy with an orientated visible columnar cell edge and goblet cells seen obliquely or *en face*. Normal cytology. (Papanicolaou × LP)

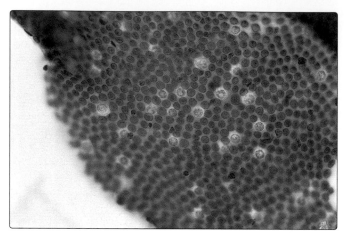

Fig. 13.3 Cytospin preparation of disposable duodenal brush including a single flat sheet of small intestinal epithelium with goblet cells *en face* every four or five cells and intraepithelial lymphocytes every eight epithelial cells. Normal cytology. (Papanicolaou × HP)

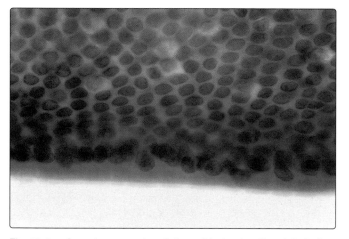

Fig. 13.2 Cytospin preparation of disposable duodenal brush including a cytologically well seen brush border. Goblet cells with intervening mucin and deep out of plane nuclei are also present. Normal cytology. (Papanicolaou × HP)

the basal nuclei are either closer to or further from the observer with the faintly opalescent mucus either behind or in front of the basally positioned nucleus. The microvillous brush border of the adjacent enterocytes is, perhaps surprisingly, more difficult to see in cytological preparations. The probable explanation is that the continuously superimposed, variably thick and orientated, three-dimensional microvillous cell edge, has less optical resolution than in the simple single plane of a histological section. The amalgamated 'terminal bar-like' insertions of the microvilli are often more easily identified, though considerably less clearly than in bronchial epithelial cells (Figs 13.1, 13.2). These small intestinal type epithelial sheets, additionally, have recognizable accompanying intraepithelial small lymphocytes (Fig. 13.3), which are interposed out of plane, reminiscent of the pattern of myoepithelial cells in aspirates of benign breast epithelial

cells. Gastric type mucosal epithelial sheets of mucinous columnar type may be present in intestinal brushes either as a result of contamination in pyloroduodenal brushes, particularly after gastric resection where the anatomical border is confused, as a consequence of apparent gastric heterotopia or as a type of metaplasia usually accompanied in the latter case by inflammation.

Inflammatory conditions

Peptic ulceration or ulcerative duodenitis

The cellular changes are similar to those described in ulcerative gastritis and are accompanied by ulcer slough. The appearances are usually present within brush smears from the first or second parts of the duodenum. Gastric type epithelial cells may be present, representing metaplasia, together with *Helicobacter pylori*. The cellularity is highly variable and not necessarily increased by comparison with 'normal' brush specimens.

Granulomatous jejunitis or ileitis

All of the cases of granulomatous inflammation in small intestinal brushes that the author has seen have been due either to atypical mycobacterial infection with *Mycobacterium avium intracellulare* in HIV patients or, in a few cases, to Crohn's disease (Figs 13.4, 13.5).

Viral duodenitis/jejunitis

Brushes of small intestine have revealed characteristic, but atypical cytomegalovirus inclusion bearing cells of probable endothelial origin in HIV and liver transplant patients in this laboratory (Figs 13.6, 13.7). These appearances are similar to those described in the oesophagus (see Chapter 12) and are accompanied by ulcer slough.

Fungal intestinal inflammation

In immunosuppressed patients, mycoses of either Mucorales or histoplasma type may occur. The author has

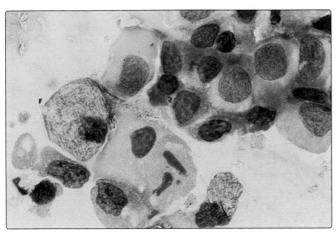

Fig. 13.4 Cytospin preparation of disposable jejunal brush including small intestinal epithelial cells and accompanying histiocytes with intracellular 'negatively stained' mycobacteria. *Mycobacterium avium intracellulare* infection in an AIDS patient. (MGG × HP)

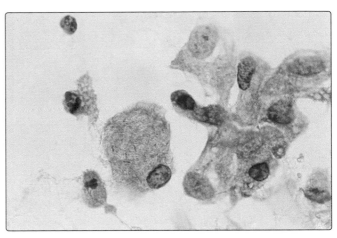

Fig. 13.5 Cytospin preparation of same case as **Fig. 13.4** showing interrupted red staining of intracellular atypical mycobacteria. (Ziehl-Neelsen × HP)

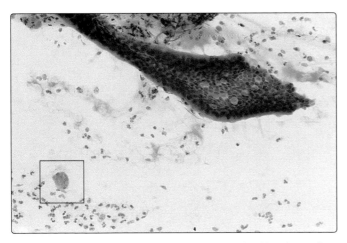

Fig. 13.6 Cytospin preparation of disposable duodenal brush revealing mucopus, a large sheet of small intestinal type epithelial cells and a single, large atypical CMV infected probable endothelial cell. CMV infection in post-liver transplant patient. (Papanicolaou × MP)

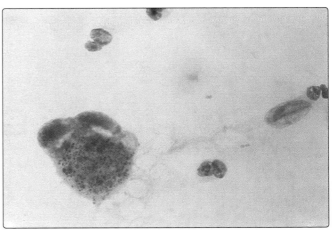

Fig. 13.7 Cytospin preparation of disposable duodenal brush of same case as in **Fig. 13.6**, showing a degenerate and therefore atypical binucleate, CMV infected cell. Smudged intranuclear and granular cytoplasmic inclusions are well seen ('frog eye' appearance). (Papanicolaou × HP)

seen a single instance of subsequent mucormycosis in a jejunal brush specimen from a liver transplant recipient following earlier infection by cytomegalovirus[11]. The appearances of the characteristic large ribbon-like orangeophilic, infrequently septate, fungal hyphae (5–20 μm diameter) embedded in ulcer slough were accompanied by necrotic cellular debris, fresh blood and inflamed epithelial sheets showing reactive, regenerative and degenerative cellular changes (Fig. 13.8). *Aspergillus* and *Candida* infections are rarer.

Parasitic inflammation

The least uncommon varieties of intestinal infestations include strongyloidiasis (hookworm), where adult worms may be incidentally identified in the upper small intestinal biopsy or brush specimens, and *Giardia lamblia*[12].

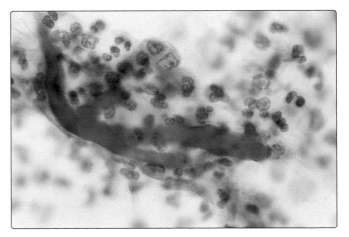

Fig. 13.8 Cytospin preparation of disposable duodenal brush showing exudate incorporating a few epithelial cells, pus cells and orangeophilic ribbon-like branched hyphal fragments of 20 μm diameter. Mucor infection in post-liver transplant patient. (Papanicolaou × HP)

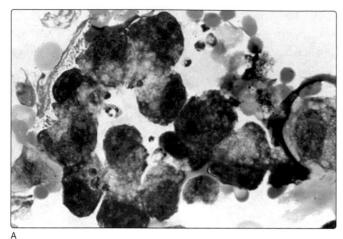

A

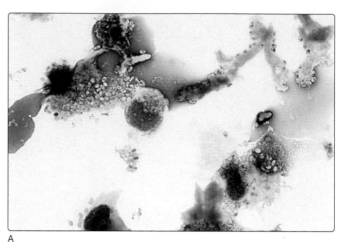

A

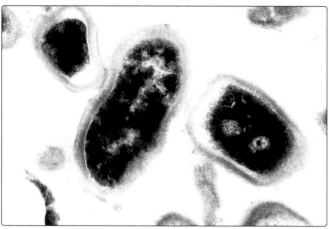

B

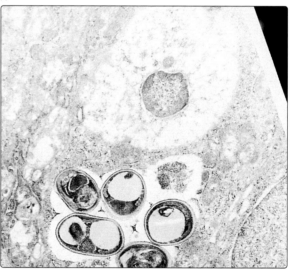

B

Fig. 13.9 (A) Cytospin preparation of ampullary brush (at ERCP) from an AIDS patient including a group of epithelial cells with closely associated *Cryptosporidia*. (MGG × HP); (B) Electron micrograph of *Cryptosporidial* organisms. Same case as **Fig. 13.9A**

Fig. 13.10 (A) Cytospin preparation of bile fluid (at ERCP) including intracellular *Microsporidia* within biliary epithelial cells. Biliary microsporidiosis in AIDS patient. (MGG × HP); (B) Electron micrograph of epithelial cell with intracellular *Microsporidia*. Same case as **Fig. 13.10A**

In immunosuppressed individuals *Cryptosporidia* (Figs 13.9A and B) and the intracellular protozoan *Isospora* (microsporidia; Figs 13.10A and B) occur and are increasingly seen in intestinal specimens, mainly from AIDS patients[8,11]. They are initially more difficult to recognize cytologically because of the increased detail not met in biopsy specimens and the lack of necessary association with cell surfaces.

Benign epithelial tumours
Benign polyps, hamartomas, adenomas

Various hamartomatous and polyposis syndromes may involve the small bowel, but all are rare and adenomatous or neoplastic change is very rare. Adenomas with various degrees of dysplasia are described in the ampulla of Vater[13]. Similarly, infiltrating carcinoma may occur in the stomach or small bowel as part of familial polyposis, otherwise involving mainly the large bowel. None is described cytologically though the author and others have reported high-grade adenomatous dysplasia (neoplasia or intramucosal carcinoma) in ampullary brushes[5].

Malignant epithelial tumours
Adenocarcinoma

These occur rarely, often in association with pre-existing adenomas and are pathologically similar in most respects to large bowel carcinomas ([Fig. 13.11]). The author is aware of a few cytological case reports as part of a published series[5]. Stomal cancers after gastric resection, dysplasia and carcinoma in Crohn's disease strictures, long standing coeliac disease associated with subsequent carcinoma and ureteric ileostomies and later stomal cancer are all described in small bowel. Endosonography combined with fine needle aspiration has proved useful in the evaluation of ulcerative lesions and surgical anastomoses of the gastro-intestinal tract when conventional biopsy and brush cytology has been unsuccessful[9].

Endocrine cell tumours

Carcinoid tumours of foregut or duodenal origin are similar to gastric or pancreatic carcinoids, may or may not be

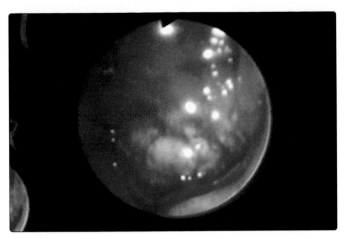

Fig. 13.11 Ampullary carcinoma photographed at ERCP. (Courtesy of Dr J S Dooley, London, UK)

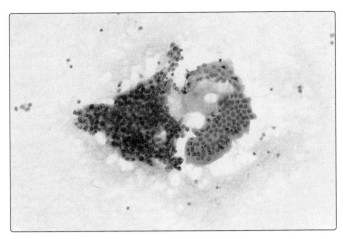

Fig. 13.12 Cytospin preparation of disposable duodenal brush revealing a loose aggregate of spheroidal intermediate size tumour cells (left) alongside a flat intestinal type epithelial sheet (right). Pancreatic islet cell tumour in duodenum. (Papanicolaou × MP)

functional, are commonly malignant and metastasizing and occur in equal numbers in both sexes, pre-eminently in the fifth and sixth decades. Midgut carcinoids (jejunum and ileum) present a decade later, are commoner in men, show a similar metastatic potential, but are more often functional (usually producing 5-hydroxytryptamine – 5-HT). They may be multiple. All begin in the deep mucosa or submucosa and may protrude luminally without ulceration.

Cytological findings

Neuroendocrine tumours have been cytologically described in bronchial exfoliative or brush specimens (see Chapter 3) and occasionally in the upper intestinal tract within fine needle aspirates[14]. The appearances in an intestinal brush specimen were reported as a single representative case in the previous edition of this text. The primary tumour in this young woman proved to be an islet cell tumour in the head of pancreas, which was visible to the endoscopist as a submucosal bulge in the second part of the duodenum. A disposable brush was used as described previously, in Chapter 12, to sample the mass. The head of the brush was collected in cell culture fluid and the particles teased by forceps and subsequent vortexing from the bristles. Cytocentrifuge preparations from the liquid medium revealed tumour cells that were arranged in loose structureless aggregates of variable size and then dissociated in trails (Figs 13.12, 13.13). The cellular appearances were homogeneous, spheroidal or oval with a plasmacytoid form owing largely to three particular features. First, they possessed an eccentric or polar nucleus. Secondly, the nucleoplasm was coarsely clumped with a 'cartwheel' or 'clockface' peripheral dispersion. Lastly (and emphasized by the MGG stain), there was a sometimes striking crescentic band of dark, granular, peripheral cytoplasm lending the cells an evident amphophilia. These granules were stained with Grimelius silver stain. A limited

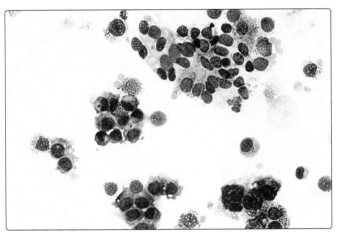

Fig. 13.13 Cytospin preparation of disposable duodenal brush of same case as in **Fig. 13.12** demonstrating scattered cuboidal intestinal type epithelial cells and discohesive admixed, sometimes vacuolated, plasmacytoid neuroendocrine tumour cells. Pancreatic islet cell tumour in duodenum. (MGG × HP) See also **Figs 13.1**4 and **13.15** on following page.

immunocytochemical panel employed in this instance, where the specimen was a disposable brush, revealed CAM 5.2 and PGP 9.5 positivity (Figs 13.14, 13.15). More specific markers for granule content were not employed.

Multiple small fine lipid-like vacuoles (most easily seen in MGG stains) have been described within the cytoplasm of the tumour cells of islet cell neoplasms[15]. Such vacuoles are seen very clearly in the examples of islet cell tumours in Chapter 16. These might distinguish them from carcinoid tumours, cytomorphologically. The author has not seen such vacuoles in carcinoid tumours of pulmonary or intestinal origin.

Non-epithelial tumours
Lymphoma
Lymphomas of the small bowel are not common in Western populations, but in the presence of few epithelial

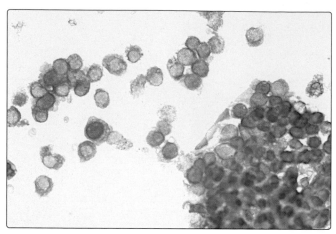

Fig. 13.14 Cytospin preparation of disposable duodenal brush of same case as in **Fig. 13.12** showing immunostaining for cytokeratin 8 (CAM 5.2). (CAM 5.2 (Dako) × HP)

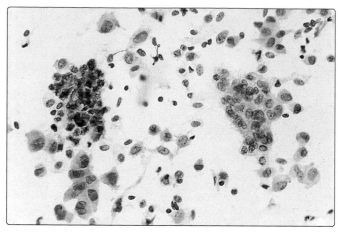

Fig. 13.16 Cytospin preparation of CT guided transabdominal intestinal fine needle aspirate, including microbiopsies, aggregates and trails of variably microvacuolated epithelioid and plump spindle cells exhibiting some hyperchromasia but otherwise bland nuclear features. Intestinal malignant stromal tumour. (Papanicolaou × MP)

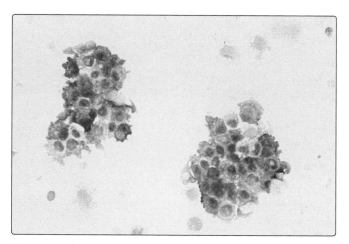

Fig. 13.15 Cytospin preparation of disposable duodenal brush of same case as in **Fig. 13.12** showing immunostaining for neuroendocrine marker PGP 9.5. (PGP 9.5 (Dako) × HP)

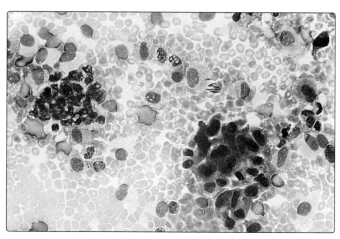

Fig. 13.17 Cytospin preparation of CT guided aspirate as in **Fig. 13.16**, including similar microbiopsies exhibiting more clearly seen lipidic vacuolation abutting on and invaginating nuclear envelopes. Other epithelioid cells without vacuolation are well seen. Intestinal malignant stromal tumour. (MGG × MP)

tumours at this site, form a relatively large percentage of all primary tumours. Premalignant conditions include primary hypogammaglobulinaemia, nodular lymphoid hyperplasia, acquired immune deficiency syndrome (AIDS), immunoproliferative small intestinal disease (IPSID) and coeliac disease. Most lymphomas are of B cell type, though some involve T cells. The tumours may mimic benign inflammatory disease and are associated with fissuring and ulceration. There are no reports of their diagnosis in the cytological literature. Secondary lymphoma in the intestine is probably more common. Tumours may be associated with perforation, which is also a particular risk of treatment.

Leukaemic infiltration of the small intestine is a common occurrence in patients dying of acute leukaemia and is particularly likely to be complicated by superinfection and perforation.

Stromal tumours

Tumours of soft tissue are of similar type, at this site, to those in the stomach. Differentiation may be variable as defined by panels of antibodies. Behaviour is not necessarily related to immunophenotype or indeed mitotic or proliferative activity. Cytological reporting of such tumours is limited to a few case reports and retrospective diagnostic reviews[16] that do not necessarily take account of advances in histological classification or nomenclature.

Cytological findings

To exemplify the complexities of such tumours, an aspirate of a jejunal tumour is illustrated here (Figs 13.16–13.19). A percutaneous aspirate was performed upon a young

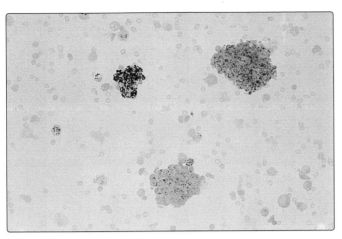

Fig. 13.18 Cytospin preparation of the same CT guided aspirate as in **Fig. 13.16** revealing stained lipid within the cytoplasmic vacuoles of the tumour cells. Intestinal malignant stromal tumour. (Sudan IV/oil red-O × MP)

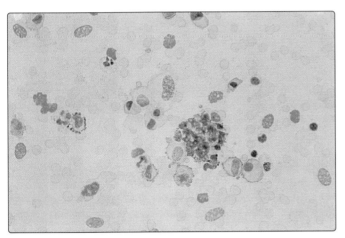

Fig. 13.19 Cytospin preparation of the same CT guided aspirate as in **Fig. 13.16** showing α-smooth muscle actin staining of some of the epithelioid tumour cells. Intestinal malignant stromal tumour. (α-smooth muscle actin immunostain (Dako) × MP)

woman under ultrasonic image guidance, aimed at a mass in the region of the tail of the pancreas. The aspirate was collected into cell culture fluid, density separated, washed, spun, resuspended, cytospun and stained to reveal several populations of cells. Microbiopsies and loose aggregates were present, composed of admixtures of epithelioid and spindle cells with varying amounts of fibrillary 'myxoid' stromal mucin. The nuclei of cells were variably plump spheroidal, plump oval or thin spindle, sometimes strikingly invaginated by cytoplasmic vacuoles (lipoblasts). Conventional cytochemistry revealed lipid in these vacuoles. Isolated cells of all morphologies and stripped nuclei of variable shape were also present. Few mitoses were seen.

The possible nature of the previously observed cytoplasmic vacuolation common to these tumours has been debated and relegated to histological degeneration[17,18]. The demonstration of lipid in this instance is unique, but was subsequently independently confirmed in frozen

section of the histological material. Immunocytochemistry revealed α-actin and S 100 positivity in both the epithelioid and spindle cell components. Similar variability was observed in the final paraffin sections. The tumour was resected together with an isolated liver metastasis found in the left lobe of the liver. The primary tumour measured 6 cm diameter and arose in the wall of the jejunum. Neither the mucosal nor the serosal surfaces were breached. The metastasis measured 10 cm and was entirely beneath the liver capsule. Clearly, such stromal tumours should be identified, at least descriptively. Their immunophenotype should be attributed only cautiously. Their behaviour or prognosis is not predictable.

Appendix

The author is unaware of cytological reports of any pathology directly involving the appendix.

Large intestine

Normal anatomy and histology

The large bowel is approximately 1.5 m in length at autopsy and consists of the caecum (Latin: *caecus*, blind), ascending, transverse, descending and sigmoid colon (Greek: *sigma*, the eighteenth, S-shaped alphabetic letter), rectum (Latin: *rectus*, straight) and anus (Latin: *anus*, ring).

The mucosa is thrown into folds or plicae by the contractile tone present in the outer longitudinal bands of muscularis propria and is composed of columnar cells, mucinous goblet cells, Paneth cells (in the right colon) and endocrine cells arranged as surface and crypt lining cells. The columnar brush border is not evident by light microscopy and intraepithelial lymphocytes are not present. There is a *muscularis mucosae*, a submucosa bearing blood vessels, lymphatics and nerves and, lying astride both at frequent intervals, lymphoglandular complexes. The muscularis propria has two layers: an internal circular muscle layer and external longitudinal layer as indicated above. A serosa of vessels and connective tissue is variably invested by peritoneal mesothelium.

Cytological sampling methods and applications

In the past, rectal washings and, later, colonic lavage techniques were described and advocated in the investigation of suspected epithelial cancers[19,20]. The development of colonoscopy had largely eliminated exfoliative cytological sampling except for a few active centres[21,22]. In immunosuppressed patients with anal intraepithelial squamous abnormalities, traditional methods of cytological screening are being employed[23,24]. The use of colonic brush and aspiration cytology has a relatively short, but encouraging history[3,25-29]. In the experience of this laboratory, the value of colonic brush cytology is particularly demonstrated in the investigation of tight strictures where biopsy forceps may not pass, in procuring enhanced exfoliative specimens in the presence

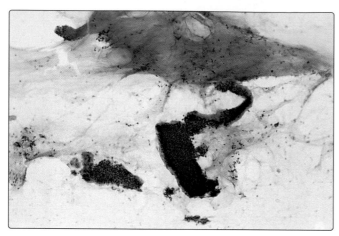

Fig. 13.20 Cytospin preparation of disposable colonic brush, including mucus, particulate faecal material and microbiopsies of tall columnar mucinous large intestinal type epithelial cells. Normal colonic cytology. (Papanicolaou × LP)

of wide or multifocal ulceration, where selective biopsy may be unproductive (ulcerative colitis) and in the identification of particular infective agents.

Normal components of large intestinal brushes

The author's first 'cytological contact' with large bowel epithelium was in Franzén needle aspirates of prostate, present as one of the inevitable contaminants.

Brush specimens in this laboratory are all now disposable brush specimens and are dealt with by the liquid based methods described earlier. The content of normal colonic brushes depends on the degree of large bowel preparation, on which part of the bowel is sampled and chaotic factors such as whether a 'lymphoglandular body' (lymphoid aggregate) has been incidentally brushed.

There are usually: mucus, recognizable polymorphs, more or less degenerate food debris with varied vegetable cells and striated animal muscle fibres, mixed mainly bacillary bacteria, yeast spores, perhaps *Entamoebae coli*, actinomycetes colonies and often variable numbers of lymphocytes, histiocytes (few), plasma cells and eosinophils from the normal lamina propria. Among the epithelial elements present, there are always some squamous cells (from anal contamination) and sheets of columnar, vacuolated intermediate columnar and evident mucinous goblet cells (Fig. 13.20). Stripped epithelial nuclei are usually present within strands of mucus.

Inflammatory conditions

Ulcerative colitis

The author is not aware of any specific cytological features of this condition in brush specimens. There is, or may be, evidence of ulceration and more or less marked regenerative and degenerative epithelial changes associated with the inflammation. These nuclear changes are not dissimilar to those seen in comparable inflammation in the stomach (see Chapter 12). Changes that might be expected, such as

a reduction in the numbers of goblet cells, are not specific or dependable. Lymphoid cells, together with increased numbers of follicle centre cells, may be striking but can be a normal constituent. Dysplasia in ulcerative colitis is similar to that described as occurring in Barrett's oesophagus under gastric dysplasia. It has been reported that such dysplasia can effectively be cytologically distinguished from frank carcinoma[26]. There are considerable similarities in the cytology of early neoplastic lesions in the glandular epithelium of several sites. These are: gastro-oesophageal junction in Barrett's oesophagus, colon in both ulcerative colitis and within adenomatous polyps, *in situ* biliary neoplasia in sclerosing cholangitis, adenomatous ampullary lesions and endocervical glandular intraepithelial neoplasia/adenocarcinoma *in situ*.

Granulomatous colitis

The presence of aggregates of histiocytes and giant multinucleate histiocytes of both Langhans' type and foreign body type within otherwise inflammatory brush smears is virtually diagnostic of Crohn's disease (Figs 13.21, 13.22). Nonetheless, tuberculosis is a possibility, particularly in brush specimens from the right colon. Endoscopic fine needle aspiration cytology has been shown to be particularly useful in achieving a diagnosis of ileo-caecal tuberculosis in populations where the disease is endemic and where previous biopsy and brush cytology have been negative[30].

Radiation changes

Radiation changes are common in large bowel after treatment for gynaecological and sometimes urological, prostatic or other malignancies. The changes are similar to those described in the stomach. Carcinoma may be an unusual and late consequence.

Infective colitis

Specific, sometimes exotic or opportunistic infections are all increasingly seen within colonic brush specimens, either as a result of increased foreign travel, or because of the rise in numbers of immunosuppressed patients. All depend on the correct identification of the organism or cytopathic effect. The ability to perform a battery of special stains is only routinely possible in brush specimens if handled as described above.

Benign epithelial tumours
Benign polyps

There are no cytological descriptions of hamartomatous, hyperplastic or juvenile or inflammatory polyps in brush specimens.

Adenomatous polyps

There have been previous attempts at cytological classification of glandular neoplasia in colorectal adenomas, based on small biopsy impression smear appearances[31]. A traditional three-grade system has been suggested. The highest grade of cellular neoplastic changes appeared to correlate with

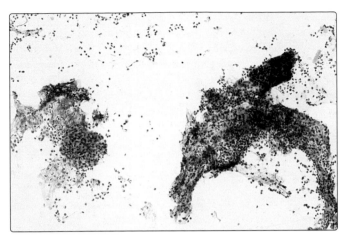

Fig. 13.21   Cytospin preparation of disposable colonic brush including mucopus, inflamed, sometimes degenerate large intestinal epithelial cells and histiocytic aggregates admixed with small lymphocytes indicating underlying granulomatous inflammation. Crohn's colitis. (Papanicolaou × MP)

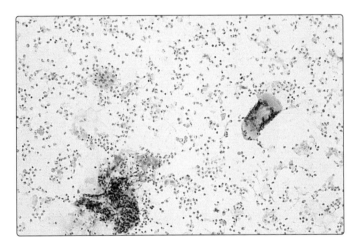

Fig. 13.22   Cytospin preparation of disposable colonic brush from same case as **Fig. 13.21**, showing Langhans' type giant histiocytes in addition. Crohn's colitis. (Papanicolaou × MP)

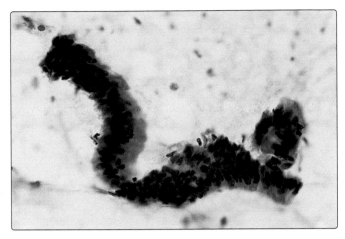

Fig. 13.23   Cytospin preparation of disposable colonic brush containing a strip of edge-on colonic epithelium, with crowding of elongated columnar cells and with hyperchromatic, overlapped, polarized, enlarged nuclei. Adenomatous colonic intraepithelial neoplasia (ACIN). (Papanicolaou × MP)

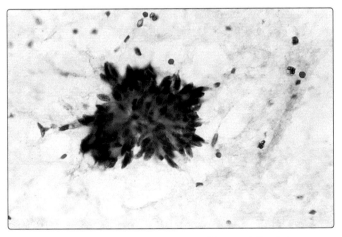

Fig. 13.24   Cytospin preparation of disposable colonic brush from same case as **Fig. 13.23**, including a single papilliform microbiopsy with feathered, drawn out, elongated, hyperchromatic columnar cells. There is crowding of nuclei, overlapping of enlarged nuclei and increased nuclear chromatin. Adenomatous colonic intraepithelial neoplasia. Histologically, a villous adenoma with severe dysplasia. (Papanicolaou × HP)

invasive malignancy. On the other hand, Koss[32] stated that in his experience 'benign polyps' could not be identified with certainty. Ehya and O'Hara[28] identified 71 of 88 (82%) neoplastic polyps (adenomas) in their reported series of 234 colonic brush specimens performed in the late 1980s. Three adenomas with 'severe dysplasia' or *in situ* carcinoma were diagnosed as frank adenocarcinoma. This author's experience of over 100 adequate disposable brush specimens from adenomatous polyps reveals 100% specificity (i.e. no false assertions of invasive malignancy).

Cytological findings

Two patterns of brushings seem to emerge, as previously suggested when discussing Barrett's oesophagus and gastric dysplasia. The patterns should be considered separately and not strictly traded or contrasted.

The first pattern (Figs 13.23, 13.24) corresponds to histological adenomatous dysplasia up to and including severe dysplasia and can be summarized as follows:

▶ Papilliform microbiopsies, cribriform microbiopsies, strips of edge-on epithelium, tufts and tubules of crowded columnar cells
▶ Feathered, drawn-out, elongated columnar cells of increased cell size within such microarchitectural configurations
▶ Hyperchromatic, overlapped, oval, similarly directed or polarized enlarged nuclei within such cells
▶ Regularly irregular chromatin, micronucleolation and mitoses

The second pattern (Figs 13.25, 13.26) corresponds either to high-grade histological adenomatous dysplasia, flat non-adenomatous dysplasia as encountered in ulcerative colitis,

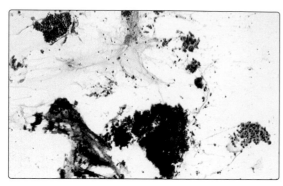

Fig. 13.25 Cytospin preparation of disposable colonic brush including, mucopus, benign sheets of large intestinal epithelial cells and small irregular microbiopsies and clusters of enlarged glandular epithelial cells exhibiting nuclear enlargement and hyperchromasia. Colonic intraepithelial neoplasia with associated ulcerative changes. (Papanicolaou × LP)

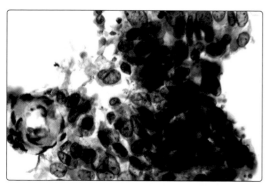

Fig. 13.26 Cytospin preparation of disposable colonic brush from same case as **Fig. 13.25**, revealing a cluster of neoplastic cells with hyperchromasia, irregular nuclear envelopes and dispersed micro- and macronucleolation. There is loss of polarity and cellular discohesion at the margins of the cluster. A small coiled vessel can be seen to the left. Colonic intraepithelial neoplasia with associated ulcerative changes. Histologically, a villous adenoma with severe dysplasia and focal ulceration. No evidence of invasion. (Papanicolaou × HP)

or possible invasive malignancy. The appearances of the neoplastic cells are coupled with either: extra features of pleomorphic invasive malignancy, or else confounding inflammatory ulceration and superimposed regenerative and degenerative cellular changes, despite the presence of only *in situ* disease:

▶ Background mucopus, cell debris and ulcer slough
▶ Papilliform, solid or cribriform microbiopsies composed of crowded, overlapped and occasionally focally clustered enlarged epithelial cells
▶ Less cohesive clusters or aggregates of enlarged epithelial cells
▶ Hyperchromatic, enlarged, variably polar nuclei within such cells
▶ Irregular dispersed micro- and macronucleolation.

The two patterns are quite distinctive, but do not have similarly distinctive histological implications. The second pattern appears to reflect that cellular changes associated with ulceration may imitate several cytological features

normally associated with invasive malignancy. The first pattern is more hyperplasia than neoplasia. The second pattern requires a cytological diagnosis of 'at least *in situ* adenocarcinoma' (as high-grade histological dysplasia). Further problems might occur where the two patterns are present within a brush specimen of the same lesion. Then the second pattern takes priority, though the lesion may prove to be a severely dysplastic adenoma with focal ulceration.

Malignant epithelial tumours
Adenocarcinoma

The incidence of colorectal carcinoma exhibits one of the most striking of contrasts for any glandular malignancy, revealing a 50-fold difference in incidence between high risk areas, such as Northern Europe and low risk areas, such as Southern Africa. Much is guessed, but little is known of the aetiological factors involved in cancer evolution at this site. Familial polyposis syndromes have directed attention to the adenoma–carcinoma sequence and have encouraged study of possible genetic mechanisms. Epidemiological studies, however, have provided few causal insights with which to focus such potential genetic modes.

Almost 75% of large bowel carcinoma occur in the sigmoid colon and rectum. Many of the tumours are ulcerated flat tumours with raised margins, although some are annular and constricting or else polypoid. These last types are more prevalent in the right colon. The tumours are usually localized and, unlike stomach, diffuse infiltrating spread is very uncommon. A detailed histological grading system has been suggested, which has prognostic impact[33]. The simultaneous presence of adenomas and carcinomas is common[34].

Cytological findings

Colonoscopic brush smears are mostly received from ulcerating and stenotic cancers and therefore reflect these growths. This ensures that appearances in smears will include ulcer slough, necrotic cell debris, papilliform and solid clusters and perhaps tubular arrangements of atypical glandular epithelial cells (Figs 13.27, 13.28). The cell size of these adenocarcinomas is usually smaller than that seen in gastric adenocarcinoma, though it may be similar. Crowded tufts or clusters of cells with aligned, polarized, tall columnar cells are a particular feature of papillary tumours and recall adenomatous growths. Mucinous patterns are not common, but can imitate the appearance of mucinous ('colloid') breast carcinoma in aspirates. Isolated islands of centrifugally orientated columnar cells embedded in mucin or else broken tubular strands of similar cells encompassing mucin lakes or clumps can be identified. Signet ring cell cancers are very uncommon, although rare examples do occur, often in young patients (Fig. 13.29).

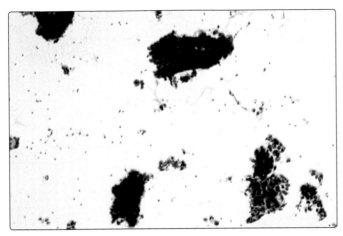

Fig. 13.27 Cytospin preparation of disposable colonic brush including papilliform, solid and cribriform clusters of malignant glandular epithelial cells. The cells are of intermediate size, have irregular nuclear envelopes, prominent irregular macronucleolation and have superimposed degenerative changes. Adenocarcinoma, colon. (Papanicolaou × MP)

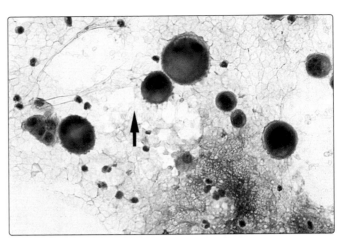

Fig. 13.29 Cytospin preparation of disposable colonic brush including fresh blood, scattered inflammatory cells and dispersed, single, anaplastic, mucinous, large signet ring cells with textured cytoplasmic mucin. Signet ring cell carcinoma of colon. (MGG × HP)

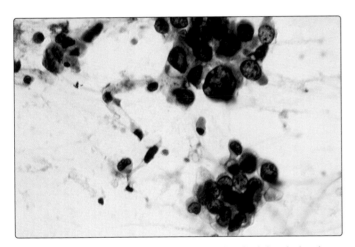

Fig. 13.28 Cytospin preparation of disposable colonic brush showing clearer cellular details of the same tumour as in **Fig. 13.27**. Adenocarcinoma, colon. (Papanicolaou × HP)

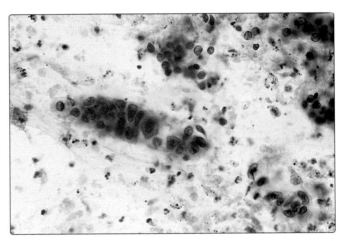

Fig. 13.30 Cytospin preparation of urine revealing background necrotic cellular debris, papilliform microbiopsies, and strips of partly orientated, intermediate sized, malignant columnar epithelial cells with a large intestinal pattern. Adenocarcinoma of colon in urinary tract. (Papanicolaou × MP)

The cell size and tendency to dyshesive cell dispersion is similar to that of these tumours in the stomach.

Not infrequently, it is possible to recognize the rather uniform arrangements typical of large bowel adenocarcinoma in metastatic sites (Fig. 13.30).

Endocrine cell tumours

These occur less commonly in the large bowel, usually in the midgut-derived right colon and are probably most often detected as already metastatic tumours in liver core or needle biopsies. Undifferentiated 'oat cell' carcinomas are also described. The features are similar to such tumours in other sites, but there are no cytological reports. Mixed neuroendocrine and typical glandular epithelial tumours may be expected in the colon but the author has not encountered any cytologically.

Non-epithelial tumours
Lymphoma

Lymphoma is a relatively uncommon primary tumour in the colon and rectum and when present either forms a single mass or multiple polypoid masses or nodules. This latter pattern is distinctive, referred to as malignant lymphomatous polyposis and may involve other parts of the intestine[35]. The tumour cells in this distinctive subtype appear centrocytic or centrocyte-like and might be compared with maltoma in stomach. Considering other mainly right-sided discrete caecal lymphomas, or rectal lymphomas, these apparently type as low- or high-grade B-cell lymphomas in roughly equal numbers[36]. There may be a particular association with chronic ulcerative colitis[36]. There are no cytological reports of lymphoma diagnosis at this site by colonoscopic brush, though abdominal

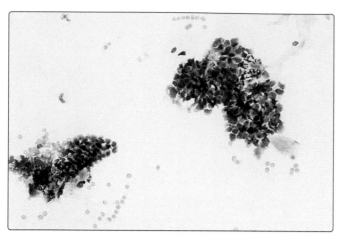

Fig. 13.31 Cytospin preparation of anal scrape specimen including microbiopsies of malignant small, oval cohesive, basaloid squamous cells, recalling basal cell carcinoma of skin, but with some nucleolation. Basaloid squamous carcinoma of anal canal. (MGG × MP)

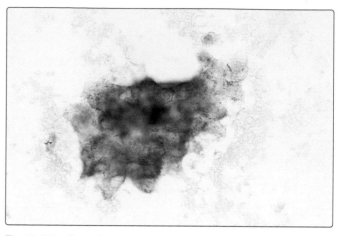

Fig. 13.32 Cytospin preparation of anal scrape sample from same case as in **Fig. 13.31** immunostained for CEA (carcinoembryonic antigen). Tumour cells are positive. (CEA immunostain (Dako) × HP)

aspirates, infrequently, have included such primary tumours.

Stromal tumours

Leiomyomas, leiomyosarcomas, vascular hamartomas, neuromas, neurosarcomas and lipomas are all possibilities that are unlikely to be suggested by brush specimens. Abdominal image guided aspiration may occasionally encounter them.

Anal canal

Anal dysplasia

Brush specimens might rarely be taken from anal squamous

carcinoma. The similarity of the most typical type of these tumours to basal cell carcinomas of skin cannot be overstressed.

Malignant epithelial tumours

The small cell pattern is most common cytologically; the tumour cells are essentially indistinguishable from those of basal cell carcinoma (Figs 13.31, 13.32). An example has already been illustrated (see Fig. 12.11).

Other important tumours that might appear in cytological specimens from this zone include melanoma and 'oat cell' carcinoma. Diverse management considerations for these tumour types emphasizes the need to separate them.

References

1 Kurzawinski T, Deery A, Davison B R. Diagnostic value of cytology for biliary stricture (Review). *Br J Surg* 1993; **80**(4): 414–421

2 Petrelli N J, Letourneau R, Webber T *et al*. Accuracy of biopsy and cytology for the pre-operative diagnosis of colo-rectal adenocarcinoma. *J Surg Oncol* 1999; **71**(1): 46–49

3 Heriot A G, Kumar D, Thomas V *et al*. Ultrasonographically-guided fine-needle aspiration cytology in the diagnosis of colonic lesions. *Br J Surg* 1998; **85**: 1713–1715

4 Jergens A E, Andreasen C B, Hagemoser W A *et al*. Cytologic examination of exfoliative specimens obtained during endoscopy for diagnosis of gastro-intestinal tract disease in dogs and cats. *J Am Vet Med Assoc* 1998; **213**(12): 1755–1759

5 Bardales R H, Stanley M W, Simpson D D *et al*. Diagnostic value of brush cytology in the diagnosis of duodenal, biliary and ampullary neoplasms. *Am J Clin Pathol* 1998; **109**(5): 540–548

6 Vamosi-Nagy I, Koves I, Sapi Z. Aspiration cytology in the diagnosis of gastro-intestinal tumours (article in Hungarian). *Orv Hetil* 1996; **137**(44): 2455–2457

7 Wang H H, Sovie S, Trawinski G *et al*. ThinPrep processing of endoscopic brushing specimens. *Am J Clin Pathol* 1996; **105**(2): 163–167

8 Orenstein J M, Lew E, Poles M A, Dieterich D. The endoscopic brush cytology specimen in the diagnosis of intestinal microsporidiosis. *AIDS* 1995; **9**(10): 1199–1201

9 Wiersema M J, Wiersema L M, Khusro Q *et al*. Combined endosonography and fine needle aspiration cytology in the evaluation of gastro-intestinal lesions. *Gastrointest Endosc* 1994; **40**(2Pt1): 199–206

10 Shah N, Deery A. Cytomegalovirus infection in mesothelial cells detected cytologically in ascitic fluid following liver transplantation. *J Pathol* 1993; **170**: 398A

11 Silverman J F, Levine J, Finley J L *et al*. Small-intestinal brushing cytology in the diagnosis of cryptosporidiasis in AIDS. *Diagn Cytopath* 1990; **6**(3): 193

12 Bendig D W. Diagnosis of Giardiasis in infants and children by endoscopic brush cytology. *J Paediatr Gastroenterol Nutr* 1989; **8**(2): 204–206

13 Yamaguchi K, Enjoji M. Adenoma of the ampulla of Vater: putative precancerous lesion. *Gut* 1991; **32**(12): 1558–1561

14 Benya R V, Metz D C, Hijayi Y J *et al*. Fine needle aspiration cytology of submucosal nodules in patients with Zollinger-Ellison syndrome. *Am J Gastroenterol* 1993; **88**(2): 258–265

15 Stormby B A, Akerman M. Cytodiagnosis of pancreatic lesions by means of fine needle biopsy during operation. *Acta Chir Scand* 1972; **138**: 363–369

16 Tao L, Davidson D D. Aspiration biopsy cytology of smooth muscle tumours. A cytologic approach to the differentiation between leiomyosarcoma and leiomyoma. *Acta Cytol* 1993; **37**(3): 300–308

17 Koss L G. The stomach. In Koss ed. *Diagnostic Cytology*, 4th edn. Philadelphia: J B Lippincott, 1992

18 Enzinger F M, Weiss S W. eds. *Soft Tissue Tumours*. St Louis: C V Mosby, 1983; 298–324

19 Bader G M, Papanicolaou G N. Application of cytology in the diagnosis of cancer of the rectum, sigmoid and descending colon. *Cancer* 1952; **5**: 307–314

20 Raskin H R, Pleticka S. The cytologic diagnosis of cancer of the colon. *Acta Cytol* 1964; **8**: 131–140

21 Bardawil R G, D'Ambrosio F G, Hajdu S I. Colonic cytology. A retrospective study with histopathologic correlation. *Acta Cytol* 1990; **34**(5): 620–626

22 Rozen P, Tobi M, Darmon E, Kaufman L. Exfoliative colonic cytology. A simplified method of collection and initial results. *Acta Cytol* 1990; **34**(5): 627–631

23 Melbye M, Palefsky J, Gonzales J et al. Immune status as a determinant of human papillomavirus detection and its association with anal abnormalities. *Internat J Cancer* 1990; **46**(2): 203–206

24 Caussy D, Goedert J J, Palefsky J et al. Interaction of human immunodeficiency and papilloma viruses: association with anal epithelial abnormality in homosexual men. *Internat J Cancer* 1990; **46**(2): 214–219

25 Jeevanandam V, Treat M R, Forde K A. A comparison of direct brush cytology and biopsy in the diagnosis of colorectal cancer. *Gastrointest Endosc* 1987; **33**(5): 370–1182

26 Melville D M, Richman P, Shepherd N A et al. Brush cytology of the colon and rectum in ulcerative colitis: an aid to cancer diagnosis. *J Clin Pathol* 1988; **41**: 1180–1186

27 Isbister W H, Gupta R K. Colonoscopy, mucosal biopsy and brush cytology in the assessment of patients with colo-rectal inflammatory bowel disease. *Surg Endosc* 1989; **3**(3):159–163

28 Ehya H, O'Hara B J. Brush cytology in the diagnosis of colonic neoplasms. *Cancer* 1990; **66**(7): 1563–1567

29 Zargar S A, Khuroo M S, Mahajan R et al. Endoscopic fine needle aspiration cytology in the diagnosis of gastro-oesophageal and colorectal malignancies. *Gut* 1991; **32**(7): 745–748

30 Kochhar R, Rajwanshi A, Goenka M K et al. Colonoscopic fine needle cytology in the diagnosis of ileo-caecal tuberculosis. *Am J Gastroenterol* 1991; **86**(1): 102–104

31 Tidbury P J, Tate J J T, Herbert A. Cytology of colorectal adenomas. *Cytopathol* 1990; **1**: 73–78

32 Koss L G. The gastrointestinal tract. In: Koss ed. *Diagnostic Cytology*, 4th edn. Philadelphia: J B Lippincott, 1992

33 Jass J R, Atkins W S, Cuzick J et al. The grading of rectal cancer. Historical perspectives and a multivariate analysis of 447 cases. *Histopathol* 1986; **10**: 437

34 Chu D Z J, Giacco G, Martin R E, Guinee V F. The significance of synchronous carcinoma and polyps in the colon and rectum. *Cancer* 1986; **57**: 445

35 Isaacson P G, MacLennon K A, Subbuswamy S G. Multiple lymphomatous polyposis of the gastrointestinal tract. *Histopathol* 1984; **8**: 641

36 Shepherd N A, Hall P A, Coates P J, Levison D A. Primary malignant lymphoma of the colon and rectum. A histopathological and immunohistochemical analysis of 45 cases with clinicopathological correlation. *Histopathol* 1988; **12**: 235–252

Hepatobiliary system and pancreas

14 Disorders of the liver

W. Bastiaan de Boer and Elaine Waters

The liver is an organ with a wide range of metabolic, regulatory and other important functions performed by hepatocytes. The complexity and sensitivity of these cells make them vulnerable to many noxious agents. At rest, one fifth of the cardiac output flows through the liver, much of it via the portal vein, so that it is constantly exposed to drugs, toxins and infections. In addition, circulating malignant cells carried by both the portal and systemic circulation lodge within the parenchyma and grow readily. Resultant diseases are many and varied. Fine needle aspiration (FNA) is principally used in the investigation of focal liver lesions and offers a useful diagnostic procedure in combination with information derived from clinical examination, other laboratory tests and radiology. It is hoped that the following information will provide a basic framework for the investigation of hepatic disorders using the fine needle aspiration technique.

The history of needle aspiration of the liver

Hepatic aspiration was performed as long ago as 1833 when Roberts and Biett reported its use in the treatment of hepatic suppuration and hydatid disease[1,2]. Needle biopsy using aspiration was first employed in 1883 by Paul Ehrlich (cited in Schupfer 1907) in a study of glycogen content of diabetic liver[3]. Aspiration using very fine needles to evaluate cytological specimens was first used by Lucatello in 1895 (cited in Lundquist 1971)[4]. At the beginning of the twentieth century, needle biopsy was accompanied by a high mortality rate[5,6]. In 1935 Frola in France tried to reduce complications by using a needle which measured 0.5 mm in diameter[7]. After the work in 1939 of Iversen and Roholm in Denmark[8] and Baron in the USA[9], cytological methods were investigated by other workers from northern continental Europe[10–13] and they subsequently gained a prominent role in diagnosis of liver disease from the middle of the twentieth century.

In 1966 Nils Soderstrom[14] published a series of 500 samples in which his observations on metastatic carcinoma and myeloid metaplasia proved diagnostic. Lundquist, a pupil of Soderstrom, published several papers[15,16] including a thesis[4] on his experience of intrahepatic tumours, acute hepatitis, cirrhosis, iron overload, fatty infiltration and other conditions. The material was gathered over 7 years

from 2600 FNA liver specimens obtained with only one serious complication: a haematoma requiring surgery. Meanwhile in 1967 Sherlock et al.[17] showed what has been confirmed by others[18,19], that more neoplasms are detected when cytological examination is performed in addition to histology. This included fluid from needles and syringes and touch preparations of biopsy tissue.

In 1972, Rasmussen et al..[20] described a method for FNA of liver metastases under direct guidance by ultrasonic scanning. They found that FNA cytology had a higher diagnostic rate than routine liver biopsy using the Menghini method. Then in 1976 Haaga et al.[21] described a method for precise localization of lesions by computed tomography (CT). This allowed accurate positioning of the needle when lesions were very small or deep.

Over the last 15 to 20 years of the twentieth century, it became increasingly clear that percutaneous FNA of single or multiple focal liver lesions demonstrated by palpation, nuclear scan, ultrasonography or CT and at laparoscopy, is both accurate and safe[22–28].

The discipline of FNA of the liver
Value and limitations of cytology in diagnosis

The principal use of liver FNA is in the diagnosis of focal liver lesions. With the use of ultrasonography and CT to screen for disease, and with their routine use in the investigation of patients with cancer, increasing numbers of focal liver lesions are being detected. FNA is used to confirm or rule out malignancy, either primary or secondary. Many primary and metastatic tumours exhibit characteristic cellular patterns and morphologies, which lead to a diagnosis on smear preparations alone: others require added information obtained from a combination of cell blocks, cytochemistry and immunocytochemistry or electron microscopy.

The aim of FNA is to provide a diagnosis of neoplasia and tumour type with a degree of accuracy similar to, if not superior to, that attainable on biopsy material thus avoiding a more complex and costly diagnostic procedure. In the investigation of single or multiple focal lesions, directed FNA, using one of several radiological techniques, can be performed safely at any site within the liver, even close to large blood vessels, dilated bile ducts and the gall bladder. Multiple passes can be performed sampling a wide area or multiple sites. Adequacy of the sample can be checked immediately. If thought necessary, concurrent thin core biopsy can be performed. A cytological diagnosis can be made quickly, accurately and safely. With cystic lesions, aspiration may be therapeutic as well as diagnostic[29]. Most procedures cause the patient very little discomfort and serious complications are rare. The procedure is economical, as hospitalization is not required.

Although principally used for the diagnosis of focal lesions, FNA can also sample benign diffuse liver disease. There are publications describing the features in smears from normal liver, non-specific hepatocellular degeneration and necrosis, pigments, acute and chronic hepatitis, cirrhosis, fatty change and alcoholic liver disease, granulomas, cholestasis, iron overload, amyloidosis and myeloid metaplasia[30–37]. Some authors report that, in their experience, aspiration smears of non-neoplastic disorders determine or at least suggest correct diagnoses in most cases[30,33]. Others, however, comment on the inability of cytology to replace biopsy diagnosis in diffuse liver disease[37].

Technique of aspiration

Most FNA samples are taken under radiological guidance, although palpable lesions can be aspirated directly. Various imaging modalities have been used including ultrasound, CT scanning, image intensifier, angiography and radioisotope scanning. The aspiration is most often performed under ultrasound guidance, which is done without exposure to radiation and is less expensive and faster than CT. The latter is used for deep, small or difficult lesions or when aspiration with ultrasonography has failed to obtain diagnostic material.

Local anaesthetic is generally given down to the liver capsule. Aspiration is performed using a syringe, with or without a holder. In our experience, generally a 22 gauge, 90 mm lumbar puncture needle is used although this can vary. The FNA technique in liver is similar to that used in other sites. Forward and backward movement of the needle is performed with the tip remaining in the lesional tissue to avoid contamination by non-lesional cells. Some advocate moving the needle at different angles to sample more widely or simultaneous rotation of the needle to facilitate 'cutting' of the tissue. Suction increases the amount of material obtained but may give rise to excess blood. Some authors advocate aspiration without suction, as it is performed more easily, generally avoids gross blood contamination and it allows excellent transmitted sensation of tissue penetration via the needle[38]. This can give good results in solid tumours without a significant stromal component, however when tumour cells are unusually cohesive or mixed with fibrous tissue, or a quantity of fluid or pus is to be collected, suction is essential. Sometimes the cytopathologist may recommend additional thin core biopsy, particularly if assessment of architecture is required.

Approach to diagnosis

The combination of a dedicated radiology team working in close association with the cytopathologist results in a high degree of diagnostic accuracy. For best results it is recommended that a cytopathologist or experienced cytotechnician is present at the time of aspiration to assess the adequacy of the sample and to allocate part of it for appropriate ancillary studies if thought necessary.

Aspirated material is used to prepare thin smears, which are air dried and/or wet-fixed in 95% ethyl alcohol or Carnoy's fixative, the latter useful for lysing red blood cells. For rapid assessment at the time of FNA an air-dried smear can be stained with Diff-Quik or a wet-fixed one with rapid H&E. Otherwise the smears are stained by May-Grünwald-Giemsa (MGG) and Papanicolaou stain, respectively. After adequate smears have been made and the diagnostic problem is defined, any remaining or additional aspirated material together with saline rinses from needles and syringes[39] should be allocated for appropriate ancillary studies, taking the available laboratory facilities into consideration.

Material collected in normal saline can be processed into cytospin preparations or into a cell block for histology, histochemistry and immunohistochemistry. Material for a cell block can also be collected directly into formalin. The importance of a good cell block cannot be over emphasized. Additional architectural information is provided which may be central to the final cytodiagnosis. It also allows the performance of multiple immunohistochemical tests. With the increasingly sophisticated range of antibodies available, it is often possible to type tumours more accurately and suggest the primary site when dealing with metastatic malignancy.

If lymphoma is suspected, this material can be sent for flow cytometry. If electron microscopy is likely to be contributory, a portion of the aspirate should be flushed gently into 10 ml of 2.5% glutaraldehyde in 0.15 molar cacodylate buffer, pH 7.2. When infection is a possibility, material should be reserved for microbiological examination.

A multimodal approach to diagnosis utilizing smears, cytochemistry and immunocytochemistry, flow cytometry and electron microscopy is ideal, if laboratory facilities and the quantity and quality of the aspirate allow.

In benign disease oil red-O on air dried smears for fat, Perls' stain for iron or Congo red for amyloid may be performed. Small amounts of bile, which stain intensely green, can be demonstrated using Fouchet's reagent[40]. PAS and PAS-D are useful for demonstrating glycogen and confirmating mucin. A reticulin stain has been reported as useful in distinguishing benign from malignant hepatocellular lesions[41–44]. Various ancillary techniques have been reported as useful in distinguishing malignant from benign hepatocytic lesions but are not routinely used. These include nucleolar organizer regions, immunostaining for p53 or CD34, telomerase activity, flow cytometry, and DNA ploidy[45-52]. These techniques will be further discussed in the section on hepatocellular carcinoma.

In typing tumours, immunoperoxidase staining may be of assistance[40,53-58]. The technique may be applied to smears, cytocentrifuge preparations and on cell blocks from which multiple sections can be obtained, allowing testing for a variety of antigens. Although a mercury-based fixative can be used, formalin is the more commonly used fixative[58,59].

Various markers are used to confirm hepatocytic differentiation and aid in the distinction from other malignancies including cholangiocarcinoma and metastases[53,54,56,58,60-72]. Alpha-fetoprotein is a marker for hepatocellular carcinoma (HCC) if germ cell tumour can be excluded. Reports in the literature of positivity for this marker in HCC tissue vary between 25–75%. Interestingly, alpha-fetoprotein positivity in tumour tissue and the serum level of the marker do not always correlate. Alpha-1-antitrypsin is a similar but less sensitive marker. Recently more specific and sensitive hepatocytic markers have been reported. Polyclonal CEA demonstrates bile canaliculi, Hep Par 1 is a marker of hepatocytic differentiation, MOC-1 is a marker for adenocarcinoma, negative in HCC and vimentin has been reported to highlight Kupffer cells. Hepatitis B surface antigen (HBsAg) can be found within HCC in the setting of chronic hepatitis B virus infection in a proportion of cases. *In-situ* hybridization can be carried out on cell block material for albumin mRNA, which is hepatocyte specific.

Due to the considerable cost of electron microscopy, it is only used if diagnostic questions remain. Semi-thin sections may show tissue architecture, and ultrastructural features reveal the origin of most tumours[73-76]. Distinctive ultrastructural patterns revealed by electron microscopy in well preserved specimens provide a basis for cell type identification independent of the standard cytological criteria. This can be helpful particularly when unusual, pleomorphic or bizarre neoplastic cells are encountered. It has also proved useful in distinguishing between various primary liver malignancies and rare metastatic deposits, and in the latter may point to likely primary sites. Collaboration between the cytopathologist and electron microscopist is crucial for optimal integration of electron microscopy into FNA.

Contraindications and complications

A co-operative patient and a safe access route are always necessary for FNA. As with conventional liver biopsy most serious complications involve bleeding. Bleeding diathesis is a definite contraindication. Prothrombin time and platelet count should be performed routinely. Occasional cases of severe and fatal haemorrhage have been reported[77,78]. The likelihood of this outcome depends on size of needle, the site of lesion and the type of lesion. Aspiration of haemangiomas, without complication has

been reported by several workers[79,80]. The theoretical risk of rupture with subsequent anaphylaxis or spread of disease while aspirating hydatid cysts is always present. Bret *et al.*[81] reported a mild allergic reaction in two of 13 patients on aspiration of hydatid disease. Langlois[82] has reviewed the literature on haemangiomas and hydatid cysts and concludes that danger resulting from puncturing either is little greater than the overall risk of FNA if precautionary measures are taken. Bile leakage may occur, usually in the presence of biliary obstruction but with FNA, in contrast to biopsy, bile peritonitis is apparently rare, with only a few reported cases[83]. Several instances of needle tract seeding by tumour have been reported[84-86] and FNA is best avoided if curative surgery for a suspected malignant neoplasm is contemplated. Rare complications of FNA have included lymphorrhoea and carcinoid crisis[87,88]. Minor complications include pain and tenderness at the puncture site, transient hypotension, small haematomas and pneumothorax. The relative safety of FNA is such that it may be used in very sick patients to obtain information when biopsy carries too high a risk.

Accuracy of diagnosis

Accuracy of diagnosis in FNA of liver lesions depends on the precision of the instruments used to obtain the specimen, the skill of the radiologist and the diagnostic acumen and experience of the cytopathologist[89]. With the use of CT and ultrasound by experienced operators, virtually every lesion has become accessible to aspiration. The needle can be visualized within the lesion so that there are few sampling errors and false negative results are minimized. Careful attention to detail in preparation of smears and cell blocks from aspirates as well as from needle and syringe rinses, the use of cytochemical and immunocytochemical stains and electron microscopy all play an important role in arriving at a correct diagnosis.

Sensitivity for the diagnosis of malignant disease within the liver, according to the literature, ranges from 84 to 100% and the specificity from 45 to 100%. The reported positive predictive value is 93–100%[28,42,90,91]. Typing of tumours is less successful, ranging between 50% and 90%[39,92-94] but when enough material is obtained for special stains and electron microscopy, the cytological diagnosis should approach or equal that of biopsy or autopsy. Nevertheless, a proportion of metastatic tumours will still defy all attempts to identify the tissue of origin and remain 'metastatic malignancy of unknown primary site'.

False positive results are uncommon and should not occur in experienced hands[95].

Diffuse malignant infiltration occurs notably with lymphoma and leukaemia, melanoma and with certain carcinomas, particularly those metastatic from lung and breast. Grossman *et al.* showed that such diffuse tumours are diagnosed more readily by cytology than by histology[19].

Normal liver

The individual hepatocyte is a polyhedral epithelial cell approximately 30 μm in diameter. The sinusoidal surface is covered with abundant microvilli, not visible by light microscopy. The canalicular surface is joined to that of neighbouring hepatocytes to form a bile canaliculus. The canalicular surface is also covered unevenly with microvilli. The cell surface, which lies between the sinusoid and the canaliculus is specialized for cell attachment and for cell-to-cell communication.

The hepatocyte nucleus generally occupies 5–10% of cell volume. There can be considerable variation in both number and size of nuclei. Hepatocyte nuclei come in various size classes with volumes in the ratio 1:2:4:8, a variation reflecting polyploidy. Mitotic figures are rare in hepatocytes from normal liver.

The cytoplasm of the liver cell is granular and may contain fine brown lipofuscin pigment, a normal 'wear and tear' pigment, which remains undigested within lysosomes over long periods. Lipofuscin is distinguishable from abnormal accumulations of bile or haemosiderin. It is PAS positive to a variable extent and diastase fast. Glycogen, which is usually present, may be demonstrated in the cytoplasm of all normal hepatocytes by the PAS stain. A small amount of glycogen may be seen normally in some hepatocyte nuclei.

Ultrastructural features, which typify the hepatocyte and are of diagnostic value include a dense but small nucleolus inside a regular spherical nucleus; numerous rather dense rounded mitochondria, glycogen rosettes, profiles of smooth and rough endoplasmic reticulum, lysosomal dense bodies and lipid droplets. Surface membranes have multiple intercellular junctions, but hepatocytes lack a basal lamina.

Endothelial cells form a slender flat smooth cytoplasmic sheet, which lines the wall of sinusoids. Their nuclei are elongated and flattened but bulge a little from attenuated cytoplasm. Kupffer cells, on the other hand, are stellate and irregular in shape and usually rest on the endothelial lining with which they do not form junctions. They show many of the structural features of macrophages, reflecting their function to remove and degrade particulate and solid matter from portal and arterial blood. They may be packed with ingested material. Kupffer cells divide when stimulated by local liver injury and are increased in number in many liver diseases. Bile duct cells range from low cuboidal to columnar with increasing size of the duct. Their nuclei are basal, the chromatin fine and evenly dispersed, nucleoli inconspicuous, and the cytoplasm rather pale staining.

Cytology of normal liver

▶ Polygonal hepatocytes, mainly in clusters or sheets
▶ Uniform round nuclei with small central nucleoli
▶ Regular, finely granular chromatin
▶ Cytoplasmic lipofuscin pigment
▶ Kupffer cells inconspicuous
▶ Bile duct epithelial cells in sheets
▶ No inflammatory cell infiltrate

In well-preserved smears made from FNA of normal liver, the smear background is blood-stained but otherwise clean and hepatocytes predominate, arranged in small clusters or in cohesive flat sheets which can show a trabecular architecture with a sinusoidal network (Fig. 14.1). Single cells are uncommon and stripped nuclei should not be seen.

Hepatocytes are polygonal with rather ill-defined cytoplasmic borders, that become more distinct in disease states. Cytoplasm may be eosinophilic or slightly basophilic (grey-blue with MGG) and granular. Microvilli cannot be seen. Fine round lipofuscin pigment granules may be plentiful (Fig. 14.2).

The similarity of nuclei in all hepatocytes from normal liver aspirates is striking. They are round and central and

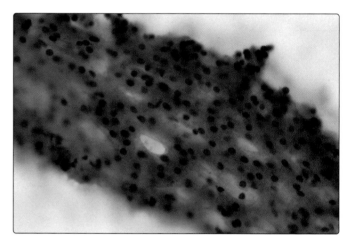

Fig. 14.1 A sheet of benign hepatocytes showing a trabecular architecture. Sinusoidal spaces are seen between the trabeculae. (H&E × MP)

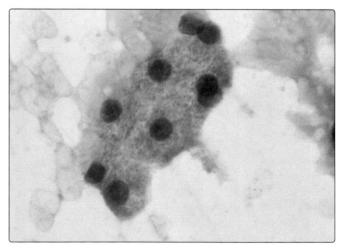

Fig. 14.2 Normal liver cell plate. Hepatocytes are polygonal and contain one or two round nuclei with a single central nucleolus. The cytoplasm is granular and the cell borders indistinct. (Papanicolaou × HP)

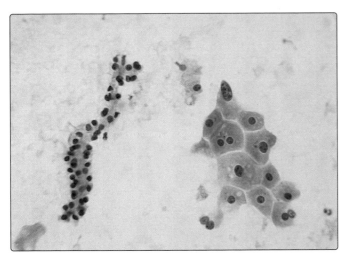

Fig. 14.3 Epithelial cells from a bile duct seen in profile as low columnar cells with regular basal nuclei. Compare with the cluster of benign hepatocytes. (Papanicolaou × HP)

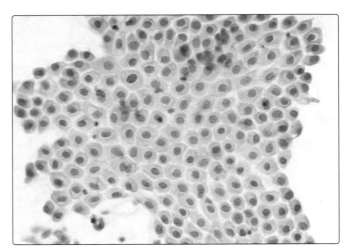

Fig. 14.4 Mesothelial cells in aspirate of liver. A flat sheet of evenly spaced, regular mesothelial cells in honeycomb pattern. Nuclei are round and chromatin finely granular. (Papanicolaou × HP)

two identical nuclei may be present in one cell. The chromatin is finely granular, pale staining and evenly distributed with a single small, but prominent, central nucleolus. Nuclear size varies exponentially, reflecting variation in ploidy, but irregular variation in nuclear size and chromatin pattern denotes disease. Clear intranuclear inclusions of cytoplasmic material occur occasionally, enclosed by the nuclear membrane.

Kupffer cells may be identified in close proximity to hepatocytes. Generally their nuclei are somewhat elongated, plump and irregular in outline; chromatin is coarsely granular and cytoplasm is comparatively clear. When Kupffer cells proliferate in response to liver cell injury, cytoplasmic borders become evident and the cells are more easily identified. Occasionally endothelial cells with their spindle-shaped nuclei and attenuated cytoplasm may be identified, closely applied to one edge of a liver cell plate.

In normal smears at least a few small aggregates of bile ductal cells should be seen (Fig. 14.3). The cells are evenly spaced and occur in small monolayered sheets or in tubular profile. Bile duct epithelium should not be confused with small fragments of mesothelium from the liver capsule (Fig. 14.4). Characteristically, mesothelial cells are seen in honeycomb pattern with regular round vesicular nuclei containing granular chromatin and a small nucleolus surrounded by a relatively constant amount of cytoplasm, but they may form atypical cell balls or contain reactive nuclei, particularly in the presence of ascites.

Benign diseases of the liver

Non-specific benign changes

In benign conditions changes in hepatocytes are frequently non-specific but, when considered in combination with the presence or absence of other cytological features, may point to a specific diagnosis. Johansen and Myren[96] observed

striking cytological alterations in patients with both acute and chronic liver disease as well as a large variety of extrahepatic diseases.

Cytological findings

► Marked non-specific hepatocellular degeneration known as ballooning degeneration has been described in acute hepatitis[33] and in cirrhosis[37]
► Apoptosis is a form of cell death that occurs particularly in viral hepatitis, cholestasis, drug-induced liver injury and graft-*vs*-host disease, and is most marked in yellow fever
► Mallory bodies (or hyaline) are a classic finding in alcoholic liver disease but may be seen in other conditions including drug toxicity, dietary deficiencies and HCC
► Regeneration may follow acute cell destruction or slow degeneration. There is cell enlargement with vesicular nuclei, prominent nucleoli and binucleation. Lipofuscin is generally absent
► Atrophy is often present around space-occupying lesions
► Necrosis is not infrequently associated with tumours

Ballooning degeneration, which results mainly from swelling of endoplasmic reticulum, is recognized by enlarged, round hepatocytes with enlarged nuclei and swollen pale cytoplasm that becomes even paler towards the cell membrane which is sharp and accentuated. Apoptosis or programmed cell death is represented by acidophilic Councilman bodies with smaller than normal hepatocytes that exhibit deeply staining cytoplasm and degenerating nuclei which eventually become pyknotic (Fig. 14.5)[97].

Reports of Mallory bodies vary. Suen[98] describes them as ropey eosinophilic strands that appear to condense into irregular discrete masses of waxy, amorphous material in the cytoplasm; Tao[99] as round or elongated acidophilic clumps located in a perinuclear position; and Brits[30] as large

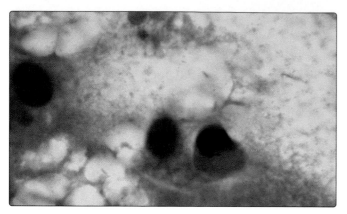

Fig. 14.5 Apoptosis. Acidophilic Councilman bodies where the hepatocytes are smaller than normal with deeply staining cytoplasm and degenerating pyknotic nuclei. (H&E × HP)

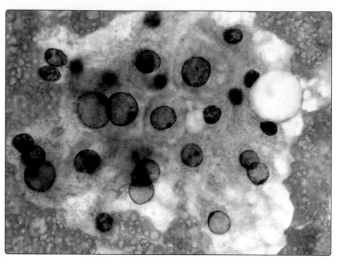

Fig. 14.6 Nuclear glycogenation in diabetes mellitus. Hepatocytes exhibiting swollen, pale nuclei. Nucleoli are peripheral and nuclear membranes intact. (Papanicolaou × HP)

irregular bluish-grey granules or bodies which may be confluent.

Smears showing evidence of regeneration contain hepatocytes in which both nucleus and nucleolus are enlarged but chromatin pattern is normal. Lipofuscin is absent from the newly formed cytoplasm of regenerating cells. In addition, mitoses and increased numbers of binucleate cells are seen. Multinucleate cells may be seen in acute hepatitis[30] and in liver cell dysplasia[100] and are not confined to hepatocellular carcinoma (HCC). Smears reflecting atrophy show small hepatocytes exhibiting reduced cytoplasm and smaller nuclei, which stain more darkly than those of normal cells. Atrophy surrounding space-occupying lesions may be accompanied by features of intrahepatic biliary stasis with accumulation of bile pigment in liver cells and canaliculi. According to Brits[30], when atrophy is due to venous congestion or veno-occlusive disease, the smear background contains many erythrocytes. When necrosis occurs, sheets of shrunken hepatocytes are seen, which vary in size. Cytoplasm becomes increasingly eosinophilic and granular and nuclei pyknotic or karyolytic. Fragments of frayed cytoplasm devoid of nuclei are present in the background. Nuclear glycogenation results in a swollen, clear or vacuolated hepatocyte nucleus (Fig. 14.6). This cleared or vacuolated appearance must be distinguished from intranuclear cytoplasmic invaginations, which may be seen in both normal and malignant hepatocytes. Glycogenated nuclei are found in 75% of diabetics, particularly in type II diabetes, but are not specific as they can also occur in normal liver, Wilson's disease, sepsis, tuberculosis, biliary tract disease, cirrhosis and chronic active hepatitis.

In addition to changes in hepatocytes, an increase in the amount of bile duct epithelium, increased inflammatory cells including polymorphonuclear leucocytes and lymphocytes, activated proliferating Kupffer cells, fibrous tissue and evidence of bile stasis are seen in different proportions in various diseases.

Common specific benign conditions
Steatosis/steatohepatitis

Steatosis or fatty change is one of the commonest morphological abnormalities seen in liver and can be caused by a large number of agents. It develops by accumulation of triglycerides in the hepatocyte cytoplasm. Two patterns are described: microvesicular and macrovesicular. In the microvesicular form, the cytoplasm is filled with many small lipid droplets that do not displace the nucleus. Alcohol and other drugs, namely tetracycline, salicylates and valproic acid cause microvesicular steatosis. These changes are also seen in Reye's syndrome, fatty liver of pregnancy and aflatoxin-induced microvesicular steatosis in Thai children.

Much more frequent is macrovesicular steatosis, which is commonly associated with excessive alcohol intake. Other associations include diabetes mellitus, obesity, drugs and heavy metals and infections, particularly hepatitis C virus. In macrovesicular steatosis the hepatocyte contains one or several large fat droplets displacing the nucleus to the periphery and indenting it. If cell necrosis occurs the lipid may coalesce to form fatty cysts. The cause of fatty change cannot be determined on morphological grounds. Lundquist[4] showed good correlation between histological and cytological scores of fatty vacuolation for roughly estimating fat content of liver parenchyma and also demonstrated correlation between cytological estimates of lipid on FNA and chemical determination of triglycerides.

Cytological findings

▶ Reduced cell cohesion
▶ Cells rounded; nuclei eccentric and may be indented
▶ Variable-sized lipid vacuoles

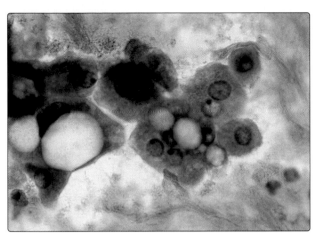

Fig. 14.7 Fatty change in benign hepatocytes (macrovesicular steatosis). Cluster of liver cells showing large cytoplasmic vacuoles displacing nuclei. (Papanicolaou × HP)

▶ Positive staining with oil red-O and Sudan III, PAS-negative
▶ Kupffer cells active

In smears from fatty liver, there is usually at least some loss of cell cohesion and fatty change is readily appreciated by recognition of fine or large lipid-containing vacuoles within the cytoplasm of hepatocytes (Fig. 14.7). In severe macrovesicular degeneration, many cells are almost completely filled with large lipid-laden vacuoles, causing peripheral displacement of the nucleus, which may remain vesicular or become pyknotic. Non-specific marginal vacuoles, which do not contain fat, may be seen in MGG-stained smears, in conditions such as cirrhosis and they should not be confused with steatosis. In doubtful cases a specific fat stain such as oil red-O is useful on air dried smears.

Steatohepatitis is most commonly a manifestation of alcoholic liver injury although 'non-alcoholic steatohepatitis' or NASH is now a recognized entity. The microscopic findings are steatosis with associated liver cell damage as indicated by altered nuclear chromatin pattern, cytoplasmic degeneration and the presence of Mallory bodies, inflammation including polymorphonuclear leucocytes and, in late stages, fibrosis with increased amounts of bile duct epithelium[30,101]. Some authors claim that a reliable cytological diagnosis of pure steatosis can be made when steatosis is seen in smears without cell necrosis, inflammatory cells and fibrous tissue[35]. Steatosis and steatohepatitis will disappear after 2–4 weeks of abstinence. With continuing alcohol abuse micronodular cirrhosis may evolve and this may become inactive and macronodular if alcohol consumption ceases. When FNA is performed on macronodular alcoholic cirrhosis, if the needle enters a large regenerating nodule, the smears may show only regenerating hepatocytes. If the needle enters a large tract of scar tissue the smears may be poorly cellular and show only microfragments of fibrous tissue. As well as steatosis (described above) there are features of cell degeneration or necrosis with an accompanying inflammatory reaction. If there is progression to fibrosis and cirrhosis, stromal elements and proliferating bile ductules can be found.

In focal fatty liver, steatosis is localized and presents as a focal lesion on both CT and ultrasound imaging[102]. The differential diagnosis includes benign and malignant hepatocytic tumours, metastases, haemangiomas, angiomyolipomas, and granulomatous disease. Focal fatty change may be associated with the same conditions known to accompany diffuse fatty liver but in many patients no cause is found. The focal nature of the disease is postulated to be due to regional ischaemia of unknown aetiology with hypoxia of contiguous portal lobules. Lesions may be solitary, or multiple, and round or oval in contour with sharp boundaries, and a diameter up to 11 cm. Accurate placement of the needle is important for a confident diagnosis. Caturelli *et al.*[103], reported 21 patients with focal fatty liver. Most of the FNA smears revealed hepatocytes affected by fatty change. In his series two lesions disappeared on ultrasound follow-up.

Hepatitis

Hepatitis in its broadest sense means inflammation of the liver. There are many diseases that include a component of inflammation. Even on histology these can be difficult, if not impossible, to separate without correlating the clinical setting and the laboratory test results. The appearance in smears is generally non-specific and FNA is rarely if ever used in the diagnosis of diffuse inflammatory liver disease. Sometimes when sampling focal lesions, material from the surrounding liver may be included and this can show an inflammatory disease process.

Viral hepatitis

Acute hepatitis caused by the hepatitis viruses is characterized by necrosis, regeneration of hepatocytes and inflammation. Cytological morphology alone cannot distinguish reliably between disease caused by the different viruses. Electron microscopy may reveal typical viral particles in the cytoplasm of hepatocytes and/or Kupffer cells[104].

Cytological findings

▶ Smear cellularity increases with severity of infection
▶ Ballooning degeneration and apoptosis
▶ Multinucleation, pleomorphism, mitoses
▶ Inflammatory cells
▶ Kupffer cells with lipofuscin and iron
▶ Bile pigment

Features vary in acute viral hepatitis according to the severity of disease[30,105]. Smears in severe acute viral hepatitis are very cellular and show a pleomorphic population of hepatocytes. There is ballooning degeneration, apoptosis, regeneration and inflammatory changes. Hepatocytes vary greatly in size, cytoplasmic staining is uneven, nucleoli vary in size and chromatin pattern and large nucleoli are present in regenerating cells. Multinucleated cells and mitoses may be present. Increased numbers of inflammatory cells are seen consisting of lymphocytes and neutrophil granulocytes, the latter intermingled with damaged hepatocytes. Kupffer cells may contain impressive amounts of iron, lipofuscin and PAS positive cellular debris. Cholestasis with bile pigment in liver cells and bile plugs between cells is a common finding but fatty change rarely occurs. In mild cases smears may appear almost normal, but Wasastjerna[37] has found disrupted or dilated canaliculi revealed by naphthylamidase staining highly sensitive in detecting minimal hepatocyte damage. These changes in hepatocyte morphology are seen in both acute and chronic hepatitis due to virus infection but in chronic disease smears also contain variable amounts of fibrous tissue and increased bile duct epithelium as seen in cirrhosis. Findings similar to those of viral hepatitis may be seen in drug-induced hepatitis but neutrophils and eosinophils constitute part of the inflammatory cell population.

Other viral diseases

Four members of the herpesvirus group of DNA viruses may involve the liver by blood-borne spread from other sites and can result in changes recognizable by cytology. These are Herpesvirus hominis, Herpesvirus varicellae (the varicella–zoster virus), cytomegalovirus and Epstein Barr virus. Cytopathic effects of Herpesvirus hominis and Herpesvirus varicellae are similar and are the same as those seen elsewhere in the body. In histology, coagulative necrosis of hepatocytes with little inflammatory response is seen. Typical Cowdry type B and Cowdry type A bodies are present in surviving liver cells and no doubt could be recognized in smears. Similarly, cytomegalovirus presenting the typical owl's eye appearance has been seen in tissue sections in hepatocytes, bile duct epithelium and endothelial cells. The very large central amphophilic nuclear inclusion surrounded by a large clear zone and prominent chromatinic rim may be accompanied by small basophilic cytoplasmic inclusions, which are PAS positive.

Epstein Barr virus causes infectious mononucleosis. When the liver is involved, histology shows small foci of parenchymal necrosis and an infiltrate of atypical mononuclear cells. Smears of aspirates from all affected tissues contain large atypical lymphocytes, their relatively abundant cytoplasm often showing plasmacytoid features, sharply delineated oval, round or indented nuclei, granular chromatin and prominent nucleoli. It is important to distinguish atypical lymphocytes of infectious mononucleosis from leukaemia and lymphoma cells.

Cirrhosis

Cirrhosis is the end result of a combination of changes: liver cell death, regenerative activity of surviving hepatocytes and fibrous tissue production. The result is architectural distortion of the liver with structurally abnormal hepatocyte nodules surrounded and separated by fibrous bands. Piecemeal necrosis of hepatocytes over a long period is usually necessary to produce this change. Bile ducts proliferate in newly formed fibrous tissue in response to bile stasis resulting from the architectural disturbance. Inflammation is also present, with leucocyte infiltration and activation and proliferation of Kupffer cells. Inflammation persists as long as damage to hepatocytes continues, but if causal factors are alleviated the cirrhosis becomes inactive and is characterized by fibrosis and abnormal nodules without an accompanying inflammatory cell response.

Micronodular cirrhosis (defined as nodules <3 mm in diameter) is typically associated with alcohol, haemochromatosis, drugs, chronic hepatic venous outflow obstruction, chronic biliary disease and rare metabolic disorders of infancy including Indian childhood cirrhosis.

Macronodular cirrhosis (defined as nodules >3 mm in diameter) is more varied and typically evolves from viral hepatitis and autoimmune chronic active hepatitis. It may also evolve when the insult to the liver is stopped, e.g. when patients with alcoholic cirrhosis reduce their intake. Liver cell dysplasia and HCC may complicate cirrhosis.

Cytological findings

- ▶ Variable cellularity and discohesion
- ▶ Mixture of irregular sheets of hepatocytes, fibrous tissue and increased bile duct epithelium
- ▶ Normal hepatocytes mixed with atypical hepatocytes
- ▶ Occasional multinucleated forms
- ▶ Degenerate and regenerating liver cells
- ▶ Inflammation

Cholestasis

Because of the complexity of bile secretion, the term cholestasis is difficult to define. Literally it means 'stand-still in bile'. It is caused by an obstruction, which may be located at any point along the pathway taken by excretory products from their site of production inside the hepatocyte to the duodenal lumen. The causes are many.

To the morphologist, cholestasis means visible stagnation of bile pigment in hepatocytes, bile canaliculi and Kupffer cells. During histological preparation and processing a considerable amount of accumulated bile pigment may wash out of sections. In cytological preparations, however, this loss does not occur; bile is readily seen and the degree of cholestasis is in general proportional to the amount of bile in the smear. As in histology, separation of cases of obstructive jaundice from those of non-obstructive jaundice can be difficult[32,37,106].

Cytological findings

- ▶ Cytoplasmic feathery degeneration
- ▶ Smooth intracytoplasmic droplets of varying size

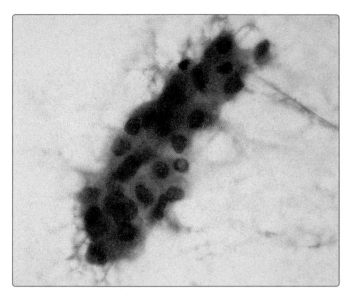

Fig. 14.8   Cholestasis. Golden brown pigment is present as bile plugs in dilated canaliculi between liver cells. (H&E × HP)

▶ Bile in canaliculi between liver cells and in Kupffer cells
▶ Proliferating bile duct epithelium may be present

Cholestasis in hepatocytes can manifest as diffuse cytoplasmic feathery degeneration with a subtle tinge of bile staining or else as smooth droplets of varying size, occasionally obscuring the nucleus (Fig. 14.8). In Papanicolaou stained smears it is yellow-green in colour. Bile is also seen in Kupffer cells and in canaliculi between liver cells. In obstructive jaundice, pigment is usually present in the form of bile plugs or branching thrombi in dilated canaliculi and free bile is seen in the smear background. Distinction between bile and haemosiderin in hepatocytes is usually not a problem. Haemosiderin is yellow-brown and granular; the granules are usually discrete and do not obscure the liver cell nucleus except in heavy iron overload, and histochemical stains for iron are positive. Brits[30] found evidence of cholestasis in cases of alcoholic hepatitis, viral hepatitis, biliary atresia, liver cell necrosis, obstructive jaundice and cholangitis. She suggested that when both bile duct cells and liver cells show signs of necrosis and many leucocytes are present in smears, the cause of cholestasis may be cholangitis.

Liver granulomas

Many diseases, which are manifested wholly or in part by a granulomatous reaction, involve the liver. Some are intrinsic hepatic diseases but most are systemic conditions in which the liver is only one of many affected organs. For more details the reader is directed to other texts[107]. Causes may be grouped into those due to infectious diseases, drug sensitivities, foreign bodies, neoplasms, specific immunodeficiency diseases and others such as sarcoidosis, primary biliary cirrhosis and granulomatous hepatitis with

prolonged fever. In establishing the cause a detailed clinical history, appropriate skin testing and microbiological and biochemical screening are essential.

Sarcoidosis is one of the commonest causes of non-caseating hepatic granulomas. They are well circumscribed and consist of aggregations of large epithelioid histiocytes often with multinucleated giant cells of Langhans' type, which may contain asteroid bodies. Lymphocytes and macrophages are also present.

In hepatic tuberculosis the granulomas show central caseation. Acid fast bacilli should be sought using Ziehl-Neelsen stains and when present, are diagnostic[30]. As well as culture to identify the organism, PCR for mycobacteria can be performed on fresh or fixed material. Hepatic tuberculoma is an uncommon but important lesion because it may be confused clinically, on ultrasonography and on CT with pyogenic abscess or hepatic tumour[108,109]. The tuberculoma consists of central caseation surrounded by epithelioid cells and fibrous tissue. If lysis occurs the space-occupying lesion may be referred to as a tuberculous 'abscess'[108,110].

Schistosome ova elicit a granulomatous response in addition to an infiltrate of neutrophils and eosinophils. The ova of *S. mansoni* and *S. japonicum* are acid fast.

Granulomas caused by drug sensitivity are accompanied by eosinophils; systemic eosinophilia usually develops; liver cell injury and cholestasis are also common.

Granulomas may be found in liver and lungs of intravenous drug users. They are caused by starch and talc, which are present as a 'filler' with injected drugs. Both are birefringent, starch particles being identified by their 'Maltese cross' appearance. Talc crystals are also refractile. Foreign body giant cells are usually seen in reaction to starch but are exceptionally rare in response to talc, however the latter are taken up by Kupffer cells and portal macrophages which may cluster to form granulomatous foci[107].

The aetiology and pathogenesis of granulomas in liver in patients with Hodgkin's disease are unknown. Granulomas can occur in focal nodular hyperplasia and liver cell adenoma and are confined to the tumour[107].

Granulomatous hepatitis is an entity occurring typically in middle aged men with prolonged fever, abdominal pain, hepatosplenomegaly and non-specific liver granulomas for which no cause can be found. In primary biliary cirrhosis essential features in addition to granulomas are evidence of cholestasis, fibrosis and inflammation.

Cytological findings

▶ Aggregates or small groups of epithelioid histiocytes
▶ Langhans' and/or foreign body type giant cells occasionally seen
▶ Variable, non-specific inflammation
▶ Necrosis may be present

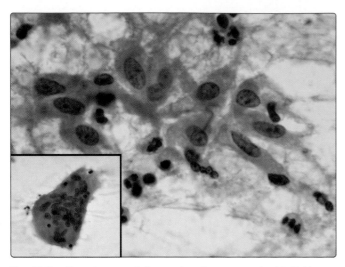

Fig. 14.9 Granulomatous inflammation. Aggregates of epithelioid histiocytes with an elongated plump nucleus showing finely granular chromatin and a small but distinct nucleolus. The cytoplasm is abundant and pale staining. Multinucleated giant cells may be present (inset). (H&E × HP)

For the cytopathologist, relatively few distinctive features are found and diagnosis hinges on identification of an organism or other aetiological agent. Stormby and Akerman[111] found seven cases containing granulomas in 1435 aspirations, of which two were due to sarcoidosis, two as part of Hodgkin's disease, one in which the patient had both sarcoidosis and Hodgkin's disease, one drug induced and one in which the cause remained unknown.

Features of liver granulomas in smears are similar to those seen in other sites. Diagnosis is made by recognition of aggregates of epithelioid histiocytes, which may be well defined, or consist of a few clusters of easily overlooked cells. The epithelioid cell is large with rather abundant, pale-staining cytoplasm and an eccentric, usually elongated nucleus, often plump and sharply curved. Chromatin is finely granular and there are small but distinct nucleoli (Fig. 14.9). Multinucleated giant cells of both Langhans' and foreign body type (Fig. 14.9 inset) are sometimes seen in smears with other inflammatory cells and necrotic material may be present. In the seven cases reported by Stormby and Akerman[111], all contained aggregates of epithelioid cells but multinucleated giant cells were seen only in one.

In examining smears containing granulomas it is important to observe the nature of inflammatory cells associated with the granuloma. Granulomas accompanied by many neutrophils, i.e. biphasic inflammatory reaction, are likely to be related to infections caused by bacteria or higher bacteria such as actinomyces organisms. The presence of any aetiological foreign body within the granuloma, microorganisms, which may be demonstrated by special stains and evidence of any hepatic parenchymal change may be helpful in differential diagnosis. The term lipogranuloma should be restricted to those lesions that contain many vacuolated macrophages resulting from extrusion of neutral lipid from hepatocytes, e.g. in alcoholic liver disease. Lesions of lepromatous leprosy are also composed of collections of vacuolated cells, which contain many lepra bacilli demonstrable by stains for acid fast bacilli. Well-formed granulomas of tuberculoid leprosy are seldom seen in viscera. In 518 smears from leprosy patients Brits[30] found cells containing bacilli in 88 but gave no further details.

Iron overload/iron storage disease

Normal iron balance in the body is maintained by regulation of its absorption via the duodenum and proximal jejunum, since man possesses no natural pathway for excretion of excess iron. Approximately one third of total body iron (about 5 g) is present as storage iron. Increase in iron absorption or parenteral administration of iron, or both, results in excess iron stores, much of the excess accumulating in the liver. From the earliest stages of disorders of excessive iron storage, both ferritin and haemosiderin accumulate and are found on electron microscopy within cytoplasmic 'siderosomes' in both hepatocytes and Kupffer cells. Both give a positive Perls' Prussian blue reaction and are seen as intense blue granules within cell cytoplasm, the granules becoming larger with increasing amounts of iron. In the hepatocytes 'siderosomes' are characteristically aligned along bile canaliculi. Whilst chemical determination of tissue iron concentration is the ultimate criterion of iron overload, visual assessment of the amount of iron revealed by Perls' stain in liver sections can provide information about the level of iron stores in a particular patient.

FNA has been shown to provide a reliable indication of increased liver iron concentration and is useful in screening for iron overload. However, it does not replace formal biopsy for histology and chemical analysis of liver iron[34]. Although biochemical estimation of iron has been accurately performed on FNA material in an animal model[112]. Clinicopathological consultation is required to reach a microscopic diagnosis beyond haemosiderosis.

Iron overload is seen mainly in the following conditions:

Genetic (idiopathic) haemochromatosis

The gene and the mutation responsible for the vast majority of genetic haemochromatosis cases was identified in 1996, although the basic metabolic defect that leads to excessive absorption of iron remains unknown. In the majority of homozygous subjects, parenchymal cell loading with iron results in functional failure of different organs leading to cirrhosis, heart failure, diabetes mellitus and gonadal atrophy. In homozygotes iron accumulation is considerable in hepatocytes by the mid-teens, young males being more affected than females who are partly protected by monthly iron loss due to menstruation. With advancing age, iron storage increases and hepatocyte turnover and fibrosis increase with eventual cirrhosis and an increased risk of developing HCC. In up to 25% of heterozygotes a limited increase in hepatic iron concentration develops, but cirrhosis and hepatic failure never occur.

Iron overload associated with anaemia

With increased iron absorption due to a mild increase in erythropoiesis, hepatic iron storage is predominantly parenchymal and cirrhosis may occur, albeit rarely. With transfusional overload, haemosiderin accumulates in hepatocytes at an early stage and later in Kupffer cells and macrophages. In thalassaemia major, cirrhosis is present in a heavily iron-laden liver by the age of 10 years.

Iron overload due to ingestion of excessive dietary iron

In the black South African (Bantu) population, the source of surplus iron in the diet has proved to be cooking pots and containers used for brewing beer, the iron being in a form particularly suitable for absorption. In late stages of disease, haemosiderin is seen predominantly in macrophages in portal tracts and fibrous tissue and there are smaller amounts in hepatocytes and Kupffer cells.

Iron overload in cirrhosis

A mild degree of hepatic siderosis is present in most cirrhotic patients. It is more commonly found in cases of hepatitis C virus infection, or steatohepatitis.

Cytological findings

- ▶ Fine and coarse granular yellow-brown pigment in hepatocytes and Kupffer cells
- ▶ Blue granules with Perls' stain
- ▶ Evidence of fibrosis, regeneration and bile duct proliferation if fibrotic or cirrhotic

Depending on the route and mechanism of iron loading, excess iron may be found in hepatocytes, biliary epithelial cells, Kupffer cells, macrophages and connective tissue cells or combinations of these (Fig. 14.10). In genetic haemochromatosis preferential loading of iron within hepatocytes is seen whereas in most other types it occurs mainly in Kupffer cells and macrophages. The excess iron may be associated with minimal to advanced fibrosis or with cirrhosis. Thus morphological appearances of iron overload vary depending on the stage of disease as well as the cause.

In smears, haemosiderin is seen as yellow-brown cytoplasmic pigment in hepatocytes and Kupffer cells and is readily identified as blue granules with Perls' stain. The granules may be small or large, tending to appear on the canalicular side of the nucleus in hepatocytes. Except where massive aggregates have formed, granules seldom obscure the nucleus. Extracellular aggregates of pigment may be seen, particularly in heavy overload. Evidence of fibrosis and bile duct proliferation, which would indicate cirrhosis,

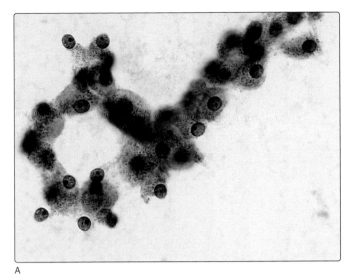

A

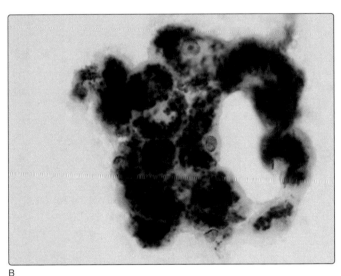

B

Fig. 14.10 Genetic haemochromatosis. (A) Heavy iron overload in hepatocytes, all of which are packed with yellow-brown granules of haemosiderin pigment. (B) Granules stain blue with Perls' stain. (A, Papanicolaou × HP; B, Perls' × HP)

should be looked for in smears. Lipofuscin pigment, which may be confused with haemosiderin, does not occur outside intact cells, is PAS positive and according to Perry and Johnston[35] is usually perinuclear and rarely clumped.

The absence of iron from malignant hepatocytes in contrast to heavy deposits in benign cells may be helpful in the diagnosis of HCC in patients with haemochromatosis.

Alpha-1-antitrypsin deficiency

Alpha-1-antitrypsin deficiency (A-1 AT) is the commonest of the inborn errors of metabolism. A-1 AT is a circulating glycoprotein and the major protease inhibitor in normal serum. There are a number of different phenotypes of the polymorphic glycoprotein. The abnormal phenotype associated with liver disease is called Pi ZZ. Possession of this phenotype may be associated with various clinical courses. Some patients present in the neonatal period with cholestatic liver disease from which they may recover. Others present in late childhood or adolescence with cirrhosis, while some young adults may suffer from chronic bronchitis and emphysema in addition to cirrhosis. About 10% of homozygotes may present for the first time in adult life with fully developed cirrhosis and there is an increased risk of HCC in these patients. The livers of all these patients show variable numbers of hepatocytes, which contain cytoplasmic inclusion bodies. These are pale with H&E stains in sections but bright magenta with PAS after diastase digestion. Inclusions are globular, may be single or multiple and reach 40 μm in diameter. Ultrastructurally, the material accumulates in distended cisternae of the endoplasmic reticulum. The globules are antigenically identical to A-1 AT and should be confirmed as such, or a serum test should be done for confirmation of the disease since not all PAS-D positive globules are composed of A-1 AT. Similar structures may be seen in other conditions, e.g. alcoholic cirrhosis.

Amyloidosis

Amyloidosis occurs in a heterogenous group of diseases all showing extra-cellular deposition of hyaline amorphous material. It is classified according to the chemical composition of the amyloid fibrils of which there are up to 15 types, the principal two being amyloid light chain (AL) or amyloid A protein (AA). It may be associated with plasma cell dyscrasias (AL) or chronic inflammation of longstanding, such as rheumatoid arthritis and bronchiectasis (AA) or heredofamilial disease. The deposition may be localized or systemic and hepatic involvement is common in the latter. In the liver, amyloid may be deposited in walls of blood vessels, in portal tract fibrous tissue or in the parenchyma within the space of Disse where accumulation causes compression atrophy of hepatocytes.

Cytological findings

▶ Extracellular amorphous material which is pink or green (Papanicolaou stain) or pink to purple (MGG)
▶ Apple green birefringence on polarizing a Congo red stained smear
▶ Liver cell atrophy

In smears, amyloid appears as extracellular amorphous material, vaguely fibrillary, glassy or waxy and staining pale pink or green with the Papanicolaou method (Fig. 14.11A) or pink to purple with MGG. Some hepatocytes in the smear may appear small and atrophic. Amyloid should be confirmed with special stains. A congo red stain shows characteristic apple-green birefringence under polarized light (Fig. 14.11B)[113-115]. Under the electron microscope, amyloid has a distinctive appearance of confluent extracellular deposits comprising networks of unbranched rigid microfilaments 7–10 nm in thickness.

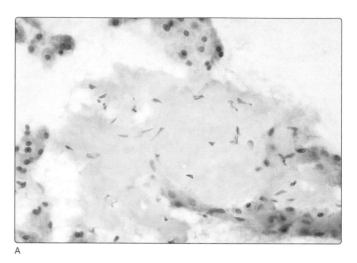

A

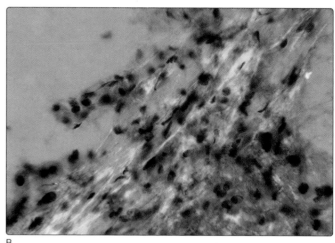

B

Fig. 14.11 Amyloidosis of liver. (A) Cloudy pale blue mass of amyloid and atrophic hepatocytes. (B) Apple-green birefringence on examination under polarized light. (A, Papanicolaou × HP; B, Congo red × HP)

Myeloid metaplasia (extramedullary haemopoiesis)

Myeloid metaplasia occurs in liver or spleen when there is replacement of the normal bone marrow and may present as a solid mass lesion. It is classically associated with myeloproliferative disease, such as polycythaemia vera, thrombocythaemia or myeloid leukaemia which may result in myelofibrosis. Other causes include metastatic carcinoma, multiple myeloma and some granulomatous lesions. It occurs regularly within hepatoblastomas and angiosarcomas of liver.

Cytological findings

▶ Normoblasts, myelocytes and megakaryocytes present
▶ Megakaryocytes are absent in myeloid leukaemia
▶ Myeloma cells present in cases of multiple myeloma

In smears showing evidence of extramedullary haemopoiesis, normoblasts, myelocytes and megakaryocytes may be seen[116-118]. They occur as single cells, sometimes clustered, separate from hepatocytes and other elements. Normoblasts are small cells with relatively small, round, central hyperchromatic nuclei and homogeneous eosinophilic or amphophilic cytoplasm. Megakaryocytes are large cells with abundant granular cytoplasm and lobated nuclei. In myelofibrosis they may be present in large numbers and have a bizarre appearance however in myeloid leukaemia, megakaryocytes are usually scarce or absent. In some cases of multiple myeloma in which myeloid metaplasia occurs the percentage of myeloma cells is the same in the liver aspirate as in the bone marrow. In cases of genuine metastatic growth, however, only myeloma cells are seen in the liver aspirate.

Other specific infections and infestations
Fungal infections
Histoplasmosis

Histoplasmosis, which occurs world-wide, is caused by *Histoplasma capsulatum*. Disseminated disease occurs in immunosuppressed patients and the liver is usually affected. The small spores 2–5 μm in diameter, are taken up by Kupffer cells, which become swollen and compress liver cells causing liver cell necrosis. There may be little inflammatory reaction or poorly formed granulomas may develop in which epithelioid cells may contain asteroid or Schaumann bodies. Diagnosis is based on identification of the organism in Kupffer cells. Methenamine silver is the stain of choice.

Candidosis, aspergillosis and phycomycosis

Not infrequently, the liver is involved when fungal infections, especially of the lungs, disseminate via the blood. The infection is usually opportunistic and occurs in immunosuppressed patients. In candidosis, abscesses form and the fungus presents in both pseudomycelial and yeast-like phases. In both aspergillosis and phycomycosis, the fungi may invade blood vessels causing thrombosis and infarction. Granulomatous lesions may be present. Diagnosis depends on identification of the aetiological agent. Hyphae of aspergillus measure 8–10 μm in diameter, are septate and show dichotomous branching. Fungi of phycomycosis have hyphae, which are broad, non-septate and branch at right angles and are readily seen with H&E and Papanicolaou stains. Special stains, such as methenamine silver, demonstrate mycelial elements and are particularly useful when the organisms are non-viable.

Parasitic diseases
Schistosomiasis

This disease is discussed in the section dealing with liver granulomas.

Liver fluke infestation

Infestation with *Clonorchis sinensis* and *Opisthorchis viverrini*, both trematode worms, is endemic in the Far East including China, Taiwan, Japan, Korea and South East Asia.

Immigrants and travellers from these areas may be infected. The hermaphrodite adult flukes live in the bile ducts and produce ova, which are passed in the stools. Clinical symptoms and signs tend to reflect the number of worms inhabiting the bile ducts, worm numbers increasing with repeated ingestion of infected fish. Eosinophilia may occur, less frequently neutrophil leucocytosis. Complications of infestation include cholangitis, cholelithiasis, acute pancreatitis and cholangiocarcinoma. Diagnosis is made by identification of ova either in stools or in bile specimens obtained at endoscopic retrograde cholangiopancreatogram (ERCP) or percutaneous transhepatic cholangiogram (PTC) or on FNA. Ova of *C. sinensis* and *O. viverrini* are indistinguishable. They are oval and measure approximately 30×15 μm. An operculum with a prominent shoulder is present at one end with a spine-like prominence at the other end.

Cytological findings

▶ Liver fluke ova may be seen
▶ Granular necrotic debris
▶ Neutrophils, eosinophils and Charcot-Leyden crystals

There are several case reports of cytological findings in clonorchiasis in material obtained at ERCP, PTC and FNA. Smears may reveal liver fluke ova in a background of granular necrotic debris, neutrophils and eosinophils with Charcot-Leyden crystals. Bile duct epithelium may be present and is often atypical. Ova averaged 24×16 μm, exhibited distinct bilaminar walls, prominent shoulders (operculum) and occasionally spinous processes at the operculum[99,119,120].

Liver transplantation

Needle core biopsy is considered the 'gold standard' in monitoring liver allografts, however, several liver transplant centres in Europe and the USA routinely use FNA for diagnosis and monitoring of acute allograft rejection. The investigation is simple and atraumatic, may be repeated daily and the findings correspond well with those in core biopsies[121–124]. Distinction between acute rejection, hepatitis C virus reactivation and cytomegalovirus infection has been reported[125]. Chronic rejection, in which the primary diagnostic features are primarily vascular and bile duct changes with variable inflammatory cell infiltration, cannot be assessed other than by biopsy or autopsy[126]. A detailed account of the role of cytology in the management of liver transplant patients is given in the chapter on organ transplantation. FNA can be used to investigate mass lesions in liver transplant patients with the differential diagnosis usually between infections and neoplastic processes including posttransplant lymphoproliferative disorders[127]. The latter is discussed in more depth in the section on primary lymphomas.

Table 14.1 Tumours and tumour-like lesions of the liver

Cysts and cystic lesions
  Congenital
  Infective
Tumour-like lesions
  Mesenchymal hamartoma
  Inflammatory pseudotumour
  Focal nodular hyperplasia
  Macro-regenerative nodule
Benign epithelial tumours
  Liver cell adenoma (hepatocellular adenoma)
  Bile duct adenoma
  Bile duct cystadenoma
Benign non-epithelial tumours
  Haemangioma
  Angiomyolipoma
Malignant epithelial tumours
  Hepatocellular (liver cell) carcinoma
    Fibrolamellar variant
    Clear cell variant
    Pleomorphic or giant cell variant
    Spindle cell variant
  Hepatoblastoma
  Bile duct carcinoma (intrahepatic cholangiocarcinoma)
    Variants: Intraduct papillary carcinoma
  Bile duct cystadenocarcinoma
  Mixed hepatocellular and bile duct carcinoma
  Other carcinomas
  Carcinoid tumour
Malignant non-epithelial tumours
  Haemangiosarcoma (angiosarcoma)
  Epithelioid haemangioendothelioma
  Undifferentiated (embryonal) sarcoma
  Other sarcomas of the liver
Other rare tumours
Metastatic tumours

Tumours and tumour-like lesions of the liver

Classification

A classification scheme is shown in Table 14.1. A wide range of neoplasms and tumour-like conditions occur in the liver and the reader is referred to other texts for further details[128–131]. Hepatocellular carcinoma (HCC) is probably the most common malignant tumour in males in the world[132,133]. Its incidence in China, Taiwan, Korea and sub-Saharan Africa is as high as 150 cases per 1 000 000 population. However HCC is relatively rare in the United States, Europe and Australia where metastatic liver disease is by far the commonest form of liver cancer and at the present time its management is one of the most challenging problems in clinical oncology. In the great majority of cases both primary and secondary tumours present as single or multiple focal lesions and the method of choice for their diagnosis is FNA guided by CT or ultrasonography[27,92,134–140].

Cysts and cystic lesions

Cysts develop as focal, usually single, masses. The differential diagnosis of cystic lesions in liver includes congenital cysts, rare causes such as endometriosis[141], cysts caused by parasites such as hydatid disease and amoebic abscess. Bacterial abscesses may present as fluid-containing space-occupying lesions. Haemangiomas and cystic primary and metastatic tumours may present as cysts[142,143]. Percutaneous FNA is used in conjunction with sonography to provide a definitive diagnosis in such lesions[144]. Congenital and infective cysts will be described here. Cystic tumours will be discussed in the section on tumours.

Congenital (developmental) cysts

Congenital cystic lesions of liver comprise a complex group of disorders, the classification and terminology of which is evolving.

Solitary (non-parasitic) cysts

Solitary cysts occur at all ages, although the majority present in the fourth to sixth decades of life. The aetiology and pathogenesis are unknown. The female to male ratio is 4:1. The cyst may be unilocular or multilocular and vary in size from 8–10 cm to a large pedunculated cyst, which may fill the abdominal cavity. Cyst fluid may be clear, milky, mucoid, purulent, bloody or bile stained. The epithelial lining can be cuboidal or columnar, ciliated or squamous in type. Those with ciliated epithelial lining are of foregut origin, i.e. a ciliated hepatic foregut cyst. Rarely, malignant tumours arise in unilocular and multilocular solitary cysts. These are usually adenocarcinomas and rarely squamous cell carcinomas[145]. In multiloculated cysts malignant change may not be detected in smears unless the locule showing malignant change is aspirated.

Cytological findings

► Smears made from aspirated cyst contents are typically sparsely cellular
► A variety of epithelial cell types including cuboidal, columnar, ciliated or squamous
► The ciliated cells have basal nuclei without prominent nucleoli, abundant apical cytoplasm, terminal plates and fine delicate cilia
► Macrophages are often present and mucin may be plentiful[146–148].

Caroli's disease

In Caroli's disease there are multiple congenital dilatations of intrahepatic and extrahepatic bile ducts. The entire liver is generally involved, but the condition may be lobar or segmental. Cystic dilatations are 1.0–4.5 cm in diameter and usually contain bile elements and soft bilirubin calculi (Fig. 14.12). The cuboidal or columnar lining epithelium may be normal or focally hyperplastic. Rarely, foci of adenocarcinoma *in situ* or invasive adenocarcinoma occur.

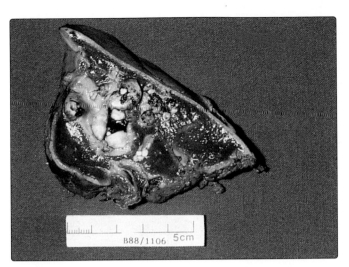

Fig. 14.12 Caroli's disease, segmental involvement. Partial lobectomy specimen showing dilated bile ducts containing biliary mud and soft bilirubin calculi.

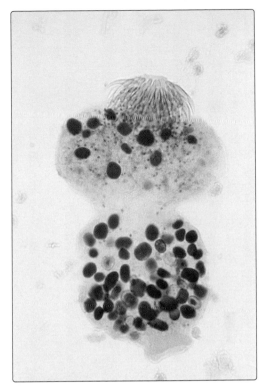

Fig. 14.14 Hydatid disease of liver. Smear from aspiration of cyst shows everted scolex of *E. granulosus* with crown of hooklets resembling miniature head of tapeworm. (Papanicolaou × HP)

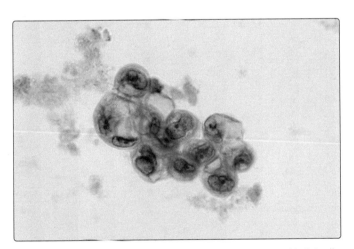

Fig. 14.13 Caroli's disease. Cluster of neoplastic bile duct epithelial cells in smear made from CT guided aspiration of lesion. The background contains bile elements. Neoplastic cells exhibit large, irregular, vesicular nuclei, nucleoli and vacuolated cytoplasm. (Papanicolaou × HP)

In smears made from aspirations of the cystic dilatations, abundant bile pigment is mixed with glandular epithelial cells, which may be normal, hyperplastic, dysplastic or, rarely, malignant (Fig. 14.13)

Adult polycystic disease

Adult polycystic disease is inherited as an autosomal dominant character and the female to male ratio is about 4:1. Average age at presentation is around 50 years. The liver is diffusely cystic, the cysts varying in diameter from 0.1–12 cm. The cyst fluid is clear and colourless, or light yellow. The cysts are lined by columnar, cuboidal or attenuated epithelium. Diagnosis and treatment of a benign, simple symptomatic hepatic cyst by percutaneous aspiration and subsequent instillation of Pantopaque was first described by Goldstein *et al.*[149].

Smears are sparsely cellular and contain a few columnar, cuboidal or attenuated epithelial cells and occasional lymphocytes.

Hydatid cyst

The cyst wall developed by the larval form of *Echinococcus granulosus* consists of an external chitinous laminated membrane surrounded by fibrous tissue and compressed liver. The inner germinal layer of the cyst gives rise to brood capsules, which enlarge to form numerous scolices or heads of future tapeworms. Each scolex contains suckers and rows of hooklets. Brood capsules separate from the cyst wall and settle as hydatid 'sand'. As the cyst enlarges, invaginations of the wall give rise to daughter cysts. The occurrence of anaphylaxis secondary to spillage is seldom reported[82].

The aspirated fluid may be clear or turbid. Smears made from aspirated hydatid cyst fluid may show scolices, hooklets or remnants of laminated membrane with the latter feature most common[150-152]. Scolices exhibiting suckers and rows of hooklets resemble miniature blunt heads of tapeworms (Fig. 14.14). Hooklets, which often float free within the fluid, are refractile and birefringent and stain brilliant purple with a Ziehl-Neelsen stain. Laminated membrane stains pink in Papanicoloau smears (Fig. 14.15), black with Gomori's methenamine silver, pink with Best's carmine and is well demonstrated with a PAS stain[153].

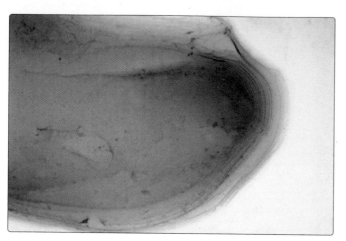

Fig. 14.15 Hydatid disease of liver. Fragment of laminated membrane, the chitinous external layer of the cyst wall. (Papanicolaou × HP)

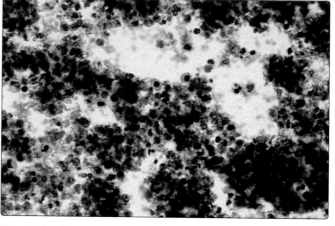

Fig. 14.16 Pyogenic abscess of liver. Smear of aspirated pus shows polymorphonuclear leucocytes and necrotic shrunken single liver cells with eosinophilic cytoplasm and pyknotic nuclei. (Papanicolaou × HP)

Pyogenic abscess

Most abscesses of liver are caused by pyogenic bacteria, which seed liver in sufficient numbers to create a focus of suppuration. Abscesses may be single or multiple, varying in size from very small to up to 20 cm in diameter. Causative organisms are usually *Escherichia coli*, but *Streptococcus milleri*, is now thought to be a major aetiological agent. The lesion is detected by CT scan or ultrasonography and FNA frequently produces pus. A portion of the aspirate should be reserved for microbiological investigations. *Actinomyces israelii*, which is found world-wide, may rarely be a cause of liver abscess. Infection may occur anywhere within the gastrointestinal tract or female genital tract, whence it may be carried by the portal vein to the liver[154,155]. Multiple microabscesses in a honeycomb arrangement are surrounded by a wall of granulation and fibrous tissue accompanied by lipid laden foamy macrophages. Characteristically, colonies of filamentous bacteria matted together with fibrin may be seen macroscopically as 'sulphur granules'.

Smears from a pyogenic abscess show neutrophil leucocytes in varying degrees of preservation, fibrin and perhaps necrotic liver cells and bacteria (Fig. 14.16). Special stains may reveal a causative organism. In actinomycosis foamy macrophages are prominent with aggregates of gram-positive filamentous organisms. *Actinomyces israelii* should be distinguished from *Nocardia asteroides*, which is also a gram-positive actinomycete and rarely may cause abscess. Actinomyces sp. gives a negative reaction to Ziehl-Neelsen stain in contrast to Nocardia sp. which are weakly acid fast.

Amoebic abscess

The parasite *Entamoeba histolytica* reaches the liver from the colon via the portal vein. The right lobe, particularly in the posterior portion of the dome, is most often affected. Amoebae secrete enzymes, which lyse liver tissue and elicit very little inflammatory cell response. The initial lesion is an area of coagulative necrosis, which enlarges and forms a cavity. This cavity contains reddish-brown blood-stained paste or fluid resembling anchovy sauce. Amoebae are rarely seen in the fluid but are present in the necrotic lining, granulation tissue or adjacent liver tissues, which form the wall of the abscess. The therapeutic value of sonographically guided FNA in conjunction with medical treatment of amoebic abscesses has been reported[156,157].

Cytological findings

▶ Thick reddish-brown aspirate
▶ Lysed tissues and blood
▶ Amoebae with eccentric nuclei, marginated chromatin
▶ Ingested red blood cells within amoebae

FNA produces characteristic thick reddish-brown semifluid anchovy sauce-like material which, on smears, is seen to consist of lysed tissues and blood, sometimes with admixed bile. Inflammatory cells, if present, are degenerate. Amoebae in Papanicolaou stained smears are characterized by an eccentric nucleus showing a central clear zone and margination of chromatin. A definite karyosome may be demonstrated by an iron haematoxylin stain. The cytoplasm is vacuolated and contains ingested red blood cells. It is weakly positive with a PAS stain[158]. Identification of amoebae in anchovy paste-like material aspirated from a liver abscess has been reported[159]. Kobayashi *et al.* demonstrated amoebae using an immunoperoxidase technique in a cell block prepared from FNA of a multiloculated liver abscess[160]. In the absence of the parasite the macroscopic appearance of the aspirate and the distinctive lysed nature of cells in smears allow a provisional cytological diagnosis of amoebic abscess and the highly sensitive indirect haemagglutination test can be used for confirmation.

Tumour-like lesions and benign neoplasms
Tumour-like lesions
Inflammatory pseudotumour of liver

The liver is probably the second most common site for the occurrence of inflammatory pseudotumour, which is also found in the lung, stomach and kidney[161]. It is seen in all age groups and is common in children and young adults. The commonest presenting symptoms are a long history of low-grade fever, abdominal pain, vomiting and diarrhoea, and some weight loss. The tumour may cause biliary obstruction with jaundice. Clinically, the liver is enlarged. Lesions may be solitary or multiple, measuring between 2 to 25 cm and have been mistaken for neoplasms on both histology and cytology[162]. It is characterized histologically by a predominant population of non-neoplastic polyclonal plasma cells with variable fibrosis containing plump spindle cells, histiocytes and other inflammatory cells[161,163,164].

Cytological findings

► Many polymorphonuclear leucocytes +/− eosinophils
► Degenerate mononuclear cells, lymphocytes, plasma cells
► Fibrous tissue with plump fibroblasts
► Hepatocytes and bile duct epithelium

The findings on smears are varied and non-specific with a mixture of acute and chronic inflammatory cells, including a prominent population of plasma cells, which are polyclonal in nature. Fragments of fibrous tissue may be cellular with plump spindled fibroblasts[165–168].

Mesenchymal hamartoma

Mesenchymal hamartoma occurs almost exclusively in infancy, particularly in the first 2 years and is twice as common in males. It presents as a painless enlarging mass, which is heterogenous and cystic on imaging. Macroscopically, multiple cystic spaces contain mucoid material and the intervening solid areas are white, yellow or brown. Microscopically, the predominant component is mesenchyme showing cystic degeneration. Scattered throughout are blood vessels, bile ducts and hepatocyte nodules. Extramedullary haemopoiesis may be seen[169].

Cytological findings

► Myxoid stroma with spindle cells either in small groups or singly
► Normal ductal epithelial cells
► Benign hepatocytes
► Background of basophilic mucoid material
► Cytology shows a mixture of bile duct epithelium, hepatocytes arranged in clusters and abundant myxoid stroma containing bland spindle cells lying singly or in ill-defined networks. The background may be mucoid[170–172].

Benign hepatocytic tumours

Focal nodular hyperplasia (FNH), macroregenerative nodule and liver cell adenoma are grouped together as each represents a proliferation of benign hepatocytes and distinction between them on FNA cytology alone is not reliable. Inadvertent sampling of adjacent, non-lesional liver parenchyma can further confuse the issue. Accurate diagnosis requires good correlation between clinical, radiological and pathological findings and even then, a histological sample is usually required. They also are the main differential diagnoses of a well-differentiated HCC[173].

Focal nodular hyperplasia

Focal nodular hyperplasia (FNH) occurs at any age, but most are seen in middle life. Female to male ratio is about 2:1. Most lesions are detected incidentally or go undetected, but a few cases present with pain and an abdominal mass. Size and vascularity of the lesion increase in women taking the contraceptive pill, but there is little evidence to support an aetiological role for contraceptive steroids. FNH is found in otherwise normal livers as a round mass, usually solitary and less than 5 cm in diameter (Fig. 14.17). It is firm and consists most commonly of a central stellate scar with fibrous septa separating nodules of normal appearing hepatocytes. Septa contain proliferating bile ducts, lymphocytes, large veins and unusually thick walled and prominent arteries (Fig. 14.18). Radiological and cytological distinction between FNH, LCA and HCC may be difficult[174].

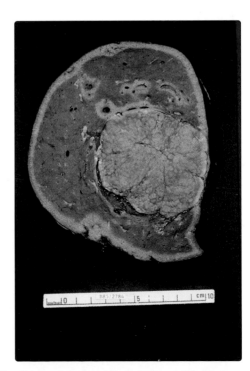

Fig. 14.17 Focal nodular hyperplasia. Solitary solid globular mass which appears nodular due to bands of pale fibrous tissue radiating from the centre of the lesion.

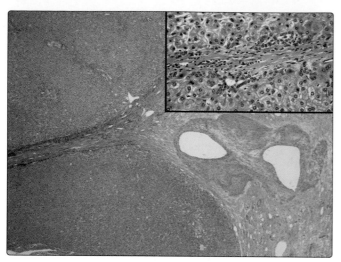

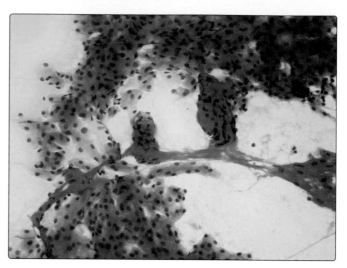

Fig. 14.18 Focal nodular hyperplasia. Section shows an abnormal thick walled arterial vessel and a radiating fibrous tissue septum containing proliferating bile ducts (inset) separating nodules of benign hepatocytes. (H&E × MP)

Fig. 14.19 Focal nodular hyperplasia. Sheets of benign polygonal hepatocytes separated by septa of fibrous tissue. (Papanicolaou × HP)

Cytological findings

► Cellular smears
► Cohesive uniform benign hepatocytes in sheets or clusters
► Trabecular/sinusoidal architecture
► No dispersal or stripped nuclei
► Fragments of fibrous tissue with lymphocytes
► Bile duct epithelium

Smears have a uniform appearance with microfragments and clusters composed of apparently normal liver cells. Sheets of cohesive benign hepatocytes traversed by parallel rows of fibroblasts are diagnostic but not always found (Fig. 14.19). Small fragments of isolated fibrous tissue sometimes infiltrated by lymphocytes or adjacent to bile duct epithelial cells may be seen. The hepatocytes are not associated with inflammatory cells[175]. A reticulin stain shows normal sinusoidal architecture.

Macroregenerative nodule

Macroregenerative nodules are found in the cirrhotic liver and are arbitrarily defined as regenerating nodules >8 mm. Accurate FNA diagnosis is important, as this is a principal differential diagnosis of well-differentiated HCC, which also arises in this setting.

Cytological findings

► Variable cellularity
► Disturbances in the normal regularity of liver cell plates
► Fragments of fibrous tissues
► Proliferating bile duct epithelium
► Polymorphous hepatocyte population
► Hepatocytes occur singly or in loose aggregates and may focally show atypia

► Degenerating liver cells may be swollen or shrunken
► Regenerating hepatocytes are large, with vesicular nuclei, prominent nucleoli and binucleation
► There may be neutrophils, lymphocytes and increased numbers of activated Kupffer cells

The cytological findings are those of cirrhosis with hepatocyte trabeculae 1–2 cells thick, separated by sinusoids. The hepatocytes may show focal atypia. Bile ducts proliferate in newly formed fibrous tissue in response to bile stasis resulting from the architectural disturbance. Inflammation is also present, with leucocyte infiltration and activation and proliferation of Kupffer cells. Hepatocyte dysplasia may complicate the cytological findings and this is discussed later under hepatocellular carcinoma.

Benign epithelial tumours
Liver cell adenoma (hepatocellular adenoma)

Benign epithelial tumours of the liver are all uncommon but, of these, liver cell adenoma (LCA) is the most important[176], particularly since its incidence has been shown to be associated with the use of oral contraceptives[177,178]. The first description by Baum *et al.* in 1973[179] of this association followed closely on the report of liver cell tumours initially thought to be HCCs arising in patients on androgenic anabolic steroids[180]. The tumours induced by either female or male synthetic gonadal steroids are now known to be similar; they are mainly LCAs and HCC is rare. Spontaneous regression may occur after discontinuation of the causative drugs[181,182]. LCA also occurs in association with type I glycogen storage disease, familial diabetes and in otherwise normal livers. Although frequently asymptomatic, symptoms include a tender right upper quadrant mass or abdominal pain, due to haemorrhagic necrosis possibly with rupture and haemoperitoneum. The tumour is usually solitary and subcapsular with a diameter of 8–15 cm. Histologically, LCA consists of thickened sheets

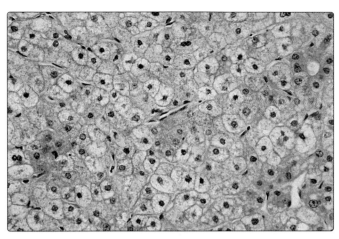

Fig. 14.20   Adenoma of liver. Section showing sheets of pale-staining hepatocytes and thin vascular septa. Nuclei are small and regular. (H&E MP)

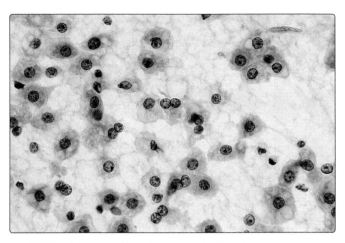

Fig. 14.21   Adenoma of liver. Smear showing loosely cohesive hepatocytes exhibiting regular, small, round nuclei, inconspicuous nucleoli and pale staining cytoplasm. The single elongated bare nucleus is interpreted as endothelial. (Papanicolaou × HP)

of normal appearing or slightly enlarged hepatocytes with no well-defined central veins or portal tracts (Fig. 14.20). Occasional thin fibrous septa are seen; bile ducts are absent and Kupffer cells reduced in number, or absent.

Cytological findings

- ▶ Moderate to high cellularity
- ▶ Single or clustered hepatocytes or tissue fragments
- ▶ Uniformity of polygonal cells with central round nuclei
- ▶ Low nuclear:cytoplasmic ratio
- ▶ Pale or vacuolated cytoplasm
- ▶ Absence of bile duct epithelium

In FNA specimens, normal appearing hepatocytes, possibly somewhat enlarged, are seen occurring singly, in clusters or tissue fragments in a clear or lightly blood-stained background (Fig. 14.21). All cells are similar in size, exhibit similar nuclear features and present a characteristic uniform pattern. Cytoplasm is usually pale staining or vacuolated because of increased amounts of glycogen or lipid. Bile duct epithelial cells are absent. Mitotic figures are rare[183]. Haemorrhage or necrosis may be seen. Differentiation from normal liver in smears depends on the absence of bile duct epithelium and appreciation of the pale-staining cytoplasm and uniformity of hepatocytes. Distinction from well-differentiated HCC can be problematical and this is discussed in the section HCC: diagnostic pitfalls.

Bile duct adenoma

These excessively rare tumours are characteristically solitary, situated just beneath Glisson's capsule and measure up to 2 cm. However, they may be multiple and located within the parenchyma where the proliferating small ducts lined by cuboidal epithelium within fibrous tissue infiltrated by lymphocytes or granulocytes, can be mistaken histologically for metastatic adenocarcinoma[184].

Cystadenoma

The majority of bile duct cystadenomas occur in women as painful epigastric masses with a peak incidence in the fifth decade[185,186]. They are usually seen in the right lobe, are multiloculated and may grow to a large size. Tumours contain mucoid fluid and are lined by cuboidal or columnar mucin-secreting epithelium, generally as a single layer. In women the surrounding mesenchymal stroma may be compact, resembling ovarian stroma. Tumours in both males and females have a tendency to recur if inadequately excised and they have definite malignant potential[187,188]. FNA may be performed as an aid to diagnosis. Raised CEA levels may be found on biochemical testing of the cyst fluid[55,189,190]. The correct treatment is surgical excision.

One case report of percutaneous aspiration of a bile duct cystadenoma detected by ultrasonography yielded clear yellow fluid without cells or crystals191.

Benign non-epithelial tumours

Haemangioma

Benign non-epithelial tumours are rare, except for haemangioma, which is the most common of all benign liver neoplasms[192]. Haemangiomas occur at all ages and in both sexes. They are usually small and of no consequence. It has been suggested that they develop at an earlier age in women and they may enlarge rapidly in pregnancy. When greater than 5 cm, they may cause symptoms. Histologically, haemangiomas are usually cavernous and are composed of dilated endothelial-lined channels supported by fibrous stroma (see Fig. 14.22B). There is increasing confidence in the diagnosis of haemangioma by radiologists using imaging techniques with contrast enhancement and therefore FNA is usually not necessary. However aspiration of haemangiomas are still done inadvertently[193]. At least one fatality from FNA of a hepatic haemangioma has been reported[78]. However, after reviewing the literature,

Langlois[82] concluded that the danger associated with needling haemangiomas is little greater than the overall risk of FNA providing appropriate precautionary measures are taken.

Cytological findings

▶ Blood-stained aspirate with few cells
▶ Bland spindled cells arranged in three-dimensional arcades or in compact dense coils
▶ Smooth muscle fragments

Cell yield tends to be scanty. In many cases, smears contain only blood or a few hepatocytes mixed with blood but even these findings in our experience are helpful when malignant disease is being investigated. Smears may, however, also contain endothelial cells, capillaries in three dimensional arcades and fragments of smooth muscle (Fig. 14.22A). A definitive cytological diagnosis of haemangioma using these features has been made in 27–91% of cases reported in the literature[79,80,194–197].

Angiomyolipoma

Angiomyolipoma (AML) of the liver was first described in 1976[198] and is a benign mesenchymal tumour with three components: blood vessels, adipose tissue and smooth muscle cells (Fig. 14.23). These are present in varying proportions and show a range of morphologies[199,200]. Extramedullary haematopoiesis is also sometimes present. The histogenesis is uncertain but it is thought to arise from a pluripotent mesenchymal cell. HMB 45, a melanoma specific antibody, is consistently positive and this has become a defining feature[201]. Bonetti et al.[202] have suggested AMLs arise from a 'perivascular epithelioid cell' and have designated it a PEComa and linked it with other benign neoplasms found in the tuberose sclerosis complex. The diagnosis of AML is problematic because of its varied appearance and the differential diagnosis includes malignant lesions such as metastatic melanoma, hepatocellular carcinoma and various sarcomas.

Cytological findings

▶ Cellular smears with irregular fragments, dissociation and stripped nuclei
▶ Thick- and thin-walled blood vessels
▶ Spindled and epithelioid smooth muscle cells, intranuclear inclusions, fibrillary cytoplasm
▶ Mature adipocytes
▶ Variable pleomorphism with giant cells
▶ No mitoses or necrosis
▶ Inflammatory cells

The smears are usually cellular with individual cells and irregular fragments. Stroma as well as thick- and thin-walled blood vessels are noted. There are a mixture of epithelioid and spindled cells with round to oval nuclei,

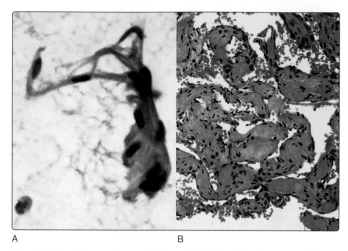

Fig. 14.22 Haemangioma. (A) The cell yield tends to be scanty with scattered endothelial cells either singly or as clusters in a background of blood. (B) Corresponding core biopsy, showing the typical appearance of a cavernous haemangioma. (A, H&E × HP; B, H&E × HP)

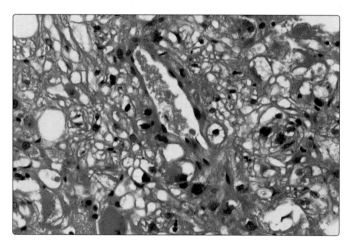

Fig. 14.23 Angiomyolipoma. Three components are present: blood vessels, adipose tissue and smooth muscle cells. (H&E × HP)

occasional nucleoli and intranuclear inclusions. The cytoplasm is fibrillar or granular and may contain vacuoles (Fig. 14.24). Mature adipocytes may feature. Focal pleomorphism may be marked but mitotic activity and necrosis is unusual. Inflammation and sometimes extramedullary haemopoiesis may be present. A PAS stain will highlight glycogen within some of the epithelioid cells. Immunohistochemistry consistently shows positivity for HMB 45 as well as occasional staining for vimentin, desmin and actin (smooth muscle cells), endothelial markers, e.g. factor VIII (blood vessels), and S 100 (adipocytes)[203–206].

Malignant epithelial tumours
Hepatocellular carcinoma

Hepatocellular carcinoma (HCC) is the most common primary liver cell malignancy. Its incidence is relatively low in western countries, however in the regions of the Far

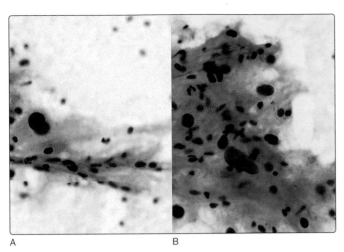

Fig. 14.24 Angiomyolipoma. (A) An irregular tissue fragment containing a branching thin walled blood vessel. (B) There is a mixture of epithelioid and spindled cells. The cytoplasm is granular and contains vacuoles. Focal pleomorphism is marked. (A, H&E × MP; B, H&E × MP)

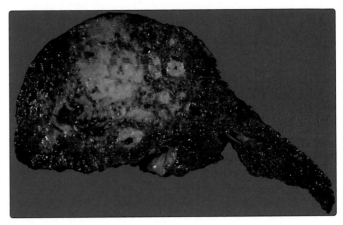

Fig. 14.25 Hepatocellular carcinoma. A poorly-defined large mass with several smaller satellite nodules.

East, Southern Africa, and Southern and Eastern Europe it is a major health problem[132,207].

Aetiology

The striking geographical differences in the incidence of HCC are attributed to various environmental factors, principally hepatitis B virus infection where integration of the viral DNA into the host genome results in a BHsAg carrier state. Other risk factors include carcinogens such as aflatoxins and thorotrast, alcohol, hormones, metabolic disorders such as tyrosinaemia and cirrhosis of any cause. The latter is thought to be the major risk factor in regions of low incidence[132,208,209].

Clinical features

Although HCC has been reported in children as young as two, its incidence increases with age; it commonly affects adults and is 4–8 times more common in males. HCC usually presents late due to large functional reserve of the liver and its location in the abdomen, beneath the rib cage, which allows expansion without detection by palpation. The classic presenting symptoms are abdominal pain, weight loss and hepatomegaly. If underlying chronic liver disease is present there may be ascites, oesophageal varices, encephalopathy and possibly jaundice. Survival is uniformly poor due to the advanced presentation, with 5-year survivals between 0 and 20%. At present only surgery is considered curative although techniques such as chemo-embolization, cryoablation and electrocoagulation can prolong survival with good quality of life.

Raised alpha-fetoprotein levels have been used as a screening and a diagnostic test for HCC. The serum levels are increased above normal in 40–90% of tumours and increased to a significant level in 25–40%. The lower levels are not specific and can be found in benign conditions such as hepatitis and liver failure. A level of greater than

415 kU/l (500 ng/ml) in the presence of a liver mass is diagnostic of HCC[210,211]. Increasing sophistication of imaging equipment and the increased use of abdominal imaging for routine investigation of non-specific abdominal signs and symptoms as well as surveillance of high risk populations has resulted in improved sensitivity with detection of smaller lesions.

Differential diagnosis

In the setting of chronic liver disease, the major differential diagnosis is of a macro-regenerative nodule as part of the cirrhotic process. For patients without chronic liver disease, focal nodular hyperplasia or hepatocellular adenoma should be considered. In either setting, metastatic malignancy, for which the liver is a common site, needs to be considered.

Macroscopic appearance

The most common macroscopic finding is that of a large mass associated with smaller satellite nodules (Fig. 14.25). Tumour tissue is soft, haemorrhagic and occasionally bile stained and has a tendency to undergo necrosis. Alternatively the tumour is multinodular or less commonly diffusely infiltrative. In the past most tumours presented late and anything less than 5 cm was considered small, but with improved and more frequent imaging, lesions as small as 1.5–2.0 cm are regularly being detected[132,212,213].

Microscopic features

Histologically the characteristics of hepatocellular carcinoma relate to its resemblance to normal liver tissue in that most tumours exhibit a trabecular growth pattern formed by plates of liver cells which vary in thickness from a few to many (2–20) cells (Fig. 14.26A). Blood supply to the tumour cells is through branches of the hepatic artery only. Sinusoids are identified, lined by endothelial cells but the presence of Kupffer cells is debated. Pseudo-acinar structures may be seen. Some resemble dilated canaliculi, which may contain bile; others appear as cystic spaces, apparently formed by degeneration and necrosis within

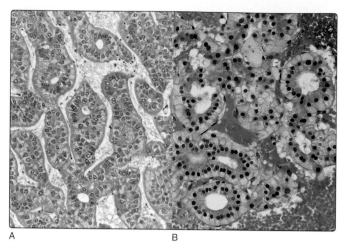

Fig. 14.26 Hepatocellular carcinoma. (A) Most tumours exhibit a trabecular growth pattern and acinar formations may be present. (B) Pseudoglandular formations in a cell block preparation. (A, H&E × MP; B, H&E × MP)

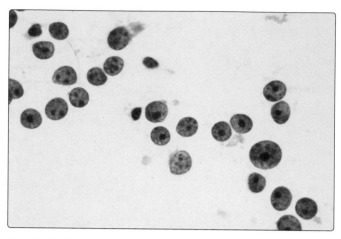

Fig. 14.27 Hepatocellular carcinoma, bare atypical nuclei. As well as dissociated single cells there are bare atypical nuclei. (H&E × HP)

solid trabeculae. As the tumour progresses the trabeculae may be replaced by solid sheets. A reticulin stain may highlight the widened trabeculae and acinar structures but in the solid sheets the amount of reticulin is decreased and fragmented or totally absent. The cells resemble normal hepatocytes to varying extents depending on their degree of differentiation. They are polygonal with vesicular nuclei, central single nucleoli and granular cytoplasm. They may surround canaliculi and bile may be present within cells or in canaliculi. Intranuclear inclusions and fat vacuoles may be seen in HCC tumour cells and are similar to those in normal hepatocytes. Mallory bodies are uncommon but seem to be relatively specific for HCC having been rarely documented in other tumours[214]. HCC arising in the setting of haemochromatosis characteristically does not show iron within tumour cells.

This is the common pattern, readily recognized in well- and moderately-differentiated HCC. It is also present in poorly-differentiated lesions but may be more difficult to discern. All other patterns of HCC are derived from this basic trabecular and sinusoidal architecture and a mixture of patterns is frequently seen. However different growth patterns and cellular variants occur, which are reflected in smears, and some authors have chosen specific terms to describe them[215-218].

Since Edmondson in 1954 published a four-tier grading system, there has been no further attempt to refine the criteria for grading[219]. This probably reflects the heterogenous nature of most HCCs and the lack of prognostic relevance of grading. The degree of differentiation is reflected in cell size, nuclear shape and size, prominence of the nucleolus and in the amount and staining character of cytoplasm. Well-differentiated tumour cells are polygonal, have central round vesicular nuclei, a central nucleolus and granular cytoplasm. Cells of poorly-

differentiated liver cell carcinoma tend to be round and smaller; nuclei are large and irregular, central or eccentric; nucleoli are prominent and cytoplasm is relatively scanty and pale staining. Of greater clinical relevance is the size of the HCC and small tumours (<2 cm) are usually well-differentiated[220,221].

Cytological findings

▶ Highly cellular smears with both large fragments and dispersed cells
▶ Widened trabeculae and/or acinar structures, best appreciated on cell block sections
▶ Capillaries traversing the fragments or endothelial cells rimming the trabeculae and acini
▶ Polygonal cells with central nuclei
▶ Increased nuclear size and atypia which tends to be monotonous
▶ Increased nuclear: cytoplasmic ratio
▶ Macronucleoli and multinucleation
▶ Numerous stripped atypical nuclei
▶ Mitotic activity
▶ Necrosis

Smears are highly cellular with many microfragments of tumour, loose clusters of cells, dissociated single cells and bare atypical nuclei (Fig. 14.27). The microfragments are large, thick and anastomosing or pseudopapillary and ball-like, corresponding to long or short trabeculae respectively (Fig. 14.28). Pseudoglandular formations are sometimes seen (Fig. 14.26B). Microfragments of tumour may be surrounded by a distinctive single layer of sinusoidal endothelial cells (Fig. 14.29) and flat disorderly sheets of tumour cells may be traversed by arborizing sinusoidal capillaries, seen as rows of endothelial cells with attenuated cytoplasm and dark oval nuclei (Fig. 14.30). A good cell block is invaluable in showing these architectural features which can be highlighted by a reticulin stain. Necrosis is

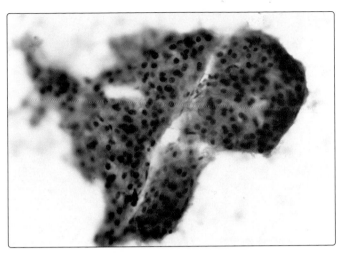

Fig. 14.28 Hepatocellular carcinoma, trabecular pattern. Microfragments have the appearance of thickened trabeculae with a smooth edge. (H&E × HP)

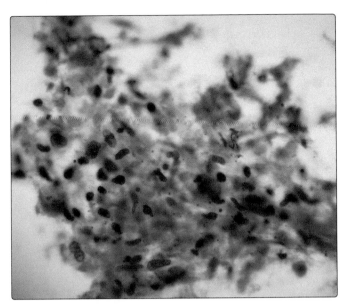

Fig. 14.31 Hepatocellular carcinoma, necrosis. (H&E × HP)

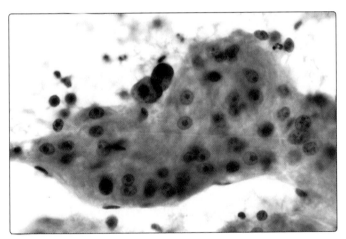

Fig. 14.29 Hepatocellular carcinoma, endothelial rimming. Tissue fragments composed of malignant hepatocytes containing enlarged nuclei and central nucleoli with a rim of elongated sinusoidal endothelial cells. (H&E × HP)

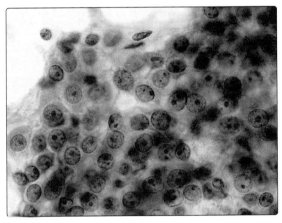

Fig. 14.32 Hepatocellular carcinoma; increased nuclear/cytoplasmic ratio. A crowded sheet of malignant hepatocytes is seen exhibiting round nuclei and prominent central nucleoli. (Papanicolaou × HP)

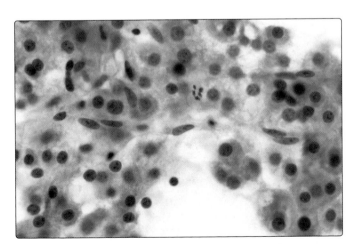

Fig. 14.30 Hepatocellular carcinoma, sinusoidal capillaries. Groups of tumour cells may be traversed by sinusoidal capillaries, seen as rows of elongated nuclei with attenuated cytoplasm. (H&E × MP)

present in a minority of cases (Fig. 14.31). Tumour cells are polygonal, very similar to normal hepatocytes, but the nuclear size and nuclear/cytoplasmic ratio are increased (Fig. 14.32) and the nuclei show increased atypia, macronuclei (Fig. 14.33) and intranuclear inclusions (Fig. 14.34). Intracytoplasmic fat and glycogen may be demonstrated and bile may be seen as coarse granules staining green or yellow in Papanicolaou-stained smears (Fig. 14.35) and greenish-black with MGG. Lipofuscin and iron pigment are usually absent. Intracytoplasmic globules (Fig. 14.36) are sometimes seen. Mallory bodies are irregular and have a somewhat fibrillary appearance (Fig. 14.37)[222-224]. Mitoses and multinucleated cells may be seen. Non-neoplastic hepatocytes and bile duct epithelium are usually not present but may be picked up from the surrounding non-neoplastic liver, particularly in the setting

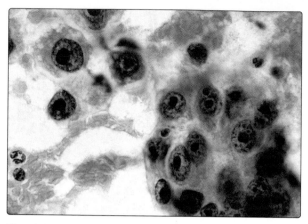

Fig. 14.33 Hepatocellular carcinoma, macronucleoli. The cells have granular cytoplasm, central large nuclei varying in size and very large, single, central nucleoli. (Papanicolaou × HP)

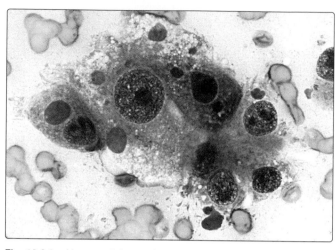

Fig. 14.36 Hepatocellular carcinoma, globular hyaline bodies. Malignant hepatocytes containing smooth, red, large cytoplasmic globules. (MGG × HP)

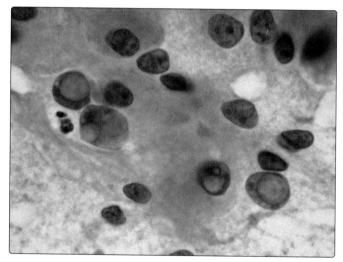

Fig. 14.34 Hepatocellular carcinoma, intra-nuclear inclusions. (H&E × HP)

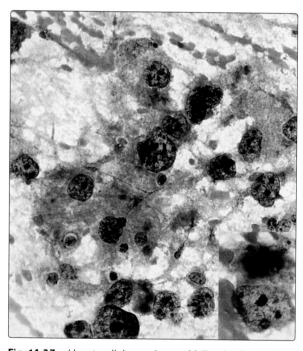

Fig. 14.37 Hepatocellular carcinoma; Mallory bodies. Malignant cells containing irregular, pleomorphic nuclei, large nucleoli and delicate cytoplasm. Several irregular, fibrillary, blue cytoplasmic inclusions are interpreted as Mallory bodies (inset). (Papanicolaou × HP)

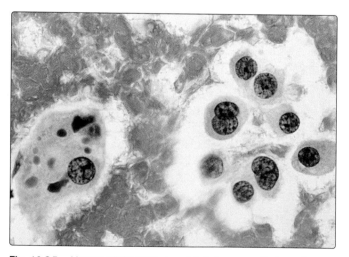

Fig. 14.35 Hepatocellular carcinoma, bile in tumour cells. Irregular globules of yellow-green bile are seen in the cytoplasm of this large malignant hepatocyte. (Papanicolaou × HP)

of cirrhosis. They are usually separate from the tumour cells. As the degree of differentiation decreases the cells become more obviously malignant and their hepatocytic features decrease while the frequency of necrosis, mitotic activity and multinucleation increases.

FNA assessment of portal vein thrombosis in the setting of chronic liver disease, known HCC or metastatic malignancy to the liver has been reported[156,215,225,226]. It has resulted in a primary diagnosis of malignancy or has documented involvement of the vein by a previously diagnosed malignancy. The latter is important in the staging of the tumour and may influence therapy and prognosis. The results showed high sensitivity and a low risk of complications.

Sub-types of hepatocellular carcinoma
Fibrolamellar hepatocellular carcinoma

This rare tumour is a distinct type of HCC. It more often affects adolescents and young adults with a slight female predilection. It is said to have a better (though still grave) prognosis than other forms of HCC, perhaps because, occurring in the absence of cirrhosis, it is usually resectable. There is no association with cirrhosis, HBV or alcoholism and the serum alpha-fetoprotein level is normal or only slightly raised. Its imaging characteristics may be confused with the more common forms of HCC or may be indistinguishable from focal nodular hyperplasia (FNH). Macroscopically, also, fibrolamellar carcinoma (FL-HCC) resembles FNH in that the tumour is well defined, often multinodular and on cut surface shows a central scar with radiating fibrous bands (Fig. 14.38). Light microscopic features of FL-HCC are characteristic. Tumour cells are very large and polygonal with macronucleoli and abundant granular eosinophilic cytoplasm, which is packed with mitochondria on ultrastructural examination. Parallel bands or lamellae of fibrous stroma divide the cells into cords and nodules (Fig. 14.39)[227,228]. In smears, cytological features of FL-HCC are diagnostic allowing its differentiation from other liver cell carcinomas[229,230].

Cytological findings

▶ Variable cellularity with discohesion
▶ Large polygonal tumour cells
▶ Abundant eosinophilic granular cytoplasm with distinct borders
▶ Intracytoplasmic hyaline and pale inclusions
▶ Intranuclear inclusions
▶ Uniform round nuclei with large central single nucleoli
▶ Fragments of fibrous lamellae

Smears vary in cellularity, at times being extremely cellular and the cell population is rather uniform. Cells generally occur singly but are also seen in loose aggregates. They are polygonal and large, three or four times the size of normal hepatocytes and have abundant eosinophilic granular cytoplasm, definite cell borders and resemble oncocytes (Fig. 14.40 inset). Nuclei are uniform, vesicular, large, round or oval with a sharp nuclear membrane and a distinctive large central nucleolus. Two or more nuclei may be seen within one cell. Intracytoplasmic hyaline globules

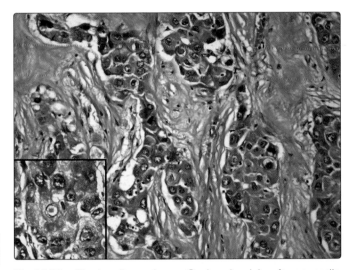

Fig. 14.39 Fibrolamellar carcinoma. Cords and nodules of tumour cells separated by parallel bands or lamellae of fibrous stroma. Tumour cells are very large and polygonal with macronucleoli and abundant granular eosinophilic cytoplasm (inset), which is packed with mitochondria on ultrastructural examination. (H&E × MP)

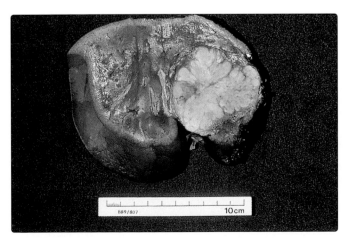

Fig. 14.38 Fibrolamellar carcinoma. Partial hepatectomy specimen of a teenage female. Well-defined tumour with a nodular appearance and fibrous bands on the cut surface.

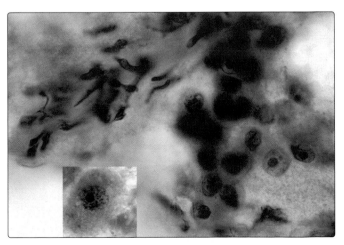

Fig. 14.40 Fibrolamellar carcinoma. Smears show fragments of fibrous tissue and large oncocyte-like hepatocytes. (Papanicolaou × HP)

which may be PAS positive or negative and distinct pale bodies which may be the canalicular inclusions seen on electron microscopy have been described. Bile pigment may be seen; mitoses are few. Parallel rows of elongated fibroblasts may intermingle with tumour cells (Fig. 14.40) or isolated fragments of hyalinized fibrous tissue forming lamellae may be seen. This finding is unusual in conventional HCC[229-231].

Clear cell hepatocellular carcinoma

This is a subtype only on morphological grounds as its biological behaviour is similar to conventional HCC. The change may involve the whole tumour but more commonly small areas of clear cells are seen in tumours that are otherwise composed of hepatocyte-like cells. The cells occur in a trabecular pattern. The clear cytoplasm is due to accumulation of glycogen or fat[232,233]. Mucin stains are usually negative. Nuclei are usually indented and are eccentric. Bile pigment or Mallory's hyaline may be present. The importance of recognizing clear cell HCC lies in distinguishing it from metastatic clear cell malignancies including carcinomas of renal, adrenal, pancreatic and ovarian origin, and sarcomas[234].

Cytological findings

▶ Cellular smears with discohesion
▶ Abundant pale cytoplasm, homogenous, multiple small vacuoles, a single large vacuole
▶ Well-defined cell borders
▶ Eccentric nuclei, hyperchromatic, irregular, prominent nucleoli

Clear cell HCC is usually moderately differentiated. The smears are hypercellular with loose groups showing a honeycomb pattern, as well as single cells. The cells show anisonucleosis, nuclear hyperchromasia and irregularity and prominent central nucleoli. They have abundant pale cytoplasm, which is finely vacuolated or clear with a large vacuole, which may displace the nucleus[235]. Hyaline bodies may be present and the cell borders are well-defined[236,237]. (Fig. 14.41) The cytoplasm is PAS positive and immunohistochemical stains for pCEA, AFP and alpha-1-antitrypsin may be positive as in conventional HCC.

Clear cell HCC may be confused with metastatic renal cell carcinoma. Both tumours may have a vascular stroma and, rarely, fragments of renal cell carcinoma (RCC) surrounded by vascular fibrous stroma mimic the trabeculae and sinusoids of HCC. Weir and Pitman found that although RCC commonly contained transgressing blood vessels, they lacked peripherally wrapping endothelium[238]. Electron microscopy will reveal basement membrane surrounding tumour cells in RCC and sinusoidal endothelium in HCC.

Spindle cell (sarcomatoid) hepatocellular carcinoma

A spindle cell or sarcomatoid variant of HCC has been described[217,239,240]. Pleomorphic spindle cells may be associated with bizarre giant cells. In one such case the original diagnosis was of a sarcoma. The differential diagnosis includes spindle cell sarcomas, sarcomatoid renal cell carcinoma, spindle cell squamous cell carcinoma or melanoma.

Cytological findings

▶ Pleomorphic spindle cells
▶ An epithelioid component with hepatocytic features may be present
▶ Increased stroma
▶ Giant cells may be seen

One of the authors has had experience with one spindle cell HCC (Fig. 14.42) which defied diagnosis until electron microscopy disclosed the hepatocytic nature of the cells.

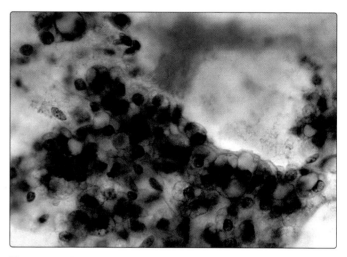

Fig. 14.41 Hepatocellular carcinoma, clear cell variant. A tumour fragment composed of neoplastic cells with eccentric indented nuclei, nucleoli and cytoplasm containing one or more large vacuoles. (Papanicolaou × HP)

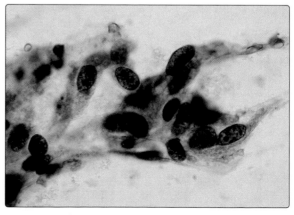

Fig. 14.42 Hepatocellular carcinoma, spindle cell variant. Spindle cells containing pleomorphic nuclei. The hepatocytic nature of the cell is not apparent. (Papanicolaou × HP)

A subsequent immunoperoxidase stain for alpha-fetoprotein was unequivocally positive.

Pleomorphic (giant cell) hepatocellular carcinoma

This variant represents the more poorly-differentiated end of the HCC spectrum. Pleomorphic cells are very large (4–5 times normal) but vary in size and shape as do their nuclei, which may be anywhere in the cytoplasm with prominent nucleoli. Bizarre multinucleated cells are seen. Glycogen and bile may be identified. These cells are often mixed with better-differentiated cells with recognizable hepatocytic differentiation[239], and occasionally are associated with a sarcomatoid element[217]. The architecture may be solid without trabeculae in which case the tumour may be difficult to differentiate from adrenal cortical carcinoma or amelanotic melanoma[224,239,241].

Cytological findings

- ▶ Cellular smears with loose groups and single cells
- ▶ Large pleomorphic cells with macronucleoli, some hepatocytic in appearance
- ▶ Multinucleated tumour giant cells

Smears are cellular, containing loose groupings and single cells, which vary greatly in size and shape, some being of giant size (Fig. 14.43). Cytoplasm is abundant, well-defined and dark staining. Nuclei also vary in size and shape and may be located anywhere within the cytoplasm. Multinucleated tumour cells are common and may be osteoclastic in type[242,243]. Nucleoli are usually prominent. A sinusoidal or trabecular pattern does not occur but the cells sometimes contain bile or intracytoplasmic hyaline globules, which are diagnostic[241].

Diagnostic pitfalls in the diagnosis of HCC in FNA cytology

Difficulty in the cytodiagnosis of HCC arises at both ends of the malignant spectrum, i.e. in distinguishing well-differentiated HCC from benign lesions, and separating poorly-differentiated HCC from metastatic malignancies or other unusual tumours[24,244]. In addition the entity of hepatocellular dysplasia, although largely accepted in the histological literature as a precursor to HCC, is a difficult diagnosis to make cytologically and its distinction from HCC is problematical.

Well-differentiated HCC

Well-differentiated HCC can be very difficult to recognize as malignant and to differentiate from benign hepatocellular lesions. The differential diagnosis includes focal nodular hyperplasia and liver cell adenoma in non-cirrhotic livers and a macroregenerative nodule +/− dysplasia in a background of cirrhosis. The subtle cytological changes may be insufficient to reach a diagnosis of malignancy and

architectural abnormalities are of greater importance (Fig. 14.44).

Cytological features

- ▶ Increased cellularity with single cells and bare atypical nuclei
- ▶ Blood vessels traversing cell groups and endothelial lining of cell groups
- ▶ Increased nuclear/cytoplasmic ratio, though the cells are small
- ▶ Monotonous appearance of atypical cells
- ▶ Macronucleoli and multinucleation
- ▶ Tumour giant cells and mitoses

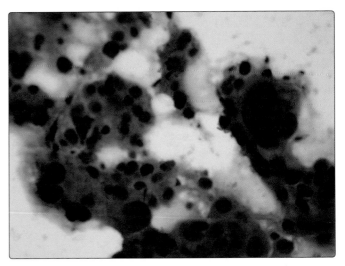

Fig. 14.43 Hepatocellular carcinoma, pleomorphic variant. Very large single sometimes multinucleated malignant cells varying in size and containing central or eccentric nuclei and large nucleoli are mixed with smaller malignant cells showing more obvious hepatocytic differentiation. (H&E × MP)

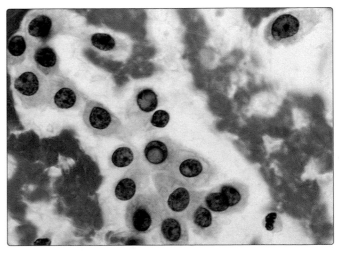

Fig. 14.44 Well-differentiated HCC. Loosely cohesive hepatocytes containing round to oval, regular nuclei, small prominent nucleoli and variable amounts of cytoplasm. Intranuclear inclusions are seen in two malignant hepatocytes. (Papanicolaou × HP)

Various criteria have been reported as useful in separating well-differentiated HCC from benign hepatocellular lesions on smears and cell block material[24,28,42,56,90,91,140,216,217,244 252]. Highly cellular smears with cell dispersal are typical features of malignancy. Many authors emphasize architectural arrangements such as acini, widened trabeculae, or sinusoidal blood vessels, which intersect or outline groups of tumour cells. The groups show irregular arrangement of cells with loss of polarity. Cytological features include increased nuclear/cytoplasmic ratio, monotony of nuclear atypia, small cell size, macronucleoli, stripped atypical nuclei, tumour giant cells, multinucleation, and mitoses.

Several ancillary techniques have been found useful in separating benign from malignant hepatocellular lesions. A reticulin stain is commonly used on histopathology sections to identify the loss of normal architecture. Ferrell *et al.*, in proposing standardized criteria for the histologic diagnosis of benign, borderline and malignant hepatocytic lesions, placed emphasis on the absence of an intact reticulin pattern as an important criterion for malignancy[253]. Several recent publications have applied this principal to smear[44] and cell block preparations[42,100]. The reticulin stain highlights loss of a normal sinusoidal architecture and shows widened trabeculae, rounded islands, pseudoglands or just a reduction or total absence of reticulin (Fig. 14.45). One confounding factor is steatosis, where lipid droplets widen the trabeculae and separate the reticulin framework. This appears as a reduction in the amount of reticulin in areas of severe fatty change. Another area of diagnostic difficulty is very small or early HCC where the reticulin pattern may not be of value, even in resected specimens. Several histologic studies have found that a proportion of small (<2 cm) well-differentiated HCCs are normotrabecular and show an intact reticulin pattern[221,254]. The recent International Working Party on the terminology

of nodular hepatocellular lesions states in respect to small (well-differentiated) HCCs 'Reticulin is occasionally less than normal in amount but this is usually a feature of moderately differentiated HCC'[220,255].

Immunohistochemical staining for CD34 antigen highlights the 'capillarisation' of the hepatic sinusoids in HCCs by staining the endothelial cells (Fig. 14.46). Sinusoidal endothelial cells are negative in normal liver and only focally positive in benign hepatocellular lesions[69,256–261]. Several recent reports comment on its usefulness in FNA samples although there is some overlap between smaller, well-differentiated HCCs and benign lesions[262–265]. Staining for CD34 is also generally negative in metastatic adenocarcinoma[264].

Several markers including immunoreactivity for mutant p53 protein[46,266], PCNA[267] and staining for nucleolar organizer regions[50], have been reported to show some success separating benign from malignant hepatocellular lesions.

Ploidy performed on FNA material either by flow cytometry or cytomorphometry has shown that most HCCs are aneuploid with the remainder euploid (either diploid or polyploid) whereas all benign samples are euploid[48,49,52,268]. Nuclear features such as nuclear size, nuclear/cytoplasmic ratio, large nucleoli and nuclear cleavage also allow fairly accurate division into benign and malignant groups[47,49,269]. It remains to be seen if any of these techniques will become clinically relevant.

There has been increasing interest in measuring telomerase activity as a means of distinguishing between benign and malignant lesions involving sites throughout the body[270]. Telomeres are a sequence of DNA at the end of chromosomes, which protect against degradation or fusion with other chromosomes. The progressive loss of telomeres is thought to play a crucial role in cell ageing and death. Telomerase is the enzyme that rebuilds telomeres and is

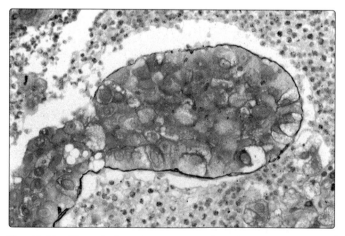

Fig. 14.45   The reticulin stain demonstrates loss of normal sinusoidal architecture and highlights widened trabeculae, rounded islands and pseudoglands and may even show a reduction or total absence of reticulin. (Gordon and Sweet's reticulin × HP)

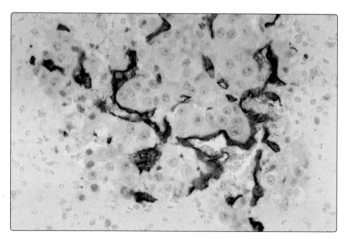

Fig. 14.46   Immunohistochemical staining for CD34 antigen stains the sinusoidal endothelial cells hepatocellular carcinomas. (Immunoperoxidase stain: CD34 antibody × HP)

necessary for normal replication of chromosomes. It is usually suppressed in normal cells; however, it is 'reactivated' in malignant cells leading to repair of any telomere loss, allowing unlimited division without programmed cell death. The degree of telomerase activity can be measured and used to differentiate between benign and malignant hepatocellular processes[69,271,272].

Liver cell dysplasia in cirrhosis

Striking morphological changes in hepatocytes in cirrhotic livers had been noted for many years by workers such as Edmondson and Steiner[219], also Scheuer[131] who made his observations on macronodular posthepatic cirrhosis, before the term 'liver cell dysplasia' was coined. This was defined in 1973 by Anthony et al.[273] as cellular enlargement, nuclear pleomorphism and multinucleation of liver cells. In their original study of 552 African patients Anthony et al. found there was a strong relationship between liver cell dysplasia, male sex, macronodular cirrhosis and the presence of HBsAg, and concluded that liver cell dysplasia was a premalignant change. The findings are supported by some workers[274–276], while others have disputed the premalignant nature of dysplasia[277–280]. The matter remains a subject of controversy.

Recent authors have divided dysplasia into large cell and small cell types. The former is represented by enlarged hepatocytes with irregular nuclei, prominent nucleoli and a normal nuclear to cytoplasmic ratio. The latter is defined by small cells in a zone of 'crowding' where the nuclei are close together. The cells are not atypical and also have a normal nuclear/cytoplasmic ratio[281–283].

Cytological findings

► Variable cellularity and discohesion
► Mixture of irregular sheets of hepatocytes, fibrous tissue and increased bile duct epithelium
► Normal hepatocytes mixed with atypical (dysplastic) hepatocytes
► Dysplastic hepatocytes which are enlarged and polygonal with enlarged atypical nuclei but a normal nuclear/cytoplasmic ratio, prominent nuclear membranes, abnormally clumped chromatin, enlarged multiple nucleoli and intranuclear inclusions
► Occasional multinucleated forms
► Degenerate and regenerating liver cells
► Inflammation

The importance of liver cell dysplasia in cytology lies in its distinction from HCC. Many of the criteria for dysplasia are also criteria for malignancy and dysplastic hepatocytes may be indistinguishable from malignant cells. In cytological material the atypia of HCC is present throughout and that of dysplasia is polymorphous, with a mixture of atypical cells and normal hepatocytes (Fig. 14.47). The dysplastic hepatocytes show a normal nuclear/cytoplasmic ratio. FNA

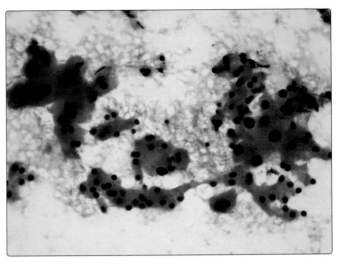

Fig. 14.47   Dysplasia. The smear contains groups of hepatocytes showing a spectrum of atypia with some enlarged irregular nuclei. Note that the nuclear:cytoplasmic ratio is not significantly increased. (H&E × MP)

smears from dysplastic nodules often show increased bile duct epithelium and inflammatory cells as part of the background cirrhosis[24,98–100,105,244,284].

Poorly-differentiated HCC

Difficulty in cytological diagnosis arises in separating poorly-differentiated HCC from cholangiocarcinoma, metastatic malignancies or other unusual primary tumours because of the loss of architectural and cytological features of hepatocellular differentiation[24,244]. The range of metastatic tumours includes various adenocarcinomas from the gastrointestinal tract (particularly colo-rectal), pancreas, breast, lung, small cell neuroendocrine carcinoma of the lung, melanoma, and neuroendocrine tumours of the gastrointestinal tract and pancreas. Less commonly the differential includes lymphoma, and thyroid and prostate carcinoma. If the tumour has a spindled morphology the differential includes sarcomatous change in cholangiocarcinoma, primary and metastatic soft tissue tumours, metastatic melanoma, metastatic sarcomatoid RCC and metastatic spindle cell squamous carcinoma.

The most common problem is differentiating between poorly-differentiated HCC and metastatic adenocarcinoma. Most poorly-differentiated HCCs show a range of atypia and the diagnosis can often be reached when the better-differentiated cells are recognized as hepatocytic.

Cytological findings

► The presence of trabeculae versus true acinar/glandular structures[216,249,285,286]
► Sinusoidal capillaries separating the malignant cells or endothelial cells arranged around cell clusters[24,252,287,288]

► Cell dissociation[244] and atypical stripped nuclei[24,249,285,286]
► Polygonal cells with central nuclei rather than columnar or cuboidal cells[24,216,249,252,286]
► Nuclei with one or more large nucleoli[244,285,286] or intranuclear cytoplasmic inclusions[249,252,285,286]
► Eosinophilic granular cytoplasm versus cytoplasmic vacuolation[216,249,286]
► Positive staining for glycogen particularly if metastatic renal cell carcinoma and adreno-cortical carcinoma can be excluded[224,289]
► The presence of bile[24,249,252,290], lipid[249], cytoplasmic hyaline globules or Mallory bodies

Immunohistochemical stains

Alpha-fetoprotein is a marker of hepatocellular differentiation (Fig. 14.48A). Its reported sensitivity ranges from 44% to 61%[53,54,56,58,60] but it has good specificity despite also staining some germ cell tumours and very occasional gastrointestinal tract adenocarcinomas including pancreatic adenocarcinoma.

Other hepatocyte products including C-reactive protein and alpha-1-antitrypsin also show low sensitivity and variable specificity[53,54]. *In-situ* hybridization for albumin mRNA has been shown to be useful even in high-grade, pleomorphic tumours[56,61–63].

Staining for specific cytokeratins (CK) shows that HCCs are positive for CK8 and CK18 but negative for CK7, CK19 and CK20 as well as CK1, CK5, CK10, CK11[53]. Using a panel of CK7, CK19 and CK20; HCC is negative for all three, cholangiocarcinoma is positive for CK7 and CK19 in most cases but for CK20 in only approximately 50% cases and metastatic colonic adenocarcinoma is CK7 and CK19 negative and CK20 positive. Of commonly available antibodies to cytokeratins, CAM 5.2 is non-discriminatory, as it is positive in both HCC and adenocarcinoma. AE1&3

has been reported to be negative in HCC but positive in adenocarcinomas although Guindi reports HCCs to be AE3 positive and AE1 negative[60], and Johnson (1992) reports 15% of HCCs positive for AE1[54].

Polyclonal CEA is positive in HCC highlighting a bile canalicular pattern due to cross-reactivity with biliary glycoprotein I (Fig. 14.48B). Reported sensitivity ranges from 47% to 90%[54,56,64–67], with a reported PPV of 100% and NPV 87%[65]. Metastatic adenocarcinomas may show diffuse cytoplasmic positivity for polyclonal CEA as well as monoclonal CEA, which is negative in HCC. Although this phenomenon decreases with increasing anaplasia it is useful in the HCC variants.

Staining for naphthylamidase on air-dried smears can also highlight the biliary canaliculi[66,291,292]. OCH1E5 (hepatocyte paraffin 1 (Hep Par 1)) is a recently described hepatocyte specific antibody used on histological material, which may have application in FNA samples[68]. Hepatitis B surface antigen is also a specific marker but only present in the tumours associated with Hepatitis B virus infection[58]. MOC-31 is an antibody originally raised against small cell undifferentiated carcinoma of the lung. It is a membrane glycoprotein of unknown function and has been shown to differentiate between adenocarcinoma metastatic to the liver (diffuse cytoplasmic positivity) and HCC (negative or weak focal positive) in histological and cytological preparations[69–71].

Vimentin staining of Kupffer cells has been used as evidence of the hepatocellular nature of a tumour[72] although this has not been substantiated by others[293].

The contribution of electron microscopy

Electron microscopy can furnish the definitive diagnosis in hepatocellular tumours, which do not show typical liver-like cells or sinusoidal stroma, as many distinctive hepatocytic ultrastructural features are still expressed (although to variable degree). In HCC gross nucleolar expansion and elaboration, reflecting neoplastic functional activation, are a frequent but not invariable finding. Assessment of mitochondrial character, glycogen status, intercellular junctions and levels of lysosomal and endoplasmic reticulum expression together serve as indicators of hepatocytic derivation (Fig. 14.49). On the other hand, diagnosis of metastatic tumours is aided by recognition of subcellular details that are characteristic of particular extrahepatic tissues of origin but which are not expressed in hepatocytes. These include specific secretory granules (e.g. zymogen or neuroendocrine), mucins, rows of classical microvilli, tonofibrils or basal lamina formations. FLHCC is distinguished readily at the ultrastructural level as the cytoplasm exhibits typical oncocytic changes, i.e. it is occupied by abundant swollen and misshapen mitochondria with abnormally stacked cristae. There are also canalicular inclusions containing hyaline accretions.

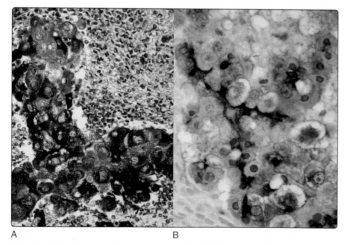

A   B

Fig. 14.48 Immunohistochemical stains. (A) Tumour cells show cytoplasmic positivity for alpha-fetoprotein. (Immunoperoxidase stain: alpha-fetoprotein antibody × HP). (B) Polyclonal CEA antibody highlights a bile canalicular pattern. (Immunoperoxidase stain: polyclonal CEA antibody × HP)

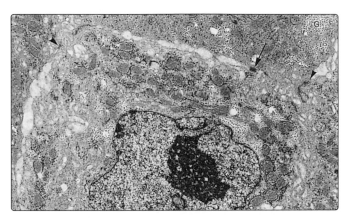

Fig. 14.49 Tumour cell ultrastructure in a poorly-differentiated HCC. Notable features include nuclear irregularity and a large dense nucleolus, dark rounded mitochondria with associated endoplasmic reticulum profiles and particulate cytoplasmic glycogen (G). There are also occasional intercellular (arrow) and pericanalicular (arrow head) junctions. (Electron micrograph × 5600)

Hepatoblastoma

Hepatoblastoma, although a rare tumour, is the most common primary liver malignancy in children. It occurs most often before the age of 3 years although isolated cases have been reported[294] in older children and adults. Absolute incidence is the same all over the world and there is up to a 50% association with various congenital anomalies. It is not associated with cirrhosis or hepatitis B virus infection. The alpha-fetoprotein level is usually very high. Microscopically, most tumours are composed exclusively of immature hepatocytes and are referred to as pure or epithelial. The degree of differentiation in epithelial hepatoblastomas varies from cells resembling fetal hepatocytes (smaller than mature hepatocytes, with slightly larger nuclei and therefore a higher nuclear/cytoplasmic ratio) arranged in laminae two cells thick to smaller more immature embryonal cells (more primitive cells with an even higher nuclear/cytoplasmic ratio) growing in a predominantly solid pattern, but also exhibiting rosettes and papillary formations. Transitions between these patterns are common. About one quarter of hepatoblastomas contain, in addition to epithelial cells, a component of malignant undifferentiated stroma, bone or cartilage and are referred to as hepatoblastoma of mixed type. Foci of extramedullary haemopoiesis are often seen and are invariably associated with the fetal pattern. Some tumours are made up largely of anaplastic cells. The differential diagnosis includes the 'small blue cell' malignancies of childhood, i.e. neuroblastoma, lymphoma, Ewing's sarcoma and rhabdomyosarcoma.

Cytological findings

▶ Clusters, ribbons and rosettes of small tumour cells
▶ Fetal epithelial cells, slightly smaller than hepatocytes with granular or clear cytoplasm and little pleomorphism, may contain fat, bile or glycogen
▶ Embryonal cells, small, oval to spindled, nuclei round to oval with prominent nucleoli, high N:C ratio, mitotic activity
▶ Malignant mesenchymal tissue; may resemble osteoid
▶ Extramedullary haemopoiesis.

In addition to isolated case reports there have been several small series reporting the FNA findings of hepatoblastoma[239,295-300]. Distinctive findings included highly cellular smears with small to intermediate size malignant cells in small clusters, rosettes or trabeculae. The nuclei are round to oval and hyperchromatic with occasional nucleoli. The cytoplasm is usually scanty, although in better-differentiated tumours it may approach that of a hepatocyte, sometimes containing bile[301]. In one case, a few intracytoplasmic eosinophilic round bodies which stained positively for alpha-fetoprotein were seen[239,295]. Malignant mesenchymal tissues may be present and in one report irregular fragments of osteoid-like tissue were apparent in smears and cell blocks[295]. Extramedullary haemopoiesis is common.

Bile duct carcinoma (cholangiocarcinoma)

Intrahepatic cholangiocarcinoma (CC) is a solid malignant tumour of intrahepatic bile duct origin (Fig. 14.50). It is much less common than HCC and is seen in an older age group, without sex predilection and without association with cirrhosis or HBV infection. It is more common in parts of South East Asia, where liver fluke infestation is responsible for an absolute as well as a relative increase in incidence. Other aetiological factors include exposure to thorotrast, ulcerative colitis, primary sclerosing cholangitis, anabolic steroids and intrahepatic lithiasis and the tumour may arise in congenitally dilated intrahepatic ducts of Caroli's disease, in simple and in multiple liver cysts[302-305]. Tumours that occur at the hilum of the liver near the bifurcation of the main hepatic ducts are referred to as

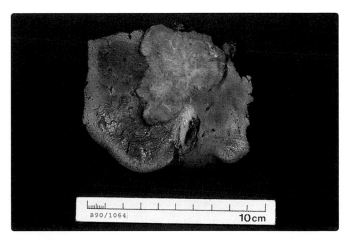

Fig. 14.50 Cholangiocarcinoma. Partial hepatectomy specimen shows a large, solid, pale, irregular tumour within the liver. There is no evidence of haemorrhage or necrosis.

Klatskin's tumour. They may be quite small and difficult to diagnose[306]. CCs are usually tough scirrhous growths, because of an abundant fibrous stroma from which aspiration of malignant epithelial cells may be difficult. Histologically, glandular differentiation is usually obvious and mucin is demonstrable in most tumours. Cytological diagnosis depends not only on cellular evaluation of the aspirate, but also on clinical and radiological findings, which should exclude adenocarcinoma arising from an extrahepatic site.

Variation in growth pattern of CC also occurs. The adenosquamous variant contains glandular and squamous elements but not in an intimate admixture, while the mucoepidermoid variant contains nests of intimately mixed glandular and squamous cells[307,308]. Squamous elements of these tumours show tonofilament bundles and classical intercellular desmosomes under the electron microscope. Rare papillary, mucinous and signet ring tumours occur. Sarcomatous change has been reported[309]. Intraduct papillary carcinoma (intraduct papillomatosis) is a rare tumour, which forms multiple cauliflower-like papillomata within intrahepatic and extrahepatic bile ducts and gall bladder. Histology reveals cuboidal or columnar cells on thin fibrous stalks without nuclear atypia or mitoses. Metastasis to periportal lymph nodes has been reported. The cells are positive for both high and low molecular weight keratin and specifically for CK7 and CK19. Monoclonal and polyclonal CEA both show diffuse cytoplasmic positivity with accentuation of the luminal brush border. EMA is also positive. Distinction from metastatic adenocarcinoma can be impossible.

Cytological findings

- ▶ Smears variably cellular
- ▶ Sheets or tubular arrangements of tumour cells
- ▶ Columnar cells with eccentric large regular nuclei and prominent nucleoli
- ▶ Delicate cytoplasm with fine vacuolization
- ▶ Mucin secretion not always obvious but mucin stains usually positive

In most cases, smears contain variable, but always considerable, numbers of neoplastic bile duct cells, exhibiting relatively large rather regular round nuclei and delicate cytoplasm. Variation in nuclear size occurs but is usually not marked; chromatin is fine and nucleoli inconspicuous. Tumour cells are usually loosely cohesive, form tube-like structures, or occur in crowded sheets. Occasionally they form ductular structures closely associated with fragments of fibrous tissue (Fig. 14.51). When cholangiocarcinoma tumour cells show overtly malignant nuclear features they may not be readily distinguished from metastatic adenocarcinoma, particularly from pancreas, but electron microscopy may help in this regard (Fig. 14.52). When papillary formations are

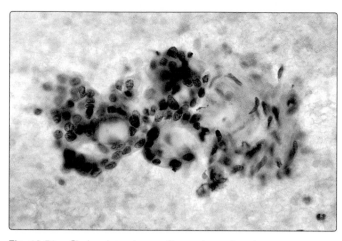

Fig. 14.51   Cholangiocarcinoma. Smear shows ductular structures formed by cuboidal cells with rather bland nuclei attached to fragment of fibrous tissue. (Papanicolaou × HP)

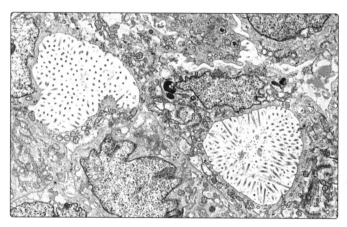

Fig. 14.52   Ultrastructural detail reveals acinar structures with intraluminal villiform projections and secretions, small indented nuclei, small vesicular mitochondria and poorly formed desmosomal junctions between cells. The features are non-hepatocytic and indicative of adenocarcinoma in keeping with cholangiocarcinoma. (Electron micrograph × 3700)

identified the possibility of an intraductal or intracystic adenocarcinoma, which may, or may not, be invasive should be considered. This can occur in the background of Caroli's disease, as illustrated in Figures 14.12 and 14.13 and as previously reported[310]. One of the authors recently had a case of non-invasive papillary intraductal/intracystic cholangiocarcinoma without good evidence of a pre-existing congenital duct abnormality (Fig. 14.53 & Fig. 14.54). A recent report outlined the FNA findings in three cases of intrahepatic biliary papillomatosis[311].

Bile duct cystadenocarcinoma

Bile duct cystadenocarcinoma is the malignant counterpart of bile duct cystadenoma and there is evidence to suggest that the carcinoma may arise in a pre-existing benign tumour[312]. It is a very uncommon tumour and distinction from adenocarcinoma, squamous carcinoma and adenosquamous carcinoma arising in various non-neoplastic cysts and cystic malformations of liver is

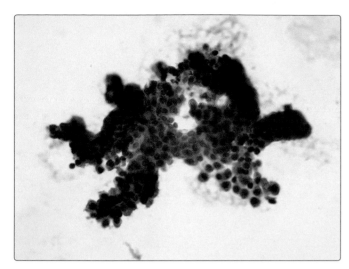

Fig. 14.53 Papillary intraductal/intracystic cholangiocarcinoma. A cohesive three dimensional aggregate, showing a papillary architecture. (H&E × HP)

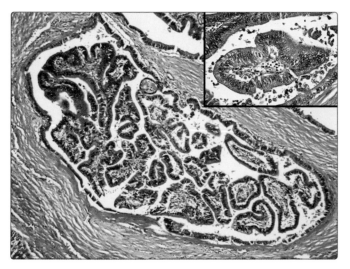

Fig. 14.54 Papillary intraductal/intracystic cholangiocarcinoma. Papillary formations confined within a dilated duct. Fibro-vascular cores are lined by columnar epithelium (inset). Cell block preparations show similar features. (H&E × MP)

difficult[313]. Cytological examination of aspirated fluid from cystic lesions should always be performed for detection of malignant cells, particularly if the fluid is blood-stained. Reported findings include clusters of malignant glandular cells, some with a papillary growth pattern, in a background of mucin and cellular debris. In sections from biopsies or autopsies, invasion of the capsule is seen and tumour may invade adjacent viscera or metastasize[187]. False negative cytology results have been reported[314-316]. In addition to cytological examination of the cyst fluid, FNA should be performed on any solid, nodular or polypoid region seen on ultrasound. Early resection may be curative.

Mixed hepatocellular carcinoma and cholangiocarcinoma

Collision tumours of these two types of primary carcinoma of liver occur, but rarely. During embryological development the same immature cell gives rise to bile duct epithelium and mature hepatocytes[317,318], so the concept of biphasic differentiation within an epithelial tumour is acceptable. Goodman *et al.* reviewed 24 cases of combined HCC–CC[319]. There were 12 cases (which they called transitional tumours) in which there were areas of intermediate differentiation and an identifiable transition between HCC and CC. Another four cases were collision tumours and eight were FL–HCCs, which contained mucin-producing pseudoglands. There have been several reports of FNA findings in 9 cases of combined hepatocellular carcinoma and cholangiocarcinoma. All mention the presence of hepatocytic and glandular elements, the latter comprising cohesive columnar cells with ovoid, basal nuclei arranged in palisades, acini or papillary structures. Intracytoplasmic, intraluminal or brush border mucin positivity was noted. One report commented on a transitional or intermediate cell with features of both cell types. Immunohistochemistry showed variable staining patterns for cytokeratins, CEA and alpha-fetoprotein between the two cell types[320-322].

Squamous carcinoma

Pure squamous cell carcinoma has been reported arising from a congenital cyst, in association with intrahepatic lithiasis and as a component of teratoma[323-325].

Neuroendocrine tumours

A few cases of primary carcinoid tumour have been reported[326-328]. They probably arise from bile ducts. Their slow growth and resectability offer potential for cure. Metastases from a primary tumour elsewhere are more common and only when this possibility has been thoroughly excluded can a diagnosis of primary carcinoid of liver be justified. The differential diagnosis includes metastatic neuroendocrine tumour, i.e. carcinoid or islet cell, metastatic small cell undifferentiated carcinoma[329], Merkel cell carcinoma, small cell adenocarcinoma (breast/prostate/stomach), cholangiocarcinoma, HCC[330,331], sarcoma and lymphoma[332,333]. Some mixed tumours comprise carcinoid features accompanied by hepatocellular or cholangiocellular elements[330,334,335].

Cytological findings

- ▶ Medium size, round, polygonal or spindle tumour cells with round nuclei
- ▶ Loosely cohesive cells
- ▶ Finely punctate chromatin, small nucleoli
- ▶ Organoid pattern (vascular) and rosettes
- ▶ Red cytoplasmic granules with MGG

In smears, regular, medium sized cells, exhibiting round regular nuclei with finely punctate chromatin, inconspicuous nucleoli and organoid pattern, are characteristic of carcinoid tumours, no matter where they arise. In MGG stained smears, cytoplasm shows a striking red granularity and indistinct cell borders. Malignant tumours show atypical cytological features and mitoses. Neurosecretory granules can sometimes be demonstrated by Grimelius's silver stain and by electron microscopy. Neuroendocrine differentiation can be identified immunohistochemically with markers such as NSE, chromogranin and synaptophysin.

Malignant neoplasms: non-epithelial tumours

Angiosarcoma

This is a rare tumour of liver. It occurs in association with certain carcinogenic agents, notably thorotrast, vinyl chloride, industrial and therapeutic arsenic, copper sulphate in sprays in vineyard workers, androgenic/anabolic steroids, stilboestrol, oral contraceptive steroids and phenelzine[305,336-338]. It may occur, however, without a known association with any of these compounds. Cirrhosis is present in approximately one-third of cases. The majority of patients are adults and elderly, symptoms and signs are non-specific, and a wide spectrum of haematological disturbances may be present[339]. Biopsy is often associated with severe or fatal haemorrhage and cases of massive bleeding after FNA have been reported[77,340,341]. At autopsy, the tumour is usually multicentric, appearing as haemorrhagic nodules. Microscopically, tumour cells line sinusoids and cavernous spaces with tufting or form solid masses. They are elongated and exhibit pleomorphic, hyperchromatic nuclei, which are occasionally multiple, surrounded by ill-defined cytoplasm. Extramedullary haemopoiesis may occur. Endothelial markers including Factor VIII, CD31, CD34, Ulex europaeus may be detected in some tumour cells[342].

Cytological findings

- ▶ Smears are highly cellular or hypocellular with abundant blood
- ▶ Fragments, loose clusters and single cells
- ▶ Spindle shaped tumour cells as vessels, papillae or solid groups
- ▶ Larger round tumour cells with abundant cytoplasm containing vacuoles or lumina
- ▶ Nuclei, oval to elongated, with variably prominent nucleoli, may be naked
- ▶ Cytoplasm is ill defined and lacy
- ▶ Bizarre cells with erythrophagocytosis and intracytoplasmic haemosiderin
- ▶ Necrosis
- ▶ Polymorphs

Smears are cellular and show endothelial cells as spindle shaped cells exhibiting oblong hyperchromatic nuclei and chromatin clumping occurring singly and in small groups (Fig. 14.55). In some reports, a second population consisting of irregular groups of large round or oval cells with abundant cytoplasm, central hyperchromatic vesicular

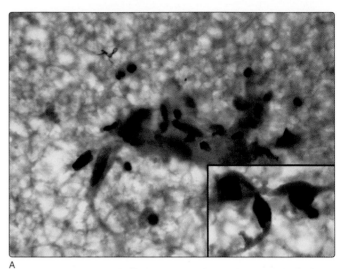

A

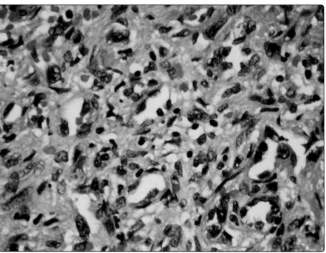

B

Fig. 14.55 Angiosarcoma. (A) Smears show spindle cells occurring singly and in small groups exhibiting elongated hyperchromatic nuclei. (B) Histology shows tumour cells lining vascular spaces and exhibiting pleomorphic, hyperchromatic nuclei surrounded by ill-defined cytoplasm. (A, H&E × HP; B, H&E × HP)

nuclei and prominent nucleoli, showed vague lumina. In addition, large bizarre malignant cells exhibiting elongate hyperchromatic nuclei and abundant cytoplasm containing phagocytosed erythrocytes were noted[343-346]. Immunocytochemistry for endothelial markers, factor VIII, CD31, CD34 and Ulex europaeus often show some focal positivity[347].

Epithelioid haemangioendothelioma

This distinctive vascular tumour occurs mostly in adult females at an average age of about 50 years. The tumour is usually multiple and involves both lobes, raising the possibility of origin elsewhere in the vascular system. It is white, of firm consistency and with time, becomes progressively more sclerotic. Growth is slow and patients survive for 5 years or more. Microscopically, tumour cells form small irregular spaces and are 'epithelioid' in appearance, being irregularly shaped, often with abundant cytoplasm and vesicular nuclei. There is subtle permeation of sinusoids at the margins and central sclerosis. There have been several reports of the cytopathologic features describing dispersed and anastomosing epithelioid and spindled cells showing some pleomorphism and containing intracytoplasmic lumens. Some tumour giant cells were noted[343,348]. Factor VIII-related antigen can usually be demonstrated in tumour cells.

Undifferentiated (embryonal) sarcoma

This rare primary liver tumour has a poor prognosis. It occurs predominantly in children between 6–10 years but occasional cases have been reported in middle and old age. Patients present with a rapidly growing abdominal mass. Microscopically, the tumour resembles embryonic mesenchyme with spindle, stellate and pleomorphic cells which are occasionally bizarre and multinucleate.

Cytological findings

- ► Cellular smears
- ► Polygonal and spindle tumour cells
- ► The polygonal cells are larger and pleomorphic, with a round or lobated nucleus, occasional multinucleation, one or several nucleoli and variable poorly-defined cytoplasm
- ► Cytoplasmic vacuoles and eosinophilic globules
- ► Myxoid material

Several case reports of the cytopathological findings have been published[349–352], including the FNA specimen of a metastatic deposit from primary undifferentiated sarcoma of liver[353]. Aspiration yielded abundant blood-stained mucoid material containing clusters and single polygonal or spindled cells exhibiting oval or irregular, often lobated nuclei with finely granular chromatin and nucleoli; cytoplasm was variable and pale staining and often contained poorly defined vacuoles; occasional bizarre multinucleated tumour cells were present and mitoses were seen. Myxoid matrix was present in the background.

Other sarcomas of the liver

All histological varieties occur but are very rare, and a primary tumour elsewhere must be excluded. The tumours are similar to those occurring in other sites of the body (see Chapter 40). Embryonal rhabdomyosarcoma can arise from major hepatic or common bile ducts presenting as progressive obstructive jaundice.

Leiomyosarcoma

Hepatic leiomyosarcoma is a rare primary malignancy, but appears to be on the increase in young HIV infected patients[354,355]. Leiomyosarcoma metastatic to the liver is more common. As in other sites, it comprises spindle cells arranged in fascicles. The cells have elongated, blunt-ended nuclei and clear perinuclear vacuoles. Occasionally the tumour cells are epithelioid with a polygonal shape. The

smears may be paucicellular with small irregular clusters of cells with blunt-ended, overlapping nuclei[356].

Malignant fibrous histiocytoma

One of the first malignant tumours encountered by the author in diagnostic liver FNA was a primary malignant fibrous histiocytoma, inflammatory variant. The patient was a middle-aged medical practitioner who presented with pain, an enlarged liver and hepatic rub. The tumour was inoperable at laparotomy and the patient died with local spread and pulmonary metastases.

Smears and sections showed large malignant histiocyte-like cells with abundant cytoplasm containing multiple small vacuoles, spindle cells and inflammatory cells (Figs 14.56, 14.57). Electron microscopy revealed a range of bizarre histiocytic and fibroblastoid neoplastic cells in loose supporting stroma, with widespread leucocytic infiltration.

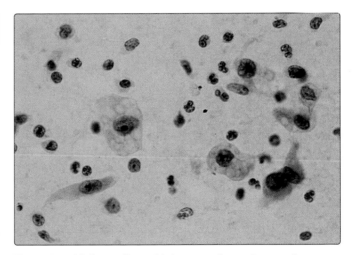

Fig. 14.56 Malignant fibrous histiocytoma. Smear shows malignant histiocyte-like cells, which vary greatly in size and exhibit abundant cytoplasm containing multiple small vacuoles, spindle cells and an inflammatory cell background. (Papanicolaou × HP)

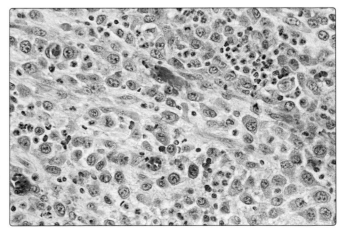

Fig. 14.57 Malignant fibrous histiocytoma. The section shows mesenchymal cells, both histiocyte-like and spindled, leucocytes and plasma cells. (H&E × MP)

Malignant lymphoma

The liver is commonly involved by disseminated malignant lymphoma: both Hodgkin's disease and non-Hodgkin's lymphoma. With systemic disease the liver is involved in 25% of cases in liver biopsies and in 50% of cases at post-mortem. Occurrence of primary lymphoma in liver is extremely rare. Reported cases have usually been non-Hodgkin's lymphoma of large B cell type (high-grade)[357–359]. Disease is usually confined to the liver until late in the course and usually responds to therapy, therefore having a good prognosis.

Primary hepatic lymphoma usually presents as one or more mass lesions. It has been associated with a range of systemic and hepatic diseases including hepatitis B and C virus, primary biliary cirrhosis, primary sclerosing cholangitis, chronic liver disease NOS, systemic lupus erythematosus, ITP, HIV[359,360]. Unless there is high index of suspicion the diagnosis may not be considered.

Cytological findings

▶ Cellular aspirates with dispersed cells and lymphoglandular bodies
▶ Cells have a high nuclear/cytoplasmic ratio
▶ Cell size variable, depending on whether it is a small cell or large cell lymphoma
▶ Small cell lymphomas usually polymorphous, large cell type usually monomorphous
▶ Necrosis and mitoses present

Aspirates are usually markedly cellular with dispersed cells and scattered small aggregates without true cohesion. In the more common large cell lymphoma, the cells are medium to large with round to oval pale vesicular nuclei, irregular nuclear membranes and one or more nucleoli. The nuclear/cytoplasmic ratio is high with a thin rim of cytoplasm. Necrosis and mitoses may be identified and lymphoglandular bodies are usually present[361]. Occasional hepatocytes may be seen. In small cell lymphomas the nuclei are only slightly larger than normal and are hypochromatic, with or without irregular contours. The cytoplasm is again scanty and lymphoglandular bodies are usually present. Immunohistochemistry is useful in excluding non-lymphoid differential diagnoses and in phenotyping the lymphoma including confirming monoclonality. Flow cytometry and molecular studies can provide similar information, but the appropriate sample is less often collected. The differential diagnosis includes inflammatory processes, extramedullary haemopoiesis, poorly-differentiated carcinoma, melanoma and small cell neoplasms. In the setting of organ transplantation, either liver or other organs, the differential diagnosis of a post transplant lymphoproliferative disorder should be considered for a mass lesion. The aspirates can show either a polymorphous smear with a spectrum of mature and immature lymphocytes, scattered plasma cells and

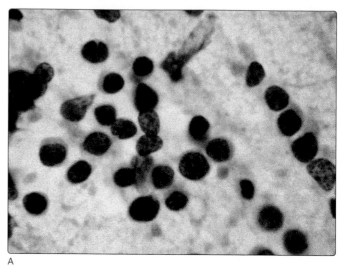

A

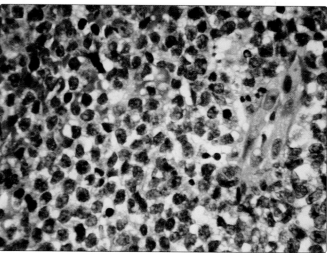

B

Fig. 14.58 Post transplant lymphoproliferative disorder. A fifty-year-old female with a bilateral lung transplant for 5 years presented with multiple liver masses. (A), A monomorphous population of large atypical lymphocytes. Flow cytometry demonstrated B lymphocyte monoclonality. (B) Core biopsy confirming a monomorphous population of atypical large lymphocytes. (A, Papanicolaou × HP; B, H&E × HP)

histiocytes or a monomorphous population of large atypical lymphocytes (Fig. 14.58). Material should always be collected for immunocytochemistry, flow cytometry or molecular studies for demonstrating B lymphocyte monoclonality and the presence of Epstein-Barr virus DNA[362–364].

Teratoma

As with lymphoma, germ cell tumours not uncommonly metastasize to liver but may rarely be primary[365,366]. These usually occur in children, with a female predilection.

Malignant neoplasms: metastatic tumours

Metastatic tumour is present in the liver in over 50% of patients who die from malignant disease. With the exception of primary brain tumours, virtually all malignant neoplasms may metastasize to the liver[367]. Spread occurs via the portal vein, hepatic artery, lymphatic channels or by direct extension. Metastatic tumours may be solitary or multiple and form small or large nodules which are usually solid but less commonly cystic or diffusely infiltrative[142,368]. The six commonest primary sites are bronchus, colon, pancreas, breast, stomach and 'primary of unknown origin'.

On imaging, many benign lesions and primary tumours present with appearances similar to metastases. FNA of focal liver lesions is therefore a most important diagnostic procedure in the management of malignant disease[369]. The presence of documented metastatic tumour to the liver may radically alter management in the individual case.

Any available previous histology or cytology should be reviewed. Morphological features similar to those of the metastasis will confirm its origin, but if different may lead to discovery of a second unsuspected primary tumour as the source of the liver metastasis. Review of previous material may also be helpful in confirming rare, though morphologically distinctive metastases, such as thymic tumours, neuroblastoma or adenoid cystic carcinoma[370].

The primary site of metastases may be indicated by immunocytochemistry as carcinoma of the prostate reacts with prostatic specific antigen, follicular carcinoma of thyroid with thyroglobulin and malignant teratoma with beta-human chorionic gonadotrophin. Differential staining for keratins of various molecular weights can provide direction for possible primary sites of adenocarcinomas, e.g. colonic adenocarcinoma is generally CK7 negative and CK20 positive. Markers, such as neurone specific enolase, chromogranin and synaptophysin can confirm neuroendocrine differentiation. Lymphoid markers, either using immunocytochemistry or flow cytometry, can confirm monoclonality of the lymphoid population and provide a degree of classification. Studies for hormone receptors can be performed if metastatic breast carcinoma is suspected. Markers to confirm melanoma include S 100, HMB 45, MART-1 and Melan-A.

Electron microscopy may be necessary to distinguish between spindle cell sarcomas, spindle cell HCC, sarcomatoid renal cell carcinoma (Fig. 14.59) and spindle cell squamous cell carcinoma or melanoma.

Metastases that can be identified confidently on FNA because their distinct morphological features include large bowel adenocarcinoma, small cell anaplastic carcinoma, carcinoid and islet cell tumours, some melanomas and lymphomas.

Adenocarcinoma of the colon

This has been the most frequently diagnosed metastasis in our case series. It often presents a characteristic pattern in which columnar cells form crypts and exhibit enlarged, elongated nuclei, palisading and stratification (Fig. 14.60). Necrosis commonly occurs inciting an acute inflammatory reaction and single necrotic cells with eosinophilic cytoplasm and irregular pyknotic nuclei may predominate

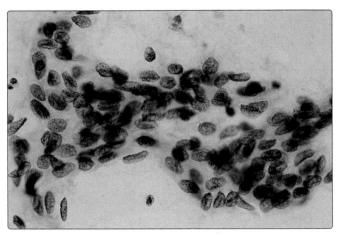

Fig. 14.59 Metastatic sarcomatoid renal cell carcinoma (RCC). Cohesive plump malignant spindle cells. (Papanicolaou × HP) Electron microscopy revealed ultrastructural features most consistent with RCC.

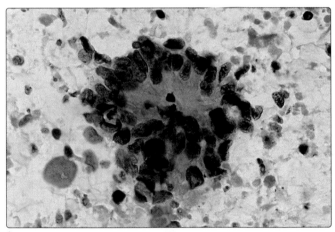

A

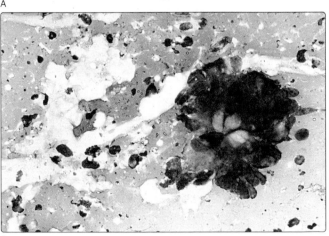

B

Fig. 14.60 Metastatic colonic carcinoma. (A) A crypt formed by palisading stratified malignant columnar cells showing elongated, hyperchromatic nuclei. (B) Similar crypt also containing goblet cells. (A, Papanicolaou × HP; B, MGG × HP)

giving a false impression of squamous cell carcinoma. Careful examination of such smears usually reveals at least a few characteristic formations of viable tumour cells.

Small cell carcinoma

Small cell carcinoma presents as dispersed small cells with round, irregular nuclei and little or no cytoplasm. Cell clusters and nuclear moulding are important features (Fig. 14.61) which distinguish small cell carcinoma from lymphomas, as the latter never form cell junctions and therefore do not occur in cohesive clusters. Small cell carcinoma of lung shows a few characteristic dense core granules on electron microscopy.

Other neuroendocrine tumours

Most patients with the carcinoid syndrome have metastases of neuroendocrine tumour in the liver. These tumours are readily recognized. Smears show a uniform population of small tumour cells dispersed or forming rosettes with regular round nuclei, punctate chromatin, small nucleoli

and delicate cytoplasm. In MGG stained smears the cytoplasm of neuroendocrine cells contains red granules, which are strikingly distinctive (Fig. 14.62) and have been described by Wilander *et al.* who applied silver stains to these granules[371]. Neuroendocrine markers such as neurone specific enolase, chromogranin and synaptophysin will often be positive. Specific dense core granules are demonstrated on electron microscopy (Fig. 14.63).

Melanoma

Melanoma has a high propensity for spread to the liver and involvement has occurred as long as 20 years after removal of the primary lesion. If well differentiated, melanomas present as a population of single cells possessing loose junctions, an eccentric nucleus, well stained cytoplasm, definite cell borders and intranuclear inclusions (Fig. 14.64). Melanin pigment provides a definitive diagnosis but it should be confirmed on a special stain, e.g. Masson Fontana, to distinguish it from other pigments within macrophages and liver cells. Because of extreme variability in cell morphology, common lack of melanin or the absence of a suggestive history, the diagnosis of metastatic melanoma can be difficult. Immunohistochemistry for S 100 or other, more specific melanoma markers (HMB 45, MART-1 or Melan-A) is often useful. Electron microscopy may disclose numerous cytoplasmic primitive melanosomes and occasional pigment-bearing cells (Fig. 14.65).

Adenocarcinoma of the breast

This entity often shows a rather uniform population of clustered polygonal epithelial cells of medium size with round nuclei, fine chromatin, a predictable single nucleolus and a small amount of dense cytoplasm. Given a history of previous breast carcinoma, this appearance is consistent with metastatic breast cancer. Immunohistochemistry for oestrogen and progesterone hormone receptors can provide confirmatory evidence.

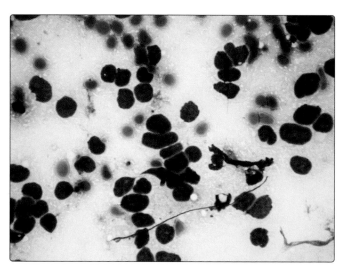

Fig. 14.61 Metastatic small cell neuroendocrine carcinoma. Small cells in a dispersed pattern with some clumping where nuclear moulding is noted. The cells have round, irregular nuclei and little or no cytoplasm. (MGG × HP)

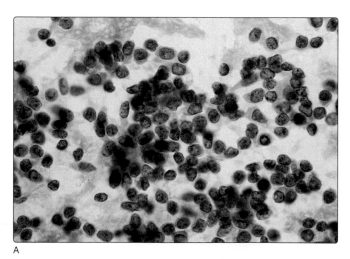

A

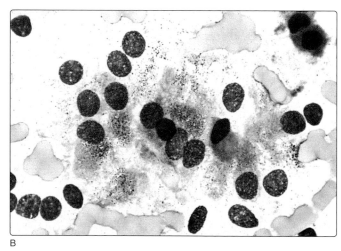

B

Fig. 14.62 Metastatic carcinoid tumour. (A) Dispersed, uniform, small tumour cells and at least one rosette; round, regular nuclei and punctate chromatin; delicate cytoplasm. (B) Rounded tumour cells with red cytoplasmic granularity and indistinct cell borders. (A, Papanicolaou × HP; B, MGG × HP)

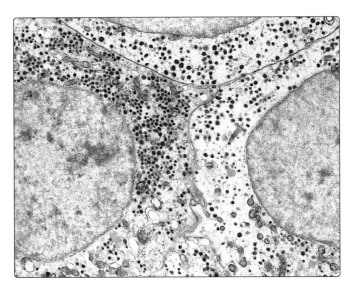

Fig. 14.63 Metastatic neuroendocrine-type cells in an aspirated liver specimen from a patient with carcinoid syndrome. Abundant spherical dense core cytoplasmic granules (100–200 nm diam.), rather bland rounded nuclei and rare intercellular junctions are typical of most carcinoid tumours. (Electron micrograph × 6150)

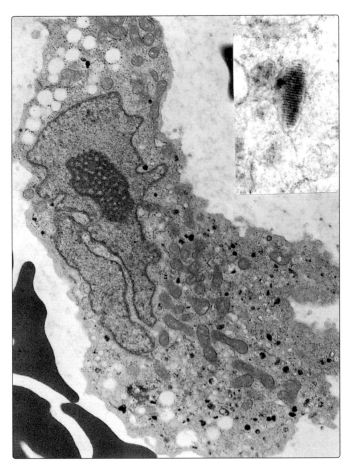

Fig. 14.65 Metastatic melanoma. Non-cohesive cells with folded nuclei and complex nucleoli. A minority of cells exhibited pigment-laden cytoplasmic melanosomes (main figure). The predominant amelanotic cells contained only rare examples of distinctive immature melanosomes (elliptical organelles with periodic cross-striations) which also identify the melanocytic cell type (inset). (Electron micrograph × 7840; inset × 73 500)

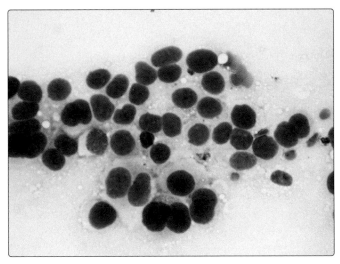

Fig. 14.64 Metastatic melanoma. A smear from a liver aspirate shows dispersed, small to medium round cells with delicate cytoplasm and no distinguishing features. (MGG × HP)

Gastrointestinal stromal tumour

Gastrointestinal stromal tumours are a heterogenous group of mesenchymal tumours excluding those with typical smooth muscle or Schwannian differentiation.

They arise anywhere along the gastrointestinal tract with a predilection for the stomach and show a spectrum of behaviour from benign to highly malignant. They can have a spindled or an epithelioid morphology and are typically positive for CD34 and C-kit protein (CD117) (Fig. 14.66) using immunohistochemical staining[372]. When malignant they may metastasize to the liver.

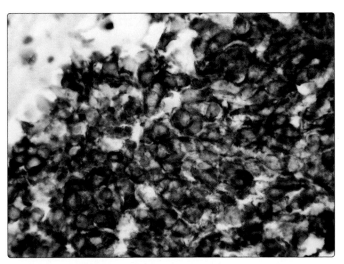

Fig. 14.66 Gastrointestinal stromal tumours. One of the defining features of these tumours is positive immunochemical staining for C-kit protein (CD117). (Immunoperoxidase stain: C-kit antigen on cell block × HP)

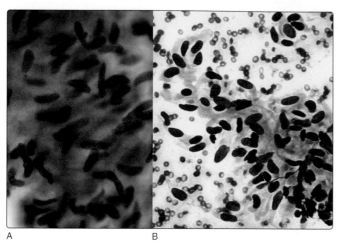

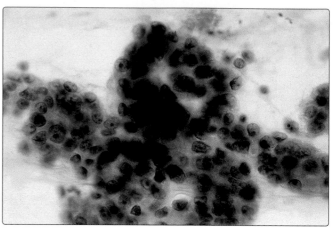

A   B

Fig. 14.67   Gastrointestinal stromal tumours. (A) and (B) The cells are spindled and arranged in cohesive fascicles or looser clusters. The nuclei are cigar shaped with even chromatin and an indistinct nucleolus. (A, Papanicolaou × HP; B, MGG × HP)

Fig. 14.68   Metastatic renal cell carcinoma. Tumour cells exhibit round nuclei and conspicuous single, often central nucleoli. A tubular pattern suggests metastatic renal cell carcinoma (RCC) and electron microscopy confirmed this diagnosis. (Papanicolaou × HP)

The smears are cellular and may include stroma. The cells are usually spindled although epithelioid cells have been reported, and are arranged in clusters or fascicles (Fig. 14.67). The nuclei are cigar shaped or tapered with even chromatin and an indistinct nucleolus. Dispersed stripped nuclei may be present. In malignant cases, features such as necrosis, mitoses and atypia may be present[373–376].

Renal cell carcinoma

Metastatic well-differentiated renal cell carcinoma (RCC) may present special difficulties. The spindle cell variant has already been discussed. In the more typical tumours smears show many small fragments of tumour encased in vascular stroma, appearing as a single layer of elongated cells and resembling the trabecular/sinusoidal pattern of HCC. Features, which are not typical of HCC, are columnar cells on the edge of tumour fragments or forming tubules, absence of central large nucleoli and abundant fibrous stroma (Fig. 14.68). On electron microscopy metastatic RCC not infrequently exhibits giant central nucleoli and clear cytoplasm containing glycogen or lipid accumulations not unlike those of HCC. Tubular-like profiles, basal laminae surrounding malignant epithelial cells and regular microvilli are present. Absence of typical organelles such as dense rounded mitochondria, profiles of endoplasmic reticulum and canaliculi argue against a diagnosis of HCC.

Metastases from other sites

Mucin-secreting signet ring cells in a background of medium-sized tumour cells showing no particular pattern suggests carcinoma of the stomach. If not obviously squamous, large cell carcinoma of the lung is usually unremarkable in smears but electron microscopy may reveal tumour cells showing squamous or glandular features and even neuroendocrine dense core granules may be present.

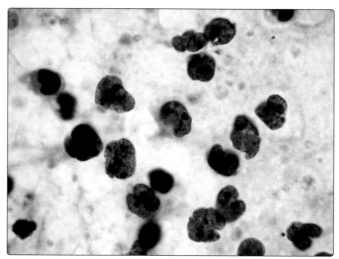

Fig. 14.69   Lymphoma. A dispersed population of large atypical lymphoid cells with irregular lobated nuclei. CD20 positivity supported a diagnosis of non-Hodgkin's B-cell lymphoma. (Papanicolaou × HP)

Lymphoma within the liver is almost always metastatic. Microscopic features of deposits resemble those in lymph nodes (Fig. 14.69). Jansson *et al.* found that 25% of patients with non-Hodgkin's lymphoma had clinically silent infiltration of the liver on routine FNA[377]. Carcinomas of thyroid and prostate tend to spread to liver comparatively less frequently than do many other tumours.

We have seen metastatic poorly-differentiated squamous cell carcinoma of the cervix on a number of occasions in younger women in whom the disease progressed rapidly. Hepatic metastases occur infrequently from ovarian carcinomas, except for granulosa cell tumours[378,379]. Morphological features of metastatic sarcomas are similar to those of the primary tumours.

References

1 Biett. Hydatides du foie avec développement considerable, de cet organe; ponction explorative; incision; sortie d'une grande quantité d'acephalocystes;guérison. *Gaz d hop* 1833; **7**: 383

2 Roberts. Abscess of the liver, with hydatids; Operation. *Lancet* 1833; **1**: 189–190

3 Schupfer F. De la possibilité de faire intravitum un diagnostic histopathologique précis de maladies du foie et de la rate. *Sem Med* 1907; **27**: 229

4 Lundquist A. Fine-needle aspiration biopsy of the liver. Applications in clinical diagnosis and investigation. *Acta Med Scand Suppl* 1971; **520**(4): 1–28

5 Bingel A. Uber die parenchympunktion der leber. *Verh Dtsch Ges Inn Med* 1923; **35**: 210

6 Olivet J. Die diagnostische leberparenchympunktion. *Med Klin* 1926; **22**: 1440

7 Frola E. Etude clinique de l'état fonctionnel du foie par la ponction hépatique. *Presse Med* 1935; **2**: 1198

8 Iverson P, Roholm K. On aspiration biopsy of the liver with remarks on its diagnostic significance. *Acta Med Scand* 1939; **102**: 1–6

9 Baron E. Aspiration for removal of biopsy material from the liver; a report of 35 cases. *Arch Intern Med* 1939; **63**: 276–289

10 Lopes Cardoso P. *Clinical Cytology*. Leiden: Staflen, 1954

11 Myren J. Levercytologi. *Nord Med* 1969; **82**: 1152

12 Nieburgs H E, Paretz A D, Perez V, Reisman H. Cytologic study of liver smears and its clinical value. *Trans Seventh Annual Meeting of Intersociety Cytology Council*, 1959

13 Weil P E, Isch-Wall P, Perles S. La ponction du foie dans la maladie du sang. *Presse Med* 1938; **46**: 1707

14 Sonderstrom N. *Fine needle aspiration biopsy. Used as a direct adjunct in clinical diagnostic work*. New York: Grune & Stratton, 1966

15 Lundquist A. Liver biopsy with a needle of 0.7 mm outer diameter. Safety and quantitative yield. *Acta Med Scand* 1970; **188**(6): 471–474

16 Lundquist A. Fine-needle aspiration biopsy for cytodiagnosis of malignant tumour in the liver. *Acta Med Scand* 1970; **188**(6): 465–470

17 Sherlock P, Kim Y S, Koss L G. Cytologic diagnosis of cancer from aspirated material obtained at liver biopsy. *Am J Dig Dis* 1967; **12**(4): 396–402

18 Carney C N. Clinical cytology of the liver. *Acta Cytol* 1975; **19**(3): 244–250

19 Grossman E, Goldstein M J, Koss L G, Winawer S J, Sherlock P. Cytological examination as an adjunct to liver biopsy in the diagnosis of hepatic metastases. *Gastroenterology* 1972; **62**(1): 56–60

20 Rasmussen S N, Holm H H, Kristensen J K, Barlebo H. Ultrasonically-guided liver biopsy. *BMJ* 1972; **2**(812): 500–502

21 Haaga J R, Alfidi R J. Precise biopsy localization by computer tomography. *Radiology* 1976; **118**(3): 603–607

22 Babb R R, Jackman R J. Needle biopsy of the liver. A critique of four currently available methods. *West J Med* 1989; **150**(1): 39–42

23 Bedenne L, Mottot C, Courtois B et al. Is the Tru-Cut needle more efficient than the fine needle in the diagnosis of hepatic lesions? Comparative study of 45 echography-guided punctures. *Gastroenterol Clin Biol* 1990; **14**(1): 62–66

24 Bottles K, Cohen M B. An approach to fine-needle aspiration biopsy diagnosis of hepatic masses. *Diagn Cytopathol* 1991; **7**(2): 204–210

25 Glenthoj A, Sehested M. Histological and cytological fine needle biopsies from focal liver lesions. Intra- and interobserver reproducibility of diagnoses. *APMIS* 1989; **97**(7): 611–618

26 Jacobsen G K, Gammelgaard J, Fuglo M. Coarse needle biopsy *vs* fine needle aspiration biopsy in the diagnosis of focal lesions of the liver. Ultrasonically guided needle biopsy in suspected hepatic malignancy. *Acta Cytol* 1983; **27**(2): 152–156

27 Sbolli G, Fornari F, Civardi G et al. Role of ultrasound guided fine needle aspiration biopsy in the diagnosis of hepatocellular carcinoma. *Gut* 1990; **31**(11): 1303–1305

28 Zainol H, Sumithran E. Combined cytological and histological diagnosis of hepatocellular carcinoma in ultrasonically guided fine needle biopsy specimens. *Histopathol* 1993; **22**(6): 581–586

29 Mauro M A, Parker L A. Percutaneous drainage of a cystic tumor for relief of pain. *South Med J* 1987; **80**(11): 1466

30 Brits C J. Liver aspiration cytology. *S Afr Med J* 1974; **48**(53): 2207–2214

31 Dominis M, Cerlek S, Solter D. Cytology of diffuse liver disorders. *Acta Cytol* 1973; **17**(3): 205–208

32 Henriques U V, Hasselstrom K. Evaluation of jaundice: fine-needle aspiration liver cytology as a discriminating tool. *Dan Med Bull* 1977; **24**(3): 104–108

33 Linsk J A, Franzen S. *Clinical Aspiration Cytology*, 2nd edn. Philadelphia: Lippincott, 1989

34 Lundin P, Lundquist A, Lundvall O. Evaluation of fine-needle aspiration biopsy smears in the diagnosis of liver iron overload. *Acta Med Scand* 1969; **186**(5): 369–373

35 Perry M D, Johnston W W. Needle biopsy of the liver for the diagnosis of nonneoplastic liver diseases. Acta Cytol 1985; **29**(3): 385–390

36 Wasastjerna C, Reissell P, Karjalainen J, Ekelund P. Fatty liver in diabetes. A cytological study. *Acta Med Scand* 1972; **191**(3): 225–228

37 Wasastjerna C. Liver. In: Zajicek J ed. *Aspiration Biopsy Cytology. Part 2 Cytology of Infradiaphragmatic Organs*. Basel: Karger, 1979; 167–193

38 Fagelman D, Chess Q. Nonaspiration fine-needle cytology of the liver: a new

technique for obtaining diagnostic samples. *Am J Roentgenol* 1990; **155**(6): 1217–1219

39 Axe S R, Erozan Y S, Ermatinger S V. Fine-needle aspiration of the liver. A comparison of smear and rinse preparations in the detection of cancer. *Am J Clin Pathol* 1986; **86**(3): 281–285

40 Orell S R, Sterrett G F, Walters M N-I, Whitaker D. *Manual and Atlas of Fine Needle Aspiration Cytology*, 3rd edn. Edinburgh: Churchill Livingstone, 1999

41 Bergman S, Graeme-Cook F, Pitman M B. The usefulness of the reticulin stain in the differential diagnosis of liver nodules on fine-needle aspiration biopsy cell block preparations. *Mod Pathol* 1997; **10**(12): 1258–1264

42 de Boer W B, Segal A, Frost F A, Sterrett G F. Cytodiagnosis of well differentiated hepatocellular carcinoma: can indeterminate diagnoses be reduced? *Cancer* 1999; **87**(5): 270–277

43 Ferrell L. Liver pathology: cirrhosis, hepatitis, and primary liver tumors. Update and diagnostic problems. *Mod Pathol* 2000; **13**(6): 679–704

44 Gagliano E F. Reticulin stain in the fine needle aspiration differential diagnosis of liver nodules [letter]. *Acta Cytol* 1995; **39**(3): 596–598

45 Ojanguren I, Ariza A, Llatjos M et al. Proliferating cell nuclear antigen expression in normal, regenerative, and neoplastic liver: a fine-needle aspiration cytology and biopsy study. *Hum Pathol* 1993; **24**(8): 905–908

46 Ojanguren I, Ariza A, Castella E M et al. p53 immunoreactivity in hepatocellular adenoma, focal nodular hyperplasia, cirrhosis and hepatocellular carcinoma. *Histopathol* 1995; **26**(1): 63–68

47 Pietron M. Cytomorphometry of fine-needle aspiration biopsy material from the liver tumours. *Patol Pol* 1993; **44**(4): 193–201

48 Russo A, Bazan V, Plaja S et al. Flow cytometric DNA analysis of hepatic tumours on ultrasound-guided fine-needle aspirates. *J Surg Oncol* 1992; **51**(1): 26–32

49 Sampatanukul P, Mikuz G, Israsena S et al. Cytomorphologic and DNA cytometric features of hepatocellular carcinoma in fine needle aspirates. *Acta Cytol* 1997; **41**(2): 435–442

50 Siddiqui M S, Soomro I N, Kayani N et al. Assessment of nucleolar organizer regions (NORs) in proliferative conditions of the liver. *Pathol Res Pract* 1999; **195**(6): 421–426

51 Zeppa P, Zabatta A, Fulciniti F et al. The role of morphometry in the cytology of well-differentiated hepatocarcinoma and cirrhosis with atypia. *Anal Quant Cytol Histol* 1988; **10**(5): 343–348

52 Zeppa P, Benincasa G, Troncone G et al. Retrospective evaluation of DNA ploidy of hepatocarcinoma on cytologic samples. *Diagn Cytopathol* 1998; **19**(5): 323–329

53 Hurlimann J, Gardiol D. Immunohistochemistry in the differential

diagnosis of liver carcinomas. *Am J Surg Pathol* 1991; **15**(3): 280–288

54 Johnson D E, Powers C N, Rupp G, Frable W J. Immunocytochemical staining of fine-needle aspiration biopsies of the liver as a diagnostic tool for hepatocellular carcinoma. *Mod Pathol* 1992; **5**(2): 117–123

55 Pinto M M, Monteferrante M, Kaye A D. Carcinoembryonic antigen in fine-needle aspirate of liver: a diagnostic adjunct to cytology. *Diagn Cytopathol* 1991; **7**(1): 23–26

56 Salomao D R, Lloyd R V, Goellner J R. Hepatocellular carcinoma: needle biopsy findings in 74 cases. *Diagn Cytopathol* 1997; **16**(1): 8–13

57 Yam L T. Immunocytochemistry of fine needle aspirates. A tactical approach. *Acta Cytol* 1990; **34**(6): 789–796

58 Bedrossian C W, Davila R M, Merenda G. Immunocytochemical evaluation of liver fine-needle aspirations. *Arch Pathol Lab Med* 1989; **113**(11): 1225–1230

59 Kung I T M, Chan S-K, Lo E S F. Application of the immunoperoxidase technique to cell block preparations from fine needle aspirates. *Acta Cytol* 1990; **34**: 297–303

60 Guindi M, Yazdi H M, Gilliatt M A. Fine needle aspiration biopsy of hepatocellular carcinoma. Value of immunocytochemical and ultrastructural studies. *Acta Cytol* 1994; **38**(3): 385–391

61 Stephen M R, Oien K, Ferrier R K, Burnett R A. Effusion cytology of hepatocellular carcinoma with *in situ* hybridisation for human albumin. *J Clin Pathol* 1997; **50**(5): 442–444

62 Papotti M, Pacchioni D, Negro F *et al.* Albumin gene expression in liver tumors: diagnostic interest in fine needle aspiration biopsies. *Mod Pathol* 1994; **7**(3): 271–275

63 Krishna M, Lloyd R V, Batts K P. Detection of albumin messenger RNA in hepatic and extrahepatic neoplasms: a marker of hepatocellular differentiation. *Am J Surg Pathol* 1997; **21**(2): 147–152

64 Wee A, Nilsson B. Fine needle aspiration biopsy of hepatic leiomyosarcoma. An unusual epithelioid variant posing a potential diagnostic pitfall in a hepatocellular carcinoma-prevalent population. *Acta Cytol* 1997; **41**(3): 737–743

65 Wolber R A, Greene C A, Dupuis B A. Polyclonal carcinoembryonic antigen staining in the cytologic differential diagnosis of primary and metastatic hepatic malignancies. *Acta Cytol* 1991; **35**(2): 215–220

66 Wong M A, Yazdi H M. Hepatocellular carcinoma *vs* carcinoma metastatic to the liver. Value of stains for carcinoembryonic antigen and naphthylamidase in fine needle aspiration biopsy material. *Acta Cytol* 1990; **34**(2): 192–196

67 Rishi M, Kovatich A, Ehya H. Utility of polyclonal and monoclonal antibodies against carcinoembryonic antigen in hepatic fine-needle aspirates. *Diagn Cytopathol* 1994; **11**(4): 358–361; discussion 361–362

68 Wennerberg A E, Nalesnik M A, Coleman W B. Hepatocyte paraffin 1: a monoclonal antibody that reacts with hepatocytes and can be used for differential diagnosis of hepatic tumors. *Am J Pathol* 1993; **143**(4): 1050–1054

69 Stahl J, Voyvodic F. Biopsy diagnosis of malignant *vs* benign liver 'nodules': new helpful markers. An update. *Adv Anat Pathol* 2000; **7**(4): 230–239

70 De Young B, Proca D, Porcell A, Niemann T. MOC31 immunoreactivity in primary and metastatic carcinoma of the liver. *Mod Pathol* 1998; **11**: 151A

71 Niemann T H, Hughes J H, De Young B R. MOC-31 aids in the differentiation of metastatic adenocarcinoma from hepatocellular carcinoma. *Cancer* 1999; **87**(5): 295–298

72 Wu H H, Tao L C, Cramer H M. Vimentin-positive spider-shaped Kupffer cells. A new clue to cytologic diagnosis of primary and metastatic hepatocellular carcinoma by fine-needle aspiration biopsy. *Am J Clin Pathol* 1996; **106**(4): 517–521

73 Barsu M, Ghiurca V, Porutiu D, Badea R. Ultrastructural aspects of human liver tumours collected by thin needle aspiration biopsy. *Morphol Embryol (Bucur)* 1989; **35**(4): 279–283

74 Berkman W A, Chowdhury L, Brown N L, Padleckas R. Value of electron microscopy in cytologic diagnosis of fine-needle biopsy. *Am J Roentgenol* 1983; **140**(6): 1253–1258

75 Sehested M, Juul N, Hainau B, Torp-Pedersen S. Electron microscopy of ultrasound-guided fine-needle biopsy specimens. *Br J Radiol* 1987; **60**(712): 351–353

76 Wills E J, Carr S, Philips J. Electron microscopy in the diagnosis of percutaneous fine needle aspiration specimens. *Ultrastruct Pathol* 1987; **11**(4): 361–387

77 Hertzanu Y, Peiser J, Zirkin H. Massive bleeding after fine needle aspiration of liver angiosarcoma. *Gastrointest Radiol* 1990; **15**(1): 43–46

78 Terriff B A, Gibney R G, Scudamore C H. Fatality from fine-needle aspiration biopsy of a hepatic hemangioma. *Am J Roentgenol* 1990; **154**(1): 203–204

79 Brambs H J, Spamer C, Volk B *et al.* Histological diagnosis of liver hemangiomas using ultrasound-guided fine needle biopsy. *Hepatogastroenterology* 1985; **32**(6): 284–287

80 Nakaizumi A, Iishi H, Yamamoto R *et al.* Diagnosis of hepatic cavernous hemangioma by fine needle aspiration biopsy under ultrasonic guidance. *Gastrointest Radiol* 1990; **15**(1): 39–42

81 Bret P M, Fond A, Bretagnolle M *et al.* Percutaneous aspiration and drainage of hydatid cysts in the liver. *Radiology* 1988; **168**(3): 617–620

82 Langlois S L. Fine-needle biopsy of hepatic hydatids and haemangiomas: an overstated hazard. *Australas Radiol* 1989; **33**(2): 144–149

83 Schulz T B. Fine-needle biopsy of the liver complicated with bile peritonitis. *Acta Med Scand* 1976; **199**(1–2): 141–142

84 Glaser K S, Weger A R, Schmid K W, Bodner E. Is fine-needle aspiration of tumours harmless? *Lancet* 1989; **1**(8638): 620

85 McGrath F P, Gibney R G, Rowley V A, Scudamore C H. Cutaneous seeding following fine needle biopsy of colonic liver metastases. *Clin Radiol* 1991; **43**(2): 130–131

86 Scheele J, Altendorf-Hofmann A. Tumor implantation from needle biopsy of hepatic metastases. *Hepatogastroenterology* 1990; **37**(3): 335–337

87 Bissonnette R T, Gibney R G, Berry B R, Buckley A R. Fatal carcinoid crisis after percutaneous fine-needle biopsy of hepatic metastasis: case report and literature review. *Radiology* 1990; **174**(3 Pt 1): 751–752

88 Damascelli B, Spagnoli I, Garbagnati F *et al.* Massive lymphorrhoea after fine needle biopsy of the cystic haemolymphangioma of the liver. *Eur J Radiol* 1984; **4**(2): 107–109

89 Leiman G, Leibowitz C B, Dunbar F. Fine-needle aspiration of the liver: out of the ivory tower and into the community. *Diagn Cytopathol* 1989; **5**(1): 35–39

90 Cohen M B, Haber M M, Holly E A *et al.* Cytologic criteria to distinguish hepatocellular carcinoma from nonneoplastic liver. *Am J Clin Pathol* 1991; **95**(2): 125–130

91 Sole M, Calvet X, Cuberes T *et al.* Value and limitations of cytologic criteria for the diagnosis of hepatocellular carcinoma by fine needle aspiration biopsy. *Acta Cytol* 1993; **37**(3): 309–316

92 Glenthoj A, Sehested M, Torp-Pedersen S. Diagnostic reliability of histological and cytological fine needle biopsies from focal liver lesions. *Histopathol* 1989; **15**(4): 375–383

93 Lin B P, Chu J M, Rose R A. Ultrasound-guided fine needle aspiration biopsy of the liver. *Pathology* 1987; **19**(2): 173–177

94 Pilotti S, Rilke F, Claren R *et al.* Conclusive diagnosis of hepatic and pancreatic malignancies by fine needle aspiration. *Acta Cytol* 1988; **32**(1): 27–38

95 Sautereau D, Vire O, Cazes P Y *et al.* Value of sonographically guided fine needle aspiration biopsy in evaluating the liver with sonographic abnormalities. *Gastroenterology* 1987; **93**(4): 715–718

96 Johansen S, Myren J. Fine-needle aspiration biopsy smears in the diagnosis of liver diseases. *Scand J Gastroenterol* 1971; **6**(7): 583–588

97 Kerr J F, Wyllie A H, Currie A R. Apoptosis: a basic biological phenomenon with wide-ranging implications in tissue kinetics. *Br J Cancer* 1972; **26**(4): 239–257

98 Suen K C. Liver. *Atlas and text of aspiration biopsy cytology.* Baltimore: Williams & Wilkins, 1990; 166–184

99 Tao L C. Liver and pancreas. In: Bibbo M ed. *Comprehensive Cytopathology.* Philadelphia: Saunders, 1991; 822–859

100 Berman J J, McNeill R E. Cirrhosis with atypia. A potential pitfall in the interpretation of liver aspirates. *Acta Cytol* 1988; **32**(1): 11–14

101 Tao L C. Oral contraceptive-associated liver cell adenoma and hepatocellular carcinoma. Cytomorphology and mechanism of malignant transformation. *Cancer* 1991; **68**(2): 341–347

102 Layfield L J. Focal fatty change of the liver: cytologic findings in a radiographic mimic of metastases. *Diagn Cytopathol* 1994; **11**(4): 385–387; discussion 387–389

103 Caturelli E, Rapaccini G L, Sabelli C et al. Ultrasonography and echo-guided fine-needle biopsy in the diagnosis of focal fatty liver change. *Hepatogastroenterology* 1987; **34**(4): 137–140

104 Tanikawa K. The liver. In: Papadimitriou JM, Henderson DW, Spagnolo DV eds. *Diagnostic Ultrastructure of Non-Neoplastic Diseases*. Edinburgh: Churchill Livingstone, 1992

105 Lundquist A, Akerman M. Fine-needle aspiration biopsy in acute hepatitis and liver cirrhosis. *Ann Clin Res* 1970; **2**(3): 197–203

106 Wasastjerna C, Thoden C J, Ekelund P, Haltia K. The bile canaliculi in cytological aspiration biopsies from patients with liver disorders. *Scand J Gastroenterol* 1970; **5**(5): 327–331

107 Ishak K G. Granulomas of the liver. In: Toacham H L ed. *Pathology of Granulomas*. New York: Raven Press, 1983; 307–369

108 Wee A, Nilsson B, Wang T L et al. Tuberculous pseudotumor causing biliary obstruction. Report of a case with diagnosis by fine needle aspiration biopsy and bile cytology. *Acta Cytol* 1995; **39**(3): 559–562

109 Xing X, Xia S. [Diagnosis and treatment of hepatic tuberculoma]. *Chung Hua Chieh Ho Ho Hu Hsi Tsa Chih* 1997; **20**(3): 169–171

110 Rosen R D. Tuberculoma of the liver. *Tubercle* 1978; **59**: 47–54

111 Stormby N, Akerman M. Aspiration cytology in the diagnosis of granulomatous liver lesions. *Acta Cytol* 1973; **17**(3): 200–204

112 Olynyk J, Williams P, Fudge A et al. Fine-needle aspiration biopsy for the measurement of hepatic iron concentration. *Hepatology* 1992; **15**(3): 502–506

113 Bose S, Kapila K, Verma K. Amyloidosis of the liver diagnosed by fine needle aspiration cytology. *Acta Cytol* 1989; **33**(6): 935–936

114 Srinivasan R, Nijhawan R, Gautam U, Bambery P. Potassium permanganate resistant amyloid in fine-needle aspirate of the liver. *Diagn Cytopathol* 1994; **10**(4): 383–384

115 Yebra M, Albarran F, Durantez A et al. Diagnosis of hepatic amyloidosis by fine needle aspiration biopsy. *Am J Med* 1987; **82**(6): 1275–1276

116 Lemos L B, Baliga M, Benghuzzi H A, Cason Z. Nodular hematopoiesis of the liver diagnosed by fine-needle aspiration cytology. *Diagn Cytopathol* 1997; **16**(1): 51–54

117 Navarro M, Crespo C, Perez L et al. Massive intrahepatic extramedullary hematopoiesis in myelofibrosis. *Abdom Imaging* 2000; **25**(2): 184–186

118 Raab S S, Silverman J F, McLeod D L, Geisinger K R. Fine-needle aspiration cytology of extramedullary hematopoiesis (myeloid metaplasia). *Diagn Cytopathol* 1993; **9**(5): 522–526

119 Hartley J P, Douglas A P. A case of clonorchiasis in England. *BMJ* 1975; **3**(5983): 575

120 Papillo J L, Leslie K O, Dean R A. Cytologic diagnosis of liver fluke infestation in a patient with subsequently documented cholangiocarcinoma. *Acta Cytol* 1989; **33**(6): 865–869

121 Lautenschlager I. Fine needle aspiration biopsy in liver transplants. *Transplant Proc* 1989; **21**(4): 3618–3620

122 Lautenschlager I, Hockerstedt K, Hayry P. Fine-needle aspiration biopsy in the monitoring of liver allografts. *Transpl Int* 1991; **4**(1): 54–61

123 Carbonnel F, Samuel D, Reynes M et al. Fine-needle aspiration biopsy of human liver allografts. Correlation with liver histology for the diagnosis of acute rejection. *Transplantation* 1990; **50**(4): 704–707

124 Kubota K, Ericzon B G, Reinholt F P. Comparison of fine-needle aspiration biopsy and histology in human liver transplants. *Transplantation* 1991; **51**(5): 1010–1013

125 Lautenschlager I, Nashan B, Schlitt H J et al. Different cellular patterns associated with hepatitis C virus reactivation, cytomegalovirus infection, and acute rejection in liver transplant patients monitored with transplant aspiration cytology. *Transplantation* 1994; **58**(12): 1339–1345

126 Hayry P, von Willebrand E, Lautenschlager I et al. Diagnosis of rejection: role of fine-needle aspiration biopsy. *Transplant Proc* 1990; **22**(6): 2597–2600

127 Gattuso P, Castelli M J, Peng Y, Reddy V B. Post transplant lymphoproliferative disorders: a fine needle aspiration biopsy study. *Diagn Cytopathol* 1997; **16**(5): 392–395

128 Anthony P P. Tumours and tumour-like lesions of the liver and biliary tract. In: MacSween R N M, Anthony P P, Scheuer P J, Burt A D, Portmann B C eds. *Pathology of the Liver*, 3rd edn., Edinburgh: Churchill Livingstone, 1994; 635–712

129 Craig J R, Peters R L, Edmonson H A. Tumours of the liver and intrahepatic bile ducts. *Atlas of Tumour Pathology*, 2nd series. Washington, DC: Armed Forces Institute of Pathology, 1989

130 Gibson J B, Sobin L H. *Histological Typing of Tumours of the Liver, Biliary Tract and Pancreas*. Geneva: World Health Organization, 1978

131 Scheuer P J, Lefkowitch J H. *Liver Biopsy Interpretation*, 6th edn. New York: WB Saunders, 2000

132 Leong A S-Y, Liew C-T, Lau J W Y, Johnson P J. *Hepatocellular Carcinoma: Diagnosis, Investigation and Management*, 1st edn. London: Arnold, 1999

133 Rustgi V K. Epidemiology of hepatocellular carcinoma. *Gastroenterol Clin North Am* 1987; **16**(4): 545–551

134 Bell D A, Carr C P, Szyfelbein W M. Fine needle aspiration cytology of focal liver lesions. Results obtained with examination of both cytologic and histologic preparations. *Acta Cytol* 1986; **30**(4): 397–402

135 Cochand-Priollet B, Chagnon S, Ferrand J et al. Comparison of cytologic examination of smears and histologic examination of tissue cores obtained by fine needle aspiration biopsy of the liver. *Acta Cytol* 1987; **31**(4): 476–480

136 Farnum J B, Patel P H, Thomas E. The value of Chiba fine-needle aspiration biopsy in the diagnosis of hepatic malignancy: a comparison with Menghini needle biopsy. *J Clin Gastroenterol* 1989; **11**(1): 101–109

137 Fornari F, Civardi G, Cavanna L et al. Ultrasonically guided fine-needle aspiration biopsy: a highly diagnostic procedure for hepatic tumors. *Am J Gastroenterol* 1990; **85**(8): 1009–1013

138 Houn H Y, Sanders M M, Walker E M, Pappas A A. Fine needle aspiration in the diagnosis of liver neoplasms: a review. *Ann Clin Lab Sci* 1991; **21**(1): 2–11

139 Roget L, Richard P, Selles M et al. Value of ultrasound-guided cytopuncture in the diagnosis of hepatocellular carcinoma. *J Radiol* 1989; **70**(2): 75–78

140 Sangalli G, Livraghi T, Giordano F. Fine needle biopsy of hepatocellular carcinoma: improvement in diagnosis by microhistology. *Gastroenterology* 1989; **96**(2 Pt 1): 524–526

141 Finkel L, Marchevsky A, Cohen B. Endometrial cyst of the liver. *Am J Gastroenterol* 1986; **81**(7): 576–578

142 Min-Hau C. Ultrasonography and guided fine needle aspiration cytology in the diagnosis of fluid-containing masses in the liver. *Chin J Intern Med* 1985; **24**: 317

143 Roemer C E, Ferrucci J T, Mueller P et al. Hepatic cysts: diagnosis and therapy by sonographic needle aspiration. *Am J Roentgenol* 1981; **136**(6): 1065–1070

144 Chen M H. Ultrasonography and guided fine-needle aspiration cytology in the diagnosis of fluid-containing masses in the liver. *Zhonghua Nei Ke Za Zhi* 1985; **24**(5): 266–268, 317

145 Weimann A, Klempnauer J, Gebel M et al. Squamous cell carcinoma of the liver originating from a solitary non-parasitic cyst case report and review of the literature. *HPB Surg* 1996; **10**(1): 45–49

146 Hornstein A, Batts K P, Linz L J et al. Fine needle aspiration diagnosis of ciliated hepatic foregut cysts: a report of three cases. *Acta Cytol* 1996; **40**(3): 576–580

147 Selig A M, Chang C D, Galvanek E G, Bardawil R G. Fine needle aspiration of hepatic foregut cysts. *Mod Pathol* 1994; **7**: 41A

148 Zaman S S, Langer J E, Gupta P K. Ciliated hepatic foregut cyst. Report of a case with findings on fine needle aspiration. *Acta Cytol* 1995; **39**(4): 781–784

149 Goldstein H M, Carlyle D R, Nelson R S. Treatment of symptomatic hepatic cyst by percutaneous instillation of Pantopaque. *Am J Roentgenol* 1976; **127**(5): 850–853

150 Das D K, Bhambhani S, Pant C S. Ultrasound guided fine-needle aspiration cytology: diagnosis of hydatid disease of the abdomen and thorax. *Diagn Cytopathol* 1995; **12**(2): 173–176

151 Singh A, Singh Y, Sharma V K *et al*. Diagnosis of hydatid disease of abdomen and thorax by ultrasound guided fine needle aspiration cytology. *Indian J Pathol Microbiol* 1999; **42**(2): 155–156

152 von Sinner W N, Nyman R, Linjawi T, Ali A M. Fine needle aspiration biopsy of hydatid cysts. *Acta Radiol* 1995; **36**(2): 168–172

153 Vercelli-Retta J, Manana G, Reissenweber N J. The cytologic diagnosis of hydatid disease. *Acta Cytol* 1982; **26**(2): 159–168

154 Granger J K, Houn H Y. Diagnosis of hepatic actinomycosis by fine-needle aspiration. *Diagn Cytopathol* 1991; **7**(1): 95–97

155 Shurbaji M S, Gupta P K, Newman M M. Hepatic actinomycosis diagnosed by fine needle aspiration. A case report. *Acta Cytol* 1987; **31**(6): 751–755

156 Dusenbery D, Dodd G D, Carr B I. Percutaneous fine-needle aspiration of portal vein thrombi as a staging technique for hepatocellular carcinoma. Cytologic findings of 46 patients. *Cancer* 1995; **75**(8): 2057–2062

157 Le Bras Y, Gervez F, Abraham E *et al*. Value of the echo-guided needle aspiration in the treatment of amebic liver abscess. Apropos of 70 cases. *J Radiol* 1991; **72**(1): 43–47

158 Clark A H, McKee E E, Dixon D C. Identification of trophozoite form of Entamoeba histolytica by cytologic techniques. *Acta Cytol* 1972; **16**(5): 429–432

159 Walsh T J, Berkman W, Brown N L *et al*. Cytopathologic diagnosis of extracolonic amebiasis. *Acta Cytol* 1983; **27**(6): 671–675

160 Kobayashi T K, Koretoh O, Kamachi M *et al*. Cytologic demonstration of Entamoeba histolytica using immunoperoxidase techniques. Report of two cases. *Acta Cytol* 1985; **29**(3): 414–418

161 Anthony P P, Telesinghe P U. Inflammatory pseudotumour of the liver. *J Clin Pathol* 1986; **39**(7): 761–768

162 Lupovitch A, Chen R, Mishra S. Inflammatory pseudotumor of the liver. Report of the fine needle aspiration cytologic findings in a case initially misdiagnosed as malignant. *Acta Cytol* 1989; **33**(2): 259–262

163 Horiuchi R, Uchida T, Kojima T, Shikata T. Inflammatory pseudotumor of the liver. Clinicopathologic study and review of the literature. *Cancer* 1990; **65**(7): 1583–1590

164 Shek T W, Ng I O, Chan K W. Inflammatory pseudotumor of the liver. Report of four cases and review of the literature. *Am J Surg Pathol* 1993; **17**(3): 231–238

165 Chen I. Inflammatory pseudotumour of the liver. *Hum Pathol* 1984; **15**: 694–696

166 Isobe H, Nishi Y, Fukutomi T *et al*. Inflammatory pseudotumor of the liver associated with acute myelomonocytic leukemia. *Am J Gastroenterol* 1991; **86**(2): 238–240

167 Malhotra V, Gondal R, Tatke M, Sarin S K. Fine needle aspiration cytologic appearance of inflammatory pseudotumor of the liver. A case report. *Acta Cytol* 1997; **41**(4 Suppl): 1325–1328

168 Yavuz E, Buyukbabani N, Cevikbas U. Inflammatory pseudotumor of the liver. Report of two cases. *Pathologica* 1998; **90**(5): 463–466

169 Stocker J T, Ishak K G. Mesenchymal hamartoma of the liver: a report of 30 cases and review of the literature. *Pediatr Pathol* 1983; **1**: 245–267

170 al-Rikabi A C, Buckai A, al-Sumayer S *et al*. Fine needle aspiration cytology of mesenchymal hamartoma of the liver. A case report. *Acta Cytol* 2000; **44**(3): 449–453

171 Drachenberg C B, Papadimitriou J C, Rivero M A, Wood C. Distinctive case. Adult mesenchymal hamartoma of the liver: report of a case with light microscopic, FNA cytology, immunohistochemistry, and ultrastructural studies and review of the literature. *Mod Pathol* 1991; **4**(3): 392–395

172 Jimenez-Heffernan J A, Vicandi B, Lopez-Ferrer P *et al*. Fine-needle aspiration cytology of mesenchymal hamartoma of the liver. *Diagn Cytopathol* 2000; **22**(4): 250–253

173 Koelma I A, Nap M, Huitema S *et al*. Hepatocellular carcinoma, adenoma, and focal nodular hyperplasia. Comparative histopathologic study with immunohistochemical parameters. *Arch Pathol Lab Med* 1986; **110**(11): 1035–1040

174 Casarella W J, Knowles D M, Wolff M, Johnson P M. Focal nodular hyperplasia and liver cell adenoma: radiologic and pathologic differentiation. *Am J Roentgenol* 1978; **131**(3): 393–402

175 Ruschenburg I, Droese M. Fine needle aspiration cytology of focal nodular hyperplasia of the liver. *Acta Cytol* 1989; **33**(6): 857–860

176 Gold J H, Guzman I J, Rosai J. Benign tumors of the liver. Pathologic examination of 45 cases. *Am J Clin Pathol* 1978; **70**(1): 6–17

177 Fechner R E. Benign hepatic lesions and orally administered contraceptives. A report of seven cases and a critical analysis of the literature. *Hum Pathol* 1977; **8**(3): 255–268

178 Klatskin G. Hepatic tumors: possible relationship to use of oral contraceptives. *Gastroenterology* 1977; **73**(2): 386–394

179 Baum J K, Bookstein J J, Holtz F, Klein E W. Possible association between benign hepatomas and oral contraceptives. *Lancet* 1973; **2**(7835): 926–929

180 Johnson F L, Lerner K G, Siegel M *et al*. Association of androgenic-anabolic steroid therapy with development of hepatocellular carcinoma. *Lancet* 1972; **2**(7790): 1273–1276

181 Edmondson H A, Reynolds T B, Henderson B, Benton B. Regression of liver cell adenomas associated with oral contraceptives. *Ann Intern Med* 1977; **86**(2): 180–182

182 Westaby D, Portmann B, Williams R. Androgen related primary hepatic tumors in non-Fanconi patients. *Cancer* 1983; **51**(10): 1947–1952

183 Nguyen G K. Fine-needle aspiration biopsy cytology of hepatic tumors in adults. *Pathol Annu* 1986; **21**(Part1): 321–349

184 Cho C, Rullis I, Rogers L S. Bile duct adenomas as liver nodules. *Arch Surg* 1978; **113**(3): 272–274

185 Iemoto Y, Kondo Y, Nakano T *et al*. Biliary cystadenocarcinoma diagnosed by liver biopsy performed under ultrasonographic guidance. *Gastroenterology* 1983; **84**(2): 399–403

186 Woods G L. Biliary cystadenocarcinoma: Case report of hepatic malignancy originating in benign cystadenoma. *Cancer* 1981; **47**(12): 2936–2940

187 Ishak K G, Willis G W, Cummins S D, Bullock A A. Biliary cystadenoma and cystadenocarcinoma: report of 14 cases and review of the literature. *Cancer* 1977; **39**(1): 322–338

188 Wheeler D A, Edmondson H A. Cystadenoma with mesenchymal stroma (CMS) in the liver and bile ducts. A clinicopathologic study of 17 cases, 4 with malignant change. *Cancer* 1985; **56**(6): 1434–1445

189 Pinto M M, Kaye A D. Fine needle aspiration of cystic liver lesions. Cytologic examination and carcinoembryonic antigen assay of cyst contents. *Acta Cytol* 1989; **33**(6): 852–856

190 Adam Y G, Nonas C J. Hepatobiliary cystadenoma. *South Med J* 1995; **88**(11): 1140–1143

191 Frick M P, Feinberg S B. Biliary cystadenoma. *Am J Roentgenol* 1982; **139**(2): 393–395

192 Ishak K G, Rabin L. Benign tumors of the liver. *Med Clin North Am* 1975; **59**(4): 995–1013

193 Taavitsainen M, Kivisaari L. Is fine-needle biopsy of liver hemangioma hazardous? *Am J Roentgenol* 1987; **148**(1): 231–232

194 Caturelli E, Rapaccini G L, Sabelli C *et al*. Ultrasound-guided fine-needle aspiration biopsy in the diagnosis of hepatic hemangioma. *Liver* 1986; **6**(6): 326–330

195 Solbiati L, Livraghi T, De Pra L *et al*. Fine-needle biopsy of hepatic hemangioma with sonographic guidance. *Am J Roentgenol* 1985; **144**(3): 471–474

196 Taavitsainen M, Airaksinen T, Kreula J, Paivansalo M. Fine-needle aspiration biopsy of liver hemangioma. *Acta Radiol* 1990; **31**(1): 69–71

197 Layfield L J, Mooney E E, Dodd L G. Not by blood alone: diagnosis of hemangiomas by fine-needle aspiration. *Diagn Cytopathol* 1998; **19**(4): 250–254

198 Ishak K G. Mesenchymal tumours of the liver. In: Okuda K P, Peters R L eds. *Hepatocellular Carcinoma*. New York: John Wiley, 1976; 247–304

199 Nonomura A, Mizukami Y, Kadoya M. Angiomyolipoma of the liver: a collective review. *J Gastroenterol* 1994; **29**(1): 95–105

200 Tsui W M, Colombari R, Portmann B C et al. Hepatic angiomyolipoma: a clinicopathologic study of 30 cases and delineation of unusual morphologic variants. *Am J Surg Pathol* 1999; **23**(1): 34–48

201 Pea M, Bonetti F, Zamboni G et al. Melanocyte-marker HMB-45 is regularly expressed in angiomyolipoma of the kidney. *Pathology* 1991; **23**(3): 185–188

202 Bonetti F, Pea M, Martignoni G et al. The perivascular epithelioid cell and related lesions. *Adv Anat Pathol* 1997; **4**: 343–358

203 Cha I, Cartwright D, Guis M et al. Angiomyolipoma of the liver in fine-needle aspiration biopsies: its distinction from hepatocellular carcinoma. *Cancer* 1999; **87**(1): 25–30

204 Ma T K, Tse M K, Tsui W M, Yuen K T. Fine needle aspiration diagnosis of angiomyolipoma of the liver using a cell block with immunohistochemical study. A case report. *Acta Cytol* 1994; **38**(2): 257–260

205 Sawai H, Manabe T, Yamanaka Y et al. Angiomyolipoma of the liver: case report and collective review of cases diagnosed from fine needle aspiration biopsy specimens. *J Hepatobiliary Pancreat Surg* 1998; **5**(3): 333–338

206 Sempoux C, Weynand B, van Beers B E et al. Angiomyolipoma of the liver: an unusual benign tumour identifiable on cytological material. *Cytopathol* 1997; **8**(3): 196–202

207 Anthony P P. Primary carcinoma of the liver: a study of 282 cases in Ugandan Africans. *J Pathol* 1973; **110**(1): 37–48

208 Weinberg A G, Mize C E, Worthen H G. The occurrence of hepatoma in the chronic form of hereditary tyrosinemia. *J Pediatr* 1976; **88**(3): 434–438

209 Messner M, Deugnier Y, Bernard-Griffiths I et al. Value of ultrasound-guided cytopuncture in the diagnosis of tumors in cirrhosis. Study of 29 cases. *Gastroenterol Clin Biol* 1985; **9**(1): 42–46

210 Jones D B, Koorey D J. Screening studies and markers. *Gastroenterol Clin North Am* 1987; **16**(4): 563–573

211 Pannall P, Kotesak D. *Cancer and Clinical Biochemistry*. London: ABC Venture Publications, 1997

212 Ebara M, Ohto M, Shinagawa T et al. Natural history of minute hepatocellular carcinoma smaller than three centimeters complicating cirrhosis. A study in 22 patients. *Gastroenterology* 1986; **90**(2): 289–298

213 Livraghi T, Sangalli G, Giordano F et al. 240 hepatocellular carcinomas: ultrasound features, tumor size, cytologic and histologic patterns, serum alpha-fetoprotein and HBs Ag. *Tumori* 1987; **73**(5): 507–512

214 Michel R P, Limacher J J, Kimoff R J. Mallory bodies in scar adenocarcinoma of the lung. *Hum Pathol* 1982; **13**(1): 81–85

215 Adeyanju M O, Dodd G D, Madariaga J R, Dekker A. Ultrasonically guided fine-needle aspiration biopsy of portal vein thrombosis: a cytomorphological study of

14 patients. *Diagn Cytopathol* 1994; **11**(3): 281–285

216 Greene C A, Suen K C. Some cytologic features of hepatocellular carcinoma as seen in fine needle aspirates. *Acta Cytol* 1984; **28**(6): 713–718

217 Noguchi S, Yamamoto R, Tatsuta M et al. Cell features and patterns in fine-needle aspirates of hepatocellular carcinoma. *Cancer* 1986; **58**(2): 321–328

218 Tao L C, Donat E E, Ho C S, McLoughlin M J. Percutaneous fine-needle aspiration biopsy of the liver. Cytodiagnosis of hepatic cancer. *Acta Cytol* 1979; **23**(4): 287–291

219 Edmondson H A, Steiner P E. Primary carcinoma of the liver: a study of 100 cases amongst 48,900 necropsies. *Cancer* 1954; **7**: 462–503

220 Kondo F, Hirooka N, Wada K, Kondo Y. Morphological clues for the diagnosis of small hepatocellular carcinomas. *Virchows Arch A Pathol Anat Histopathol* 1987; **411**(1): 15–21

221 Nagato Y, Kondo F, Kondo Y et al. Histological and morphometrical indicators for a biopsy diagnosis of well-differentiated hepatocellular carcinoma. *Hepatology* 1991; **14**(3): 473–478

222 Ali M A, Akhtar M, Mattingly R C. Morphologic spectrum of hepatocellular carcinoma in fine needle aspiration biopsies. *Acta Cytol* 1986; **30**(3): 294–302

223 Grimelius L, Stenram U, Westman J, Westman-Naeser S. Hyaline cytoplasmic inclusions in human hepatoma. A case report. *Acta Cytol* 1977; **21**(3): 469–476

224 Gupta S K, Das D K, Rajwanshi A, Bhusnurmath S R. Cytology of hepatocellular carcinoma. *Diagn Cytopathol* 1986; **2**(4): 290–294

225 Dodd G D, Carr B I. Percutaneous biopsy of portal vein thrombus: a new staging technique for hepatocellular carcinoma. *Am J Roentgenol* 1993; **161**(2): 229–233

226 De Sio I, Castellano L, Calandra M et al. Ultrasound-guided fine needle aspiration biopsy of portal vein thrombosis in liver cirrhosis: results in 15 patients. *J Gastroenterol Hepatol* 1995; **10**(6): 662–665

227 Berman M A, Burnham J A, Sheahan D G. Fibrolamellar carcinoma of the liver: an immunohistochemical study of nineteen cases and a review of the literature. *Hum Pathol* 1988; **19**(7): 784–794

228 Craig J R, Peters R L, Edmondson H A, Omata M. Fibrolamellar carcinoma of the liver: a tumor of adolescents and young adults with distinctive clinico-pathologic features. *Cancer* 1980; **46**(2): 372–379

229 Davenport R D. Cytologic diagnosis of fibrolamellar carcinoma of the liver by fine-needle aspiration. *Diagn Cytopathol* 1990; **6**(4): 275–279

230 Suen K C, Magee J F, Halparin L S et al. Fine needle aspiration cytology of fibrolamellar hepatocellular carcinoma. *Acta Cytol* 1985; **29**(5): 867–872

231 Perez-Guillermo M, Masgrau N A, Garcia-Solano J et al. Cytologic aspect of fibrolamellar hepatocellular carcinoma in fine-needle aspirates. *Diagn Cytopathol* 1999; **21**(3): 180–187

232 Buchanan T F, Huvos A G. Clear-cell carcinoma of the liver. A clinicopathologic study of 13 patients. *Am J Clin Pathol* 1974; **61**(4): 529–539

233 Mathew T, Affandi M Z. Fine needle aspiration biopsy of a hepatic mass. An example of a near error. *Acta Cytol* 1989; **33**(6): 861–864

234 Jensen C S, Donnelly A D, Silverman J F et al. The role of fine needle aspiration cytology in the work up of metastatic clear cell tumours. *Mod Pathol* 1995; **8**: Abstract 41A

235 Gupta R K, AlAnsari A G, Fauck R. Aspiration cytodiagnosis of clear cell hepatocellular carcinoma in an elderly woman. A case report. *Acta Cytol* 1994; **38**(3): 467–469

236 Donat E E, Anderson V, Tao L C. Cytodiagnosis of clear cell hepatocellular carcinoma. A case report. *Acta Cytol* 1991; **35**(6): 671–675

237 Singh H K, Silverman J F, Geisinger K R. Fine-needle aspiration cytomorphology of clear-cell hepatocellular carcinoma. *Diagn Cytopathol* 1997; **17**(4): 306–310

238 Weir M, Pitman M B. The vascular architecture of renal cell carcinoma in fine-needle aspiration biopsies. An aid in its distinction from hepatocellular carcinoma. *Cancer* 1997; **81**(1): 45–50

239 Suen K C. Diagnosis of primary hepatic neoplasms by fine-needle aspiration cytology. *Diagn Cytopathol* 1986; **2**(2): 99–109

240 Tatsuta M, Yamamoto R, Kasugai H et al. Cytohistologic diagnosis of neoplasms of the liver by ultrasonically guided fine-needle aspiration biopsy. *Cancer* 1984; **54**(8): 1682–1686

241 Chetty R, Learmonth G M, Taylor D A. Giant cell hepatocellular carcinoma. *Cytopathol* 1990; **1**(4): 233–237

242 Hood D L, Bauer T W, Leibel S A, McMahon J T. Hepatic giant cell carcinoma. An ultrastructural and immunohistochemical study. *Am J Clin Pathol* 1990; **93**(1): 111–116

243 McCluggage W G, Toner P G. Hepatocellular carcinoma with osteoclast-like giant cells. *Histopathol* 1993; **23**(2): 187–189

244 Wee A, Nilsson B, Tan L K, Yap I. Fine needle aspiration biopsy of hepatocellular carcinoma. Diagnostic dilemma at the ends of the spectrum. *Acta Cytol* 1994; **38**(3): 347–354

245 Kung I T, Chan S K, Fung K H. Fine-needle aspiration in hepatocellular carcinoma. Combined cytologic and histologic approach. *Cancer* 1991; **67**(3): 673–680

246 Pitman M B, Szyfelbein W M. Significance of endothelium in the fine-needle aspiration biopsy diagnosis of hepatocellular carcinoma [see comments]. *Diagn Cytopathol* 1995; **12**(3): 208–214

247 Tao L C, Ho C S, McLoughlin M J et al. Cytologic diagnosis of hepatocellular carcinoma by fine-needle aspiration biopsy. *Cancer* 1984; **53**(3): 547–552

248 Abendroth C S, Grenko R T, Welch D R. Features distinguishing cirrhosis from

hepatocellular carcinoma by fine needle aspiration. *Acta Cytol* 1994; **38**(5): Abstract 16, p. 800

249 Das D K. Cytodiagnosis of hepatocellular carcinoma in fine-needle aspirates of the liver: its differentiation from reactive hepatocytes and metastatic adenocarcinoma. *Diagn Cytopathol* 1999; **21**(6): 370–377

250 Wee A, Nilsson B, Chan-Wilde C *et al.* Cytological diagnosis from fine needle aspiration biopsy of the liver. *Ann Acad Med Singapore* 1991; **20**(2): 208–214

251 Pedio G, Landolt U, Zobeli L, Gut D. Fine needle aspiration of the liver. Significance of hepatocytic naked nuclei in the diagnosis of hepatocellular carcinoma. *Acta Cytol* 1988; **32**(4): 437–442

252 Bottles K, Cohen M B, Holly E A *et al.* A step-wise logistic regression analysis of hepatocellular carcinoma. An aspiration biopsy study. *Cancer* 1988; **62**(3): 558–563

253 Ferrell L D, Crawford J M, Dhillon A P *et al.* Proposal for standardized criteria for the diagnosis of benign, borderline, and malignant hepatocellular lesions arising in chronic advanced liver disease. *Am J Surg Pathol* 1993; **17**(11): 1113–1123

254 Ferrell L, Wright T, Lake J *et al.* Incidence and diagnostic features of macroregenerative nodules *vs.* small hepatocellular carcinoma in cirrhotic livers. *Hepatology* 1992; **16**(6): 1372–1381

255 International Working Party. Terminology of nodular hepatocellular lesions. *Hepatology* 1995; **22**(3): 983–993

256 Dhillon A P, Colombari R, Savage K, Scheuer P J. An immunohistochemical study of the blood vessels within primary hepatocellular tumours. *Liver* 1992; **12**(5): 311–318

257 Ruck P, Xiao J C, Kaiserling E. Immunoreactivity of sinusoids in hepatocellular carcinoma. An immunohistochemical study using lectin UEA-1 and antibodies against endothelial markers, including CD34. *Arch Pathol Lab Med* 1995; **119**(2): 173–178

258 Scott F R, el-Refaie A, More L *et al.* Hepatocellular carcinoma arising in an adenoma: value of QBend 10 immunostaining in diagnosis of liver cell carcinoma. *Histopathol* 1996; **28**(5): 472–474

259 Tanigawa N, Lu C, Mitsui T, Miura S. Quantitation of sinusoid-like vessels in hepatocellular carcinoma: its clinical and prognostic significance. *Hepatology* 1997; **26**(5): 1216–1223

260 Maeda T, Adachi E, Kajiyama K *et al.* CD34 expression in endothelial cells of small hepatocellular carcinoma: its correlation with tumour progression and angiographic findings. *J Gastroenterol Hepatol* 1995; **10**(6): 650–654

261 Cui S, Hano H, Sakata A *et al.* Enhanced CD34 expression of sinusoid-like vascular endothelial cells in hepatocellular carcinoma. *Pathol Int* 1996; **46**(10): 751–756

262 de Boer W B, Segal A, Frost F A, Sterrett G F. Can CD34 discriminate between benign and malignant hepatocytic lesions in fine-

needle aspirates and thin core biopsies? *Cancer* 2000 Oct 25; **90**(5): 273–278

263 Abraham S, Sack M, Furth E E. The utility of CD34 in distinguishing hepatocellular carcinoma from non-neoplastic lesions in fine needle aspirates of the liver. *Mod Pathol* 1999; **12**(1): Abstract 211 p39A

264 Gottschalk-Sabag S, Ron N, Glick T. Use of CD34 and factor VIII to diagnose hepatocellular carcinoma on fine needle aspirates. *Acta Cytol* 1998; **42**(3): 691–696

265 Kong C S, Appenzeller M, Ferrell L D. Utility of CD34 reactivity in evaluating focal nodular hepatocellular lesions sampled by fine needle aspiration biopsy. *Acta Cytol* 2000; **44**(2): 218–222

266 Ojanguren I, Castella E, Llatjos M *et al.* p53 immunoreaction in hepatocellular carcinoma and its relationship to etiologic factors. A fine needle aspiration study. *Acta Cytol* 1996; **40**(6): 1148–1153

267 Adachi E, Hashimoto H, Tsuneyoshi M. Proliferating cell nuclear antigen in hepatocellular carcinoma and small cell liver dysplasia. *Cancer* 1993; **72**(10): 2902–2909

268 Ng I O L, Lai E C S, Ho J C W *et al.* Flow cytometric analysis of DNA ploidy in hepatocellular carcinoma. *AJCP* 1994; **102**(1): 80–86

269 Deprez C, Vangansbeke D, Fastrez R *et al.* Nuclear DNA content, proliferation index, and nuclear size determination in normal and cirrhotic liver, and in benign and malignant primary and metastatic hepatic tumors [see comments]. *Am J Clin Pathol* 1993; **99**(5): 558–565

270 Vasef M A, Ross J S, Cohen M B. Telomerase activity in human solid tumors. Diagnostic utility and clinical applications. *Am J Clin Pathol* 1999; **112**(1suppl 1): S68–S75

271 Nagao K, Tomimatsu M, Endo H *et al.* Telomerase reverse transcriptase mRNA expression and telomerase activity in hepatocellular carcinoma. *J Gastroenterol* 1999; **34**(1): 83–87

272 Nakashio R, Kitamoto M, Tahara H *et al.* Significance of telomerase activity in the diagnosis of small differentiated hepatocellular carcinoma. *Int J Cancer* 1997; **74**(2): 141–147

273 Anthony P P, Vogel C L, Barker L F. Liver cell dysplasia: a premalignant condition. *J Clin Pathol* 1973; **26**(3): 217–223

274 Borzio M, Bruno S, Roncalli M *et al.* Liver cell dysplasia is a major risk factor for hepatocellular carcinoma in cirrhosis: a prospective study. *Gastroenterology* 1995; **108**(3): 812–817

275 Mion F, Grozel L, Boillot O *et al.* Adult cirrhotic liver explants: precancerous lesions and undetected small hepatocellular carcinomas. *Gastroenterology* 1996; **111**(6): 1587–1592

276 Ganne-Carrie N, Chastang C, Chapel F *et al.* Predictive score for the development of hepatocellular carcinoma and additional value of liver large cell dysplasia in Western patients with cirrhosis. *Hepatology* 1996; **23**(5): 1112–1118

277 Cohen C, Berson S D. Liver cell dysplasia in normal, cirrhotic, and hepatocellular

carcinoma patients. *Cancer* 1986; **57**(8): 1535–1538

278 Henmi A, Uchida T, Shikata T. Karyometric analysis of liver cell dysplasia and hepatocellular carcinoma. Evidence against precancerous nature of liver cell dysplasia. *Cancer* 1985; **55**(11): 2594–2599

279 Hytiroglou P, Theise N D, Schwartz M *et al.* Macroregenerative nodules in a series of adult cirrhotic liver explants: issues of classification and nomenclature. *Hepatology* 1995; **21**(3): 703–708

280 Ballardini G, Groff P, Zoli M *et al.* Increased risk of hepatocellular carcinoma development in patients with cirrhosis and with high hepatocellular proliferation. *J Hepatol* 1994; **20**(2): 218–222

281 Roncalli M, Borzio M, de Biagi G *et al.* Liver cell dysplasia and hepatocellular carcinoma: a histological and immunohistochemical study. *Histopathol* 1985; **9**(2): 209–221

282 Schwartz M R. Liver cell dysplasia and other atypical lesions: new insights and applications. *Adv Anat Pathol* 1998; **5**(2): 99–105

283 Watanabe S, Okita K, Harada T *et al.* Morphologic studies of the liver cell dysplasia. *Cancer* 1983; **51**(12): 2197–2205

284 Silverman J F, Geisinger K R. *Fine Needle Aspiration Cytology of the Thorax and Abdomen*, 1st edn. Hong Kong: Churchill Livingstone, 1996

285 Pedio G, Zobeli L, Landolt U. Cytological diagnosis of hepatocellular carcinoma based on ultrasonically guided fine needle biopsy. *Schweiz Med Wochenschr* 1988; **118**(7): 239–243

286 Shariff S, Thomas J A, Kaliaperumal V G. An experience with ultrasonically guided liver aspirates from south India. *Cytopathol* 1993; **4**(5): 291–298

287 Domagala W, Lasota J, Weber K, Osborn M. Endothelial cells help in the diagnosis of primary *vs* metastatic carcinoma of the liver in fine needle aspirates. An immunofluorescence study with vimentin and endothelial cell-specific antibodies. *Anal Quant Cytol Histol* 1989; **11**(1): 8–14

288 Pitman M B. Fine needle aspiration biopsy of the liver. Principal diagnostic challenges. *Clin Lab Med* 1998; **18**(3): 483–506

289 Bret P M, Labadie M, Bretagnolle M *et al.* Hepatocellular carcinoma: diagnosis by percutaneous fine needle biopsy. *Gastrointest Radiol* 1988; **13**(3): 253–255

290 Whitlatch S, Nunez C, Pitlik D A. Fine needle aspiration biopsy of the liver. A study of 102 consecutive cases. *Acta Cytol* 1984; **28**(6): 719–725

291 Ekelund P, Wasastjerna C. Cytological identification of primary hepatic carcinoma cells. *Acta Med Scand* 1971; **189**(5): 373–375

292 Wasastjerna C, Ekelund P. The amino acid naphthylamidase reaction of the bile canaliculi in liver smears. *Acta Cytol* 1974; **18**(1): 23–29

293 Sharifi S, Hayek J, Khettry U, Nasser I. Immunocytochemical staining of Kupffer and endothelial cells in fine needle

aspiration cytology of hepatocellular carcinoma. *Acta Cytol* 2000; **44**(1): 7–12

294 Carter R. Hepatoblastoma in the adult. *Cancer* 1969; **23**(1): 191–197

295 Dekmezian R, Sneige N, Popok S, Ordonez N G. Fine-needle aspiration cytology of pediatric patients with primary hepatic tumors: a comparative study of two hepatoblastomas and a liver-cell carcinoma. *Diagn Cytopathol* 1988; **4**(2): 162–168

296 Ersoz C, Zorludemir U, Tanyeli A *et al.* Fine needle aspiration cytology of hepatoblastoma. A report of two cases. *Acta Cytol* 1998; **42**(3): 799–802

297 Kaw Y T, Hansen K. Fine needle aspiration cytology of undifferentiated small cell ('anaplastic') hepatoblastoma. A case report. *Acta Cytol* 1993; **37**(2): 216–220

298 Cangiarella J, Greco M A, Waisman J. Hepatoblastoma. Report of a case with cytologic, histologic and ultrastructural findings. *Acta Cytol* 1994; **38**(3): 455–458

299 Wakely P E, Silverman J F, Geisinger K R, Frable W J. Fine needle aspiration biopsy cytology of hepatoblastoma. *Mod Pathol* 1990; **3**(6): 688–693

300 Sola Perez J, Perez-Guillermo M, Bas Bernal A B, Mercader J M. Hepatoblastoma. An attempt to apply histologic classification to aspirates obtained by fine needle aspiration cytology. *Acta Cytol* 1994; **38**(2): 175–182

301 Bhatia A, Mehrotra P. Fine needle aspiration cytology in a case of hepatoblastoma. *Acta Cytol* 1986; **30**(4): 439–441

302 Akwari O E, Van Heerden J A, Foulk W T, Baggenstoss A H. Cancer of the bile ducts associated with ulcerative colitis. *Ann Surg* 1975; **181**(3): 303–309

303 Imamura M, Miyashita T, Tani T *et al.* Cholangiocellular carcinoma associated with multiple liver cysts. *Am J Gastroenterol* 1984; **79**(10): 790–795

304 Kasai Y, Sasaki E, Tamaki A *et al.* Carcinoma arising in the cyst of the liver – report of three cases. *Jpn J Surg* 1977; **7**(2): 65–72

305 Winberg C D, Ranchod M. Thorotrast induced hepatic cholangiocarcinoma and angiosarcoma. *Hum Pathol* 1979; **10**(1): 108–112

306 Karstrup S. Ultrasound diagnosis of cholangiocarcinoma at the confluence of the hepatic ducts (Klatskin tumours). *Br J Radiol* 1988; **61**(731): 987–990

307 Barr R J, Hancock D E. Adenosquamous carcinoma of the liver. *Gastroenterology* 1975; **69**(6): 1326–1330

308 Ho J C. Two cases of mucoepidermoid carcinoma of the liver in Chinese. *Pathology* 1980; **12**(1): 123–128

309 Sasaki M, Nakanuma Y, Nagai Y, Nonomura A. Intrahepatic cholangiocarcinoma with sarcomatous transformation: an autopsy case. *J Clin Gastroenterol* 1991; **13**(2): 220–225

310 Tarroch X, Tallada N, Castells C, Garcia M. Fine-needle aspiration biopsy of hepatic papillary cystadenocarcinoma in Caroli's disease. *Diagn Cytopathol* 1992; **8**(2): 167–170

311 Tsui W M, Lam P W, Mak C K, Pay K H. Fine-needle aspiration cytologic diagnosis of intrahepatic biliary papillomatosis (intraductal papillary tumor): report of three cases and comparative study with cholangiocarcinoma. *Diagn Cytopathol* 2000; **22**(5): 293–298

312 Wee A, Nilsson B, Kang J Y *et al.* Biliary cystadenocarcinoma arising in a cystadenoma. Report of a case diagnosed by fine needle aspiration cytology. *Acta Cytol* 1993; **37**(6): 966–970

313 Azizah N, Paradinas F J. Cholangiocarcinoma coexisting with developmental liver cysts: a distinct entity different from liver cystadenocarcinoma. *Histopathol* 1980; **4**(4): 391–400

314 Ameriks J, Appleman H, Frey C. Malignant nonparasitic cyst of the liver: case report. *Ann Surg* 1972; **176**(6): 713–717

315 Dean D L, Bauer H M. Primary cystic carcinoma of the liver. *Am J Surg* 1969; **117**(3): 416–420

316 Kanamori H, Kawahara H, Oh S *et al.* A case of biliary cystadenocarcinoma with recurrent jaundice. Diagnostic evaluation of computed tomography. *Cancer* 1985; **55**(11): 2722–2724

317 Bloom W. The embryogenesis of human bile duct capillaries and ducts. *Am J Anat* 1925–1926; **36**: 451–466

318 Shiojiri N. The origin of intrahepatic bile duct cells in the mouse. *J Embryol Exp Morphol* 1984; **79**(2): 25–39

319 Goodman Z D, Ishak K G, Langloss J M *et al.* Combined hepatocellular-cholangiocarcinoma. A histologic and immunohistochemical study. *Cancer* 1985; **55**(1): 124–135

320 Gibbons D, de las Morenas A. Fine needle aspiration diagnosis of combined hepatocellular carcinoma and cholangiocarcinoma. A case report. *Acta Cytol* 1997; **41**(Suppl 4): 1269–1272

321 Kilpatrick S E, Geisinger K R, Loggie B W, Hopkins M B D. Cytomorphology of combined hepatocellular-cholangiocarcinoma in fine needle aspirates of the liver. A report of two cases. *Acta Cytol* 1993; **37**(6): 943–947

322 Wee A, Nilsson B. Combined hepatocellular-cholangiocarcinoma. Diagnostic challenge in hepatic fine needle aspiration biopsy. *Acta Cytol* 1999; **43**(2): 131–138

323 Gresham G A, Rue L W. Squamous cell carcinoma of the liver. *Hum Pathol* 1985; **16**(4): 413–416

324 Lynch M J, McLeod M K, Weatherbee L *et al.* Squamous cell cancer of the liver arising from a solitary benign nonparasitic hepatic cyst. *Am J Gastroenterol* 1988; **83**(4): 426–431

325 Song E, Kew M C, Grieve T *et al.* Primary squamous cell carcinoma of the liver occurring in association with hepatolithiasis. *Cancer* 1984; **53**(3): 542–546

326 Gupta R K, Naran S, Lallu S, Fauck R. Fine needle aspiration diagnosis of neuroendocrine tumors in the liver. *Pathology* 2000; **32**(1): 16–20

327 Miura K, Shirasawa H. Primary carcinoid tumor of the liver. *Am J Clin Pathol* 1988; **89**(4): 561–564

328 Sioutos N, Virta S, Kessimian N. Primary hepatic carcinoid tumor. An electron microscopic and immunohistochemical study. *Am J Clin Pathol* 1991; **95**(2): 172–175

329 Nakasuka H, Okada S, Okusaka T *et al.* Undifferentiated carcinoma of the liver with neuroendocrine features: a case report. *Jpn J Clin Oncol* 1998; **28**(6): 401–404

330 Barsky S H, Linnoila I, Triche T J, Costa J. Hepatocellular carcinoma with carcinoid features. *Hum Pathol* 1984; **15**(9): 892–894

331 Piatti B, Caspani B, Giudici C, Ferrario D. Fine needle aspiration biopsy of hepatocellular carcinoma resembling neuroendocrine tumor. A case report. *Acta Cytol* 1997; **41**(2): 583–586

332 Pisharodi L R, Bedrossian C. Diagnosis and differential diagnosis of small-cell lesions of the liver. *Diagn Cytopathol* 1998; **19**(1): 29–32

333 Wee A, Nilsson B, Yap I. Fine needle aspiration biopsy of small/intermediate cell tumors in the liver. Considerations in a southeast Asian population. *Acta Cytol* 1996; **40**(5): 937–947

334 Alpert L I, Zak F G, Werthamer S, Bochetto J F. Cholangiocarcinoma: a clinicopathologic study of five cases with ultrastructural observations. *Hum Pathol* 1974; **5**(6): 709–728

335 Primack A, Wilson J, GT O C *et al.* Hepatocellular carcinoma with the carcinoid syndrome. *Cancer* 1971; **27**(5): 1182–1189

336 Baxter P J, Anthony P P, Macsween R N, Scheuer P J. Angiosarcoma of the liver: annual occurrence and aetiology in Great Britain. *Br J Ind Med* 1980; **37**(3): 213–221

337 Falk H, Thomas L B, Popper H, Ishak K G. Hepatic angiosarcoma associated with androgenic-anabolic steroids. *Lancet* 1979; **2**(8152): 1120–1123

338 Thomas L B, Popper H, Berk P D *et al.* Vinyl-chloride-induced liver disease. From idiopathic portal hypertension (Banti's syndrome) to angiosarcomas. *N Engl J Med* 1975; **292**(1): 17–22

339 Locker G Y, Doroshow J H, Zwelling L A, Chabner B A. The clinical features of hepatic angiosarcoma: a report of four cases and a review of the English literature. *Medicine (Baltimore)* 1979; **58**(1): 48–64

340 Koss L G, Woyke S, Olszewski W. *Aspiration Biopsy; Cytologic Interpretation and Histologic Basis*, 1st edn. Tokyo: Igaku-Shoin, 1984

341 Ludwig J, Hoffman H N. Hemangiosarcoma of the liver. Spectrum of morphologic changes and clinical findings. *Mayo Clin Proc* 1975; **50**(5): 255–263

342 Orchard G E, Zelger B, Jones E W, Jones R R. An immunocytochemical assessment of 19 cases of cutaneous angiosarcoma. *Histopathol* 1996; **28**(3): 235–240

343 Cho N H, Lee K G, Jeong M G. Cytologic evaluation of primary malignant vascular tumors of the liver. One case each of angiosarcoma and epithelioid hemangioendothelioma. *Acta Cytol* 1997; **41**(5): 1468–1476

344 Liu K, Layfield L J. Cytomorphologic features of angiosarcoma on fine needle aspiration biopsy. *Acta Cytol* 1999; **43**(3): 407–415

345 Nguyen G K, Husain M. Fine-needle aspiration biopsy cytology of angiosarcoma. *Diagn Cytopathol* 2000; **23**(2): 143–145

346 Saleh H A, Tao L C. Hepatic angiosarcoma: aspiration biopsy cytology and immunocytochemical contribution. *Diagn Cytopathol* 1998; **18**(3): 208–211

347 Wong J W, Bedard Y C. Fine-needle aspiration biopsy of hepatic angiosarcoma: report of a case with immunocytochemical findings. *Diagn Cytopathol* 1992; **8**(4): 380–383

348 Gambacorta M, Bonacina E. Epithelioid hemangioendothelioma: report of a case diagnosed by fine-needle aspiration. *Diagn Cytopathol* 1989; **5**(2): 207–210

349 Sola-Perez J, Perez-Guillermo M, Gimenez-Bascunana A, Garre-Sanchez C. Cytopathology of undifferentiated (embryonal) sarcoma of the liver. *Diagn Cytopathol* 1995; **13**(1): 44–51

350 Garcia-Bonafe M, Allende H, Fantova M J, Tarragona J. Fine needle aspiration cytology of undifferentiated (embryonal) sarcoma of the liver. A case report. *Acta Cytol* 1997; **41**(4 Suppl): 1273–1278

351 Krishnamurthy S C, Datta S, Jambhekar N A. Fine needle aspiration cytology of undifferentiated (embryonal) sarcoma of the liver: a case report. *Acta Cytol* 1996; **40**(3): 567–570

352 Pollono D G, Drut R. Undifferentiated (embryonal) sarcoma of the liver: fine-needle aspiration cytology and preoperative chemotherapy as an approach to diagnosis and initial treatment. A case report. *Diagn Cytopathol* 1998; **19**(2): 102–106

353 Pieterse A S, Smith M, Smith L A, Smith P. Embryonal (undifferentiated) sarcoma of the liver. Fine-needle aspiration cytology and ultrastructural findings. *Arch Pathol Lab Med* 1985; **109**(7): 677–680

354 McLoughlin L C, Nord K S, Joshi V V et al. Disseminated leiomyosarcoma in a child with acquired immune deficiency syndrome. *Cancer* 1991; **67**(10): 2618–2621

355 Mueller B U, Butler K M, Higham M C et al. Smooth muscle tumors in children with

human immunodeficiency virus infection. *Pediatrics* 1992; **90**(3): 460–463

356 Smith M B, Silverman J F, Raab S S et al. Fine-needle aspiration cytology of hepatic leiomyosarcoma. *Diagn Cytopathol* 1994; **11**(4): 321–327

357 DeMent S H, Mann R B, Staal S P et al. Primary lymphomas of the liver. Report of six cases and review of the literature. *Am J Clin Pathol* 1987; **88**(3): 255–263

358 Jaffe E S. Malignant lymphomas: pathology of hepatic involvement. *Semin Liver Dis* 1987; **7**(3): 257–268

359 Rappaport K M, DiGiuseppe J A, Busseniers A E. Primary hepatic lymphoma: report of two cases diagnosed by fine-needle aspiration. *Diagn Cytopathol* 1995; **13**(2): 142–145

360 Ellenrieder V, Beckh K, Muller D et al. Intrahepatic high-grade malignant non-Hodgkin lymphoma in a patient with chronic hepatitis C infection. *Z Gastroenterol* 1996; **34**(5): 283–285

361 Blandamura S, Boccato P. Primary isolated lymphoma of the liver: rapid cytological diagnosis by fine needle aspiration biopsy. *Pathologica* 1991; **83**(1083): 81–88

362 Collins K A, Geisinger K R, Raab S S, Silverman J F. Fine needle aspiration biopsy of hepatic lymphomas: cytomorphology and ancillary studies. *Acta Cytol* 1996; **40**(2): 257–262

363 Gattuso P, Reddy V B, Kizilbash N et al. Role of fine-needle aspiration in the clinical management of solid organ transplant recipients: a review. *Cancer* 1999; **87**(5): 286–294

364 Raymond E, Tricottet V, Samuel D et al. Epstein-Barr virus-related localized hepatic lymphoproliferative disorders after liver transplantation. *Cancer* 1995; **76**(8): 1344–1351

365 Wakely P E, Jr., Krummel T M, Johnson D E. Yolk sac tumor of the liver. *Mod Pathol* 1991; **4**(1): 121–125

366 Heaton G E, Matthews T H, Christopherson W M. Malignant trophoblastic tumors with massive hemorrhage presenting as liver primary. A report of two cases. *Am J Surg Pathol* 1986; **10**(5): 342–347

367 Cady B. Natural history of primary and secondary tumors of the liver. *Semin Oncol* 1983; **10**(2): 127–134

368 Dent G A, Feldman J M. Pseudocystic liver metastases in patients with carcinoid tumors: report of three cases. *Am J Clin Pathol* 1984; **82**(3): 275–279

369 Adson M A. Mass lesions of the liver. *Mayo Clin Proc* 1986; **61**(5): 362–367

370 Plafker J, Nosher J L. Fine needle aspiration of liver with metastatic adenoid cystic carcinoma. *Acta Cytol* 1983; **27**(3): 323–325

371 Wilander E, Norheim I, Oberg K. Application of silver stains to cytologic specimens of neuroendocrine tumors metastatic to the liver. *Acta Cytol* 1985; **29**(6): 1053–1057

372 Miettinen M, Sarlomo-Rikala M, Lasota J. Gastrointestinal stromal tumours: recent advances in understanding of their biology. *Hum Pathol* 1999; **30**(10): 1213–1220

373 Cheuk W, Lee K C, Chan J K. C-kit immunocytochemical staining in the cytologic diagnosis of metastatic gastrointestinal stromal tumor. A report of two cases. *Acta Cytol* 2000; **44**(4): 679–685

374 Dodd L G, Nelson R C, Mooney E E, Gottfried M. Fine-needle aspiration of gastrointestinal stromal tumors. *Am J Clin Pathol* 1998; **109**(4): 439–443

375 Isimbaldi G, Santangelo M, Cenacchi G et al. Gastrointestinal autonomic nerve tumor (plexosarcoma): report of a case with fine needle aspiration biopsy and histologic, immunocytochemical and ultrastructural study. *Acta Cytol* 1998; **42**(5): 1189–1194

376 Seidal T, Edvardsson H. Diagnosis of gastrointestinal stromal tumor by fine-needle aspiration biopsy: a cytological and immunocytochemical study. *Diagn Cytopathol* 2000; **23**(6): 397–401

377 Jansson S E, Bondestam S, Heinonen E et al. Value of liver and spleen aspiration biopsy in malignant diseases when these organs show no signs of involvement in sonography. *Acta Med Scand* 1983; **213**(4): 279–281

378 Benda J A, Zaleski S. Fine needle aspiration cytologic features of hepatic metastasis of granulosa cell tumor of the ovary. Differential diagnosis. *Acta Cytol* 1988; **32**(4): 527–532

379 Margolin K A, Pak H Y, Esensten M L, Doroshow J H. Hepatic metastasis in granulosa cell tumor of the ovary. *Cancer* 1985; **56**(3): 691–695

15 Gall bladder and extrahepatic bile ducts

Gregory F. Sterrett, Felicity A. Frost and Darrel Whitaker

Introduction and historical perspective

Carcinoma of the gall bladder is the fifth most common tumour of the gastrointestinal tract and constitutes about two-thirds of biliary tract tumours[1]. There is considerable geographical and racial variation in prevalence; the tumour is also much more common in females[1]. Pre-operative diagnosis is seldom made; diagnosis is usually established at laparotomy for presumed cholecystitis. The disease is associated with cholelithiasis and chronic cholecystitis in about 70% of cases. Calcification of the wall of the so-called 'porcelain' gall bladder was said to be associated with carcinoma in the past but this is now disputed[2].

Approximately 70% of tumours are unresectable and the overall prognosis remains poor. Radical surgery together with radiotherapy and chemotherapy may be of value for small numbers of patients with advanced disease. Secondary spread occurs to the liver, to adjacent cystic or common bile ducts and peripancreatic lymph nodes, and diffuse carcinomatosis is the usual final outcome. The median survival is around 8 months and the 5-year survival is less than 10%. Papillary adenocarcinoma is the only histological subtype with a significantly better survival, related in part to the lower stage at diagnosis.

Although studies of the progression and the development of gall bladder cancer have shown passage through stages of atypical hyperplasia and carcinoma *in situ*, similar to those in other epithelial tissues[3-6], no easy way of detecting these early lesions has been discovered in life. Owing to the risks of bile extravasation, particularly in the presence of bile duct stenosis[7], gall bladder puncture with bile aspiration is more suited to the immediate preoperative period[4]. The procedure is not appropriate for large scale screening, except perhaps in areas of particularly high prevalence such as reported in Mexico[8].

Cytological diagnosis is therefore generally restricted to percutaneous or intraoperative FNA of malignant mass lesions[9-12]. There have also been suggestions that the diagnosis of benign lesions by FNA may be of value intraoperatively, in order to reduce the need for resection[13]. Some authors report value in diagnosing malignancy by way of preoperative FNA or ultrasound guided FNA of the gall bladder for bile collection[8,14-16].

Carcinoma of the extrahepatic bile ducts constitutes one-third of biliary tract cancers[1]. In contrast to gall bladder cancer, gallstones are present in only 20% of cases[1]. There is however an association between carcinoma and sclerosing cholangitis or chronic suppurative cholangitis, biliary parasites such as liver flukes, ulcerative colitis and choledochal cysts[1]. A proportion of carcinomas may arise in pre-existing benign papillary neoplastic lesions, which may be localized or multifocal; papillary tumours have a better prognosis[1].

Clinical investigations are usually prompted by evidence of bile duct obstruction with elevated serum bilirubin, alkaline phosphatase and gamma glutamyl transferase and reduced albumin levels. Imaging techniques, such as ultrasound, and percutaneous transhepatic cholangiography (PTC) or endoscopic retrograde cholangiopancreatography (ERCP) are generally required for diagnosis. Fewer than 30% of cases are resectable locally and there is a mean survival of less than 30 months. More recently, radical liver and bile duct resection and liver transplantation have been performed, but in most cases, stenting of the obstructed segment is employed for palliation.

Hilar cholangiocarcinomas, so-called 'Klatskin' tumours[17], are a particular clinical problem because of difficulty in their diagnosis and a tendency to cause symptoms relating to obstruction and associated infection out of proportion to their size. They present with jaundice in 90–98% of cases, but may not if only a single intrahepatic duct is involved. Clinical diagnosis is very difficult because of the sclerosing or submucosal growth pattern, which closely mimics inflammatory processes, such as sclerosing cholangitis. Moreover, carcinoma may supervene in cases previously diagnosed as sclerosing cholangitis. Associated infection, inflammatory changes and fibrosis often obscure tumour tissue, and the well-differentiated nature of many of these cancers renders even histological diagnosis 'excruciatingly onerous' at times[18]. The overall prognosis is poor, but has improved somewhat with more radical approaches to surgery.

A range of other neoplastic and tumour-like processes occurs in the region (Table 15.1)[1,19].

Between the 1940s and 1960s per-oral duodenal aspiration of bile for cytology was an accepted method of diagnosis of malignancy[20-25]. The procedure was associated with significant patient discomfort and this limited its use,

Table 15.1   Primary tumours of the gall bladder and extrahepatic bile ducts[1,19]

Epithelial neoplasms	Carcinoid–adenocarcinoma (mixed)	Malignant melanoma
Benign	Paraganglioma, Gangliocytic	Malignant lymphoma
Adenoma	paraganglioma	Germ cell tumours
Papillomatosis		
Cystadenoma	**Non-epithelial neoplasms**	**Tumour-like lesions**
Epithelial dysplasia and carcinoma *in situ*	Benign	Regenerative epithelial atypia
Malignant	Leiomyoma	Papillary hyperplasia
Adenocarcinoma:	Lipoma	Squamous metaplasia
Papillary, intestinal, gastric foveolar,	Haemangioma	Adenomyomatous hyperplasia
clear cell, mucinous, signet ring,	Lymphangioma	Mucocoele
cystadenocarcinoma	Osteoma	Heterotopias
Adenosquamous carcinoma	Granular cell tumour	Cholesterol polyp
Squamous cell carcinoma	Neurofibroma	Inflammatory polyp
Small cell carcinoma (neuroendocrine,	Ganglioneuroma	Fibrous polyp
undifferentiated)	Malignant	Myofibroblastic proliferations
Large cell neuroendocrine carcinoma	Rhabdomyosarcoma	Xanthogranulomatous cholecystitis
Large cell undifferentiated carcinoma:	Malignant fibrous histiocytoma	Cholecystitis with lymphoid hyperplasia
Spindle and giant cell/Sarcomatoid	Angiosarcoma	Malacoplakia
With osteoclast-like giant cells	Leiomyosarcoma	Congenital cyst
Neuroendocrine neoplasms	Kaposi's sarcoma	Amputation neuroma
Carcinoid		Primary sclerosing cholangitis
Adenocarcinoid (goblet-cell carcinoid)	**Miscellaneous**	
	Carcinosarcoma	

though excellent results could be obtained and some reported a high sensitivity of detection of cancer[26,27].

In the 1970s, the development of endoscopic retrograde cholangiopancreatography (ERCP) and percutaneous transhepatic cholangiography (PTC) allowed direct aspiration of pancreatic and bile duct contents[28–32], and aspiration of bile from within the liver[33–35], techniques which are still finding their place in cytodiagnosis[36–43]. In addition, in the 1980s, various duct brushing and washing procedures were devised[14–16,18,42,44–47]. Also in the 1980s, percutaneous transcatheter brushing[47–53] and fine needle aspiration directed at masses imaged by ultrasound[54–56], fluoroscopy[55,56], CT[57], ducts opacified by contrast media, stent tubes or PTC tubes within obstructed ducts[33,39], either alone or in combinations of the above[38,55,56,58], became more widely used.

In the late 1980s and 1990s, transductal and transcatheter fine needle aspiration were introduced[59,60]. In the last decade of the twentieth century, there was more widespread use of brush and guidewires designed for multiple lumen catheters and endoscopes, allowing more effective sampling of strictures[61,62]. Endoscopic ultrasound guided FNA is now used in some centres[63]. Our own experience has mirrored this trend. The highest yield of positive diagnoses has been from duct brushings and percutaneous FNA samples directed at masses, opacified ducts or the sites of stent tubes. Small numbers of cases are diagnosed on aspirated bile, or by intra-operative FNA, or transductal FNA samples. Despite these technical efforts the overall accuracy is still described as 'modest'[64–66].

Other modalities have been used to increase the sensitivity of cytological diagnosis. DNA ploidy analysis may increase sensitivity but with increased false positives[67].

Mutations in p53 and ras oncogenes are a common finding in biliary carcinomas[68], however the diagnostic value of their detection in cytological preparations either by PCR or immunocytochemistry is debated. Some workers found no increase in sensitivity over cytology for p53 immunocytochemistry[69,70]. Others were able to increase the sensitivity over cytological diagnosis alone, but with a relatively low overall sensitivity[71]. Assessing Ki-ras mutations by PCR of brushings may be limited by the presence of such changes in hyperplasias, by intratumoural heterogeneity and by low frequency in bile duct compared to pancreatic carcinoma[72]. Telomerase activity has also been associated with bile duct carcinoma and can be measured in cytological samples[73].

Value and limitations of cytological diagnosis

Diagnosis of malignant tumours of this region is a continuing challenge to medicine. Although technical advances have resulted in improved endoscopic diagnosis and simple by-pass procedures have been developed to relieve bile duct obstruction, neither endoscopic nor cytological methods have resulted in a significant improvement in the ultimate clinical outcome. For example, in the 1980s, Yamada was able to diagnose 21 of 23 bile duct cancers on bile cytology mainly at percutaneous transhepatic cholangiography (PTC); 12 of these were considered operable but cure was likely in only three cases, including one apparently *in situ* lesion and one minimally invasive carcinoma[43]. There has been little change in overall outcomes since that time.

The role of cytology in this area is therefore mainly to provide a definitive diagnosis of malignancy to support a clinical or endoscopic diagnosis. This will allow palliative therapy, particularly for bile duct obstruction by tumour, and it will ensure the avoidance of more extensive investigations. Cytodiagnosis by a single technique or on a single sample has a lower sensitivity in the detection of malignancy here than in some other sites and the area is one of acknowledged difficulty in diagnosis. Cellular degeneration in bile or duodenal contents and the well differentiated and fibrosing growth pattern of many cancers render obtaining sufficient material for unequivocal diagnosis difficult. A large number of technical variations have been developed to help overcome these limitations (Table 15.2). They are dependent on the skill, enthusiasm and experience of the gastroenterologist and radiologist[33], no less than the skill necessary to interpret the cytological features.

Definitive diagnosis of benign processes is limited, although FNA diagnosis of xanthogranulomatous cholecystitis[74,75], cholesterol polyps[76], abscess[13], and even Pneumocystis infection[77] are reported. Liver fluke infestation may be recognized in bile. This is an important clinical problem in some geographic areas or in areas with high South East Asian immigration[78,79].

These reservations do not negate the value of cytology in these situations, as cytological methods may be the only way of establishing a diagnosis. Large needle biopsy of this area is usually contraindicated because of the higher rate of complications and low sensitivity[55]. In up to 20% of patients with carcinoma of extrahepatic bile ducts even laparotomy may not provide a definitive diagnosis[41,56]; the presence of tumour in such cases may only be proven subsequently[56].

Diagnostic procedures and cytological techniques

The main procedures providing material for cytodiagnosis are listed in Table 15.2. A number of authors have suggested protocols to maximize diagnostic yield[18,38,40,41].

1. *For bile sampling*: three bile samples should be obtained on successive days from any patient undergoing percutaneous drainage; as large a volume as can be aspirated should be collected and sent promptly to the laboratory.

2. *For brush or catheter samples*: The stricture is first negotiated with a guide wire, and a brush passed over the wire and drawn back and forth along the stricture. Multiple samples improve sensitivity. In our experience having cytology staff on site optimizes smear preparation and allows confirmation of adequacy of material.

3. *For FNA samples*: multiple sampling may be necessary and multiple imaging procedures are of value in combination. The presence of the pathologist at the procedure for rapid reporting can reduce the number of needle passes. Transcatheter brush sampling is preferred for hilar lesions of the liver and biliary strictures, whereas FNA

Table 15.2 Biliary tract cytology: diagnostic procedures and accuracy

Aspiration of gastric/duodenal contents
1. Simple catheter aspiration
2. Double lumen tubes
3. Stimulation of bile/pancreatic flow by $MgSO_4$, cholecystokinin, pancreozymin, secretin[20-27]

Sensitivity of malignant diagnosis:	40–78%
Predictive value of malignant diagnosis:	91.5–100%

Direct collection of bile
1. At outflow of ampulla of Vater or by catheterization of ampulla[28-32]

Sensitivity of malignant diagnosis:	20–77%
Predictive value of malignant diagnosis:	~100%

2. Selective bile duct catheterization at ERCP[29,31]
3. Percutaneous bile drainage:
   (a) T-tube aspiration or drainage[34,40]
   (b) Percutaneous transhepatic cholangiography (PTC)[37-43]

Sensitivity of malignant diagnosis:	34–73%
Predictive value of malignant diagnosis:	94–100%

4. Transhepatic puncture of bile ducts during laparotomy[35]
5. Gall bladder puncture[4,14,16]

Sensitivity of malignant diagnosis:	53–91.3%

Bile duct brushings or washings
1. Direct brushing of ducts during ERCP[18,41,44-46]

Sensitivity of malignant diagnosis:	18–60%
Predictive value of malignant diagnosis:	~100%

2. Transcatheter brushing +/− guidewire bypass of obstruction:
   (a) Retrograde at ERCP[47,48,50,61,62,64,66,82,98]
   (b) Percutaneous at PTC[49,51-53,61,62]

Sensitivity of malignant diagnosis:	35–82%
Predictive value of malignant diagnosis:	92–100%

3. Saline irrigation of ducts at ERCP[12,13]

Fine needle aspiration
1. Percutaneous FNA of mass; guidance by combinations of:
   (a) Ultrasound[9-12,54-56,76]
   (b) Fluoroscopy[55,56]
   (c) CT[57]
   (d) Angiography[33]

Sensitivity of malignant diagnosis:	40–91.2%
Predictive value of malignant diagnosis:	~100%

2. Percutaneous FNA of:
   (a) Site of stent tube
   (b) Ducts opacified by contrast media (PTC)[33,39,55]

Sensitivity of malignant diagnosis:	53–87.5%
Predictive value of malignant diagnosis:	~100%

3. Transductal, transcatheter FNA or transduodenal during ERCP or PTC[59,60]
4. Intra-operative FNA[39]
5. Endoscopic ultrasound-guided FNA[63]

Cell block preparations
1. Material retrieved from obstructed stent tube[81]
2. Cell deposit from bile or FNA samples[56]

samples are probably more sensitive for pancreatic head masses. Intraoperative FNA is useful when less invasive procedures have proved negative to prove a diagnosis before major surgery.

Preparation of samples from this region requires some flexibility on the part of the cytology laboratory. Bile samples and duodenal contents containing gastroduodenal and pancreatic secretions provide a hostile cell medium, and necessitate rapid transport to the laboratory to reduce degeneration. Ice baths are used to cool bile collected during drainage procedures, but transport to the laboratory within 1 hour gives quite satisfactory cell preservation without cooling[37,40]. Where delay is unavoidable, alcohol prefixation may aid in cell preservation, though this renders membrane filter preparations unsatisfactory.

Bile obtained from drainage bags shows bacterial overgrowth and loss of cell detail and is not suitable for cytological assessment. In patients with external biliary drains, bile for cytology should be aspirated directly from the drainage catheter[37], or collected over a short period. Some authors suggest that samples that contain contrast medium, e.g. following ERCP, encourage cell degeneration and may not be as satisfactory. Washing the brushes in saline and cytocentrifuging the elutant may increase the yield from ductal brush samples as may 'salvage' cytology of endoscopic brush sheaths[18,80].

Approach to cytodiagnosis

Familiarity with the degenerative and regenerative changes seen in cells from this site is necessary. There is a risk of false positive diagnosis of malignancy in regenerating bile duct epithelium associated with cholangitis, stones, following procedures such as PTC or ERCP and in association with catheter or stent by-pass of obstruction. The higher prevalence of false positive diagnosis in samples obtained from the duodenum in early reports reflected the greater degree of degenerative change in this medium together with the pioneering nature of this work. It has not occurred in later studies, or in material from other sources and close to 100% predictive value of malignant diagnosis is now achieved (see Table 15.2).

Contrasting abnormal epithelium with the benign epithelium included in most samples is among the most useful exercises in establishing a malignant diagnosis[22]. Cell block preparations allow an appreciation of tissue architecture and are a valuable addition to the range of techniques applied to the cell harvest[81]. Some authors found more value in cell blocks than in smears[56]. Brush samples may allow the highest yield of satisfactory samples[82].

Complications and contraindications

Percutaneous FNA may rarely result in biliary peritonitis, peritonitis due to bowel perforation and haemorrhage (see Chapters 14, 16). FNA sampling of normal pancreas is said to be associated with a higher risk of pancreatitis[56]. ERCP with or without brushing is commonly associated with amylasaemia but in only a very small proportion of cases is there pancreatitis or sepsis. In Ryan's ERCP series[47], only 3% of patients developed mild pancreatitis, which resolved within 48 hours and only one patient developed sepsis. Rabinowitz reported some complications relating to the ERCP procedure as a whole but not to brushings *per se*: these were transient haemobilia in three patients, bile leaks around the catheter and procedure-associated infection in a few cases[18].

Gall bladder puncture can result in bile leaks, particularly in association with common bile duct obstruction[7]. This technique is thus not usually advised except in the immediate pre-operative period[13] or unless special precautions are taken. However, ultrasound or laparoscopically guided FNA of gall bladder for collection of bile, apparently without significant complications, has been described[8]. Brush, catheter or FNA sampling might perhaps be associated with tumour seeding along a catheter tract but this is of largely theoretical importance in view of the inoperability of most lesions of the site.

Cytological findings: normal

Duodenal aspirates

▶ Biliary epithelium in monolayered sheets
▶ Duodenal cells with brush borders or goblet cell forms
▶ 'Matchstick' cells of gall bladder origin
▶ Cuboidal pancreatic acinar cells
▶ Degenerate cells of indeterminate origin

The normal cell components of this site include cells from the stomach, duodenum and those shed from bile ducts and the pancreas. Most often, specific identification of the epithelium of origin will not be possible. Ductal cells from all sites are shed as small monolayered sheets with moderately dense cytoplasm (Fig. 15.1). Duodenal cells have a more prominent brush border and are taller columnar cells with a goblet cell component; gall bladder cells are described as 'matchstick' cells[32] with a columnar morphology and bulging terminal nuclei[23]. Pancreatic acinar

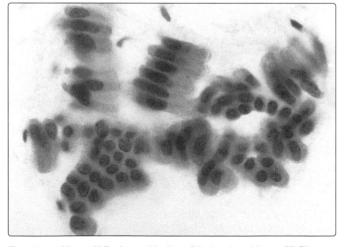

Fig. 15.1 Normal bile duct epithelium. Bile duct brushing at ERCP. (H&E × OI)

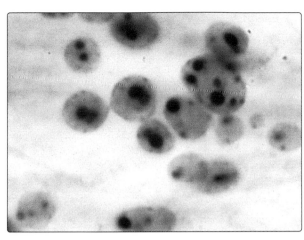

Fig. 15.2 Degenerate cells, most likely epithelial in origin. Fluid aspirated from ampulla of Vater at ERCP. (Papanicolaou × OI)

cells are cuboidal and lie in small clusters. Cells showing round densely hyperchromatic nuclear fragments within rounded-up cell bodies (Fig. 15.2) have been the subject of considerable controversy[20–23,25,83,84], though they are considered to be degenerate epithelial cells by most authors[15,21,83]. We have obtained some electron microscopic evidence for this view (unpublished). Gibbs attributed the name 'mercury droplet' cells to Hemming's original observation, which likened the nuclear fragments to small mercury drops[83,84]. A number of authors have commented that these cells are present only in pancreatic duct or duodenal aspirates but not in selective bile duct aspirates and that they are, therefore, of pancreatic acinar or ductal origin[30,32], but we have observed them in bile duct brushings.

Bile
▶ Scanty cellular material
▶ Background of bile pigment and crystals
▶ Cholesterol crystals in some conditions
▶ Sheets of gall bladder epithelium, especially after saline irrigation

Normal bile contains little cellular material, though bile and pancreatic secretion stimulated by secretin, pancreozymin, cholecystokinin or magnesium sulphate result in increased cell shedding. Bile pigment and crystals are observed in the background. Cholesterol crystals are present in patients with a variety of disorders of the biliary tree including cholelithiasis or cholecystitis; they are said to be absent from patients with diseases of the liver or pancreas[85,86]. Gall bladder epithelium presents in sheets or aggregates with dense cytoplasm; saline irrigated samples are more cellular[15] and contain better preserved abraded sheets.

Bile duct brushings
Normal bile duct or pancreatic ductal epithelium appears as distorted cohesive sheets of regular cells with a honeycomb structure, a columnar form when seen on edge, and having small rounded or oval nuclei (Fig. 15.1).

FNA samples
▶ Different types of cells depending on organs traversed.

As with percutaneous FNA of other intra-abdominal sites, epithelium of multiple types may be encountered as the needle traverses tissues such as bowel mucosa, liver or pancreatic acinar and ductal tissue.

Cytological findings: benign conditions

Inflammatory and reactive processes
▶ Variable inflammatory cell component
▶ Degenerative and regenerative changes in epithelial cells
▶ Extreme reactive changes may simulate malignancy

Chronic calcific pancreatitis will be discussed later in Chapter 16. Inflammatory changes and organisms have been demonstrated in bile by gall bladder puncture preoperatively[13] in cholecystitis. Intraoperative FNA has been used to diagnose abscess[13] and xanthogranulomatous cholecystitis by finding a mixed inflammatory cell component in company with large numbers of foamy histiocytes and surrounding capillary blood vessels[74]. Krishnani *et al.* suggest that sheets of mesothelium-like cells, multinucleate histiocytes, and a pink granular background in Giemsa preparations were additional useful criteria[75].

Changes due to sclerosing cholangitis, stent placement and postoperative effect are similar in all types of cytological samples and include a range of regenerative and degenerative alterations in bile duct epithelium, with cells reminiscent of squamous metaplasia[82], nuclear enlargement, nuclear size variation, prominent nucleoli and cellular disorganization (Figs 15.3, 15.4)[52].

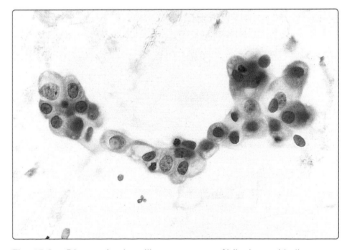

Fig. 15.3 Disorganized papillary aggregate of bile duct epithelium showing moderate anisokaryosis and nuclear enlargement but a low nuclear/cytoplasmic ratio. In this case it was difficult to distinguish between reactive epithelium and well-differentiated adenocarcinoma. Catheter sample of bile at ERCP. (H&E × HP)

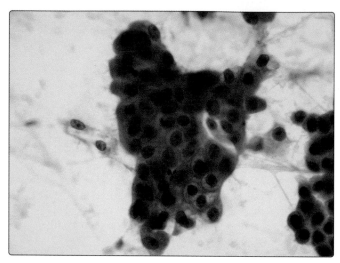

Fig. 15.4   Monolayered sheet with enlarged nuclei and prominent nucleoli, but retained honeycomb structure and low nuclear/cytoplasmic ratio. Presumed reactive changes. Bile duct brushings. (H&E × HP)

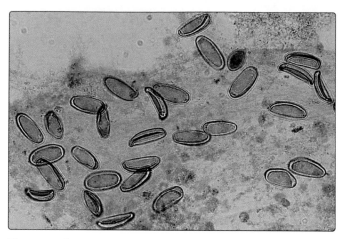

Fig. 15.5   Ova of *Clonorchis sinensis* in bile. (Papanicolaou × HP)

More extreme changes have been reported in parasitic infestation[79]. Reactive papillary clusters may be seen; a lack of nuclear irregularity, nuclear hyperchromasia, or high nuclear/cytoplasmic ratio will generally allow a distinction from neoplastic change. Nevertheless, in our experience, and in that of most authors the need for caution leads to a number of 'inconclusive' diagnoses in cases eventually proven to be carcinoma (Fig. 15.3).

Parasitic infestation
▶ Parasitic ova
▶ Inflammatory and necrotic debris
▶ Worms, fragmented or entire
▶ Epithelial hyperplasia, metaplasia
▶ Late risk of cholangiocarcinoma

In PTC-obtained bile submitted for cytological examination, ova of liver flukes (for example *Clonorchis sinensis* and *Opisthorchis viverrini*) may be identified against a background of granular necrotic debris, neutrophils and eosinophils[79]. *Fasciola hepatica* infestation may also be identified. We have seen one such case, where ova compatible with Fasciola were observed in T-tube drainage specimens from a 12-year-old African girl who presented with obstructive jaundice. Ova were also present within inflamed intrahepatic ducts in a wedge biopsy of the liver. Criteria for recognition of Clonorchis ova include small size, (24 µm × 16 µm) laminated walls, opercula with prominent shoulders and spinous processes (Fig. 15.5). Whole worms, or parts thereof, may also be seen[78]. Biliary infestation with Clonorchis is also associated with epithelial hyperplasia, goblet cell metaplasia, squamous metaplasia and adenomatous hyperplasia. The high mucin content of the bile is associated with bacterial superinfection, stone formation and later, cholangiocarcinoma may supervene. All these conditions may coexist[78,79].

Cytological findings: malignancy

Adenocarcinoma of gall bladder and extrahepatic bile ducts
Bile samples
▶ Single and clustered tumour cells
▶ Moulding and cell-in-cell patterns
▶ Enlarged pleomorphic nuclei
▶ Single cell pattern and giant tumour cells in poorly-differentiated types
▶ Inflammatory and degenerative changes with necrosis

Adenocarcinoma of gall bladder, bile duct or pancreatic origin presents as single cells and small three-dimensional clusters showing moulding, cell-in-cell arrangements, nuclei with irregular nuclear outlines and pleomorphism, prominent nucleoli and increased nuclear/cytoplasmic ratio (Fig. 15.6, inset). Poorly-differentiated tumours show more dispersal and, occasionally, a purely single cell pattern, or marked pleomorphism including giant cell forms. In

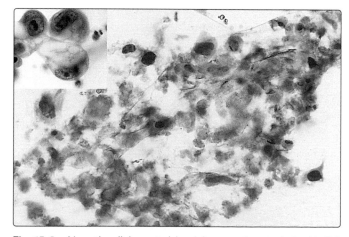

Fig. 15.6   Necrotic cellular material and degenerating atypical epithelial cells. Inset: a small cluster of malignant cells from a common bile duct adenocarcinoma. Catheter sample of bile at ERCP. (Papanicolaou × HP; inset: Papanicolaou × HP)

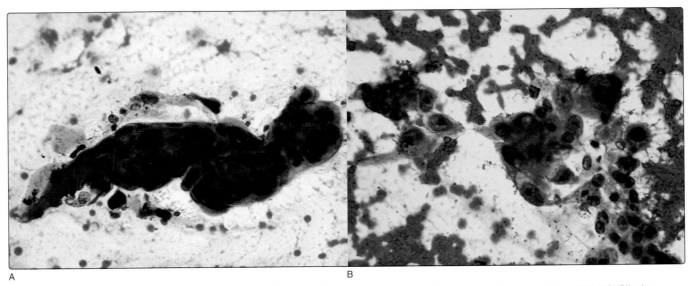

A   B

Fig. 15.7   (A) Irregular disorganized sheet of malignant cells from a bile duct adenocarcinoma. Nuclear moulding. Associated cell debris. Bile duct brushings. (Papanicolaou × HP) (B) Loose aggregate and dispersed malignant epithelial cells associated with a small sheet of benign ductal epithelium. Marked nuclear enlargement, and irregular nuclear outlines. Bile duct brushings. (Papanicolaou × HP)

contrast, benign reactive cells present as larger more cohesive sheets[4,14,26]. The background may show variable numbers of inflammatory cells and histiocytes, necrotic material and degenerating cells (Fig. 15.6). Screening for abnormal cells is mandatory.

Brush samples

▶ Disorganized sheets, loose aggregates, small acinar groups and single pleomorphic cells
▶ Nuclear enlargement, moulding and irregular nuclear outlines
▶ Nuclear crowding and high nuclear/cytoplasmic ratio
▶ Background of necrotic debris

Architectural features of malignancy include disorganization within clusters, loss of cohesion, small acinar groups and single cells (Figs 15.7, 15.8)[82]. Marked nuclear enlargement within sheets, nuclear crowding, moulding, irregularity of nuclear outline and nuclear pleomorphism permit a definitive diagnosis of malignancy when there is adequate well preserved material (Figs 15.7, 15.8)[82]. A background of necrotic debris may be helpful in some cases. Very well-differentiated tumours present as cohesive monolayered sheets which are much more difficult to evaluate and unequivocal nuclear criteria of malignancy may not be present (Fig. 15.9A). Cell block assessment of architecture may allow a diagnosis of malignancy in well-differentiated tumours (Fig. 15.9B). Cohen et al. considered nuclear moulding, chromatin clumping and increased N/C ratio to be the most important criteria in diagnosing malignancy[87]. In Renshaw's study either an 'overall assessment of malignancy' or chromatin clumping, increased N/C ratio, nuclear moulding and loss of honeycombing had an equally high predictive value and reproducibility between pathologists; an 'overall

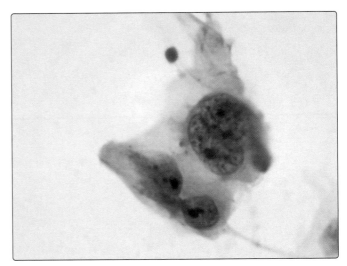

Fig. 15.8   Malignant epithelial cells showing marked nuclear pleomorphism, irregularity of nuclear outlines and multinucleation. Bile duct brushings. (Papanicolaou × OI)

assessment' had the highest sensitivity[88]. This finding was an interesting validation of the usual approach to diagnosis taken by cytopathologists. Layfield et al. demonstrated a spectrum of cytological atypia in cases with proven carcinoma, including cases without fully developed criteria of malignancy[65].

FNA samples

▶ Large aggregates of malignant cells
▶ Small clusters of crowded atypical cells
▶ Monolayered sheets with marked nuclear enlargement and pleomorphism
▶ Irregular nuclei with some multinucleation
▶ Apoptotic debris in tumour cell sheets.

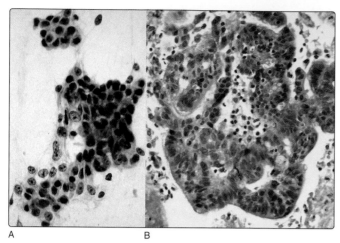

Fig. 15.9 (A) Sheet of ductal epithelial cells with slight disorganization and loss of honeycomb structure, some nuclear pleomorphism and enlargement, and hyperchromasia; suspicious of malignancy. Bile duct brushings (Papanicolaou × HP). (B) Cell block showing well-differentiated adenocarcinoma. Complex architecture allowing a diagnosis of malignancy. Bile duct brushings. (H&E × MP)

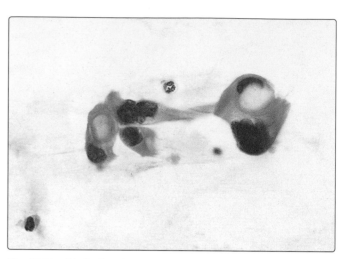

Fig. 15.11 Markedly enlarged multinucleate malignant cells, with dense cytoplasm but showing focal mucin vacuolation. Poorly differentiated bile duct adenocarcinoma. Percutaneous FNA sample at site of stent tube. (Papanicolaou × HP)

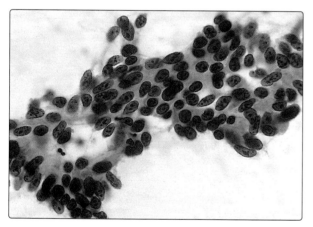

Fig. 15.10 Disorganized aggregate of malignant cells but with some nuclear palisading and a loose gland structure. Bile duct adenocarcinoma. Percutaneous fluoroscopically guided FNA sample from the region of a stent tube. (H&E × HP)

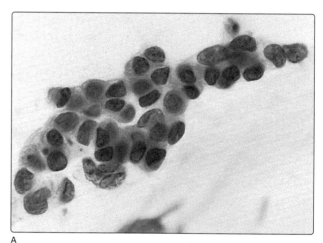

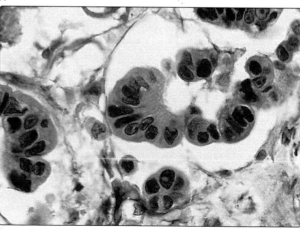

Large disorganized aggregates of cells with overt features of malignancy are often obtained (Figs 15.10–15.12). Small three-dimensional clusters of atypical cells with overlapping nuclei, which are irregular and show moderate anisokaryosis, are also useful criteria of malignancy. Multinucleation involving atypical cells is another important feature in our opinion (Fig. 15.11). Monolayered sheets in which there is marked nuclear enlargement, anisokaryosis and nuclear crowding in the absence of associated inflammation are seen in well-differentiated carcinoma and are most likely to be misinterpreted as benign because of a retained honeycomb arrangement. Apoptotic nuclear debris may be visible in association with tumour cells (Fig. 15.12A) and is not a feature of regenerating epithelium.

Fig. 15.12 (A) Disorganized malignant cells: pleomorphic, hyperchromatic and showing nuclear moulding; small amount of intracytoplasmic apoptotic debris. Bile duct adenocarcinoma. Transductal FNA. (H&E × HP) (B) Palisades and loose gland structures of neoplastic epithelium. Cell block prepared from transductal FNA sample. (H&E × HP)

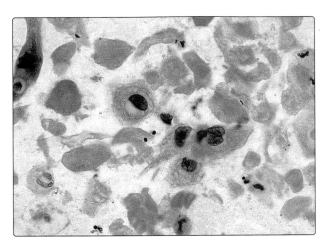

Fig. 15.13 Keratinous debris and malignant cells from a keratinizing squamous cell carcinoma of gall bladder. Percutaneous FNA of gall bladder mass. (H&E × HP)

Identification of a tumour as glandular is difficult in less differentiated cases where cell clusters are disorganized and the cytoplasm is dense and squamoid. Degenerative change may add to a squamous appearance by producing pyknotic, spindle or oval nuclei and dense eosinophilic cytoplasm.

Adenosquamous and squamous cell carcinoma

The region of the gall bladder, extrahepatic bile ducts and pancreas is well known for mixed tumours and, more rarely, pure squamous cell carcinoma (SCC) (Fig. 15.13). Gupta *et al.* diagnosed two cases of pure SCC of gall bladder by CT-guided FNA[89].

Premalignant changes in bile ductal or gall bladder epithelium

Gall bladder puncture or bile removed during PTC may show premalignant cellular changes of biliary duct epithelium. Alonso-de-Ruiz *et al.* reported on a large series of 250 cytological and histological samples from operatively removed gall bladders[4]. Dysplastic cell changes manifested in aspirated bile with enlarged, round nuclei, a higher nuclear/cytoplasmic ratio than in normal or hyperplastic epithelium, and looser, more disorganized sheets. Carcinoma *in situ* demonstrated more numerous abnormal cells, forming loose syncytia with considerable variation in nuclear size. In invasive cancers there was more complete loss of cohesion and tumour diathesis. Alonso-de-Ruiz *et al.*[4] showed a high correlation between cytological and histological diagnosis of carcinoma *in situ* and invasive carcinoma but lower correlation for cytological diagnosis of hyperplasia and dysplasia. Other authors have used the term 'dysplasia' for the purposes of classification of cases in studies of the accuracy of bile duct brushings in the diagnosis of malignancy[64,65,66] and found that a diagnosis of 'high grade dysplasia' was generally associated with invasive adenocarcinoma[65]. Most authors do not consider it possible to diagnose precursors of carcinoma accurately or

to distinguish between intraepithelial and invasive tumours in brush samples[82,90,91].

Papillary and intraductal bile duct lesions

Villous adenoma and well-differentiated papillary carcinoma with a predominantly exophytic growth are rare, albeit well described. Ahsan and Berman[36] suggest that identification of papillary aggregates of malignant cells in bile would be more suggestive of this lesion than pancreatic carcinoma where such a growth pattern is less common, but others have not been able to make such a distinction[52]. We have seen an intrahepatic intracystic papillary cholangiocarcinoma where the diagnosis of a bile duct neoplasm was suggested on CT guided percutaneous FNA (see Chapter 14).

Brush samples of villous adenoma are described as yielding cellular specimens with pavement-like sheets and some three-dimensional papillary clusters with elongated columnar cells[41,90,92]. Bardales *et al.*[90] observed that some cases showed features indistinguishable from invasive adenocarcinoma. Stewart *et al.* reported on brush findings in three patients with adenomas of bile duct or ampulla with sufficient cytological atypia for a 'positive' diagnosis[82]. There was a general preservation of architectural arrangement although some small acinar clusters were seen in two, and the overall findings were similar to cases of confirmed invasive adenocarcinoma. In some other reported cases the changes were difficult to distinguish from benign bile duct epithelium[47].

Tsui *et al.* reported the FNA findings in three cases of intrahepatic, intraductal biliary papillomatosis[93]. Distinctive features were hypercellular smears, broad double-layered sheets of ductal epithelium, papillary structures, preserved honeycomb pattern and dysplastic, but not overtly malignant nuclear features. The authors have seen a case in extrahepatic ducts in a 65-year-old man who presented with a long history of abdominal symptoms and abnormal liver function tests followed by obstructive jaundice, irregularly stenotic bile ducts on ERCP, and dilated intrahepatic bile ducts. A villous adenoma of the ampulla of Vater had been resected some time previously. The bile duct brushings showed abundant abnormal ductal epithelium in sheets, palisaded clusters and three-dimensional groups in a background of debris (Fig. 15.14A). The findings were reported as suspicious of adenocarcinoma. Choledochoscopy revealed a carpet-like growth with abundant mucin in ducts. Biopsy/curettings confirmed multiple papillary adenomatosis with no obvious invasive tumour (Fig. 15.14B). Following photodynamic therapy, symptoms resolved and previously high serum levels of CA 19-9 returned to normal. Symptoms have since returned, along with high serum CA 19-9 levels.

Cystadenoma and cystadenocarcinoma

Cystic mucinous neoplasms of extrahepatic bile duct origin are morphologically identical to those described in the pancreas and intrahepatic ducts (Chapter 16).

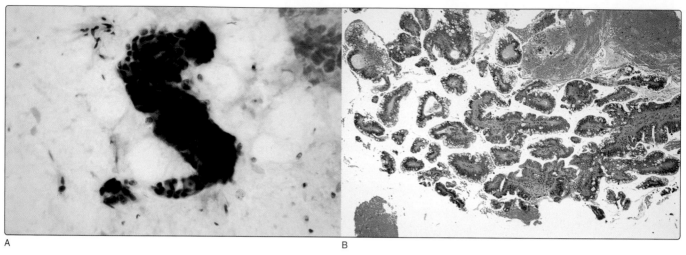

Fig. 15.14 (A) Disorganized sheet of hyperchromatic cells. Biliary papillomatosis. Bile duct brushings. (Papanicolaou × HP). (B) Neoplastic epithelium in papillary aggregates with fibrovascular cores. Biliary papillomatosis. Bile duct biopsies. (H&E × LP)

Other neoplasms

Dusenbery[94], Nilsson et al.[95] and Stewart et al.[96] diagnosed hepatocellular carcinoma in bile duct brushings. Metastatic carcinomas from the upper and lower gastrointestinal tract, are diagnosed by all the methods described above[95,82], although brush and bile samples have a lower reported sensitivity than percutaneous or direct intraoperative FNA. As with other sites, a comparison with the original tumour will be of most value in confirming metastasis rather than a new primary lesion. The diagnosis of sarcoma in this site is exceptional.

The cytological diagnosis of lymphoma in the retroperitoneum or region of the gall bladder and bile ducts is only easy when the tumours are monotonous and of high-grade. Mixed cell lymphomas and those of low-grade are extremely difficult to distinguish from reactive processes without flow cytometry or immunocytochemical analysis. In the experience of Hall-Craggs and Lees[55], the identification of lymphoma of this site ranks with well-differentiated adenocarcinoma in difficulty of diagnosis, and these tumours were a major cause of misdiagnosis.

Diagnostic pitfalls

The difficulty of distinguishing reactive bile duct epithelium from well-differentiated adenocarcinoma has been emphasized (Figs 15.3, 15.4, 15.9A). Stewart et al., in reviewing previous series of duct brushings, quote misinterpretation of low-grade dysplasia, reactive papillary changes with epithelial atypia, intestinal metaplasia of biliary epithelium and the effects of previous bile duct stenting as causes of false positive reports[82]. These authors describe in detail three cases leading to presumed false positive diagnoses, in patients with sclerosing cholangitis, bile duct stones and pancreatitis. In one case there were crowded three-dimensional clusters, nuclear moulding, a coarse chromatin pattern and distinct nucleoli. Pronounced degenerative changes were seen in some of the atypical epithelium and in associated normal epithelium. In a second case, small numbers of highly atypical but somewhat degenerate cell groups were reported as consistent with adenocarcinoma, and in the third there were small numbers of highly atypical cells with some degenerative changes. The degenerative changes present and the small amounts of material in two of the specimens were features that might have led to an equivocal rather than definite malignant diagnosis[82]. Rupp et al.[52] reported on a characteristic case in which highly atypical epithelial cells were present in brushings from a bile duct in which a catheter had been in place for a week. There was marked cellular and nuclear enlargement but the lack of nuclear hyperchromasia, nuclear membrane irregularity or high nuclear/cytoplasmic ratio were features against a diagnosis of malignancy. De Peralta et al.[91] describe a benign case with large papillary tissue fragments showing architectural disarray and marked nuclear overlapping, resulting in a false positive diagnosis. Parasitic infestation of ducts may be a source of similar difficulty[79] as may papillitis or inflammatory changes in the region of ampulla of Vater. Primary sclerosing cholangitis often gives rise to worrying regenerative change[18] and inflammatory changes associated with other benign lesions such as bile duct cysts may also afford diagnostic difficulty. Yamada[43], Ryan[47] and Bardales[90] report 'false positive' diagnoses of malignancy from cytology of adenoma of the duodenal papilla. Stewart et al.[82] argue, correctly in our view, that such diagnoses are not 'false positive' because the lesions need to be identified as neoplastic and to proceed to operative resection. Nevertheless, the inability of cytology to reliably distinguish intraductal from invasive lesions means that other modalities must be used to identify cases that might benefit from resection rather than palliative management.

Underdiagnosis of malignancy may result from inexperience, particularly in duct brushings, whereby an overcautious approach in an area of known diagnostic difficulty leads to 'suspicious' reports on material with nuclear criteria of malignancy. Concentration of experience will reduce this problem, although for many centres, the number of cases seen may not be enough to acquire expertise. In FNA samples, well-differentiated carcinomas presenting in monolayered sheets with a retained honeycomb structure may be underdiagnosed. The presence of nuclear enlargement (compared with benign epithelium) and focal marked pleomorphism with multinucleation is helpful in establishing the diagnosis in our experience. Tumours of unusual type such as mucinous and papillary intraductal lesions may have a particularly bland appearance[64].

Accuracy of diagnosis

Table 15.2 includes the reported range of sensitivities and positive predictive values in the diagnosis of malignancy for the various techniques used. Many of the series quoted include pancreatic carcinoma in the calculation of results.

False positive diagnoses of malignancy are infrequent, but occasionally occur even for very experienced workers[82,91]. The difficulty in diagnosis in this region and the frequency of reactive changes, which may resemble malignancy, also lead to a proportion of 'atypical' or inconclusive reports. Stewart et al. report 10.1% such reports in their series, with no reduction over the course of the study. Two-thirds of patients with these reports were shown later to have carcinoma[82].

A combination of techniques in a given case allows a higher sensitivity for a malignant diagnosis[55], and the selection of which to apply first depends on the individual case. Single bile samples are of inherently lower sensitivity than brush or FNA specimens; the latter can be accurately directed to the site of abnormality[55,62]. For example, intraoperative FNA, even of small tumours at the confluence of the biliary tree, has a high sensitivity. Dalton-Clarke et al.[39] were able to diagnose 10 out of 11 such carcinomas cytologically.

The reasons for false negative results for bile samples include enzymatic digestion and degeneration of tumour cells, and obstruction of ducts by external compression, which prevents cell shedding. A lower sensitivity is reported in the diagnosis of pancreatic carcinoma compared with bile duct cancers, when PTC samples are used. Some find the distance of a tumour from a bile sampling site to be a factor in the low yield of diagnostic samples[28,38], whereas others found no difference in the detection rate for hilar or more distal extrahepatic bile duct tumours in PTC samples or brushings. Where there is concentrated experience, bile aspirates from patients with percutaneous bile drainage

give sensitivities of the order of 60% for diagnosing malignancy[97].

Brush cytology during ERCP is the most useful method of cytological diagnosis in pancreato-biliary strictures. Stewart et al. in a study of 406 patients found an overall sensitivity of 60% in the diagnosis of neoplasm, and a 70% sensitivity in the last-third of their experience[82]. Other recent smaller studies found somewhat lower sensitivities ranging from 35–48%[64,66,72,98]. Ryan[47] achieved a higher sensitivity for ERCP brush/guidewire diagnosis in bile duct tumours (68.8%) than pancreatic lesions (30%) or metastases (50%) and some other workers have shown similar results[71,99] but Stewart et al. found similar sensitivities for pancreatic carcinoma (59.6%) and cholangiocarcinoma (62.5%)[82]. Satisfactory samples can be obtained in up to 94.7% of brushings[82]. Failure to cannulate the desired duct is now less often a usual cause of unsatisfactory specimens due to improvements in guidewire bypass instruments. The absence of a luminal component may be the cause in some cases[82]. Poor sampling, lack of criteria for the distinction between dysplasia/carcinoma in situ and invasive carcinoma, difficulties in recognizing special tumour types and underestimating the significance of the smear background were quoted by Kocjan and Smith, as other reasons for the 'modest' sensitivity of bile duct brushings in diagnosing malignancy[64]. In 36 false negative cases, Logrono et al. found sampling to be the cause of error in 24, however there were interpretive errors related to small numbers of malignant cells or subtle atypia in six cases, and errors related to poor slide preparation, such as air-drying in six[66]. Some workers are able to achieve a very high degree of accuracy. In the series by Rupp et al., the sensitivity of cancer diagnosis by brush sampling was 82%[52]. In another large study[18], although a single brush sample had low sensitivity, in patients in whom three separate brush samples were performed there were very few false negative reports overall. Stewart et al. improved their sensitivity of diagnosis of malignancy from 44.3% in the initial third of the study to 70.7% in the final third[82]. In our view, this area of diagnosis perhaps more than any other, requires concentration of experience for optimal results.

For FNA samples, false negative results may result from various sources. Necrosis and accompanying inflammation may obscure malignant cells. Vascular lesions may yield inadequate, blood-stained samples. Desmoplastic tumours, which are common in this site, and peritumoral fibrosis, where, e.g. a fine needle may not be placed in the tumour tissue, may not yield the neoplastic elements. Well-differentiated or unusual tumours may not be recognized. Closer attention to target definition and biopsy needle placement by combining, e.g. radiographic and ultrasonic needle guidance, and heavier patient sedation and analgesia, have improved accuracy[55]. A higher sensitivity for FNA of pancreatic tumours compared to bile duct lesions is reported[33] (see also Chapter 16).

Cell block preparations of aspirated material or material expressed from obstructed stent tubes[81] have yielded a diagnosis in several of our cases when previous procedures were unhelpful (Fig. 15.15). Material adherent to stent removers may also be diagnostic[97]. Teplick *et al.* noted that cell blocks prepared from other types of sample were as important as smears in arriving at a diagnosis[56].

Larger needle biopsy techniques are generally contraindicated in this anatomical region, mainly due to the higher rate of complications. When feasible, core needle samples are better for tumour typing and diagnosis of rare or unusual tumours; however, overall, they are probably less sensitive in diagnosing malignancy than fine needle samples.

Endoscopic biopsy provides a high yield of definite malignant diagnoses in the region of the ampulla and can provide evidence of invasion which, in turn, may determine the extent of the resection necessary[45,90]. Biopsies are also feasible from further along the duct system (Fig. 15.14B)[98]. Some authors consider them complementary to cytology[98,99], whereas others found no increase in sensitivity over cytology alone[100].

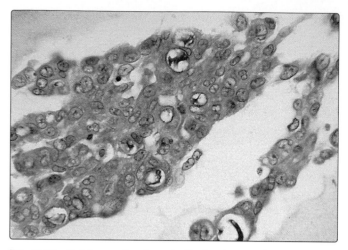

Fig. 15.15 Solid mass of malignant cells, showing prominent intracytoplasmic mucin. Poorly differentiated bile duct adenocarcinoma. Cell block preparation from material aspirated from obstructed stent tube. (PAS/diastase × HP)

References

1 Albores-Saavedra J G, Henson D E, Klimstra D S. Tumours of the gallbladder, extrahepatic bile ducts and ampulla of Vater. *Atlas of Tumour Pathology*, 3rd Series, Fascicle 27. Washington DC: Armed Forces Institute of Pathology, 2000

2 Towfigh S, McFadden D W, Cortina G R et al. Porcelain gallbladder is not associated with gallbladder carcinoma. *Am Surg* 2001; **67**: 7–10

3 Albores-Saavedra J G, Alcantra-Vazquez A, Cruz-Ortiz H, Herrera-Goepfert R. The precursor lesions of invasive gall bladder carcinoma. *Cancer* 1980; **45**: 919–927

4 Alonso-de-Ruiz P, Albores-Saavedra J G, Henson D E, Monroy M N. Cytopathology of precursor lesions of invasive carcinoma of the gall bladder. *Acta Cytol* 1982; **26**: 144–152

5 Ojeda V J, Shilkin K B, Walters M N-I. Premalignant epithelial lesions of the gall bladder: a prospective study of 120 cholecystectomy specimens. *Pathol* 1985; **17**: 451–454

6 Strom B L, Iliopoulos D, Atkinson B et al. Pathophysiology of tumour progression in human gall bladder: flow cytometry CEA and CA 19–9 levels in bile and serum in different stages of gall bladder disease. *J Natl Cancer Inst* 1989; **81**: 1575–1580

7 Yamada T. Early diagnosis of gall bladder cancer. *Acta Cytol* 1985; **29**: 498 (letter)

8 Alonso de Ruiz P, Monroy M N. Early diagnosis of gall bladder cancer. *Acta Cytol* 1985; **29**: 496 (letter)

9 Das D K, Tripathi R P, Bhambhani S et al. Ultrasound-guided fine-needle aspiration cytology diagnosis of gallbladder lesions: a study of 82 cases. *Diagn Cytopathol* 1998; **18**: 258–264

10 Dodd L G, Moffatt E J, Hudson E R, Layfield L J. Fine-needle aspiration of primary gallbladder carcinoma. *Diagn Cytopathol* 1996; **15**: 151–156

11 Shukla V K, Pandey M, Kumar et al. Ultrasound-guided fine needle aspiration cytology of malignant gallbladder masses. *Acta Cytol*. 1997; **41**: 1654–1658

12 Venkataramu N K, Sood B P, Gupta S et al. Ultrasound-guided fine needle aspiration biopsy of gall bladder malignancies. *Acta Radiol* 1999; **40**: 436–439.

13 Philips G, Bank S, Kumari-Subaiya S, Kurtz, L M. Percutaneous ultrasound-guided puncture of the gall bladder (PUPG). *Radiol* 1982; **145**: 769–772

14 Ishikawa O, Ohhigashi H, Sasaki Y O et al. The usefulness of saline-irrigated bile for the intraoperative cytologic diagnosis of tumors and tumor-like lesions of the gall bladder. *Acta Cytol* 1988; **32**: 475–481

15 Nishimura A, Den N, Sato H, Takeda B. Exfoliative cytology of the biliary tract with the use of saline irrigation under choledochoscopic control. *Ann Surg* 1973; **178**: 594–599

16 Yamagata S, Miura K, Ishioka K et al. Cytological diagnosis of cancer of the liver, bile duct and gall bladder by bile juice aspirated directly under laparoscopic observation. *J Jpn Soc Clin Cytol* 1968; **7**: 15–16

17 Klatskin G. Adenocarcinoma of the hepatic duct at its bifurcation within the porta hepatis. *Am J Med* 1965; **38**: 241–256

18 Rabinowitz M, Zajko A B, Hassanein T et al. Diagnostic value of brush cytology in the diagnosis of bile duct carcinoma: a study in 65 patients with bile duct strictures. *Hepatology* 1990; **12**: 747–752

19 Albores-Saavedra J, Henson D E, Sobin L H. The WHO histological classification of tumours of the gall bladder and extrahepatic bile ducts. *Cancer* 1992; **70**: 410–414

20 Drieling D A, Nieburgs H E, Janowitz H D. The combined secretin and cytology test in the diagnosis of pancreatic and biliary tract cancer. *Med Clin North Am* 1960; **44**: 801–815

21 Fidler A, Innes J, Davidson L S P. Duodenal intubation; significance of the cellular contents of bile in the diagnosis of diseases of the biliary tract. *BMJ* 1941; **4229**: 865–869

22 Lemon H M, Byrnes W W. Cancer of the biliary tract and pancreas; diagnosis from cytology of duodenal aspirations. *JAMA* 1949; **241**: 254–257

23 Nieburgs H E, Dreiling D A, Rubio C, Reisman H. The morphology of cells in duodenal-drainage smears: histologic origin and pathologic significance. *Am J Dig Dis* 1962; **7**: 489–505

24 Raskin H F, Wenger J, Sklar M et al. The diagnosis of cancer of the pancreas, biliary tract and duodenum by combined cytologic and secretory methods I. Exfoliative cytology and description of a rapid method of duodenal intubation. *Gastroenterol* 1958; **34**: 996–1008

25 Wenger J, Raskin H F. The diagnosis of cancer of the pancreas, biliary tract and duodenum by combined cytologic and secretory methods II. The secretion test. *Gastroenterol* 1958; **34**: 1009–1017

26 Kline T S, Joshi L P, Goldstein F. Preoperative diagnosis of pancreatic malignancy by the cytologic examination of duodenal secretions. *Am J Clin Pathol* 1978; **70**: 851–854

27   Vilardell F. Cytological diagnosis of digestive cancer. *Am J Gastroenterol* 1978; **70**: 357–364

28   Endo Y, Morii T, Tamura H, Okuda S. Cytodiagnosis of pancreatic malignant tumours by aspiration under direct vision using a duodenal fiberscope. *Gastroenterol* 1974; **67**: 944–951

29   Harada H, Sasaki T, Yamamoto N et al. Assessment of endoscopic aspiration cytology and endoscopic retrograde cholangio-pancreatography in patients with cancer of the hepato-biliary tract. *Gastroenterol Japonica* 1977; **12**: 59–64

30   Hatfield A R W, Smithies A, Wilkins R, Levi A J. Assessment of endoscopic retrograde cholangiopancreatography (ERCP) and pure pancreatic juice of cytology in patients with pancreatic disease. *Gut* 1976; **17**: 14–21

31   Roberts-Thomson I C, Hobbs J B. Cytodiagnosis of pancreatic and biliary cancer by endoscopic duct aspiration. *Med J Aust* 1979; **1**: 370–372

32   Smithies A, Hatfield A R W, Brown B E. The cytodiagnostic aspects of pure pancreatic juice obtained at the time of endoscopic retrograde cholangiopancreatography (ERCP). *Acta Cytol* 1977; **21**: 191–195

33   Evander A, Ihse I, Lunderquist A et al. Percutaneous cytodiagnosis of carcinoma of the pancreas and bile duct. *Ann Surg* 1978; **188**: 90–92

34   Cressman F K. Carcinoma of the common bile duct. Diagnosis by cytological examination of T-tube drainage contents. *Acta Cytol* 1977; **21**: 496–497 (letter)

35   Wertlake P T, Del Guercio L R M. Cytopathology of intrahepatic bile as a component of integrated procedure ('Minilap') for hepatobiliary disorders. *Acta Cytol* 1976; **20**: 42–45

36   Ahsan N, Berman J J. Papillary carcinoma of the common bile duct. Diagnosis by bile drainage cytology. *Acta Cytol* 1988; **32**: 471–474

37   Cobb C J, Floyd W N. Usefulness of bile cytology in the diagnostic management of patients with biliary tract obstruction. *Acta Cytol* 1985; **29**: 93–100

38   Cohan R H, Illescas F F, Newman G E et al. Biliary cytodiagnosis; bile sampling for cytology. *Invest Radiol* 1985; **20**: 177–179

39   Dalton-Clarke H J, Pease E, Krause T et al. Fine needle aspiration cytology and exfoliative biliary cytology in the diagnosis of hilar cholangiocarcinoma. *Eur J Surg Oncol* 1986; **12**: 143–145

40   Harell G S, Anderson M F, Berry P F. Cytologic bile examination in the diagnosis of biliary duct neoplastic strictures. *AJR* 1981; **137**: 1123–1126

41   Howell L P, Chow H-C, Russell L A. Cytodiagnosis of extrahepatic biliary duct tumours from specimens obtained during cholangiography. *Diagn Cytopathol* 1988; **4**: 328–334

42   Muro A, Mueller P R, Ferrucci J T, Taft P P. Bile cytology. A routine addition to percutaneous biliary drainage. *Radiology* 1983; **149**: 846–847

43   Yamada T, Murohisa B, Muto Y et al. Cytologic detection of small pancreatoduodenal and biliary cancers in the early developmental stages. *Acta Cytol* 1984; **28**: 435–442

44   Aabakken L, Karesen R, Serck-Hanssen A, Osnes M. Transpapillary biopsies and brush cytology from the common bile duct. *Endoscopy* 1986; **18**: 49–51

45   Gmelin E, Weiss H D. Tumours in the region of the papilla of Vater. *Eur J Radiol* 1981; **1**: 301–306

46   Osnes M, Serck-Hanssen A, Myren J. Endoscopic retrograde brush cytology (ERBC) of the biliary and pancreatic ducts. *Scand J Gastroenterol* 1975; **10**: 829–831

47   Ryan M E. Cytologic brushings of ductal lesions during ERCP. *Gastrointest Endoscopy* 1991; **37**: 139–142

48   Cropper L D, Gold R E. Simplified brush biopsy of the bile ducts. *Radiology* 1983; **148**: 307–308

49   Elyaderani M K, Gabriele O. Brush and forceps biopsy of biliary ducts via percutaneous transhepatic catheterization. *Radiology* 1980; **135**: 777–778

50   Foutch P G, Harian J R, Kerr D, Sanowski R A. Wire-guided brush cytology: a new endoscopic method for diagnosis of bile duct cancer. *Gastrointest Endosc* 1989; **35**: 243–247

51   Mendez G, Russell E, Levi J V et al. Percutaneous brush biopsy of internal drainage of biliary tree through endoprosthesis. *AJR* 1980; **134**: 653–659

52   Rupp M, Hawthorne C M, Ehya H. Brushing cytology in biliary tract obstruction. *Acta Cytol* 1990; **34**: 221–226

53   Yip C K Y, Leung J W C, Chan M K M, Metreweli C. Scrape biopsy of malignant biliary structure through percutaneous transhepatic biliary drainage tracts. *AJR* 1989; **152**: 529–530

54   Bondestam S, Jansson S-E, Taavitsainen M, Standersjold-Nordenstam C-G. Ultrasound guided fine-needle biopsy of mass lesions affecting the hepatobiliary tract. *Acta Radiol Diagn* 1981; **22**: 549–551

55   Hall-Craggs M A, Lees W R. Fine needle aspiration biopsy: pancreatic and biliary tumours. *AJR* 1986; **147**: 399–403

56   Teplick S K, Haskin P H, Kline T S et al. Percutaneous pancreatobiliary biopsies in 173 patients using primarily ultrasound or fluoroscopic guidance. *Cardiovasc Intervent Radiol* 1988; **11**: 26–28

57   Geng J Z, Qin P R, Hui L D, Po P D. CT guided fine needle aspiration biopsy of biliopancreatic lesions: report of 30 cases. *Jap J Surg* 1987; **17**: 461–464

58   Cohan R H, Illescas F F, Braun S D, Newman G E. Fine needle aspiration biopsy in malignant obstructive jaundice. *Gastrointest Radiol* 1986; **11**: 145–150

59   Howell D A, Beveridge R, Bosco J, Jones M. Endoscopic needle aspiration biopsy at ERCP in the diagnosis of biliary strictures. *Gastrointest Endosc* 1991; **37**: 271

60   Kuroda C, Yoshioka H, Tokunaga K et al. Fine needle aspiration biopsy via percutaneous transhepatic catheterization: technique and clinical results. *Gastrointest Radiol* 1986; **11**: 81–84

61   Foutch P G. Diagnosis of cancer by cytologic methods performed during ERCP. *Gastrointest Endosc* 1994; **40**: 249–252

62   Kurzawinski T R, Deery A, Dooley J S et al. A prospective study of biliary cytology in 100 patients with bile duct strictures. *Hepatology* 1993; **18**: 1399–1403

63   Fritscher-Ravens A, Broering D C, Sriram P V et al. EUS-guided fine-needle aspiration cytodiagnosis of hilar cholangiocarcinoma: a case series. *Gastrointest Endosc* 2000; **52**: 534–540

64   Kocjan G, Smith A N. Bile duct brushings cytology: potential pitfalls in diagnosis. *Diagn Cytopathol* 1997; **16**: 358–363

65   Layfield L J, Wax T D, Lee J G, Cotton P B. Accuracy and morphologic aspects of pancreatic and biliary duct brushings. *Acta Cytol* 1995; **39**: 11–18

66   Logrono R, Kurtycz D F, Molina C P et al. Analysis of false-negative diagnoses on endoscopic brush cytology of biliary and pancreatic duct strictures: the experience at 2 university hospitals. *Arch Pathol Lab Med* 2000; **124**: 387–392

67   Ryan M E, Baldauf M C. Comparison of flow cytometry for DNA content and brush cytology for detection of malignancy in pancreaticobiliary strictures. *Gastrointest Endosc* 1994; **40**: 133–139

68   Itoi T, Takei K, Shinohara Y et al. K-ras codon 12 and p53 mutations in biopsy specimens and bile from biliary tract cancers. *Pathol Int* 1999; **49**: 30–37

69   Stewart C J, Burke G M. Value of p53 immunostaining in pancreatico-biliary brush cytology specimens. *Diagn Cytopathol* 2000; **23**: 308–313

70   Ponsioen C Y, Vrouenraets S M, van Milligen de Wit A W et al. Value of brush cytology for dominant strictures in primary sclerosing cholangitis. *Endoscopy* 1999; **31**: 305–309

71   Tascilar M, Sturm P D, Caspers E et al. Diagnostic p53 immunostaining of endobiliary brush cytology: preoperative cytology compared with the surgical specimen. *Cancer* 1999; **87**: 306–311

72   Sturm P D, Hruban R H, Ramsoekh T B et al. The potential diagnostic use of K-ras codon 12 and p53 alterations in brush cytology from the pancreatic head region. *J Pathol* 1998; **186**: 247–253

73   Niiyama H, Mizumoto K, Kusumoto M et al. Activation of telomerase and its diagnostic application in biopsy specimens from biliary tract neoplasms. *Cancer* 1999; **85**: 2138–2143

74   Hales M S, Miller T R. Diagnosis of xanthogranulomatous cholecystitis by fine needle aspiration biopsy. A case report. *Acta Cytol* 1987; **31**: 493–496

75   Krishnani N, Shukla S, Jain M et al. Fine needle aspiration cytology in xanthogranulomatous cholecystitis, gallbladder adenocarcinoma and coexistent lesions. *Acta Cytol*. 2000; **44**: 508–514

76   Wu S S, Lin K C, Soon M S, Yeh K T. Ultrasound-guided percutaneous transhepatic fine needle aspiration cytology

study of gallbladder polypoid lesions. *Am J Gastroenterol* 1996; **91**: 1591–1594

77 Yang G C. Pneumocystis carinii infection presents as common bile duct mass biopsied by fine-needle aspiration. *Diagn Cytopathol* 2000; **22**: 25–26

78 Leung J W C, Sung J Y, Banez V P *et al*. Endoscopic cholangiopancreatography in hepatic clonorchiasis–a follow-up study. *Gastrointest Endosc* 1990; **36**: 360–363

79 Papillo J L, Leslie K O, Dean R A. Cytologic diagnosis of liver fluke infestation in a patient with subsequently documented cholangiocarcinoma. *Acta Cytol* 1989; **33**: 865–869

80 Baron T H, Lee J G, Wax T D *et al*. An in vitro, randomized, prospective study to maximize cellular yield during bile duct brush cytology. *Gastrointest Endosc* 1994; **40**: 146–149

81 Leung J W C, Sung J Y, Chung S C S, Chan K M. Endoscopic scraping biopsy of malignant biliary structures. *Gastrointest Endosc* 1989; **35**: 65–66

82 Stewart C J, Mills P R, Carter R *et al*. Brush cytology in the assessment of pancreatico-biliary strictures: a review of 406 cases. *J Clin Pathol* 2001; **54**: 449–455

83 Gibbs P D. Degenerating cells in bile stained gastric aspirates. *Acta Cytol* 1963; **7**: 311–314

84 Hemming N, Witte S. *Atlas der Gastroenterologischen Cytodiagnostik*. Stuttgart: Georg Thieme, 1957

85 Prolla J C, Kirsner J B. *Handbook and Atlas of Gastrointestinal Exfoliative Cytology*. Chicago: University of Chicago Press, 1972; 48–54

86 Koss L G. *Diagnostic cytology and Its Histopathologic Bases*, 4th edn. Philadelphia: Lippincott, 1992; 1063–1081

87 Cohen M B, Wittchow R J, Johlin F C *et al*. Brush cytology of the extrahepatic biliary tract: comparison of cytologic features of adenocarcinoma and benign biliary strictures. *Mod Pathol* 1995; **8**: 498–502

88 Renshaw A A, Madge R, Jiroutek M, Granter S R. Bile duct brushing cytology: statistical analysis of proposed diagnostic criteria. *Am J Clin Pathol* 1998; **110**: 635–640

89 Gupta R K, Naran S, Lallu S *et al*. Fine needle aspiration cytodiagnosis of primary squamous cell carcinoma of the gallbladder. Report of two cases. *Acta Cytol* 2000; **44**: 467–471

90 Bardales R H, Stanley M W, Simpson D D *et al*. Diagnostic value of brush cytology in the diagnosis of duodenal, biliary, and ampullary neoplasms. *Am J Clin Pathol* 1998; **109**: 540–548

91 de Peralta-Venturina M N, Wong D K, Purslow M J, Kini S R. Biliary tract cytology in specimens obtained by direct cholangiographic procedures: a study of 74 cases. *Diagn Cytopathol* 1996; **14**: 334–348

92 Veronezi-Gurwell A, Wittchow R J, Bottles K, Cohen M B. Cytologic features of villous adenoma of the ampullary region. *Diagn Cytopathol* 1996; **14**: 145–149

93 Tsui W M, Lam P W, Mak C K, Pay K H. Fine-needle aspiration cytologic diagnosis of intrahepatic biliary papillomatosis (intraductal papillary tumor): report of three cases and comparative study with cholangiocarcinoma. *Diagn Cytopathol* 2000; **22**: 293–298

94 Dusenbery D. Biliary stricture due to hepatocellular carcinoma: diagnosis by bile duct brushing cytology. *Diagn Cytopathol* 1997; **16**: 55–56

95 Nilsson B, Wee A, Yap I. Bile cytology. Diagnostic role in the management of biliary obstruction. *Acta Cytol* 1995; **39**: 746–752

96 Stewart C J, Stephen M R, Ferrier R K. Hepatocellular carcinoma diagnosis in bile duct brush cytology. *Diagn Cytopathol* 1998; **19**: 149–150

97 Mansfield J C, Griffin S M, Wadehra V, Matthewson K. A prospective evaluation of cytology from biliary strictures. *Gut* 1997; **40**: 671–677

98 Ponchon T, Gagnon P, Berger F *et al*. Value of endobiliary brush cytology and biopsies for the diagnosis of malignant bile duct stenosis: results of a prospective study. *Gastrointest Endosc* 1995; **42**: 565–572

99 Schoefl R, Haefner M, Wrba F *et al*. Forceps biopsy and brush cytology during endoscopic retrograde cholangiopancreatography for the diagnosis of biliary stenoses. *Scand J Gastroenterol* 1997; **32**: 363–368

100 Cozzi G, Alasio L, Civelli E *et al*, Percutaneous intraductal sampling for cyto-histologic diagnosis of biliary duct strictures. *Tumori* 1999; **85**: 153–156

16 Pancreas

Vikram Deshpande*

Introduction

The incidence of pancreatic malignancies is increasing in the Western world. There are 29 000 new cases of pancreatic cancer diagnosed in the USA each year and pancreatic cancer is now the 4th leading cause of cancer deaths in both men and women[1]. The majority of patients have advanced unresectable disease at the time of diagnosis. In one series, only 14 of 253 patients were found to have resectable tumours[2]. The prognosis is abysmal, with only 8% of patients surviving for more than 2 years[2]. Modern imaging tests such as high-resolution spiral computed tomography, transcutaneous ultrasonography, magnetic resonance imaging, and endoscopic ultrasound have improved our ability to recognize and delineate pancreatic masses and secondary deposits if any. A tissue diagnosis is necessary in most cases because a variety of non-neoplastic and benign neoplasms of the pancreas can mimic pancreatic cancer both clinically and on imaging studies. Fine needle aspiration (FNA) biopsy of the pancreas is now a well-established technique for obtaining a tissue diagnosis in both solid and cystic lesions of the pancreas.

Value and limitations of cytology in diagnosis

Traditional surgical biopsies using wedge resection or a Vim Silverman needle have a high complication rate of between 5–20%[3–5]. The complications include fistula formation, haemorrhage and pancreatitis. Fatalities have been recorded in 2–3% of cases[3,6,7]. However, a wedge biopsy is regarded as safe, provided the biopsy can be kept as superficial as possible and is limited to abnormal tissue on the pancreatic surface[8]. Needle biopsies are recommended for lesions deep in the pancreas. By comparison there have been very few serious complications reported with FNA.

Intraoperative FNA biopsy allows the surgeon to take multiple passes through the mass safely. Repeated fine needle insertions improve the cytological success rate, leading to a diagnostic accuracy of between 71–100%[9–18]. The sensitivity is higher than that reported with histology and frozen section[19]. Adjacent lymph nodes and omental deposits can also be sampled at laparotomy. An experienced cytopathologist can provide a cytological report within minutes if required.

Fine needle aspiration is well accepted in non-operable pancreatic carcinoma. However, some authors oppose performing FNAs in small potentially resectable cancers unless preoperative chemotherapy, radiation or intraoperative radiotherapy is part of the treatment[8]. This is to avoid potential dissemination of the tumour, which although rare, cannot be ignored. If practised in centres with documented low operative mortality, the strategy of waiving a biopsy is logical, as chronic pancreatitis is an accepted indication for resection[8].

Percutaneous fine needle aspiration biopsy has been shown to be highly reliable in diagnosing pancreatic cancer, with a specificity of 100% in most series[8]. Percutaneous fine needle aspirates are more sensitive than percutaneous core biopsies[20,21]. There have been very few reports of false positive[22–24] or false suspicious results[9,25–27]. Most of the errors have occurred in differentiating regenerative atypia seen in chronic pancreatitis from well-differentiated adenocarcinoma[9,25–27]. The inaccuracies of pancreatic fine needle aspirates appear to be due almost entirely to false negative reports. The sensitivity of pancreatic FNA is variable, ranging from 45% to 97%[13,24,27–36]. One study found that the diagnostic sensitivity of FNA decreases significantly with decreasing tumour size[12]. It is, however, difficult to compare the sensitivity of FNA among studies because of the variability regarding factors, such as needle size, operator experience and improvement in radiological equipment. Additionally, the atypical and suspicious categories have been variably interpreted as negative or positive for the purposes of these studies. The sensitivity for cystic neoplasms is lower than that for solid neoplasms[36–38].

Experience has shown that endoscopic ultrasound directed fine needle aspiration (EUS-FNA) also has a variable sensitivity for solid malignancies of the pancreas, varying from 59.9% to 92%[39–41]. In fine needle aspiration of the pancreas only a positive cytological diagnosis is of clinical value, since a negative result does not exclude malignancy.

False positive results have been reported with exfoliative cytology specimens. Cobb and Floyd report an average false positive rate of 6.2% with samples of bile obtained from duodenal drainage[42]. Interpretative difficulties relate to degenerative cell changes. This technique is now obsolete.

*The author gratefully acknowledges his debt to Merle L Greenberg, whose contribution to the previous edition of this chapter provided a substantial basis for this revised edition.

Diagnostic procedures

A major problem in diagnosing pancreatic cancer is accurately locating the lesion to obtain representative tissue. Prior to the advent of modern imaging techniques, cytological samples were obtained by duodenal intubation and suction, with limited success[43–45]. Since the Scandinavians first utilized FNA in the 1970s, it has become the method of choice in obtaining representative tissue for diagnosis, either at exploratory laparotomy or under imaging guidance[9,22,33,46–48]. Currently ultrasound and computerized tomography are generally the preferred guidance techniques for FNA in the pre-operative evaluation of pancreatic masses[49].

Selection of a diagnostic procedure depends on the size and location of the lesion, and on whether it is solid or cystic. The radiologist's personal preference and expertise with a particular modality are also important factors in determining which technique is used. FNA using ultrasound guidance is technically more difficult but allows for real-time imaging of the needle tip. Computerized Tomography (CT) is technically easier, is not affected by bowel gas or obesity (as ultrasound is), but does not allow real time imaging, making the procedure more time consuming[49]. The type of needle used and details of the procedure are similar to that of other deep seated FNA and will not be repeated here.

Endoscopic retrograde cholangiopancreatography (ERCP) allows visualization of the pancreatic duct[4,50]. This permits sampling of pancreatic juice by cannulation of the main pancreatic duct via the ampulla of Vater, with or without secretin stimulation[43,50,51]. Brushings and FNA can also be performed at ERCP to enhance the diagnosis of small pancreatic cancers[4,52,53].

FNA material obtained through endoscopic ultrasound guidance is a relatively new and rapidly growing technique. It now plays a valuable role in the evaluation of pancreatic masses and the staging of pancreatic malignancy[40]. There are several advantages of endoscopic ultrasonography-guided fine needle aspiration (EUS-FNA) over percutaneous FNA[54]. Perhaps the greatest advantage is that it allows biopsy of small lesions that are not evident by conventional imaging studies. The second advantage is the close proximity of the echoendoscope to the target tissue. The short needle path decreases potential complications. The tissue around the needle path is resected at the time of definitive surgery. This greatly reduces the possibility of tumour dissemination by FNA. The equipment consists of an image guidance system, such as Pentax FG-32US (Pentax Precision Instruments Corporation, Orangeburg, NY), which has a linear array ultrasound transducer mounted distal to the viewing optics of the endoscope[55]. A 2 mm-biopsy channel is part of the equipment and is oriented so that the biopsy needle is advanced into the imaging plane, allowing for real time imaging of the actual biopsy. After endoscopic and ultrasound examination, the biopsy needle is advanced through the stomach or duodenum into the pancreatic mass under real time imaging. The procedure commonly uses a 22G disposable needle. Once in the lesion, the stylet is removed, and suction is applied using a syringe and the needle is moved to and fro within the lesion[54]. The procedure can be repeated until diagnostic tissue is obtained. EUS allows for more accurate staging including assessment of tumour size, invasion of local structures such as the common bile duct, metastasis to lymph nodes (including sampling by FNA) and venous involvement. This simultaneous staging reduces the number of laparotomies for non-resectable pancreatic carcinomas[56].

Pancreatic cysts can be aspirated both percutaneously and by EUS[57]. In addition to routine cytology, analysis of cyst fluid can provide valuable data and is discussed later in this chapter. Rapid microscopic examination, Gram stains and culture of fluid samples may help to distinguish pancreatic inflammatory masses from a pancreatic abscess[58].

Rapid interpretation of selected smears is routinely performed at our institution by a cytologist at the time of the aspiration. This has been shown to be of great benefit by reducing the number of inadequate specimens[30].

Complications and contraindications

From a literature review, Neuerburg and Gunther[59] report a 0.05% risk of major complications using fine 20–23 gauge needles as compared with a 5–20% risk with conventional surgical biopsies[3]. The most common complications arising from FNA of the pancreas are haemorrhage and pancreatitis. One of three documented intra-abdominal haematomas was noted incidentally at surgery 2 months after FNA of a pancreatic pseudocyst[3,60,61]. Although the relative risk of pancreatitis is low, six of the 14 cases reported were fatal[62–68]. Two reported cases of fatal septic shock, both thought to be due to bacterial contamination by colonic contents, followed aspiration of a pseudocyst[69] and a cancer[70]. A fatal pancreatic fistula followed blockage of a pancreatic duct by blood clot after intraoperative FNA on a patient with Crohn's disease[71]. Bile peritonitis and postoperative abscess are other potential hazards[72].

Spread of tumour along the needle tract is considered rare. Thousands of pancreatic FNAs have been performed since 1972 and have generated only 10 documented cases of cutaneous or abdominal wall seeding by tumour, 2–5 months following biopsy[73–79]. At our centre, patients scheduled for potential curative surgery on the basis of imaging findings receive 1000 Gy of local radiotherapy before FNA to prevent needle tract seeding[49]. This does not affect interpretation of the FNA material.

Fornari[80] described a case of peritoneal dissemination following aspiration biopsy. One study suggested that peritoneal washings of patients with pancreatic cancer who have undergone pancreatic FNA, are more likely to be positive for malignant cells and the survival is significantly shorter than that of patients who have not undergone a FNA procedure[81]. However, this was not confirmed by a subsequent study[82] and it is now felt that presence of cancer cells in peritoneal washings is an indicator of advanced disease rather than a consequence of prior percutaneous fine needle aspiration of the pancreas[8]. As mentioned earlier EUS-FNA lessens this potential complication. There are several other minor and self limiting complications, such as abdominal discomfort and pain during the procedure, hypotension, vasovagal attack and minor bleeding[34,60]. These are easily dealt with as long as the patient is carefully monitored during the procedure and in the immediate post-operative period. Additional complications unique to EUS include perforation associated with luminal stenosis[54].

The contraindications to aspiration of the pancreas are relative rather than absolute. Caution is advisable with patients who have a haemorrhagic diathesis unless the defect is corrected[83,84]. Aspiration of a suspected hydatid cyst is considered a contraindication by some because of the risk of an anaphylactic reaction. Additional contraindications for EUS-FNA would be the same as those for upper endoscopy.

Normal structure

Normal anatomy and histology

The bulk of the pancreas consists of an exocrine portion comprising acini arranged in lobules, secreting their digestive enzymes into an excretory duct system. The main duct traverses the length of the gland and empties into the duodenum together with the common bile duct at the ampulla of Vater. Ductal epithelium varies from tall columnar to cuboidal depending on the calibre of the duct. Goblet cells may be seen in the epithelium from the main duct. Islets of Langerhans form the endocrine component and are more concentrated in the body and tail of the gland. A dense zone of connective tissue surrounds the islets and probably accounts for the absence of endocrine cells in most aspirate smears. The different cell types present are classified according to the hormones that are secreted into the adjacent capillary circulation. These are: alpha cells (glucagon), beta cells (insulin), delta cells (somatostatin), enterochromaffin cells (5-hydroxytryptamine), pancreatic polypeptide cells (pancreatic polypeptide).

Acinar epithelium

Aspirates from normal pancreas are of scant to moderate cellularity and comprise mainly acinar cells. These are arranged in tight clusters or balls. Less commonly they occur as single cells, in tissue fragments with ill-defined fibrovascular stroma, or as bare nuclei. The cells are pyramidal in shape with ample cytoplasm, which is usually dense and granular and stains blue green with the standard Papanicolaou stain (Fig. 16.1). The prominent coarse granularity is probably the most characteristic feature of acinar cells. Air-dried, May-Grünwald-Giemsa-stained preparations enhance the abundance and granularity of the

cytoplasm. Nuclei are round and eccentrically placed with finely stippled chromatin. Small nucleoli are often easily identified.

PAS-trichrome stains the zymogen granules of acinar cells bright orange and distinguishes acinar cells from endocrine cells[85]. Acinar cells tend to be absent in exfoliative samples and brushings from the pancreatic duct.

Ductal epithelium

Ductal cells tend to be sparse in aspirate smears from normal pancreas, but are more noticeable in the presence of duct obstruction secondary to tumour or chronic pancreatitis. They are readily identified in pancreatic brushings. Depending on the calibre of the ducts, the cells may be tall columnar or cuboidal. They are larger than acinar cells and are often arranged as monolayer sheets or strips of cells with luminal cytoplasm. Viewed *en face* the sheets may have a honeycomb appearance with well-defined cell borders (Fig. 16.2). The nuclei are round to

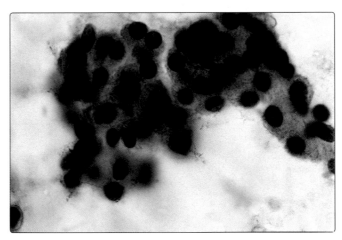

Fig. 16.1 Pancreatic acinar cells. Clusters of cells with acinar arrangement. Eccentric small round uniform nuclei, small nucleoli with abundant granular cytoplasm. (Papanicolaou × HP)

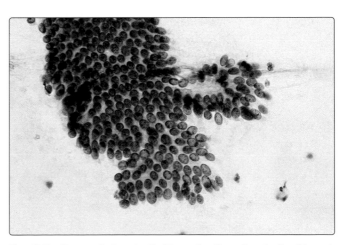

Fig. 16.2 Pancreatic ductal cells. Sheet of uniform ductal cells with a strip displaying luminal cytoplasm. (Papanicolaou × HP)

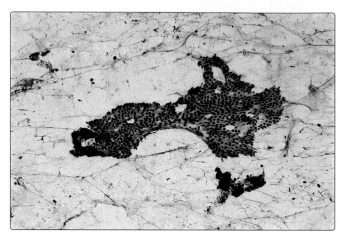

Fig. 16.3   Gastrointestinal contamination. Monolayered honeycombing sheet with crypt openings. (Papanicolaou × MP)

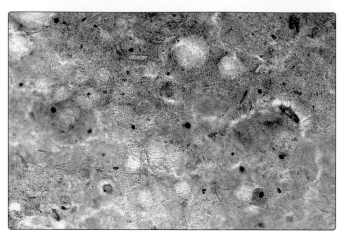

Fig. 16.4   Acute pancreatitis with fat necrosis. Foamy macrophages and degenerate fat cells in a dirty background. (Papanicolaou × MP)

oval, with evenly distributed finely granular chromatin. Nucleoli, if present, are small but may become enlarged and prominent with ductular proliferation. Cytoplasm varies in amount from scanty to moderate. There may be a luminal border but cilia are absent.

Islet cells

These are not usually visualized with routine stains, requiring special stains for identification[85,86].

Contaminants

Percutaneous fine needle biopsies may traverse liver, transverse colon, duodenum, bile duct and mesothelium. Contamination from these tissues may pose a diagnostic problem if one is not familiar with their morphology. Contamination by duodenal or gastric mucosal cells is a significant problem when dealing with EUS-FNA. Gastrointestinal contamination is typically present as flat monolayer sheets with a honeycomb pattern (Fig. 16.3). These large sheets of mucin producing cells could resemble a mucinous cystic neoplasm of the pancreas. These contaminating sheets may be folded and appear crowded and atypical. Identifying gastric pits or crypts of Lieberkuhn (both seen as small rosettes) helps to differentiate gastrointestinal contamination from lesional and pancreatic tissue. However, in some cases this distinction may not be possible. Reactive hepatocytes may appear atypical with enlarged nuclei and prominent nucleoli and may be mistaken for tumour. The presence of cytoplasmic lipofuscin pigment may indicate the origin of these cells.

Reactive and inflammatory processes

Pancreatitis commonly involves the parenchyma diffusely and is a relative contraindication for aspiration biopsy, as there is a slight risk of exacerbation of the pancreatitis. However, the sequelae of acute pancreatitis, such as pseudocyst and abscess formation, and the hard nodular gland of chronic pancreatitis, may simulate cancer. Thus tissue diagnosis may be necessary.

Acute pancreatitis

Acute pancreatitis is a debilitating disease of sudden onset, which may follow episodes of alcoholic abuse, trauma or obstruction of the pancreatic duct by stones or tumour. Liberation of destructive digestive enzymes causes extensive necrosis and inflammation of the parenchyma and surrounding tissue. Aspirates from patients with acute pancreatitis are only rarely seen. Occasionally a focal mass lesion is simulated on imaging and an FNA is performed to rule out tumour.

Cytological findings *(Fig. 16.4)*

- ▶ Acute inflammatory cells predominate
- ▶ Cellular debris
- ▶ Macrophages and lipophages
- ▶ Degenerate epithelial cells
- ▶ Granulation tissue including capillaries and reactive fibroblasts are seen in the healing phase

Diagnostic pitfalls

- ▶ Regenerative epithelial atypia
- ▶ Irritated mesothelial cells
- ▶ Atypical lipophages seen in association with fat necrosis
- ▶ Attention to the prominent inflammatory component seen should prevent potential pitfalls

Chronic pancreatitis

The most important disease to be distinguished from chronic pancreatitis is pancreatic adenocarcinoma, which it can mimic clinically, on imaging, intraoperatively, and importantly, on fine needle aspiration cytology. Focal pancreatic enlargement has been reported in 30% of cases on imaging, thus raising the possibility of malignancy. The

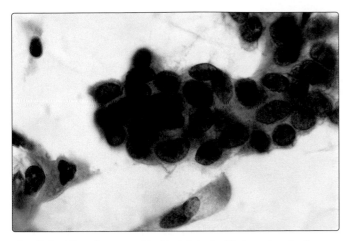

Fig. 16.5 Chronic pancreatitis: Ductal atypia. Clusters of markedly atypical ductal cells. (Papanicolaou × HP)

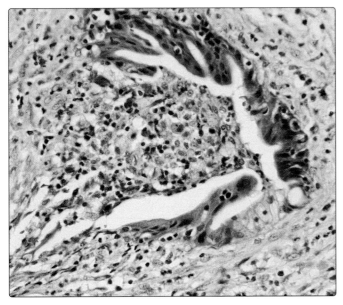

Fig. 16.6 Chronic pancreatitis. Tissue section: inflammatory changes with severe regenerative epithelial atypia. (H&E × LP)

atrophic pancreas may show extensive loss of the exocrine portion. A relative prominence of the endocrine component is seen on histology. Replacement fibrosis may complicate sampling with a fine needle. Prominent epithelial regeneration of ducts and acini with varying degrees of atypia may simulate a well-differentiated adenocarcinoma (Figs 16.5, 16.6)[3,87,88].

Cytological findings

- ► Scant to moderate cellularity
- ► Variable chronic inflammatory cell infiltrate
- ► Ductal epithelial cells with varying degrees of atypia
- ► No necrosis and only rare mitoses
- ► Rare single cells
- ► Admixture with other elements including acinar epithelium
- ► Occasional fragments of fibroblastic tissue

Diagnostic pitfalls

- ► Regenerative epithelial atypia simulating adenocarcinoma
- ► Non-representative or scanty tissue
- ► Islet cell hyperplasia versus islet cell tumour[89]

When the smear shows a predominantly inflammatory background with scant benign appearing ductal epithelium, the diagnosis is relatively easy. However, a relatively pure population of ductal cells with even mild atypia raises the possibility of a well-differentiated adenocarcinoma. Cell blocks can be useful in making this distinction, as they can show invasion of stroma and nerves. Additionally, marked reactive atypia can simulate a high-grade carcinoma. The distinction between these two entities is addressed in the section on ductal carcinoma.

Cystic lesions of the pancreas (Tables 16.1 and 16.2)

Abscess

Abscess formation may result from infected necrotic pancreatic tissue or superinfection of a pseudocyst secondary to acute pancreatitis. Clinical features, CT and ultrasound findings cannot confidently distinguish inflammatory pancreatic masses from necrotic cancers[90–92]. Also, CT cannot distinguish sterile inflammation from infection. Fine needle aspiration of the fluid collection under aseptic conditions has become the procedure of choice for verification of bacterial infection[93]. Drainage of a pancreatic abscess is a surgical emergency with a mortality rate of up to 67% if treatment is delayed. Immediate cytological examination may support the clinical diagnosis of an abscess if the smears consist of a marked acute inflammatory exudate and necrotic cellular debris[90,91]. Identification of bacteria with a rapid Gram stain is sufficient evidence for prompt surgical intervention and drainage. Aerobic and anaerobic culture of the aspirated material is obligatory, as a negative Gram stain is not completely reliable[92,94].

Pseudocyst

Pseudocysts, secondary to attacks of acute pancreatitis, are the commonest non-neoplastic cystic lesions of the pancreas[95]. Cytological confirmation for patient management is often necessary to differentiate these cysts from cystic neoplasms and other fluid collections in this region (Table 16.2). Over a 12-year period, more than one-third of patients referred to the Massachusetts General Hospital with cystic neoplasms were misdiagnosed as having pseudocysts on clinical and radiological grounds[96,97]. Misdiagnosis has lead to inappropriate therapy and fatal results for some patients. Errors have occurred on frozen sections because large portions of the epithelium can be denuded in cystic pancreatic tumours. Percutaneous aspiration is safe and efficient and can be of both diagnostic and therapeutic benefit[58]. Although surgery remains the standard therapy for drainage of pseudocysts, recently

Table 16.1 WHO histological classification of tumours of the exocrine pancreas

Benign	Borderline	Malignant
Serous cystadenoma		Serous cystadenocarcinoma
Mucinous cystadenoma	Mucinous cystic neoplasm with moderate dysplasia	Mucinous cystadenocarcinoma
Intraductal papillary-mucinous adenoma	Intraductal papillary- mucinous neoplasm with moderate dysplasia	Intraductal papillary- mucinous carcinoma
Mature teratoma		
	Solid-pseudopapillary neoplasm	
		Ductal adenocarcinoma
		Subtypes-mucinous noncystic carcinoma, signet ring cell carcinoma, adenosquamous carcinoma, undifferentiated (anaplastic) carcinoma, undifferentiated carcinoma with osteoclastic giant cells, mixed ductal-endocrine carcinoma
		Acinar cell carcinoma
		Mixed acinar-endocrine carcinoma
		Pancreatoblastoma

Table 16.2 Key features of common pancreatic cystic lesions

Lesion	Clinical features	Cytological criteria
Pseudocyst	History of pancreatitis	Hypocellular
		Debris, blood, histiocytes
		Absence of epithelium
		Diagnosis of exclusion
Lymphoepithelial cysts		Anucleate squames and keratinous debris
Serous cystadenoma	Elderly females	Hypocellular
		Small honeycombing cell clusters
		Clear cytoplasm containing glycogen
Mucinous cystic neoplasms	Females, 4th decade	Abundant background mucin
		Columnar mucinous epithelium
		Variable atypia
Intraductal papillary-mucinous neoplasms	Males, 7th to 8th decade	Same as mucinous cystic neoplasm
Solid-pseudopapillary tumour	Adolescent girls and young women	Highly cellular
		Globules and papillary structures with myxoid stroma
		Monomorphic nuclei with occasional grooves

endoscopic ultrasound (EUS) has been used for this purpose[98]. Cyst fluid aspirated during this procedure helps confirm the diagnosis of pseudocyst. The fluid aspirated varies in amount and appearance. It may be clear and translucent, or turbid and brown if there has been prior bleeding, or creamy if inflamed. Cyst fluid analysis is useful in distinguishing pseudocysts from neoplastic cysts, particularly mucinous neoplasms and will be addressed at the end of this section.

Cytological findings *(Fig. 16.7)*

► Hypocellular
► Background of granular debris, blood and bile pigments
► Scattered foamy macrophages
► Flecks of calcification
► Possible necrotic fat cells
► Inflammatory cells may be present
► Absence of epithelial cells

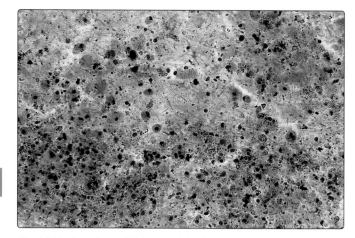

Fig. 16.7 Pseudocyst. Histiocytes, bile pigment and debris. Note the absence of mucinous epithelium. (Papanicolaou × MP)

Diagnostic pitfalls

▶ The presence of extracellular mucin, mucinous epithelium or muciphages in a percutaneous aspirate excludes the diagnosis of a pseudocyst and suggests a mucinous lesion instead. A mucicarmine stain is useful in identifying mucin

▶ Gastrointestinal (GI) contamination is a major problem when dealing with samples obtained by EUS-FNA. Typical monolayered sheets of gastrointestinal epithelium may be disregarded. However in some cases the distinction between GI contamination and a mucinous lesion may not be possible, and a differential diagnosis may have to be offered. A mucicarmine stain would not help in this situation

▶ The diagnosis of pseudocyst is one of exclusion.

Lymphoepithelial cysts

Lymphoepithelial cysts are uncommon, with only 39 documented cases in the literature[99]. They are more common in males, and on radiology are seen as macrocystic lesions that are sharply demarcated from the adjacent pancreas. Because of this sharp demarcation, and their benign nature, they are amenable to cystectomy, surgery that might not be considered for most other cystic neoplasms. Macroscopically they can be multilocular or unilocular and are filled with 'cheesy' material. On microscopy these cysts are lined by stratified squamous epithelium that may show prominent keratinization. Dense lymphoid tissue, including germinal centres, is present in the wall. The cytological features of lymphoepithelial cysts have recently been described[100,101].

Cytological findings (Fig. 16.8)

▶ Anucleate squames and abundant keratinous debris
▶ Mature superficial squamous cells
▶ Lymphocytes may or may not be present
▶ Cholesterol clefts

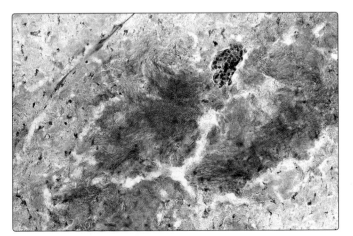

Fig. 16.8 Lymphoepithelial cyst. Keratin and keratinaceous debris. A fragment of gastrointestinal epithelial contaminant is also present. (Papanicolaou × MP)

Diagnostic pitfalls

▶ Other squamous lined cysts in the region of the pancreas such as dermoid cysts and epidermoid cysts
▶ The distinction between these entities may frequently not be possible, and may not be clinically relevant.

Retention cysts

These are small cysts that form from cystically dilated segments of pancreatic ducts as a consequence of focal duct obstruction. They are typically unilocular, small (<1 cm), and are lined by ductal epithelium, which is often denuded[102]. The cytologic features are non-diagnostic, showing few ductal epithelial cells and inflammatory cells. They are unlikely to be confused with a mucinous neoplasm either clinically and/or on imaging studies. It is however conceivable that aspirates of these lesions, when focally lined by metaplastic mucinous epithelium, may show a few mucinous epithelial cells and muciphages[103].

Cystic neoplasms

The vast majority of pancreatic tumours are solid. Cystic tumours of the pancreas constitute about 1–2% of pancreatic neoplasms and occur predominantly in women, in the body and tail of the pancreas.

Serous cystadenoma

Serous cystadenomas (microcystic or glycogen-rich cystadenoma) are estimated to account for about 25% of all cystic tumours and occur more frequently in elderly females. Almost all cases are benign. However 11 cases of serous cystic tumour of the pancreas with features that have been interpreted as malignant or that have behaved in a malignant fashion have been reported in the literature[104]. The tumour has been further subclassified into microcystic and oligocystic subtypes, depending on the number and size of the cysts. Both types are composed of cysts lined by monomorphic cuboidal cells with central bland nuclei and clear cytoplasm. Although imaging studies can be diagnostic, misdiagnosis on EUS or CT occurs in as many as 25% to 50% of cases[105–107]. Fine needle aspirates may aid in the preoperative diagnosis of these lesions[38,95,108–112]

Cytological findings (Fig. 16.9A)

▶ Usually hypocellular
▶ Epithelial cells are cuboidal or low columnar
▶ Cellular arrangement may include flat sheets with a honeycomb pattern, small flat clusters or single cells
▶ Bland, round or oval nuclei
▶ Clear cytoplasm with well-defined borders
▶ Indistinct nucleoli
▶ Nuclear grooves and intracytoplasmic inclusions
▶ Cytoplasmic glycogen demonstrated by PAS with and without diastase
▶ No intracellular or extracellular mucin

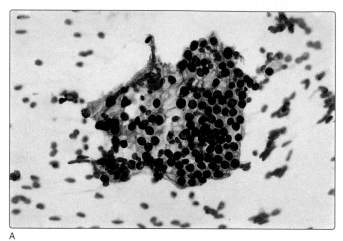

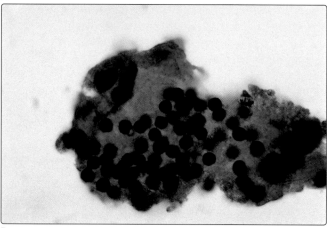

Fig. 16.9 (A) Serous cystadenoma (intraoperative scrape smear). Monolayered sheet with bland nuclei and clear cytoplasm. (Papanicolaou × HP) (B) Serous cystadenoma (ThinPrep from EUS guided aspirate). Monolayered sheet with bland nuclei. Marked ThinPrep artefacts of both the nucleus and cytoplasm are evident. (Papanicolaou × HP)

Pitfalls

Most aspirates from these lesions are hypocellular and thus non-diagnostic. In ThinPrep smears the nuclear details may not be appreciated (Fig. 16.9B).

Mucinous cystic neoplasms

Mucinous cystic neoplasms (MCN) of the pancreas comprise approximately 1% to 2% of all pancreatic tumours and 9.7% of all cystic pancreatic tumours[113]. They typically affect women in their late 40s[114]. Grossly, MCNs are usually multiloculated large cystic neoplasms, filled with tenacious mucin. The cysts are lined by tall mucin-producing columnar cells and are surrounded by a dense stroma that resembles ovarian stroma. This latter feature and the lack of communication of these tumours with the ductal system help in distinguishing MCN from intraductal papillary-mucinous neoplasms (IPMN). Depending on the degree of architectural and cytological atypia, the lesions are categorized in the WHO classification[115] as mucinous

cystadenoma, mucinous cystic neoplasm with moderate dysplasia and mucinous cystadenocarcinoma (these may be non-invasive or invasive). Mucinous cystadenomas contain a single layer of epithelium lacking significant cytological and architectural atypia. The carcinomas are characterized by severe atypia, mitotic activity, and/or cribriforming or bridging structures without fibrovascular cores. In borderline mucinous cystic neoplasms the cells show significant, but lesser degrees of cytological atypia with or without architectural atypia. A single mucinous cystic neoplasm can show a range of atypia, and areas of carcinoma may be very focal. In FNA material, because the cyst lining is heterogeneous, malignancy cannot be excluded[38,108,116]. Indeed in a recent study the presence of a mass on echoendoscopy was more sensitive (but less specific) for malignancy in MCN than cytology[57]. Fortunately, distinguishing between borderline lesions and carcinoma is not clinically necessary, as all MCN are treated with resection. It is, however, important to distinguish mucinous from non-mucinous lesions and FNA can reliably make this distinction[38]. Completely resected mucinous cystadenomas, borderline MCN, or MCN with *in-situ* carcinoma follow a benign course[117]. The 5-year survival for invasive mucinous cystadenocarcinomas in this series was 31%.

Mucinous cystadenoma

Cytological findings

► Abundant mucin
► Variable cellularity with columnar mucinous epithelium
► Sheets, papillary groups, and single cells
► Absence of atypia, necrosis or mitosis

Mucinous cystadenocarcinoma

Cytological findings (*Figs 16.10A, 16.10B*)

In addition to the above findings

► Abundant cellularity with prominent cell dyshesion
► Prominent cytological atypia and prominent nucleoli
► Mitosis and necrosis

Diagnostic pitfalls

► Scant and under-representative sample. A mucin stain will help identify rare mucin-containing cells and muciphages. These may not be diagnostic of a MCN, but can alert the surgeon to this possibility
► Obscuring inflammation, necrosis and debris
► Gastrointestinal contamination in EUS guided aspirates. The presence of flat, innocuous sheets of cells may help identify contamination
► IPMN cannot be distinguished from MCN. Imaging studies may help to make this distinction.

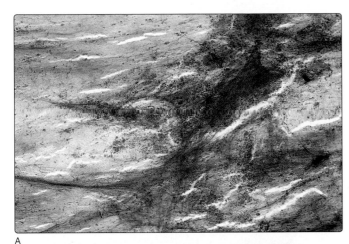

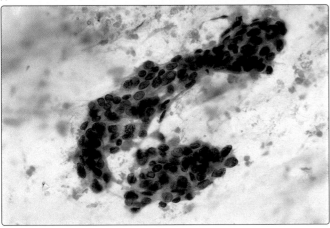

Fig. 16.10   (A) Mucinous cystic tumour. Abundant mucin with coagulative tumour necrosis. (Papanicolaou × MP) (B) Mucinous cystic tumour at least borderline. The two epithelial fragments show overlapping cells with nuclear membrane irregularities and a single mitotic figure. Streaks of mucin are also present. (Papanicolaou × HP)

▶ Pseudocysts do not contain background mucin, mucin containing cells or muciphages

Intraductal papillary-mucinous neoplasms (IPMN)

IPMN usually afflict elderly patients (7th and 8th decade) with a slight male predominance. These tumours are not uncommon, and accounted for 30.6% of cystic pancreatic neoplasms in one series[113]. IPMN is characterized by ectasia of the main pancreatic duct (and sometimes the branch ducts), which is filled with tenacious mucin. The ectatic ducts are lined by papillary mucinous epithelium. Because of cystic dilatation of the main or branch ducts IPMN may resemble true cystic pancreatic lesions clinically, radiographically and on gross examination[118]. Histologically, the proliferation may show a spectrum of cytoarchitectural atypia similar to MCN. Based on the degree of atypia these neoplasms are classified into intraductal papillary-mucinous adenoma, intraductal papillary-mucinous neoplasm with moderate dysplasia, and intraductal

papillary-mucinous carcinoma (invasive or non-invasive)[115]. Mucin extrusion from the ampulla and a radiographic finding of ectasia of the ducts is virtually diagnostic of these tumours[119]. However, these features are not seen in all cases.

Experience with the preoperative cytological diagnosis of these neoplasms is very limited. Using cytological material obtained by EUS guided catheter, Uehara et al. were able to correctly diagnose 10 of 11 intraductal papillary-mucinous carcinomas[120]. The cytological features overlap with those of MCN. The smears show abundant extracellular mucin with sheets and clusters of mucinous epithelium. The atypia mirrors that seen in mucinous cystic tumours, with carcinomas showing small papillary clusters and single cells with marked atypia, necrosis and mitosis[103]. As with MCN, assessment of the degree of atypia, although useful, is not clinically necessary, nor is it necessarily accurate (given the marked heterogeneity of the atypia). All cystic mucinous neoplasms need to be completely resected. The potential pitfalls are similar to those of MCN.

Solid-pseudopapillary tumour (SPT)

This tumour, also referred to as papillary, papillary-cystic and Frantz's tumour, occurs predominantly in adolescent girls and young women. This tumour can be both solid and cystic. However, since larger lesions tend to undergo cystic degeneration, this neoplasm must be considered in the differential diagnosis of cystic pancreatic lesions. SPT has been shown to be of low malignant potential with metastasis present in 10 to 15% of cases, usually at the time of first presentation[121]. This is an indolent tumour and long-term survival has been reported even in patients with metastases to the liver and peritoneum[122,123].

As the name suggests, the predominant histologic patterns are solid and pseudopapillary, with the papillary areas resulting from degenerative change occurring in a fundamentally solid tumour with rich vasculature. The tumour is composed of small uniform tumour cells that surround fibrovascular cores composed of myxoid mucinous stroma (Fig. 16.11, 16.12 and 16.13). The cytological features of SPT are highly characteristic, and accurate preoperative diagnosis is possible by using fine needle aspiration cytology[124–126].

Cytological findings[95,127–132] (Figs 16.11, 16.12)
(*denotes key features)

▶ Extremely cellular
▶ *Balls or globules of myxoid (metachromatic with Giemsa stains) stroma with or without a surrounding thick layer of neoplastic cells
▶ *Numerous large branching papillary clusters with slender central fibrovascular cores with myxoid stroma
▶ *Monomorphic round to oval nuclei with occasionally nuclear grooves and only slight pleomorphism
▶ *Finely granular chromatin and small nucleoli

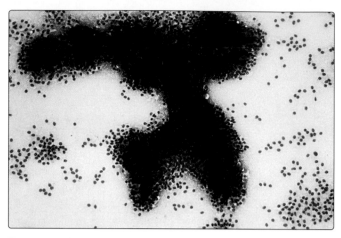

Fig. 16.11   Solid-pseudopapillary tumour. Branching papilliform fragment. Metachromatic material in centre of vascular stalk. (Diff-Quik × LP)

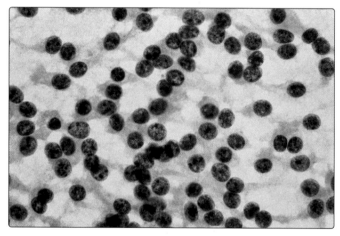

Fig. 16.12   Solid-pseudopapillary tumour. Uniform, bland tumour cell nuclei, fine nuclear chromatin, and small nucleoli. Cytoplasm absent or scanty. (Papanicolaou × HP)

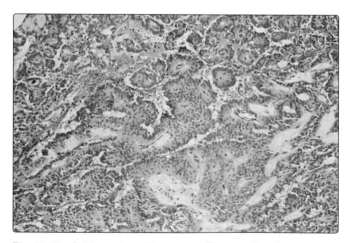

Fig. 16.13   Solid-pseudopapillary tumour. Tissue section of same case as **Fig. 16.10**. Several layers of tumour cells are orientated around vascular spaces imparting a pseudopapillary and pseudoacinar appearance. Areas of central cystic change. (H&E × MP)

► Cytoplasm is pale and moderate in amount
► Acinar arrangements with central metachromatic material may impart an adenoid cystic appearance
► Foamy macrophages and necrosis (evidence of cystic change)

Differential diagnoses include other tumours with low-grade, relatively monomorphic nuclei including acinar cell carcinoma and pancreatic endocrine tumours (Table 16.3). SPT do not show the atypia seen in ductal adenocarcinoma.

Cystic forms of typically solid pancreatic tumour

Rarely other tumours that are typically solid can undergo cystic change. These include pancreatic endocrine tumours, acinar cell carcinoma, large-duct type ductal carcinoma, invasive ductal adenocarcinoma with cystic change and cystic metastatic tumours.

Other pancreatic cysts

These include congenital cysts, para-ampullary duodenal wall cysts, enteric duplication cysts and endometrial cysts.

Non-pancreatic cysts masquerading as pancreatic cysts

In a study from the Massachusetts General Hospital, six of 28 cysts, submitted by the radiologist as a pancreatic cyst, were non-pancreatic on surgical excision[38]. They included intestinal papillary cystadenocarcinoma, retroperitoneal mesenteric inclusions cyst, a lymphoma with cystic degeneration, retroperitoneal leiomyoma with cystic degeneration, retroperitoneal serous cystadenoma and an adrenal cyst. The cytology in five of the six cases was non-diagnostic. Only the intestinal papillary cystadenocarcinoma yielded diagnostic cytology material, and this was interpreted as adenocarcinoma. It is important to remember that a radiologically identified 'pancreatic cyst' may not be pancreatic in origin.

Analysis of cyst fluid in pancreatic cysts

The biochemical analysis of fluid from cystic lesions of the pancreas may be very helpful in distinguishing cystic tumours from pseudocysts, serous cystadenomas from mucinous cystic tumours, and benign from malignant mucinous cystic tumours[113]. Pseudocysts usually have a relative viscosity less than that of serum, contain low levels of CEA, pS2, mucin-like carcinoma-associated antigen (MCA), CA72-4, and CA125. Mucinous tumours are typically are associated with high viscosity and elevation of the markers mentioned above[113]. Two additional markers, NB/70K and leucocyte esterase, when elevated, favour the diagnosis of pseudocyst over serous cystadenoma[133]. Serous cystadenomas have low levels of CEA (<25 ng/ml), distinguishing them from mucinous cystic neoplasms, which typically are associated with high levels of CEA. High levels of CA72-4, pS2 and tissue polypeptide antigen (TPA) have both been shown to correlate with malignancy in mucinous cystic neoplasms. Sampling may be an issue, as both retention cysts and pseudocysts may be associated

Table 16.3 Pancreatic neoplasms with monomorphic cells

	Pancreatic endocrine tumour	Acinar cell carcinoma	Solid-pseudopapillary tumour
Cytological features	Single cells, loosely cohesive clusters and branching fibrovascular stroma with attached cells	Single cells and loosely cohesive clusters	Cell balls and papillary clusters with myxoid stroma
	Monomorphic plasmacytoid cells with 'salt and pepper' nuclear chromatin	Monomorphic cells with granular cytoplasm and prominent nucleoli	Monomorphic cells with nuclear grooves
Immunocytochemistry	Positive for cytokeratin, chromogranin, synaptophysin and other specific endocrine hormones	Positive for trypsin, chymotrypsin and lipase	Positive for alpha-1-antitrypsin, alpha-1-chymotrypsin and NSE. Generally negative for other neuroendocrine and acinar cell carcinoma markers
Electron microscopy	Neuroendocrine granules	Electron dense zymogen granules	Abundant mitochondria and zymogen-like granules

with cystic neoplasms. Although a panel of cyst fluid markers is useful, the analysis is not diagnostic in isolation and is best viewed in conjunction with clinical, radiological and cytology findings.

Solid malignant neoplasms

Ductal adenocarcinoma of pancreas

Adenocarcinomas arising from the exocrine pancreas (Table 16.1) constitute 80–90% of all pancreatic cancers, with more than 60% located in the head region. They are highly aggressive tumours occurring mainly in the 5th to 7th decades of life. On histology most tumours are well- to moderately-differentiated. Poorly-differentiated adenocarcinomas are infrequent, and are composed predominantly of solid tumour cell nests and sheets. There may be small squamoid, spindle cell or anaplastic foci. By definition these areas constitute less than 20% of the tumour[134]. Almost all adenocarcinomas are associated with chronic pancreatitis due to obstruction.

The majority of moderately differentiated adenocarcinomas and all poorly-differentiated

adenocarcinomas are easily diagnosed as malignant. However well-differentiated adenocarcinomas are more problematic. The under diagnosis of well-differentiated adenocarcinoma as reactive epithelial changes is probably the single most influential reason for the relative low sensitivity of FNA in diagnosing pancreatic adenocarcinoma[135]. Several studies over the last two decades have addressed this issue[135–139]. In one of these series application of improved criteria resulted in an increase in sensitivity from 70% to 90%[135]. The same authors suggest that at least six clusters of tumour cells need to be identified before a definitive diagnosis of malignancy is reached.

Cytological findings in well-differentiated adenocarcinoma (Figs 16.14, 16.15)
(*denotes key features)

▶ Cellular smears
▶ *Monolayer sheets with nuclear overlapping

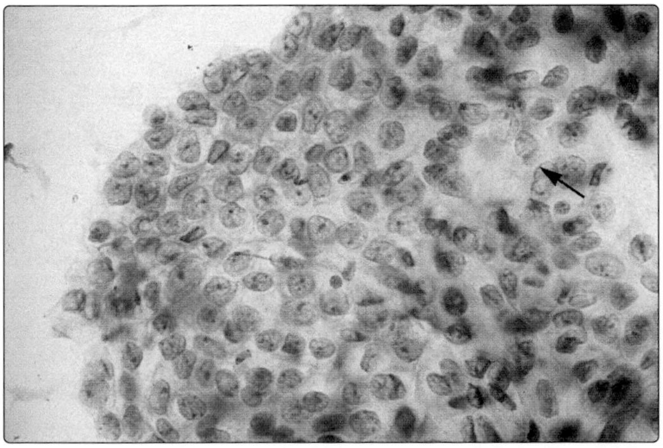

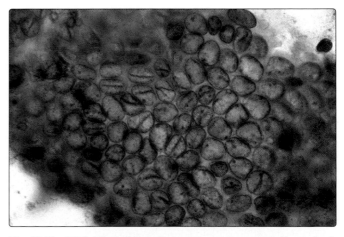

Fig. 16.14 Well-differentiated adenocarcinoma (pancreas). Cohesive sheet with enlarged atypical nuclei, well-defined cell borders. Tendency to acinar pattern (arrow). (Papanicolaou × HP)

Fig. 16.15 Well-differentiated adenocarcinoma (pancreas). Sheet of cells showing marked crowding of nuclei, 'washed out' nuclear chromatin, and nuclear membrane irregularities, including several nuclear grooves. (Papanicolaou × HP)

▶ *Subtle nuclear contour irregularities
▶ *Chromatin clearing and/or clumping
▶ 'Washed-out' nuclear chromatin with rimming of the nuclear membrane
▶ *Nuclear area variation (>4:1)
▶ Mitosis, necrosis and dyshesion with single cells are useful but rarely present

As the cytological criteria for the diagnosis of pancreatic adenocarcinomas rely more on nuclear criteria and cellular relationships[139,140], alcohol-fixed Papanicolaou stained smears are preferable to air dried smears.

Robin et al.[135] published a comprehensive study on the FNA findings in ductal adenocarcinoma. They identified three major criteria (nuclear crowding and overlap, irregular chromatin distribution and nuclear contour irregularity) and four minor criteria (nuclear enlargement, single malignant cells, necrosis and mitosis) that assist in making a diagnosis of adenocarcinoma. The presence of two or more major criteria or one major and three minor criteria were diagnostic of malignancy. Lin and Staerkel[137] identified four criteria that were consistently present in well-differentiated adenocarcinoma: (1) nuclear volume variation of cells within the same group (positive if found to exceed 4:1), (2) nuclear membrane abnormalities, (3) nuclear crowding/overlap/three-dimensional fragments and (4) nuclear enlargement ($>1.5 \times$ RBC).

Diagnostic pitfalls

▶ Overdiagnosis of chronic pancreatitis. These aspirates contain flat monolayered sheets that may show significant nuclear overlap, but lack the other nuclear features of carcinoma listed above. Additionally, aspirates from chronic pancreatitis tend to be less cellular, are associated with an inflammatory component, and show admixed acinar cells
▶ Underdiagnosis of adenocarcinoma. Relatively pure populations of ductal cells should be viewed with suspicion, and careful attention paid to nuclear detail
▶ Gastrointestinal contamination. This is present as flat honeycombing sheets, with well-defined cytoplasmic outlines and without the nuclear features of malignancy

Cytological findings in moderately to poorly-differentiated adenocarcinoma (Figs 16.16–16.18)

▶ Three-dimensional groups, 'drunken honeycomb pattern', easily identified single cells
▶ Obvious nuclear membrane irregularities, hyperchromasia and coarse chromatin
▶ Mitosis and necrosis
▶ There is no difficulty in diagnosing malignancy in moderately and poorly-differentiated adenocarcinomas, as the cytological criteria for malignancy are readily identified. Some poorly-differentiated adenocarcinomas may present mainly as a dispersed cell population.

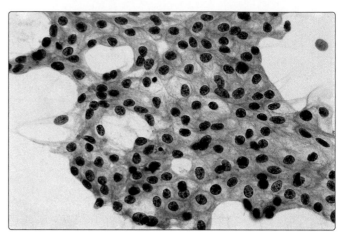

Fig. 16.16   Adenocarcinoma (pancreas). Sheet of tumour cells showing disordered honeycomb (drunken honeycomb) pattern. (Papanicolaou × HP)

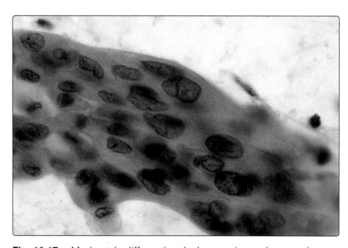

Fig. 16.17   Moderately-differentiated adenocarcinoma (pancreas). Obviously malignant features with pleomorphism, nuclear overlapping and nuclear grooves. (Papanicolaou × HP)

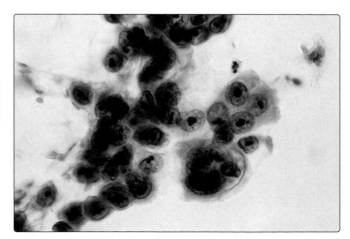

Fig. 16.18   Poorly-differentiated adenocarcinoma (pancreas). Loose aggregate of malignant cells with cellular dissociation. Some cells have a columnar shape. (Papanicolaou × HP)

Diagnostic pitfalls

▶ Chronic pancreatitis with reactive atypia. Ductal cells tend to be cohesive and lack the necrosis and frequent mitoses associated with carcinoma
▶ Neuroendocrine tumours
▶ Metastatic adenocarcinomas
▶ Lymphoma

A definite diagnosis of primary pancreatic adenocarcinoma should not be made when only a few atypical cells are seen, especially if they are admixed with benign exocrine elements[139]. Immunohistochemical stains such as cytokeratin, chromogranin and leucocyte common antigen may be necessary to differentiate carcinomas from neuroendocrine tumours and lymphoma. Cell block preparations from needle rinses of the aspirate are useful for assessing tumour architecture and for performing special stains.

Carcinomas of extra hepatic bile duct origin cannot be distinguished on morphology from those that arise in the pancreas.

Variants of ductal adenocarcinoma

Undifferentiated carcinoma (anaplastic carcinoma) *(Fig. 16.19)*

This is a rare and rapidly fatal variant of ductal carcinoma. The majority of patients die within 2–3 months of diagnosis[141–144]. Haematogeneous spread to the lungs and liver is common, compared with lymphatic metastases with ductal adenocarcinoma[143].

The tumour is composed of large eosinophilic pleomorphic cells and/or ovoid to spindle shaped cells that form poorly cohesive groups supported by scant fibrous stroma. This tumour is fundamentally a carcinoma. Positive staining with cytokeratin and electron microscopic findings support this fact[143,145].

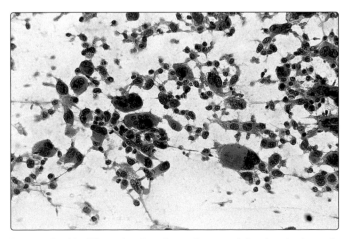

Fig. 16.19   Undifferentiated carcinoma (pancreas). Poorly cohesive and bizarre malignant cells. Also seen are a few osteoclast type giant cells. (Papanicolaou × MP)

Cytological findings

▶ Marked cellularity with prominent tumour diathesis
▶ Predominantly isolated and poorly cohesive cells with only rare clusters
▶ Numerous bizarre, multinucleated malignant cells
▶ Malignant mononucleated and spindle cells with numerous bizarre mitotic figures
▶ Focal squamous differentiation and occasional osteoclastic-type giant cells may be present.

Immunohistochemical stains and electron microscopy may be required to differentiate this neoplasm from metastatic melanoma, pleomorphic soft tissue sarcoma, hepatocellular carcinoma and germ cell tumours.

Undifferentiated carcinoma with osteoclast-like giant cells

This is a rare neoplasm, and as the name suggests is a carcinoma composed of pleomorphic to spindle shaped cells and numerous scattered osteoclast-like giant cells[134,146]. With immunohistochemical stains, at least some of the neoplastic cells express cytokeratin. A mean survival of 12 months has been suggested[134].

Cytological findings[147–149]

(*denotes key features)

▶ *Dual cell population
▶ *Bland multinucleated osteoclastic giant cells
▶ Spindled to ovoid malignant cells
▶ Osteoid may be present

Benign and malignant processes in which multinucleated giant cells are a prominent feature should be distinguished from this tumour[148]. Malignant tumours that may yield bizarre multinucleated malignant cells include pleomorphic carcinoma of the pancreas, metastatic anaplastic carcinoma, malignant melanoma, hepatocellular carcinoma, sarcomas and trophoblastic tumours. Granulomatous inflammation, fat necrosis and foreign body giant cell reactions are among the benign lesions in which multinucleated giant cells may be found[148].

Adenosquamous carcinoma

This is a rare neoplasm characterized by the presence of a variable proportion of mucin-producing glandular elements and squamous components. The squamous component should account for at least 30% of the tumour[134]. A few reports have described the FNA findings of adenosquamous carcinoma[150–153]. As in histology, the proportion of squamous and glandular elements vary. The squamous element may dominate or may be the only element seen, and single cells with cytoplasmic mucin vacuoles may be the only evidence of glandular differentiation (Figs 16.20, 16.21). Pure squamous cell carcinomas of the pancreas are very rare. It is important to remember that neoplastic squamous cell can

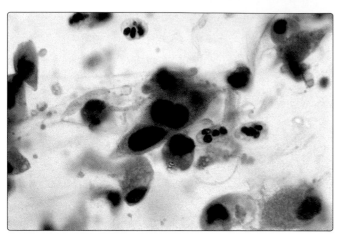

Fig. 16.20 Adenosquamous carcinoma (pancreas). Cluster of malignant squamous cells and neoplastic mucin-containing glandular cells. (Papanicolaou × HP)

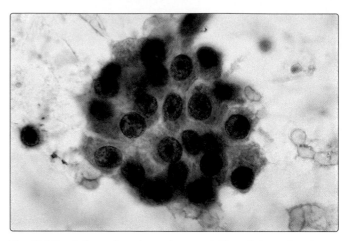

Fig. 16.22 Acinar cell carcinoma (pancreas). The cells have abundant granular cytoplasm. The tumour cells can be distinguished from normal acinar cells (**Fig. 16.1**) by their prominent nucleoli and high nuclear cytoplasmic ratio. (Papanicolaou × HP)

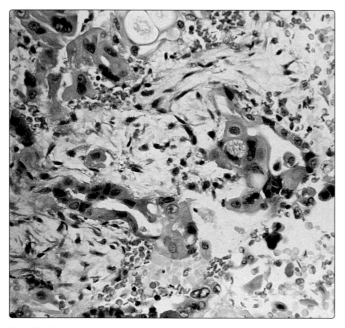

Fig. 16.21 Adenosquamous carcinoma (pancreas). Tissue section. (H&E × MP)

also be seen in undifferentiated carcinomas and in metastatic squamous cell carcinomas.

Signet ring carcinoma

This is an extremely rare carcinoma composed almost exclusively of mucin filled signet ring cells[154]. Metastasis from a gastric primary should be excluded before making this diagnosis[134].

Mucinous non-cystic carcinoma

This is an uncommon carcinoma in which mucin accounts for >50% of the tumour[134]. The aspirates resemble those from colloid carcinoma of the breast with groups of well-differentiated tumour cells floating in pools of mucin. Cytologically, the aspirates resemble mucinous cystic

neoplasms and imaging studies may have to be relied upon to make this distinction. However, the distinction is important because mucinous cystic tumours have a better prognosis than mucinous non-cystic tumours[117].

Other primary tumours

Acinar cell carcinoma

These are rare tumours that occur predominantly in adults, with a mean age of 62 years. However, paediatric cases have been reported[134]. A few patients reportedly develop a syndrome characterized by subcutaneous fat necrosis and polyarthralgia[155], caused by excessive lipase in the serum secreted by this type of tumour. Because of their large size and relatively sharp circumscription, acinar cell carcinomas can be distinguished from ductal carcinomas radiologically. Occasionally multicystic masses are seen[156]. These tumours are aggressive with a median survival of 18 months and a 5-year survival of less than 10%. On histology the most common patterns are acinar (composed of small glandular units) and solid. Acinar cell carcinoma resembles acinic cell carcinoma of the salivary gland.

Cytological findings[157–159] *(Fig. 16.22)*

- ▶ Cellular smears
- ▶ Single cells, including stripped naked nuclei
- ▶ Loosely cohesive clusters and vague acini
- ▶ Monomorphic cells with round to oval nuclei and prominent nucleoli
- ▶ Scant to moderate cytoplasm with granularity (best seen on air-dried smears)

Diagnostic pitfalls

- ▶ Pancreatic endocrine tumour and solid-pseudopapillary tumour: both of these tumours have monomorphic nuclei.

These three tumours are compared in Table 16.3. Immunohistochemistry and electron microscopy studies can be diagnostic

▶ Normal acinar cells may be mistaken for acinar cell carcinoma. Normal acinar cells form small cohesive grape-like clusters. The cell clusters in acinar cell carcinoma are larger and less cohesive and contain significantly larger nucleoli.

Pancreatoblastoma

This is a rare malignant epithelial tumour generally affecting young children, with a mean age of 4 years. It accounts for 30–50% of pancreatic neoplasms in children[160]. Grossly these neoplasms have a solid fleshy cut surface, intersected by fibrous bands. On histology they are composed of solid nests of polygonal cells, with acinar differentiation and intervening cellular fibrous bands. One of the characteristic features is aggregates of cells with squamous differentiation (squamoid corpuscles). The FNA features in one report described a hypercellular specimen composed of predominantly dissociated primitive cells and some cell groupings. The cells were oval to cuboidal cells with coarse, evenly distributed chromatin and moderate amounts of granular cytoplasm[161]. Spindle shaped, elongated and triangular shaped cells were also seen with abundant fragments of stroma. Squamous corpuscles were not seen. Immunohistochemistry and electron microscopy confirm acinar differentiation. The differential diagnosis includes acinar cell carcinoma.

Endocrine tumours

Primary pancreatic endocrine tumours are uncommon lesions that constitute less than 5% of all primary pancreatic tumours. Included in the spectrum are benign and malignant islet cell tumours, and carcinoid tumours. These endocrine tumours commonly arise as solitary lesions in the body and tail of the pancreas. Less than 10% are multiple.

Pancreatic endocrine tumour

Pancreatic endocrine tumour (PET) can occur at any age, but is uncommon in children. The majority of clinically relevant PET are functional[162]. Among the functional tumours, insulinomas are the most common, followed by gastrinomas, VIPomas, glucagonomas and somatostatinomas[163]. Unequivocal evidence of malignancy is gross invasion of adjacent organs, or metastasis to lymph nodes, liver or other sites. It is possible to identify prognostic subgroups within PET and several prognostic markers have been proposed. The Capella classification divides PET into four categories: benign, benign or low-grade malignant, low-grade malignant and high-grade malignant tumours based on functional status of the tumour, tumour size, presence or absence of angioinvasion and tumour differentiation[164,165]. Generally, most insulinomas less than 2 cm and other PET less than 1 cm behave in a benign fashion. In the largest study of non-

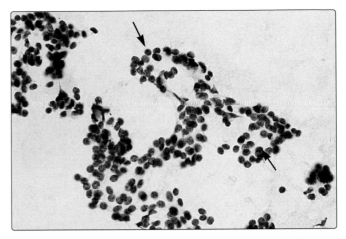

Fig. 16.23 Islet cell tumour (pancreas). Loose aggregates of uniform tumour cells with tendency to rosette arrangements (arrows). (Papanicolaou × HP)

functional PET, vascular or perineural invasion and Ki67 proliferation index (>2%) were found to be the two best markers that correlated with malignancy[164].

Grossly PET are generally solid, well-circumscribed and fleshy tumours. Rarely they can present as cystic masses[156]. On histology the most common patterns are trabecular or gyriform, glandular and solid. The cells are generally monomorphic with moderate to abundant eosinophilic cytoplasm. Vacuolated and oncocytic variants have been described[166]. The nuclei are characterized by salt and pepper type chromatin and nucleoli are generally not prominent.

Cytological findings[86,167–174]

(*denotes key features)

▶ Highly cellular smears
▶ *Predominantly single cells, some with stripped nuclei
▶ Loose or more rarely tightly cohesive clusters and rosettes (Fig. 16.23)
▶ Branching fibrovascular stroma surrounded by loosely attached tumour cells
▶ *Monomorphic population of small to medium sized cells with occasional larger cells
▶ *Nuclei commonly round, with finely stippled chromatin and smooth nuclear membrane (Figs 16.24A,16.24B)
▶ *Plasmacytoid cells with eccentrically placed nuclei and scant to moderate amounts of delicate cytoplasm (Fig. 16.25)
▶ Metachromatic cytoplasmic granules (on air dried material)
▶ Nucleoli small and inconspicuous or rarely prominent
▶ Bi- and multinucleation sometimes seen
▶ Mitoses and nuclear pleomorphism uncommon
▶ Tumour diathesis usually absent

Diagnostic pitfalls

▶ Acinar cell carcinoma (see Table 16.3)
▶ Misinterpreting the islets present in islet cell hyperplasia islets as neoplastic. Islet cell hyperplasia is associated with an

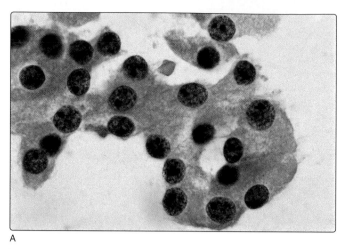
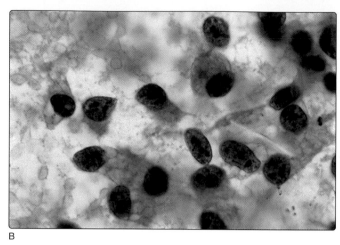

Fig. 16.24 (A) Pancreatic endocrine tumour. Plasmacytoid cells with 'salt and pepper' nuclear chromatin and small nucleoli. (Papanicolaou × HP) (B) Pancreatic endocrine tumour. Note the vacuolated cytoplasm. (Papanicolaou × HP)

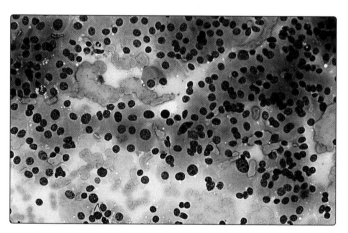

Fig. 16.25 Islet cell tumour (pancreas). Dispersed population of large tumour cells with eccentric nuclei. Some variation in nuclear size. Stippled nuclear chromatin. Cytoplasm dense and granular (plasmacytoid). (Diff-Quik × HP)

admixture of exocrine and endocrine cells. Also, the endocrine cells appear more cohesive than in PET[89,175]. However, in scantily cellular specimens it may be difficult to differentiate between the two.

► Other plasmacytoid tumours such as plasmacytoma and malignant melanoma
► Metastatic or primary small cell undifferentiated carcinoma shows prominent tissue necrosis, nuclear moulding and scanty cytoplasm, features not associated with PET.
► Oncocytic[176] and vacuolated[166] PET
► Immunohistochemistry and electron microscopy can play a significant role in confirming the diagnosis (Table 16.3). It is not possible to predict the outcome of PET based on cytology[169].

Carcinoid tumours

There are no morphological or ultrastructural features that distinguish carcinoid tumours from islet cell neoplasms. Elevated levels of 5-hydroxytryptamine or its precursors in association with the carcinoid syndrome are prerequisites for this diagnosis.

Small cell carcinoma

Primary undifferentiated small cell carcinoma of the pancreas is extremely rare. The histological features are indistinguishable from small cell carcinomas of the lung[177,178]. The cytological features of these neuroendocrine neoplasms are the same as described for other sites[174]. Nuclear moulding, finely granular chromatin, inconspicuous nucleoli and scant cytoplasm are characteristic features. The differential diagnosis includes metastatic neuroendocrine carcinomas.

Metastatic tumours

Isolated cases of metastases from lung, breast, bladder, colon, kidney, prostate, testes and other organs have been reported[9,34,48,140,179]. Renal cell carcinoma is unique as a primary site since it can give rise to late solitary metastasis[180]. Direct extension from cancer of the stomach, duodenum, gall bladder, liver and retroperitoneum may also occur. Differentiation from a primary pancreatic neoplasm requires correlation with clinical and imaging findings as well as special investigations for accurate interpretation.

Cytological monitoring of pancreatic allograft rejection

During the last decade the role of pancreatic transplantation in type I diabetes has expanded, and it can now induce a normoglycemic insulin-independent state. The results have dramatically improved, with a 1-year survival of 70% to 80%[181]. The procedure is done either as a solitary pancreatic transplant, or more commonly as a combined renal and pancreatic transplant.

Cellular rejection is still a major cause of graft failure. In a combined kidney and pancreatic transplant, the status of the co-transplanted kidney is a reliable indicator of rejection. The diagnosis of rejection in solitary pancreatic transplant is currently performed on biopsy material in most centres. The presence of septal inflammation composed of large and small-activated lymphocytes with associated venous endotheliitis is diagnostic for rejection[182]. Fine needle aspiration cytology has been used to monitor a graft for rejection. The diagnosis of rejection

in cytology material is based on the presence of activated inflammatory cells, including lymphoblasts and plasmablasts and other inflammatory cells including lymphocytes, plasma cells and macrophages[183,184]. Pancreatic juice secretion has also been used in the detection of acute rejection[185].

References

1 Landis S H, Murray T, Bolden S, Wingo P A. Cancer statistics, 1998. *CA Cancer J Clin* 1998; **48**: 6–29

2 Cooperman A M. Pancreatic cancer: the bigger picture. *Surg Clin North Am* 2001; **81**: 557–574

3 Lightwood R, Reber H A, Way L W. The risk and accuracy of pancreatic biopsy. *Am J Surg* 1976; **132**: 189–194

4 Moossa A R, Altorki N. Pancreatic biopsy. *Surg Clin North Am* 1983; **63**: 1205–1214

5 McLoughlin M J, Ho C S, Langer B et al. Fine needle aspiration biopsy of malignant lesions in and around the pancreas. *Cancer* 1978; **41**: 2413–2419

6 Arnejo B, Stormby N, Akerman M. Cytodiagnosis of pancreatic lesions by means of fine-needle biopsy during operation. *Acta Chir Scand* 1972; **138**: 363–369

7 Schultz N J, Sanders R. Evaluation of pancreatic biopsy. *Acta Surg* 1963; **158**: 1053–1057

8 Ihse I, Axelson J, Dawiskiba S, Hansson L. Pancreatic biopsy: why? When? How? *World J Surg* 1999; **23**: 896–900

9 Forsgren L, Orell S. Aspiration cytology in carcinoma of the pancreas. *Surgery* 1973; **73**: 38–42

10 Koivuniemi A, Lempinen M, Pantzar P. Fine-needle aspiration biopsy of pancreas. *Ann Chir Gynaecol Fenn* 1972; **61**: 273–280

11 Nieberg RK. Peroperative pancreatic aspirations. *Ann Clin Lab Sci* 1979; **9**: 11–15

12 Schadt M E, Kline T S, Neal H S et al. Intraoperative pancreatic fine needle aspiration biopsy. Results in 166 patients. *Am Surg* 1991; **57**: 73–75

13 Soreide O, Skaarland E, Pedersen O M et al. Fine-needle biopsy of the pancreas: results of 204 routinely performed biopsies in 190 patients. *World J Surg* 1985; **9**: 960–965

14 Earnhardt R C, McQuone S J, Minasi J S et al. Intraoperative fine needle aspiration of pancreatic and extrahepatic biliary masses. *Surg Gynecol Obstet* 1993; **177**: 147–152

15 Hyoty M K, Mattila J J, Salo K, Nordback I H. Intraoperative fine needle aspiration cytologic examination of pancreatic lesions. *Surg Gynecol Obstet* 1991; **173**: 193–197

16 Keighley M R, Moore J, Thompson H. The place of fine needle aspiration cytology for the intraoperative diagnosis of pancreatic malignancy. *Ann R Coll Surg Engl* 1984; **66**: 405–408

17 Parsons L, Jr., Palmer C H. How accurate is fine-needle biopsy in malignant neoplasia of the pancreas? *Arch Surg* 1989; **124**: 681–683

18 Smith R C, Lin B P, Loughman N T. Operative fine needle aspiration cytology of pancreatic tumours. *Aust NZ J Surg* 1985; **55**: 145–148

19 Cote J, Dockerty M B, Priestley J T. An evaluation of pancreatic biopsy with Vim-Silverman needle. *Arch Surg* 1959; **79**: 588–596

20 Wittenberg J, Mueller P R, Ferrucci J T, Jr. et al. Percutaneous core biopsy of abdominal tumors using 22 gauge needles: further observations. *Am J Roentgenol* 1982; **139**: 75–80

21 Glenthoj A, Sehested M, Torp-Pedersen S. Ultrasonically guided histological and cytological fine needle biopsies of the pancreas. Reliability and reproducibility of diagnoses. *Gut* 1990; **31**: 930–933

22 Hancke S, Holm HH, Koch F. Ultrasonically guided percutaneous fine needle biopsy of the pancreas. *Surg Gynecol Obstet* 1975; **140**: 361–364

23 Mitchell M L, Bittner C A, Wills J S, Parker F P. Fine needle aspiration cytology of the pancreas. A retrospective study of 73 cases. *Acta Cytol* 1988; **32**: 447–451

24 Luning M, Kursawe R, Schopke W et al. CT guided percutaneous fine-needle biopsy of the pancreas. *Eur J Radiol* 1985; **5**: 104–108

25 Cubilla A L, Fitzgerald P J. Morphological patterns of primary non-endocrine human pancreas carcinoma. *Cancer Res* 1975; **35**: 2234–2248

26 Luning M, Kursawe R, Schopke W et al. CT guided percutaneous fine needle biopsy of the pancreas. *Eur J Radiol* 1985; **5**: 104–108

27 Soudah B, Fritsch R S, Wittekind C et al. Value of the cytologic analysis of fine needle aspiration biopsy specimens in the diagnosis of pancreatic carcinomas. *Acta Cytol* 1989; **33**: 875–880

28 Brandt K R, Charboneau J W, Stephens D H et al. CT- and US-guided biopsy of the pancreas. *Radiology* 1993; **187**: 99–104

29 Lerma E, Musulen E, Cuatrecasas M et al. Fine needle aspiration cytology in pancreatic pathology. *Acta Cytol* 1996; **40**: 683–686

30 Paksoy N, Lilleng R, Hagmar B, Wetteland J. Diagnostic accuracy of fine needle aspiration cytology in pancreatic lesions. A review of 77 cases. *Acta Cytol* 1993; **37**: 889–893

31 Enayati P G, Traverso L W, Galagan K et al. The meaning of equivocal pancreatic cytology in patients thought to have pancreatic cancer. *Am J Surg* 1996; **171**: 525–528

32 Rodriguez J, Kasberg C, Nipper M et al. CT-guided needle biopsy of the pancreas: a retrospective analysis of diagnostic accuracy. *Am J Gastroenterol* 1992; **87**: 1610–1613

33 Evander A, Ihse I, Lunderquist A et al. Percutaneous cytodiagnosis of carcinoma of the pancreas and bile duct. *Ann Surg* 1978; **188**: 90–92

34 Hajdu E O, Kumari-Subaiya S, Phillips G. Ultrasonically guided percutaneous aspiration biopsy of the pancreas. *Semin Diagn Pathol* 1986; **3**: 166–175

35 Kocjan G, Rode J, Lees W R. Percutaneous fine needle aspiration cytology of the pancreas: advantages and pitfalls. *J Clin Pathol* 1989; **42**: 341–347

36 Sperti C, Pasquali C, Di Prima F et al. Percutaneous CT-guided fine needle aspiration cytology in the differential diagnosis of pancreatic lesions. *Ital J Gastroenterol* 1994; **26**: 126–131

37 Carlson S K, Johnson C D, Brandt K R et al. Pancreatic cystic neoplasms: the role and sensitivity of needle aspiration and biopsy. *Abdom Imaging* 1998; **23**: 387–393

38 Centeno B A, Warshaw A L, Mayo-Smith W et al. Cytologic diagnosis of pancreatic cystic lesions. A prospective study of 28 percutaneous aspirates. *Acta Cytol* 1997; **41**: 972–980

39 Chang K J, Nguyen P, Erickson R A et al. The clinical utility of endoscopic ultrasound-guided fine-needle aspiration in the diagnosis and staging of pancreatic carcinoma. *Gastrointest Endosc* 1997; **45**: 387–393

40 Brandwein S L, Farrell J J, Centeno B A, Brugge W R. Detection and tumor staging of malignancy in cystic, intraductal, and solid tumors of the pancreas by EUS. *Gastrointest Endosc* 2001; **53**: 722–727

41 Gress F, Gottlieb K, Sherman S, Lehman G. Endoscopic ultrasonography-guided fine-needle aspiration biopsy of suspected pancreatic cancer. *Ann Intern Med* 2001; **134**: 459–464

42 Cobb C J, Floyd W N, Jr. Usefulness of bile cytology in the diagnostic management of patients with biliary tract obstruction. *Acta Cytol* 1985; **29**: 93–100

43 Goodale R L, Gajl-Peczalska K, Dressel T, Samuelson J. Cytologic studies for the diagnosis of pancreatic cancer. *Cancer* 1981; **47**: 1652–1655

44 Goldstein H M, Zornoza J. Percutaneous transperitoneal aspiration biopsy of pancreatic masses. *Am J Dig Dis* 1978; **23**: 840–843

45 Dreiling D A, Nieburgs H E, Janowitz H D. The combined secretin and cytology test in diagnosis of cancer and biliary tract cancer. *Med Clin North Am* 1960; **44**: 801–815

46 Ekberg O, Bergenfeldt M, Aspelin P et al. Reliability of ultrasound-guided fine-needle biopsy of pancreatic masses. *Acta Radiol* 1988; **29**: 535–539

47 Oscarson J, Stormby N, Sundgren R. Selective angiography in fine-needle aspiration cytodiagnosis of gastric and pancreatic tumours. *Acta Radiol Diagn (Stockh)* 1972; **12**: 737–750

48 Dickey J E, Haaga J R, Stellato T A et al. Evaluation of computed tomography guided percutaneous biopsy of the pancreas. *Surg Gynecol Obstet* 1986; **163**: 497–503

49 Ryan M J, Hahn P R, Meuller P R. Pancreatic fine needle aspiration biopsy: imaging, equipment, and technique. In: Centeno B A, Pitman M B eds. *Fine Needle Aspiration Biopsy of the Pancreas*. Boston: Butterworth-Heinemann, 1999: 5–11

50 Endo Y, Morii T, Tamura H, Okuda S. Cytodiagnosis of pancreatic malignant tumors by aspiration, under direct vision, using a duodenal fiberscope. *Gastroenterology* 1974; **67**: 944–951

51 Kasugai T, Kobayashi S, Kuno N. Endoscopic cytology of the esophagus, stomach and pancreas. *Acta Cytol* 1978; **22**: 327–330

52 Schwamberger K, Bodner E. Diagnosis of resectable pancreatic carcinomas by means of ERCP and intraoperative fine-needle biopsy. *Endoscopy* 1979; **11**: 172–174

53 Sawada Y, Gonda H, Hayashida Y. Combined use of brushing cytology and endoscopic retrograde pancreatography for the early detection of pancreatic cancer. *Acta Cytol* 1989; **33**: 870–874

54 Quirk D M, Brugge W R. Endoscopic ultrasonography-directed fine needle aspiration. In: Centeno B A, Pitman M B eds. *Fine Needle Aspiration Biopsy of the Pancreas*. Boston: Butterworth-Heinemann, 1999: 13–30

55 Ahmad N, Kochman M L. EUS instrumentation and accessories: a primer. *Gastrointest Endosc* 2000; **52**: S2–S5

56 Harewood G C, Wiersema M J. A cost analysis of endoscopic ultrasound in the evaluation of pancreatic head adenocarcinoma. *Am J Gastroenterol* 2001; **96**: 2651–2656

57 Brugge W R. The role of EUS in the diagnosis of cystic lesions of the pancreas. *Gastrointest Endosc* 2000; **52**: S18–22

58 Barkin J S, Pereiras R, Hill M et al. Diagnosis of pancreatic abscess via percutaneous aspiration. *Dig Dis Sci* 1982; **27**: 1011–1014

59 Neuerburg J, Gunther R W. Percutaneous biopsy of pancreatic lesions. *Cardiovasc Intervent Radiol* 1991; **14**: 43–49

60 Holm H H, Pedersen J F, Kristensen J K et al. Ultrasonically guided percutaneous puncture. *Radiol Clin North Am* 1975; **13**: 493–503

61 Goldstein H M, Zornoza J, Wallace S et al. Percutaneous fine needle aspiration biopsy of pancreatic and other abdominal masses. *Radiology* 1977; **123**: 319–322

62 Phillips V M, Hersh T, Erwin B C et al. Percutaneous biopsy of pancreatic masses. *J Clin Gastroenterol* 1985; **7**: 506–510

63 Livraghi T, Damascelli B, Lombardi C, Spagnoli I. Risk in fine-needle abdominal biopsy. *J Clin Ultrasound* 1983; **11**: 77–81

64 Evans W K, Ho C S, McLoughlin M J, Tao L C. Fatal necrotizing pancreatitis following fine-needle aspiration biopsy of the pancreas. *Radiology* 1981; **141**: 61–62

65 Dzieniszewski G P, Neher M, Linhart P, Frank K. Necrotising pancreatitis after ultrasonically guided fine-needle aspiration biopsy. *Dtsch Med Wochenschr* 1982; **107**: 1438–1440

66 Levin D P, Bret P M. Percutaneous fine-needle aspiration biopsy of the pancreas resulting in death. *Gastrointest Radiol* 1991; **16**: 67–69

67 Morton A L, Taylor E W. Fatal clostridial pancreatitis following transduodenal biopsy of the pancreas. *J R Coll Surg Edinb* 1990; **35**: 254

68 Mueller P R, Miketic L M, Simeone J F et al. Severe acute pancreatitis after percutaneous biopsy of the pancreas. *AJR Am J Roentgenol* 1988; **151**: 493–494

69 Ulich T R, Layfield L J. Fatal septic shock after fine needle aspiration of a pancreatic pseudocyst. *Acta Cytol* 1985; **29**: 879–881

70 Ferrucci J T, Jr., Wittenberg J, Mueller P R et al. Diagnosis of abdominal malignancy by radiologic fine-needle aspiration biopsy. *AJR Am J Roentgenol* 1980; **134**: 323–330

71 Simms M H, Tindall N, Allan R N. Pancreatic fistula following operative fine-needle aspiration. *Br J Surg* 1982; **69**: 548

72 Alpern G A, Dekker A. Fine needle aspiration cytology of the pancreas. An analysis of its use in 52 patients. *Acta Cytol* 1985; **29**: 873–878

73 Ferrucci J T, Wittenberg J, Margolies M N, Carey R W. Malignant seeding of the tract after thin-needle aspiration biopsy. *Radiology* 1979; **130**: 345–346

74 Smith F P, Macdonald J S, Schein P S, Ornitz R D. Cutaneous seeding of pancreatic cancer by skinny-needle aspiration biopsy. *Arch Intern Med* 1980; **140**: 855

75 Rashleigh-Belcher H J, Russell R C, Lees W R. Cutaneous seeding of pancreatic carcinoma by fine-needle aspiration biopsy. *Br J Radiol* 1986; **59**: 182–183

76 Frohlich E, Fruhmorgen P, Seeliger H. Cutaneous implantation metastasis after fine needle puncture of a pancreatic cancer. *Ultraschall Med* 1986; **7**: 141–144

77 Hall-Craggs M A, Lees W R. Fine-needle aspiration biopsy: pancreatic and biliary tumors. *AJR Am J Roentgenol* 1986; **147**: 399–403

78 Caturelli E, Rapaccini G L, Anti M et al. Malignant seeding after fine-needle aspiration biopsy of the pancreas. *Diagn Imaging Clin Med* 1985; **54**: 88–91

79 Bergenfeldt M, Genell S, Lindholm K et al. Needle-tract seeding after percutaneous fine-needle biopsy of pancreatic carcinoma. Case report. *Acta Chir Scand* 1988; **154**: 77–79

80 Fornari F, Civardi G, Cavanna L et al. Complications of ultrasonically guided fine-needle abdominal biopsy. Results of a multicenter Italian study and review of the literature. The Cooperative Italian Study Group. *Scand J Gastroenterol* 1989; **24**: 949–955

81 Warshaw A L. Implications of peritoneal cytology for staging of early pancreatic cancer. *Am J Surg* 1991; **161**: 26–29

82 Leach S D, Rose J A, Lowy A M et al. Significance of peritoneal cytology in patients with potentially resectable adenocarcinoma of the pancreatic head. *Surgery* 1995; **118**: 472–478

83 Edoute Y, Lemberg S, Malberger E. Preoperative and intraoperative fine needle aspiration cytology of pancreatic lesions. *Am J Gastroenterol* 1991; **86**: 1015–1019

84 Nguyen G K. Percutaneous fine-needle aspiration cytology of the pancreas. *Pathol Annu* 1985; **20**: 221–238

85 Hidvegi D, Nieman H L, DeMay R M, Janes W. Percutaneous transperitoneal aspiration of pancreas guided by ultrasound: morphologic and cytochemical appearance of normal and malignant cells. *Acta Cytol* 1979; **23**: 181–184

86 Tao L C. Liver and pancreas. In: Bibbo M ed. *Comprehensive Cytopathology* 2nd edn. Philadelphia: Saunders, 1997: 827–863

87 Bowden M. The fallibility of pancreatic biopsy. *Ann Surg* 1954; **139**: 403–408

88 Goldman M L, Naib Z M, Galambos J T et al. Preoperative diagnosis of pancreatic carcinoma by percutaneous aspiration biopsy. *Am J Dig Dis* 1977; **22**: 1076–1082

89 Nguyen G K, Rayani N A. Hyperplastic and neoplastic endocrine cells of the pancreas in aspiration biopsy. *Diagn Cytopathol* 1986; **2**: 204–211

90 Hill M C, Dach J L, Barkin J et al. The role of percutaneous aspiration in the diagnosis of pancreatic abscess. *AJR Am J Roentgenol* 1983; **141**: 1035–1038

91 Pinto M M, Kaye A D, Brogan D A, Criscuolo E H. Diagnosis of cystic lesions of the pancreas: a biochemical and cytologic analysis of material obtained utilizing radiographic or intraoperative technique. *Diagn Cytopathol* 1986; **2**: 40–45

92 Stiles G M, Berne T V, Thommen V D et al. Fine needle aspiration of pancreatic fluid collections. *Am Surg* 1990; **56**: 764–768

93 Mithofer K, Mueller P R, Warshaw A L. Interventional and surgical treatment of pancreatic abscess. *World J Surg* 1997; **21**: 162–168

94 Freeny P C, Kidd R, Ball T J. ERCP-guided percutaneous fine-needle pancreatic biopsy. *West J Med* 1980; **132**: 283–287

95 Young N A, Villani M A, Khoury P, Naryshkin S. Differential diagnosis of cystic neoplasms of the pancreas by fine-needle aspiration. *Arch Pathol Lab Med* 1991; **115**: 571–577

96 Warshaw A L, Compton C C, Lewandrowski K et al. Cystic tumors of the

pancreas. New clinical, radiologic, and pathologic observations in 67 patients. *Ann Surg* 1990; **212**: 432–443

97 Warshaw A L, Rutledge P L. Cystic tumors mistaken for pancreatic pseudocysts. *Ann Surg* 1987; **205**: 393–398

98 Chak A. Endosonographic-guided therapy of pancreatic pseudocysts. *Gastrointest Endosc* 2000; **52**: S23–27

99 Adsay N V, Hasteh F, Cheng J D, Klimstra D S. Squamous-lined cysts of the pancreas: lymphoepithelial cysts, dermoid cysts (teratomas), and accessory-splenic epidermoid cysts. *Semin Diagn Pathol* 2000; **17**: 56–65

100 Mandavilli S R, Port J, Ali S Z. Lymphoepithelial cyst (LEC) of the pancreas: cytomorphology and differential diagnosis on fine-needle aspiration (FNA). *Diagn Cytopathol* 1999; **20**: 371–374

101 Liu J, Shin H J, Rubenchik I et al. Cytologic features of lymphoepithelial cyst of the pancreas: two preoperatively diagnosed cases based on fine-needle aspiration. *Diagn Cytopathol* 1999; **21**: 346–350

102 Kloppel G. Pseudocysts and other non-neoplastic cysts of the pancreas. *Semin Diagn Pathol* 2000; **17**: 7–15

103 Centeno B A. Cystic lesion. In: Centeno B A, Pitman M B eds. *Fine Needle Aspiration Biopsy of the Pancreas.* Boston: Butterworth-Heinemann, 1999: 53–108

104 Compton C C. Serous cystic tumors of the pancreas. *Semin Diagn Pathol* 2000; **17**: 43–55

105 Ooi L L, Ho G H, Chew S P et al. Cystic tumours of the pancreas: a diagnostic dilemma. *Aust NZ J Surg* 1998; **68**: 844–846

106 Procacci C, Graziani R, Bicego E et al. Serous cystadenoma of the pancreas: report of 30 cases with emphasis on the imaging findings. *J Comput Assist Tomogr* 1997; **21**: 373–382

107 Torresan F, Casadei R, Solmi L et al. The role of ultrasound in the differential diagnosis of serous and mucinous cystic tumours of the pancreas. *Eur J Gastroenterol Hepatol* 1997; **9**: 169–172

108 Centeno B A, Lewandrowski K B, Warshaw A L et al. Cyst fluid cytologic analysis in the differential diagnosis of pancreatic cystic lesions. *Am J Clin Pathol* 1994; **101**: 483–487

109 Hittmair A, Pernthaler H, Totsch M, Schmid K W. Preoperative fine needle aspiration cytology of a microcystic adenoma of the pancreas. *Acta Cytol* 1991; **35**: 546–548

110 Nguyen G K, Vogelsang P J. Microcystic adenoma of the pancreas. A report of two cases with fine needle aspiration cytology and differential diagnosis. *Acta Cytol* 1993; **37**: 908–912

111 Jones E C, Suen K C, Grant D R, Chan N H. Fine-needle aspiration cytology of neoplastic cysts of the pancreas. *Diagn Cytopathol* 1987; **3**: 238–243

112 Laucirica R, Schwartz M R, Ramzy I. Fine needle aspiration of pancreatic cystic epithelial neoplasms. *Acta Cytol* 1992; **36**: 881–886

113 Adsay N V, Klimstra D S, Compton C C. Cystic lesions of the pancreas. Introduction. *Semin Diagn Pathol* 2000; **17**: 1–6

114 Wilentz R E, Albores-Saavedra J, Hruban R H. Mucinous cystic neoplasms of the pancreas. *Semin Diagn Pathol* 2000; **17**: 31–42

115 Zamboni G, Kloppel G, Hruban R et al. Mucinous cystic neoplasms of the pancreas. In: Aaltonen L A, Hamilton S R, World Health Organization, International Agency for Research on Cancer eds. *Pathology and Genetics of Tumours of the Digestive System.* Lyon; Oxford: IARC Press, **2000**: 234–236

116 Dodd L G, Farrell T A, Layfield L J. Mucinous cystic tumor of the pancreas: an analysis of FNA characteristics with an emphasis on the spectrum of malignancy associated features. *Diagn Cytopathol* 1995; **12**: 113–119

117 Wilentz R E, Albores-Saavedra J, Zahurak M et al. Pathologic examination accurately predicts prognosis in mucinous cystic neoplasms of the pancreas. *Am J Surg Pathol* 1999; **23**: 1320–1327

118 Adsay N V, Longnecker D S, Klimstra D S. Pancreatic tumors with cystic dilatation of the ducts: intraductal papillary mucinous neoplasms and intraductal oncocytic papillary neoplasms. *Semin Diagn Pathol* 2000; **17**: 16–30

119 Hyde G L, Davis J B, Jr., McMillin R D, McMillin M. Mucinous cystic neoplasm of the pancreas with latent malignancy. *Am Surg* 1984; **50**: 225–229

120 Uehara H, Nakaizumi A, Iishi H et al. Cytologic examination of pancreatic juice for differential diagnosis of benign and malignant mucin-producing tumors of the pancreas. *Cancer* 1994; **74**: 826–833

121 Klimstra D S, Wenig B M, Heffess C S. Solid-pseudopapillary tumor of the pancreas: a typically cystic carcinoma of low malignant potential. *Semin Diagn Pathol* 2000; **17**: 66–80

122 Ogawa T, Isaji S, Okamura K et al. A case of radical resection for solid cystic tumor of the pancreas with widespread metastases in the liver and greater omentum. *Am J Gastroenterol* 1993; **88**: 1436–1439

123 Sclafani L M, Reuter V E, Coit D G, Brennan M F. The malignant nature of papillary and cystic neoplasm of the pancreas. *Cancer* 1991; **68**: 153–158

124 Kashima K, Hayashida Y, Yokoyama S et al. Cytologic features of solid and cystic tumor of the pancreas. *Acta Cytol* 1997; **41**: 443–449

125 Naresh K N, Borges A M, Chinoy R F et al. Solid and papillary epithelial neoplasm of the pancreas. Diagnosis by fine needle aspiration cytology in four cases. *Acta Cytol* 1995; **39**: 489–493

126 Pelosi G, Iannucci A, Zamboni G et al. Solid and cystic papillary neoplasm of the pancreas: a clinico-cytopathologic and immunocytochemical study of five new cases diagnosed by fine-needle aspiration cytology and a review of the literature. *Diagn Cytopathol* 1995; **13**: 233–246

127 Greenberg M L, Rennie Y, Grierson J M et al. Solid and papillary epithelial tumour

of the pancreas: cytological case study with ultrastructural and flow cytometric evaluation. *Diagn Cytopathol* 1993; **9**: 541–546

128 Chen K T, Workman R D, Efird T A, Cheng A C. Fine needle aspiration cytology diagnosis of papillary tumor of the pancreas. *Acta Cytol* 1986; **30**: 523–527

129 Katz L B, Ehya H. Aspiration cytology of papillary cystic neoplasm of the pancreas. *Am J Clin Pathol* 1990; **94**: 328–333

130 Stachura J, Popiela T, Pietron M et al. Cytology of solid and papillary epithelial neoplasms of the pancreas: a case report. *Diagn Cytopathol* 1988; **4**: 339–341

131 Foote A, Simpson J S, Stewart R J et al. Diagnosis of the rare solid and papillary epithelial neoplasm of the pancreas by fine needle aspiration cytology. Light and electron microscopic study of a case. *Acta Cytol* 1986; **30**: 519–522

132 Bondeson L, Bondeson A G, Genell S et al. Aspiration cytology of a rare solid and papillary epithelial neoplasm of the pancreas. Light and electron microscopic study of a case. *Acta Cytol* 1984; **28**: 605–609

133 Yang J M, Lee J, Southern J F, Warshaw A L et al. Measurement of pS2 protein in pancreatic cyst fluids. Evidence for a potential role of pS2 protein in the pathogenesis of mucinous cystic tumors. *Int J Pancreatol* 1998; **24**: 181–186

134 Kloppel G, Hruban R, Longnecker D et al. Ductal adenocarinoma of the pancreas. In: Aaltonen LA, Hamilton SR, World Health Organization, International Agency for Research on Cancer eds. *Pathology and Genetics of Tumours of the Digestive System.* Lyon; Oxford: IARC Press, **2000**: 221–230

135 Robins D B, Katz R L, Evans D B et al. Fine needle aspiration of the pancreas. In quest of accuracy. *Acta Cytol* 1995; **39**: 1–10

136 Francillon Y J, Bagby J, Abreo F, Turbat-Herrera E. Criteria for predicting malignancy in fine needle aspiration biopsies of the pancreas and biliary tree. *Acta Cytol* 1996; **40**: 1084

137 Lin F, Staerkel G. Cytologic criteria for well-differentiated adenocarcinoma of pancreas diagnosed by fine needle aspiration. *Acta Cytol* 2000; **13**: 49A

138 Hejka A G, Bernacki E G. Cytopathology of well-differentiated columnar adenocarcinoma of the pancreas diagnosed by fine needle aspiration. *Acta Cytol* 1990; **34**: 716

139 Mitchell M L, Carney C N. Cytologic criteria for the diagnosis of pancreatic carcinoma. *Am J Clin Pathol* 1985; **83**: 171–176

140 Fekete P S, Nunez C, Pitlik D A. Fine-needle aspiration biopsy of the pancreas: a study of 61 cases. *Diagn Cytopathol* 1986; **2**: 301–306

141 Cubilla A, Fitzgerald P J. Pancreatic cancer 1. Ductal adenocarcinoma. A clinical-pathologic study of 380 patients, part 1. *Pathology Annual* 1978; **13**: 241–289

142 Silverman J F, Dabbs D J, Finley J L, Geisinger K R. Fine-needle aspiration biopsy of pleomorphic (giant cell)

carcinoma of the pancreas. Cytologic, immunocytochemical, and ultrastructural findings. *Am J Clin Pathol* 1988; **89**: 714–720

143 Pinto M M, Monteiro N L, Tizol D M. Fine needle aspiration of pleomorphic giant-cell carcinoma of the pancreas. Case report with ultrastructural observations. *Acta Cytol* 1986; **30**: 430–434

144 Tschang T P, Garza-Garza R, Kissane J M. Pleomorphic carcinoma of the pancreas: an analysis of 15 cases. *Cancer* 1977; **39**: 2114–2126

145 Hoorens A, Prenzel K, Lemoine N R, Kloppel G. Undifferentiated carcinoma of the pancreas: analysis of intermediate filament profile and Ki-ras mutations provides evidence of a ductal origin. *J Pathol* 1998; **185**: 53–60

146 Nojima T, Nakamura F, Ishikura M *et al.* Pleomorphic carcinoma of the pancreas with osteoclast-like giant cells. *Int J Pancreatol* 1993; **14**: 275–281

147 Manci E A, Gardner L L, Pollock W J, Dowling E A. Osteoclastic giant cell tumor of the pancreas. Aspiration cytology, light microscopy, and ultrastructure with review of the literature. *Diagn Cytopathol* 1985; **1**: 105–110

148 Walts A E. Osteoclast-type giant-cell tumor of the pancreas. *Acta Cytol* 1983; **27**: 500–504

149 Silverman J F, Finley J L, MacDonald K G, Jr. Fine-needle aspiration cytology of osteoclastic giant-cell tumor of the pancreas. *Diagn Cytopathol* 1990; **6**: 336–340

150 Gupta R K, Wakefield S J, Fauck R, Stewart R J. Immunocytochemical and ultrastructural findings in a case of rare carcinoma of the pancreas with predominance of malignant squamous cells in an intraoperative needle aspirate. *Acta Cytol* 1989; **33**: 153–156

151 Wilczynski S P, Valente P T, Atkinson B F. Cytodiagnosis of adenosquamous carcinoma of the pancreas. Use of intraoperative fine needle aspiration. *Acta Cytol* 1984; **28**: 733–736

152 Leiman G, Markowitz S, Svensson L G. Intraoperative cytodiagnosis of pancreatic adenosquamous carcinoma: a case report. *Diagn Cytopathol* 1986; **2**: 72–75

153 Lozano M D, Panizo A, Sola I J, Pardo-Mindan F J. FNAC guided by computed tomography in the diagnosis of primary pancreatic adenosquamous carcinoma. A report of three cases. *Acta Cytol* 1998; **42**: 1451–1454

154 Tracey K J, O'Brien M J, Williams L F *et al.* Signet ring carcinoma of the pancreas, a rare variant with very high CEA values. Immunohistologic comparison with adenocarcinoma. *Dig Dis Sci* 1984; **29**: 573–576

155 Klimstra D S, Heffess C S, Oertel J E, Rosai J. Acinar cell carcinoma of the pancreas. A clinicopathologic study of 28 cases. *Am J Surg Pathol* 1992; **16**: 815–837

156 Adsay N V, Klimstra D S. Cystic forms of typically solid pancreatic tumors. *Semin Diagn Pathol* 2000; **17**: 81–88

157 Labate A M, Klimstra D L, Zakowski M F. Comparative cytologic features of pancreatic acinar cell carcinoma and islet cell tumor. *Diagn Cytopathol* 1997; **16**: 112–116

158 Villanueva R R, Nguyen-Ho P, Nguyen G K. Needle aspiration cytology of acinar-cell carcinoma of the pancreas: report of a case with diagnostic pitfalls and unusual ultrastructural findings. *Diagn Cytopathol* 1994; **10**: 362–364

159 Samuel L H, Frierson H F, Jr. Fine needle aspiration cytology of acinar cell carcinoma of the pancreas: a report of two cases. *Acta Cytol* 1996; **40**: 585–591

160 Grosfeld J L, Vane D W, Rescorla F J *et al.* Pancreatic tumors in childhood: analysis of 13 cases. J Pediatr Surg 1990; **25**: 1057–1062

161 Silverman J F, Holbrook C T, Pories W J *et al.* Fine needle aspiration cytology of pancreatoblastoma with immunocytochemical and ultrastructural studies. *Acta Cytol* 1990; **34**: 632–640

162 Kloppel G, Heitz P U. Pancreatic tumors in man. In: Polak J M ed. *Diagnostic histopathology of neuroendocrine tumors.* Edinburgh: Churchill Livingstone, 1993: 91–121

163 Solcia E, Capella C, Klöppel G. *Tumors of the Pancreas.* Washington, DC: Armed Forces Institute of Pathology, 1997

164 La Rosa S, Sessa F, Capella C *et al.* Prognostic criteria in nonfunctioning pancreatic endocrine tumours. *Virchows Arch* 1996; **429**: 323–333

165 Capella C, Heitz P U, Hofler H *et al.* Revised classification of neuroendocrine tumours of the lung, pancreas and gut. *Virchows Arch* 1995; **425**: 547–560

166 Ordonez N G, Silva E G. Islet cell tumour with vacuolated lipid-rich cytoplasm: a new histological variant of islet cell tumour. *Histopathol* 1997; **31**: 157–160

167 Bell D A. Cytologic features of islet-cell tumors. *Acta Cytol* 1987; **31**: 485–492

168 Al-Kaisi N, Siegler E E. Fine needle aspiration cytology of the pancreas. *Acta Cytol* 1989; **33**: 145–152

169 Collins B T, Cramer H M. Fine-needle aspiration cytology of islet cell tumors. *Diagn Cytopathol* 1996; **15**: 37–45

170 Hsiu J G, D'Amato N A, Sperling M H *et al.* Malignant islet-cell tumor of the pancreas diagnosed by fine needle aspiration biopsy. A case report. *Acta Cytol* 1985; **29**: 576–579

171 Leiman G, Mair S. Aspiration cytology of neuroendocrine tumors below the diaphragm. *Diagn Cytopathol* 1989; **5**: 263–268

172 Sneige N, Ordonez N G, Veanattukalathil S, Samaan N A. Fine-needle aspiration cytology in pancreatic endocrine tumors. *Diagn Cytopathol* 1987; **3**: 35–40

173 Shaw J A, Vance R P, Geisinger K R, Marshall R B. Islet cell neoplasms. A fine-needle aspiration cytology study with immunocytochemical correlations. *Am J Clin Pathol* 1990; **94**: 142–149

174 Banner B F, Myrent K L, Memoli V A, Gould V E. Neuroendocrine carcinoma of the pancreas diagnosed by aspiration cytology. A case report. *Acta Cytol* 1985; **29**: 442–448

175 Nguyen G K. Cytology of hyperplastic endocrine cells of the pancreas in fine needle aspiration biopsy. *Acta Cytol* 1984; **28**: 499–502

176 Pacchioni D, Papotti M, Macri L *et al.* Pancreatic oncocytic endocrine tumors. Cytologic features of two cases. *Acta Cytol* 1996; **40**: 742–746

177 O'Connor T P, Wade T P, Sunwoo Y C *et al.* Small cell undifferentiated carcinoma of the pancreas. Report of a patient with tumor marker studies. *Cancer* 1992; **70**: 1514–1519

178 Reyes C V, Wang T. Undifferentiated small cell carcinoma of the pancreas: a report of five cases. *Cancer* 1981; **47**: 2500–2502

179 Gupta R K, Lallu S, Delahunt B. Fine-needle aspiration cytology of metastatic clear-cell renal carcinoma presenting as a solitary mass in the head of the pancreas. *Diagn Cytopathol* 1998; **19**: 194–197

180 Butturini G, Bassi C, Falconi M *et al.* Surgical treatment of pancreatic metastases from renal cell carcinomas. *Dig Surg* 1998; **15**: 241–246

181 Sutherland D E, Gruessner R W, Gruessner A C. Pancreas transplantation for treatment of diabetes mellitus. *World J Surg* 2001; **25**: 487–496

182 Drachenberg C B, Papadimitriou J C, Klassen D K *et al.* Evaluation of pancreas transplant needle biopsy: reproducibility and revision of histologic grading system. *Transplantation* 1997; **63**: 1579–1586

183 Egidi M F, Shapiro R, Khanna A *et al.* Fine-needle aspiration biopsy in pancreatic transplantation. *Transplant Proc* 1995; **27**: 3055–3056

184 Egidi M F. Fine-needle aspiration biopsy in renal transplantation: a review of cytologic features. *Diagn Cytopathol* 1990; **6**: 330–335

185 Klima G, Margreiter R. Pancreatic juice cytology in the monitoring of pancreas allografts. *Transplantation* 1989; **48**: 980–985

Kidney and urinary tract

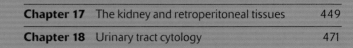

17 The kidney and retroperitoneal tissues

Grace McKee

The kidney

Introduction

The kidneys are paired bean-shaped organs measuring approximately $12 \times 5 \times 2.5$ cm. Each kidney is covered by a thick capsule, which is perirenal fat which, in turn, is covered by thickened connective tissue known as Gerota's fascia. The renal sinus on the medial aspect of the kidney has no capsule but contains the renal calyces, part of the renal pelvis and the major blood vessels of the kidney. The lymphatic channels of the kidney (located in the cortex only, not the medulla) drain into the hilar and para-aortic lymph nodes.

Embryologically the kidney is derived from the primitive mesenchyme of the nephric ridge, from tissue called the nephrogenic blastema. The kidney is prone to congenital and acquired diseases, both non-neoplastic and neoplastic, many of which can be diagnosed by cytology.

Sampling of renal lesions

Urine cytology is not an efficient method of detecting renal pathology. Most renal inflammatory processes and tumours do not shed diagnostic cells into urine. Rarely, tumour cells from a renal neoplasm may be found in urine samples[1]. The most effective method of sampling renal lesions is by fine needle aspiration (FNA) cytology, a technique which has been in use for almost 50 years[2] and has proved to be extremely useful[3–10]. The diagnostic accuracy of FNAs has been shown to reach 91.3%[11] while the specificity ranges from 91.9%[10] to 99%[12] and the sensitivity between 91.6%[4] - 92.5%[10]. The reported complications of fine needle aspiration of kidney include transient haematuria[13], post-biopsy haemorrhage with severe pain[2], perirenal haemorrhage, pneumothorax, infection, arteriovenous fistula and urinoma[14], also cutaneous seeding following the use of a Chiba needle[15,16].

Fine needle aspiration of the kidney is best accomplished under radiological imaging guidance for accuracy of needle placement. There are several methods in use for radiological investigation of renal lesions including intravenous pyelography, angiography, ultrasonography, computed tomography and magnetic resonance imaging. Each has its place, advantages and limitations. Excretory urography is useful in demonstrating kidney function but is of no use in detecting small tumours. Renal arteriography is no longer the procedure of choice in the evaluation of renal masses. Ultrasonography (US) is a satisfactory method of detecting and sampling cysts[17]. US can also be used for aspirating non-neoplastic lesions[18]. Computed tomography (CT), on the other hand, is more useful for complex renal masses[17], and is extremely helpful in detecting small tumours and providing information about tumour spread to adjacent structures[19]. Magnetic resonance imaging (MRI) is useful for complex renal cysts, although not always able to distinguish benign from malignant lesions[20], other renal lesions and for staging of tumours[21]. The earliest report of renal sampling under radiological guidance dates back to 1946[2]. At present, the most commonly used modalities are ultrasonography and computed tomography for the procurement of FNAs.

The attendance of a cytotechnologist or cytopathologist at radiologically-guided FNAs where possible is of importance, not merely for preparation of the smears but to provide a rapid preliminary diagnosis and to decide whether material should be saved for ultrastructural examination, flow cytometry or for special stains such as immunocytochemistry. Cyst fluid is collected into a clean container and sent to the cytology laboratory for processing. Other material is smeared on to slides and either fixed in 95% alcohol or air dried. The needle is usually rinsed into saline to retrieve any remaining cells. This needle rinse may be used for cytospin smears or thin-layer cytology, or even for cell block preparations. The latter are particularly useful if immunocytochemical stains need to be performed to determine the type of tumour. A useful procedure when only core biopsies are performed is to transfer the cores into a fresh container of formalin and to spin down the saline in which they were first placed, for a rapid cytological diagnosis.

Histology of the kidney

On cut section, the kidney displays an inner medulla and outer cortex (Fig. 17.1). The functional unit of the kidney, the nephron, consists of the glomerulus, the proximal convoluted tubule, the loop of Henle, distal convoluted tubule and the collecting ducts. The glomerulus is composed of endothelial and epithelial cells with specialized mesangial cells (Fig. 17.2). The proximal convoluted tubule is lined by columnar cells with numerous microvilli and mitochondria, the latter imparting an

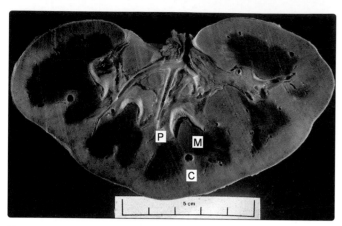

Fig. 17.1   Section of kidney. Photograph of adult human kidney cut longitudinally to show the arrangement of the (C) cortex, (M) medulla and (P) papilla. (Illustration courtesy of Alan Stevens and James Lowe, *Histology*, Mosby, London)

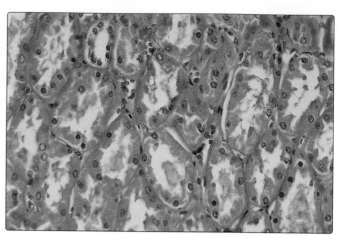

Fig. 17.3   Histology: Proximal convoluted tubule. The columnar cells lining these tubules have abundant eosinophilic cytoplasm. (H&E × HP)

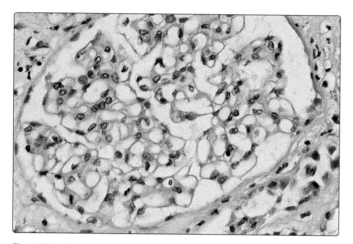

Fig. 17.2   Histology: Glomerulus. This section of kidney shows a normal glomerulus composed predominantly of capillaries. (H&E × HP)

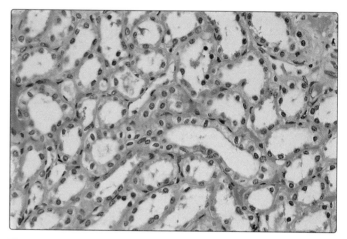

Fig. 17.4   Histology: Distal convoluted tubule. These tubules are lined by cuboidal cells with less cytoplasm than in cells of the proximal convoluted tubule. (H&E × HP)

acidophilic, granular appearance to the cytoplasm of the cells (Fig. 17.3). The cells lining the loop of Henle and the distal convoluted tubule are of both columnar and cuboidal types with fewer microvilli and mitochondria (Fig. 17.4). The collecting ducts are composed of cuboidal cells with central nuclei, few organelles and, occasionally, prominent lipofuscin granules. Some cells exhibit microvilli and most show a single apical cilium, best seen on scanning electron microscopy. These cells show strong positivity with antibodies to high molecular weight keratins unlike the cells of the proximal and distal tubules, which are negative with these antibodies. This may be of use in identifying the site of origin of some renal tumours.

Cytology of the kidney

An aspirate of a renal lesion not infrequently includes normal kidney; hence it is important to recognize normal structures. Glomeruli are visualized as fairly tight, three-dimensional groups of small cells with a lobulated appearance (Figs 17.5, 17.6). The cells contain little

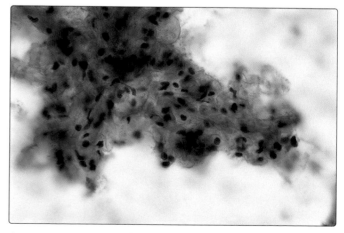

Fig. 17.5   Fine needle aspirate: Glomerulus. The glomerulus seen in this field is a three-dimensional structure with a lobulated appearance. (Papanicolaou × HP)

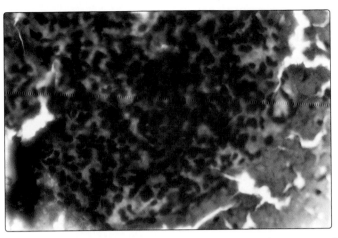

Fig. 17.6   Fine needle aspirate: Glomerulus. The lobulated appearance of the glomerulus is well demonstrated in this illustration. (MGG × HP)

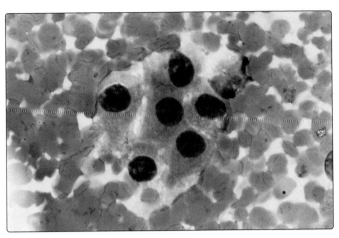

Fig. 17.8   Fine needle aspirate: Proximal convoluted tubule. Note the granularity of the cytoplasm and the uniform round nuclei of these proximal convoluted tubule cells. (MGG × OI)

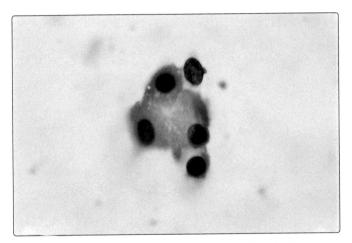

Fig. 17.7   Fine needle aspirate: Proximal convoluted tubule. The cells seen here have abundant granular cytoplasm and fairly well-defined cell borders. (Papanicolaou × OI)

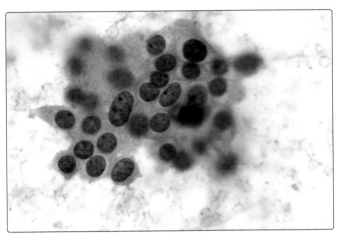

Fig. 17.9   Fine needle aspirate: Distal convoluted tubule. These cells have much less cytoplasm than those from the proximal convoluted tubule. (Papanicolaou × HP)

cytoplasm and rarely, tiny blood vessels may be identified containing erythrocytes. Proximal convoluted tubule cells are fairly large, usually single or in small flat sheets, with abundant granular cytoplasm that is usually a greenish blue with the Papanicolaou stain and violet-blue with May-Grünwald-Giemsa (Figs 17.7, 17.8). Microvilli are not identifiable on fine needle aspiration material. Distal convoluted tubule and collecting duct cells are smaller with central nuclei and cytoplasm that is not as granular as that of the convoluted tubules (Figs 17.9, 17.10). These cells may also be seen singly or in small flat sheets. With the H&E stain, it might be difficult to distinguish between convoluted tubule and collecting tubule cells as the granularity of the cytoplasm is not easily identifiable.

Pathological processes involving the kidney include non-neoplastic lesions such as infection and inflammation, also renal cysts and neoplasms, which may be benign or malignant.

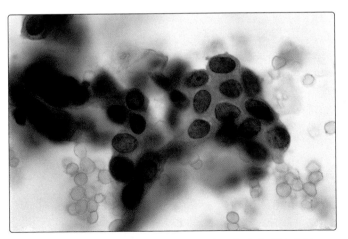

Fig. 17.10   Fine needle aspirate: Distal convoluted tubule: This field illustrates the uniform cells with little cytoplasm, originating from the distal convoluted tubule. (H&E × HP)

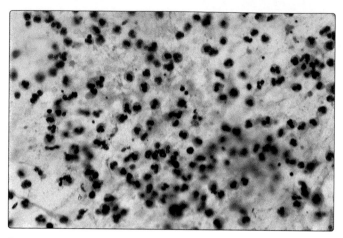

Fig. 17.11   Fine needle aspirate: Perinephric abscess. Numerous neutrophil polymorphs are present. (Papanicolaou × HP)

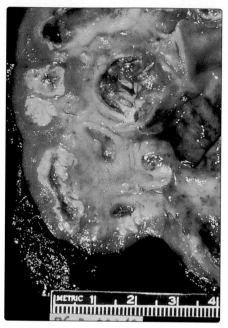

Fig. 17.12   Kidney: Xanthogranulomatous pyelonephritis. This section of kidney shows the macroscopic appearance of this lesion, with obvious necrosis. (Courtesy of Dr E. Brogi, Massachusetts General Hospital, Boston)

Infective and inflammatory processes

Acute pyelonephritis

This is a bacterial infection, usually caused by *E. coli*, less commonly by other enteric bacteria, and often following a lower urinary tract infection. Abundant acute inflammatory cells are present surrounding the renal tubules and within them. Untreated infections may lead to abscess formation. These lesions are diagnosable clinically and fine needle aspiration is usually unnecessary. The aspirate contains numerous neutrophil polymorphs and histiocytes with variable numbers of lymphocytes. Bacteria may be identified using a Gram stain.

Perinephric abscess

This is located within the perinephric fat and may follow rupture of an untreated renal abscess or, rarely, following surgery. The abscess contains acute inflammatory cells, histiocytes and debris (Fig. 17.11). Organisms may be present.

Cytological findings

▶ Abundant inflammatory cells including histiocytes
▶ Debris is present
▶ Organisms may be identified using the Gram stain

Xanthogranulomatous pyelonephritis

Chronic inflammatory disease (pyelonephritis) usually follows repeated bouts of bacterial infection. Xanthogranulomatous pyelonephritis (Fig. 17.12) develops in this fashion, the combination of obstruction and infection leading to a necrotic mass containing neutrophils, surrounded by xanthomatous cells in foamy macrophages, with an outer layer of fibroblasts. Fine needle aspirates contain necrotic debris, inflammatory cells, foamy macrophages, multinucleated giant histiocytes and, occasionally, fibroblasts (Fig. 17.13). The foamy macrophages have abundant, finely vacuolated cytoplasm

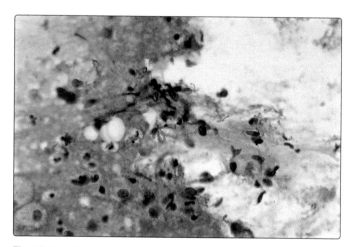

Fig. 17.13   Fine needle aspirate: Xanthogranulomatous pyelonephritis. Delicate stromal fragments and degenerating foamy macrophages are seen in this aspirate. (Papanicolaou × HP)

and can be mistaken for the clear cells of renal cell carcinoma. The fibroblasts may appear atypical and thus raise the possibility of a spindle cell tumour. This is compounded by the clinical and radiological features of this entity, which can mimic a renal neoplasm. The foamy macrophages do not form cohesive clusters, however, and their cytoplasm is finely vacuolated rather than clear. The nuclei are predominantly bean-shaped and nucleoli are not prominent. Xanthogranulomatous pyelonephritis also occurs in childhood, mimicking neoplastic and other inflammatory processes, and is frequently associated with renal calculi[22].

Diagnostic pitfalls

Renal cell carcinoma cells with abundant, finely vacuolated cytoplasm may mimic xanthoma cells. However, carcinoma cells are usually seen in clusters. The typical blood vessels of renal cell carcinoma are not visualized in xanthogranulomatous pyelonephritis. Inflammatory cells are not a common feature of renal cell carcinoma. . It may be necessary to resort to immunocytochemistry to differentiate between the two lesions.

The multinucleated giant cells of xanthogranulomatous pyelonephritis may be mistaken for Langhans-type giant cells of tuberculosis. Culture and a Ziehl Neelsen stain can help differentiate between the two conditions.

Malakoplakia is rarely seen in the kidney but is much more common in the urinary bladder (see Chapter 18). Renal malakoplakia may follow repeated bouts of infection in middle-aged women. The clinical and radiological findings often suggest a neoplasm. The lesions are soft, yellowish nodules composed of numerous large eosinophilic histiocytes containing basophilic inclusions known as Michaelis-Gutmann bodies. These inclusions are believed to be bacillary in origin with a mineral content and can be stained with PAS as well as with stains for calcium and iron. Malakoplakia can be diagnosed on fine needle aspiration cytology, the smears showing large, foamy granular macrophages containing round inclusions with a laminated appearance[23].

Cytological findings

- ▶ Large eosinophilic histiocytes
- ▶ Characteristic laminated inclusions (Michaelis-Gutmann bodies) within the histiocytes

Renal infarcts

The cytology sample shows necrotic debris. Renal epithelial cells may be present and can show degenerative changes. The necrosis and atypia that is sometimes seen can mimic malignancy[24].

Post-transplant changes

These may be monitored either by fine needle aspiration cytology[25] or by examining urine samples (see Chapter 18). A full description of changes seen on aspiration cytology may be found in Chapter 21.

Cystic lesions of the kidney

Renal cysts may be congenital or acquired. They comprise several entities, not all of which have specific diagnostic features, including acquired cystic kidney, simple benign cyst, multilocular renal cyst, complex renal cyst and cystic hamartoma of renal pelvis. Renal cysts are often discovered as incidental findings in the course of investigation of lower urinary tract symptoms. These lesions can be evaluated by ultrasonography (US) as well as CT and MRI. Ultrasonography is useful in detecting simple benign cysts while computed tomography and magnetic resonance imaging are useful in the detection and diagnosis of complex or multilocular renal cysts. Benign cysts appear spherical and homogeneous on imaging, with smooth internal margins while neoplastic lesions may show nodules projecting from the internal border into the cysts. In a study of complex renal cysts using MRI, the majority of cysts with irregular walls, and mural thickening or nodules in the walls, proved to be malignant on pathological examination[26]. However, the features of benign and malignant cysts may overlap. The cytological appearance of complex renal cysts may mimic that of angiomyolipoma[27]. Benign cysts contain clear straw-coloured fluid whereas neoplastic cysts contain necrotic debris, blood and tissue fragments.

Cytological findings

- ▶ Abundant foamy macrophages (xanthoma cells)
- ▶ Varying numbers of chronic inflammatory cells including multinucleated giant cells
- ▶ Necrotic debris
- ▶ Fibroblasts

Benign cyst fluid, on cytological examination, shows foamy macrophages (Figs 17.14, 17.15), haemosiderin-laden macrophages if there has been haemorrhage into the cyst (Fig. 17.16), scanty epithelial lining cells, renal tubular cells, neutrophils occasionally[28], and Liesegang rings (Fig. 17.17). These rings are concentric rings morphologically similar to those seen in benign breast lesions and to corpora amylacea in the prostate. They are believed to form by precipitation in supersaturated cyst fluids. Transmission electron microscopy shows that they are composed of an electron-dense core surrounded by fibrillary concentric

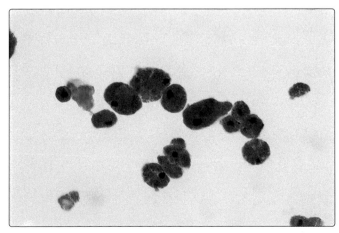

Fig. 17.14   Fine needle aspirate: Renal cyst. Foamy macrophages are present in varying numbers in renal cyst fluid. (Papanicolaou × HP). (Courtesy of Dr S. Granter, Brigham & Womens' Hospital, Boston)

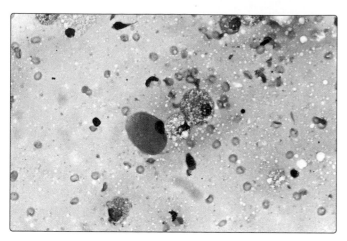

Fig. 17.15   Fine needle aspirate: Renal cyst. Foamy macrophages with vacuolated cytoplasm are seen in this field. (MGG × HP)

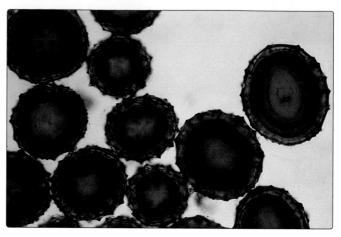

Fig. 17.18   Fine needle aspirate: Renal cyst calcospherites. (Courtesy of Dr P. Trott, Royal Marsden Hospital, London)

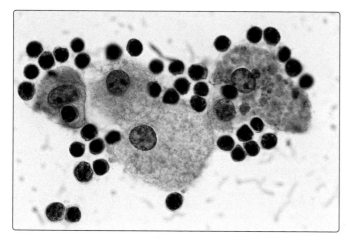

Fig. 17.16   Fine needle aspirate: Renal cyst siderophages. Greenish-brown haemosiderin granules are present in the cytoplasm of one of these foamy macrophages. (Papanicolaou × OI)

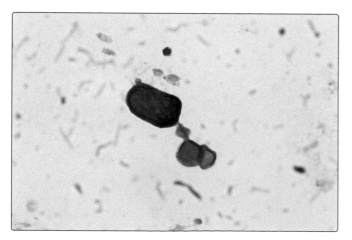

Fig. 17.17   Fine needle aspirate: Renal cyst Liesegang rings. These deposits are laminated, resembling corpora amylacea from the prostate. The laminated structure is better visualized on wet-fixed smears. (MGG × HP)

rings[29]. Rarely, the fluid in a benign cyst may contain numerous calcific concretions or calcospherites which are also laminated (Fig. 17.18). These are too small to appear as calcifications on imaging, but the fluid in these cases appears dense. Malignant renal cysts may arise in a neoplasm but tumours may also develop in the wall of a simple renal cyst[30], 1% of renal carcinomas arise in this manner[31].

Neoplastic lesions in adults

Benign renal neoplasms

Angiomyolipoma (AML)

This benign renal tumour is believed to be derived from perivascular epithelioid cells[32] and is composed of three elements: thick-walled blood vessels, smooth muscle and fat. 50% of these neoplasms are associated with tuberose sclerosis, the tumours being multiple, small and incidental. 80% of patients with tuberous sclerosis may have angiomyolipomas. The other 50% of AMLs occur sporadically and are commonly symptomatic and large. The male to female ratio is 1:2. Although these tumours are benign, they can extend into the vena cava and spread to regional lymph nodes[32]. AML in the kidney can undergo sarcomatous change, invade the liver and metastasize to the lung[33]. These neoplasms can be detected by imaging but the findings are not always diagnostic. Renal cell carcinomas with a fatty component may mimic AML on imaging[34] while both imaging and fine needle aspiration cytology findings of AML can be misdiagnosed as carcinoma[35].

Grossly these tumours appear yellow and slightly oily but may be firm and grey if there is a preponderance of smooth muscle[36], with a well-circumscribed border (Fig. 17.19). Haemorrhage into the tumour is a common occurrence, especially in larger tumours. Histologically, the tumour is composed largely of mature fat, smooth muscle and thick-walled blood vessels arranged in a disorderly fashion (Fig. 17.20). The fat sometimes exhibits fat necrosis with

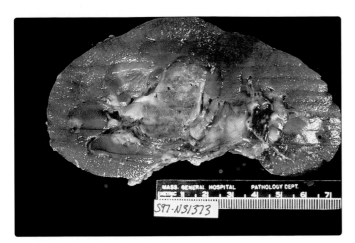

Fig. 17.19   Kidney: Angiomyolipoma, gross appearance. Multiple angiomyolipomas are seen in this specimen. (Courtesy of Dr Edi Brogi, Massachusetts General Hospital, Boston)

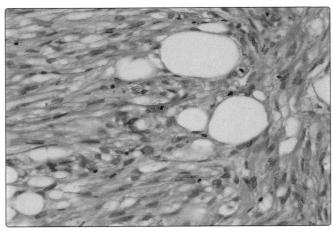

Fig. 17.21   Histology: Angiomyolipoma. Spindle shaped smooth muscle cells and adipocytes are seen in this field. (H&E × HP)

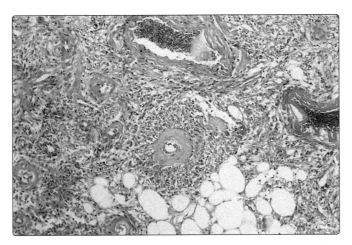

Fig. 17.20   Histology: Angiomyolipoma. The various components of this lesion are demonstrated here: fat, smooth muscle and thick-walled blood vessels. (H&E × LP)

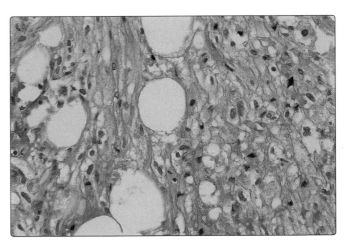

Fig. 17.22   Histology: Angiomyolipoma. Leiomyoblasts with clear cytoplasm are a feature of this lesion. (H&E × HP)

accompanying foamy macrophages and multinucleated giant cells. The smooth muscle cells appear to be derived from the walls of the blood vessels and are usually spindle shaped (Fig. 17.21), but may be epithelioid in appearance with abundant cytoplasm. There are variable numbers of immature smooth muscle cells (leiomyoblasts) with clear cytoplasm (Fig. 17.22) which react positively with HMB 45[35,37–39]. The smooth muscle cells may demonstrate marked pleomorphism, hyperchromasia and mitoses.

Cytological findings

- ► Abundant smooth muscle cells
- ► Abundant adipocytes
- ► Foamy macrophages, giant histiocytes and inflammatory cells may be seen
- ► Smooth muscle cells may be vacuolated
- ► HMB 45 is a useful immunocytochemical test

Fine needle aspiration cytology findings in AML are well described and can be diagnostic[40], especially when combined with imaging. Clusters of adipocytes are common (Fig. 17.23), sometimes accompanied by features of fat necrosis. Smooth muscle cells are usually present, either singly or in groups (Figs 17.24, 17.25), and these may show the vacuolation noted in histological sections, mimicking lipoblasts[40]. These smooth muscle cells may also display spindling and nuclear pseudoinclusions[41]. A certain degree of pleomorphism may be seen in the smooth muscle cells[42] (Fig. 17.26). Blood vessels are also noted in the aspirate. The cytological diagnosis is made more difficult if the radiological diagnosis is unclear[43].

Diagnostic pitfalls

Angiomyolipomas can be mistaken for renal cell carcinoma both on imaging and on fine needle aspirates. Immunocytochemical stains for HMB 45 and smooth muscle actin are useful in distinguishing between the two

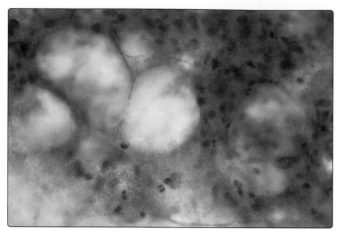

Fig. 17.23   Fine needle aspirate: Angiomyolipoma. Adipocytes are seen surrounded by smooth muscle cells in this fragment of aspirated tissue. (Papanicolaou × HP)

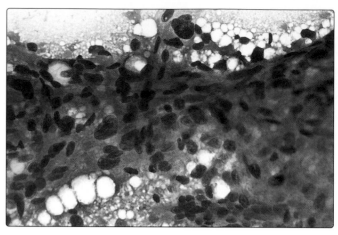

Fig. 17.26   Fine needle aspirate: Angiomyolipoma. Plump spindle-shaped smooth muscle cells are seen in this air-dried smear. (MGG × HP)

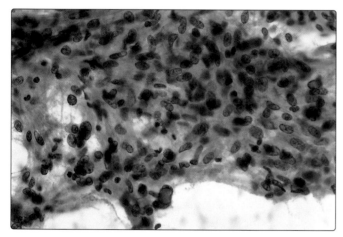

Fig. 17.24   Fine needle aspirate: Angiomyolipoma. Thick clusters of smooth muscle cells are seen in this field. (Papanicolaou × HP)

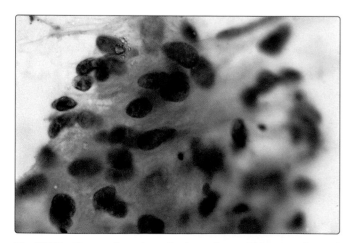

Fig. 17.25   Fine needle aspirate: Angiomyolipoma. This group of smooth muscle cells demonstrates variability in nuclear size and shape. (H&E × OI)

lesions. Aspirates of renal cell carcinomas contain less fat than do angiomyolipomas.

Renal cortical adenoma

There is much controversy about whether renal cortical adenoma can be distinguished from renal cell carcinoma apart from the presence of metastasis. There are no histological, ultrastructural or immunohistochemical differences[44,45]. Tumour size has been used as a criterion but tumours under 3 cm in size have metastasized while very large ones have remained non-invasive. There is no evidence at this time that these tumours will not metastasize if not surgically excised, especially if they are of the clear cell type[46]. Reported sizes vary from 2 to 10 cm[47]. Papillary renal adenomas occur in up to 40% of adults, and typically have papillary, tubular or tubulopapillary architecture and a diameter equal to or less than 5 mm[48]. They have been reported associated with a renal cyst, the histology showing papillary, benign features[49]. Renal cortical adenomas are often an incidental finding at post-mortem or in surgically-excised kidneys. They are usually pale grey or pale yellow and arise in subcapsular areas of the kidney. Histologically they show densely packed tubules, and are circumscribed though not encapsulated. They may demonstrate a papillary pattern, may contain psammoma bodies and xanthoma cells.

Cytological findings

► Cellular aspirate
► Cells with clear abundant cytoplasm
► Small nuclei, nucleoli variable
► No pleomorphism
► No mitoses

Metanephric adenoma

These rare benign tumours of the kidney occur in children and young adults in the form of a well-circumscribed mass.

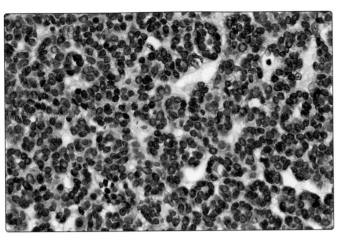

Fig. 17.27 Histology: Metanephric adenoma. This neoplasm is composed of small uniform cells forming small acinar structures. (H&E × HP)

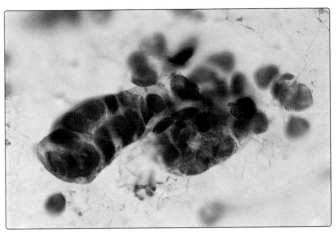

Fig. 17.29 Fine needle aspirate. Metanephric adenoma. A small tubular structure is seen, composed of cells with little cytoplasm. (H&E × OI)

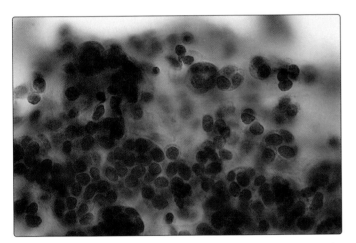

Fig. 17.28 Fine needle aspirate: Metanephric adenoma. This tumour is composed of small, uniform cells with indiscernible cytoplasm. (H&E × HP)

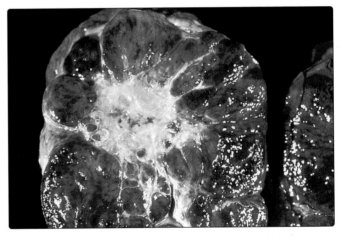

Fig. 17.30 Kidney: Renal oncocytoma. The cut surface of this tumour displays a central scar. (Courtesy of Dr Edi Brogi, Massachusetts General Hospital, Boston)

The histological appearance is of a cellular tumour (Fig. 17.27) composed of small cells with little cytoplasm, forming closely packed acinar structures[50]. Occasionally papillary structures and psammoma bodies are seen[51]. A variant, metanephric adenofibroma has been described, composed partly of a fibroblastic component with a small immature epithelial area, which could be mistaken for a Wilms' tumour[52]. Fine needle aspirates of this metanephric adenoma demonstrate the small dark-staining cells and the acinar pattern seen in the histological sections. The cells are the size of lymphocytes with small nucleoli (Fig. 17.28), contain scant cytoplasm and are arranged as tubules (Fig. 17.29), rosettes and glomeruloid structures[53].

Diagnostic pitfalls

Wilms' tumour contains small, closely packed epithelial cells that are mitotically active, often in large sheets, but occasionally displaying loss of cohesion. The nucleoli are small and the cytoplasm is scanty, making cell borders indistinct.

Renal oncocytoma

These are benign neoplasms composed of cells with abundant, acidophilic, granular cytoplasm, the granularity being due to the presence of abundant mitochondria. They account for about 3% of all renal tumours that result in nephrectomy and are commoner in men than in women with a median age of 62 years, whereas renal cell carcinomas have a median age of 55 years. Most oncocytomas are incidental findings[54], but some are symptomatic with flank pain, a mass and haematuria. They are solitary, mahogany brown due to the lipochrome pigment in the mitochondria and large tumours often display a central scar (Fig. 17.30). Rarely, oncocytomas show cystic degeneration and necrosis, also calcium, but these features should always raise the suspicion of a renal cell carcinoma. The tumour is usually well demarcated although involvement of the pericapsular fat has been

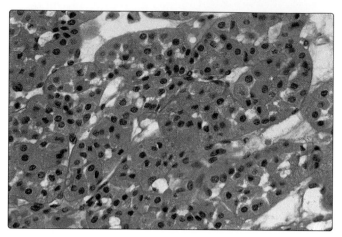

Fig. 17.31 Histology: Renal oncocytoma. This tumour is composed of cells with abundant pink cytoplasm. (H&E × HP)

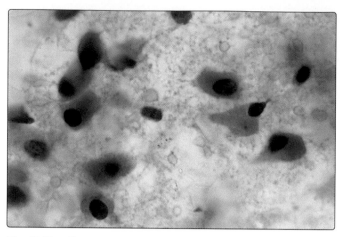

Fig. 17.32 Fine needle aspirate: Renal oncocytoma. Single epithelial cells with abundant cytoplasm are seen in this field. (Papanicolaou × OI)

reported[54,55]. Histologically the tumour is composed of a uniform population of cells with granular, pink cytoplasm in alveolar groups, trabeculae or tubules (Fig. 17.31). Occasionally cells with bizarre hyperchromatic nuclei may be seen[54]. The macroscopic central scar consists of tumour nests and hyalinized connective tissue. There may be areas suggestive of blastema with smaller cells with less abundant cytoplasm and denser nuclei. Small basophilic cells with a high nuclear-cytoplasmic ration and hyperchromatic nuclei have been reported, these cells being designated as ëoncoblastsí[55]. RCC was found coexisting with oncocytoma in 10% cases in a large series of 139 patients[56].

Cytological findings

▶ Large eosinophilic cells with moderate to abundant cytoplasm
▶ Cytoplasm is granular and eosinophilic
▶ Nuclei small with even chromatin may be binucleate
▶ Nucleoli may be prominent
▶ Some cytologic atypia may be noted

On FNA, large eosinophilic cells with prominent nucleoli, some binucleate and granular cytoplasm are seen[57], (Figs 17.32, 17.33). Careful search should be made for any evidence of renal cell carcinoma in the aspirate as the latter may contain areas of oncocytic change. Computed tomography in such cases displays inhomogeneity of composition of the lesion[58].

Diagnostic pitfalls

Oncocytomas should be distinguished from chromophobe and renal cell carcinoma showing granular cells. Renal cell carcinomas should contain, in addition to the oncocytic cells, typical features such as abundant clear cytoplasm and numerous small blood vessels. Chromophobe renal cell

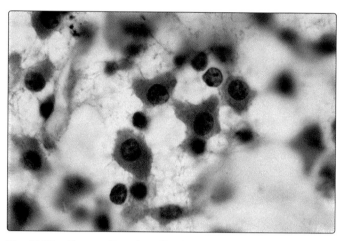

Fig. 17.33 Fine needle aspirate: Renal oncocytoma. In this field similar cells are noted, showing abundant, granular cytoplasm and round nuclei with visible nucleoli. (H&E × OI)

carcinomas have wrinkled nuclei and coarse chromatin and typically demonstrate perinuclear haloes[59].

Other benign renal tumours

Renal tumours of other types are occasionally encountered, usually as incidental findings. They include lipomas, fibromas, leiomyomas and haemangiomas. The cytological findings are identical to those seen in these tumours in other organs (see Chapter 39).

Renal cell carcinoma

Renal cell carcinomas (RCC) are adenocarcinomas and account for 3% of malignant tumours in adults, with a male to female ratio of 1.6:1, and a peak incidence in the 6th decade. The most important risk factor is tobacco. Most tumours exhibit chromosomal abnormalities, commonly chromosome 3 in the clear cell type but 17 and 7 in the papillary type. This neoplasm may arise in kidneys affected by other lesions such as cysts and occurs in 38–55% of patients with von Hippel-Lindau disease. The tumour may

Table 17.1   Fuhrman grading system

Grade	Features
I	Nuclei round, uniform, approx. 10 μm, nucleoli inconspicuous or absent
II	Nuclei slightly irregular, approx. 15 μm, nucleoli evident (at × 400)
III	Nuclei very irregular, approx. 20 μm, nucleoli large and prominent (at × 100)
IV	Nuclei bizarre, multilobated, 20 μm or more, nucleoli prominent, chromatin clumped

remain occult for a long period; when advanced, the symptoms include haematuria and flank pain accompanied by a mass in the flank. Non-specific symptoms such as fever, weight loss, nausea and tiredness are common. Polycythaemia is seen in up to 6% of patients. Radiographic imaging is accurate in detection of these tumours. CT localizes small tumours well, US is useful for fine needle aspiration and core biopsies. MRI provides a three-dimensional picture of the tumour and is useful in planning surgery.

Grading schemes for renal cell carcinoma are related to cytological features, the preferred one being the Fuhrman grading system[60] (Table 17.1).

Renal cell carcinomas are classified into the following types:

Clear cell (hypernephroid)
Chromophil (papillary)
Chromophobe
Collecting duct type (Carcinoma of Bellini's collecting ducts).

Granular cell renal cell carcinoma is a term that is no longer used as even clear cell carcinomas may have cells with granular cytoplasm. The majority of renal cell carcinomas can be typed on fine needle aspiration cytology, but tumours with a predominantly cystic component may be non-diagnostic[61].

Renal cell carcinoma, clear cell type

This is the commonest histological type (75%). It occurs usually as a solitary tumour but may be multiple, often coexisting with an adenoma. In diseases such as von Hippel-Landau syndrome the lesions may be multiple and bilateral. The tumours that are detected by radiological techniques tend to be smaller than those that are symptomatic. Clear cell tumours are well-differentiated and usually well-demarcated from the adjacent kidney. The lesions are usually necrotic and haemorrhagic with cystic degeneration and calcification. The cystic changes may be marked. Often the tumours are golden yellow due to the accumulation of lipid droplets (Fig. 17.34).

Histologically clear cell renal carcinoma is composed of cells which appear clear but which can be shown to contain lipids and glycogen using Oil red-O and the periodic acid-

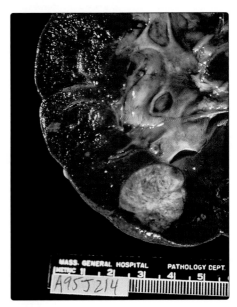

Fig. 17.34   Kidney: Renal cell carcinoma, clear cell type. The tumour appears to be well-circumscribed in this section of kidney. (Courtesy of Dr Edi Brogi, Massachusetts General Hospital, Boston)

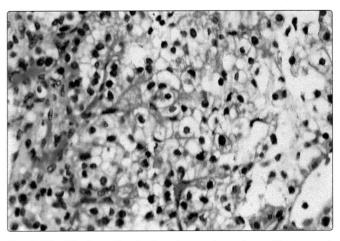

Fig. 17.35   Histology: Renal cell carcinoma, clear cell type. The tumour is composed of clear cells with relatively small nuclei, separated by delicate blood vessels. (H&E × HP)

Schiff (PAS) stains. In addition, the cells often contain cytoplasmic globules that are 5-7 μm in diameter, resemble Mallory's hyaline and stain pink with PAS. The tumour cell groups are separated by delicate blood vessels (Fig. 17.35). Cells with eosinophilic granular cytoplasm may also be seen. The nuclei are round and uniform with finely granular evenly distributed chromatin and inconspicuous nucleoli but some cells may contain pleomorphic nuclei with large, prominent nucleoli.

Cytological findings

► Cellular aspirates containing cells with abundant clear cytoplasm
► Low nuclear/cytoplasmic ratio

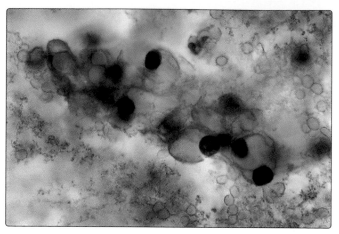

Fig. 17.36   Fine needle aspirate: Renal cell carcinoma, clear cell type. This cluster of neoplastic cells has clear cytoplasm and uniform, round nuclei. (Papanicolaou × OI)

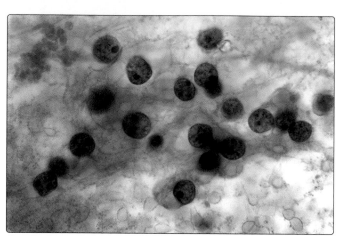

Fig. 17.38   Fine needle aspirate: Renal cell carcinoma, clear cell type. This cluster of cells shows round nuclei with visible nucleoli and finely-vacuolated cytoplasm. (Papanicolaou × OI)

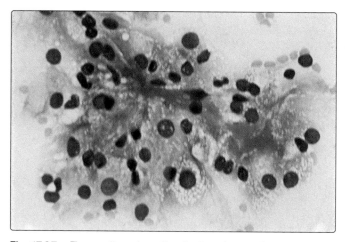

Fig. 17.37   Fine needle aspirate: Renal cell carcinoma, clear cell type. The finely-vacuolated cytoplasm of the tumour cells is clearly seen in this air-dried smear. (Diff-Quik × HP). (Courtesy of Dr S. Granter, Brigham & Womens' Hospital, Boston)

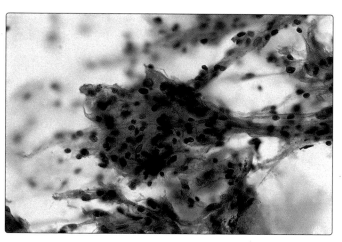

Fig. 17.39   Fine needle aspirate: Renal cell carcinoma, clear cell type. Small blood vessels are seen merging with the cluster of epithelial cells. (H&E × HP)

▶ Small nuclei, nucleoli may be small or more prominent depending on the degree of differentiation
▶ Occasional very large nuclei may be seen
▶ Eosinophilic globules may be noted in the cytoplasm
▶ An air-dried smear stains positive for lipid with Oil red-O

A fine needle aspirate shows features similar to the histological findings, namely clusters of cells with abundant, finely vacuolated or clear cytoplasm and small nucleoli with visible nucleoli (Figs 17.36–17.38). The eosinophilic cytoplasmic globules in neoplastic cells in histological sections may also be seen in aspirates[62]. Branching capillaries are usually evident, either traversing groups of neoplastic cells or unaccompanied by cells (Fig. 17.39). The appearance of vessels passing through clusters of cells is similar to that seen in hepatocellular carcinoma, but differs from it in that there are no peripherally-wrapping endothelial cells around tumour cell groups[63].

Renal cell carcinomas may contain intracellular haemosiderin[64].

Diagnostic pitfalls

Urothelial (transitional cell) carcinoma of the renal pelvis may be difficult to differentiate from renal cell carcinoma. However, urothelial cells usually have denser cytoplasm and sharply defined cytoplasmic borders. Nuclear grooves are sometimes seen in urothelial carcinomas. The presence of capillaries is a pointer to renal cell carcinoma. Oncocytoma should be distinguished from renal cell carcinoma as the prognosis and surgical treatment are different. Wilms' tumour in children may be mistaken for renal cell carcinoma; the presence of blastema is a clue to the diagnosis. Xanthogranulomatous pyelonephritis may be misdiagnosed as renal cell carcinoma, but xanthoma cells

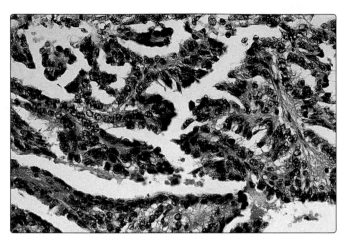

Fig. 17.40   Histology: Renal cell carcinoma, papillary type. The papillary architecture of this tumour is seen in this field, with epithelial cells overlying fibrovascular cores. (H&E × HP). (Courtesy of Dr Edi Brogi, Massachusetts General Hospital, Boston)

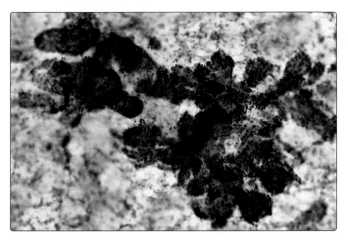

Fig. 17.41   Fine needle aspirate: Renal cell carcinoma, papillary type. This low power field demonstrates papillary architecture on cytology. (Papanicolaou × LP)

have foamy, not clear cytoplasm, the vascular pattern is missing, and inflammatory cells are present. Adrenocortical carcinomas may be difficult to differentiate from renal cell carcinoma cytologically. The cells in the former are not vacuolated, show focal pleomorphism and spindling, and also have eccentric nuclei[65].

Renal cell carcinoma, papillary type (chromophil type)

Some 10–12% of tumours are of this type. The smaller ones must be distinguished from renal cortical adenomas. These neoplasms are well circumscribed and are eccentrically placed in the renal cortex. They are often found in the walls of cysts, are often multiple and associated with renal cortical adenomas. The colour of the gross tumour may be grey but is often yellow due to xanthomatous foamy macrophages in the stroma. Necrosis and haemorrhage are not uncommon.

Microscopically the tumour consists of a single layer of epithelial cells overlying fibrovascular cores containing variable numbers of xanthomatous foamy macrophages (Fig.17.40). Cholesterol clefts, psammoma bodies and haemosiderin granules within tumour cells are often present. The tumour cell nuclei are small and regular; cells range from those with little cytoplasm to others with abundant eosinophilic cytoplasm. The prognosis of papillary RCCs is related to their histopathological characteristics, being significantly better in cases demonstrating infiltration by foam cells, those with a pseudocapsule and in those with basophilic cells. Tumour grade affects survival but there is no significant difference between patients with papillary RCC and those with clear cell RCC[66].

Cytological findings

▶ Cellular aspirates
▶ Papillary clusters with fibrovascular cores

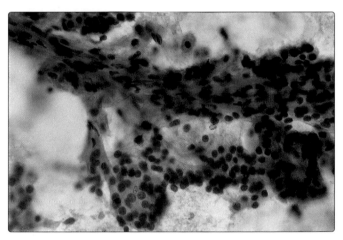

Fig. 17.42   Fine needle aspirate: Renal cell carcinoma, papillary type. A blood vessel crosses this field horizontally, part of a fibrovascular core. (Papanicolaou × HP)

▶ Cells contain small nuclei with prominent grooves
▶ Histiocytes and psammoma bodies may be present
▶ Haemosiderin may be present in the cytoplasm

Fine needle aspirates of papillary renal cell carcinoma display abundant papillary clusters of cells arranged along vascular cores, with few single cells (Figs 17.41–17.43). The neoplastic cells contain small nuclei with prominent nuclear grooves. Haemosiderin may be present in the cytoplasm of neoplastic cells. Foamy histiocytes and siderophages may be noted. Psammoma bodies have been reported in aspirates[67].

Diagnostic pitfalls

These tumours may be misdiagnosed as clear cell carcinoma. Papillary transitional cell carcinoma of the renal pelvis also demonstrates papillary clusters of cells in the aspirate. Urothelial carcinoma cells usually have well-

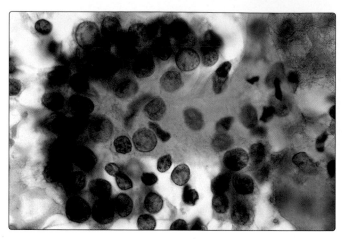

Fig. 17.43 Fine needle aspirate: Renal cell carcinoma, papillary type. This cluster of neoplastic cells at the tip of a fibrovascular core contains fairly uniform nuclei with occasional nuclear grooves. (Papanicolaou × OI)

defined cytoplasmic borders and denser cytoplasm than those of renal cell carcinoma. Squamous differentiation is occasionally present in transitional cell carcinomas of the renal pelvis, as in the bladder.

Renal cell carcinoma, chromophobe type

This recently described tumour[68] affects males and females equally, with a mean age of 55 years and may have a better prognosis than the clear cell type. These carcinomas constitute about 5% of renal neoplasms, are well circumscribed and solitary. Grossly they are solid, tan to brown and typically do not show haemorrhage or necrosis.

Microscopically the cells show an alveolar pattern and demonstrate well-defined cytoplasmic borders and abundant cytoplasm (Fig. 17.44). Some cells have pale cytoplasm while others contain more flocculent or granular cytoplasm. The pale cytoplasm is due to an abundance of microvesicles[69] which are located near the nucleus whereas

the granularity is due to increased numbers of mitochondria, located more peripherally. The nuclei are somewhat pleomorphic with coarse chromatin and occasionally, prominent nucleoli. The microvesicles contain mucopolysaccharides unique to renal cell carcinomas[69]. These can be stained by Hale's colloidal iron. Chromophobe type tumour cells are vimentin negative whereas the cells of clear cell type are vimentin positive.

Cytological findings

▶ Cellular aspirate with single cells and small groups
▶ Cytoplasm varies from flocculent to granular
▶ Thickened cells borders and perinuclear haloes impart a koilocytic appearance
▶ Nuclear variability from wrinkled to binucleate to multinucleate
▶ Coarse nuclear chromatin
▶ Intranuclear inclusions
▶ Hales colloidal iron positive

The cytological appearances of this tumour are characteristic. Fine needle aspirates are cellular, showing single cells as well as small groups of cells with granular to flocculent cytoplasm[70] (Figs 17.45, 17.46). Intranuclear inclusions are not uncommon (Fig. 17.47). Occasional bizarre, multinucleated large cells are present (Fig. 17.48). Nuclear hyperchromasia with variable nuclear size, thickened cytoplasmic membranes and a resemblance to vegetable cells or koilocytes is typical (Fig. 17.49). Hale's colloidal iron is strongly positive in this tumour. The presence of microvesicles can be confirmed ultrastructurally using fine needle aspiration material[71]. Two variants of this tumour have been described: the *atypical variant* resembling a clear cell renal cell carcinoma and the *eosinophilic variant*, which resembles an oncocytoma[72].

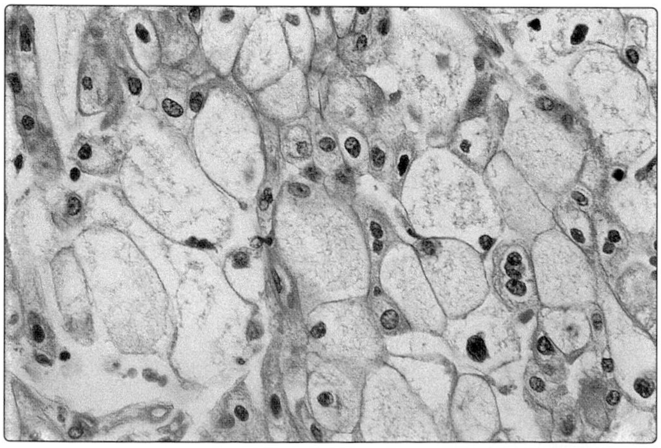

Fig. 17.44 Histology: Renal cell carcinoma, chromophobe type. This section shows the abundant cytoplasm and well-defined borders of the epithelial cells in this tumour. (H&E × HP). (Courtesy of Dr S. Granter, Brigham & Womens' Hospital, Boston)

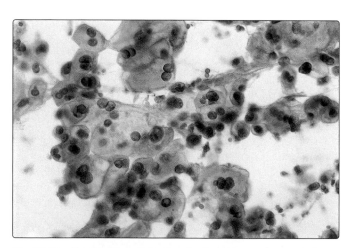

Fig. 17.45 Fine needle aspirate: Renal cell carcinoma, chromophobe type. The cells in this smear show abundant cytoplasm, varying from pale to flocculent. The nuclei are mildly pleomorphic and many of the cells display prominent cytoplasmic borders. (Papanicolaou × HP). (Courtesy of Dr S. Granter, Brigham & Womens' Hospital, Boston)

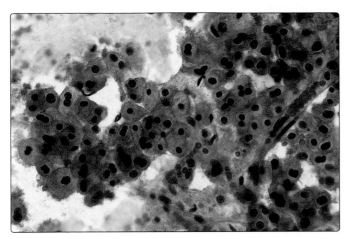

Fig. 17.46   Fine needle aspirate: Renal cell carcinoma, chromophobe type. This field shows cells with abundant cytoplasm and some clearing around the nuclei. (H&E × HP)

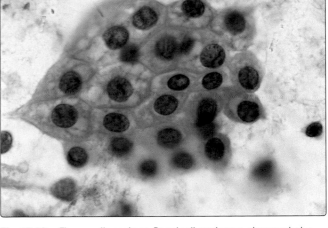

Fig. 17.49   Fine needle aspirate: Renal cell carcinoma, chromophobe type. The resemblance to vegetable cells and/or koilocytes is well demonstrated in this field. (Papanicolaou × OI)

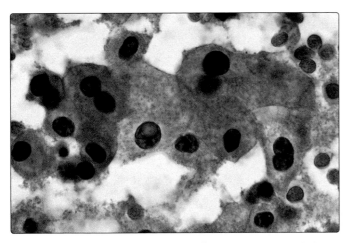

Fig. 17.47   Fine needle aspirate: Renal cell carcinoma, chromophobe type. This high power view shows the flocculent appearance of the cytoplasm in this tumour. Note the intranuclear inclusion. (H&E × OI)

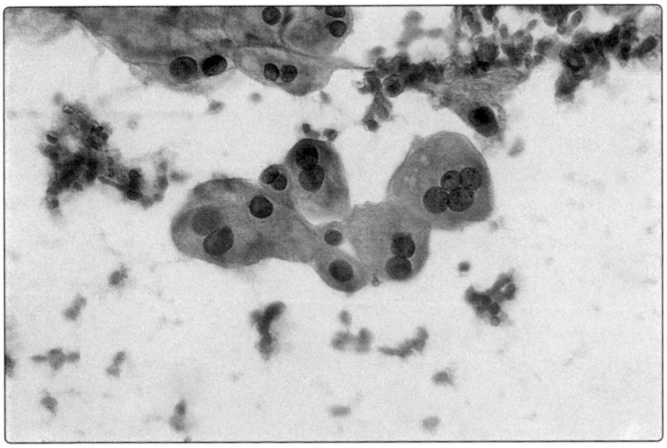

Diagnostic pitfalls

The main differential diagnosis is oncocytoma. Chromophobe RCC has cells with wrinkled nuclei, bi- and multi-nucleation with coarse chromatin and perinuclear haloes while renal oncocytoma has round, uniform nuclei and nucleoli are more commonly seen.

Clear cell carcinoma may be diagnosed if the typical vegetable cell appearance is not conspicuous.

'Sarcomatoid transformation' in renal cell carcinoma

The sarcomatoid type of renal cell carcinoma is no longer classified as a separate entity. A total of 5% renal cell carcinomas contain areas of sarcomatoid appearance and are believed to have a worse prognosis. Although the tumour may look sarcomatoid or have a variable mixture of carcinomatous and sarcomatoid features, light microscopic, ultrastructural and immunocytochemical features invariably show epithelial differentiation[73]. Some reported cases show areas of chondro- or osteosarcoma[74]. The gross appearance is variable, often firm and fibrous. Histologically interlacing bundles of spindle cells, sometimes in a storiform pattern, with areas of carcinoma composed of clear, granular, mixed or oncocyte cells or even a papillary pattern. Some tumours resemble malignant fibrous histiocytoma. Chromophobe carcinoma is probably the most frequent epithelial type associated with sarcomatoid transformation[75]. In summary, sarcomatoid renal cell carcinoma results from de-differentiation of renal epithelial malignancy[76]. On fine needle aspiration the sarcomatoid component cells are spindle shaped. (Fig. 17.50)

Diagnostic pitfalls

Sarcoma of the kidney shows similar cytological features to renal cell carcinoma with sarcomatoid features. The

Fig. 17.48   Fine needle aspirate: Renal cell carcinoma, chromophobe type. Multinucleation is a fairly frequent feature of this tumour. (Papanicolaou × HP). (Courtesy of Dr S. Granter, Brigham & Womens' Hospital, Boston)

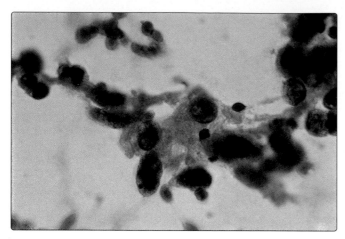

Fig. 17.50 Fine needle aspirate: Renal cell carcinoma with sarcomatoid features. Some of the neoplastic cells in this illustration are spindle shaped. The rest of the tumour showed the typical features of clear cell carcinoma. (Papanicolaou × OI). (Courtesy of Dr S. Granter, Brigham & Womens' Hospital, Boston)

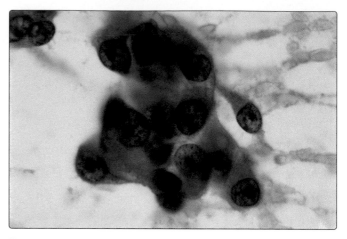

Fig. 17.51 Fine needle aspirate: Transitional cell carcinoma, renal pelvis. Transitional cells display fairly dense cytoplasm and well-defined cell borders as shown in this field. The nuclear-cytoplasmic ratio is high. (Papanicolaou × OI)

distinguishing test is immunocytochemistry, using antibodies to cytokeratin. These are negative in sarcoma.

Renal cell carcinoma, collecting duct type

This type of renal cell carcinoma comprises less than 1% of cases. There are features that are similar to those of papillary RCC but collecting duct carcinomas are located in the medulla and are predominantly tubular. They may have a multicystic appearance but haemorrhage and necrosis are not typical. Histologically the neoplasm shows a mixture of dilated tubules and papillae, both lined by a single layer of cuboidal cells with a hobnail appearance. Tubules may give the tumour a sponge-like appearance. Nuclear pleomorphism is minimal in well-differentiated lesions but pleomorphism is very occasionally seen. The adjacent collecting ducts may show atypical hyperplasia. The cells are positive for high and low molecular weight cytokeratins and epithelial membrane antigen.

Cytological findings

► Round to oval cells in clusters and single cells
► Large, hyperchromatic nuclei
► Moderate amounts of well-defined, vacuolated cytoplasm
► Chromatin clearing

Fine needle aspirates of a collecting duct carcinoma show round to oval cells, single and in clusters with well-defined cytoplasm and large hyperchromatic nuclei with prominent single nucleoli and chromatin clearing. The morphologic features resemble those of a carcinoma derived from breast, ovary or pancreas rather than a renal cell carcinoma[77]. These tumours have malignant features, which are not distinctive and overlap with those of high-grade renal cell carcinoma and transitional cell carcinoma[78].

Renal cell carcinomas spread by direct extension, spreading along the renal vein and involving regional lymph nodes as well. Distant metastases have been diagnosed by fine needle aspirates, the most frequently reported secondary sites being thyroid[79–82], lung[83,84], breast[85,86], pancreas[87,88], adrenal[89], Bartholin's glands[90], vagina[91], and testis[92].

Other renal tumours

Rare tumours of the kidney include leiomyosarcoma, carcinoid (neuroendocrine) tumour, and lymphoma[93]. Leiomyosarcomas, although very rare, have distinctive features that enable a diagnosis on fine needle aspiration cytology[94–96]. The aspirates contain polygonal to spindle-shaped cells, either closely packed or loosely arranged in myxoid stroma, often displaying marked pleomorphism.

Transitional cell (urothelial) carcinoma of the renal pelvis

Urothelial carcinoma of the renal pelvis is similar to that occurring in the urinary bladder. It is commoner in males, in older people and is linked to tobacco and phenacetin use. Patients present with haematuria and occasionally, flank pain. In keeping with urothelial carcinomas arising at other sites such as the bladder, the tumours may be multifocal. Most presenting tumours are low grade, the grading scheme being identical to that for the bladder. The histological appearances are also similar to those in the bladder and may demonstrate squamous differentiation. Cytologically it may be difficult in some cases to differentiate between renal cell and transitional cell carcinoma of the renal pelvis. Transitional cell tumours tend to have well-defined cytoplasmic borders and denser cytoplasm (Fig. 17.51)

Squamous cell carcinoma of the renal pelvis

These tumours comprise about 10% of those occurring in the renal pelvis. The cytological features are similar to those seen in squamous cell tumours occurring at other sites.

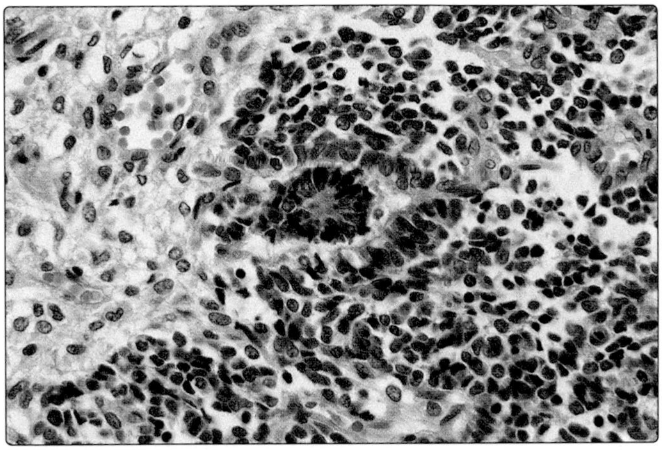

Fig. 17.52 Histology: Wilms' tumour. This section shows small neoplastic cells, some forming tubules. (H&E × LP)

Fig. 17.53 Fine needle aspirate: Wilms' tumour. Small undifferentiated cells are seen here, some in small clusters. Very little cytoplasm is seen. (Papanicolaou × HP)

Tumours in infancy and childhood

Renal tumours occurring in children are usually mesenchymal in composition, those in adults more often epithelial. However, either type of differentiation may be seen in tumours in both age groups.

Nephroblastoma (Wilms' tumour)

This is a neoplasm derived from blastemal cells and may therefore demonstrate epithelial, blastemal and stromal differentiation. It is a tumour of young children, most commonly between the ages of 1 and 3 years, is uncommon in infancy, and rarely occurs in adults. The tumour may be bilateral and multicentric It is well-visualized by ultrasonography, computed tomography and magnetic resonance imaging. Macroscopically these tumours are soft and friable, often displaying necrotic areas and haemorrhage. Microscopically there are variable proportions of three types of cells: blastemal cells, cells showing epithelial differentiation and those showing stromal differentiation. Blastemal cells are small and closely packed with round or oval nuclei, coarse but even chromatin and small nucleoli. The epithelial component may be composed of rosettes, tubules and primitive glomerular structures (Fig. 17.52). Skeletal muscle, adipose tissue, cartilage, bone and neural tissue may be seen.

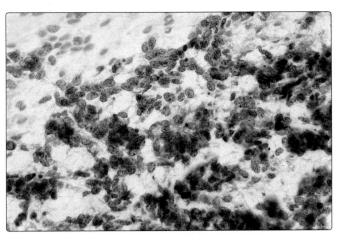

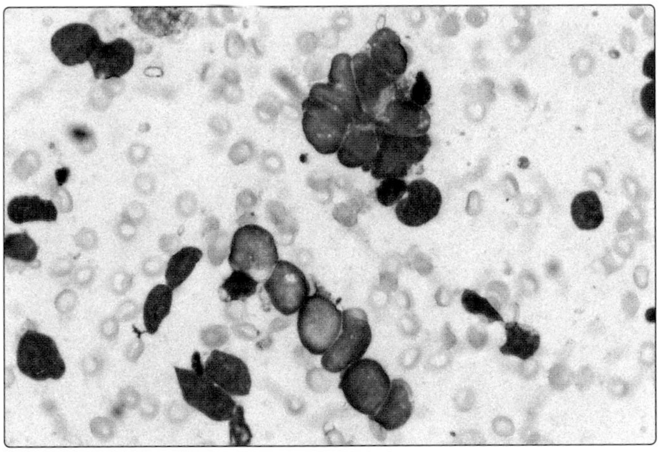

Fig. 17.54 Fine needle aspirate: Wilms' tumour. In air-dried smears the cells appear small with no visible cytoplasm and may be mistaken for lymphoid cells, except that they are in small clusters. (MGG × OI)

blastemal cells (Figs 17.53, 17.54), epithelial cells, tubular and glomeruloid differentiation are identifiable on aspirates[97,98]. Rosettes, tightly grouped spherical cellular clusters and groups with peripheral palisading have been noted[99], as has necrosis[100].

Cytological findings

▶ Small hyperchromatic, closely packed blastemal cells with little cytoplasm, and small nucleoli
▶ Primitive tubules resembling rosettes
▶ Primitive glomeruloid structures
▶ Myxoid material and spindle cells
▶ Necrosis
▶ Adipose tissue, muscle and cartilage may be seen

The cytological features seen on fine needle aspirates correlate well with the histological pattern. Small round

Diagnostic pitfalls

Aspirates of neuroblastoma demonstrate classic Homer Wright rosettes with nuclei around a fibrillary zone. However, Wilms' tumour may also display rosettes and neurone-specific enolase positivity[101]. Lymphoma can resemble Wilms' tumour, the use of immunocytochemical stains assists in the diagnosis.

Cystic nephroma

In children, both this entity and cystic, partially differentiated nephroblastoma are thought to be cystic

Wilms' tumours with no or little metastatic potential[102]. Cystic nephroma in adults usually occurs in females and follows a benign course. The cytological features of this tumour include clusters and rows of cells with occasional discrete blastemal cells[103].

Mesoblastic nephroma

This is a congenital tumour, usually occurring in the first few months of life. Haemorrhage, necrosis and cystic change are common. They are composed of spindle cells of mesenchymal origin. Cytological features that have been described in fine needle aspirates include mildly atypical spindle cells, mostly cohesive, also tadpole cells with small nuclei and dense cytoplasm in a background of mucoid fibrillary material[104,105].

Clear cell sarcoma

This is a rare aggressive tumour composed predominantly of clear cells separated by small blood vessels. Cytological findings include cellularity, a monomorphic cell population with round to oval nuclei, fragile cytoplasm[104] and prominent nuclear grooves and indentations[106,107]. A mucoid background may be present[108].

Rhabdoid tumour

This is a rare malignant neoplasm with a very poor prognosis, occurring in infants. The neoplastic cells resemble tumours of skeletal muscle, hence the name. The cytological features are fairly diagnostic showing round, polygonal and irregularly-shaped cells, with large nuclei and prominent nucleoli and light pink to purple dense cytoplasmic inclusions[109–110].

The retroperitoneum

Retroperitoneal lesions encompass proliferative lesions such as retroperitoneal fibrosis, as well as a variety of tumours from lymphoma to metastatic carcinoma and neuroblastoma, also infective processes such as tuberculosis. In infants and children the most frequent tumour is non-Hodgkin's lymphoma, followed by neuroblastoma, then nephroblastoma[111]. Fine needle aspiration cytology is a safe, and reliable procedure, usually performed under CT guidance. Aspirates of retroperitoneal lymph nodes may be performed under ultrasonographic guidance.

Retroperitoneal fibrosis

This inflammatory process associated with proliferation can lead to obstruction of retroperitoneal structures including the ureters. The process may be primary or secondary to drugs, radiation, inflammatory disease of the bowel, or to neoplasms. Histologically, inflammation and fibrosis are seen. Fine needle aspirates may show similar features (Fig. 17.55), but are often non-diagnostic.

Other benign conditions of the retroperitoneum may be diagnosed on fine needle aspiration cytology. In malakoplakia, aspirates show large numbers of bacilli

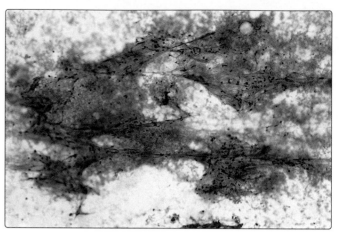

Fig. 17.55 Fine needle aspirate: Retroperitoneal fibrosis. These fragments of stroma with inflammatory cells are non-diagnostic, but are the usual findings in aspirates from these lesions. (Papanicolaou × LP)

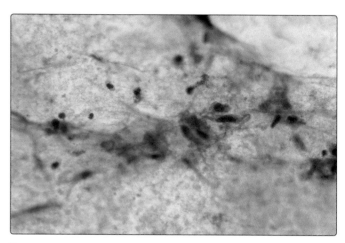

Fig. 17.56 Fine needle aspirate: Schwannoma. This neoplasm is composed of thin, spindle-shaped cells, usually in groups as seen here. (Papanicolaou × HP)

within histiocytes, the numbers decreasing during treatment and increasing with relapse of the disease[112]. Extra-adrenal myelolipomas; tumours which are most commonly found in the retroperitoneal area, show a mixture of mature fat cells and normal haematopoietic cells and should be distinguished from liposarcoma[113]. Schwannomas display characteristic spindly, wavy nuclei, some in a palisading arrangement (Fig. 17.56). Haemangiopericytomas are more difficult to diagnose on fine needle aspirates (Fig. 17.57). *Taenia echinococcus* has been diagnosed unexpectedly on fine needle aspirates of retroperitoneum and para-renal areas[114,115], as has dirofilariasis[116]. Extramedullary haemopoesis should not be mistaken for malignancy[117].

Lymphomas of various types are recognizable on fine needle aspirates of the retroperitoneum (Figs 17.58, 17.59). Immunohistochemical stains and flow cytometry are essential in the classification of these neoplasms, therefore

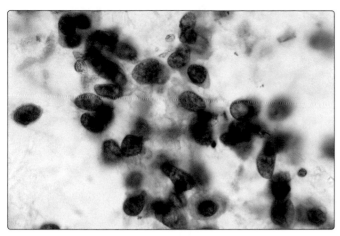

Fig. 17.57 Fine needle aspirate: Haemangiopericytoma: This photomicrograph demonstrates the cells seen in a malignant haemangiopericytoma. The cells are fairly small with little cytoplasm and irregular nuclear margins. (Papanicolaou × OI)

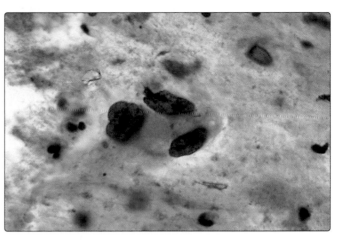

Fig. 17.60 Fine needle aspirate: Leiomyosarcoma. Markedly pleomorphic cells are seen in this field. Immunocytochemical tests are necessary for diagnosis of the tumour type. (Papanicolaou × OI)

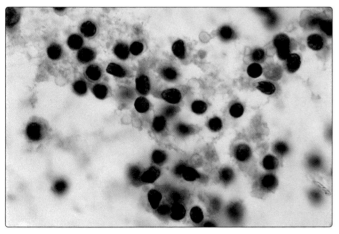

Fig. 17.58 Fine needle aspirate: Small lymphocytic B-cell lymphoma. The lymphoid cells seen in this aspirate are monomorphic, raising the suspicion of lymphoma. Immunocytochemistry and flow cytometry are essential for an accurate diagnosis. (Papanicolaou × HP)

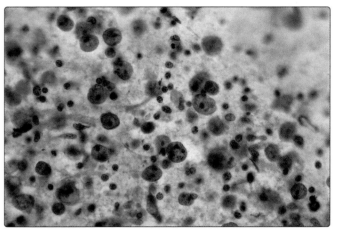

Fig. 17.61 Fine needle aspirate: Seminoma. This tumour is composed of large neoplastic cells with round nuclei and prominent nucleoli. The cytoplasm is very fragile and difficult to discern on wet-fixed smears. Note the lymphocytes in the background. (H&E × OI)

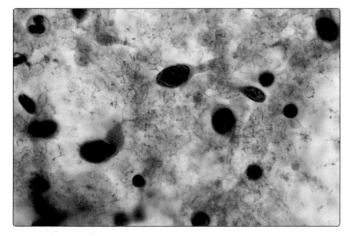

Fig. 17.59 Fine needle aspirate. Large B-cell lymphoma. Large abnormal lymphoid cells are noted in this aspirate, with a few small lymphocytes in the background. Immunocytochemistry and flow cytometry confirmed the diagnosis. (Papanicolaou × OI)

a dedicated pass is recommended to obtain material for these tests when lymphoma is suspected clinically. Diagnosis and classification of lymphoma at this site is discussed in Chapter 19.

A variety of metastatic tumours are seen in the retroperitoneum. These include adenocarcinomas, squamous carcinoma and transitional cell carcinoma, the features of which are similar to those seen in other sites. Sarcomas of various types are also found in the retroperitoneum, liposarcoma, chondrosarcoma and leiomyosarcoma (Fig. 17.60), neuroblastoma, extragonadal germ cell tumours including seminoma (Fig. 17.61), yolk sac tumour, choriocarcinoma and embryonal carcinoma. Details of the identifying cytological features of these tumours are described in the chapters dealing with the common primary site (Chapters 26, 36 and 40).

References

1 Lindblom K. Percutaneous puncture of renal cysts and tumours. *Acta Radiol* 1946; **27**: 66

2 Orell S R, Langlois S L L, Marshall V R. Fine needle aspiration cytology in the diagnosis of solid renal and adrenal masses. *Scand J Urol Nephrol* 1985; **19**(3): 211–216

3 Pilotti I, Rilke F, Alasia L, Garbagnati F. The role of fine needle aspiration in the assessment of renal masses. *Acta Cytol* 1988; **32**(1): 1–10

4 Leiman G. Audit of fine needle aspiration cytology of 120 renal lesions. *Cytopathol* 1990; **1**(2): 65–72

5 Cristallini E G, Paganelli C, Bolis G B. Role of fine-needle aspiration biopsy in the assessment of renal masses. *Diagn Cytopathol* 1991; **7**(1): 32–35

6 Haubek S, Lundorf E, Laudsen K N. Diagnostic strategy in renal mass lesions. *Scand J Urol Nephrol Suppl* 1991; **137**: 35–39

7 Kelley C M, Cohen M B, Raab S S. Utility of fine-needle aspiration biopsy in solid renal masses. *Diagn Cytopathol* 1996; **14**(1): 14–19

8 Renshaw A A, Granter S R, Cibas E S. Fine needle aspiration of the adult kidney. *Cancer* 1997; **8**(2): 71–88

9 Nguyen G-K, Akin M-R. Fine needle aspiration cytology of the kidney, renal pelvis, and adrenal. *Clinics in Laboratory Medicine* 1998; **18**(3): 429–459

10 Zardawi I M. Renal fine needle aspiration cytology. *Acta Cytol* 1999; **43**(2): 184–190

11 Mondal A, Ghosh E. Fine needle aspiration cytology (FNAC) in the diagnosis of solid renal masses – a study of 92 cases. *Indian J Pathol Microbiol* 1992; **35**(4): 333–339

12 Katz R L. Kidneys, adrenals and retroperitoneum. In: Bibbo M ed. *Comprehensive Cytopathology*, 2nd edn. Philadelphia: WB Saunders, 1997; p 781

13 Nguyen G K. Percutaneous fine needle aspiration biopsy cytology of the kidney and adrenal. *Pathol Annu* 1987; **22**: 115

14 Lang E K. Renal cyst puncture and aspiration. A survey of complications. *Am J Roentgenol* 1997; **128**: 723

15 Shenoy P D, Lakhkar B N, Ghosh M K, Patil U D. Cutaneous seeding of renal carcinoma by Chiba needle aspiration biopsy. Case report. *Acta Radiol* 1991; **32**(2): 50–52

16 Slwotzky C, Maya M. Needle tract seeding of transitional cell carcinoma following fine-needle aspiration of a renal mass. *Abdom Imaging* 1994; **19**(2):

17 Wolf J S Jr. Evaluation and management of solid and cystic renal masses. *J Urol* 1998; **159**(4): 1120–1133

18 De Boisgisson P, Roussel F, Leclerc D, Picquenot J M. Granulomatous renal mass during endovesical BCG therapy for bladder carcinoma. Diagnosis by fine-needle aspiration. *Urol* 1991; **37**(6): 557–560

19 Lang E K. Angio-computed tomography and dynamic computed tomography in staging of renal cell carcinoma. *Radiol* 1984; **151**: 149–155

20 Balci N C, Semelka R C, Patt R H et al. Complex renal cysts: findings on MR imaging. *Am J Roentgenol* 1999; **172**(6): 1495–1500

21 Karstaedt N, McCullough D L, Wolfman N T, Dyer R B. Magnetic resonance imaging of the renal mass. *J Urol* 1986; **136**: 566–570

22 Quinn F M, Dick A C, Corbally M T et al. Xanthogranulomatous pyelonephritis in childhood. *Arch Dis Child* 1999; **81**(6): 483–486

23 Kapasi H, Robertson S, Futter N. Diagnosis of renal malacoplakia by fine needle aspiration cytology. A case report. *Acta Cytol* 1998; **42**(6): 1419–1423

24 Silverman J R, Gurley A M, Harris J P et al. Fine needle aspiration cytology of renal infarcts: cytomorphologic findings and potential diagnostic pitfalls in two cases. *Acta Cytol* 1991; **35**: 736–741

25 Pasternack A. Fine needle aspiration biopsy in the diagnosis of human renal allograft rejection. *J Urol* 1973; **109**: 167–172

26 Balci N C, Semelka R C, Patt R H et al. Complex adrenal cyst: findings on MR imaging. *Am J Roentgenol* 1999; **172**(6): 1495–1500

27 Morgan C, Greenberg M L. Multilocular renal cyst: a diagnostic pitfall on fine-needle aspiration cytology. *Diagn Cytopathol* 1995: **13**(1): 66–70

28 Todd D T, Dhurandhar B, Mody D et al. Fine-needle aspiration of cystic lesions of the kidney. Morphologic spectrum and diagnostic problems in 41 cases. *Am J Clin Pathol* 1999; **11**(3): 317–328

29 Raso D S, Greene W B, Finley J L, Silverman J F. Morphology and pathogenesis of Liesegang rings in cyst aspirates: report of two cases with ancillary studies. *Diagn Cytopathol* 1998; **19**(2): 116–119

30 Varma K R, Tiamson E, Golman S M, Tankin L H. Papillary carcinoma in wall of simple renal cyst. *Urol* 1974; **3**: 762–765

31 Eble J. Neoplasms of the kidney. In: Bostwick D and Eble JN eds. *Urologic Surgical Pathol* 1997, St. Louis: Mosby, p 87

32 Eble J. Angiomyolipoma of kidney. *Semin Diagn Pathol* 1998; **15**(1): 21–40

33 Ferry J A, Malt R A, Zamboni G. Renal angiomyolipoma with sarcomatous transformation and pulmonary metastases. *Am J Surg Pathol* 1991; **15**(11): 1083–1088

34 Roy C, Tuchmann C, Linder V et al. Renal cell carcinoma with a fatty component mimicking angiomyolipoma on CT. *Br J Radiol* 1998; **71**(849): 977–979

35 Benzanini M, Pea M, Martignoni G et al. Preoperative diagnosis of renal angiomyolipoma: fine needle aspiration cytology and immunocytochemical characterization. *Pathol* 1994; **26**(2): 170–175

36 Murphy W M, Beckwith J B, Farrow G M eds. Tumors of the kidney. In: *Atlas of Tumor Pathology, Tumors of the Kidney, Bladder, and Related Urinary Structures*. Washington, DC: Armed Forces Institute of Pathology 1994, p 168

37 Kaiserling E, Lepber S, Xiao J-C et al. Angiomyolipoma of the kidney. Immunoreactivity with FMB-45, light and electron-microscopic findings. *Histopathol* 1994; **25**: 41–48

38 Sturtz C L, Dabbs D J. Angiomyolipomas. The nature and expression of the HMB45 antigen. *Mod Pathol* 1994; **7**: 842–845

39 Gupta R K, Mowitz M, Wakefield S J. Fine-needle aspiration cytology of renal angiomyolipoma: report of a case with immunocytochemical and electron microscopic findings. *Diagn Cytopathol* 1998; **18**(4): 297–300

40 Wadih G E, Raab S S, Silverman J F. Fine needle aspiration cytology of renal and retroperitoneal angiomyolipoma. Report of two cases with cytologic findings and clinicopathologic pitfalls in diagnosis. *Acta Cytol* 1995; **39**(5): 945–950

41 Sangawa A, Shintaku M, Nishimura M. Nuclear pseudoinclusions in angiomyolipoma of the kidney. A case report. *Acta Cytol* 1998; **42**(2): 425–429

42 Tallada N, Martinez S, Rowentos A. Cytologic study of renal angiomyolipoma by fine-needle aspiration biopsy: report of four cases. *Diagn Cytopathol* 1994; **10**(1): 37–40

43 Granter S R, Renshaw A A. Cytologic analysis of renal angiomyolipoma: a comparison of radiologically classic and challenging cases. *Cancer* 1999; **89**(3): 135–140

44 Bennington J L. Specimen of renal adenoma and carcinoma. *Am J Surg Pathol* 1981(Abstract); **5**: 194

45 Fisher E R, Horvat B. Comparative ultrastructural study of so-called renal adenoma and carcinoma. *J Urol* 1972; **108**: 382–386

46 Bostwick D G and Eble J N eds. Renal tumors in adults. In: *Urologic Surgical Pathology*. St. Louis: Mosby, 1997, p 84

47 Murphy W M, Beckwith J B, Farrow G M eds. Tumors of the kidney. In: *Atlas of Tumor Pathology, Tumors of the Kidney, Bladder, and Related Urinary Structures*. Washington, DC: Armed Forces Institute of Pathology 1994, p 133

48 Grignon D J, Eble J N. Papillary and metanephric adenomas of the kidney. *Semin Diagn Pathol* 1998; **15**(1): 1–41

49 Itoh Y, Okamura T, Sasaki S et al. Renal adenoma associated with renal cyst formation. *Int J Urol* 1999; **5**(10): 604–605

50 Imamoto T, Furuya Y, Ueda T, Ito H. Metanephric adenoma of the kidney. *Int J Urol* 1999; **6**(4): 200–202

51 Bostwick D G and Eble J N eds. Renal tumors. In: *Urologic Surgical Pathology*. St. Louis: Mosby, 1997, p 120

52 Shek T W, Luk I S, Peh W C et al. Metanephric adenofibroma: report of a case and review of the literature. *Am J Surg Pathol* 1999; **23**(6): 727–733

53 Granter S R, Fletcher J A, Renshaw A A. Cytologic and cytogenetic analysis of metanephric adenoma of the kidney:

a report of 2 cases. *Am J Clin Pathol* 1997;
108(5): 544–549

54 Amin M B, Crotty T B, Tickoo S K, Farrow
G M. Renal oncocytoma: a reappraisal of
morphologic features with
clinicopathologic findings in 80 cases. *Am J
Surg Pathol* 1997; **21**(1): 1–12

55 Perez-Ordonez B, Hamed G, Campbell S *et
al*. Renal oncocytoma: a clinicopathologic
study of 70 cases. *Am J Surg Pathol* 1997;
21(8): 871–883

56 Dechet C B, Bostwick D G, Blute M L *et al*.
Renal oncocytoma: multifocality,
bilateralism, metachronous development
and coexistent renal cell carcinoma. *J Urol*
162(1); 40–42

57 Alanen K A, Tyrkko J E, Nurmi M J.
Aspiration biopsy cytology of renal
oncocytoma. *Acta Cytol* 1985; **29**(5):
859–862

58 Talja M R, Kinsaari L M, Koivuniemi A P
et al. Diagnostic difficulties in oncocyte-
containing renal carcinoma. *Scand J Urol
Nephrol* 1986, **20**(1): 77–80

59 Tickoo S K, Amin M B. Discriminant
nuclear features of renal oncocytoma and
chromophobe renal cell carcinoma.
Analysis of their potential utility in the
differential diagnosis. *Am J Clin Pathol* 1999;
110(6): 782–787

60 Fuhrman S A, Lasky L C, Limas C.
Prognostic significance of morphologic
parameters in renal cell carcinoma. *Am J
Surg Pathol* 1982; **6**: 655–663

61 Renshaw A A, Lee K R, Madge R,
Granter S R. Accuracy of fine-needle
aspiration in distinguishing subtypes of
renal cell carcinoma. *Acta Cytol* 1997;
41(4): 987–994

62 Unger P, Hague K, Klein G *et al*. Fine needle
aspiration of a renal cell carcinoma with
eosinophilic globules. A case report. *Acta
Cytol* 1993; **37**(2): 201–204

63 Weir M, Pitman M. The vascular
architecture of renal cell carcinoma in fine-
needle aspiration biopsy. An aid in its
distinction from hepatocellular carcinoma.
Cancer 1997; **81**(1): 45–50

64 Weaver M G, al-Kaisi N, Abdul-Karim F N.
Fine needle aspiration cytology of a renal
cell carcinoma with massive intracellular
hemosiderin accumulation. *Diagn Cytol*
1991; **7**(2): 147–149

65 Scharfe A T, Yokajama M, Alken P *et al*.
Immunoperoxidase staining of fine-needle
aspiration biopsies of renal cell carcinoma
using tumor-specific monoclonal antibody.
Eur Urol 1987; **13**(5): 331–333

66 Onishi T, Onishi Y, Goto H *et al*. Papillary
renal cell carcinoma: clinicopathologic
characteristics and evaluation of prognosis
in 42 patients. *ABJU Int* 1999; **83**(9):
937–943

67 Dekmezian R, Sneige N, Shabb N. Papillary
renal cell carcinoma: fine needle aspiration
of 15 cases. *Diagn Cytopathol* 1991; **7**(2):
198–203

68 Thoenes W, Stoerkel S, Rumpelt H-J *et al*.
Human chromophobe renal carcinoma.
Virchows Arch B 1985; **48**: 207–217

69 Murphy W M, Beckwith J B, Farrow G M
eds. Tumors of the kidney. In: *Atlas of Tumor

Pathology, Tumors of the Kidney, Bladder, and
Related Urinary Structures*. Washington, DC:
Armed Forces Institute of Pathology, p 113

70 Granter S R, Renshaw A A. Fine-needle
aspiration of chromophobe renal cell
carcinoma. Analysis of 6 cases. *Cancer* 1997;
81(2) 122–128

71 Akhtar M, Ali M F. Aspiration cytology of
chromophobe cell carcinoma of the kidney.
Diagn Cytopathol 1995; **13**(4): 287–294

72 Renshaw A A, Granter S R. Fine needle
aspiration of chromophobe renal cell
carcinoma. *Acta Cytol* 1996; **40**(5):
867–877

73 Murphy W M, Beckwith J B, Farrow G M
eds. Tumors of the kidney. In: *Atlas of Tumor
Pathology, Tumors of the Kidney, Bladder, and
Related Urinary Structures*. Washington, DC:
Armed Forces Institute of Pathology, 1994,
p 117

74 Auger M, Katz R L, Sella A *et al*. Fine-
needle aspiration cytology of sarcomatoid
renal cell carcinoma: a morphological and
immunocytochemical study of 15 cases.
Diagn Cytopathol 1993; **9**(1): 46–51

75 Akhtar A M, Tulbah A, Karbar A H, Ali M A.
Sarcomatoid renal cell carcinoma: the
chromophobe connection. *Am J Surg Pathol*
1997; **21**(10): 1188–1195

76 Delahunt B. Sarcomatoid renal carcinoma:
the final common dedifferentiation
pathway of renal epithelial malignancies.
Pathol 1999; **31**(3): 185–190

77 Layfield L J. Fine-needle aspiration biopsy
of renal collecting duct carcinoma. *Diagn
Cytopathol* 1994; **11**(1): 74–78

78 Raway N P, Wojcik E M, Katz R L *et al*.
Cytologic findings of collecting duct
carcinoma of the kidney. *Diagn Cytopathol*
1995; **13**(4): 304–309

79 Dal Fabbro S, Monari G, Barbazza R.
A thyroid metastasis revealing an occult
renal clear-cell carcinoma. *Tumori* 1987;
73(2):197–190

80 Halbauer M, Kodama T, Skelin L *et al*.
Aspiration cytology of renal-cell carcinoma
metastatic to the thyroid. *Acta Cytol* 1991;
35(4): 443–446

81 Rikabi A C, Yound A E, Wilson C.
Metastatic renal clear cell carcinoma in the
thyroid gland diagnosed by fine needle
aspiration cytology. *Cytopathol* 1991; **2**(1):
47–49

82 Bertin J, Rhamani D, Maurice H, Pujol H.
Intrathyroid metastasis of kidney cancer. A
rare case and diagnostic trap. *Ann Endocrinol
(Paris)* 1999; **60**(1): 45–47

83 Piscioli F K, Pojer A, Pusiol T, Luciani L.
Diagnosis by aspiration biopsy of lung
metastasis of renal cell carcinoma 24 years
after nephrectomy. *Eur Urol* 1984; **10**(5):
358–360

84 Yoshida J, Nagai K, Hasebi T *et al*.
Pulmonary metastasis of renal cell
carcinoma resected sixteen years after
nephrectomy. *Jpn J Clin Oncol* 1995; **25**(1):
20–24

85 Ferrera G, Mappi O. Metastatic neoplasms
of the breast fine-needle aspiration cytology
of two cases. *Diagn Cytopathol* 1996; **15**(2):
139–143

86 Kannan V. Fine-needle aspiration of
metastatic renal-cell carcinoma
masquerading as primary breast carcinoma.
Diagn Cytopathol 1998; **18**(5): 343–345

87 Derias N Q, Chong W H. Fine needle
aspiration diagnosis of a late solitary
pancreatic metastasis of renal
adenocarcinoma. *Cytopathol* 1993; **4**(6):
369–372

88 Gupta R K, Delahunt B. Fine-needle
aspiration cytology of metastatic clear-cell
renal carcinoma presenting as a solitary
mass in the head of the pancreas. *Diagn
Cytopathol* 1998; **19**(3): 194–197

89 Duggan Mak, Forestwell C F, Hanley D A.
Adrenal metastasis of renal-cell carcinoma
19 years after nephrectomy. Fine needle
aspiration cytology of a case. *Acta Cytol*
1987; **431**(4): 512–516

90 Leiman G, Markowitz S, Veiga-Ferreira M M,
Margoluis K A. Renal adenocarcinoma
presenting with bilateral metastases to
Bartholin's glands: primary diagnosis by
aspiration cytology. *Diagn Cytopathol* 1986;
2(3): 252–255

91 Queiroz C, Bachchi C E, Oliveira C *et al*.
Cytologic diagnosis of vaginal metastasis
from renal cell carcinoma. A case report.
Acta Cytol 1999; **43**(6): 1098–1100

92 Steiner G, Heimbach D, Pakos E, Muller S.
Simultaneous testicular metastases from a
renal cell carcinoma. *Scand J Urol Nephrol*
199; **33**(2); 136–137

93 Fernandez-Acenero M J, Galendo M,
Bengochea O *et al*. Primary malignant
lymphoma of the kidney: case report and
literature review. *Gen Diagn Pathol* 1998;
143(5–6): 317–320

94 Akhtar M, Ali M A, Sackey K, Burgess A.
Fine-needle aspiration biopsy of clear-cell
sarcoma of the kidney: light and electron
microscopic features. *Diagn Cytopathol*
1989; **5**(2): 181–187

95 Chow L T, Chen S K, Chow W H. Fine
needle aspiration cytodiagnosis of
leiomyosarcoma of the renal pelvis. A case
report with immunohistochemical study.
Acta Cytol 1994; **38**(3):759–763

96 Villanueva R R, Nguyen-Ho P, Nguyen G K.
Leiomyosarcoma of the kidney. Report of a
case diagnosed by fine needle aspiration
cytology and electron microscopy. *Acta
Cytol* 1994; **38**(1): 568–572

97 Dey P, Radhika S, Rajwanshi A *et al*.
Aspiration cytology of Wilms' tumor. *Acta
Cytol* 1993; **37**(4): 477–482

98 Ellison D A, Silverman J F, Strausbauch P H
et al. Role of immunocytochemistry,
electron microscopy, and DNA analysis in
fine-needle aspiration biopsy diagnosis of
Wilms' disease. *Diagn Cytopathol* 1996;
14(2): 101–107

99 Hazarika D, Narasimhamurthy K N,
Rao C R, Gopinath K S. Fine needle
aspiration cytology of Wilms' tumor.
A study of 17 cases. *Acta Cytol* 1994;
38(3): 355–360

100 Sharifah N A. Fine needle aspiration
cytology characteristics of renal tumors in
children. *Pathol* 1994; **26**(4): 359–364

101 Drut A R. Neuron-specific enolase-positive
rosettes in nephroblastoma: a possible

diagnostic pitfall in aspiration cytology. *Diagn Cytopathol* 1987; **3**(1): 74–76

102 Eble J N, Bonsi B S M. Extensively cystic renal neoplasms with cystic nephroma, cystic partially differentiated nephroblastoma, multiloculated cystic renal cell carcinoma and cystic hamartoma of renal pelvis. *Semin Diagn Pathol* 1998; **15**(1): 2–20

103 Dey P, Das A, Radhika S. Fine needle aspiration cytology of cystic partially differentiated nephroblastoma. A case report. *Acta Cytol* 1996; **40**(4): 770–772

104 Sharifah N A. Fine needle aspiration cytology characterization of renal tumors in children. *Pathol* 1994; **26**(4): 359–364

105 Dey P, Srinivasan R, Nijhawan R *et al*. Fine needle aspiration cytology of mesoblastic nephroma. A case report. *Acta Cytol* 1992; **36**(3): 404–406

106 Drut R, Pomar M. Cytologic characteristics of clear-cell sarcoma of the kidney (CCSK) in fine-needle aspiration biopsy (FNAB): a report of 4 cases. *Diagn Cytopathol* 1991; **7**(6): 611–614

107 Krishnamurthy S, Bharadwaj R. Fine needle aspiration cytology of clear cell sarcoma of the kidney. A case report. *Acta Cytol* 1998; **42**(6): 1444–1446

108 Akhtar M, Ali M A, Sackey K, Burgess A. Fine needle aspiration biopsy of clear-cell sarcoma of the kidney. *Diagn Cytopathol* 1989; **5**(2): 181–187

109 Akhtar M, Ali M A, Sackey K *et al*. Fine-needle aspiration biopsy diagnosis of malignant rhabdoid tumor of the kidney. *Diagn Cytopathol* 1991; **7**(1): 36–40

110 Drut R. Malignant rhabdoid tumor of the kidney diagnosed by fine-needle aspiration cytology. *Diagn Cytopathol* 1990; **6**(2): 124–126

111 Valkow I, Bojikin B. Fine-needle aspiration biopsy of abdominal and peritoneal tumors in infants and children. *Diagn Cytopathol* 1987; **3**(2): 129–133

112 Akhtar M, Ali M A, Robinson C, Harfi H. Role of fine needle aspiration biopsy in the diagnosis and management of malacoplakia. *Acta Cytol* 1985; **29**(3): 457–460

113 Prahlow J A, Loggie B W, Cappellari J O *et al*. Extra-adrenal myelolipoma: report of two cases. *South Med J* 1995; **88**(6): 639–643

114 Kapila K, Verma K. Aspiration cytology diagnosis of echinococcosis. *Diagn Cytopathol* 1990; **6**(5): 301–303

115 Guiffre G, Mondello P, Inferrera A *et al*. Unexpected cytological diagnosis of two cases of echinococcosis. *Pathologica* 1993; **85**(1100): 747–753

116 Roussel F, Delaville A, Campos H *et al*. Fine needle aspiration of retroperitoneal human dirofilariases with a pseudotumoral presentation. *Acta Cytol* 1990; **34**(4): 533–535

117 Jan Y J, Chen J T, Chang M C, Ho W L. Fine-needle aspiration cytology of retroperitoneal extramedullary hematopoiesis: a case report. *Kao Hsiung I Hsueh Ko Hsueh Tsa Chih* 1998; **14**(10): 659–553

18 Urinary tract cytology

Grace McKee

Introduction

Cytological examination of urine is a simple diagnostic procedure which can reveal evidence of disease anywhere in the urinary tract from the kidneys, ureters and bladder to the urethra and its related structures. The earliest mention of urine cytology for diagnosis of bladder cancer is Sanders' report of finding neoplastic tissue in urine in 1864[1]. The results of cytological examination of urinary sediment for diagnosis of urinary tract carcinomas were later published by Papanicolaou in 1945[2] and the procedure is now established as part of the routine investigation of patients with haematuria, prostatism and suspected urinary tract neoplasia. Cytological evaluation of urine can detect most high-grade bladder cancers and is especially useful for carcinoma-*in-situ* which is difficult to identify cystoscopically. However, it has limited success in the diagnosis of low-grade urothelial carcinoma because the cells do not exhibit the usual features of malignancy. Cytology may also contribute to investigation of certain aspects of renal parenchymal disease such as acute interstitial nephritis[3] and glomerular haematuria[4-7]. It has been recently shown that urine cytology can be used to detect renal allograft rejection. One method involves testing urine with specific markers such as ICAM-1, TGF-alpha and interferon-gamma receptor[8]. If renal tubular cells are positive with the first two and negative with the third, this is an indicator of acute rejection. Negative ICAM-1 and TGF-alpha with positive interferon-gamma receptor are not associated with allograft rejection. Urine can also be examined for evidence of interstitial nephritis caused by polyoma virus, which can provoke damage to the transplanted kidney[9]. Systemic diseases may manifest with urinary symptoms and urine cytology also plays a part in the diagnosis of uncommon infections[10].

Urinary cytology has become an established industrial screening procedure for workers exposed to carcinogens such as aniline dyes and coal tar volatiles. In addition, cytology can be used to follow up patients treated for neoplasia with topical therapy. More recently, new techniques have been developed such as DNA measurements by flow cytometry and image analysis. Immunocytochemical studies to detect the presence or loss of various antigens can contribute to identification of cells and other molecular biological techniques are proving helpful as research tools. These procedures are discussed briefly at the end of this chapter.

Anatomy of the urinary tract

The kidneys are bean-shaped organs which produce and excrete urine. Their investigation by direct cytological sampling with fine needle aspiration is dealt with in Chapter 17. Blood entering the glomeruli is filtered and the filtrate passes through the convoluted and distal tubules where its composition is altered by resorption and excretion of various ions and absorption of water until it becomes concentrated urine. Urine passes from the renal calyces via the renal pelves into the ureters and thence into the urinary bladder; here it is stored until voided via the urethra, which traverses the prostate gland in males (Fig. 18.1). The muscular sphincter between the bladder and the urethra is under voluntary control, allowing the bladder to function as a reservoir. The ureters and urethra are tubular structures with muscular walls, lined by epithelium similar to that lining the bladder, formerly called transitional

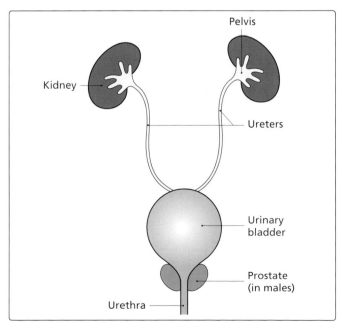

Fig. 18.1 Diagrammatic representation of the urinary tract. Urine passes from the kidney into the calyces, the renal pelvis, via the ureter into the bladder and is finally voided through the urethra.

471

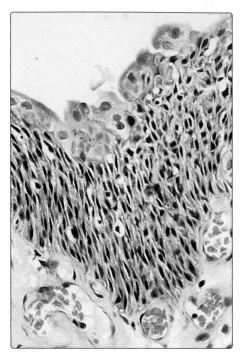

Fig. 18.2 Histology: section of urinary bladder. Urothelium is composed of several layers of small cells with a superficial layer of large 'umbrella' cells. Each superficial cell overlies several deeper layer cells. Polarity is a striking feature. (H&E × HP)

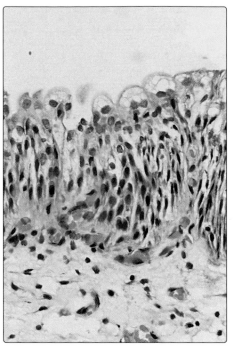

Fig. 18.3 Histology: distended bladder. The urothelium in this section appears to have fewer layers of epithelial cells than that in **Fig. 18.2**. Note the superficial umbrella cells. (H&E × HP)

epithelium but now more commonly referred to as urothelium.

Histology of urothelium

The mucosa of the urinary tract is deceptively simple in appearance, being in fact highly adapted to the changing demands of its function, namely to form a waterproof lining for the structures involved in the storage and excretion of urine. This is achieved by a multilayered epithelium with an average of 5–7 layers of specialized cells resting on a basement membrane (Fig. 18.2).

The thickness of bladder mucosa varies with the state of the bladder: when distended, there are few layers of urothelial cells (Fig. 18.3), while an empty bladder appears to have a thickly layered epithelium. The cells of the deeper layers are small, each with a single nucleus and a smaller amount of cytoplasm than present in cells of the most superficial layer. Superficial cells are larger and are multinucleated, with from 2–55 nuclei. Each superficial cell overlies two or three deeper layer cells and hence is called an 'umbrella' cell. On electron microscopy superficial cells are seen to be adherent to each other by tight junctions and to the deeper layer cells by desmosomes and also have a special asymmetrical membrane over their luminal surface. The surface of the urothelium is covered by a layer of glycoprotein. The urothelium lining the ureter is thicker than bladder urothelium (Fig. 18.4).

The basal area of the bladder between the insertion of the ureters and the urethra is called the trigone. This is often

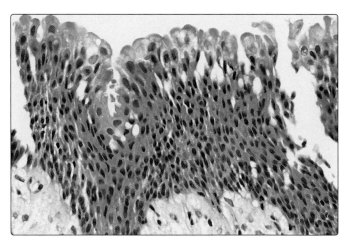

Fig. 18.4 Histology: section of ureter. The urothelium is thicker than that of bladder but is composed of identical cells. (H&E × HP)

lined by squamous epithelium, which, in females, can show similar cyclical changes to those that occur in the epithelium of the ectocervix. Sometimes the bladder epithelium includes areas of mucin-secreting columnar cells. In most normal bladders the urothelium forms several cup-shaped or goblet-shaped depressions. These are known as von Brunn's nests (Fig. 18.5). They are occasionally lined by mucin secreting columnar cells rather than urothelium and become distended with mucin, a finding referred to as cystitis cystica or cystitis glandularis (Fig. 18.6). The cystoscopic appearances of cystitis glandularis can give novice urologists an erroneous impression of neoplasia.

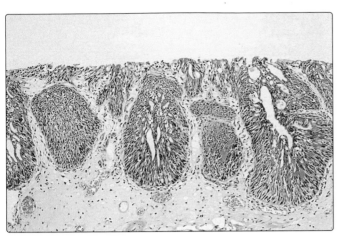

Fig. 18.5   Histology: von Brunn's nests. In this section of bladder several nests or buds of epithelium are seen dipping into the underlying stroma. These nests are lined by urothelial cells. (H&E × MP)

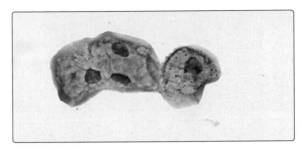

Fig. 18.7   Urine: urothelial cells containing glycogen. This is a small group of benign, deeper layer urothelial cells, all containing cytoplasmic glycogen. (Papanicolaou × HP)

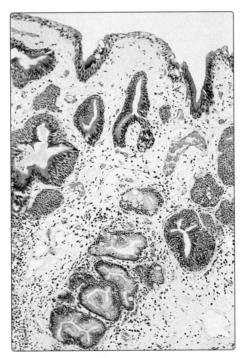

Fig. 18.6   Cystitis glandularis. The von Brunn's nests seen in the section are lined by mucin secreting tall columnar cells. (H&E × MP)

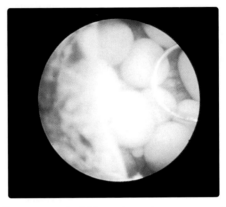

Fig. 18.8   Cystoscopy: calculi. The cystoscopic appearance of typical bladder stones, which are smooth and round, probably formed of urates. (Courtesy of Mr R G Notley, Guildford, UK)

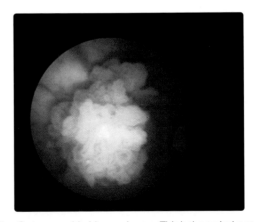

Fig. 18.9   Cystoscopy: bladder carcinoma. This is the typical cystoscopic appearance of a well-differentiated non-invasive papillary urothelial carcinoma. (Courtesy of Mr R G Notley, Guildford, UK)

Urothelial cells contain varying amounts of glycogen (Fig. 18.7).

Technical procedures

Investigative methods other than urinary cytology that are used in diagnosing urinary tract diseases include cystoscopy and intravenous or retrograde pyelography. Cystoscopy can identify inflammatory lesions, diverticula, obstruction, calculi (Fig. 18.8), tumours (Fig. 18.9) and even cystitis cystica (Fig. 18.10). Pyelograms are useful in identifying both tumours and calculi. However, the sheer simplicity of urinary tract cytology justifies its early use, the results of which may then determine the nature and extent of disease and the need for other more invasive tests. The specificity of urine cytology is high but the sensitivity is poor overall[11]. Urine cytology reporting may not always be straightforward. The reliability of cytological diagnosis of primary bladder tumours depends on the reporting pathologist and marked variability between pathologists has been demonstrated[12].

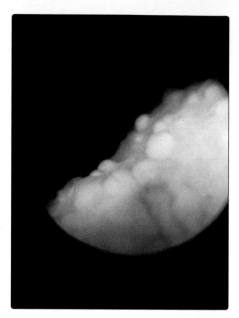

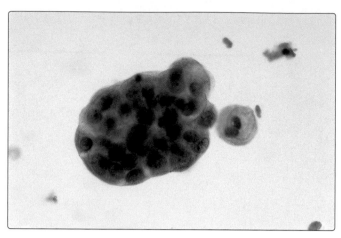

Fig. 18.11   Catheterized urine sample: A cluster of benign urothelial cells that has been dislodged by the procedure. The outline of the group is smooth and the cells are uniform. (Papanicolaou × HP)

Fig. 18.10   Cystoscopy: cystitis glandularis. Illustrated here is the macroscopic appearance of dilated von Brunn's nests. This can prove a confusing picture to the inexperienced urologist. (Courtesy of Mr R G Notley, Guildford, UK)

Collection of specimens

Voided urine is the simplest method of collection. Although an early morning urine specimen is the most useful one for other pathological investigations such as microbiology, it is next to useless for cytological evaluation. Exfoliated cells lying in urine for several hours are usually too degenerate for accurate assessment. A mid-morning or random specimen is recommended, with the sample being sent to the laboratory quickly for processing. If a short delay is inevitable the container may be placed in a refrigerator; with an unavoidable longer delay, alcohol should be added to the sample to fix the cells.

In many centres only one sample of urine is examined. It has been shown however, that the sensitivity of urine cytology for bladder neoplasia rises from 97% with a single voided specimen to 100% when two or more specimens are examined[13]. At least three urine specimens should be examined ideally[14]. Fractionated urine specimens have been studied cytologically to assess the initial, midstream and final parts of the voided specimen, but did not demonstrate improved diagnostic accuracy[15].

The advantage of voided urine examination is that it is a readily repeatable, simple procedure. One disadvantage is that there is usually contamination by cells from the genital tract in females. Furthermore, in men with urinary obstruction large residual volumes mean that exfoliated cells show severe degenerative changes[15]. Normal voided urine samples usually contain few epithelial cells.

Catheterized specimens. These are collected only when clinically indicated, as catheterization is an invasive procedure that can produce much discomfort. The advantages are that contamination is avoided and

specimens can be collected from precise locations such as either ureter. The cells of such samples are usually well preserved, but an important pitfall is that sheets of epithelial cells may be dislodged by the tip of the catheter, and these can mimic papillary neoplasia (Fig. 18.11). It is therefore essential that clinicians indicate the nature of the sample when catheterized urine is sent for cytological assessment.

Bladder washings. This is performed by irrigating the bladder with saline or an electrolyte solution and sending the lavage specimen to the laboratory. The disadvantages are the same as those for catheterized specimens, but the cellular yield and preservation are usually good, making this method of collection superior to voided urine[16]. The sensitivity for detection of neoplasia in one reported study was 100% for bladder washings[17]. Again, the laboratory must be informed of the method of specimen collection for accurate interpretation.

Brushings. These are carried out via a cystoscope. The epithelial cells are removed with a brush, smeared on to slides and sent to the laboratory. The cellular yield is good and the urothelial cells tend to stay in cohesive flat sheets (Fig. 18.12). Lubricant is often seen in smears prepared from catheterization specimens and bladder washings (Fig. 18.13).

Preparation techniques

Urine specimens are processed for microscopy by centrifugation followed by cytocentrifugation, then fixed in alcohol before staining with the Papanicolaou technique. This produces a monolayer of cells 6 mm in diameter. A large volume cytocentrifuge method has been described which has the advantage of a larger number of cells on the slide. Direct smears are easier to prepare but show scanty cellularity[18].

Membrane filter preparations are difficult to prepare but show good cellularity. Staining should always be done on

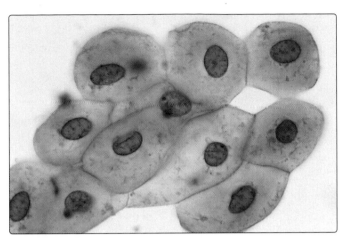

Fig. 18.12   Bladder cytology: brush sample. In brush samples urothelial cells tend to stay attached to each other in flat sheets. Smears are more cellular than those from voided urine samples. (Papanicolaou × OI)

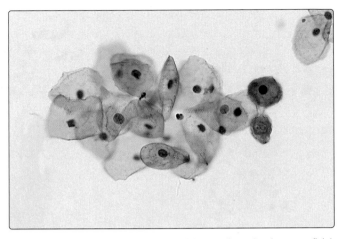

Fig. 18.14   Urine: vaginal cells. Most of these cells are benign superficial cells representing vaginal contamination in the female. (Papanicolaou × HP)

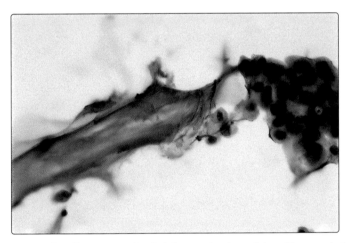

Fig. 18.13   Cystoscopy urine: Lubricant stains deep pink and is somewhat similar to mucin but is denser. Note the cluster of benign urothelial cells in this field. (Papanicolaou × HP)

wet-fixed material using the Papanicolaou stain. Experience is necessary in the interpretation of filter preparations because of the background staining of the filter itself.

Monolayer preparations such as ThinPrep (Cytyc Corporation, Boxborough, MA, USA) are increasingly being used for preparation of urine samples. The specimen passes through a processor, which uses gentle suction to collect almost all the cells present, and applies them to a glass slide, within a defined area. The preservation of the cells is usually excellent and the number of cells obtained is greater than that found in Millipore filter preparations[19].

Normal urine

Cytological findings

▶ Scanty cellularity in voided samples
▶ Cells are usually single in voided urine

▶ Clusters or sheets of urothelial cells in cystoscopy urine and bladder washings
▶ Umbrella cells, deeper layer cells, squamous cells seen
▶ A few polymorphs may be present
▶ Spermatozoa and corpora amylacea may be present in males

Normal urine usually contains very little cellular material. There are usually a few epithelial cells, mainly of deeper urothelial origin, with occasional superficial cells. In women urine samples can contain large numbers of squamous cell contaminants from the vagina (Fig. 18.14). Urine from men may also contain some squamous cells as the trigone can undergo squamous metaplasia. A small number of polymorphs and a few macrophages may be seen.

Spermatozoa may be noted in normal urine (Fig. 18.15) as may seminal vesicle cells. The latter are large cells with hyperchromatic nuclei, which have occasionally been mistakenly identified as malignant cells in view of their high nuclear/cytoplasmic ratio. A helpful distinguishing feature is the presence of pigment granules, thought to be lipofuscin, in the cytoplasm of seminal vesicle cells (Fig. 18.16).

Superficial urothelial cells, the 'umbrella cells' of histology, are large binucleate or multinucleated cells with clear hyaline or vacuolated cytoplasm (Figs 18.17, 18.18). They are much larger than urothelial cells derived from the deeper layers (Fig. 18.19). These superficial cells are sometimes seen to have one convex and one flattened or concave surface, the former corresponding to the luminal edge[17]. The deeper layer cells are smaller with denser deep blue cytoplasm and round nuclei (Fig. 18.20). These cells have sharp nuclear and cytoplasmic margins.

Urothelial cells often show degenerative changes in the form of vacuolation of the cytoplasm (Fig. 18.21), crinkling and hyperchromasia of nuclei (Fig. 18.22) and red intracytoplasmic inclusions of varying sizes, seen best in Papanicolaou stained preparations (Fig. 18.23).

475

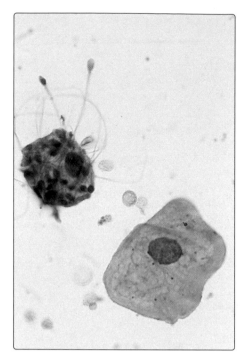

Fig. 18.15   Urine: spermatozoa. A number of spermatozoa are seen clustered over a benign urothelial cell. A few erythrocytes are seen in the background. (Papanicolaou × HP)

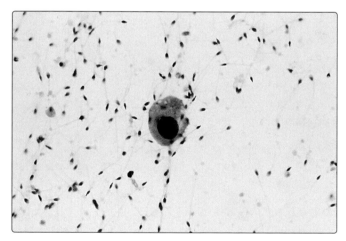

Fig. 18.16   Urine: seminal vesicle cell. This large cell with its hyperchromatic nucleus and abundant cytoplasm is a seminal vesicle cell. Note the pigment in the cytoplasm. (Papanicolaou × OI)

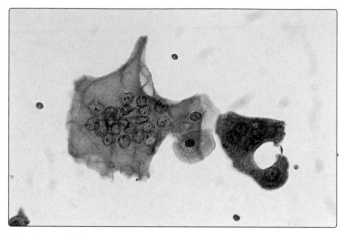

Fig. 18.17   Urine: superficial or 'umbrella' cells. There are two large umbrella cells in this field, one with over 15 nuclei. (Papanicolaou × OI)

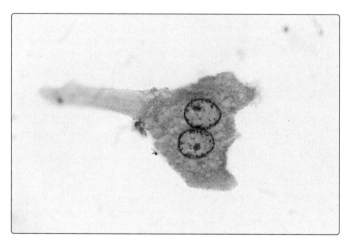

Fig. 18.18   Urine: superficial cell. This superficial cell is large, with abundant cytoplasm but only two nuclei. (Papanicolaou × OI)

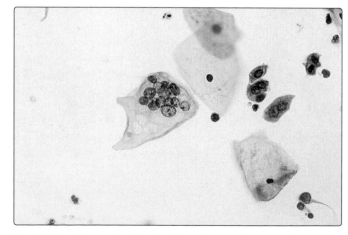

Fig. 18.19   Urine: epithelial cells. This field shows the range of normal epithelial cells seen in urine, superficial and intermediate squamous cells, a large multinucleated superficial urothelial cell and several small deeper layer urothelial cells. (Papanicolaou × HP)

Increased numbers of urothelial cells are seen in bladder washings and catheterized specimens. The cells are often cohesive, leading to a false impression of a papillary structure. However, the morphological details are those of benign urothelial cells (Fig. 18.24). A helpful feature of cell clusters dislodged by catheterization is the presence of a smooth outer contour (Fig. 18.25), in contradistinction to the ragged or irregular margins seen in papillary clusters from well-differentiated urothelial tumours[20].

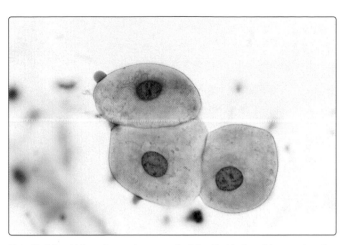

Fig. 18.20 Urine: deeper layer urothelial cells. Under oil immersion these cells are seen to have sharp cytoplasmic borders, abundant cytoplasm and clearly defined nuclear margins. (Papanicolaou × HP)

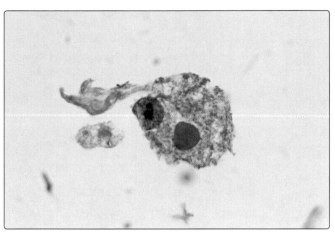

Fig. 18.23 Urine: degenerative changes. This cell shows advanced degenerative changes with disintegrating cytoplasm, nuclear pyknosis and a large red inclusion. (Papanicolaou × OI)

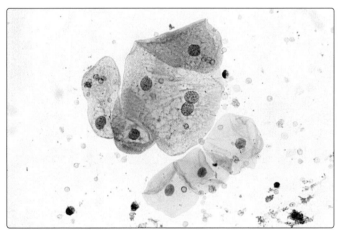

Fig. 18.21 Urine: degenerative changes. The longer urothelial cells stay in urine the more they tend to degenerate. The large umbrella cell and some of the deeper layer cells seen here show finely vacuolated cytoplasm indicative of degenerative changes. (Papanicolaou × HP)

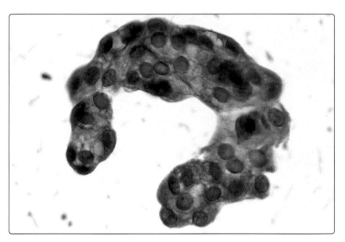

Fig. 18.24 Urine: benign urothelial cells. This group of cells may be mistaken for a papillary cluster under lower magnification. However this is not a true papillary cluster and the cells are all benign. (Papanicolaou × HP)

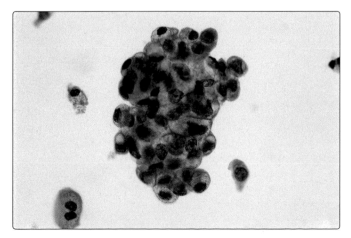

Fig. 18.22 Urine: degenerative changes. Here, in addition to cytoplasmic vacuolation, we see early degenerative changes in the nuclei, namely hyperchromasia and wrinkling of the margin. (Papanicolaou × OI)

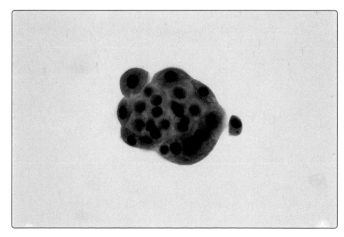

Fig. 18.25 Catheterized urine: A cluster of benign urothelial cells with a smooth outer contour. (Papanicolaou × HP)

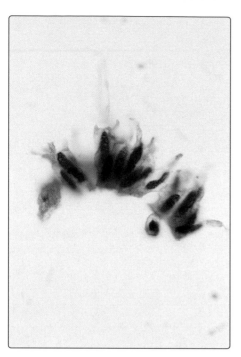

Fig. 18.26   Urine: tall columnar cells. This strip of somewhat degenerate cells shows the wedge-shaped cytoplasm associated with columnar cells. This type of cell is occasionally seen in urine. (Papanicolaou × HP)

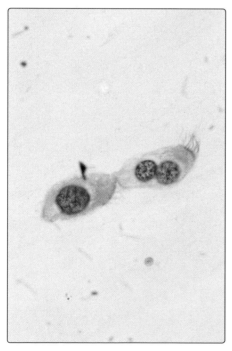

Fig. 18.27   Urine: tall columnar ciliated cells. These two cells are columnar in type. Note the pink cilia in one of the cells. (Papanicolaou × OI)

Occasionally, tall columnar cells, both ciliated and non-ciliated are seen in voided urine and in bladder washings (Figs 18.26, 18.27). These may be cells lining areas of cystitis glandularis, but may possibly have arisen from the genital tract. Small amounts of mucin are occasionally

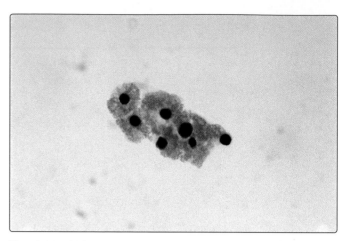

Fig. 18.28   Urine: Renal tubular cells: These are small cells with dark, degenerate nuclei and granular cytoplasm. The cytoplasmic markings are indistinct. (Papanicolaou × OI)

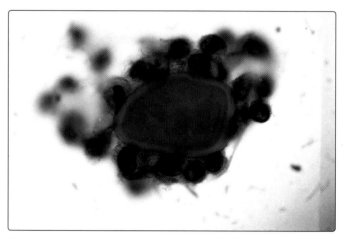

Fig. 18.29   Urine: corpora amylacea. These are laminated structures seen in the urine of males. They usually stain pale blue but this one is orange and is surrounded by histiocytes. (Papanicolaou × HP)

noted in urine samples, in some cases associated with cystitis glandularis. Degenerate renal tubular cells are a common finding (Fig. 18.28). Corpora amylacea from the prostate gland may also be seen in urine specimens. They stain pale blue and appear as almost translucent laminated structures (Fig. 18.29).

Inflammation

Inflammation of the bladder, clinically termed cystitis, is a common condition at all ages although the underlying causes vary in different age groups. Cytology is unlikely to be employed in the investigation of cystitis in children or in relation to pregnancy, but is an important step in assessment of symptoms of cystitis in other patients, especially if recurrent. Not infrequently, cystitis is secondary to the presence of other pathology, a neoplasm or calculus in the urinary tract. Xanthogranulomatous cystitis, for example, has been seen adjacent to or surrounding bladder tumours[21]. Other predisposing conditions, such as diabetes mellitus, prostatism and immunosuppression increase the likelihood of infection and influence the type of infecting organism.

The inflammatory process may be acute or chronic and is usually bacterial in origin, although viruses, fungi and parasites are also recognized causes. Organisms from the large bowel, such as *Escherichia coli* are the most frequent pathogens, but other important, less common, bacteria such as *Mycobacterium tuberculosis* are also encountered. Non-infective causes of cystitis include radiation effects and chemical irritation, to be considered later in this chapter.

Cytological findings

► Hazy or turbid urine specimen
► Numerous polymorphs, histiocytes, occasionally eosinophils
► Reactive changes in epithelial cells
► Organisms may be present, bacterial or parasitic
► Evidence of associated pathology may be seen such as debris in the presence of calculi

The diagnosis of cystitis is often apparent on receipt of the sample, the urine appearing turbid or even blood-stained to the naked eye. Microscopically, polymorphs are present in abundance (Fig. 18.30), often accompanied by histiocytes (Fig. 18.31). On occasion, eosinophils may be identified (Fig. 18.32) and may even be the predominant finding in cases of eosinophilic cystitis, usually accompanied by blood eosinophilia with an allergic diathesis. The symptoms include dysuria, frequency, haematuria and sometimes urinary retention[22]. Eosinophils are also seen in urine in several other conditions such as acute interstitial nephritis, acute tubular necrosis and chronic renal failure[23]. Eosinophiluria of >5%, accompanied by eosinophilia accompanies *Schistosoma haematobium* infection[24]. Urothelial cells appear reactive in cystitis samples (Fig. 18.33).

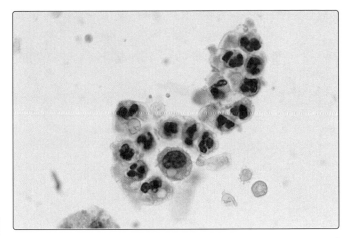

Fig. 18.31 Urine: cystitis. Shown here are some polymorphs and a small histiocyte. (Papanicolaou × OI)

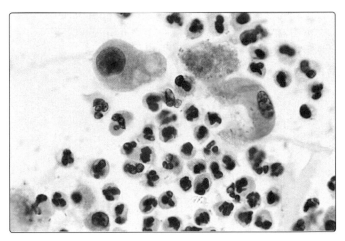

Fig. 18.32 Urine: cystitis. The polymorphs are indicative of cystitis, which often produces reactive change in urothelial cells as pictured here. A single eosinophil with cytoplasmic granules is seen between the epithelial cells. (Papanicolaou × OI)

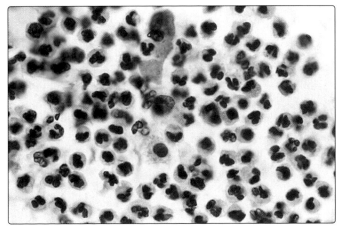

Fig. 18.30 Urine: acute cystitis. The whole field is covered by inflammatory cells, mainly neutrophil polymorphs, which obscure all cellular detail. (Papanicolaou × OI)

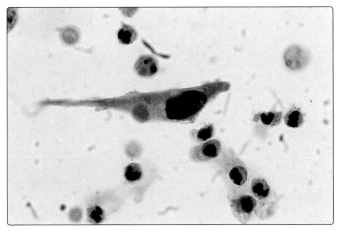

Fig. 18.33 Urine: cystitis. The urothelial cell in the centre of this field shows reactive changes including slight nuclear enlargement and hyperchromasia.

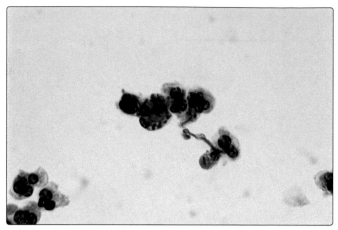

Fig. 18.34   Urine: organisms. These neutrophils have engulfed numerous bacteria. Bacterial organisms cannot be reliably identified in cytology samples. (Papanicolaou × OI)

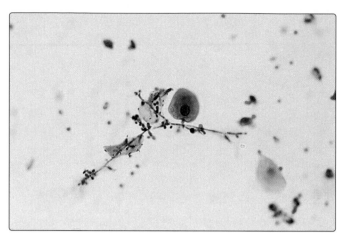

Fig. 18.36   Urine: *Candida albicans*. Candida is quite commonly seen in urine specimens. Here we see both hyphae and spores adjacent to a deeper layer urothelial cell. (Papanicolaou × HP)

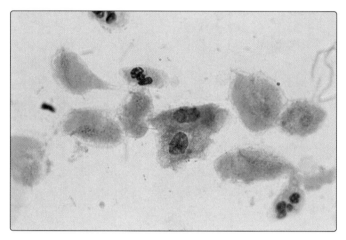

Fig. 18.35   Urine: *Trichomonas hominis*. The blue blobs in the background with elongated pale nuclei are *Trichomonas hominis*, which are infrequently seen in urine samples. (Papanicolaou × OI)

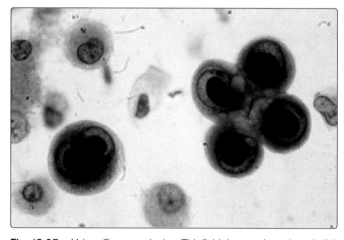

Fig. 18.37   Urine: *Cytomegalovirus*. This field shows enlarged urothelial cells with nuclei, each containing a large homogeneous basophilic cytomegalovirus inclusion body. (Papanicolaou × OI)

In acute cystitis, the causative organism cannot be identified reliably by cytology, although it is possible to detect bacteria under oil immersion (Fig. 18.34). Delay in transit of the sample to the laboratory invariably leads to overgrowth of bacteria, but this must be disregarded as a cytological finding in the absence of a significant increase in inflammatory cells. All cases of cystitis should have a midstream urine sent to the Microbiology department for culture and sensitivity, this being the appropriate method for establishing the diagnosis. Tuberculosis of the urinary tract is an important cause of sterile pyuria, requiring appropriate culture methods for diagnosis.

Specific infections
Organisms that may be detected cytologically in urine are the unicellular protozoan *Trichomonas hominis* in males, *Trichomonas vaginalis* contaminant in females (Fig. 18.35) and the yeast *Candida albicans*, both spores and hyphae

(Fig. 18.36), seen especially in debilitated and immunosuppressed patients. Mucor has been diagnosed in a single urine sample in a patient with mucor pyelonephritis[25].

Viral changes are rarely seen in normal urine, though much has been written about the cytopathic changes induced by human polyomavirus[26-28]. The importance of these findings is that they should not be mistaken for malignancy since the nuclear changes are similar to those of high-grade urothelial neoplasia[27] (Fig. 18.37). Polyomavirus-infected cells are sometimes referred to as 'decoy cells' for this reason (Fig. 18.38). Large numbers of infected cells are associated with acute renal allograft dysfunction[29]. Herpesvirus and human papillomavirus can also induce cytopathic effects in urine samples, the changes being similar to those found in infection at other sites (see Chapter 28). Cytomegalovirus infection is seen with increasing frequency in immunosuppressed patients.

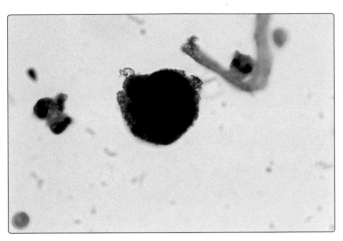

Fig. 18.38 Urine: *Polyomavirus*. This polyomavirus-infected cell has a high nuclear-cytoplasmic ratio and smudged chromatin. Cells in the early stages of infection often show a network of degenerate chromatin. (Papanicolaou × OI)

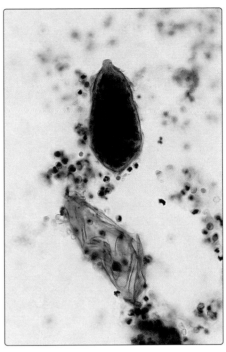

Fig. 18.40 Urine: *Schistosoma haematobium* ovum. This schistosome ovum is not well preserved and the typical spine is not clearly visible. The background contains inflammatory cells. (Papanicolaou × HP)

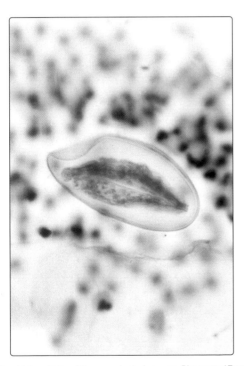

Fig. 18.39 Urine: *Enterobius vermicularis* ovum. Pinworm (*Enterobius vermicularis*) ova are typical in that they have one flat edge and one convex edge with a fold. Note the inflammatory cells in the background. (Papanicolaou × OI)

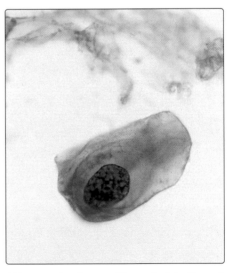

Fig. 18.41 Urine: reactive changes. The urothelial cell seen here shows some nuclear enlargement and granular chromatin. These changes are often seen in inflammatory conditions. (Papanicolaou × OI)

In this country, an occasional cause of cystitis is the pinworm *Enterobius vermicularis* (Fig. 18.39). The ova are accompanied by erythrocytes, polymorphs, eosinophils and histiocytes. In Egypt, a common cause of cystitis and indeed of carcinoma of the bladder is schistosomiasis, usually due to *Schistoma haematobium*. These schistosome ova are recognizable in urine samples by their characteristic terminal spine (Fig. 18.40).

Diagnostic pitfalls

The urothelial cells in inflammatory conditions generally show reactive changes such as nuclear enlargement and some hyperchromasia (Fig. 18.41), but the nuclear abnormalities are not as severe as those seen in malignant cells. There may also be a non-specific increase in the number of epithelial cells due to greater exfoliation in the

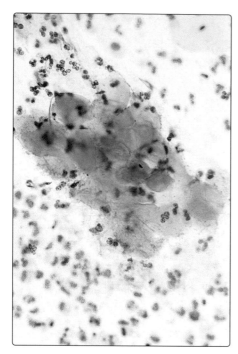

Fig. 18.42 Urine: anucleate squames. Keratinized anucleate squamous cells may be seen in urine samples in inflammatory processes. (Papanicolaou × HP)

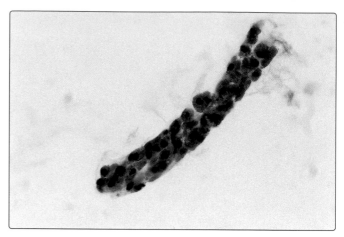

Fig. 18.43 Urine: renal tubular cast. This cast is composed of renal tubular cells. (Papanicolaou × HP)

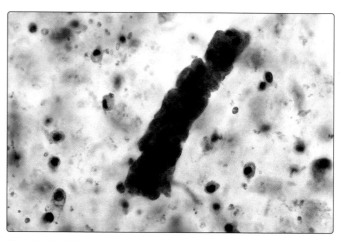

Fig. 18.44 Urine: granular cast. This cast is coated with red cells. (Papanicolaou × HP)

presence of infection. Anucleate squames are occasionally seen (Fig. 18.42). Abundant inflammatory cells may also be seen in urine in the presence of high-grade urothelial carcinoma. If there is doubt about interpretation of nuclear changes in the presence of cystitis, cytology should be repeated after treatment of the infection, to exclude an underlying neoplasm.

The overgrowth of organisms resulting from delay in transit of a specimen should not present diagnostic problems if there is no significant increase in inflammatory cells.

Haematuria

Haematuria is a common clinical problem. The blood in the urine may be macroscopic or microscopic. It is accompanied by pain when associated with inflammation, cystitis, calculi or the passage of clots, but is otherwise usually painless. There are numerous causes for the appearance of blood in urine, the commonest being inflammation, either infective or chemical, calculi and neoplastic processes. When urine cytology is employed as a diagnostic tool in patients with haematuria, it is essential to evaluate the urothelial cells carefully as heavy blood-staining can obscure cellular abnormalities.

It is helpful to divide patients with haematuria into those with a renal origin and those with urinary tract causes, the cytological findings in the latter group relating to the various lesions in renal pelvis, ureters, bladder or urethra that are liable to present as haematuria.

Renal haematuria

Apart from the nowadays quite rare event of a renal neoplasm presenting in this way, renal haematuria generally results from renal glomerular disease leading to leakage of red blood cells through the glomerular capillary tuft. This may be accompanied by the formation of casts of cell debris in the renal tubules, renal tubular casts, fragments of which are sometimes found in urine specimens (Fig. 18.43). In renal haematuria, the casts are sometimes coated with red blood cells and described as granular casts (Fig. 18.44), in contrast to the hyaline casts seen in other conditions.

Renal haematuria can be investigated in several ways using cytology preparations:

Normal voided urine cytology. Erythrocytes originating in the glomeruli are dysmorphic when examined in urine, a finding attributed to processes occurring as the cells travel along the nephron. Other reports show that only 15% of patients with glomerular disease have dysmorphic erythrocytes in urine specimens examined after cytocentrifugation and staining by the Papanicolaou method[30].

Phase contrast microscopy This is the method most commonly used to assess red cells in urine of patients with glomerulonephropathy and is extremely effective in identifying dysmorphic erythrocytes[3,31,32].

Immunocytochemical/immunofluorescent staining can be used to identify Tamm–Horsfall protein-coated dysmorphic erythrocytes[33].

Scanning electron miscroscopy will reveal the characteristic forms of the abnormal red blood cells[34].

Urinary calculi

Patients with calculi generally present with pain accompanied by haematuria. Cystitis may supervene or may precede the formation of the stones. Diagnosis can be made by intravenous pyelogram (IVP), which shows whether the calculus is situated in the calyx of the kidney, the ureter or bladder. Calculi appear as filling defects on IVPs and can be clearly visualized on cystoscopy when in the bladder (Fig. 18.45). It is important that clinicians provide the cytopathologist with the relevant clinical information as cytological changes accompanying calculi can quite easily be mistaken for malignancy.

The urine sample usually contains many erythrocytes, often accompanied by neutrophil polymorphs. The red blood cells seen in urine samples from patients with calculi are morphologically normal.

Cytological findings

▶ Cloudy urine or grossly blood-stained sample
▶ Erythrocytes are often seen
▶ Variable inflammatory cell component
▶ Papillary clusters of urothelial cells with slightly increased nuclear/cytoplasmic ratio and small nucleoli, smooth or irregular borders
▶ The cells may be very reactive and suspicious of malignancy

The epithelial changes can be quite alarming. A combination of trauma and inflammation produced by calculi causes marked atypia in urothelial cells. The cells are frequently exfoliated in papillary clusters (Fig. 18.46) and their cytoplasm shows degenerative vacuolation. The nuclei may be somewhat enlarged with hyperchromasia. Small nucleoli may be visible (Fig. 18.47). In addition to these features, a bandlike thickening of the cytoplasmic rim of the cell clusters has been described[35]. The atypia in these cells is often worse than that seen in clusters of cells shed from a grade 1 papillary urothelial carcinoma (Fig. 18.48).

In a study comparing cytological changes due to calculus and transitional cell carcinoma, Highman and Wilson[36] showed that in patients with calculi there were two types of papillary clusters, a smooth-bordered type and irregular clusters of cells with ragged borders and abnormal nuclei. The latter, which were seen in a minority of cases, showed features similar to those of a low-grade urothelial carcinoma. However, in the presence of calculi the urine contained fewer single urothelial cells compared with the urine of patients with transitional cell carcinoma. Another important differentiating feature is the greater morphological variability of the cells in urine from patients with carcinoma. However, morphological features alone may not be reliable in distinguishing between the two lesions.

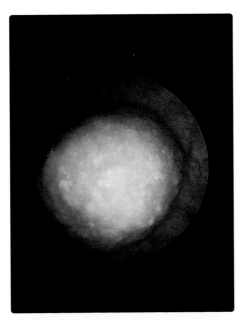

Fig. 18.45   Cystoscopy: calculus. Illustrated here is a large round bladder stone. This type of calculus is usually associated with infection. (Courtesy of Mr R G Notley, Guildford, UK)

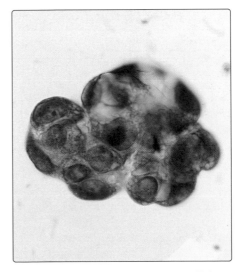

Fig. 18.46   Urine: papillary cluster of urothelial cells. This type of papillary cluster of urothelial cells with a rounded edge and degenerative vacuolation is commonly seen in the presence of calculi. (Papanicolaou × OI)

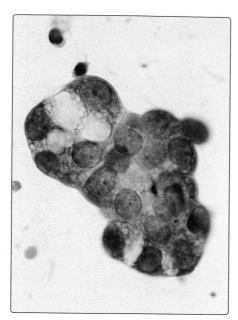

Fig. 18.47   Urine: papillary cluster. The bland chromatin and small nucleoli in these cells indicate that they are not malignant. (Papanicolaou × OI)

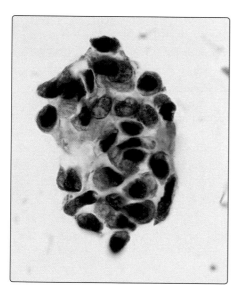

Fig. 18.48   Urine: papillary cluster. This cluster of cells shows hyperchromasia, lack of cohesion and some irregularity of nuclear outline. This atypia, which is quite frequently seen in urine associated with calculi, can lead to a suspicious cytology report. (Papanicolaou × OI)

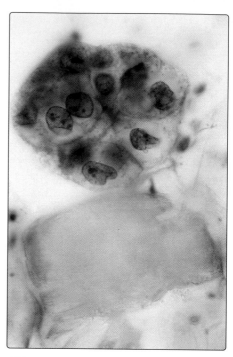

Fig. 18.49   Urine: papillary cluster. Illustrated here is a cluster of well preserved reactive urothelial cells adjacent to a matrix crystal. (Papanicolaou × OI)

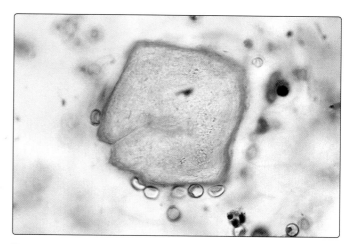

Fig. 18.50   Urine: matrix crystal. These large crystals are transparent and are not birefringent. (Papanicolaou × OI)

Crystalluria

Crystal formation in urine can accompany the presence of bladder calculi (Fig. 18.49) or occur independently. An important component of urinary calculi is organic matrix, which is composed of urinary microproteins. Crystals composed of matrix are clear and transparent and are not birefringent (Fig. 18.50). It has been postulated that bacterial infection leads to increased production of matrix, thus predisposing to crystalluria[37]. Several other types of crystals are seen in urine specimens, some identifiable by their shape. These include triple phosphate crystals (Fig. 18.51) and cholesterol crystals (Fig. 18.52). Others are only identifiable by chemical examination of the urine (Fig. 18.53).

Other non-neoplastic conditions
Malakoplakia

Malakoplakia is a condition that occurs more often in the bladder than in any other genitourinary site and is more common in women. It forms nodules consisting of histiocytes and other inflammatory cells, the diagnostic feature being Michaelis-Gutmann bodies. These are extra-

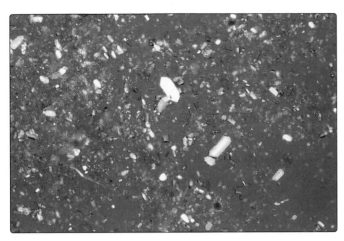

Fig. 18.51   Urine: triple phosphate crystals. These small crystals are birefringent. (Papanicolaou × HP)

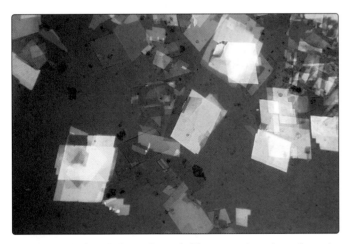

Fig. 18.52   Urine: cholesterol crystals. These crystals are large, flat and square or rectangular with one corner chipped off. (Papanicolaou × HP)

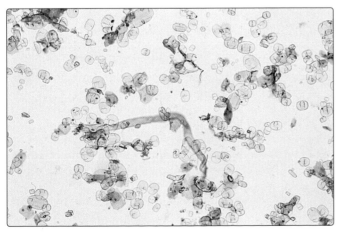

Fig. 18.53   Urine: crystals. Non-birefringent crystalline structures are occasionally seen in urine. These cannot be typed on cytology but would need biochemical examination for identification. (× LP)

or intracellular structures composed of incompletely digested bacteria covered by iron and phosphates[38].

Endometriosis

In women of reproductive age, the bladder may be involved by endometriosis leading to the shedding of clusters of crowded small dark glandular cells similar to those seen in cervical smears taken at the time of menstruation. The cytological appearance of endometrial cells in urine may arouse the suspicion of transitional cell carcinoma[39].

Neoplasms of the urinary tract

Both benign and malignant tumours may arise in any portion of the excretory system of the body, but historically cytologists have concentrated on recognition of the common malignant epithelial tumours since benign tumours do not generally exfoliate readily and have fewer diagnostic features.

Benign epithelial neoplasms

Urothelial papilloma

The WHO classification of urothelial tumours includes benign urothelial papilloma, which has a tendency to recur, does not invade or metastasize, but may subsequently be associated with the development of urothelial carcinoma[40]. The hotly-debated controversy about the diagnosis of this entity has been well documented[41]. Exophytic transitional cell papillomas are considered to be benign neoplasms by some authorities and as low-grade carcinomas by others. These lesions are usually diploid. The tumours are usually small, single and are composed of benign urothelial cells covering fibrovascular cores. A clue to the diagnosis is the increased cellularity of the urine sample although the cells are morphologically normal.

Inverted urothelial papilloma

This lesion, of unknown aetiology, is believed to be reactive by some authors[42], and as a neoplastic process by others[43] and are usually found in the trigone. Histology demonstrates trabecular downgrowths of transitional cells into the stroma. There are no diagnostic features on urine cytology.

Urothelial carcinoma

Carcinoma of the urinary tract is usually urothelial in origin, 90% of bladder tumours being of this type. High-grade urothelial carcinomas often show areas of squamous or glandular metaplasia but these are limited in extent. Pure squamous carcinomas occur occasionally, usually associated with *Schistosoma haematobium* infection, and primary adenocarcinoma of the bladder is rare.

Transitional cell or urothelial carcinoma usually develops in late middle age and is commoner in men than women. Young adults and children are not totally exempt from risk. The tumour can arise anywhere in the urinary tract from the calyx of the kidney to the urethra, although the bladder is the most common site. Tumours may be multiple and they have a tendency to recur.

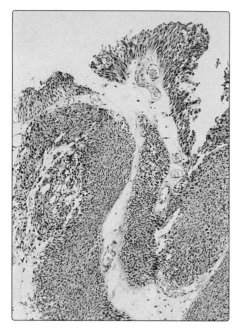

Fig. 18.54 Histology: papillary carcinoma. This low power field shows a fragmented papillary carcinoma of bladder displaying a fronded arrangement of multilayered epithelium on a delicate branching fibrovascular core. (H&E × LP)

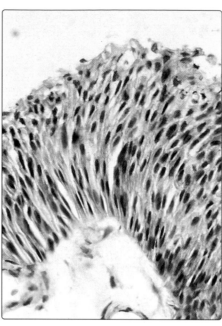

Fig. 18.55 Histology: papillary carcinoma. On higher magnification the tip of the papilla shows well-differentiated cells which maintain their polarity. (H&E × HP)

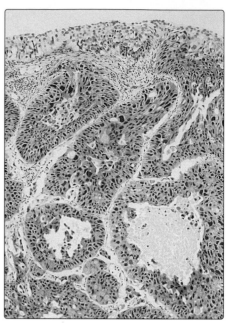

Fig. 18.56 Histology: infiltrative carcinoma. This section shows an invasive carcinoma of bladder. The surface epithelium at this magnification appears to show a grade II carcinoma. (H&E × LP)

Aetiological factors in bladder cancer include exposure to carcinogens such as aniline dyes, including beta naphthylamines and other chemicals used in the textile, printing, rubber and water industries. Other factors associated with an increased risk include phenacetin and benzidine[44]. Therapeutic drugs, such as cyclophosphamide and busulphan are known to increase the risk of developing bladder cancer. Cigarette smokers also have a higher risk of the disease. Schistosoma haematobium infection is associated with the development of bladder cancer,

Bladder cancer is frequently multicentric, suggesting that a field change has occurred as a result of the action of carcinogens on the urinary tract. Dysplastic lesions may coexist with *in situ* and invasive urothelial carcinoma. The larger the tumour the greater the likelihood of malignant cells being found in urine[45], but the relationship between the number of tumours present and cytological evidence of neoplasia is not as reliable.

The presenting symptoms of bladder cancer include haematuria, dysuria and frequency. In tumours related to schistosomiasis, the symptoms include those of chronic irritation as well as haematuria.

Urothelial carcinomas may be papillary (Figs 18.54, 18.55), infiltrative (Fig. 18.56) or flat (*in situ*) (Fig. 18.57). Low-grade lesions are papillary and diploid while high-grade tumours may be nodular, flat or papillary and the majority are aneuploid[46]. Invasive carcinomas are especially prone to develop from flat abnormalities such as atypical hyperplasia and carcinoma *in situ*[47].

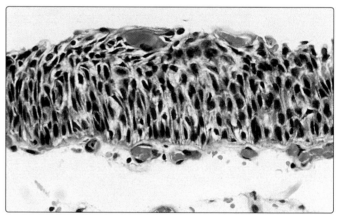

Fig. 18.57 Histology: carcinoma *in situ* (flat carcinoma). The carcinoma involves the whole thickness of the urothelium and is composed of hyperchromatic pleomorphic cells. The basement membrane is intact. (H&E × HP)

Grade I papillary carcinoma

About 80% of grade I carcinomas are non-invasive. They tend to recur and eventually may become invasive solid carcinomas, which tend to be of higher grade and have the potential to metastasize.

Papillary carcinomas are composed of fibrovascular stalks covered by delicate branching fronds of well-differentiated transitional cells. The number of cell layers is greater than that seen in normal urothelium, but there is very little cytological atypia and few mitoses are present (Fig. 18.58).

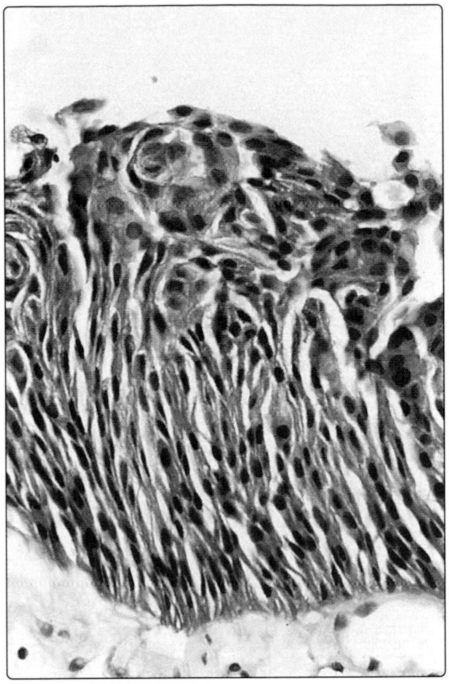

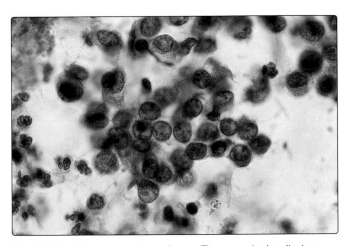

Fig. 18.59 Urine: low-grade carcinoma. These neoplastic cells show some nuclear enlargement but are fairly uniform. This type of appearance is often reported as suspicious because typical features of malignancy are not identifiable. (Papanicolaou × HP)

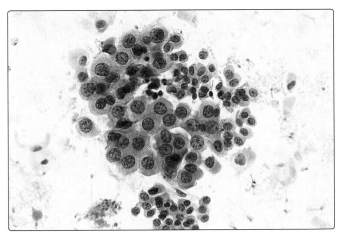

Fig. 18.60 Urine: low-grade carcinoma. In this field we see sheets of loosely cohesive cells with enlarged hyperchromatic nuclei. The chromatin is granular and the cells are variable in size. (Papanicolaou × HP)

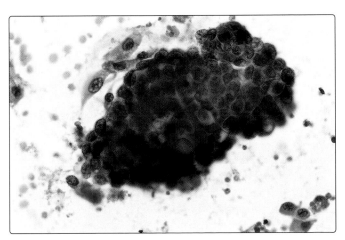

Fig. 18.61 Urine cytology: low-grade carcinoma. This smear of a grade I urothelial carcinoma shows a cluster of mildly pleomorphic carcinoma cells. Note the irregular edge of the cluster. (Papanicolaou × OI)

Fig. 18.58 Histology: grade I urothelial carcinoma. This section of bladder shows well-differentiated carcinoma cells. There are more layers of cells than are seen in normal bladder urothelium. No mitoses are evident. (H&E × HP)

The cells are closely packed together and maintain some sense of polarity in low-grade tumours.

Cytological findings

▶ Tumour cells resemble normal urothelial cells
▶ Increased cellularity with many single cells
▶ Cells may be in loose clusters
▶ Vesicular chromatin
▶ Nucleoli usually absent
▶ Clean background

These carcinomas can be very difficult to diagnose on urine cytology. Only 30–60% of grade I carcinomas exfoliate carcinoma cells[48]. The neoplastic cells in voided urine samples closely resemble normal urothelial cells. The samples show many single cells, not uncommonly columnar or spindled in appearance, as well as clusters of mildly pleomorphic epithelial cells (Fig. 18.59). Some of the clusters may be loosely cohesive, unlike the tighter papillary clusters seen with calculi. The chromatin pattern is vesicular or finely granular (Fig. 18.60). Nucleoli are not prominent (Fig. 18.61). There is often an overall increase in cellularity due to the exfoliation of rather small single urothelial cells but the background is generally clean. These urine samples are usually reported either as benign or suspicious rather than positive as they cannot be distinguished reliably from cellular changes due to calculi or instrumentation.

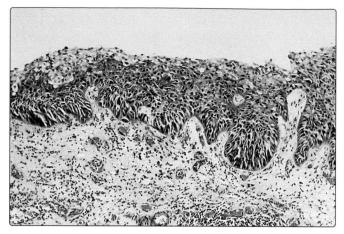

Fig. 18.62   Histology: grade II urothelial carcinoma. This section of bladder tumour shows an increased number of cell layers, moderate pleomorphism and loss of polarity. (H&E × LP)

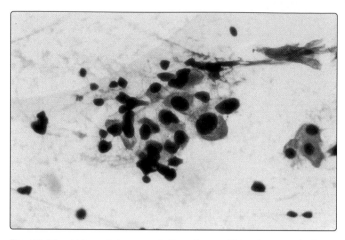

Fig. 18.63   Urine cytology: grade II carcinoma. This urine sample shows moderately pleomorphic carcinoma cells with enlarged, irregular nuclei. (Papanicolaou × HP)

Grade II urothelial carcinoma

Grade II urothelial carcinomas are less differentiated than grade I neoplasms. Some grade II carcinomas exhibit a papillary growth pattern but these tumours have a more solid infiltrative component than their grade I counterparts. Histological sections show a greatly increased number of cell layers in the malignant epithelium, with some loss of polarity of cells, pleomorphism and an increased number of mitoses (Fig. 18.62).

Cytological findings

► Much cellularity with single cells and groups
► Nuclear enlargement and crowding
► Some irregularity of nuclear outlines
► Coarse chromatin
► Clean background

Because the cells are more pleomorphic than in grade I carcinomas and exfoliate more freely, grade II tumours are easier to diagnose on cytology. The cytological features include large irregular tissue fragments composed of abnormal urothelial cells (Fig. 18.63) as well as many dissociated cells. The cytoplasm is usually dense but is often degenerate. The nuclei show granular chromatin (Fig. 18.64) and somewhat irregular margins (Fig. 18.65). The background again is usually clean.

Grade III urothelial carcinoma

Grade III carcinomas are usually invasive and readily detectable in urine samples. They are rarely papillary, generally showing a solid infiltrating pattern of growth with surface ulceration and necrosis. Histological sections reveal irregular epithelial masses composed of extremely pleomorphic cells showing marked loss of polarity and much mitotic activity (Fig. 18.66). Foci of squamous differentiation may be present. Glandular and small cell differentiation may also occur[49].

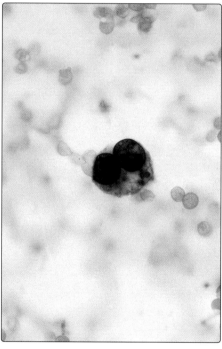

Fig. 18.64   Urine: urothelial carcinoma. This malignant cell is binucleate with granular chromatin. (Papanicolaou × OI)

Cytological findings

► Markedly increased cellularity
► Malignant cells, singly, clustered and in syncytial groups
► Cell-in-cell arrangements
► Pleomorphic nuclei with coarse abnormal chromatin
► Large nucleoli
► Mitotic figures
► Dirty background

On cytological examination the most striking feature is often the dirty background, with many polymorphs, histiocytes and erythrocytes (Fig. 18.67). Lying within this,

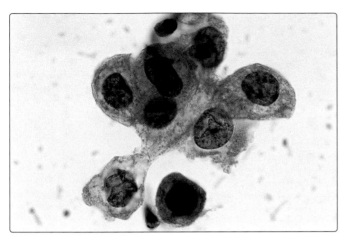

Fig. 18.65   Urine: urothelial carcinoma. The neoplastic cells show irregularity of the nuclear margin and an abnormal chromatin pattern. (Papanicolaou × OI)

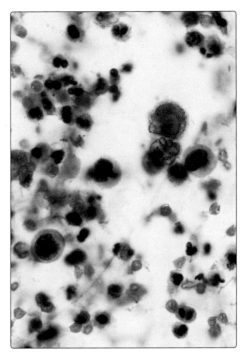

Fig. 18.67   Urine: grade III carcinoma. Notice the small carcinoma cells showing markedly increased nuclear/cytoplasmic ratios. The background is messy with blood and degenerate cells. (Papanicolaou × OI)

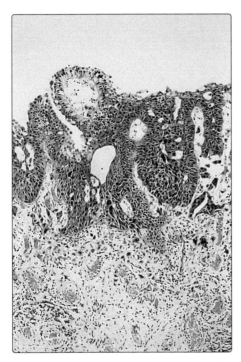

Fig. 18.66   Histology: grade III carcinoma. This section of bladder tumour shows thickened epithelium composed of pleomorphic cells showing loss of polarity. Early invasion is also seen. (H&E × LP)

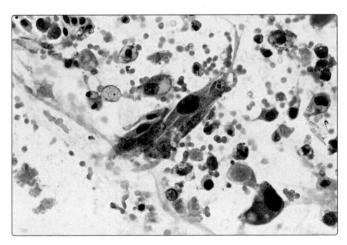

Fig. 18.68   Urine: grade III carcinoma. In this field there is a cluster of pleomorphic carcinoma cells as well as single cells. Some cells have prominent nucleoli while others have pyknotic degenerate nuclei. The background shows blood and cellular debris. (Papanicolaou × OI)

carcinoma cells are seen singly as well as in clusters (Fig. 18.68). Marked pleomorphism (Fig. 18.69) is present with some syncytial formations and cell-in-cell arrangements, referred to as cannibalism (Fig. 18.70)[50]. Clumping and clearing of chromatin is frequently seen (Fig. 18.71), as are huge nucleoli (Fig. 18.72). Keratinized malignant cells may be present, indicating squamous differentiation.

Carcinoma *in situ*

This flat lesion may occur adjacent to urothelial carcinoma or on its own, either as a single lesion or involving much of the urothelium[51]. In the latter case the abnormal epithelium may even extend into von Brunn's nests, a feature worth remembering when topical chemotherapy is used, as it may not penetrate these structures. Similarly, cystoscopy is not helpful, as the bladder mucosa shows no visible tumour. The clinical presentation may mimic that of interstitial cystitis.

Histologically, the lesion is confined to the epithelium and may consist of a few to several layers of pleomorphic carcinoma cells (Fig. 18.73). Numerous mitotic figures may be seen, including abnormal forms. It has been shown that 55% of patients with flat carcinoma *in situ* lesions develop invasive carcinoma within five years[48,52].

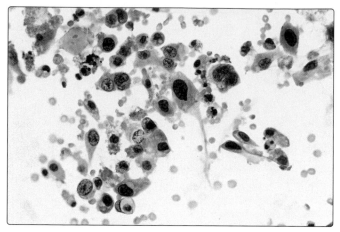

Fig. 18.69 Urine: grade III carcinoma. This field contains carcinoma cells, which exhibit marked pleomorphism. (Papanicolaou × HP)

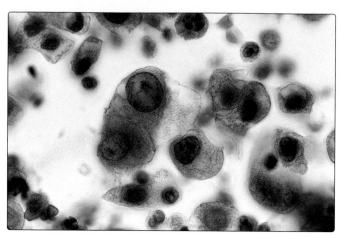

Fig. 18.72 Urine: grade III carcinoma. These carcinoma cells contain visible nucleoli. The chromatin pattern is also abnormal. (Papanicolaou × OI)

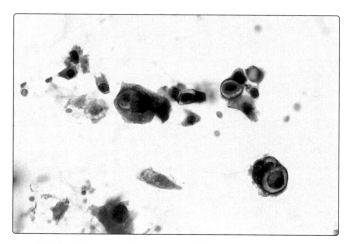

Fig. 18.70 Urine: grade III carcinoma. A feature that may be seen in high-grade urothelial carcinoma is 'cannibalism' or a 'cell-in-cell' appearance. The cells show features of malignancy. (Papanicolaou × HP)

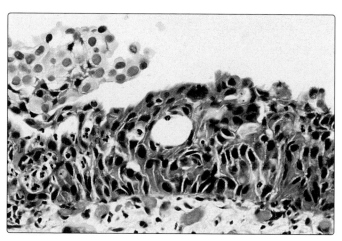

Fig. 18.73 Histology: carcinoma *in situ*. Several layers of pleomorphic carcinoma cells are seen in this section of bladder. The lesion is confined to the epithelium. (H&E × LP)

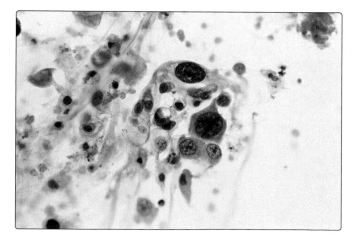

Fig. 18.71 Urine: grade III carcinoma. These pleomorphic carcinoma cells show marked chromatin clumping with clear spaces between the clumps, a nuclear feature seen in high-grade neoplasia. (Papanicolaou × HP)

Cytological findings

► Somewhat increased cellularity with mainly single cells
► Pleomorphic cells and nuclei
► Abnormal chromatin pattern
► Nucleoli not usually seen
► Clean background

Cytology reveals abnormal transitional cells both in small flat sheets and lying singly in a clear background. The nuclei are enlarged and contain either coarsely granular (Fig. 18.74) or dark structureless chromatin (Fig. 18.75). The cells show marked pleomorphism suggestive of high-grade malignancy, similar to the hyperchromatic, nucleolated cells seen in biopsy specimens (Figs 18.76, 18.77). However nucleoli are not prominent. Carcinoma *in situ* is diagnosed as a grade III transitional cell carcinoma in 50% of cases[50].

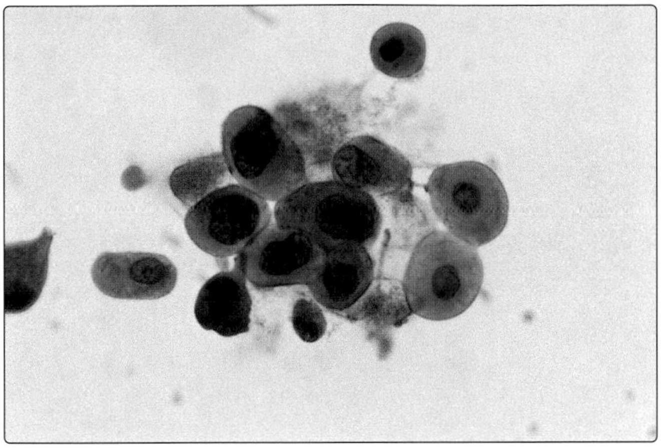

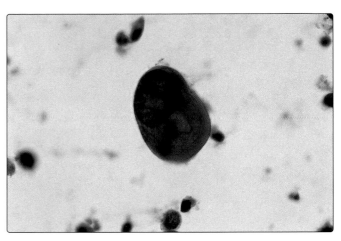

Fig. 18.74 Urine: carcinoma *in situ*. These loosely cohesive malignant cells show nuclear hyperchromasia and coarsely granular chromatin. Note the clean background. (Papanicolaou × OI)

Fig. 18.77 Urine: carcinoma *in situ*. A large malignant cell with abnormal chromatin is seen in this field. (Papanicolaou × HP)

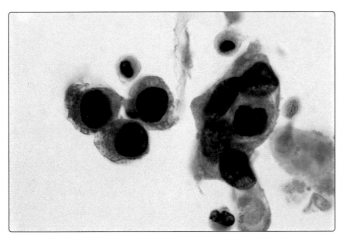

Fig. 18.75 Urine: carcinoma *in situ*. This cluster of carcinoma cells shows dark structureless chromatin within some of the nuclei. (Papanicolaou × OI)

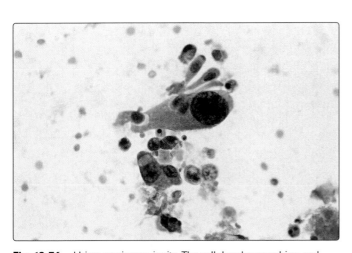

Fig. 18.76 Urine: carcinoma *in situ*. The cellular pleomorphism and abnormal chromatin would make it difficult to distinguish carcinoma *in situ* from grade III carcinoma, as there is some blood in the background. (Papanicolaou × HP)

Diagnostic accuracy of cytology for urothelial tumours

The reliability of urine cytology in the detection of urothelial neoplasia depends on various factors including tumour size and number, tumour grade, the quality of the sample, preparation method and experience in interpretation. Small tumours, even though multiple, may result in negative cytology. The higher-grade urothelial carcinomas are more frequently diagnosed on cytology while grade I tumours are more frequently missed by this method. Carcinoma *in situ* is almost always identified as malignant, 50% of cases are diagnosed as a high-grade tumour.

In a series of patients followed up by urine cytology, Highman demonstrated that cytology reflects the development of invasive and more extensive tumours[53]. Low-grade invasive tumours were associated with shedding of smaller, less pleomorphic cells in cohesive clusters. High-grade tumours tended to exfoliate single pleomorphic cells with larger nuclei and prominent nucleoli.

The cytological diagnosis of carcinoma *in situ*, or indeed of urothelial carcinoma, may be associated with negative cystoscopy and histology. Multiple random biopsy specimens may be required to detect this lesion histologically. In some cases, investigations other than cytology remain negative for months before tumour becomes apparent[46,54]. All patients with positive or suspicious cytology confirmed on review should be carefully followed up, as positive cytology may precede clinically obvious bladder tumours by a considerable interval.

Urinary cytology has been shown to be a good predictor of recurrent tumour following resection. It is of particular value since negative pre-selected site biopsies from these patients are not always reliable[53]. Urine cytology is also useful in the follow up of patients treated by non-surgical methods such as chemotherapy or immunotherapy. The presence of malignant cells in urine reliably identifies a negative response to treatment (Figs 18.78, 18.79)[55].

Positive urinary cytology may be related to urothelial tumours in the upper urinary tract rather than in the bladder. These constitute 5–8% of all urothelial cancers[56]. In a reported series 67% of such tumours were diagnosed and 20% suspected on urinary cytology, again with diagnosis being easier in higher-grade tumours[57]. Selective catheterization or brush cytology are useful methods of obtaining representative samples.

Diagnostic pitfalls

False positive cytology is most often due to misinterpretation of the cellular atypia, that accompanies calculi and inflammation, or sometimes follows catheterization. Features favouring neoplasia include greater cellularity in the centrifuged deposit, with more cell dissociation, pleomorphism of nuclei and irregularity of chromatin pattern. Smooth bordered papillary clusters favour reactive or inflammatory processes. Where the diagnosis is in doubt, as may happen especially with well-differentiated papillary tumours, it is advisable to request further samples and check whether there has been any recent instrumentation or urinary tract infection.

On the other hand, repeated positive cytology in the face of normal cystoscopy and biopsies should not be ignored, as it may be an indicator of new or recurrent tumour elsewhere in the urinary tract. Occult sites such as within a bladder diverticulum should also be considered. The risk of neoplasia is higher in diverticula, where stasis of urine and formation of calculi may enhance the likelihood of tumour formation.

A further potential source of false positive results is intravesical chemotherapy. This can produce enlarged, degenerate urothelial cells with hyperchromatic nuclei, which can be mistaken for malignancy, especially if full clinical details are not included on the request form. These findings and other related iatrogenic changes are discussed more fully later in this chapter.

Other neoplasms

Although only 5% of bladder tumours are pure primary **squamous carcinomas**, squamous metaplasia is frequently seen in urothelial carcinomas. True squamous carcinomas are usually invasive and are associated with chronic schistosomiasis of the bladder in countries where this infection is endemic. Chronic irritation due to bladder stones or an indwelling catheter is another risk factor. The cytological features include cytoplasmic keratinization in well-differentiated tumours (Fig. 18.80), but poorly-differentiated types may show only bizarre malignant giant cells.

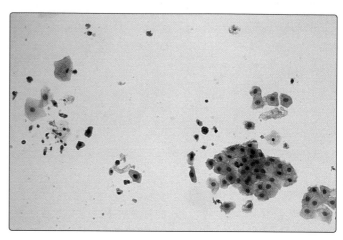

Fig. 18.78 Urine: post-treatment degenerative changes. The deposit is moderately cellular and includes small degenerate single cells as well as reactive groups. No evidence of malignancy is seen. (Papanicolaou × MP)

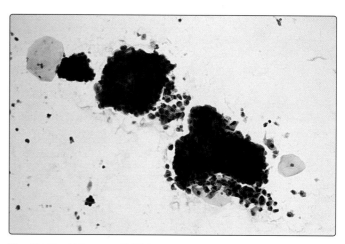

Fig. 18.79 Urine: post-BCG therapy recurrence. Degenerate papillary tumour and a few dissociated abnormal cells are recognizable, in contrast to the preceding illustration. (Papanicolaou × MP)

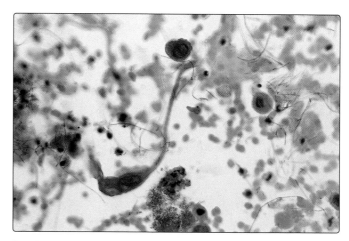

Fig. 18.80 Urine: squamous carcinoma. Pleomorphic malignant cells are shown, with keratinized cytoplasm and densely hyperchromatic nuclei. Inflammatory cells are seen in the background. This case of squamous carcinoma of bladder was not associated with schistosomiasis. (Papanicolaou × OI)

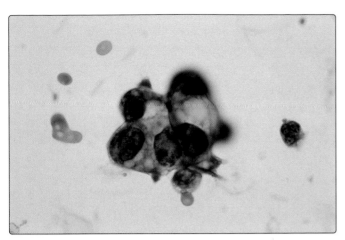

Fig. 18.81 Urine: metastatic carcinoma. This cluster of adenocarcinoma cells with prominent nuclei and cytoplasmic vacuoles was seen in the urine of a patient who had widespread metastases from carcinoma of the breast. (Papanicolaou × OI)

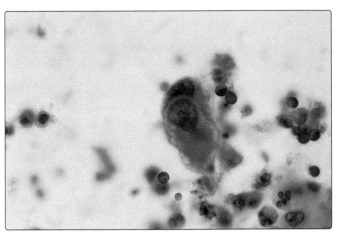

Fig. 18.82 Urine: renal cell carcinoma. Large pleomorphic malignant cells, one of which shows a rounded nucleus and prominent nucleolus. There is a background of red blood cells and inflammatory debris. (Papanicolaou × OI)

Primary **adenocarcinoma** of the bladder is uncommon, constituting approximately 2% of bladder tumours. Some are derived from the glandular mucosa of von Brunn's nests and the presence of cystitis glandularis. Others arise from urachal remnants or occur in bladders with exstrophy. The cells may be recognized cytologically by the presence of glandular differentiation, especially if mucin secretion is seen. Clear cell[58] and signet ring cell variants of adenocarcinoma are also encountered[59], but are rare.

Small cell carcinoma of neuroendocrine origin[60–61], oat cell carcinoma[62] and less aggressive carcinoid tumours are also extremely rare. **Lymphomas** of the urinary tract are described and may be solitary or multifocal. The overlying bladder mucosa is often intact, reducing the likelihood of detection by urine cytology. Primary **malignant melanoma** of bladder is a rarity but the appearance of melanin pigment in urine from widespread malignant melanoma elsewhere in the body is a well recognized occurrence. Other rare neoplasms of urinary tract include sarcomas and sarcomatoid carcinomas, germ cell tumours and choriocarcinoma. A pitfall that may be encountered is the cytology of inflammatory pseudotumour of the bladder, a lesion that exfoliates spindle cells into urine, mimicking sarcoma[63].

Direct tumour spread to the bladder from an adjacent squamous carcinoma of the cervix can occur and malignant squamous cells may be seen in urine specimens from these patients. A vaginal examination and cervical smear will confirm the site of the primary tumour in such cases. Prostatic adenocarcinoma may extend by direct growth into the bladder or may shed malignant cells in urine if invading the urethral mucosa. In such cases the malignant cells usually show evidence of glandular differentiation. Distant **metastatic spread** is most often derived from a primary carcinoma of breast (Fig. 18.81) or malignant melanoma, sometimes from ovarian carcinoma[64].

Renal cell carcinomas rarely shed tumour cells into urine. This is only possible in locally advanced disease with direct invasion of the renal pelvis by tumour. If a renal cell neoplasm is suspected, and unclassifiable tumour cells are found in urine samples (Fig. 18.82), it can be helpful to stain preparations with oil red-O stain. This will distinguish the lipid containing cells of renal cell carcinoma from malignant urothelial cells that do not contain lipid.

Iatrogenic changes

Apart from the unusual pattern of exfoliation of epithelial cells produced by catheterization and other types of instrumentation, iatrogenic changes encountered in urinary cytology are usually the result of various forms of therapy, most commonly cytotoxic drugs or irradiation of the bladder. Therapeutic procedures such as fashioning an ileal conduit after total cystectomy also cause changes in urine cytology.

Drugs such as cyclophosphamide, busulphan and cyclosporin are widely used in the treatment of cancer as well as for non-neoplastic conditions such as systemic lupus erythematosus. These agents can cause renal tubular cell toxicity as well as haemorrhagic cystitis and urothelial carcinoma. Changes in urothelial cells may be seen 13–20 days after starting treatment[65]. They include cellular and nuclear enlargement without prominent nucleoli or mitoses and with much background debris[66]. Cytoplasmic degeneration and multinucleation may be seen. Distinction from urothelial malignancy can be difficult, but although the nuclei are hyperchromatic their chromatin pattern is generally smudged and structureless.

Haemorrhagic cystitis develops much more rapidly in patients treated with intravenous cyclophosphamide than in those on oral therapy. The clinical symptoms include haematuria and irritative symptoms due to mucosal

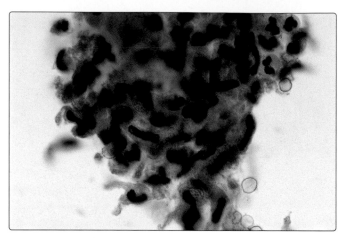

Fig. 18.83 Urine: post-BCG therapy. A collection of epithelioid-type histiocytes with a few lymphocytes and polymorphs is illustrated in this urine sample from a patient who had received BCG therapy. (Papanicolaou × OI)

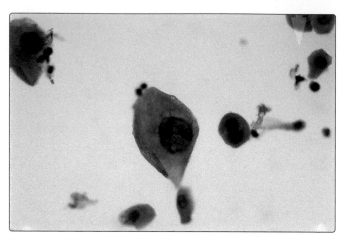

Fig. 18.84 Urine: post-radiation therapy. The transitional cell in the centre of the field shows both nuclear and cytoplasmic enlargement and a prominent nucleolus but evidence of degeneration is seen in the incomplete nuclear membrane.

inflammation and ulceration, necessitating cystectomy in some extreme cases. Urothelial carcinoma developed in 5% of cases of haemorrhagic cystitis following cyclophosphamide therapy in one series[67].

Laser treatment is sometimes used for treating superficial urothelial carcinomas. Post-laser bladder wash specimens contain spindle cells both singly and in stacked groups that are difficult to evaluate for malignancy. Heat from diathermy produces similar spindling in surgical biopsies taken at the same time as the urine samples[68]. On the other hand, bizarre spindle cells may be seen in urine from patients with low-grade papillary carcinomas[69].

A much used form of treatment for widespread carcinoma *in situ* of the bladder is **immunotherapy** using intravesical *Bacillus Calmette-Guerin* (BCG)[70]. It is also used for treatment of residual superficial papillary tumours, prophylactically after resection of tumours[71], and is of value in patients who do not respond to chemotherapy. The complications include cystitis with haematuria and distant infections. The urine contains blood and numerous inflammatory cells, mainly histiocytes (Fig. 18.83) and lymphocytes[72]. Lymphocytes in urine are increased in number after repeated instillations of BCG, suggesting a specific immune response. Collections of histiocytes resembling granulomas may be present[73] and multinucleated giant cells have been noted[74]. Urine cytology is advocated as a useful follow-up test in patients treated with BCG as it is useful in assessing recurrence[75,76]. Surveillance is recommended for 5 years[70].

Radiation treatment is used for some inoperable cases of urothelial carcinoma and may result in a scarred fibrosed bladder. Urinary tract complications can also occur following radiotherapy to carcinoma of the cervix, as long as 30 years after cessation of treatment. These include haematuria, incontinence and irritable bladder symptoms[77]. Cytological changes seen in voided urine include cellular swelling with multinucleation, nuclear enlargement,

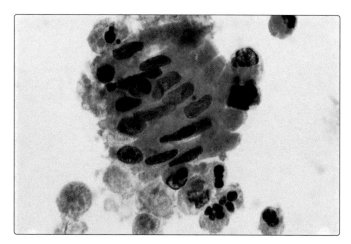

Fig. 18.85 Urine: ileal conduit sample. A cluster of degenerating columnar epithelial cells is seen in the centre of the field with scattered inflammatory cells. (Papanicolaou × OI)

variable hyperchromasia and prominent nucleoli (Fig. 18.84). The nuclear/cytoplasmic ratio generally remains low and the changes tend to be present in all cells in contrast to the mixed population of benign and malignant cells found in cases of recurrent carcinoma.

Construction of an **ileal conduit** following total cystectomy is usually performed for patients with multifocal recurrences of bladder carcinoma or widespread carcinoma *in situ*. The possibility of further recurrences in the remaining upper urinary tract can subsequently be monitored by regular cytological examination of urine obtained from the ileal conduit. Samples from these patients show inflammatory cells, especially macrophages and leucocytes, many exfoliated cells from the lining ileal mucosa and much cellular debris (Fig. 18.85). Malignant transitional cells from a recurrence either above or directly involving the conduit are usually recognizable amongst these cells since the tumours are generally of high-grade malignancy[57,78]. Rectosigmoid segments may be used in preference to ileal loops. There are reported complications following these procedures, many occurring years after surgery. They include ileal conduit stenosis due to severe inflammation and fibrosis[79], the development of adenomas and adenocarcinomas at or close to the anastomosis site in rectosigmoid bladders[80–82] and squamous cell carcinoma[81].

Occupational bladder cancer is known to be a hazard for workers in the textile, dyeing and printing industries, also in primary aluminium production workers and in the rubber industry. The implicated carcinogens are aniline dye intermediates such as β–naphthylamine and benzidine congeners. In aluminium production, benzene soluble coal tar pitch volatiles are responsible. Annual screening of urine samples from workers in these industries is undertaken in some countries. The average latent period from onset of exposure to diagnosis is 23.3 years[83].

New techniques

Immunocytochemical techniques have been used to aid detection of bladder cancer and some have been reported to be superior to cytology[84]. Carcinoembryonic antigen is detectable in most urothelial neoplasms and can be used as a tumour marker in urine. However, it is of limited value since many other carcinomas also show positive staining. A new marker that has been found to be more sensitive than urine cytology is cytokeratin 20[85]. An even more recent test is Immunocyt, which detects cellular markers specific for transitional cell carcinoma in urine[86]. It is highly sensitive and, when combined with cytology, may possibly replace cystoscopy for follow-up of low-grade transitional cell carcinomas.

The BTA (bladder tumour antigen) is another new method of detecting malignant cells in urine. It has been described as being superior to voided urine cytology in detecting low-grade tumours[87,88], but has a relatively high false positive rate and is therefore best used as an adjunct to urine cytology[89]. ELISA-like assays have been used to measure urinary hyaluronic acid and hyaluronidase markers that are highly sensitive and specific for bladder carcinoma cells and can even grade the tumour[90]. A method that has been compared with urine cytology is the TRAP assay (telomeric repeat amplification protocol)[91]. Urine cytology has greater sensitivity than TRAP.

Flow cytometry is becoming a widely used method for detecting bladder carcinoma and for monitoring treatment[92]. In combination with urine cytology the detection rate for bladder cancers is 90–94%[93], especially after intravesical therapy[94]. Bladder wash flow cytometry has a greater sensitivity than urine flow cytometry[95–97]. Microfluorometry is another new technique, which is used on bladder washings. Unlike flow cytometry, microfluorometry is able to focus on individual cells in a field, assessing the amount of fluorescent activity within the nucleus. Unfortunately, the false positive rate is very high[98]. The sensitivity of fluorescence *in situ* hybridization (FISH) has been demonstrated to be better than cytology for urine specimens but not as good with bladder washings[99]. The most promising new test seems to be NMP22 with a sensitivity of 100% and a specificity of 90% for detecting bladder carcinoma[100]. A recent article reviews all the current methods that are available for early detection of urothelial carcinoma[101], cytology being the yardstick against which all new methods are measured.

References

1 Sanders W R. Cancer of the bladder. Fragments forming urethral plugs discharged in the urine, concentric colloid bodies. *Edin J Med* 1864; **10**: 273

2 Papanicolaou G N, Marshall V F. Urine sediment: a diagnostic procedure in cancers of the urinary tract. *Science* 1945; **101**: 519–521

3 Cornin H L, Bray R A, Naber M H. The detection and interpretation of urinary eosinophils. *Arch Pathol Lab Med* 1989; **113**: 1256–1258

4 Kitamoto Y, Tomita M, Akamine M *et al*. Differentiation of haematuria using a uniquely-shaped red cell. *Nephron* 1993; **64**: 32–36

5 Goldwasser P, Antiguani A, Mittman N *et al*. Urinary red cell size: diagnostic value and determinants. *Am J Nephrol* 1990; **10**: 148–156

6 Tsukahara H, Yoshimoto M, Morikawa K *et al*. Mean cellular volume of urinary red blood cells in investigation of haematuria. *Acta Paediatr Jpn* 1989; **31**: 476–479

7 Trott P A. Cytological screening for cancer of the bladder. *Proc Roy Soc Med* 1976; **69**: 496

8 Corey H E, Alfonso F, Hamele-Bena D *et al*. Urine cytology and the diagnosis of renal allograft rejection. II. Studies using immunostaining. *Acta Cytol* 1997; **41**: 1742–1746

9 Howell A D N, Smith S R, Butterly D Q *et al*. Diagnosis and management of BK polyomavirus interstitial nephritis in renal transplant recipients. *Transplantation* 1999; **68**: 1279–1288

10 Harris M J, Schwinn C P, Morrow J W *et al*. Exfoliative cytology of the urinary bladder irrigation specimen. *Acta Cytol* 1971; **15**: 385–399

11 Brown F M. Urine cytology. Is it still the gold standard for screening? *Urol Clin North Am* 2000; **27**(1): 25–27

12 Paez A, Coba J M, Murillo N *et al*. Reliability of the routine cytological diagnosis in bladder cancer. *Eur Urol* 1999; **35**(1): 228–232

13 Geisse L J, Tweeddale D N. Pre-clinical cytological diagnosis of bladder cancer. *J Urol* 1978; **120**: 51–56

14 Pask C H, Britsch C, Uson A G, Veenema R J. Reliability of positive exfoliative cytology study of the urine in urinary tract malignancy. *J Urol* 1969; **102**: 91

15 Hastie K J, Ahmad R, Moisey Ch. Fractionated urine cytology in the follow-up of bladder cancer. *Brit J Urol* 1990; **66**: 40–41

16 Trott P A, Edwards L. Comparison of bladder washings and urine cytology in the diagnosis of bladder cancer. *J Urol* 1973; **110**: 664–666

17 Matzkin H, Moinuddin S, Soloway M. Value of urine cytology vs. bladder washings in bladder cancer. *Urology* 1992; **39**: 201–203

18 Farrow G M. Urine cytology in the detection of bladder cancer: a critical approach. *J Occup Med* 1990; **32**: 817–821

19 Luthra U K, Dey P, George J *et al*. Comparison of ThinPrep and conventional preparations: urine cytology evaluation. *Diagn Cytopathol* 1999; **21**(5): 364–465

20 Kannan V, Bose S. Low grade transitional cell carcinoma and instrument artefact: a challenge in urinary cytology. *Acta Cytol* 1993; **37**: 899–902

21 Bates A W, Fegan A W, Baithun S I. Xanthogranulomatous cystitis associated with neoplasms of the bladder. *Histopathol* 1998; **33**(3): 212–215

22 Devasia A, Kekre N S, Date A et al. Eosinophilic cystitis – not that uncommon! *Scand J Urol Nephrol* 1999; **33**(6): 396–399

23 Koss L G. *Diagnostic Cytology and its Histopathologic Basis*, 4th edn. Philadelphia: JB Lippincott Co., 1992; 896

24 Issa R M, Shalaby M A. Eosinophilia as a diagnostic value in patients suffering from schistosomiasis haematobium comparing to eosinophiluria and egg count in the urine. *J Egupt Soc Parasitol* 1999; **29**(2): 431–449

25 Florentine B D, Carriere C, Abdul-Karim F W. Mucor pyelonephritis. Report of a case diagnosed by urine cytology, with diagnostic considerations in the workup of funguria. *Acta Cytol* 1997; **41**(6): 1797–1800

26 Coleman D V. The cytodiagnosis of human polyoma virus infection. *Acta Cytol* 1975; **19**: 93–96

27 Kupper T, Stoffels U, Pawlita M et al. Morphological changes in urothelial cells replicating human polyomavirus BK. *Cytopathol* 1993; **4**: 361–368

28 Minassian H, Schinella R, Reilly J C. Polyomavirus in the urine: follow-up study. *Diagn Cytopathol* 1994; **10**: 209–211

29 Drachenberg C B, Beskow C O, Cangro C B et al. Human polyomavirus in renal allograft biopsies: morphological findings and correlation with urine cytology. *Hum Pathol* 1999; **30**(8): 970–977

30 Thal S M, DeBellis C C, Iversm S A, Schumann G B. Comparison of dysmorphic erythrocytes with other urinary sediment parameters of renal bleeding. *Am J Clin Pathol* 1986; **86**: 784–787

31 Pellet H, Buenerd A, Mirairie E et al. Clinical prevalence of glomerular haematuria: a nine year retrospective study. *Diagn Cytopathol* 199; **7**: 27–31

32 Fassett R G, Morgan B A, Mathew T H. Detection of glomerular bleeding by phase-contrast microscopy. *Lancet* 1982; 1432–1434

33 Janssens P M W, Kornaat N, Tieleman F, Willems J L. Localising the site of haematuria by immunochemical staining of erythrocytes in urine. *Chemical Chemistry* 1992; **38**: 216–222

34 Pollock C, Pei-Ling L, Gijory A Z et al. Dysmorphism of urinary red blood cells – value in diagnosis. *Kidney International* 1989; **36**: 1045–1049

35 Kannan V, Gupta D. Calculus artefact. A challenge in urinary cytology. *Acta Cytol* 1999; **43**(5): 794–800

36 Highman W, Wilson E. Urine cytology in patients with calculi. *J Clin Pathol* 1982; **35**: 350–356

37 Zaharopoulus P, Wong J Y, Wen J W. Matrix crystals in cytologic urine specimens. *Diagn Cytopathol* 1990; **6**: 390–395

38 Murphy W M, Beckwith J B, Farrow G M. Tumors of the urinary bladder. In: Rosai J and Sobin LH eds. *Tumors of the Kidney,* *Bladder, and Related Urinary Structures. Atlas of Tumor Pathology*, Fascicle 11, Washington: Armed Forces Institute of Pathology 1994, p 282

39 Bohlmeyer T J, Shroyer K R. Endometriosis of the bladder: cytologic findings and differentiation from transitional cell carcinoma. *Acta Cytol* 1996; **40**(2): 382–384

40 Jordan M M, Weingarten J, Murphy W M. Transitional cell neoplasms of the urinary bladder: can biologic potential be predicted from histologic grading? *Cancer* 1987; **60**: 2766–2774

41 Eble J N, Young R H. Benign and low-grade papillary lesions of the urinary bladder: a review of the papilloma-papillary carcinoma controversy and a report of 5 typical papillomas. *Diagn Pathol* 1989; **6**: 351–371

42 Kunze E, Schauer A, Schmitt M. Histology and histogenesis of two different types of inverted urothelial papilloma. *Cancer* 1983; **51**: 348–358

43 Cameron K M, Lupton CH. Inverted papilloma of the lower urinary tract. *Br J Urol* 1976; **48**: 567–577

44 Murphy W M. Diseases of the urinary bladder, urethra, ureters, and renal pelves. In: Murphy W M ed. *Urological Pathology*. Philadelphia: WB Saunders, 1989: 64–96

45 Rife C C, Farrow G M, Utz D C. Urine cytology of transitional cell neoplasms. *Urol Clin North Am* 1979; **6**: 599–612

46 Murphy W M, Beckwith J B, Farrow G M. Tumors of the Urinary Bladder. In: Rosai J and Sobin L H, eds. *Tumors of the Kidney, Bladder, and Related Urinary Structures. Atlas of Tumor Pathology*, Fascicle 11, Washington DC: Armed Forces Institute of Pathology 1994, p 200

47 Koss L G. Mapping of the urinary bladder: its impact on the concepts of bladder cancer. *Hum Pathol* 1979; **10**: 533–548

48 Murphy W M. Current status of urinary cytology in the evaluation of bladder neoplasms. *Hum Pathol* 1990; **21**: 886–895

49 Chodak G W, Straus F W, Schoenberg H W. Simultaneous occurrence of transitional, squamous and adenocarcinoma of the bladder. After 15 years of cyclophosphamide ingestion. *J Urol* 1981; **125**: 424–426

50 Shenoy U A, Colby T V, Schumann G B. Reliability of urinary cytodiagnosis in urothelial neoplasms. *Cancer* 1985; **56**: 2041–2045

51 Ro J Y, Staerkel G A, Ayala A G. Cytologic and histologic features of superficial bladder cancer. *Urol Clin North Am* 1992; **19**: 435–453

52 Cotran R, Kumar V, Robbins S L, eds. Urinary bladder. In: *Robbins Pathologic Basis of Disease*, 4th edn. Philadelphia: WB Saunders, 1989; 1086–1097

53 Highman W. Flat *in situ* carcinoma of the bladder: cytological examination of urine in diagnosis, follow-up and assessment of response to chemotherapy. *J Clin Pathol* 1988; **41**: 540–546

54 Keney W M, Szyfelbein W M, Daly J J. Positive urinary cytology in patients without evident tumour. *J Urol* 1977; **117**: 223–224

55 Harving N, Wolf H, Melsen F. Positive urinary cytology after tumour resection: an indicator for concomitant carcinoma-in-situ. *J Urol* 1988; **140**: 495–497

56 Kannan V. Papillary transitional cell carcinoma of the upper urinary tract: a cytological review. *Diagn Cytopathol* 1990; **6**: 204–209

57 Highman W J. Transitional carcinoma of the upper urinary tract: a histological and cytological review. *J Clin Pathol* 1986; **39**: 297–305

58 Doria M I Jr, Saint Martin G, Wang H H et al. Cytologic features of clear cell carcinoma of the urethra and urinary bladder. *Diagn Cytopathol* 1996; **14**(2): 150–154.

59 Shinagawa T, Atadokoro M, Abe M et al. Papillary urothelial carcinoma of the urinary bladder demonstrating prominent signet-ring cells in a smear. A case report. *Acta Cytol* 1998; **42**(2): 407–412

60 Ali S Z, Reuter Vek Zakowski M F. Small cell neuroendocrine carcinoma of the urinary bladder. A clinicopathologic study with emphasis on cytologic features. *Cancer* 1997; **79**: 356–361

61 Borghi L, Bianchini E, Atlavilla G. Undifferentiated small-cell carcinoma of the urinary bladder: report of two cases with a primary urinary cytodiagnosis. *Diagn Cytopathol* 1995; **13**(1): 61–65

62 McRae S, Garcia B M. Cytologic diagnosis of a primary pure oat cell carcinoma of the bladder in voided urine. A case report. *Acta Cytol* 1997; **41**(4 Suppl): 1279–1283

63 Sonobe H, Okada Y, Sudo S et al. Inflammatory pseudotumor of the urinary bladder with aberrant expression of cytokeratin. Report of a case with cytologic, immunocytochemical and cytogenetic findings. *Acta Cytol* 1999; **43**(2): 257–262

64 Edgerton M E, Hoda R S, Gupta P K. Cytologic diagnosis of metastatic ovarian adenocarcinoma in the urinary bladder: a case report and review of the literature. *Diagn Cytol* 1999; **20**(3): 156–159

65 Stella F, Battistelli S, Marcheggianni F et al. Urothelial cell changes due to Busulphan and Cyclophosphamide treatment in bone marrow transplantation. *Acta Cytol* 1990; **34**: 885–890

66 Stella F, Battistelli S, Marcheggianni F et al. Urothelial toxicity following conditioning therapy in bone marrow transplantation and bladder cancer: morphologic and morphometric comparison using exfoliation urinary cytology. *Diagn Cytopathol* 1992; **8**: 216–221

67 Stillwell T J, Benson R C. Cyclophosphamide-induced haemorrhagic cystitis. A review of 100 patients. *Cancer* 1988; **61**: 451–457

68 Fanning C V, Staerkl G A, Sneige N et al. Spindling artefact of urothelial cells in post-laser treatment urinary cytology. *Diagn Cytopathol* 1993; **9**: 279–281

69 Fontana P, Baiocco R. Bizarre spindle cells in urine cytology specimens. *Diagn Cytopathol* 1993; **9**: 605 (letter)

70 Lebret T, Bohin D, Kassardjian Z et al. Recurrence, progression and success in stage Ta grade 3 bladder tumours treated

with low dose Bacillus Calmett-Guerin installation. *J Urol* 2000; **163**(1): 63–67

71 Sharma N, Prescott S. BCG vaccine in superficial bladder cancer. *BMJ* 1994; **308**: 801–802 (editorial)

72 De Beer E C, De Jong W H, Van der Meijden A P M *et al*. Presence of activated lymphocytes in the urine of patients with superficial bladder cancer after intravesical immunotherapy with Bacillus Calmette-Guerin. *Cancer Immunol Immunother* 1991; **33**: 411–416

73 Betz S A, See W A, Cohen M B. Granulomatous inflammation in bladder wash specimens after intravesical Bacillus Calmette-Guerin therapy for transitional cell carcinoma of the bladder. *Am J Clin Pathol* 1993; **99**: 244–249

74 Cohen J-M, Szporn A J, Unger P *et al*. Noncaseatring granulomata of the bladder following intravesical administration of Bacille Calmette-Guerin. *Acta Cytol* 1991; **35**: 600

75 Dalbagni G, Rechtschaffen T, Herr H W. Is transurethral biopsy of the bladder necessary after 3 months to evaluate response to Bacillus Calmette-Guerin therapy? *J Urol* 1999; **162**(3, part 1): 708–709

76 Bhan R, Pisharodi L R, Gudlaugsson E, Bedrossian C. Cytological, histological and clinical correlations in intravesical Bacillus Calmette-Guerin immunotherapy. *Ann Diagn Pathol* 1998; **2**(1): 55–60

77 Zonbik J, McGuire E J, Noll F, Delancey J O L. The late occurrence of urinary tract damage in patients successfully treated by radiotherapy for cervical carcinoma. *J Urol* 1989; **141**: 1347–1349

78 Wolinska W H, Melamed M R. Urinary conduit cytology. *Cancer* 1973; **32**: 100–106

79 Magnusson B, Carlen B, Bak-Jensen B *et al*. Ileal conduit stenosis – an enigma. *Scan J Urol Nephrol* 1996; **30**(3): 193–197

80 Malone M J, Izes J K, Hurley L J. Carcinogenesis: The fate of intestinal segments used in urinary reconstruction. *Urol Clin North Am* 1997; **34**(4): 723–725

81 Shokeir A A, Smama M, el-Mekresh M M *et al*. Late malignancy in bowel segments exposed to urine without fecal stream. *Urol* 1995; **46**(5): 657–661

82 Stewart M. Urinary diversion and bowel cancer. *Ann R Coll Surg Engl* 1986; **68**(2): 98–102

83 Frumin E, Velez H, Bingham E *et al*. Occupational bladder cancer in textile dyeing and printing workers: 6 cases and their significance for screening programs. *J Occup Med* 1990; **32**: 887–890

84 Lin C–W, Kirley A–H *et al*. Detection of exfoliated bladder cancer cells by monoclonal antibodies to tumour-associated cell surface antigen. *J Occup Med* 1990; **32**: 910–916

85 Buchumensky V, Klein A, Zemer R *et al*. Cytokeratin 20: a new marker for early detection of bladder carcinoma? *J Urol* 1998; **160**(6, part 1): 1971–1974

86 Mian C, Pycha A, Wiener H K *et al*. Immunocyt: a new tool for detecting transitional cell cancer of the urinary tract. *J Urol* 1999; **161**(5): 1486–1489

87 Heino A, Aaltoman S, Ala-Opas M. BTA test is superior to voided urine cytology in detecting malignant bladder tumours. *Ann Chir Gynaecol* 1999; **84**(4): 304–307

88 Leigh H, Marberger M, Conort P *et al*. Comparison of the BTA stat test with voided urine cytology and bladder wash cytology in the diagnosis and monitoring of bladder cancer. *Eur Urol* 1999; **35**(2): 52–56

89 Nasuti J F, Gomella L G, Ismail M, Bibbo M. Utility of the BTA stat test for bladder cancer screening. *Diagn Cytol* 1999; **21**(1): 27–29

90 Lokeshwar V B, Obek C, Pham H T *et al*. Urinary hyaluronic acid and hyaluronidase markers for bladder cancer detection and evaluation of grade. *J Urol* 2000; **1**: 348–356

91 Dalbagri G, Han W, Zlang A F *et al*. Evaluation of the telomeric repeat amplification protocol (TRAP) assay for telomerase as a diagnostic modality in recurrent bladder cancer. *Clin Cancer Res* 1997; **3**(9): 1593–1598

92 Melamed M R, Klein F A. Flow cytometry of urinary bladder irrigation specimens. *Hum Pathol* 1984; **15**: 362–365

93 Deitch A D, Andersen K A, de Vere White R W. Evaluation of DNA flow cytometry as a screening test for bladder cancer. *J Occup Med* 1990; **32**: 898–903

94 Giella J G, Ring C, Olsson C A. The predictive value of flow cytometry and urinary cytology in the follow up of patients with transitional cell carcinoma of the bladder. *J Urol* 1992; **148**: 293–296

95 Mellon K, Shenton B K, Neal D E. Is voided urine suitable for flow cytometric DNA analysis? *Brit J Urol* 1991; **67**: 48–53

96 Hermansen D C, Badalament R A, Bretton R R *et al*. Voided flow cytometric in screening high-risk patients for the presence of bladder cancer. *J Occup Med* 1990; **32**: 894–897

97 Koss L G, Wersto R P, Simmons D A *et al*. Predictive value of DNA measurements in bladder washings. *Cancer* 1989; **64**: 916–924

98 Gerber W L, Lenahan P J, Kendall A R, Mercer W E. Computer-assisted microfluorometric detection of individual malignant bladder cells. *Urology* 1991; **38**: 466–472

99 Junker K, Werner W, Mueller C *et al*. Interphase cytogenetic diagnosis of bladder cancer on cells from urine and bladder washings. *Int J Oncol* 1999; **14**(2): 309–313

100 Zippe C, Pandrangi L, Potto J M *et al*. NMP22: a sensitive cost-effective test in patients at risk for bladder cancer. *AntiCancer Res* 1999; **19**(4A): 2621–2623

101 Ross J S, Cohen M B. Ancillary methods for the detection of recurrent urothelial neoplasia. *Cancer* (*Cancer Cytopathlogy*) 2000; **90**:75–86

Lymphoreticular system

Lymph nodes

Lambert Skoog and Edneia Tani*

Introduction

Enlarged lymph nodes were the first organs to be biopsied by fine needle aspiration (FNA); today, they are one of the most frequently sampled tissues. In 1904, Greig and Gray reported that trypanosomes could be demonstrated in smears from lymph node aspirates[1], and for some years afterwards, the technique was used to identify various organisms in infected lymph nodes. The earliest report of a wider application of needle aspiration came from the USA in 1921 when Guthrie described using aspirated material to diagnose a variety of diseases causing lymphadenopathy[2]. Over the next 30 years the technique was slowly adopted by clinicians and pathologists, resulting in a number of reports on its usefulness. The first study to show a convincingly high sensitivity was presented by Morrison et al. in 1952[3].

We now have a large body of evidence supporting the use of aspiration cytology as a primary method of diagnosis in reactive, infective and metastatic lymphadenopathy, but the diagnosis of malignant lymphoma by FNA has been much more controversial. However, several recent studies have shown conclusively that a combined cytological and immunological evaluation of aspirated lymphoid cells results in distinctly improved diagnostic accuracy in cases of lymphoma[4-22]. This will inevitably lead to acceptance of FNA cytology as a method, which is comparable with histopathology in diagnostic significance.

The role of cytology in lymph node diagnosis

Lymph nodes react to a variety of micro-organisms and non-specific stimuli by expansion of the follicle centres and/or interfollicular tissue. This results in enlargement of nodes, which may sometimes be considerable. The clinical management of patients with enlarged lymph nodes varies with factors such as age, the presence of known infection and the previous medical history. For example, children can present with massive local lymphadenopathy even after mild infections. Accordingly, medical treatment and a period of observation usually precede the request for FNA in a child with persistent lymph nodes after a recent history of infection.

In contrast, adult or elderly patients often react to infections with only slight to modest lymph node enlargement: therefore distinct lymphadenopathy in an elderly patient will arouse suspicion of malignancy and justify immediate needle biopsy. For patients between these two extreme clinical settings, it is more difficult to decide which patient is more likely to have a reactive or neoplastic lymphadenopathy.

FNA biopsy was introduced in most medical centres with a view to reducing the number of excisional biopsies of nodes. Although a routine procedure, surgical excision is considerably more expensive and time consuming, and is afflicted with a distinctly higher morbidity than FNA. Using cytomorphology alone, it is often possible to decide if the lymphadenopathy has resulted from reactive lymphadenitis, metastatic malignancy or lymphoma. Patients with reactive lymph node enlargement or metastasis from a known malignancy can thus be spared lymph node excision. In cases with a cytological diagnosis or suspicion of lymphoma, surgical excision has usually been regarded as mandatory.

Today, this still seems to be the prevailing application of FNA cytology in patients with lymphadenopathy. There has however been a trend towards accepting cytomorphology alone as sufficient for diagnosis in patients with abdominal or mediastinal lymphomas. Obviously, this is not because lymphomas at these sites are easier to diagnose than those found in superficial sites, but results rather from clinical considerations. The laparotomy and mediastinotomy or mediastinoscopy otherwise required have a distinct morbidity and can also lead to delay in therapy.

Aspirated cells perform excellently in immunocytochemistry, flow cytometry and gene rearrangement analysis, as has been demonstrated by a number of authors[4-29]. This has increased the accuracy of lymphoma diagnosis on FNA material to the same level as histopathology in some series[7-11]. However, it should be pointed out that the correct subclassification of lymphomas on cytological material requires experience and optimal material, both of which may be difficult to obtain at centres with relatively few lymphoma patients. In principle this variation in reliability of cytological diagnosis means that FNA cytology can be exercised in the management of patients with lymphadenopathy either at a basic or an advanced level.

*The authors gratefully acknowledge their debt to the late Torsten Löwhagen, whose contribution to the previous edition of this chapter provided a substantial basis for this revised edition.

At a basic level, aspirated cells are evaluated on routine smears alone. This will allow a conclusive diagnosis in the majority of patients with metastatic tumours and in many cases of reactive lymphadenopathy. Most high-grade lymphomas should also be recognizable, while many of the low-grade lymphomas and some cases of reactive lymphadenopathy will not be identified reliably. From this it is clear that conventional FNA cytology should be used to select patients for open biopsy where tissue is needed for histology and immunological evaluation.

At an advanced level, aspirated cells are evaluated on smears and the diagnosis is then substantiated by immunocytochemistry, flow cytometry and/or gene rearrangement analysis. This approach allows a conclusive diagnosis in the vast majority of metastatic tumours, reactive processes and lymphomas. Confirmation by histology is then only necessary in a minority of lymphomas, namely those in which choice of treatment is based on growth pattern, such as whether nodular or diffuse. Even at this advanced diagnostic level some cases of lymphadenopathy cannot be diagnosed conclusively. In such cases our experience is that lymph node excision with subsequent histology will rarely be of additional diagnostic value. It is accordingly advisable to perform a repeat FNA biopsy after 2–3 weeks. This time is obviously not fixed but will be determined by various factors including any active infection, the condition of the patient and patient anxiety.

In the opinion of the authors, all laboratories involved in the diagnosis of patients with lymphadenopathy should use FNA cytology in conjunction with immunological characterization. This diagnostic approach will have a substantial impact on the clinical management of such patients.

Technical aspects

Smear making

Aspiration biopsies of lymph nodes should preferably be performed with a 23 gauge (0.6 mm) needle. In most cases this will provide enough cells for smears as well as cytospin preparations. The use of larger needles usually results in admixture of peripheral blood, which may preclude cytological and immunological evaluation of the lymphoid cells.

Lymph node aspirates are usually cellular, making it difficult to prepare smears of good quality. The smear should be thin to ensure instant fixation, which will allow an optimal evaluation of cytological details. However, care must be exercised not to use too much pressure in preparing such thin smears. Lymphoid cells are fragile and readily lose their cytoplasm. Fragmented cytoplasm will appear as small pale grey structures with Romanowsky stains, and these are often called 'lymphoglandular bodies'. Sometimes identical structures can also be seen in smears from other fragile cells; they are thus not pathognomonic for cells of lymphoid origin.

Whenever possible, both air-dried and alcohol-fixed smears should be prepared for May-Grünwald-Giemsa (MGG) and Papanicolaou staining, respectively. These stains complement each other and allow an optimal evaluation of cytological details. If mycobacterial or fungal infections are suspected, extra smears should be prepared for special stains.

Cytospin preparations

After using parts of the aspirates for smear making, the remainder should be suspended in a buffered balanced salt (BBS) solution at pH 7.4 for cytospin preparations. An ordinary aspirate from an enlarged lymph node will yield several millions of cells. The number of suspended cells should therefore be calculated and the concentration adjusted to $1-2 \times 10^6$ cells/ml. Cell-rich suspensions can be diluted to optimal concentration by adding BBS solution. Vigorous mixing should be avoided since it can destroy lymphoid cells, particularly the large immature cells seen in high-grade lymphomas. If the cell concentration is low the cells can be concentrated by centrifugation at 700 rpm for 3–5 min. The resulting pellet is then gently resuspended in a reduced volume of BBS solution. The suspension is spun in a cytocentrifuge at 700 rpm for 3 min. Each cytospin should contain $1-2 \times 10^5$ nucleated cells.

One of the cytospins should always be stained with MGG and compared with the smears to monitor recovery of all cell components. If the suspension contains a rich admixture of red blood cells, it is possible to purify the lymphoid cells by density gradient centrifugation. Normally this procedure does not result in any significant cell loss except in some cases of large cell lymphomas, which may be fragile and therefore lost in density gradient centrifugation.

Air-dried cytospin preparations can be stored at room temperature for up to 1 week without detrimental effect on the immunological staining. Alternatively the cytospin can be stored at –20°C either in a plastic box or wrapped in aluminium foil. Under these conditions lymphoid cells retain their immunological and morphological characteristics for at least 1–2 years. It is important that the slides are kept wrapped until fully thawed when brought out for use otherwise the cells are prone to disintegration. Both immunoalkaline phosphatase and immunoperoxidase methods are suitable for cytospin preparations.

Flow cytometry

Aspirated cells can also be immunologically characterized by flow cytometry[9,11,14–20]. As in the case of immunocytochemistry on cytospin preparations one part of the aspirate should be used for smear making. The second part should be suspended in BBS solution at pH 7.4. A cell concentration of 1–2 million cells/ml buffer will be sufficient for a complete characterization of reactive lesions as well as most B- and T-cell lymphomas. A simultaneous four-colour staining technique is preferred.

Molecular biology

Aspirated cells also perform well in PCR rearrangement analysis[23-29]. Aspirated cells suspended in BBS at pH 7.4 should be pelleted immediately, snap frozen and stored at −70°C until used for rearrangement analysis.

Normal lymph node histology and cytology

Knowledge of the structural, histological and cytological features of normal lymph nodes is essential in the evaluation of FNA smears from enlarged nodes, whether the pathology is reactive, infective or due to a lymphoproliferative disorder. A brief outline of the structure of a normal lymph node is therefore included, followed by a more detailed description of the normal cell population.

The lymph node parenchyma is surrounded and divided by a fibrous capsule with attached septa. The parenchyma is composed of the cortex, medulla and paracortex. B cells predominate in the cortex and medulla whereas T cells are mainly found in the paracortical tissues.

The cortex contains primary and secondary follicles, the proportions varying with the state of activity of the node. Primary follicles, composed of aggregates of small resting B cells, are found in the unstimulated node. Secondary follicles develop after antigen stimulation and are composed of a narrow mantle zone of small B lymphocytes surrounding a germinal centre. Several types of cells are found in the germinal centre, the vast majority being B cells in the form of centroblasts and centrocytes. Macrophages containing phagocytosed cellular debris are also present.

Mature immunoglobulin secreting B cells, familiar as plasma cells, are the principal cell types found in the medulla. The paracortex contains many small lymphoid cells, which are of T phenotype. In addition, activated T cells and immunoblasts are present.

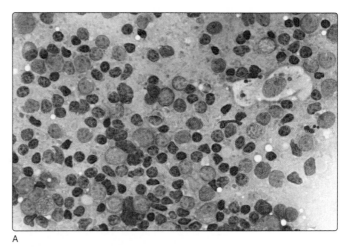

A

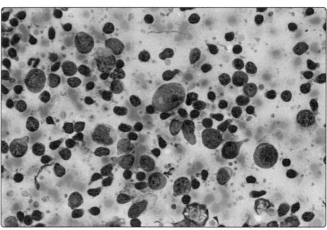

B

Fig. 19.1   Lymph node aspirates with normal lymphoid cells. (A) A macrophage with plentiful clear cytoplasm containing 'tingible bodies' is surrounded by large round centroblasts with sparse cytoplasm. Medium sized centrocytes with irregular nuclei and smooth chromatin and small mature lymphocytes with condensed chromatin are also present. (MGG × OI) (B) One large immunoblast with an eccentrically placed nucleus and well developed basophilic cytoplasm is surrounded by smaller immunoblasts and mature plasma cells. (MGG × OI)

Cytological findings *(Fig. 19.1)*

As could be predicted from the description of the normal histology, aspirates from normal lymph nodes and from some reactive nodes are dominated by different types of lymphocytes, but plasma cells, macrophages and granulocytes are also found.

► Mature lymphocytes of either B or T phenotype measure around 8 μm in air-dried smears. They have a dense nucleus with coarse chromatin and a pale blue rim of cytoplasm
► Plasma cells are characterized by their eccentrically placed nucleus with its chromatin arranged in a cartwheel-like pattern. The abundant cytoplasm often shows a less intense basophilic staining in the paranuclear area
► Centrocytes are B cells which measure around 10 μm and have sparse, weakly stained basophilic cytoplasm. The

nucleus has a fine chromatin pattern, is usually irregular in shape and may be cleaved
► Centroblasts are larger than centrocytes and have a characteristic round nucleus usually with several marginal nucleoli. The cytoplasm is sparse and may contain some vacuoles
► Immunoblasts of either B or T phenotype are the largest of the lymphoid cells and measure 20–30 μm. They have a round nucleus, often eccentrically placed, with 1–3 large strongly basophilic nucleoli. The cytoplasm is usually also intensely basophilic
► Macrophages have a round to oval nucleus with evenly distributed chromatin and an inconspicuous nucleolus. The poorly defined cytoplasm varies markedly in size but may measure up to 45 μm. In stimulated lymph nodes the macrophages contain phagocytosed cellular debris consisting of darkly stained particles, often referred to as tingible bodies

Reactive lymphadenopathy

Lymph nodes respond to many different agents by enlarging and becoming more active. Depending on the type of stimulus, a node may react with one of three basic histological and cytological patterns: reactive hyperplasia, suppurative lymphadenitis or granulomatous lymphadenitis. In some cases it is possible to identify the causative agent, either in routine preparations or by special stains such as those for mycobacteria, leishmania, histoplasma and trypanosomes, but the majority of reactive nodes show non-specific changes.

Reactive hyperplasia

Histologically, this response may take the form of enlargement of the lymphoid follicles, which develop active germinal centres. These are characterized by numerous centroblasts and centrocytes, a rich admixture of macrophages with a poorly defined pale cytoplasm containing tingible bodies, and a surrounding cuff of small lymphocytes. Alternatively, there may be expansion of the interfollicular tissue by numerous mature lymphocytes, lymphoplasmacytoid cells, plasma cells and varying numbers of immunoblasts. A mixture of both patterns is present in some cases. Nodes draining tumour or other sources of tissue breakdown may be further expanded by the presence of numerous histiocytes in the sinusoids, a picture referred to as sinus histiocytosis.

Cytological findings (Figs 19.2, 19.3)

Non-specific hyperplasia

Non-specific hyperplasia yields a cytological pattern on FNA, which depends on the proportions of follicular and interfollicular tissue in the aspirate, and this in turn usually correlates with the histological findings described above. Thus, smears from a node composed predominantly of large follicles with active germinal centres contain many centroblasts and centrocytes, while the interfollicular tissue is comparatively sparsely represented by mature lymphocytes, plasma cells and immunoblasts (Fig. 19.2).

In extreme cases the pattern may mimic a mixed lymphoma of centroblastic/centrocytic type. The presence or absence of tingible body macrophages is of little diagnostic value. Immunocytochemical evaluation of the lymphoid population may be the only way to resolve this diagnostic problem.

In contrast, when interfollicular tissue predominates, the smears are rich in lymphocytes, plasma cells, lymphoplasmacytoid cells and some immunoblasts. Such smears are difficult to differentiate from those of a low-grade lymphoma. Analysis of light chain immunoglobulin restriction is usually required to arrive at a conclusive diagnosis.

Some conditions lead to a cytological pattern, which clearly deviates from the general types described above. A description of the best recognized of these follows. It is important to remember that definitive diagnosis is dependent on good clinical correlation.

Viral and postvaccinial lymphadenitis

These conditions cause intense reactivity in the interfollicular tissue, which presents with a prominent immunoblastic proliferation in addition to lymphoplasmacytoid cells and plasma cells.

HIV infection

Generalized lymphadenopathy is common in patients with acquired immunodeficiency syndrome (AIDS)[30,31].

There is a florid follicular hyperplasia with immature follicle centre cells in a background of mature lymphocytes, plasma cells and macrophages. Immunoblasts are always present. The pattern is non-specific and thus not diagnostic for AIDS. A majority of the lymphoid cells are polyclonal B cells.

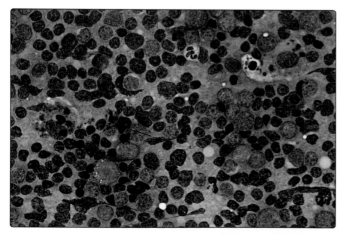

Fig. 19.2   Reactive lymphadenitis. Mixed lymphoid cells, granulocytes, plasma cells and tingible body macrophages. (MGG × OI)

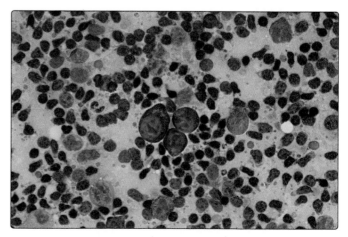

Fig. 19.3   Infectious mononucleosis. Several atypical immunoblasts are present in a background of small lymphocytes. (MGG × OI)

Infectious mononucleosis

Infectious mononucleosis can also cause lymphadenitis, which is mainly confined to the interfollicular tissue (Fig. 19.3). Cytologically, it is characterized by numerous immunoblasts, some of which are atypical with large irregular nuclei[32,33]. In rare cases, the pattern may even be suggestive of Hodgkin's disease[32,33]. Serological tests can be helpful, but phenotyping of the atypical cell population may be the only way to rule out a lymphoma.

Rheumatoid arthritis, systemic lupus erythematosus and secondary syphilis

All of these conditions can cause massive lymphadenopathy. Cytologically, there is a reactive pattern with numerous plasma cells, some containing Russell bodies, which may lead to a suspicion of a low-grade lymphoma with plasmacytic differentiation. In such cases, it may be impossible to arrive at a conclusive diagnosis without resorting to immunocytochemistry.

Dermatopathic lymphadenopathy

This is a special variant of reactive lymphadenitis, which is observed in patients with chronic skin disorders such as psoriasis or dermatitis. The germinal centres are hyperplastic and the interfollicular tissue is expanded by cells of histiocytic appearance[34]. Smears from such lymph nodes show numerous small lymphocytes, plasma cells, eosinophils and occasional blast cells. There are numerous histiocyte-like cells, also known as interdigitating reticulum cells, with pale indistinct cytoplasm. Macrophages containing brown melanin pigment from the damaged skin are always present.

Immunocytochemistry *(Figs 19.4, 19.5)*

In reactive lymphadenitis, the small lymphocytes are mostly T cells of which the helper type predominate. The B cells are of various sizes and are polyclonal, expressing both kappa and lambda light chains. Atypical immunoblasts are either of T or B phenotype, some of which may also express CD30 (Ki-1). They do not express CD15 (Leu M1). This phenotype can be misinterpreted to represent that of the neoplastic cells in Hodgkin's lymphoma.

Sinus histiocytosis

It is a very common finding in reactive lymph nodes and often associated with follicular hyperplasia but may also be seen in its absence. Characteristic is dilatation of subcapsular and trabecular sinuses, which are partially or completely filled with histiocytes/macrophages. This type of hyperplasia is observed in lymph nodes, which drain areas with cancer as well as inflammatory lesions but in many cases, the cause is unknown.

Cytological findings

The sinus histiocytosis is characterized by a mixture dominated by small lymphocytes, some blasts and numerous, sometime multinucleated, macrophages with

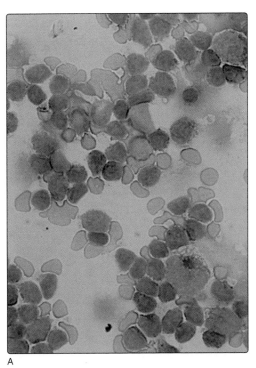
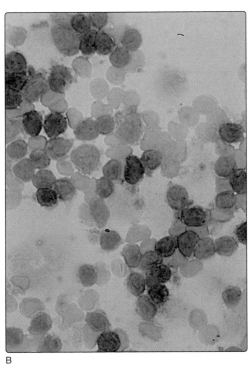

A   B

Fig. 19.4 Immunocytochemistry in reactive lymphadenopathy. Cytospin material from the aspirate shown in **Fig. 19.2** using B and T-cell markers reveals a mixed population of lymphoid cells. (A) B cells of varying sizes. (B) Small mature T cells. (Alkaline phosphatase × OI)

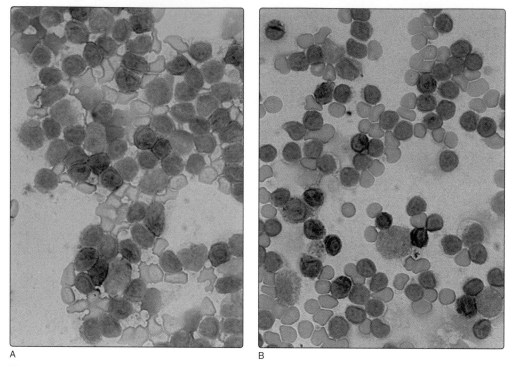

A   B

Fig. 19.5 Immunocytochemistry in reactive lymphadenopathy showing polyclonal light chain expression with no predominance of either kappa or lambda to suggest lymphoma. (A) Kappa. (B) Lambda. (Alkaline phosphatase × OI)

abundant foamy cytoplasm and round, oval or kidney shaped nuclei.

Sinus histiocytosis with massive lymphadenopathy

This is a rare, extreme form of sinus histiocytosis that was first described by Rosai and Dorfman in 1969[35]. The disorder is seen most often in black children and adolescents. Most patients are in good health and develop massive bilateral non-tender enlargement of the cervical lymph nodes followed by fever. Extra nodal involvement has also been described. The cause is unknown but the disorder has a prolonged course and spontaneous regression of the nodes usually takes place.

Cytological findings *(Fig. 19.6)*

There are numerous lymphocytes and large pale histiocytes, which have vesicular nuclei with small nucleoli and an abundant vacuolated cytoplasm. The histiocytes often have well preserved lymphocytes in the cytoplasm which is referred to as lymphocytophagocytosis or emperipolesis[36–38].

Immunocytochemistry

Some mature T cells are present. The B cells and plasma cells are polyclonal. A strong S 100 positivity and lack of lysozyme reactivity is characteristic for the large histiocytes.

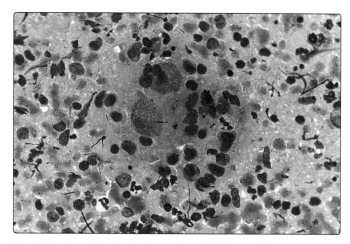

Fig. 19.6 Rosai-Dorfman's disease. Large histiocyte with prominent nucleoli and lymphophagocytosis. (MGG × OI)

Kikuchi's disease

Histiocytic necrotizing lymphadenitis is a rare well-defined clinical entity, which was first described by Kikuchi and Fujimoto *et al.* in 1972[39,40]. It affects chiefly, young women presenting with fever and enlargement of one or more cervical nodes. It is a benign, self limiting disease and its aetiology is still unknown.

Cytological findings

Numerous foamy macrophages, as well as 'tingible body' macrophages containing karyorrhectic debris in a background of necrotic material; small lymphocytes, as well as activated lymphocytes are found. Neutrophils, epithelioid cells and plasma cells, when present, are in few numbers[41–43].

Infective and granulomatous lymphadenopathy

A more definitive morphological categorization of lymph node disease is sometimes possible in certain infections directly involving nodes and in the group of inflammatory or infective disorders associated with granuloma formation. It is of the utmost importance in these conditions, however, that microbiological culture is undertaken for confirmation of the infectious agent.

Acute suppurative lymphadenitis

Lymph nodes draining or adjacent to a focus of bacterial infection, may be directly invaded by the organisms, causing acute lymphadenitis followed in some cases by suppuration. Initially a light infiltrate of neutrophil polymorphs is present but as the tissues undergo necrosis the node becomes a suppurative mass. Appropriate treatment may result in resolution or scarring.

Cytological findings

► In the initial phase slightly turbid fluid is aspirated
► Smears show a proteinaceous background with cell debris, mixed lymphocytes and sparse granulocytes
► Later the aspirate becomes purulent with many degenerate neutrophils in a thick background of cell debris

Granulomatous lymphadenopathy

The most common cause of granulomatous lymphadenitis in developed countries is sarcoidosis, but in many tropical areas, and in patients with immunodeficiency, other aetiologies are more common. Infections are a particularly important group and tuberculosis is the commonest of these, although many other organisms can present with granulomatous lymphadenopathy, such as leprosy, cat scratch disease, paracoccidioidomycosis, histoplasmosis, leishmaniasis, lymphogranuloma venereum, brucellosis and tularaemia. Granulomatous lymphadenitis can also be caused by foreign bodies such as talc or silica. Furthermore, granulomas may form part of a reactive background in the presence of malignant lymphoma or may occur in nodes draining a carcinoma.

The general cytological picture of granulomatous lymphadenitis is characterized by clusters of epithelioid cells which have elongated nuclei, picturesquely described as banana, footprint or carrot shaped, arranged in a syncytial fashion with abundant ill-defined cytoplasm. A variable number of multinucleated Langhans giant cells

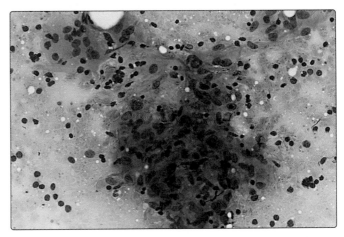

Fig. 19.7 Sarcoidosis. Cluster of epithelioid cells forming a granuloma, with a multinucleated giant cell upper left. (MGG × MP)

may be present, their nuclei polarized in an arc at one part of the cell border. The presence or absence of pale amorphous necrosis is of diagnostic significance in establishing the aetiology of the granulomatous reaction.

Sarcoidosis *(Fig. 19.7)*

This systemic disorder of young adults is characterized histologically by the presence of non-caseating giant cell granulomata and tends to affect lungs and lymph nodes most commonly. A similar reaction is sometimes seen in nodes draining a primary carcinoma whether or not metastases to the node have occurred. This finding is referred to as a sarcoidal reaction.

Cytological findings

► The aspirate contains cohesive clusters of epithelioid cells and numerous small mature lymphocytes
► In most cases multinucleated giant cells are present
► The background is free from necrosis, a finding strongly suggestive of sarcoidosis

Diagnostic pitfalls

If Langhans giant cells are absent the differential diagnosis should include tuberculosis, Hodgkin's disease and low-grade T-cell lymphoma. Techniques such as PCR and special stains for organisms, such as mycobacteria and fungi, as well as immunocytochemistry to characterize the lymphoid cells are of value in reducing the number of diagnostic alternatives. In sarcoidosis the lymphoid population is dominated by T cells, with a normal ratio of helper to suppressor cells, while the B cells are polyclonal. This contrasts with the lymphocytic alveolitis of pulmonary sarcoidosis in which CD4 positive T lymphocytes predominate.

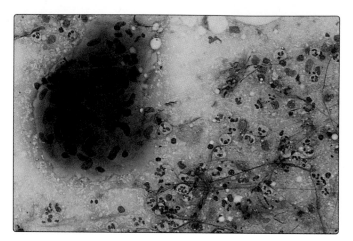

Fig. 19.8 Tuberculosis. A granuloma composed of epithelioid cells is present in a background of necrosis with numerous granulocytes. (MGG × MP)

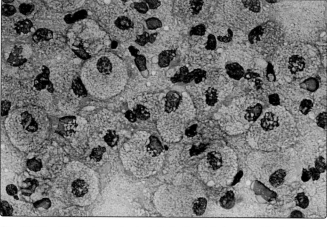

Fig. 19.10 Atypical mycobacterial infection. Histiocytes with abundant 'foamy' cytoplasm are seen. In an immunocompromised patient this picture should arouse suspicion of the presence of an atypical mycobacterial organism. (MGG × OI)

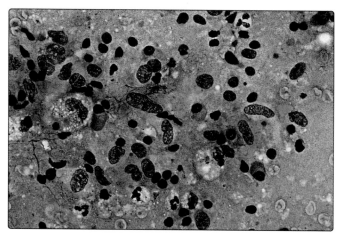

Fig. 19.9 Tuberculosis. This field contains a mixture of epithelioid cells, plasma cells, lymphocytes and macrophages. (MGG × OI)

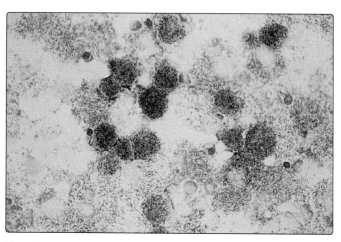

Fig. 19.11 Ziehl-Neelsen staining of the aspirate shown in **Fig. 19.10**, revealing numerous acid fast bacilli distending the histiocytic cells. (× OI)

Tuberculous lymphadenitis *(Figs 19.8, 19.9)*

Infection of lymph nodes by *Mycobacterium tuberculosis* is usually the result of spread from primary lung infection and can present clinically with massive generalized lymphadenopathy, especially of the cervical nodes, even to the extent of simulating lymphoma. The hallmark of tuberculosis histologically is the presence of caseating necrosis associated with epithelioid giant cell granulomata. Early diagnosis is particularly important since the condition is treatable.

Cytological findings[44-47]

Aspiration smears from tuberculous lymphadenitis show three major cell patterns:

▶ Epithelioid granulomas without necrosis, in which there are small clusters of epithelioid histiocytes and single forms, mixed with reactive lymphocytes, but Langhans' giant cells are not often seen

▶ Epithelioid granulomas with necrosis, showing similar features, but in addition there is a variable amount of pale stained amorphous material in the background
▶ Necrosis without epithelioid granuloma. This type shows thin necrotic debris containing large numbers of polymorphonuclear cells and scattered histiocytes

For definitive diagnosis, acid fast bacilli should be identified using the Ziehl-Neelsen stain or other stains for acid fast bacilli[47]. These stains have a relatively low sensitivity and are nowadays often replaced by PCR techniques to identify the mycobacteria.

Atypical mycobacterial infection *(Figs 19.10, 19.11)*

Immunodeficient patients, including those with AIDS, suffer from many of the infectious causes of lymphadenitis and are especially predisposed to tuberculosis, but may also be infected by less common organisms, which are rarely encountered in the general population. Infection due to *Mycobacterium avium-intracellulare* is an example of this type of lymphadenitis and is recognized with increasing frequency in this group of patients.

Histologically, the lymphoid tissue is replaced by large histiocytes with voluminous finely vacuolated, ill-defined cytoplasm containing numerous bacilli. Further details of this condition may be found in Chapter 22.

Cytological findings

▶ Smears show histiocytic cells with abundant pale cytoplasm
▶ In MGG stained preparations the mycobacteria present as cylindrical non-stained 'negative images' of bacilli that are diagnostic of mycobacterial infection[48]
▶ The presence of bacilli is readily demonstrated using the ZN stain. Characteristically, they are arranged randomly within the cytoplasm

Other types of infectious granulomatous lymphadenopathy
Leprosy

Leprosy is a chronic destructive systemic infection due to *Mycobacterium leprae* and is now mainly seen in Third World countries. As in the histology of this disease, two different types of reaction are seen cytologically in affected lymph nodes, referred to as lepromatous and tuberculoid[49].

In the lepromatous or Virchow's form of leprosy, the enlarged lymph nodes yield syncytial histiocytes with abundant clear cytoplasm containing numerous acid fast bacilli. In leprosy, the bacilli are present in parallel disposition in the form of globi in the cytoplasm of the histiocytes, which are sometimes referred to as Virchow's or globus cells. The arrangement of organisms is important in distinguishing leprosy from atypical mycobacterial infection[49,50].

In the tuberculoid form of leprosy, the predominant cytological picture is a granulomatous process, containing epithelioid histiocytes in a background of lymphocytes. Organisms are present in low numbers, and are more difficult to identify than in the lepromatous form.

Paracoccidioidomycosis *(Figs 19.12, 19.13)*

Paracoccidioidomycosis is a fungal infection endemic in South America. *P. brasiliensis* often causes massive

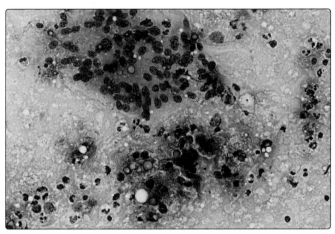

Fig. 19.12 Paracoccidioidomycosis. Multinucleated giant cell and histiocytes in a necrotic background with granulocytes. The spores are seen as rounded structures with birefringent capsules. (MGG × MP) (Courtesy Dr Viero RM, Dept Pathology, Faculdade de Medicina de Botucato UNESP, Brazil)

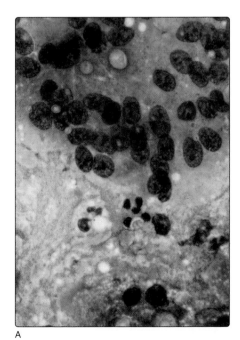

A

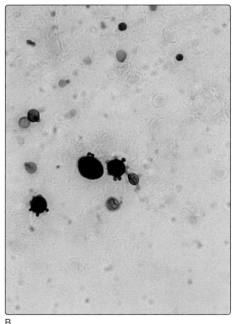

B

Fig. 19.13 Paracoccidioidomycosis. (A) Multinucleated giant cell with spores visible in the cytoplasm. (MGG × OI) (B) Spores with pathognomonic multiple budding. (Gomori × OI) (Courtesy Dr Viero RM, Dept Pathology, Faculdade de Medicina de Botucato UNESP, Brazil)

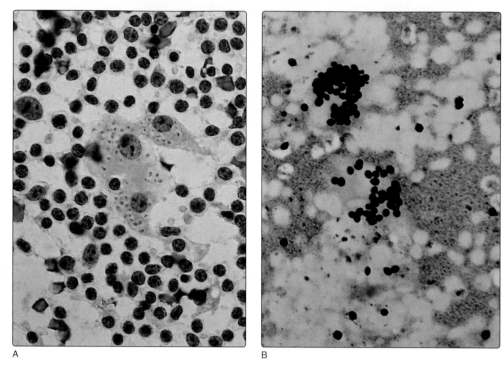

A   B

Fig. 19.14   Histoplasmosis. (A) Several histiocytes with tiny oval spores characteristically within the cell cytoplasm. (Shorr × OI) (B) Multiple spores identified by Gomori × 160. (Courtesy Dr Viero RM, Dept Pathology, Faculdade de Medicina de Botucato UNESP, Brazil)

lymphadenopathy, which results from a granulomatous reaction. Epithelioid cells, multinucleated giant cells, neutrophils and eosinophils are found in varying numbers. The diagnosis is established by identification of multiple budding spores, 5–15 μm in diameter, with birefringent cell membranes[51]. A Gomori-Grocott silver stain will readily identify the spores.

Histoplasmosis *(Fig. 19.14)*

Histoplasmosis is another fungal infection that can give rise to a granulomatous reaction. The yeast form is oval and 2–3 μm in diameter and resides in the cytoplasm of macrophages.

Cryptococcosis

Cryptococcosis is also one of the fungal infections that may lead to a granulomatous reaction in lymph nodes. However most cases present with an inflammatory infiltrate dominated by neutrophils and histiocytes.

Actinomycosis

Actinomycosis, the condition caused by filamentous bacterial organisms of the Actinomyces species, is a further source of granulomatous inflammation to be considered in the differential diagnosis[52]. The organisms are best shown by Gram stain.

Foreign body granulomas

Talc, silicone or beryllium can induce massive lymphadenopathy which is clinically impossible to differentiate from metastatic lymph node disease. The aspirated material consists mainly of giant cells containing foreign body particles, together with lymphocytes of mature type and mononuclear histiocytes[53,54]. Antibodies to vimentin, and epithelial, lymphoid, melanocytic and myogenic differentiation markers should be used to corroborate the diagnosis.

Malignant lymphomas

Introduction

Malignant lymphomas are divided into two major categories: Hodgkin's disease and non-Hodgkin's lymphomas. They can be further divided into several subgroups, which are important to identify because of their different clinical behaviour. Hodgkin's disease is most commonly subclassified according to the Rye scheme which was proposed in 1966[55] which also is followed in the recent REAL classification[56].

The classification of non-Hodgkin's lymphomas has been more controversial. The Kiel classification propounded in 1975 and the 1982 Working Formulation have been the two most commonly used schemes for this group of tumours[57,58]. Histological assessment of architectural and cytological features has traditionally formed the basis for all of the classifications. The updated Kiel classification, published in 1988, also incorporated data from immunophenotypic analysis[59]. In the REAL (revised European-American classification of lymphoid neoplasms) an attempt was made to define clinical relevant subgroups of lymphomas that could be recognized with available morphological, immunological and genetic techniques[56].

The role of cytology in lymphoma diagnosis

Much effort has been spent on the diagnosis of malignant lymphomas by FNA, attempts which have until recently been only partially successful. One major reason for this is that most neoplastic lymphoid cells lack the traditional cytological features of malignancy. Such cells are close replicas of their benign counterparts. In many instances the cytological diagnosis therefore rests on evaluation of whether or not the smears show a spectrum of cells in proportions typical of benign conditions.

If the aspirate is composed of only one cell type a confident diagnosis of non-Hodgkin's lymphoma can usually be made. However, some lymphomas are composed of several types of neoplastic cells, while others contain a confusing admixture of benign lymphoid cells with neoplastic elements, which obviously obscures the picture. The complexity of such smears may be an overwhelming task even for the most experienced cytopathologist. In the case of Hodgkin's lymphoma the finding of large atypical cells with multilobated nuclei has been considered diagnostic.

At present, no system of classification has been constructed for aspiration cytology material. From published data, it seems clear that histological diagnosis based on the Kiel classification correlates very well with FNA findings[60]. This partly results from the fact that the Kiel classification has only two subgroups in which growth pattern is of importance for diagnosis and choice of therapy. In contrast, the Working Formulation uses growth pattern as a diagnostic criterion for six subgroups, making correlation with FNA material more difficult to achieve. In the REAL classification system there is much greater emphasis on cytomorphology, immunophenotyping and molecular studies. Growth pattern, whether nodular or diffuse, contributes to diagnosis in only one subtype. Thus this system will allow a conclusive diagnosis and subtyping of most lymphomas on cytological material if the morphological evaluation is combined with immunophenotypic studies.

The diagnosis and subclassification of Hodgkin's disease have been attempted on aspirated material[61-63]. Again, the classification schemes in current use are based on both architectural and cytological features in excised tissue, making their application to FNA material somewhat difficult.

The reported accuracy of cytological diagnosis and classification of lymphomas on FNA samples varies between 10–90%[64,65]. Not surprisingly, this degree of variation has impeded the acceptance of FNA cytology as the sole diagnostic modality in patients with suspected lymphoma. However, as previously pointed out, FNA cytology is more readily accepted for evaluation of patients with suspected recurrent lymphoma, or deep-seated primary lymphomas. This attitude is somewhat puzzling since the diagnostic difficulties encountered in these special circumstances are identical irrespective of the fact that the lymphoma is primary or recurrent, superficial or deep-seated.

The recent use of adjunctive techniques such as immunocytochemistry, cytogenetics and DNA hybridization has greatly increased the utility of cytological material for conclusive diagnosis of lymphoma. In fact, cytology specimens seem ideal for immunological evaluation; recent studies indicate great diagnostic accuracy if the cytological findings are combined with immunophenotyping and clonal restriction analysis[7-11].

Hodgkin's disease

Clinical background

Hodgkin's disease accounts for approximately 1% of all malignancies in the Western world. It shows a bimodal age incidence curve with the first peak between 20–30 years of age, followed by a decline to about 50 years. After this there is a distinct rise in old age. This bimodal pattern, together with differences in histological subtype, has led to the suggestion that Hodgkin's disease is, in fact, two malignancies. Speculations about the aetiology have included environmental agents, Epstein-Barr virus infection and genetic factors such as impaired immunocompetence.

Most patients present with lymphadenopathy which affects cervical nodes in approximately 60% of cases. Axillary or inguinal nodes are less often the primary site, accounting for 15% of cases each. Systemic symptoms such as weight loss, fever, itching and night sweats are relatively common.

The histological diagnosis of Hodgkin's disease rests on the identification of mononuclear Hodgkin's cells and giant cells with lobated nuclei, the so-called Reed-Sternberg cells. These two cell types can occur in different background settings, and it is the settings that form the basis for subtyping. Histologically the subtypes acknowledged in the REAL classification are[56]:

I   Lymphocyte predominance
II   Nodular sclerosis
III Mixed cellularity
IV   Lymphocyte depletion
V   Provisional entity: lymphocyte rich classical Hodgkin's disease

These subgroups can often be identified in smears of aspirates by evaluation of the proportion of large atypical cells and reactive cells[61-64,66].

The subtyping of Hodgkin's disease has clinical relevance with respect to prognosis. The nodular variant of the lymphocyte predominant type has an excellent prognosis sometimes even when untreated. This favourable prognosis, and recent findings that the Reed-Sternberg-like cells in this subgroup are B cells with polytypic light chain expression, strongly suggest that this entity is not a neoplastic disorder[67]. Of the other subtypes, nodular sclerosis has been reported to have the best and lymphocyte depletion the worst prognosis.

It is important to realize that the histopathological identification of Hodgkin's disease can be difficult. Cases of non-Hodgkin's lymphoma may be misdiagnosed as Hodgkin's disease. This problem seems to occur most often in the diffuse lymphocyte predominant and the lymphocyte depleted subgroups. If cases of non-Hodgkin's lymphoma can be completely excluded, the prognostic differences between the subgroups of Hodgkin's disease diminishes. In addition, recent studies suggest that stage of disease, i.e. the extent of spread, rather than subtype is the most important prognostic factor[68]. As a consequence, the current choice of treatment is often based on tumour extension, irrespective of histological subtype.

Several other neoplasms both of lymphoid and non-lymphoid origin may present with a morphological picture indistinguishable from that of Hodgkin's disease. It is therefore important that the morphological diagnosis is confirmed by immunocytochemistry.

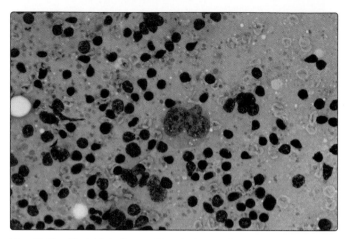

Fig. 19.15   Hodgkin's disease. Note the large mirror-image binucleated lymphoid cell of Reed-Sternberg type with a mixed population of lymphoid cells in the background. (MGG × OI)

Cytological findings *(Figs 19.15–19.19)*

▶ Hodgkin's cells are large mononuclear cells with a prominent nucleolus and abundant cytoplasm
▶ The Reed-Sternberg cell has variable cytology, with abundant pale grey cytoplasm on MGG. Characteristically, the nucleus is bilobed or multilobated with distinct nucleoli. The identification of Hodgkin's and Reed-Sternberg cells is highly suggestive of Hodgkin's lymphoma
▶ In smears, the lymphocyte predominant form can be identified by the large number of small lymphocytes with few diagnostic atypical cells. Reed-Sternberg cells are rarely seen
▶ In nodular sclerosis the smears are often poorly cellular and contain fibroblasts, eosinophils and collagen fragments, in addition to the diagnostic Hodgkin's and Reed-Sternberg cells
▶ Mixed cellularity Hodgkin's disease has a more complex cell pattern with lymphocytes, eosinophils, histiocytes and plasma cells along with a varying number of atypical cells
▶ The lymphocyte depleted subtype demonstrates a paucity of lymphocytes with a relative predominance of large atypical cells

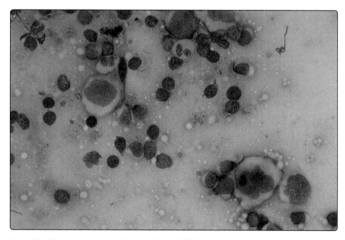

Fig. 19.16   Hodgkin's disease. This field includes large mononuclear cells with abundant cytoplasm and prominent nucleoli. These are Hodgkin's cells. A Reed-Sternberg cell is also seen. (MGG × OI)

Diagnostic pitfalls

The differential diagnosis includes non-Hodgkin's lymphoma, infectious mononucleosis and metastatic lymph node involvement. The greatest of these diagnostic dilemmas occurs with large cell anaplastic Ki-1 positive lymphomas, T cell-rich B-cell lymphomas and peripheral T-cell lymphomas of mixed type. Each of these can present with large atypical cells, some of which are binucleate or multinucleated, in a background of lymphocytes and eosinophils. Using cytomorphology alone, these lymphomas may be indistinguishable from Hodgkin's

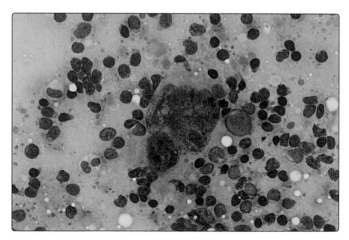

Fig. 19.17   Hodgkin's disease. At the centre there is a giant cell with a large multilobated nucleus with many huge nucleoli. This is a variant of the Reed-Sternberg cell. (MGG × OI)

disease. However, phenotyping will disclose their true nature. The importance of separating these lymphomas from Hodgkin's disease lies in their differing clinical courses.

The cytological identification of infectious mononucleosis can be exceedingly difficult. Immunocytochemistry should therefore always supplement the cytological diagnosis. Metastasis from non-lymphoid tumours such as poorly-differentiated carcinomas from nasopharynx or the tonsil, melanomas, large cell carcinomas or seminomas can occasionally cause diagnostic problems. However, knowledge of the existence and type of a primary malignancy will be helpful in selecting antibodies for immunological confirmation.

The rare suppurative variant of Hodgkin's disease can be difficult to diagnose on FNA smears due to the paucity of tumour cells in a heavy background of granulocytes and cell debris[69-71].

Immunocytochemistry *(Fig. 19.20)*

Both Hodgkin's and Reed-Sternberg cells are CD30 (Ki-1) and CD15 (Leu-M1) positive[66]. No positivity should be observed for antibodies to CD45 which is the leucocyte common antigen (LCA), nor to pan-T and pan-B markers. Demonstrating the antigenic profile of the large atypical

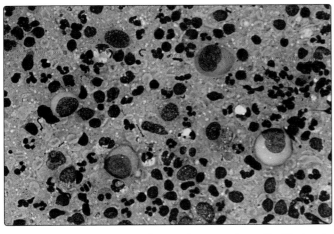

Fig. 19.18 Hodgkin's disease. Scattered mononuclear cells with abundant cytoplasm and indistinct nucleoli can be seen. These are variants of the Hodgkin's cell. (MGG × OI)

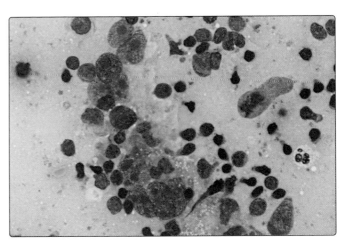

Fig. 19.19 Infectious mononucleosis. Large atypical lymphoid cells with prominent nucleoli present. Cytologically, these cells are indistinguishable from those observed in Hodgkin's lymphoma. (MGG × OI)

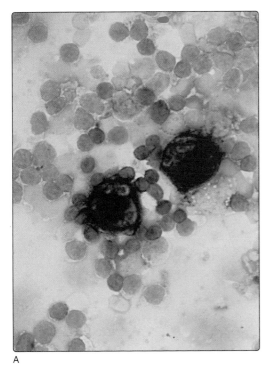

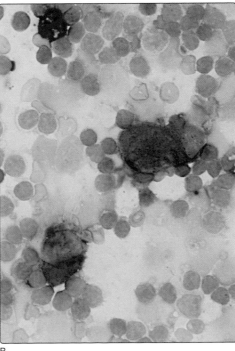

Fig. 19.20 Hodgkin's disease. Immunocytochemistry on cytospin preparations of lymph node FNA. The large atypical cells are positive for: (A) CD30/Ber H2 and (B) CD15/Leu M1. (× OI)

A

B

513

cells is sometimes difficult in cytospin preparations, because the diagnostic cells are fragile and often occur in low numbers. Careful scrutiny of the immunological stains should reveal the phenotype of the diagnostic cells in a majority of cases.

Large cell anaplastic Ki-1 lymphomas are CD30 (Ki-1) and CD45 (LCA) positive but CD15 (Leu-M1) negative. Many of these lymphomas are also positive for pan-T markers and EMA. The large atypical cells in T cell-rich B-cell lymphomas are monoclonal B cells. They do not express CD15 (Leu-M1). In infectious mononucleosis the large atypical cells are either T cells or polytypic B cells.

Non-Hodgkin's lymphoma

Clinical background

The non-Hodgkin's lymphomas comprise 2–3% of all malignancies in developed countries. They represent a spectrum of neoplasms ranging from indolent to aggressive tumours, the latter having a rapidly fatal course. The age specific incidence increases throughout life. Their aetiology remains unknown but environmental factors, virus infections and genetic abnormalities are all considered of importance.

The clinical presentation of non-Hodgkin's lymphoma shows an extremely variable pattern. Many patients seek medical advice because of a tumour mass which may be nodal or extranodal. General symptoms such as weight loss, fever, infections and lethargy are common and may be the initial complaint. Often, patients have widespread disease with bone marrow involvement at the time of diagnosis.

The histological diagnosis and method of classification has long been a matter of debate. Today most pathologists use the REAL classification[56] which is summarized in Table 19.1. The subheadings used in this chapter in the descriptions of the different lymphomas refer to the REAL classification. Its various elements are correlated with comparable terms from the Kiel classification, given in brackets underneath the main headings.

The REAL classification is based both on morphology, immunocytochemistry and sometimes genetic techniques as well as clinical features. B and T cell derived lymphomas are morphologically subclassified in entities which also have clinical relevance. Thus some subtypes tend to follow an indolent course but are usually ultimately fatal, while others are rapidly progressive, but potentially curable if vigorously treated.

General cytological approach

Cytological evaluation of FNA smears from non-Hodgkin's lymphomas includes:

▶ *Identification of the various cell types present.* To evaluate a lymph node smear it is essential to recognize normal lymphoid cells at all stages of development. Figure 19.1 depicts the lymphoid cell types as seen in an air-dried, MGG stained FNA smear of a benign lymph node

Table 19.1 The Revised European American Lymphoma (REAL) classification of non-Hodgkin's lymphoma and corresponding Kiel classification

REAL classification	Kiel classification
Precursor B-lymphoblastic lymphoma/leukaemia	B-lymphoblastic
Small lymphocytic (SLL/CLL)	Lymphoplasmacytic immunocytoma
Mantle cell lymphoma	Centrocytic
Follicular centre lymphoma, follicular (grade1, 2)	Centroblastic-centrocytic, follicular
Follicular centre lymphoma, follicular (grade 3)	Centroblastic, follicular
Marginal zone/MALT	Monocytoid, immunocytoma
Hairy cell leukaemia	Hairy cell leukaemia
Plasmacytoma/myeloma	Plasmacytic
Diffuse large B-cell lymphoma	Centroblastic, B-immunoblastic
Burkitt's; Burkitt's like lymphoma	Burkitt's lymphoma
Precursor T lymphoblastic lymphoma/leukaemia	T-lymphoblastic
T-cell CLL	T-lymphocytic, CLL type
Mycosis fungoides/ Sezary syndrome	Mycosis fungoides/ Sezary syndrome
Peripheral T-cell lymphomas	T-zone, pleomorphic T-cell lymphomas
Angioimmunoblastic T-cell lymphoma	Angioimmunoblastic
Adult T-cell lymphoma/leukaemia	Pleomorphic T-cell, HTLV1+
Anaplastic large cell lymphoma	T-large cell anaplastic (Ki-1)

▶ *Estimation of the proportion of the various cell types.* A monotonous pattern is present when one cell type predominates but even so, additional cell types can be found in low numbers. Such a monotonous composition indicates abnormal expansion of one, or at the most two subtypes of the lymphoid population. This pattern is seen in almost all B-cell lymphomas and some T-cell neoplasms. A heterogeneous mixture of lymphocytes indicates stimulation of the entire lymphoid cell population. This suggests reactive lymphadenitis, but a few B-cell neoplasms and some T-cell lymphomas show a similar pattern

▶ *Evaluation of individual cell characteristics, such as size and nuclear atypia.* It should, however, be pointed out that most lymphoma cells are faithful replicas of their normal counterparts. Distinct nuclear atypia is thus relatively rare and most often seen in large cell lymphomas

Immunocytochemistry

As previously mentioned, it is important that the morphological assessment of a lymph node aspirate is accompanied by an immunological work-up. In the authors' laboratory this approach has led to an improvement in the rate of conclusive diagnosis from approximately 70% to over 95%.

Cytospin preparations or suspensions for flow cytometry are used for assessment of phenotype to establish whether the cells are T or B in origin, and whether clonal restriction of light chain production is present. In Western countries most lymphomas are of B-cell lineage with immunoglobulin light chain expression restricted to either kappa or lambda. Clonal expansion in T-cell lymphomas is more difficult to demonstrate. Loss of pan-T cell subtype antigen or anomalous expression of T cell subset antigens can be taken as evidence of clonality.

The initial immunological work-up should be based on a preliminary cytological evaluation. A diagnosis of reactive hyperplasia or B-cell lymphoma should entail a limited panel of antibodies to include pan-T and pan-B antibodies as well as antibodies to the light chains, Bcl-2 and the cALLa (common acute lymphoblastic leukaemia antigen). A kappa:lambda ratio below 6:1 or lambda:kappa ratio not exceeding 3:1 strongly favours a polyclonal reactive B-cell population. Values exceeding these figures suggest a monoclonal malignant expansion of B cells. The subclassification of the B-cell lymphomas sometimes requires the additional staining with antibodies to CD5, CD23 and CD43[56].

The common acute lymphoblastic leukaemia antigen (cALLa or CD10) is expressed in some mixed cell lymphomas and large cell tumours. A majority of high-grade lymphomas are readily diagnosed as large cell neoplasms in cytological preparations, and in these cases immunocytochemistry is needed only to phenotype the neoplastic cells.

In contrast, a conclusive cytological diagnosis of many low-grade T-cell lymphomas is extremely difficult. The lack of strict immunological criteria for monoclonality further compounds this diagnostic dilemma. As in histopathology, such cases will require T-cell receptor (TCR) gene rearrangement analysis to prove that the process is neoplastic.

Gene rearrangement analysis

Immunoglobulin (Ig) or TCR gene rearrangement is present in almost all lymphoid malignancies. Tumours which display an immunological B-cell phenotype most often show rearrangements of Ig genes. A pattern of TCR rearrangements is consistent with a T-cell lineage. FNA material from both B and T-cell lymphomas has been used for analysis of gene rearrangement[23–29].

The sensitivity of these techniques allows the detection of a neoplastic population as low as 1–5% of the total cell sample[23,72]. Such methods are thus important in the diagnosis of some lymphoid malignancies. Some authorities would argue that they should be part of the diagnostic armamentarium in all laboratories that evaluate patients with lymphoproliferative disorders.

Proliferation rate

The fraction of proliferating cells in non-Hodgkin's lymphomas is correlated to prognosis and response to chemotherapy. Several methods are available to estimate the proliferation rate. Mitotic counting is time consuming and inaccurate. Flow cytometry is a rapid and accurate technique but is not available in all laboratories. Staining with Ki-67 antibody or antibodies to proliferating cell nuclear antigen (PCNA) offers a highly sensitive procedure which can be performed in most laboratories. The Ki-67 antibody stains cells in late G, S, M and G2 phase[73]. It thus gives a figure which is approximately three times higher than methods which are selective for cells in S phase or mitosis.

Diagnostic criteria for B-cell lymphomas (REAL classification)

Lymphocytic lymphoma and chronic lymphatic leukaemia (B-lymphocytic, CLL)

Cytological findings *(Fig. 19.21)*

The smears are composed of round lymphoid cells with a small rim of cytoplasm. The nucleus is somewhat larger than that of a mature lymphoid cell. The chromatin pattern is irregular and clumped. Mitoses are rare. A few prolymphocytes as well as blasts and macrophages may be present.

The differential diagnosis includes reactive hyperplasia, immunocytoma, CLL of T cell type and centroblastic/centrocytic lymphoma with a predominance of centrocytes. In patients without bone marrow involvement a correct diagnosis is often impossible without the aid of immunocytochemistry.

Immunocytochemistry *(Fig. 19.22)*

The expression of B-cell antigens and light chain restriction are usually weak. CD5, CD23 and CD43 are positive. The fraction of proliferating cells is low — less than 10% as measured by Ki-67 antibody staining.

Lymphoplasmacytoid lymphoma, immunocytoma (Immunocytoma)

Cytological findings *(Fig. 19.23)*

The predominant cell is slightly larger than a mature lymphocyte. It has an eccentric nucleus with a plasma cell-like chromatin pattern. The cytoplasm is basophilic and more abundant than that seen in CLL. Additional cells such as plasma cells, mast cells and a few immunoblasts are regularly observed. On morphology alone, this subtype is difficult to differentiate from some reactive conditions as well as CLL.

In some variants a substantial fraction of mature plasma cells are seen. The distinction from an extramedullary plasmacytoma can thus be difficult, but if more than 50% of the population consists of plasma cells it is likely to be a plasmacytoma.

Some lymphomas may show an admixture of plasma cells; such cases are classified according to major features in the REAL classification.

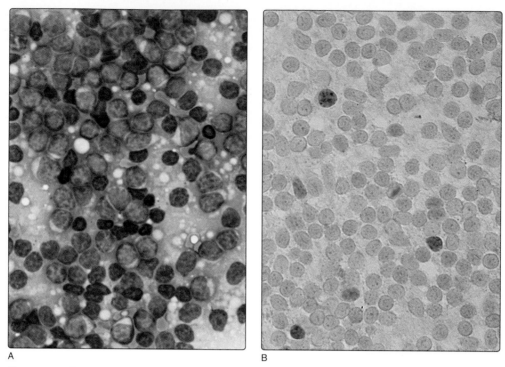

A   B

Fig. 19.21   Chronic lymphatic leukaemia. (A) Small to medium sized cells with sparse cytoplasm are present. (MGG × OI) (B) Ki-67 staining shows a low proliferation rate. (Immunoperoxidase × OI)

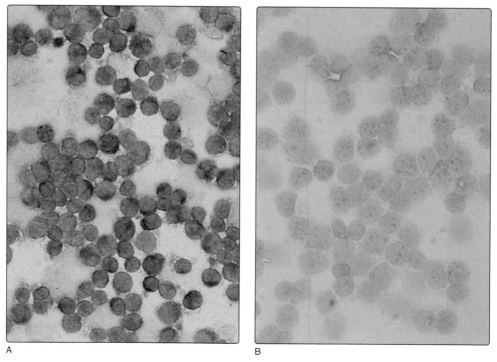

A   B

Fig. 19.22   Chronic lymphatic leukaemia. Immunocytochemistry on cytospin preparation from aspirate shown in **Fig. 19.21**. (A) The cells are monoclonal for kappa. (B) No positivity for lambda staining. (Alkaline phosphatase × OI)

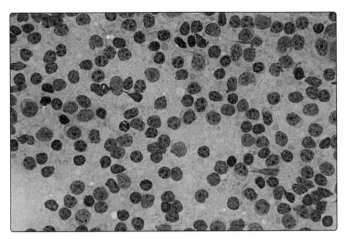

Fig. 19.23 Lymphoplasmacytoid lymphoma/Immunocytoma. Small monotonous cells with eccentric nuclei and typical chromatin pattern. (MGG × OI)

Immunocytochemistry

The expression of B-cell antigens varies, and some cases react with only weak positivity, but light chain restriction is readily demonstrated. CD5 and CD10 are not expressed. The fraction of proliferating cells varies from a few per cent to as high as 20%. Plasmacytomas usually have between 25–50% proliferating cells.

Mantle cell lymphoma (centrocytic/mantle cell lymphoma)

Cytological findings (Fig 19.24)

The smears are monotonous composed of small to medium-sized lymphoid cells, slightly larger than lymphocytes. The nuclei are cleaved and have a dispersed chromatin, inconspicuous nucleoli and a thin pale cytoplasm[74,75].

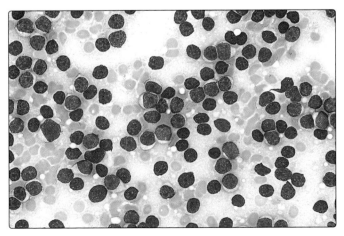

Fig. 19.24 Mantle cell lymphoma. Small to medium sized cells with round nucleus and pale cytoplasm. (MGG × OI)

In rare cases the cells are immature with larger nuclei and high proliferation rate. Because of resemblance to lymphoblastic lymphoma the term 'lymphoblastoid' or 'blastoid' variant has been proposed[56,76].

Immunocytochemistry (Fig 19.25)

The cells are of B phenotype (CD20) with light chain restriction. In addition the cells are consistently CD5 and CD43 positive and most often CD10 negative. The fraction of proliferating cells is usually low, around 10% as measured by Ki-67 (Mib-1). The 'blastoid' variant has a high proliferation rate.

Cytogenetics

Translocation t(11;14) is observed in a majority of cases.

Follicle centre lymphoma (centroblastic–centrocytic and centroblastic follicular pattern)

Cytological findings (Fig. 19.26)

The predominating cell is the medium sized centrocyte which has little cytoplasm and an irregular cleaved or angulated nucleus. These cells often lack cytoplasm and may seem to form aggregates. Centroblasts are present but the proportion varies. It has been suggested that follicular centre lymphomas are subdivided into grades I, II and III based on the proportion of large cells present[56]. However no criteria for this grading was given which obviously will severely reduce its reproducibility.

Other cell types present in CB/CC lymphomas are small mature non-neoplastic lymphoid cells and macrophages. A smear with a high number of non-neoplastic cells may be impossible to differentiate from reactive lymphadenopathy unless cytomorphology is complemented by immunocytochemical evaluation.

Immunocytochemistry (Figs 19.27, 19.28)

The B-cell lineage of these tumour cells is readily identified by light chain restriction. Light chain restriction can usually be demonstrated as well as positive staining for CD10 (cALLa). Mature reactive T cells are present, and may constitute up to 50% of the lymphoid population. The proliferation fraction in the neoplastic B-cells varies considerably from case to case. Figures below 5% are seldom seen but in occasional cases up to 50% of the neoplastic population may react positively to proliferation markers. Such cases show aggressive behaviour and should be treated as high-grade lymphomas irrespective of their cytological classification.

Cytogenetics

A majority of these lymphomas show a t(14;18) translocation.

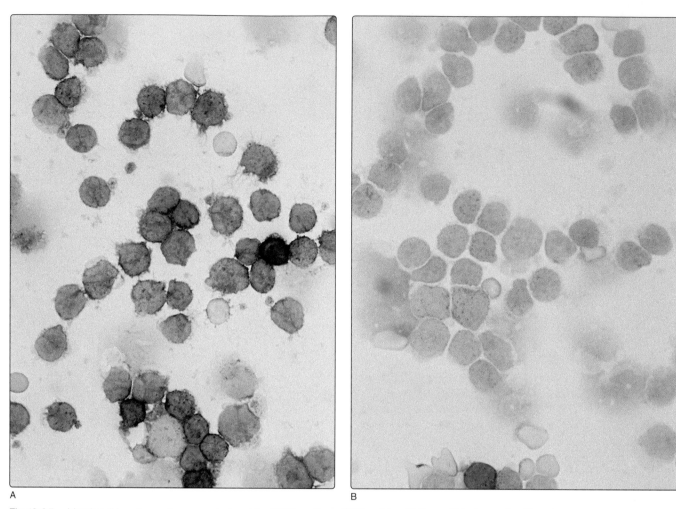

A

B

Fig 19.25   Mantle cell lymphoma. Immunocytochemistry. (A) The cells are CD5 positive. (B) No positivity is seen for CD10. (Alkaline phosphatase × OI)

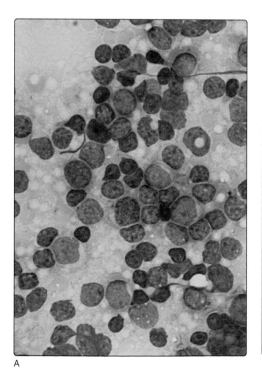

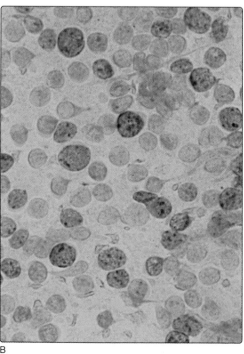

A

B

Fig. 19.26   Follicle centre lymphoma. (A) There is a predominance of medium sized cells with irregular cleaved nuclei. Some larger centroblasts are seen. (MGG × OI) (B) Ki-67 shows proliferation of both centrocytes and centroblasts. (Immunoperoxidase × OI)

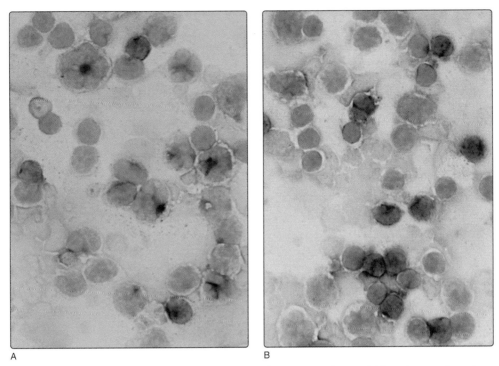

A

B

Fig. 19.27 Follicle centre lymphoma. Immunocytochemistry on cytospin material from the case shown in **Fig. 19.26**. (A) The cleaved centrocytes and centroblasts are of B phenotype. (B) Small mature cells of T phenotype are relatively frequent. (Alkaline phosphatase × OI)

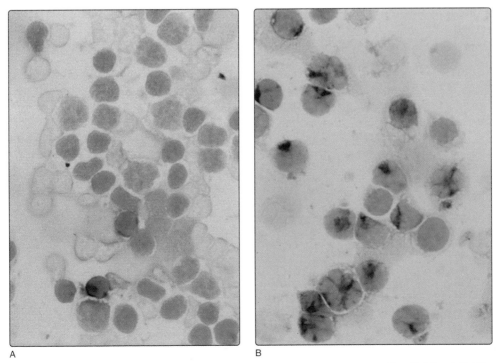

A

B

Fig. 19.28 Follicle centre lymphoma. Immunocytochemistry from the same case as Figs **19.26** and **19.27**. (A) Only a few mature cells are kappa positive. (B) Monoclonal expression of lambda light chain. (Alkaline phosphatase × OI)

Marginal zone B-cell lymphoma (monocytoid B-cell, immunocytoma)

Cytological findings

The tumour cell population is dominated by small to medium sized cells, the marginal zone cell, which is centrocyte-like but with indistinct nucleoli and a more abundant cytoplasm[77]. Plasma cells, centroblasts and some monocytoid B cells are often present.

Immunocytochemistry

The tumour cells are of B phenotype and show light chain restriction but no expression of CD5, CD10, CD23 or CD43. The plasma cells are often monoclonal. The proliferation rate is usually low.

Plasmacytoma/myeloma

Cytological findings (Fig. 19.29)

The neoplastic cell may have a morphology almost identical to that of a normal plasma cell but usually show atypia such as enlarged pleomorphic nuclei, double nuclei and large irregular cytoplasm.

Immunocytochemistry (Fig. 19.30)

The cells lack expression of most B-cell antigens but show light chain restriction and are CD38 positive.

Diffuse large B-cell lymphoma (centroblastic, immunoblastic and large cell anaplastic)

Cytological findings (Figs 19.31–19.33)

The most common type of this subgroup is composed of large round centroblasts. The nuclei are only slightly irregular and show several small nucleoli, often at the nuclear membrane. The cytoplasm is scanty and may contain a few vacuoles. In addition, a number of other cells such as centrocytes, small mature lymphocytes and macrophages may be found.

Another type in this subgroup is the polymorphic centroblastic lymphoma which contains immunoblasts in addition to centroblasts. Some centrocytes and small mature cells are regularly observed.

In some lymphomas of this subgroup the cell population is composed of mostly immunoblasts. These are large cells with an eccentric nucleus with unevenly distributed chromatin and a central distinct nucleolus. The cytoplasm is abundant with a greyish blue staining in MGG. Rarely, poorly-differentiated carcinomas or melanomas may on cytomorphology be misdiagnosed as this variant of lymphoma.

An uncommon variant is the multilobated centroblastic lymphoma, in which the cells are polymorphic with multilobated, sometimes bizarre nuclei. Such cases may be difficult to identify as lymphoid in origin, and to distinguish from other high-grade neoplasms.

T-cell rich B-cell lymphomas are also included in this subgroup[56]. They can be mistaken morphologically for Hodgkin's lymphoma but immunological characterization will identify the monotypic B phenotype of the large atypical cells[78]

Immunocytochemistry (Figs 19.34–19.38)

The cells often express several B antigens such as CD19, CD20 and CD22. Kappa or lambda light chains are expressed in most cases and CD10 positivity is common in the centroblastic variants. A population of mature T cells is regularly present. The fraction of proliferating cells is usually around 50% or more, which predicts relatively aggressive clinical behaviour. The multilobated subtype often runs a rapid clinical course which is reflected in a proliferation fraction often exceeding 80%.

The immunoblasts are CD38 (OKT 10) negative, which differentiates them from those of a polymorphic myeloma (plasmacytosarcoma). The fraction of proliferating cells is usually above 75%.

Burkitt's lymphoma (Burkitt's or Burkitt-like lymphoma)

Cytological findings (Fig. 19.39)

The Burkitt cells have a low nuclear/cytoplasmic ratio. They have deep blue cytoplasm on MGG staining which contains many punched out vacuoles.

The nuclei are convoluted or lobated and the chromatin is fine and nucleoli are often absent.

Immunocytochemistry

The B-cell lineage of Burkitt's lymphoma is often revealed by light chain restriction and expression of IgM. Some cases are of B-cell lineage but may not express light chains. The CD10 antigen (cALLa) is usually expressed. The fraction of Ki-67 positive cells is above 75%.

Cytogenetics

Most cases have a t(8;14) translocation but t(2;8) and t(8;22) translocations also occur.

Diagnostic criteria for T-cell lymphomas (REAL Classification)

Peripheral T-cell lymphomas (chronic lymphocytic leukaemia, T cell CLL)

Cytological findings

The cytological presentation in smears is similar to that of the B cell type, but the cells show more nuclear irregularity

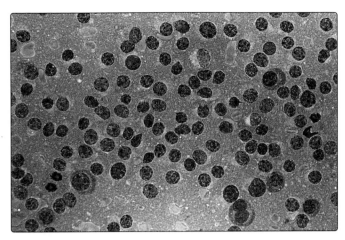

Fig. 19.29 Plasmacytoma. Many naked nuclei and some eccentric nucleus and distinct basophilic cytoplasm. (MGG × OI)

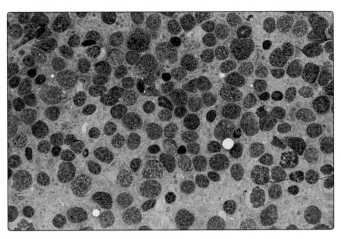

Fig. 19.31 Large B-cell lymphoma. Centroblastic variant. Note the predominance of large rounded centroblasts. (MGG × OI)

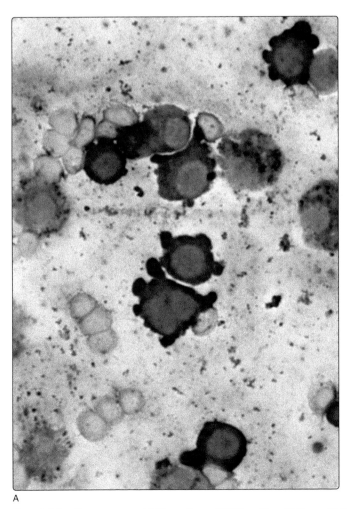

A

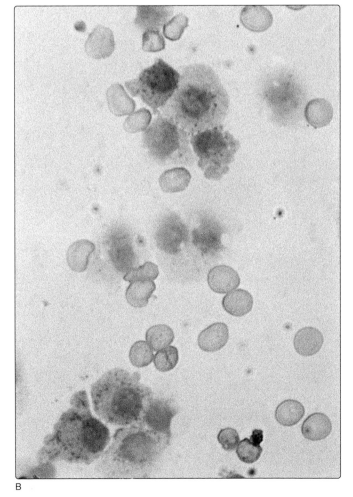

B

Fig. 19.30 Plasmacytoma. (A) The cells are CD38 positive. (B) No positivity for CD20. (Alkaline phosphatase × OI)

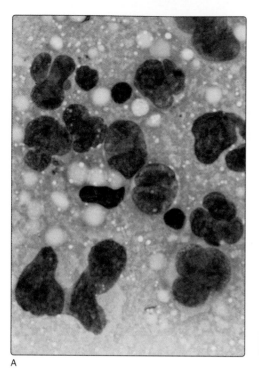
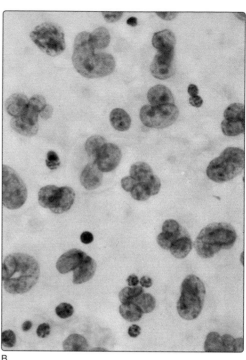

A   B

Fig. 19.32   Large B-cell lymphoma of multilobated type. There are large cells with characteristic polymorphic multilobated nuclei. ((A) MGG and (B) Papanicolaou × OI)

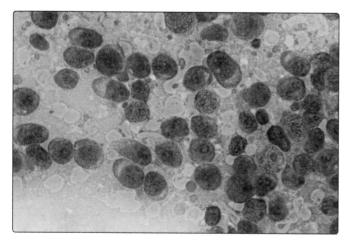

Fig. 19.33   Large B-cell lymphoma of immunoblastic type. The field consists almost entirely of large cells with eccentric nuclei and strongly basophilic cytoplasm. (MGG × OI)

and more abundant cytoplasm. The differential diagnostic considerations are the same as for the B cell variant.

Immunocytochemistry

T-cell antigens (CD2,3,5,7) are readily demonstrated. In most cases less than 10% of cells are Ki-67 positive.

Cytogenetics

Clonal rearrangement of TCR genes can be demonstrated.

Mycosis fungoides

Cytological findings *(Fig. 19.40)*

Lymph node involvement usually occurs late in this disease which initially affects the skin. In lymph node FNAs the predominant cells are small to medium sized and have irregular 'folded' nuclei. Large atypical cells resembling Hodgkin's cells can occasionally be observed. CLL, centrocyte predominant follicle centre lymphoma and Hodgkin's lymphoma may all simulate mycosis fungoides. However, the clinical presentation as well as the immunologic characterization should prevent mistakes.

Immunocytochemistry *(Figs 19.41, 19.42)*

The cells are of T helper phenotype and only a few suppressor cells can be found. The large atypical cells are also of T helper phenotype and express the CD30 (Ki-1) antigen, which sometimes makes them difficult to distinguish from true Ki-1 lymphoma cells. The proliferation rate is low in the population of small cells.

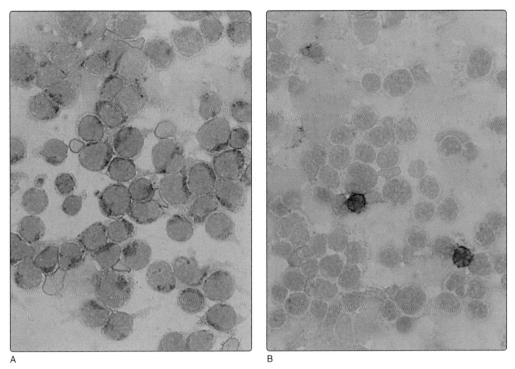

A   B

Fig. 19.34   Large B-cell lymphoma, centroblastic variant. Immunocytochemistry on aspirate shown in **Fig. 19.31**. (A) All large cells are of B phenotype. (B) A few small mature T cells are also present. (Alkaline phosphatase × OI)

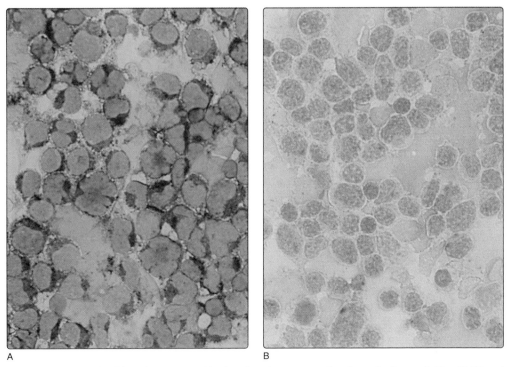

A   B

Fig. 19.35   Large B-cell lymphoma, centroblastic variant. Immunocytochemistry of cells seen in **Figs 19.31** and **19.33**. (A) Monoclonal kappa expression (B) No lambda positivity. (Alkaline phosphatase × OI)

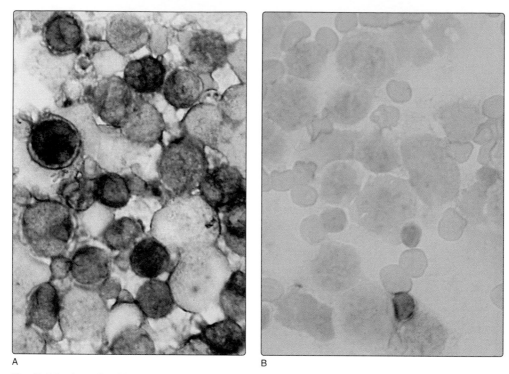

A

B

Fig. 19.36 Large B-cell lymphoma of multilobated type (case shown in **Fig. 19.34**). (A) Immunocytochemistry shows intense kappa expression in all cells. (B) One small mature lambda positive cell is seen. (Alkaline phosphatase × OI)

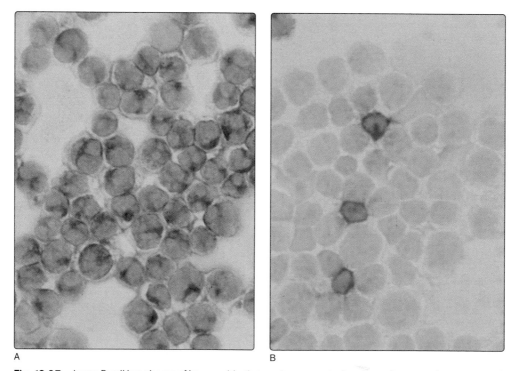

A

B

Fig. 19.37 Large B-cell lymphoma of immunoblastic type. Immunocytochemistry of same aspirate presented in **Fig. 19.34**. (A) The immunoblasts are of B-cell phenotype. (B) Only few small mature T cells are shown. (Alkaline phosphatase × OI)

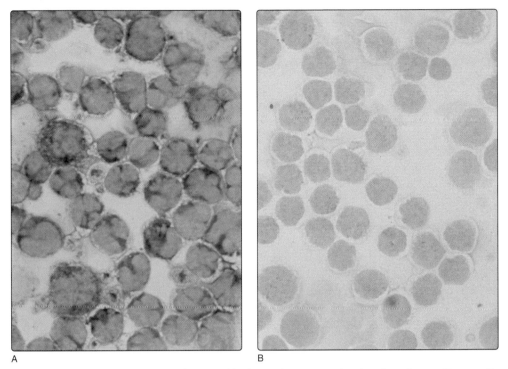

A

B

Fig. 19.38 Large B-cell lymphoma of immunoblastic type. Immunocytochemistry from the case illustrated in **Figs 19.34** and **19.37**. (A) Monoclonal kappa expression (B) No lambda positive cells are present. (Alkaline phosphatase × OI)

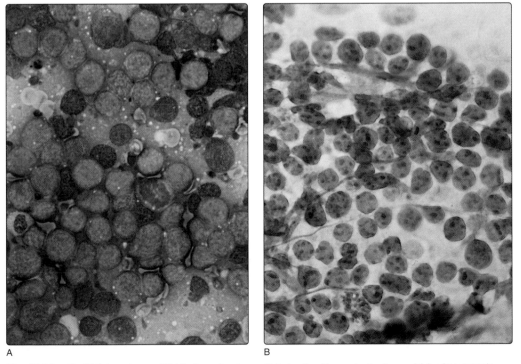

A

B

Fig. 19.39 Burkitt's lymphoma. (A) Medium sized round blast cells with scant cytoplasm which often contain small vacuoles. (MGG × OI) (B) Almost all cells are proliferating as shown by Ki-67 staining. (Immunoperoxidase × OI)

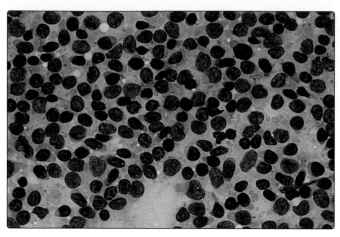

Fig. 19.40 Mycosis fungoides. Small to medium sized cells with irregular nuclei. (MGG × OI)

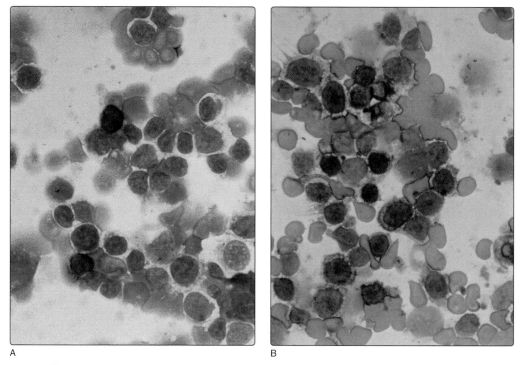

A

B

Fig. 19.41 Mycosis fungoides. Immunocytochemistry on cytospin material from the aspirate shown in **Fig. 19.40** (A) A few small mature B cells are present. (B) The neoplastic cells are of T phenotype. (Alkaline phosphatase × OI)

Peripheral T-cell lymphomas unspecified (T-cell lymphoma/small, medium and large cell, AILD, T-immunoblastic)

Cytological findings (Figs 19.43–19.45)

Aspirates from these lymphomas show a spectrum of atypical cells ranging from small to large. The cells have irregular nuclei often with marked nucleoli and coarse chromatin. Occasional large cells with multilobated or multiple nuclei are often seen. The cytoplasm of the atypical cells is also variable but the medium sized and large cells have a rich cytoplasm which commonly stains pale grey in MGG. Epithelioid cells, plasma cells and eosinophils are present in varying proportions. Fragments of vessels are often found. The cytological presentation of the individual subgroups seems to vary considerably. The rarity of these disorders also contributes to the difficulty of making a conclusive diagnosis on cytological smears alone.

Immunocytochemistry (Fig 19.46)

A majority of the cases are CD4 (T helper) positive.

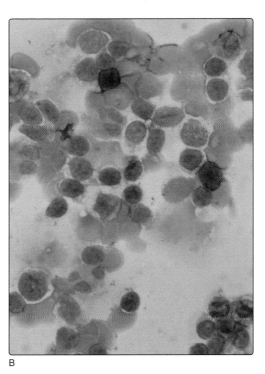

A B

Fig. 19.42 Mycosis fungoides. Immunocytochemistry from the case shown in **Figs 19.40** and **19.41**. (A) The tumour cells are of T helper phenotype. (B) Few T suppressor cells are present. (Alkaline phosphatase × OI)

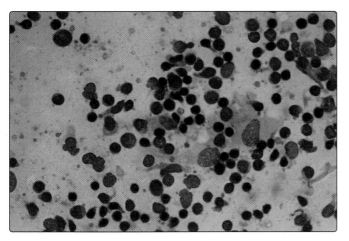

Fig. 19.43 Peripheral T-cell lymphoma. The field illustrated shows small and medium sized irregular lymphoid cells and several histiocytes. (MGG × OI)

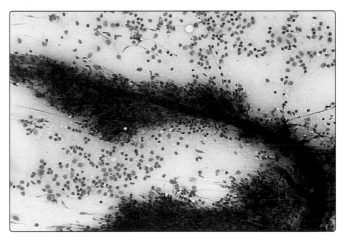

Fig. 19.44 Peripheral T-cell lymphoma of medium to large cell type. The smear shows fragments of vessels in a background of lymphoid cells. (MGG × LP)

Aberrant T-cell antigen expression and deletion of pan-T-antigens strongly indicate a neoplastic lymphoid population. The plasma cells, being reactive, are polyclonal. In keeping with their varying clinical behaviour of this process the proliferation rate varies between 10%-50%.

Cytogenetics
The TCR genes are rearranged in most cases.

Precursor T-lymphoblastic lymphoma/leukaemia (T-lymphoblastic)

Cytological findings

The tumour cells have a round or convoluted nuclei with inconspicuous nucleoli and scant cytoplasm. These cells cannot with certainty be distinguished from those of B-lymphoblastic lymphoma.

Immunocytochemistry

Most cells are CD3, CD7 and TdT positive. The expression of CD2 and CD5 is variable.

Analplastic large cell lymphoma (Large cell anaplastic Ki-1 positive type)

Cytological findings (Fig. 19.47)

The large cells are markedly pleomorphic with multilobated, horseshoe or ring shaped nuclei[79–81]. Their abundant pale grey (MGG) cytoplasm is vacuolated. There is always an admixture of reactive lymphoid cells. The anaplastic large cell lymphoma can be misdiagnosed as Hodgkin's disease, true histiocytic lymphoma or anaplastic carcinoma. However, the cytological presentation of this rare lymphoma is relatively typical and should initiate selection of an appropriate antibody panel to confirm the morphologic impression.

Immunocytochemistry (Fig. 19.48)

The tumour cells show a strong expression of CD30 (Ki-1) antigen. They are also CD45 (LCA) positive and of T helper subtype[82,83]. CD15 (Leu-M1) is characteristically absent.

Some tumours may express EMA but are cytokeratin negative. The ALK protein can be detected in many cases. The reactive background population contains a mixture of T cells and polyclonal B cells. Almost all tumour cells are proliferating, as shown by Ki-67 staining.

Cytogenetics

A t(2;5) translocation seems to be present in 2/3 of the cases.

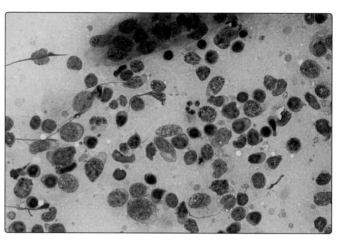

Fig. 19.45 Peripheral T-cell lymphoma of medium to large cell type. Polymorphic lymphoid cells are seen together with a fragment of vessel. (MGG × OI)

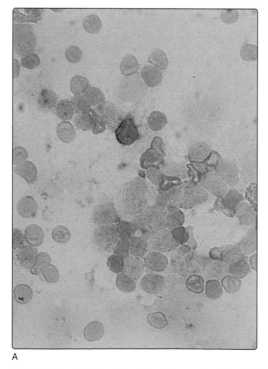

A

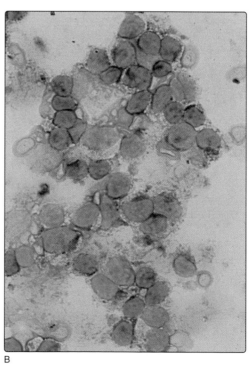

B

Fig. 19.46 Peripheral T-cell lymphoma of medium to large cell type. This illustrates the immunocytochemistry on the aspirate shown in **Fig. 19.45**. (A) One small B cell. (B) The larger polymorphic cells are of T phenotype. (Alkaline phosphatase × OI)

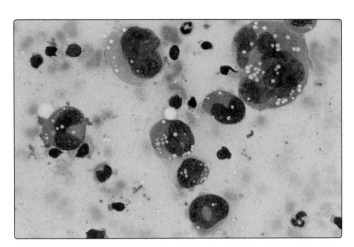

Fig. 19.47 Anaplastic large cell lymphoma. Note the large pleomorphic cells with multilobated or ring-form nuclei and abundant vacuolated cytoplasm. (MGG × OI)

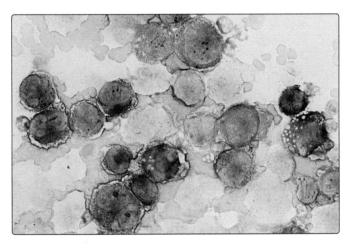

Fig. 19.48 Anaplastic large cell lymphoma. Immunocytochemistry performed on the aspirate shown in **Fig. 19.47**. The cells strongly express CD30/Ki-1. (Alkaline phosphatase × OI)

Metastatic lymph node disease

Introduction

Lymph nodes enlarged by metastatic tumour spread often show diffuse involvement, therefore an FNA biopsy from an involved node will almost invariably result in diagnostic cells. Such foreign cells are in most instances readily identified in a background of lymphoid cells. The diagnostic accuracy of FNA cytology in lymph node metastatic malignancy is high and figures above 90% are usually quoted[84,85].

In previously healthy patients, the cytological identification of a lymph node metastasis results in a search for the primary tumour. This investigation will be focused on various organs depending on factors such as age, sex, site of metastatic node and the cytological features. Table 19.2 summarizes the most frequent metastatic sites for some of the most common malignancies.

Table 19.2 Most frequent metastatic sites of commonest malignancies

Lymph node metastasis in:	Primary tumour most likely in:
Supraclavicular fossa	Breast, lung, gastrointestinal tract, ovary, prostate
Neck (excl. supraclavicular fossa)	Oral cavity, pharynx, salivary glands, thyroid, lung, breast
Axilla	Breast, lung, ovary
Groin	Gynaecological tract, penis, prostate

Table 19.3

Carcinoma CK profile	Possible primary
CK7 + CK20 +	Bladder, pancreas, ovary (mucinous)
CK7 + CK20 −	Breast, ovary, endometrium, thyroid (papillary ca), lung (non small cell)
CK7 − CK20 +	Colorectal
CK7 − CK20 −	Hepatocellular, prostate, renal, lung (squamous and small cell ca).

The search for a primary tumour can be facilitated by immunological characterization of the aspirated cells. In metastases from epithelial tumours the CK7, CK20 profile can often be helpful to focus on possible sites of the primary tumour (Table 19.3). Using an additional limited panel of antibodies it is then often possible to obtain correct information about the primary site (Table 19.4). Unfortunately, some metastases defy all diagnostic efforts and their origin remains obscure. The cytological presentation of different tumours is relatively independent of metastatic site. Hence the following description of various metastases will focus on identification of tumour cell type.

Metastatic epithelial tumours

Cytological findings

Squamous carcinomas *(Figs 19.49, 19.51)*

Squamous carcinomas often yield a mixed pattern. In the well-differentiated type, keratinized cells with blue cytoplasm on MGG staining are the commonest seen. These cells have hyperchromatic nuclei and may show squamous pearl formation. The cellular atypia is often minimal and in such cases the diagnosis may rest on the knowledge that the cells were aspirated from a lymph node.

Some keratinizing carcinomas show liquefaction and a yellow turbid thick material is aspirated from metastatic nodes of this kind. The smears consist largely of inflammatory cells and debris and malignant cells may be sparse, requiring careful search of Papanicolaou stained smears. If such material is aspirated from a neck tumour

Table 19.4   Tumour diagnostic algorithm (cytologically unclassified tumour)

Marker positivity	CK, EMA		LC		HMB 45, S 100, VIM	VIM	
Tumour	Carcinoma		Lymphoma		Melanoma	Sarcoma	
	Marker	*Subtype*	*Marker*	*Subtype*		*Marker*	*Subtype*
	ER	Breast	pan B	B-LY		DESMIN	Rhabdomyo-
	THYROG	Thyroid	pan T	T-LY		NB84	Neuroblastoma
Subtype	PSA	Prostate	Ki-1	Ki-1 LY		CK	Epithelioid cell
	α-FETOP	Liver	α-1-anti-	Histiocyte-LY		FACT-8	Angio-
	CALCITON	Medullary	trypsin			CD99	Ewing/PNET
	NSE	Merkel, Oat cell					
	VIM	Renal cell,					
		Epithelioid sarcoma					
		Spindle cell					
	Ki-1	Embryonal					

CK, Cytokeratin; EMA, Epithelial membrane antigen; LC, Leucocyte common; VIM, Vimentin; ER, Estrogen receptor; THYROG, Thyroglobulin; PSA, Prostate specific antigen; α-FETOP, alpha-fetoprotein; CALCITON, Calcitonin.

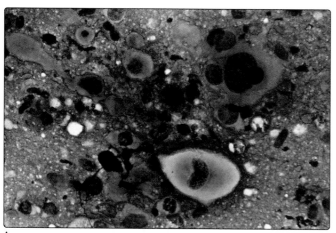

A

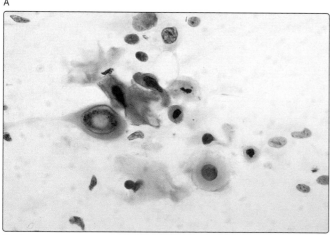

B

Fig. 19.49   Metastatic squamous carcinoma. (A) There are several atypical squamous cells with hyperchromatic nuclei and blue cytoplasm. (MGG × OI) (B) Same aspirate alcohol fixed and Papanicolaou stained. (MGG × OI)

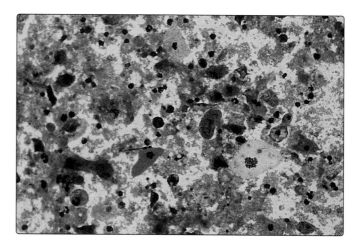

Fig. 19.50   Branchial cyst. Atypical squamous cells and inflammatory cells in a background of cell debris. (MGG × MP)

the possibility of a branchial cleft cyst should be considered (Fig. 19.50). This inflamed epithelium can show some degree of atypia. In the case of a metastatic carcinoma a repeat biopsy from the periphery of the tumour may yield clusters of more immature carcinoma cells.

Aspirates from poorly-differentiated squamous carcinomas yield cohesive fragments of hyperchromatic polymorphic cells. Occasional small keratinized cells can point toward a diagnosis of squamous cell carcinoma but in their absence the cytological picture may be that of an undifferentiated malignant tumour which defies further categorization (Fig. 19.51).

Adenocarcinoma *(Figs 19.52, 19.53)*

These metastases will often disclose their nature by gland formation. The diagnosis of such typical metastases does not present significant problems, but their site of origin may be difficult to determine. In this process additional features might be helpful, for instance, mucin production is often seen in gastrointestinal and lung carcinomas. In metastases from lobular breast carcinomas, some cells may have cytoplasmic lumina with pinkish purple inclusions,

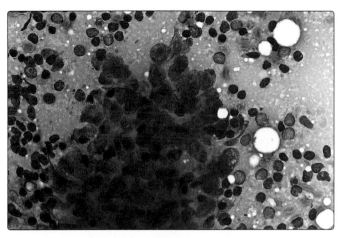

Fig. 19.51 Lymph node metastasis from an undifferentiated squamous cell carcinoma of nasopharynx. Poorly- differentiated cohesive cells with an indistinct cytoplasm. (MGG × OI)

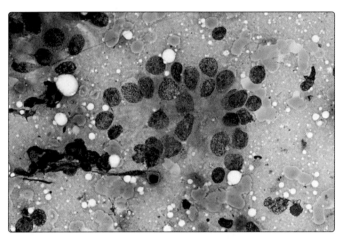

Fig. 19.52 Metastatic adenocarcinoma. The glandular arrangement of the malignant epithelial cells is obvious. This is a deposit from a well-differentiated prostatic carcinoma. (MGG × OI)

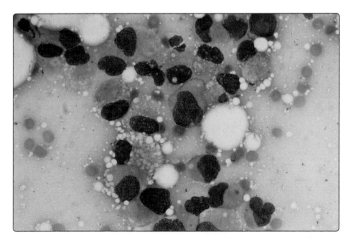

Fig. 19.53 Metastatic adenocarcinoma. The tumour deposit in this case shows poorly-differentiated adenocarcinoma cells which originated from a breast carcinoma. (MGG × OI)

magenta bodies on MGG. Cells with pale grey vacuolated cytoplasm on MGG and a nucleus with a central nucleolus are suggestive of a renal cell carcinoma.

Papillary carcinoma

Metastases of papillary carcinoma usually have their origin in the ovary, thyroid, breast or lung. Psammoma bodies are most frequent in metastases originating from ovarian and thyroid carcinomas. Seropapillary ovarian carcinomas often spread to lymph nodes in the groin, lower axilla and supraclavicular fossa. In contrast a papillary carcinoma of the thyroid seldom spreads outside the regional nodes.

Breast carcinoma

Atypical apocrine cells suggest origin in a breast carcinoma. In this context, it is important to point out that aspirates from an axillary node may contain apocrine cells without atypia. Such cells probably stem from accidentally aspirated sweat glands. Smears of aspirates from poorly-differentiated adenocarcinomas can be impossible to differentiate from other poorly-differentiated tumours.

Small cell anaplastic carcinoma

Small cell anaplastic carcinoma metastases yield crowded ragged clusters of tumour cells with scanty cytoplasm, nuclear moulding, coarse chromatin, frequent mitoses and a background of necrosis. They may resemble lymphoma cells, but the presence of cohesive clumps of tumour cells is strong evidence against a diagnosis of lymphoma.

Immunocytochemistry (Fig. 19.54)

Epithelial markers are readily detected and cytokeratin can be used to confirm the epithelial nature of the tumour deposits. Evaluation of CK7 and CK20 expression can substantially reduce the number of possible primary sites[86,87]. Positive staining for prostate specific antigen (PSA), thyroglobulin or calcitonin will conclusively identify the primary site in appropriate cases. Carcinoid tumours show staining for chromogranin A.

The presence of oestrogen or progesterone receptors strongly favours metastatic breast carcinoma[88,89]. In addition, positivity for these receptors suggests responsiveness to hormonal treatment which will aid the choice of treatment[90,91]. CA125 positivity strongly favours an ovarian origin[92]. Antibodies directed to other antigens such as carcinoembryonic antigen (CEA) for gastrointestinal tract or neurone specific enolase (NSE) for neuroendocrine tumours can be helpful in reducing the number of possible primary tumours.

Small cell anaplastic carcinoma cells show positive staining with cytokeratin, albeit sometimes irregular or dot-like in distribution. They stain positively with some neural markers, and, in particular, the neural cell adhesion molecule marker (N-CAM or UJ13A) is usually positive.

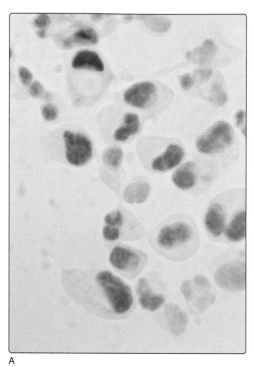

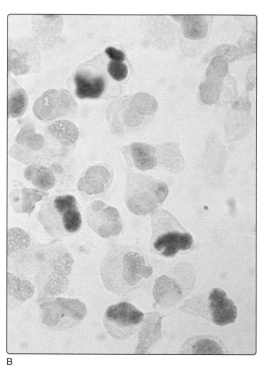

A

B

Fig. 19.54 Oestrogen (A) and progesterone (B) receptor staining of the aspirate shown in **Fig. 19.53**. (Immunoperoxidase × OI)

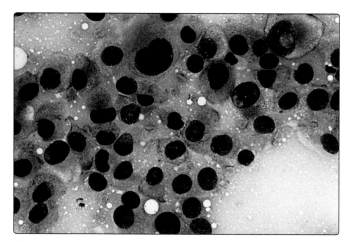

Fig. 19.55 Metastatic malignant melanoma. The aspirate shows polymorphic dissociated cells containing pigment. Note the intranuclear inclusion, which is seen as a circumscribed area of pallor within the nucleus of the cell in the top right corner. (MGG × OI)

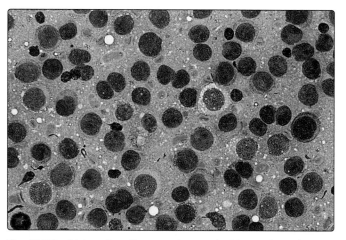

Fig. 19.56 Metastatic malignant melanoma. In this case the aspirate consists of dissociated relatively monotonous round cells. This rare variant is difficult to differentiate from other round cell tumours. (MGG × OI)

Metastatic malignant melanoma *(Figs 19.55, 19.56)*

Aspirates from metastatic melanoma often have quite typical features, with polymorphic dissociated cells which may contain fine pigment granules staining darkly on MGG. However, the cytoplasm often shows vacuoles only and this is referred to as 'negative pigmentation'. The nuclei have large nucleoli which occasionally may be replaced by cytoplasmic invaginations into the nucleus. The cytology of metastatic melanoma may mimic either carcinoma or sarcoma, or even sometimes lymphoma[93]. Even if the patient has a history of melanoma it can be virtually impossible in some cases to arrive at a conclusive diagnosis based on cytomorphology alone.

Immunocytochemistry *(Figs 19.57, 19.58)*

A panel of antibodies to epithelial and lymphoid antigens, S 100 and vimentin, together with antibody HMB 45, should be used. Positivity for vimentin, S 100 and HMB 45 will conclusively identify a metastatic melanoma[93].

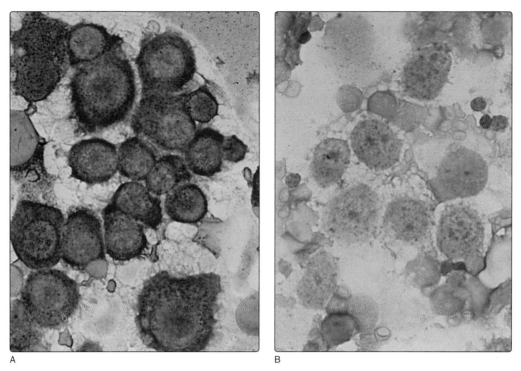

A B

Fig. 19.57 Immunocytochemistry of melanoma cells in cytospin material from aspirate shown in **Fig. 19.55**. The tumour cells are HMB 45 positive (A) and cytokeratin negative (B), confirming their origin. (Alkaline phosphatase × OI)

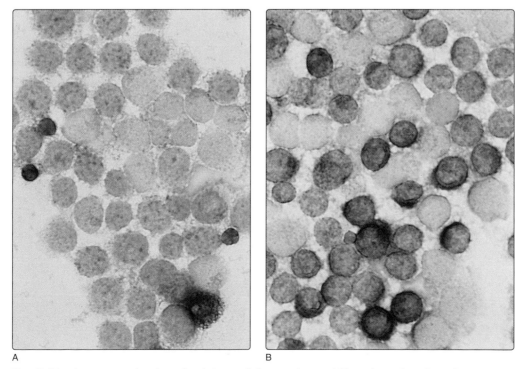

A B

Fig. 19.58 Immunocytochemistry of melanoma cells in cytospin material from the aspirate shown in **Fig. 19.56**. The cells are leucocyte common antigen negative (A) and HMB 45 positive (B). (Alkaline phosphatase × OI)

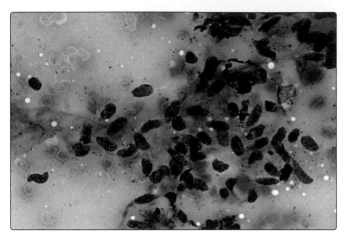

Fig. 19.59   Metastatic sarcoma. Lymph node deposit of abnormal spindle cells from a Kaposi's sarcoma occurring in an HIV positive patient. (MGG × OI)

However, it is important to remember that positivity for HMB 45 is lacking in approximately 20% of melanomas. Melan-A, recently described, is providing to be a reliable marker for melanoma cells.

Metastatic sarcomas *(Fig. 19.59)*

Sarcomas may occasionally spread to lymph nodes. The findings in FNA material mirror the diversity of histological appearances encountered in primary sarcomas of different types. A metastasis from a spindle cell sarcoma, such as Kaposi's sarcoma, should not cause any diagnostic difficulties. In contrast, round cell sarcomas such as childhood rhabdomyosarcomas or epithelioid sarcomas, in particular alveolar soft part sarcoma, can be difficult to diagnose in a lymph node aspirate without the use of immunocytochemistry. However, in such cases knowledge of the clinical history will often lead to a correct diagnosis.

Immunocytochemistry

Antibodies to epithelial, melanocytic and lymphoid cells give negative staining reactions in sarcomatous metastases. Vimentin and markers for neural, vascular and myogenic differentiation will confirm the diagnosis of metastatic sarcoma.

References

1   Greig E D W, Gray A C H. Note on lymphatic glands in sleeping sickness. *Lancet* 1904; **1**: 1570

2   Guthrie C G. Gland puncture as a diagnostic measure. *Bull Johns Hopkins Hosp* 1921; **32**: 266–269

3   Morrison M, Samwick A A, Rubinstein J *et al.* Lymph node aspiration. Clinical and hematologic observations in 101 patients. *Am J Clin Pathol* 1952; **22**: 255–262

4   Martin S E, Zhang H Z, Magyarosy E *et al.* Immunologic methods in cytology: definitive diagnosis of non-Hodgkin's lymphoma using immunologic markers for T and B cells. *Am J Clin Pathol* 1984; **80**: 666–673

5   Tani E M, Christensson B, Porwit A, Skoog L. Immunocytochemical analysis and cytomorphologic diagnosis on fine-needle aspirates of lymphoproliferative disease. *Acta Cytol* 1988; **32**: 209–215

6   Oertel J, Oertel B, Kastner M *et al.* The value of immunocytochemical staining of lymph node aspirates in diagnostic cytology. *Br J Haematol* 1988; **70**: 307–316

7   Tani E, Liliemark J, Svedmyr E *et al.* Cytomorphology and immunocytochemistry of fine-needle aspirates from blastic non-Hodgkin's lymphomas. *Acta Cytol* 1989; **33**: 363–371

8   Liliemark J, Tani E, Christensson B *et al.* Fine-needle aspiration cytology and immunocytochemistry of abdominal non-Hodgkin's lymphomas. *Leuk Lymphoma* 1989; **1**: 65–69

9   Cafferty L L, Katz R L, Ordonez N G *et al.* Fine-needle aspiration diagnosis of intra-abdominal and retroperitoneal lymphomas by a morphologic and immunocytochemical approach. *Cancer* 1990; **65**: 72–77

10   Skoog L, Tani E. The role of fine needle aspiration cytology in the diagnosis of non-Hodgkin's lymphoma. *Diagn Oncol* 1991; **1**: 12–18

11   Cartagena N, Katz R L, Hirsch-Ginsberg C *et al.* Cabanillas F. Accuracy of diagnosis of malignant lymphoma by combining fine-needle aspiration cytomorphology with immunocytochemistry and in selected cases. Southern blotting of aspirated cells: a tissue controlled study of 86 patients. *Diagn Cytopathol* 1992; **8**: 456–464

12   Katz R L, Caraway N P. FNA lymphoproliferative diseases: myths and legends. *Diagn Cytopathol* 1995; **12**: 99–100

13   Leong A S Y, Stevens M. Fine-needle aspiration biopsy for the diagnosis of lymphoma: a prospective. *Diagn Cytopathol* 1996; **15**: 352–357

14   Saddik M, el Dabbagh L, Mourad W A. Ex vivo fine-needle aspiration cytology and flow cytometric phenotyping in the diagnosis of lymphoproliferative disorders: a proposed algorithm for maximum resource utilisation. *Diagn Cytopathol* 1997; **16**(2): 126–131

15   Dunphy C H, Ramos R. Combining fine-needle aspiration and flow cytometric immunophenotyping in evaluation of nodal and extranodal sites for possible lymphoma: a retrospective review (Review). *Diagn Cytopathol* 1997; **16**(3): 200–206

16   Clatch R J, Foreman J R, Walloch J L. Simplified immunophenotypic analysis by laser scanning cytometry (Review). *Cytometry* 1998; **34**: 3–16

17   Horii A, Yoshida J, Hattori K *et al.* DNA ploidy, proliferative activities, and immunophenotype of malignant lymphoma: application of flow cytometry. *Head Neck* 1998; **20**(5): 392–398

18   Liu K, Mann K P, Vitellas K M *et al.* Fine-needle aspiration with flow cytometric immunophenotyping for primary diagnosis of intra-abdominal lymphomas. *Diagn Cytopathol* 1999; **21**(2): 98–104

19   Ravinsky E, Morales C, Kutryk E, Chrobak A, Paraskevas F. Cytodiagnosis of lymphoid proliferations by fine needle aspiration biopsy. Adjunctive value of flow cytometry. *Acta Cytol* 1999; **43**(6): 1070–1078

20   Young N A, Al-Saleem T I, Ehya H, Smith M R. Utilization of fine needle aspiration cytology and flow cytometry in the diagnosis and subclassification of primary and recurrent lymphoma. *Cancer (Cancer Cytopathol)* 1998; **84**: 252–261

21   Young N A, Al-Saleenil. Diagnosis of lymphoma by fine-needle aspiration cytology using the Revised European-American classification of lymphoid neoplasms. *Cancer (Cancer Cytopathol)* 1999; **87**: 325–345

22   Wakely P E. Aspiration cytopathology of malignant lymphoma. *Cancer Cytopathology* 1999; **87**: 322–324

23   Hu E, Homing S, Flynn S *et al.* Diagnosis of B cell lymphoma by analysis of immunoglobulin gene rearrangements in biopsy specimens obtained by fine needle aspiration. *J Clin Oncol* 1986; **4**(3): 278–283

24   Kube M J, McDonald D A, Quin J W, Greenberg M L. Use of archival and fresh cytologic material for the polymerase chain reaction. Detection of the bcl-2 oncogene in lymphoid tissue obtained by fine needle

biopsy. *Anal Quant Cytol Histol* 1994; **16**(3): 174–182

25 Aiello A, Delia D, Giardini R et al. PCR analysis of IgH and BCL2 gene rearrangement in the diagnosis of follicular lymphoma in lymph node fine-needle aspiration. A critical appraisal. *Diagn Mol Pathol* 1997; **6**(3): 154–160

26. Jeffers M D, McCorriston J, Farquharson M A et al. Analysis of clonality in cytologic material using the polymerase chain reaction (PCR). *Cytopathology* 1997; **8**(2): 114–120

27 Lovchik J, Lane M A, Clark D P. Polymerase chain reaction-based detection of B-cell clonality in the fine aspiration biopsy of a thyroid mucosa-associated lymphoid tissue (MALT) lymphoma. *Hum Pathol* 1997; **28**(8): 989–992

28 Vianello F, Tison T, Radossi P et al. Detection of B-cell monoclonality in fine needle aspiration by PCR analysis. *Leuk Lymphoma* 1998; **29**(1–2): 179–185

29 Grosso L E, Collins B T. DNA polymerase chain reaction using fine needle aspiration biopsy smears to evaluate non Hodgkin's lymphoma. *Acta Cytol* 1999; **43**(5): 837–841

30 Grossl N A, Mosunjac M I, Wallace T M. Utility of fine needle aspiration in HIV-positive patients with corresponding CD4 counts. Four years experience in a large inner city hospital. *Acta Cytol* 1997; **41**: 811–816

31 Reid A J, Miller R F, Kocjan G I. Diagnostic utility of fine needle aspiration (FNA) cytology in HIV-infected patients with lymphadenopathy. *Cytopathology* 1998; **9**: 230–239

32 Kardos T F, Kornstein M J, Frable W J. Cytology and immunocytology of infectious mononucleosis in fine needle aspiration of lymph nodes. *Acta Cytol* 1988; **32**: 722–726

33 Stanley M W, Steeper T A, Horwitz C A et al. Fine-needle aspiration of lymph nodes in patients with acute infectious mononucleosis. *Diagn Cytopathol* 1990; **6**: 323–329

34 Schnitzer B. Reactive lymphoid hyperplasia. In: Jaffe E S ed. *Surgical Pathology of the Lymph Nodes and Related Organs*. Philadelphia: WB Saunders, 1985; 22

35 Rosai J, Dorfman R F. Sinus histiocytosis with massive lymphadenopathy. *Arch Pathol* 1969; **87**: 63–70

36 Layfield L. Fine-needle aspiration cytology findings in a case of sinus histiocytosis with massive lymphadenopathy. *Acta Cytol* 1990; **34**: 767–770

37 Pettinato G, Manivel C, d'Amore E, Petrella G. Fine needle aspiration cytology and immunocytochemical characterization of the histiocytes in sinus histiocytosis with massive lymphadenopathy (Rosai-Dorfman syndrome). *Acta Cytol* 1990; **34**: 771–777

38 Schmitt F. Sinus histiocytosis with massive lymphadenopathy (Rosai-Dorfman Disease): cytomorphologic analysis on fine needle aspirates. *Diagn Cytopathol* 1992; **8**: 596–599

39 Kikuchi M. Lymphadenitis showing focal reticulum cell hyperplasia with nuclear debris and phagocytosis. *Nippon Ketsueki Gakkai Zasshi* 1971; **35**: 379–380

40 Fujimoto Y, Kozima Y. Yamazuchi K. Cervical subacute necrotizing lymphadenitis. A new clinicopathologic entity. *Naika* 1972; **20**: 920–927

41 Kung I T M, Ng W F, Yue R W S, Chan J K C. Kikuchi's histiocytic necrotizing lymphadenitis: diagnosis by fine needle aspiration. *Acta Cytol* 1990; **34**: 323–328

42 Greenberg M, Cartwright L, McDonald D. Histiocytic necrotizing lymphadenitis (Kikuchi's disease). Cytologic diagnosis by fine needle aspiration cytology. *Diagn Cytopathol* 1993; **9**: 444–447

43. Hsueh E-J, Ko W S, Hwang W S, Yam L T. Fine needle aspiration of histiocytic necrotizing lymphadenitis (Kikuchi's disease). *Diagn Cytopathol* 1993; **9**: 448–452

44 Sadanah-Metre M, Jayaram G. Acid-fast bacilli in aspiration smears from tuberculous lymph nodes. An analysis of 255 cases. *Acta Cytol* 1981; **31**: 17–19

45 Bailey T M, Akhtar M, Ali M A. Fine needle aspiration biopsy in the diagnosis of tuberculosis. *Acta Cytol* 1985; **29**: 732–736

46 Rajwanshi A, Bhambhani S, Das D K. Fine needle aspiration cytology diagnosis of tuberculosis. *Diagn Cytopathol* 1987; **3**: 13–16

47 Das D K, Pant J N, Chachra K L et al. Tuberculous lymphadenitis: correlation of cellular components and necrosis in lymph node aspirate with AFB positivity and bacillary count. *Indian J Pathol Microbiol* 1990; **33**: 1–10

48 Stanley M W, Horwitz C A, Burton L G, Weisser J A. Negative images of bacilli and mycobacterial infection: a study of fine-needle aspiration smears from lymph nodes in patients with AIDS. *Diagn Cytopathol* 1990; **6**: 118–121

49 Gupta S K, Kumar B, Kaur S. Aspiration cytology of lymph nodes in leprosy. *Int J Lepr* 1981; **49**: 9–15

50 Cavett J R III, McAfee R, Ramzy I. Hansen's disease (leprosy). Diagnosis by aspiration biopsy of lymph nodes. *Acta Cytol* 1986; **30**: 189–193

51 Tani E M, Franco M. Pulmonary cytology in paracoccidioidomycosis. *Acta Cytol* 1984; **28**: 571–575

52 Das D K, Bhatt N C, Khan V A, Luthra U K. Cervicofacial actinomycosis: diagnosis by fine needle aspiration cytology. *Acta Cytol* 1989; **33**: 278–280

53 Housini I, Dabbo D J, Coyne L. Fine needle aspiration cytology of talc granulomatosis in a peripheral lymph node in a case of suspected intravenous drug abuse. *Acta Cytol* 1990; **34**: 342–344

54 Tabatowski K, Elson C E, Johnston W W. Silicone lymphadenopathy in a patient with a mammary prosthesis. Fine needle aspiration cytology, histology and analytical electron microscopy. *Acta Cytol* 1990; **34**: 10–14

55 Lukes R J, Craver L F, Hall T C et al. Report of the nomenclature committee. *Cancer Res* 1966; **26**: 311

56 Harris N, Jaffee E, Stein H et al. A revised European-American classification of lymphoid neoplasms: a proposal from the International Lymphoma Study Group. *Blood* 1994; **84**: 1361–1392

57 Lennert K, Mohri N, Stein H, Kaiserling E. The histopathology of malignant lymphoma. *Br J Hematol* 1975; **31**: 193–203

58 The non-Hodgkin's lymphoma pathological classification project. National Cancer Institute sponsored study of lymphomas: summary and description of a working formulation of clinical usage. *Cancer* 1982; **49**: 2112–2135

59 Stansfeld A G, Diebold J, Kapanci Y et al. Updated Kiel classification for lymphomas. *Lancet* 1988; **i**: 292–293

60 Orell S R, Skinner J M. The typing of non-Hodgkin's lymphoma using fine needle aspiration cytology. *Pathology* 1982; **14**: 389–394

61 Lopes-Cardozo P. In: Lopes-Cardozo P ed. *Atlas of Clinical Cytology*. The Netherlands: Verlag Chemi, 1975

62 Moriarty A T, Banks E R, Bloch T. Cytological criteria for subclassification of Hodgkin's disease using fine-needle aspiration. *Diagn Cytopathol* 1989; **5**: 122–125

63 Das D K, Gupta S K. Cytodiagnosis of Hodgkin's disease: a study of its subtypes by differential cell count in fine needle aspiration smear. *Acta Cytol* 1990; **34**: 337–341

64 Godwin J T. Cytology diagnosis of aspiration biopsies of solid or cystic tumors. Symposium on diagnostic accuracy of cytologic techniques. *Acta Cytol* 1964; **8**: 206

65 Frable W J, Kardos T F. Fine needle aspiration biopsy: applications in the diagnosis of lymphoproliferative diseases. *Am J Surg Pathol* 1988; **12**: 62–72

66 Grosso L E, Collins B T, Dunphy C H, Ramos R R. Lymphocyte-depleted Hodgkin's disease: diagnostic challenges by fine needle aspiration. *Diagn Cytopathol* 1998; **19**(1): 66–69

67 Fulciniti F, Zeppa P, Vetrani A et al. Hodgkin's disease mimicking suppurative lymphadenitis: a possible pitfall in fine-needle aspiration biopsy cytology. *Diagn Cytopathol* 1989; **5**(3): 282–285

68 Tani E, Ersoz C, Svedmyr E, Skoog L. Fine-needle aspiration cytology and immunocytochemistry of Hodgkin's disease suppurative type. *Diagn Cytopathol* 1998; **18**(6): 437–440

69 Vicandi B, Jimenez-Heffernan J A, Lopez-Ferrer P et al. Hodgkin's disease mimicking suppurative lymphadenitis: a fine-needle aspiration report of five cases. *Diagn Cytopathol* 1999 ; **20**(5): 302–306

70 Wright D H. Hodgkin's disease. In: McGee J O'D, Isaaccson P G, Wright N A eds. *Oxford Textbook of Pathology*. Oxford: Oxford University Press 1992; 1789

71 Masik A S, Weisenburger D D, Vose J M et al. Histologic grade does not predict prognosis in optimally treated advanced stage nodular sclerosing Hodgkin's disease. *Cancer* 1992; **69**: 228–232

72 Davey D D, Kamat D, Zaleski S et al. Analysis of immunoglobulin and T cell receptor gene rearrangement in cytologic specimens. *Acta Cytol* 1989; **33**: 583–590

73 Gerdes J, Schwab U, Lemke H, Stein H. Production of a mouse monoclonal antibody reactive with a human nuclear antigen associated with cell proliferation. *Int J Cancer* 1987; **31**: 13–20

74 Wojcik E M, Katz R L, Fanning T V *et al.* Diagnosis of mantle cell lymphoma on tissue acquired by fine needle aspiration in conjunction with immunocytochemistry and cytokinetic studies. Possibilities and limitations *Acta Cytol* 1995; **39**(5): 909–915

75 Rassidakis G Z, Tani E, Svedmyr E *et al.* Diagnosis and subclassification of follicle center, and mantle cell lymphomas on fine needle aspirates: A cytologic and immunocytochemical approach based on REAL classification. *Cancer (Cancer Cytopathology)* 1999; **87**: 216–223

76 Hughes J H, Caraway N P, Katz R L. Blastic variant of mantle-cell lymphoma: cytomorphologic, immunocytochemical and molecular genetic features of tissue obtained by fine-needle aspiration biopsy. *Diagn Cytopathol* 1998; **19**(1): 59–62

77 Matsushima A Y, Hamele-Bena D, Osborne B M. Fine-needle aspiration biopsy findings in marginal zone B cell lymphoma. *Diagn Cytopathol* 1999; **20**: 190–198

78 Tani E, Johansson B, Skoog L. T-cell-rich B-cell lymphoma: fine-needle aspiration cytology and immunocytochemistry. *Diagn Cytopathol* 1998 **18**(I): 1–4

79 Tani E, Löwhagen T, Nasiell K *et al.* Fine-needle aspiration cytology and immunocytochemistry of large-cell lymphomas expressing the Ki-1 antigen. *Acta Cytol* 1989; **331**: 359–362

80 Akhtar M, Ali M A, Haider A *et al.* Fine needle aspiration biopsy of Ki-1 positive anaplastic large cell lymphomas. *Diagn Cytopathol* 1992; **8**: 242–247

81 Bizjak-Schwarzbartl M. Large anaplastic Ki-1+ non-Hodgkin's lymphoma vs. Hodgkin's disease in fine needle aspiration biopsy samples. *Acta Cytol* 1997; **41**: 351–356

82 Agnarsson B A, Kadin M E. Ki-1 positive large cell lymphoma. A morphologic and immunologic study of 19 cases. *Am J Surg Pathol* 1988; **12**: 264–274

83 Burns B F, Dardick I. Ki-1 positive non-Hodgkin's lymphomas. An immunophenotypic, ultrastructural and morphometric study. *Am J Clin Pathol* 1990; **93**: 327–332

84 Engzell U, Jakobsson P A, Sigurdsson A, Zajicek J. Aspiration biopsy of metastatic carcinoma in lymph nodes of neck: a review of 1101 consecutive cases. *Acta Otolaryngol* 1971; **72**: 138–147

85 Hsu C, Leung B S, Lau S K *et al.* Efficacy of fine needle aspiration and sampling of lymph nodes in 1484 Chinese patients. *Diagn Cytopathol* 1990; **6**: 154–159

86 Wang N P, Zarbo R J, Gown A M. Coordinate expression of cytokeratins 7 and 20 define carcinoma. *Applied Immunohistochem* 1995; **3**: 99–107

87 Miettinen M. Keratin 20: Immunohistochemical marker for gastrointestinal, urothelial, and Merkel cell carcinomas. *Mod Pathol* 1995; **8**: 384–388

88 Skoog L, Humla S, Isaksson S, Tani E. Immunocytochemical analysis of receptors for estrogen and progesterone in fine needle aspirates from human mammary carcinomas. *Diagn Cytopathol* 1990; **6**: 95–98

89 Tani E M, Borregon A, Humla S, Skoog L. Estrogen receptors in fine needle aspirates from metastatic lesions of gynecologic tumors. *Gynecol Oncol* 1989; **32**: 365–367

90 Coombes R C, Berger U, McClelland R A *et al.* Prediction of endocrine response in breast cancer by immunocytochemical detection of estrogen receptor in fine-needle aspirates. *Lancet* 1987; **ii**: 701–703

91 Skoog L, Wilking N, Humla S *et al.* Estrogen and progesterone receptors and modal DNA value in tumor cells obtained by fine-needle aspiration from primary breast carcinomas during tamoxifen treatment. *Diagn Oncol* 1991; **1**: 282–287

92 Kabawat S E, Bast RC, Welch WR *et al.* Immunopathologic characterization of a monoclonal antibody that recognizes common surface antigens of human ovarian tumors of serous, endometrioid, and clear cell types. *Amer J Clin Pathol* 1983; **79**: 98–104

93 Nasiell K, Tani E, Skoog L. Fine needle aspiration cytology and immunocytochemistry of metastatic melanoma. *Cytopathology* 1991; **2**: 137–147

Other lymphoreticular organs

Edneia Tani and Lambert Skoog*

Introduction

Lymph nodes form only part of the immunological defence system distributed throughout the body. Other organs and anatomical sites also harbour lymphoid tissue, which participates in primary and secondary immune responses. The term 'extranodal lymphoid tissue' is used to refer to lymphoid tissue situated other than in lymph nodes. This tissue includes organs such as spleen, thymus and the nasopharyngeal lymphoid aggregations known as Waldeyer's ring. In addition, extranodal lymphoid tissue exists as mucosa associated lymphoid tissue (MALT) in the gastrointestinal tract, lung, salivary gland, thyroid and orbit[1].

Inflammation, autoimmune disorders and malignant lymphomas can involve any of the extranodal collections of lymphoid tissue or lymphoreticular organs, as well as lymph nodes. In contrast, however, the extranodal lymphoid tissue is rarely the seat of metastatic tumour spread, which is so frequently seen in lymph nodes.

This chapter will consider the main cytological findings in disease processes at the different anatomical sites of extranodal lymphoid tissue, highlighting any contrasting features with the conditions found in lymph nodes.

Waldeyer's ring

Lymphoid tissue in the tonsils, base of the tongue and epipharynx compose Waldeyer's ring. These extranodal sites are often affected by inflammatory disorders, but are rarely the target of FNA biopsy. Waldeyer's ring is a relatively frequent site for B cell derived non-Hodgkin's lymphomas, a high proportion arising particularly in the tonsils[1,2]. In contrast, T-cell lymphomas and Hodgkin's disease are rarely encountered at this site.

All subtypes of B-cell neoplasms can occur in any part of Waldeyer's ring, but follicle centre cell lymphomas appear to be the most frequent. At the time of diagnosis, most patients have cervical node involvement as well.

The tonsil and epipharynx may also be the primary sites for undifferentiated carcinomas. In these cases distinction from blastic lymphomas may pose a problem.

FNA procedure

The aspiration technique is similar to that of most palpable lesions, but an 8 cm long 25 gauge (0.5 mm) needle will be necessary in most cases. Occasionally, a Franzén prostate needle guide is needed to reach targets not otherwise accessible. Aspiration with a 25 G needle usually gives sufficient material for both smears and immunological evaluation. Local anaesthesia is seldom required but when needed it should be administered in spray form.

Cytological findings

Reactive lymphoid hyperplasia

Reactive lymphoid hyperplasia is common in the lymphoid tissue of Waldeyer's ring, as elsewhere, and is characterized by a spectrum of lymphoid cells ranging from small mature lymphocytes to immunoblasts. In addition, granulocytes, plasma cells and macrophages containing tingible body material are present.

Non-Hodgkin's lymphomas

The cytological patterns of the different non-Hodgkin's lymphomas are identical to those seen in lymph nodes as described in detail in the preceding chapter. Briefly, the smears are composed of a relatively uniform cell population apart from the mixed lymphomas, which include neoplastic follicle centre cells as well as some benign lymphocytes. The most common high-grade lymphoma is the large B-cell follicle derived lymphoma (Fig. 20.1). The cells have round nuclei with 1–4 small nucleoli often at the nuclear membrane. The cytoplasm is sparse and may contain small vacuoles. Hodgkin's disease does not generally involve lymphoid tissue in this area.

Poorly-differentiated carcinoma

Poorly-differentiated carcinoma cells may superficially mimic those of a high-grade malignant lymphoma. However carcinomas show a tendency to form aggregates in which the individual cells have poorly defined cytoplasm (Fig. 20.2). In rare cases a confident distinction is only possible by immunocytochemistry.

*The authors gratefully acknowledge their debt to the late Torsten Löwhagen, whose contribution to the previous edition of this chapter provided a substantial basis for this revised edition.

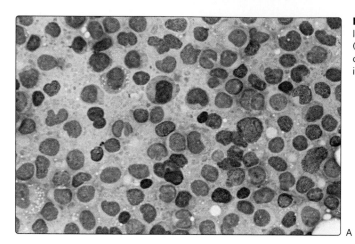

Fig. 20.1 Centroblastic lymphoma of tonsil. (A) FNA smear consisting of large centroblasts with round nuclei and a thin rim of cytoplasm. (MGG × HP) (B) Immunocytochemistry showing positive reactivity for B-cell marker in centroblasts. (C) Monoclonal lambda light chain expression in centroblasts, indicating neoplasia. (Alkaline phosphatase × HP)

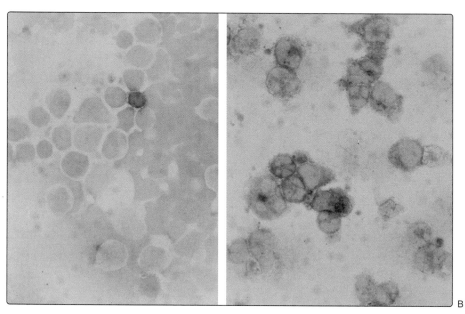

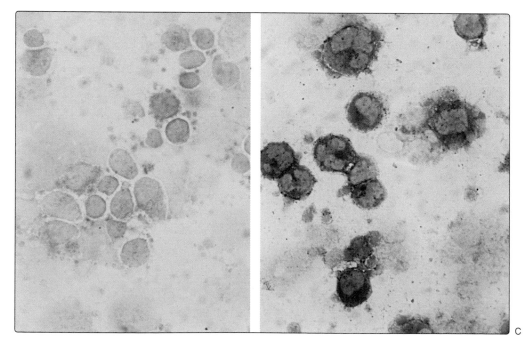

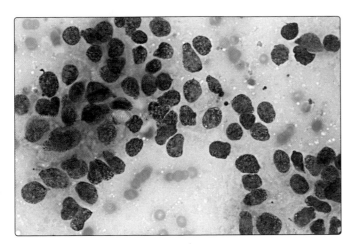

Fig. 20.2 Poorly-differentiated carcinoma of tonsil with pleomorphic tumour cells in loose clusters. (MGG × HP)

Immunocytochemistry

In reactive hyperplasia, polytypic B cells predominate. The vast majority of the lymphomas in this area are of B-cell phenotype with readily detectable light chain restriction. Positive staining for cytokeratin or EMA will allow identification of an undifferentiated carcinoma.

Thymus

The thymus is a lymphoepithelial organ that has a vital role in the production of T cells derived from bone marrow. It lies in the anterior part of the mediastinum and reaches its greatest size in childhood. In old age the gland is almost indiscernible.

The thymus undergoes hyperplasia in the autoimmune disease myasthenia gravis, and is occasionally affected by primary neoplasms. These include thymomas, lymphomas and germ cell tumours which arise in the epithelial, lymphoid or germinal crest tissue respectively[3,4].

The relative incidence of tumours differs in childhood and adult life. Thus, in childhood, lymphomas account for 50% of the neoplasms, while germ cell and mesenchymal tumours represent 20% each. In adults, thymomas are the most common neoplasm, representing approximately 50% of all primary tumours. Lymphomas are second and germ cell tumours third in frequency with a relative frequency of 25% and 15%, respectively. Carcinoids are rare as thymic tumours and are usually aggressive.

Tumours in the anterior mediastinum, such as thymomas, can be reached by puncture through the sternum or the intercostal space close to the sternum with the help of radiological guidance. This can often be performed under local anaesthesia.

Lymphomas

The thymus appears to be the primary site for two types of lymphoma. The T cell lymphoblastic subtype occurs predominantly in males, almost exclusively in children and is exceedingly uncommon after adolescence. The second type is the recently described large B-cell lymphoma, which frequently involves the thymus[5]. This variant shows a predilection for women in the third or fourth decades. The tumour cells, which resemble centroblasts or immunoblasts, are of B phenotype and are thought to be of thymic origin. With aggressive chemotherapy this lymphoma has a relatively good prognosis. In addition to these two subtypes almost all other variants of lymphoma can affect the thymus in rare instances.

Cytological findings

Lymphoblastic lymphoma

Lymphoblastic lymphoma is composed of small to medium sized cells with moderately basophilic cytoplasm (Fig. 20.3). The chromatin is fine and nucleoli are inconspicuous. There is usually a high mitotic rate.

Large B-cell lymphoma (primary mediastinal)

Aspirates from large B-cell lymphoma of adults show large atypical cells, which may superficially resemble centroblasts or immunoblasts (Fig. 20.4). Other tumours to be considered in the differential diagnosis include primary germ cell tumours of the mediastinum and seminoma. Immunophenotyping will be distinctive.

Immunocytochemistry

Lymphoblastic lymphoma is a T-cell neoplasm with expression of the lymphoblastic marker terminal deoxynucleotidyl transferase (TdT). The fraction of proliferation cells as analysed by Ki-67 staining is often over 90%.

The large B-cell lymphomas express B-cell associated antigens (CD19, CD20, CD22, CD79a) and the tumour cells rarely express surface immunoglobulin.

Germ cell tumours

In the mediastinum, these rare neoplasms are thought to arise in the primordial germinal crest of the thymus. The most common one is the benign teratoma, which accounts for over 80% of germ cell tumours. They grow to a large size and may be cystic. The malignant teratomas are almost exclusively seen in males in the second and third decade of life[3]. In patients with these tumours it is important to exclude metastasis from a primary gonadal neoplasm, which, however, is extremely uncommon.

Cytological findings

Benign teratoma; seminoma

Aspirates from benign teratomas may contain stratified

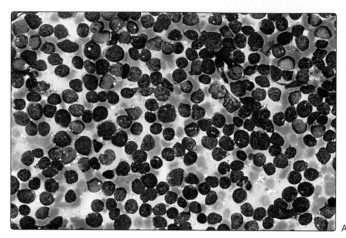

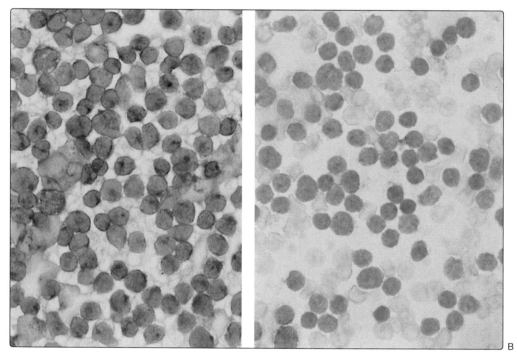

Fig. 20.3 Lymphoblastic lymphoma of thymus. (A) Aspirate from mediastinum composed of small to medium sized blast cells. (MGG × 160) (B) Immunocytochemistry shows T-cell lineage with positive staining on the left and no reaction to the B-cell marker on the right. (Alkaline phosphatase × HP)

squamous epithelium, sebaceous material and a variety of benign cells from all germinal layers. Smears from seminomas show dispersed fragile cells in a characteristic lace like, or 'tigroid' background due to fragmentation of the glycogen-laden cytoplasm (Fig. 20.5). The tumour cell nuclei are pale and have evenly distributed chromatin. Small lymphocytes may be present reflecting the histological presence of a lymphoid or granulomatous infiltrate in these neoplasms.

Embryonal carcinoma

Embryonal carcinoma is a pleomorphic tumour. The cells are usually in tight clusters and have a high nuclear/cytoplasmic ratio (Fig. 20.6). Individual cells may simulate immature lymphoid cells but their epithelial origin is identified by the finding of large nucleoli and the formation of cell clusters.

Teratocarcinoma

Teratocarcinoma may be well differentiated and the smears then look deceptively benign. However, a majority of the cases are composed of sheets of poorly-differentiated epithelial cells and stromal fragments (Fig. 20.7).

Metastases from any poorly-differentiated carcinoma may be impossible to differentiate from embryonal carcinoma or teratocarcinoma by cytomorphology.

Immunocytochemistry

Germ cell tumours are positive for placental alkaline phosphatase (PLAP). Embryonal carcinomas and terato-carcinomas may show positivity for cytokeratin, human chorionic gonadotrophin (HCG) and alpha fetoprotein (AFP), while seminomas are negative. These features allow

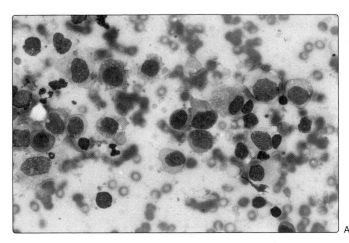

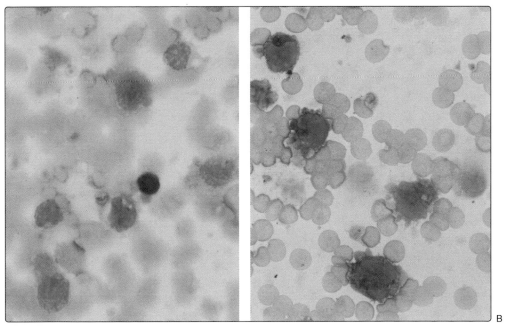

Fig. 20.4 Large B-cell lymphoma of thymus. (A) The immature tumour cells have irregular nuclei and large cytoplasm. (MGG × 160) (B) Immunocytochemistry: B cell positivity in tumour cells. (Alkaline phosphatase)

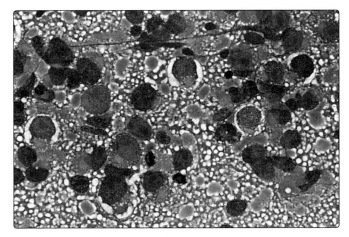

Fig. 20.5 Mediastinal seminoma. Dispersed fragile cells with poorly defined cytoplasm in typical 'tigroid' background. (MGG × HP)

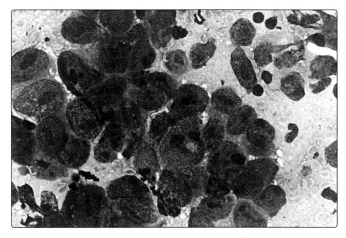

Fig. 20.6 Embryonal carcinoma of mediastinum. Clusters of large malignant cells with distinct nucleoli. (MGG × HP)

differentiation between carcinomas of germ cell type and those of other origin.

Occasionally mediastinal involvement by small cell anaplastic carcinoma of lung may present diagnostic difficulties in distinguishing the cells from those of other poorly-differentiated tumours involving the mediastinum. The neural cell adhesion molecule marker (N-CAM or UJ13 A) is usually positive in cells from small cell anaplastic carcinoma.

Thymomas

These are tumours of middle age and are exceedingly rare in children. Approximately half of the cases have symptoms related to the tumour mass but a substantial number of patients present with myaesthenia gravis. Most thymomas are benign but some may show invasive growth and may even metastasize. This malignant behaviour is not reflected in the cytology of the tumour.

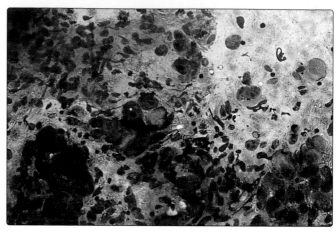

Fig. 20.7   Mediastinal teratocarcinoma. Note the malignant epithelial cell cluster and fragment of undifferentiated mesenchymal tissue. (MGG × HP)

Cytological findings *(Fig. 20.8)*

By definition, the epithelial cells in thymomas are neoplastic. There are, however, always a variable number of benign mature T cells accompanying the tumour cells. In extreme cases lymphoid cells predominate and the lesion is difficult to distinguish from a lymphoma. The epithelial cells are oval to spindle shaped with homogeneous chromatin. They are cohesive, and rarely seen as isolated cells[6-8]. The *spindle cell variant* can be misdiagnosed as a true neoplasm of connective tissue. Thymic *carcinomas* are distinguished from thymomas on the basis of marked cytological atypia[9]. These tumours behave aggressively.

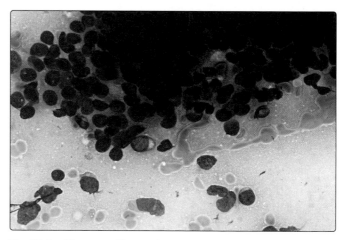

Fig. 20.8   Thymoma. Cluster of monotonous epithelial cells with indistinct cytoplasm. Few lymphoid cells present. (MGG × HP)

Immunocytochemistry

The epithelial cells may be difficult to identify when the lymphoid component predominates. Staining for cytokeratin, epithelial membrane antigen and for T and B-cell markers helps to identify the cellular component[10-12]. The CDI (Leu 6) antigen is expressed by thymic lymphocytes. The spindle cell variant also expresses epithelial markers, which allows distinction from connective tissue lesions. Carcinoid tumours can be identified by their positive staining reaction with chromogranin A.

Spleen

The spleen is relatively rarely subjected to FNA. Needle biopsy is usually requested for a patient with splenomegaly of unknown cause. If the enlargement is marked a palpable mass is found in the left upper quadrant. It then becomes an easy target for FNA. A non-palpable spleen can often be successfully biopsied via a direct intercostal puncture but

ultrasound guidance gives a higher success rate, with less risk of pneumothorax.

Technical procedure

A few remarks concerning the technique may be useful. Infiltration of local anaesthetic is carried out as far as the peritoneum. This significantly reduces the risk of a vasovagal reaction. A 25 gauge, 8 cm spinal needle with a stylet offers maximum adaptability. The patient is instructed to maintain apnoea after several deep breaths. The needle is inserted, the mandrel removed and the syringe attached. Suction of approximately 5 ml is applied and the needle moved back and forth. As soon as blood is seen in the needle hub the suction is stopped and the needle withdrawn. The aspirated material is used for smears and sometimes cytospin preparations.

After the biopsy, the patient should be supervised for approximately 1 h to exclude complications. Patients with coagulopathies can be punctured but blood-typing and hospitalization are obligatory.

Non-neoplastic splenomegaly

Splenomegaly occurs in a number of aetiologically different conditions such as congestion, haematological disorders, storage diseases and inflammatory lesions. In the majority of such cases the underlying disorder is known and there is no need for FNA of the enlarged spleen. However, splenic cytology can be an important method of diagnosis for some disorders, which primarily manifest themselves as splenomegaly.

Haematophagocytic syndrome

This occurs in patients with immunosuppression resulting from a variety of disorders such as infections, most commonly of viral type, familial erythrophagocytic lymphohistiocytosis, AIDS and treatment with immunosuppressive drugs[13,14]. The splenomegaly is usually marked.

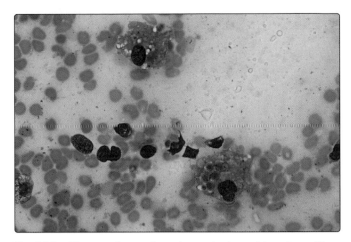

Fig. 20.9 Haematophagocytic syndrome. Aspirate of the spleen with histiocytic cells containing phagocytosed erythrocytes and cell debris. (MGG × HP)

Cytological findings (Fig. 20.9)

A spectrum of lymphoid cells is present in a background of abundant blood and platelet aggregates. There are numerous histiocytic cells with abundant vacuolated cytoplasm. The histiocytes are cytologically benign but often contain phagocytosed erythrocytes.

Myeloid metaplasia

Myelofibrosis of the bone marrow and chronic myeloid leukaemia are accompanied by splenomegaly. This results from population of the spleen by blood forming cells normally confined to bone marrow, leading to the development of foci of extramedullary haemopoiesis[15].

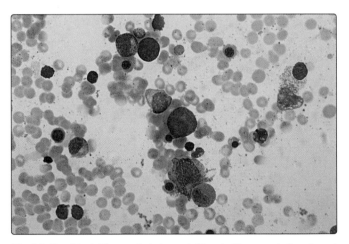

Fig. 20.10 Myeloid metaplasia in myelofibrosis. Haemopoietic cells and some lymphoid cells. (MGG × HP)

Cytological findings (Fig. 20.10)

Normal splenic cells are in a minority, and haemopoietic cells dominate the smears. Megakaryocytes may be mistaken for malignant cells by those not familiar with their appearance in cytological specimens.

Granulomatous processes

The causes of granulomatous splenitis are numerous. The commonest of these are infections such as tuberculosis, but sarcoidosis and malignant lymphomas sometimes produce a granulomatous reaction.

Cytological findings (Fig. 20.11)

Numerous epithelioid histiocytes with ill-defined cytoplasm and pale elongated nuclei are present and often form granulomatous clusters. Multinucleated giant cells may be found in granulomas of any cause and are likely to be seen in *sarcoidosis*[16] and *tuberculosis*. Caseation necrosis is sometimes identifiable in cases of tuberculosis as pale amorphous inflammatory debris. Mycobacteria are best

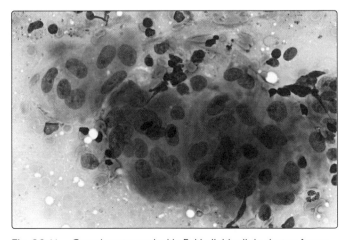

Fig. 20.11 Granulomatous splenitis. Epithelioid cells in clusters from a patient with sarcoidosis. (MGG × HP)

identified by PCR technique. The diagnostic criteria for *lymphomas* associated with granulomatous splenomegaly are the same as those in node based disease and these have been described in Chapter 19.

Storage disorders

Massive splenomegaly results from pathological accumulation of macrophages laden with glucocerebrosides and sphingolipids in Gaucher's and Nieman-Pick's disease, respectively.

Cytological findings *(Fig. 20.12)*

The smears contain numerous large histiocytes with foamy cytoplasm. The nuclei are monotonous and without nucleoli.

Neoplastic splenomegaly

Metastases to the spleen are relatively rare and seldom of clinical significance. In contrast, lymphomas frequently involve the spleen[17-20]. Usually, splenic involvement reflects generalized disease, but primary lymphoma of the spleen does occur.

Non-Hodgkin's lymphoma (NHL)

All types of NHL can affect the spleen and the cytological findings are identical to those of the lymphoma type in lymph node FNA. As in aspiration of lymphomatous nodes, the cytological diagnosis should be confirmed by immunocytochemistry. Small lymphocytic lymphoma and hairy cell leukaemia are the most common lymphomatous entities to cause splenomegaly.

Cytological findings *(Fig. 20.13)*

Smears of *small lymphocytic lymphomas* are similar to those from other sites. *Hairy cell leukaemia* presents a monotonous cytological pattern. The cells are small but have relatively abundant pale cytoplasm, which may show fine hair-like cytoplasmic processes. Bone marrow aspirates and peripheral blood smears show the same cells.

Immunocytochemistry

Small lymphocytic lymphoma and hairy cell leukaemia are both monoclonal B-cell neoplasms.

Hodgkin's disease

The spleen is rarely the only site affected in cases of Hodgkin's disease and the diagnosis is therefore usually known prior to FNA. Suspicion of residual or recurrent disease can, however, lead to an FNA biopsy. Involvement may be nodular, and when Hodgkin's disease is suspected multiple biopsies are recommended. Ultrasound guidance may be of value in targeting involved areas.

Cytological findings

The diagnosis rests on the identification of Hodgkin's or Reed-Sternberg cells in a polymorphic cellular background. Epithelioid cells and granulomas may be present but do not represent involvement by Hodgkin's disease if diagnostic cells are absent.

Primary malignancies

Few primary malignant tumours have been documented in the spleen. The commonest of these are *angiosarcomas* and *fibrosarcomas*. Their cytological characteristics are the same as those seen at other sites, as described in Chapter 39.

Mucosa associated lymphoid tissue (MALT)

Expansion of the MALT can be diffuse or tumorous. In both events it offers an easy target for FNA when present in the thyroid, orbit and salivary gland[21-27]. Accordingly, this

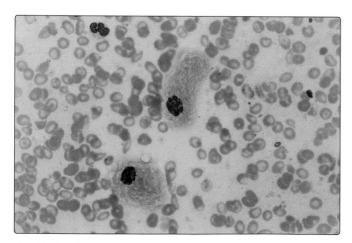

Fig. 20.12 Gaucher's disease. Histiocytes with abundant foamy cytoplasm are typical of this storage disorder. (MGG × HP)

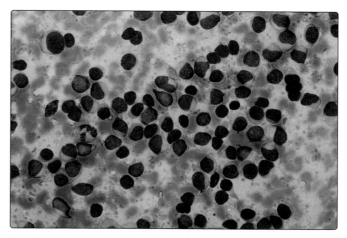

Fig. 20.13 Hairy cell leukaemia. Small to medium sized lymphoid cells with pale distinct cytoplasm. (MGG × HP)

chapter will focus on disorders affecting MALT in these organs.

Granulomatous disorders

In western countries, *sarcoidosis* is probably the most common cause of a granulomatous process in MALT. The infiltrate is predominantly diffuse, consisting of non-caseating epithelioid granulomata, and is symptomatic only when massive enlargement has occurred. The salivary gland and orbit are more often affected than the thyroid.

Cytological findings

The normal tissue components are mixed with small mature lymphocytes and epithelioid cells in clusters. Giant cells are present in varying numbers. Necrosis is not seen.

Autoimmune disorders

Sjögren's syndrome is an autoimmune disease affecting MALT, with multiple organ involvement. Dryness of the mouth and eyes are caused by lymphoid infiltration and atrophy of glandular tissue. Hashimoto's thyroiditis falls into the same category, with a diffuse or nodular infiltration of lymphocytes in the thyroid gland resulting in hypothyroidism accompanied by raised microsomal antibody titres in blood. Both of these conditions are commoner in females.

Cytological findings

Sjögren's sialadenitis

Sjögren's sialadenitis is characterized by glandular atrophy and a spectrum of lymphoid cells including plasma cells. Small mature lymphocytes predominate. Separation from a neoplastic lymphoid infiltrate requires immunocytochemistry to exclude a monomorphic infiltration. Further descriptions of the cytological findings in Sjögren's syndrome can be found in Chapter 10.

Hashimoto's disease

In Hashimoto's disease, thyroid follicular epithelium shows Hurthle cell transformation. The lymphoid population consists largely of small mature cells but centrocytes, centroblasts and plasma cells are also present (Fig. 20.14). When the follicular cells are few or without distinct Hurthle cell transformation, the possibility of a non-Hodgkin's lymphoma must be considered. Further discussion of the cytological findings in Hashimoto's disease can be found in Chapter 23.

Immunocytochemistry

Marker studies on the lymphoid cells in Sjögren's disease and Hashimoto's thyroiditis will identify both T and polyclonal B cells.

Malignant lymphomas (Fig. 20.15)

MALT can be the site of both primary and secondary malignant lymphomas. In general, lymphomas arising de novo in MALT tend to remain localized for many years, and therefore deserve special attention[1,28]. Orbital lymphomas usually do not show this behaviour and have a tendency to disseminate even though they are morphologically low-grade. Node-based lymphomas, which secondarily involve MALT, are more aggressive than primary MALT lymphomas. The cytology and immunology of these initially node-based lymphomas are described in Chapter 19.

Cytological findings (Fig. 20.16)

MALT lymphomas are composed of small to medium sized cells resembling centrocytes and reactive B cell follicles. The tumour cells may show lymphoplasmacytoid features and mature plasma cells are relatively frequent. Transformation into high-grade lymphoma may evolve from these low-grade neoplasms. Smears from low-grade MALT

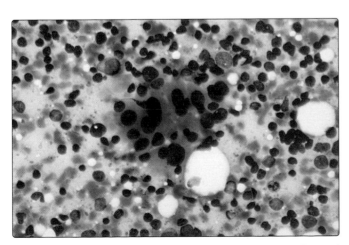

Fig. 20.14   Hashimoto's thyroiditis. Hurthle cell follicular epithelium and mixed lymphoid cells. (MGG × HP)

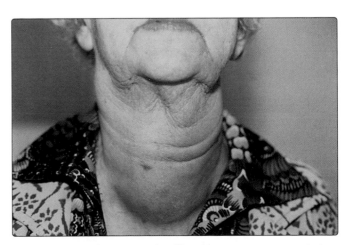

Fig. 20.15   Lymphomatous goitre. Note the enormous asymmetrical enlargement of the thyroid gland in an elderly woman.

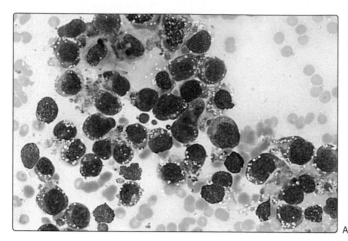

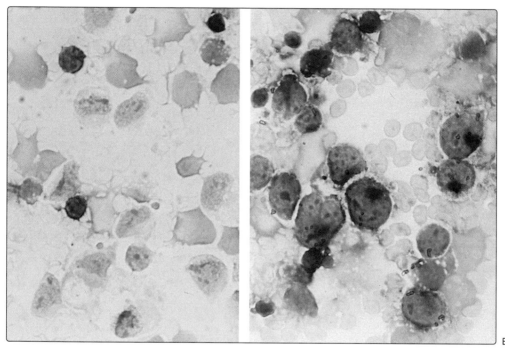

Fig. 20.16 Aspirate from the patient in Fig. 20.15 (A) Large atypical cells consistent with high-grade lymphoma. (MGG × HP) (B) Immunocytochemistry shows B-cell lineage of the neoplastic cells. Few mature T cells present. (Alkaline phosphatase × HP)

lymphomas are in most cases impossible to differentiate from reactive infiltrates using cytomorphology alone.

Immunocytochemistry

The neoplastic cells are of B phenotype and show monotypic expression of immunoglobulin chains and the tumour cells are CD5–, CD10–, CD23–, CD43–/+, CD11c+/–. A high proportion of reactive cells in the aspirate will sometimes obscure identification of the monoclonal cell fraction.

Diagnostic value of FNA in assessment of extranodal lymphoid tissue

The contribution made by FNA cytology to the management of patients with diseases of extranodal lymphoid tissue cannot be represented by a single statistical calculation based on correlations with histology. Such a figure would be meaningless in view of the widespread distribution of the tissues and the great diversity of disease processes to be found. Furthermore, the value of a cytological diagnosis in the clinical setting does not bear a simple relationship to histological correlation since the cytological diagnosis may obviate the need for surgery in the case of infection and may be the only feasible procedure in debilitated patients.

Undoubtedly, the commonest conditions investigated cytologically are those arising in MALT, particularly thyroid and salivary swellings where ease of access is an encouragement to FNA sampling. The diagnostic accuracy of these procedures is considered in the relevant chapters on thyroid and salivary gland disorders (Chapters 23 and 10, respectively).

Mediastinal tumours are sampled by FNA under radiological guidance with increasing frequency and achieve a high diagnostic rate in experienced hands. The diagnostic accuracy in this group of tumours is reviewed in Chapter 3.

References

1 Isaacson P G. Extranodal lymphomas. In: McGee J O'D, Isaacson P G, Wright N A eds. *Oxford Textbook of Pathology*. Oxford: Oxford University Press, 1992; 1787

2 Lennert K. *Histopathology of Non-Hodgkin Lymphomas*. Berlin: Springer, 1984

3 Rosai J, Levine G D, eds. Tumors of the thymus. In: *Atlas of Tumor Pathology*, 2nd series, Fascicle 13. Washington: Armed Forces Institute of Pathology, 1975

4 Ritter M A, Lampert I A. The thymus. In: McGee J O'D, Isaacson P G, Wright N A eds. *Oxford Textbook of Pathology*. Oxford: Oxford University Press, 1992; 1807

5 Addis B J, Isaacson P G. Large cell lymphomas of the mediastinum: a B-cell tumor of probable thymic origin. *Histopathol* 1986; **10**: 379–390

6 Dahlgren S, Sandstedt B, Sundstrom C. Fine needle aspiration cytology of thymic tumors. *Acta Cytol* 1983; **27**: 1–6

7 Tao L C, Pearson F C, Cooper J D et al. Cytopathology of thymoma. *Acta Cytol* 1984; **28**: 165–170

8 Shin H J, Katz R L. Thymic neoplasia as represented by fine needle aspiration biopsy of anterior mediastinal masses. A practical approach to the differential diagnosis. *Acta Cytol* 1998; **42**: 855–864

9 Finley J L, Silverman J F, Strausbach P M et al. Malignant thymic neoplasms: diagnosis by fine-needle aspiration biopsy with histology, immunocytochemical and ultrastructural confirmation. *Diagn Cytopathol* 1986; **2**: 118–126

10 Chan W G, Zaatari G S, Tabei S et al. Thymoma: an immunohistochemical study. *Am J Clin Pathol* 1984; **82**: 160–166

11 Battifora H, Sun T T, Bahv R M, Rao S. The use of antikeratin antiserum as a diagnostic tool: thymoma versus lymphoma. *Hum Pathol* 1980; **11**: 635–641

12 Ali S Z, Erozan Y S. Thymoma. Cytopathologic features and differential diagnosis on fine needle aspiration. *Acta Cytol* 1998; **42**: 845–854

13 Risdall R J, McKenna R W, Nesbit M E et al. Virus-associated hemophagocytic syndrome — a benign histiocytic proliferation distinct from malignant histiocytosis. *Cancer* 1979; **44**: 993–1002

14 Jaffe E S. Malignant histiocytosis and true histiocytic lymphomas. In: Jaffe E S ed. *Surgical Pathology of the Lymph Node and Related Organs*. Philadelphia: WB Saunders, 1985; 397

15 Soderstrom N. How to use spleen puncture. *Acta Med Scand* 1976; **199**: 1–5

16 Taavitsainen M, Koivuniemi, Helminen J et al. Aspiration biopsy of the spleen in patients with sarcoidosis. *Acta Radiol* 1987; **28**: 723–725

17 Kaplan H S. *Hodgkin's Disease*, 2nd edn. Cambridge, MA: Harvard University Press, 1980

18 Goffinet D R, Warnke R, Dunnick N R et al. Clinical and surgical (laparotomy) evaluation of patients with non-Hodgkin's lymphomas. *Cancer Treat Rep* 1977; **61**: 981–992

19 Zeppa P, Vetrani A, Luciano L et al. Fine needle aspiration biopsy of the spleen. A useful procedure in the diagnosis of splenomegaly *Acta Cytol* 1994; **38**(3): 299–309

20 Silverman J F, Geisinger K R, Raab S S, Stanley M W. Fine needle aspiration biopsy of the spleen in the evaluation of neoplastic disorders. *Acta Cytol* 1993; **37**: 158–162

21 Stewart C J, Jackson R, Farquharson M, Richmond J. Fine-needle aspiration cytology of extranodal lymphoma. *Diagn Cytopathol* 1998; **19**: 260–266

22 Tennvall J, Cavallin-Stahl E, Akerman M. Primary localized non-Hodgkin's lymphoma of the thyroid. *Eur J Surg Oncol* 1987; **13**: 297–302

23 Das D K, Gupta S K, Francis I M, Ahmed M S. Fine-needle aspiration cytology diagnosis of non-Hodgkin lymphoma of thyroid: a report of four cases. *Diagn Cytopathol* 1993; **9**: 639–645

24 Tani E M, Skoog L. Fine needle aspiration cytology and immunocytochemistry in the diagnosis of lymphoid lesions of the thyroid. *Acta Cytol* 1989; **33**: 48–52

25 Skoog L, Löwhagen T, Astarita R et al. Fine needle aspiration cytology and immunocytochemistry of ocular adnexal lymphoid tumours. *Diagn Oncol* 1992; **2**: 136–140

26 Chhieng D C, Cangiarella J F, Cohen J M. Fine-needle aspiration cytology of lymphoproliferative lesions involving the major salivary glands. *Am J Clin Pathol* 2000; **113**: 563–571

27 Allen E A, Ali S Z, Mathew S. Lymphoid lesions of the parotid. *Diagn Cytopathol* 1999; **21**: 170–173

28 Isaacson P G, Spencer J. Malignant lymphoma of mucosa-associated lymphoid tissue. *Histopathol* 1987: **11**: 445–462

Section 9

Transplantation and immunosuppression

21 Organ transplantation

Eva von Willebrand and Irmeli Lautenschlager

Introduction

Over the course of the last 15 years of the twentieth century, cytological methods and diagnosis established their role in the monitoring of organ transplants and are used today in transplantation centres around the world. Kidney and liver transplantation are the commonest procedures subjected to cytological monitoring but the techniques have been used for pancreas as well, and recently for lung transplantation.

Cytological specimens from solid organ transplants are usually obtained either by fine needle aspiration (FNA), the method mostly used in monitoring kidney and liver transplants, or by collecting urine or bile for cytological analysis. In lung transplantation bronchoalveolar lavage specimens are used for cytological assessment.

The aspiration biopsy technique itself is old. In modern clinical practice it was developed by Franzen in 1960[1] to diagnose urological malignancies and applied to renal transplants in humans for the first time in 1968 by Pasternack[2]. The cytology of allograft rejection was at the time practically unknown and during the following decade, experimental work on rat and human kidney allografts[3-6] helped to elucidate the immunological and cytological sequence of events in allograft rejection. This experimental work revealed that the inflammation indicative of activation of the immune system associated with rejection is seen earlier and is more specific in the transplanted organ than in the peripheral blood of the recipient.

The advantage of cytological methods is that the risk of complications to graft and patient is minimal, the specimens can be obtained daily if necessary, and the methods are quick to perform. In 1982 the FNA method was also applied in liver transplantation[7,8]. Experience of over 17 000 FNAs in kidney transplants and over 5000 FNAs in liver transplants has shown that cytological analysis of aspiration biopsies is well suited to monitoring the transplant during the early postoperative period when the risk of acute rejection is highest. The main limitation of cytology is that the information obtained is limited in certain respects compared to histology, especially with regard to the architectural structure of the transplant.

In this chapter, we discuss the cytology of kidney and liver transplantation based on aspiration cytology methods and also summarize briefly the experiences of bronchoalveolar lavage (BAL) cytology in lung transplantation. Details of the findings in pancreatic transplants are discussed in Chapter 16.

Kidney transplant cytology

Sampling and processing of cytological specimens

In renal transplantation the method most often used to obtain cytological specimens from the transplant is a modification of Franzen's fine needle aspiration[9,10].

Aspiration biopsies are taken using a 20–22 gauge spinal needle connected to a 20 ml syringe which contains 5 ml of RPMI-1640 tissue culture medium supplemented with 5% human serum albumin, 50 IU/ml heparin and 1% Hepes buffer. An aspiration biopsy pistol may be used, but is not necessary for the procedure. The transplant is usually located easily by palpation. When necessary, ultrasound guidance can be used.

The biopsy is performed percutaneously without local anaesthesia in aseptic conditions. The needle is inserted into the renal cortex, full suction is applied and the needle is moved back and forth three or four times through a distance of 1–2 cm. In this way the needle traverses the entire cortex and reaches several periglomerular and perivascular areas. Sampling is complete when the colour of cellular fluid can be seen in the needle hub. The needle is then rapidly withdrawn after releasing suction and the sample of 10–50 μl inside the needle is flushed immediately with tissue culture medium to get the whole sample into the syringe. The syringe with sample inside is then sent to the laboratory for immediate processing. If necessary, samples can be kept overnight in syringes containing culture medium in a refrigerator.

To compare the relative leucocyte distribution between peripheral blood and graft, simultaneous samples of blood, usually 2–3 drops, are taken from the fingertip into another syringe containing 5 ml of the same RPMI medium.

The FNA and blood samples are processed in parallel. The cells are centrifuged, resuspended, counted and 100–200 μl aliquots are spun on to microscope slides using a cytocentrifuge. The smears are air dried for routine diagnostic use and stained with May-Grünwald-Giemsa (MGG). Parallel preparations can be used for other cytological stains or immunocytochemical staining techniques.

Table 21.1 FNAB report

Inflammatory cells	FNAB	Blood	Increment	Correction factor	Corrected increment
Lymphoid blast cells	3	0	3	1.0	3.0
Activated lymphocytes	4	0	4	0.5	2.0
Lgl lymphocytes	1	1		0.2	
Lymphocytes	40	13	27	0.1	2.7
PMN:					
Juvenile forms	0	0		0.1	
Neutrophils	35	62		0.1	
Basophils	0	2		0.1	
Eosinophils	7	14		0.1	
Monoblast	0	0		1.0	
Monocytes	10	8	2	0.2	0.4
Macrophages	0	0		1.0	
Total corrected increment					7.1
Total blast cells/cytoprep		22			
Parenchymal cells		Normal	Swelling	Swelling vacuolation	Necrosis
Morphology score		1	2	3	4
Parenchymal cells			2		
Parenchymal cells per 100 inflammatory cells				20	

Conclusions: Clear blastogenic rejection. Some swelling and degeneration in parenchymal cells

Interpretation of cytological specimens

MGG stained cytospin smears of the graft and blood are examined microscopically and the findings reported on a standard report form (Table 21.1), derived from the First International Workshop on Transplant Aspiration Cytology in Munich in 1982. The three most important features to be evaluated are specimen adequacy, the leucocyte differential and the morphological features of the parenchymal cells.

Specimen adequacy

To be evaluated, the aspirate must be representative. The inevitable but variable contamination of renal and liver aspirates by blood makes assessment of specimen adequacy of utmost importance in interpretation of the findings.

Since the cellular infiltration of acute rejection is always most pronounced in the renal cortex, representative specimens must include sufficient cortical material. Cytological samples taken from the medulla are usually not diagnostic[11,12], as is also the case in histology. The presence of glomeruli cannot be used as a criterion for adequacy since glomeruli do not always appear in aspirates and many of them are lost in processing. Instead, adequacy of

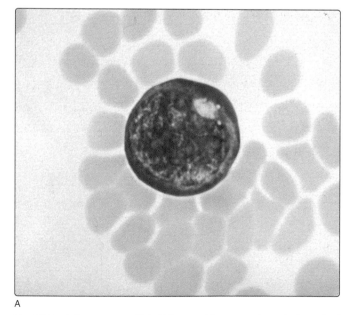

A

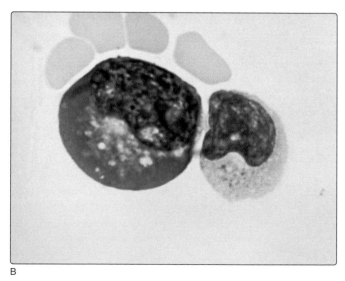

B

Fig. 21.1 Inflammatory cells in kidney and liver transplants during rejection. Giemsa stained cytocentrifuge preparations. (A) A lymphoid blast cell with immature nucleus and cytoplasmic basophilia, (B) a blast cell with plasmacyroid morphology and a large granular lymphocyte with cytoplasmic granulation.

representation is assessed by calculating the ratio of tubular cells to inflammatory leucocytes.

Cytological criteria for representative samples and reproducibility of transplant aspirate specimens have been established by analysing duplicate aspirates[13], where a correlation coefficient of 0.95 was obtained if both specimens contained at least seven tubular cells per 100 inflammatory leucocytes. When the ratio of tubular cells to leucocytes in either sample fell below this, the correlation coefficient fell accordingly. Other groups have reported similar results for double aspirate biopsy analysis[14,15].

Inflammatory cells

Most of the inflammatory leucocytes in cytological preparations can be identified readily according to standard haematological criteria[6,10] in routine MGG stained smears (Fig. 21.1). These include small lymphocytes, activated lymphocytes with increased cytoplasmic basophilia, and large granular lymphocytes, which are the morphological form of natural killer cells[16]. The appearance of blast cells is diagnostic of acute rejection.

Lymphoid blast cells are characterized by their large size (15–25 μm in diameter), their large immature nuclei and intense cytoplasmic basophilia. Approximately 50% of the lymphoid blast cells are B blasts containing intracytoplasmic immunoglobulins, as identified by immunofluorescence staining. The other half of the blast cells are T blasts, characterized by T cell surface antigens, and identified with monoclonal antibodies using immunoperoxidase staining.

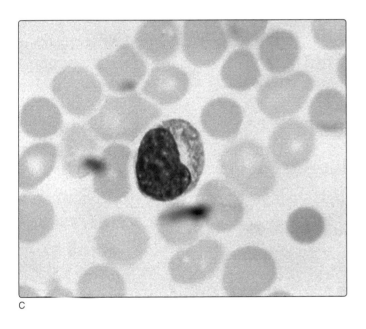

C

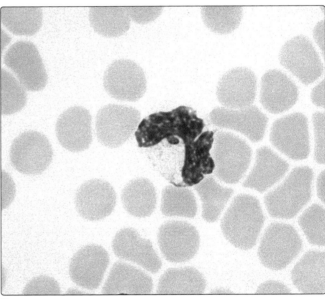

D

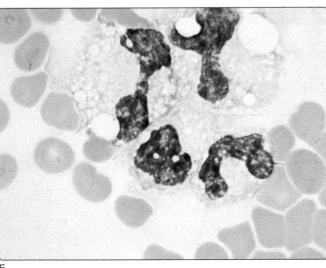

E

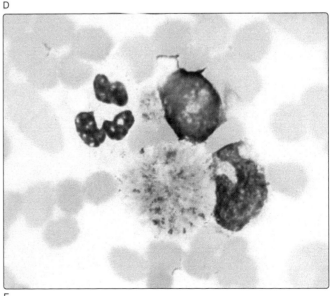

F

Fig. 21.1 *(cont'd)*   (C) an activated lymphocyte, (D) a monocyte with irregular nuclear contours, (E) macrophages with cytoplasmic vacuolation and elongated nuclei, (F) a thrombocyte aggregate with a monocyte.

Different forms of monocyte-macrophage cells can also be seen, including small monocytes, large monocytes with irregular, multilobulated nuclei and macrophages in different stages of maturation. Macrophages are large cells, up to 60 μm in diameter, usually showing vacuolated cytoplasm and pyknotic elongated nuclei lying at the periphery of the cell. They are usually seen in abundance in the later phases of severe and irreversible rejection and in acute vascular rejection in the early phase.

Eosinophils are usually more frequent at the beginning of immunological reactivation, and are seen both in aspirates and in peripheral blood, indicating generalized immune response to the graft[17]. Platelets are also seen during rejection in excess in the graft[18,19]. Small loose platelet aggregates disappear during successful rejection treatment, but large aggregates on endothelial cells seem to indicate a worse prognosis[19]. Neutrophils are usually seen in excess in the graft only when there is irreversible rejection with necrotic changes. In cases with bacterial infection of the graft, neutrophil aggregates with intracellular bacteria can be seen.

Cytological characteristics of renal parenchymal cells

Aspiration biopsy specimens consist mainly of single parenchymal cells, although clumps of renal tubular cells or even parts of tubules and whole glomeruli may often be encountered in the specimens. The parenchymal cells most commonly seen are tubular cells from different parts of the nephron, and endothelial cells from the renal vascular endothelium, usually from capillary blood vessels (Fig. 21.2).

For more detailed characterization of the parenchymal cells, immunocytochemistry can be used. With monoclonal antibodies different parenchymal cell types can be identified precisely. Cytokeratin antibodies are used for tubular cell characterization, since these antibodies do not stain endothelial cells or leucocytes. Endothelial cells can be stained with antibodies to Factor VIII-related antigens or with vimentin antibodies, which do not stain tubular cells[20].

Morphological changes in parenchymal cells in different graft complications

Changes in the parenchymal cells are scored from 1–4, 1 being normal and 4 representing necrosis, and this score is

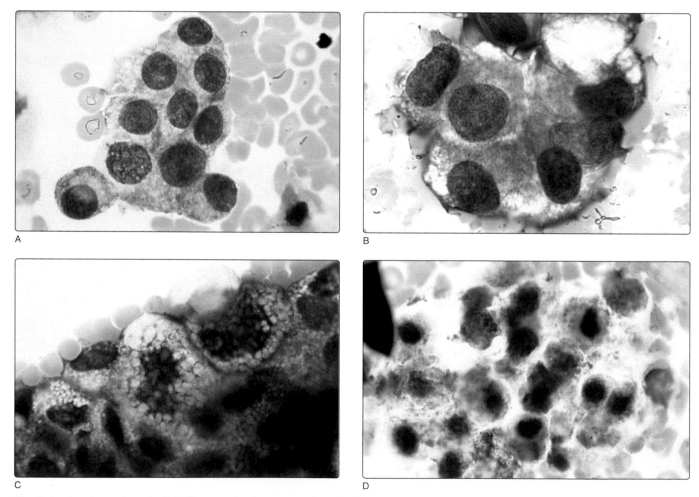

Fig. 21.2 Renal parenchymal cells in Giemsa stained cytopreparations. (A) A group of normal tubular cells, (B) swelling, degeneration and vacuolation in tubular cells in ATN, (C) pronounced isometric vacuolation and swelling in tubular cells during CyA toxicity, (D) necrotic tubular cells in graft necrosis.

recorded in the report (Table 21.1). Although typical findings in parenchymal cells can be seen in several different graft complications, the findings are basically non-specific. Degenerative changes can be seen in tubular cells in acute tubular necrosis (Fig. 21.2), in advancing rejection, in cyclosporin A (CyA) nephrotoxicity and also in urological complications. The information derived from graft parenchymal cell morphology is useful in the differential diagnosis of graft complications, but interpretation of the changes requires concomitant evaluation of the inflammation and also knowledge of the clinical data.

In acute tubular necrosis (ATN) tubular cells are swollen, with cytoplasmic degeneration and irregular vacuolation. In very severe cases necrotic tubular cells may also be seen, but usually only a few. These changes are due to prolonged cold ischaemia and return to normal with improving graft function in 1–2 weeks. In pure ATN there are no signs of immunoactivation.

Similar, but more pronounced changes are seen in the tubular cells in acute CyA toxicity. The cells are swollen, with increased cytoplasmic basophilia and prominent isometric vacuolation[21–23]. Toxic isometric vacuolation is quite typical of acute CyA toxicity, although it is a non-specific phenomenon. It has also been reported in experimental kidney transplantation models[24]. The deposits of CyA and its metabolites can be demonstrated by specific monoclonal antibodies and immunofluorescence techniques[25]. Isometric vacuolation is not seen in chronic CyA toxicity, where tubular atrophy and degeneration with interstitial fibrosis are the dominating features. Today, with triple drug immunosuppressive treatment and rather low CyA doses, acute CyA toxicity is not a very common complication.

At the beginning of acute rejection, tubular and endothelial cells usually have normal morphology and also retain normal morphology in short easily treated rejections. In severe and prolonged rejection, on the other hand, there are progressive degenerative changes in tubular cells and even necrosis in irreversible rejection.

Severe necrotic changes in tubular cells are also seen in graft infarction[25], which is usually due to renal vein thrombosis. This clinical complication is often fulminant with rapidly progressing necrosis, but fortunately it is not a frequent event.

Quantitation of inflammation in the transplant
Increment method
As all aspiration biopsies are contaminated with variable amounts of blood, the inflammation in the graft is evaluated against the blood background by increment analysis: differential counts of 100–200 leucocytes from the aspirate and blood specimens are performed and the blood values are subtracted from aspirate values to obtain the increment of inflammatory cells (Table 21.1). As all

inflammatory cells in allograft rejection do not have equal diagnostic significance[3,4], correction factors are used in calculating the corrected increment[10]. The cells with greatest significance in acute rejection, blast cells and macrophages, have a full correction factor of 1.0. Correction factors for all inflammatory cells are given in Table 21.1.

The sum of the corrected increment values, known as corrected increment units (CIU), represents the total corrected increment (TCI), which describes the intensity of inflammation in the graft. Usually, a TCI higher than 3.0 and a blast cell increment of 1.0 indicates acute rejection[26,27]. The presence of blast cells is in itself suggestive of immunological activation in the graft: therefore the total number of blast cells per cytopreparation is also counted. In a stable graft no blasts are seen, but during immune activation the number of blast cells rises up to 10–50 per cytopreparation and may be even higher[26]. In the analysis of Helderman et al.[28] a total count of >6 blast cells per slide proved representative of rejection independent of the TCI score. With the increment method it is possible to describe the aspirate findings with a single numerical value instead of by description only, although the description is also important.

Cytology in monitoring of the transplant
Sequential follow-up of the transplant with regular aspiration biopsies and cytological samples permits definition of the course of intragraft events.

In a stable graft lymphocytic/monocytic infiltration in the aspirates is either absent or minimal. When acute rejection begins increasing numbers of lymphoid and monocytic cells infiltrate the graft, and blast cells in particular appear in the aspirate. Lymphoid blast response is the hallmark of acute rejection together with an elevated TCI, usually also associated with deteriorating graft function. With successful rejection treatment inflammatory cells disappear from the graft and graft function improves. In unresponsive severe rejections macrophages begin to infiltrate the graft, tubular cell degeneration increases and graft necrosis ensues. Macrophage accumulation during rejection usually indicates a poor prognosis.

In most cases of acute cellular rejection, the inflammation follows the cytological pattern described above. However, individual patients may have different inflammatory profiles. Sometimes mild transient lymphocytic/monocytic infiltrates with some blast cells can be seen in the graft around 1 week after transplantation. These usually resolve without any further treatment and without deterioration in transplant function. In these cases of mild immunological activation the existing immunosuppressive treatment is efficient enough to keep the inflammation below the threshold of clinical rejection[29].

Evidence of acute vascular rejection (AVR) is a major feature of rejections that do not respond to steroid treatment[30,31]. Diagnosis of AVR is always based on histology: however characteristic cytological findings in acute vascular rejection have been defined[32-34]. These include accumulation of monocytes and macrophages in the graft. Lymphocytic infiltrates, especially of blast cells, are not prominent in AVR, at least not in the pure forms[35]. Combinations of ACR and AVR are also common[31,35] and are often resistant to ordinary steroid rejection treatment. Monoclonal or polyclonal antibodies, OKT3 or ATG, are used in the treatment of these rejections[30,31].

The immunosuppressive protocol used clearly modifies the aspiration cytology profiles. Today, when most centres use triple treatment, a combination of cyclosporin, azathioprine and steroids, only approximately 30% of cadaver kidney grafts have any acute rejection episodes during the first postoperative month[36], compared with 70% with the older treatment protocols using azathioprine and steroids[37,38]. The onset of rejection is also delayed and the inflammation is milder, with fewer blast cells. Regular monitoring by cytology thus also allows assessment of the impact of different immunosuppressive drugs on the graft.

Immunocytochemistry

Using immunocytological techniques, such as immunoperoxidase or immunofluorescence staining with monoclonal antibodies, it is possible to evaluate in even greater detail the state of the transplant and the nature of the inflammatory infiltrates in the graft[39-43] The different T and B lymphocyte subsets can be analysed, including their state of activation. Mononuclear phagocytes can be differentiated, as can parenchymal cells. Expression of adhesion molecules on parenchymal cells can also be evaluated with relevant monoclonal antibodies.

Lymphocyte populations in graft rejections

In most acute cellular rejections CD8 T lymphocytes outnumber CD4 cells in the graft, although at the beginning of the rejection episode CD4 T cells seem to be frequent[40,44,45]. In severe irreversible rejections, persistence of CD4 dominance in the graft has been seen[46].

Usually the sum of CD4 and CD8 cells in the transplant is greater than the total number of CD2 or CD3 positive T cells. A minority of lymphocytes are positive for both CD4 and CD8. The number of B lymphocytes is usually rather low during rejection, forming approximately 5–20% of the lymphocytes, but the number of B blast cells is relatively high; of the blast cells in rejection infiltrates approximately 50% are B blast cells and 50% T blast cells.

Different forms of mononuclear phagocytes can be stained and identified with relevant monoclonal antibodies. Lymphocyte subpopulations in grafts are however variable, both during different phases of rejection and also during viral infections, and cannot as such be used as diagnostic findings. Nevertheless, analysis of the different inflammatory subsets gives important additional information on the state of the transplant.

Activation markers and adhesion molecules in acute rejection

Analysis of activation markers and the adhesion molecules of inflammatory cells infiltrating the graft and parenchymal cells has proved to be useful in rejection diagnosis. In acute rejection induction of interleukin-2 (IL-2) receptors (CD25) on activated lymphoid cells has been demonstrated[47,48] and HLA-class II antigens are induced on the tubular cells[49,50,51]. With successful rejection treatment CD25 positive lymphoid cells disappear rapidly and class II expression diminishes to background level[48,52]. In stable grafts there is no induction of activation markers.

Adhesion molecules are also induced during rejection on different transplant components. Constitutively normal kidneys express several adhesion molecules on the endothelial cells of vessels, such as intercellular adhesion molecule-1 (ICAM-1) and vascular cell adhesion molecule (VCAM-1)[53]. Tubular cells do not normally express these molecules, or only in small quantities on the luminal surfaces, but during rejection these adhesion molecules are induced on cells of tubular origin. The induction of ICAM-1 on tubular cells occurs early in rejection and disappears rapidly with successful rejection treatment[54]. The role of these molecules in the rejection process is at present under intensive investigation.

Viral infections

Viral infections often cause differential diagnostic problems in transplant patients. Cytomegalovirus (CMV) infections can induce generalized immunological activation in the patient; lymphoid blast cells, activated lymphocytes and large granular lymphocytes are found in the patient's blood and also in the transplant aspirate[55-58]. CMV infections are also related to rejection, patients with frequent rejections having more CMV infections, while patients with CMV infection have more rejections. CMV infection has been shown to induce HLA class II antigens on kidney transplant tubular cells[59]. Apparently this is the link to the rejection process. Specific virological methods, such as antigen detection, viral culture or PCR are, however, necessary to diagnose CMV or other viral infections[60,61].

Correlation with histology

The correlation between aspiration cytology and histology in renal transplantation has been assessed in several studies[10,14,33]. A high concordance between simultaneous cytology and histology findings has been reported, particularly in acute cellular rejection, ATN, acute CyA toxicity and also when the graft situation is stable[34,62-66]. It has been shown that there is a relation between the histological severity of acute rejection, whether mild, moderate or severe, and the level of inflammation in cytology[67]. Diagnostic sensitivities and specificities of >90% have been reported in a prospective study comparing cytology and histology in monitoring of kidney transplant patients[28] and in a blind study comparing cytology and histology in 200 patients[27].

Recently, a prospective, randomized study[68] compared cytology, histology and immunohistology in the rejection diagnosis, using clinical evaluation of rejection as the gold standard. The respective specificities were 96%, 87% and 80%, with sensitivities of 59%, 75% and 77%. In this analysis cytology had an increased tendency to miss clinical rejection episodes but proved most reliable in monitoring non-functioning or stable grafts.

Diagnostic value of cytology in organ transplant failure

The value of cytology in the differential diagnosis of graft complications is presented in Table 21.2.

Liver transplant cytology

As a result of experimental studies[7,69] and the experience gained in monitoring kidney allografts, FNA transplant cytology has also been applied to hepatic transplantation[8,70,71]. Liver FNA has been used as a routine clinical procedure since 1982[8]. It has proved to be a reliable method of diagnosing inflammation associated with acute liver rejection and for monitoring the response to antirejection therapy[71-74]. A good correlation with biopsy histology in the diagnosis of acute rejection has been reported from several centres[75-77]. FNA monitoring is therefore accepted as a routine diagnostic tool in liver transplantation.

Technical aspects

Liver allograft recipients are monitored with frequent FNAs from the day of transplantation, usually at 3–5 day intervals. Specimens should be obtained through the medial aspect of the right costal margin, to minimize the risk of complications or contamination from the intraperitoneal cavity[78]. The technique for performing and processing FNAs of liver and corresponding blood

---

Table 21.2   Cytology in the differential diagnosis of graft complications

Good
Acute cellular rejection
Normal graft
Parenchymal damage
Acute CyA toxicity
Necrosis of the graft

Satisfactory
Lymphocele, haematoma
Bacterial infection in the graft
Acute vascular rejection (kidney)
Viral infection, CMV (I.P staining)

Not satisfactory
Chronic rejection
Chronic CyA toxicity
Recurrence of the original disease

---

specimens is similar to that described for renal allografts[10]. The quantitation of inflammation by the increment method is also similar[10].

Cytological findings in acute liver allograft rejection

Diagnosis of liver allograft rejection is difficult, as clinical signs or biochemical markers are rather non-specific and the findings cannot be distinguished from conditions such as cholangitis, infections or cholestasis. Thus, invasive methods are necessary for the evaluation of liver rejection. However, conventional core needle biopsy always creates some risk of complications, such as bleeding or infection.

In biopsy histology, the hallmark of acute liver allograft rejection is infiltration of the portal areas by mononuclear cells[79,80]. The inflammatory infiltrate consists mainly of lymphocytes and a few plasma cells. In addition, the cellular infiltrate often contains eosinophils, neutrophil polymorphs and mononuclear phagocytes. Portal inflammation with bile duct and vascular involvement, together with cholestasis, are characteristic histological findings in acute rejection.

In FNA material, the emergence of lymphoid blast cells and an increase in lymphocytes in the graft are typical findings at the beginning of acute liver rejection[69,71]. The first day on which FNA reveals inflammation with >3.0 CIU and the presence of lymphoid blast cells is considered as the onset of immune activation in the graft[71]. In the advanced stages of rejection the blastogenic response subsides and the cellular infiltrate becomes dominated by mononuclear phagocytes. Large numbers of macrophages are associated with irreversible rejection and parenchymal necrosis[69,71]. The neutrophil or eosinophil infiltration of the graft described in biopsy histology cannot usually be evaluated against the background blood in FNA material. However, blood eosinophilia correlates with immune activation in the graft[71].

The clinical diagnosis of rejection is based not only on FNA findings, but also on other laboratory parameters and clinical signs. It is well known from biopsy histology and FNA cytology that a few days after liver transplantation, some inflammatory infiltrate may appear in portal areas without tissue damage, and disappear without any clinical sign of rejection or additional immunosuppression[81-83]. This type of immune activation may be initiated by donor cells in the graft representing an *in situ* graft-versus-host (GVH) reaction, or alternatively could be an incomplete or subclinical form of the alloresponse under certain immunosuppressive conditions[77]. Thus, the typical findings on FNA or in biopsy histology, together with graft dysfunction are needed for the clinical diagnosis of acute liver allograft rejection.

Activation markers and cellular findings of rejection

Although hardly necessary, immunological activation marker analysis may be performed on FNA specimens to confirm the cytological findings. An increase in MHC class II positive lymphocytes and the appearance of IL-2 receptor expressing cells in the graft correlate with immune activation and blast response in the FNA.[84]

Expression of class II antigens on liver parenchymal cells has also been shown to correlate with acute cellular rejection[85,86]. However, various infections, especially viral infections, also induce class II expression. Induction of adhesion molecules, such as in the graft ICAM-1, is an early marker for immune activation[87,88]. Induction of ICAM-1 on liver parenchymal cells can be regarded as even less specific than class II, since it is expressed on liver parenchymal cells not only during rejection and viral infections[89,90], but also during bacterial infections[90].

Liver transplant cytology and infections

Systemic infections, such as bacterial sepsis or various viral infections, have practically no effect on FNA findings of intragraft inflammation[91]. In bacteraemia, a prominent neutrophilia is seen in the blood specimen, and characteristic findings in viral infections are either lymphocytosis or, after long lasting viraemia, lymphopenia.

During CMV infection, which is the most common of the viral infections, mild lymphoid activation with a few lymphoid blasts is recorded in both FNA and the corresponding blood sample[92]. However, immune activation in the graft simply reflects the haematological changes in the background blood and the total inflammation seldom exceeds 3.0 CIU. Other characteristic findings for CMV infection are blood eosinophilia and increased numbers of large granular lymphocytes. This generalized immune response against CMV subsides with successful antiviral treatment[92]. Not only CMV, but also the other members of the herpesvirus family, such as human herpesvirus-6, are associated with lymphocyte dominated immune response, which can be falsely interpreted[93].

Any infection located in the graft may lead to cellular changes in the FNA specimen. Large numbers of neutrophils in the aspirate, often with hypersegmented nuclei, indicate either a bacterial infection in the graft, an abscess or contamination from a wound infection. Intracellular bacteria are sometimes seen. Viral hepatitis may generate lymphocyte infiltration in the graft and cause differential diagnostic problems[83]. Hepatitis C virus (HCV) is common among liver transplant recipients, and recurrence of the infection is associated with graft lymphocytosis[94]. Because of the high incidence of infections in liver transplant patients, careful microbiological investigations, especially virological, should be included in patient monitoring.

Liver parenchymal cell cytology

Normal liver transplant FNAs contain hepatocytes in clusters and in single cell form (Fig. 21.3A). The number of parenchymal cells is evaluated, and the specimens are considered representative according to the same principles as for renal FNAs[13]. In addition to hepatocytes, other parenchymal components such as bile duct cells (Fig. 21.3B) and endothelial cells are, occasionally seen in FNA specimens.

Degenerative changes in hepatocytes with swelling and irregular vacuolation (Fig. 21.3C) are recorded in FNA during the inflammatory episodes of acute rejection[71]. Necrotic cells (Fig. 21.3D) in the FNA indicate severe tissue damage. Degeneration of hepatocytes without inflammation in the graft is due to other causes, such as vascular complications or drug toxicity. There are characteristic morphological changes associated with CyA hepatotoxicity[71,95] with isometric vacuolation of hepatocytes (Fig. 21.3E). Deposits of CyA or its metabolites can be demonstrated in the cells by immunofluorescence.

Cholestasis is often recorded in association with an inflammatory episode or rejection (Fig. 21.3F). Bile droplets in hepatocytes or between the cells indicate either impaired graft function or extracellular cholestasis during rejection[71]. Cholestasis without inflammation indicates biliary complications or impaired graft function for reasons other than rejection[71,73].

The role of aspiration cytology in liver transplantation

Although a close correlation between FNA and liver biopsy histology has been reported by several groups[75-77], cytology is not intended to replace biopsy histology. In general, FNA is used for frequent monitoring, even daily, especially during the first 3–4 weeks after transplantation, when 95% of acute liver rejections occur. During this time core needle biopsy may be obtained, if needed, to diagnose various complications other than rejection, to confirm the diagnosis or to assess the degree of liver damage and need for retransplantation. After the first postoperative months, when chronic pathology of the liver graft supervenes, the diagnostic value of FNA decreases. If there is a suspicion of chronic rejection, as evidenced by the development of the vanishing bile duct syndrome or any other late complications, core needle biopsy histology is the only dependable diagnostic method.

Biochemical markers of graft dysfunction such as increased serum values of transaminases, alkaline phosphatase and bilirubin, correlate with inflammatory episodes in FNA, but the cytological diagnosis of acute rejection, based on lymphoid activation and blast response, can be recognized 1–3 days earlier by FNA. However, as has already been stated, graft dysfunction, together with cytological or histological findings are needed for the clinical diagnosis of liver rejection. However, monitoring of viral infections is necessary because of differential diagnostics.

In addition to diagnostic purposes, the FNA method can also be used for further studies on the mechanisms of liver allograft rejection[96–99].

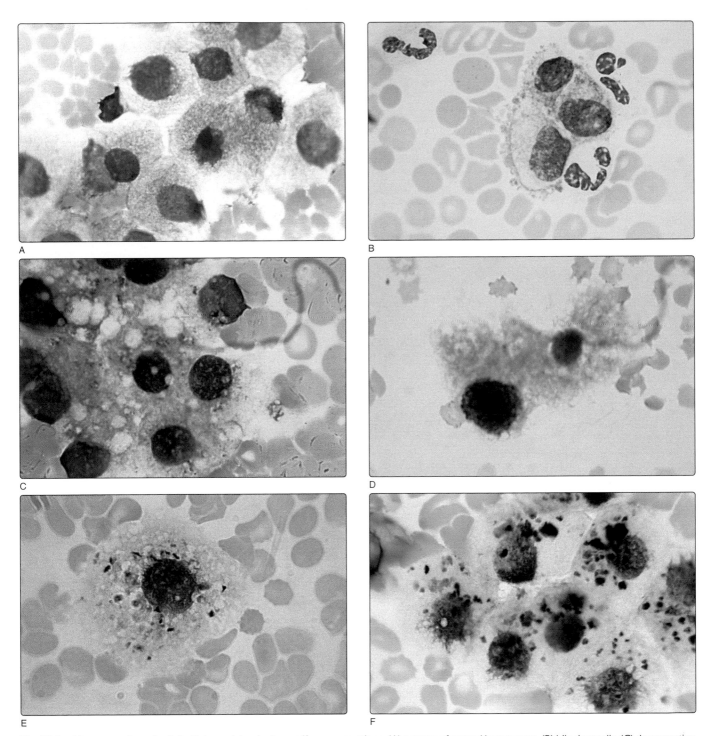

Fig. 21.3 Liver parenchymal cells in Geimsa stained cytocentrifuge preparations: (A) a group of normal hepatocytes, (B) bile duct cells, (C) degenerative changes in hepatocytes during rejection, (D) necrotic liver parenchymal cells, (E) fine isometric vacuolation in a hepatocyte during high dose CyA treatment, (F) accumulation of bile in hepatocytes indicating cholestasis.

Lung transplant cytology

Lung transplant rejection and other intragraft complications can only be reliably diagnosed by biopsy histology[100] and the criteria for diagnosing and grading of lung rejection have been established[101]. Because of the high mortality associated with open lung biopsy, less dangerous procedures, such as transtracheal biopsies, are more often used for routine diagnosis[100]. Bronchoalveolar lavage (BAL) and cytological analysis of BAL fluid provide diagnostic tools suitable for frequent monitoring of lung allografts.

BAL cytology

Cellular analysis of BAL fluid provides a useful method for monitoring the intragraft events after lung and heart-lung transplantation[102–105]. An increase in total cell count indicates either rejection or infection. Patients undergoing rejection demonstrate a predominance of lymphocytes and macrophages, but also some neutrophils in the BAL fluid. Additional immunological studies can be performed on BAL specimens, but the results of lymphocyte subtype analysis have been controversial and are probably influenced by various infections.

The cellular picture of bacterial infection is neutrophil dominated, but protozoal infections, such as *Pneumocystis carinii*, or viral infections, especially CMV, may cause differential diagnostic problems, because of the lymphocyte and macrophage response in the lungs during these complications[100]. Functional analysis of BAL lymphocytes may provide some help in the differential diagnosis of rejection[106].

In addition to BAL cytology, parallel microbiological monitoring is necessary. Thus, the current clinical use of BAL after lung transplantation consists of cytological and possibly immunological studies combined with investigation of various infections.

Pancreatic transplant cytology

This subject is considered in Chapter 16, which also deals with other aspects of the cytopathology of the pancreas.

Conclusions

Cytological methods allow frequent monitoring of intragraft events in organ transplantation. Aspiration biopsies can be performed daily if necessary, without risk to the graft or to the patient. Monitoring of the cytological and immunological sequence of events gives a dynamic picture of the progress of the graft and makes it possible to evaluate the effect of immunosuppressive treatment of the transplant.

The main limitation of the method is that cytology does not allow evaluation of the architectural structures of the transplant. Therefore acute cellular rejection can be diagnosed with certainty, and in renal transplants identification of normal grafts or the presence of acute tubular necrosis or acute cyclosporin toxicity can be made. The most important conditions in which cytology can only be suggestive, are acute vascular rejection in kidney transplants, chronic rejection, chronic cyclosporin toxicity and recurrent or *de novo* diseases in the transplant.

In liver transplantation, FNA cytology is a reliable method for diagnosing acute rejection. It also reveals cholestasis and parenchymal damage associated either with rejection or with biliary or vascular complications is during the first months after transplantation. The diagnosis of chronic rejection and other late complications is based on histology, cytology being best suited for monitoring the transplant during the early postoperative period.

References

1 Franzen S, Giertz G, Zaijcek J. Cytological diagnosis of prostatic tumors by transrectal aspiration biopsy. *Br J Urol* 1960; **32**: 193–196

2 Pasternack A. Fine-needle aspiration biopsy of human renal homografts. *Lancet* 1968; **ii**: 82–84

3 von Willebrand E, Häyry P. Composition and in vitro cytotoxicity of cellular infiltrates in rejecting human kidney allografts. *Cell Immunol* 1978; **41**: 358–372

4 von Willebrand E, Soots A, Häyry P. In situ effector mechanisms in rat kidney allograft rejecting I. Characterization of the host cellular infiltrate in rejecting allograft parenchyma. *Cell Immunol* 1979; **46**: 309–326

5 Häyry P, von Willebrand E, Soots A. In situ effector mechanisms in rat kidney allograft rejection III. Kinetics of the inflammatory response and generation of donor-directed killer cells. *Scand J Immunol* 1979; **10**: 95–108

6 von Willebrand E. Fine needle aspiration cytology of human renal transplants. *Clin Immunol Immunopathol* 1980; **17**: 309–322

7 Lautenschlager I, Höckerstedt K, Taskinen E et al. Fine-needle aspiration cytology of liver allografts in pig. *Transplantation* 1984; **38**: 330–334

8 Lautenschlager I, Höckerstedt K, von Willebrand E et al. Aspiration cytology of

human liver allograft. *Transplant Proc* 1984; **16**: 1243–1246

9 Häyry P, von Willebrand E. Monitoring of human renal allograft rejection with fine-needle aspiration cytology. *Scand J Immunol* 1981; **13**: 87–97

10 Häyry P, von Willebrand E. Practical guidelines for fine needle aspiration biopsy of human renal allografts. *Ann of Clin Res* 1981; **13**: 288–306

11 Belitsky P, Gupta R, Campbell J. Diagnosis of acute cellular rejection in kidney allografts by fine needle aspiration cytology. *Transplant Proc* 1984; **16**: 1076–1079

12 Gupta R, Om A, Ghose T, Belitsky P. Distinction between cortex and medulla in kidney transplant aspiration cytology and relevance to interpretation of results. *Transplant Proc* 1987; **19**: 1641–1643

13 von Willebrand E, Häyry P. Reproducibility of the fine needle aspiration biopsy. Analysis of 93 double biopsies. *Transplantation* 1984; **38**: 314–316

14 Belitsky P, Campbell J, Gupta R. Serial biopsy controlled evaluation of fine needle aspiration in renal allograft rejection. *Lab Invest* 1985; **53**: 580–585

15 Vereerstraeten P, Romasco F, Monsieur R et al. Representativeness and reproducibility of WBC counts in fine needle aspiration specimens from kidney transplants. *Transplant Proc* 1985; **17**: 2106–2107

16 Saksela E, Timonen T, Ranki A, Häyry P. Morphological and functional characterization of isolated effector cells responsible for human natural killer cell activity to fetal fibroblasts and to cultured cell line targets. *Immunol Rev* 1979; **44**: 71–123

17 Lautenschlager I, von Willebrand E, Häyry P. Blood eosinophilia, steroids and rejection. *Transplantation* 1985; **40**: 354–357

18 Smith N, Chandler S, Hawker R J et al. Indium-labelled autologous platelets as diagnostic aid after renal transplantation. *Lancet* 1979; **ii**: 1241–1242

19 von Willebrand E, Zola H, Häyry P. Thrombocyte aggregates in renal allografts. Analysis by the fine needle aspiration biopsy and monoclonal anti-thrombocyte antibodies. *Transplantation* 1985; **39**: 258–262

20 von Willebrand E, Lautenschlager I, Inkinen K et al. Distribution of the major histocompatibility complex antigens in human and rat kidney. *Kidney Int* 1985; **27**: 616–621

21 von Willebrand E, Häyry P. Cyclosporin A deposits in renal allografts. *Lancet* 1983; **ii**: 189–192

22 Egidi F, De Vecchi A, Pagliari B et al. Lack of relationship between blood cyclosporine levels and nephrotoxicity as assessed by

fine needle aspiration biopsy of renal allografts. *Transplant Proc* 1985; **17**: 2096–2097

23 Santelli G, Ouziala M, Charpentier B, Fries D. Predictive value of fine needle aspiration biopsy for cyclosporine nephrotoxicity. *Transplant Proc* 1985; **17**: 2094–2095

24 Whiting P H, Thomson A W, Blair J T, Simpson J G. Experimental cyclosporin A nephrotoxicity. *Br J Pathol* 1982; **63**: 88–94

25 Hughes D A, Rapoport J, Roake J A *et al.* Confirmation of renal allograft infarction using fine-needle aspiration cytology. In: Yussim A, Hammer C eds. *Contributions to Transplantation Medicine: Transplant Monitoring.* Wolfgang Pabst Verlag, 1992; 52–56

26 von Willebrand E. Long-term experience with fine needle aspiration in kidney transplant patients. *Transplant Proc* 1989; **21**: 3568–3570

27 Reinholt F P, Bohman S-O, Wilczek H *et al.* Fine needle aspiration cytology and conventional histology in 200 renal allografts. *Transplantation* 1990; **49**: 910–912

28 Helderman J H, Hernandez J, Sagalowsky A *et al.* Confirmation of the utility of fine needle aspiration biopsy of the renal allograft. *Kidney Int* 1988; **34**: 376–381

29 Häyry P, von Willebrand E. Transplant aspiration cytology. *Transplantation* 1984; **38**: 7–12

30 Salmela K, von Willebrand E, Kyllönen L *et al.* The association of HLA-DR antigens with acute steroid resistant rejection and poor kidney graft survival. *Transplantation* 1991; **51**: 768–771

31 Salmela K, von Willebrand E, Kyllönen L *et al.* Acute vascular rejection in renal transplantation ó diagnosis and outcome. *Transplantation* 1992; **54**: 858–862

32 von Willebrand E, Taskinen E, Ahonen J, Häyry P. Recent modifications in the fine needle aspiration biopsy of human renal allografts. *Transplant Proc* 1983; **15**: 1195–1197

33 Cooksey G, Reeve R S, Wenham P W *et al.* Comparison of fine needle aspiration cytology with histology in the diagnosis of renal allograft rejection. In: Kreis H, Droz D eds. *Renal Transplant Cytology.* Milan: Wichtig Editore, 1984; 73–78

34 Reeve R S, Cooksey G, Wenham P W *et al.* A comparison of fine needle aspiration cytology and tru-cut tissue biopsy in the diagnosis of acute renal allograft rejection. *Nephron* 1986; **42**: 68–71

35 von Willebrand E, Salmela K, Isoniemi H *et al.* Induction of HLA class II antigen and interleukin 2 receptor expression in acute vascular rejection of human kidney allografts. *Transplantation* 1992; **53**: 1077–1081

36 Isoniemi H, Ahonen J, Eklund B *et al.* Renal allograft immunosuppression: early inflammatory and rejection episodes in triple drug treatment compared to double drug combinations or cyclosporin monotherapy. *Transplant Int* 1990; **3**: 92–97

37 Häyry P, von Willebrand E, Ahonen J, Eklund B. Glucocorticosteroids in renal transplantation I. Impact of high vs. low dose postoperative methyl-prednisolone administration on the first episode(s) of rejection. *Scand J Immunol* 1982; **16**: 39–49

38 Häyry P, von Willebrand E, Ahonen J *et al.* Effects of cyclosporine, azathioprine and steroids on the renal transplant, on the cytological patterns of intra-graft inflammation and on concomitant rejection-associated changes in the recipient blood. *Transplant Proc* 1988; **20**: 153–162

39 Wood R F M, Bolton E M, Thompson J F, Morris P J. Monoclonal antibodies and fine needle aspiration cytology in detecting renal allograft rejection. *Lancet* 1982; **ii**: 278

40 von Willebrand E. OKT 4/8 ratio in the blood and in the graft during episodes of human allograft rejection. *Cell Immunol* 1983; **77**: 196–201

41 Bolton E M, Thompson J F, Wood R F, Morris P J. Immunoperoxidase staining of fine needle aspiration biopsies and needle core biopsies from renal allografts. *Transplantation* 1983; **36**: 728–731

42 Cooksey G, Reeve R S, Paterson A D *et al.* Lymphocyte subpopulations in cytologic aspirates from human renal allografts. *Transplant Proc* 1985; **17**: 630–632

43 Hughes D A, Kempson M G, Carter N P, Morris P J. Immunogoldsilver/ Romanowsky staining: simultaneous immunocytochemical and morphological analysis of fine-needle aspirate biopsies. *Transplant Proc* 1988; **20**: 575–576

44 Vereerstraeten P, Romasco F, Kinnaert P *et al.* T cell subset patterns in peripheral blood and in fine needle aspiration lymphocytes after kidney transplantation. *Transplant Proc* 1985; **17**: 2115–2116

45 Waugh J, Bishop G A, Hall B *et al.* T cell subsets in fine needle aspiration biopsies from renal transplant recipients. *Transplant Proc* 1985; **17**: 1701–1703

46 Lautenschlager I, von Willebrand E, Häyry P. Does T4 predominance in the graft signify severe rejection? *Transplant Proc* 1986; **18**: 1311–1313

47 Hancock W W, Gee D, De Moerloose P *et al.* Immunohistological analysis of serial biopsies taken during human renal allograft rejection. Changing profile of infiltrating cells and activation of the coagulation system. *Transplantation* 1985; **39**: 430–438

48 von Willebrand E, Häyry P. Relationship between cellular and molecular markers on inflammation in human kidney allograft rejection. *Transplant Proc* 1987; **19**: 1644–1645

49 Häyry P, von Willebrand E, Ahonen J, Eklund B. Do well-to-do and repeatedly rejecting renal allografts express the transplantation antigens similarly on their surface? *Scand J Urol Nephrol* 1981; **64**(suppl): 52–55

50 Hall B M, Duggin G G, Philips J *et al.* Increased expression of HLA-DR antigens on renal tubular cells in renal transplants: relevance to the rejection response. *Lancet* 1984; **ii**: 247–251

51 Fuggle S V, McWhinnie D L, Chapman J R *et al.* Sequential analysis of HLA-class II antigen expression in human renal allografts. Induction of tubular class II antigens and correlation with clinical parameters. *Transplantation* 1986; **42**: 144–150

52 Häyry P, von Willebrand E. The influence of the pattern of inflammation and administration of steroids on class II MHC antigen expression in renal transplants. *Transplantation* 1986; **42**: 358–363

53 Bishop G A, Hall B M. Expression of leucocyte and lymphocyte adhesion molecules in the human kidney. *Kidney Int* 1989; **36**: 1078–1085

54 von Willebrand E, Loginov R, Salmela K *et al.* Relationship between intercellular adhesion molecule-1 and HLA class II expression in acute cellular rejection of human kidney allografts. *Transplant Proc* 1993; **25**: 870–871

55 Nguyen L, Hammer C, Dendorfer U *et al.* Changes in large granular lymphocyte size and number in kidney transplant patients during rejection and viral infection. *Transplant Proc* 1985; **17**: 2110–2111

56 Ouziala M, Santelli G, Charpentier B, Fries D. Diagnostic value of fine needle aspiration biopsy during viral infections in renal transplant recipients. *Transplant Proc* 1985; **17**: 2098–2099

57 Hammer C. Diagnosis of inflammatory events. In: Hammer C ed. *Cytology in Transplantation.* West Germany: Verlag R S Schulz, 1989; 127–154

58 von Willebrand E, Lautenschlager I, Ahonen J. Cellular activation in the graft and in the blood during CMV disease. *Transplant Proc* 1989; **21**: 2080–2081

59 von Willebrand E, Pettersson E, Ahonen J, Häyry P. CMV infection, class II antigen expression, and human kidney allograft rejection. *Transplantation* 1986; **42**: 364–367

60 Smith T F. Rapid methods for diagnosis of viral infections. *Lab Med* 1987; **18**: 16–20

61 Van der Bij W, Toresma R, van Son W J *et al.* Rapid immunodiagnosis of active cytomegalovirus infection by monoclonal antibody staining of blood leucocytes. *J Med Virol* 1988; **25**: 179–188

62 Droz D, Campos H, Noel L H *et al.* Renal transplant fine needle aspiration cytology: correlations to renal histology. In: Kreis H, Droz D eds. *Renal Transplant Cytology.* Milan: Wichtig Editore, 1984; 59–65

63 De Vecchi A, Egidi F, Banfi G *et al.* Comparison of fine needle aspiration biopsy and needle biopsy in renal transplantation. In: Kreis H, Droz D eds. *Renal Transplant Cytology.* Milan: Wichtig Editore, 1984; 67–72

64 Koller C, Hammer C, Gokel J M *et al.* Correlation between core biopsy and aspiration cytology. *Transplant Proc* 1984; **16**: 1298–1300

65 Egidi F, De Vecchi A, Banfi G *et al.* Comparison of renal biopsy and fine needle aspiration biopsy in renal transplantation. *Transplant Proc* 1985; **17**: 61–63

66 Gupta R, Campbell J, Om A, Belitsky P. Serial monitoring of cellular rejection by

simultaneous histology and fine needle aspiration cytology. *Transplant Proc* 1985; **17**: 2123–2124

67 Hughes D A, McWhinnie D L, Sutton R *et al*. Can incremental scoring of fine-needle aspirates predict histopathologic renal allograft rejection? *Transplant Proc* 1988; **20**: 690–691

68 Gray D W R, Richardson A, Hughes D *et al*. A prospective, randomized, blind comparison of three biopsy techniques in the management of patients after renal transplantation. *Transplantation* 1992; **53**: 1226–1232

69 Lautenschlager I, Höckerstedt K, Taskinen E *et al*. Fine-needle aspiration biopsy in the monitoring of liver allografts I. Correlation between aspiration biopsy and core biopsy in experimental pig liver allografts. *Transplantation* 1988; **46**: 41–46

70 Vogel W, Margreiter R, Schmalzl F, Judmaier G. Preliminary results with fine needle aspiration biopsy in liver grafts. *Transplant Proc* 1984; **16**: 1240–1242

71 Lautenschlager I, Höckerstedt K, Ahonen J *et al*. Fine-needle aspiration biopsy in the monitoring of liver allografts II. Applications to human allografts. *Transplantation* 1988; **46**: 47–52

72 Hammerer P, Kraemer-Hansen H, Kremer B *et al*. Aspiration cytology of liver transplants. *Transplant Proc* 1988; **20**: 640–641

73 Höckerstedt K, Lautenschlager I, Ahonen J *et al*. Diagnosis of rejection in liver transplantation. *J Hepatol* 1988; **2**: 217–221

74 Greene C L, Fehrman I, Tillery G W *et al*. Liver transplant aspiration cytology is a useful tool for identifying and monitoring allograft rejection. *Transplant Proc* 1988; **20**: 657–658

75 Kirby R M, Young J A, Hubscher S G *et al*. The accuracy of aspiration cytology in the diagnosis of rejection following orthotopic liver transplantation. *Transplant Int* 1988; **1**: 119–126

76 Carbonel F, Samuel D, Reynes M *et al*. Fine needle aspiration biopsy of human liver allografts. Correlation with liver histology for the diagnosis of acute rejection. *Transplantation* 1990; **50**: 704–707

77 Schlitt J, Nashan B, Krick P *et al*. Intragraft immune events after human liver transplantation. Correlation with clinical signs of acute rejection and influence of immunosuppression. *Transplantation* 1992: **54**: 273–278

78 Lautenschlager I, Höckerstedt K, Häyry P. Fine-needle aspiration biopsy in the monitoring of liver allografts. *Transplant Int* 1991; **4**: 54–61

79 Porter K A. Pathology of liver transplantation. *Transplant Rev* 1969; **2**: 129–170

80 Wight D G D, Portman B. Pathology of rejection. In: Calne R Y ed. *Liver Transplantation*. London: Grune & Stratton, 1987; 385–410

81 Snover D C, Freese D K, Sharp H L *et al*. Liver allograft rejection. An analysis of the use of biopsy determining outcome of rejection. *Am J Surg Pathol* 1987; **11**: 1–10

82 Nashan B, Schlitt H J, Wittekind C W *et al*. Patterns of immune activation during the first four weeks in liver transplant patients. *Transplant Proc* 1989; **21**: 3623–3624

83 Schlitt H J, Nashan B, Ringe B *et al*. Differentation of liver graft dysfunction by transplant aspiration cytology. *Transplantation* 1991; **51**: 786–792

84 Lautenschlager I, Höckerstedt K, Häyry P. Activation markers in acute liver allograft rejection. *Transplant Proc* 1988; **20**: 646–647

85 Zannier A, Faure J L, Neidecker J *et al*. Monitoring of liver allografts using fine-needle aspiration biopsy: value of hepatocyte MHC-DR expression in the diagnosis of acute rejection. *Transplant Proc* 1987; **19**: 3810–3811

86 Vogel W, Wohlfahrter P, Then P *et al*. Longitudinal study of major histocompatibility complex antigen expression on hepatocytes in fine-needle aspiration biopsies from human liver grafts. *Transplant Proc* 1988; **20**: 648–649

87 Lautenschlager I, Höckerstedt K, Häyry P. ICAM-1 induction on hepatocytes is an early marker of acute liver allograft rejection. *Transplant Int* 1992; **5**: S283–S285

88 Lautenschlager I, Höckerstedt K. ICAM-1 induction on hepatocytes as a marker for immune activation of acute liver allograft rejection. *Transplantation* 1993; **56**: 1495–1499

89 Lautenschlager I, Höckerstedt K. Induction of ICAM-1 on hepatocytes precedes the lymphoid activation of acute liver allograft rejection and cytomegalovirus infection. *Transplant Proc* 1993; **25**: 1429–1430

90 Steinhoff G, Wonigeit K, Pichlmayer R. Induction of ICAM-1 on hepatocyte membranes during liver allograft rejection and infection. *Transplant Proc* 1990; **22**: 2308–2309

91 Höckerstedt K, Lautenschlager I, Ahonen J *et al*. Differentiation between acute rejection and infection in liver transplant patients. *Transplant Proc* 1989; **21**: 2317–2318

92 Lautenschlager I, Höckerstedt K, Salmela K *et al*. Fine-needle aspiration biopsy (FNAB) in the monitoring of liver allografts; different cellular findings during rejection and CMV infection. *Transplantation* 1990; **50**: 798–803

93 Lautenschlager I, Höckerstedt K, Linnavuori K, Taskinen E. Human herpesvirus-6 infection after liver transplantation. *Clin Infect Dis* 1998; **26**: 702–707

94 Lautenschlager I, Nashan B, Schlitt HJ *et al*. Different cellular patterns associated with hepatitis C virus reactivation, cytomegalovirus infection and acute rejection in liver transplant patients monitored with transplant aspiration cytology. *Transplantation* 1994; **58**: 1339–1345

95 Ciardi A, Pecorella I, Rossi M *et al*. Morphologic features in liver transplantation. *Transplant Proc* 1988; **20**: 637–639

96 Lautenschlager I, Nashan B, Schlitt H J *et al*. Early intragraft inflammatory events of liver allografts ending up with chronic rejection. *Transplant Int* 1995; **8**: 446–451

97 Kiuchi T, Schlitt H J, Oldhafder K J *et al*. Backgrounds of early intragraft immune activation and rejection in liver transplant recipients. Impact of graft reperfusion quality. *Transplantation* 1995; **60**: 49–55

98 Martelius T, Mäkisalo H, Höckerstedt K *et al*. A rat model of monitoring liver allograft rejection. *Transplant Int* 1997; **10**: 103–108

99 Lautenschlager I, Höckerstedt K, Meri S. Complement membrane attack complex and protectin (CD59) in liver allografts during acute rejection. *J Hepatol* 1999; **31**: 537–541

100 Griffith B P. Detection of rejection in the transplanted lungs and immunology. In: Wallwork J ed. *Heart and Heart-lung Transplantation*. Philadelphia: W B Saunders, 1989; 507–521

101 Yousem S A, Berry G J, Brunt E M *et al*. A working formulation for the standardization of nomenclature in the diagnosis of heart and lung rejection: lung rejection study group. *J Heart Lung Transplant* 1990; **9**: 593–601

102 Gryzan S, Paradis I L, Hardesty R L *et al*. Bronchoalveolar lavage in heart-lung transplantation. *J Heart Transplant* 1985; **4**: 4114–4116

103 Maurer J R, Gough E, Chamberlain D W *et al*. Sequential bronchoalveolar lavage studies from patients undergoing double lung and heart-lung transplant. *Transplant Proc* 1989; **21**: 2585–2587

104 Prior C, Klima G, Gattringer C *et al*. Serial bronchoalveolar lavage in heart-lung transplant recipients: cytological and microbiologic findings. *Transplant Proc* 1989; **21**: 2588–2589

105 Clelland C A, Higgenbottam T W, Monk J A *et al*. Bronchoalveolar lavage lymphocytes in relation to transbronchial lung biopsy in heart-lung transplants. *Transplant Proc* 1990; **22**: 1479

106 Zeevi A, Fung J J, Paradis I L *et al*. Lymphocytes of bronchoalveolar lavages from heart-lung transplant recipients. *J Heart Transplant* 1985; **4**: 417–421

22 Cytological investigation of immune suppressed patients

Jennifer A. Young and Rebecca F. Harrison

Introduction

Acquired immunodeficiency syndrome (AIDS) accounts for a high percentage of immunosuppressed individuals but other causes, as shown in Table 22.1 are numerous. Some of the patient groups, e.g. transplant recipients, have also increased in number.

Illness in immunosuppressed individuals is progressive, atypical in clinical presentation and not infrequently multifactorial. Speedy, accurate diagnosis is essential if prompt and appropriate treatment is to be instigated. Cytopathological techniques can make a valuable contribution in this field especially by the rapid diagnosis of certain opportunistic infections and neoplastic diseases.

This chapter specifically addresses the role of cytopathology in the management of patients with immunosuppression. However, the diagnostic problems encountered in such cases may also arise when there is no known background of immunodeficiency. The initial approach to diagnosis is similar in these patients although the long-term management is likely to be different.

Opportunistic infection

Bacterial infection

Mycobacteria (*Fig. 22.1*)

Mycobacterium avium intracellulare (MAI) is not generally considered a pathogen in the non-immunocompromised, but is a common cause of illness in patients with AIDS[1,2]. Organisms are usually widespread but lymph nodes, liver and spleen are most frequently involved and infection of the respiratory and gastrointestinal tracts is less common. The diagnosis is often not suspected clinically and may be encountered unexpectedly in fine needle aspiration (FNA) of lymph nodes. There is little granulomatous reaction in MAI[1] and epithelioid cells, giant cells or evidence of caseation are unlikely. Macrophages are numerous and when stained with Ziehl-Neelsen (ZN) are seen to be filled with mycobacteria (see Figs 19.10, 19.11). The organisms can also be visualized with Giemsa, Grocott and periodic acid-Schiff (PAS) stains. Culture is necessary to distinguish MAI from *Mycobacterium tuberculosis* (MTB).

MTB occurs in persons other than immune suppressed, lung and lymph nodes being the commonest sites, although other organs are also affected. An excellent account of the

Table 22.1	Conditions causing immune suppression

AIDS
Chemotherapy
Steroid therapy
    Organ transplantation
    Collagen vascular diseases
Malignant disease
    Leukaemia
    Lymphoma
    Hodgkin's disease
    Myeloma
Congenital immunodeficiency syndromes

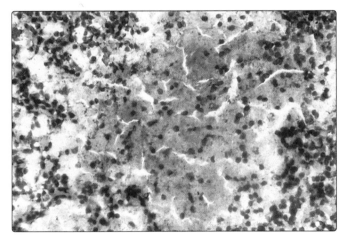

Fig. 22.1 Tuberculosis. Caseous necrosis in FNA of lymph node.

FNA diagnosis of 574 cases is given by Das *et al.*[3] Evidence of epithelioid granulomata without necrosis was seen in 31.5% of aspirates and granulomata with necrosis in 31.9%. In the remaining cases (36.6%) the material consisted of acellular caseous debris. Acid fast bacilli were identified in 160 specimens and varied from an occasional organism to vast numbers.

Respiratory disease remains the commonest type in the immunodeficient and the clinical distinction from *Pneumocystis carinii* pneumonia (PCP) and fungal infection is sometimes difficult. Extrapulmonary disease and disseminated MTB are not uncommon, and frequently associated with lymphadenopathy, when FNA may be diagnostic[4]. Intraoperative imprint cytology may aid in the

563

diagnosis of unexpectedly encountered suspected mycobacterial infection[5].

Other mycobacterial infections such as *Mycobacterium kansasii, M. scrofulaceum, M. bovis* and *M. xenopi* occur in the immune suppressed in whom clinical presentation resembles MTB. Acid-fast-positive *Legionella pneumophilia* is a potential pitfall[6]. Culture is necessary for classification.

Investigation of the donor lung by means of bronchoalveolar lavage (BAL) may be a useful adjunct to the assessment of potential donor organs. Mycobacteria present in the lavage fluid, and sputum post-lung transplantation may be donor acquired and thus the patient may require antituberculous drug therapy post-transplantation as a necessary precaution. However, mycobacterial infections in lung allografts are uncommon when compared with other infections and may be typical or atypical[7].

Other bacterial infections

Staphylococcus aureus, Haemophilus pneumoniae, Streptococcus pneumoniae, Pseudomonas aeruginosa and *Legionella pneumophilia* all cause numerous episodes of pulmonary infection in immunosuppressed patients. In lung-allografted patients, such bacterial infections are a particular problem as those transplanted for cystic fibrosis may be colonized with multiple resistant *Pseudomonas aeruginosa* and *Barkholderia cepacia*[8]. None is amenable to cytological identification but must be considered in the differential diagnosis of pneumonia especially in cases where BAL is cytologically non-diagnostic. Nocardia can be morphologically recognized in BAL fluid[9], but is uncommon (see Chapter 2).

Severe Salmonella and Shigella gastrointestinal infections are associated with AIDS[10] but cytological investigation does not contribute to diagnosis.

Viral infection

Cytomegalovirus *(Figs 22.2, 22.3)*

Cytomegalovirus (CMV) is a DNA virus of the herpes virus group. It is a widely distributed opportunistic infectious agent in all classes of immunocompromised persons, particularly those with AIDS and transplant recipients, and usually involves many organs. CMV interstitial pneumonitis is associated with a mortality rate of over 80% in bone marrow transplant patients[11] and is the most common cause of opportunistic infection in lung allograft recipients in the four to eight week postoperative period[12]. Indeed, in those who survive for two or more weeks, the prevalence of CMV infection may exceed 75%[13]. However this is not always associated with a pneumonitis. PCR on BAL fluid and peripheral blood is a sensitive method of detecting active infection, but together with cytological investigations cannot distinguish between simple and pathological infection. CMV is second only to *Pneumocystis carinii* pneumonia as the most frequent AIDS associated infection found at autopsy[14].

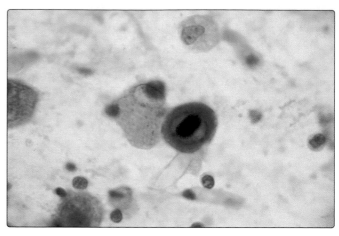

Fig. 22.2 Cytomegalovirus infection. Large cell showing characteristic 'owl's eye' cytopathic effect. BAL fluid. (Papanicolaou × OI)

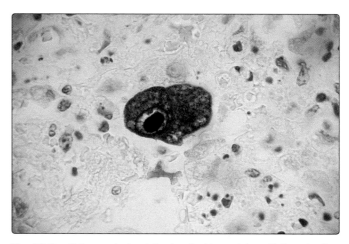

Fig. 22.3 Cytomegalovirus infection. Positive staining of infected cell. (Anticytomegalovirus monoclonal antibody (Dako), × OI)

Culture of CMV for diagnostic purposes is slow and expensive and estimation of serological titres is not particularly helpful and has been superceded by PCR on blood, fluid and sputum. Early diagnosis and aggressive treatment improve survival[11]. Identification of the characteristic viral cytopathic effects by light microscopy of histological or cytological material from the respiratory or gastrointestinal tract still provides the most rapid and certain means of diagnosis.

Pathognomonic 'owl's eye' viral inclusions can be identified in pneumocytes and alveolar macrophages in BAL fluid. In Papanicolaou stained material the diagnostic cells contain round or oval basophilic intranuclear inclusions, each surrounded by a clear halo due to margination of chromatin. Granular, occasionally eosinophilic, small inclusions can sometimes be seen in the cytoplasm[15-17]. Similar cells indicative of CMV oesophagitis have been identified in oesophageal brushings[18] and in FNA from the salivary glands[19].

Sensitivity of detection of CMV is enhanced by special

techniques such as monoclonal antibody studies[20], *in situ* hybridization[21] and PCR, which is now mainstream[22]. *In situ* hybridization has been successfully carried out on decolourized Papanicolaou stained slides[23].

Herpes simplex and *Herpes zoster*

Recurrent *Herpes simplex* types I and II infections are very troublesome to the immune suppressed, but are seldom life threatening. Mucocutaneous oral and facial lesions, oesophageal and cervical infection in women and anorectal involvement in homosexual men present similar clinical features to *H. simplex* infection in non-immunocompromised persons. In the earlier years of heart lung transplantation, 10% of patients could develop HSV pneumonia and ulcerative tracheobronchitis, but this has been minimized more recently by the introduction of prophylactic antiviral therapy with Acyclovir[24,25].

The characteristic multiple, moulded, 'ground glass' nuclei can be seen in cervical smears and in scrapings from cutaneous vesicles. Similar cytopathic effects are identifiable in squamous cells in oesophageal brushings in cases of herpetic oesophagitis. Large infected squamous cells, which may be of bizarre shape as well as multinucleated, can be found in sputum or bronchial brushings in herpetic tracheobronchitis. The classical multiple moulded nuclei are particularly a feature of squamous cell infection but in herpetic pneumonia, the result of haematogenous viral dissemination, this cytopathological effect may not be evident. Diagnosis by morphological appearance alone is therefore difficult on BAL material and *in situ* hybridization is helpful in suspected cases[26].

Skin lesions due to *Herpes zoster* follow a dermatomal distribution and seldom present a clinical diagnostic problem. Scrapings from the vesicles contain the characteristic multinucleated squamous cells.

Other viral infections

Both Epstein-Barr virus (EBV) and human papillomavirus (HPV) are associated with the condition of hairy leukoplakia, which produces a white raised lesion on the lateral surface of the tongue[27]. Oesophageal lesions are also possible. Koilocytosis and herpetic-type nuclear inclusions are reported to occur and coexisting candidosis is common. Genital HPV infection is linked with cervical dyskaryosis and neoplasia in women and anorectal and penile lesions in homosexual men. Infection with HIV is associated with 'high-risk' HPV types which suggests that immunodepression favours the likelihood of oncogenic progression[28]. The cytomorphological features are no different to those described in non-immunosuppressed individuals. EBV is associated with post-transplant lymphoproliferative disorders and possibly other malignant tumours, such as gastric carcinoma.

Intranuclear inclusions due to polyoma virus may occasionally be identified in exfoliated cells in urine from immunosuppressed patients, particularly transplant recipients, but the pathological effects of this virus are unknown. Nested PCR is the most reliable means of diagnosis of polyoma virus in the urine and molecular biology remains the only means of distinguishing BK virus and JC virus[29]. Recurrent viral infections are common, especially in liver transplant patients allografted for Hepatitis B (HBV) and Hepatitis C (HCV) disease. Currently antiviral therapy including lamivudine and its analogues my be affective in recurrent HBV disease, but therapy is not available for recurrent HCV.

Fungal infection

Pneumocystis carinii *pneumonia (PCP)* (Figs 22.4, 22.5)

Pneumocystis carinii pneumonia is the most common and most life threatening opportunistic infection in individuals with AIDS. Approximately 80% of patients have at least one episode and recurrent disease is associated with a particularly poor prognosis[30]. The incidence of PCP in other immune suppressed groups, particularly transplant recipients, has been greatly reduced by the administration of prophylactic trimethoprim-sulphamethoxazole.

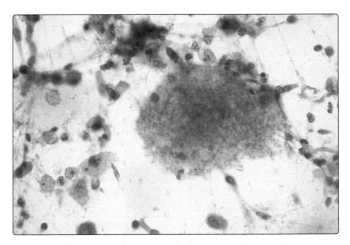

Fig. 22.4 Pneumocystis pneumonia. Foamy alveolar cast with honeycomb texture. BAL fluid. (Papanicolaou × OI)

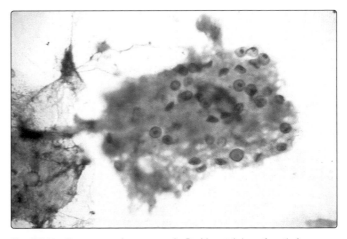

Fig. 22.5 Pneumocystis pneumonia. Positive staining of cystic forms within alveolar cast. (Grocott × OI)

Definitive diagnosis of PCP still requires the demonstration of *P. carinii* morphologically as serological tests are not a reliable indicator of disease and culture of the human strain of the organisms does not appear to be feasible. Diagnosis by cytological examination of induced sputum or BAL fluid is the method of choice as both procedures are safe.

Percutaneous fine needle aspiration (PCFNA) also yields diagnostic material[31] but is generally considered to be associated with an unacceptable level of complications, especially pneumothorax. Transbronchial biopsy (TBB) is a sensitive method for diagnosis of PCP but is also associated with a high risk of pneumothorax[32]. In lung allograft recipients and other transplant patients, immunosuppression modifies the morphological response to PCP infection. Characteristically, there is a granulomatous response with small numbers of cysts, and so very few organisms may be seen on TBB[33]. As TBB adds little to the diagnostic yield of BAL, which is a safer procedure, it is seldom now carried out during bronchoscopy on suspected cases of PCP. If neither induced sputum nor BAL are diagnostic, open lung biopsy is preferable. Imprint smears prepared from the tissue can be helpful and are quick to process, providing a useful technique when examination is required out of routine laboratory hours. Extrapulmonary dissemination of *P. carinii* is documented[34] but is very unusual.

Specimen collection and processing

Prior to the collection of *induced sputum* the patient should rinse the mouth and gargle with water. Neither toothpaste nor mouthwash should be used. Expectoration is induced by 15–20 min inhalation of a mist of 3% saline from an ultrasonic nebulizer. Specimens are collected in sterile plastic containers for both cytology and microbiology.

For BAL, dedicated bronchoscopes for AIDS and non-AIDS patients are required. Several small aliquots are sequentially instilled and aspirated. The first aliquot frequently only contains bronchial debris and diagnostic material may not be recovered until later samples. Part of each specimen should be sent for microbiological evaluation. Processing in the cytology laboratory is by standard techniques[35] but strict attention to safety precautions are mandatory. Because of the wide range of possible diagnoses and coexisting conditions material should be stained by the Papanicolaou, May-Grünwald-Giemsa (MGG), Gram, ZN and Perls' methods and additional slides prepared and retained for immunocytochemistry and other special techniques.

Cytological findings

Examination of Papanicolaou stained material is highly sensitive and specific for the detection of PCP providing lower respiratory tract sampling is adequate and the patient has not received prior empirical therapy. Characteristic foamy alveolar casts are present[15,17], some of which usually display biphasic staining. By focusing up and down on these casts clear circular areas representing cystic forms of the organism and tiny dense staining specks indicative of the trophozoites within are identifiable. With the Grocott stain, the walls of the cysts stain black and characteristic clusters can be visualized within the casts. Two 'mirror image' reniform structures are visible within intact cysts. Collapsed empty cysts are cup shaped. Fungal spores also stain with Grocott but they have thicker walls, may show budding and are not concentrated within foamy casts. The trophozoites of *P. carinii* stain weakly with Giemsa and with Gram.

The sensitivity of induced sputum examination using light microscopy is in the region of 55–79%[36,37]. The method is non-invasive but collection can be problematical[38]. Sensitivity of detection by BAL is high, ranging from 79–98%[32,39,40]. Special techniques enhance detection. Fluorescence microscopy of Papanicolaou stained material shows the pneumocysts present as green-yellow circular structures 5 µm in diameter with the two reniform bodies present in intact cysts[41]. Wehle *et al.*[42] also noted fluorescent inclusions 1–3 µm diameter within alveolar macrophages which they interpreted as the remnants of pneumocysts. Using this additional criterion PCP was identified in 100% of cases. By comparison TBB permitted the correct diagnosis in only 62.5% of the same patients. Immunofluorescence staining using a murine monoclonal antibody directed against *P. carinii* cysts (Northumbria Biological Ltd) also improves diagnosis from both sputum[43] and BAL[44,45]. DNA amplification by PCR is also applicable and more sensitive than immunofluorescence[34,35]. Even PCR, however, may be negative if prior treatment has been given[46].

Diagnostic pitfalls

CMV, MTB and other bacterial and fungal opportunistic infections may be difficult to distinguish clinically from PCP. Even if morphological evidence of *P. carinii* is identified, a search for additional infectious agents must be carried out as the aetiology of pneumonia is not uncommonly multifactorial.

Table 22.2 summarizes the numerous conditions that can be associated with respiratory distress in the immune suppressed and which should be considered in the differential diagnosis of PCP. Alveolar haemorrhage, is indicated by blood-stained BAL, and haemosiderin-laden Perls' positive macrophages on microscopy. Drug and radiation toxicity, graft-versus-host disease (GVHD) in appropriate cases, and diffuse malignant infiltration must all be considered, especially in non-AIDS patients (see Chapter 2). Very occasionally, PCP is associated with lipoproteinosis (Fig. 22.6), usually in patients with leukaemia. Then, much non-staining lipoid debris and large vacuolated macrophages are found in the BAL fluid.

Candidosis

The commonest species are *Candida albicans, C. tropicalis* and *C. parapsiliosis.* All appear similar morphologically and culture is necessary for speciation but *C. albicans* is encountered most frequently in clinical practice. Mucocutaneous and genital candidosis are widespread in the community and many healthy people harbour saprophytic oral Candida spp. Candidosis of the gastrointestinal[46], respiratory and urinary tracts as well as disseminated infection occur in debilitated and immunosuppressed patients. Although invasive oesophageal candidosis is an indicator disease of AIDS and 'oral thrush' very common, systemic candidosis occurs in only a small percentage of cases. Invasive fungal infections, including candidosis, are among the most common life threatening opportunistic infections in transplant recipients and in patients with leukaemia, lymphoma and allied conditions. Drug regimes that lead to bone marrow depletion or steroid and immunosuppressive drug therapy also predispose to invasive candidosis.

Cytological findings

Microscopically, Candida spp are seen as showers of small discrete oval spores mixed with filamentous pseudohyphae. Unlike Aspergillus spp, the filamentous elements of Candida spp do not display dichotomous branching or true septation. Budding spores arising at points of constriction along the pseudohyphae are a helpful morphological feature[17].

Aspergillus *(Fig. 22.7)*

Aspergillus spp are responsible for several different forms of illness, including bronchocentric granulomatosis, non-invasive aspergillosis (mycetoma) and invasive aspergillosis leading to pneumonia or abscess formation and granulomatous manifestations in any part of the body. Disseminated invasive infection is a potentially lethal complication of immunosuppression in transplant recipients and patients with lymphoma. It is relatively uncommon in AIDS. Clinically, Aspergillus infection may be a problem in lung-allografted patients, especially at the donor-recipient bronchial anastomosis, where ischaemic cartilage predisposes to invasion[47].

Aspergillus fumigatus, A. flavus and *A. niger* are usually indistinguishable in cytological and histological preparations as the characteristic conidiophore vesicles are uncommonly present[48] and culture is necessary for

Table 22.2	Principal causes of pulmonary dysfunction in the immune suppressed

Infection	Neoplasia
Bacterial	Lymphoproliferative disorders
Staph. aureus	Leukaemia
Strep. pneumoniae	Hodgkin's disease
H. influenzae	Myeloma
P. aeruginosa	Kaposi's sarcoma
L. pneumophilia	Bronchial carcinoma
M. tuberculosis	Secondary carcinoma
M. avium-intracellulare	**Iatrogenic processes**
Viral	Irradiation
Cytomegalovirus	Drug toxicity
Herpes simplex	Oxygen toxicity
Adenovirus	Graft versus host disease
Fungal	Rejection of lung allograft
P. carinii	**Idiopathic and miscellaneous**
Candida spp.	**processes**
Aspergillus spp.	Lipoproteinosis
C. neoformans	Alveolar haemorrhage
H. capsulatum	Lymphocytic interstitial
C. immitis	pneumonia
Parasitic	Non-specific interstitial
T. gondii	pneumonia
S. stercoralis	

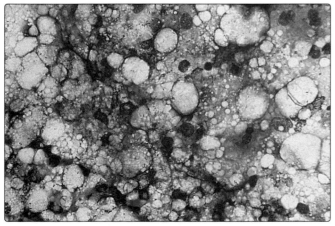

Fig. 22.6 Lipoproteinosis. Non-staining globules of lipoid material in BAL fluid from a patient with *P. carinii* pneumonia. (MGG × MP)

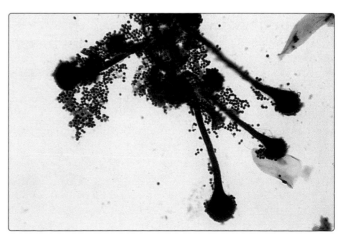

Fig. 22.7 *Aspergillus fumigatus.* Flask-shaped conidiophore vesicles. (Grocott × MP)

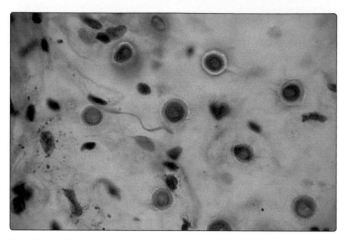

Fig. 22.8   Cryptococcosis. Numerous encapsulated forms of *C. neoformans*. PCFNA of lung. (× OI)

speciation. Aspergillus is seldom a saprophyte and the finding of hyphae in sputum, BAL[48] or PCFNA[49,50] specimens is indicative of clinical infection. Hyphae of Aspergillus spp are larger than those of Candida spp, are septate and display dichotomous branching, i.e. branching into two equal divisions at approximately 45°.

Cryptococcus *(Fig. 22.8)*

Infection with *Cryptococcus neoformans* is quite common in both AIDS and non-AIDS cases. The clinical presentation is generally meningitis or pneumonitis but in disseminated disease cryptococci can be identified in lymph nodes, genitourinary tract and liver. The gastrointestinal tract is very seldom involved.

Cryptococci are spherical budding yeasts, each of which is surrounded by a characteristic mucoid capsule, although non-encapsulated strains do occur, particularly in AIDS patients. The capsule is pale and translucent with Papanicolaou[17,51] or MGG stains but a diagnostic bright magenta with Mayer's mucicarmine. The 'central nuclei' stain with Grocott and periodic acid-Schiff and the non-encapsulated forms can be mistaken for spores of Candida spp. The single buds are attached by a narrow isthmus to the parent cell, which distinguishes them from *Blastomyces dermatitidis,* in which the connection is broader. In cytological laboratories, cryptococci are most likely to be encountered in cerebrospinal fluid (CSF) or PCFNA of the lung[51].

Other fungal infections

Morphologic identification of other types of fungi is possible from cytological material[52] although precise speciation is not always feasible. Those described below are illustrated in Chapter 2.

The class Zygomycetes includes many genera, which are morphologically indistinguishable. All have broad non-septate hyphae, which stain lightly with Grocott and resemble 'tangled cellophane ribbons'. Mucor spp is the commonest form.

Blastomyces dermatidis is virtually confined to North America and the similar *B. brasiliensis* to South America. Blastomycosis is very uncommon in Europe. Disseminated disease can occur in immune suppressed individuals, but is rare outside endemic areas. The mother and daughter yeast cells of *B. dermatidis* and *B. brasiliensis* are attached to each other by a broader base than those of *C. neoformans* (see Figs 2.41A, B, 2.37).

Histoplasma capsulatum is a dimorphic fungus, the yeast phase of which is the invasive form. Distribution is world-wide, but is most prevalent in the southern states of North America and portions of Central and South America. Disseminated histoplasmosis is usually due to reactivation of a latent infection as a result of the onset of immunocompromised status. Many of the clinical features of the disease resemble tuberculosis. The yeast forms are intracellular and have been reported in alveolar macrophages in BAL[53], in sputum[17] and in FNA of lymph nodes[54] (see Figs 2.39, 2.40, 19.14).

Coccidioides immitis is a soil borne fungus mainly found in south and west North America, Mexico and South America. Disseminated coccidioidomycosis occasionally follows pulmonary disease in non-immune suppressed individuals but is uncommon even in endemic areas. Acute coccidioidal pneumonia occurs in immunocompromised patients and is generally followed by disseminated infection. It is included in the definitional criteria for AIDS but is unlikely to be seen in Europe. Diagnosis is made by identification of large thick-walled spherules containing endospores[17,54] (see Fig. 2.38).

Parasitic infestation

Toxoplasmosis

Infection with *Toxoplasma gondii* can present perinatally as a congenital infection in the absence of immune suppression but otherwise is uncommon except in association with AIDS or lymphoma and allied conditions. The central nervous system (CNS) is involved in most cases. Extracerebral *T. gondii* infection is unusual but disease in lungs, gastrointestinal tract, heart or other sites may be found at autopsy. Toxoplasmosis was common in heart transplantation until the advent of prophylaxis. Since then it has become very rare. Diagnosis of cerebral toxoplasmosis is by identification of the characteristic cysts filled with tiny organisms in CSF, brain biopsy or stereotactic FNA material. Cytological diagnosis is reviewed by Strigle and Gal[55]. Serological investigation is helpful but raised titres occur in subclinical infection.

Strongyloidiasis *(Fig. 22.9)*

Hyperinfestation and disseminated strongyloidiasis can occur in patients with lowered host resistance. *Strongyloides stercoralis* is a nematode with a complex and variable life-cycle.

The adult female lives in the intestine and produces eggs, which hatch into rhabditiform larvae. These are passed in

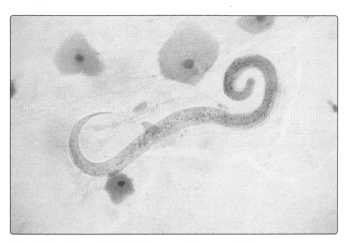

Fig. 22.9   Strongyloidiasis. Larvum of *S. stercoralis*. Sputum. (Papanicolaou × MP)

the faeces and develop into filariform larvae, which then reinfect via penetration of the skin.

In immunosuppressed and severely debilitated patients, the complete life-cycle can be accomplished in the intestine and the filariform larvae reach the lungs and can be coughed up in sputum[17]. Patients not uncommonly develop bacteraemia and meningitis as the result of intestinal bacteria carried by the migrating larvae[56]. Infestation with *S. stercoralis* may be subclinical for very many years and only become apparent when disseminated disease follows the onset of immunosuppression. Patients from endemic areas seem to be at particular risk of explosive hyperinfestation when put on immunosuppressive therapy prior to transplantation.

Intestinal protozoal infections

Enteritis is a severe problem in many patients with AIDS. Cryptosporidium causes fulminating diarrhoea[57]. The small protozoal organisms, 2–4 μm in diameter, cling to the mucosal brush border of the intestine (see Chapter 13). They stain with Grocott which is excellent on biopsy material but not very suitable for stool specimens as the organisms are difficult to distinguish from fungal spores. Modified Ziehl-Neelsen or auramine-phenol stains are preferable for the identification of oocysts in faeces[57]. Endoscopic sampling for cytological diagnosis is sometimes helpful[47]. Other protozoa include *Entamoeba histolytica* and *Giardia lamblia*, both of which are recognizable in routine cytologically stained specimens. *Isospora belli* is another unusual cause of enteritis. The differential criteria of *I. belli* and Cryptosporidium are well summarized by Strigle *et al.*[58].

Cytological investigation of rejection

The lymphoid component of BAL fluid has been assessed in a bid to diagnose acute rejection and distinguish it from infection. However, no correlation with the biopsy findings has been demonstrated[59]. Assessment of rejection of renal and liver transplants by FNA has also been largely discontinued in many units.

Neoplastic disease

Kaposi's sarcoma

Kaposi's sarcoma (KS) occurs in various forms but is particularly associated with AIDS. It develops, however, most frequently in white, homosexual HIV-seropositive men and is very uncommon in haemophiliacs with AIDS. It is also uncommon in patients with other forms of immunosuppression, such as transplant recipients. Various aetiological co-factors in addition to HIV, such as Herpes virus 8, have been suggested as a cause for this variation in incidence[60] but none is reliably proven.

The skin is involved in 75% of patients but visceral lesions are present in many cases especially of the lungs (see Chapter 3), gastrointestinal tract and lymph nodes. The clinical presentation of pulmonary KS may be indistinguishable from that of pneumonia due to opportunistic infection. Antemortem identification is difficult, as bronchial brushings or biopsies are seldom reliably diagnostic and even open lung biopsy may fail to reveal focal lesions[61].

In the alimentary tract, as KS is a subepithelial tumour, cytological sampling of even endoscopically visible lesions is also seldom diagnostic (see Chapter 11).

Several reports describe the diagnostic appearance of KS in fine needle aspirates[54,62–64], based on the presence of cohesive clusters of spindle cells with overlapping nuclei and little pleomorphism or mitotic activity. However, the cytological diagnosis should be advanced with caution except in recurrent or metastatic disease, as distinction from granulation tissue, reparative process and other types of spindle-cell tumour is problematical.

Lymphoproliferative disorders (*Figs 22.10–22.13*)

Patients with both congenital and acquired immunodeficiency have an increased incidence of lymphoproliferative disorders, particularly transplant recipients[65] and AIDS cases[66,67]. Any organ may be involved but the CNS, lymph nodes and gastrointestinal tract are the most common sites. Cytological diagnosis is most likely to be required from examination of CSF[55], serous fluids or fine needle aspirates of lymph nodes[54,63] or other sites. Definitive diagnosis from gastric brushings is seldom possible due to the mainly submucosal nature of the lesion and the likelihood that only Papanicolaou stained material will be available[58].

Transplant patients, in particular heart/lung recipients, who receive relatively large amounts of immunosuppression may develop a spectrum of post-transplant lymphoproliferative disorders (PTLDs)[68]. These range from the benign hyperplastic conditions, which are likely to regress with reduction in immunosuppression,

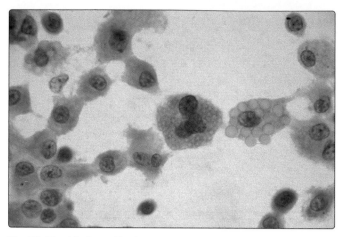

Fig. 22.10 Myeloma. Two large and one small Mott cell with yellow staining retained immunoglobulin surrounded by plasma cells. BAL fluid. (Papanicolaou × OI)

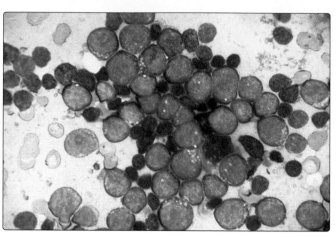

Fig. 22.12 Non-Hodgkin's lymphoma. Monomorphic population of immunoblasts. FNA of parotid from liver transplant recipient. (MGG × OI)

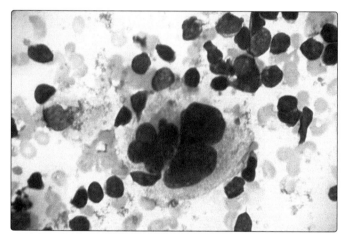

Fig. 22.11 Hodgkin's disease. Multinucleated Reed-Sternberg cell with lymphocytes. FNA cervical lymph node. (MGG × OI)

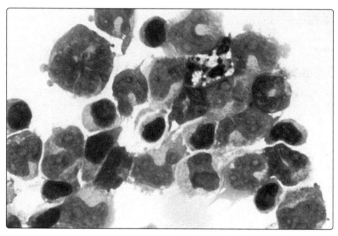

Fig. 22.13 Non-Hodgkin's lymphoma. Malignant cells from a high-grade lymphoma (unclassified). CSF from a patient with AIDS. (MGG × OI)

through polyclonal and oligoclonal proliferations to overt lymphoma, which may not respond to withdrawal of immunosuppression. The PTLD may occur either within the graft or elsewhere, with gastrointestinal involvement being common. Both T and B cell types may be associated with EBV infection[68].

Non-Hodgkin's lymphoma in the immunosuppressed is high-grade, which facilitates cytological detection, and is invariably of B-cell lineage. Burkitt's lymphoma with or without plasmablastic differentiation and diffuse large B-cell lymphoma (REAL classification) types predominate. Strigle et al.[54] identified a lymphoproliferative lesion in 186 of 396 FNA specimens obtained from HIV positive patients. They diagnosed by immunocytochemistry B-cell lymphoma in 22 of 186 aspirates. The remaining 141 showed evidence of persistent generalized lymphadenopathy (PGL). The cytomorphological features of these lymphomas are similar to those seen in non-immunosuppressed individuals (see Chapter 19).

Other malignant tumours

A wide range of other tumours apart from Kaposi's sarcoma and lymphoma are prone to develop in individuals with AIDS and those on immunosuppressive therapy. Patients with lymphoma, leukaemia and allied conditions are also at risk of secondary malignancy. Aetiology is multifactorial but it is probable that the high incidence of infection with HPV and hepatitis B virus are contributory factors in the development of squamous neoplasia and hepatocellular carcinoma respectively. In the study by Strigle et al.[54], 12 of 396 FNA specimens showed malignant processes other than lymphoma or KS. These included three cases of metastatic melanoma. An increase in intraepithelial neoplasia of the cervix has been reported in both organ recipients[69] and AIDS patients[70]. Cervical cytology and the cellular appearances of carcinoma, melanoma and other tumours are similar to those of the non-immunosuppressed population and descriptions will be found elsewhere in this book (Chapters 28–32).

Miscellaneous conditions

Drug therapy and irradiation can induce marked cytological alterations, which at times may produce changes virtually indistinguishable from malignant transformation[71]. Knowledge of the history of irradiation and/or the administration of antineoplastic drugs in particular is vital for the cytopathologist if correct interpretation is to be achieved.

Toxic iatrogenic effects causing diagnostic difficulties are most likely to be encountered in the examination of BAL fluid (Fig. 22.14)[72]. In addition to drugs and irradiation, graft versus host disease, rejection of lung allograft and non-specific pneumonitis may all cause exfoliation of bizarre cells. Nuclei are frequently greatly enlarged, hyperchromatic and contain macronucleoli but commonly also display degenerative changes with patchy chromatin and discontinuous nuclear membranes. Multinucleation is prominent. Cytoplasm may be dense or show evidence of vacuolation. Affected bronchial epithelial cells may retain their cilia, which is a helpful feature and mitigates against an erroneous diagnosis of adenocarcinoma. Cells, arising from areas of atypical squamous metaplasia, however, can show cytomorphological changes almost identical to squamous cell carcinoma and are a particular pitfall[71]. Bizarre squamous cells may be seen in obliterative bronchiolitis of the lung allograft[47] especially following total lymphoid irradiation.

Other pulmonary lesions listed in Table 22.2 include alveolar haemorrhage, when numerous haemosiderin-laden Perls' positive macrophages will be found. Small numbers occur in other conditions and diagnosis again requires correlation with clinical history.

Lipoproteinosis may very occasionally be associated with PCP and sudanophilic macrophages are then recovered in the BAL fluid. Lymphocytic interstitial pneumonia (LIP) is a common complication of HIV infection in children but is much less common in adults. The clinical presentation is

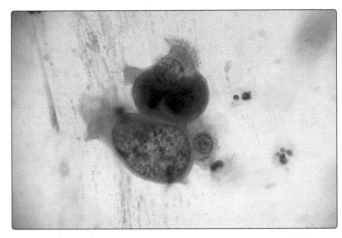

Fig. 22.14   Drug and irradiation toxicity. Bizarre ciliated bronchial epithelial cells. BAL fluid from a marrow transplant recipient. (Papanicolaou × OI)

similar to PCP[73]. The aetiology is unknown but it is believed to be a tissue response to EBV and HIV infection or both. High levels of CD8 T cells have been reported in BAL fluid[73] but this finding is not diagnostic as a CD8 lymphocytosis is typical of AIDS even in the absence of LIP. Open biopsy is usually necessary for diagnosis[73].

The urinary tract is the other system that is most likely to give rise to interpretive problems. Post-radiation effect and alterations due to chemotherapy are extensively reviewed by Koss[74]. Cyclophosphamide-induced atypia in exfoliated cells in urine can be particularly severe. Bizarre cells with hyperchromatic nuclei can be numerous and give rise to false suspicion of malignancy if the history of chemotherapy is unknown. Long-term follow-up of patients who have received cyclophosphamide is prudent, however, as there is an associated risk of transitional and squamous cell carcinoma. Immunosuppression can activate polyoma virus infection and the morphological effects of this, combined with other iatrogenic changes can be pronounced[74].

References

1 Klatt E C, Jensen D F, Meyer P R. Pathology of Mycobacterium avium-intracellulare infection in patients with AIDS. *Hum Pathol* 1987; **18**: 709–714

2 Horsburgh C R Jr. Mycobacterium avium complex infection in the acquired immunodeficiency syndrome. *N Engl J Med* 1991; **324**: 1644–1650

3 Das D K, Bhambhani S, Pant J N et al. Superficial and deep-seated tuberculous lesions: fine needle aspiration cytology diagnosis of 574 cases. *Diagn Cytopathol* 1992; **8**: 211–215

4 Barnes P F, Bloch A B, Davidson D T, Snider D E Jr. Tuberculosis in patients with human immunodeficiency virus infection. *N Engl J Med* 1991; **324**: 1644–1650

5 Jannotta F S, Sidawy M R. The recognition of mycobacterial infections by intraoperative

cytology in patients with acquired immunodeficiency syndrome. *Arch Pathol Lab Med* 1989; **113**: 1120–1123

6 Bentz J S, Carroll K, Ward J H et al. Acid-fast-positive Legionella pneumophilia a possible pitfall in the cytologic diagnosis of myobacterial infection in pulmonary specimens. *Diagn Cytopathol* 2000; **22**: 45–48

7 Trulock G P, Bolman R M, Gentou R. Pulmonary disease caused by Mycobacterium chetonae in a heart-lung transplant recipient with obliterative bronchiolitis. *Am Rev Respir Dis* 1989; **140**: 802–805

8 Maurer J R, Frost A E, Estenne M et al. International guidelines for the selection of lung transplant candidates. *J Heart-Lung Transplant* 1998; **17**: 703–709

9 Rodriquez J L, Barrio J L, Pitchenik A E. Pulmonary nocardiosis in the acquired

immunodeficiency syndrome. *Chest* 1986; **90**: 912–914

10 Profeta S, Forrester C, Eng R H et al. Salmonella infections in patients with acquired immunodeficiency syndrome. *Arch Intern Med* 1985; **145**: 670–672

11 Ljungman P, Englehard D, Link H et al. Treatment of interstitial pneumonitis due to cytomegalovirus with ganciclovir and intravenous immune globulin: experience of European Bone Marrow Transplant Group. *Clin Infectious Dis* 1992; **14**: 831–835

12 Dawber J H, Paradis I L, Dummer J S. Infectious complications in pulmonary allograft recipients. In: Grossman R F, Maurer J R eds. *Pulmonary Considerations in Transplantation. Clinics in Chest Medicine* 1990; **11**: 291–308

13 Duncan S R, Paradis I L, Yousein SA et al. Sequelae of CMV pulmonary infections in lung allograft recipients. *Am Rev Respir Dis* 1992; **146**: 1419–1425

14 Klatt E C, Shibata D. Cytomegalovirus infection in the acquired immunodeficiency syndrome: clinical and autopsy findings. *Arch Pathol Lab Med* 1988; **122**: 540–544

15 Young J A, Hopkin J M, Cuthbertson W P. Pulmonary infiltrates in immunocompromised patients: diagnosis by cytological examination of bronchoalveolar lavage fluid. *J Clin Pathol* 1984; **37**: 390–397

16 Young J A, Stone J W, McGonigle R J S et al. Diagnosing Pneumocystis carinii pneumonia by cytological examination of broncho-alveolar lavage fluid: report of 15 cases. *J Clin Pathol* 1986; **39**: 945–949

17 Young J A. *Colour Atlas of Pulmonary Cytology*. London: Harvey Miller Publishers and Oxford University Press, 1985; 37–51

18 Teot L A, Ducatman B S, Geisinger K R. Cytologic diagnosis of cytomegaloviral oesophagitis: a report of three acquired immunodeficiency syndrome related cases. *Acta Cytol* 1993; **37**: 93–96

19 Santiago K, Rivera A, Cabanas D et al. Fine needle aspiration of cytomegalovirus sialadenitis in a patient with acquired immunodeficiency syndrome: pitfalls of Diff-Quik staining. *Diagn Cytopathol* 2000; 22; 101–103

20 Martin W J, Smith T F. Rapid detection of cytomegalovirus in bronchoalveolar lavage specimens by a monoclonal antibody method. *J Clin Microbiol* 1986; **23**: 1006–1008

21 Hilborne H L, Nieberg R K, Chen L, Lewin K L. Direct *in situ* hybridization for rapid detection of cytomegalovirus in bronchoalveolar lavage. *Am J Clin Pathol* 1987; **87**: 766–769

22 Olive D M, Simek M, Al-Mufti S. Polymerase chain reaction assay for detection of human cytomegalovirus. *J Clin Microbiol* 1989; **27**: 1238–1242

23 Iwa N, Sasaki M, Yutani C, Wakasa K. Detection of cytomegalovirus DNA in pulmonary specimens: confirmation by *in situ* hybridization in two cases. *Diagn Cytopathol* 1992; **8**: 357–360

24 Smyth R L, Higenbottom T W, Scott J P et al. Herpes simplex virus infection in heart-lung transplant recipients. *Transplantation* 1990; **49**: 735–739

25 Smyth R L, Higenbottom T W, Scott J P et al. Herpes simplex virus infection in heart-lung transplant recipients. *Transplantation* 1990; **49**: 735–739

26 Grosby J H, Pantazis C G, Stigall B. *In situ* hybridization for confirmation of herpes simplex virus in bronchoalveolar smears. *Acta Cytol* 1991; **35**: 248–250

27 Fraga F J, Chaves B M A, Burgos L E, Araques M H. Oral hairy leucoplakia, a histopathologic study of 32 cases. *Am J Dermatopathol* 1990; **12**: 571–578

28 Gomousa-Michael M, Gialama E, Gourmousas N, Gialama G. Genital human papillomavirus infection and associated penile intraepithelial neoplasia in males infected with human immunodeficiency virus. *Acta Cytol* 2000; **44**: 305–309

29 Boldorini R, Zarini E O, Vigano P et al. Cytologic and biomolecular diagnosis of HIV-positive patients. *Acta Cytol* 2000; **44**: 205–210

30 Mitchell D M, Johnson M A. Treatment of lung disease in patients with the acquired immunodeficiency syndrome. *Thorax* 1990; **45**: 219–224

31 Wallace J M, Batra P, Gong H et al. Percutaneous needle lung aspiration for diagnosing pneumonitis in patients with acquired immunodeficiency syndrome. *Am Rev Respir Dis* 1985; **131**: 382–392

32 Broaddus C, Daka M D, Stulbarg M S et al. Bronchoalveolar lavage and transbronchial biopsy for the diagnosis of pulmonary infections in the acquired immunodeficiency syndrome. *Ann Intern Med* 1985; **102**: 747–752

33 Travis W D, Pithluga S, Lipschick G Y et al. Atypical pathologic manifestation of Pneumocystis carinii pneumonia in the required immune deficiency syndrome. *Am J Surg Pathol* 1990; **14**: 615–625

34 Radin D R, Baker E L, Klatt E V et al. Visceral and nodal calcification in patients with AIDS-related Pneumocystis carinii infections. *AJR* 1990; **154**: 27–31

35 Young J A. Pulmonary cytology. ACP Broadsheet. *J Clin Pathol* 1993; **46**: 589–595

36 Biagby T D, Margolskee D, Curtis J L. The usefulness of induced sputum in the diagnosis of Pneumocystis carinii pneumonia in patients with the acquired immunodeficiency syndrome. *Am Rev Respir Dis* 1986; **133**: 515–518

37 Pitchenik A E, Ganfei P, Torres A et al. Sputum examination for the diagnosis of Pneumocystis pneumonia in the acquired immunodeficiency syndrome. *Am Rev Respir Dis* 1986; **133**: 226–229

38 Miller R F, Semple Sjg, Kocjan G. Difficulties with sputum induction for diagnosis of Pneumocystis carinii pneumonia. *Lancet* 1990; **i**: 112

39 Orenstein M, Webber C A, Cash M et al. Value of bronchoalveolar lavage in the diagnosis of pulmonary infection in acquired immune deficiency syndrome. *Thorax* 1986; **41**: 345–349

40 Golden J A, Holland H, Stulbarg M S et al. Bronchoalveolar lavage as the exclusive diagnostic modality for Pneumocystis carinii pneumonia. *Chest* 1986; **90**: 18–21

41 Ghali V S, Garcia R L, Skolom J. Fluorescence of Pneumocystis carinii in Papanicolaou smears. *Hum Pathol* 1984; **15**: 907–909

42 Wehle K, Blanke M, Koenig G, Pfitzer P. The cytological diagnosis by fluorescence microscopy of Papanicolaou stained bronchoalveolar lavage specimens. *Cytopathol* 1991; **2**: 133–120

43 Carmichael A, Bateman N, Nayagam M. Examination of induced sputum in the diagnosis of Pneumocystis carinii pneumonia. *Cytopathol* 1991; **2**: 61–66

44 Leigh T R, Wakefield A E, Peters S E et al. Comparison of DNA amplification and immunofluorescence for detecting Pneumocystis carinii in patients receiving immunosuppressive therapy. *Transplantation* 1992; **54**: 468–470

45 Leigh T R, Gazzard B G, Rowbottom A, Collins J V. Quantitative and qualitative comparison of DNA application by PCR with immunofluorescence staining for diagnosis of Pneumocystis carinii pneumonia. *J Clin Pathol* 1993; **46**: 140–144

46 Young J A, Elias E. Gastro-oesophageal candidiasis; diagnosis by brush cytology. *J Clin Pathol* 1985; **38**: 293–296

47 Stewart S. *Lung transplantation in Practical Pulmonary Pathology*. London: Edward Arnold Publisher, 1995; 88–109

48 Stanley M W, Davies S, Deike M. Pulmonary aspergillosis: an unusual cytologic presentation. *Diagn Cytopathol* 1992; **8**: 585–587

49 McCalmont T H, Silverman J F, Geisinger K R. Fine needle aspiration cytology. Application in cardiac transplantation for the diagnosis of pulmonary aspergillosis. *Arch Surg* 1991; **126**: 394–396

50 Stanley M W, Deike M, Knoedler J, Iber C. Pulmonary mycetomas in immunocompetent patients: diagnosis by fine needle aspiration. *Diagn Cytopathol* 1992; **8**: 577–579

51 Young J A. Lung, pleura and chest wall. In: Young J A ed. *Fine Needle Aspiration Cytopathogy*. Oxford: Blackwells, 1993; 97–121

52 Johnston W W. Cytopathology of mycotic infections. *Lab Med* 1971; **2**: 34–40

51 Blumenfeld W, Gan G L. Diagnosis of histoplasmosis in bronchoalveolar lavage fluid by intracytoplasmic localization of silver-positive yeast. *Acta Cytol* 1991; 710–712

54 Strigle S M, Rarwick M V, Cosgrove M M, Martin S E. A review of fine-needle aspiration cytology findings in human immunodeficiency virus infection. *Diagn Cytopathol* 1992; 41–42

55 Strigle S M, Gal A A. Review of central nervous system cytopathology in human immunodeficiency virus infection. *Diagn Cytopathol* 1991; **7**: 387–401

56 Smallman L A, Young J A, Carey M, Shortland-Webb W. Strongyloides stercoralis hyperinfestation syndrome: a report of two cases. *J Clin Pathol* 1986; **39**: 366–370

57 Casemore D P, Sands R L, Curry A. Cryptosporidium species: 'new' human pathogen. *J Clin Pathol* 1985; **38**: 1321–1336

58 Strigle S M, Gal A A, Martin S E. Alimentary tract cytopathology in human immunodeficiency virus infection: a review of experience in Los Angeles. *Diagn Cytopathol* 1990; **6**: 409–420

59 Paradis I L, Marrairi M, Zeevi A et al. HLA phenotype of lung lavage cells following heart-lung transplantation. *Heart Transplant* 1985; **4**: 422–425

60 Halmberg S D. Possible cofactors for the development of AIDS-related neoplasms. *Cancer Detect Prev* 1990; **22**: 311–336

61 Ognibene F P, Shelhamer J H. Kaposi's sarcoma. In: White D A, Slover D E eds. *Pulmonary effects of AIDS. Clinics in Chest Medicine* 1988; **9**: 459–465

62 Hales M, Bottles K, Miller T et al. Diagnosis of Kaposi's sarcoma by fine needle

aspiration biopsy. *Am J Clin Path* 1987;
88: 20–25

63 Martin-Bates E, Tanner A, Suvarna S K *et al.*
Use of fine needle aspiration cytology for
investigating lymphadenopathy in HIV
positive patients. *J Clin Pathol* 1993;
46: 564–566

64 Al-Rikabi A C, Haidar Z, Arif M *et al.* Fine
needle aspiration cytology of primary
Kaposi's sarcoma of lymph nodes in an
immunocompetent man. *Diagn Cytopathol*
1998; **19**: 451–454

65 Wilkinson A H, Smith J L, Hunsicker L G *et
al.* Increased frequency of post-transplant
lymphomas in patients treated with
cyclosporine, azathioprine, and prednisone.
Transplantation 1989; **47**(2): 293–296

66 Levine A M. Reactive and neoplastic
lymphoproliferative disorders and other
miscellaneous cancers associated with HIV
infection. In: DeVita V T, Hellman S,

Rosenberg S A eds. *AIDS: aetiology, treatment
and prevention*. Philadelphia:
J B Lippincott 1988; 263–275

67 Raphael M, Gentilhomme O, Tulliez M *et al.*
Histopathologic features of high-grade non-
Hodgkin's lymphomas in acquired
immunodeficiency syndrome. *Arch Pathol
Lab Med* 1991; **155**: 15–20

68 Swerdtow S. Post-transplant
lymphoproliferative disorders, a
morphologic, phenotypic and genotypic
spectrum of disease. *Histopathology* 1992;
20: 373–385

69 Porreco R, Penn I, Droegemueller W
et al. Gynecologic malignancies in
immunosuppressed organ homograft
recipients. *Obstet Gynecol* 1975; **45**: 359–364

70 Henry M J, Stanley M W, Cruikshank S,
Carson L. Association of human
immunodeficiency virus-induced
immunosuppression with human papilloma

virus infection and cervical intraepithelial
neoplasia. *Am J Obstet Gynecol* 1989;
160: 352–353

71 Walloch J L, Hong H Y, Bibb L M. Effects
of therapy on cytologic specimens. In:
Bibbo M ed. *Comprehensive Cytopathology*.
Philadelphia: WB Saunders, 1991;
860–877

72 Huang M-S, Colby T V, Goellner J R,
Martin W J. Utility of bronchoalveolar
lavage in the diagnosis of drug-induced
pulmonary toxicity. *Acta Cytol* 1989; **33**:
533–538

73 Teirstein A S, Rosen M J. Lymphocytic
interstitial pneumonia. In: White D A,
Stover D E eds. Pulmonary effects of AIDS.
Clinics in Chest Medicine 1988; **9**: 467–471

74 Koss L C. The urinary tract in the absence
of cancer. *Diagnostic Cytology and its
Histopathology Bases*, 4th edn. Philadelphia:
J B Lippincott, 1992; 890–933

Endocrine system

23 The thyroid gland

Ian D. Buley

Introduction

Historical perspective and clinical indications

Fine needle aspiration (FNA) of the thyroid was documented in the Martin and Ellis paper of 1934[1] and further developed in papers by Tempka *et al.* and Piaggio-Blanco *et al.* in 1948 (given in Grunze and Spriggs[2]). The use of the technique was established subsequently by Scandinavian workers[3,4]. FNA is now recognized to be the first-line investigation for a solitary thyroid nodule, has a valuable role in the diagnosis of the diffuse non-toxic goitre and can be used to confirm the diagnosis of clinically obvious malignancy, enabling the separation of treatable lymphomas from poor prognosis anaplastic carcinomas.

Anatomy and physiology

The adult thyroid weighs approximately 20–25 g. It is a bilobed endocrine organ situated on either side of the trachea and oesophagus. The lobes are joined anteriorly by an isthmus extending over the trachea. Each lobe is about 5 cm in length and extends from the oblique line of the thyroid cartilage to the sixth tracheal ring. The gland's relationship to other neck structures is indicated in Figure 23.1. It is invested by the pretracheal fascia, which is firmly attached posteriorly to the second to fourth tracheal rings. For this reason, the gland and tumours arising from it characteristically move with the larynx on swallowing.

The gland produces thyroxine under the control of thyroid stimulating hormone (TSH) secreted by the pituitary, and also contains neuroendocrine parafollicular cells, which produce calcitonin. The thyroid is derived embryologically as a downgrowth from the base of the tongue. The site of this origin is marked by a vestigial pit, the foramen caecum. A tubular evagination of endodermally derived cells, the thyroglossal duct, extends inferiorly in front of the laryngeal cartilage and the trachea. The distal end proliferates, forming the adult organ, and the path of descent should be obliterated. The calcitonin secreting cells are thought to arise as a separate contribution to the embryonic thyroid gland from the fourth and fifth pharyngeal pouches (ultimobranchial body).

Histologically, the gland consists of numerous follicles (Fig. 23.2), which are the functional units capable of synthesizing, storing and secreting triiodothyronine and tetraiodothyronine (T_3 and T_4); hormones having a wide

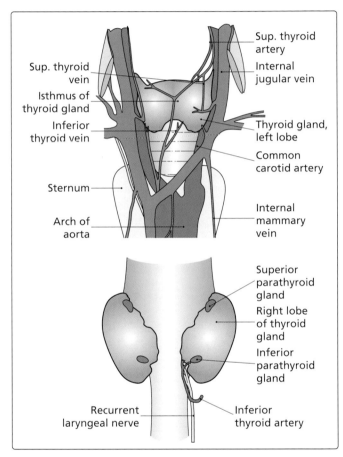

Fig. 23.1 The anterior and posterior relationships of the thyroid.

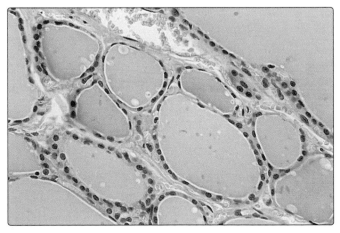

Fig. 23.2 Normal thyroid histology. (H&E × MP)

range of actions stimulating metabolism. The follicles are spheroidal structures lined by a single layer of cuboidal follicular cells. The cells have microvillous processes embedded in the central store of thyroglobulin or colloid, which is a large iodinated glycoprotein from which T_3 and T_4 are subsequently split after endocytosis. In the euthyroid state the follicles vary in size but average 200 μm in diameter. Secretion of thyroid hormones takes place directly into the rich network of capillaries seen in this vascular organ. Longstanding stored thyroglobulin may accumulate calcium oxalate crystals and ageing follicular cells accumulate lipofuchsin.

The parafollicular or C cells are part of the diffuse neuroendocrine system. Although termed parafollicular, these cells are incorporated into follicles. They secrete calcitonin. This hormone has a hypocalcaemic action but its physiological importance in man is unclear. The C cells are immunoreactive to other peptides, including somatostatin, and it is possible that these substances are involved in local paracrine control of T_3 and T_4 production and secretion. These cells are extremely difficult to distinguish from follicular cells using conventional histological stains. The cells are slightly larger, paler and spindle or polyhedral in shape with a faintly granular cytoplasm. They are preferentially localized in the thyroid to the central regions of the lateral lobes and are particularly seen in proximity to solid cell nests, which are thought to be ultimobranchial body remnants.

Technique

Aspiration by the pathologist with immediate staining and interpretation allows the preparation of optimal specimens and the best appreciation of the clinical history, examination findings and the results of biochemical and imaging data. The procedure should be preceded by clinical examination of the neck from the front and behind the seated patient. The differential diagnostic possibilities of lumps in the neck should be considered (Table 23.1).

Thyroid aspiration should be carried out with the patient lying flat, positioned with a pillow beneath the shoulders and neck. This enables the head to fall back in a relaxed position, which separates the sternomastoid muscles, uncovering more of the lateral lobes of the thyroid. Patients will need reassurance as needle aspiration of the neck is one of the more alarming sites for aspiration cytology. They should also be asked not to speak or swallow during the procedure to avoid movement of the gland. Local anaesthetic injection is not recommended. When aspiration is performed in children topical anaesthetic cream is valuable but its use requires forethought, as the cream must be applied under an occlusive dressing for at least an hour to ensure anaesthesia. The vascularity of the thyroid means that a 23 or 25 gauge needle should be used. For the majority of thyroid lesions at most only three passes of the needle in a single plane should be carried out. Persisting

Table 23.1	Fine needle aspiration of lumps in the neck
Structure	**Pathology**
Thyroid	Multinodular goitre and colloid nodules
	Thyroiditis and hyperplasia
	Neoplasms
Lymph nodes	Reactive
	Malignant – lymphomas and metastases
Salivary gland	Sialadenitis
	Neoplasms
Branchial arch remnant	Branchial cyst
Carotid bifurcation	Carotid body tumour and aneurysm
Lymphatics	Cystic hygroma
Pharynx	Pharyngeal pouch
Thymus	Ectopic thymoma
Bone	Cervical rib, hyoid bone
Skin and soft tissues	Skin tumours including dermoid cysts, lipoma, haemangioma, sarcomas, fasciitis and fibromatosis
Parathyroid	Cyst or carcinoma

beyond this results in blood contamination of the sample and the dilution or loss of diagnostic features. An exception to this is in sclerosing malignancies where multiple passes may be necessary to obtain sufficient material. Traversing the sternomastoid should be avoided as it is painful, obscures the depth of the lesion and muscle spasm makes directional control of the needle difficult.

Needle puncture without the use of an aspirating syringe may be of use. Holding the needle alone allows fine and controlled passes. Numerous studies have shown that this technique is particularly valid in the thyroid[5–7] and achieves adequate specimens at least as often as conventional aspiration. In the experience of the author and other workers, blood contamination is reduced but the yield of diagnostic material is also reduced[8]. The technique does not facilitate the diagnostic and therapeutic aspiration of cysts in the thyroid and is recommended only where previous aspirates have been heavily blood contaminated.

The careful sampling necessary in the thyroid because of its vascularity means that at least two aspirates should be taken at any one time from lesions to reduce the risk of false negative diagnosis. In the author's practice, a minimum of four aspirates are taken during the course of initial presentation and subsequent clinical follow-up before a lesion is assumed to be benign and the patient discharged.

Material should be spread by a conventional one step technique but a two stage spreading technique may be used where there is heavy blood contamination[9]. May-Grünwald-Giemsa (MGG) or a rapid Romanowsky-type stain such as Diff-Quik[10] is recommended as this allows the visualization of colloid and can be used alone in thyroid fine needle aspiration. Wet fixation and Papanicolaou staining can provide complementary information in a minority of cases. Thin layer preparations can facilitate examination of poor quality blood-stained specimens but it is not clear whether this technique allows the level of diagnostic accuracy possible with good quality conventional preparations[11].

There are no absolute contraindications to needle aspiration of the thyroid in cooperative patients. The main risk is haematoma formation in those with large goitres or malignant tumours in the neck causing marked tracheal compression. Care should be exercised in those who are anticoagulated and clotting status checked prior to neck aspiration. Puncture of the carotid requires the aspirator to occlude the puncture site for five minutes. Puncture of the trachea may lead to transient coughing. Temporary laryngeal nerve paresis has been recorded post aspiration, as has haemorrhagic necrosis of thyroid tumours, particularly adenomas[12–17]. Needle track implantation by a thyroid malignancy is extraordinarily rare[18,19]. Infection following FNA is very rare but has been recorded[20]. Worrisome histological alterations such as regenerative nuclear changes, vascular proliferations, metaplasias and capsular pseudo-invasion may occur in approximately 10% of thyroid excisions following FNA but awareness of these artefacts by histopathologists avoids misdiagnosis[21].

Impalpable thyroid lesions are a less common clinical presentation. It is possible to take multiple blind aspirates from the area in question, but if there is doubt as to whether the aspirates are representative of the lesion, ultrasound-guided FNA should be carried out. Where a thyroid tumour coexists with regional adenopathy, both the thyroid and the lymph node should be aspirated to rule out coexisting pathology and to allow preoperative staging in the case of thyroid malignancies[22].

Normal cytological findings

Aspiration of normal thyroid tissue yields colloid and sheets of follicular cells together with similar dissociated cells (Fig. 23.3). The colloid stains blue/mauve with MGG or the Diff-Quik stain and is seen as a wash of background colour. The Papanicolaou method does not stain colloid well. If the aspirate is contaminated by blood the diluted colloid may be difficult to distinguish from serum. Follicular cells are relatively small with regular round or slightly oval nuclei of a similar size to those of lymphocytes. The chromatin pattern is even and single small nucleoli are just discernible. Where aspirated in a sheet, the nuclei appear evenly spaced in a honeycomb pattern, each with a small amount of pale cytoplasm. The cytoplasm of dissociated cells is disrupted and the cells usually appear as bare nuclei. Occasionally whole follicles may be aspirated and these appear as pseudo-giant cells. The central colloid is usually inapparent (Fig. 23.4).

The follicular cells may contain deep blue intracytoplasmic paravacuolar granules (Fig. 23.5). These consist of lysosomal accumulations of lipofuscin and haemosiderin. The former arises from degradation of endogenous cellular material and the latter due to the erythrophagocytic capability of follicular cells. Their name derives from the association of these degradative materials with small degenerative paranuclear vacuoles formed by dilated rough endoplasmic reticulum. These granules can occur in normal thyroid but are more frequently seen in functional pathology, such as in a multinodular goitre where there are cystic and

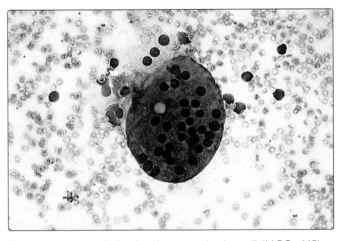

Fig. 23.4 An intact follicle forming a pseudo-giant cell. (MGG × MP)

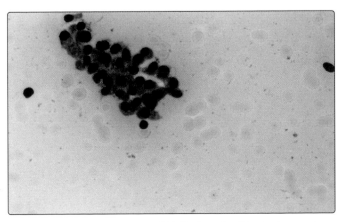

Fig. 23.3 Sheet of normal thyroid follicular cells with a background 'wash' of colloid. (MGG × MP)

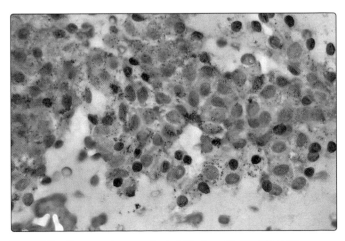

Fig. 23.5 Paravacuolar granules in follicular cells. (MGG × HP)

haemorrhagic changes. They also occur occasionally in neoplasms[23]. Other pigments may accumulate in the thyroid and prolonged use of minocycline for acne results in a black thyroid with accumulation of lipofuscin and a pigment derived from the breakdown of the antibiotic[24].

Extraneous cells can be obtained by the passage of the needle through the strap muscles of the neck or sternomastoid muscle. Striated muscle fibres stain a characteristic deep blue colour and cross-striations can be seen. Puncture of the trachea yields respiratory epithelial cells, mucus and occasionally fragments of cartilage. Adipose tissue is not usually obtained except in the very obese and its presence should raise the possibility of a lipoma of the neck[25] although there are other possibilities including aspiration of a thyrolipoma[26] and adipose metaplasia in a nodular goitre.

Developmental abnormalities
Lingual thyroid
Failure of descent of the organ leads to the formation of a lingual thyroid, the presence of mature functional thyroid tissue at the base of the tongue. Presentation may be with dysphonia, dysphagia or respiratory obstruction. This may necessitate surgical removal but the nature of the tongue mass can be diagnosed by needle aspiration, hence avoiding untreated postoperative hypothyroidism in the 70% of cases who have no thyroid tissue at the normal site. Less acute cases can be treated with exogenous thyroxine, which will shrink the lingual mass. Incomplete descent leads to thyroid tissue placed high in the neck and this subhyoid thyroid presents as a mass in the neck. A normal variation present in up to 40% of individuals is formed by a persistence of the distal extremity of the thyroglossal duct and this pyramidal lobe extends superiorly from the isthmus and lies over the second and third tracheal rings. It may lie slightly to the left of the midline. Excessive descent of thyroid tissue into the superior mediastinum forms a retrosternal thyroid which may manifest as a mediastinal mass with compression symptoms, particularly if nodularity should supervene on the gland.

Thyroglossal cyst
Should the thyroglossal duct persist partially or *in toto* a thyroglossal cyst or sinus may form. This is a characteristically midline swelling most often present immediately below the hyoid bone. Presentation typically occurs in children or young adults with a history of a painless mass of long duration. The cyst may become infected and present with an inflamed mass, which is prone to spontaneous rupture through the skin and the formation of a sinus. Histologically, the cyst is lined by respiratory-type or squamous epithelium with lymphoid tissue in the wall. There may be small amounts of adjacent thyroid tissue. Fine needle aspiration yields clear or mucoid fluid with degenerate foamy cells and respiratory or squamous

cells. The possibility of skin or tracheal contamination should be considered. Some reactive lymphoid tissue may be obtained. The presence of thyroid follicular cells or colloid is less common. Cholesterol crystals may be seen. Rarely, carcinomas arise in a thyroglossal cyst or duct. These are usually papillary in type[27,28] and follicular tumours are exceptionally rare. Squamous carcinoma and anaplastic carcinoma have been recorded but medullary carcinomas are unknown and this is thought to be a consequence of the embryological derivation of the parafollicular cells.

Cytological findings
▶ Clear or mucoid fluid on aspiration
▶ Respiratory epithelial and/or squamous cells are present
▶ Reactive lymphoid cells may be seen
▶ Follicular cells or colloid are less frequently seen

Lateral aberrant thyroid
Lateral aberrant thyroid was once thought to represent developmental inclusions of thyroid tissue positioned lateral to the jugular veins. It is now recognized that most if not all such cases represent follicular pattern metastases in cervical lymph nodes arising from occult papillary carcinomas of the thyroid.

Thymus
The thymus develops from the third pharyngeal pouch and a thymoma may arise in ectopic tissue incorporated into the lower pole of the thyroid, mimicking a thyroid mass[29,30].

Acquired non-neoplastic conditions
Multinodular goitre, colloid nodules and cysts
The thyroid gland is in a state of constant but varying activity, becoming more active at puberty, in pregnancy and with physiological stress. It even changes in size and activity during the normal menstrual cycle. These changes may lead to a sporadic goitre. Whether the goitre is sporadic or due to a well-defined cause (Table 23.2), with persistence of a goitrogenic stimulus the gland may cease to behave in an homogeneous fashion. The mechanism of this is not fully understood. While the patient is usually euthyroid, parts of the gland are hyperplastic whereas other areas are inactive and accumulate colloid. The latter areas

Table 23.2 Goitres – diffuse enlargement of the thyroid

Simple non-toxic goitre
   Physiological (including endemic, due to dietary iodine deficiency)
   Dietary goitrogens, goitrogenic drugs and chemicals
   Dyshormonogenetic: inborn errors of thyroxine synthesis
Multinodular goitre
syn: colloid goitre, nodular goitre, adenomatous goitre
Toxic goitre
Thyroiditis

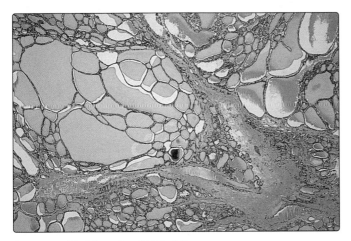

Fig. 23.6   Nodular goitre. (H&E × LP)

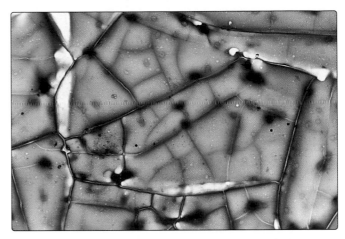

Fig. 23.7   Thick varnish-like coat of colloid with 'crazy paving' pattern. (MGG × MP)

form enlarged colloid nodules and the structure of these may break down, particularly after spontaneous haemorrhage, to form cysts. Radioiodine studies show the enlarged inactive follicles and cysts as radioactively cold areas, a characteristic shared with most thyroid neoplasms. Occasionally a hyperplastic focus within a nodular goitre may cause clinical hyperthyroidism. Autoimmune thyroiditis or hyperplasia may also supervene on a multinodular goitre and these cases may become respectively hypo- or hyperthyroid.

Histologically, a multinodular goitre is characterized by nodularity with fibrosis, calcification and deposition of haemosiderin and cholesterol as evidence of previous haemorrhage (Fig. 23.6). Within the areas of fibrosis and haemorrhage, groups of follicular cells may show regenerative and degenerative changes.

Multinodular goitre presents clinically in approximately 5% of the population and the female to male ratio is at least three. It presents as a mass in the neck which may cause tracheal or oesophageal compression. Haemorrhage into a colloid nodule causes the sudden and painful appearance or enlargement of a mass in the neck. A dominant nodule in the context of a multinodular goitre is the most frequent indication for fine needle aspiration and correct diagnosis of a colloid nodule or cyst with the exclusion of malignancy allows the avoidance of surgery in most cases.

Cytological findings

Aspiration of a small colloid goitre with little nodularity may yield normal findings. Aspiration of a colloid nodule yields abundant colloid and this may be recognized as a thick transparent yellow fluid. It forms a varnish-like coat over the slide and tends to develop a crazy paving pattern of cracks (Fig. 23.7). This thick coat of colloid may be lost on staining if the slide has not been allowed to dry thoroughly. This can occur in a fine needle aspiration clinic setting where immediate staining and interpretation is carried out

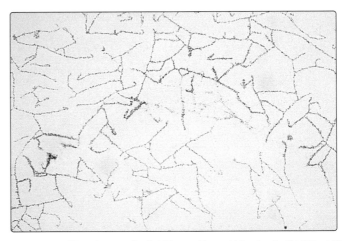

Fig. 23.8   Ghost-image of colloid formed by red blood cells. (MGG × LP)

and in this circumstance drying the slide in a warm stream of air, e.g. from a hairdryer, is particularly recommended. Loss of colloid may result in a ghost image of the colloid being formed by red blood cells in the aspirate (Fig. 23.8). The colloid consistency is variable and may appear thin and diffuse but inspissated dense fragments of colloid may also be seen.

Degenerate foamy cells containing both haemosiderin and lipofuscin will be seen scattered amongst the colloid (Fig. 23.9). Conventionally these are considered to be histiocytes although some may be degenerate follicular cells. Follicular cells are also seen. These vary from being few in number to being numerous and most frequently occur in monolayered sheets. Follicular cells in multinodular goitre more frequently contain paravacuolar bodies. An appreciation of the ratio between the quantities of colloid and follicular cells is crucial to the distinction of the benign functional abnormality in a multinodular goitre from a potentially malignant follicular neoplasm. This distinction is subjective and repeat aspiration can be helpful. In cases of continuing doubt excision biopsy should

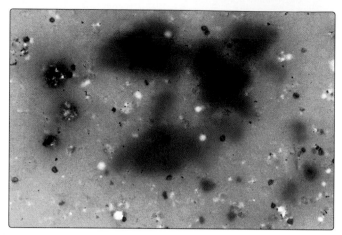

Fig. 23.9   Aspirate from a colloid nodule. (MGG × MP)

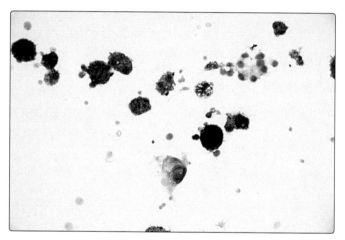

Fig. 23.10   Aspirate from a nodular goitre with debris-laden macrophages and follicular cells, one of which shows marked regenerative and degenerative change. (MGG × HP)

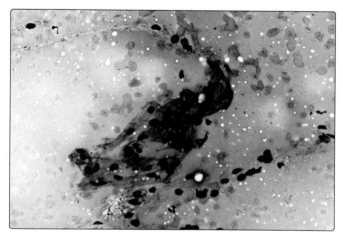

Fig. 23.11   Aspirate from a nodular goitre showing a fragment of fibrous stroma. (MGG × HP)

be recommended. The presence of abundant colloid indicates a low likelihood of neoplasia.

The number of follicular cells is likely to be increased where a hyperplastic nodule has been included in the aspiration and the cytological features of hyperplasia need to be searched for. These may be florid with the formation of marginal fire flares (see Fig. 23.13), or may be more subtle with an increase in the amount of cytoplasm and mild nuclear enlargement with small single nucleoli. The latter changes are seen in cells originating from smaller, more active, follicles and foci of microfollicular architecture may be recognized in such cases. Features of hyperplasia are suggestive of a functional abnormality but occasionally tumours may show hyperplastic changes[31,32]. Reactive lymphocytes and Hürthle cell change in follicular cells may be seen where there is coexisting thyroiditis. In a multinodular goitre degenerative and regenerative changes in follicular epithelium may be marked (Fig. 23.10) and care must be taken not to mistake these cells for anaplastic carcinoma cells either of the spindle cell or giant cell form. The clinical and cytological context of these cells, which are usually few in number and show degenerative changes, must be taken into account.

Aspiration also yields small fragments of loose fibrous stroma containing groups of follicular cells (Fig. 23.11). Fragments of calcification and rarely psammoma bodies, which are regarded as strongly indicative of papillary carcinoma, may be seen in multinodular goitre[33]. Nuclear grooves and inclusions, also regarded as indicative of papillary carcinoma, are occasionally seen[34].

Where haemorrhage has occurred into a colloid nodule the aspirate is of chocolate-brown fluid with disappearance or shrinkage of the mass. The fluid requires centrifugation for proper examination. Degenerate red blood cells are present and in longstanding cysts cholesterol crystals are seen. Debris-containing foamy histiocytes may be numerous and follicular cells tend to be few and appear degenerate. The main differential diagnosis is with cystic degeneration in a tumour, particularly papillary carcinoma[35]. If there is a residual mass this should be aspirated and the thyroid adjacent to a cyst should also be sampled. Almost half of benign cysts are cured by the first aspiration. Recurrent cysts should be excised for cure and to exclude an underlying neoplasm[36]. Other differential diagnoses include thyroglossal cyst and parathyroid cyst.

Cytological findings

▶ Abundant colloid
▶ Debris-containing histiocytes
▶ Cystic degeneration results in aspirates of brown fluid containing degenerate red blood cells, cholesterol crystals, debris-containing histiocytes and degenerate follicular cells
▶ Follicular cells often with paravacuolar bodies
▶ Follicular cells may show degenerative and regenerative changes
▶ Fragments of fibrous stroma
▶ Hürthle cells, hyperplastic changes and lymphoid cells may be seen

Hyperplasia

Primary hyperplasia of the thyroid, or Graves disease, results from the presence of autoantibodies to the TSH receptor on follicular cells. These IgG antibodies mimic the action of TSH at the receptor site. Separate antibodies, which stimulate the cellular hyperplasia of the thyroid, are also present together with blocking antibodies to both groups of immunoglobulins. Similar antibodies are present in autoimmune thyroiditis and differences in the clinical manifestations of these diseases may relate to the degree of activity of the blocking antibodies. Thyroid hyperplasia is one component of the syndrome of Graves disease which also includes exophthalmos and pretibial myxoedema. The condition affects females at least five times as often as males and has a peak age distribution in the third and fourth decades. The clinical features are a consequence of the hypermetabolic state induced by excess thyroxine and are summarized in Table 23.3.

Histologically, there is diffuse hyperplasia with small follicles containing pale-staining colloid. The follicular cells appear crowded and may protrude as papillary projections into the follicle. The follicular cells are enlarged and columnar with pale cytoplasm and scalloping of the colloid adjacent to the cells. Foci of Hürthle cell change may be seen and the thyroid interstitium may contain a reactive lymphoid infiltrate (Fig. 23.12).

Diagnosis is achieved by clinical examination, biochemical and serological tests. Fine needle aspiration is not necessary for primary diagnosis. Hyperplastic changes can be seen in other clinical situations (Table 23.4) and particularly as a focal change in multinodular goitre and in thyroiditis.

Cytological findings

▶ Blood-stained aspirates
▶ Little colloid
▶ Moderate cellularity
▶ Dispersed follicular cells with an enlarged round nucleus and single nucleolus
▶ Cytoplasmic marginal vacuolation

Aspiration of the thyroid yields blood-stained material due to the vascularity of the gland. Colloid may not be recognized and where it is seen it appears as a thin pink wash with MGG stains. Amongst the blood is a dispersed population of thyroid follicular cells of moderate cellularity with enlarged round nuclei and an easily discernible single nucleolus. There may be some variation in nuclear size. The cytoplasm is increased in amount and is fragile with a faintly frothy texture. It stains pale blue/grey with MGG stains. Bare nuclei may be present. Flat sheets of cells may be seen and in these groups the characteristic marginal vacuolation of cells is present. These pink soap bubble, colloid suds, flame or fire flare appearances (Fig. 23.13) are a manifestation of the active pinocytosis of thyroglobulin

Table 23.3   Manifestations of Graves disease

Psychological	– nervousness, emotional lability, heat intolerance, tiredness
Nervous system	– tremor, eye changes
Cardiovascular	– arrhythmias, tachycardia, cardiomegaly
Gastrointestinal	– good appetite, weight loss, diarrhoea
Musculoskeletal	– weakness (proximal myopathy), osteoporosis
Skin	– hot and sweaty

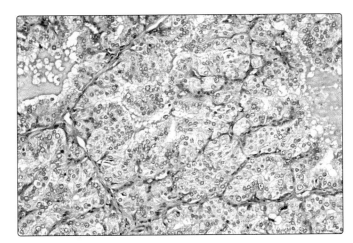

Fig. 23.12   Thyroid hyperplasia. (H&E × LP)

Table 23.4   Causes of hyperthyroidism

Common
  Graves disease (diffuse toxic goitre)
  Toxic multinodular goitre
  Toxic adenoma
Uncommon
  Acute phase of thyroiditis
  Hyperfunctioning thyroid carcinoma
  Choriocarcinoma, hydatidiform mole (TSH like activity)
  TSH secreting pituitary tumour
  Neonatal thyrotoxicosis (mother with Graves disease)
  Struma ovarii (ovarian teratoma – no thyroid hyperplasia)
  Iatrogenic (exogenous – no thyroid hyperplasia)

from the small follicles found in thyroid hyperplasia. They are found in the majority but not all cases of hyperplasia. Occasional small follicular structures and papillary formations may be seen. Small numbers of lymphocytes may be recognized although these are often inapparent due to dilution by blood. The pathogenic overlap between Graves disease and Hashimoto's thyroiditis results in the recognition of Hürthle cell changes, epithelioid histiocytes and multinucleate giant histiocytes in some cases[37].

Caution needs to be exercised in the interpretation of aspirates from Graves disease which has failed to respond to medical therapy. The drugs used, which interfere with

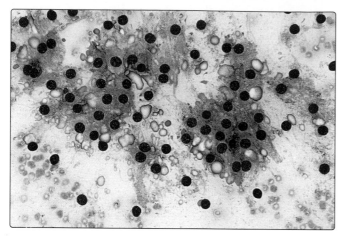

Fig. 23.13   Thyroid hyperplasia showing florid 'fire flare' appearances. (MGG × HP)

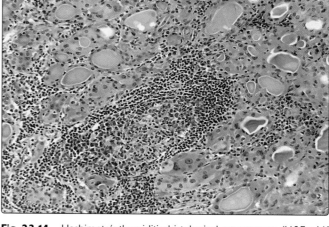

Fig. 23.14   Hashimoto's thyroiditis: histological appearances. (H&E × MP)

thyroid hormone biosynthesis, can cause marked nuclear atypia as can the previous use of ablative radioactive iodine[38,39]. Dyshormonogenetic goitres similarly show florid hyperplastic features often with papillary architecture and also show nuclear atypia.

Thyroiditis

Inflammation of the thyroid can be subdivided into lymphocytic and autoimmune (Hashimoto's) thyroiditis, de Quervain's thyroiditis, Riedel's thyroiditis and acute bacterial thyroiditis. Fine needle aspiration in this situation is usually carried out to exclude neoplasia as rapid enlargement of the gland, firmness, nodularity and fixation to surrounding structures may occur in inflammatory conditions. Additionally, thyroiditis may coexist with a neoplasm and indeed primary lymphoma of the thyroid is predisposed to by underlying autoimmune thyroiditis. Needle aspiration can also contribute to the primary diagnosis of Hashimoto's thyroiditis, particularly in the minority of cases which do not have classical serological changes.

Lymphocytic and autoimmune thyroiditis

A non-specific lymphocytic infiltrate may be found focally in the thyroid adjacent to neoplasms but the majority of cases of lymphocytic thyroiditis are due to autoimmune disease. A lymphocytic infiltrate and even germinal centre formation may occur in Graves disease but the classical destructive autoimmune thyroiditis is Hashimoto's thyroiditis. In 95% of cases the patient is female and typically middle-aged although the disease can occur in other age groups including children. The disease is often familial and may be associated with other organ-specific autoimmune disorders. The patient usually presents with a smooth and moderately enlarged painless goitre. In the acute initial phase of the disease there may be mild thyrotoxicosis (Hashitoxicosis). The majority of patients progress to hypothyroidism over a period of a few years

although the time course may be much longer and such low-grade thyroiditides account for the idiopathic myxoedema of the elderly. Microsomal antibodies are present in high titre in 95% of cases. Approximately 10% of the normal female population has low titres of the same antibody. Hashimoto's thyroiditis is a clinicopathological diagnosis depending on clinical, serological and morphological findings.

The typical gross pathology is a diffuse firm enlargement of the thyroid gland with a pale grey lobulated cut surface. Occasionally the proliferation is nodular and peripherally placed nodules containing lymphoid and epithelial cells may be mistaken for malignancy in a cervical lymph node. Histologically (Fig. 23.14), there is a lymphoplasmacytic infiltrate with germinal centre formation. This is associated with destruction of the follicles and fibrosis. Occasional epithelioid histiocytes and multinucleate histiocytes are seen. The residual follicular cells show an oxyphilic metaplastic change termed Askanazy or Hürthle cell change. These cells may also show mixed hyperplastic features and form papillary infoldings. They show nuclear enlargement and variability. Squamous metaplasia may be seen. In a minority of cases, Hashimoto's thyroiditis may be predominantly a fibrosing process and can be confused clinically with malignancy.

Cytological findings

► Reactive lymphoid cells
► Hürthle cells
► Multinucleate and epithelioid histiocytes
► Little colloid

Aspiration cytology yields numerous lymphoid cells. These appear reactive and polymorphous with a mixed cell population of lymphocytes, centrocytes, centroblasts, immunoblasts, plasma cells and occasional tingible-body

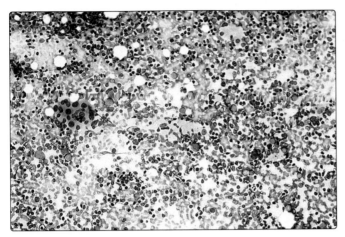

Fig. 23.15 Hashimoto's thyroiditis: cytological appearances. (MGG × LP)

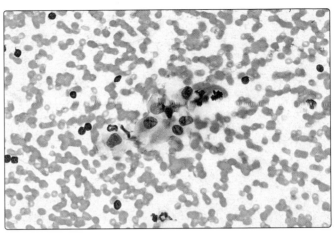

Fig. 23.17 Hashimoto's thyroiditis. Epithelioid histiocytes. (MGG × HP)

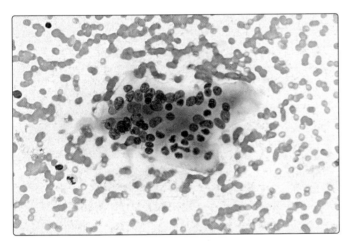

Fig. 23.16 Hashimoto's thyroiditis. Multinucleate histiocyte. (MGG × HP)

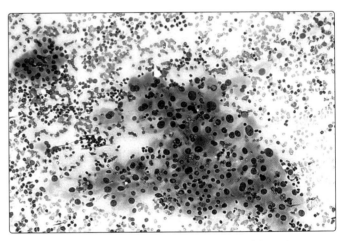

Fig. 23.18 Hashimoto's thyroiditis. Hürthle cells. (MGG × MP)

macrophages (Fig. 23.15). Large multinucleate histiocytes (Fig. 23.16) and small groups of epithelioid histiocytes (Fig. 23.17) may be seen. The latter can be distinguished from epithelial cells by the more delicate quality of their cytoplasm and the presence of footprint shaped nuclei. The lymphoid cells may be seen admixed within groups of epithelial cells. The epithelial cells show Hürthle cell change manifested by an increase in the size of the cell and nucleus. The cytoplasm is moderately dense and blue-grey with a fine granularity. Cell-to-cell boundaries within the groups are not particularly well-defined. Some of the cell groups have a vaguely papillary outline. The nuclei appear enlarged, sometimes grossly so, and hyperchromatic and may appear atypical with variation in size and shape. Nucleoli can be prominent. Rarely, intranuclear inclusions are seen. In Hashimoto's thyroiditis mixed Hürthle cell and hyperplastic appearances are commonly seen within individual cells (Fig. 23.18). The exact appearances in an aspirate are dependent on the phase of the disease. Early in the disease abundant lymphocytes are present and later Hürthle cell change and fibrosis predominate[40].

Diagnostic pitfalls

Hürthle cell groups can be confused with those of papillary carcinoma; points of distinction include the granular quality of the cytoplasm and the presence of more distinct cell-to-cell boundaries in the latter. The other main differential diagnostic problem is the distinction from a Hürthle cell neoplasm. Hürthle cell nodules with a less intense inflammatory component may occur in later phase Hashimoto's thyroiditis and the appearances may mimic a neoplasm both histologically and cytologically[41]. Paradoxically, the extent of nuclear variability may be less in a Hürthle cell neoplasm. The groups of cells in neoplasms may present a more papillary or trabecular outline and are not usually associated with a reactive lymphoid infiltrate. The mixed Hürthle cell–hyperplasia appearance rarely occurs in neoplasms.

There is an increased risk of lymphoma in Hashimoto's thyroiditis and recognition of this coexisting pathology relies upon the appreciation of a monomorphic pattern amongst the lymphoid cells. In addition, Hürthle cells are

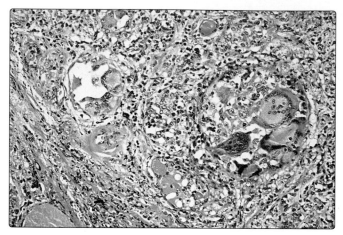

Fig. 23.19   de Quervain's thyroiditis: histological appearances. (H&E × MP)

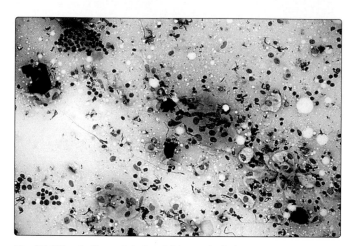

Fig. 23.20   de Quervain's thyroiditis: cytological appearances. (MGG × MP)

likely to be sparse or absent. The lymphomas are most often high-grade and of B cell type. Immunocytochemistry to demonstrate monoclonality of light chain expression may be helpful particularly in the low-grade lymphomas which can be more difficult to diagnose[42].

de Quervain's thyroiditis (granulomatous thyroiditis)

This condition is a rare form of thyroid inflammation probably due to viral infection in genetically predisposed individuals. Mumps, measles, adenovirus, Epstein-Barr virus, Coxsackie and influenza viruses have been implicated. Typically, it presents in adults following an upper respiratory infection with fever and diffuse tender enlargement of the thyroid. There is a female predominance. The usual time course of the illness is a few months. There may be initial mild hyperthyroidism but this is followed by hypothyroidism, which is usually transient. Asymmetric involvement of the gland may raise the question of neoplasia and hence cases come to cytological attention. Histopathologically, there is an initial infiltration of the follicles by mixed inflammatory cells. This appears to result in damage and the release of thyroglobulin to which there is a foreign-body granulomatous reaction (Fig. 23.19). Subsequently there is follicular regeneration and interfollicular fibrosis.

Cytological findings

► Numerous multinucleate histiocytes
► Mixed inflammatory cells including epithelioid histiocytes and lymphocytes
► Degenerative changes in follicular cells – cell debris and colloid

The cytological findings (Fig. 23.20) are of numerous multinucleate histiocytes together with mixed inflammatory cells. These include epithelioid histiocytes and lymphocytes. Degenerating follicular cells may be seen together with a dirty background including cell debris and

colloid. Ingested colloid can occasionally be seen within the multinucleate histiocytes. The presence of apparent necrosis and degenerative atypia in follicular cells may lead to an inappropriate suspicion of malignancy[43].

Granulomatous changes may also arise in the thyroid as a histiocytic response to haemorrhage, as a reaction to spilled colloid adjacent to a neoplasm following clinical examination (palpation thyroiditis), with mycobacterial[44] or fungal infections, in sarcoidosis, in some forms of vasculitis and as a foreign body reaction. The latter has been recorded in a case of Teflon injection into the vocal cord with contamination of the adjacent thyroid[45]. All of these conditions might mimic the appearances of de Quervain's thyroiditis on needle aspiration. Multinucleate giant cells are also seen in autoimmune thyroiditis and aspiration of intact follicles (pseudo-giant cells) should not be confused with multinucleate histiocytes. Osteoclast-like giant cells may occur as a reactive population in anaplastic carcinoma of the thyroid. If these cells predominate in an aspirate they may cause diagnostic confusion with a granulomatous process[46].

Riedel's thyroiditis

This is a very rare inflammatory fibrosis of unknown aetiology involving the thyroid and adjacent tissues of the neck. It therefore presents with a very firm (ligneous) mass, which appears to be fixed to surrounding structures and hence mimics malignancy. It occurs in adults and shows a female predominance. There may be pressure symptoms with dysphagia or stridor. The gland can be focally involved or totally involved, and in the latter case there may be hypothyroidism. Histologically, fibrous tissue replaces the gland. The follicles are obliterated and appear atrophic. Hürthle cell change is not seen. The fibrosis is dense and hyaline but may also contain an inflammatory infiltrate chiefly of lymphocytes and plasma cells. The inflammatory infiltrate has a perivascular distribution and vasculitis, particularly affecting veins, may be seen. The findings on

Table 23.5   Thyroid neoplasms

Primary neoplasms
Benign
    Adenoma
    Atypical adenoma
Malignant
    Angioinvasive follicular carcinoma
    Follicular carcinoma
    Papillary carcinoma
    Mixed follicular and medullary carcinoma
    Medullary carcinoma
    Anaplastic carcinoma
    Lymphoma
    Sarcomas
Secondary neoplasms

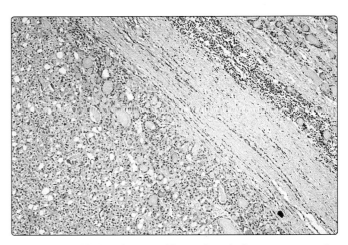

Fig. 23.21   Follicular adenoma with capsule and adjacent compressed and atrophic thyroid follicles. (H&E × LP)

fine needle aspiration are non-specific. The aspirate is poorly cellular and may include a few fibroblasts and inflammatory cells. Where there is clinical suspicion biopsy will be necessary to exclude a sclerosing malignancy of the thyroid.

Other forms of thyroiditis

Infection by mycobacteria, fungi and viruses have been mentioned in the context of granulomatous or de Quervain's thyroiditis. In addition cytomegalovirus and *Pneumocystis carinii* infection of the thyroid are recorded in the immunocompromised[47]. Microfilaria of various species have been visualized as incidental findings in aspirates from cystic degeneration in multinodular goitres[48,49]. Acute bacterial infection also occurs, particularly in the debilitated, with resultant acute inflammation and abscess formation.

Thyroid neoplasms (Table 23.5)

Carcinomas of the thyroid show great differences in their epidemiology, pathogenesis, presentation, natural history, management and prognosis depending upon the histological subtype. Overall thyroid cancer is more common in females with an approximate predominance of 2.5:1. It also shows marked geographical variation but accounts for approximately 0.5% of cancer deaths in the UK. Known risk factors include irradiation to the head and neck area and residence in an endemic goitre region.

Follicular neoplasms
Follicular adenoma

Follicular adenomas are the most common of thyroid neoplasms. Autopsy series have shown an incidence of the order of 3% of the adult population. They are slow-growing and show morphological and biochemical evidence of follicular cell differentiation. There is a range of appearances with microscopic features recapitulating the embryology and functional states of the thyroid. Hence, there are embryonal, foetal, normofollicular and macrofollicular patterns. Adenomas may also demonstrate

various metaplasias and degenerative changes and hence there are Hürthle cell, clear cell, signet-ring cell adenomas, the adenolipoma showing adipose metaplasia in its stroma and the adenochondroma with cartilaginous metaplasia. Atypical adenomas show nuclear atypia. Common to these tumours, however, are the presence of a well circumscribed and complete fibrous capsule with compression of the surrounding thyroid gland and a relatively uniform appearance of the tumour within the capsule which differs from the surrounding thyroid (Fig. 23.21). Adenomas are usually solitary masses in contrast to colloid nodules in a multinodular goitre. Larger tumours may show degenerative changes with areas of fibrosis and calcification. In the extreme they may undergo cystic degeneration. Irrespective of their histological pattern they are benign and usually asymptomatic. Occasionally haemorrhage occurs into an adenoma and the patient presents with a painful and tender mass. A small minority of adenomas behave autonomously and cause hyperthyroidism. The majority of adenomas are hypofunctional and appear as cold nodules on radioisotope scanning.

Follicular carcinoma

Follicular carcinoma is the second most common type of thyroid carcinoma, constituting approximately 25% of the total. It shows a female predominance in the ratio of 2.5:1 and presents most commonly in the 40–60 age range. The tumour characteristically metastasizes haematogenously with secondaries predominantly in the skeleton and lungs.

These malignant thyroid epithelial tumours show evidence of follicular differentiation with no features to suggest any of the other subtypes. They range from well-differentiated to poorly-differentiated (Figs 23.22, 23.23). Well-differentiated carcinomas may be cytologically bland and resemble adenomas, indeed well-differentiated follicular carcinoma may appear cytologically less atypical than the benign atypical adenoma. The carcinoma is characterized by the architectural features of local and

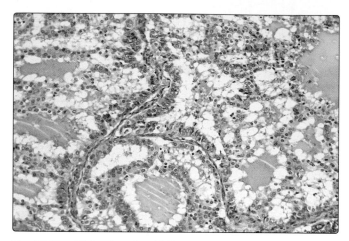

Fig. 23.22 Well-differentiated follicular carcinoma of the thyroid. (H&E × MP)

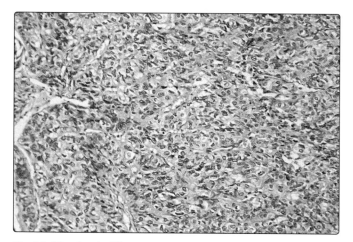

Fig. 23.23 Poorly-differentiated follicular carcinoma of the thyroid. (H&E × MP)

vascular invasion. This may be obvious but some carcinomas appear totally encapsulated and are so defined on the basis of vascular invasion in capsular vessels. Such lesions can be difficult to diagnose, requiring the examination of multiple histological blocks of the capsule[50,51]. Treatment for encapsulated or minimally invasive lesions can be by lobectomy and isthmusectomy; widely invasive lesions require total thyroidectomy followed by ablative radioactive ^{131}I and thyroxine replacement therapy. The overall prognosis gives a 5-year survival of approximately 70%, dependent on the grade, invasiveness and stage of the tumour. The angioinvasive encapsulated follicular carcinoma however metastasizes in only approximately 5% of cases. Well-differentiated skeletal metastases can be very indolent with survival for many years. Hürthle cell variants of follicular carcinoma constitute approximately 5% of the total. These have been thought to be intrinsically more aggressive than other follicular carcinomas but the consensus view is that these lesions behave similarly according to their invasiveness, grade and stage. Hürthle cell tumours are prone to undergo

clear cell change caused by swelling of the numerous mitochondria which they contain and this is one of the derivations of clear cell variants of follicular carcinoma.

Fine needle aspiration of follicular lesions serves as a screening tool for the selection of cases requiring excision and histological examination to make the definitive diagnosis of an adenoma or carcinoma on the basis of the architectural features. The selection of such cases relies primarily on the appreciation of the degree of cellularity of the specimen and its relationship with the amount of colloid present. Since these observations are also dependent on the technical quality of the smear, reliable diagnosis requires good quality specimens from a consistent aspirator, preferably the pathologist in person.

Cytological findings

▶ Cellular aspirates with little colloid, microfollicles
▶ Cytological features of hyperplasia usually absent
▶ Atypical features may be present: nuclear crowding, increased nuclear size, frequency and number of nucleoli raised, nuclear membrane irregularity and irregular chromatin distribution

Aspirates from follicular neoplasms are apt to be blood-stained due to the vascularity of the tumour. With the exception of thyroid hyperplasia, most neoplasms are more cellular than functional abnormalities and also contain less colloid. Colloid, where present, may occur as small inspissated globules which can superficially resemble psammoma bodies (Fig. 23.24). The follicular cells, which occur dispersed and in groups, may appear cytologically bland and similar to those seen in aspirates from a multinodular goitre. The cells tend to show less variation of appearance in follicular neoplasms with a repetitive pattern of cell groups. Cytological features of hyperplasia are usually absent in neoplasms[31,32]. The presence of numerous microfollicular aggregates (Fig. 23.25) implies a follicular

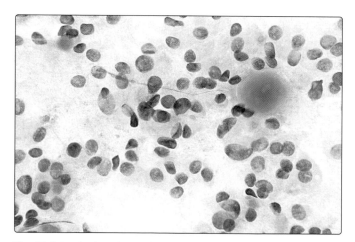

Fig. 23.24 Aspirate from a follicular neoplasm including an inspissated globule of colloid. (Papanicolaou × HP)

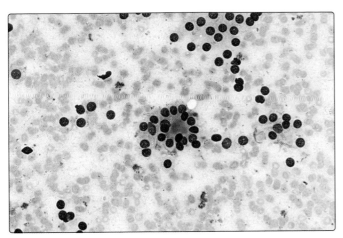

Fig. 23.25 Aspirate from a follicular neoplasm including a microfollicular aggregate. (MGG × MP)

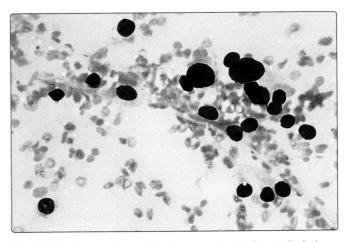

Fig. 23.26 Aspirate from a follicular neoplasm showing cytological atypia. The subsequent histology showed a benign atypical adenoma. (MGG × HP)

neoplasm as such structures are uncommon in nodular goitre aspirates. There may be nuclear enlargement and crowding in the cell groups. The presence of one or more nucleoli may be appreciated.

Diagnostic pitfalls

The cytological appearances of a benign functional nodule in a goitre and the appearances of a follicular neoplasm can overlap. Hence one diagnostic problem is the distinction between a macrofollicular follicular neoplasm and a nodule in a multinodular goitre. Few of the former are carcinomas and this is an uncommon though potential source of false negative diagnosis in practice. The clinical context may be helpful and the policy of clinical follow-up and repeat aspiration minimizes the possibility of a missed well-differentiated malignancy.

The major diagnostic problem is the distinction between an adenoma and a carcinoma. The presence of cytological atypia is common to many benign endocrine tumours including thyroid adenomas. This is exemplified by the aspirate illustrated in Figure 23.26 from an atypical adenoma. Absolute distinction between a benign adenoma and a well-differentiated follicular carcinoma on simple morphological grounds is realized to be impossible. Methods used to try and resolve this difficulty include nuclear DNA content[52–55] and nuclear morphometry. Adenomas can be diploid, aneuploid or polyploid in common with follicular carcinoma and hence DNA content does not appear helpful. The results of nuclear morphometry studies to distinguish well-differentiated follicular carcinoma from adenoma have been conflicting[56] but generally show the technique to be unhelpful[57–60]. The conflicting results and lack of general applicability of the technique may be due to the influence of other factors on nuclear size including fixation and the flattening of nuclei which occurs under different spreading conditions[61].

The proportion of cells with nucleoli and the number of nucleoli per cell appear helpful but do not discriminate absolutely, three or more nucleoli per cell being rare in follicular adenomas and occurring in occasional cells in 70% of follicular carcinomas[62]. Some studies have shown that the combination of nuclear diameter, percentage of nucleolated cells and numbers of nucleoli improves the distinction between adenoma and carcinoma above that achieved by subjective evaluation[63]. Silver staining nucleolar organizer region area and number have also been investigated but there is overlap between benign lesions and the higher values seen with malignancies[64,65]. A wide range of cell surface antigens, enzymes and oncogene products have also been investigated as potential discriminants. Recent candidates have included CD44, Galectin-3, the antibody HBME-1 and telomerase[66]. Distinction between a follicular adenoma and follicular carcinoma remains problematical and a report of follicular neoplasm should be given in appropriate cases. It must be ensured that the physician or surgeon understands the meaning of the phrase and the need for excision in all such cases. A comment may be added as regards the presence of atypia. The most discriminant atypical features are high cellularity, crowding in cell groups, increased nuclear size, more than 75% of cells with nucleoli, cells with three or more nucleoli, nuclear membrane irregularity and irregular chromatin distribution[62,63,67]. The presence of necrotic debris also supports the suspicion of malignancy[68]. In a minority of cases where the clinical findings suggest malignancy and the aspirates show marked cytological atypia, it is appropriate to diagnose malignancy just as one may with the anaplastic carcinomas. Intraoperative frozen section has an important role in separating widely invasive follicular carcinomas requiring total thyroidectomy from follicular adenomas and minimally invasive carcinomas, which can be managed by local resection[69].

Variant follicular neoplasms

Insular carcinoma

The insular carcinoma is a poorly-differentiated follicular carcinoma. Histologically, it consists of well-defined nests of fairly uniform cells and small follicles. These cells often show prominent mitotic activity and the tumour is infiltrative and aggressive in behaviour. Cytologically, smears are hypercellular with sheets of cells, occasional microfollicular aggregates and dispersed cells. The sheets of cells typically show nuclear crowding. The cells are relatively uniform with no gross pleomorphism. Intracytoplasmic vacuoles containing thyroglobulin may be seen. Necrosis may be present. The nuclear to cytoplasmic ratio is high with moderate anisokaryosis and nuclear atypia. Intranuclear inclusions and nuclear grooving can be seen together with a papillary configuration to some of the cell groups and this can cause confusion with papillary carcinoma[70–73].

Hyalinizing trabecular adenoma

Another follicular tumour, which causes difficulties in cytological diagnosis, is the hyalinizing trabecular adenoma. This is a benign tumour but a malignant variant has been described. The tumour is well circumscribed and encapsulated with polygonal or spindled cells arranged in trabeculae and small islands. Scattered follicles containing thyroglobulin are present. Occasionally small papillary projections occur into cystic spaces. The trabeculae are surrounded by hyaline fibrosis and basement membrane material. This eosinophilic material may mimic amyloid although it is Congo red negative. Elongated epithelial cells may be arranged radially around the basement membrane material. Prominent vascular sinusoids are present within the stroma. Intranuclear inclusions and nuclear grooving can be seen. Calcification and the occasional formation of psammoma bodies may be present (Fig. 23.27)[74–76]. The tumour cells stain immunocytochemically for thyroglobulin and are negative for calcitonin. Histologically and cytologically[77–79], these tumours can be mistaken for both papillary carcinoma by virtue of the nuclear characteristics and medullary carcinoma due to the eosinophilic stroma and the paragangliomatous appearance of the islands of cells. Figure 23.28 illustrates such a case[80], which was misdiagnosed as suspicious of papillary carcinoma, on the basis of the nuclear characteristics, but differed from a typical papillary carcinoma aspirate by the poor cellularity, a haemorrhagic aspirate, the lack of clear papillae and viscous colloid, and the spindling of some of the cells. The rarity of this tumour and its misleading cytological features mean that correct diagnosis on fine needle aspiration is unlikely.

Clear cell tumours

Clear cell and signet-ring cell variants of follicular neoplasms may cause diagnostic difficulty. Clear cell change can occur in nodular goitre, follicular neoplasms, papillary carcinoma and medullary carcinoma[81]. Frequently it represents clear cell metaplasia in a Hürthle cell neoplasm (Fig. 23.29). This change may be focal or extensive. Cytologically (Fig. 23.30) there is abundant pale diffusely vacuolated cytoplasm superimposed on the features of the

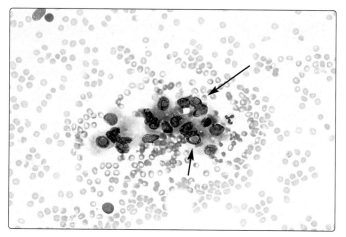

Fig. 23.28 Hyalinizing trabecular adenoma. Cytological appearances with intranuclear inclusions (arrows). (MGG × HP)

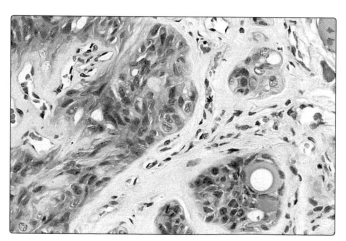

Fig. 23.27 Hyalinizing trabecular adenoma. Histology. (H&E × MP)

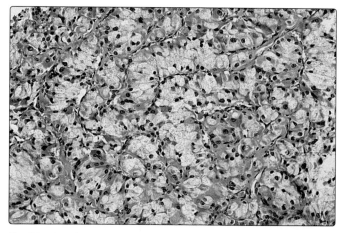

Fig. 23.29 Hürthle cell adenoma with focal clear cell change. (H&E × MP)

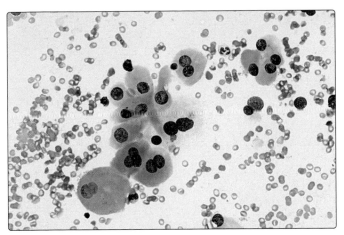

Fig. 23.30 Aspirate from a Hürthle cell tumour showing the characteristic appearances together with the central binucleate cell which shows clear cell change. (MGG × HP)

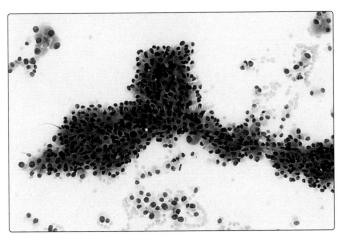

Fig. 23.31 Aspirate from a Hürthle cell tumour illustrating a papillaroid architecture. (MGG × MP)

underlying neoplasm. Where the clear cell change is extensive the possibility of a non-thyroid neoplasm should be considered, in particular a parathyroid tumour or metastatic carcinoma of the kidney[82].

Hürthle cell tumours

Hürthle cell tumours present particular difficulties. The differential diagnoses are with autoimmune thyroiditis and nodular goitre. The neoplasm aspirates are cellular and generally lack an associated chronic inflammatory infiltrate. There is not the polymorphic cell population seen in thyroiditis or in nodular goitre. The tumour cells have the characteristic abundant finely granular blue-grey cytoplasm in large polygonal or oval cells. The cells may be single, in loose groups or a papillaroid/trabecular architecture may be seen. The characteristic nuclear enlargement and pleomorphism of Hürthle cells is seen with prominent nucleoli. Intranuclear inclusions may be present. Binucleation is common (Figs 23.30–23.32)[83–85]. Distinction between adenoma and carcinoma is unreliable and the diagnosis of a Hürthle cell neoplasm requiring surgical excision should be made.

Papillary carcinoma

Papillary carcinoma is the most common malignancy of the thyroid and constitutes 70% of the clinically apparent carcinomas. There is a female sex predominance of approximately 3:1. It can occur at any age but presents most commonly in the 30–50 age range. Cases in young adults and children are not uncommon. Thorough post mortem studies and examination of thyroids removed for functional abnormalities have shown a high incidence, of between 6–35% of the population, of clinically unsuspected, occult, papillary carcinoma. These are small tumours of less than 1 cm diameter. The significance of this finding and the metastatic potential of such cases is as yet unknown. A well-established risk factor for papillary carcinoma is exposure of the thyroid to irradiation during childhood

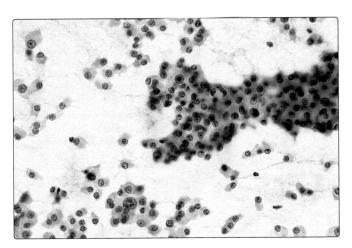

Fig. 23.32 Hürthle cell tumour aspirate showing nuclear enlargement, pleomorphism and prominent nucleoli. (Papanicolaou × HP)

either therapeutically or due to radioactive fall-out. The region surrounding Chernobyl in the Ukraine, which sustained a nuclear accident in 1986, has shown a significant increase in childhood cases[86].

Patients present with a lump in the thyroid or adjacent neck, the latter due to cervical node metastases. This carcinoma generally has a better prognosis than follicular carcinoma, with a 10- year survival of the order of 80%. The majority of cases can be managed by thyroidectomy. Spread of the tumour is by lymphatics and early blood vessel spread is uncommon. So long as involved lymph nodes can be excised, lymphatic spread does not significantly worsen the prognosis.

Histologically, most cases lack a capsule and intraglandular metastases (multicentricity) are seen in one quarter of cases. The presence of true papillae appears to imply a malignant potential and a benign counterpart, papillary adenoma, is not recognized. The tumour consists of papillae with a central fibrovascular core covered by cuboidal or columnar cells. These cells have distinctive

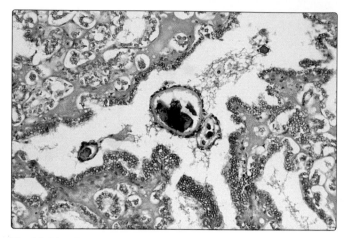

Fig. 23.33 Papillary carcinoma of the thyroid illustrating the characteristic overlapping 'ground-glass' nuclei and psammoma bodies. (H&E × MP)

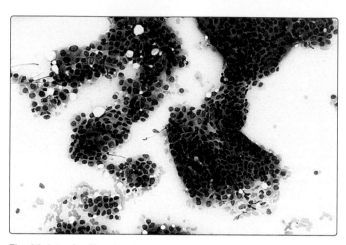

Fig. 23.34 Papillary fronds in papillary carcinoma. (MGG × MP)

nuclear features. The nuclei are large and pale staining with a ground glass appearance due to peripheral displacement of the chromatin. Typically the nuclei overlap. Small nucleoli are seen peripherally. A proportion of nuclei show cytoplasmic inclusions and longitudinal nuclear grooving. Some papillae in approximately 50% of cases contain concentrically laminated calcified concretions or psammoma bodies (Fig. 23.33).

These tumours are not exclusively papillary: trabecular and follicular areas are common. Indeed purely follicular variants of papillary carcinoma are recognized, diagnosis being dependent on the nuclear characteristics. Such tumours have been shown to have the behaviour and prognosis of typical papillary carcinomas[87]. Papillary carcinoma is the most common of several conditions in which focal squamous metaplasia may occur in the thyroid[88]. There are some subtypes of papillary carcinoma, which carry a poorer prognosis. These include the diffuse sclerosing variant, which may present as a diffuse painful enlargement of the gland mimicking thyroiditis, the tall cell and columnar cell variants. Other variants include Hürthle cell forms, clear cell forms, the Warthin like tumour and papillary carcinoma with a nodular fasciitis-like stromal component.

Cytological findings

- ▶ Cellular aspirate
- ▶ Papillary fronds and sheets of cells
- ▶ Dense blue-grey cytoplasm with well-defined cell boundaries
- ▶ Intranuclear inclusions
- ▶ Nuclear grooves
- ▶ Psammoma bodies
- ▶ Multinucleate histiocytes
- ▶ Chewing-gum colloid

Cytologically, papillary carcinoma is the least difficult of the thyroid malignancies to diagnose. Aspirates are cellular and the tumour is characterized by the presence of papillary

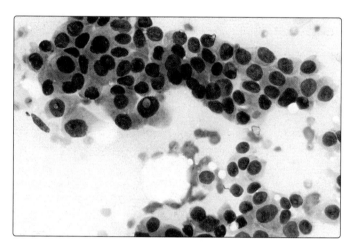

Fig. 23.35 Intranuclear inclusions and well-defined cell boundaries in papillary carcinoma. (MGG × HP)

fronds. These are of varying shapes and sizes but show a smooth surface contour and peripheral palisading of the surface cells (Fig. 23.34). The core, which is less often visualized, is made up of a small amount of fibrous tissue and a small blood vessel. More often the connective tissue core is not aspirated and only papillaroid groups of epithelial cells are seen. Monolayered sheets may be seen. The cells in these sheets are relatively large with a polygonal shape. The cytoplasm appears dense and blue-grey with Giemsa stains. It has characteristically well-defined cell-to-cell boundaries unlike groups of Hürthle cells, with which there may be a superficial resemblance. The nuclei are enlarged and oval with mild to moderate nuclear pleomorphism. The chromatin pattern may or may not be coarsened. Multiple nucleoli are usually evident. Intranuclear cytoplasmic inclusions are found without difficulty in 90% of cases (Fig. 23.35). These are well-defined, faintly pink staining round or oval areas of pallor in the nucleus. They usually occupy at least one third of the nuclear area. Nuclear grooves and clefts are present in a

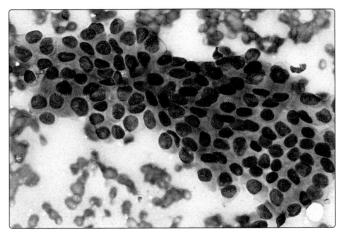

Fig. 23.36 Papillary carcinoma. Nuclear grooving. (MGG × HP)

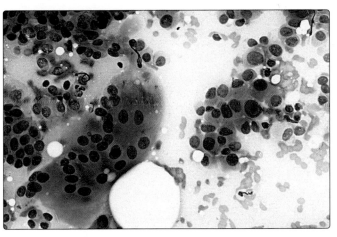

Fig. 23.38 Papillary carcinoma. Multinucleate histiocyte. (MGG × HP)

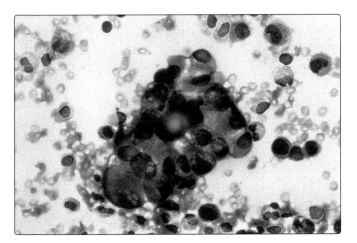

Fig. 23.37 Papillary carcinoma. Psammoma body. (MGG × HP)

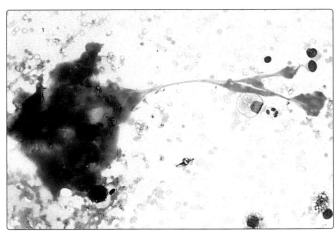

Fig. 23.39 Papillary carcinoma. 'Chewing-gum' colloid. (MGG × HP)

similar proportion but are a little more difficult to visualize on air-dried and MGG stained preparations (Fig. 23.36).

Psammoma bodies are seen in approximately one third of aspirates from papillary carcinomas. They appear as deep blue staining laminated structures in the tips of the papillary fragments (Fig. 23.37). Aspirates from approximately half of the cases of papillary carcinoma also contain large multinucleate histiocytes (Fig. 23.38). They are inapparent on histological examination but originate from the interpapillary space. In some cases dense chewing-gum colloid may be present but this is not a particularly constant or specific feature in the author's experience (Fig. 23.39)[89–94].

An infiltrate of lymphocytes may be seen due to non-specific focal thyroiditis in association with a papillary carcinoma but lymphoid cells may be prominent in the diffuse sclerosing and Warthin-like variants of papillary carcinoma[95,96]. Cytological findings have been described for the columnar cell variant which shows hyperchromatic and elongated nuclei in the absence of intranuclear inclusions[97], the tall cell variant[98], the diffuse sclerosing variant which as well as the inflammatory element is characterized by

abundant psammoma bodies and squamous metaplasia[99] and for the variant with a nodular fasciitis-like stroma[100]. Aspirates from the follicular and macrofollicular variants tend to show more colloid and a follicular architectural pattern which may lead to a false negative diagnosis if the nuclear features are not appreciated[101–103].

Diagnostic pitfalls

In practice, the nuclear inclusions, abundant nuclear grooves, the quality of the cytoplasm and the presence of papillae are found to be of most use in diagnosis. These are all strong indicators of papillary carcinoma but it should be remembered that rarely intranuclear inclusions can be seen in other lesions including multinodular goitre, hyalinizing trabecular adenoma, Hürthle cell tumours, follicular tumours, including insular carcinoma, and medullary carcinoma[34,70–72,77–79,85,89,94,104–106]. Occasional nuclear grooves are seen in nodular goitres, Hashimoto's thyroiditis, follicular adenomas, hyalinizing trabecular adenoma, insular carcinoma and in medullary carcinoma[34,70–72,77,92,93,105,107].

Psammoma bodies are a very valuable finding but are seen in only one third of cases. Their presence in any thyroid aspirate is always suspicious of papillary carcinoma and an indication for surgery. They can nonetheless very rarely be seen in thyroid hyperplasia, multinodular goitres, Hashimoto's thyroiditis and in hyalinizing trabecular adenomas[33,74,75,77,108] and can also be confused with inspissated balls of colloid. Papillae are valuable but may be absent if a predominantly follicular area of the tumour is sampled[101,102] and can also occur in hyperplasia and in a nodular goitre. Accurate diagnosis of papillary carcinoma therefore depends upon recognition of the combination of the most common features.

Cystic degeneration in a papillary carcinoma alters cytological appearance. These cases are generally less cellular and show degenerative features with a background of debris and macrophages. The tumour cells may show cytoplasmic foamy vacuolation. Such cases may require centrifugation of the fluid aspirate in order to distinguish the findings from cystic degeneration in a colloid nodule.

Medullary carcinoma

Medullary carcinoma of the thyroid is a malignant epithelial tumour showing parafollicular cell differentiation. It constitutes 5–10% of thyroid carcinomas. 75% of the cases are sporadic, the peak of the age distribution being in the fifth decade. The remaining 25% occur in a younger population, particularly in the third and fourth decades, in the context of the multiple endocrine neoplasia syndromes (Table 23.6). There is a slight female preponderance. The tumour invades locally and tends to metastasize early to local lymph nodes. Bloodstream spread is common. Treatment is primarily surgical and prognosis is dependent upon the stage and completeness of excision. There is an overall 5-year survival of approximately 70%.

The tumour usually lacks a capsule and is clearly infiltrative histologically with frequent blood vessel and lymphatic invasion. The tumour occurs in the central and upper parts of the thyroid lobes. It is characterized by amyloid deposition (Fig. 23.40) but this is not invariable, occurring in 80% of cases. The amyloid shows some positivity with antibodies to calcitonin and is believed to be derived from this secretory product. The amyloid may calcify and metaplastic bone formation can occur. The carcinoma cells are tremendously variable. They are usually polyhedral in shape but may show spindling, be small ovoid carcinoid-like cells or may mimic oat cell carcinoma cells. Giant cell, clear cell, melanotic, mucinous and oncocytic forms are also recognized. Architecturally common patterns are trabecular and an alveolar paragangliomatous arrangement. Rarer patterns include the angiomatous, tubular and papillary forms. The cells contain neurosecretory granules, are argyrophilic and immunocytochemically 80% of cases stain positively for calcitonin. There is a rare group of tumours, which show

Table 23.6   Multiple endocrine neoplasia (MEN) syndromes

MEN type I (Werner's syndrome)
Pituitary adenoma
Parathyroid hyperplasia
Pancreatic islet cell tumours

MEN type IIa (Sipple's syndrome)
Phaeochromocytoma – often bilateral
Medullary carcinoma of the thyroid – usually bilateral in association with parafollicular cell hyperplasia
Parathyroid hyperplasia or adenoma

MEN type IIb
Phaeochromocytoma – often bilateral
Medullary carcinoma of the thyroid – usually bilateral in association with parafollicular cell hyperplasia
Multiple mucosal neuromas
Skeletal abnormalities

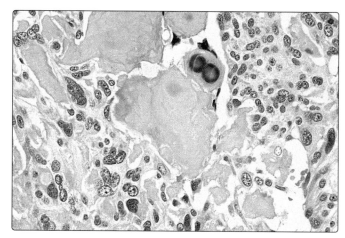

Fig. 23.40   Medullary carcinoma. Amyloid showing calcification. (H&E × MP)

features of both medullary and follicular differentiation with immunocytochemical positivity for both calcitonin and thyroglobulin.

Cytological findings

▶ Dispersed cellular aspirate
▶ Variable cell size and shape
▶ Cytoplasmic granularity
▶ Amyloid
▶ Calcitonin positivity

Cytologically, the aspirates are moderately to highly cellular depending on the degree of stromal fibrosis and amyloid deposition. The cells are poorly cohesive often with a dispersed pattern and vary from case to case in size and shape as would be expected from the histological description given. Most commonly the cells are polygonal, ovoid or spindled in shape (Fig. 23.41). There may be pleomorphism of cell size and shape within a single aspirate and the presence of a mixed cell population is a diagnostic

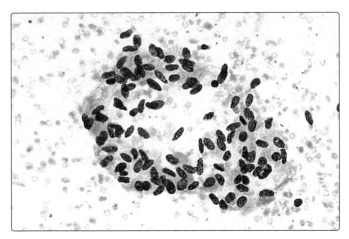

Fig. 23.41 Medullary carcinoma. Spindled cells with pink granules in the cytoplasm. (MGG × HP)

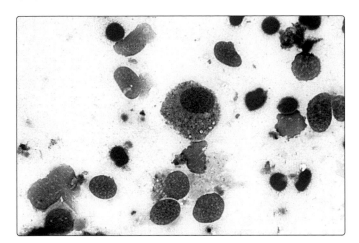

Fig. 23.42 Medullary carcinoma. Ovoid cells with pink granules in the cytoplasm. (MGG × HP)

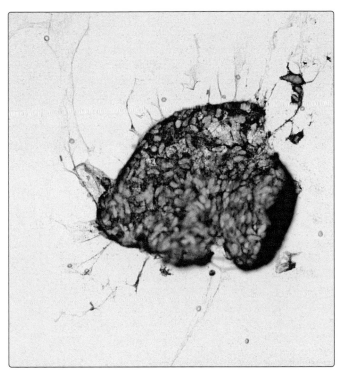

Fig. 23.43 Immunoalkaline phosphatase staining for calcitonin. Medullary carcinoma aspirate. (× MP)

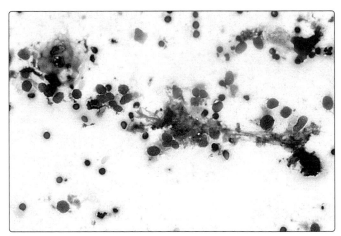

Fig. 23.44 Amyloid in a medullary carcinoma. (MGG × MP)

pointer to medullary carcinoma. The nuclei in the polygonal or ovoid cell types are often eccentrically placed within the cytoplasm, giving a plasmacytoid appearance. Multinucleate cells and nuclear pleomorphism may be present with occasional bizarre giant cells. Nucleoli are small and inconspicuous. Occasional nuclear grooves and intranuclear cytoplasmic inclusions may be present. The chromatin pattern is typically speckled. Mitoses are rare. MGG staining shows a proportion of the cells to have a fine, typically pink, cytoplasmic granularity (Fig. 23.42). This granularity may also be recognized in Papanicolaou stained smears but with less ease. Immunocytochemical staining, which can be carried out on spare or destained preparations, substantiates the diagnosis and confirms that the granules contain calcitonin (Fig. 23.43).

Other special techniques which may be helpful, particularly for the minority of cases which are calcitonin negative, are immunocytochemical positivity for chromogranin A, the histochemical demonstration of argyrophilia and electron microscopy for the detection of neurosecretory granules. These techniques avoid confusion

of the cytoplasmic granularity with that seen in Hürthle cell neoplasms. Other points of distinction are the denser cytoplasm and presence of prominent nucleoli in Hürthle cell tumours. Amyloid appears as amorphous or fibrillar blue-magenta material (Fig. 23.44). With Papanicolaou staining it is pink/orange. It can be confused with small fragments of loose connective tissue or colloid, is often present in small amounts and may be absent in up to 50% of cases. Occasionally it may appear in discrete blobs surrounded by tumour cells giving a follicular pattern. Congo red staining, which can be carried out on spare or destained material, helps confirm its nature. Rarely, fragments of calcification and even psammoma bodies may be seen[109–112]. It should also be noted that amyloid can also be seen in thyroid aspirates from the rare amyloid goitre[113]. Mixed follicular and medullary carcinomas are defined by the presence of calcitonin positivity. Their cytological appearances may be very misleading and the diagnosis of a follicular neoplasm may be made. The author has experience of one case[80] misdiagnosed as a papillary carcinoma due to the presence of abundant intranuclear inclusions and the confusion of amyloid with chewing-gum colloid. The cytological appearances of mucinous[114] and melanotic[115] variants of medullary carcinoma have been described.

Anaplastic carcinoma

Anaplastic carcinomas are a group of tumours that include at least a component of undifferentiated carcinoma. They constitute approximately 10% of thyroid carcinomas and occur in the elderly with a female predominance. They are highly aggressive tumours presenting with a rapidly advancing hard mass in the thyroid. At presentation there is often hoarseness, stridor and dysphagia. Death is usually as a result of local invasion although nodal and haematogenous spread also occurs. Most cases are inoperable at presentation; radiotherapy and chemotherapy are generally ineffective. Survival in most cases is limited to a few months.

Histologically, the appearances are variable with principally giant cell, spindle cell and squamoid forms. A small cell subtype has been recognized but immunocytochemical studies have revealed that the majority of these tumours are lymphomas. Anaplastic carcinomas are highly pleomorphic with a high mitotic index. Foci of necrosis may be present. About 10% of cases contain admixed osteoclast-like giant cells. The spindle cell form may be associated with a prominent stromal response and can mimic a variety of sarcomas. With the exception of angiosarcoma in endemic goitre regions, true sarcomas of the thyroid are extremely rare. Occasionally foci of well-differentiated thyroid carcinomas may be observed amongst the anaplastic carcinoma suggesting that these tumours arise by dedifferentiation of all the major subtypes of carcinoma. Immunocytochemically there is usually low molecular weight cytokeratin expression although this may be lost during the course of dedifferentiation. Thyroglobulin expression is frequently lost. Vimentin expression and coexpression with cytokeratins is common, particularly in spindle cell areas[116,117].

Fine needle aspiration has a particularly valuable role enabling the confirmation of what is usually clinically obvious malignancy without recourse to traumatic large bore needle biopsy or surgery. This enables the immediate adoption of appropriate palliative care. Most importantly, however, FNA allows the identification of treatable thyroid lymphomas, which may present in an identical fashion to anaplastic carcinoma.

Cytological findings

- ► Elderly patients with a rapidly advancing hard mass in the neck
- ► Bizarre giant, squamoid or spindle cells
- ► Necrosis may be present

Aspirates show bizarre giant or spindle cells (Figs 23.45, 23.46) which may be isolated or in small clusters. The cellularity of the specimen is variable: the spindle cell variant may be paucicellular due to the fibrosis associated with this subtype. The cells have pleomorphic nuclei and may be multinucleate. Multiple nucleoli are usually present. The chromatin pattern is coarse and clumped. Necrosis may be observed and there may be an inflammatory component. Osteoclast-like giant cells may be seen. Occasionally elements of better-differentiated areas are present and if sampling is poor only these areas might be aspirated, giving a tumour diagnosis which may be at odds with the aggressive clinical behaviour. In the differential diagnosis pleomorphic and spindle cells may

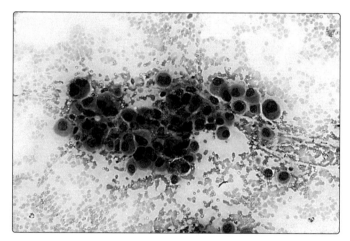

Fig. 23.45　Anaplastic carcinoma. Giant cell form. (MGG × HP)

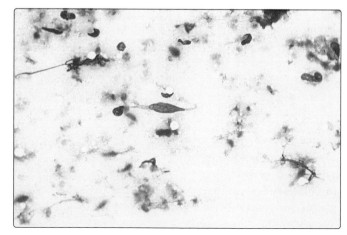

Fig. 23.46　Anaplastic carcinoma. Spindle cell form with necrosis. (MGG × HP)

also be seen in medullary carcinoma. Occasional bizarre cells may be seen as a degenerative change in multinodular goitre, in follicular adenomas and following irradiation or chemotherapy but in the appropriate clinical and cytological setting there should be no difficulty with diagnosis. The possibility of a metastatic carcinoma should also be considered[118–121].

Lymphoma

Lymphomas of the thyroid may either originate in that site or affect the thyroid secondarily as a manifestation of systemic disease. Primary lymphoma constitutes approximately 5% of thyroid malignancies. This tumour occurs predominantly in middle-aged and elderly women presenting with a rapidly enlarging firm mass. Local compression effects with dysphagia, stridor and voice change are not uncommon and hence the mode of presentation is very similar to that of anaplastic carcinoma. There is a strong association between primary thyroid lymphoma and preceding Hashimoto's thyroiditis.

The lymphomas are predominant of B cell non-Hodgkin's type. The morphology and behaviour of these neoplasms suggests that they arise as tumours of the mucosa associated lymphoid tissues (MALT lymphomas). Hodgkin's disease presenting in the thyroid is rare and always associated with cervical or mediastinal lymphadenopathy[122].

Lymphoma cells diffusely infiltrate the thyroid parenchyma and, after involving the entire gland, then affect the surrounding soft tissues. The lymphoid cells characteristically invade the lumina of thyroid follicles giving rise to lymphoepithelial lesions. Blood vessel wall invasion may also be seen. The lymphomas can be divided broadly into low-grade and high-grade types. At presentation most cases are diffuse large B-cell high-grade lesions. Low-grade lymphomas are small cell in type classified as marginal zone B-cell lymphomas (MALT type) using the REAL classification. In 80% of cases a background of autoimmune thyroiditis can be seen. Treatment is usually by radiotherapy and surgical decompression if necessary. If there is evidence of dissemination, chemotherapy is appropriate. The prognosis for localized disease is good with approximately 75% 10-year survival. If recurrence occurs it tends to be local. Where dissemination occurs it tends to be to other sites where mucosa associated lymphoid tissue occurs, such as the gastrointestinal tract.

Cytological findings

Cytologically, the large cell lymphomas consist of a population of dissociated large blastic lymphoid cells usually with the typical background of pale blue fragments of cytoplasm (lymphoglandular bodies) (Fig. 23.47). These appearances usually present no difficulty in distinguishing anaplastic carcinoma and lymphoma but if necessary

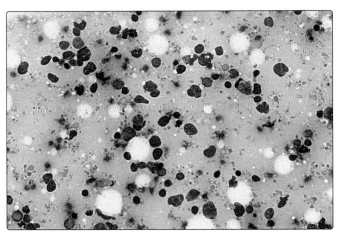

Fig. 23.47 High-grade non-Hodgkin's lymphoma aspirate from the thyroid. Note the 'lymphoglandular bodies'. (MGG × HP)

immunostaining for leucocyte common antigen and the absence of cytokeratin staining can be demonstrated.

The low-grade lymphomas are more difficult to diagnose, particularly if the aspirates also harvest cells from the surrounding autoimmune thyroiditis. There may therefore be a rather mixed cell population of reactive and neoplastic lymphoid cells together with Hürthle cells. Multiple aspirates may be necessary to clarify the situation. Low-grade lymphomas can be recognized by the more monotonous lymphoid population with a predominance of small centrocyte-like cells. Plasmacytic differentiation may be seen. If a mixture of reactive and neoplastic elements is obtained the cytological appearances may only be suspicious. Immunocytochemistry for light chain restriction may be difficult to interpret, flow cytometry may be helpful but diagnosis may require biopsy. The small malignant cells are usually readily recognizable as lymphoid in type. The differential diagnostic possibilities of a small cell medullary carcinoma and the poorly differentiated insular carcinoma should be considered. The author's own practice is to recommend core-biopsy confirmation of the diagnosis of low-grade NHL in the thyroid in view of the diagnostic difficulties prior to radiotherapy whereas this is generally not necessary for high-grade lymphomas[123–126].

Metastatic malignancies

Careful post-mortem examination reveals metastatic carcinoma in the thyroid in approximately 10% of cases of malignancy. The most common sites of origin are breast, kidney, lung, the gastrointestinal tract and squamous carcinomas of the head and neck region. Metastatic melanoma also occurs. Clinical presentation with a secondary malignancy in the thyroid is, however, rare. One series of nearly 25 000 fine needle aspirates of the thyroid revealed only 25 cases of metastases. Eleven of these cases had a known history of previous malignancy and in the absence of such a history only five cases were identified as metastatic[127]. Secondary malignancies cause difficulty in diagnosis, as they may be confused with primary thyroid neoplasms.

Clear cell carcinoma of the kidney mimics clear cell tumours of the thyroid. PAS and oil red-O positivity are features in favour of a renal origin. Thyroglobulin immunostaining is generally unreliable, as a renal secondary aspirate may be contaminated by thyroglobulin from the surrounding thyroid and some clear cell tumours of the thyroid are thyroglobulin negative[128–130]. It should be remembered that statistically, a clear cell tumour of the thyroid is more likely to be a secondary than a primary thyroid neoplasm, particularly if there is a past history or current radiological evidence of a renal tumour. Carcinomas from the breast or lung may mimic anaplastic or papillary carcinoma of the thyroid. Pure squamous carcinomas of the thyroid are rare and are more likely to represent local spread from an oesophageal, pharyngeal, laryngeal or tracheal primary or metastasis from the bronchus. Cases of carcinoid and amelanotic melanoma metastatic to the thyroid simulating medullary carcinoma have been recorded. In general, when a neoplasm is recognized in an aspirate from the thyroid of a patient with a history of a cancer elsewhere in the body, it should be considered a metastasis rather than a second primary neoplasm. Biopsy confirmation should be considered where there is any cytological or clinical doubt to avoid unnecessarily poor prognostication in those with previous malignancy and to ensure appropriate treatment of a primary thyroid neoplasm[131–133].

The diagnostic accuracy of thyroid cytology

Before discussion of the diagnostic accuracy of fine needle aspiration of the thyroid some consideration must be given to what constitutes an adequate aspirate. The need for multiple aspirates has been discussed. It has been proposed, on the basis of reviewing large numbers of known false negative cases, that the minimum criteria for adequacy in the examination of thyroid nodules and exclusion of neoplasia should be the presence of at least six clusters of cells on each of at least two slides taken from separate aspirates. Even with these criteria, false negatives will still occur and a further reduction in that rate will result from further aspirations[134]. The unsatisfactory and false negative rate is, of course, dependent on the underlying pathology and upon the skills of the aspirator and interpreter. Inadequate samples in most studies account for about 15% of the total. Aspiration by the pathologist with access to all of the clinical information together with immediate staining and interpretation reduces false negative rates and allows the best judgement as to whether an aspirate is adequate or not and whether further aspirates are advisable.

The most important role of thyroid aspiration is in the diagnosis of solitary or dominant nodules. Fewer than 5% of palpable nodules are malignant. The use of needle aspiration reduces the use of surgery by approximately one third, doubles the proportion of malignancies amongst surgical resections and increases cost effectiveness[135]. FNA is substantially more accurate in the preoperative evaluation of a thyroid mass than clinical, biochemical or radiological assessment. Serious diagnostic delay due to false negative needle aspiration is uncommon where there is an appreciation of the false negative rate for a single aspirate. In some studies up to 10% of carcinomas, particularly cystic carcinomas, of the thyroid are missed as a result of false negative needle aspiration. Other studies show a false negative rate of only 1–3%. The false negative rate is minimized by the policy of clinical follow-up and repeat aspiration of apparently benign lesions before patients are discharged from a clinic[136]. False positive diagnoses are rare, less than 1% of cases, where the convention of diagnosing follicular neoplasia rather than always attempting to specify adenoma or carcinoma is used. The use of clear and consistent reporting categories with defined follow-up or therapeutic actions ensures appropriate interpretation of needle aspiration results by surgical colleagues[36,63,69,137–145].

References

1 Martin H E, Ellis E B. Aspiration biopsy. *Surg Gynaecol Obstet* 1934; **59**: 578–589

2 Grunze H, Spriggs A I. *History of Clinical Cytology: A Selection of Documents*, 2nd edn. Darmstadt: G-I-T Verlag Ernst Giebeler, 1983; 132

3 Söderström N. Puncture of goiters for aspiration biopsy. A preliminary report. *Acta Med Scand* 1952; **144**: 237–244

4 Einhorn J, Franzén S. Thin-needle biopsy in the diagnosis of thyroid disease. *Acta Radiol* 1962; **58**: 321–336

5 Santos J E C, Leiman G. Nonaspiration fine needle cytology: application of a new technique to nodular thyroid disease. *Acta Cytol* 1988; **32**: 353–356

6 Ciatto S, Iossa A, Cicchi P *et al.* Nonaspiration fine needle cytology of thyroid tumours (letter). *Acta Cytol* 1989; **33**: 939

7 Rajasekhar A, Sundaram C, Chowdhary T *et al.* Diagnostic utility of fine-needle sampling without aspiration: a prospective study. *Diagn Cytopathol* 1991; **7**: 473–476

8 Mair S, Dunbar F, Becker P J, Du Plessis W. Fine needle cytology – is aspiration suction necessary? A study of 100 masses in various sites. *Acta Cytol* 1989; **33**: 809–813

9 Abele J S, Miller T R, King E B, Lowhagen T. Smearing techniques for the concentration of particles from fine needle aspiration biopsy. *Diagn Cytopathol* 1985; **1**: 59–65

10 Silverman J F, Frable W J. The use of the Diff-Quik stain in the immediate interpretation of fine-needle aspiration biopsies. *Diagn Cytopathol* 1990; **6**: 366–369

11 Scurry J P, Duggan M A. Thin layer compared to direct smear in thyroid fine needle aspiration. *Cytopathol* 2000; **11**: 104–115

12 Gordon D L, Gattuso P, Castelli M *et al.* Effect of fine needle aspiration biopsy on the histology of thyroid neoplasms. *Acta Cytol* 1993; **37**: 651–654

13 Keyhani-Rofagha S, Kooner D S, Keyhani M, O'Toole R V. Necrosis of a Hürthle cell tumour of the thyroid following fine needle aspiration: case report and literature review. *Acta Cytol* 1990; **34**: 805–808

14 Layfield L J, Lones M A. Necrosis in thyroid nodules after fine needle aspiration biopsy: report of two cases. *Acta Cytol* 1991; **35**: 427–430

15 Alejo M, Matias-Guiu X, de las Heras Duran P. Infarction of papillary thyroid carcinoma after fine needle aspiration (letter). *Acta Cytol* 1991; **35**: 478–479

16 Us Krasovec M, Golouh R, Auesperg M, Pogacnik A. Tissue damage after fine needle aspiration biopsy (letter). *Acta Cytol* 1992; **36**: 456–457

17 Jones J D, Pittman D L, Sanders L R. Necrosis of thyroid nodules after fine needle aspiration. *Acta Cytol* 1985; **29**: 29–32

18 Hales M S, Hsu F S F. Needle tract implantation of papillary carcinoma of the thyroid following aspiration biopsy. *Acta Cytol* 1990; **34**: 801–804

19 Panunzi C, Palliotta D S, Papini E *et al*. Cutaneous seeding of a follicular thyroid cancer after fine-needle aspiration biopsy? *Diagn Cytopathol* 1994; **10**: 156–158

20 Isenberg S F. Thyroid abscess resulting from fine-needle aspiration. *Otolaryng Head Neck Surg* 1994; **111**: 832–833

21 Pandit A A, Phulpager M D. Worrisome histologic alterations following fine needle aspiration of the thyroid. *Acta Cytol* 2001; **45**: 173–179

22 Guarda L A. Simultaneous fine-needle aspiration of thyroid lesions and regional cervical lymph nodes: clinicopathologic implications. *Diagn Cytopathol* 1992; **8**: 377–379

23 Sidawy M K, Costa M. The significance of paravacuolar granules of the thyroid: a histologic, cytologic and ultrastructural study. *Acta Cytol* 1989; **33**: 929–933

24 Keyhani-Rofagha S, Kooner D S, Landas S K, Keyhani M. Black thyroid: a pitfall for aspiration cytology. *Diagn Cytopathol* 1991; **7**: 640–643

25 Butler S L, Oertel Y C. Lipomas of anterior neck simulating thyroid nodules: diagnosis by fine-needle aspiration. *Diagn Cytopathol* 1992; **8**: 528–531

26 Rollins S D, Flinner R L. Thyrolipoma: diagnostic pitfalls in the cytologic diagnosis and review of the literature. *Diagn Cytopathol* 1991; **7**: 150–154

27 Pitts W C, Tani E M, Skoog L. Papillary carcinoma in fine needle aspiration smears of a thyroglossal duct lesion. *Acta Cytol* 1988; **32**: 599–601 (letter)

28 Kashkari S. Identification of papillary carcinoma in a thyroglossal cyst by fine-needle aspiration biopsy. *Diagn Cytopathol* 1990; **6**: 267–270

29 Vengrove M A, Schimmel M, Atkinson B F *et al*. Invasive cervical thymoma masquerading as a solitary thyroid nodule: report of a case studied by fine needle aspiration. *Acta Cytol* 1991; **35**: 431–433

30 Oertel Y C. Thymoma mimicking papillary carcinoma: another pitfall in fine needle aspiration. *Diagn Cytopathol* 1997; **17**(1): 61–63

31 Pitts W C, Berry G J. Marginal vacuoles in metastatic thyroid carcinoma: a case report. *Diagn Cytopathol* 1989; **5**: 200–202

32 Kaur A, Jayaram G. Thyroid tumours: cytomorphology of follicular neoplasms. *Diagn Cytopathol* 1991; **7**: 469–472

33 Riazmontazer N, Bedayat G. Psammoma bodies in fine needle aspirates from thyroids containing nontoxic hyperplastic nodular goiters. *Acta Cytol* 1991; **35**: 563–566

34 Harach H R, Zusman S B, Day E S. Nodular goiter: a histocytological study with some emphasis on pitfalls of fine-needle aspiration cytology. *Diagn Cytopathol* 1992; **8**: 409–419

35 Jayaram G, Kaur A. Cystic thyroid nodules harboring malignancy: a problem in fine needle aspiration cytodiagnosis (letter). *Acta Cytol* 1989; **33**: 941–942

36 Sarda A K, Bal S, Gupta S D, Kapur M M. Diagnosis and treatment of cystic disease of the thyroid by aspiration. *Surgery* 1988; **103**: 593–596

37 Jayaram G, Singh B, Marwaha R K. Graves disease: appearance in cytologic smears from fine needle aspirates of the thyroid gland. *Acta Cytol* 1989; **33**: 36–40

38 Oz F, Urgancioglu I, Uslu I *et al*. Cytologic changes induced by ^{131}I in the thyroid glands of patients with hyperthyroidism: results of fine needle aspiration cytology. *Cytopathol* 1994; **5**: 154–163

39 Centeno B A, Szyfelbein W M, Daniels G H, Vickery A L. Fine needle aspiration biopsy of the thyroid gland in patients with prior Graves disease treated with radioactive iodine. *Acta Cytol* 1996; **40**: 1189–1197

40 Poropatich C, Marcus D, Oertel Y C. Hashimoto's thyroiditis: fine needle aspiration cytology of 50 asymptomatic cases. *Diagn Cytopathol* 1994; **11**: 141–145

41 Carson H J, Castelli M J, Gattuso P. Incidence of neoplasia in Hashimoto's thyroiditis: A fine needle aspiration study. *Diagn Cytopathol* 1996; **14**: 38–42

42 Tani E, Skoog L. Fine needle aspiration cytology and immunocytochemistry in the diagnosis of lymphoid lesions of the thyroid gland. *Acta Cytol* 1989; **33**: 48–52

43 Offner C, Hittmair A, Kroll I *et al*. Fine needle aspiration cytodiagnosis of subacute (de Quervain's) thyroiditis in an endemic goitre area. *Cytopathol* 1994; **5**: 33–40

44 Das D K, Pant C S, Chachra K L, Gupta A K. Fine needle aspiration cytology diagnosis of tuberculous thyroiditis: a report of eight cases. *Acta Cytol* 1992; **36**: 517–522

45 Wilson R A, Gartner W S Jr. Teflon granuloma mimicking a thyroid tumor. *Diagn Cytopathol* 1987; **3**: 156–158

46 Berry B, MacFarlane J, Chan N. Osteoclastoma-like anaplastic carcinoma of the thyroid: diagnosis by fine needle aspiration cytology. *Acta Cytol* 1990; **34**: 248–250

47 Walts A E, Pitchon H E. Pneumocystis carinii in FNA of the thyroid. *Diagn Cytopathol* 1991; **7**: 615–617

48 Das D K, Khanna C M, Tripathi R P *et al*. Microfilaria of Wuchereria bancrofti in fine needle aspirate from a colloid goitre (letter). *Diagn Cytopathol* 1989; **5**: 114–115

49 Sodhani P, Nayar M. Microfilariae in a thyroid aspirate smear: an incidental finding (letter). *Acta Cytol* 1989; **33**: 942–943

50 Lang W, Georgii A, Stauch G, Kienzle E. The differentiation of atypical adenomas and encapsulated follicular carcinomas in the thyroid gland. *Virchows Arch A Path Anat Histol* 1980; **385**: 125–141

51 Yamashina M. Follicular neoplasms of the thyroid: total circumferential evaluation of the fibrous capsule. *Am J Surg Pathol* 1992; **16**: 392–400

52 Sprenger E, Löwhagen T, Vogt-Schaden M. Differential diagnosis between follicular adenoma and follicular carcinoma of the thyroid by nuclear DNA determination. *Acta Cytol* 1977; **21**: 528–530

53 Backdahl M, Auer G, Forsslund G *et al*. Prognostic value of nuclear DNA content in follicular thyroid tumours. *Acta Chir Scand* 1986; **152**: 1–7

54 Greenbaum E, Koss L G, Elequin F, Silver C E. The diagnostic value of flow cytometric DNA measurements in follicular tumours of the thyroid gland. *Cancer* 1985; **56**: 2011–2018

55 Joensuu H, Klemi P, Eerola E. DNA aneuploidy in follicular adenomas of the thyroid gland. *Am J Pathol* 1986; **124**: 373–376

56 Boon M E, Löwhagen T, Willems J-S. Planimetric studies on fine needle aspirates from follicular adenoma and follicular carcinoma of the thyroid. *Acta Cytol* 1980; **24**: 145–148

57 Luck J B, Mumaw V R, Frable W J. Fine needle aspiration biopsy of the thyroid: differential diagnosis by Videoplan image analysis. *Acta Cytol* 1982; **26**: 793–796

58 Bondeson L, Bondeson A-G, Lindholm K *et al*. Morphometric studies on nuclei in smears of fine needle aspirates from oxyphilic tumours of the thyroid. *Acta Cytol* 1983; **27**: 437–440

59 Wright R G, Castles H, Mortimer R H. Morphometric analysis of thyroid cell aspirates. *J Clin Pathol* 1987; **40**: 443–445

60 Fadda G, Rabitti C, Minimo C *et al*. Morphologic and planimetric diagnosis of follicular thyroid lesions on fine needle aspiration cytology. *Anal Quant Cytol Histol* 1995; **17**: 247–256

61 Boon M E, Kok L P. An explanation for the reported variability of nuclear areas in air-dried Romanowsky-Giemsa-stained smears of follicular tumours of the thyroid. *Acta Cytol* 1987; **31**: 527–530 (letter)

62 Montironi R, Braccischi A, Scarpelli M *et al*. The number of nucleoli in benign and malignant thyroid lesions: a useful diagnostic sign in cytological preparations. *Cytopathol* 1990; **1**: 153–161

63 Montironi R, Braccischi A, Scarpelli M *et al*. Well-differentiated follicular neoplasms of the thyroid: reproducibility and validity of a decision tree classification based on nucleolar and karyometric features. *Cytopathol* 1992; **3**: 209–222

64 Karmakar T, Dey P. Role of AgNOR in diagnosis of thyroid follicular neoplasms in fine-needle aspiration smears. *Diagn Cytopathol* 1995; **12**: 148–151

65 Solymosi T, Toth V, Sapi Z et al. Diagnostic value of AgNOR method in thyroid cytopathology: Correlation with morphometric measurements. *Diagn Cytopathol* 1996; **14**: 140–144

66 Aogi K, Kitahara K, Buley I et al. Telomerase activity in lesions of the thyroid: Application to diagnosis of clinical samples including fine needle aspirates. *Clin Cancer Res* 1998; **4**: 1965–1970

67 Suen K C. How does one separate cellular follicular lesions of the thyroid by fine-needle aspiration biopsy? *Diagn Cytopathol* 1988; **4**: 78–81

68 Harach H R, Zusman S B. Necrotic debris in thyroid aspirates: a feature of follicular carcinoma of the thyroid. *Cytopathol* 1992; **3**: 359–364

69 Schmid K W, Ladurner D, Zechmann W, Feichtinger H. Clinicopathologic management of tumors of the thyroid gland in an endemic goitre area: combined use of preoperative fine needle aspiration biopsy and intraoperative frozen section. *Acta Cytol* 1989; **33**: 27–30

70 Zakowski M F, Schlesinger K, Mizrachi H H. Cytologic features of poorly differentiated insular carcinoma of the thyroid: a case report. *Acta Cytol* 1992; **36**: 523–526

71 Sironi M, Collini P, Cantaboni A. Fine needle aspiration cytology of insular thyroid carcinoma: a report of four cases. *Acta Cytol* 1992; **36**: 435–439

72 Pietribiasi F, Sapino A, Papotti M, Bussolati G. Cytologic features of poorly differentiated insular carcinoma of the thyroid, as revealed by fine-needle aspiration biopsy. *Am J Clin Pathol* 1990; **94**: 687–692

73 Pereira E M, Maeda S A, Alves F et al. Poorly differentiated carcinoma (insular carcinoma) of the thyroid diagnosed by fine needle aspiration (FNA). *Cytopathol* 1996; **7**: 61–65

74 Carney J A, Ryan J, Goellner J R. Hyalinizing trabecular adenoma of the thyroid gland. *Am J Surg Pathol* 1987; **11**: 583–591

75 Katoh R, Jasani B, Williams E D. Hyalinizing trabecular adenoma of the thyroid. A report of three cases with immunohistochemical and ultrastructural studies. *Histopathol* 1989; **15**: 211–224

76 McCluggage W G, Sloan J M. Hyalinising trabecular carcinoma of thyroid gland. *Histopathol* 1996; **28**: 357–362

77 LiVolsi V A, Gupta P K. Thyroid fine-needle aspiration: intranuclear inclusions, nuclear grooves and psammoma bodies – paraganglioma-like adenoma of the thyroid. *Diagn Cytopathol* 1992; **8**: 82–84

78 Goellner J R, Carney J A. Cytologic features of fine-needle aspirates of hyalinizing trabecular adenoma of the thyroid. *Am J Clin Pathol* 1989; **91**: 115–119

79 Strong C J, Garcia B M. Fine needle aspiration cytologic characteristics of hyalinizing trabecular adenoma of the thyroid. *Acta Cytol* 1990; **34**: 359–362

80 Kulacoglu S, Ashton-Key M, Buley I. Pitfalls in the diagnosis of papillary carcinoma of the thyroid. *Cytopathol* 1998; **9**: 193–200

81 Harach H R, Virgili E, Soler G et al. Cytopathology of follicular tumours of the thyroid with clear cell change. *Cytopathol* 1991; **2**: 125–135

82 Jayaram G. Cytology of clear cell carcinoma of the thyroid (letter). *Acta Cytol* 1989; **33**: 135–136

83 Kini S R, Miller J M, Hamburger J I. Cytopathology of Hürthle cell lesions of the thyroid gland by fine needle aspiration. *Acta Cytol* 1981; **25**: 647–652

84 Kaur A, Jayaram G. Thyroid tumours: Cytomorphology of Hurthle cell tumours including an uncommon papillary variant. *Diagn Cytopathol* 1993; **9**: 135–137

85 Chen K T K. Fine-needle aspiration cytology of papillary Hürthle-cell tumours of thyroid: a report of three cases. *Diagn Cytopathol* 1991; **7**: 53–56

86 Furmanchuk A W, Averkin J I, Egloff B et al. Pathomorphological findings in thyroid cancers of children from the Republic of Belarus: a study of 86 cases occurring between 1986 (post-Chernobyl) and 1991. *Histopathol* 1992; **21**: 401–408

87 Rosai J, Zampi G, Carcangiu M L. Papillary carcinoma of the thyroid: a discussion of its several morphologic expressions, with particular emphasis on the follicular variant. *Am J Surg Pathol* 1983; **7**: 809–817

88 LiVolsi V A, Merino M J. Squamous cells in the human thyroid gland. *Am J Surg Pathol* 1978; **2**: 133–140

89 Kini S R, Miller J M, Hamburger J I, Smith M J. Cytopathology of papillary carcinoma of the thyroid by fine needle aspiration. *Acta Cytol* 1980; **24**: 511–521

90 Akhtar M, Ali M A, Huq M, Bakry M. Fine-needle aspiration biopsy of papillary thyroid carcinoma: cytologic, histologic and ultrastructural correlations. *Diagn Cytopathol* 1991; **7**: 373–379

91 Kaur A, Jayaram G. Thyroid tumours: cytomorphology of papillary carcinoma. *Diagn Cytopathol* 1991; **7**: 462–468

92 Rupp M, Ehya H. Nuclear grooves in the aspiration cytology of papillary carcinoma of the thyroid. *Acta Cytol* 1989; **33**: 21–26

93 Bhambhani S, Kashyap V, Das D K. Nuclear grooves: valuable diagnostic feature in May-Grünwald-Giemsa-stained fine needle aspirates of papillary carcinoma of the thyroid. *Acta Cytol* 1990; **34**: 809–812

94 Miller T R, Bottles K, Holley E A et al. A stepwise logistic regression analysis of papillary carcinoma of the thyroid. *Acta Cytol* 1986; **30**: 285–293

95 Pai R R, Lobo F D, Upadhyay K, Muniappa M. Warthin-like tumour of the thyroid – the fine needle aspiration cytology features. *Cytopathol* 2001; **12**: 127–129

96 Fadda G, Mule A, Zannoni G F et al. Fine needle aspiration of a Warthin-like thyroid tumour. Report of a case with differential diagnostic criteria vs other lymphocyte rich thyroid lesions. *Acta Cytol* 1998; **42**: 998–1002

97 Hui P-K, Chan J K C, Cheung P S Y, Gwi E. Columnar cell carcinoma of the thyroid: fine needle aspiration findings in a case. *Acta Cytol* 1990; **34**: 355–358

98 Harach H R, Zusman S B. Cytomorphology of the tall cell variant of thyroid papillary carcinoma. *Acta Cytol* 1992; **36**: 895–899

99 Caruso G, Tabarri B, Lucchi I, Tison V. Fine needle aspiration cytology in a case of diffuse sclerosing carcinoma of the thyroid. *Acta Cytol* 1990; **34**: 352–354

100 Us-Krasovec M, Golouh R. Papillary carcinoma with exuberant nodular fasciitis-like stroma in a fine needle aspirate. A case report. *Acta Cytol* 1999; **43**: 1101–1104

101 Harach H R, Zusman S B. Cytologic findings in the follicular variant of papillary carcinoma of the thyroid. *Acta Cytol* 1992; **36**: 142–146

102 Hugh J C, Duggan M A, Chang-Poon V. The fine-needle aspiration appearance of the follicular variant of thyroid papillary carcinoma: a report of three cases. *Diagn Cytopathol* 1988; **4**: 196–201

103 Martinez-Parra D, Fernandez J C, Hierro-Guilman C C et al. Follicular variant of papillary carcinoma of the thyroid: To what extent is fine needle aspiration reliable. *Diagn Cytopathol* 1996; **15**: 12–16

104 Glant M D, Berger E K, Davey D D. Intranuclear cytoplasmic inclusions in aspirates of follicular neoplasms of the thyroid: a report of two cases. *Acta Cytol* 1984; **28**: 576–580

105 Gould E, Watzak L, Chamizo W, Albores-Saavedra J. Nuclear grooves in cytologic preparations: a study of the utility of this feature in the diagnosis of papillary carcinoma. *Acta Cytol* 1989; **33**: 16–20

106 Lew W, Orell S, Henderson D W. Intranuclear vacuoles in nonpapillary carcinoma of the thyroid: a report of three cases. *Acta Cytol* 1984; **28**: 581–586

107 Francis I M, Das D K, Sheikh Z A et al. Role of nuclear grooves in the diagnosis of papillary thyroid carcinoma. *Acta Cytol* 1995; **39**: 409–415

108 Dugan J M, Atkinson B F, Avitabile A et al. Psammoma bodies in fine needle aspirate of the thyroid in lymphocytic thyroiditis. *Acta Cytol* 1987; **31**: 330–334

109 Mendonça M E, Ramos S, Soares J. Medullary carcinoma of thyroid: a re-evaluation of the cytological criteria of diagnosis. *Cytopathol* 1991; **2**: 93–102

110 Zeppa P, Vetrani A, Marino M et al. Fine needle aspiration cytology of medullary thyroid carcinoma: a review of 18 cases. *Cytopathol* 1990; **1**: 35–44

111 Bose S, Kapila K, Verma K. Medullary carcinoma of the thyroid: a cytological, immunocytochemical, and ultrastructural study. *Diagn Cytopathol* 1992; **8**: 28–32

112 Das A, Gupta S K, Banerjee A K et al. Atypical cytologic features of medullary carcinoma of the thyroid: a review of 12 cases. *Acta Cytol* 1992; **36**: 137–141

113 Nijhawan U S, Marwaha R K, Sahoo M, Ravishankar L. Fine needle aspiration cytology of amyloid goitre. A report of 4 cases. *Acta Cytol* 1997; **41**: 830–834

114 Haleem Akthar M, Ali M A, Iqbal Z. Fine needle aspiration biopsy of mucus producing medullary carcinoma of the thyroid. Report of a case with cytologic, histologic and ultrastructural correlations. *Diagn Cytopathol* 1990; **6**: 112–117

115 Kimura N, Ishioka K, Miura Y *et al.* Melanin-producing medullary thyroid carcinoma with glandular differentiation. *Acta Cytol* 1988; **33**: 61–66

116 Rosai J, Saxén E A, Woolner L. Session III: undifferentiated and poorly differentiated carcinoma. *Seminars in Diagnostic Pathology* 1985; **2**: 123–136

117 Carcangiu M L, Steeper T, Zampi G, Rosai J. Anaplastic thyroid carcinoma: a study of 70 cases. *Am J Clin Pathol* 1985; **83**: 135–158

118 Guarda L A, Peterson C E, Hall W, Baskin H J. Anaplastic thyroid carcinoma: cytomorphology and clinical implications of fine-needle aspiration. *Diagn Cytopathol* 1991; **7**: 63–67

119 Vinette D S J, MacDonald L L, Yazdi H M. Papillary carcinoma of the thyroid with anaplastic transformation: diagnostic pitfalls in fine-needle aspiration biopsy. *Diagn Cytopathol* 1991; **7**: 75–78

120 Luze T, Tötsch M, Bangerl I *et al.* Fine needle aspiration cytodiagnosis of anaplastic carcinoma and malignant haemangioendothelioma of the thyroid in an endemic goitre area. *Cytopathol* 1990; **1**: 305–310

121 Us-Krasovec M, Golouh R, Auersperg M *et al.* Anaplastic thyroid carcinoma in fine needle aspirates. *Acta Cytol* 1996; **40**: 953–958

122 Granados R, Pinkus G S, West P, Cibas E S. Hodgkin's disease presenting as an enlarged thyroid gland: report of a case diagnosed by fine needle aspiration. *Acta Cytol* 1991; **35**: 439–442

123 Detweiler R E, Katz R L, Alapat C *et al.* Malignant lymphoma of the thyroid: a report of two cases diagnosed by fine-needle aspiration. *Diagn Cytopathol* 1991; **7**: 163–171

124 Matsuda M, Sone H, Koyama H, Ishiguro S. Fine-needle aspiration cytology of malignant lymphoma of the thyroid. *Diagn Cytopathol* 1987; **3**: 244–249

125 Jayaram G, Rani S, Raina V *et al.* B cell lymphoma of the thyroid in Hashimoto's thyroiditis monitored by fine-needle aspiration cytology. *Diagn Cytopathol* 1990; **6**: 130–133

126 Sangalli G, Serio G, Zampatti C *et al.* Fine needle aspiration cytology of primary lymphoma of the thyroid. A report of 17 cases. *Cytopathol* 2001; **12**: 257–263

127 Schmid K W, Hittmair A, Öfner C *et al.* Metastatic tumours in fine needle aspiration biopsy of the thyroid. *Acta Cytol* 1991; **35**: 722–724

128 Gritsman A Y, Popok S M, Ro J Y *et al.* Renal-cell carcinoma with intranuclear inclusions metastatic to thyroid: a diagnostic problem in aspiration cytology. *Diagn Cytopathol* 1988; **4**: 125–129

129 Rikabi A C A, Young A E, Wilson C. Metastatic renal clear cell carcinoma in the thyroid gland diagnosed by fine needle aspiration cytology. *Cytopathol* 1991; **2**: 47–49

130 Halbauer M, Kardum-Skelin I, Vranesic D, Crepinko I. Aspiration cytology of renal-cell carcinoma metastatic to the thyroid. *Acta Cytol* 1991; **35**: 443–446

131 Chacho M S, Greenebaum E, Moussouris H F *et al.* Value of aspiration cytology of the thyroid in metastatic disease. *Acta Cytol* 1987; **31**: 705–712

132 Cristallini E G, Bolis G B, Francucci M. Diagnosis of thyroid metastasis of colonic adenocarcinoma by fine needle aspiration biopsy. *Acta Cytol* 1990; **34**: 363–365

133 Michelow P M, Leiman G. Metastases to the thyroid gland. Diagnosis by aspiration cytology. *Diagn Cytopathol* 1995; **13**: 209–213

134 Hamburger J I, Husain M, Nishiyama R *et al.* Increasing the accuracy of fine-needle biopsy for thyroid nodules. *Arch Pathol Lab Med* 1989; **113**: 1035–1041

135 Hamberger B, Gharib H, Melton L J *et al.* Fine-needle aspiration biopsy of thyroid nodules: impact on thyroid practice and cost of care. *Am J Med* 1982; **73**: 831–384

136 Dwarakanathon A A, Staren E D, D'Amore M J *et al.* Importance of repeat fine-needle biopsy in the management of thyroid nodules. *Am J Surg* 1993; **166**: 350–352

137 Harach H R. Usefulness of fine needle aspiration of the thyroid in an endemic goiter region. *Acta Cytol* 1989; **33**: 31–35

138 Goellner J R, Gharib H, Grant C S, Johnson D A. Fine needle aspiration cytology of the thyroid, 1980 to 1986. *Acta Cytol* 1987; **31**: 587–590

139 Altavilla G, Pascale M, Nenci I. Fine needle aspiration cytology of thyroid gland diseases. *Acta Cytol* 1990; **34**: 251–256

140 Hsu C, Boey J. Diagnostic pitfalls in the fine needle aspiration of thyroid nodules: a study of 555 cases in Chinese patients. *Acta Cytol* 1987; **31**: 699–704

141 Cusick E L, MacIntosh C A, Krukowski Z H *et al.* Management of isolated thyroid swellings: a prospective six year study of fine needle aspiration cytology in diagnosis. *BMJ* 1990; **301**: 318–321

142 Klemi P J, Joensuu H, Nylamo E. Fine needle aspiration biopsy in the diagnosis of thyroid nodules. *Acta Cytol* 1991; **35**: 434–438

143 Friedman M, Shimaoka K, Getaz P. Needle aspiration of 310 thyroid lesions. *Acta Cytol* 1979; **23**: 194–203

144 Willems J-S, Löwhagen T. Fine-needle aspiration cytology in thyroid disease. *Clinics in Endocrinology and Metabolism* 1981; **10**: 247–266

145 Orell S R, Phillips J, eds. The role of fine needle biopsy in the investigation of thyroid disease and its diagnostic accuracy. In: The thyroid, fine needle biopsy and cytological diagnosis of thyroid lesions. *Monographs in Clinical Cytology*, vol 14, chap. 3. Basel: Karger, 1997

24 Other endocrine organs

Ian D. Buley

The parathyroid

Anatomy and physiology

There are usually four parathyroid glands arranged as two pairs. The upper pair, which develop as a dorsal diverticulum of the fourth pharyngeal pouch, are present at the posterolateral border of the thyroid just beneath the upper poles. The lower pair, derived from the third pharyngeal pouch, are located at the lower poles of the thyroid. They are situated within the pretracheal fascia either on the surface or just within the thyroid tissue. Anomalies of position in the neck and anterior mediastinum may occur. A fifth supernumerary gland occurs in approximately 5% of individuals and is usually present in thymic tissues inferior to the thyroid. Rarely, more than five glands may occur. The glands are ovoid in shape. The weights of individual glands are variable but in the adult the total glandular weight averages 120 mg in males and 142 mg in females. Any single gland weighing more than 60 mg is likely to be abnormal. The average maximal dimension is 5 mm although the normal range of size extends up to 1 cm.

Histologically, the parathyroid cells are arranged in cords and sheets set within a richly vascular stroma. Small follicles containing colloid-like material may be seen and the appearances can mimic those of the thyroid gland. During puberty and early adult life the glands accumulate adipose tissue, fat cells insinuating themselves amongst the endocrine cells. The endocrine cells have two main histological subtypes: the chief cell and the oxyphil cell. The former predominate and are rounded cells with pale granular or vacuolated cytoplasm. They are rich in glycogen and lipid. Oxyphil cells increase in number with age and may form discrete nodules. These cells are larger with abundant eosinophilic cytoplasm containing numerous mitochondria. Transitional forms between chief cells and oxyphil cells also occur.

The parathyroid glands produce and secrete parathyroid hormone (PTH). This single chain polypeptide contributes to the maintenance of calcium ion homeostasis together with vitamin D metabolites. A fall in the level of extracellular calcium ion concentration cause the release of PTH which promotes the renal excretion of the phosphate ion, enhances renal tubular reabsorption of calcium, stimulates bone resorption and stimulates the synthesis of the active metabolite of vitamin D, 1,25 dihydroxycholecalciferol. The latter promotes intestinal calcium absorption and increases its release from bone. The resulting increase in extracellular calcium ion has a negative feedback action on the parathyroid, decreasing the release of PTH.

Primary hyperparathyroidism

The most common pathology of the parathyroid is primary hyperparathyroidism. This is a common cause of hypercalcaemia, occurring in approximately 0.25% of the population. It is more common in middle aged and elderly women. It occurs sporadically, can also be familial and may be associated with the multiple endocrine neoplasia syndromes (Table 23.6). The disease may be detected incidentally on routine laboratory tests or may present clinically with painful bones, renal stones, abdominal pain from peptic ulceration or pancreatitis and with fatigue and depression. The underlying pathology is either parathyroid hyperplasia, which affects all of the glands, or an adenoma or carcinoma, which nearly always affects only a single gland. The most common pathology is an adenoma, which gives rise to approximately 80% of cases of primary hyperparathyroidism. Traditional treatment is surgical removal of the affected gland. Hyperplasia requires the removal of three glands and partial removal of the fourth gland. As the histological appearances of a single hyperplastic gland and a gland containing an adenoma may be similar, distinction may require perioperative frozen section examination of two glands. In the case of an adenoma, the second gland will be normal or atrophic whereas in hyperplasia the glands will show similar changes.

Parathyroid adenoma

Parathyroid adenomas usually weigh between 200 mg and 1 g. The weight of the gland correlates with the clinical symptomatology and in patients with severe hyperparathyroid bone disease adenomas frequently weigh 10 g or more. Some 90% of adenomas occur in the upper or lower parathyroids, with the lower glands more frequently involved, and 10% occur in other sites in the neck and mediastinum. They are brown in colour and may show areas of haemorrhage, cystic degeneration, fibrosis or calcification. Microscopically, the adenoma (Fig. 24.1) is a

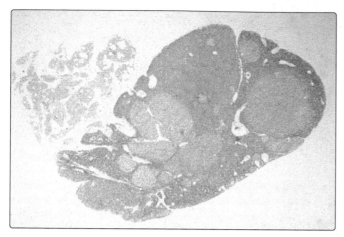

Fig. 24.1 Parathyroid adenoma with adjacent normal parathyroid tissue. (H&E × LP)

well-circumscribed proliferation of cells within a thin fibrous capsule. Usually, residual compressed atrophic parathyroid is seen adjacent to the adenoma. This is most commonly seen at the vascular hilum of the gland. The cell population of the adenoma may consist of dark granular or pale vacuolated chief cells, oxyphil cells or transitional-type cells. Some chief cells show extreme vacuolation and form 'water-clear' cells. Frequently, the cell population is mixed. Adenomatous chief cells contain less cytoplasmic lipid than normal or atrophic chief cells. Architecturally, the cells may be arranged in sheets, nodules, nests, cords, in rosettes or follicles and may even form a papillary pattern. Adenomas contain few stromal fat cells except in the case of the rare lipoadenoma. In common with many other benign endocrine tumours parathyroid adenomas may show marked nuclear pleomorphism. Mitoses are however rare. In the follicular pattern, calcification of the intraluminal secretion gives rise to structures resembling psammoma bodies.

Parathyroid hyperplasia

Parathyroid hyperplasia affects the chief cells of all of the glands giving rise to the common chief cell hyperplasia and the rare water-clear cell hyperplasia. Involvement of the glands is often uneven both between and within glands, giving rise to nodular proliferations, which may be difficult to distinguish from an adenoma if only a single gland is available for examination. Classically, the parenchyma is dense with closely packed cells and a decrease in the number of stromal fat cells. There is no compressed rim of normal parathyroid tissue. Hyperplastic chief cells show a decrease in their content of lipid. The cells in hyperplasia also show variable architecture, being arranged in sheets, trabeculae, alveoli or in follicles. Cystic change may occur rarely. Marked nuclear pleomorphism is rare.

Parathyroid carcinoma

Parathyroid carcinoma is rare, causing only approximately 1% of cases of primary hyperparathyroidism. Most cases have severe hypercalcaemia and the parathyroid tumour is large and may be palpable. Classically, at operation the tumour is hard and invasive with adherence to surrounding structures. Microscopically, there is a thick fibrous capsule, which may be invaded by the malignant cells. Fibrous bands often extend into the parenchyma of the tumour. Blood vessel invasion may be seen. The tumour cells are usually of chief cell type although oxyphil carcinomas have been described. The cells are arranged in sheets or trabeculae. They show some nuclear enlargement, coarsening of the chromatin pattern and prominent nucleoli but paradoxically lack the bizarre pleomorphism, which may be seen in some adenomas. Mitoses are usually seen. The prognosis depends on successful surgical removal, as the tumour is not very sensitive to radiotherapy or current chemotherapy.

Parathyroid cysts

Parathyroid cysts may develop as a result of degeneration of a hyperplastic or adenomatous gland but most are pharyngeal pouch remnants. They usually occur in relation to the inferior parathyroids and may measure up to 10 cm in diameter. They are lined by a layer of chief cells and the wall may contain nodules of parathyroid, thymic or lymphoid tissue.

The role of fine needle aspiration of the parathyroid

Parathyroid lesions may be aspirated as masses in the neck clinically believed to be of thyroid origin and earlier reports of parathyroid cytology indicated the difficulty in distinguishing the findings from thyroid lesions[1]. These include follicular lesions, papillary carcinoma and medullary carcinoma[2]. The distinction may be complicated on occasion by the observation that parathyroid tumours and thyroid carcinomas may coexist as they share the common aetiological factor of radiation to the neck[3]. Distinguishing between thyroid and parathyroid cells may require the use of special techniques to identify the neurosecretory granules in the parathyroid cells. These include demonstrating argyrophilia and immunocytochemistry for PTH or chromogranin A together with a lack of immunostaining for thyroglobulin or calcitonin as appropriate. Radioimmunoassay for PTH can be carried out on material obtained by FNA[4,5]. The morphological distinguishing features are dense nuclear chromatin and lack of a regular architecture in the cell groups of parathyroid lesions. The absence of characteristic features of thyroid tissue, colloid, macrophages and follicular structures may also be helpful, although all of these features may be seen in parathyroid lesions. In one comprehensive survey colloid-like material was seen in 21%, macrophages in 10% and follicular arrangements in 15% of parathyroid smears[6].

The refinement of ultrasonography and other imaging techniques has enabled planned fine needle aspiration of

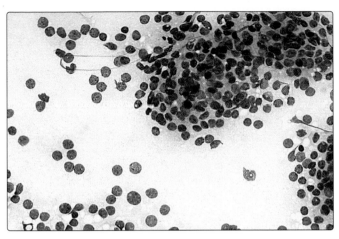

Fig. 24.2 Aspirate from a parathyroid adenoma. (MGG × MP)

Cytological findings

▶ Crowded cell groups with surrounding bare nuclei
▶ Monomorphic cells with granular cytoplasm
▶ Round hyperchromatic nuclei
▶ Occasional pleomorphic cells especially in adenomas
▶ Mitoses suggest carcinoma
▶ Oxyphil cells, colloid-like material and follicular arrangements may be seen

A parathyroid cyst aspiration characteristically yields clear watery fluid but occasionally cloudy golden-brown fluid is obtained, resembling that aspirated from thyroid cysts. Follicular and papillary cell arrangements which may be seen can cause further diagnostic confusion. Most parathyroid cysts are clinically 'non-functional' but assay of the fluid for parathyroid hormone as well as immunocytochemical staining of the aspirated cells may be useful in diagnosis[20,21].

The adrenal
Anatomy and physiology
The adrenal glands are situated superomedial to each of the kidneys. On the right side the adrenal capsule is usually fused with the overlying liver capsule and occasionally the gland may be embedded within the liver. Each adrenal weighs between 5–6.5 g and measures approximately 4 × 3 × 0.5 cm.

The adrenal is composed of two distinct parts. The medulla is derived from the neural crest and is a sympathetic paraganglion responsible for the secretion of adrenaline and noradrenaline. The cortex, which constitutes 90% of the gland, is mesodermally derived. It is divided into three concentric regions. The outer zona glomerulosa secretes mineralocorticoids, which are responsible for the conservation of sodium ions and water and the excretion of potassium ions. The inner zona fasciculata and reticularis secrete glucocorticoids, which have a wide range of effects on carbohydrate, protein and lipid metabolism, and sex hormones.

Histologically (Fig. 24.3), the zona glomerulosa consists of clumps of endocrine cells surrounded by a delicate but richly vascular connective tissue stroma. The cytoplasm has a poorly staining, clear cell appearance due to the presence of abundant lipid and smooth endoplasmic reticulum. The zona fasciculata consists of cords of secretory cells with abundant clear and foamy appearing cytoplasm. The cells of the zona reticularis are arranged in a network of branching cords and are smaller with a more compact cytoplasm, which may contain lipofuscin granules. The cells, phaeochromocytes, of the adrenal medulla are arranged in clumps in a vascular stroma of sinusoids and larger venous channels. They have abundant granular basophilic cytoplasm and large nuclei. Some sympathetic ganglion cells are also present.

the enlarged parathyroid gland[7–9]. Non-surgical destructive techniques for parathyroid adenomas rely on accurate identification of parathyroid tissue and needle aspiration also has a role in the identification of residual parathyroid tissue in patients who remain hypercalcaemic after surgery for hyperparathyroidism[10]. FNA can also contribute to diagnosis of parathyroid cysts and carcinomas. A potential complication of needle aspiration, particularly applicable to parathyroid tissue, is needle tract implantation. This has not been associated with aspiration of benign parathyroid lesions[11] but cutaneous spread after FNA of a parathyroid carcinoma has been recorded[12].

No clear cytological criteria for the distinction between hyperplastic and adenomatous parathyroid cells have been defined. Aspirates from parathyroids yield thick, crowded cell groups with irregular borders sometimes clustering around branching vascular cores. The cells are usually monomorphic. A moderate amount of finely granular cytoplasm is present and occasional small vacuoles are seen. Around the cell groups numerous bare nuclei are present. Nuclei are round and hyperchromatic with granular chromatin. Small nucleoli may be present (Fig. 24.2). In adenomas, occasional larger and pleomorphic nuclei may occur. Oxyphil cells have abundant granular cytoplasm and variable nuclear size resembling thyroid Hürthle cells. Fragments of hyaline colloid-like material may be seen together with follicular arrangements particularly in some parathyroid adenomas. Intranuclear inclusions, mast cells, lymphocytes and amyloid are occasional features[13,14,6].

As might be expected from the histological findings, the cytological findings in parathyroid carcinoma do not enable reliable distinction from an adenoma or even hyperplasia but with the appropriate clinical and radiological information the identification of parathyroid cells enables the diagnosis of primary[15–17] or secondary[18] malignancy to be suggested. FNA may be particularly helpful in distinguishing between a bony metastasis and bone changes, resulting from hyperparathyroidism[19].

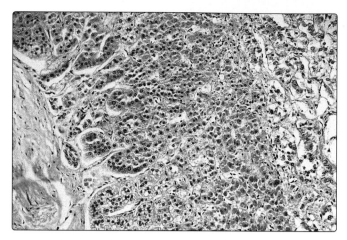

Fig. 24.3 Adrenal gland. Normal histology. (H&E × MP)

The role of fine needle aspiration of the adrenal

Adrenal cells may be encountered in attempted aspirates of surrounding structures such as the liver and kidney. Modern imaging techniques with CT and ultrasound guided aspiration enables investigation of adrenal masses. Interpretation of an aspirate must be in the light of a full knowledge of the clinical and radiological findings, e.g. the cytological findings from an adrenal adenoma may be identical to those from a normal adrenal, diffuse hyperplasia or nodular hyperplasia. The findings may be very similar in adrenocortical carcinoma and even in a renal clear cell adenocarcinoma. FNA allows the diagnosis of metastases in the adrenal, adrenocortical tumours, phaeochromocytomas, ganglioneuromas and neuroblastomas. It can also be of use in the diagnosis of some infections affecting the adrenal such as tuberculosis and histoplasmosis, allows confirmation of the presence of a simple adrenal cyst and the diagnosis of myelolipoma of the adrenal. Several large studies have shown greater than 90% accuracy in the diagnosis of adrenal masses. The principal indication for adrenal FNA is a consequence of the frequency of nodular hyperplasia and non-functioning adenomas in the population resulting in the need to investigate incidental adrenal masses in patients who have had abdominal imaging. This is particularly important in patients with known malignancy to clarify their staging and hence treatment[22–26].

Normal findings

Needle aspiration yields cortical cells and medulla cells are seen only occasionally. The cortical cells are present in loose aggregates and cords. The cytoplasm is delicate, foamy and pale staining. The nuclei are small and round with an even chromatin pattern and a small nucleolus. Occasional cells from the zona reticularis with denser cytoplasm containing lipofuscin are seen. Intranuclear cytoplasmic inclusions may be seen. Occasional small spindle shaped stromal cells are present.

Adrenal cyst

Adrenal cysts are increasingly detected as radiological incidental findings although they may present with a mass or with flank pain. Their aetiology is unclear. They may arise as a result of adrenal haemorrhage, or may arise from lymphangiomas, haemangiomas or vascular malformations. Occasionally they are bilateral. Histologically, they are lined by fibrous tissue which may show calcification.

Clear, turbid or bloody fluid is aspirated. The samples are poorly cellular with occasional inflammatory cells and debris. Occasional adrenal cortical cells are seen. If haemorrhage has occurred into the cyst erythrocytes and haemosiderin-containing macrophages are present.

The possibility of cystic degeneration in an adrenal tumour should be considered and the appropriate cytological features sought.

Adrenal myelolipoma

This is a rare benign tumour of the adrenal which is usually asymptomatic and an incidental finding in up to 0.8% of autopsies. Occasionally it presents clinically with abdominal pain or a mass. Increasingly, small tumours are being detected in staging CT scans in patients with malignancy. They are usually detected in the middle-aged and elderly and can measure up to 34 cm in diameter and weigh more than 5 kg. The tumour has been associated with hypertension, atherosclerosis, diabetes mellitus, adrenal cortical tumours and hyperplasia, chronic inflammatory states and various malignancies. It may be, however, that the presence of some of these conditions merely increases the chance of detection of the lesion. The radiographic appearances are of a low density mass with areas of punctate calcification. The radiographic differential diagnosis lies between myelolipoma, metastatic carcinoma, adenoma, granulomatous disease, renal angiomyolipoma and for larger tumours would include retroperitoneal liposarcoma.

Aspiration yields adipose tissue with haematopoietic elements. Granulocytic elements and megakaryocytes are readily identified[27–29].

Granulomatous infectious disease

Tuberculosis of the adrenal gland is the classical cause of adrenal insufficiency, Addison's disease (see Table 24.1). Aspiration of the bilaterally enlarged adrenals yields granulomatous material together with caseous necrosis. Ziehl-Neelsen staining usually reveals mycobacteria. Disseminated histoplasmosis has also been diagnosed by needle aspiration of the adrenal with recognition of the silver-staining intracytoplasmic yeasts in clusters of histocytes[30,31]. Cases of North American blastomycosis and cryptococcosis diagnosed by adrenal FNA are also recorded[32,33].

Adrenal adenomas

Adrenal adenomas are benign adrenocortical tumours. Some may be functional, leading to Cushing's syndrome or

Table 24.1 Addison's disease

Aetiology
Primary adrenal
(a) Autoimmune
(b) Tuberculous
(c) Congenital adrenal hypoplasia
(d) Adrenal haemorrhage. Waterhouse-Friederichsen syndrome
(e) Others: amyloidosis, sarcoidosis, haemochromatosis, metastatic carcinoma, surgical, other infections
Features
Chronic: weakness, hypoglycaemia, weight loss, hyperpigmentation, vitiligo (in autoimmune cases), anorexia, nausea, salt and water depletion
Acute: adrenal crisis: circulatory collapse, vomiting and abdominal pain

Table 24.2 Cushing's syndrome

Aetiology
(a) Pituitary basophil adenoma
(b) Benign and malignant adrenocortical tumours
(c) Exogenous ACTH secretion by other tumours, e.g. oat cell carcinoma of the bronchus
(d) Bilateral adrenal hyperplasia
(e) Iatrogenic, i.e. steroid therapy
Features
Truncal obesity, 'moon face', 'buffalo hump'
Muscle wasting and weakness, osteoporosis, thin skin, striae, bruising, acne, low resistance to infection
Diabetes, hypertension, amenorrhoea, hirsutism, steroid psychosis

Table 24.3 Conn's syndrome

Aetiology
(a) Approximately 80% of cases are due to an adrenal adenoma Rarely, adrenocortical carcinoma causes pure hyperaldosteronism
(b) Multinodular adrenal hyperplasia
Features
Hypertension, polydipsia, nocturia, muscle weakness, cramps and tetany
Biochemically, there is a hypokalaemic alkalosis with a high aldosterone level and low renin and angiotensin

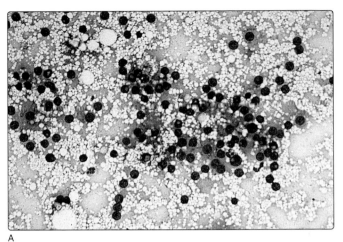

A

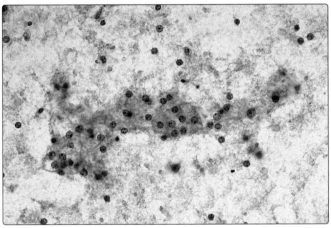

B

Fig. 24.4 Aspirate from an adrenal adenoma. (A, MGG; B, Papanicolaou × MP)

Conn's syndrome if glucocorticoids or mineralocorticoids, respectively, are being secreted (Tables 24.2, 24.3). If sex hormones are secreted these tumours may cause precocious puberty or virilism. Clinically unsuspected 'non-functioning' adenomas are found in approximately 2% of adult autopsies. Typical adrenal adenomas weigh less than 50 g and measure up to 5 cm in diameter. They are well-circumscribed solitary tumours and are usually bright yellow due to their lipid content. They may be brown or black if they have accumulated lipofuscin. Histologically, they consist of a proliferation of clear and compact type cells similar or identical to their normal counterparts.

Occasional enlarged nuclei are present but atypia and mitotic activity are very rare.

Aspiration yields numerous adrenal cortical cells with small regular nuclei and abundant lipid-containing foamy cytoplasm. Cells with more compact cytoplasm and cells containing lipofuscin may be seen. They are arranged in sheets, cords and as dispersed single cells. Binucleate cells may be seen. The chromatin pattern is dispersed and only occasional small nucleoli are seen. There is occasional nucleomegaly but no or only minimal atypia. Necrosis and mitotic activity are absent (Fig. 24.4)[22,23,34,35]. The fragility of the cytoplasm may lead to its disruption and the presence of numerous bare nuclei on a foamy background of disrupted cytoplasm. This appearance may resemble that of a small round cell tumour or even oat cell carcinoma as an appearance resembling nuclear moulding may be seen[36].

Adrenocortical carcinoma

Adrenocortical carcinomas are rare. They usually present in middle age and show an equal sex distribution. Approximately half of the cases have hormonal abnormalities, principally due to an excess of glucocorticoids, and this abnormal secretion is not suppressed by high dose dexamethasone therapy. The tumour may also present with an abdominal mass, abdominal pain, fever and weight loss.

Carcinomas are larger than adenomas, usually weighing more than 100 g and having a diameter of at least 6 cm. Macroscopically, there may be areas of haemorrhage and necrosis. Microscopically, the appearances may closely resemble those of an adenoma but atypia, mitotic activity and necrosis can be seen. The tumour is often poorly circumscribed with an infiltrative margin and invasion of large veins may be present. In well-differentiated carcinomas the size and weight of the tumour are of great importance in the prediction of malignancy. Overall this carcinoma has a poor prognosis, is often recurrent after surgery and responds poorly to radiotherapy or chemotherapy.

Cytologically, aspirates are cellular and show loss of cohesion. The appearances of a well-differentiated tumour are similar to those of an adenoma but some nuclear enlargement, atypia and mitoses may be seen. Less-differentiated tumours show increasing atypia with coarsened chromatin, a thickened nuclear membrane and the presence of prominent nucleoli. The cytoplasm tends to contain less lipid. Poorly-differentiated carcinomas show extreme cellular pleomorphism with often bizarre multinucleated cells[22,37,38]. Spindle cell forms may be seen[39]. These appearances in conjunction with clinical data have allowed the diagnosis of this tumour following the aspiration of metastases[40].

Cytological findings – adrenal cortical tumours

► Sheets, cords and dispersed cells
► Abundant foamy fragile cytoplasm
► Bare nuclei
► Uniform small nuclei with occasional nucleomegaly
► Large tumours, nuclear atypia, mitoses and spindled cells suggest malignancy

---

Diagnostic pitfalls

The separation of adrenocortical carcinomas from adenomas may be helped by special techniques including flow cytometry for the estimation of ploidy[41] and the determination of proliferation[42]. These techniques are applicable to FNA samples. The differential diagnosis also includes clear cell carcinoma of the kidney, hepatocellular carcinoma, phaeochromocytoma and metastases of other carcinomas, particularly clear cell tumours. Further investigations may help to resolve these diagnostic pitfalls. Clinical or biochemical evidence of steroid secretion should be ascertained. Electron microscopy of adrenocortical tumours usually reveals mitochondria with the tubular or vesicular cristae characteristically seen in steroid secreting cells together with an extensive smooth endoplasmic reticulum, lamellar stacks of rough endoplasmic reticulum and lipid droplets. Neurosecretory granules are present in phaeochromocytomas and they may be visualized by electron microscopy or their presence demonstrated by their argentaffin properties or immunocytochemically. Glycogen and mucin stains may also contribute to the distinction between adrenocortical carcinoma and renal cell carcinoma or another secondary carcinoma respectively.

Clear cell carcinoma of the superior pole of the kidney may mimic radiologically an adrenal neoplasm, and ipsilateral adrenal metastases of renal adenocarcinoma are not uncommon. Cytologically, renal adenocarcinoma cells may mimic an adrenocortical neoplasm[43]. The presence of papillary or tubular structures suggests a renal tumour. Adrenocortical carcinomas have been cited as having certain features more frequently than renal adenocarcinomas. These include focal dramatic anisonucleosis and crushed spindled fragments[44]. Adrenocortical cells are also negative for epithelial membrane antigen (EMA), which is present on renal carcinomas, and renal carcinomas are usually glycogen rich. Melan A, which is usually negative in carcinomas may be a useful marker of steroidogenic cells[45] and anti alpha inhibin has been reported as staining adrenal cells but not renal carcinomas[46].

Metastatic carcinoma

The most common metastasis to the adrenal is from bronchogenic carcinoma. Metastases from the breast, kidney, melanoma and lymphoma are also not uncommon. Metastases are more frequently bilateral and particularly with an appropriate history may present no diagnostic difficulty. However some metastases may mimic an adrenal tumour and where initial presentation is with the adrenal mass, diagnosis may be problematic[47]. The differential diagnostic problem can usually be resolved by clinical and biochemical data with appropriate use of special stains as indicated in the previous section.

Tumours of the adrenal medulla

Neuroblastoma, ganglioneuroblastoma and ganglioneuroma

Neuroblastoma arises from primitive neuroblasts. Some 70% of cases occur in children under 4 years of age and the majority of cases arise in the adrenal, although they may also arise elsewhere in the retroperitoneum, in the chest and in the neck. Approximately 70% of cases have metastases at presentation. Catecholamines and breakdown products may be found in the urine but hypertension is rare. Histologically, the tumour consists of a diffuse growth of uniform small cells which focally show the formation of rosette structures arranged around a central zone of neurofibrils (Fig. 24.5). Treatment is primarily chemotherapy and prognosis is generally poor but dependent on the age of the patient, stage and grade of tumour. Particularly in younger patients, the tumour may

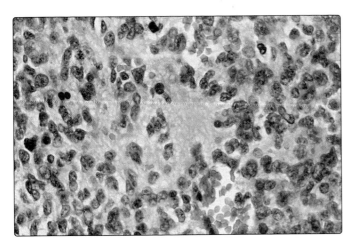

Fig. 24.5 Neuroblastoma. (H&E × HP)

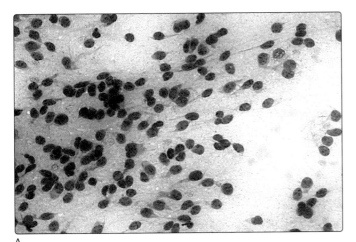

A

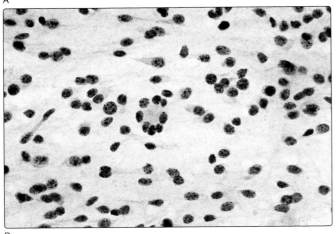

B

Fig. 24.6 Aspirate from a neuroblastoma. (A, MGG; B, Papanicolaou × MP)

spontaneously regress or mature to a ganglioneuroma.

Needle aspiration yields a cellular aspirate with numerous loosely cohesive small oval tumour cells with little cytoplasm. Some bipolar cells with cytoplasmic processes may be seen. The nuclei appear hyperchromatic with a granular chromatin pattern. Small nucleoli are visible. Occasional rosette arrangements can be seen. Characteristically, a fine pink (with MGG) fibrillar background is present due to the production of neurofibrils (Fig. 24.6). The differential diagnosis is that of small round cell tumours of childhood including Wilms' tumour, Ewing's sarcoma, embryonal rhabdomyosarcoma and lymphoblastic lymphoma. The differential diagnosis between these tumours can be aided by glycogen staining, electron microscopy, immunocytochemistry and cytogenetic analysis[48,49] and hence, in appropriate cases, some material should be reserved for these investigations. In the context of an adrenal neuroblastoma the differential diagnosis with a Wilms tumour (nephroblastoma) may arise. Morphologically, the nephroblastoma differs by the presence of three elements representing blastemal cells, epithelial differentiation with tubular and glomeruloid arrangements and spindle cells originating from the stromal element. Electron microscopy reveals neurosecretory granules, neurofilaments and microtubules in neuroblastoma and immunocytochemically there is positivity for neurone specific enolase, neural cell adhesion molecule and neurofilaments. Approximately 70% of neuroblastomas have cytogenetically visible deletions in the short arm of chromosome 1[50].

Ganglioneuroblastomas are partially-differentiated neuroblastomas. They have a better prognosis than neuroblastomas and occur more frequently in the retroperitoneum than in the adrenal. Histologically, they show gangliocytic differentiation and this is reflected in the aspiration cytology findings where neuroblasts are seen admixed with large ganglion cells. These have abundant granular cytoplasm and large eccentrically placed nuclei with prominent nucleoli. The cells may be bi- or multi-nucleate. Intermediate cell forms between the neuroblast and ganglion cell are also present[51,52].

The ganglioneuroma is a benign tumour occurring most frequently in adults. The tumour is usually found in the retroperitoneum or posterior mediastinum though may occur in the adrenal. Aspiration yields groups of spindle cells with narrow undulating nuclei, similar to those found in peripheral nerve sheath tumours (neurilemmomas and neurofibromas), together with occasional ganglion cells.

Phaeochromocytoma and other paraganglionomas

Paraganglia consist of scattered collections of neuroendocrine cells thought to be derived from the neural crest. They exist in proximity to branches of both the sympathetic and parasympathetic autonomic nervous system. The adrenal medulla is an example of a sympathetic paraganglion and the carotid body is a parasympathetic paraganglion.

The phaeochromocytoma is a paraganglionoma of the adrenal medulla. It is a rare tumour which may occur at any age. The peak age distribution is between the ages of 20–50. The sex distribution is approximately equal. The tumour occurs sporadically but in up to 10% of cases is associated with familial disorders. This is chiefly the MEN II syndrome but there are also associations with neurofibromatosis, Von Hippel–Lindau syndrome and Sturge–Weber syndrome. Familial cases are frequently bilateral, arise on a background of hyperplasia of the medulla, and present in a younger age group.

Phaeochromocytomas secrete catecholamines, giving rise to the classical clinical features of paroxysmal hypertension with associated headache, sweating, anxiety, tremor, fatigue, nausea and vomiting, abdominal pain and visual disturbance. Paroxysms may be precipitated by stress, exercise, posture changes or even abdominal palpation. In practice, paroxysmal features are often absent and patients may present with sustained hypertension only. A small minority of tumours may be clinically non-functional. Diagnosis is by the measurement of urinary catecholamines and their metabolites, vanillylmandelic acid and metadrenalines. Surgical handling and removal of phaeochromocytomas is associated with a risk of precipitating massive secretion of catecholamines and a hypertensive crisis. Accordingly patients are treated with alpha and beta adrenoceptor blocking drugs preoperatively.

Macroscopically, the tumour is well circumscribed and yellow or brown in colour. Larger tumours show areas of haemorrhage, necrosis and cystic degeneration. Histologically, the tumour is highly vascular with numerous vascular sinusoids surrounding tumour cells. The tumour cells are arranged in nests although these may be poorly defined and may form sheets or cords of cells (Fig. 24.7). The cells have well-defined granular cytoplasm and nuclei with prominent nucleoli. There may be marked nuclear pleomorphism. Approximately 10% of phaeochromocytomas behave in a malignant fashion. The diagnosis of malignancy, which is often retrospective, depends on the demonstration of local invasion and metastasis and cannot be made definitively on the basis of cytological features. Phaeochromocytomas can show

gangliocytic differentiation and mixed phaeochromocytomas and ganglioneuromas and ganglioneuroblastomas occur.

Diagnosis of phaeochromocytoma depends on clinical features, imaging techniques and measurements of catecholamines and their metabolites. Needle aspiration should not be carried out where these parameters suggest the diagnosis in view of the risk of provoking a hypertensive crisis or haemorrhage. Nonetheless, phaeochromocytomas are now frequently aspirated as part of the investigation of an adrenal or retroperitoneal mass and the risks appear to be small. Radiologists have been recommended to use no larger than a 22 gauge needle, to restrict the number of needle passes to minimize haemorrhage and to be aware of the emergency treatment of severe changes in blood pressure[53].

Aspiration produces bloody but cellular smears with numerous poorly cohesive cells. Groups of cells are arranged in loose alveolar clusters. Large bizarre nuclei may be seen with bi- and multinucleate forms. Intranuclear inclusions are usually easily found. Mitoses are rare. Nucleoli are often prominent and the chromatin appears hyperchromatic but even. There is a variety of cell shapes including polygonal, pleomorphic and occasional spindle cells. The larger cells show some resemblance to ganglion cells. The cytological pleomorphism provides no information as to the likely benignity or malignancy of the tumour. Characteristically for this neuroendocrine tumour there is abundant cytoplasm in which red granules (MGG) can be seen (Fig. 24.8). The cytoplasm appears fragile with poor definition of its boundaries. Lipid may accumulate in the cytoplasm in this tumour and on occasion there may be difficulty in distinguishing the findings from those of an adrenal cortical tumour. This problem may be resolved by the histochemical, immunocytochemical or electron microscopic demonstration of neurosecretory granules[54]. Rarely, phaeochromocytomas may accumulate lipofuscin or a melanin like pigment, which may cause confusion with malignant melanoma[55]. Ganglioneuromatous differentiation in a phaeochromocytoma yields ganglion cells and spindle cells in addition to phaeochromocytes[56].

Other paraganglionomas

Paraganglionomas may also arise in the retroperitoneum or pelvis and in these sites have been termed extraadrenal phaeochromocytomas. Paraganglionomas associated with the parasympathetic nervous system are usually non-functional and most frequently present in the neck as a carotid body tumour. Jugulotympanic paraganglionomas have been termed glomus jugulare and glomus tympanicum tumours according to their sites of origin within the temporal bone. Similar tumours rarely occur in the mediastinum.

Carotid body tumours are located at and firmly attached to the carotid bifurcation. Classically on examination they can be moved horizontally but not vertically. They are extremely vascular and may pulsate. They occur in patients

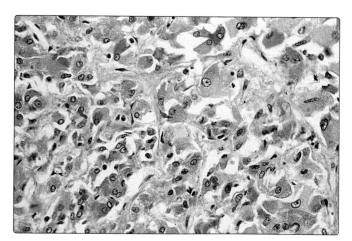

Fig. 24.7 Phaeochromocytoma. (MGG × HP)

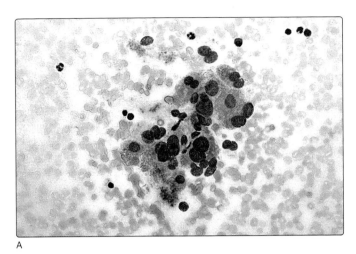

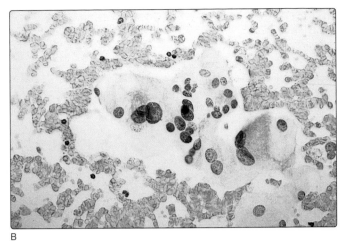

A

B

Fig. 24.8 Aspirate from a phaeochromocytoma. (A, MGG; B, Papanicolaou × MP)

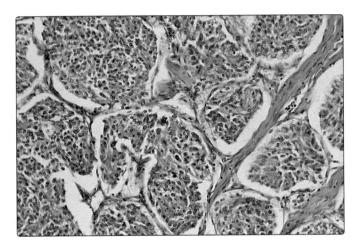

Fig. 24.9 Carotid body tumour. (H&E × LP)

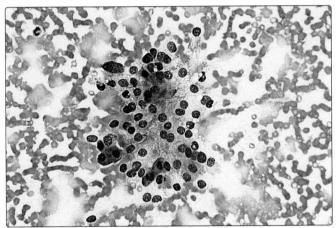

Fig. 24.10 Aspirate from a carotid body tumour. (MGG × HP)

of all ages with a slight preponderance in females. Some cases are familial and these cases are more likely to be bilateral. Patients present with a mass in the neck which may cause local compression and hence hoarseness, dysphagia or carotid sinus syndrome. The majority are benign, but approximately 10% behave in a malignant fashion. Histologically (Fig. 24.9), they consist of well-defined nests of cuboidal cells separated by vascular fibrous septa. Wrapped around the cuboidal cells are spindle shaped sustentacular cells. Again there are no absolutely reliable histological features to separate benign from malignant tumours. The cells contain neurosecretory granules, are argyrophil, but non-chromaffin and only weakly argentaffin.

Jugulotympanic paraganglionomas usually arise within the temporal bone and present as a mass in the middle ear, external auditory meatus or as a mass at the base of the skull. They may occur at any age and there is a strong female predeliction. Some cases are familial, may be bilateral and may coexist with carotid body tumours. These slow growing tumours may produce auditory disturbances

and cranial nerve palsies. They rarely metastasize but may cause death if intracranial extension occurs.

Preoperative diagnosis of a carotid body tumour is important to forewarn the surgeon of the possibility of severe haemorrhage and damage to the carotid artery at diagnostic excisional biopsy. Fine needle aspiration should be carried out cautiously in view of the risk of haemorrhage and the possibility of precipitating compression of the underlying carotid artery. The cytological findings in jugulotympanic and carotid body paragangliomas are identical and very similar to those of a phaeochromocytoma. Aspiration yields blood-stained samples with tumour cells both singly and in loose clusters. Blood contamination may be severe with relatively few tumour cells. There may be an acinar or follicular arrangement. There is abundant poorly-defined cytoplasm with a red granularity. Nuclei vary from round to spindle shaped; the chromatin pattern appears uniform although there may be some variation in nuclear size, and intracytoplasmic nuclear inclusions may be present. Single or multiple nucleoli may be present (Fig. 24.10). Nuclear pleomorphism, as in most endocrine tumours, does not signify malignancy, which is defined by architectural features although the presence of necrosis and frequent mitoses is suspicious.

The presence of acinar or follicular structures, cytoplasmic granularity and intranuclear inclusions may cause confusion with a range of thyroid pathologies. Immunocytochemical or histochemical methods can demonstrate the presence of neurosecretory granules enabling distinction from metastatic follicular or papillary carcinoma. There still may be confusion with medullary carcinoma of the thyroid and the clinical presentation and location of the lesion should be considered together with the immunocytochemical absence of calcitonin[57-60]. Rarely ectopic parathyroid glands can also be located at the carotid bifurcation causing diagnostic confusion[6].

Cytological findings – paraganglionomas

► Haemorrhagic aspirates
► Acinar groups of cells with some dissociation
► Cells may be pleomorphic with prominent nucleoli especially in phaeochromocytoma
► Intranuclear inclusions
► Abundant poorly-defined cytoplasm with red granularity (MGG)
► Cellular pleomorphism does not imply malignancy but necrosis and mitotic activity does

References

1 Löwhagen T, Sprenger E. Cytologic presentation of thyroid tumors in aspiration biopsy smear: a review of 60 cases. *Acta Cytol* 1974; **18**: 192–197

2 Friedman M, Shimaoka K, Lopez C A, Shedd D P. Parathyroid adenoma diagnosed as papillary carcinoma of thyroid on needle aspiration smear. *Acta Cytol* 1983; **27**: 337–340

3 Beecham J E. Coexistent disease as a complicating factor in the fine needle aspiration diagnosis of papillary carcinoma of the thyroid. *Acta Cytol* 1986; **30**: 435–438

4 Winkler B, Gooding G A W, Montgomery C K et al. Immunoperoxidase confirmation of parathyroid origin of ultrasound-guided fine needle aspirates of the parathyroid glands. *Acta Cytol* 1987; **31**: 40–44

5 Abati A, Skarulis M C, Shawker T, Soloman D. Ultrasound-guided fine-needle aspiration of parathyroid lesions: a morphological and immunocytochemical approach. *Hum Pathol* 1995; **26**: 338–343

6 Bondeson L, Bondeson A-G, Nissborg A, Thompson N W. Cytopathological variables in parathyroid lesions: a study based on 1,600 cases of hyperparathyroidism. *Diagn Cytopathol* 1997; **16**: 476–482

7 Halbauer M, Crepinko I, Brzac H T, Simonovic I. Fine needle aspiration cytology in the preoperative diagnosis of ultrasonically enlarged parathyroid glands. *Acta Cytol* 1991; **35**: 728–735

8 Karstrup S, Glenthøj A, Torp-Pedersen S et al. Ultrasonically guided fine needle aspiration of suggested enlarged parathyroid glands. *Acta Radiol* 1988; **29**: 213–216

9 Gutekunst R, Valesky A, Borisch B et al. Parathyroid localization. *J Clin Endocrinol Metabol* 1986; **63**: 1390–1393

10 MacFarlane M P, Fraker D L, Shawker T H et al. Use of preoperative fine needle aspiration in patients undergoing reoperation for primary hyperparathyroidism. *Surgery* 1994; **116**(6): 959–965

11 Kendrick M L, Charboneau J W, Curlee K J et al. Risk of parathyromatosis after fine needle aspiration. *Am Surg* 2001; **67**(3): 290–294

12 Spinelli C, Bonadio A G, Berti P et al. Cutaneous spreading of parathyroid carcinoma after fine needle aspiration cytology. *J Endocrinol Invest* 2000; **23**(4): 255–257

13 Davis Davey D, Glant M D, Berger E K. Parathyroid cytopathology. *Diagn Cytopathol* 1986; **2**: 76–80

14 Mincione G P, Borrelli D, Cicchi P et al. Fine needle aspiration cytology of parathyroid adenoma: a review of seven cases. *Acta Cytol* 1986; **30**: 65–69

15 Hara H, Oyama T, Kimura M et al. Cytologic characterisation of parathyroid carcinoma: A case report. *Diagn Cytopathol* 1998; **18**(3); 192–198

16 Nasser G, Loberant N, Salameh A et al. Oxyphil cell carcinoma of the parathyroid: a rare cause of hyperparathyroidism. *Clin Oncol* 1995; **7**(5): 323–324

17 Guazzi A, Gabrielli M, Guadagni G. Cytologic features of a functioning parathyroid carcinoma: a case report. *Acta Cytol* 1982; **26**: 709–713

18 Saikia B, Dey P, Saikia UN, Das A. Fine needle aspiration of metastatic scalp nodules. *Acta Cytol* 2001; **45**(4): 537–541

19 Sulak L E, Brown R W, Butler D B. Parathyroid carcinoma with occult bone metastases diagnosed by fine needle aspiration cytology. *Acta Cytol* 1989; **33**: 645–648

20 Layfield L J. Fine needle aspiration cytology of cystic parathyroid lesions: a cytomorphologic overlap with cystic lesions of the thyroid. *Acta Cytol* 1991; **35**: 447–450

21 Birnbaum J, Van Herle A J. Immunoheterogeneity of parathyroid hormone in parathyroid cysts: diagnostic implications. *J Endocrinol Invest* 1989; **12**: 831–836

22 Katz R L, Patel S, Mackay B, Zornoza J. Fine needle aspiration cytology of the adrenal gland. *Acta Cytol* 1984; **28**: 269–282

23 Saboorian M H, Katz R L, Charnsangarej C. Fine needle aspiration cytology of primary and metastatic lesions of the adrenal gland. A series of 188 biopsies with radiologic correlation. *Acta Cytol* 1995; **39**: 843–851

24 Wu H H J, Cramer H M, Kho J, Elsheikh T M. Fine needle aspiration cytology of benign adrenal cortical nodules: a comparison of cytologic findings with those of primary and metastatic adrenal malignancies. *Acta Cytol* 1998; **42**: 1352–1358

25 De Augustin P, Lopez-Rios F, Albert N, Perez-Barios A. Fine needle aspiration biopsy of adrenal glands: a ten year experience. *Diagn Cytopathol* 1999; **21**(2): 92–97

26 Fassina A S, Borsato S, Fedeli U. Fine needle aspiration cytology (FNAC) of adrenal masses. *Cytopathol* 2000; **11**: 302–311

27 Pinto M M. Fine needle aspiration of myelolipoma of the adrenal gland: report of a case with computed tomography. *Acta Cytol* 1985; **29**: 863–866

28 Dunphy C H. Computed tomography-guided fine needle aspiration biopsy of adrenal myelolipoma: case report and review of the literature. *Acta Cytol* 1991; **35**: 353–356

29 Belezini E, Daskalopoulou D, Markidou S. Fine needle aspiration of adrenal myelolipoma: a case report. *Cytopathol* 1992; **3**: 31–34

30 Valente P T, Calafati S A. Diagnosis of disseminated histoplasmosis by fine needle aspiration of the adrenal gland. *Acta Cytol* 1989; **33**: 341–343

31 Anderson C J, Pitts W C, Weiss L M. Disseminated histoplasmosis diagnosed by fine needle aspiration biopsy of the adrenal gland: a case report. *Acta Cytol* 1989; **33**: 337–340

32 Heaston D K, Handel D B, Ashton P R, Korobkin M. Narrow gauge needle aspiration of solid adrenal masses. *Am J Radiol* 1982; **138**: 1143–1148

33 Kawamura M, Miyazaki S, Mashiko S et al. Disseminated cryptococcosis associated with adrenal masses and insufficiency. *Am J Med Sci* 1998; **316**(1): 60–64

34 Dusenbery D, Dekker A. Needle biopsy of the adrenal gland: retrospective review of 54 cases. *Diagn Cytopathol* 1996; **14**: 126–134

35 Wadih G E, Nance K V, Silverman J F. Fine needle aspiration cytology of the adrenal gland. Fifty biopsies in 48 patients. *Arch Pathol Lab Med* 1992; **116**: 841–846

36 Min K-W, Song J, Boesenberg M, Acebey J. Adrenal cortical nodule mimicking small round cell malignancy on fine needle aspiration. *Acta Cytol* 1988; **32**: 543–546

37 Levin N P. Fine needle aspiration and histology of adrenal cortical carcinoma: a case report. *Acta Cytol* 1981; **25**: 421–424

38 Cochand-Priollet B, Jacquenod P, Warnet A *et al.* Adrenal cortical carcinoma: a case diagnosed by fine needle aspiration cytology (letter). *Acta Cytol* 1988; **32**: 128–130

39 Nance K C, McLeod D L, Silverman J F. Fine needle aspiration cytology of spindle cell neoplasms of the adrenal gland. *Diagn Cytopathol* 1992; **8**: 235–241

40 Varma S, Amy R W. Adrenal cortical carcinoma metastatic to the lung: report of a case diagnosed by fine needle aspiration biopsy (letter). *Acta Cytol* 1990; **34**: 104–105

41 Remmelink M, Salmon I, Passteels J L *et al.* Nuclear DNA content, proliferation index and nuclear size determination in normal and tumoral adrenal tissue, phaeochromocytomas and metastases. *Acta Cytol* 1995; **39**: 416–422

42 Öz B, Dervisoglu S, Dervisoglu M, Öz Ö. Silver binding nucleolar organizer regions in adrenocortical neoplasia. *Cytopathol* 1992, **3**: 93–99

43 Duggan M A, Forestell C F, Hanley D A. Adrenal metastases of renal-cell carcinoma 19 years after nephrectomy: fine needle aspiration cytology of a case. *Acta Cytol* 1987; **31**: 512–516

44 Sharma S, Singh R, Verma K. Cytomorphology of adrenal carcinoma and comparason with renal cell carcinoma. *Acta Cytol* 1997; **41**: 385–392

45 Shin S J, Hoda R S, Ying L, De Lellis R A. Diagnostic utility of the monoclonal antibody A103 in fine needle aspiration biopsies of the adrenal. *Am J Clin Pathol* 2000; **113**(2): 295–302

46 Fetsch P A, Powers C N, Zakowski M F, Abati A. Anti alpha inhibin: marker of choice for the consistent distinction between adrenocortical carcinoma and renal cell carcinoma in fine needle aspiration. *Cancer* 1999; **87**(3): 168–172

47 Mitchell M L, Ryan F P Jr, Shermer R W. Pulmonary adenocarcinoma metastatic to the adrenal gland mimicking normal adrenal cortical epithelium on fine needle aspiration. *Acta Cytol* 1985; **29**: 994–998

48 Triche T J, Askin F B, Kissane J M eds. Neuroblastoma, Ewing's sarcoma, and the differential diagnosis of small-, round-, blue-cell tumors. In: *Pathology of Neoplasia in Children and Adolescents*. Philadelphia: WB Saunders, 1986; 145

49 Akhtar M, Bedrossian C W M, Ali M A, Bakry M. Fine-needle aspiration biopsy of pediatric neoplasms: correlation between electron microscopy and immunocytochemistry in diagnosis and classification. *Diagn Cytopathol* 1992; **8**: 258

50 Heim S, Mitelman F (eds). Cytogenetics of solid tumours. In: *Recent Advances in Histopathology*. Edinburgh: Churchill Livingstone, 1992; 37–67

51 Kumar P V. Fine needle aspiration cytologic diagnosis of ganglioneuroblastoma. *Acta Cytol* 1987; **31**: 583–586

52 Otal-Salaverri C, González-Cámpora R, Hevia-Vazquez A *et al.* Retroperitoneal ganglioneuroblastoma: report of a case

diagnosed by fine needle aspiration cytology and electron microscopy. *Acta Cytol* 1989; **33**: 80–84

53 Casola G, Nicolet V, van Sonnenberg E *et al.* Unsuspected pheochromocytoma: risk of blood-pressure alterations during percutaneous adrenal biopsy. *Radiol* 1986; **159**: 733–735

54 Nguyen G-K. Cytopathologic aspects of adrenal pheochromocytoma in a fine needle aspiration biopsy: a case report. *Acta Cytol* 1982; **26**: 354–358

55 Rupp M, Ehya H. Fine needle aspiration cytology of retroperitoneal paraganglioma with lipofuscin pigmentation. *Acta Cytol* 1990; **34**: 84–88

56 Layfied L J, Glasgow B J, Du Puis M H, Bhuta S. Aspiration cytology and immunohistochemistry of a pheochromocytoma–ganglioneuroma of the adrenal gland. *Acta Cytol* 1987; **31**: 33–39

57 Engzell U, Franzén S, Zajicek J. Aspiration biopsy of tumours of the neck II. Cytologic findings in 13 cases of carotid body tumour. *Acta Cytol* 1971; **15**: 25–30

58 González-Cámpora R, Otal-Salaverri C, Panea-Flores P *et al.* Fine needle aspiration cytology of paraganglionic tumors. *Acta Cytol* 1988; **32**: 386–390

59 Fleming M V, Oertel Y C, Rodriguez E R, Fidler W J. Fine-needle aspiration of six carotid body paragangliomas. *Diagn Cytopathol* 1993; **9**: 510–515

60 Jacobs D M, Waisman J. Cervical paraganglioma with intranuclear vacuoles in a fine needle aspirate. *Acta Cytol* 1987; **31**: 29–32

Section 11

Male genital tract

25 Prostate: benign and malignant

Svante R. Orell

Introduction

Transrectal fine needle aspiration biopsy (FNA) was introduced in Sweden in 1960 by Franzén, Giertz and Zajicek[1] as a minimally invasive cytological method to confirm a clinical diagnosis of carcinoma of the prostate. It has now been in use for 40 years and has proved to be a simple, safe and accurate method of investigation of palpable lesions in the prostate gland[2-8].

Epidemiology of prostatic cancer

Cancer of the prostate has become the most common cancer in males in western countries. It accounts for approximately 20% of all cancers and for 11–12% of all cancer deaths, thus ranking second only to lung cancer in men in the USA and Australia[9-11]. The incidence of prostatic cancer shows a marked geographical/racial variation and is highest among American black males; high in some European countries, particularly in Scandinavia, and low in Asia and Africa. It increases rapidly with age and a further overall increase can be expected as the average age of the population is rising. A recent study from Denmark[12] found an almost 3-fold increase in incidence and a 25% increase in mortality of prostatic cancer between the periods 1943–47 and 1988–92 without any major change in age distribution or diagnostic procedures.

A number of autopsy studies have shown an extremely high prevalence of occult clinically undetected cancer of the prostate. In this respect prostatic cancer is unique among human cancers. On careful examination, cancerous foci have been found at autopsy in approximately 30% of men over the age of 50 years. It has been estimated that four-fifths of these cancers are truly occult but that one-fifth have the potential to become clinically manifest and eventually lethal. Yet the incidence of clinical cancer, i.e. the new cases of cancer diagnosed per year, equals only just over 1% of the prevalence found in autopsy studies[11].

Thus, a large proportion of clinically significant cancers remain undetected. At the time of diagnosis, almost half of the cancers are advanced and a little over half are localized and potentially curable. These data emphasize the need for improvement in the diagnosis and detection of prostatic cancer. Some improvement may already have occurred. Rietbergen et al.[13] found that among cancers detected by screening, 78% had organ confined disease.

Aetiology and pathogenesis

The aetiology and pathogenesis of prostatic cancer are not known. A genetic susceptibility is suggested by the striking racial variation in incidence and by an increased frequency among relatives of prostatic cancer patients. Most prostatic cancers respond to a reduction in androgen stimulation, and hormonal changes probably play an important role in carcinogenesis, but the exact mechanisms are still unknown. Environmental and dietary factors are also likely to contribute[10].

Clinical features

Clinical symptoms develop only late in the disease. They are mainly related to bladder outlet obstruction. Such symptoms are non-specific and may be caused by prostatic enlargement of whatever nature, including benign prostatic hyperplasia and some forms of prostatitis. Haematuria or haemospermia are sometimes the first symptoms. However, most cancers are asymptomatic and detected by routine rectal palpation, abnormal transrectal ultrasound examination or by a raised serum prostate-specific antigen. Not infrequently, secondary deposits cause the presenting symptoms while the primary tumour is silent, e.g. supraclavicular lymph node enlargement or pain from bone secondaries.

Diagnostic procedures

Three methods are currently available for the detection and diagnosis of carcinoma of the prostate: digital rectal examination (DRE), measurement of serum prostate-specific antigen (PSA) levels and transrectal ultrasonography (TRUS). Each method alone has limited sensitivity and specificity, but combination of the three has significantly improved the cancer detection rate. If there is no palpable abnormality, a serum PSA level over 4 ng/ml in combination with an abnormal TRUS, or a PSA level over 10 ng/ml alone, are highly suggestive of clinically significant cancer[11].

If cancer is suggested by one or more of these diagnostic methods, preoperative morphological confirmation of the diagnosis is the next step. This can be done by needle biopsy, either by transrectal fine needle aspiration (FNA) for cytological diagnosis, or by transrectal or transperineal core needle biopsy for histological examination. The diagnostic accuracy of FNA compared with that of core needle biopsy will be discussed at the end of this chapter.

Core needles in use today are usually 18 gauge or less. Some workers claim that with needles of this size, the complication rate is similar to that of FNA.[14]. Others find that the risk of complications is higher and patient discomfort is greater with core needles and recommend they be used selectively[15]. Tumour implantation in the needle track has not been reported for prostatic FNA but does occur, albeit rarely, following transperineal core needle biopsy[16,17]. Transrectal FNA remains the simplest, quickest and least expensive method to confirm clinically palpable cancer[2,3]. Ultrasound directed core needle biopsy is more appropriate in the investigation of non-palpable malignancy suggested by either a high serum PSA or by an abnormal transrectal ultrasonogram[18–21].

Technique of transrectal FNA of prostate

Biopsy is guided by transrectal palpation. The Franzén guide cannula was designed to make it possible to position the needle accurately in the abnormal area felt with the fingertip. It is secured by a metal ring fixed to the fingertip and a plate in the palm of the hand. A rubber fingerstall is pulled over it. The needles are 23 gauge (Figs 25.1, 25.2) and are now available in a disposable version. Other devices have been designed and used in a similar way with similar results[22,23]. The key to successful biopsy is to develop a fingertip sensitivity projected to the tip of the needle. The operator should be able to feel when the needle passes through the capsule of the prostate and if it enters normal or abnormal tissue. The aspiration technique is otherwise similar to that applied to any other site. Up to six passes can be made in one session but two to four are usually sufficient.

FNA of the prostate is an office procedure that needs no patient preparation and no anaesthesia. Prophylactic administration of antibiotics should be considered in patients who have active symptomatic prostatitis or urinary tract infection and in patients at increased risk to infection, such as diabetics, since septic reactions can occur[24]. Post biopsy haematuria is not an infrequent occurrence and patients should be warned that this may happen, but significant haemorrhagic complications do not occur even in patients on anticoagulant treatment[25].

Whether to use air-dried smears stained with a Romanowsky stain, such as May-Grünwald-Giemsa (MGG) or Diff-Quik, or wet-fixed smears for Papanicolaou or haematoxylin and eosin staining, is a matter of personal preference. Ideally, the two methods should be used in parallel since they highlight different features. For example, nuclear enlargement, cytoplasmic texture and secretory products are best seen in air-dried smears, chromatin pattern and nucleoli in wet-fixed smears.

Air-dried smears are more dependent on correct smearing technique. Wet-fixed smears are therefore usually preferred when smears prepared by clinicians are received in the laboratory. Highly cellular smears from a cancer make good air-dried preparations; the thin liquid aspirate often obtained from benign prostatic hyperplasia is more suitable for alcohol fixation.

Special stains are rarely used in prostatic cytology. However, immunocytochemical staining can be of considerable value in some cases. Staining for PSA and for prostate-specific acid phosphatase (PSAP) is helpful in the recognition of primary prostatic adenocarcinoma[26] and in the distinction between adenocarcinoma and transitional cell carcinoma. Staining for cytokeratins, which are present in the prostate only in basal cells, has been found helpful in differentiating benign proliferative processes from well-differentiated adenocarcinoma[27–29]. Immune markers are essential in the recognition of small cell carcinoma of neuroendocrine type. Finally, macrophage markers and PSA/PSAP can be used in distinguishing granulomatous prostatitis from poorly differentiated carcinoma, which is occasionally also a problem histologically[30].

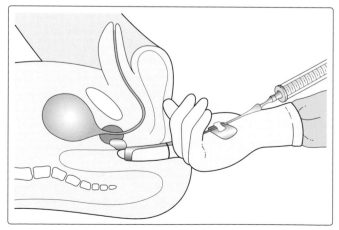

Fig. 25.1   Diagram of fine needle aspiration of prostate using the Franzén instrumentarium.

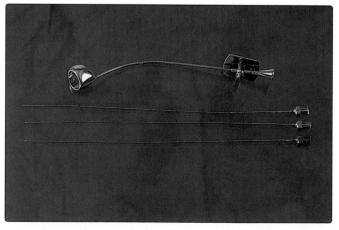

Fig. 25.2   The Franzén instrumentarium: guide cannula and 23 gauge needles.

Pathologists who do not feel confident making definitive diagnoses on cytological smears may use special needles of 21–22 gauge to obtain tiny tissue cores or fragments for cell blocks for histological sectioning. These fine calibre core needles are claimed to be as safe as the usual 23 gauge needles[31].

Causes of prostatic enlargement

The purpose of FNA is to confirm a clinical suspicion of cancer and to decide the nature of a palpable abnormality. Any condition that can cause prostatic enlargement, firmness and irregularity therefore enters the differential diagnosis. The most common cause is nodular benign prostatic hyperplasia. Prostatitis may also cause a palpable abnormality, in particular granulomatous prostatitis can clinically mimic cancer. An enlarged seminal vesicle can occasionally feel suspicious.

Most prostatic neoplasms are adenocarcinomas. A few uncommon types such as prostatic duct (endometrioid) adenocarcinoma and mucinous adenocarcinoma can be separated from the usual adenocarcinoma. Neuroendocrine tumours and transitional cell carcinomas are uncommon and so are mesenchymal tumours. A classification of prostatic tumours modified from Murphy[32] is presented in Table 25.1.

Benign prostatic hyperplasia

It is usually not difficult to obtain cellular material from a case of benign prostatic hyperplasia (BPH). However, the cells may be diluted by a large amount of thin secretion and may need to be concentrated by two-step smearing.

Table 25.1 Neoplasms of the prostate

1. Epithelial neoplasms
   Adenocarcinoma:
   (a) Usual type
   (b) Prostatic duct (endometrioid/papillary) type
   (c) Mucinous type
   Neuroendocrine (small cell) tumours
   Transitional cell carcinoma
   Others:
   (a) Squamous cell carcinoma
   (b) Adenosquamous carcinoma
   (c) Adenoid cystic carcinoma
   (d) Basal cell carcinoma
2. Carcinosarcoma
3. Non-epithelial tumours
   Benign:
   (a) Leiomyoma
   (b) Haemangioma, etc.
   Sarcoma:
   (a) Rhabdomyosarcoma
   (b) Leiomyosarcoma
   (c) Cystosarcoma phyllodes
   Malignant lymphoma
   Germ cell tumours

Admixture with blood is rarely a problem. In general, smears of BPH aspirates contain many fewer cells than smears from adenocarcinoma.

Cytological findings

- ▶ Monolayered sheets of bland glandular epithelial cells
- ▶ Abundant pale cytoplasm, sometimes with red (MGG) cytoplasmic granules
- ▶ Distinct cell membranes producing a honeycomb pattern
- ▶ Uniformly distributed round or oval nuclei
- ▶ Bland granular chromatin, inconspicuous nucleoli
- ▶ Background of abundant thin and thick secretion
- ▶ Inflammatory cells variable

Benign glandular epithelial cells are cohesive and occur mainly as large monolayered sheets, reflecting the relatively large size of the glands in BPH. The cells are seen on end and are therefore polygonal in shape with central round nuclei. The cytoplasm is abundant, thin and pale and cell membranes are distinctly visible, giving the epithelial sheets a honeycomb pattern. At the margins of the sheets there may be a row of columnar cells seen in profile. Single cells are uncommon unless too much pressure at smearing has caused the sheets to break up. However, it has been pointed out that small groups of cells suggestive of loss of cohesion occur in prostatic smears from men younger than 40 years[33].

The nuclei of benign epithelial cells are evenly distributed without overlapping or crowding. There is little variation in size or shape. The chromatin is uniformly finely granular. Nucleoli are inconspicuous (Fig. 25.3). In MGG-stained smears, coarse dark red cytoplasmic granules are commonly present in benign glandular epithelial cells (Fig. 25.3A). They are less obvious in Papanicolaou stained smears. The granules are a strong indicator of benignity although they can occasionally be found also in well-differentiated carcinoma.

Smears have a background of secretion, which may be thin and watery or thick with a high protein content condensed to dark staining clumps, amyloid bodies or concretions. A small number of histiocytes, lymphocytes and neutrophils are frequently seen in the absence of prostatitis. The fibromuscular stroma is only rarely represented by tiny tissue fragments of spindle smooth muscle cells (Fig. 25.4).

Other elements that may be found in smears of BPH are metaplastic or mature squamous epithelial cells from the mucosa of the bladder neck or urethra, mucin secreting columnar cells from the rectal mucosa, and cells from the seminal vesicles. Metaplastic squamous epithelial cells may be prominent around infarcted adenomatous nodules. They are cytologically bland and should not raise a suspicion of malignancy. Rectal mucosal cells and cells from the seminal vesicle, however, may cause diagnostic

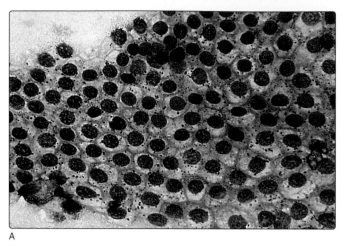

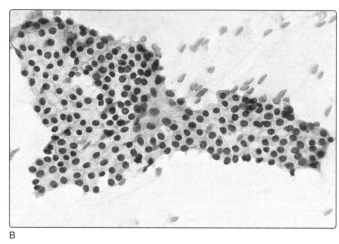

A
B

Fig. 25.3 Benign prostatic glandular epithelium. Monolayered sheets with regular distribution of nuclei, visible cell membranes and coarse red cytoplasmic granules visible in (A). (A, MGG; B, Papanicolaou; both × HP)

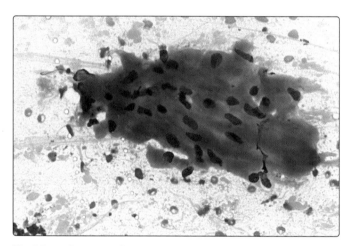

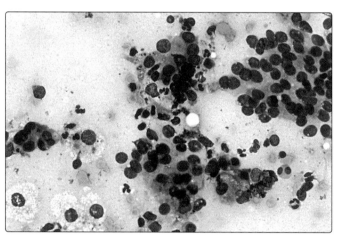

Fig. 25.4 Fragment of smooth muscle stroma in smear from case of BPH. (MGG × HP)

Fig. 25.5 Chronic prostatitis. Note irregular distribution and some overlapping of nuclei in glandular epithelium. (MGG × HP)

problems. This will be discussed in the section on adenocarcinoma.

Prostatitis

Cytological findings

▶ Numerous inflammatory cells including neutrophils
▶ Benign glandular epithelial cells which may show mild atypia

Inflammatory cells are commonly present in smears of BPH. They should be present in large numbers before a cytological diagnosis of prostatitis is made. The glandular epithelial cells may appear mildly atypical. The nuclei may be irregularly distributed, cell membranes may be less distinct and there may be a slight reduction in cell cohesion with more frequent single cells. Neither multilayering of cells in aggregates nor microacinar groupings of epithelial cells are seen, the chromatin is bland and nucleoli remain inconspicuous (Fig. 25.5).

Granulomatous prostatitis

Cytological findings

▶ Large multinucleated histiocytic giant cells
▶ Many histiocytes, some of epithelioid type
▶ Various inflammatory cells
▶ Degenerate or mildly atypical glandular epithelium

When present, large multinucleated histiocytic giant cells, which often contain clumps of phagocytosed secretion, render the diagnosis of granulomatous prostatitis obvious. Cytological diagnosis is important since there is often a high level of suspicion of cancer clinically. Histiocytes are frequent, most are of epithelioid type and may form granulomatous clusters. There is a dirty background of secretion, debris and various inflammatory cells.

The diagnosis may be less obvious if spindled histiocytes predominate and giant cells are absent (Fig. 25.6). In the presence of granulomatous prostatitis, mild epithelial

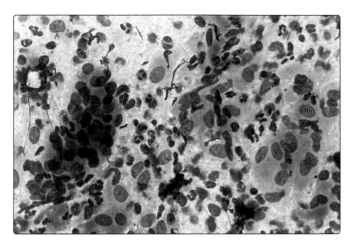

Fig. 25.6 Granulomatous prostatitis. Characteristic large multinucleated giant cells not shown; note epithelioid histiocytes, inflammatory cells in background and fragment of mildly atypical glandular epithelium. (MGG × HP)

atypia should not be a cause for concern. Histiocytes may sometimes appear rather atypical, particularly in MGG smears. If this causes diagnostic problems, immunocytochemical staining for macrophage markers are helpful[30].

Cytological findings in malakoplakia of the prostate have been reported[34].

Seminal vesicle

Cytological findings

▶ Glandular epithelial cells with atypical, pleomorphic nuclei
▶ Coarse intracytoplasmic pigment granules
▶ Spermatozoa in background

The epithelial cells of the seminal vesicle may display a degree of nuclear atypia and pleomorphism not seen in any other benign epithelium, except perhaps in the pregnancy-related Arias Stella reaction of the endometrium. Nuclei may be huge, of irregular shape, hyperchromatic and have large nucleoli, and may be indistinguishable from malignant cells. The clue to the correct diagnosis lies in the presence, in many of the cells, of coarse pigment granules, which stain dark black/green with MGG and brown with Papanicolaou staining (Fig. 25.7). Other helpful features are the presence of heads of spermatozoa in the background and a knowledge that the biopsy derives from the upper lateral corner of the prostate[35,36].

Adenocarcinoma

Several architectural criteria apply in the diagnosis of adenocarcinoma of the prostate. The quantity of cells obtained at biopsy clearly varies with the technique and with the amount of tumour stroma. Nevertheless, a very large number of cells is in itself suggestive of cancer and may be one of the most important signs in very well-

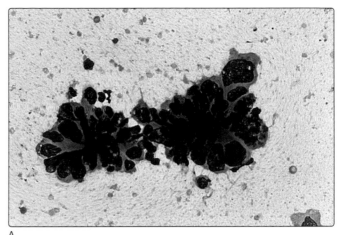

A

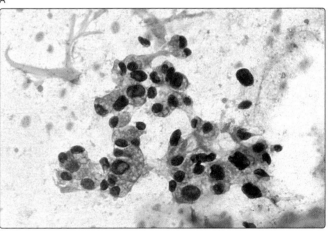

B

Fig. 25.7 Seminal vesicle epithelial cells. Note nuclear pleomorphism and the presence of coarse cytoplasmic pigment. (A, MGG; B, Papanicolaou; both × HP)

differentiated tumours. The orderly monolayered sheets of benign glandular epithelium are replaced by multilayered aggregates of cells showing nuclear crowding and overlapping and loss of visible cell borders.

Within the aggregates, the cells have a tendency to form multiple microacinar groupings (Fig. 25.8). Although this feature may be less obvious at both extremes of differentiation, it is generally so characteristic that a prostatic origin may be suggested when it is seen in a metastasic site. Loss of cell cohesion and dissociation of cell aggregates also indicate malignancy, except perhaps in young patients[33]. This phenomenon increases with decreasing differentiation and is one of the features on which cytological grading is based.

Standard cytological criteria of malignancy such as nuclear pleomorphism and chromatin abnormalities are obvious in less well-differentiated carcinoma (Fig. 25.9). In well-differentiated tumours, nuclear abnormalities are more subtle (Fig. 25.10). The two most important criteria are increases in nuclear size and in nucleolar size. Differences in nuclear size are exaggerated and therefore more obvious in air-dried smears due to flattening of cells

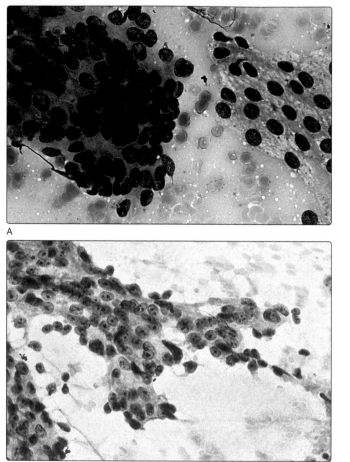

A

B

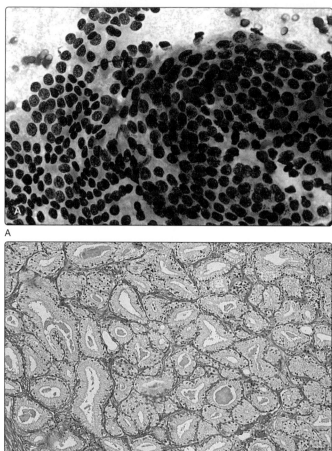

A

B

Fig. 25.8 Moderately-differentiated adenocarcinoma (grade II). Note nuclear enlargement, crowding and overlapping and contrasting benign epithelium in (A), nucleolar enlargement and chromatin clumping in (B), microacinar pattern in both. (A, MGG; B, Papanicolaou; both × HP)

Fig. 25.10 Well-differentiated adenocarcinoma (grade I). Abundance of cells showing nuclear crowding and mild enlargement but a bland chromatin. (A, MGG × HP; B, tissue section; H&E × HP)

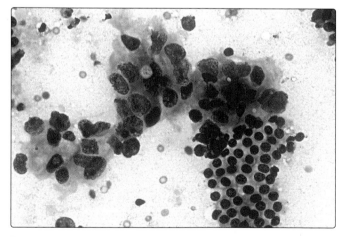

Fig. 25.9 Poorly-differentiated adenocarcinoma (grade III). Note severe nuclear atypia and striking contrast with benign epithelium. (MGG × HP)

and nuclei. Chromatin coarseness and nucleoli, on the other hand, are more clearly shown in Papanicolaou stained smears (Fig. 25.11). The cytoplasm of adenocarcinoma cells is pale and poorly defined and cell borders are indistinct. Sometimes the cytoplasm is finely vacuolated, resembling that of renal cell carcinoma, sometimes it is dispersed in the background leaving the nuclei stripped.

The diagnosis of adenocarcinoma in FNA smears of the prostate is facilitated by the fact that, contrary to most other sites, there is usually a mixture of benign and malignant cells. The contrast between the orderly, monolayered sheets of benign glandular epithelium and the irregular, multilayered aggregates and dispersed cells of carcinoma is readily appreciated (Figs 25.8–25.10). Nuclear enlargement in malignant cells is also easy to assess by comparison with benign epithelial cells present in the same smear.

It is important to recognize the cytological pattern of prostatic adenocarcinoma in FNA samples from metastatic sites so that appropriate palliative treatment can be administered. For example, supraclavicular lymphadenopathy not infrequently is the first manifestation of a clinically silent prostatic cancer. The cytological pattern described above is usually suggestive enough to raise this possibility which can be confirmed by immunostaining for PSA[37,38].

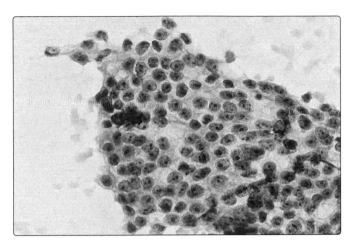

Fig. 25.11 Relatively well-differentiated adenocarcinoma (grade I–II). Note cohesive monolayered sheet and fairly regular distribution of nuclei but also nuclear enlargement, prominent nucleoli and mild chromatin irregularity. (Papanicolaou × HP)

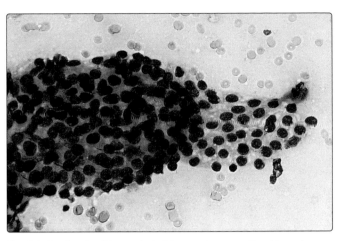

Fig. 25.12 Basal cell hyperplasia. Note nuclear crowding. Normal epithelium to the right. (MGG × HP)

Cytological grading of prostatic carcinoma

Most workers have found cytological grading to be less reliable than histological grading. This is one important reason why most urologists prefer core needle biopsy to FNA in the diagnosis of prostatic cancer. The problem is in part related to selective sampling by the minimal biopsy, partly to the relative absence of architectural patterns. However, a simple three grade system based on cell cohesion/dissociation and nuclear atypia proposed by Esposti in 1971 has shown a good correlation with survival[39,40]. More recent authors have also found cytological grading to be of clinical value[41].

Aspirated cell material is eminently suitable for DNA analysis, e.g. by flow cytometry or video image analysis. Ploidy levels have been found to be superior to morphological grading and clinical stage as a prognostic indicator, particularly in combination with proliferation index[42–45]. The expression of PSA and PSAP by the tumour cells has shown no correlation with histological grade[26].

Diagnostic pitfalls

The main problem is the distinction of well-differentiated carcinoma from basal cell hyperplasia and prostatic intraepithelial neoplasia (PIN). In basal cell hyperplasia, nuclear crowding and overlapping and loss of visible cell membranes may raise a suspicion of malignancy, but there is neither nuclear nor nucleolar enlargement (Fig. 25.12)[29,46]. Immunocytochemical staining for cytokeratins present only in the basal cells has been found to be useful in distinguishing benign epithelial proliferation and well-differentiated carcinoma[27–29].

So far, the correlation between cytology and histology of PIN has not been well documented. Cells of high-grade PIN are unlikely to be easily distinguished from cells of well-differentiated adenocarcinoma, neither are cells originating from microscopic foci of occult low-grade carcinoma. In a case of extensive high-grade PIN associated with a minor component of invasive carcinoma recently seen in our laboratory, FNA smears contained numerous, poorly cohesive relatively uniform columnar epithelial cells which showed only mild to moderate nuclear atypia (Fig. 25.13). The pattern was distinctly different from both BPH and usual adenocarcinoma and resembled low-grade papillary and cribriform ductal carcinoma *in situ* of the breast both cytologically and histologically. To avoid overdiagnosis of PIN and microscopical, occult low-grade carcinoma, which does not require treatment, a cytological diagnosis of well-differentiated adenocarcinoma may need to be supported by clinical findings or a raised serum PSA, particularly if the atypical cells constitute only a small proportion of the cell population. In the absence of supportive evidence, repeat biopsies to confirm the diagnosis may be advisable if less than some 20% of the cell population show malignant features. In doubtful and borderline cases, core needle biopsy for histological examination should be performed[47].

Distinguishing poorly-differentiated adenocarcinoma from transitional cell carcinoma and neuroendocrine tumours can cause problems. This distinction is of clinical importance since the latter tumours are unresponsive to hormonal treatment. The differential diagnosis may require the use of immunocytochemical markers and will be discussed in relation to the respective tumour types.

The greatest risk to a beginner of making a false positive diagnosis is in mistaking epithelial cells from the seminal vesicle for malignant cells. If one is aware of the bizarre nuclear pleomorphism that can occur in seminal vesicle cells and pays attention to the characteristic cytoplasmic pigment granules and other features mentioned above, misinterpretation should be avoided (see Fig. 25.7).

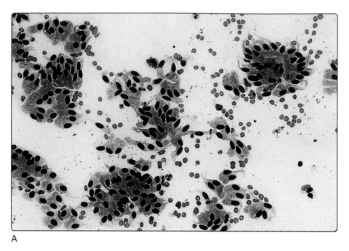

A

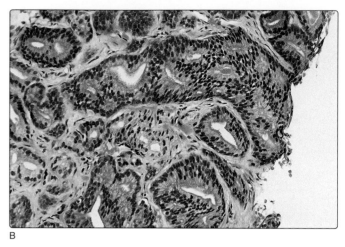

B

Fig. 25. 13   Prostatic intraepithelial neoplasia (PIN). Cellular smear of moderately atypical columnar epithelial cells. Intraglandular cribriform atypical epithelial proliferation seen in sections. (A, MGG × IP; B, tissue section; H&E × IP)

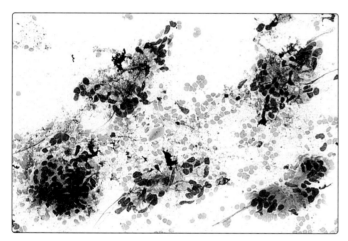

Fig. 25.14   Rectal mucosal epithelium in FNA of prostate. Clusters of columnar epithelial cells, some goblet cells. Prostatic glandular epithelium lower left. (MGG × MP)

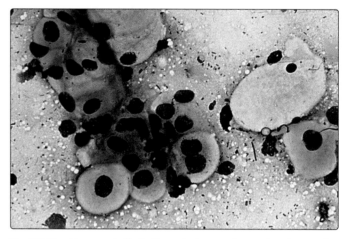

Fig. 25.15   Hormonal effects. Case of adenocarcinoma showing good response clinically. Note glycogenization and squamous metaplasia and absence of clearly malignant cells. (MGG × HP)

Epithelial cells from the rectal mucosa can occur as small glandular structures and may raise a suspicion of adenocarcinoma. However, the cells are tall columnar and palisading, with goblet cell forms, and there is usually abundant mucus in the background (Fig. 25.14).

The main cause of false negative diagnosis is inadequate or non-representative sampling. Very well-differentiated adenocarcinoma may not show any obvious cytological criteria of malignancy, and the large quantity of cells obtained may be the only feature suggestive of malignancy (see Fig. 25.10). Histological confirmation may be necessary in such cases.

An adenocarcinoma responding well to hormonal treatment may no longer be recognizable as malignant in smears taken after commencement of treatment. The typical features of hormonal response are squamous metaplasia, a marked increase in pale cytoplasm due to 'glycogenization' of many epithelial cells, both benign and malignant, and shrinkage of the nuclei of neoplastic cells

(Fig. 25.15). Similar changes may be seen as a response to irradiation[48-50].

Subtypes of adenocarcinoma

Ductal (endometrioid) adenocarcinoma

The cytological findings in the uncommon ductal or papillary adenocarcinoma of the prostate have been described in a few case reports[51,52]. Cytological atypia may be subtle, the diagnosis being based on the presence of abnormal papillary fragments. One of the reports describes longitudinal nuclear grooves similar to those of papillary carcinoma of thyroid.

The hypothesis that these tumours are of Mullerian origin has been abandoned since tumour cells are strongly positive for PSA. The tumour appears to arise from the larger, periurethral ducts and is seen as a papillary growth at the verumontanum at cystoscopy. Whether its clinical behaviour differs from that of the usual adenocarcinoma is not clear and it has recently been suggested this is not a separate entity but a growth pattern of typical adenocarcinoma spreading into periurethral ducts[53].

Mucinous adenocarcinoma

Some mucin is not uncommonly seen in prostatic adenocarcinoma. A predominantly mucinous pattern is rare, however. In such a case the possibility of an adenocarcinoma invading the prostate from the bowel or the bladder must be considered. The problem can be solved by immunoperoxidase studies since primary mucinous carcinoma of the prostate stains positively for PSA and PSAP.

Neuroendocrine (small cell) tumours

Neuroendocrine cells are not infrequently found in prostatic adenocarcinoma in variable numbers. In some cancers, a small cell anaplastic pattern is seen focally or throughout the tumour. The cells stain positively for chromogranin, synaptophysin and other neuroendocrine markers, but negatively for PSA and PSAP.

These tumours are highly malignant and do not respond to hormonal treatment[54,55]. The smear pattern is similar to neuroendocrine cancers in other sites, such as the lung[56]. The tumour cells are partly dispersed and partly seen in tight clusters with nuclear moulding. The cytoplasm is scanty and nuclei are hyperchromatic with inconspicuous nucleoli and tend to be elongated (Fig. 25.16). Part of the tumour cell population may show the usual adenocarcinoma pattern.

Transitional cell carcinoma

Transitional cell carcinoma (TCC) constitutes less than 3% of prostatic cancers and only a quarter of these are not preceded by carcinoma of the urinary bladder[57]. Its distinction is important since treatment is different from adenocarcinoma. TCC and adenocarcinoma not infrequently occur together.

Primary TCC of the prostate arises from periurethral ducts and infiltrates the deep parts of the posterior lobe. Since it is infiltrating the glandular tissue, the malignant cells are mixed with benign cells in FNA smears and may constitute only a minority of the population.

Cytological findings

▶ Malignant cells single and in multilayered aggregates, no obvious microacinar pattern
▶ Single cells with dense (squamoid) cytoplasm and distinct cell borders
▶ Prominent nuclear pleomorphism and hyperchromasia
▶ Negative staining for PSA and PSAP

TCC of the prostate, whether infiltrating from the bladder or primary, is usually high-grade and solid. The neoplastic cells are single or form irregular multilayered aggregates without obvious papillary or glandular structures. Sometimes, palisading of cells at the periphery of solid cords can give an impression of glandular groupings in smears. Cell borders are indistinct in cell aggregates but are well defined in single cells. The cytoplasm is also denser than that of adenocarcinoma cells and may appear squamoid. Variation in nuclear size is much more prominent than that in adenocarcinoma and nuclear chromatin is also more variable; some nuclei are intensely hyperchromatic (Fig. 25.17). Immunoperoxidase staining for PSA and PSAP is helpful in difficult cases.

Rare epithelial tumours
Squamous cell carcinoma

Squamous cell carcinoma of the prostate is rare, forming less than 1% of prostatic cancer[58]. It may be pure squamous or mixed adenosquamous. It is highly aggressive and responds poorly to treatment. Some patients have a history of hormonal treatment, radiotherapy or Schistosomiasis.

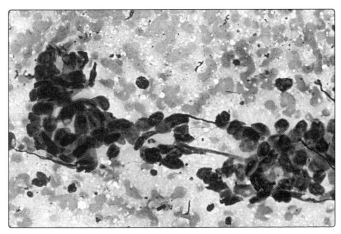

Fig. 25.16 Small cell (neuroendocrine) carcinoma of prostate. Cluster of closely packed cells with scanty cytoplasm, ovoid hyperchromatic nuclei with some moulding; nucleoli not visible. Confirmed by TURP, staining for chromogranin positive, PSA negative. (MGG × HP)

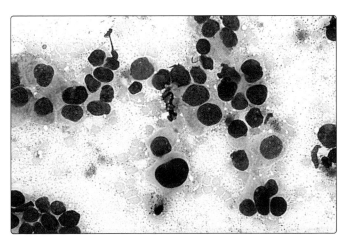

Fig. 25.17 Transitional cell carcinoma of prostate. Note dense cytoplasm, pleomorphic hyperchromatic nuclei and lack of architectural pattern. (MGG × HP)

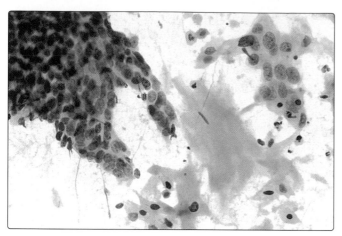

Fig. 25.18   Squamous cell carcinoma of prostate. The fragment to the left shows no obvious squamous differentiation, to the right keratinizing atypical cells. (Papanicolaou × HP)

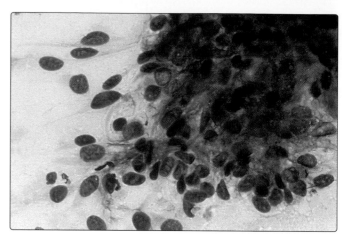

Fig. 25.19   Leiomyosarcoma of prostate. Tissue fragment of atypical spindle cells separated by intercellular collagen. Note attenuated strands of grey (eosinophilic) cytoplasm. (MGG × HP)

Like TCC, it arises from the bladder or urethral mucosa or from periurethral ducts. Cytological criteria are the same as for squamous carcinoma at other sites (Fig. 25.18). Squamous metaplasia, e.g. occurring in relation to infarcted adenomatous nodules, lacks nuclear atypia and should not cause any suspicion of malignancy.

Adenoid cystic carcinoma

This tumour rarely occurs in the prostate. It is histologically and cytologically similar to adenoid cystic carcinoma of salivary glands and may be associated with adenocarcinoma of the usual type. PSA and PSAP are negative in these tumours, which have a better prognosis than the common adenocarcinoma.

Non-epithelial neoplasms

Only embryonal rhabdomyosarcoma[59–61] and leiomyosarcoma (Fig. 25.19)[62] occur with some frequency, the former mainly in young patients, the latter in older patients[63]. For a detailed account of diagnostic criteria see Chapter 40.

Malignant lymphoma, whether a manifestation of systemic disease or rarely primary, may present as a prostatic tumour. All subtypes, non-Hodgkin's or Hodgkin's, may occur. Diagnostic criteria are the same as in other sites, the main differential diagnoses are small cell carcinoma of neuroendocrine type and embryonal rhabdomyosarcoma.

Diagnostic accuracy

It is more difficult to calculate the true diagnostic accuracy of FNA of the prostate than for most other sites. Material available for histological correlation has usually been obtained by transurethral resection, which often does not include the subcapsular parts of the gland. The problem is further complicated by the lack of morphological criteria

to distinguish latent cancer from clinically significant cancer.

The false negative rate is likely to be higher than the average of 10% reported in the literature[6,64–66]. In this aged patient population, many may die of other disease before a prostatic cancer missed by FNA has become clinically manifest. Statistical results drawn from a series of patients must clearly be influenced by patient selection. If the majority of cases have advanced disease and palpable abnormalities, sensitivity will be much higher than if there is a major proportion of cases of early, nonpalpable cancers. However, sensitivity can be improved in the latter group by multiple biopsies covering all accessible parts of the gland. Many reported series also give a small false positive rate. This is likely to reflect cases of truly latent cancer or PIN, a hypothesis, supported by long term follow up studies[67].

From a practical point of view, studies comparing the diagnostic accuracy of transrectal FNA with histological examination of core needle biopsies are of particular interest as a basis for the choice of diagnostic method. The results of such studies are conflicting[2,15,19,20,67–69]. It is almost impossible to exclude bias and results are likely to be influenced by the investigator's level of experience with and personal preference for either method.

A proportion of biopsies is unsatisfactory and nondiagnostic with both methods and account for the majority of the false negative results. This proportion decreases considerably with increasing experience and practice. It appears that an absolute diagnostic sensitivity of 90–95% is achievable with either method. Transrectal FNA has the advantage of being, faster, less expensive and causing less patient discomfort whereas most histopathologists feel more comfortable with core needle biopsy, which is easier to interpret and allows more accurate tumour grading. The two techniques should not be mutually exclusive but should be applied in a selective manner. In the author's opinion, transrectal FNA is the method of choice in patients with a palpable prostatic lesion, in older patients who are not candidates for radical surgery and in the diagnosis of disseminated disease. Multiple transrectal core needle biopsies guided by US is the appropriate method in patients with a raised serum PSA or abnormal US but no palpable abnormality[21]. It is the obvious second step when cytology is indeterminate, for example in some cases of very well-differentiated adenocarcinoma. From having been practically replaced by core needle biopsy for a few years, FNA of the prostate has made a certain come back in Australia in the last couple of years, and is now being used along the lines mentioned above.

References

1 Franzén S, Giertz G, Zajicek J. Cytological diagnosis of prostatic tumours by transrectal aspiration biopsy: a preliminary report. *Br J Urol* 1960; **32**: 193–196

2 Al-Abadi H. Fine needle aspiration biopsy vs. ultrasound-guided transrectal random core biopsy of the prostate. Comparative investigations in 246 cases. *Acta Cytol* 1997; **41**: 981–986

3 Anderson L, Hagmar B, Ljung B-M, Skoog L. Fine needle aspiration biopsy for diagnosis and follow-up of prostatic cancer. *Scand J Urol Nephrol* 1994; **162**(suppl): 43–49

4 Cohen M B, Ljung B M. Fine needle aspiration biopsy of the prostate. *Pathol Annu* 1991; **26**(part 2): 89–108

5 Esposti P L, Franzén S. Transrectal aspiration biopsy of the prostate. A re-evaluation of the method in the diagnosis of prostatic carcinoma. *Scand J Urol Nephrol* 1980; **55**(suppl): 49–52

6 Kline T S. *Guides to Clinical Aspiration Biopsy: Prostate.* New York: Igaku-Shoin, 1985

7 Leistenschneider W, Nagel R. *Atlas of Prostatic Cytology.* Berlin: Springer, 1984

8 Staehler W, Ziegler H, Volter D, Schubert G E. *Zytodiagnostic der Prostata – Grundriss und Atlas.* Stuttgart: Schattauer, 1975

9 Bonnett A, Roder D, McCaul K, Milliter L. *Epidemiology of Cancer in South Australia.* Adelaide: South Australian Cancer Registry, 1992

10 Nomura A M Y, Kolonel L N. Prostatic cancer: a current perspective. *Epidemiol Rev* 1991; **13**: 200–207

11 Scardino P T, Weaver R, Hudson M A. Early detection of prostate cancer. *Hum Pathol* 1992; **23**: 211–222

12 Brasso K, Friis S, Krüger Kjaer S et al. Prostate cancer in Denmark: a 50-year population-based study. *Urol* 1998; **51**: 590–594

13 Rietbergen J, Hoedemaeker R, Boeken Kruger A et al. The changing pattern of PC at the time of diagnosis: characteristics of screen detected PC in a population based screening study. *J Urol* 1999; **161**: 1192–1198

14 Renfer L G, Vaccaro J A, Kiesling V J et al. Digitally-directed transrectal biopsy using biopty gun versus transrectal needle aspiration: comparison of diagnostic yield and comfort. *Urol* 1991; **38**: 108–122

15 Dearnaley D P, Kirby R S, Malone P et al. Diagnosis and management of early prostatic cancer. Report of a British Association of Urological Surgeons Working Party. *BJU International* 1999; **83**: 18–33

16 Bastacky S S, Walsh P C, Epstein J I. Needle biopsy associated tumor tracking of adenocarcinoma of the prostate. *J Urol* 1991; **145**: 1003–1007

17 Moul J W, Miles B J, Skoog S J, McLeod D G. Risk factors for perineal seeding of prostate cancer after needle biopsy. *J Urol* 1989; **142**: 86

18 American Cancer Society/American Urological Association. International workshop on prostatic cancer and hyperplasia. *Cancer* 1992; **70**(suppl): 207–378

19 Eble J N, Angermeier P A. The roles of fine needle aspiration and needle core biopsies in the diagnosis of primary prostatic cancer. *Hum Pathol* 1992; **23**: 249–257

20 Engelstein D, Mukamel E, Cytron S et al. A comparison between digitally-guided fine needle aspiration and ultrasound-guided transperineal core needle biopsy of the prostate for the detection of prostatic cancer. *Br J Urol* 1994; **74**: 210–213

21 Waisman J, Adolfsson J, Löwhagen T, Skoog L. Comparison of transrectal prostate digital aspiration and ultrasound-guided core biopsies in 99 men. *Urol* 1991; **37**: 301–307

22 Maksem J A, Galang C F, Johenning P W et al. Aspiration biopsy of the prostate: a brief review of collection, fixation and pattern recognition with special attention to benign and malignant prostatic epithelium. *Diagn Cytopathol* 1990; **6**: 258–266

23 Norming U, Gustafsson O, Nyman C R et al. Fine needle aspiration biopsy with a new automatic fine-needle gun versus histologic core in ultrasonically-guided transrectal biopsy for detection of prostatic cancer. *Acta Oncol* 1991; **30**: 155–157

24 Esposti P L, Elman A, Norlen H. Complications of transrectal aspiration biopsy of the prostate. *Scand J Urol Nephrol* 1975; **9**: 208–213

25 Gustafsson O, Norming U, Nyman R, Ohström M. Complications following combined transrectal aspiration and core biopsy of the prostate. *Scand J Urol Nephrol* 1990; **24**: 249–251

26 Katz R L, Raval P, Brooks T E, Ordonez N G. Role of immunocytochemistry in diagnosis of prostatic neoplasia by fine needle aspiration biopsy. *Diagn Cytopathol* 1985; **1**: 28

27 Ostrzega N, Cheng L, Layfield L J. Keratin immunoreactivity in fine needle aspiration of the prostate: an aid in the differentiation of benign epithelium from well-differentiated adenocarcinoma. *Diagn Cytopathol* 1988; **4**: 38–41

28 Shah I A, Schlageter M-O, Stirenett P, Lechago J. Cytokeratin immunohistochemistry as a diagnostic tool for distinguishing malignant from benign epithelial lesions of the prostate. *Mod Pathol* 1991; **4**: 220–224

29 Van de Voorde W, Baldewijns M, Lauweryns J. Florid basal cell hyperplasia of the prostate. *Histopathol* 1994; **24**: 341–348

30 Presti B, Weidner N. Granulomatous prostatitis and poorly differentiated prostate carcinoma: their distinction with the use of immunohistochemical methods. *Am J Clin Pathol* 1991; **95**: 330–334

31 Mohler J L, Erozan Y S, Walsh P C, Epstein J I. Fine needle core and aspiration biopsy. A new method for diagnosis of prostatic carcinoma. *Cancer* 1989; **63**: 1846–1855

32 Murphy W M. *Urological Pathology.* Philadelphia: Saunders, 1989

33 Howell L P, Arnott T R, de Vere-White R. Aspiration biopsy cytology of the prostate in young adult men. *Diagn Cytopathol* 1990; **6**: 89–94

34 Cazzaniga M G, Tommasini-Degna A, Negri R, Pioselli F. Cytologic diagnosis of prostatic malakoplakia. Report of three cases. *Acta Cytol* 1987; **31**: 48–52

35 Droese M, Voeth C. Cytologic features of seminal vesicle epithelium in aspiration biopsy smears of the prostate. *Acta Cytol* 1976; **20**: 120–125

36 Koivuniemi A, Tyrkko J. Seminal vesicle epithelium in fine needle aspiration biopsies of the prostate as a pitfall in the cytologic diagnosis of carcinoma. *Acta Cytol* 1976; **20**: 116–119

37 Carson H J, Candel A G, Gattuso P, Castelli M J. Fine-needle aspiration of supraclavicular lymph nodes. *Diagn Cytopathol* 1996; **14**: 216–220

38 Reyes C V, Thompson K S, Jensen J D, Choudhury A M. Metastasis of unknown origin: the role of fine-needle aspiration cytology. *Diagn Cytopathol* 1998; **18**: 319–322

39 Esposti P L. Cytologic malignancy grading of prostatic carcinoma by transrectal aspiration biopsy. *Scand J Urol Nephrol* 1971; **5**: 119–209

40 Willems J S, Löwhagen T. Transrectal fine needle aspiration biopsy for cytologic diagnosis and grading of prostatic carcinoma. *Prostate* 1981; **2**: 381–395

41 Jacobs D M, Vago J F, Weiss M A. Gleason grading of prostatic adenocarcinoma on fine-needle aspiration. *Diagn Cytopathol* 1989; **5**: 126–133

42 Ahlgren G, Lindblom K, Falkmer U, Abrahamsson P A. A DNA cytometric

proliferation index improves the value of the DNA ploidy pattern as a prognosticating tool in patients with carcinoma of the prostate. *Urology* 1997; **50**: 379–384

43 Hardt N S, Hendricks J B, Sapi Z *et al*. Ploidy results in prostatic carcinoma vary with sampling method and with cytometric technique. *Mod Pathol* 1994; **7**: 44–48

44 Tribukait B. DNA flow cytometry in carcinoma of the prostate for diagnosis, prognosis and study of tumor biology. *Acta Oncol* 1991; **30**: 187–192

45 Visakorpi T, Kallioniemi O-P, Paronen I Y I *et al*. Flow cytometric analysis of DNA ploidy and S-phase fraction from prostatic carcinomas: implications for prognosis and response to endocrine therapy. *Br J Cancer* 1991; **64**: 578–582

46 De Gaetani C F, Trentini G P. Atypical hyperplasia of the prostate. A pitfall in the cytologic diagnosis of carcinoma. *Acta Cytol* 1978; **22**: 483–486

47 Ritchie A W, Layfield L J, Turcillo P, deKernion J B. The significance of atypia in fine needle aspiration cytology of the prostate. *J Urol* 1988; **140**: 761–765

48 Böcking A, Auffermann W. Cytological grading of therapy-induced tumor regression in prostatic carcinoma: proposal of a new system. *Diagn Cytopathol* 1987; **3**: 108–111

49 Spieler P, Gloor F, Egle N, Bandhauer K. Cytological findings in transrectal aspiration biopsy of hormone- and radio-therapy treated carcinoma of the prostate. *Virchow's Arch (Pathol Anat)* 1976; **372**: 149–159

50 Tomic R, Angstrom T, Ljungberg B. Cellular changes in prostatic carcinoma after treatment with orchidectomy, estramustine phosphate and medroxyprogesterone acetate. *Scand J Urol Nephrol* 1997; **31**: 255–258

51 Masood S, Swartz D A, Meneses M *et al*. Fine needle aspiration cytology of papillary endometrioid carcinoma of the prostate. The grooved nucleus as a cytologic marker. *Acta Cytol* 1991; **35**: 451–455

52 Vandersteen D P, Wiemerslage S J, Cohen M B. Prostatic duct adenocarcinoma: a cytologic and histologic case report with review of the literature. *Diagn Cytopathol* 1997; **17**: 480–483

53 Bock B J, Bostwick D G. Does prostatic ductal adenocarcinoma exist? *Am J Surg Pathol* 1999; **23**: 781–785

54 Oesterling J E, Hanzeur C G, Farrow G M. Small cell anaplastic carcinoma of the prostate: a clinical, pathological and immunohistochemical study of 27 patients. *J Urol* 1992; **147**: 804–807

55 Téta B, Ro J Y, Ayala A G *et al*. Small cell carcinoma of prostate: a clinicopathological study of 20 cases. *Cancer* 1987; **59**: 1803–1809

56 Caraway N P, Fanning C V, Shin H J C, Amato R J. Metastatic small-cell carcinoma of the prostate diagnosed by fine-needle aspiration biopsy. *Diagn Cytopathol* 1998; **19**: 12–16

57 Matzkin H, Soloway M S, Hardeman S. Transitional cell carcinoma of the prostate. *J Urol* 1991; **146**: 1207–1212

58 Sarma D P, Weilbaecher T G, Moon T D. Squamous cell carcinoma of prostate. *Urol* 1991; **37**: 260–262

59 Henkes D N, Stein N. Fine needle aspiration cytology of prostatic embryonal rhabdomyosarcoma: a case report. *Diagn Cytopathol* 1987; **3**: 163–165

60 Moroz K, Crespo P, de las Morenas A. Fine needle aspiration of prostatic rhabdomyosarcoma. A case report

demonstrating the value of DNA ploidy. *Acta Cytol* 1995; **39**: 785–790

61 Yao J C, Wang W C, Tseng H H, Hwang W A. Primary rhabdomyosarcoma of the prostate. Diagnosis by needle biopsy and immunocytochemistry. *Acta Cytol* 1988; **32**: 509–512

62 Cookingham C L, Kumen N B. Diagnosis of prostatic leiomyosarcoma with fine needle aspiration cytology. *Acta Cytol* 1985; **29**: 170–173

63 Muller H A, Wunsch P H. Features of prostatic sarcomas in combined aspiration and punch biopsies. *Acta Cytol* 1981; **25**: 480–484

64 Benson M C. Fine needle aspiration of the prostate. *NCI Monogr* 1988; **7**: 19–24

65 Graham J B, Ignatoff J M, Holland J M, Christ M L. Prostatic aspiration biopsy: an assessment of accuracy based on long-term observations. *J Urol* 1988; **139**: 971–974

66 Ljung B M, Cherrie R, Kaufman J J. Fine needle aspiration biopsy of the prostate gland: a study of 103 cases with histological follow up. *J Urol* 1986; **135**: 955–959

67 Suhrland M J, Deitch D, Schreiber K *et al*. Assessment of fine needle aspiration as a screening test for occult prostatic carcinoma. *Acta Cytol* 1988; **32**: 495–498

68 Narayan P, Jajodia P, Stein R, Tanagho E A. A comparison of fine needle aspiration and core biopsy in diagnosis and preoperative grading of prostatic cancer. *J Urol* 1989; **141**: 560–563

69 Narayan P, Jajodia P, Stein R. Core biospy instrument in the diagnosis of prostate cancer: superior accuracy to fine needle aspiration. *J Urol* 1991; **145**: 795–797

Cytology of testis and scrotum

Russell Smith, David Melcher and Margaret Ashton-Key

Introduction

Cytological examination of material obtained from the testis and scrotum by needle is by no means a modern technique[1-3]. Max Huhner, a urologist working in America, published on the subject in 1913, using the method in evaluation of infertility and as a way of excluding surgery for clearing blockages in the vas or epididymis. The patients seen by Dr Huhner must indeed have been men of steel!

> The technique of aspiration of the testicle is quite simple. A small area of the skin of the scrotum is painted with iodine. The testicle is held firmly against its skin and a rather large bore needle attached to an ordinary hypodermic syringe is plunged through the skin into the body of the testicle and epididymis. Aspiration is started immediately and kept up while the needle is being slowly withdrawn. A small amount of collodium is poured over the puncture and this completes the entire operation. Although I have done 78 aspirations, I have never had any bad results following this procedure. The pain is quite sharp at times and is testicular in nature, i.e. anaesthetizing the skin has no effect on the pain. After, it is felt more in the region of the inguinal canal than in the testicle itself. Pain disappears within a short time, though on one occasion it lasted the entire day[3].

In the authors' experience, fine needle cytology of the testis is an acceptable technique with no complications. However the investigation is not widely used in routine diagnostic practice despite its potential advantages. This chapter documents the role of FNA in patient management, the main cytological findings in the conditions most commonly encountered and the pitfalls in diagnosis for the cytologist.

Microanatomy of the testis

Knowledge of the normal structure of the testis is essential for accurate assessment of cells obtained by aspiration, regardless of the indication for the procedure, since normal cells may also be obtained by FNA along with the abnormal.

The adult testis is composed of a compact mass of long thin seminiferous tubules, forming the body of the testis, which is enclosed by a tough tunica albuginea. Each tubule is connected to a system of channels, the rete testis, situated on the posterior surface of the body of the testis. These drain by efferent ductules into the epididymis, where testicular fluid is concentrated prior to entering the vas deferens in the spermatic cord and passing into the seminal vesicles for storage.

Seminiferous tubules (Fig. 26.1) are lined by germinal epithelium, which matures towards the lumen by a process of spermatocytogenesis, from large rounded primitive spermatogonia resting on the basement membrane to smaller primary spermatocytes. Meiotic division then occurs, the resulting haploid cells or secondary spermatocytes subsequently undergoing a further meiotic division to spermatids. This step and the transformation of spermatids to tiny motile spermatozoa is known as spermiogenesis and takes place at the brink of the lumen of the seminiferous tubule.

There is a second population of cells within seminiferous tubules, which give support to the fragile germinal cells just described. These Sertoli cells are secretory and phagocytic in function and have a role in testosterone management. They are elongated columnar cells attached to the basement membrane, extending between the spermatogenic cells to the lumen. They form the predominant cell type up to the age of puberty, after which germinal cells comprise about 90% of the lining epithelium. Detailed description of each of these cell types is to be found in the following section.

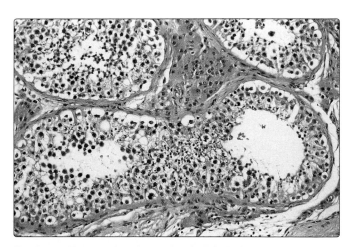

Fig. 26.1 Tissue section of normal testis. Tubule showing abundant sperm production with a cluster of Leydig cells seen lying between tubules. Note the coarse chromatin pattern in the primary spermatocytes, the softer chromatin of the spermatogonia at the periphery and the abundant 'fluffy' cytoplasm of the Sertoli cells. (H&E × HP)

There is a delicate vascular connective tissue stroma around the seminiferous tubules and within this, small groups of interstitial cells, Leydig cells, are found.

The epididymis and rete testis are lined by columnar epithelium with microvilli at the luminal surface. Efferent ductules have ciliated cells mingling with the microvillous type. Smooth muscle and connective tissue envelop all of these ductular structures.

Within the scrotum, the testis and its appendages are partially surrounded by a potential space formed by the two opposed layers of peritoneum which accompany the testis as it migrates from the retroperitoneum into the scrotum in embryological development. This double layer of mesothelial cells, the tunica vaginalis, can communicate with the peritoneal cavity and, if patent, provides a route for tracking of ascitic fluid around the testis.

Clinical indications for FNA of testis

Indications for the procedure are divided into three main areas:

1. Assessment of testicular activity in the infertile male
2. Investigation of clinically demonstrable lesions within the scrotum or testis
3. Monitoring the testis for evidence of recurrent disease in cases of treated leukaemia or lymphoma.

In the first case, surgical intervention may or may not be indicated depending upon the presence or absence of spermatogenesis/spermiogenesis, while in the second, only presurgical diagnosis of malignancy may be obtained, providing useful guidance in case management. For the third group of patients, a rapid cost-effective diagnostic test is available which may obviate the need for testicular biopsy[4].

Technical procedure

Investigation of infertility

The skin of the scrotum is cleaned, e.g. with an isopropyl alcohol swab, and a 25 gauge fine needle is rapidly plunged into the body of the testis. Aspiration has been found to be unnecessary as, presumably due to the friable nature of testicular tissue, material from the testis forms a minute plug within the lumen of the needle. The needle is then attached to a syringe filled with air, the specimen gently blown on to a slide and lightly spread with the needle. The slide is then waved in the air to dry the material obtained and stained by May-Grünwald-Giemsa (MGG). Wet fixation may, of course, be applied if Papanicolaou staining is preferred, but in our hands the material obtained, although adequate for the investigation, tends to be sparse and therefore dries very rapidly, which does not lend itself easily to wet fixation.

Investigation of palpable lesions within the scrotum

If cytology is to be used in the identification of palpable lesions within the scrotum then traditional fine needle aspiration techniques, well described in the literature, are applicable[3,5–9]. The needle of choice becomes 21 gauge and aspiration of the mass is usually indicated, using a 10 ml syringe. The material obtained may then of course be air-dried or wet-fixed depending on the staining method preferred by the user.

Monitoring for leukaemia relapse

Both testes must be sampled and sedation or general anaesthesia is usually required. An aspiration technique is generally advised, using a 22–23 gauge needle, the material then being wet-fixed or air-dried and stained appropriately[4].

Infertility

Fine needle cytology of the testis is a useful procedure in the investigation of azoospermia. The method does not of course deliver as much information as formal testicular biopsy but is obviously less invasive. Studies have shown good correlation between FNA and biopsy findings and an abnormal finding on fine needle aspiration can be followed up and evaluated further with a formal testicular biopsy[10,11].

The technique is most useful either when spermatocytogenesis/spermiogenesis is totally absent or when the full range of spermatozoa production is present[12–14]. If spermatogenesis is absent then surgical intervention in the transmission of spermal fluid would not be indicated. If, however, morphologically normal spermatocytogenesis and spermiogenesis is present, then surgery to correct a blockage in the epididymis or spermatic duct is likely to be considered. As the technique is simple, low cost and relatively non-invasive, several 'punctures' may be performed on each testis in order to obtain a truly representative yield[12–14].

Cytological findings

Diagnosis is made by identification of the cell types present and the proportion of the cell population represented by each. Thus accurate recognition of the normal cytological findings in FNA of testis is the key to diagnosis (see Figs 26.1–26.11). The MGG staining method is used throughout for the following descriptions.

Sertoli cells (Figs 26.2–26.4)

▶ A round or oval nucleus with a rather smooth chromatin pattern. Large pale or blue nucleoli are usually present. The cytoplasm is abundant, pale slate blue and is usually foamy with poorly-defined borders. Although occurring singly, these cells usually form sheets or a loose matrix. When spermatogenesis is present the spermatogenic cells are interposed within the matrix. Bare nuclei presumably extruded from the matrix are common. Sertoli cells are invariably present even in the total absence of spermatogenesis. Their presence therefore gives the cytologist confidence that the testis has been sampled correctly.

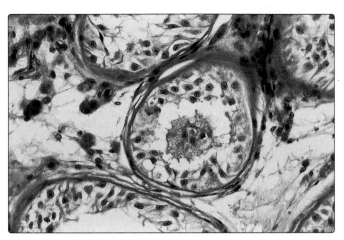

Fig. 26.2 Tissue section of testis in azoospermia. Testicular tubules containing Sertoli cells only. Leydig cells are also demonstrated lying between the tubules. (H&E × MP)

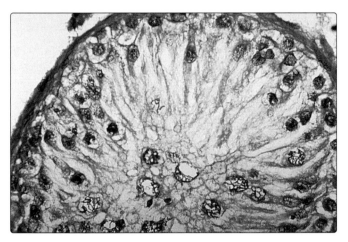

Fig. 26.3 Tissue section of testis in azoospermia. A high power view of tubule showing a severe left shift. Spermatogenesis is absent but the coarse chromatin pattern identifies a few primary spermatocytes scattered within the abundant cytoplasm of the Sertoli cells. (H&E × HP)

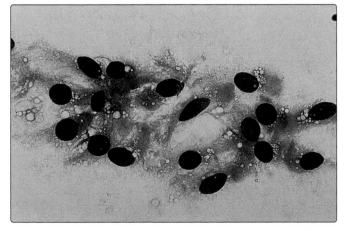

Fig. 26.4 Testicular cytology: azoospermia. A sheet of Sertoli cells lying in a matrix of fluffy cytoplasm with poorly-defined cell borders. Sperm precursors are absent. (MGG × OI)

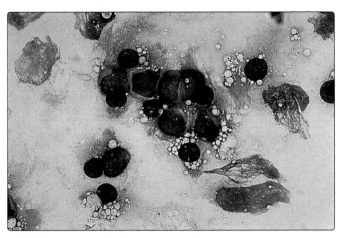

Fig. 26.5 Testicular cytology: a group of spermatogonia intermingled Sertoli cells. Note the rather smooth chromatin and the small amount of basophilic cytoplasm. (MGG × OI)

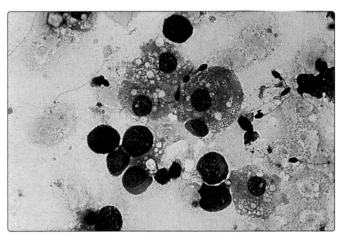

Fig. 26.6 Testicular cytology: primary spermatocytes admixed with Sertoli cells and spermatozoa. Note the coarse chunky nuclear chromatin pattern and moderate amount of hyperbasophilic cytoplasm. (MGG × OI)

Spermatogenic cells (in order of maturation)

Spermatogonia *(Fig. 26.5)*

▶ A round 16–20 μm nucleus with smooth finely woven pale staining nuclear chromatin. Nucleoli are not usually seen. The cytoplasm is scanty, smooth and pale blue. Spermatogonia are outnumbered by spermatocytes in normal spermatogenesis and may only occur in relatively small numbers. When, however, a maturation arrest is present they are often abundant

Primary spermatocytes *(Fig. 26.6)*

▶ A round nucleus, 14–20 μm, the size depending upon the state of maturation, with a heavy, coarse chromatin pattern. The nuclear chromatin shows a 'chunky' appearance with a clear dark/light effect. The cytoplasm stains deeply hyperbasophilic and is moderate in amount. Nucleoli are not seen

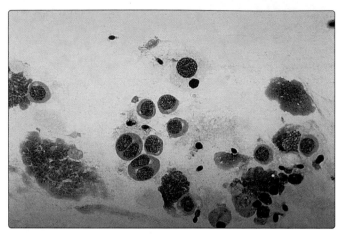

Fig. 26.7 Testicular cytology: secondary spermatocytes mixed with spermatozoa (spermiogenesis). The cells are smaller than the primary spermatocytes and although nuclear chromatin continues to exhibit a coarse pattern this is less striking than that of primary spermatocytes. The cytoplasm remains basophilic but is not hyperbasophilic. Degenerate cells are also a feature of testicular cytology and are presumably due to the rapid turnover within the process of spermatogenesis, some unable to complete and dying along the way. (MGG × OI)

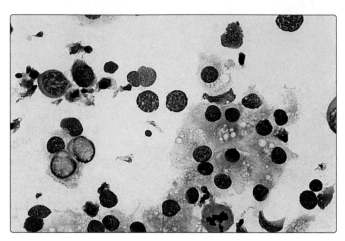

Fig. 26.9 Testicular cytology: spermatocytogenesis/spermiogenesis. An admixture of Sertoli cells, spermatogonia, primary and secondary spermatocytes, spermatids and spermatozoa. (MGG × OI)

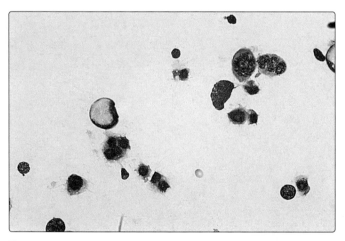

Fig. 26.8 Testicular cytology: secondary spermatocytes and spermatids. One spermatogonia is also present. The 'ragged' cytoplasm of the spermatids is a common but not unique feature. Sperm tails are seen projecting from the spermatids. (MGG × OI)

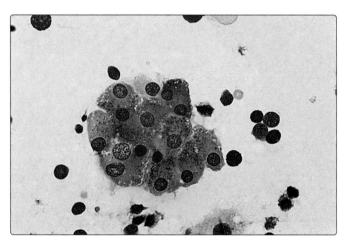

Fig. 26.10 Testicular cytology: a group of Leydig cells with dense cytoplasm and deeper basophilic granules. (MGG × OI)

Secondary spermatocytes *(Fig. 26.7)*

▶ A round nucleus, variable in size depending on maturation, from 8–16 μm. Binucleate forms are common. The chromatin pattern is coarse but to a lesser extent than that seen in the primary spermatocytes and exhibits a similar pattern. The cytoplasm is moderate in amount, basophilic but not hyperbasophilic as seen in the primary spermatocyte. As the cell matures towards spermatid the cytoplasm is often reasonably abundant. Nucleoli are not seen

Spermatids *(Fig. 26.8)*

▶ A small cell, although the size is variable. The nucleus is less than 8 μm depending, as in the other spermatogenic cells, upon maturation stage. In the 'close to mature' stage, the nucleus of course resembles a sperm head. The nuclear chromatin is darkly staining and smooth. The cytoplasm is

grey blue and often shows a ragged, uneven border. Sperm tails are commonly seen either in or protruding from the cytoplasm

Mature spermatozoa *(Fig. 26.9)*

▶ Mature, morphologically normal spermatozoa must be identifiable if natural spermatogenesis is taking place. This end point is proof that spermiogenesis, the transformation of spermatid to spermatozoa, is functional. A maturation arrest at this stage of the process is not uncommon which would of course produce azoospermia and infertility and therefore a cytological conclusion that the testis is functioning normally must include observation of all stages of maturation

Leydig (interstitial) cells *(Fig. 26.10)*

▶ Leydig cells are relatively uncommon in testicular cytology when compared with the other cellular components. They are however usually present in small numbers if careful scrutiny is applied. The nucleus is 10–12 μm, round, darkly staining with a relatively smooth chromatin. The cytoplasm is abundant and stains basophilic. The cell borders are usually clearly defined in contrast to the poorly defined Sertoli cell

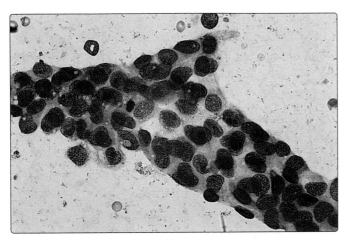

Fig. 26.11 Testicular cytology: a sheet of mesothelial cells. Mesothelium is an expected finding 'picked up' during the sampling procedure. The cells are arranged in confluent sheets with a moderately high nuclear/cytoplasmic ratio. Mesothelial cells must not be confused with Sertoli cells as, if present alone within the specimen, they obviously indicate a sampling failure and not azoospermia. (MGG × OI)

borders. The cytoplasm is also cleaner and smoother when compared with Sertoli cells. Scattered green/blue granules are seen lying within the cytoplasm. These cells can occur singly but are usually seen in small sheets, similar in pattern to those seen in tissue sections lying between the tubules of the testis in clusters

Mesothelial cells *(Fig. 26.11)*

▶ Sheets of mesothelial cells are an expected finding, picked up on the way in from the scrotal lining. It is important to identify the mesothelial cell and to differentiate from Sertoli cells in order to be certain that the sample is indeed from the testis and not a failure

Large numbers of degenerate autolysing cell forms are a feature of testicular cytology. This effect is presumed to be due to the rapid 'turnover' of the spermatogenic cells within the organ and consequent loss of many, not an artefact produced by the heavy handedness of the sampler.

Cytology of the testis in infertility gives useful information but has obvious limitations. Impaired function is easily recognized with a maturation arrest demonstrable at various stages of the process and including total absence of spermatogenesis. Morphological abnormality of spermatozoa may also be identified but traditional methods of semen analysis, etc., must also be applied (see Chapter 27). When spermatogenesis is absent, cytology is unable to specify the cause, but when morphologically natural spermatogenesis/spermiogenesis is present then a failure in the spermatic fluid transport system may be assumed.

Testicular lesions

Fine needle aspiration is a useful 'first time' approach in the identification of palpable testicular lesions[5,6,8]. In the authors' opinion, with few exceptions, cytological

Table 26.1	Tumours of testis
Germ cell tumours	Sex cord stromal tumours
Seminoma	Sertoli cell tumour
Teratoma	Leydig cell tumour
Mixed tumour	
Haemopoietic tumours	Adnexal tumours
Non-Hodgkin's lymphoma	Benign adenomatoid tumour
Leukaemia	Rhabdomyosarcoma

Table 26.2   Main classifications of germ cell tumours of testis

WHO	British Testicular Tumour Panel
Seminoma	Seminoma
typical	classical
spermatocytic	spermatocytic
Embryonal carcinoma	Malignant teratoma, undifferentiated
Embryonal carcinoma with teratoma (teratocarcinoma)	Malignant teratoma, intermediate
Teratoma, mature	Malignant teratoma, differentiated
Choriocarcinoma	Malignant teratoma, trophoblastic
Yolk sac tumour	Yolk sac tumour

assessment of the lump should not try to establish a definitive diagnosis as tissue section is the method of choice for this. FNA cytology does, however, have the ability to distinguish a neoplasm from a benign inflammatory lesion such as a spermatic granuloma (see Fig. 26.26), and is also able, for the most part, to establish that a lesion is malignant.

The majority of testicular masses are malignant germ cell tumours, as described below. Cytological assessment of these neoplasms enables the pathologist to indicate the malignant nature of the lesion, but possibly not to specify the tumour type with certainty. There are of course exceptions, such as seminoma or lymphoma, where a specific diagnosis is achievable[5,6,8,15].

Neoplasms

Testicular neoplasia is a rare event, but of major significance because it is prone to develop in young males and is, in many cases, responsive to treatment. Early accurate diagnosis is therefore of paramount importance. Tumours can develop from virtually any of the cells forming the testis, as shown in Table 26.1, but in fact over 95% are derived from the germ cells lining the seminiferous tubules[16].

Little is known with certainty about pathogenesis but there is evidence of heightened risk of malignancy in the undescended testis. Most neoplasms present in a similar way, as a painless localized or diffuse testicular swelling, easily accessible to FNA[17].

Germ cell tumours

Classification of these tumours is still debated but two main schemes are in general use and are compared in Table

26.2[16]. The majority of germ cell neoplasms are seminomas and mixed tumours are next in frequency, either mixed types of teratoma or seminoma combined with teratomatous elements.

Malignant teratoma

Teratomas most commonly present in males before the age of 30 years and show a range of histologically differentiating features, leading to a subclassification closely related to prognosis. Definitive categorization requires widespread sampling and can only be achieved by histological examination of the entire tumour. FNA cytology is able to identify those components sampled but, of course, lack of poor prognostic features in a cytology specimen does not guarantee their absence[17].

If additional material is available for immunocytochemistry it may be possible, in appropriate cases, to stain smears with markers for human chorionic gonadotrophin or alpha fetoprotein, thus revealing trophoblastic or yolk sac elements respectively.

Teratoma differentiated *(Fig. 26.12A,B)*

Cytological findings

- ▶ Scanty aspirates
- ▶ Squamous or columnar cells may be present
- ▶ Mesenchymal elements not commonly seen

Aspirates from a mature teratoma tend to be scanty and yield little material when compared with the undifferentiated lesion. Occasionally, some fluid is obtained, presumably from cystic areas. Diagnosis depends upon the presence of differentiated epithelial components such as squamous or columnar cells. Mesodermal elements, muscle, cartilage or stromal tissue cells do not aspirate easily.

Teratoma undifferentiated *(Figs 26.13A,B; 26.14A,B)*

Cytological findings

- ▶ Aspirate is usually cellular
- ▶ Loose clusters of large pleomorphic cells
- ▶ Coarse, granular chromatin, macro- and multiple nucleoli
- ▶ Ill-defined cytoplasmic margins
- ▶ Clean background

Aspirates usually yield a cellular sample with large undifferentiated cells, which have obviously malignant characteristics. The cells occur in loose clusters and are moderately pleomorphic with single cells breaking away from the edges. The nuclear chromatin is coarse and granular with huge, often multiple, nucleoli. A moderate amount of cytoplasm is present, often with an ill-defined border. The background is clean and lymphocytic infiltrate is absent.

Seminoma *(Figs 26.15, 26.16)*

Seminomas tend to present at a slightly older age than teratomas, usually in early middle age. Classical seminomas are composed of sheets of immature germ cells with clear cytoplasm, vesicular nuclei and prominent nucleoli. The connective tissue stroma is characteristically infiltrated by lymphoid cells, sometimes associated with epithelioid granuloma formation. This is an important diagnostic feature both in the primary tumour and in metastases.

A few seminomas show a more mature pattern histologically — a subgroup known as spermatocytic seminoma — consisting of pleomorphic tumour cells resembling a range of spermatogenic cells. The granulomatous inflammation seen in classical seminomas is noticeably absent. The prognosis is extremely good.

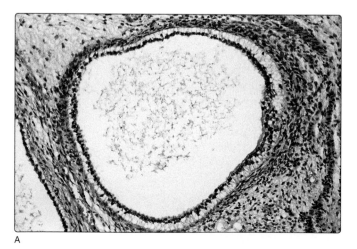

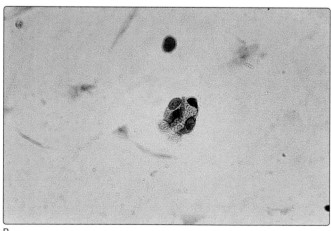

A   B

Fig. 26.12   (A) Tissue section: mature teratoma of the testis. A small cyst lined by columnar epithelium lying within a fibrous stroma. (H&E × HP) (B) Testicular cytology: mature teratoma. A small cluster of ciliated columnar cells, including a goblet cell, is seen. (Papanicolaou × OI)

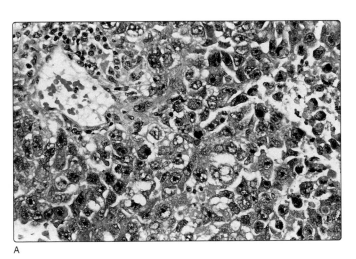

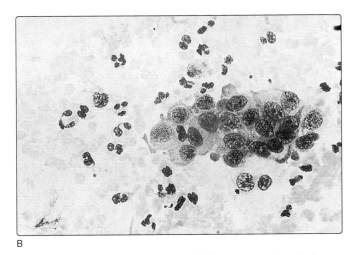

Fig. 26.13 (A) Tissue section: malignant teratoma. A sheet of undifferentiated tumour cells with prominent macronucleoli is seen, together with dense fibrous stroma. (H&E × OI) (B) Cytology: a loose cluster of undifferentiated malignant cells is demonstrated with coarse nuclear chromatin and prominent nucleoli. (MGG × OI)

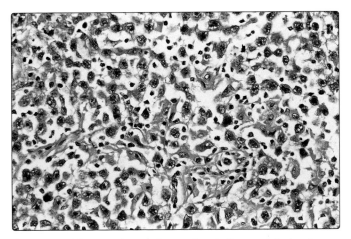

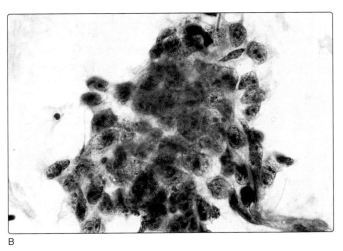

Fig. 26.14 (A) Tissue section: undifferentiated germ cell tumour (teratoma) showing marked pleomorphism, prominent macronucleoli and mitotic activity. (H&E × HP) (B) Cytology: a cluster of malignant cells aspirated from the case seen in **Fig. 26.14A**. The cells show similar features, coarse clumped chromatin, macronucleoli and pleomorphism. (H&E × HP)

Fig. 26.15 Tissue section: seminoma of testis. Tumour cells showing pleomorphism and prominent nucleoli. Cords of lymphocytes are seen running throughout the lesion. (H&E × HP)

Cytological findings

► Cellular aspirates, many disrupted cells
► Cells mostly dissociated, large and pleomorphic
► Nucleoli are prominent
► Cytoplasm not well-defined, forms a 'wash' in the background
► Numerous lymphocytes in the background

FNA of seminoma produces a high cell yield. The tumour cells are large pleomorphic, and in contrast to teratomas, are almost totally dissociated. The nuclear chromatin is softer and has an 'interwoven' appearance. Prominent multiple nucleoli are a feature and the nuclear borders are markedly irregular. Many disrupted forms are common, presumably due to increased fragility of the cells. Cytoplasm is often absent but, if seen, is clear blue.

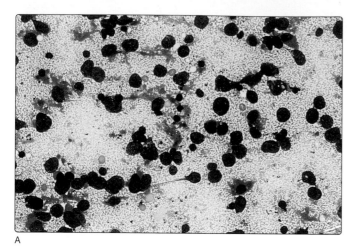
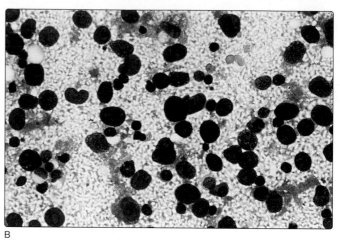

A   B

Fig. 26.16   (A) Cytology: seminoma. Scattered dissociated cells with irregular nuclear outline. Frequent often multiple prominent nucleoli are seen. Cytoplasm is wispy and often absent. Nuclear disruption is a common feature, presumably due to the fragility of the cells. Scattered lymphocytes are present intermingled with the tumour cells. A wash of fine grained background material is present. (MGG × HP) (B) Cytology: seminoma. A higher power view demonstrating the rather coarse chromatin pattern and multiple macronucleoli. Scattered lymphocytes are invariably present. (MGG × HP)

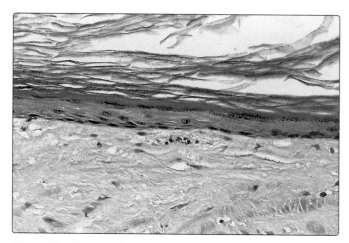

Fig. 26.17   Tissue section of an epidermoid cyst of the testis. Showing a cyst lined by stratified squamous epithelium. (H&E × HP)

Excluding the rare spermatocytic variant[18], diagnosis is also dependent on the presence of frequent lymphocytes admixed with the tumour cells. The background to the specimen characteristically shows a 'wash' of finely granular grey/blue staining material, which is considered to be cytoplasmic remnants.

Other testicular tumours

Epidermoid cyst *(Fig. 26.17)*

These are rare benign lesions of the testis that may be treated with local excision, rather than orchidectomy if diagnosed preoperatively. The aspirate shows features identical to that from cutaneous epidermoid cysts with superficial squamous cells. The presence of other elements such as adnexal structures is suggestive of a teratoma, which would require more radical treatment. Careful histopathological examination of the excised cyst wall is recommended to exclude any teratomatous elements[19].

Sertoli cell tumour

The authors do not have experience of this rare neoplasm, but a palpable mass yielding a pure population of Sertoli cells is expected on fine needle aspiration. Confusion with azoospermia testis may occur. A pre-operative cytological diagnosis may allow a conservative surgical approach[20].

Leydig (interstitial) cell tumour *(Figs 26.18–26.22)*

Cytological findings

► Mostly single cells with single prominent nucleoli
► Nuclear pseudo-inclusions present
► Intracytoplasmic Reinke's crystalloids

The aspirated cells occur singly, exhibit marked pleomorphism and have single prominent nucleoli. A background 'wash' of material is present similar to that found in seminoma but the lymphocyte infiltrate is absent. Two identifying features for the tumour are the presence of large, pale pseudo-nucleoli and oblong crystalline cytoplasmic inclusions known as Reinke's crystalloids. Both of these entities are expected but may be very scanty and the material needs careful scrutiny to establish their presence[21,22].

Malignant lymphoma *(Figs 26.23–26.25)*

Malignant lymphoma of the testis may occur as a primary tumour or the testis may be involved by lymphoma originating elsewhere. The patients are usually elderly and have widespread disease at presentation. The majority are non-Hodgkin's lymphomas of B cell type and most are high-grade[17].

The testis sometimes contains deposits of leukaemic cells, e.g. in chronic lymphatic leukaemia or in childhood acute leukaemia, but it is rare for these deposits to form a tumour mass. The role of FNA in monitoring the latter group of patients for recurrence has already been described.

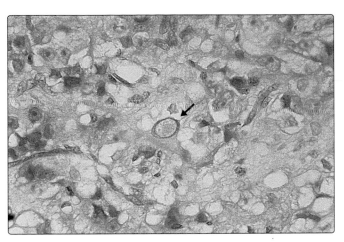

Fig. 26.18 Tissue section: Leydig (interstitial) cell tumour. Pleomorphic cell population with variable amounts of cytoplasm. The featured nucleus in the centre shows a large pseudonucleolus. (H&E × OI) (Figs 26.18–26.22 Courtesy of the late Dr V Crucioli, Oxford, UK)

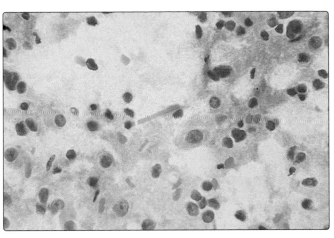

Fig. 26.21 Cytology: Leydig (interstitial) cell tumour. Scattered pleomorphic tumour cells together with one large and several smaller Reinke's crystalloids. Same case as **Fig. 26.18**. (Papanicolaou × OI)

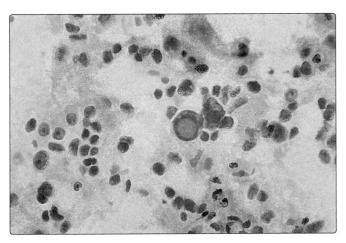

Fig. 26.19 Cytology: Leydig (interstitial) cell tumour. A pleomorphic population of cells. A large cell with a prominent pseudonucleolus is present. Same case as **Fig. 26.18**. (Papanicolaou × OI)

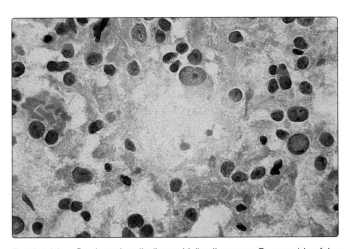

Fig. 26.22 Cytology: Leydig (interstitial) cell tumour. On one side of the picture a nucleus containing a large pseudonucleolus is seen with, above, a Reinke's crystalloid. Same case as **Fig. 26.18**. (Papanicolaou × OI)

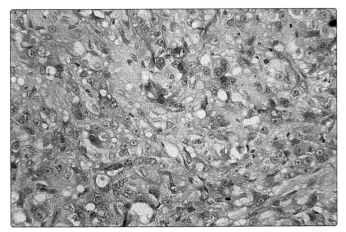

Fig. 26.20 Tissue section: Leydig (interstitial) cell tumour. Marked nuclear variation is seen. Lying near the centre of the field a Reinke's crystalloid is demonstrated. Same case as **Fig. 26.18**. (H&E × OI)

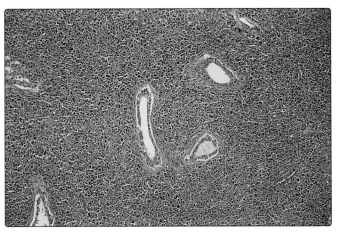

Fig. 26.23 Tissue section: malignant lymphoma. A low power view to show testicular tissue invaded by large numbers of small lymphocytes from a high-grade malignant lymphoma. (H&E × LP)

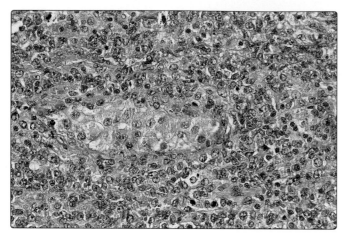

Fig. 26.24 Tissue section: malignant lymphoma (high-grade) involving the testis. The testicular tubules are partially obliterated by the invading lymphocytes. (H&E × HP)

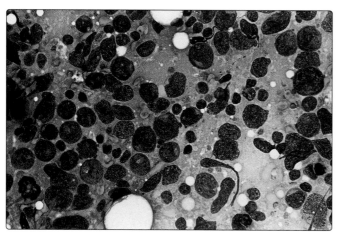

Fig. 26.25 Cytology of the testis: a population of lymphocytes in which large cells predominate from a high-grade malignant lymphoma infiltrating the testis. Testicular tissue was not identified in this aspirate. (MGG × HP)

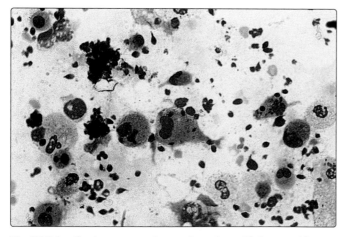

Fig. 26.26 Cytology: spermatic granuloma. Large histiocytes with abundant cytoplasm in which sperm heads and debris are phagocytosed. Numerous degenerate sperm heads and cellular debris scattered throughout. (MGG × OI)

For detailed classification of non-Hodgkin's lymphomas and their immunophenotyping by immunocytochemical methods, the reader is referred to Chapter 19.

Cytological findings

As lymphomas of testis are generally high-grade, the diagnosis of malignancy is usually straightforward. Large numbers of dissociated lymphoid blasts are present producing a rather monotonous low power picture, although at high magnification the cells are obviously pleomorphic.

Separation from seminoma depends upon:

▶ Lack of the background material seen in seminoma which is replaced in cases of lymphoma by the presence of lymphoglandular bodies, recognizable as scattered small blue/grey blobs of cytoplasmic material
▶ The nuclear chromatin of the malignant blast cells is softer and smoother
▶ The nucleoli of the lymphoblasts are less prominent
▶ The typical clear blue cytoplasm of the lymphoblast will be seen in the majority of the tumour cells, whereas in seminoma cells cytoplasm is usually absent

The diagnosis of low-grade malignant lymphoma is more difficult to establish but a population of small lymphocytes must produce suspicion. In this situation tissue diagnosis must be obtained with the use of appropriate markers for immunophenotyping.

Inflammatory and cystic lesions

Spermatic granuloma (Fig. 26.26)

This granulomatous lesion is the result of leakage of sperm in the region of the epididymis into the surrounding tissues. Aspirated material contains a mixture of neutrophils, lymphocytes, degenerate sperm and histiocytes. Giant cells may be present but are rare. The histiocytes contain phagocytosed degenerate sperm heads and debris. The background is dirty due to the presence of extensive degeneration[23,24].

Orchitis

Acute inflammation is painful and does not lend itself to aspiration. Chronic granulomatous orchitis yields leucocytes, histiocytes and giant cells mixed with spermatogenic cells, Sertoli and interstitial cells.

Hydrocele (Fig. 26.27)

This common condition, accumulation of serous fluid in the potential space between the two mesothelial layers of the peritoneum around the body of the testis, requires aspiration for treatment as well as diagnosis. There is usually an underlying inflammatory condition of the testis or epididymis, but occasionally a testicular tumour is present.

Hydrocele fluid is clear and has a relatively low cell content. Following centrifugation, histiocytes, occasional lymphocytes and mesothelial cells are seen. Spermatozoa

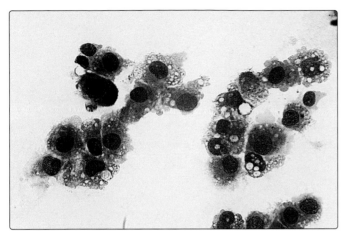

Fig. 26.27 Cytology: hydrocoele fluid. Centrifuged deposit containing histocytes and a few mesothelial cells. Fluid drained from a hydrocoele usually contains few cells and spermatocytes and spermatozoa are absent. (MGG × OI)

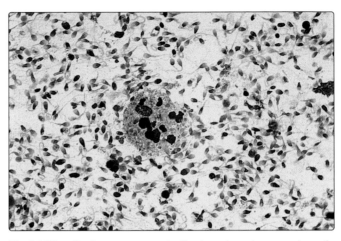

Fig. 26.28 Cytology: spermatocele. Cytology shows large numbers of mature spermatozoa with scattered, usually poorly preserved spermatocytes. Histiocytes are also frequently observed, many of which will contain phagocytosed sperm material. (MGG × OI)

and spermatogenic cells are absent unless the body of the testis has been punctured in the process of collecting the sample[25].

Spermatocele *(Fig. 26.28)*

Fluid from a spermatocele is opaque, resembling thin chylous fluid. Microscopy reveals many mature, often degenerate spermatozoa with sperm precursors and histiocytes scattered throughout. Many of the histiocytes

will contain engulfed spermatozoa and degenerate sperm material[25].

Conclusion

Testicular cytology has obvious limitations but is able to add useful information to patient management at little cost to the patient in terms of discomfort. In some instances the technique removes the need for surgical intervention.

References

1 Posner C. Die diagnostiche hodenpunktoin. *Berl Klin Wschr* 1905; **24**: 119

2 Huhner M. *Sterility in the Male and Female and its Treatment.* New York: Rebman, 1913

3 Huhner M. Aspiration of the testicle in the diagnosis and prognosis of sterility. *J Urol* 1928; **19**: 31

4 Mendes de Almeida M, Chagas M, Valenca de Sousa J, Evelina Mendonca M. Fine needle aspiration cytology as a tool for the detection of testicular relapse of acute lymphoblastic leukaemia in children. *Diagn Cytopathol* 1994; **10**: 44–46

5 Zajicek J. *Aspiration Biopsy Cytology.* Basel: Kargem, 1979; 104–128

6 Linsk J A, Franzen S, eds. Aspiration biopsy of the testis. In: *Clinical Aspiration Cytology.* Philadelphia: J B Lippincott, 1983; 267–279

7 Nseyo U O, Englander L S, Huben R P, Pontes J E. Aspiration biopsy of testis: another method for histologic examination. *Fertil and Steril* 1984; **42**: 2

8 Melcher D, Linehan J, Smith R. *Practical Aspiration Cytology.* Edinburgh: Churchill Livingstone, 1986; 158–163

9 Coburn M, Wheeler T, Lipshultz L I. Testicular biopsy. *Urol Clin North Am* 1987; **14**: 3

10 Mahajan A D, Ali N I, Walwalker S J *et al.* The role of fine-needle aspiration cytology in

the diagnostic evaluation of infertility. *BJU International* 1999; **84**: 485–488

11 Batra V V, Khadgawat R, Agarwal A *et al.* Correlation of cell counts and indices in testicular FNAC with histology in male infertility. *Acta Cytol* 1999; **43**: 617–623

12 Charney C N. Testicular biopsy: its value in male sterility. *JAMA* 1940; **115**: 1429

13 Persson P S, Ahren C, Obrant K O. Aspiration biopsy smear of testis in azoospermia. *Scand J Urol Nephrol* 1971; **5**: 22–26

14 Cohn M S, Fryes, Warner R S, Veiter E. Testicular needle biopsy in diagnosis of infertility. *Urology* 1984; XXIV

15 Balslev E, Francis D, Jacobsen G K. Testicular germ cell tumours: classification based on fine needle aspiration biopsy. *Acta Cytol* 1990; **34**: 690–694

16 True L D, Rosai J. Tumours of the testis. In: McGee J O'D, Issacson P G, Wright N A eds. *Oxford Textbook of Pathology.* Oxford: OUP, 1992; 2a: 1554–1562

17 Verma K, Ram T R, Kapila K. Value of fine needle aspiration in the diagnosis of testicular neoplasms. *Acta Cytol* 1989; **33**: 631–634

18 Lopez J I, Aranda F I. Fine needle aspiration cytology of spermatic seminoma. *Acta Cytol* 1984; **33**: 627–630

19 Berner A, Franzen S, Helio A. Fine needle aspiration (FNA) cytology in the diagnosis of epidermoid cyst in testis. *Cytopathol* 1998; **9**: 126–129

20 Sironi M, Assi A, DiBella C *et al.* Cytological, histological and ultrastructural findings of a pure benign Sertoli cell tumour. *Archivio Italiano di Urologia, Andrologia* 1995; **67**: 265–267

21 Crucioli V, Fuciniti F. Fine needle aspiration of interstitial-cell tumour of the testis. *Acta Cytol* 1987; **31**: 578–582

22 Assi A, Sironi M, Bacchioni A M *et al.* Leidig cell tumour of the testis: a cytological, immunohistochemical, and ultrastructural case study. *Diagn Cytopathol* 1997; **16**: 262–266

23 Perez-Guillermo M, Thor A, Lowhagen T. Spermatic granuloma: diagnosis by fine needle aspiration cytology. *Acta Cytol* 1989; **33**: 1–5

24 Classy F S, Mostofi F K. Spermatic granulomas of the epididymis. *Am J Clin Path* 1956; **26**: 1303–1313

25 Haddon M. Semen analysis, and the cytology of hydroceles and spermatoceles, and the prostatic gland. In: Coleman D V, Chapman P A eds. *Clinical Cytopathology.* London: Butterworths, 1989; 327–338

27 Laboratory semen analysis and sperm function testing

Mathew J. Tomlinson, Denny Sakkas and Christopher L. R. Barratt

Introduction

Infertility is usually defined as an absence of conception after 1 year of unprotected intercourse. Without contraception, around 75% of couples conceive within 12 months and a further 10% may conceive in the subsequent year. Thereafter, the conception rate is relatively low and the remaining 10–15% of couples within the reproductive age may present for treatment. In the UK, one in six couples have failed to conceive after 12 months of trying for a child.

Male factors are now recognized as the single most common cause of infertility, with sperm defects accounting for around 30–50% of cases presenting to the clinic[1]. A high quality standard semen analysis is therefore viewed as a mandatory test for inclusion in the investigation of the infertile couple[2,3].

Assessment of the semen

Detection of male fertility problems relies heavily on the assessment of conventional parameters, namely sperm concentration, motility, morphology, viability, volume and pH[3]. A carefully performed semen analysis will help to identify clearly abnormal semen samples and provide us with broad diagnostic categories. Unfortunately, an accurate prediction of whether an individual will achieve a pregnancy or not, is still some way off[4]. This particular problem is complicated by the multifactorial nature of infertility, the discrepancy between centres as to what constitutes a 'standard' semen analysis and indeed between individuals at performing the various diagnostic tests. It is therefore widely accepted that the use of standardized protocols for basic semen tests and the reduction of error and intra-operator variation by implementing strict quality control schemes will increase the predictive power of semen analysis. A gold standard is laid down by the WHO[5]. This is the best laboratory manual available, and is recommended reading for everybody performing or interpreting semen analysis. It explains which tests should be performed and provides details of how to conduct them. In addition to the WHO manual there are several papers and textbooks which provide more detailed information[6–9]. Current diagnostic terminology is defined in Table 27.1.

Table 27.1 Diagnostic terminology

WHO Classification	Definition
Normozoospermia	Normal semen profile
Oligozoospermia	Sperm concentration $< 20 \times 10^6$/ml
Severe oligozoospermia	Sperm concentration $< 5 \times 10^6$/ml
Cryptozoospermia	Few sperm in pellet after centrifugation
Asthenozoospermia	Progressive motility $< 50\%$
Teratozoospermia	Morphologically ideal forms $< 15\%$*
Azoospermia	No sperm in ejaculate
Aspermia	No ejaculate
	Low ejaculate volume
Globozoospermia	No acrosome 'round head defect'
Necrozoospermia	No viable (living) sperm
Leucocytospermia	Leucocyte concentration $> 1 \times 10^6$/ml

* Suggested threshold. From WHO *Laboratory Manual for the Examination of Human Semen and Semen-Cervical Mucus Interaction*, 4th edn., 1999.

Standard procedures for semen analysis

The basic rules of semen analysis

From booking the appointment with the laboratory to delivering the sample, properly standardized procedures need to be established to ensure that the semen analysis result is clinically meaningful. Understandably, the production of a semen sample for many men is often embarrassing and it is important to make the man feel as relaxed as possible about the procedure. The specimen should therefore be produced at the laboratory and to this end, a quiet, secure room must be provided (Human Fertilisation and Embryology Authority, Code of Practice, 1991)[10]. This also helps to ensure that samples are collected in an identical manner, controlling both the temperature at which the sample is kept and indeed the ejaculation-analysis interval. If facilities are not available for production 'on-site', then appropriate instruction should be given on: (a) abstinence from sexual activity. This should be for at least 2, but for no longer than 6 days. It should be stressed that abstinence for longer periods will not improve the sperm quality; (b) hygiene (wash hands and genitals prior to ejaculation). It is important to note that contamination of the semen sample with either soap or water may also adversely affect sperm quality; (c) specimen pots (only sterile, non-toxic, wide-necked pots should be used). Samples should not be obtained by withdrawal (*coitus interruptus*) or by using a contraceptive condom. In exceptional circumstances only, should a couple be provided with a special non-toxic silastic condom.

There can be considerable variation in semen quality between ejaculates from the same individual for a variety of reasons. In order to have a complete semen evaluation, ideally a repeat analysis should be performed on a second sample collected between 7 days and 3 months after the initial analysis, particularly if the first semen result shows one, or multiple abnormalities. Discrepancies in results can occur for a number of reasons. The sperm count itself can be viewed as a 'health marker', typically being lowered in times of stress, chronic illness, e.g. malignancy or recent febrile ('flu-like') illness. Other common causes can be attributed to incomplete collection of the ejaculate (the first portion of an ejaculate contains the majority of the spermatozoa), clearly illustrating the need to document all relevant information at the time of collection. If there are conflicting results from the two analyses, giving different diagnoses, then further semen assessments should be undertaken.

Semen sample appearance, volume, pH, viscosity, liquefaction

After ejaculation the seminal secretions form a coagulum, which gradually liquefies due to the action of prostatic enzymes. Most samples are fully liquefied after 1 h. An hour is therefore a useful 'benchmark' for the time at which the semen analysis should proceed. The overall appearance (normally greyish/opalescent) should be recorded, taking note particularly of any strong odour; discolouration or any other deviation from the norm, e.g. jelly like grains and mucoid streaks. Seminal fluid appearance can immediately highlight signs of a problem, for example a brown or red tint suggests red blood cell contamination.

Normal pH of semen is slightly alkaline (7.2–8.0) but this does increase with time. pH alone gives us little prognostic information. However, in certain urogenital conditions, pH may be abnormally high or low, e.g. azoospermia, and gives a clue as to the cause. pH should be performed 60 min after ejaculation, either by: using pH test paper range 6.5–10 and noting the colour change or a pH meter.

The presence of urine in semen is detected not so much by a faint yellow discolouration, as by a strong ammonia smell. Direct observation should show a very poor or absent motility as urine has a very toxic effect on sperm. Urine contamination can be due to disturbances in bladder neck function and ejaculation, pH will be lowered with significant urine contamination.

The ejaculate volume should be measured using either a disposable wide-mouthed pipette or a plastic (toxicity tested) syringe. Semen volumes 'normally' lie between 1.5 and 5 ml, however, volumes as low as 1 ml or as high as

10 ml are sometimes recorded. Reductions in volume and increases in pH can indicate an infection in the prostate gland or seminal vesicles causing a reduction in secretion. Ejaculatory disorders such as retrograde ejaculation (where the ejaculate goes into the bladder) will also result in a low volume sample (see below). It should also be remembered that artificial anomalies such as incomplete sample collection or long periods of sexual abstinence can affect both volume and pH.

Normal samples can be poured drop by drop from a container or pipette, whereas viscous samples will form a long strand of semen of 2 cm or more. Excessive viscosity can affect sample mixing, therefore accurate estimation of sperm concentration and motility may be impossible. A sample that has not liquefied may form a coagulum, contain mucus streaks or, if it is partially liquefied, will contain small clots. Absence of clotting or liquefaction may therefore indicate problems with the secretory function of the accessory glands. Gelatinous bodies are also a common finding but evidence to date suggests they are no great clinical significance.

Retrograde ejaculation (RE)

Any interference with the integrity of the bladder neck and posterior urethra (anatomical, trauma, neurogenic, drug induced) may result in abnormal function of the internal sphincter of the urethra and favour ejaculation into the bladder (retrograde) as the path of least resistance. Amongst patients attending an infertility clinic, it is most commonly found in men with: (a) diabetes; (b) post-traumatic paraplegia and (c) post bladder-neck surgery. Classically, RE presents as a complete absence or extremely low ejaculate volume, while orgasmic sensation is preserved. Confirmation of diagnosis is by identification of significant numbers of sperm in post-orgasmic urine. As urine, particularly of low osmolarity and low pH, has such a rapid deleterious effect on sperm, treatment of RE by sperm preparation will nearly always require further intervention, e.g. alkalinization of the bladder using sodium bicarbonate. Flushing of the bladder with media is commonly used as a treatment for RE.

Microscopic evaluation of semen

Phase contrast optics with $\times 20$, $\times 40$ objectives must be used for all examinations of unstained fresh spermatozoa. Initial assessment includes measurement of sperm motility, sperm agglutination and round cell concentration, sperm concentration (sperm count), and morphological assessment of prepared slides. Further assessment should include antisperm antibody testing.

Motility

As sperm motility is one of the most useful indicators of a man's fertility[11-13] it is extremely important that it is assessed quickly, at a consistent time post-ejaculation and with as much care as possible to ensure accurate and

Table 27.2 Motility

Rapid forward progression	Sperm swims forwards at > 5 times the distance of its own head in 1 s
Medium forward progression	Sperm moves forwards between 1 and 5 head-lengths/s
Non progressive	Flagellum is beating or sperm is shaking on the spot, but not progressing
Static/immotile	Sperm are stationary

reliable results. Both motility and velocity are highly temperature sensitive, therefore measures must be taken to ensure a consistent temperature under the microscope. The most practical way to do this is to use a heated microscope stage, set to 37°C. Motility is assessed according to WHO guidelines with sperm graded into four categories of motion and expressed as a percentage (Table 27.2). Normally 100–200 sperm are categorized using a 4-way bench tally and results are expressed as a percentage.

Agglutination and other cells in semen

Agglutination is the term given when motile sperm stick to each other whether it be by the head, midpiece or tail and may be suggestive of immunological infertility, i.e. the presence of antisperm antibodies. Large clumps of agglutination will obviously have a significant affect on sperm motility and make accurate assessment of sperm concentration very difficult.

The presence of other cell types in human semen other than spermatozoa is common and should always be noted. They include: bacteria; protozoa; red blood cells (erythrocytes); white blood cells (leucocytes); epithelial cells and immature germ cells (IGCs). Both WBCs and IGCs are often collectively referred to as 'round cells' and are difficult to tell apart. It is firmly believed that large numbers of leucocytes ($>1 \times 10^6$ million/ml), known as leucocytospermia may indicate an infection within the reproductive tract[5], either a urethritis or infection in the accessory glands. Consistent leucocytospermia may also indicate a chronic subclinical infection. A count of this magnitude should be reported to the clinician, and if found to be associated with protozoa or bacteria and/or clinical symptoms, further investigation at a genitourinary medicine clinic may be warranted. Leucocytes are also known to be powerful generators of reactive oxygen species (ROS) or free oxygen radicals, which are widely believed to have severe detrimental effects on sperm function. Although not usually a problem in semen due to protective enzymes within seminal plasma, sperm samples prepared for assisted conception may have reduced fertilizing capacity if contaminated by ROS producing leucocytes[14,15]. The finding of large numbers of immature germ cells (IGCs) (> 5 RC per high power field at ×400 magnification) may be an indication of a spermatogenic problem. Indeed,

very high concentrations of IGCs are often associated with poor sperm morphology and motility. Epithelial cells, usually derived from the lining of the urethra are thought to be of little clinical significance.

The number of non sperm cells can be estimated in wet preparations using a Neubauer counting chamber. Further discrimination between leucocytes and germinal cells requires the use of immunocytochemistry as certain phenotypes are morphologically similar[16].

Sperm concentration

Sperm concentration, sometimes known as the 'sperm count' or 'sperm density' is usually measured using a haemocytometer, such as the improved Neubauer chamber. Under the microscope the Neubauer chamber contains a central grid of a known area and, used with the correct coverslip, holds a fixed volume of semen. To assist in the count, sperm are usually immobilized and diluted using a buffer containing 3.5% formalin. When settled, only whole sperm are counted, ignoring headless sperm, 'pin-heads' or tail-less heads. Where possible, and for an accurate count, at least 200 sperm should be counted from both sides of the haemocytometer. If the difference between the two counts is greater than 10%, the chamber must be re-loaded and the count repeated. The mean should be reported. The sperm concentration is expressed in millions per millilitre ($\times 10^6$/ml) of semen and the total sperm/ejaculate is reported in millions ($\times 10^6$) per ejaculate.

Examination of azoospermic and severely oligozoospermic samples

In cases of severe oligozoospermia (very low sperm concentration), where very few sperm are present in each microscope field, accurate assessment of sperm concentration may be impossible. In which case 'concentrating' the sperm within the sample by centrifugation and removal of the bulk of the seminal fluid may help. The final sperm concentration should be reported based on the original total ejaculate volume, and motility and morphology assessment can be made on the pellet. If no sperm are observed in a wet semen preparation, it is extremely important to confirm the presence or absence of sperm, since such an azoospermic sample may in reality be very severely oligozoospermic. The observation of only a few sperm in a semen sample is therapeutically extremely important since it is now possible to treat such patients by intra-cytoplasmic sperm injection (ICSI). Similarly, in patients who have elected vasectomy as a method of sterilization, the detection of any sperm in the semen sample is critical, particularly since sperm from such patients remain functionally competent for long periods of time. Such samples again should be examined following centrifugation as described above. The pellet of material obtained should be carefully examined and if possible a stained preparation of the pellet material should be obtained as a permanent record.

Assessment of sperm morphology

The classification of normal and abnormal semen samples based on sperm morphology, has been, and remains controversial[4]. The lack of universal standardized criteria for normal/abnormal sperm have in the past led to varying conclusions about the predictive value of morphology with regard to conception. However, a degree of uniformity has been established with the adoption by many centres of the Tygerberg 'strict' criteria for morphology evaluation[17]. In doing so, centres are beginning to report sperm morphology with significant prognostic value in relation to both natural and assisted conception[17–19].

Normal sperm morphology has been defined from studies of spermatozoa recovered from the female tract, especially those found at the endocervix, and are defined as follows: (a) head — should be uniformly oval with a length of between 4.0 and 5.0 µm and width of 2.5–3.5 µm. The acrosomal region should occupy about 40% of the head region; (b) midpiece — should be slender <1/3 width of the head and about the same length. There should be no cytoplasmic droplets of larger than a third of the head size, around the head and midpiece; (c) tail — should be single, thin and uncoiled and about 50 µm long (Fig. 27.1).

Common morphological defects include: (a) head shape/size defects, such as large, small, tapering, pyriform, amorphous, vacuolated, multiple heads or any combination of these (Fig. 27.1); (b) neck and midpiece defects, such as non-inserted or bent tail, distended/irregular/bent midpiece, thin midpiece (no mitochondrial sheath), absent tail (free or loose heads) or any combination of these; (c) tail defects, such as short, multiple, hairpin, broken, irregular width, coiled tails, tails with terminal droplets or any combination of these; (d) cytoplasmic droplets, retained cytoplasm, which is greater than one-third the size of a normal sperm head.

Differential counts should be performed on a fixed-stained preparation, using bright-field microscopy and ×100 oil immersion objectives. Most classification systems have been devised using this method and it does have the major advantage that a permanent record of an individual sample can be made. The most commonly used stain is the Papanicolaou stain (Pap stain) which permits clear definition between acrosomal and post acrosomal regions of the head, midpiece and tail (Fig. 27.1).

Sperm vitality

A sperm which is moving, no matter how feebly, is clearly 'alive'. However, without a specific test, it is unknown whether immotile sperm are alive or dead. If the percentage of immotile sperm exceeds 50%, then the proportion of live spermatozoa should be determined. This is important since certain conditions exist (e.g. immotile cilia syndrome/Kartagener's syndrome) where all the sperm are immotile, may be viable and able to achieve a pregnancy using assisted reproductive techniques such as ICSI.

Sperm vitality is assessed, using tests which determine the functional integrity of the plasma membrane, such as the hypo-osmotic swelling (HOS) test or by dye exclusion or using supra-vital stains such as eosin. Live spermatozoa with intact plasma membranes will swell in the presence of a hypo-osmotic solution as a result of an influx of water. In contrast, dead cells fail to swell. Live sperm are then identified by the coiling of the tail. This method is of particular use in embryology laboratories, which may not wish to use potentially hazardous dyes in an assisted reproduction setting.

Antisperm antibodies (ASAs)

As spermatozoa are first produced at puberty, many years after the induction of immunological tolerance, they are not recognizable as 'self' and can therefore elicit an immune response in the reproductive male. In the male, antibodies usually of immunoglobulin classes IgA and/or IgG, can manifest themselves in the seminal plasma, on spermatozoa and in the blood. Their incidence in men attending infertility clinics is between five and ten[20].

Surface sperm antibodies, usually of the IgG and IgA classes, have been found to affect sperm function in a number of ways (see below), although conflicting results show that their impact on conception rates is yet to be fully determined. It is thought that sperm antibodies can cause agglutination of the sperm, reduce their motility[21]; impede progression of the sperm through the cervical mucus (male antibodies)[22], interfere with the sperm/egg binding process[23] and/or enhance sperm killing by phagocytic leucocytes[24].

Testing for the presence of ASAs is therefore recommended as an adjunct to the conventional semen analysis. The basic principal behind the ASA testing involves the use of anti-IgG and anti-IgA coated particles, which bind to the ASA coating the spermatozoa. These can be simply visualized and enumerated (usually as a percentage) under phase contrast microscopy. The simplest and most commonly used method for the detection of ASAs is the MAR (mixed antiglobulin reaction) test and can be

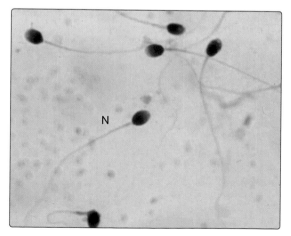

Fig. 27.1   Papanicolaou-stained semen smear. N denotes normal spermatozoa. (Courtesy of R. Menkveld)

carried out using a commercially available kit (Conception Technologies, San Diego USA, or Fertipro, Belgium). Alternatives, such as the immunobead test (IBT), are also widely used, producing comparable results. Motile spermatozoa (preferably 200) should be scored for adherence to the latex particles and those bound expressed as a percentage. ASAs adhering to one region of the sperm (head, midpiece or tail) should be noted. It is widely accepted that unless the titre is at least 50%, the result is unlikely to be clinically significant[5]. Severely oligozoospermic and/or severely asthenozoospermic semen samples are therefore often unsuitable for testing, in which case, it may be wise to use an indirect ASA test. The basic principle of the indirect ASA test involves the incubation of highly motile sperm in a test fluid, e.g. serum, seminal plasma and cervical mucus. If antibodies are present in the test fluid they will coat the (already proven) ASA negative donor sperm which can then be tested using the Sperm Mar test as before.

External quality assurance

With the increasing requirement for laboratory accreditation and the emphasis placed on QA by the World Health Organisation[5], a comprehensive programme in the andrology laboratory should be mandatory. In order to obtain meaningful information from the laboratory, careful consideration must be given to: the nature of the laboratory methods employed, the technical competence of the operator and the systems in place for monitoring the effectiveness of both, i.e. quality assurance (QA). Many andrology laboratories still ignore the need for QA despite an increasingly large body of evidence suggesting that there is considerable variation in results within and between technicians and within the same laboratory, as well as significant differences between laboratories[25,26].

The experience of the UKNEQAS (UK National External Quality Assurance Scheme) quality control scheme (below), suggests that after an initial learning curve, laboratories improve, once centres receive feedback from the scheme organizers and re-evaluate their own methods. The UKNEQAS is one of the few national andrology quality assessment schemes operating in the world. There is still, however, a high degree of variability between centres examining the same semen sample, although the vast majority use WHO criteria[27] but this is not particular to the UK[28]. These are international issues and hopefully the problems identified can be used as a basis for improving the quality of semen assessments world-wide.

Sperm preparation methods

Sperm preparation is an essential component of the work carried out in the modern assisted conception laboratory. Effective sperm preparation aims not only to separate seminal fluid from spermatozoa but also to enrich the sample with more rapidly motile and morphologically normal sperm, specifically for use in procedures such as intra-uterine insemination (IUI), gamete intra-fallopian

transfer (GIFT), *in-vitro* fertilization (IVF) and intra-cytoplasmic sperm injection (ICSI). In many centres, sperm preparation is also used as an adjunct to the basic semen analysis, often helping to decide upon the most appropriate treatment group for the patient.

The two most widely used methods for sperm preparation are: the swim-up, which as it implies, separates sperm purely on their ability to swim; and density gradient centrifugation, in which the highly motile sperm fraction is separated from the dysfunctional sperm by virtue of its density[29].

Swim-up or sperm migration

Semen is simply covered by a layer of medium, e.g. Earle's balanced salt solution (EBSS), into which highly motile sperm migrate, leaving behind other cell contamination, e.g. leucocytes, germinal cells, immotile/dead sperm. Although it remains a very popular method in some assisted reproduction centres, the swim-up has been largely superseded by density gradient centrifugation (see below). The basic method is described in Table 27.3 (Fig. 27.2).

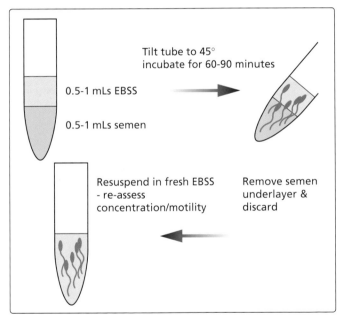

Fig. 27.2 Sperm swim-up.

Table 27.3 Swim-up or sperm migration method

1. Gently layer 1 ml of medium (EBSS), supplemented with 5% serum and 0.1% HEPES over fresh semen (if a clean preparation is not obtained try centrifugation for 20 s). This has a layering effect and allows clean separation between the two layers.
2. Incubate for 1 h at 37°C.
3. Remove supernatant, and place in a fresh tube. If very highly viscous, remove the bottom seminal layer by placing a fine pipette at the bottom of the tube. This will result in a cleaner preparation.
4. Mix well, assess sperm density, motility and morphology.
5. A wash step is recommended at the end if a clean preparation is not obtained.

Table 27.4   Density gradient centrifugation method

1. Pipette 1 ml 90% Percoll into a clean sterile tube (those with a conical base give the best pellet).
2. Gently layer 1 ml 45% Percoll on top of the above, taking care not to disturb the 45%/90% interface between the two.
3. Layer 1–2 ml fresh liquefied semen over the top of the 45% and centrifuge at 500 g for 20 min.
4. Discard supernatant and resuspend pellet at base of the 90% fraction in 1 ml fresh culture media (EBSS).

Density gradient centrifugation

A density gradient is formed usually by layering a 45% solution of a density gradient medium over one of 90% (or alternatively 40% and 80% layers). Percoll, a colloidal suspension of PVP coated silica particles has been used extensively. However, as it is licensed for *in-vitro* use only, it can only be used for diagnostic purposes. Alternatives are available specifically for clinical use, using silane instead of PVP in colloidal suspension. Functionally normal, motile sperm which have higher density, pellet at the base of the 90% fraction, at the bottom of the tube/flask, whereas abnormal spermatozoa (with low density) and round cells are trapped at the interface between the 45% and 90% layers. There is evidence to suggest that for poorer sperm samples, density gradients are more flexible and should be the method of choice, with sperm concentration in a series of 'mini-preps', a widely used technique in many laboratories. In addition, sperm collected from the 90% fraction appear to have fewer nuclear DNA anomalies, as measured by *in situ* nick translation, and a lower percentage of Chromomycin A_3 positive sperm, which indirectly correlates with the presence of protamine in the nuclear chromatin[30], than those harvested by swim-up, when compared with the raw, unprepared sample (see Table 27.4 and Fig. 27.3).

Sperm function tests

There is a plethora of putative sperm function tests[31,32]. However, many suggested assays of sperm function have been shown, with subsequent rigorous testing, to be of little clinical value. There are three assays, which have stood the test of time and can be regarded as robust and reliable tests of sperm function: zona-binding assay, acrosome reaction and cervical mucus penetration test.

The zona-binding assay examines the ability of human sperm to bind to the human zona. This is regarded as the ultimate test of sperm function and a large number of studies have shown it to be reliable. In fact, one cause of sperm dysfunction is an inability of the cells to bind to the zona. Often this occurs in men with otherwise normal semen and thus the zona-binding assay is particularly useful. While an excellent test of sperm function, the limited availability of spare human zona to perform the experiments means this assay can only be of limited use on a routine basis. The acrosome reaction assay is also

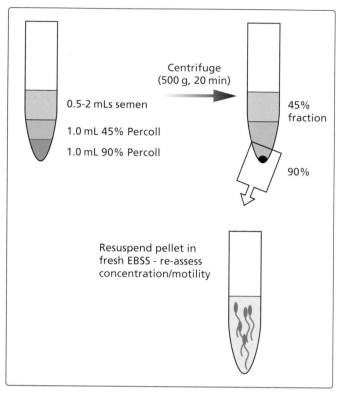

0.5-2 mLs semen

1.0 mL 45% Percoll

1.0 mL 90% Percoll

Centrifuge (500 g, 20 min)

45% fraction

90%

Resuspend pellet in fresh EBSS - re-assess concentration/motility

Fig. 27.3   Density gradient centrifugation.

diagnostic of sperm function. Basically a spermatozoon that cannot undergo the acrosome reaction cannot fertilize an egg. This assay is technically difficult to perform and requires specialized materials/equipment nevertheless it is a good assay of sperm function with a number of studies supporting its use in a clinical setting. The last of the three sperm function tests is the oldest one, i.e. the penetration of sperm into cervical mucus. Many formats of this test exist including post-coital test and Kremer test. The ability of sperm to successfully penetrate cervical mucus is critical to subsequent fertility. In some cases men can have apparently normal semen yet their sperm are unable to penetrate cervical mucus. The difficulty in obtaining cervical mucus and the problems standardizing testing makes the assay confined to specialist laboratories, however, substitutes for mucus, such as hyaluronic acid make routine testing a reality and this test remains the most cost effective and easy sperm function test to perform.

New methods of semen analysis

In order to determine the functional capacity of the sperm it is necessary to use specific tests. A greater understanding of how spermatozoa are formed and function will lead to the investigation of spermatozoa at different levels, nuclear, organelle and cytoskeletal, using new diagnostic methods. A number of defects have already been reported in human sperm mitochondria centrioles, however, there are few patients in these categories. One form of analysis, which is likely to be of widespread use, is analysis of the integrity of the sperm nuclear chromatin. Links between sperm chromatin defects and decreased fertilization have been reported in the context of assisted reproduction techniques[33–37]. In addition, numerous studies have shown that spermatozoa with abnormal nuclear chromatin organization are more frequent in sub-fertile or infertile men[33,35,37–39].

Evidence of a relationship between sperm nuclear DNA integrity and fertility has recently been reported in two studies, which have used the sperm chromatin structure assay (SCSA), proposing its future use as a prognostic factor[40,41]. The SCSA measures the susceptibility of sperm nuclear DNA to heat or acid induced denaturation *in situ*. The Evenson study[40] found that men who had an SCSA value of greater or equal to 30%, had difficulties in achieving a pregnancy. The Spano study[41] reported similar results showing that the SCSA was highly indicative of male subfertility, regardless of the concentration, motility and morphology of spermatozoa. This type of test is still in the developmental stages.

Summary

A comprehensive high quality semen analysis is the cornerstone of infertility investigations. However, it is important to recognize, that at least in the UK and USA, where detailed information is available, many laboratories are simply incapable of performing a basic accurate semen assessment as their quality control and assurance methods are completely inadequate. It is imperative that high standards of laboratory practice are followed when performing a semen analysis.

Acknowledgements

The authors would like to thank Julie Edwards for typing assistance with this chapter and the Assisted Conception Unit, Birmingham Women's Hospital, for its support.

References

1. Hull M G R. Infertility treatment: relative effectiveness of conventional and assisted conception methods. *Hum Reprod* 1992; **7**: 785–796

2. World Health Organization 1992 *WHO Laboratory Manual for the Examination of Human Semen and Semen–Cervical Mucus Interaction*. 3rd edn: Cambridge: Cambridge University Press

3. Royal College of Obstetricians & Gynaecologists 1992 *Infertility: Guidelines for Practice*. London: RCOG Press

4. Tomlinson M J, Kessopoulou E, Barratt C L R. The Diagnostic and Prognostic Value of Traditional Semen Parameters. *J Androl* 1999; **20**: 588–593

5. World Health Organization 1999 *WHO Laboratory Manual for the Examination of Human Semen and Semen–Cervical Mucus Interaction*, 4th edn. Cambridge: Cambridge University Press

6. Barratt C L R, Cooke I D 1993 *Donor Insemination*. Cambridge: Cambridge University Press, p 231

7. Mortimer D 1994 *Practical Laboratory Andrology*, New York: Oxford University Press

8. Glover T D, Barratt C L R. 1999 *Male Fertility and Infertility*. Cambridge: Cambridge University Press, p 320

9. Barratt C L R, Kessopoulou E, Thompson L A, Tomlinson M T. The functional significance of leukocytes in human reproduction. *Repro Med Rev* 1992; **1**: 115–129

10. Human Fertilisation and Embryology Authority 1991 *Code of Practice*. London: HFEA

11. Hargreave T B, Elton R A. Is conventional sperm analysis of any use? *Br J Urol* 1983; **55**: 774–779

12. Barratt C L R, Tomlinson M J, Cooke I D. The prognostic significance of computerised motility analysis for in vivo fertility. *Fertil Steril* 1993; **60**: 520–525

13. Tomlinson M J, Amissah-Arthur J B, Thompson K A et al. Prognostic indicators for intra-uterine insemination: Statistical model for IUI success. *Hum Reprod* 1996; **11**: 1892–1896

14. Aitken J, Kraus C, Buckingham D. Relationships between biochemical markers for residual sperm cytoplasm, reactive oxygen species generation and the presence of leukocytes and precursor germ cells in human sperm suspensions. *Mol Reprod Devel* 1994; **39**(3): 268–279

15. Gomez E, Aitken J. Impact of in vitro fertilisation culture media on peroxidative damage to human spermatozoa. *Fertil Steril* 1996; **65**: 880–882

16. Tomlinson M J, Barratt C L R, Cooke I D. Prospective study of leukocytes and leukocyte subpopulations in semen suggests they are not a cause of male infertility. *Fertil Steril* 1993; **60**: 1069–1075

17. Eggert-Kruse W, Schwarz H, Rohr G et al. Sperm morphology assessment using strict criteria and male fertility under in-vivo conditions of conception. *Hum Reprod* 1996; **11**: 139–146

18. Kruger T F, Menkveld R, Stander F S H et al. Sperm morphologic features as a prognostic factor in in vitro fertilization. *Fertil Steril* 1986; **46**: 1118–1122

19. Kruger T F, Acosta A A, Simmons K F et al. Predictive value of abnormal sperm morphology in in vitro fertilization. *Fertil Steril* 1988; **49**: 112–117

20. Matson P L 1994 Detection and clinical significance of sperm antibodies. In: Grudzinskas J G, Yovich J L, Chart T eds. *Cambridge Reviews in Human Reproduction*. Cambridge: Cambridge University Press

21. Barratt C L R, Havelock L M, Harrison P E, Cooke I D. Antisperm antibodies are more prevalent in men with low sperm motility. *Int J Androl* 1989; **12**: 110–116

22. Menge A C, Beitner O. Interrelationships among semen characteristics, antisperm antibodies and cervical mucus penetration assays in infertile human couples. *Fertil Steril* 1989; **51**: 486–492

23. Lui D Y, Clark G N, Baker H W G. Inhibition of human sperm-zona pellucida and sperm-oolemma binding by antisperm antibodies. *Fertil Steril* 1991; **55**: 440–442

24. London S N, Haney A F, Weinberg J F. Macrophages and infertility: enhancement of human macrophage-mediated sperm killing by antisperm antibodies. *Fertil Steril* 1985; **43**: 274–278

25. Matson P L. External quality assessment for semen analysis and sperm antibody detection: results of a pilot scheme. *Hum Reprod* 1995; **10**: 620–625

26. Clements S, Cooke I D, Barratt C L R. Implementing comprehensive quality control in the andrology laboratory. *Hum Reprod* 1995; **10**: 2096–2106

27. World Health Organization 1992 *WHO Laboratory Manual for the Examination of Human Semen and Semen–Cervical Mucus Interaction*, 5th edn. Cambridge: Cambridge University Press

28. Keel B A, Quinn P, Schmidt C F Jr et al. Results of the American Association of Bioanalysts national proficiency testing programme in andrology. *Hum Reprod* 2000; **15**: 680–686

29. Mortimer D. Sperm preparation methods. *J Androl* 2000; **21**: 357–366

30. Sakkas D, Manicardi G C, Tomlinson M et al. The use of density gradient centrifugation techniques and the swim-up method to separate spermatozoa with chromatin and nuclear DNA anomalies. *Hum Reprod* 2000; **15**: 1112–1116

31. Muller C H. Rationale, interpretation, validation, and uses of sperm function tests. *J Androl* 2000; **21**: 10–30

32 Oehninger S, Franken D R, Sayed E *et al.* Sperm function assays and their predictive value for fertilization outcome in IVF therapy: a meta-analysis. *Hum Reprod Update* 2000; **6**: 160–168

33 Bianchi P G, Manicardi G C, Urner F *et al.* Chromatin packaging and morphology in ejaculated human spermatozoa: evidence of hidden anomalies in normal spermatozoa. *Mol Hum Reprod* 1996; **2**:139–144

34 Sakkas D, Urner F, Bianchi P G *et al.* Sperm chromatin anomalies can influence decondensation after intracytoplasmic sperm injection. *Hum Reprod* 1996; **11**: 837–843

35 Sun J G, Jurisicova A, Casper R F. Detection of deoxyribonucleic acid fragmentation in human sperm: correlation with fertilization in vitro. *Biol Reprod* 1997; **56**: 602–607

36 Lopes S, Sun J G, Jurisicova A *et al.* Sperm deoxyribonucleic acid fragmentation is increased in poor-quality semen samples and correlates with failed fertilization in intracytoplasmic sperm injection. *Fertil Steril* 1998; **69**: 528–532

37 Esterhuizen A D, Franken D R, Lourens J G *et al.* Sperm chromatin packaging as an indicator of in-vitro fertilization rates. *Hum Reprod* 2000; **15**: 657–661

38 Evenson D P, Darzynkiewicz Z, Melamed M R. Relation of mammalian sperm chromatin heterogeneity to fertility. *Science* 1980; **210**: 1131–1133

39 Irvine D S, Twigg J P, Gordon E L *et al.* DNA integrity in human spermatozoa: relationships with semen quality. *J Androl* 2000; **21**: 33–44

40 Evenson D P, Jost L K, Marshall D *et al.* Utility of the sperm chromatin structure assay as a diagnostic and prognostic tool in the human fertility clinic. *Hum Reprod* 1999; **14**:1039–1049

41 Spano M, Bonde J P, Hjollund H I *et al.* Sperm chromatin damage impairs human fertility. The Danish First Pregnancy Planner Study Team. *Fertil Steril* 2000; **73**: 43–50

Female genital tract

28 Normal vulva, vagina and cervix: hormonal and inflammatory conditions

Mathilde E. Boon and Winifred Gray

Introduction

A dramatic development in the history of cytology took place in the first half of the twentieth century, with the discovery that cancer of the cervix could be recognized by the presence of tumour cells in cytological samples from the vagina. As described in the Introduction to this book, the finding was reported independently in 1927 by Professor Aurel Babeş in Romania, and in the following year in the USA by Dr George Papanicolaou[1]. It was clear that in some cases the tumour was at a very early stage clinically, but the significance of this observation in relation to prevention of cervical carcinoma was not pursued, largely because the concept of preinvasive cancer was not widely accepted.

When Papanicolaou and Traut published their treatise *Diagnosis of Uterine Cancer by the Vaginal Smear* in 1943[2], the work was viewed more favourably. Shortly thereafter, screening for precancerous cervical mucosal changes in normal women was actively promoted in North America and parts of Europe. Improvements in sampling of cells by taking smears directly from the cervix soon followed, aided by the introduction of Ayre's spatula in 1947[3].

Initially there was a feeling that the problem of deaths from cervical cancer would be solved quite easily. However mortality did not fall as quickly as expected, even in countries with well organized screening programmes[4]. Factors such as the need to achieve full population coverage, the problems of sampling in smear taking, and the standard of screening in laboratories had all been underestimated[5]. Added to this, there has been a rise in the incidence of precancerous lesions of the cervix from the late 1960s, making screening programmes appear ineffective.

Now that the difficulties associated with cervical screening are more widely recognized, there is evidence of falling mortality in most countries with well developed screening programmes as problems are addressed[6,7]. Tragically, in many of the third world countries where the incidence of cervical cancer is much higher, the resources for comprehensive population screening are simply not available.

Cytological examination of material from the female genital tract is not confined to the diagnosis of precancerous changes in the cervix. Reactive and infective conditions of the cervix and vagina can be recognized, as can tumours other than the commonest type, squamous cell carcinoma and its precursors. Cervical smears may include cells exfoliated from the body of the uterus, and even at times from the fallopian tubes and ovaries when pathology is present. Although other sampling methods are now in use for diagnosis of conditions at these more remote sites, the cervical smear procedure still dominates the field of investigation of gynaecological patients by cytology.

Cell samples from the lower genital tract are usually obtained directly by scraping or brushing the lining epithelium. The cells collected in this way are a mixture of those which have been mechanically dislodged by smear taking, and cells exfoliated spontaneously as part of the continuous shedding of superficial layers of normal mucosa.

The epithelial surfaces of the vagina, cervix and endometrium are influenced by the concentration of circulating ovarian hormones. Surface mucosal cells undergo regular cyclical changes throughout a woman's reproductive life and for longer if hormone replacement therapy is given. Thus a thorough knowledge of the gross and microscopic anatomy of the female genital tract and the effect of hormones is essential for interpretation of the cytological findings.

This chapter will discuss the normal findings in smears from the cervix, vulva and vagina, the cyclical variations and the changes induced by infections, reactive processes or iatrogenic effects. Cytological findings in neoplasia of the cervix are the subjects of chapters to follow.

Gross and microscopic anatomy

The basic structure of the female genital tract is depicted diagrammatically in Figure 28.1, illustrating the different types of lining epithelium seen in cytological samples from various sites.

Vulva

The labia majora and minora of the vulva are covered by keratinizing squamous epithelium (Fig. 28.2A), which undergoes very little hormonal change during the menstrual cycle. The outer surfaces of the labia majora are hair-bearing. The inner surfaces are free of hair, but have many sebaceous glands and apocrine sweat glands, the secretions of which provide protection against infection and local damage to the skin.

The clitoris is also covered by epidermis, and is devoid of skin appendages, being instead richly supplied with sensory nerve endings. The labia show pigmentation from the age of puberty, diminishing on the inner aspect of the labia minora where only a thin layer of keratin is present. This epithelium extends to cover the vestibule as far as the hymen. The vagina and the urethra open on to the vestibule of the vulva. Mucin secreting glands are present on either side of the vaginal introitus, including Bartholin's glands, which are situated in the lower vaginal wall, providing protection and lubrication.

Vagina

Developmentally, the upper two thirds of the vagina is formed by fusion of the two mullerian ducts *in utero*. The tube thus formed differentiates into the uterus and cervix above and unites distally with the urogenital sinus to form the vagina. Thus the lower third of the vagina has a different embryological origin from the upper two-thirds. The importance of this dual derivation lies in the fact that the mullerian epithelium in the upper two-thirds is initially columnar in type, but undergoes metaplasia *in utero* to squamous mucosa on exposure to the acid pH of the vagina. Normally, the change to squamous epithelium is complete, but the process may be interrupted, leading to persistence of glandular tissue in the adult vagina, a condition known as vaginal adenosis (see Fig. 28.105).

Under normal conditions, the vagina is lined by stratified squamous non-keratinizing epithelium throughout (Fig. 28.2B), usually showing no hair follicles, sweat glands or sebaceous glands to weaken its surface. The mucosa is subject to cyclical changes under the influence of the sex hormones.

Cervix

The cervix is a cylindrical fibromuscular structure of variable length, within which lies the endocervical canal connecting the body of the uterus at the internal os with the vagina at the external os. The lower portion of the cervix protrudes into the vagina, forming the anterior, posterior and two lateral fornices in the upper vagina where pooling of secretions and exfoliated cells occurs. The outer aspect of

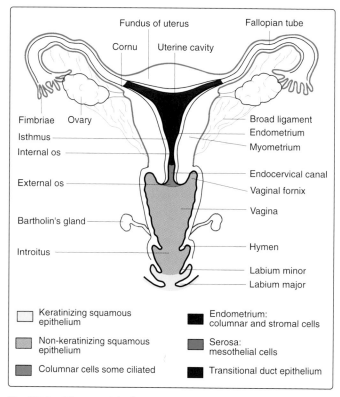

Fig. 28.1 Diagram of the female genital tract demonstrating the main structures and the types of epithelium covering the surface accessible to sampling directly or indirectly by exfoliative cytology. (Courtesy of Professor D Coleman and Mrs P Chapman, with permission from Butterworths, London)

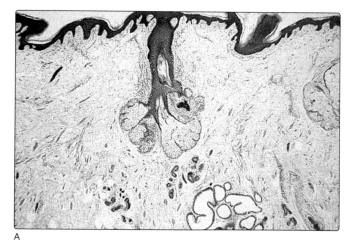
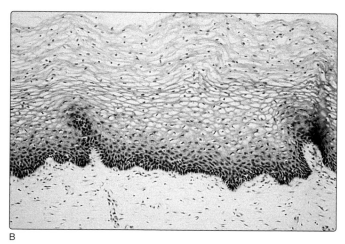

Fig. 28.2 (A) Vulval skin showing stratified squamous keratinizing epithelium with skin appendages. (H&E × LP) (B) Vaginal squamous mucosa is not normally keratinized and is hormone sensitive, in contrast to vulval skin. The squamous cell cytoplasm is clear in this section due to the presence of glycogen. (H&E × MP)

the cervix, known as the ectocervix or portio vaginalis, is covered by squamous mucosa in continuity with vaginal epithelium distally and with the lining of the endocervix at or near the external os (Fig. 28.3).

The endocervical canal is not exposed to the vaginal pH and therefore retains its glandular lining of tall columnar epithelium, with an inconspicuous layer of reserve cells beneath. The glandular mucosa forms branching crypts that extend into the stroma of the cervix in a racemose pattern for a distance of up to 5 mm, their orifices facing distally. The canal itself is narrow, being only a few millimetres wide, and in health is filled by a plug of mucus. During the menstrual cycle the physical properties of the cervical mucus change. Prior to ovulation the mucus is dilute, and when spread on to a slide and dried it forms a fern-like pattern (see Fig. 28.17). After ovulation the mucus becomes thicker and no longer demonstrates ferning.

It will be apparent from the above description that there is a point of junction between the squamous epithelium of the ectocervix and the lining of the endocervical canal. This meeting point is referred to as the squamocolumnar junction. The changes that occur in this area are of crucial significance in cervical pathology.

Squamocolumnar junction and transformation zone

Major changes in the size and shape of the cervix take place during reproductive life. Before puberty, the squamocolumnar junction forms the outer boundary of the endocervical glands, known as the 'original' squamocolumnar junction, coinciding with the site of the external os.

After puberty, the location of the squamocolumnar junction changes as the cervix alters in shape. The endocervical mucosa of the lower canal, including the underlying crypts, is everted and comes to lie on the ectocervical aspect of the cervix, resulting in an ectropion or ectopy (Fig. 28.4). An ectropion is clinically visible as a reddened zone extending out from the external os. It is sometimes mistakenly called an erosion although no actual ulceration is present and the condition is physiological.

Endocervical eversion is followed by progressive metaplasia of the exposed mucosa to less specialized more protective squamous epithelium under the influence of the vaginal pH. The term metaplasia refers to a change from one type of epithelium to another. The metaplastic process arises in the reserve cell population that normally replenishes the columnar epithelium. Instead, these reserve cells differentiate as immature squamous metaplastic cells beneath the single layer of columnar cells on the surface (Fig. 28.5A).

The metaplastic layers increase and mature progressively to form a new normal squamous mucosa indistinguishable from the original squamous epithelium of the ectocervix. The underlying endocervical crypts remain facing on to the ectocervix as a permanent marker of the site of the original

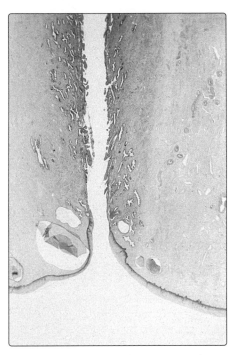

Fig. 28.3 Section of adult cervix showing the ectocervix covered by non-keratinizing squamous epithelium, the external os and the endocervical canal running up towards the body of the uterus. Endocervical crypts face downwards and are lined by a single layer of columnar epithelial cells. (H&E × LP)

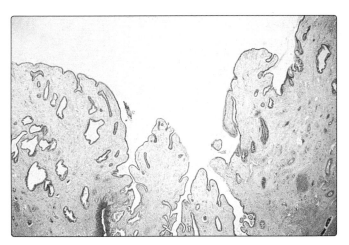

Fig. 28.4 Ectropion. At menarche and during certain phases of reproductive life, the squamocolumnar junction is everted so that the endocervical glands come to lie on the outer aspect of the cervix, producing an ectropion. (H&E × MP)

squamocolumnar junction, which can be recognized colposcopically as well as in histological section (Fig. 28.5B). Glands with orifices obstructed by the metaplastic process are prone to distend with mucus, even becoming visible macroscopically as rounded nodules on the ectocervix, known as nabothian follicles.

The extent to which eversion of the endocervix occurs varies in different women and the new junction may be asymmetrical in relation to the external os, with ectropion

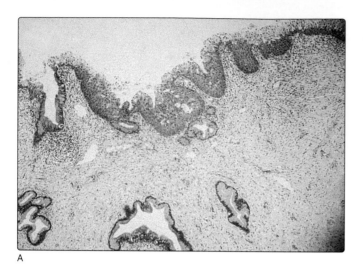

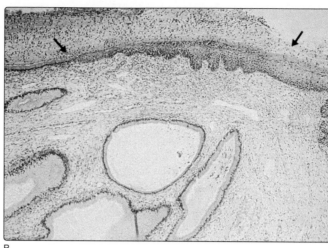

A

B

Fig. 28.5 (A) Reserve cell hyperplasia is seen beneath everted columnar epithelium. The cells are starting to show multilayered immature squamous metaplasia, forming a transformation zone. (H&E × MP) (B) The transformation zone (between arrows) is now maturing but its site of origin is marked by the position of the first endocervical gland. Note the plug of mucus covering the surface. (H&E × MP)

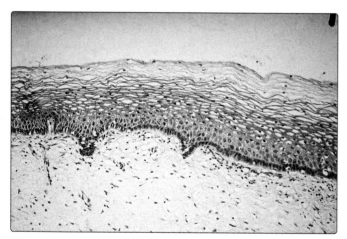

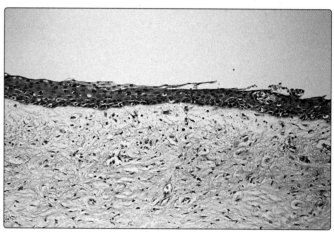

Fig. 28.6 Stratified squamous mucosa from the cervix during reproductive life shows a distinct row of primitive basal cells resting on a thin basement membrane. Above this there is progressive maturation from 3–4 parabasal cell layers to an intermediate cell layer with more cytoplasm and preserved nuclear structure, while the uppermost superficial cells have condensed pyknotic nuclei and voluminous cytoplasm. (H&E × HP)

Fig. 28.7 Post-menopausal atrophy of ectocervical squamous mucosa. The epithelium is thinned, with crowding of squamous cells due to their reduced cytoplasm. The basal layer is still distinct and polarization of cells is visible. (H&E × HP)

covering one or both sides of the ectocervix, even extending on to the vaginal walls. Ectropion is liable to recur with certain hormonal events. The most obvious of these is pregnancy, during which ectopy is a common finding due to enlargement of the cervix under the influence of progesterone. Some types of oral contraceptive therapy have a similar effect. After the menopause the cervix shrinks and the squamocolumnar junction migrates into the endocervical canal.

The area of metaplastic epithelium proximal to the original squamocolumnar junction is referred to as the transformation zone since it is an area of epithelial instability. Immature metaplastic cells appear to carry an extra risk of neoplastic change. It is said that the

transformation zone 'precisely defines the field of neoplastic potential'.

Structure of stratified squamous epithelium
(Figs 28.6, 28.7)

The germinal layer is composed of a single layer of small regular cells adhering to a basement membrane and showing signs of active growth. These undifferentiated cells are referred to as the basal cells. Above this layer it is possible to distinguish parabasal cells, immature and crowded, lying two to three cells deep. These cells mature into an intermediate layer of variable thickness in which the cells have more cytoplasm and the nuclei still show a recognizable chromatin pattern. The cells in this layer are bound to each other by intercellular cytoplasmic bridges.

In fully mature cervical squamous mucosa there is a superficial layer consisting of cells that do not normally mature any further. Intercellular bridges are not highly developed at this level so that the cell bonds are weaker. Superficial cells are actually dead or dying and exfoliate spontaneously. Sometimes a thin layer of cells with dark cytoplasmic keratohyaline granules may be present in histological sections, formed of the cells that precede keratinization, but a keratinized layer is not seen under normal conditions.

Mucosal thickness depends upon hormonal status as the parabasal, intermediate and superficial layers are all hormonally responsive. Under the influence of oestrogen a superficial layer develops in about four days. This multilayered epithelium provides a barrier against external injuries and stores nutrients in the form of glycogen.

Keratinization

Keratin and keratinization are terms that cause confusion. Keratin refers to a group of fibrous proteins that occur in epidermal derivatives such as hair and nails. Keratin proteins were used by Corey and Pauling[8] in 1955 to establish the first three-dimensional model of a biochemical substance in the form of an alpha helix. Since then considerable progress has been made concerning the biochemical and immunological characterization of keratin.

It is now known that this family of proteins form part of the cytoskeleton of all epithelial cells. Molecular weights of these proteins range from 40–68 kD. Based on their molecular size and isoelectric point, they have been divided into acidic and basic subfamilies and given numbers from 1 to 19[9,10]. Members of the acidic subfamily have a corresponding member in the basic subfamily, usually expressed as keratin pairs. The expression of keratins in epithelial cells depends on cell type, the degree of differentiation and the pattern of growth (Table 28.1).

Commercially available antibodies directed against these different keratin proteins have offered the pathologist an approach to tumour classification, since their cell specific distribution is in general, well preserved in neoplasms. Thus, with the immunoperoxidase technique, keratins 1, 2 and 10 are found in keratinizing squamous cell carcinoma

of the skin and keratins 8 and 18 are detected in all adenocarcinomas. Non-keratinizing cervical squamous cell carcinoma may express keratins 5, 6, 7, 8, 13, 14, 15, 17, 18 and 19. Keratinizing cervical squamous cell carcinoma lacks keratins 7, 8 and 18. In cervical adenocarcinomas expression of keratins 7, 8, 17, 18 and 19 is found[11].

Confusion arises because pathologists refer to 'keratinization' as a morphological process in which cells synthesize large amounts of cytoplasmic keratin, while the nucleus of the cell becomes pyknotic and disappears, leaving the husk of the cell behind as an anucleate squame. In stratified squamous epithelium, synthesis of keratin fibres actually begins when cells are still in the basal layers[10]. As epithelial cells differentiate and proceed to migrate to the upper layers of an epithelial surface, increasing amounts of keratin are produced.

The amount of keratin in a cell relates to how rapidly the cell differentiates and the type of epithelium in which it occurs. Cells of mucous membranes, such as the mouth, usually show little keratinization whereas the cells of intensely cornified epidermis may consist almost entirely of keratin fibres[12]. We have retained the pathological description of keratinization in this chapter, but on the understanding that the difference is quantitative and that all epithelial cells contain keratin in some form.

Cytological identification of epithelial cells

Identification of squamous cells from the various layers described above is a basic step in the interpretation of cervical smears. The Papanicolaou stain is ideally suited for this purpose, having been devised originally to assess hormonal status according to the degree of cytoplasmic maturation in vaginal squamous cells. Columnar and metaplastic cells are identified by a combination of morphology and staining reactions.

Two of the components of the Papanicolaou stain are cytoplasmic stains: eosin, which stains superficial cells pink or orange, and light green, which is taken up by the cytoplasm of all of the less mature cells. Because they are alcohol-based, the cytoplasmic staining is particularly delicate and translucent, unless keratinization is present, when the staining becomes densely orangeophilic. Thus the full range of squamous cells can be identified by a combination of morphological and tinctorial features. The nuclei are stained by haematoxylin. Good fixation is an essential prerequisite for successful use of the Papanicolaou stain, particularly for revealing nuclear detail. The smears illustrated in this chapter are all stained by the Papanicolaou method except where stated otherwise.

Basal cells

These small primitive cells are parent to all the cells in the squamous mucosa that migrate to the surface, die and exfoliate. They are difficult to recognize in a smear with

Table 28.1   Keratin expression in various epithelia

Epithelia	Acidic	Basic
Keratinization (skin)	10	1, 2
Sweat duct epithelium	9	–
Corneal epithelium	12	3
Non-keratinized squamous epithelium	13	4
All stratified epithelia	14, 15	5
Hyperplastic keratinocytes	16	6
Simple and some stratified epithelia	17	7
Simple epithelia	18, 19	8

confidence and are likely to be sampled only rarely due to their deep position in the mucosa and their firm attachment to the basement membrane. They are said to occur in short rows of small regular cells with sparse green cytoplasm, oval nuclei and a high nuclear/cytoplasmic (N/C) ratio. The chromatin pattern is fine and several chromocentres may be present[13].

Parabasal cells *(Fig. 28.8)*

▶ Round to oval cells with fairly dense green cytoplasm
▶ Nuclei occupy about one half of the cell, with fine chromatin pattern
▶ Nuclear area 45–90 μm², cell area 105–1200 μm², giving a low N/C ratio

Immature parabasal cells generally lie in sheets while the more mature cells are usually dissociated.

Parabasal cells may predominate in atrophic smears from post-menopausal women. In younger women, postnatal atrophy or high dose progesterone oral contraception produce similar changes. With poor fixation and in some inflammatory states parabasal cytoplasm may appear amphophilic, taking up eosin staining centrally while retaining peripheral cyanophilia.

Intermediate cells *(Fig. 28.9)*

▶ Large polygonal cells, ample pale green filmy cytoplasm often folded at periphery
▶ Nucleus round or ovoid, vesicular, fine chromatin pattern
▶ Nuclear area 25–75 μm², cellular area 1200–3000 μm², giving a low N/C ratio

The cells lie in tight groups or discretely in the smear, depending upon the hormonal state. In the second half of the cycle, when cell clumping is greatest, the cytoplasm becomes ragged and may disintegrate altogether, leaving bare nuclei (see Figs 28.42, 28.48). Under the influence of high levels of progesterone, intermediate cells tend to accumulate glycogen, forming an irregular central deposit of pale yellow stained material. With poor fixation the cytoplasm may take on amphophilic staining or may stain uniformly orange while retaining its other characteristics.

Superficial cells *(Fig. 28.9)*

▶ Large polygonal cells, pink to orange flat cytoplasm, rarely folded
▶ Cellular area 2500–4500 μm²
▶ Nuclei small (10–25 μm²), condensed or pyknotic; no visible internal structure

Normal superficial cells are usually discrete in contrast to intermediate cells. Cells from the granular layer, if formed, display small dark blue keratohyaline granules, probably cytolysosomes, evenly distributed in the cytoplasm. Nests of benign squamous cells known as epithelial pearls are sometimes seen in normal smears (Fig. 28.10A). The cells may be artefactually squashed and distorted by the smear taking (Fig. 28.10B).

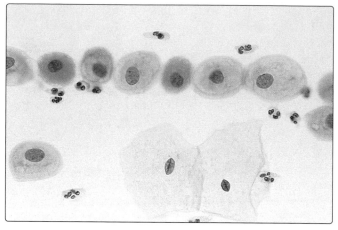

Fig. 28.8   A row of parabasal cells, rounded or polygonal in shape, dissociated and in small groups. The cytoplasm is dense and cyanophilic, the nuclei stain darkly and the nuclear/cytoplasmic ratio is high compared with the intermediate cells at lower edge. (× HP)

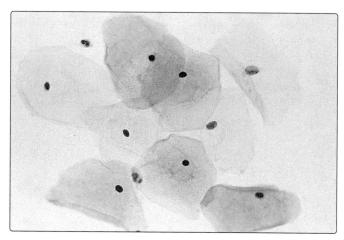

Fig. 28.9   Intermediate and superficial squamous cells. The former have translucent green cytoplasm with a tendency to fold at the periphery; the nuclei show a vesicular chromatin pattern and the nuclear/cytoplasmic ratio is low. The superficial cells are large, flat, polygonal and dissociated, with pinkish orange cytoplasm. The tiny dark nuclei have lost their chromatin pattern. (× HP)

Anucleate squames

▶ Mature superficial squamous cells with loss of nuclei
▶ Stain with the dimer of eosin producing orange or yellow stained cytoplasm (Fig. 28.11)
▶ Site of nucleus may be recognizable as a lighter central area or nuclear ghost

Anucleate squames are often present in combination with granular cells, indicating completion of keratinization. The cells are a normal finding in vulval scrapes. Numerous anucleate squames in cervical smears suggest keratinization of the cervix (hyperkeratosis) due to irritation from, for instance, a prolapse or the wearing of a pessary. Hyperkeratosis also occurs in human papillomavirus infection, leukoplakia and in some cases of cervical carcinoma. The presence of anucleate squames is,

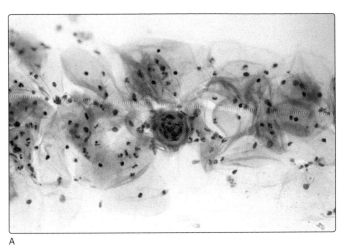

A

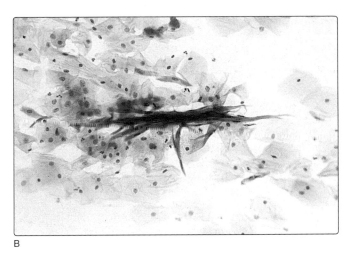

B

Fig. 28.10 (A) Concentric epithelial pearls can be seen in normal smears and in benign reactive conditions. (× HP) (B) Compression artefact of squamous cells induced by the smear-taking procedure is not infrequent. (× HP)

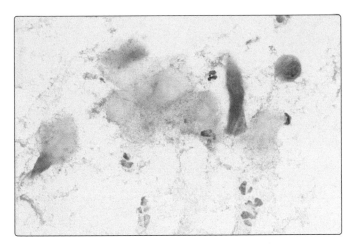

Fig. 28.11 Vulval contamination of a cervical smear is suggested by these yellowish orange anucleate squames. They are also seen in direct vulval scrapes. (× HP)

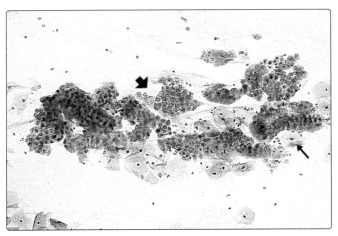

Fig. 28.12 Endocervical cells in sheets and groups, their columnar form giving a picket-fence (arrow) or honeycomb appearance (arrowhead). The cytoplasm is delicate and nuclei are rounded with a vesicular chromatin pattern. (× MP)

however, of low predictive value for these conditions. Less mature cells from the deeper layers may also become anucleate, usually in association with degenerative changes.

Endocervical cells *(Fig. 28.12)*

► Columnar cells with basal nuclei, in flat variable sized sheets or loosely associated
► Cyanophilic translucent cytoplasm or vacuolated
► Viewed from above, sheets have a honeycomb appearance
► In profile, cells in 'picket-fence' palisades with basal nuclei and columnar cytoplasm
► From above, nuclei rounded, from the side, the nuclei are oval
► Nuclear area 25–45 μm², cell area 150–300 μm²
► The chromatin pattern is fine, and one or more small nucleoli may be identified
► Bare nuclei may accompany groups of degenerate endocervical cells (Fig. 28.13)

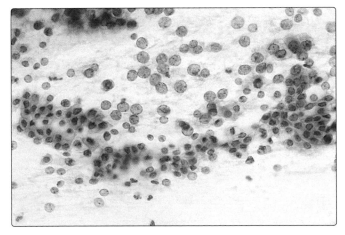

Fig. 28.13 Bare nuclei are frequently seen around endocervical cell groups. The nuclei become swollen and flattened like a fried egg when unsupported by cytoplasm, with pale but uniform chromatin. These nuclei may be of reserve cell origin. (× HP)

Occasionally cilia are visible, staining pink with eosin, attached to the terminal bar at the luminal pole of the cell (Fig. 28.14). Ciliated columnar epithelial cells are more common post-menopausally when the cell and nuclear sizes are usually smaller than in the reproductive period. Ciliated cells may also arise from areas of metaplasia to a tubal type of epithelium, which can occur in the process of healing of the cervical mucosa after injury.

Mucin-secreting goblet cells, with cytoplasm distended above the nucleus by a globule of mucin, (Fig. 28.15, also see Fig. 28.61) are an infrequent finding, usually due to a reactive change. Metaplasia to a goblet cell producing intestinal instead of endocervical mucus may occur and is referred to as intestinal metaplasia. This type of goblet cell is seen in cervical glandular neoplasia and therefore has associations with precancerous changes and the risk of malignancy (see Chapter 32). Background mucus from endocervical cells stains variably, either faintly green or tinged with pink. The amount of mucus present in a smear, its quality and distribution also vary considerably (Fig. 28.16). Depending on hormonal activity, it can be transparent or dense and striped, as is seen at the time of ovulation when ferning occurs (Fig. 28.17).

Endocervical cells may show considerable variation in nuclear size within a group. Multinucleation is not uncommon especially in the event of inflammation or injury (Fig. 28.18). Cells with these reactive changes may also originate from the lining of a nabothian cyst. The appearance of these cells in a smear varies with hormonal status and method of smear taking. Aylesbury spatulas and those with an extended arm to sample the lower canal harvest more endocervical cells than the Ayre spatula, while endocervical brushes usually include many groups of endocervical cells, albeit sometimes distorted.

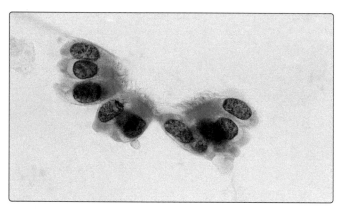

Fig. 28.14 A few ciliated endocervical cells form part of the normal glandular epithelium of the cervix but the cilia are not often seen as they are prone to undergo degenerative changes. (× HP)

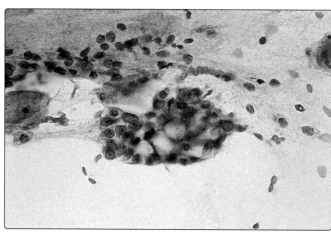

Fig. 28.15 Goblet cells distended with mucin as illustrated are an infrequent finding, usually representing reactive change. (× HP)

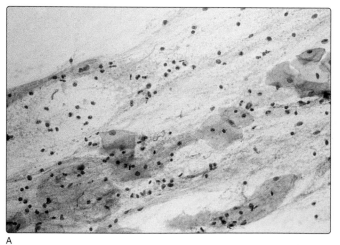

A

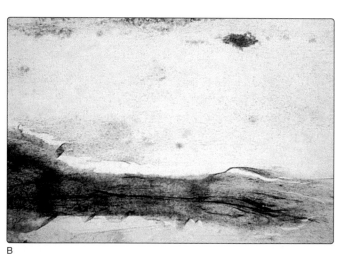

B

Fig. 28.16 (A) Background mucus stained pale pink or green is a useful indicator of sampling from the cervix. Vaginal and vulval smears usually contain little or no mucus. (× MP) (B) The mucous plug of the cervix may be spread on a smear largely intact. The plug contains inflammatory cells but the remainder of the smear will be clean, in contrast to a genuine infection. (× LP)

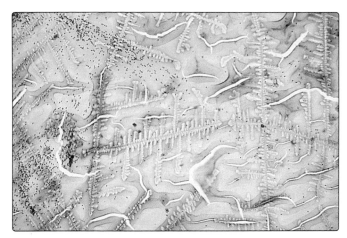

Fig. 28.17 Cervical mucus spread in a cervical smear taken at midcycle showing a ferning pattern due to the effects of oestrogen. (× MP)

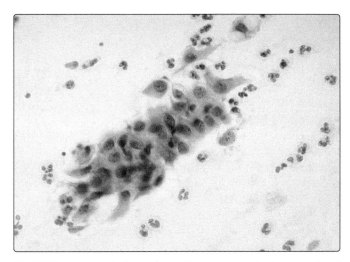

Fig. 28.19 A metaplastic group showing angular and polygonal cells with dense blue-green cytoplasm and nuclei resembling those of endocervical cells. (× HP)

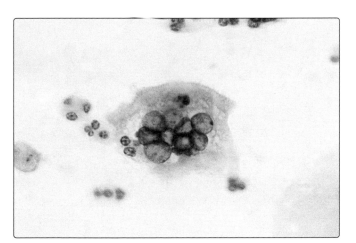

Fig. 28.18 Multinucleation of endocervical cells is common as a non-specific reactive response. The chromatin pattern remains uniform and the nucleoli regular. (× OI)

Metaplastic cells (Figs 28.19, 28.20)

► Cells the size of parabasal or early intermediate cells in small sheets
► Detached cells have cytoplasmic projections or bridges loosely connecting adjacent cells
► Delicate or dense cyanophilic cytoplasm or prematurely keratinized
► Nuclei vary in size, having vesicular chromatin and a high N/C ratio

These cells are a normal constituent of smears once the transformation zone has developed (Fig. 28.19). While immature, they do not exfoliate spontaneously but can be lifted from the surface of the cervix by the abrading action of a spatula or brush. With progressive maturation, the cells increasingly resemble intermediate and superficial cells from the original ectocervix and therefore cannot be recognized as a separate cell population in smears.

The cytoplasmic projections that give a spidery contour to the single cells result from their forcible removal during

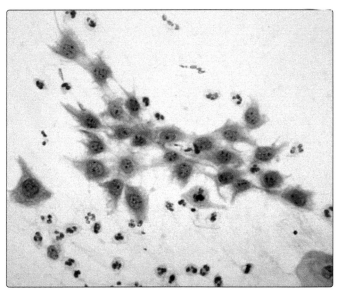

Fig. 28.20 Immature squamous metaplasia showing the typical spidery cytoplasmic projections due to forceful removal of the cells from the mucosa. (× HP)

smear taking. In metaplastic cell sheets the cytoplasmic projections may appear as fine intercellular bridges (Fig. 28.20). In the unstable environment of the transformation zone, premature keratinization of these cells may occur and the cytoplasm is then a deep orange colour. Other degenerative changes such as vacuolation and the presence of intracytoplasmic polymorphs may be seen, even in the absence of significant inflammation. Degenerative nuclear changes may also occur if maturation of the transformation zone is arrested; these include pyknosis, referring to condensation of the entire nucleus, and fragmentation or dissolution of chromatin, referred to as karyorrhexis and karyolysis respectively.

Other cellular components of cervical and vaginal smears

Endometrial cells *(Figs 28.21, 28.22)*

During menstruation and for some days following, cells from the endometrial cavity may be collected along with squamous and endocervical cells by the process of smear taking. It is generally stated that endometrial cells can be seen physiologically in smears for the first 12 days of the cycle, but that their presence may be of pathological significance at other times. Menorrhagia and other menstrual irregularities affect these times, as does the presence of an intrauterine contraceptive device, which can cause endometrial cells to exfoliation throughout the cycle.

The appearance of endometrial cells varies with the stage of the cycle and their degree of preservation. During and shortly after menstruation they are grouped in well-formed tight three-dimensional clusters with a peripheral rim of epithelial cells and a central core of stromal cells (Fig. 28.21). Degenerative changes quickly supervene, with crumpling of the nuclei and disorganization of the cells. They then stand out as small clusters of densely hyperchromatic crowded cells (Fig. 28.22), in contrast to the larger, more regular and better-preserved groups of endocervical cells. Neutrophil polymorphs are often seen within endometrial clusters.

The cellular changes in endometrial cells in cervical smears in pathological states, such as endometrial hyperplasia or neoplasia, are described in Chapter 35.

Reserve cells

Subcolumnar reserve cells are difficult to identify in cervical smears as they do not exfoliate. They could be represented by some of the bare nuclei seen in the vicinity of endocervical groups. When reactive reserve cell hyperplasia has occurred the cells can sometimes be identified as groups of small crowded cells with round darkly stained nuclei, frequently overlapping (Fig. 28.23). They may be distinguished from the cell groups of glandular dyskaryosis by the lack of architectural abnormalities, the smaller size and uniform chromatin pattern of reserve cell nuclei, and the presence of bare nuclei.

Neutrophil polymorphs

These are the commonest of the non-epithelial cells found in normal smears, their presence being physiological in the mucous plug of the cervix (see Fig. 28.17). They can be found in large numbers without necessarily implying significant infection, although they are usually increased in cases of cervicitis or vaginitis and also in malignant disease of the cervix. The clinical context and the overall smear findings are important in evaluating their significance. There may be problems in the interpretation of a smear if the epithelial cells are largely obscured by polymorphs. This problem is overcome to a considerable extent by the use of

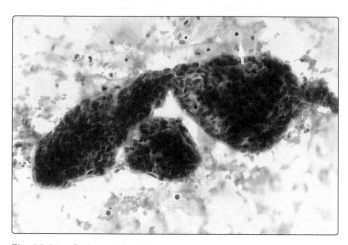

Fig. 28.21   Endometrial cells in a well preserved group showing a central core of compact stroma surrounded by a looser regimented layer of small dark epithelial cells. This is the characteristic appearance of endometrial cells shed early in menstruation. (× HP)

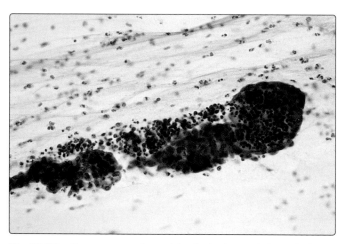

Fig. 28.22   Degenerate endometrial cells shed towards the end of menstruation are darkly stained and lie amid inflammatory debris. Cell detail is difficult to make out at this stage and awareness of the timing of smear collection in the cycle is important. (× MP)

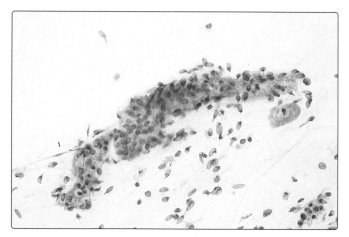

Fig. 28.23   Reserve cells forming a crowded group. Some lie at the edges of the group, having lost their scanty cytoplasm. (× HP)

liquid-based methods of preparation (see Chapter 31), whereby much of the inflammatory cell population is removed from the epithelial cell components.

Macrophages

Macrophages are sometimes seen as part of the inflammatory cell population, especially following menstruation and in post-menopausal women. They are extremely variable in size and appearance, but can generally be distinguished from parabasal or columnar cells by their ill-defined foamy cytoplasm, their eccentric bean-shaped nuclei, and the presence of ingested particulate material in some instances. However, many of them have small round central nuclei and do not contain phagocytosed particles, making identification less certain. It is helpful when in doubt to look at neighbouring cells as these frequently include other macrophages with more typical features (Fig. 28.24).

Macrophages are always dissociated cells but may be loosely aggregated, especially in postmenstrual smears. They may become multinucleated and very large, forming giant cells, a phenomenon seen particularly in smears from post-menopausal women (Fig. 28.25).

Lymphocytes

These cells are usually scanty, forming a minor component of the inflammatory cell population in some normal women. They are present in larger numbers in follicular cervicitis in association with tingible-body macrophages (see Fig. 28.63).

Other inflammatory cells

Eosinophils, basophils (mast cells) and plasma cells (see Fig. 28.54) are seen in smears occasionally, recognizable by their characteristic morphology.

Cells other than inflammatory and epithelial cells

Spermatozoa are seen in postcoital smears, even several days after intercourse (Fig. 28.26). They usually present no problem in identification, but the accompanying seminal fluid may contain large degenerate cells from the seminal vesicles and these must be distinguished from dyskaryotic cells. Nearby spermatozoa provide a clue to their origin.

Contaminants

Cytological specimens can be contaminated at any stage in the collection, transmission or laboratory preparation of the sample. Liquid-based cytology preparations are less prone to contamination from these sources. In addition, cervical smears may include extraneous material from the vagina or vulva, including parasites or their ova from the digestive tract, especially in those parts of the world where parasitic infestations are common[14]. Even outside such endemic areas parasites are encountered from time to time in cervical smears and their identification is important in patient management.

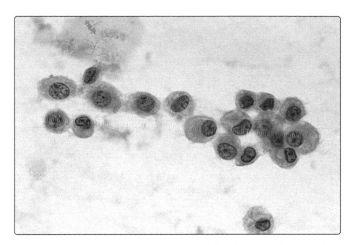

Fig. 28.24 Macrophages are always dissociated cells, varying greatly in size and appearance but often small in cervical smears. This collection includes several with bean-shaped nuclei and foamy cytoplasm, features typical of macrophages. (× HP)

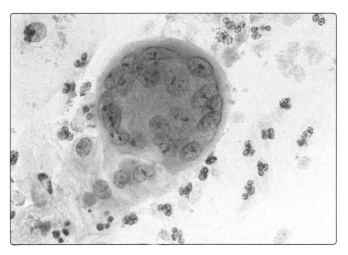

Fig. 28.25 Multinucleated macrophages or giant cells are a non-specific finding, especially after the menopause. They are also seen in granulomatous inflammation or repair and after radiotherapy. (× HP)

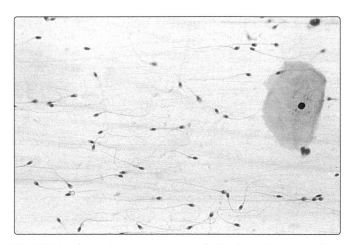

Fig. 28.26 Spermatozoa are a common finding in cervical smears. They show darkly stained ovoid sperm heads with some preserved tails. (× HP)

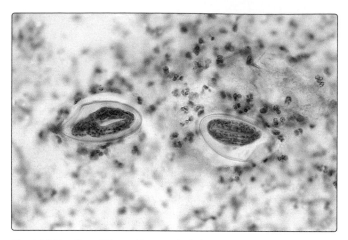

Fig. 28.27   Ova of *Enterobius vermicularis,* showing the thick glassy eosinophilic capsule and larva within. (× HP)

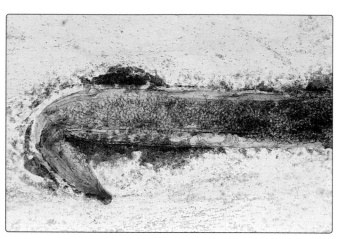

Fig. 28.28   Adult *Enterobius vermicularis* worm in a cervical smear. (× LP)

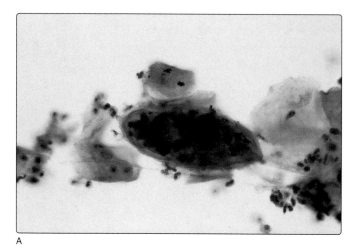

A

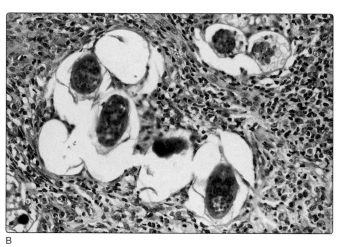

B

Fig. 28.29   (A) *Schistosoma haematobium* ovum in a cervical smear taken from a patient with vulval schistosomiasis. Note the size of the ovum compared with the squamous cells, and the terminal spine. (× HP) (B) Vulval biopsy from the same patient showing numerous ova within the dermis and a surrounding foreign body reaction. (H&E × MP)

Ova of the threadworm *Enterobius vermicularis*[15] (Fig. 28.27) are seen not infrequently in smears from infected patients, especially if there is poor personal hygiene. The eggs are oval and are smaller than schistosome ova, with a smooth double walled shell, often with one side flipped over. The larva can usually be recognized within (Fig. 28.28).

Descriptions of *Ascaris lumbricoides, Taenia coli*[16], *Trichuris trichuria, Hymenolepsis nana*[17] and the microfilaria of *Wuchereria bancrofti*[18,19] have been recorded. *Schistosoma haematobium, S. japonicum* and *S. mansoni* ova can be identified in smears as elliptical ova, larger than those of the threadworm *E. vermicularis*. The first two are the common types of schistosome ova found in cervical smears and are distinguished by the presence of a terminal or lateral spine respectively (Fig. 28.29A,B)[20]. The trophozoites of *Balantidium coli* may be seen in patients with intestinal infestation by this uncommon protozoal organism (Fig. 28.30).

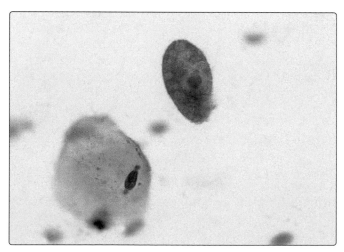

Fig. 28.30   *Balantidium coli,* a protozoal organism pathogenic in the large bowel, is a rare finding in smears and may not signify infection. In this asymptomatic patient only occasional trophozoites were seen. No treatment was given. (× HP)

Pediculus humanus, the body louse, and the pubic louse, *Phthirus pubis*, are seen occasionally in cervical smears

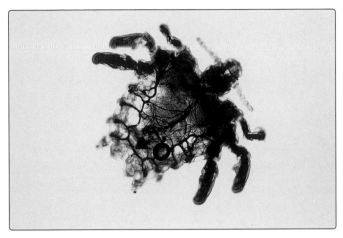

Fig. 28.31 Pubic (crab) louse found in a cervical smear. (× MP)

(Fig. 28.31). The louse may be damaged during smear preparation, with fragmentation of the tail part from head and legs.

Many external contaminants have been described, including pollen and insects due to atmospheric contamination, and also various fungi, either from contaminated laboratory solutions, the water supply or from the atmosphere (Fig. 28.32). Particulate material from sources such as tampons or glove powder is usually easily identified (Fig. 28.33)[21].

A refractile brown deposit overlying the central portion of the cytoplasm, known as 'cornflake artefact', is not uncommon in smears and may obscure nuclear detail (Fig. 28.34). This is a problem peculiar to cytological smears, thought to result from trapping of air on the surface of cells during mounting especially in thickly spread smears. Inadequate removal of spray fixative containing Carbowax may cause similar problems. The artefact may be so marked as to require a further smear for accurate assessment.

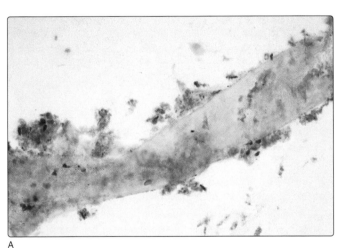

A

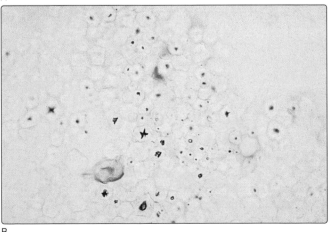

A

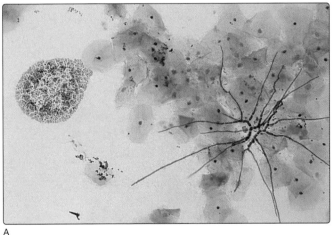

B

Fig. 28.32 (A) Contamination of a cervical smear by fungal spores and hyphae, probably from the atmosphere. (× HP) (B) A plant particle (sclerid) seen occasionally in smears due to atmospheric contamination. (× HP)

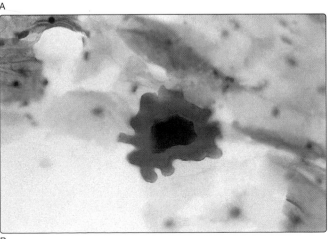

B

Fig. 28.33 (A) Cotton fibres are not infrequently seen as contaminants in smears. (× HP) (B) Glove powder can often be present in smears. Even without polarized light, the characteristic Maltese cross structure can be seen at the centre of some of the starch particles. (× HP)

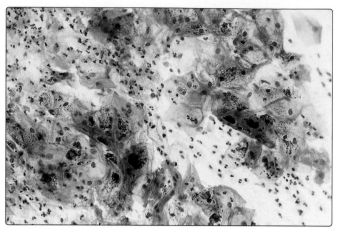

Fig. 28.34 'Cornflake' artefact refers to a brown slightly refractile deposit overlying the nuclei, sometimes obscuring nuclear detail completely. (× HP)

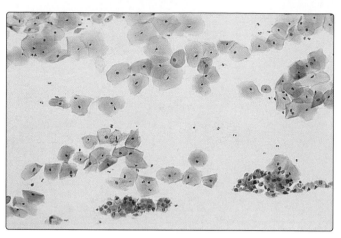

Fig. 28.35 A good quality smear consists of well-displayed cells with representative sampling of both squamous and endocervical or metaplastic epithelium. (× HP)

Carryover of cellular material from one smear to another may occur during smear preparation in the laboratory, posing difficulty in assessing the findings. The contaminant cells are often distributed along the upper or side edge of the slide and may be in a slightly different plane of focus from the rest of the cells. If there is any abnormality in the carryover it is confined to cells at this site and does not appear to relate to the morphology of other cells present.

Assessment of quality of smears

The question of adequacy of cervical smears is central to the success of cervical screening in the prevention of cervical cancer deaths. The problem of establishing exactly what constitutes an adequate sample has received increasing attention in recent years, culminating in broad guidelines from various sources, including the British Society for Clinical Cytology, which has issued criteria for acceptability of smear quality[22]. In North America, the Bethesda system of terminology advocates a mandatory statement on quality of smear, grouping specimens as adequate, less than optimal and inadequate[23]. While there is by no means unanimity over these criteria, it is important that cytologists have a degree of confidence about the threshold of acceptability of smear quality.

The feature of paramount importance in assessing smear quality is that there should be adequate numbers of epithelial cells on the slide, with evidence that they are from the appropriate area of the cervix (Fig. 28.35). In theory, the latter requirement can only be satisfied if squamous metaplastic cells, endocervical cells and mucus are present in sufficient proportions to establish that the entire circumference of the transformation zone has been scraped[24]. Clearly, however, metaplastic cells will not be firmly identifiable once the transformation zone is fully mature, and endocervical cells will not always be sampled, especially after the menopause. Recognition of a

representative sample therefore requires knowledge of the woman's age and menstrual status and of any hormonal treatment.

Formal training in smear taking is essential if the cervical smear test is to be reliable and such training is increasingly available. As a quality assurance measure, the proportion of inadequate or unsatisfactory smears in relation to the entire smear workload of a laboratory provides a valuable indication of the standard of reporting and of the level of expertise of the smear takers. The NHSCSP has set up a system in England and Wales monitoring laboratory reporting against national targets to ensure that laboratories fall within acceptable ranges for all categories of smear reports[22].

To reduce the possibility of incorrect assessment of smear tests by the laboratory, the UK has now introduced a quality control procedure for all negative and inadequate smears prior to sending out such reports. These smears are currently subjected to shortened rescreening by a different member of staff from the original screener, a method found to detect a substantial proportion of abnormalities missed on primary screening. The process, referred to as 'rapid review', has proved helpful in identifying smears wrongly assessed initially as either adequate or inadequate, as well as for finding missed abnormalities[25-27].

Criteria for assessing smear quality

► As a working principle, cervical smears should consist of clearly displayed cellular material covering at least one third of the area under the coverslip, and preferably over one half. The mere inclusion of columnar or metaplastic cells, or both, does not necessarily confirm that the entire circumference of the transformation zone has been fully sampled. The smear taker has to be relied upon for confirming the thoroughness of the sampling procedure.

▶ Squamous cells of cervical origin are usually distributed in loosely cohesive streaks along the lines of spread of the smear. This is helpful in attempting to determine whether squamous cells are cervical or vaginal in origin, the latter usually lying in a flat dispersed pattern due to the lack of background mucus. Post-menopausal smears with little or no mucus may, misleadingly, appear to be vaginal in origin.

▶ Whether smears without any endocervical cells or recognizable metaplastic cells should be accepted as representative is debatable. The presence of these cells is determined largely by the position of the squamocolumnar junction and the state of maturation of the transformation zone, factors that are hormone dependent. Thus it may not be possible to include endocervical cells or identify metaplastic cells at all times. An additional factor is the nature of the sampling device (Fig. 28.36), the Aylesbury spatula giving a greater yield from within the canal than the Ayre spatula. Brushes and broom devices provide the largest

endocervical component. There are many reports of comparative trials of the different smear taking instruments[28–32], the general conclusion being that devices with an extended arm give a more representative sample and have a greater likelihood of including abnormalities.

▶ An excess of leucocytes obscuring epithelial cells (Fig. 28.37A) may require investigation for a treatable cause, especially if a discharge is present. Recommendation to repeat the smear at midcycle often provides a better sample than at other times of the cycle. Similarly, unsatisfactory smears taken postnatally should be repeated when normal menstrual cycles are re-established.

▶ Blood-stained smears are often poorly fixed or obscured by the blood (Fig. 28.37B). Contact bleeding on smear taking may be due to an ectropion, requiring treatment before a satisfactory smear can be obtained.

▶ Post-menopausal atrophy leads to scanty or inflamed smears, often with no endocervical cells. The threshold of acceptance of smears from these women must be adjusted, but if there is cause to doubt the adequacy of sampling a short course of local oestrogen cream prior to smear taking usually ensures better sampling[33] (Fig. 28.38).

Liquid based thin layer cytological preparations reduce the rate of obscured and inadequate smears by removing much of the inflammatory debris and blood and by providing a representative sample of all of the material from the spatula, most of which is usually discarded in routine smear preparation. The preparation technique is already used in some laboratories in the USA (see Chapter 31) and is undergoing pilot studies in the UK at the time of writing.

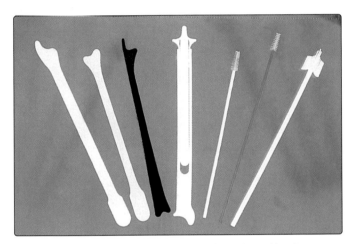

Fig. 28.36   A sample of the great variety of spatulas and brushes available for smear taking. The original Ayre spatula (second from left) is shaped without a prolongation to increase endocervical sampling. The Aylesbury spatula (far left) is in widespread use in the UK. Brushes are recommended for liquid-based cytology.

Influence of sex hormones on squamous epithelium

The diagnostic potential of cytohormonal evaluation using vaginal smears was reported as early as 1925 by Papanicolaou[34]. Hormonal cytology is a bioassay, which means that it is not the concentration of circulating

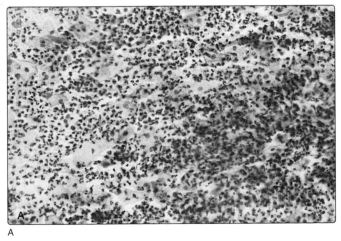

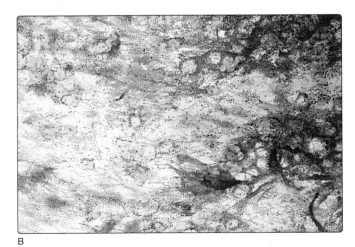

Fig. 28.37   Unsatisfactory smears due to: (A) an excess of polymorphs. (× HP) (B) an excess of blood. (× MP)

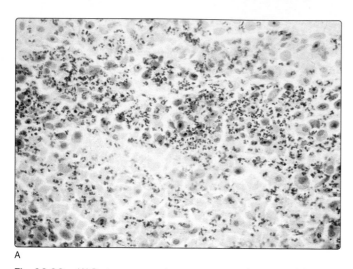
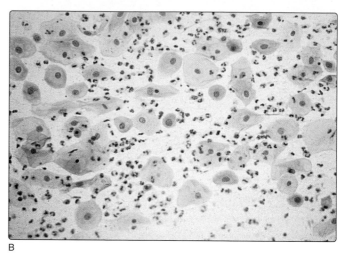

Fig. 28.38   (A) Post-menopausal smears are sometimes unsatisfactory due to the combination of atrophy and inflammatory exudate. (B) Interpretation can be improved by the use of local oestrogen cream for 1–2 weeks, then repeating the smear; the findings are then usually easily assessed. (× HP)

hormone which is being determined; rather it is the effect of the hormone on the target organ, the stratified squamous epithelium in this case, which is evaluated.

One problem here is that the sensitivity of the target organ to the hormone varies from person to person. Moreover, it is usually not the sole effect of one hormone that is registered but the combined effect of several. Also the administration of hormonal therapy can influence the cell pattern seen in a smear. It is essential to keep these facts in mind if correct cytohormonal evaluation is to be achieved.

Oestrogens

Oestrogens promote growth and maturation of stratified squamous epithelium up to and including the superficial layer. Smears contain many superficial epithelial cells when the oestrogen level is high and unopposed by progesterone, as in the first half of the menstrual cycle. These cells lie quite flat and are generally discrete; the smear background is noticeably free of polymorphs (Fig. 28.39).

A small dose of oestrogen can cause atrophic squamous epithelium to develop into epithelium with several layers of intermediate cells. When the dose of oestrogen is increased or prolonged, intermediate cells mature into superficial cells. The concept of 'oestrogen effect' should only be used when oestrogens alone circulate in the bloodstream, thus exerting a monohormonal effect.

Progesterone

Once the stratified squamous epithelium has matured under the influence of oestrogen, progesterone causes rapid desquamation of the topmost layers. The intermediate cells develop curled edges giving a folded appearance, and the cytoplasm often contains glycogen, staining yellow at the centre of the cell. Exfoliation occurs in compact clusters of cells in which the margins of individual cells are indistinct.

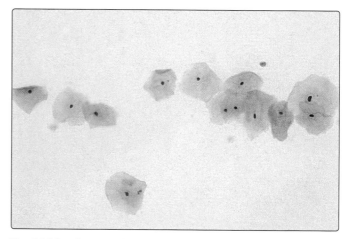

Fig. 28.39   Oestrogenic effects are manifested by the appearance of large, flat dissociated eosinophilic superficial squamous cells in a clean background. (× HP)

Many Döderlein's bacilli (lactobacilli) and leucocytes appear in the smear. They bring about cytolysis of the intermediate cells, causing dissolution of the cell cytoplasm (Fig. 28.40). As a result, numerous naked vesicular nuclei are present and the smear may appear hypocellular. Further progesterone induces the appearance of boat-shaped navicular cells (see Fig. 28.43).

When there is mild oestrogen deficiency, as may be encountered at the time of the menopause, the cytological pattern is difficult to distinguish from that of progesterone or androgen stimulation. The clusters are, however, usually slightly smaller, often containing no more than ten cells.

If progesterone is administered to patients with an atrophic mucosa, maturation of the squamous epithelium including the superficial layers is the initial result. Administration of progesterone to patients with pre-existing mature epithelium leads to disappearance of the

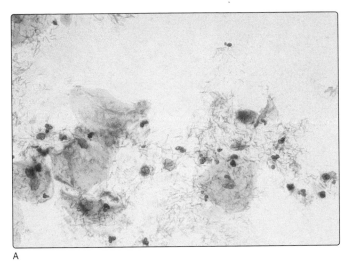

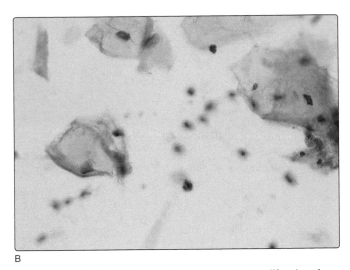

A

B

Fig. 28.40 (A, B) Progesterone effects include maturation of squamous cells to intermediate level, with increased glycogen content; proliferation of lactobacilli and cytolysis follow further exposure to progesterone. (× HP)

superficial layer and no superficial cells are found in the smear.

Androgen

Administration of this hormone when the stratified squamous epithelium is atrophic and smears are composed exclusively of parabasal cells results in a predominance of intermediate cells (Fig. 28.41). The smears are particularly rich in cells[35]. If androgens are administered to patients with fully mature stratified squamous epithelium, the opposite effect is seen: superficial cells disappear, to be replaced by intermediate cells. Prolonged administration of androgens produces a smear pattern with cytolysis.

Physiological cytohormonal patterns

These are best revealed in vaginal smears taken from the lateral vaginal wall, preferably sequentially; but the changes are mirrored by the findings in cervical smears. Vulval tissues are much less responsive to cyclical hormonal fluctuations, although subject to hormonally determined development and atrophy at the menarche and the menopause respectively.

Birth to seven days

Maternal sex hormones penetrate the placenta during pregnancy and exert an influence on the epithelial cells of the genital tract of the fetus *in utero*. The vaginal epithelium of a newborn female baby is therefore fully mature.

From the first week to puberty

In this period production of sex hormones is low. Vaginal smears normally manifest atrophy with many parabasal cells.

Puberty

Puberty marks the cyclical production of the sex hormones. The vaginal epithelium slowly reaches maturity. At first,

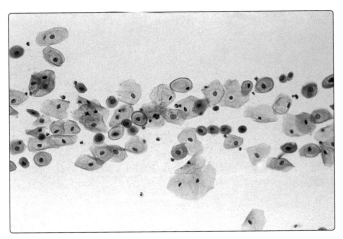

Fig. 28.41 Androgenic effects include maturation of an atrophic smear to intermediate cell level. The background is usually clean, lacking the cytolysis seen with progesterone activity. (× HP)

many intermediate epithelial cells are seen; when menstrual cycles begin, many superficial cells are also present. In the second half of these cycles, however, a true progesterone pattern is not apparent as the cycles are initially anovulatory. In the cervix the squamocolumnar junction at this stage coincides with the site of the most distal endocervical gland.

Sexual maturity

When menstrual cycles become ovulatory, the following consecutive patterns can be expected (Fig. 28.42A,B,C,D):

▶ *Menstrual phase (1st–5th day)*. The smear contains erythrocytes, leucocytes, endometrial cells, and superficial and intermediate epithelial cells.
▶ *Proliferative or follicular phase (6th–10th day)*. First the 'clean-up crew' appears in the form of a large number of histiocytes, often in loose aggregates. These are mainly derived from endometrial stromal cells shed in a process known as the

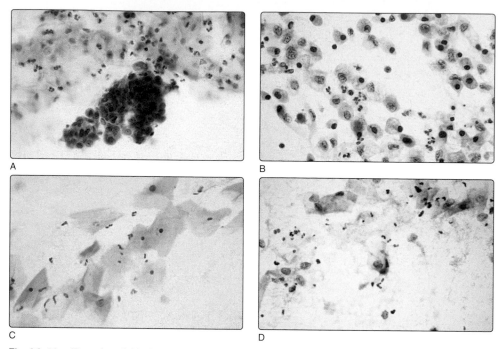

Fig. 28.42 These four fields show some of the characteristic features of smears at different stages of the menstrual cycle. (A) Menstrual phase with endometrial cells. (B) Early proliferative phase with stromal histiocytes ('exodus'). (C) Ovulation, producing a clean mature smear. (D) Late secretory phase with marked cytolysis. (× HP)

exodus. There are also many early intermediate squamous epithelial cells lacking the folding seen under the influence of progesterone. Polymorphs and endometrial cells are present, the latter decreasing in number up to the 10th–12th day. Towards the end of the proliferative phase superficial squamous cells increase in number.

▶ *Ovulation (11th–13th day)*. During this phase there are numerous superficial epithelial cells lying flat and obviously discrete. The pattern is 'clean', that is, practically without leucocytes and with very few bacteria. In some smears the endocervical mucus creates a pattern of ferning on the slide (see Fig. 28.17).

▶ *Secretory or luteal phase (14th–28th day)*. The pattern changes abruptly after ovulation: now intermediate squamous cells predominate. Within several days the characteristic progesterone pattern appears, with folding and clustering of intermediate cells, the reappearance of polymorphs and many Döderlein's bacilli.

▶ Towards the end of the cycle, marked cytolysis develops, accompanied by a further increase in polymorphonuclear leucocytes. Just before menstruation the proportion of mature epithelial cells increases once again. A few women also shed endometrial cells several days before menstruation. In some women with normal ovulatory cycles, the characteristic progesterone pattern is absent and only the midcycle peak of oestrogenic effects points to ovulation.

Hormonal effects may be monitored by taking sequential smears from the lateral vaginal wall. The ratio of superficial cells with pyknotic nuclei to less mature epithelial cells with vesicular nuclei can be estimated at intervals, giving a karyopyknotic index (KPI). Other indices occasionally still used include counting the cells with eosinophilic cytoplasm, giving an eosinophilic index (EI) and giving the ratio of parabasals, intermediates and superficial cells. All of these methods are quite unreliable, being subjective assessments and prone to variations with staining technique and fixation. Today, estimates of hormonal activity are more often made by direct measurement of serum hormone levels.

Pregnancy

In the event of pregnancy, the corpus luteum does not involute but instead grows larger, producing increasing amounts of progesterone and oestrogen. The cytological pattern of pregnancy is that of heightened progesterone activity, with clustering and folding of intermediate cells and the presence of navicular cells. These are cells distended with yellow glycogen, becoming boat shaped, with a rim of folded cytoplasm and the nucleus pushed to the periphery (Fig. 28.43). The changes are most pronounced in the third trimester, when numerous Döderlein's bacilli are seen and the accompanying cytolysis is at its height.

About three months after conception, the placenta takes over from the corpus luteum the task of producing progesterone and oestrogens. If this change does not proceed smoothly the progesterone level may drop, sometimes even far enough for the pregnancy to be threatened. Cytologically, this may be manifested as an increase in the number of superficial cells and a rise in the KPI.

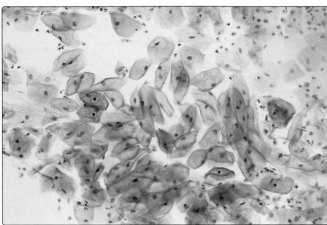

Fig. 28.43   Navicular cells containing yellow stained glycogen are characteristically boat-shaped with the nucleus pushed to the periphery of the cell and the cytoplasm folded at the cell margins. (× OI)

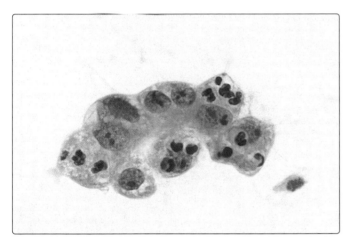

Fig. 28.44   Trophoblastic cells are difficult to identify with confidence. This group of degenerate cuboidal cells with enlarged hyperchromatic nuclei is presumed to be of cytotrophoblastic origin. The cells were present in a smear taken two weeks after a miscarriage. Follow-up smears have been normal. (× HP)

Arias-Stella changes, seen in the endometrium in some pregnancies, may also develop in endocervical glands and have been described as a rare finding in cervical or vaginal smears[36,37]. The cells have an exaggerated secretory pattern as seen in the endometrial glands, and show enlarged degenerate hyperchromatic nuclei with intranuclear inclusions. The association with pregnancy and lack of any preserved abnormal chromatin pattern, combined with awareness of this entity, should ensure correct assessment of the findings.

Syncytiotrophoblastic cells are multinucleated cells from the outer surface of the chorionic villi and hence are fetal in origin, occurring only rarely in smears from patients with placenta praevia or in the presence of a threatened miscarriage. The cells are large, with an average of 50 nuclei per cell and a characteristic coarse-grained chromatin pattern resembling coarsely ground pepper. The number of nuclei is large in relation to the amount of cytoplasm. The cytoplasm is granular, in contrast to that of a histiocytic giant cell.

Cytotrophoblastic cells also line the villi. They are cuboidal cells with central nuclei. Cytologically, these cells cannot be firmly identified and may mimic neoplastic cells due to their prominent nucleoli, coarse chromatin pattern and high nuclear/cytoplasmic ratio (Fig. 28.44).

Intact placental villi have occasionally been identified in smears taken postpartum[38]. As illustrated in (Fig. 28.45), a villus may be recognized by its size and form, with degenerate trophoblastic cells and inflammatory debris coating a long three-dimensional structure with a translucent quality internally.

Decidual cells are modified endometrial stromal cells responding to the high circulating progesterone levels in pregnancy or to high progesterone content oral contraceptives. Decidual changes may also occur in the stromal cells of the cervix and are occasionally sampled in smears taken during or shortly after pregnancy. The cells

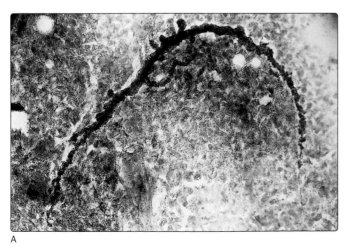

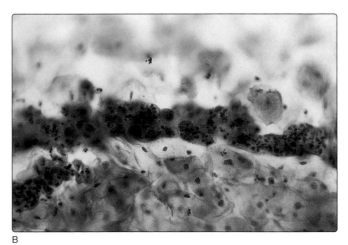

A   B

Fig. 28.45   (A) Placental villus in a cervical smear taken six weeks after delivery. The structure appears three-dimensional on low power. (B) High power magnification shows degenerate trophoblasts on the outer surface with a few adherent inflammatory cells.

are swollen and pale due to their content of glycogen. They have abundant clear, sometimes vacuolated cytoplasm and central large nuclei. The chromatin is often smudged and ill-defined and nucleoli are prominent. Decidual cells can be recognized by the fact that, in contrast to squamous epithelial cells, they are not flat but convex; the cells are round to oval and the cytoplasm appears to be less dense than that of epithelial cells (Fig. 28.46)[39].

Postpartum

With the expulsion of the placenta, the most important source of progesterone and oestrogen disappears. The smear pattern changes to one chiefly composed of parabasal epithelial cells, which are somewhat angular and contain glycogen or may undergo keratinization (Fig. 28.47). Such cells are called lactational or postpartum cells. They are derived from the parabasal epithelial layer, which becomes hyperplastic during pregnancy and exfoliates after delivery. These cells may appear in the smear until the normal ovarian cycle has resumed.

One third of women in the postpartum period do not show these typical postpartum cells; highly divergent patterns may be seen, including inflammatory and repair changes if there has been damage to the cervix in labour.

Lactation

During breast-feeding, the postpartum pattern described above may persist for as long as the ovarian cycle is suppressed. This picture can pose problems in recognition of precancerous changes since the cells are small and active, with a relatively high nuclear/cytoplasmic ratio. For this reason the postnatal period is best avoided for routine cervical screening, deferring smear taking in well-screened women until normal menstrual cycles have returned.

Pre-menopausal phase

Just before the onset of the menopause, the cycles often become anovulatory and irregular. In this period persistent ovarian follicles may be encountered when ovulation fails to occur. Unopposed oestrogen production replaces the progestogenic phase of the cycle and smears show a predominance of superficial cells or sometimes intermediate cells without glycogen storage: oestrogen withdrawal bleeding takes place after a variable interval. When both ovulatory and anovulatory cycles occur, a mixed picture is often seen, either due to progesterone effects with many Döderlein's bacilli and cytolysis, or due to early atrophy.

Post-menopausal state

Following the menopause, when ovarian cycles no longer occur, the stratified squamous epithelium undergoes no further cyclical changes. A highly variable cellular pattern may then be seen. In the early post-menopausal phase there are many flat dispersed intermediate epithelial cells. Alternatively, a 'mixed pattern' with no single cell type predominating can be found.

With advancing age, progressive atrophy usually occurs but at a variable rate. Eventually in most women parabasal cells predominate. They are arranged singly or in variable sized sheets of undifferentiated cells with scanty cytoplasm (Fig. 28.48). Endocervical cells may be absent, partly because the squamocolumnar junction has retreated into the canal out of reach of sampling; also because they are less easily distinguished from parabasal cells in sheets. The emergence of many dissociated parabasal cells with dense reddish orange cytoplasm and pyknotic nuclei is aptly termed 'red atrophy' (Fig. 28.49).

Atrophic smears may contain cyanophilic bodies known as 'blue blobs' (Fig. 28.50). They are similar in size and shape to parabasal cells. Their origin is disputed, some claiming they are degenerate cells, while others have found them to be derived from inspissated mucus. It is likely that both mechanisms are valid. Ultimately, they disintegrate into granular background material. They differ from tumour nuclei in their lack of internal structure and they evoke no inflammatory reaction[40].

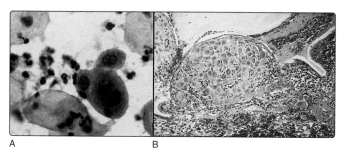

Fig. 28.46 (A) Decidual cells seen in a postnatal cervical smear taken at the same time as the accompanying biopsy. In the smear the cells have dense rather convex cytoplasm with bland nuclei, as in the biopsy (B). (HP, H&E × MP)

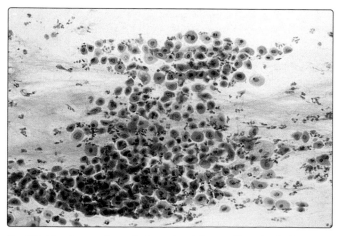

Fig. 28.47 Postnatal atrophy/lactational change. Note the darkly stained nuclei in some of these small atrophic cells. These changes can be difficult to assess and may require a further smear after menstrual cycles are re-established, for accurate interpretation. (× HP)

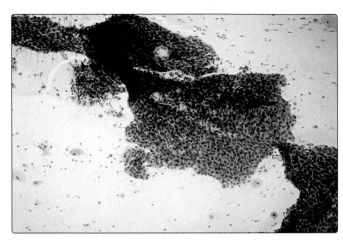

Fig. 28.48 Post-menopausal atrophy is usually more pronounced than postnatal atrophy, resulting ultimately in sheets of undifferentiated parabasal cells. (× MP)

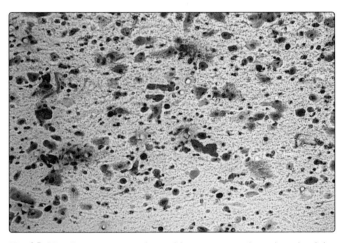

Fig. 28.49 Post-menopausal atrophic smears may show altered staining of cytoplasm producing the picture referred to as 'red atrophy'. This degree of atrophy may be difficult to assess. (× HP)

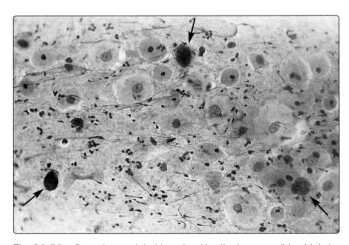

Fig. 28.50 Round or oval darkly stained bodies known as 'blue blobs' (arrows) are a feature of atrophic post-menopausal smears. They must be distinguished from bare nuclei and may raise concern about dyskaryosis, but they lack any defined chromatin pattern. (× HP)

Other hormonal effects

Some ovarian neoplasms such as hilus cell and Sertoli-Leydig cell tumours may secrete male sex hormones, and granulosa cell tumours frequently produce oestrogens. Vaginal or cervical smears from post-menopausal women who have a granulosa cell tumour may show many superficial cells, and also small groups of endometrial cells.

Oestrogen-containing drugs and cosmetics can produce oestrogenic effects, and similarly many superficial cells are found when therapeutic compounds such as digitalis and anticoagulant drugs are taken.

In post-menopausal women the adrenal glands are the main source of oestrogen. Stimulation of the adrenals, for instance in anxiety states, may result in high levels of all adrenal hormones, resulting in an increase of superficial cells. Similarly, obesity is associated with persistence of oestrogen effects since adipose tissue acts as a depot for steroid hormone production.

Inflammation and infection of the vagina and cervix

The squamous mucosa of the vagina and cervix are in continuity. Both are therefore exposed to similar risks of infection and have similar protective mechanisms. The vulva shares certain of these risks, although the presence of a surface layer of keratin ensures resistance to some of the infections seen in the adjacent vagina.

The natural protection of the vagina and cervix against infections is determined by the general state of health[41], a competent immune system[42], the presence of intact stratified squamous epithelium, the acid pH of the vagina and the equilibrium between the various micro-organisms normally present as commensals. These organisms do not cause infection in normal women since they create a stable polymicrobial vaginal milieu. If this equilibrium is disturbed, one type may overgrow the others and the vaginal milieu then becomes monomicrobial.

Thus locally, the chance of invasion by microorganisms from outside or of a commensal organism causing inflammation depends upon whether one or more of the following has occurred:

▶ Damage to the squamous epithelium by mechanical or chemical factors such as trauma or using vaginal sprays
▶ The presence of an ectropion with its thin covering of endocervical columnar epithelium, which is more easily penetrated by bacteria
▶ A decrease in thickness of squamous epithelium as seen in atrophic mucosa with only a few cell layers
▶ A change in vaginal pH from acidic to neutral or to an alkaline environment: in the course of the menstrual cycle the pH varies from 6.8 during menstruation to 3.9 during the second half of the cycle
▶ A rapid increase in or abundance of microorganisms

Clinical features of vaginal and cervical infections

Most patients with vaginitis or cervicitis complain of an excessive vaginal discharge, which may be white (leucorrhoea), discoloured or blood-stained. It cannot be assumed that this is always due to infection since hormonal changes may lead to excess mucus, as can allergies to local applications such as soaps or spermicidal ointment. In vaginitis, the main complaints are of burning and dryness of the vagina.

The mode of spread of infection is determined to a large extent by the nature of the organism. Various mechanisms by which infectious agents travel from the lower to the upper genital tract have been considered, including the possibility that trichomonads or spermatozoa act as vectors for the infectious agents, or that passive transport occurs[43]. An ascending infection may ultimately cause endometritis and salpingitis, or give rise to pain in the lower abdomen due to pelvic inflammatory disease.

Histological findings in cervicitis

An acute inflammatory process develops primarily in the stroma in close proximity to the capillaries. The local reaction consists of hyperaemia, exudation of fluid and migration of polymorphonuclear neutrophils from the bloodstream to the site of infection (Fig. 28.51). Polymorphs and macrophages are involved in phagocytosis of organisms and cell debris. Eosinophils are found particularly when the inflammation is due to allergy or parasites.

When inflammation persists, it becomes chronic in type. The cellular infiltrate then changes character. Lymphocytes, plasma cells and histiocytes now predominate (Fig. 28.52). Some inflammatory processes are chronic in type from the outset due to the nature of the factors inducing the inflammation. Granulomata composed of epithelioid histiocytes, giant cells and lymphocytes may form, particularly with certain specific infecting organisms. Eventually, scarring may ensue.

Cytological findings

In the presence of active inflammation smears usually contain many polymorphonuclear leucocytes and histiocytes, followed by lymphocytes and plasma cells if inflammation persists. The epithelial cells show various inflammatory changes and cell debris may be found. The composition of the cell population also changes. When the upper layers of the epithelium are damaged, parabasal cells from the lower layers of the epithelium are found. This phenomenon is even more pronounced when there is regeneration of already injured epithelium. On the other hand in some circumstances inflammatory irritation may increase the maturation of the squamous epithelium,

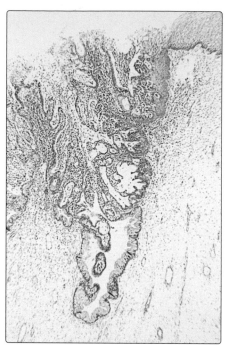

Fig. 28.51   Acute cervicitis is present in this histological section which shows many neutrophil polymorphs infiltrating the glands and stroma. (H&E × LP)

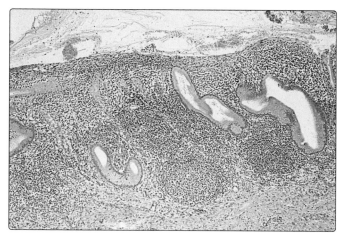

Fig. 28.52   Chronic cervicitis in a section of cervix. There is a dense infiltrate of chronic inflammatory cells in the submucosa and some lymphoid aggregates with germinal centres have formed, indicating follicular cervicitis. (H&E × LP)

leading to a smear pattern with predominantly superficial cells and sometimes even with anucleate squames due to keratinization.

Background findings in inflammatory smears:

▶ A marked increase in inflammatory cells, beyond the physiological mild to moderate leucocytosis seen in normal women

▶ Epithelial cells are covered by an exudate of polymorphs, and polymorphs may be seen permeating the cytoplasm of epithelial cells (Figs 28.53, 28.54)

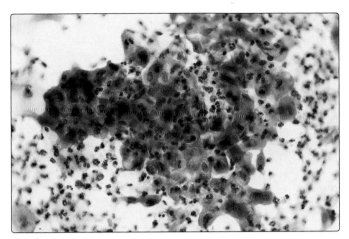

Fig. 28.53 Acute cervicitis changes in a smear from a patient with vaginal discharge. There is an acute inflammatory exudate of polymorphs around and within the epithelial group. The cells show nuclear enlargement and variable staining. (× MP)

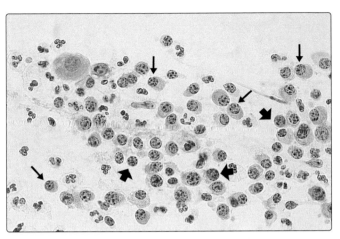

Fig. 28.55 Lymphocytes and plasma cells mingle together in this smear from a patient with chronic cervicitis. The lymphocytes (arrowheads) have smaller nuclei than the plasma cells, with condensed chromatin and very little cytoplasm. Plasma cells (arrows) have eccentric nuclei and a coarse chromatin pattern, likened to a clock face. (× HP)

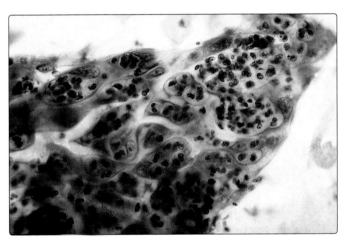

Fig. 28.54 Acute cervicitis in a sheet of vacuolated metaplastic cells permeated by neutrophil polymorphs, indicating active inflammation. (× OI)

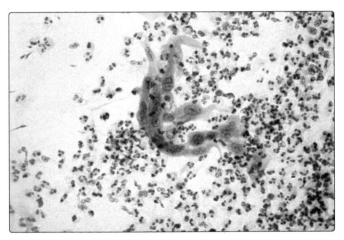

Fig. 28.56 Metaplastic cells in an inflammatory background, showing marked nuclear reactive and degenerative changes with amphophilic cytoplasmic staining. (× HP)

► Lymphocytes are present in significant numbers, with or without plasma cells (Fig. 28.55)

► Reactive and degenerative changes are seen in epithelial cells with altered maturity of cells as described below

► Fibrinous and proteinaceous material may form a granular or smooth, usually eosinophilic, background in the smear

Inflammatory changes in squamous epithelial cells

Cytoplasmic abnormalities include:

► Vacuolation
► Perinuclear haloes
► Altered staining
► Abnormal keratinization

Small vacuoles may appear in the cytoplasm, sometimes merging into a single large vacuole pushing the nucleus to one side. The thin border of cytoplasm can usually be

identified as that of a squamous cell because it retains its compact appearance. Leucocytes may be seen within vacuoles in the epithelial cells, a process known as leucophagocytosis or emperipolesis (Fig. 28.54). Condensation or thinning of cytoplasm may occur (Figs 28.56, 28.57). The cytoplasm immediately surrounding the nuclear membrane is often lighter in colour, forming a narrow zone of clearing (Fig. 28.58). The boundary of this halo is often vague.

Changes in staining reaction are seen with certain types of inflammation. Intermediate, parabasal and metaplastic cells show eosinophilia, staining pink instead of green (see Fig. 28.56). In senile vaginitis when there is inflammation of atrophic squamous mucosa parabasal cells may stain deep orange to red with eosin and the cytoplasm appears more dense than normal (see Fig. 28.49). Premature or excessive keratinization of squamous cells may occur. The

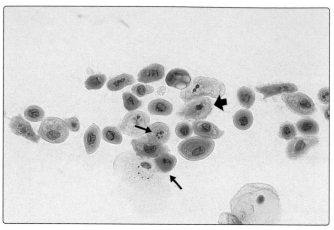

Fig. 28.57 Metaplastic cells showing variable preservation of cytoplasm with karyorrhexis (arrows) and pyknosis (arrowhead) of nuclei due to degenerative changes in the transformation zone in response to inflammation. (× HP)

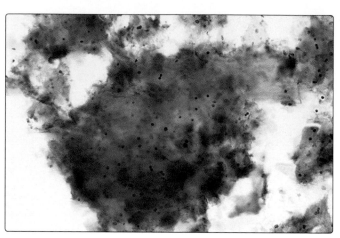

Fig. 28.59 A keratinized plaque of deep orange keratotic material with parakeratotic nuclear remnants. Cell borders cannot be discerned. (× HP)

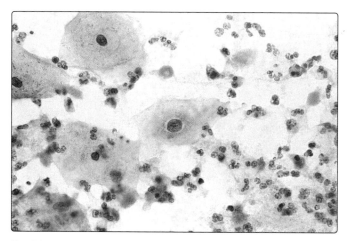

Fig. 28.58 Perinuclear haloes can be seen in two of the superficial cells, forming a narrow zone of pallor around the nucleus. This is a non-specific inflammatory response most often seen in *Trichomonas vaginalis* infection, as here, or due to Candida infection. (× HP)

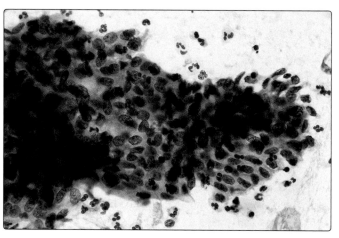

Fig. 28.60 A sheet of endocervical cells showing polymorphs within the cell group. There is loss of the regular honeycomb pattern with nuclear pleomorphism and ragged cytoplasmic borders. (× HP)

former involves individual cell keratinization and is referred to as dyskeratosis (see Fig. 28.87). Surface keratinization may retain nuclear remnants forming layers of parakeratosis (Fig. 28.59) or may consist of pure keratin. Although non-specific, these changes are most often seen in association with human papillomavirus infection.

The following changes can be seen in the nucleus:

► Swelling
► Wrinkling of nuclear membranes
► Multinucleation
► Chromatin degeneration

The nucleus commonly enlarges, with pale staining chromatin due to fluid absorption. This results in considerable variation in nuclear size (Fig. 28.56). Wrinkling of the nuclear membrane may occur, with selective condensation of chromatin at the nuclear margin and clearing of the nucleus centrally (Fig. 28.56). There is

retention of nuclear symmetry and the nucleolus can disappear altogether[44]. Multinucleation is common. Condensation of the chromatin, known as pyknosis, may occur in dying cells, or the nucleus may disintegrate and fragment in a process known as karyorrhexis (Fig. 28.57). Dissolution of the nucleus or karyolysis is another mode of cell death sometimes seen in inflamed smears. Nucleoli may be prominent and multiple (Figs 28.54, 28.56).

Inflammatory changes in endocervical cells

► Cytoplasmic degeneration
► Nuclear variation
► Ciliocytophthoria

Sometimes the delicate cytoplasm loses definition and lies in tatters around the nucleus or is permeated by polymorphs (Fig. 28.60). In other cases mucous vacuolation of cytoplasm is prominent, as in goblet cell

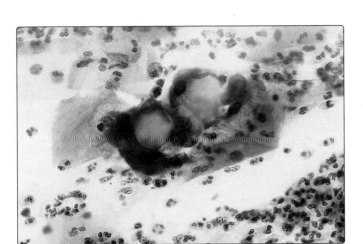

Fig. 28.61   Multinucleated endocervical cells forming goblet cells distended with mucin. The cells were seen in an inflamed smear from a patient on oral contraceptive therapy. Microglandular hyperplasia was found on cervical biopsy. (× HP)

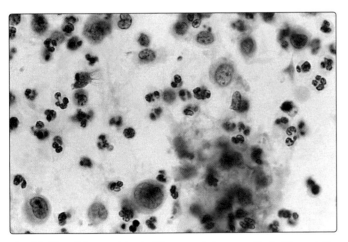

Fig. 28.62   Ciliocytophthoria. The smear is from a patient with cervicitis associated with an IUCD. A tuft of pink cilia can be seen (left), with cell debris and pyknotic nuclear remnants on the right. (× OI)

hyperplasia (Fig. 28.61). Nuclei vary markedly in size, but the shape remains round to oval. Nucleoli may be enlarged or multiple. The chromatin is often somewhat coarsened but never markedly so. Nuclear overlapping, as seen in dyskaryotic columnar cells, does not occur except when due to multinucleation, which is common in individual cells. When regeneration supervenes, mitotic figures are seen in the endocervical epithelium, but the mitoses are always morphologically normal.

Occasionally, numerous anucleate small ciliated tufts are found, consisting of the terminal plate and pink or red cilia (Fig. 28.62), mingling with vacuolated endocervical cells without cilia resembling histiocytes. Pyknotic nuclear remnants are usually also seen. This phenomenon, ciliocytophthoria (CCP), was originally thought to be due solely to viral damage, but is now recognized as a non-specific degenerative change[45].

Diagnostic pitfalls

Although several studies have shown that inflammatory changes in smears are associated with isolation of pathogenic organisms in around 40% of cases[46,47], the overall significance of inflammatory changes in smears from asymptomatic women has been called into question by other work showing lack of correlation between smear findings and identification of pathogens. One practice-based study in Canada[48] found a virtually equal rate of positive cultures (48% and 47% respectively) in women with and without cytological inflammatory changes. The authors conclude that inflammatory smears are a poor predictor of cervical infection.

Readers experienced in cytology will be aware that there are some inflammatory and degenerative characteristics shared with dyskaryotic squamous cells. These include nuclear enlargement, chromatin condensation, hyperchromasia and altered cytoplasm. Dyskaryotic cells, however, usually exhibit coarse chromatin granularity, uneven chromatin clumping, causing irregular nuclear contours, or other abnormalities of chromatin pattern, in contrast to the empty-looking nucleus with marginal chromatin condensation seen in the presence of inflammation. Nevertheless, diagnostic problems in this area should not be underestimated.

Caught between uncertainty about the significance of an inflammatory picture, the risk of under-reporting a potentially serious abnormality and the desire not to engender unnecessary anxiety for the patient, the cytologist must interpret inflammatory smear findings in the light of clinical details and the degree of confidence in establishing the absence of dyskaryosis, given that the sample is of appropriate quality. Policies on management of smears with inflammatory changes and possible dyskaryosis vary widely, but should be based on the following principles:

▶ Smears in which there are nuclear changes that might be dyskaryotic are directly reported as showing *borderline nuclear changes* ('atypical squamous cells of undetermined significance' in the Bethesda system[49]), and repeated after a short interval. Referral for colposcopy is indicated if the findings persist. Helpful guidelines have now been published in the UK[50,2] for distinguishing borderline changes from minor reactive changes and from dyskaryosis
▶ Minor inflammatory changes which are clearly not dyskaryotic and which show no evidence of a specific pathogen can be reported as within normal limits if the woman is asymptomatic and the cervix appears normal. Clinical suspicion of cervical carcinoma should always prompt gynaecological assessment and biopsy
▶ In the presence of a vaginal discharge or clinical evidence of cervicitis, a borderline smear picture should encourage the clinician to undertake microbiological investigations

Examples of smear findings from a case with simple reactive changes not requiring early repeat smears, a case with more marked nuclear abnormality reported as showing borderline nuclear changes necessitating a follow-up smear in 3–6 months and an example of definite dyskaryosis

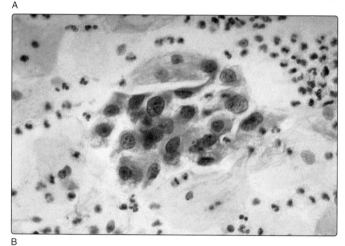

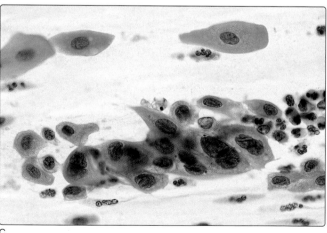

Fig. 28.63 A spectrum of nuclear changes in squamous metaplastic cells highlighting the similarity and differences between: (A) simple repair changes where there is bland nuclear enlargement in a group of immature metaplastic cells; (B) Borderline changes in metaplastic cells with some nuclear hyperchromasia but the group also includes normal nuclei (see cells on left of group) and (C) dyskaryotic nuclear changes in partially mature cells, in which the enlarged irregular nuclei show coarsely granular chromatin. (× HP)

requiring referral for colposcopy are shown in sequence in Figures 28.63 A,B,C. The diagnosis of dyskaryosis is the subject of the following chapters and the use of the term borderline change is explored further in Chapter 30.

Special types of cervicitis and vaginitis
Follicular cervicitis

This condition, also known as chronic lymphocytic cervicitis, is characterized histologically by the presence of a submucosal infiltrate of lymphocytes forming lymphoid follicles with active germinal centres (see Fig. 28.52). Although usually an incidental finding in post-menopausal women, in younger women there is an association with chlamydial infection. In the presence of ulceration or if the cervix is scraped firmly, elements of a follicle may be found in smears.

Cytological findings *(Fig. 28.64)*

► Small and large lymphocytes
► Tingible body macrophages
► Other inflammatory cells

Small mature lymphocytes with a thin rim of cytoplasm, round hyperchromatic nuclei, uniformly dense chromatin and no nucleoli predominate. Larger immature lymphocytes, several times the size of the small lymphocytes and with paler nuclei are also present.

Macrophages from the germinal centre of the lymphoid follicles confirm the diagnosis. These cells have pale nuclei and prominent nucleoli, with vague but voluminous cytoplasm. They regularly show evidence of phagocytosis, hence the term tingible body macrophages. Mitotic figures may be observed among these cells. Plasma cells and polymorphonuclear leucocytes are sometimes present.

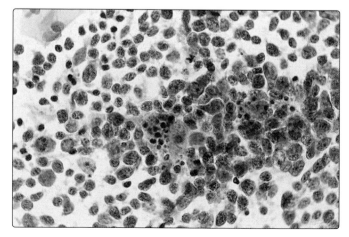

Fig. 28.64 Follicular cervicitis. An aggregate of lymphoid cells at the centre is surrounded by scattered lymphocytes of variable size. Several tingible body macrophages are present at the centre, with ingested particulate material in the cytoplasm. (× HP)

All of these cells are distributed singly, albeit closely associated: cohesive groups are not observed. The inflammatory cells are usually confined to certain areas of the smear, reflecting their focal distribution in the sampling procedure.

Diagnostic pitfalls

If this pattern is not recognized the lymphoid cells can be interpreted erroneously as undifferentiated malignant cells. The latter tend to be more regular as they are of one cell type, and they generally exfoliate in cohesive cell groups as well as singly.

The findings may also be mistaken for malignant lymphoma (see Chapter 33). In malignant lymphoma the pattern is usually rather monotonous, consisting predominantly of one type of cell with no tingible body macrophages, whereas a great variety of cells is seen in chronic lymphocytic cervicitis.

Atrophic vaginitis

Senile or atrophic vaginitis implies inflammation of the atrophic epithelium of the vagina and cervix associated with hormonal deprivation, as occurs in many post-menopausal women.

Cytological findings

▶ Poorly preserved parabasal cells, usually dissociated
▶ Numerous polymorphs covering other cells

The parabasal cells are often poorly stained with dense irregular or pyknotic or fragmented nuclei. Epithelial cells may be virtually obscured by the inflammatory exudate making it difficult to exclude dyskaryosis (Fig. 28.38). With loss of cytoplasm the nuclei may appear as dark purple nuclear streaks due to the spreading and 'blue blobs' may be noted. A change in the staining reaction of the cytoplasm of the majority of cells in the smear from green to deep orange is sometimes seen, producing appearances known as 'red atrophy' (see Fig. 28.49). There may also be a tendency for cells to form syncytia[51].

Diagnostic pitfalls

The cytological picture of senile vaginitis may be difficult to interpret as pyknotic nuclei in particular cause problems in evaluation. It is essential to note that these nuclei are dark and homogeneous without a clearly defined chromatin pattern (Figs 28.49, 28.65). When interpretation of a smear from a patient with senile vaginitis is difficult, the clinician can be requested to treat the patient with oestrogen, either applied locally or taken by mouth. A smear test one to two weeks later will have a clean background with more mature

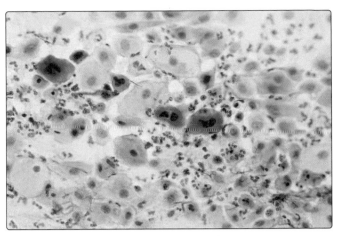

Fig. 28.65   This atrophic smear from a post-menopausal woman aged 59 shows several partially keratinized orange cells with hyperchromatic irregular nuclei. They appear degenerate and chromatin detail cannot be seen. Subsequent smears reverted to normal after use of local oestrogen cream. (× HP)

epithelial cells which are usually easily assessed (see Fig. 28.38).

If dyskaryotic cells are present they should be readily recognized after short term use of oestrogen because they do not mature[52]. In documenting this finding, however, Kashimura et al. noted that the number of *mature* dyskaryotic cells increased in smears after administration of oestrogen, possibly because dyskaryotic cells have more cytoplasmic oestrogen receptors than malignant cells.

Microorganisms of the vagina and cervix

Bacteria

In routine smears it is only possible to establish the shape and distribution of bacteria. These features may suggest a particular organism but definitive identification must be made by microbiological culture. It is essential to be fully aware of the endogenous flora of the vagina to understand the role of bacteria in vaginitis and cervicitis.

Endogenous flora of the vagina

Döderlein's bacilli or lactobacilli are rod-shaped organisms 3–6 μm in length, arranged singly or in chains (Figs 28.66, 28.67). Their enzymes are able to dissolve the cell wall of intermediate cells by cytolysis, freeing the glycogen content, which is then degraded. This change is brought about by a process of anaerobic glycolysis, not by transformation of glycogen into lactic acid by the organisms, thus accounting for the 25% of asymptomatic women without vaginal lactobacilli yet with an acid vaginal pH.

Döderlein's bacilli are not found in smears when the pH is alkaline, as they are dependent on an acid pH. Lactobacillus overgrowth with extreme cytolysis can occur during pregnancy, in the second half of the menstrual cycle, when progesterone containing contraceptive drugs are used, and sometimes at the menopause, especially in diabetics.

Corynebacteria are Gram-positive bacilli that can theoretically be distinguished from lactobacilli by their arrangement in groups. However, identification is almost impossible to achieve in a cervical smear. These bacteria can proliferate in the vagina because the mucous membrane functions as a culture medium, breakdown of the epithelial cells ensuring a continuous supply of nutrients in the form of amino acids and glycogen.

Leptothrix are non-pathogenic thread-like bacteria lying in loops or sometimes in pairs (Fig. 28.68). They are much longer than Döderlein's bacilli and the latter never lie in loops. Leptothrix are sometimes found together with trichomonads. The presence of Leptothrix in a smear is of no clinical importance and their precise microbiological identity is unclear.

Exogenous flora

Bacteria from the surrounding environment can be introduced into the vagina. If the endogenous flora is poorly developed, for instance before puberty when the epithelium is thin and contains no glycogen, local organisms from outside the vagina proliferate and may finally dominate the field.

In adults, microorganisms from without are most commonly introduced during coitus from the skin of the vulva, perineum or penis. Semen, too, can contain pathogenic microorganisms from the urethra or prostate gland of the sexual partner in cases of urethritis or prostatitis. Other sources of extrinsic infection include

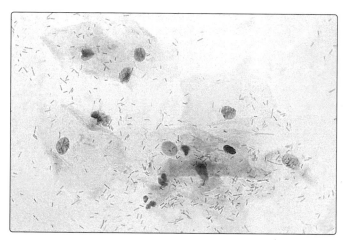

Fig. 28.66 Lactobacilli. The background of this smear shows numerous rod-shaped organisms, arranged singly and in short chains. Cytolysis of intermediate cells is also apparent, leaving bare nuclei and wisps of cytoplasm. (× HP)

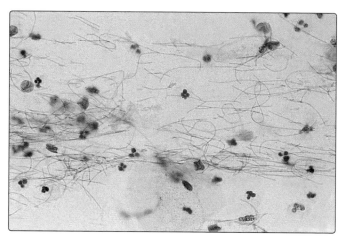

Fig. 28.68 Leptothrix organisms are seen in this smear in long strands and loops. Note the absence of any significant inflammatory infiltrate. (× HP)

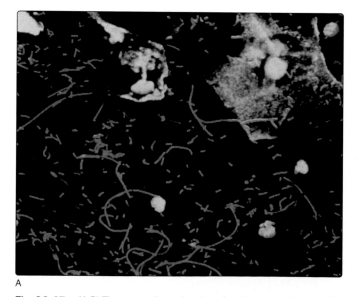
A

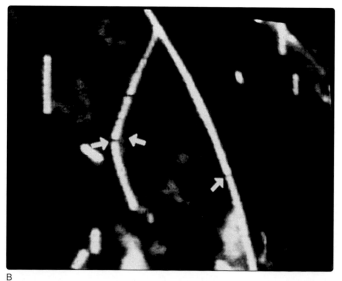
B

Fig. 28.67 (A,B) These two-dimensional confocal images of lactobacilli emphasize their structure and arrangement. (× HP)

spread of organisms from the upper genital tract and blood-borne spread.

Coccoid overgrowth

The perineal skin flora forms a heterogeneous group of organisms consisting of short rods and cocci (Fig. 28.69A). Staphylococci in groups and streptococci in chains are included in this coccoid flora and may gain access to the vagina or cervix. They are only pathogenic in the vagina when the epithelium is damaged.

Coitus influences the pH and protein concentration in the vagina since semen is alkaline and the ejaculate is rich in protein. Both factors can affect bacterial growth: coccoid organisms, in particular, need an alkaline environment for an overgrowth to occur while the altered pH inhibits the growth of lactobacilli. The presence of coccoid bacteria is not usually reported and is only significant if there is overgrowth accompanied by absence of Döderlein's bacilli. The latter reappear when vaginal irrigation fluid containing lactic acid based liquid soap is used.

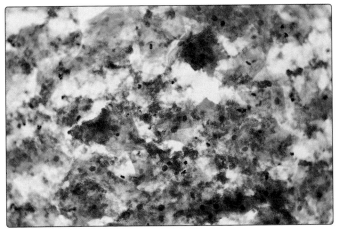

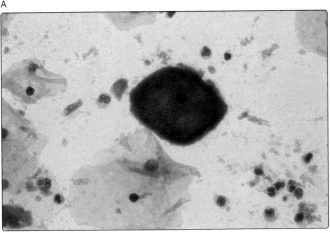

Fig. 28.69 (A) Coccoid overgrowth, creating a bacterial haze over both cells and background. An epithelial pearl is present near the centre. (× HP) (B) A typical 'clue cell' covered by a dense layer of organisms seen in a smear from a patient with bacterial vaginosis. (× HP)

Gardnerella vaginalis

Gardnerella vaginalis is a small rod-shaped bacterium. It is transmitted by sexual intercourse and can be cultured in 20% of asymptomatic women. The significance of this finding is not well understood[53], but the organism is associated with the symptomatic condition bacterial vaginitis[54], also known as bacterial vaginosis[55]. Patients with symptoms due to bacterial vaginosis have pruritus and leucorrhoea. The vagina contains a mixed population of microorganisms, including *Gardnerella vaginalis*, Bacteroides species, anaerobic cocci, Mobiluncus species and *Mycoplasma hominis*. A pH above 4.5 and interaction between Gardnerella and various Bacteroides organisms are factors in the production of symptoms.

Since the exact aetiology and pathogenesis of bacterial vaginosis is still unclear, the definition of bacterial vaginosis proposed at an international meeting held in Stockholm in 1984 is followed: 'A replacement of Döderlein bacteria by characteristic groups of bacteria accompanied by changed properties of the vaginal fluid'. Clinically, the diagnosis is based on the presence of a thin homogeneous discharge with a pH above 4.5 and a fishy amine odour, more manifest when the pH is further raised by KOH. Diagnosis is particularly important in pregnancy, as there is a risk of chorioamnionitis and preterm delivery if the condition is untreated[56,57].

Cytological findings

► Clue cells
► Mixed bacteria, mainly coccoid
► Absence of polymorphs

In a routine smear *coccoid* bacteria are seen mainly on squamous epithelial cells which, as a result, stain darkly and appear cloudy (Fig. 28.69B). In the North American literature these cells are called 'clue cells', but the term 'glue cell' may be more apt since the Gardnerella organisms seem to be glued to squamous cells. Examination of these cells under oil immersion allows detection of the different organisms present; small rods which are *Gardnerella vaginalis*, cocci and curved bacilli, Mobiluncus spp[58]. The range of organisms present can be confirmed by Gram stain[59].

Reporting the presence of Mobiluncus spp. (Fig. 28.70) in smears of women with bacterial vaginosis is thought to be clinically relevant, since it implies a need for prolonged treatment with metronidazole[47]. Mycoplasmas such as *M. hominis* are microorganisms so small that they pass through bacterial filters. They can barely be seen with the light microscope.

Actinomyces organisms

Actinomyces spp. are 'higher bacteria', capable of forming colonies, and commonly found in the cervical smears of women using various types of intrauterine devices (IUDs)[60], particularly plastic devices. The organisms are usually saprophytic and cause no symptoms. They are also found in association with vaginal pessaries, and in the presence of foreign bodies such as forgotten tampons. They are frequently present in the tonsillar crypts of the pharynx, and may therefore be transmitted to the vagina by orogenital contact. Gupta[61] reports that actinomycotic

infection can cause clinical symptoms of lower genital tract inflammation, including a malodorous brownish discharge in some cases. Dissemination of Actinomyces spp. to distant sites has also been documented[62].

Cytological findings

▶ Colonies of filamentous organisms staining dark blue
▶ Variable inflammatory exudate
▶ Variable inflammatory changes in epithelial cells

With Papanicolaou staining, actinomycotic colonies appear as dark 'bales of wool', stained blue with haematoxylin. Thin radiating filaments protrude outwards from the central tangled mass (Fig. 28.71A). The diagnostic sulphur granules seen macroscopically in sputum are seldom found in cervicovaginal smears. Special stains, such as the Gram stain or Gomori's methenamine silver, may be of help in confirming the diagnosis and in differentiating these bacteria from other organisms forming radiating colonies (Fig. 28.71B)[61]. Lactobacilli are usually absent, having been replaced by a coccoid flora.

Non-specific inflammation frequently accompanies the organisms, whether or not the woman has symptoms. The epithelial cells may show inflammatory changes in nucleus or cytoplasm, usually only minor and infrequently requiring a repeat of the smear for exclusion of dyskaryosis.

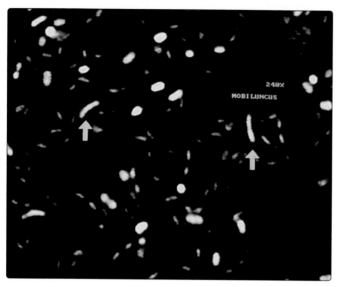

Fig. 28.70 Mobiluncus bacilli (arrows) in a mixed flora. Note their comma-like shape. Three-dimensional confocal image. (× HP)

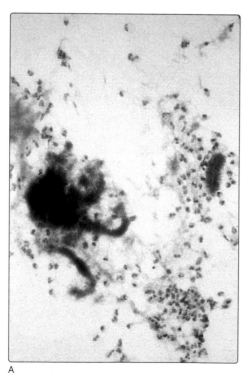

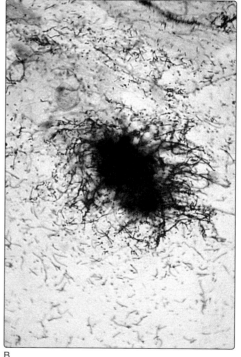

A   B

Fig. 28.71 (A) Actinomyces organisms in a smear from an asymptomatic woman with an IUCD *in situ*. The organisms form a tangled mass of filamentous bacteria projecting irregularly from the margins. (× HP) (B) Gram staining of a destained smear shows the filamentous structure of the organisms and reveals many organisms in the background. (× HP)

Actinomycotic organisms are usually commensal. However some gynaecologists advocate removal of the IUCD and treatment with antibiotics, because in rare instances certain Actinomyces spp. may cause pelvic inflammatory disease with subsequent infertility or ectopic pregnancy. It is necessary to report the presence of actinomycotic organisms in a smear to enable interpretation of the finding in the light of any clinical abnormalities, but the mere presence of the organism cannot be equated with infection.

Visualization of vaginal flora in cervical smears using the Jones-Marres silver staining method

The advantage of studying the vaginal flora for bacteria and fungi in cervical smears instead of using microbiological culture, is that they can be observed as they occur in their natural habitat[59]. They are, however, only faintly stained with the conventional Papanicolaou method and their visualization is limited. Therefore a modified microwave silver staining method has been developed, the so-called Jones-Marres method[63]. Bacteria and fungi stain distinctly black and can be studied in greater detail, and their interrelationship demonstrated.

The originally Papanicolaou-stained smears do not need to be decolourized, and can be stained directly, as described by Boon et al.[63]. The haematoxylin and EA of the Papanicolaou staining method are almost completely removed by the periodic acid staining solution of the staining method. Fungi and bacteria stain black. Bacteria can be identified as such because their shape is outlined in great detail, while protein debris, often present as background, is greyish and the particles have no specific shape.

Actinomyces in Jones-Marres-stained smears

Actinomyces are very well outlined in black, displaying the well-known arrangement into 'bales of wool' with thin radiating threads protrude outward. In addition, many single thread-like structures lying loose in the background of the smear are observed. In the silver-stained smears, it is no longer difficult to differentiate these bacteria from the so-called pseudoactinomycotic radiate granules[64], because the latter do not stain with silver.

Candida in Jones-Marres-stained smears

In the silver stain, both pseudohyphae and spores of Candida albicans, a yeast organism, stain black, the spores more intensely than the hyphae. Recurrent Candida infection is a clinical problem and antifungal treatments may have only limited success. It is therefore of interest to have a closer look at the associated bacterial flora to devise new approaches. Candida thrives on glycogen, thus it is not surprising that we see it often with overgrowth of lactobacilli (23%). The most prominent flora is that of lactobacilli, associated with a low pH. It is clear that vaginal rinses using acid solutions will not help, but alkaline rinses are helpful by stimulating the growth of coccoid bacteria[13].

The rationale behind these alkaline vaginal rinses in counteracting Candida albicans is that the adherence of Candida spores is inversely related to pH[65].

Typing of the bacterial flora in Jones-Marres-stained smears

Because the bacteria are well stained, the vaginal flora can be classified into four groups, depending on the shape and form of the bacteria, and on which type predominates.

Type 1: Lactobacillus overgrowth. In this type of flora the bacteria are rod-shaped, slender and long, sometimes arranged in long chains. There is an abundance of bacteria within and outside the epithelial cells, often with marked cytolysis of the glycogen-rich intermediate squamous cells. No coccoid bacteria are detected.

Type 2: Lactobacillus flora. The number of lactobacilli is much lower than in Type 1, and the organisms are not in chains. There is no cytolysis. In some smears, one can find a limited number of coccoid bacteria, but the lactobacilli still predominate.

Type 3: Mixed flora. In this flora a mixture of lactobacilli and various other short, plump or round bacteria including the comma-shaped Mobiluncus[66], streptococci in short rows, and other coccoid bacteria from the perineal flora[13] can be observed. Occasionally, a few 'clue cells', with coccoid Gardnerella covering epithelial cells[42] can be found in these smears. The number of bacteria is variable, but never extremely abundant such as in Type 1 and Type 4 smears.

Type 4: Coccoid overgrowth. There is an abundance of coccoid bacteria in the background of the smear and covering epithelial cells ('clue cells'). In addition, the bacteria cling to the outer edge of the epithelial cells. In silver stained preparations there may be a few lactobacilli, but most of the bacteria are coccoid in type.

Table 28.2 Vaginal flora in the presence of Candida or Actinomyces

	Candida (n = 100)	Actinomyces (n = 100)
Lactobacilli overgrowth	23%	0%
Lactobacilli	35%	4%
Mixed flora	42%	22%
Coccoid overgrowth	0%	74%

Table 28.3 Vaginal flora of symptomatic and asymptomatic women

	Symptomatic		Asymptomatic	
	n	%	n	%
Lactobacilli overgrowth	12	40.0	10	6.5
Lactobacilli	4	13.3	24	15.7
Mixed flora	4	13.3	60	38.9
Coccoid overgrowth	10	33.3	60	38.9

In Jones-Marres-stained slides there is a clear relationship between the type of vaginal flora and the presence of *Candida albicans* or Actinomyces spp. (Table 28.3). Coccoid overgrowth is never seen in the presence of Candida but is often seen in combination with actinomycotic organisms. Symptomatic women, other than those with potential pathogens such as Trichomonas vaginalis, tend to show either Lactobacillus overgrowth or coccoid overgrowth. Coccoid overgrowth has long been recognized as causing symptoms[54], but it would appear that overgrowth of lactobacilli might not always be physiological. In this context it is important to mention that Eschenbach *et al.*[67] found as many as 16 different Lactobacillus species among symptomatic women. Recent publications show that Lactobacillus species can show pathogenic potential[68]. The above findings are in keeping with the papers quoted and confirm that an overgrowth of lactobacilli is not necessarily physiological.

Neisseria gonorrhoeae

The gonococcus is the organism causing gonorrhoea, a cosmopolitan venereal disease. In women, the epithelial cells of the urethra and endocervix are infected. Infection may extend to the vestibular glands causing bartholinitis, and to the endometrium causing endometritis or salpingitis if the fallopian tubes are involved. Even the peritoneal cavity may be involved, leading to pelvic inflammatory disease.

In cervical smears the bacteria are shaped like coffee beans in a characteristic pattern of pairs (diplococci) whereby the round sides of the two beans face outward. They are slightly larger than the cocci of the perineal flora and have occasionally been identified in routine Papanicolaou stained cervical smears[69]. Gonococci may be found in smears when infection has not been suspected clinically.

Characteristic Gram-negative intracellular diplococci, best observed in the air-dried areas of the smear, are strongly suggestive of gonorrhoea, but the final diagnosis should be made by microbiological culture or by RNA–DNA *in situ* hybridization.

Mycobacterium tuberculosis

Tuberculous endometritis or cervicitis is almost always secondary to tuberculosis of the fallopian tubes, which in turn results from blood-borne infection due to primary tuberculosis of lung or intestine. The infection is now rare in Western society, while remaining a frequent occurrence in third world countries such as Africa and India.

Histological examination reveals that the stroma of the endometrium or cervix contains epithelioid giant cell granulomata or tubercles. They show central caseation necrosis, and there may be overlying ulceration with non-specific chronic inflammation. Epithelioid cells are derived from histiocytes, subsequently fusing to form the giant cells, which are of Langhan's type.

In tuberculous cervicitis, cervical smears may include elements of the granulomas[70]. Epithelioid histiocytes with slender footprint-shaped nuclei, fine chromatin and ill-defined cytoplasm have been described; Langhan's giant cells, with nuclei polarized at the periphery of the cytoplasm, are less often seen. They differ from other histiocytic giant cells, which have more central nuclei and may contain ingested material.

Granular pale pink amorphous material arising from caseous necrosis may be substantial or inconspicuous. *M tuberculosis* can be demonstrated in this material by acid- or alcohol-fast stains such as the Ziehl Neelsen technique. However the final diagnosis can only be established on the basis of histological and bacteriological studies using the Ziehl Neelsen stain and special culture media for positive identification.

The pattern of tuberculous cervicitis must be distinguished from tissue repair and ulceration, either of which may accompany the infection. Smears then show ragged sheets of reactive epithelial cells with enlarged nuclei and prominent nucleoli, and there is non-specific background inflammation.

Calymmatobacterium (Donovania) granulomatosis

This bacterium causes granuloma inguinale (donovaniasis), a venereal infection common in tropical and subtropical climates, being rare in Europe and the USA. It induces granulomatous inflammation with caseous necrosis mainly in the skin of the external genitalia and perianal region. Scrapings from ulcerated lesions of the vulva, vagina or cervix show histiocytes with multiple vacuoles containing straight or curved dumbell-shaped rods. They have prominent bipolar granules known as Donovan bodies[71,72]. Donovan bodies can be visualized very well with the Warthin-Starry silver staining method and by Giemsa staining.

Treponema pallidum

The spirochaetal organism *Treponema pallidum*, causative agent of syphilis, usually infects the vulva initially but may produce a primary chancre on the cervix. The organisms cannot be identified in Papanicolaou stained smears, although demonstrable by silver stains such as the Warthin-Starry method. The overall picture in a smear is that of non-specific inflammation.

Protozoa

Trichomonas vaginalis

Trichomonas vaginalis is a protozoan organism found in the vagina, either as a saprophyte or as a pathogenic organism[73]. A figure approaching 50% of women with vaginal trichomoniasis are symptom free. In the male, the organism can be found in the prostate gland. Infection is regarded as venereal in origin[74], requiring treatment of both partners for complete eradication. *Trichomonas vaginalis* infection can produce a variety of symptoms including a foamy or white discharge, vaginal dryness, postcoital and intermenstrual bleeding. Punctate haemorrhagic spots may develop in the mucosa, an appearance known as 'strawberry vagina'.

Trichomoniasis is usually but not invariably associated with inflammation. The vaginal pH is often alkaline, and a coccoid flora is frequently seen.

Cytological findings *(Figs 28.72–28.74)*

► Unicellular pear-shaped organisms 8–20 μm in diameter
► Pale grey-green cytoplasm with eosinophilic granules centrally
► Oval or crescentic vesicular nuclei, lightly stained
► Inflammatory changes often very pronounced

Trichomonads vary in size and shape, sometimes even occurring as giant forms measuring over 150 μm. There is some correlation between size and pathogenicity: the smaller organisms are more likely to be symptomatic. They vary from oval or triangular to comma or tadpole-shaped and move by means of trailing flagella, which are rarely seen in Papanicolaou stained smears. They multiply by binary fission and the organisms can be found in mitosis.

With a pronounced inflammatory reaction, the smear shows a characteristic purple colour caused by the pinkish red colour of mature epithelial cells and the darkly stained polymorphs. The latter are often arranged as an agglomeration around an organism. A web of fibrinous exudate may be seen in the background. Leptothrix organisms may be present as well.

Trichomonads sometimes attach to the surface of squamous cells to form a ring around the margin. They may even invade the epithelial cell cytoplasm. The nuclei of squamous epithelial cells are enlarged and hyperchromatic; the chromatin pattern can be irregular and perinuclear

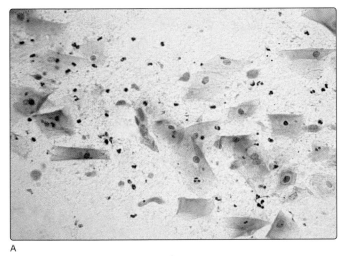

A

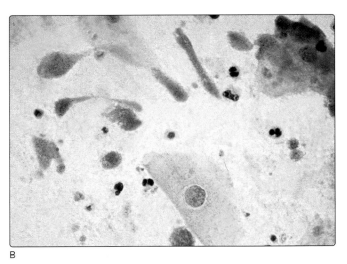

B

Fig. 28.72 (A) *Trichomonas vaginalis* organisms are rounded or ovoid cyanophilic organisms, larger than polymorphs but smaller than the parabasal cells at centre. (× MP) (B) This closer view of the protozoa shows their variable shapes. The cytoplasmic granules and outline of a nucleus can just be discerned. Note the halo around the intermediate cell nucleus. (× HP)

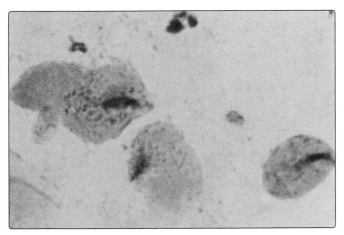

Fig. 28.73 Giant trichomonads showing obvious vesicular crescentic nuclei stained lightly by haematoxylin. (× OI)

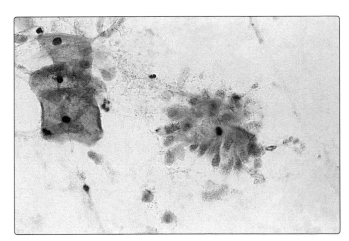

Fig. 28.74 Trichomonads attached to the margin of a squamous cell. Many free organisms are also seen. (× HP)

haloes are common[75] (see Figs 28.55, 28.70B). Secondary orangeophilia of cell cytoplasm may be seen.

Diagnostic pitfalls

In atrophic smears mucus, cell fragments and parabasal cells with karyolysis can be mistaken for trichomonads. Although similar in size and staining, they lack the crescentic nucleus and cytoplasmic granules of *T. vaginalis*.

Sometimes epithelial changes are such that mild dyskaryosis is suspected. In these cases a further smear should be taken after treatment of the infection to establish whether the changes are due to the trichomonads or represent concomitant dyskaryosis.

Entamoeba gingivalis

Entamoeba gingivalis has been reported in 10% of patients with IUCDs colonized by actinomycotic organisms[76]. This protozoan parasite is often found in the oral cavity if teeth and gums are in poor condition. Spread to the genital tract probably occurs by orogenital contact. *Entamoeba gingivalis* is unlikely to be pathogenic in this setting.

Cytological findings

▶ Rounded amoeboid organisms 10–40 µm in diameter
▶ Pale cyanophilic cytoplasm with eccentric nuclei
▶ Ingested polymorphs within cytoplasm

The organism is virtually always found in combination with actinomycotic colonies at the borders of the tangled organisms where it attaches itself to the filaments (Fig. 28.75). *E. gingivalis* can usually be differentiated from the more pathogenic *E. histolytica*: trophozoites of the former show ingestion of polymorphs, a coarser karyosome, less delicate pattern of peripheral chromatin and multidirectional pseudopodia; *E. histolytica* trophozoites

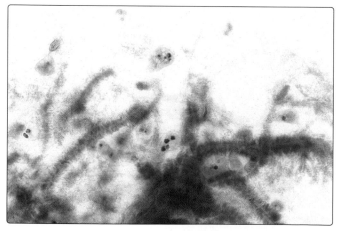

Fig. 28.75 *Entamoeba gingivalis* organisms can be seen at the margins of this colony of actinomycotic organisms in a smear from a patient with an IUCD. The protozoa have ingested fragments of leucocytes. (× HP)

show ingested erythrocytes, a fine central karyosome, delicate peripheral chromatin and unidirectional pseudopodia[77].

Entamoeba histolytica

Entamoeba histolytica infection, also known as amoebiasis, is widespread in subtropical and tropical areas. Infection begins when trophozoites invade the colonic mucosa and may remain localized for many years, or may extend to the liver and other organs, including the female genital tract. The majority of patients with genital amoebiasis have simultaneous amoebic colitis, suggesting that protozoa reach the genital tract by direct contamination due to poor hygiene.

Cytological diagnosis is based on identification of the protozoa. These small round or oval organisms have cytoplasm staining faintly with the light green component of the Papanicolaou stain. Erythrophagocytosis is frequently seen. With the aid of the PAS stain, the parasite can be readily identified because of its high glycogen content[78]. The background of the smear may contain many polymorphs and necrotic granular material.

Most European laboratories do not encounter *E. histolytica* in smears, but sporadic cases do occur in developed countries, usually imported from endemic areas.

Fungi

Fungi are microorganisms multiplying by spore formation or by division. The spores elongate to form pseudohyphae or may grow into long septate hyphae, which branch to form a mycelium. The rudimentary part derived from the spore is the thallus.

Classification of fungi is based on the nature and method of spore formation. The simplest forms of colony and spore formation are seen in the unicellular fungi: the Saccharomyces (baker's yeast) and the Cryptococci. These reproduce by budding or gemmation and do not produce a mycelium. Candida is slightly more complicated in that several germinal ducts develop from the spore. The germinal ducts form long branching hyphae in which cell division occurs. New spores develop on the hyphae.

Most of the fungal infections in the vagina are caused by *Candida albicans*, sometimes still known as monilia. A few cases are due to *Geotrichum candidum* or *Torulopsis glabrata*, which is now classified with candida. Other fungal elements seen are usually contaminants (see Fig. 28.32).

Candida albicans

This dimorphic fungus is a common cause of symptomatic infection, with a white curdy non-odorous vaginal discharge and pruritus vulvae. Candida infections are prone to occur when the progesterone level is high, as in pregnancy or when contraceptive hormones are used. Infections are also common when bacterial equilibrium is disturbed, e.g. by broad-spectrum antibiotics or chemotherapeutic drugs.

In symptomatic infections, the organisms invade the squamous cells. When saprophytic, as in 20% of cases, spores and pseudohyphae are sparse in the smear, lying between or on top of the squamous cells.

Cytological findings *(Figs 28.76, 28.77)*

► Double-contoured pale pink hyphae and pseudohyphae
► Pseudohyphae appear septate
► Spores are eosinophilic, measuring 2–4 μm
► Inflammatory changes are variable

In Papanicolaou stained smears the filaments of Candida stain faintly with eosin, sometimes with haematoxylin. They are usually pseudohyphae, formed by branching chains of elongated buds, giving an appearance of septation likened to a bamboo cane. The Jones-Marres silver stain reveals black spores and paler pseudohyphae.

The epithelial cells often lie in plaques due to progesterone effects, from which the fungal filaments protrude like thin spider's legs. Inflammatory exudate, inflammatory changes in epithelial cell cytoplasm and perinuclear haloes are often seen.

Diagnostic pitfalls

Degenerate red blood cells may be mistaken for spores and streaks of mucus for hyphae. They do not show the typical structure of Candida. Contaminant fungi are occasionally a source of confusion.

There is often little or no inflammatory exudate and the Candida may then not be relevant clinically, especially if there are no symptoms and only spores are found. The fungus should be reported, stating the extent and whether in the form of spores or hyphae, to enable clinical assessment to be made.

The squamous cells may show reactive changes such as nuclear enlargement, orange staining of cytoplasm and perinuclear haloes. If these changes are marked or the cells are obscured by polymorphs the smear may need to be repeated after treatment.

Candida glabrata

Vaginal infection by this organism, formerly known as *Torulopsis glabrata*, is much less common than *Candida albicans* infection. Slight pruritus or burning can occur but discharge is slight and there may be no symptoms. Spores of variable size (2–8 μm) with unilateral gemmation are seen in small groups with absence of filaments. Lactobacilli are often present. Cell changes are slight apart from eosinophilia[79].

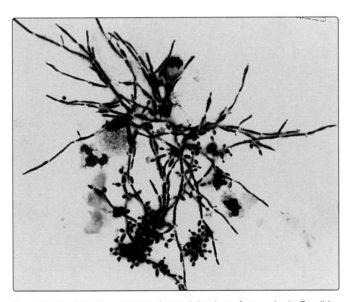

Fig. 28.76 Budding yeasts and pseudohyphae of saprophytic *Candida albicans*. (× HP)

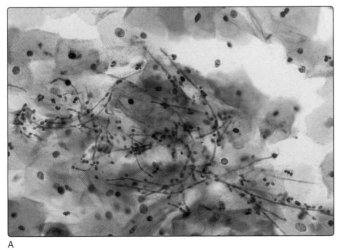

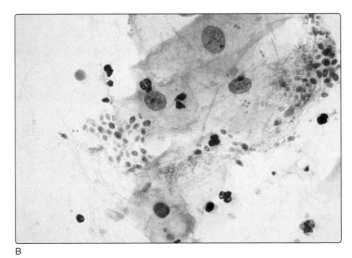

A   B

Fig. 28.77 (A) Candida hyphae forming a tangled mass overlying a plaque of squamous cells. Some spores can be seen between the hyphae. (× HP) (B) Spore forms of Candida are often seen in smears, as illustrated. They do not necessarily signify active infection in the absence of hyphae. (× HP)

Viruses

Viral infections of the female genital tract are common and important. Besides causing infections which may be painful, distressing and recurrent, there is now overwhelming evidence that the pathogenesis of cervical carcinoma is linked to certain strains of the human papillomavirus, and other viruses may act as cofactors, although their exact role in cervical carcinogenesis is not yet fully elucidated (see Chapter 29).

Herpes simplex virus

Herpes simplex type II virus (HSV II) or *herpes genitalis* and the closely related *herpes simplex* type I virus (HSV I) or *herpes labialis* belong to the neurodermotropic herpesviruses, that is they have a predilection for tissues of ectodermal origin such as skin or mucosa, and also for nervous tissue. *Herpes labialis* causes blisters on the lips. HSV infection of the genital tract, caused chiefly by HSV II and occasionally by HSV I, is acquired by sexual contact.

Primary genital HSV infection is manifested by the appearance of multiple widespread vesicles or ulcerative lesions on the external genitalia. Small pustular lesions may coalesce into large areas of ulceration. The ulcers persist from 4–15 days until crusting and healing occur.

Primary genital herpes is associated with HSV cervicitis in 90% of patients[80], and is frequently accompanied by systemic symptoms such as fever, headache, malaise and muscle pain. In addition, there are local symptoms of pain, itching, dysuria, vaginal or urethral discharge, and tender swollen inguinal lymph nodes. The disease is self-limiting. After an attack the virus assumes a state of latency, usually in the dorsal root ganglia of the lumbosacral plexus.

In some women, recurrent episodes of infection occur. Because antibodies to the virus have already been produced, recurrences are of short duration and have much milder symptoms. HSV may affect the cervix alone, without involving the external genitalia and these patients may be asymptomatic. Immunosuppressed patients are predisposed to more frequent and more severe recurrent episodes.

Cytological findings *(Fig. 28.78A,B,C)*

▶ Swollen nuclei with multinucleation
▶ Ground glass chromatin with prominent nuclear membranes
▶ Nuclear inclusions

The cytopathic effects evolve in three stages. In the first stage there is increased granularity in epithelial nuclei with fine intranuclear vacuolation. It may be difficult to distinguish these changes from those seen in degenerate cells due to other causes. The second stage is marked by further change in the chromatin pattern, which becomes indistinct, giving a so-called 'ground glass' appearance to the nucleus. This is caused by swelling of the viral material in the nucleus[81]. A distinct nuclear membrane is visible. The cytoplasm becomes dense and basophilic. In the third stage the nucleus contains an acidophilic inclusion body, which is surrounded by a clear zone[82]. The inclusion bodies have been described by virologists as 'tombstones' because they

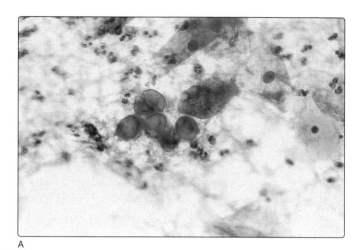

A

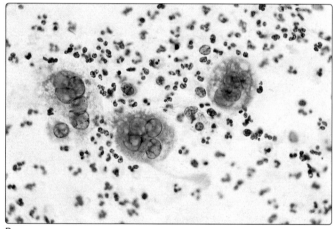

B

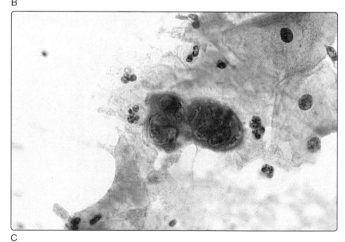

C

Fig. 28.78   (A, B, C) *Herpes simplex* virus changes in cervical epithelial cells. Initially there is swelling of the nuclei, followed by degeneration of chromatin leading to a ground glass pattern (A). Multinucleation is a prominent feature (B). Inclusion bodies appear as the cells start to die (C). (× HP)

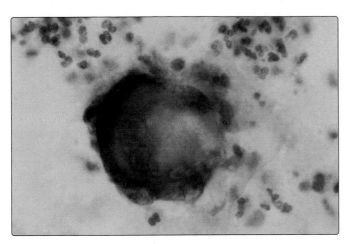

Fig. 28.79 Immunoperoxidase stain using monoclonal antibody to Herpesvirus hominis, showing positive inclusion bodies in a group of cervical epithelial cells. (× HP)

reveal the death of the cell. They are not, as some authors suggest, a sign of recurrent infection.

In the second and third stages many multinucleated cells are found. They may contain 20 or more nuclei lying close together, moulding against each other without overlapping, a point of contrast with those in reactive multinucleated endocervical cells or histiocytes. The nuclei show ground glass changes and inclusion bodies as described above. These multinucleate cells are characteristic of herpetic infection at any site.

The virus infects cells from the ectocervical and endocervical epithelium. The cell shape is usually distorted and may make identification of cell type difficult. Immunoperoxidase techniques have proved reliable for the confirmation of HSV II (Fig. 28.79)[83]. More recently, specific probes have become available for the demonstration of HSV II by means of DNA *in situ* hybridization.

Diagnostic pitfalls

Multinucleation and nuclear swelling are reactive features common to various other inflammatory and repair processes, although usually lesser in degree than in *herpes simplex* infection. Ground glass nuclear changes are more specific, as are intranuclear inclusions.

The risk of over-diagnosis of HSV in endocervical brush samples in particular has been stressed by Stowell *et al.*, who found multinucleation and margination of nuclear chromatin to be of limited value in diagnosis compared with the presence of a ground glass chromatin pattern, which had a sensitivity and specificity of 95%[84].

In 1990 in Leiden, herpesvirus was recognized in 0.02% of smears, one fifth of the frequency reported by Patten[85]. Naib and Masukawa[86] reported an incidence of 1.6:1000. The prevalence of herpes infection is almost 20 times higher in women attending genito-urinary medicine clinics than in women attending clinics for obstetrics and gynaecology[87].

The diagnosis of herpetic infection is important because the patients are at risk of having other sexually transmitted infections. Furthermore, women with herpes infection may have a concomitant *in situ* or invasive cervical carcinoma[88], and conversely, necrotic herpetic lesions of the cervix may mimic invasive cancer macroscopically. Finally, there is a risk, albeit low, that maternal herpesvirus infection may be transmitted to the foetus during vaginal delivery; this infection is potentially fatal.

Human papillomavirus (HPV): wart virus infection

Genital warts or condylomata acuminata are caused by infection with human types of papillomaviruses. These DNA viruses of the Papovavirus family now include over 80 different subtypes, exhibiting site specificity. The viruses are epidermotropic, infecting first the basal layer of cells and inducing proliferation of the infected epithelium. Productive growth with viral shedding from the surface of the lesion occurs later. Certain strains are known to have oncogenic potential, probably as initiating agents in the pathogenesis of cervical carcinoma, although it appears that cofactors are necessary for progression to invasive cancer (see Chapter 29).

The virus produces characteristic cytopathic effects in squamous cells, recognizable in tissue sections and in cervical smears. Definitive identification of the virus is, however, dependent on specific techniques. There are currently four such methods, listed in order of increasing sensitivity: identification of the virus by electron microscopy; staining of the capsule antigen with immunocytochemical techniques; identification of viral DNA by *in situ* hybridization; and most sensitive of all, the polymerase chain reaction (PCR) technique, based on DNA amplification. Each method has advantages and limitations, as discussed in Chapter 29.

It should be noted that cells showing the cytopathic effects of papillomavirus infection in a smear are often positive for the virus by immunocytochemistry, but *in situ* hybridization reveals additional evidence of the presence of the virus in cytologically normal cells.

Two major types of condylomatous lesions can be distinguished histologically, namely the papillary type, which is clinically visible as a genital wart or condyloma acuminatum, and the flat wart or condyloma planum, which may only be detectable by colposcopy or, in the male, by peniscopy (Fig. 28.80). Condylomata acuminata are usually multiple and may be present on the vulva or vagina as well as the cervix[89].

Genital warts were recognized in ancient times by Roman and Greek physicians. They occur mainly in young adults. Their transmission by sexual intercourse was firmly established in 1954[90]. In a follow-up study of American servicemen returning from the Korean War who acquired

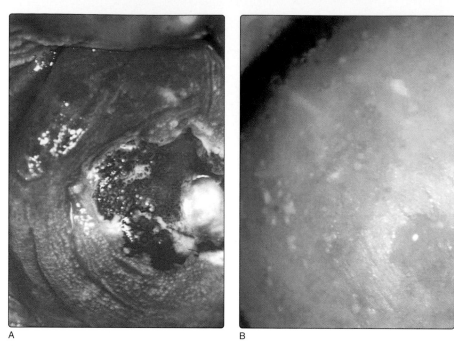

A   B

Fig. 28.80   (A) Colposcopic view of cervix with a flat HPV lesion revealed as an area of white mucosa after application of weak acetic acid. (B) Peniscopy of partner of the above patient with HPV infection. Note multiple flat lesions.

penile warts while in Korea, the study found that genital warts appeared in the wives of these servicemen after an incubation period of four to six weeks. The partners of women with colposcopically detected flat HPV lesions also show flat penile lesions[91].

Condylomata are associated with promiscuity and with the presence of other venereal diseases[92]. Alternative modes of transmission are known to occur, such as during childbirth, but are much less common. Immunosuppression, whether iatrogenic or due to natural disease, is a major risk factor for developing papillomavirus infection. A defective immune system also appears to play a part in progression of these lesions to CIN or invasive carcinoma[93].

Histological findings in HPV infection

Condylomata are composed of thickened squamous epithelium, often keratinized, arranged in numerous papillary folds supported by projecting cores of fibrovascular tissue (Fig. 28.81). Cytopathic viral effects can be seen in histological sections, consisting of a broad empty zone around the nucleus with a thick rim of residual cytoplasm at the periphery. The nucleus is enlarged, hyperchromatic and crumpled. Cells with these changes are called koilocytes, derived from the Greek word 'koilos,' meaning hollow. Multinucleation, normal mitotic figures and premature keratinization of individual cells (dyskeratosis) are also seen.

Flat condylomas or condylomata plana can only be identified with the aid of the colposcope and were not described until 1976[94] and 1977[95]. Histologically, they lack

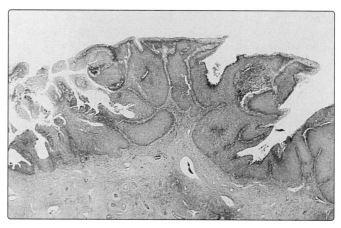

Fig. 28.81   Condyloma acuminatum of cervix in histological section. The form is that of a raised excrescence of folded hyperplastic epithelium, with a layer of keratinization on the surface and some nonspecific inflammation in the underlying stroma. (× LP)

the classical exophytic papillary epithelial proliferation of condylomata acuminata, the mucosa being only slightly thickened, but the cytopathic changes in individual cells can be seen, enabling a diagnosis of HPV infection to be made with some confidence (Fig. 28.82). Koilocytes may be difficult to distinguish from glycogen-laden cells in the upper layers of the mucosa; the focal distribution of koilocytes, accompanied by nuclear changes and other cytopathic effects, favour HPV change.

Whereas condylomata acuminata occur predominantly in the native stratified squamous epithelium of the vulva,

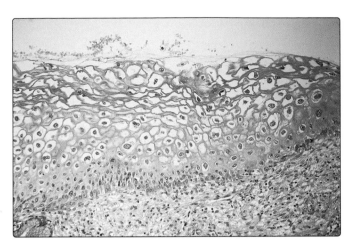

Fig. 28.82 Flat condyloma due to HPV infection of cervical mucosa. The mucosa is thickened. Koilocytosis is present in the upper layers, with dyskeratosis, enlarged crumpled or pyknotic nuclei, binucleation and a few normal mitoses. (× HP)

vagina and ectocervix, flat condylomas are most commonly found in the metaplastic epithelium of the transformation zone[96]. The condylomatous metaplastic epithelium may grow into endocervical glandular necks, replacing pre-existing columnar epithelium. The lesion is referred to as an inverted or endophytic condyloma.

Papillomavirus particles can be visualized in the cell nuclei of infected squamous cells by electron microscopy. They were first described in the papillary lesion in 1968[97] and in the flat lesion in 1978[98]. Their appearance proved to be identical to the viral particles found in skin warts. Application of DNA *in situ* hybridization has made it clear that cervical condylomata and skin warts are caused by different HPV subtypes[99].

Since these initial reports, much progress has been made in the field of papillomavirus research, with the help of molecular biological techniques[100,101]. Of the 80 or more different HPV strains capable of infecting mucosa or skin, only one quarter of these affect the female genital tract. HPV 6 and 11 are preferentially found in benign condylomatous lesions of the cervix and low-grade cervical intraepithelial neoplasia (CIN I). HPV 16, 18, 31, and 33 have been detected predominantly in high-grade lesions such as CIN II-III, formerly known as moderate to severe dysplasia or carcinoma *in situ* or as high-grade SIL in the Bethesda system, and in infiltrating carcinoma.

Most genital warts, and the changes in smears induced by the infection, regress after about two years and in general they are managed conservatively by close cytological surveillance[102] or by ablative therapy in the first place. If evidence of dyskaryosis supervenes in the smear, colposcopic examination and appropriate treatment are required. Policies on the management of HPV infection in the absence of dyskaryosis vary a great deal, however, reflecting uncertainty about its exact significance for an individual woman.

HPV subtyping of infected cervical squamous cells has been proposed as an alternative to routine cervical screening, women carrying high-risk subtypes of the virus being then investigated by colposcopy (see Chapters 29, 30 and 31). Alternatively, subtyping can be added if minor cytological abnormalities are found, thereby identifying at an early stage women at greatest risk of developing cervical cancer. Women found not to be harbouring any high-risk subtypes of HPV could then be subjected to less frequent smear testing.

Cytological findings

► Koilocytosis
► Multinucleation
► Nuclear swelling and degeneration
► Keratotic spikes, pearls and rafts
► Single dyskeratotic cells

In cervical smears, the presence of koilocytic cells provides the most reliable evidence of HPV infection. Koilocytes were first described by Koss and Durfee in 1956[103], and many other reports followed[92–94,104,105]. Koilocytes are defined as squamous cells with a large well-demarcated clear perinuclear zone surrounded by a dense peripheral cytoplasmic rim. The shape of the clear zone may be oval, rounded or scalloped (Figs 28.83–28.85). Superficial and intermediate cells are the cells most frequently showing koilocytic changes, but parabasal and metaplastic cells can also be affected.

The nucleus is enlarged and may appear crumpled or wrinkled at the margins, with loss of nuclear detail, producing a smudged effect. Some degree of hyperchromasia is usual and pyknosis or karyorrhexis is often seen. Binucleation is extremely common and sometimes multinucleation is pronounced (Fig. 28.86). These multiple nuclei show the swelling and degenerative changes described above. The cytoplasm of multinucleated cells may be koilocytic or dense and granular.

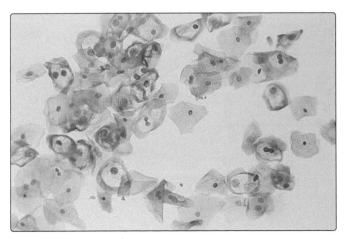

Fig. 28.83 Koilocytosis. This screening power magnification shows scattered mature squames with well-defined clearing of cytoplasm around the nuclei and slight nuclear enlargement. (× MP)

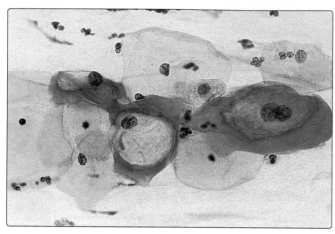

Fig. 28.84 Koilocytes in a cervical smear. These superficial cells show a wide zone of perinuclear clearing with condensed peripheral cytoplasm. Nuclei are slightly enlarged and chromatin is increased. Binucleation can be seen. (× HP)

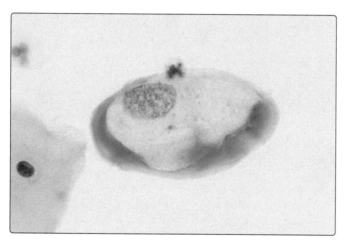

Fig. 28.85 HPV infection. Intermediate cell with typical koilocytosis. Note the swollen but bland-looking nucleus with uneven chromatin pattern. (× OI)

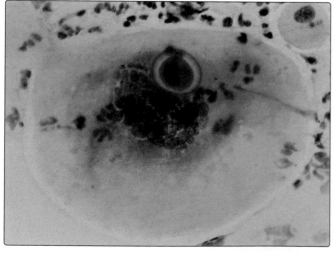

Fig. 28.86 HPV infection. Single enlarged multinucleated cell due to HPV infection. (× OI) (Courtesy of Dr J Johnson, Nottingham, UK)

Disturbances of keratinization are often seen in koilocytes, especially intermediate cells: the cytoplasm may appear cracked and amphophilic, staining partly with light green and partly with eosin. Some of these intermediate cells are extremely large, measuring 7000 μm² and over (Fig. 28.86). Hyperkeratosis and parakeratosis are frequently observed: superficial cells stain intensely orange and are arranged in plaques of variable size and shape described as pearls, rafts or spikes (Fig. 28.87). Anucleate squames are often present but are not a specific finding[106]. Dissociated dyskeratotic cells are sometimes present: these are cells of the size of a metaplastic cell (50–150 μm²), staining intensely red or orange (Fig. 28.87). The nucleus is pyknotic, measuring 45–75 μm².

Recently, Tanaka *et al.* reported the cytological findings in cervical smears in relation to HPV subtype in 150 cases positive for HPV by Southern blot analysis[107]. Their results indicate that all of the above criteria correlate well with the presence of HPV, but koilocytosis, dyskeratosis, parakeratosis and karyorrhexis are the most specific. Using the presence of two out of these three criteria alone, a diagnostic specificity of 100% was achieved, with a sensitivity of 36%.

A further recent study found that smears from women with HPV proved by PCR technique contained koilocytes in only 3% of cases, demonstrating that HPV is underdiagnosed when koilocytosis is the sole cytological criterion used[108]. Hyperkeratosis was the most frequent morphological change in these smears (66%), followed by parakeratosis (34%). Detection of HPV by DNA hybridization on reprocessed routine Papanicolaou smears[109] has shown that up to 21% of normal smears without koilocytosis contain HPV.

Diagnostic pitfalls

Koilocytosis must be distinguished from vacuolation of cells from other causes such as glycogen content, non-specific degenerative changes or the perinuclear haloes associated with inflammation. The nuclei of koilocytes differ from those of other cells, being enlarged, wrinkled and often lacking in nuclear detail, appearing smudged or pyknotic. The koilocytic zone is large and fairly empty, in contrast to the yellow staining of glycogen storage in the cytoplasm or the small neat area of pallor seen in perinuclear halo formation (see Fig. 28.58).

Multinucleation is not specific for wart virus infection as it can be seen in many reactive processes, including after irradiation. Nevertheless, it is a common feature in HPV infection, adding weight to the overall picture especially when extensive in superficial and intermediate cells. Nuclear moulding does not occur, in contrast to herpetic multinucleation.

Nuclear enlargement, chromatin disturbance and irregular nuclear contours are among the nuclear features of dyskaryosis. It is often extremely difficult or impossible

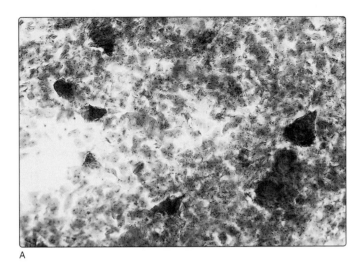

A

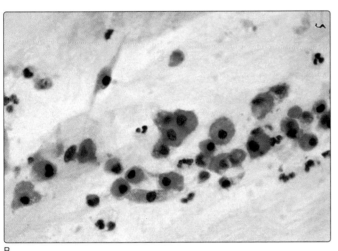

B

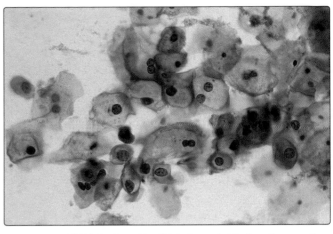

Fig. 28.88 HPV infection with mild dyskaryosis. Nuclear changes of HPV infection and mild dyskaryosis are similar and often impossible to distinguish with certainty. These cells show features of both and subsequent biopsy revealed CIN I as well as HPV infection. Note the similarity to the cells in **Fig. 28.84**, where the histology showed no evidence of CIN. (× HP)

to establish with certainty whether dyskaryosis, especially mild dyskaryosis, has developed in the presence of HPV changes (Fig. 28.88). Such cases should be managed according to the suspected grade of dyskaryosis.

Viral nuclear abnormalities with or without keratinization or parakeratosis may be present with or without koilocytosis. When the nuclear changes fall short of dyskaryosis, these smears are reported as showing *borderline nuclear changes* in current UK terminology. In the Bethesda system koilocytic HPV changes are classified with mild dyskaryosis as a low-grade squamous intraepithelial lesion (SIL) whereas nuclear abnormalities of viral type without koilocytosis generally fall into the ASCUS category. Following a terminology conference in Manchester in March 2002 the BSCC has recommended merging koilocytic changes with mild dyskaryosis as low-grade dyskaryosis, approximating to the two tier Bethesda System. Such smears are checked earlier than is done routinely, and referred for colposcopic assessment if the findings persist. A variable proportion of these persistent changes, ranging up to 20% will show CIN on investigation (see Chapter 30).

Koilocytes are a striking finding in smears from flat lesions, but in some smears from visible genital warts only anucleate squames and parakeratotic cells from the surface may be found. Thus cytology is a more sensitive test for identifying flat condylomata than macroscopically visible genital warts. Attempts at subtyping HPV by morphological changes in smears has proved to be unreliable on criteria known at present[107]. Using cellular material collected from the cervix for liquid based cytology, HPV subtyping can be performed in conjunction with screening of the thin layer preparation to establish whether high-risk subtypes of HPV are present when low-grade abnormalities are found in the smear. This adjunctive test allows rational management of the smear findings.

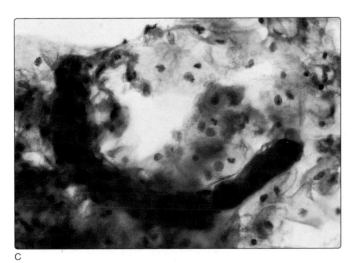

C

Fig. 28.87 HPV infection. (A) Multiple hyperkeratotic cell groups throughout the smear with small pyknotic nuclei are frequently seen in HPV infection although not specific for the virus especially when only in small numbers. (× LP) (B) Single dyskeratotic cells are small and orangeophilic with pyknotic uniform chromatin and regular nuclear contours. (× HP) (C) A spike of keratinized squamous cells with some nuclear enlargement and hyperchromasia, leading in this case to a report of borderline changes. (× HP)

Cytomegalovirus

The endocervical epithelium is susceptible to Cytomegalovirus (CMV) infection[110,111], but in spite of this, infection is uncommon and is often asymptomatic. Reactivation of latent CMV occurs in 2–4% of pregnant women, probably due to disturbance of steroid metabolism and altered immunity and also in immunosuppressed patients for other reasons, and can be recognized in transplant patients.

Cytological findings

Small irregular nuclear inclusion bodies are observed at first. Later the enlarged nuclei contain a very large single eosinophilic inclusion body surrounded by a narrow halo which gives the cells an 'owl's eye' appearance (Figs 28.89, 28.90)[111]. The cytoplasm may contain finely granular basophilic inclusions. Electron microscopy or immunocytochemistry can be used to verify the presence of the virus[87].

Cervical screening is not a practical way of detecting CMV. The number of affected cells is often very low[112]. If inclusion-bearing cells are detected in pregnancy, however, it is important to investigate the possibility of active CMV infection because this may threaten the health of the fetus.

Molluscum contagiosum

This pox virus produces crops of hyperplastic skin nodules and may therefore infect the vulval area. Large inclusion bodies fill the squamous cells at the core of the lesion, pushing the nucleus to the outer rim of the cell (Fig. 28.91). Eventually the material at the core is discharged on to the skin surface. The diagnosis can be made on scrapings from these lesions, and occasionally molluscum bodies are found in cervical smears.

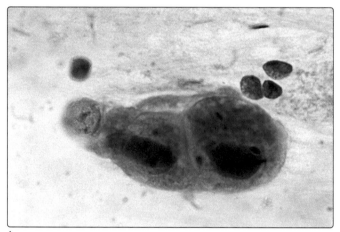

A

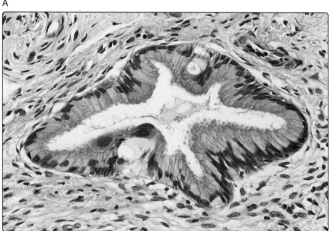

B

Fig. 28.89 (A) Cytomegalovirus infection in a renal transplant patient. The smear showed several groups of cells with enormous dense inclusion bodies surrounded by a large halo giving the characteristic owl's eye appearance. Note the granular area in the cytoplasm representing viral particles (× OI). (B) Histological section shows isolated cells in endocervical cells with similar features. (× HP)

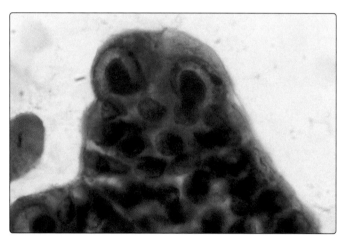

Fig. 28.90 A group of endocervical cells from the same patient as shown in **Fig. 28.89**, demonstrating the owl's eye appearance very clearly. (× HP)

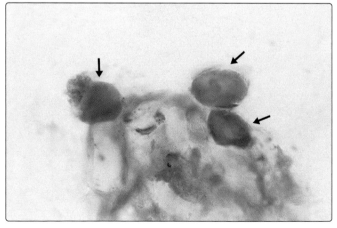

Fig. 28.91 Molluscum bodies (arrows) are seen amongst anucleate keratinized squames, filling the cells with dense orange inclusion material. This vulval smear was from a patient with Molluscum contagiosum infection. (× HP) (Courtesy of Professor B Naylor, Michigan, USA)

Adenovirus

Cells with features suggesting adenovirus infection can be of endocervical, metaplastic or parabasal type. Early in the infection they contain three or four small eosinophilic nuclear inclusions with haloes; later a large eosinophilic nuclear inclusion with an irregularly lobulated contour develops. Some chromatin deposition on the nuclear membrane may be found. Multinucleation is not seen[113].

Chlamydia trachomatis

Although they are in fact bacteria, chlamydiae are placed between bacteria and viruses because of their properties and characteristics. They contain DNA and RNA, have discrete cell walls and are sensitive to tetracycline and sulphonamides, like bacteria. On the other hand, they are obligatory intracellular organisms that multiply within the host cell by binary fission, like viruses.

Within the genus Chlamydia, two species are recognized namely *Chlamydia trachomatis* and *Chlamydia psittaci*. By serological methods different types of *Chlamydia trachomatis* can be identified. Serotypes A–C are associated with endemic blinding trachoma, serotypes D–K with sexually transmitted oculogenital infections and serotype L with lymphogranuloma venereum.

Chlamydia trachomatis infection is the commonest sexually transmitted disease (STD) in the United States and Western Europe. Diagnosis is important since infection can lead to infertility in the female many years after primary exposure. Epidemiological studies have shown that sexually active teenagers and women with other venereal disease, such as gonorrhoea, are high-risk groups for cervical chlamydial infection. The prevalence in women attending STD clinics is as high as 40%, exceeding that of gonorrhoea: in the STD detection programme in general practice in Holland, it is five times more frequent.

In women, the infection is often asymptomatic. Since columnar epithelium and metaplastic cells are the target cells for *Chlamydia trachomatis*, the cervix is the most commonly infected site in the female genital tract. Ascending infection may lead to salpingitis and pelvic inflammatory disease, both important causes of infertility and ectopic pregnancy. Pregnancy and the use of oral contraceptives promote the risk of infection because there is often an ectropion, providing an increased surface area lined by endocervical columnar cells. Follicular cervicitis is strongly associated with *Chlamydia trachomatis* infection in younger premenopausal women.

Different types of 'diagnostic' inclusion bodies have been described[114]. Studies of the accuracy of cytological diagnosis of chlamydial infection based on the detection of various inclusion bodies, however, reveal an average sensitivity of only 27% and specificity of 79%, with large numbers of false positive and false negative results[115]. The most reliable cytological evidence of chlamydial infection is the presence of so-called indicator cells[116].

Cytological findings

Indicator cells are metaplastic cells with altered cytoplasmic staining due to the presence of small ill-defined nebular inclusions, giving the cytoplasm a freckled, mottled appearance (Fig. 28.92A,B). Other inclusions and vacuoles in metaplastic cells cannot be regarded as evidence of chlamydial infection. The cytoplasmic changes can be found in endocervical cells and may also be seen in dyskaryotic cells. Follicular cervicitis may be present.

A study in Leiden of 60 patients with clinical signs of chlamydial infection, using immunofluorescence techniques and isolation of *Chlamydia trachomatis* according to Kuo *et al.*[117], demonstrated nebular inclusions in indicator cells in 20 of the 25 smears which were positive for Chlamydia on immunofluorescence (Fig. 28.93)[118]. The large inclusion bodies within vacuoles described by Gupta

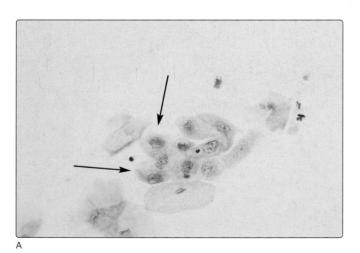

A

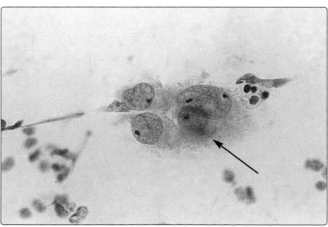

B

Fig. 28.92 (A, B) Chlamydial inclusions. Faint nebular inclusions can be made out in the cytoplasm of metaplastic cells in two cervical smears from patients with chlamydial infection (arrows). (× HP)

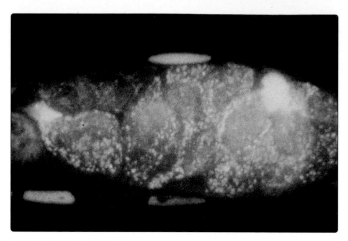

Fig. 28.93 Chlamydia infection of cervix. Intracytoplasmic organisms are visualized by immunofluorescence using antichlamydial monoclonal antibodies. (× HP)

et al.[114] were negative for Chlamydia on immunofluorescence and are therefore non-specific. Using the immunoperoxidase technique, Shiina found that only nebular inclusions in indicator cells stained positively[118], confirming the importance of these cells. For immunocytochemical staining smears must be fixed in methanol-ether[119–121]. A recent study using immunoelectron microscopy has demonstrated elementary, reticulate and intermediate bodies in nebular inclusions[122].

Definitive diagnosis of *Chlamydia trachomatis* requires confirmation by immunofluorescence[123], immunoperoxidase staining methods[124], or isolation techniques using cultured HeLa cells[117]. Recently, a PCR procedure has also been developed for cervical material suspended in transport medium[125], and has proved even more sensitive than the gold standard of isolation of Chlamydia in cultured HeLa cells.

The immunofluorescence technique can be used for confirmation of chlamydial infection in routine smears with indicator cells, follicular cervicitis or many lymphocytes[126]. In a Leiden series of 305 patients, 34% of smears with follicular cervicitis had positive fluorescence as did 48% of the smears with indicator cells, emphasizing the value of these cytological criteria.

Specific RNA–DNA probes are now available commercially for the detection of *Chlamydia trachomatis* by molecular hybridization[127]. In a pilot study of this technique Boon found that chlamydial infection in men and women is closely related to recent sexual contact with a new partner. Using this criterion as a reason to perform RNA–DNA hybridization, a positivity rate of 11.4 was found, ranging from 19% in 15–19-year-olds to 5% in the age group 40–44. The infection rate was 17.4% among prostitutes. These data illustrate that chlamydial infection is a serious health problem in the Netherlands.

Chlamydial nebular inclusions can be detected in dyskaryotic cells, suggesting that they are highly permissive

for this infective agent. The organism is also frequently encountered in cancer patients treated by radiotherapy[128].

Iatrogenic lesions

Cell patterns in cervical smears are influenced by a variety of medical treatments including the use of oral contraceptives. Surgical procedures involving the cervix may also influence the findings in smears. In this section, some aspects of these iatrogenic influences will be considered in more detail.

Changes induced by hormones

Hormonal contraceptives

Oral contraceptives influence both the squamous and glandular epithelium. Different formulations vary in their effects clinically and cytologically, depending on the balance of oestrogenic and progesterone activity and whether or not an ovulatory peak is induced. High dose progesterone oral contraception is more commonly used today than the formulations with a high level of oestrogen.

Cytological findings

▶ Scanty smears with cytolysis
▶ Atrophic changes after long-term use
▶ Goblet cells
▶ Endometrial cells due to breakthrough bleeding at midcycle

Smears from current 'pill users' are usually less cellular and more mucoid than normal, and contain fewer endocervical cells in spatula samples[13]. Cytolysis is a prominent feature in high progesterone regimes, adding to the impression of sparse material. In this situation the woman's hormonal status must be taken into account before deciding that the smear is inadequate.

Smears become atrophic while contraception is used; this is seen particularly with the injectable progesterone compound Depo-Provera. The endocervical epithelium may become hyperplastic. Histologically, the changes of microglandular hyperplasia can develop (see Chapters 32 and 33). The smear changes are variable and usually non-specific. Large vacuoles of mucus may be observed in the cytoplasm due to hypersecretion (see Fig. 28.59).

Inhibition of the hypothalamus may be marked such that when oral contraception is discontinued normal cycles are not resumed. A vaginal or cervical smear then shows an atrophic pattern. Breakthrough bleeding at midcycle during oral contraceptive use will lead to shedding of endometrial cells in cervical smears taken at this time of the cycle, potentially leading to over-investigation if clinical details are not given.

Hormone replacement treatment (HRT)

Hormone replacement can be used to treat menopausal symptoms and to protect against the long-term risks of post-menopausal osteoporosis and heart disease. The therapy may be sequential, based on a combination of oestrogen counterbalanced by the inclusion of cyclical progesterone, thus re-creating the hormonal environment of the premenopausal woman, or may consist of a continuous low dose of both hormones which is not usually associated with any withdrawal bleeding.

In either case, smears usually contain superficial and intermediate cells but may not show a fully oestrogenized picture in all women, depending on the type of hormonal preparation used. It is important to remember that regular menstruation is occurring when sequential therapy is given and that groups of endometrial cells may therefore be found within the first 12 days of the cycle, or later if breakthrough bleeding occurs. Some women experience bleeding while receiving continuous HRT.

The risk of atypical endometrial hyperplasia and development of endometrial carcinoma is increased in women on HRT, particularly if the oestrogen content is not counterbalanced by progesterone administration. The cytological recognition of clusters of atypical endometrial cells or cells outside the normal time of endometrial shedding should lead to appropriate investigation to exclude these complications.

Local administration of oestrogen per vaginam is used as intermittent HRT for short-term effect, providing, among other benefits, a helpful method of obtaining a mature cervical smear in cases where an atrophic smear has been difficult to interpret.

Tamoxifen therapy

Tamoxifen is a synthetic compound with anti-oestrogenic properties used with increasing frequency in the treatment of breast carcinoma in post-menopausal women and also in premenopausal patients if the tumour cells are shown to have oestrogen receptors[129]. Paradoxically, the effect of Tamoxifen on the female genital tract includes a weak oestrogenic action so that post-menopausal smears show increased squamous maturation in a high proportion of cases[130]. Oestrogen associated changes can be seen in the endometrium in up to 30% of women receiving the hormone, usually after several years of therapy[131]. In general, the smears have a clean background and a modestly oestrogenic picture, developing early after starting treatment[132] (Fig. 28.94A). Premenopausal women have been found to have an immature cell pattern in vaginal smears as estimated by KPI measurement[133].

There is a growing body of evidence that Tamoxifen therapy carries a heightened risk of endometrial hyperplasia and carcinoma, a rate ratio of 6.4 for endometrial carcinoma having been found in a major study in Sweden in 1989[134]. Other tumours, including benign polyps and sarcomatous tumours of uterus and cervix are also found more frequently with Tamoxifen use. Vaginal adenosis[135] and various types of metaplasia have also been ascribed to the use of Tamoxifen. The effects are apparent within about two years of treatment and are presumably related to the oestrogenic effects of the compound.

Since Tamoxifen is of established value in the management of breast cancer and most endometrial tumours usually have a good prognosis if detected early, the benefits of Tamoxifen therapy appear to outweigh the risks. More recently, Tamoxifen has been used to reduce the risk of breast carcinoma in women at extra risk of the disease; consequently there could be an increase in the number of women with endometrial tumours unless methods are available to counteract the adverse effects[131].

Meanwhile, smears from these patients require careful screening for the detection of abnormal glandular cells (Fig. 28.94B), with appropriate investigation and treatment if needed.

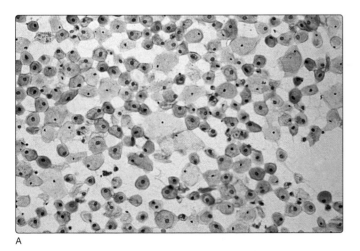

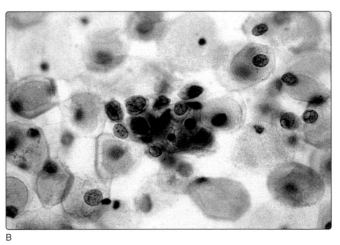

A

B

Fig. 28.94 (A) Tamoxifen therapy induces squamous maturation in cervical smears in some post-menopausal women. The smears tend to have a clean background as seen here. Maturation of the smear is dose related. (× MP) (B) A cluster of hyperchromatic glandular cells is seen at the centre, in a smear from a patient with early endometrial carcinoma who had received Tamoxifen therapy for three years. (× HP)

Other drugs with hormonal activity

Various non-hormonal preparations exert an influence on the maturation and exfoliation of squamous epithelium. Digitalis is known to stimulate mucosal maturation. Tetracyclines cause accelerated exfoliation, so that in some cases only parabasal cells are found in smears soon after starting therapy[136].

Intrauterine devices (IUDs)

IUDs are made from a variety of materials, the commonest being plastic or copper. They may be used pre-menopausally as a form of contraception or in pre- and post-menopausal women to administer HRT locally. Different designs are available. All types are prone to induce changes in the cervical mucosa and superficial endometrium, leading to changes in cervical smears.

Cytological findings

► Endometrial shedding at any stage of the cycle
► Single and clustered enlarged vacuolated glandular cells
► Neutrophilic inflammatory cell exudate
► Actinomycotic colonies

Endometrial cells may be seen at any stage of the menstrual cycle, outside the usual cyclical timespan. Occasionally groups of endometrial cells display swollen nuclei and coarse vacuolation of the cytoplasm, accompanied by inflammatory debris[137]. An erroneous diagnosis of endometrial adenocarcinoma may be made in such cases. Endocervical columnar cells, too, sometimes show pronounced enlargement, prominent nucleoli, and mitotic figures. They occur as single rounded cells associated with cell debris or in clusters (Fig. 28.95). The cytoplasm is often vacuolated and polymorphs can be seen in the cytoplasm or in vacuoles.

Smears frequently show many polymorphs, to the extent that the epithelial cells may be obscured. Histiocytes with phagocytosed spermatozoa, foreign body giant cells and even fibroblasts can also be seen[138]. Actinomycotic colonies are common, particularly with plastic devices[139] (see Fig. 28.71). Saprophytic amoebae may also be found[140] (see Fig. 28.75), together with a coccoid flora. Removal of the IUD in these circumstances should rarely be necessary, especially if the woman is asymptomatic. Misra *et al.*[141] observed that the incidence of dysplasia and endometrial hyperplasia was much higher when the IUDs had been changed than when the original devices were worn continuously. Symptoms of pelvic inflammatory disease in the presence of an IUD warrant investigation and treatment. Calcification around particles from the IUD can result in the presence of psammoma bodies in the smear (Fig. 28.96)[142,143].

Surgical intervention, ablative therapy

In the healing stages after surgical procedures such as conization, hysterectomy or curettage, smears usually show evidence of inflammation and repair. More limited procedures such as electrocoagulation, laser vaporization, cryotherapy and excision of cervical lesions by diathermy loop excision (DLE) are associated with similar changes.

The repair process is effected by regeneration of residual epithelium to cover the area of excision. This may take several weeks depending on the extent of the procedure, the presence or absence of local infection and the general health of the patient. Smear findings are also influenced by these factors.

Cytological findings

► Repair changes
► Inflammation
► Metaplasia

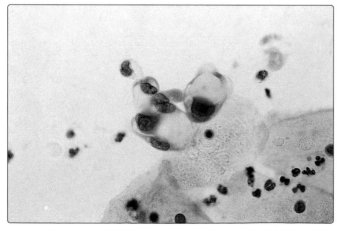

Fig. 28.95 IUCD changes in endocervical cells, showing enlarged pleomorphic cells with vacuolated cytoplasm and hyperchromatic nuclei. Repeat smears are indicated if interpretation is problematical. (× HP)

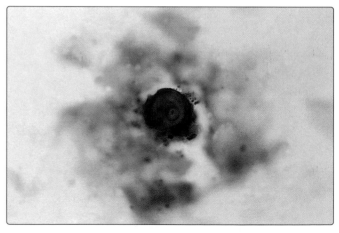

Fig. 28.96 Psammoma body in cervical smear associated with IUCD use. This was an isolated finding and there was no evidence of malignancy. (× HP)

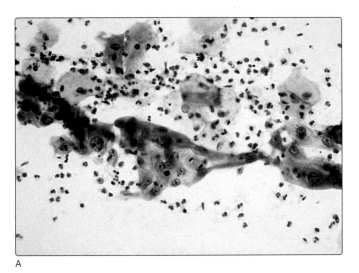

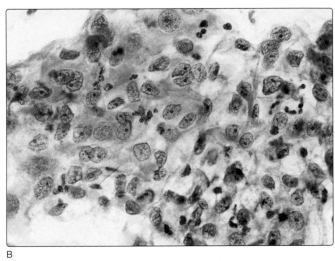

A

B

Fig. 28.97 (A) Repair changes. This group of metaplastic cells shows ill-defined cell boundaries, some nuclear variation and prominent nucleoli. (× MP) (B) A sheet of immature metaplastic cells showing repair changes with irregular pleomorphic nuclei and prominent nucleoli. (× HP)

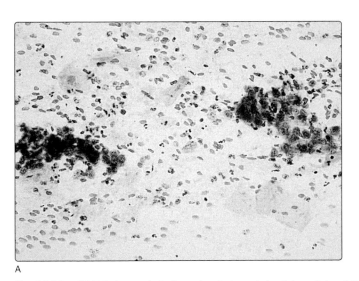

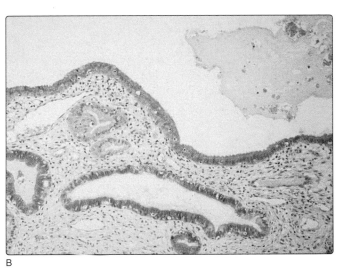

A

B

Fig. 28.98 (A) Tubal metaplasia. Irregular clusters of glandular cells in a follow up smear after excisional treatment of CIN. The cells appear crowded and irregular and include occasional larger cells with clear cytoplasm. The findings suggest tubal metaplasia, given the clinical setting. (× MP) (B) Section from the cervix of this patient shows tubal metaplasia in several of the glands and also in the surface epithelium. (× MP)

Repair cells are usually metaplastic in origin and are found in ragged sheets of rather pleomorphic cells with ill-defined cell boundaries (Fig. 28.97A,B). They may show slight or even marked nuclear atypia due to coarsening of the chromatin with condensation at the nuclear membrane, and frequently have large active or multiple nucleoli[144]. Distinction from dyskaryosis may be difficult without a full history, but the lack of significant abnormality of chromatin distribution usually enables a correct diagnosis. In cases of doubt the smear should be followed up as having borderline findings.

In most cases, atypical cells are found within the first four weeks following cryosurgery or DLE and smears return to normal within 8 weeks[145]. The healing process may lead to changes in squamous cells which mimic neoplasia[136,146,147].

Tubal and tuboendometrioid metaplasia

Follow-up smears after surgery to the cervix may contain sheets of glandular cells with crowded hyperchromatic nuclei giving an initial impression of endocervical dyskaryosis. These cells have been shown to arise from areas of tubal or tuboendometrioid metaplasia in the vicinity of the external os of the cervix at the site of previous surgical treatment (Fig. 28.98). The incidence of this regenerative phenomenon in histological sections of cervix following surgery for reactive or neoplastic conditions varies from 30–70% in different series (see Chapter 32)[148,149].

The cytological findings in tuboendometrioid metaplasia have been described by Ducatman and associates[150], and more recently by Hirschowitz et al.[151]. These authors point out that the groups of crowded hyperchromatic cells may be mistaken for dyskaryotic glandular cells, leading to unnecessary treatment.

Cytological findings *(Fig. 28.96)*

▶ Sparse groups of crowded dark epithelial cells
▶ Lack of architectural features of endocervical dyskaryosis
▶ Ciliated borders may be seen
▶ An appropriate history

At low magnification, occasional groups of darkly stained cells are readily seen in both spatula and brush samples. The groups are two or three-dimensional, consisting of small crowded cells with central hyperchromatic nuclei and very little cytoplasm. The presence of cilia or a terminal bar is not a dependable finding as these structures are prone to degenerative changes, but if found, these provide reassurance that the cell groups are likely to be metaplastic rather than neoplastic in type. A potentially useful monoclonal antibody marking the basal bodies of ciliated cells may provide a means of distinguishing tubal metaplasia from endocervical dyskaryosis[152]. No feathering or other architectural abnormalities typical of glandular neoplasia are seen in tubal or tuboendometrial metaplasia and there are no mitoses or enlarged nucleoli. In general, the cells are smaller than those of glandular dyskaryosis.

The three-dimensional groups lack the central stromal core of endometrial cell clusters shed physiologically. However, some postoperative follow-up cases show large casts of glands in the absence of tuboendometrioid metaplasia. The glandular structures are composed of uniform cells with regular nuclei and small nucleoli; mitoses may be seen and sometimes a few stromal cells or capillary fragments may be seen along the outer border of the gland. These intact glands are thought to come from the isthmic region of the endometrial cavity especially if the endocervical canal has been shortened by excisional treatment. They are referred to as lower uterine segment sampling and are commoner in brush samples than in spatula smears (Fig. 28.99)[153].

Endometriosis of the cervix is also found in a few cases following surgery, with foci of endometrial glands set in endometrial stroma (see Chapter 32). Cells from these lesions have the same appearances as groups from the endometrial cavity, although usually better preserved and present at times unrelated to the normal menstrual cycle.

Radiation changes

Radiotherapy has been used in the treatment of malignant tumours of the female genital tract, notably carcinoma of the cervix, throughout this century[154]. Follow-up vault or cervical smears may be helpful in monitoring the area for the possibility of local recurrence. Under the influence of ionizing radiation, benign as well as malignant cells change markedly and interpretation of these smears raises particular problems. The changes have been well documented by Shield *et al.*[155].

Cytological findings *(Figs 28.100, 28.101)*

▶ Swelling of cells and nuclei
▶ Bizarre cell shapes
▶ Altered cytoplasmic staining
▶ Nuclear degenerative changes

General cellular enlargement is seen, affecting both nucleus and cytoplasm so that the nuclear/cytoplasmic ratio remains largely within normal limits. Bizarre cell shapes are seen, with altered cytoplasmic staining affinity to light green at the periphery and to eosin around the nucleus, giving the two-tone effect of amphophilia. Cytoplasmic vacuolation is a prominent feature, either fine and uniformly distributed or coarse and variable in distribution. The nuclei acquire a peculiar wrinkled appearance. They are hyperchromatic, with a coarse but uniformly dense chromatin pattern. Multinucleation is common and vacuolation of nuclei may be seen. The nucleoli are often enlarged and even pleomorphic but the ratio of nucleolus to nucleus remains low. Nuclear degeneration with karyorrhexis is often seen.

During radiotherapy, smears are characterized by numerous leucocytes, with much cellular debris and blood. Many histiocytes and multinucleated giant cells may be seen, as well as repair and radiation changes. Radiosensitive malignant cells generally disappear during the course of the radiotherapy. Shortly after irradiation, smears become atrophic even in premenopausal women. Epithelial cells are shed in large fragments due to the fragility of the mucosa and stromal cells may be noted. As many as 20 years after radiotherapy an effect may still be apparent in the epithelial cells; usually, however, the changes subside over a period of time.

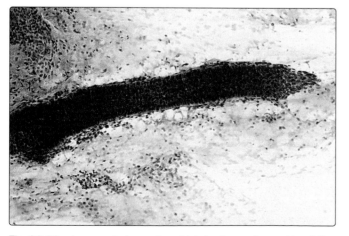

Fig. 28.99　Large cast of an endometrial gland, one of several in a follow-up endocervical brush smear after cervical surgery. (× LP)

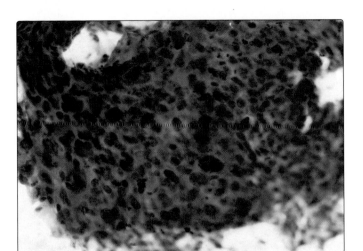
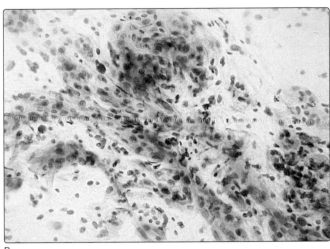

A   B

Fig. 28.100   Radiotherapy changes (A) Radiation repair. Vaginal smear six months after radiotherapy for carcinoma of the cervix. The sheet of immature epithelium shows some features of repair but there is more marked nuclear swelling and the staining is variable. (× HP) (B) Vaginal smear taken five years after radiotherapy for endometrial carcinoma. There is pronounced atrophy and the fragile cells are in large sheets. Some nuclear enlargement persists. (× MP)

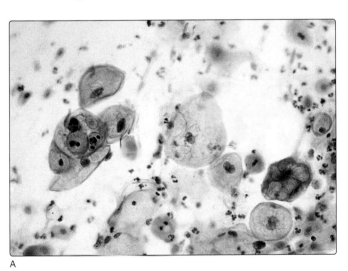
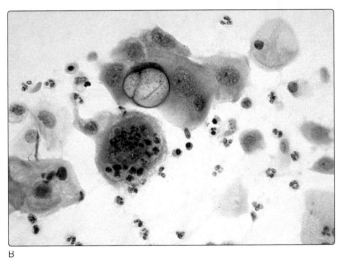

A   B

Fig. 28.101   (A, B) Radiation damage in vaginal smear from a post-menopausal woman treated for carcinoma of the ovary by surgery and radiotherapy. The cells and nuclei are swollen and deeply stained but the nuclear/cytoplasmic ratio is normal. Fine and coarse vacuolation of cytoplasm has occurred and degenerate polymorphs are seen within cells. Note also some binucleation and the prominent nucleoli. (× HP)

Diagnostic pitfalls

Residual malignant cells may undergo any or all of the above changes but in addition they fulfil the nuclear criteria of malignancy and represent a separate population from the majority of cells in the smear. Helpful features pointing to a recurrence include an irregular chromatin distribution in the nucleus, a high N/C ratio and a resemblance to the original tumour (Fig. 28.102). Differentiation of radiation effects from dyskaryosis is not, however, always possible by cytology alone. A detailed clinical history, colposcopic examination of the vaginal vault or cervix and biopsy of any visible lesion may be necessary to resolve the problem.

There are other conditions that may be confused with radiotherapy effects in treated patients. These include atrophy caused by hormonal treatment, inflammation from causes other than the radiotherapy, and the effect of cytotoxic agents given in conjunction with the radiotherapy. Folic acid deficiency during radiotherapy specifically affects the maturation of cell nuclei. In some of these conditions there may be cytomegaly, nuclear enlargement and hyperchromasia, vacuolation of cytoplasm, multinucleation and abnormal nuclear shapes[156]. Differentiation from radiation effects and from dyskaryosis may require colposcopy and biopsy of any abnormality.

Radiation dysplasia

Smears from patients who have received radiotherapy may in time develop cellular abnormalities morphologically resembling those of neoplasia. This condition, known as radiation dysplasia, can develop after a latent period varying

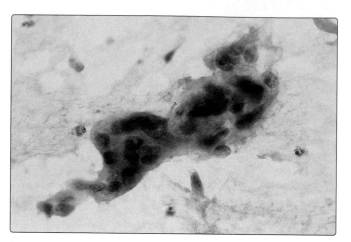

Fig. 28.102 Recurrence of adenocarcinoma of endocervix in the vaginal vault after radiotherapy. The cluster of cells has an 'anatomical border' along one margin, suggesting a glandular origin. The nuclei are large and rounded with prominent nucleoli. They closely resemble the malignant cells seen originally in this patient's diagnostic smears prior to treatment. (× HP)

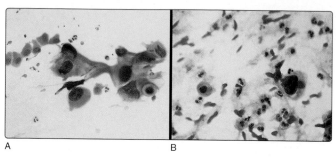

Fig. 28.103 (A, B) Radiation dysplasia. This patient had radiotherapy for endometrial carcinoma four years previously. A follow-up vault smear showed immature squamous cells with a high nuclear/cytoplasmic ratio and intense hyperchromasia. A vault biopsy showed severe dysplasia consistent with radiation induced dysplasia. (× HP)

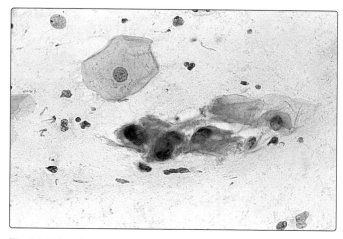

Fig. 28.104 Cytotoxic therapy effects seen in a smear from a patient with non-Hodgkin's lymphoma treated with cyclophosphamide. The cells show enlarged hyperchromatic nuclei with possible dyskaryosis. Close follow-up is necessary since the risk of CIN is increased in these patients. (× HP)

from several months to 20 years. According to the literature[155], radiation dysplasia of the vagina develops in 18.7–26% of patients who have received radiotherapy, usually within three years of treatment. Approaching 30% of cases have been found to regress[157], but the natural history of these lesions is not fully known. The majority are believed either to persist or progress.

Cytological findings *(Fig. 28.103)*

The dyskaryotic cells may be found either as isolated cells or in sheets. The shapes of the cells vary from polygonal to oval or round. The cytoplasm is usually eosinophilic but may also stain an indefinite colour[155]. The nuclei are often slightly enlarged, and oval or round. Hyperchromatism and coarsening of the chromatin are common. Sometimes there is a nucleolus, but never a macronucleolus[158].

Radiation dysplasia must be differentiated from acute radiation changes and from a new or recurrent carcinoma. The likelihood of progression of radiation dysplasia to *in situ* carcinoma or CIN III is twice that of the equivalent lower grades of CIN arising without any preceding irradiation. A distinction should be made between radiation dysplasia developing within three years of treatment and one that develops later, which has a considerably better prognosis[158].

Most studies have given a diagnostic sensitivity approaching 50% for detection of tumour recurrence in follow-up smears, with a range from 11.5–85%, probably reflecting differences in access to the recurrence for sampling. In about one quarter of cases the cytological detection precedes any clinical evidence of recurrent carcinoma[155]. False negative results are common, due to a high level of inadequate samples and also problems of access[159].

Cytotoxic drugs

Cytotoxic agents are used in the primary treatment of certain tumours such as haematological malignancies, and also as palliative treatment for advanced inoperable cancers. Their use leads to cellular changes similar to those seen in the epithelium as a result of radiotherapy. Busulfan therapy, for example, gives rise to cells with markedly enlarged abnormal nuclei and abundant cytoplasm[160]. Multinucleation is common. The histology and cytological patterns in these drug reactions may be hard to distinguish from intraepithelial neoplasia (Fig. 28.104).

An early study on the effects of prolonged cyclophosphamide administration showed enhanced development of neoplasia[161]. The finding of atypical cells associated with cytotoxic drug therapy warrants close cytological surveillance.

Immunosuppressive drugs

Drugs inhibiting the immunological defence mechanisms of the body are used increasingly as treatment for a wide

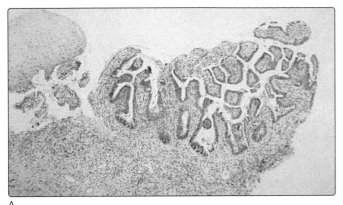

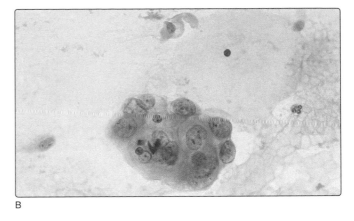

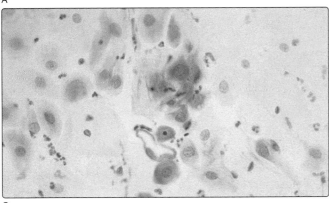

A

B

C

Fig. 28.105 Vaginal adenosis. (A) Vaginal biopsy from a 12-year-old girl whose mother was given diethylstilboestrol in pregnancy. The normal squamous mucosa is partly replaced by columnar epithelium, which has failed to undergo metaplasia *in utero* to mature squamous epithelium (× MP). (B) Vaginal smear taken directly from an area of vaginal adenosis showing a cluster of hyperplastic glandular cells with reactive nuclei. (× OI) (C) Vaginal smear with immature metaplastic epithelium from an area of persistent metaplasia in the vagina of the daughter of a woman given DES in pregnancy. (× HP)

range of conditions and also to prevent organ rejection in transplant patients. The state of immunosuppression induced by these agents increases the risk of HPV infection, precancerous changes in the cervix[162] and progression to cervical cancer. Women who are immunosuppressed due to infection by the human immunodeficiency virus (HIV) also have a higher incidence of cervical cancer and precancer[93]. Both groups of patients require annual cervical screening.

Diethylstilboestrol exposure *in utero*

The hormone diethylstilboestrol (DES) was used in the USA and some European countries earlier in this century to maintain pregnancy in cases of threatened or habitual abortion. By the 1970s, it was noted that daughters of such pregnancies had deformities of the lower genital tract including persistence of columnar epithelium in the vagina, known as vaginal adenosis, and on the ectocervix. This mucosa appears to be at risk of malignant change, either developing the rare glandular neoplasm, a clear cell adenocarcinoma, or intraepithelial neoplasia in the metaplastic epithelium. The normal process of metaplasia of the primitive glandular lining of the vagina that takes place in fetal development appears to be arrested by the hormonal treatment.

Since 1973, when the first report in the Netherlands of DES-related vaginal adenosis was published, it has become clear that there is a population of young women at risk of cervical or vaginal neoplasia. It is estimated that 40 000 pregnant women were treated with DES.

Helmerhorst and co-workers[163] published the colposcopic, cytological and histological findings of DES-exposed offspring referred to colposcopic DES clinics. Structural abnormalities of cervix and vagina such as large areas of exposed columnar epithelium were found in 30% of patients (Fig. 28.105A,B): in 9% CIN was diagnosed and in 4.5% the vaginal epithelium was dysplastic.

These increased rates are in accordance with the study in the USA performed by Robboy *et al.*[164] in which 4000 DES cases and matched controls were followed up from 1974–84. There was an increased risk of both cervical and vaginal intraepithelial neoplasia. The incidence rate correlated with the extent of metaplasia replacing the originally exposed columnar epithelium (Fig. 28.105C). The cytological findings in these conditions are described further in Chapter 32.

References

1 Grunze H, Spriggs A I, eds. Cytology in gynaecology. In: *History of Clinical Cytology*, 2nd edn. G-I-T: Verlag Ernst Giebeler, 1983; 86–93

2 Papanicolaou G N, Traut H F. *Diagnosis of Uterine Cancer by the Vaginal Smear*. New York: Commonwealth Fund, 1943

3 Ayre J E. Selective cytology smear for diagnosis of cancer. *Am J Obstet Gynecol* 1947; **53**: 609

4 Fidler H K, Boyes D A, Worth A J. Cervical cancer detection in British Columbia. *J Obstet Gynaecol Br Commonw* 1968; **75**: 392–404

5 Koss L G. The Papanicolaou test for cervical cancer detection: a triumph and a tragedy. *JAMA* 1989; **261**: 737–743

6 Quinn M, Babb P, Jones J, Allen E. Effect of screening on incidence of and mortality from cancer of cervix in England: evaluation based on routinely collected statistics. *BMJ* 1999; **318**: 904–908

7 Sasieni P, Adams J. Effect of screening on cervical cancer mortality in England and Wales: analysis of trends with an age period cohort model. *BMJ* 1999; **318**: 1244–1245

8 Corey R B, Pauling L. *Proceedings of the Wool Textile Research Conference*. Australia: 1955; 249

9 Moll R, Franke W W, Schiller D L *et al*. The catalog of human cytokeratins: patterns of expression in normal epithelia, tumors, and cultured cells. *Cell* 1982; **31**: 11–24

10 Cooper D, Schermer A, Sun T T. Classification of human epithelia and their neoplasms using monoclonal antibodies to keratins: strategies, applications and limitations. *Lab Invest* 1985; **52**: 243–256

11 Moll R, Levy R, Czernobilsky B *et al*. Cytokeratins of normal epithelia and some neoplasms of the female genital tract. *Lab Invest* 1983; **49**: 599–609

12 Fawcett D W. *The Cell: Its Organelles and Inclusions*. Philadelphia: W B Saunders, 1966

13 Boon M E, Suurmeijer A J H. *The Pap smear*, 3rd edn. Amsterdam and Tokyo: Harwood Academic Publishers, 1996

14 Yassin S M, Garret M. Parasites in cytodiagnosis. *Acta Cytol* 1980; 539–544

15 Bhambhani S, Milner A, Pant J, Luthra U K. Ova of Taenia and Enterobius vermicularis in cervicovaginal smears. *Acta Cytol* 1985; **29**: 193–194

16 Bhambhani S. Egg of Ascaris lumbricoides in cervicovaginal smear. *Acta Cytol* 1984; **28**: 92

17 Gupta P K. Microbiology, inflammation and viral infections. In: Bibbo M ed. *Comprehensive Cytopathology*. Philadelphia: W B Saunders, 1991; 115–152

18 Chandra K, Annousamy R. An unusual finding in the vaginal smear. *Acta Cytol* 1975; **19**: 403

19 Vargese R, Raghuveer C V, Pai M R, Bansal R. Microfilariae in cytological smears: a report of six cases. *Acta Cytol* 1996; **40**: 299–301

20 Learmonth G M, Murray M M. Helminths and protozoa as an incidental finding in cytology specimens. *Cytopathol* 1990; **1**: 163–170

21 Van Hoeven K H, Bertolini P K. Prevalence, identification and significance of fiber contaminants in cervical smears. *Acta Cytol* 1996; **40**: 489–495

22 Patnick J, Johnson J. Achievable standards, Benchmarks for reporting and Criteria for evaluating cervical cytopathology. *Cytopathol* 2000; **11**: 212–242

23 Schneider V. Current issues. The Bethesda system – the European perspective: report on the second conference on the Bethesda system for reporting cervical/vaginal cytological diagnoses. *Cytopathol* 1992; **3**: 27–29

24 Vooijs P G, Elias A, van der Graaf Y, Veling S. Relationship between the diagnosis of epithelial abnormalities and the composition of cervical smears. *Acta Cytol* 1985; **29**: 323–328

25 Baker A, Melcher D, Smith R S. Role of rescreening of cervical smears in internal quality control. *J Clin Pathol* 1995; **48**: 1002–1004

26 Faraker C A, Cross P A. Rapid rescreening of cervical smears as a quality control method. *Cytopathol* 1997; **8**: 79–84

27 Faraker C A. Rapid review. *Cytopathol* 1998; **9**: 71–76

28 Wolfendale M R, Howe-Guest R, Usherwood M McD, Draper G J. Controlled trial of a new cervical spatula. *BMJ* 1987; **294**: 33–35

29 Alons-van Kordelaar J J M, Boon M E. Diagnostic accuracy of squamous cervical lesions studied in spatula-cytobrush smears. *Acta Cytol* 1988; **32**: 801–804

30 Waddell C A, Rollason T P, Amarilli J M *et al*. The cervex: an ectocervical brush sampler. *Cytopathol* 1990; **1**: 171–181

31 Williamson S L H, Hair T, Wadhera V. The effects of different sampling techniques on smear quality and the diagnosis of cytological abnormalities in cervical screening. *Cytopathol* 1997; **8**: 188–195

32 Jarvi K. Cervex brush v. vaginal-cervical-endocervical (VCE) triple smear techniques in cervical sampling. *Cytopathol* 1997; **8**: 282–288

33 Waddell C A. The influence of the cervix on smear quality. 1: Atrophy: an audit of cervical smears taken post-colposcopic management of intraepithelial neoplasia. *Cytopathol* 1997; **8**: 274–281

34 Papanicolaou G N. The diagnosis of early human pregnancy by the vaginal smear method. *Proc Soc Exp Biol Med* 1925; **22**: 436

35 Boschann H W. Zytologische Untersuchungen uber die Wirkung von Androgenen am atrofischen Vagina-epithel in Abhangigkeit von Dosierung and Applikationsakt. *Arch Gynak* 1956; **187**: 39 (in German)

36 Yates W A, Persad R V, Stanbridge C M. The Arias-Stella reaction in the cervix: a case report with cervical cytology. *Cytopathol* 1997; **8**: 40–44

37 Kobayashi T K, Okamoto H. Arias-Stella changes in cervico-vaginal specimens (letter). *Cytopathol* 1997; **8**: 289–290

38 Quincey C, Persad R V, Stanbridge C M. Chorionic villi in post partum cervical smears. *Cytopathol* 1995; **6**: 149–15

39 Murad T M, Terhart K, Flint A. Atypical cells in pregnancy and postpartum smears. *Acta Cytol* 1981; **25**: 623–630

40 Ziabkowski T A, Naylor B. Cyanophilic bodies in cervico-vaginal smears. *Acta Cytol* 1976; **20**: 340–342

41 Larsen B, Galask R P. Vaginal microbial flora: composition and influences of host physiology. *Ann Intern Med* 1982; **96**(suppl 6, part 2): 926–930

42 Henry-Stanley M J, Simpson M, Stanley M W. Cervical cytology findings in women infected with the human immunodeficiency virus. *Diagn Cytopathol* 1993; **9**: 508–509

43 Keith L G, Berger G S, Edelman D A *et al*. On the causation of pelvic inflammatory disease. *Am J Obst Gynecol* 1984; **149**: 215–224

44 Gondos B. Cell degeneration: light and electron microscopic study of ovarian germ cells. *Acta Cytol* 1974; **18**: 504–510

45 Muller Kobold-Wolterbeek A C, Beyer-Boon M E. Ciliocytophthoria in cervical cytology. *Acta Cytol* 1975; **19**: 89–91

46 Kelly B A, Black A S. The inflammatory cervical smear: a study in general practice. *Br J Gen Pract* 1990; **40**: 238–240

47 Wilson J D, Robinson A J, Kinghorn S, Hicks D A. Implications of inflammatory changes on cervical pathology. *BMJ* 1990; **300**: 638–640

48 Parsons W L, Godwin M, Robbins C, Butler R. Prevalence of cervical pathogens in women with and without inflammatory changes on smear testing. *BMJ* 1993; **306**: 1173–1174

49 Bethesda Workshop. The Bethesda system for reporting cervical/vaginal cytologic diagnoses. *Acta Cytol* 1993; **37**: 115–114

50 BSCC/NCN Working Party report. Borderline changes in cervical smears. *J Clin Pathol* 1994; **47**: 481–492

51 Smolka H, Soost H J. *Grundriss und Atlas der gynakologischen Zytodiagnostik*. Stuttgart: Thieme, 1971; 111–116, 138–143 (in German)

52 Kashimura M, Baba S, Nakamura S *et al*. Short-term estrogen test for cytodiagnosis in post-menopausal women. *Diagn Cytopathol* 1987; **3**: 181–184

53 Giacomini G, Reali D, Vita D *et al*. The diagnostic cytology of non specific vaginitis. *Diagn Cytopathol* 1987; **3**: 198–204

54 Gardner H L, Dukes C D. Haemophilus vaginalis vaginitis: a newly defined specific infection previously classified as 'nonspecific' vaginitis. *Am J Obstet Gynecol* 1955; **69**: 962–976

55 Spiegel C A, Eschenbach D A, Amsel R, Holmes K K. Curved anaerobic bacteria in

bacterial (nonspecific) vaginosis and their response to antimicrobial therapy. *J Infec Dis* 1983; **148**: 817–822

56 Brennan J P, Silverman N, van Hoeven K H. Association between a shift in vaginal flora on Papanicolaou smear and acute chorioamnionitis and preterm delivery. *Diagn Cytopathol* 1999; **21**: 7–9

57 Michael C W. The Papanicolaou smear and the obstetric patient: a simple test with great benefits. *Diagn Cytopathol* 1999; **21**: 4–6

58 Schnadig V J, Davie K D, Shafer S K et al. The cytologist and bacteriosis of the vaginal-ectocervical area. Clues, commas, and confusion. *Acta Cytol* 1989; **33**: 287–297

59 Prey M. Routine Pap smears for the diagnosis of bacterial vaginosis. *Diagn Cytopathol* 1999; **21**: 10–13

60 Gupta P K, Hollander D H, Frost J K. Actinomycetes in cervicovaginal smears: an association with IUD usage. *Acta Cytol* 1976; **20**: 295–297

61 Gupta P K. Intrauterine contraceptive devices: vaginal cytology, pathologic changes and clinical implications. *Acta Cytol* 1982; **26**: 571–613

62 De la Monte S M, Gupta P K, White C L III. Systemic Actinomyces infection: a potential complication of intrauterine contraceptive devices. *JAMA* 1982; **248**: 1876–1877

63 Boon M E, Marres E M, Hoogeveen M M et al. Visualization of vaginal flora in cervical smears using a modified microwave silver-staining method. *Histochem J* 1998; **30**: 75–80

64 Bhagavan B S, Ruffier J, Shinn B. Pseudoactinomycotic radiate granules in the lower female genital tract: relationship to the Splendore-Hoeppli phenomenon. *Hum Pathol* 1982; **13**: 898–904

65 Bibel D J, Aly R, Lahti L et al. Microbial adherence to epithelial cells. *J Med Microbiol* 1987; **23**: 75–82

66 Giacomini G, Paavonen J, Rilke F. Microbiologic classification of cervicovaginal flora in Papanicolaou smears. *Acta Cytol* 1989; **33**: 276–278

67 Eschenbach D A, Davick P R, Williams B L et al. Prevalence of hydrogen peroxide-producing Lactobacillus species in normal women and women with bacterial vaginosis. *J Clin Microbiol* 1989; **27**: 251–256

68 Harty D W, Oakey H J, Patrikakis M et al. Pathogenic potential of lactobacilli. *Int J Food Microbiol* 1994; **24**: 179–189

69 Arsenault G M, Kalman C F, Sorensen K W. The Papanicolaou smear as a technique for gonorrhea detection: a feasibility study. *J Am Vener Dis Ass* 1976; **2**: 35–38

70 Angrish K, Verma K. Cytologic detection of tuberculosis of the uterine cervix. *Acta Cytol* 1981; **25**: 160–162

71 De Boer A L, de Boer F, van der Merwe J V. Cytologic identification of Donovan bodies in granuloma inguinale. *Acta Cytol* 1984; **28**: 126–128

72 Naib Z M. *Exfoliative Cytopathology*, 3rd edn. Boston: Little, Brown, 1985

73 Bridland R. Trichomoniasis. *Tskr Norske Laegoforg* 1962; **82**: 441

74 Gupta P K, Frost J K. Human urogenital trichomoniasis epidemiology, clinical and pathological manifestations. *Acta Univ Carol* 1988; **30**: 399–410

75 Frost J K. Trichomonas vaginalis and cervical epithelial changes. *Ann NY Acad Sci* 1962; **97**: 792–799

76 De Moraes-Ruehsen M, McNeill R E, Frost J K et al. Amoebae resembling Entamoeba gingivalis in the genital tracts of IUD users. *Acta Cytol* 1980; **24**: 413–420

77 Rachman R, Rosenberg M. Distinction between Entamoeba gingivalis and Entamoeba histolytica, revisited. *Acta Cytol* 1986; **30**: 82

78 Fentanes de Torres E, Benitez-Bribiesca L. Cytologic detection of vaginal parasitosis. *Acta Cytol* 1973; **17**: 252–257

79 Boquet-Jiminez E, Alvarez San Cristobal A. Cytologic and microbiological aspects of vaginal Torulopsis. *Acta Cytol* 1978; **22**: 331–334

80 Corey L, Adams H G, Brown Z A, Holmes K K. Genital herpes simplex virus infection: clinical manifestations, course and complications. *Ann Int Med* 1983; **98**: 958–972

81 Langley F H, Crompton A C. *Epithelial Abnormalities of the Cervix Uteri*. Berlin: Springer, 1973

82 Ng A B P, Reagan J W, Lindner E. The cellular manifestations of primary and recurrent herpes genitalis. *Acta Cytol* 1970; **14**: 124–129

83 Anderson G H, Matisic J P, Thomas B A. Confirmation of herpes simplex viral infection by an immunoperoxidase technique. *Acta Cytol* 1985; **29**: 695–700

84 Stowell S B, Wiley C M, Powers C M. Herpesvirus mimics: a potential pitfall in endocervical brush specimens. *Acta Cytol* 1994; **38**: 43–50

85 Patten S F Jr. *Diagnostic Cytopathology of the Uterine Cervix*, 2nd edn. Basel: Karger, 1978

86 Naib Z M, Masukawa N. Identification of condyloma acuminata cells in routine vaginal smears. *Obstet Gynecol* 1961; **18**: 735–738

87 Coleman D V, Russell W J I, Hodgson J et al. Human papovavirus in Papanicolaou smears of urinary sediment detected by transmission electron microscopy. *J Clin Pathol* 1977; **30**: 1015–1020

88 Rawls W E, Tompkins W A F, Melnick J L. The association of herpes virus type 2 and carcinoma of the uterine cervix. *Am J Epidemiol* 1969; **89**: 547–554

89 Marsh M, Brooklyn N Y. Papilloma of the cervix. *Am J Obstet Gynecol* 1952; **64**: 281–291

90 Barrett T J, Silbar J D, McGinley J P. Genital warts – a venereal disease. *JAMA* 1954; **154**: 333–334

91 Boon M E, Schneider A, Hogewoning C J A et al. Penile studies and heterosexual partners: peniscopy, cytology, histology, and immunocytochemistry. *Cancer* 1988; **61**: 1652–1659

92 Stormby N. *Morphology of Virus Induced Changes*. The Fourth European Congress of Cytology, Ljubljana, 1974

93 Henry M J, Stanley M W, Cruikshank S, Carson L. Association of human immunodeficiency virus-induced immunosuppression with human papilloma virus infection and cervical intraepithelial neoplasia. *Am J Obstet Gynecol* 1989; **160**: 352–353

94 Meisels A, Fortin R. Condylomatous lesions of the cervix and vagina I. *Acta Cytol* 1976; **20**: 64–71

95 Purola E, Savia E. Cytology of gynecologic condyloma acuminatum. *Acta Cytol* 1977; **21**: 26–31

96 Metzelaar-Venema A. *Correlation Study Between Macroscopy and Cytology of Condylomatous Lesions of the Cervix*. The Eighth European Congress of Cytology, Szczecin, 1978

97 Dunn A E G, Ogilvie M M. Intranuclear virus particles in human genital wart tissue: observations on the ultrastructure of the epidermal layer. *J Ultrastruct Res* 1968; **22**: 282–295

98 Laverty C R, Russel P, Hills E, Booth N. The significance of non-condylomatous wart virus infection of the cervical transformation zone: a review with discussion of two illustrative cases. *Acta Cytol* 1978; **22**: 195–201

99 Zur Hausen H, Meinhof W, Schreiber W, Bornkamm G W. Attempts to detect virus-specific DNA sequences in human tumors. I. Nucleic acid hybridizations with complementary RNA of human wart virus. *Int J Cancer* 1974; **13**: 650–656

100 Syrjanen S M. Basic concepts and practical applications of recombinant DNA techniques in detection of human papillomavirus (HPV) infections. *APMIS* 1990; **98**: 95–110

101 Stoler M H. Human papillomaviruses and cervical neoplasia: a model for carcinogenesis. *Int J Gynec Pathol* 2000; **19**: 16–28

102 Dudding N, Sutton J, Lane S. Koilocytosis: an indication for conservative management. *Cytopathol* 1996; **7**: 32–37

103 Koss L G, Durfee G R. Unusual patterns of squamous epithelium of the uterine cervix: cytologic and pathologic study of koilocytic atypia. *Ann NY Acad Sci* 1956; **63**: 1245–1261

104 Papanicolaou G N. *Atlas of Exfoliative Cytology*, Cambridge, Massachusetts: Harvard University Press, 1960; suppl 2

105 Meisels A. The story of a cell. The George N. Papanicolaou Award Lecture. *Acta Cytol* 1983; **27**: 584–596

106 Kern S. Significance of anucleated squames in Papanicolaou stained cervicovaginal smears. *Acta Cytol* 1991; **35**: 89–93

107 Tanaka H, Chua K-L, Lindh E, Hjerpe A. Patients with various types of human papilloma virus: covariation and diagnostic relevance of cytological findings in Papanicolaou smears. *Cytopathol* 1993; **4**: 273–283

108 Burrows D A, Howell L P, Hinrichs S, Richard O. Cytomorphologic features in

the diagnosis of human papillomavirus infection of the uterine cervix. *Acta Cytol* 1990; **34**: 737–738

109 Rakoczy P, Hutchinson L, Kulski J K et al. Detection of human papillomavirus in reprocessed routine Papanicolaou smears by DNA hybridization. *Diagn Cytopathol* 1990; **6**: 210–214

110 Vesterinen E, Leinikki P, Saksela E. Cytopathogenicity of cytomegalovirus to human ecto- and endocervico-epithelial cells in vitro. *Acta Cytol* 1975; **19**: 473–481

111 Huang A C, Naylor B. Cytomegalovirus infection of the cervix detected by cytology and histology: a report of five cases. *Cytopathol* 1993; **4**: 237–241

112 Morse A R, Coleman D V, Gardner S D. An evaluation of cytology in the diagnosis of herpes simplex virus infection and cytomegalovirus infection of the cervix uteri. *J Obstet Gynec Br Commonw* 1974; **81**: 393–398

113 Laverty C R, Russell P, Black J et al. Adenovirus infection of the cervix. *Acta Cytol* 1977; **21**: 114–117

114 Gupta P K, Lee E F, Erozan Y S et al. Cytologic investigations in Chlamydia infection. *Acta Cytol* 1979; **23**: 315–320

115 Bernal J N, Martinez M A, Dabacens A. Evaluation of proposed cytomorphologic criteria for the diagnosis of Chlamydia trachomatis in Papanicolaou smears. *Acta Cytol* 1989; **33**: 309–313

116 Boon M E, Hogewoning C J A, Tjiam K H et al. Cervical cytology and Chlamydia trachomatis infection. *Arch Gynecol* 1983; 131–140

117 Kuo C C, Wang S P, Wentworth B B, Grayston J T. Primary isolation of TRIC organisms in HeLa 229 cells treated with DEAE dextran. *J Infect Dis* 1972; **125**: 665–668

118 Shiina Y. Cytomorphologic and immunocytochemical studies of Chlamydial infections in cervical smears. *Acta Cytol* 1985; **29**: 683–691

119 Kobayashi T K, Ueda M, Araki H et al. Immunocytochemical demonstration of Chlamydia infection in the urogenital tract. *Diagn Cytopathol* 1987; **3**: 302–306

120 Gupta P K, Shurbaji M S, Mintor L J, Ermatinger S V. Cytopathologic detection of Chlamydia trachomatis in vaginopancervical (fast) smears. *Diagn Cytopathol* 1988; **4**: 224–229

121 Shiina Y, Kobayashi T K. Detection of Chlamydia trachomatis by Papanicolaou-stained smear and its limitations (letter). *Diagn Cytopathol* 1990; **6**: 148–151

122 Immunoelectron microscopic detection of chlamydial antigens in Papanicolaou-stained routine vaginal smears. *Acta Cytol* 1999; **4**: 835–837

123 Tam H, Stamm W, Handsfield H et al. Culture-independent diagnosis of Chlamydia trachomatis using monoclonal antibodies. *N Engl J Med* 1984; **310**: 1146–1150

124 Crum C P, Mitao M, Winkler B et al. Localizing Chlamydia infection in cervical biopsies with the immunoperoxidase

technique. *Int J Gynec Pathol* 1984; **3**: 191–197

125 Claas H C, Melchers W J, de Bruijn I H et al. Detection of Chlamydia trachomatis in clinical specimens by the polymerase chain reaction. *Eur J Clin Microbiol Inf Dis* 1990; **9**: 864–868

126 Lindner L E, Nettum J A. The diagnosis of Chlamydial infection in a cytology laboratory: ten months' experience using immunofluorescence with and without previous cytologic prediction. *Diagn Cytopathol* 1988; **4**: 18–22

127 Ghirardini C, Boselli F, Messi P et al. Chlamydia trachomatis infections in asymptomatic women: results of a study employing different staining techniques. *Acta Cytol* 1989; **33**: 115–119

128 Maeda M Y S, Filho A L, Shih L W S et al. Chlamydia trachomatis in cervical uterine irradiated cancer patients. *Diagn Cytopathol* 1990; **6**: 86–88

129 Legha S. Tamoxifen in the treatment of breast cancer. *Ann Int Med* 1988; **109**: 219–228

130 Eells T P, Alpern H D, Grzywacz C et al. The effect of tamoxifen on cervical squamous maturation in Papanicolaou stained cervical smears of post-menopausal women. *Cytopathol* 1990; **1**: 263–268

131 Neven P. Tamoxifen and endometrial lesions (editorial). *Lancet* 1993; **342**: 452

132 Bertolissi A, Carter G, Turrin D et al. Behaviour of vaginal epithelial maturation and sex hormone-binding globulin in post-menopausal breast cancer patients during the first year of Tamoxifen therapy. *Cytopathol* 1998; **9**: 263–270

133 Athanassiadou P P, Kyrkou K A, Antoniades L G, Athanassiades P H. Cytological evaluation of the effect of Tamoxifen in premenopausal women with primary breast cancer by analysis of the karyopyknotic indices of vaginal smears. *Cytopathol* 1992; **3**: 203–208

134 Fornander T, Cedermark B, Mattsson A et al. Adjuvant Tamoxifen in early breast cancer: occurrences of new primary cancers. *Lancet* 1989; 117–120

135 Ganesan R, Ferryman S, Waddell C A. Vaginal adenosis in a patient on Tamoxifen therapy: a case report. *Cytopathol* 1999; **10**: 127–130

136 Koss L G. *Diagnostic Cytology and its Histopathologic Bases*, 4th edn. Philadelphia: Lippincott, 1992

137 Fornari M L. Cellular changes in the glandular epithelium of patients using IUCD – a source of cytologic error. *Acta Cytol* 1974; **18**: 341–345

138 Sagiroglu N, Sagiroglu E. The cytology of intrauterine contraceptive devices. *Acta Cytol* 1970; **14**: 58–65

139 Gupta P K, Hollander D H, Frost J K. Actinomycetes in cervicovaginal smears: an association with IUD usage. *Acta Cytol* 1976; **20**: 294–298

140 Arroyo G, Quinn JA Jr. Association of amoebae and Actinomyces in an intrauterine contraceptive device user. *Acta Cytol* 1989; **33**: 298–300

141 Misra J S, Engineer A D, Tandon P. Cytopathological changes in human cervix and endometrium following prolonged retention of copper-bearing intrauterine contraceptive devices. *Diagn Cytopathol* 1989; **5**: 237–242

142 Highman W J. Calcified bodies and the intrauterine device. *Acta Cytol* 1971; **15**: 473–476

143 Boon M E, Kirk R S, de Graaff Guilloud J C. IUD pathology; psammoma bodies and some opportunistic infections detected in cervical smears of women fitted with an IUD. *Contracep Deliv Syst* 1981; **2**: 231–236

144 Bibbo M, Keebler C M, Weid G L. The cytologic diagnosis of tissue repair in the female genital tract. *Acta Cytol* 1971; **15**: 133–137

145 Hasegawa T, Tsutsui F, Kurihara S. Cytomorphologic study on the atypical cells following cryosurgery for the treatment of chronic cervicitis. *Acta Cytol* 1975; **19**: 533–538

146 Butler E B. *The Cytology of the Cervix After Cryosurgery*. The Sixth European Congress of Cytology, Weimar, 1976

147 Bukovsky A, Zidovsky J. Cytologic phenomena accompanying uterine cervix electrocoagulation. *Acta Cytol* 1985; **30**: 353–362

148 Suh K S, Silverberg S G. Tubal metaplasia of the uterine cervix. *Int J Gynecol Pathol* 1990; **9**: 122–128

149 Ismail S M. Cone biopsy causes cervical endometriosis and tuboendometrioid metaplasia. *Histopathol* 1991; **18**: 107–114

150 Ducatman B S, Wang H H, Jonasson J G et al. Tubal metaplasia: a cytologic study with comparison to other neoplastic and non-neoplastic conditions of the endocervix (Leiman G, editorial comment). *Diagn Cytopathol* 1993; **9**: 98–105

151 Hirschowitz L, Eckford S D, Philpotts B, Midwinter A. Cytological changes associated with tubo-endometrioid metaplasia of the uterine cervix. *Cytopathol* 1994; **5**: 1–8

152 Comea M T, Andrew A C, Leese H J et al. Application of a marker for ciliated epithelial cells in gynaecological pathology. *J Clin Pathol* 1999; **52**: 355–357

153 Lee K R. Atypical glandular cells in cervical smears from women who have undergone cone biopsy: a diagnostic pitfall. *Acta Cytol* 1993; **37**: 705–709

154 Cleaves M A. Radium with a preliminary note on radium rays in the treatment of cancer. *J Adv Ther* 1903; 667–682

155 Shield P W, Daunter B, Wright R G. Review. Post-irradiation cytology of cervical cancer patients. *Cytopathol* 1992; **3**: 167–182

156 Van Niekerk W A. Cervical cytological abnormalities caused by folic acid deficiency. *Acta Cytol* 1966; **10**: 67–73

157 Mclennan M T, Mclennan L E. Significance of cervicovaginal cytology after radiation therapy for cervical cancer. *Am J Obstet Gynecol* 1975; **121**: 96–100

158 Patten S F, Reagan J W, Obenauf M, Ballard L A. Postirradiation dysplasia of uterine cervix and vagina: an analytical study of the cells. *Cancer* 1963; **16**: 173–182

159   Muram D, Curry R H, Drouin P. Cytologic follow-up of patients with cervical carcinoma treated by radiotherapy. *Am J Obstet Gynecol* 1982; **142**: 350–354

160   Gureli N, Denham S W, Root S W. Cytologic dysplasia related to busulfan (myeleran) therapy. *Obstet Gynec* 1963; **21**: 466–470

161   Walker S E, Bole G G. Augmented incidence of neoplasia in female New Zealand black/New Zealand white mice treated with long-term cyclophosphamide. *J Lab Clin Med* 1971; **78**: 978–979

162   Gupta P K, Pinn V M, Taft P D. Cervical dysplasia associated with azathioprine (Imuran) therapy. *Acta Cytol* 1969; **13**: 373–377

163   Helmerhorst T J M, Wijnen J A, Tjioe G S T D *et al*. Colposcopic findings and intraepithelial neoplasia in DES-exposed offspring. In: Helmerhorst Th J M ed. Trends in management of female lower genital intraepithelial neoplasia. PhD Thesis; Amsterdam, 1988; 113–121

164   Robboy S J, Noller K L, O'Brien P C. Increased incidence of cervical and vaginal dysplasia in 3980 diethylstilbestrol-exposed young women. *Cancer* 1986; **52**: 2979–2983

29 The pathogenesis of cervical neoplasia

Simon Herrington

Introduction

The aetiology of cervical neoplasia has been studied epidemiologically for over 150 years. More recently, experimental approaches have been applied and, with the advent of molecular biology, putative infectious agents can now be studied more easily and with greater precision. This chapter will address the contribution of both epidemiological and experimental approaches to current understanding of the pathogenesis of cervical neoplasia.

Epidemiology of cervical cancer

Studies based on demographic data such as death certification are only as accurate as the information provided to cancer registries. Similarly, studies of risk factors are dependent on accurate histological and cytopathological diagnosis. Factors involved in the interpretation of cervical biopsies and smears must be considered in assessment of studies which depend on classification of cervical lesions by these means.

Incidence, prevalence and geographical variation of cervical cancer

Cervical cancer accounts for approximately 15% of all cancers diagnosed in women world-wide with approximately 400 000 cases diagnosed per annum with 190 000 deaths[1]. A total of 78% of these cases occur in developing countries, where it is the commonest cancer in women. The highest crude mortality rate is recorded for Southern Africa (15.7 per 100 000), but the highest risk of death from cervical cancer is recorded in Melanesia. North America, Western Europe and Australasia have a low incidence with cervical cancer accounting for only 4–6% of female cancer[2]. The lowest mortality rate is in China[1]. In the UK, 3450 cases of cervical cancer were diagnosed in 1995 and cervical cancer ranks sixteenth in overall incidence and tenth in incidence in females (Table 29.1).

Variation in incidence and mortality of cervical cancer with time

The incidence of cervical cancer has decreased significantly since the 1960s[3,4]. It has been suggested that this is in part due to the effect of screening by cervical cytology, which has counteracted the rise in incidence that would be predicted from analysis of risk factors. Age-specific rates, however,

Table 29.1 UK cancer incidence and mortality in women[162]

Site	Incidence (1995)	Mortality (1996)
Breast	33 040 (27%)	13 680 (18%)
Large bowel	15 360 (12%)	8710 (12%)
Lung	14 490 (12%)	13 000 (17%)
Ovary	5910 (5%)	4580 (6%)
Uterus	4090 (3%)	–
Stomach	3870 (3%)	2920 (4%)
Bladder	3820 (3%)	1720 (2%)
Non-Hodgkin's lymphoma	3720 (3%)	2140 (3%)
Pancreas	3580 (3%)	3380 (5%)
Cervix	3450 (3%)	–
Oesophagus	–	2620 (4%)
Leukaemia	–	1810 (2%)
Others	32 840 (26%)	20 550 (27%)

show an increase in young women, particularly those aged 25–29. Mortality rates have increased among young women in the UK[5], Australia[6] and New Zealand[7] and this increase has occurred on a background of an overall decrease in cervical cancer mortality at all ages. Reasons for this are unclear but the introduction of a new risk factor, which operates to a greater extent in the younger population, would explain the difference. It is not due to less effective screening of the younger population as it has been shown that screening has partially counteracted the increase in younger women[8].

Risk factors for cervical cancer: from epidemiology to aetiological theories

Sexual factors

In 1842, Rigoni-Stern reported that cervical cancer occurred only in married women[9]. Thus, the association of cervical cancer and sexual activity has been known for over 150 years. Epidemiologically, cervical cancer behaves like a sexually transmitted disease: it is more common in women who have had multiple sexual partners[10] or whose partners are promiscuous[11], and is absent in virgins[12]. The number of sexual partners and age at first intercourse are crude measures of probability of exposure to a putative infectious agent and time elapsed since earliest possible exposure respectively, indirectly suggesting involvement of an infectious agent.

The most likely source of a potential infectious agent is an infected male partner. Evidence for the existence of a 'high risk' male is compelling. First, geographical clusters of high rates of cancer of both cervix and penis have been described[13]. Second, wives of men with cancer of the penis have a three to six-fold greater risk of cervical cancer than control women[14–16]. Third, women married to men whose previous wives had cervical cancer have a two-fold increased risk of cervical cancer themselves[17]. Comparison of the husbands of women with cervical cancer with those of control women has provided more direct evidence: cases are five to seven times more likely to have husbands who have had ten or more partners than controls[18]. The relative risk (RR) of development of invasive cervical cancer is 8.62 for women whose current partner has had >10 partners[19].

Although the predominant mechanism by which human papillomaviruses are transmitted is sexual, there is now considerable evidence that vertical transmission, particularly from mother to infant, can occur. This may explain the finding of HPV DNA in lesions of the aerodigestive tract[20].

Smoking and cervical cancer

The original suggestion of a link between smoking and cervical cancer was made by Winkelstein in 1977[21]. Since then, the association has been extensively studied and possible mechanisms investigated. Several case control studies have shown that smoking is a risk factor independent of sexual parameters, with an overall two-fold increase in risk for the development of cervical intraepithelial neoplasia (CIN) and invasive cervical cancer[13,22–28]. Moreover, there is a dose response relationship[13,22,23] and the elevated risk is reduced in former smokers[13,29].

Although correction for sexual factors has been performed, these are crude measures of exposure to a potential infectious agent. Therefore, it is possible that, if correction were made for the infectious agent itself, the association with smoking could disappear. A case control study of smoking and HPV infection[30] found an increased risk associated with smoking which disappeared on multivariate analysis when HPV 16/18 infection was considered. A study performed in a high incidence area where intensive smoking among women is rare showed an age adjusted RR of 1.2 in women who had never smoked and 1.7 in those who smoked more than 30 cigarettes per day[31]. This risk virtually disappeared after adjustment for number of sexual partners and alcohol consumption. However, among women infected with HPV 16/18 as detected by filter *in situ* hybridization the RR was 5.0 for smokers compared with non-smokers. Moreover, a dose response relationship was found, with RR >5.5 for less than 10 cigarettes a day and 8.4 for greater. These studies suggest that smoking may interact with particular HPV types in cervical carcinogenesis. More recent epidemiological studies have confirmed that smoking is an independent risk factor for the development of intraepithelial as well as invasive disease operating in addition to HPV infection[32].

The mechanism by which smoking increases the risk of cervical cancer is less clear although it has been suggested to have a late stage effect[33]. Studies of DNA adduction products with polycyclic hydrocarbons have shown that these adducts are more frequent in smokers than non-smokers: this may provide a link between smoking and DNA mutation induction and hence carcinogenesis[34].

Oral contraceptives (OC) and cervical cancer

Several cross-sectional studies have suggested a link between OC use and an elevated risk of CIN[26,27,35], even when correction is made for potentially confounding variables. Other studies have however found no association[25,36,37]. Studies of invasive squamous cell carcinoma similarly produce conflicting results: some found a significant increase in risk in OC users[36,38,39] with the association stronger for patients who had never used barrier methods of contraception or who had a history of genital infection[38,39]. This may represent an interaction between infectious agents and the OC[40], either as interaction between HPV and OC in cervical carcinogenesis or increased HPV replication in the tumours of patients taking the OC[41]. However, in two studies in which correction for confounding variables was carried out, no association between invasive cervical cancer risk and OC was found[35,42] and a large study of depot medroxy-progesterone treatment showed no increased risk[43].

A large cohort study of 47 000 women followed from 1968[44] found a significantly increased risk of cervical cancer in patients who had ever used oral contraceptives, the incidence increasing with duration of use. A study of 17 032 patients followed for 16 years[45] showed a RR of 4.9 in OC users, but the 95% confidence interval for this figure was 0.7–230. A recent meta-analysis of 51 studies found a relative risk for CIN of 1.52 and for invasive carcinoma of 1.21 in users of oral contraceptives[46]. The possible interaction with infectious agents, particularly HPV, may be important in these associations, consistent with experimental evidence linking steroid hormones and enhanced HPV transcription (see below).

Other contraceptives and cervical cancer

The hypothesis that infectious agents are involved in the pathogenesis of cervical cancer predicts that barrier methods of contraception would be protective. A cohort study of 17 032 women found that the incidence of cervical cancer was lower in diaphragm users (0.17 per 1000 women years) than in IUCD users (0.85) or pill users (0.97), even after adjustment for confounding variables[47]. Several other studies have shown a protective effect and this applies to both overall use of barrier methods and the use of diaphragm[19,27] or condoms[19] specifically. From a mechanistic point of view, this is not surprising if an infectious agent is involved in cervical carcinogenesis.

Diet and cervical cancer

The effect of diet on the incidence of cancer is difficult to study as there is wide variation in dietary intake between communities, within communities and from day to day for individuals. Nevertheless, it has been suggested that several dietary factors are important in carcinogenesis in general and cervical cancer in particular[48]. Most information is available regarding vitamins A and C, some studies showing an inverse relationship between intake of these vitamins and risk of cervical cancer[49,50]. These data suggest that dietary factors may be involved in the genesis of cervical cancer, although cautious interpretation is required in the absence of correction for potential infectious agents. Some more recent studies have examined the potential confounding effect of sexual factors and HPV. In one questionnaire-based study, a weak protective effect of increased fruit consumption became non-significant after adjustment for sexual behaviour[51]. In another study, no protective effect of diet was identified for cervical intraepithelial neoplasia, with or without correction for HPV[32].

Immunosuppression and cervical cancer

Immunosuppression may be primary or secondary, systemic or local. Most data are available for secondary systemic immunosuppression, which is either physiological, pathological or iatrogenic. An increased incidence of CIN has been described in patients who have received renal transplants[52]: in one study, mean lag time to condylomatous change was 22.4 months and to CIN or invasive cancer 38.0 months[53]. During pregnancy, there is transient depression of cell mediated immunity. HPV DNA is detected more often in pregnant women[54], although this may simply be due to increased viral replication and does not necessarily imply an increase in prevalence. More recently, an increased risk of cervical neoplasia has been noted in patients infected with HIV[55]. Local immunosuppression is more difficult to investigate but is discussed below.

Host factors

Since the suggestion that the prevalence of HLA DQw3 is greater in patients with cervical carcinoma than in the control population[56], a large number of studies examining the relationship between HLA and cervical neoplasia has been published. Mechanistically, the association between some class II HLA antigens and increased susceptibility to cervical carcinoma may be related to defective clearance of viruses such as HPV and there are some data showing that the association is stronger between HLA DQw3 and HPV infection than it is with the degree of CIN or invasive carcinoma[57]. However, although numerous studies examining the relationship between HLA genotype and phenotype and cervical neoplasia have been published, the majority of the findings in these studies are not consistent, possibly reflecting population differences and complex interactions between HLA genotype, phenotype and infecting HPV types[58,59].

Infectious agents

Most attention has been focused in recent years on the role of human papillomaviruses in cervical carcinogenesis. Many other agents have been studied, however, and these will now be discussed. Evidence for the involvement of HPV will be presented later.

The epidemiological evidence for involvement of *Herpes simplex* virus (HSV) in cervical carcinogenesis is suggestive[60-63], but there is no clear experimental evidence to support it. Two hypotheses have been formulated to explain this: the 'hit-and-run' hypothesis[64,65] and synergism between HSV and HPV[66]. There is more evidence supporting the latter hypothesis (see below).

Investigation of the other herpes viruses, namely cytomegalovirus (CMV) and Epstein-Barr virus (EBV) by serological means revealed no difference in prevalence of antibodies to these agents in patients with cervical cancer compared with patients with condylomata or a control group. However, antibodies to early CMV antigens were found more commonly in patients with cervical cancer[67].

Determination of exposure by culture and special stains showed no differences between cases and controls for the following organisms: HSV2, CMV, *Chlamydia trachomatis*, *Neiserria gonorrhoeae*, *Gardnerella vaginalis*, *Ureoplasma ureolyticum*, *Mycoplasma hominis*, *Candida albicans*[68]. No association was found in one study between chlamydia and HPV infection using the polymerase chain reaction (PCR)[69] but HIV infection appears to be associated with a greater risk of development of CIN, possibly related to associated immunosuppression[56,70].

Overall, therefore, there is evidence that HIV infection, and possibly HSV infection, may interact with HPV in the process of cervical carcinogenesis.

Screening and cervical cancer

Parkin *et al.*[8] have shown that screening has reduced the incidence and mortality of cervical cancer. It is widely believed that cervical screening is responsible for the decline in overall incidence of cervical cancer and that it has attenuated the rise in incidence in younger women[3,8]. The duration of relative protection afforded by cervical screening by smear testing has been estimated to be 4–6 years in a case control study[71]. This protection is not constant for all women, varying with screening interval as well as with other epidemiological parameters. Klassen *et al.*[72] noted that patients who had had a cervical smear taken up to 4 years prior to the study had significantly greater protection than those screened more than 11 years previously or never screened. Protection was less for older women, women with earlier age of first intercourse, and non-users of barrier contraception. Similarly, van der Graaf *et al.*[73] found that the relative risk of women screened at least once compared with those never screened was 0.22 when corrected for age at first intercourse. This, together with the high incidence of cervical carcinoma in developing nations, supports the suggestion that the most effective public health measure for women in these countries would be a single cervical smear at the age of 40. Analysis of the interval since the last smear showed that the relative risk of women screened ≥5 years previously was 0.30 compared with 0.18 for women screened 2–5 years previously. Thus, even screening at intervals of greater than five years appears to be protective. With the establishment of cervical screening, it can now be viewed that the lack of screening constitutes a risk factor for cervical neoplasia.

Conclusions

There is now considerable epidemiological evidence that the risk of developing cervical cancer is in part sexually transmitted. The most likely explanation for the data discussed above is that an infectious agent is involved but much of the interpretation of the epidemiological studies quoted has of necessity been performed without knowledge of the identity of this agent. It is possible therefore that the other associations noted may simply represent confounding variables themselves and hence be reflections of the effect of an infectious agent. With the increasing evidence, both epidemiological and experimental, that HPV is the infectious agent in question, the role of other factors can now be addressed with more confidence. As has been shown above, the effects of some risk factors thought initially to be important are partially or completely negated by correction for HPV infection. However, HPV infection is not by itself responsible for cervical carcinogenesis. The epidemiological and experimental evidence implicating HPV infection in cervical carcinogenesis and its relationship to other risk factors is now discussed.

Human papillomaviruses and cervical neoplasia

Molecular classification of human papillomaviruses

The papillomaviruses are double-stranded DNA viruses (Baltimore class 1) and have been included traditionally in the Papovaviridae (papillomaviruses, polyomaviruses, SV40 related viruses). However, they are sufficiently dissimilar from the other two members to be considered as a separate group[74]. Ultrastructurally, all papillomavirus types are identical so it was thought initially that there was only one type. Molecular cloning of viral nucleic acid from human lesions demonstrated that multiple types existed and, indeed, over 80 types of HPV are now described[75]: this does not include animal papillomaviruses or other papillomavirus sequences, which have not yet been fully characterized.

Table 29.2   Classification of papillomaviruses[a]

Supergroup A (genital HPVs)
Group A1: HPV 32 and HPV 42
Group A2: HPV 3, HPV 10, HPV 28 and HPV 29
Group A3: HPV 61, HPV 62, HPV 72, CP6108, CP8304 and MM8
Group A4: HPV 2, HPV 27 and HPV 57
Group A5: HPV 26, HPV 51, HPV 69, ISO39 and MM4
Group A6: HPV 30, HPV 53, HPV 56 and HPV 66
Group A7: HPV 18, HPV 39, HPV 45, HPV 59, HPV 68 and HPV 70
Group A8: HPV 7, HPV 40 and HPV 43
Group A9: HPV 16, HPV 31, HPV 33, HPV 35, HPV 52, HPV 58, HPV 67 and RhPV
Group A10: HPV 6, HPV 11, HPV 13, HPV 44, HPV 55 and PCPV
Group A11: HPV 34, HPV 64 and HPV 73
Poorly resolved lineages within supergroup A: CgPV, CP8061, LVX82 and HPV 54

Supergroup B (EV HPVs)
Group B1: HPV 5, HPV 8, HPV 9, HPV 12, HPV 14, HPV 15, HPV 17, HPV 19, HPV 20, HPV 21, HPV 22, HPV 23, HPV 24, HPV 25, HPV 36, HPV 27, HPV 38, HPV 47 and HPV 49
Group B2: HPV 4, HPV 48, HPV 50, HPV 60 and HPV 65

Supergroup C (ungulate fibropapillomaviruses)
Group C1: BPV 1 and BPV 2
Group C2: DPV, EPV and OvPV
Isolated lineage within supergroup C with likely group rank: BPV 5

Supergroup D (BPVs causing true papillomas)
Group D1: BPV 3, BPV 4, and BPV 6

Supergroup E (animal and human cutaneous PVs)
Group E1: HPV 1 and HPV 63
Isolated lineages within supergroup E with likely group rank: COPV, CRPV and HPV 41

Poorly resolved lineages which likely represent taxa of supergroup rank

[a] Modified from[163].
HPV, human papillomavirus; RhPV, rhesus monkey papillomavirus; PCPV, pigmy chimpanzee papillomavirus; CgPV, colobus monkey papillomavirus; EV, epidermodysplasia verruciformis; BPV, bovine papillomavirus; DPV, deer papillomavirus; EPV, European elk papillomavirus; OvPV, ovine (sheep) papillomavirus; COPV, canine oral papillomavirus; CRPV, cottontail rabbit papillomavirus.
Other abbreviations refer to individual sequence designations[163]

The human papillomaviruses are classified according to their degree of molecular homology. A phylogenetic tree has been constructed and HPVs are conventionally divided into supergroups, which are in turn subdivided into individual groups (see Table 29.2). HPV types share less than 90% homology with other HPV types, sub-types share 90–98% homology and variants are >98% homologous. Thus, HPVs can vary by up to 2% from the prototype sequence and still be considered to be the same HPV type[59]. From a clinical perspective, the viruses are often classified according to their association with cutaneous or anogenital warts, intraepithelial neoplasia or invasive neoplasia. Thus, these viruses can be considered 'high risk' (e.g. HPV 16, 18, 45, 56) 'intermediate risk' (for example HPV 31, 33, 35, 39, 51, 52, 58) and 'low risk' (for example HPV 6, 11, 42, 43, 44). Many investigators now combine high and intermediate risk viruses into an

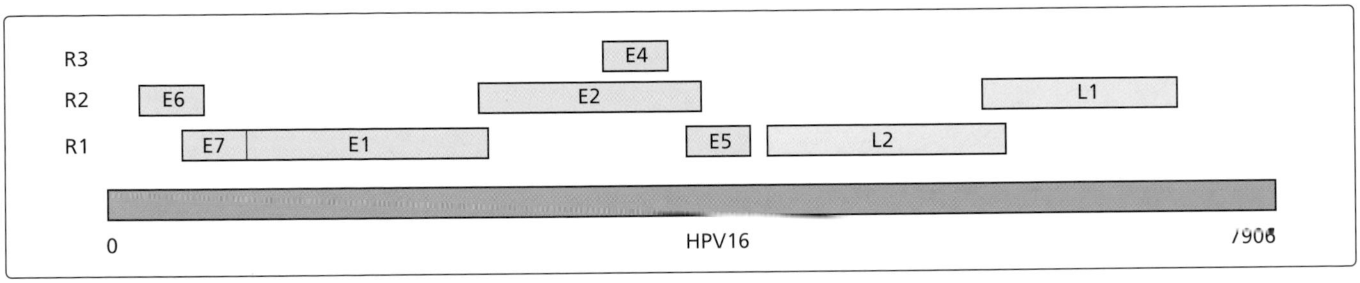

Fig. 29.1   Schematic view of the molecular organization of HPV 16. The boundaries of each gene are those of the open reading frames; HPV16 is 7906 base pairs long; E and L refer to the early and late genes respectively; three reading frames are denoted by R1, R2 and R3. Derived from data in reference no. 168.

oncogenic group, with the remainder forming a non-oncogenic group of HPVs.

Molecular organization, virology and pathology of HPVs

The molecular organization of all papillomavirus genomes described conforms to the pattern shown in Figure 29.1[76]. The viral genes are divided into two functional groups: the late (L) and early (E) genes. There are seven E genes, each of which serves a different function in viral replication (Fig. 29.1). The E1 and E2 genes tend to be disrupted in viral integration, the E6 and E7 genes (with some recent evidence implicating E5) being involved in cellular transformation[76–79]. The two L genes encode structural viral proteins and are therefore required for productive viral infection.

Viral infection involves interaction between the virus and host cells. Only certain cell types can support vegetative viral production. Cells that do not support infection are termed non-permissive, non-transformable: the majority of cells fall into this category for HPV infection. In permissive cells, HPV replication and protein synthesis are closely linked to keratinization[80]. This may explain the tropism of HPV for squamous epithelia. Thus, permissive infection of squamous epithelia only occurs in the strata spinosum and granulosum. Non-permissive transformable infection describes the situation in which viral replication and vegetative viral production does not occur but viral DNA persists within the cell either as an extra-chromosomal element or by integration into the host genome. This persistence may be associated with cellular transformation as in high-grade cervical intraepithelial neoplasia (CIN) and invasive squamous cell carcinoma (ISCC). HPV infection of columnar glandular epithelium is being increasingly described[81], and may also represent this form of infection. The cytopathic effect of HPV in squamous epithelial cells is well recognized, with koilocytosis, nuclear enlargement, dyskeratosis and multinucleation being the major changes (see Chapter 39).

Detection of HPV in clinical material

The detection of nucleic acid in clinical material is the most appropriate way of achieving a clinical diagnosis and of investigating the epidemiology and natural history of viral infections as:

1   Clinical features are not diagnostic
2   The cytopathic effect is to some extent insensitive and nonspecific
3   Viral protein production is not constitutive
4   Classification is molecular

Either DNA or RNA can be analysed but the detection of RNA is technically more difficult and is dependent on viral gene transcription. In general, therefore, viral DNA is analysed and this can be achieved in two basic ways: after extraction from tissue with or without amplification by the polymerase chain reaction (see below) or directly by *in situ* hybridization.

DNA can be extracted from peripheral blood, cellular suspensions, frozen tissue and fixed, processed embedded material. It is therefore possible to analyse the DNA content of any clinical sample encountered in everyday practice[82]. However, the amount of material required in each case varies both with the techniques used and the nature of material available. The PCR can be used to amplify a specific DNA region by as much as 10^8-fold[83] and the basic PCR can be performed on the smallest of clinical samples with simple equipment[82]. If product identity is established by restriction digestion, it is routinely applicable, but if Southern blotting or nucleotide sequencing are employed, the time and expertise required are correspondingly increased. An alternative approach to the detection of HPV DNA in extracted nucleic acids is the hybrid capture technique in which the target DNA is identified using RNA probes by 'capture' of DNA/RNA hybrids using antibodies to double-stranded nucleic acids. These 'captured' hybrids are then identified by signal amplification using a chemiluminescent read-out system[84]. *In situ* hybridization allows cellular localization of signal in both cytological and histological material, thus increasing specificity for cellular infection but with lower absolute sensitivity[85–87] (Fig. 29.2).

Detection of HPV in clinical material is therefore most appropriately achieved by DNA analysis and, with recent refinements in technology, generic PCR and hybrid capture

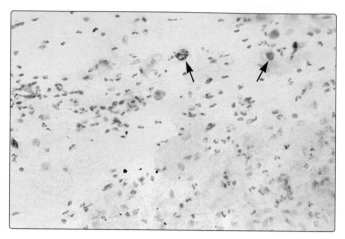

Fig. 29.2 *In situ* hybridization of a routine cervical smear with a cocktail of digoxigenin labelled probes for HPV 16, 18, 31 and 33. Note the red signal within epithelial cell nuclei (arrows).

(particularly hybrid capture II) are the most favoured techniques for routine applicability[84,88].

The role of HPV in human disease

It has been shown above that different HPVs have a predilection for different anatomical sites. HPVs are markedly epitheliotropic and have been found in squamous epithelium (both original and metaplastic) at virtually every site. Particular attention has been paid to anogenital HPV infection, in view of the association with premalignant and malignant vulval, penile and cervical lesions. The finding of HPVs in squamous cell carcinomas of the anus has extended the list of lesions related to these viruses. HPV infection is not confined to squamous epithelia. It has been demonstrated in adenocarcinoma (both invasive and *in situ*) of the cervix[81,89]. The finding that HPV18 has a particular propensity to infect endocervical epithelium suggests that individual HPV types may exhibit more specific epitheliotropism.

Clinico-molecular classification

The HPV types found in anogenital lesions are more associated with the histopathology than the site of the lesion. Thus, a condyloma acuminatum is likely to be infected with HPV 6 or 11 whether it is of anal, vulval, penile or cervical origin. Similarly, the flat condyloma of the cervix and Bowenoid papulosis of the penis are both associated with 'high risk' HPV infection (particularly HPV 16 and 18)[90,91]. Dysplastic lesions from all anogenital sites (anal dysplasia, vulval intraepithelial neoplasia (VIN), penile intraepithelial neoplasia (PIN) and cervical intraepithelial neoplasia (CIN) have been associated with HPV infection by HPV 16, 18 and related viral types analysed by both epidemiological and experimental means[92]. These clinical associations have led to the definition of 'high risk' (HPV 16 and 18 particularly), 'intermediate risk' (HPV 31 and 33 particularly) and 'low

risk' (HPV 6, 11, 42) viral types[75,93]. Invasive squamous cell carcinomas of the larynx, vulva, penis, anus and cervix are all associated with the same 'high-risk' HPV types, suggesting a common aetiological link.

In the following two sections, the epidemiological and experimental evidence linking HPV in general, and 'high risk' HPV types in particular to cervical neoplasia will be reviewed.

The role of HPV in cervical neoplasia: epidemiological evidence

In studies of CIN, analysis of the relationship between CIN and HPV is dependent on the accurate diagnosis of CIN and its distinction from the effects of HPV infection. This may be difficult in low-grade lesions. In strict terms, controls should be defined by the absence of the disease process under study, in this case CIN not HPV. Therefore, patients with pure wart virus infection should be included as controls. This is not performed in most studies. It is important to appreciate that there is considerable inter- and intra-observer variation when assessing particularly low-grade intraepithelial lesions. This is one of the factors underlying the adoption of the Bethesda classification in some countries for the assessment of intraepithelial disease. However, many studies use CIN 2 or 3, or high-grade squamous intraepithelial lesions (SILs), as their endpoint and the CIN and SIL systems are, in this regard, generally interchangeable.

Early molecular studies suggested the association of HPV 6/11 with condylomata and low-grade dysplasia (CIN 1) and of HPV 16, 31, 33, 35, etc. with high-grade dysplasia (CIN 2/3) and invasive squamous cell carcinoma of the cervix (ISCC). In view of this observation, it was postulated that HPV 16 and related viral types were causally related to the development of CIN and ISCC. The prevalence of HPV16/18 increases with the severity of the lesion, viral DNA being integrated in the majority of CIN 3 lesions and ISCC. Progression from HPV infection alone through CIN to invasive squamous cell carcinoma has been documented histopathologically[94]. Mitchell *et al.*[95] reported an almost 16-fold increased risk for the development of carcinoma *in situ* in patients with cytological evidence of wart virus infection and Syrjänen *et al.*[96] found that after a mean follow up of 35 months, regression of HPV infection occurred in 28.6% of women, persistent infection in 55.6% and progression to CIN in 13.6% (12.9% to carcinoma *in situ*). These data argue that HPV infection is a precursor lesion to the development of CIN. This has been confirmed by a recent cohort study in which the presence of HPV was determined by Southern and dot blotting, in which the relative risk of development of CIN 2 or 3 in the presence of HPV16 or 18 DNA was 11.0[97]. Analysis of eight cross-sectional studies estimated that the presence of oncogenic HPV types as determined by Southern blotting conferred an increased risk ranging from 65.1–235.7 for CIN 2/3 and 31.1–296.1 for an invasive lesion[93].

Many of the problems previously encountered in the analysis of epidemiological data regarding the prevalence of HPV infection were due to variations in methodology. This was particularly true of PCR, which has suggested that the HPV 16 carriage rate in normal women is as high as 84%[98]. However, it has become clear that a high rate of false positive results is obtained with PCR if measures are not taken to eliminate or control for sample contamination and environmental contamination from surgeons' gloves and biopsy forceps[99,100] has been described. With the appropriate precautions, however, PCR can be used fruitfully[101,102] and, although there were very high estimates of HPV16 prevalence in early studies, more recent studies have found much lower carriage rates for high risk HPV types in the community, estimates ranging from 3.5–30%[103–106]. Clearly, this depends on the population studied but there does appear to be a difference between patients with normal and dyskaryotic smears. There also appears to be an age-dependent prevalence of HPV, with women over the age of 30 to 35 showing a much reduced carriage rate of HPV DNA, and persistent HPV infection is also an important risk marker for disease progression[107]. These observations are important when considering the potential role of HPV testing.

With the increasing standardization and consistency of HPV typing systems, particularly those utilizing generic PCR and hybrid capture, a degree of consistency is appearing in the literature regarding the possible application of HPV testing in cervical screening. This potential has been underscored recently by the identification of HPV DNA in almost 100% of invasive cervical carcinomas in a multi-national study[108]. The combination of good technical reproducibility and the potential for achievement of 100% sensitivity underscores the potential benefit of HPV testing and supports further investigation of its possible use in the context of cervical screening.

The role of HPV in cervical cancer: experimental evidence

Two experimental approaches have been taken to the study of HPV:

1. Analysis of the presence and physical state of HPV DNA and RNA in human cervical lesions and cell lines
2. Analysis of the effect of introduction of viral sequences into cultured cells *in vitro*

Analysis of naturally occurring lesions and cultured cell lines

HPV sequences have been localized to epithelial cell nuclei by *in situ* hybridization[55,109,110]. Invasive cervical cancer and CIN 3 lesions often contain areas of lower grade CIN adjacent to the main lesion. Analysis of this situation by *in situ* hybridization has shown that the same HPV type is present in areas of all grades of CIN including the main lesion, suggesting that these areas represent sequential steps in the same process[55,111]. In addition, this observation suggests that HPV infection occurs early in the process of cervical carcinogenesis.

The HPV genome in high-grade lesions is transcriptionally active[112,113] and *in situ* hybridization analysis using riboprobes shows viral RNA transcripts whenever viral DNA is present[110]. The pattern of viral transcription is constant in low-grade CIN but altered and variable in high-grade CIN and invasive cancer[113]. Viral mRNA is produced by all HPV containing cervical carcinoma derived cell lines studied[112,114,115]. The major transcripts are derived from the E6 and E7 genes of both HPV16[114] and HPV18[112], although in some cell lines only E1 mRNA was found[114]. However, the continued requirement of E6/E7 transcription for maintenance of the transformed phenotype has been demonstrated[116].

The HPV genome is integrated in most cell lines either arising spontaneously[112,117,118] or induced *in vitro*[119]. This mirrors the situation in high-grade clinical lesions[120,121]. Integration of the viral genome appears to occur at random[117,119–124] at fragile sites, a pattern not exclusive to HPV[125]. The site of breakage of the viral genome is more consistent, occurring in the E1/E2 region. The E2 gene is involved in the control of viral transcription, suggesting that a break at this point might lead to enhanced transforming gene transcription.

The viral proteins found in cervical carcinoma derived cell lines are the products of E6 and E7. This correlates with the major transcripts found in these cells. These proteins bind to cellular proteins involved in the regulation of growth control (see below), thus suggesting a mechanism for the interaction between HPV infection and integration and aberrant cellular growth.

Transformation by human papillomaviruses *in vitro*
HPV DNA can transform rodent and human primary epithelial cells. Using raft culture techniques, human fetal ectocervical cells transfected with HPV 16 produced lesions morphologically indistinguishable from CIN[126,127]. It has been shown that the E7 gene of HPV16 is sufficient for immortalization of primary keratinocytes although further events are required to effect full transformation. The effect of the E6 gene has been shown to be additive in this regard[59,128].

HPV interaction with other factors
The available epidemiological and experimental evidence suggests that HPVs alone are not responsible for the development of CIN and invasive cervical cancer. Much of the data regarding cofactors have been derived by epidemiological means and this has already been discussed. The experimental evidence relevant to the interaction of HPV with other cofactors will now be reviewed.

Oncogenes and anti-oncogenes
There are several studies on the amplification and expression of c-myc in cervical tumours. c-myc

rearrangement and/or amplification (up to 185-fold) has been described in cervical carcinomas[129], both in lesions containing HPV16 sequences and in those without. This finding is, however, not consistent between workers[130,131]. Riou *et al.* demonstrated a correlation between amplification of both c-myc and H-ras-1 and advanced tumour stage and between elevated c-myc expression and poor prognosis of early cervical carcinomas[132,133]. Analysis of the H-ras-1 gene has demonstrated loss of heterozygosity in 36% of tumours, 90% of which contained HPV16 or 18 DNA. Mutations in codon 12 of the H-ras-1 gene were identified in 2% of early and 24% of advanced tumours[134]. In addition, 40% of tumours, which had a mutation, had lost the other H-ras-1 allele. In the same series, 100% of tumours with a mutation showed either over expression or amplification of the c-myc gene. Similarly, 70% of tumours with a deletion exhibited the same phenomenon. This is consistent with involvement of establishment and transforming genes in phenotypic transformation. HPV integration and amplification is described at the cytogenetic site of the c-myc protooncogene in HeLa and C4–1 cells and c-myc transcription is enhanced in both cell lines. As noted above, however, this site of viral integration is not universal.

It has been shown that E7 proteins of HPV16 and 18 bind to the retinoblastoma gene product (Rb-1)[135] and E6 proteins of these viruses bind to p53 protein, albeit with different affinities[136]. It has been suggested that binding of these proteins *in vivo* may alter cellular regulatory functions such that proliferation and transformation occur secondary to inactivation of Rb-1 and p53. This has led to the hypothesis that p53 mutation and inactivation by complexing with E6 protein are mutually exclusive events, i.e. the p53 gene is mutated in HPV negative tumours and wild type in HPV positive tumours[137]. Binding of p53 by E6 protein of HPV 16 but not that of HPV 6 leads to accelerated degradation of the complex via the ubiquitin pathway[138]. This hypothesis has been tested using cervical carcinomas with conflicting results[139–141], although it is difficult in these studies to exclude the occurrence of secondary p53 mutations in HPV containing tumours. Nevertheless, binding of Rb-1 to E7 is analogous to its binding to adenovirus E1A antigen and SV40 large T antigen, suggesting a common mechanism of transformation involving altered regulation of the cell cycle[142]. Other factors are, however, likely to be involved.

Smoking

There are limited data regarding the interaction of smoking and HPV infection but the finding of reduced numbers of Langerhans cells in cervical epithelium in smokers suggests that reduced presentation of viral antigen may occur, resulting in viral persistence[143]. Recent epidemiological studies have shown that viral persistence is associated with an increased risk of progression of CIN. The epidemiological link between smoking and HPV infection

may therefore be mechanistically explicable. Similarly, polycyclic hydrocarbon DNA adducts have been shown to be more frequent in smokers than in non-smokers as assessed by urinary nicotine:cotinine ratio[34].

Chromosome aberrations

Chromosome abnormalities, particularly of chromosomes 1 and 11, can be induced in human cells by cotransfection with HPV DNA and EJ-ras[144]. Cytogenetic analysis of cervical tumours has shown that chromosomes 1, 3, 11 and 17 are commonly abnormal[145]. Several studies have identified loss of heterozygosity on the short arm of chromosome 3 in cervical carcinoma. Moreover, gain of chromosome 3q has been identified by comparative genomic hybridization in high-grade intraepithelial disease and also in a high proportion of invasive carcinomas[59]. Abnormalities of chromosome 3 may therefore be particularly important in the progression from high-grade intraepithelial to invasive disease. It is possible that changes in gene dosage by chromosome loss, duplication or rearrangement following induction of aneuploidy might lead to inactivation of cellular antioncogenes such as p53 or activation of oncogenes as noted above. Induction of aneuploidy by HPV16 sequences[146–148] suggests that viral DNA may play a part in this process.

Hormones

The epidemiological role of oral contraceptives has been discussed above. It has been demonstrated experimentally that the upstream regulatory region of HPV16 contains a glucocorticoid regulatory element (GRE)[149]. This element permits E2 independent early gene transcription. It is therefore possible that steroid hormones may enhance viral transcription *in vivo*, as has been shown for oestrogens in SiHa cells[150]. Progesterone and dexamethasone had no effect in this study. Conversely, progestagens extracted from oral contraceptive tablets were found to cooperate with H-ras-1 and HPV16 in the transformation of primary BRK cells[151] while oestrogens had no effect. Cell lines produced in this way were capable of producing tumours in syngeneic animals. There is therefore experimental evidence to support a link between the oral contraceptive and HPV in the genesis of cervical neoplasia.

Carcinogens

There is much evidence to support involvement of methylcholanthrene in cervical carcinogenesis in mice but the role of carcinogens in human disease is less well documented.

Immunosuppression

Systemic immunosuppression is associated with an increased risk of disseminated viral infection and viral warts are more common in renal transplant patients than in normals. There are many immunocytochemical studies of immune effector cells in cervical epithelium in normal cases, CIN and invasive cancer[152]. It has been noted that the number of Langerhans cells in the cervical epithelium is reduced in smokers[143] and in association with both wart virus infection and CIN[153,154]. This may lead to reduced antigen presentation and hence defective viral clearing. Similarly, T cell numbers are reduced in patients with WVI and CIN, suggesting a local defect in cell mediated immunity. The aetiological role played by these alterations, and whether they are primary or secondary, remains to be determined.

Interaction between HPV and other infectious agents

There is little evidence for interaction between HPV and other agents except *Herpes simplex* virus. Transformation of HSV-immortalized but not primary Syrian hamster embryo cells can be achieved by HPV16 or 18 DNA sequences. HPV16 but not HPV18 sequences could be demonstrated in these cells, consistent with a 'hit-and-run' mechanism for HPV18[155]. Analysis of CIN 3 and ISCC has demonstrated HPV16 in six of eight HSV-containing lesions[131] although none of these lesions contained E6 protein by immunohistochemistry. However, it is known that HSV can induce chromosome alterations and there is evidence of concomitant infection of cervical cells by both HPV and HSV2. Nevertheless, prospective clinical studies are required to investigate the potential role of HSV2 infection in synergy with HPV, particularly given the strength of association between HPV and cervical cancer[156].

There is an increased incidence of HPV infection with associated epithelial abnormalities in HIV-positive patients who are not immunocompetent. It is also known that the HIV Tat1 protein is capable of transactivating HPV16 transcription. There are therefore two possible mechanisms by which HIV infection may act in concert with HPV, namely by altering HPV gene transcription and by inducing immunosuppression[59].

Cellular interfering factor

The study of HeLa cells/fibroblast hybrids has led to the hypothesis that cellular genes which suppress the function of viral transformation genes exist in normal human cells[66] and somatic cell hybrid experiments have localized this function to chromosome 11. This has been termed cellular interfering factor (CIF) and has been postulated to act by suppression of E6/E7 expression *in vivo*[66]. Both tumourigenic and non-tumourigenic HeLa cell/fibroblast hybrids express HPV18 E6/E7 mRNA to a high level *in vitro* but this expression is inhibited *in vivo* only in non-tumourigenic hybrids[157]. This is further evidence for the existence and role of cellular interfering factor.

Model of cervical carcinogenesis

Synthesis of the data presented suggests that HPV infection occurs early in the process of cervical carcinogenesis, followed by the effects of less well defined oncogenes, hormones, chromosomal aberrations and carcinogens,

which are interlinked and may act through viral integration and up-regulation of early gene expression[158,159]. It is of note that recent studies of 'low risk' HPV types have demonstrated that they possess similar properties to 'high risk' types (namely p53 protein binding capacity and cooperative transformation functions) but have much reduced transformation efficiency and protein binding affinity, with a reduced ability to lead to p53 protein degradation[138]. The experimental data regarding these two groups of viruses therefore demonstrate relative but not absolute differences and further exploration of these particular functions is likely to give insight into both regulation of the cell cycle and the mechanism of HPV induced transformation.

Conclusions

Experimental evidence linking HPV to cervical neoplasia is strong. The differential effects of 'high' and 'low' risk viruses can be partially explained and the epidemiological suggestion of interaction between HPV and other factors has some experimental basis. With increasing knowledge, particularly from the study of systems such as the collagen raft culture and the refinement of techniques for HPV detection in clinical material, it is likely that the mechanisms by which HPVs act in the process of carcinogenesis will be defined further.

HPV infection and clinical practice

Several studies have suggested that the presence of certain HPV types is associated with cervical neoplasia. This suggests that diagnosis of a particular HPV infection would dictate a particular clinical outcome and hence be useful in patient management. In particular, HPV18 infection has been associated with rapid clinical progression[160]. Demonstration of a carrier state for 'high risk' viruses might identify a high risk group of patients with normal cervical smears. The development of reliable and reproducible molecular techniques, particularly generic PCR and hybrid capture, has led to more consistent epidemiological data being generated from clinical studies. This has prompted a significant reassessment of the potential role of HPV testing in cervical screening, both in the context of existing cervical screening programmes and in countries where no screening programme currently exists. In the UK, a systematic review of the potential use of HPV testing in the UK Cervical Screening Programme, has recently been published[161]. This applies not only to women with cervical cytological abnormalities, particularly if they are low-grade, but also to the potential use of HPV testing in general population screening. A variety of factors need to be considered including the performance characteristics of the test together with the health economics and psychological effects of introduction of viral testing, whether testing is to be introduced in the context of a cervical screening programme or *ab initio*.

References

1 Pisani P, Parkin D M, Bray F, Ferlay J. Estimates of the worldwide mortality from 25 cancers in 1990. *Int J Cancer* 1999; **83**: 870–873

2 Parkin D M, Läärä E, Muir C S. Estimates of the worldwide frequency of sixteen major cancers in 1980. *Int J Cancer* 1988; **41**: 184–197

3 Devesa S S, Young J L Jr, Brinton L A, Fraumeni J F Jr. Recent trends in cervix uteri cancer. *Cancer* 1989; **64**: 2184–2190

4 Munoz N, Bosch F X. Epidemiology of cervical cancer. In: Munoz N, Bosch F X, Jensen O M eds. *Human Papillomaviruses and Cervical Cancer*, IARC (WHO) No. 94. Oxford: Oxford University Press, 1989; 9–39

5 Cook G A, Draper G J. Trend in cervical cancer and carcinoma *in situ* in Great Britain. *Br J Cancer* 1984; **50**: 367–375

6 Armstrong B, Holman D. Increasing mortality from cancer of the cervix in young Australian women. *Med J Aust* 1981; **1**: 460–462

7 Green G H. Rising cervical cancer mortality in young New Zealand women. *NZ Med J* 1979; **89**: 89–91

8 Parkin D M, Nguyen-Dinh X, Day N E. The impact of screening on the incidence of cervical cancer in England and Wales. *Br J Obstet Gynaecol* 1985; **92**: 150–157

9 Rigoni-Stern D. Statistical facts relating to cancer. *G Servire Progr Pathol Terap Ser* 1842; **2**: 507–517

10 Wynder E L, Cornfield J, Schroff P D, Doraiswami K R. A study of environmental factors in carcinoma of the cervix. *Am J Obstet Gynaecol* 1954; **63**: 1016–1052

11 Buckley J D, Doll R, Harris R W C *et al*. Case control study of the husbands of women with dysplasia or carcinoma of the cervix uteri. *Lancet* 1981; **ii**: 1010–1015

12 Gagnon F. Contribution to the study of the etiology and prevention of cancer of the cervix of the uterus. *Am J Obstet Gynaecol* 1950; **60**: 516–522

13 Licciardone J C, Wilkins J R 3rd, Brownson R C, Chang J. Cigarette smoking and alcohol consumption in the aetiology of uterine cervical cancer. *Int J Epidemiol* 1989; **18**: 533–537

14 Graham S, Priore R, Graham H *et al*. Genital cancer in wives of penile cancer patients. *Cancer* 1980; **44**: 1870–1874

15 Martinez I. Relationship of squamous cell carcinoma of the cervix uteri to squamous cell carcinoma of the penis. *Cancer* 1969; **24**: 777–780

16 Smith P G, Kinlen L J, White G C *et al*. Mortality of wives of men dying with cancer of the penis. *Br J Cancer* 1980; **41**: 422–428

17 Kessler I I. Venereal factors in human cervical cancer. Evidence from marital clusters. *Cancer* 1977; **39**: 1912–1919

18 Zunzunegui M V, King M-C, Coria C F, Charlet J. Male influence on cervical cancer risk. *Am J Epidemiol* 1986; **123**: 302–307

19 Slattery M L, Overall J C Jr, Abbott T M *et al*. Sexual activity, contraception, genital infections, and cervical cancer: support for a sexually transmitted disease hypothesis. *Am J Epidemiol* 1989; **130**: 248–258

20 Rice P S, Cason J, Best J M, Banatvala J E. High risk genital papillomavirus infections are spread vertically. *Rev Med Virol* 1999; **9**: 15–21

21 Winkelstein W. Smoking and cervical cancer – current status: a review. *Am J Epidemiol* 1977; **131**: 945–957

22 Brinton L A, Schairer C, Haenszel W *et al*. Cigarette smoking and invasive cervical cancer. *J Am Med Assoc* 1986; **255**: 3265–3269

23 Brock K E, MacLennan R, Brinton L A, Melnick J L, Adam E, Mock P A *et al*. Smoking and infectious agents and risk of *in situ* cervical cancer in Sydney, Australia. *Cancer Res* 1989; **49**: 4925–4928

24 Clarke E A, Morgan R W, Newman A M. Smoking as a risk factor in cancer of the cervix: additional evidence from a case control study. *Am J Epidemiol* 1982; **115**: 59–66

25 Clarke E A, Hatcher J, McKeown-Eyssen G E, Lickrish G M. Cervical dysplasia: association with sexual behaviour, smoking and oral contraceptive use? *Am J Obstet Gynaecol* 1985; **151**: 612–616

26 Harris R W C, Brinton L A, Cowdell R H *et al*. Characteristics of women with dysplasia or carcinoma *in situ* of the cervix uteri. *Br J Cancer* 1980; **42**: 359–369

27 Jones C J, Brinton L A, Hamman R F *et al*. Risk factors for *in situ* cervical cancer: results from a case-control study. *Cancer Res* 1990; **50**: 3657–3662

28 LaVecchia C, Franceschi S, Decarli A *et al*. Sexual factors, venereal diseases, and the risk of invasive cervical cancer. *Cancer* 1986; **58**: 935–941

29 Slattery M L, Robinson L M, Schuman K L *et al*. Cigarette smoking and exposure to passive smoke are risk factors for cervical cancer. *J Am Med Assoc* 1989; **261**: 1593–1598

30 Reeves W C, Caussy D, Brinton L A *et al*. Case control study of human papillomaviruses and cervical cancer in Latin America. *Int J Cancer* 1987; **40**: 450–454

31 Herrero R, Brinton L A, Reeves W C, Brenes M M, Tenorio F, de Britton R C *et al*. Invasive cervical cancer and smoking in Latin America. *J Natl Cancer Inst* 1989; **81**: 205–211

32 Kjellberg L, Hallmans G, Ahren A M *et al*. Smoking, diet, pregnancy and oral contraceptive use as risk factors for cervical intraepithelial neoplasia in relation to human papillomavirus infection. *Br J Cancer* 2000; **82**: 1332–1338

33 Daling J R, Sherman K J, Hislop T G *et al*. Cigarette smoking and the risk of anogenital cancer. *Am J Epidemiol* 1992; **135**: 180–189

34 Simons A M, Mugica van Herckenrode C, Rodriguez J A *et al*. Demonstration of smoking-related DNA damage in cervical epithelium and correlation with human papillomavirus type 16, using exfoliated cervical cells. *Br J Cancer* 1995; **71**: 246–249

35 Irwin K L, Rosero-Bixby L, Oberle M W *et al*. Oral contraceptives and cervical cancer risk in Costa Rica. *J Am Med Assoc* 1988; **259**: 59–64

36 LaVecchia C, Decarli A, Fasoli M *et al*. Oral contraceptives and cancers of the breast and of the female genital tract. Interim results from a case-control study. *Br J Cancer* 1986; **54**: 311–317

37 Thomas D B. Relationship of oral contraceptives to cervical carcinogenesis. *Obstet Gynaecol* 1972; **40**: 508–518

38 Brinton L A, Huggins G R, Lehman H F *et al*. Long-term use of oral contraceptives and risk of cervical cancer. *Int J Cancer* 1986; **38**: 339–334

39 WHO collaborative study of neoplasia and steroid contraceptives. Invasive cervical cancer and combined oral contraceptives. *BMJ* 1985; **290**: 961–965

40 Hildesheim A, Reeves W C, Brinton L A, Lavery C, Brenes M, De La Guardia M E *et al*. Association of oral contraceptive use and human papillomaviruses in invasive cervical cancers. *Int J Cancer* 1990; **45**: 860–864

41 Brinton L A. Oral contraceptives and cervical neoplasia. *Contraception* 1991; **43**: 581–595

42 Peters R K, Thomas D, Hagan D G *et al*. Risk factors for invasive cervical cancer in latinas and non-latinas in Los Angeles county. *J Natl Cancer Inst* 1986; **77**: 1063–1077

43 Thomas D B. WHO collaborative study of neoplasia and steroid contraceptives. The influence of combined oral contraceptives on risk of neoplasms in developing and developed countries. *Contraception* 1991; **43**: 695–710

44 Beral V, Hannaford P, Kay-C. Oral contraceptive use and malignancies of the genital tract. Results from the Royal College of General Practitioners' Oral Contraception Study. *Lancet* 1988; **ii**: 1331–1335

45 Vessey M P, Villard-Mackintosh L, McPherson K, Yeates D. Mortality among oral contraceptive users: 20 year follow up of women in a cohort study. *BMJ* 1989; **299**: 1487–1491

46 Delgado R M, Sillero A M, Martin M J, Galvez V R. Oral contraceptives and cancer of the cervix uteri. A meta-analysis. *Acta Obstet Gynecol Scand* 1992; **71**: 368–376

47 Wright N H, Vessey M P, Kenward B *et al*. Neoplasia and dysplasia of the cervix uteri and contraception: a possible protective effect of the diaphragm. *Br J Cancer* 1978; **38**: 273–279

48 Block G B, Patterson B, Subar A. Fruit, vegetables, and cancer prevention: a review of the epidemiological evidence. *Nutr Cancer* 1992; **18**: 1–29

49 Wassertheiler-Smoller S, Romney S L, Wylie-Rosett J et al. Dietary vitamin C and uterine cervical dysplasia. *Am J Epidemiol* 1981; **114**: 714–724

50 Romney S L, Palan P R, Dattagupta C et al. Retinoids and the prevention of cervical dysplasias. *Am J Obstet Gynaecol* 1981; **141**: 890 894

51 Cuzick J, Sasieni P, Singer A. Risk factors for invasive cervix cancer in young women. *Eur J Cancer* 1996; 32A: 836–841

52 Porreco R, Penn I, Droegemueller W et al. Gynaecologic malignancies in immunosuppressed organ homograft recipients. *Obstet Gynaecol* 1975; **45**: 359–364

53 Schneider A, Kay S, Lee H M. Immunosuppression as a high risk factor in the development of condyloma acuminatum and squamous neoplasia of the cervix. *Acta Cytol* 1983; **27**: 220–224

54 Schneider A, Oltersdorf T, Schneider V, Gissmann L. Distribution pattern of human papilloma virus 16 genome in cervical neoplasia by molecular *in situ* hybridisation of tissue sections. *Int J Cancer* 1987; **39**: 717–721

55 Mandelblatt J S, Fahs M, Garibaldi K et al. Association between HIV infection and cervical neoplasia: implications for clinical care of women at risk for both conditions. *Aids* 1992; **6**: 173–178

56 Wank R, Tomssen C. High risk of squamous cell carcinoma of the cervix for women with HLA-DQw3. *Nature (London)* **352**: 723–725

57 Mehal W Z, Lo Y M-D, Herrington C S et al. Human papillomavirus infection plays an important role in determining the HLA associated risk of cervical carcinogenesis. *J Clin Pathol* 1994; **47**: 1077–1081

58 Krul E J T, Schipper R F, Schrueder G M T et al. HLA and susceptibility to cervical neoplasia. *Hum Immunol* 1999; **60**: 337–342

59 Southern S A, Herrington C S. Molecular events in uterine cervical cancer. *Sexually Transmitted Infections* 1998; **74**: 101–109

60 Graham S, Rawls W, Swanson M, McCurtis J. Sex partners and herpes simplex virus type 2 in the epidemiology of cancer of the cervix. *Am J Epidemiol* 1982; **115**: 729–735

61 Krcmar M, Suchankova A, Kanka J, Vonka V. Prospective study on the relationship between cervical neoplasia and herpes simplex type 2 virus. III. Presence of herpes simplex type 2 antibody in sera of subjects who developed cervical neoplasia later in the study. *Int J Cancer* 1986; **38**: 161–165

62 Rawls W E, Lavery C, Marrett L D et al. Comparison of risk factors for cervical cancer in different populations. *Int J Cancer* 1986; **37**: 537–546

63 Vonka V, Kanka J, Hirsch I et al. Prospective study on the relationship between cervical neoplasia and Herpes simplex type 2 virus. II. Herpes simplex type 2 antibody presence in sera taken at enrolment. *Int J Cancer* 1984; **33**: 61–66

64 Galloway D A, McDougall J K. The oncogenic potential of herpes simplex viruses: evidence for a 'hit-and-run' mechanism. *Nature* 1983; **302**: 21–24

65 Zur Hausen H. Human genital cancer: synergism between two virus infections or synergism between a virus infection and initiating events? *Lancet* 1982; **ii**: 1370–1372

66 Zur Hausen H. Intracellular surveillance of persisting viral infections: human genital cancer results from deficient cellular control of papillomavirus gene expression. *Lancet* 1986; **ii**. 489 491

67 Munoz N, de Thé G, Aristizabal N et al. Antibodies to herpes viruses in patients with cervical cancer and controls. In: De Thé G, Epstein M A, Zur Hausen H eds. *Oncogenesis and Herpesviruses II (IARC Scientific Publications No. 11)*. Lyon: International Agency for Research on Cancer 1975; 45–51

68 Guijon F B, Paraskevas M, Brunham R. The association of sexually transmitted diseases with cervical intraepithelial neoplasia: a case-control study. *Am J Obstet Gynaecol* 1985; **151**: 185–190

69 Claas E C, Melchers W J, Niesters H G et al. Infections of the cervix uteri with human papillomavirus and Chlamydia trachomatis. *J Med Virol* 1992; **37**: 54–57

70 Palefsky J. Human papillomavirus infection among HIV-infected individuals. Implications for development of malignant tumors. *Hematol Oncol Clin North Am* 1991; **5**: 357–370

71 Celentano D D, Klassen A C, Weisman C S, Rosenshein N B. Duration of relative protection of screening for cervical cancer. *Prev Med* 1989; **18**: 411–422

72 Klassen A C, Celentano D D, Brookmeyer R. Variation in the duration of protection given by screening using the Pap test for cervical cancer. *J Clin Epidemiol* 1989; **42**: 1003–1011

73 van der Graaf Y, Zielhuis G A, Peer P G, Vooijs P G. The effectiveness of cervical screening: a population-based case-control study. *J Clin Epidemiol* 1988; **41**: 21–26

74 Tomita Y, Shirasawa H, Sekine H, Simizu B. Expression of the human papillomavirus type 6b L2 open reading frame in Escherichia coli: L2 beta-galactosidase fusion proteins and their antigenic properties. *Virology* 1987; **158**: 8–14

75 Brown D R, McClowry T L, Woods K, Fife K H. Nucleotide sequence and characterization of human papillomavirus type 83, a novel genital papillomavirus. *Virology* 1999; **260**: 165–172

76 Syrjänen K, Syrjänen S. *Papillomavirus Infections in Human Pathology*. London: Wiley, 2000; pp 11–51

77 Thierry F. Proteins involved in the control of HPV transcription. *Papillomavirus Rep* 1993; **4**: 27–32

78 Münger K, Phelps W C. The human papillomavirus E7 protein as a transforming and transactivating factor. *Biochem Biophys Acta* 1993; **1155**: 111–123

79 Banks L, Matlashewski G. Cell transformation and the HPV E5 gene. *Papillomavirus Rep* 1993; **4**: 1–4

80 Chang F. Role of papillomaviruses. *J Clin Pathol* 1990; **43**: 269–276

81 Parker M F, Arroyo G F, Geradts J et al. Molecular characterisation of

adenocarcinoma of the cervix. *Gynecol Oncol* 1997; **64**: 242–251

82 Herrington C S, McGee J O'D. *Diagnostic Molecular Pathology*, vols 1 and 2. Oxford: Oxford University Press, 1992

83 Saiki R K, Gelfand D H, Stoffel S et al. Primer directed enzymatic amplification of DNA with a thermostable DNA polymerase. *Science* 1988; **239**: 487–491

84 Peyton C L, Schiffman M, Lorincz A T et al. Comparison of PCR- and hybrid capture-based human papillomavirus detection systems using multiple cervical specimen collection strategies. *J Clin Microbiol* 1998; **36**: 3248–3254

85 Herrington C S, McGee J O'D. Principles and basic methodology of DNA/RNA detection by *in situ* hybridization. In: Herrington C S, McGee J O'D eds. *Diagnostic Molecular Pathology*, vol. 1. Oxford: Oxford University Press, 1992; 69–102

86 Herrington C S, McGee J O'D. *In situ* hybridization in diagnostic cytopathology. In: Herrington C S, McGee J O'D eds. *Diagnostic Molecular Pathology*, vol. 1, Oxford: Oxford University Press, 1992; pp 205–220

87 Syrjänen S. Viral gene detection by *in situ* hybridization. In: Herrington C S, McGee J O'D eds. *Diagnostic Molecular Pathology*, vol. 1. Oxford: Oxford University Press, 1992; 103–139

88 Jacobs M V, Snijders P J F, van den Brule A J C et al. A general primer GP5+/GP6+ mediated PCR enzyme immunoassay method for rapid detection of 14 high-risk and 6 low-risk human papillomavirus genotypes in cervical scrapings. *J Clin Microbiol* 1997 **35**: 791–795

89 Tase T, Okagaki T, Clark B A et al. Human papillomavirus types and localisation in adenocarcinoma and adenosquamous carcinoma of the uterine cervix: a study by *in situ* DNA hybridisation. *Cancer Res* 1988; **48**: 993–998

90 Dürst M, Gissmann L, Ikenberg H, Zur Hausen H. A papillomavirus DNA from a cervical carcinoma and its prevalence in cancer biopsy samples from different geographic regions. *Proc Natl Acad Sci USA* 1983; **80**: 3812–3815

91 Ikenberg H, Gissman L, Gross G et al. Human papillomavirus type 16–related DNA in genital Bowen's disease and in bowenoid papulosis. *Int J Cancer* 1983; **32**: 563–565

92 Syrjänen K, Syrjänen S. *Papillomavirus Infections in Human Pathology*. London: Wiley, 2000

93 Lorincz A T, Reid R, Jensen A B et al. Human papillomavirus infection of the cervix: relative risk associations of 15 common anogenital types. *Obstet Gynaecol* 1992; **79**: 328–337

94 Syrjänen K, De Villiers E-M, Saarikoski S et al. Cervical papillomavirus infection progressing to invasive cancer in less than three years. *Lancet* 1985; **i**: 510–511

95 Mitchell H, Drake M, Medley G. Prospective evaluation of risk of cervical cancer after cytological evidence of human

papillomavirus infection. *Lancet* 1986;
i: 573–575

96 Syrjänen K, Mäntyärvi R, Saarikoski S *et al.*
Factors associated with progression of
cervical human papillomavirus (HPV)
infections into carcinoma *in situ* during
long-term prospective follow-up. *Br J Obstet
Gynaecol* 1988; **95**: 1096–1102

97 Koutsky L A, Holmes K K, Critchlow C W
et al. A cohort study of the risk of cervical
intraepithelial neoplasia grade 2 or 3 in
relation to papillomavirus infection. *N Engl
J Med* 1992; **327**: 1272–1278

98 Tidy J A, Parry G C N, Ward P *et al.* High
rate of human papillomavirus type 16
infection in cytologically normal cervices.
Lancet 1989; i: 434

99 Ferenczy A, Bergeron C, Richart R M.
Human papillomavirus DNA in CO2
laser-generated plume of smoke and its
consequences to the surgeon. *Obstet
Gynaecol* 1990; **75**: 114–118

100 Ferenczy A, Bergeron C, Richart R M.
Human papillomavirus DNA in fomites
on objects used for the management of
patients with genital human
papillomavirus infections. *Obstet Gynaecol*
1989; **74**: 950–954

101 Shibata D. The polymerase chain reaction
and the molecular genetic analysis of tissue
biopsies. In: Herrington C S, McGee J O'D
eds. *Diagnostic Molecular Pathology: A
Practical Approach*. Oxford: Oxford
University Press, 1992; 85–112

102 van den Brule A J C, Snijders P J F,
Meijer C J L M, Walboomers J M M.
PCR-based detection of genital HPV
genotypes: an update and future
perspectives. *Papillomavirus Rep* 1993;
4: 95–99

103 Schiffman M H. Recent progress in defining
the epidemiology of human papillomavirus
infection and cervical neoplasia. *J Natl
Cancer Inst* 1992; **84**: 394–398

104 Bauer H M, Greer C E, Manos M M.
Determination of genital human
papillomavirus infection by consensus
polymerase chain reaction amplification.
In: Herrington C S, McGee J O'D eds.
Diagnostic Molecular Pathology, vol. 2.
Oxford: Oxford University Press, 1992;
131–151

105 Walboomers J M M, Melkert P W J, van den
Brule A J *et al.* The polymerase chain
reaction for human papillomavirus
screening in diagnostic cytopathology of
the cervix. In: Herrington C S, McGee J O'D
eds. *Diagnostic Molecular Pathology*, vol. 2.
Oxford: Oxford University Press, 1992;
153–171

106 Meijer C J L M, van den Brule A J, Snijders
P J *et al.* Detection of human papillomavirus
in cervical scrapes by the polymerase chain
reaction in relation to cytology: possible
implications for cervical cancer screening.
IARC Sci Publ 1992; **119**: 271–281

107 Remmink A J, Walboomers J M M,
Helmerhorst T J M *et al.* The presence of
persistent high-risk HPV genotypes in
dysplastic cervical lesions is associated
with progressive disease – natural history
up to 36 months. *Int J Cancer* 1995
61: 306–311

108 Walboomers J M, Jacobs M V, Manos M M
et al. Human papillomavirus is a necessary
cause of invasive cervical cancer worldwide.
J Pathol 1999; **189**: 12–19

109 Schiffman M H, Bauer H M, Hoover R N
et al. Epidemiologic evidence showing that
human papillomavirus infection causes
most cervical intraepithelial neoplasia.
J Natl Cancer Inst 1993; **85**: 958–964

110 Stoler M H, Broker T R. *In situ* hybridisation
detection of human papillomavirus DNAs
and messenger RNAs in genital
condylomas and a cervical carcinoma. *Hum
Pathol* 1986; **17**: 1250–1258

111 Gupta J W, Saito K, Saito A *et al.* Human
papillomaviruses and the pathogenesis
of cervical neoplasia. *Cancer* 1989;
64: 2104–2110

112 Schwarz E, Freese U K, Gissmann L *et al.*
Structure and transcription of human
papillomavirus sequences in cervical
carcinoma cells. *Nature* 1985; **314**: 111–114

113 Shirasawa H, Tomita Y, Kubota K *et al.*
Transcriptional differences of the human
papillomavirus type 16 genome between
precancerous lesions and invasive
carcinomas. *J Virol* 1988; **62**: 1022–1027

114 Baker C C, Phelps W C, Lindgren V *et al.*
Structural and transcriptional analysis of
human papillomavirus type 16 sequences
in cervical carcinoma cell lines. *J Virol* 1987;
61: 962–971

115 Pater M M, Pater A. Expression of human
papillomavirus types 16 and 18 DNA
sequences in cervical carcinoma cell lines.
J Med Virol 1988; **26**: 185–195

116 Crook T, Morgenstein J, Crawford L,
Banks L. Continued expression of HPV16
E7 protein is required for maintenance of
the transformed phenotype of cells
transformed by HPV16 plus EJ-ras. *EMBO J*
1989; **8**: 513–519

117 Mincheva A, Gissmann L, Zur Hausen H.
Chromosomal integration sites of human
papillomavirus DNA in three cervical
cancer cell lines mapped by *in situ*
hybridisation. *Med Microbiol Immunol* 1987;
176: 245–256

118 Yee C, Krishnan-Hewlett I, Baker C C *et al.*
Presence and expression of human
papillomavirus sequences in human
cervical carcinoma cell lines. *Am J Pathol*
1985; **119**: 361–366

119 Popescu N C, Amsbaugh S C, DiPaolo J A.
HPV type 18 DNA is integrated at a single
chromosome site in cervical carcinoma cell
line SW756. *J Virol* 1987; **51**: 1682–1685

120 Dürst M, Kleinheinz A, Holtz M,
Gissmann L. The physical state of human
papillomavirus type 16 DNA in benign and
malignant genital tumours. *J Gen Virol*
1985; **66**: 1515–1522

121 Wagatsuma M, Hashimoto K, Matsukura T.
Analysis of integrated human
papillomavirus type 16 DNA in cervical
cancers: amplification of viral sequences
together with cellular flanking sequences.
J Virol 1990; **64**: 813–821

122 Ambros P F, Karlic H I. Chromosomal
insertion of human papillomavirus 18
sequences in HeLa cells detected by
nonisotopic *in situ* hybridisation and

reflection contrast microscopy. *Hum Genet*
1987; **77**: 251–254

123 Popescu N C, DiPaolo J A, Amsbaugh S C.
Integration sites of HPV18 DNA sequences
on HeLa cell chromosomes. *Cytogenet Cell
Genet* 1987; **44**: 58–62

124 Popescu N C, DiPaolo J A. Integration of
human papillomavirus 16 DNA and
genomic rearrangements in immortalised
human keratinocyte lines. *Cancer Res* 1990;
50: 1316–1323

125 Popescu N C, DiPaolo J A. Preferential
sites for viral integration on mammalian
genome. *Cancer Genet Cytogenet* 1989;
42: 157–171

126 McCance D J, Kopan R, Fuchs E,
Laimins L A. Human papillomavirus type
16 alters human epithelial cell
differentiation in vitro. *Proc Natl Acad Sci
USA* 1988; **85**: 7168–7173

127 Rader J S, Golub T R, Hudson J B *et al.* In
vitro differentiation of epithelial cells from
cervical neoplasias resembles in vivo
lesions. *Oncogene* 1990; **5**: 571–576

128 Song S, Liem A, Miller J A, Lambert P F.
Human papillomavirus type 16 E6 and E7
contribute differently to carcinogenesis.
Virology 2000; **267**: 141–150

129 Gariglio P, Ocadiz R, Sauceda R. Human
papillomavirus DNA sequences and c-myc
oncogene alteration in uterine cervix
carcinoma. *Cancer Cells* 1987; **5**: 343–348

130 Di Luca D, Rotola A, Pilotti S *et al.*
Simultaneous presence of herpes simplex
and human papillomavirus sequences in
human genital tumours. *Int J Cancer* 1987;
40: 763–768

131 Di Luca D, Costa S, Rotola A *et al.* Search
for human papillomavirus, herpes simplex
and c-myc oncogene in human genital
tumours. *Int J Cancer* 1989; **43**: 570–577

132 Riou G, Barrois M, Tordjman I *et al.*
Presence de genomes de papillomavirus et
amplification des oncogenes c-myc et
c-Ha-ras dna des cancers envahissants du
col de l'uterus. *C R Acad Sci III* 1984;
299: 575–580

133 Riou G, Barrois M, Le M *et al.* C-myc
protooncogene expression and prognosis in
early carcinoma of the cervix. *Lancet* 1987;
i: 761–763

134 Riou G, Barrois M, Sheng Z-M *et al.*
Somatic deletions and mutations of
c-Ha-ras gene in human cervical cancers.
Oncogene 1988; **3**: 329–333

135 Dyson N, Howley P, Munger K, Harlow E.
The human papillomavirus-16 E7
oncoprotein is able to bind to the
retinoblastoma gene product. *Science* 1989;
243: 934–937

136 Werness B A, Levine A J, Howley P M.
Association of human papillomavirus types
16 and 18 E6 proteins with p53. *Science*
1990; **248**: 76–79

137 Crook T, Wrede D, Vousden K H. p53 point
mutation in HPV negative human cervical
carcinoma cell lines. *Oncogene* 1991; **6**:
873–875

138 Crook T, Tidy J A, Vousden K H.
Degradation of p53 can be targeted by HPV
E6 sequences distinct from those required

for p53 binding and transactivation. *Cell* 1991; **67**: 547–556

139 Borresen A L, Helland A, Holm R *et al.* Papillomaviruses, p53 and cervical cancer. *Lancet* 1992; **339**: 1350–1351

140 Crook T, Wrede D, Tidy J A *et al.* Clonal p53 mutation in primary cervical cancer: association with human papillomavirus negative tumours. *Lancet* 1992; **339**: 1070–1073

141 Helland A, Holm R, Kristensen G *et al.* Genetic alteration of the TP53 gene, p53 protein expression and HPV infection in primary cervical carcinomas. *J Pathol* 1993; **171**: 105–114

142 Southern S A, Herrington C S. Disruption of cell cycle control by human papillomaviruses with special reference to cervical carcinoma. *Int J Gynaecol Cancer* 2000; **10**: 263–274

143 Barton S E, Hollingworth A, Maddox P H *et al.* Possible cofactors in the etiology of cervical intraepithelial neoplasia. An immunopathologic study. *J Reprod Med* 1989; **34**: 613–616

144 Matlashewski G, Osborn K, Banks L *et al.* Transformation of primary human fibroblast cells with human papillomavirus type 16 DNA and EJ-ras. *Int J Cancer* 1988; **42**: 232–238

145 Teyssier J R. The chromosomal analysis of human solid tumours: a triple challenge. *Cancer Genet Cytogenet* 1989; **37**: 103–125

146 Dürst M, Ozarlieva-Petrusevska R T, Boukamp P *et al.* Molecular and cytogenetic analysis of immortalised primary keratinocytes obtained after transfection with human papillomavirus type 16 DNA. *Oncogene* 1987; **1**: 251–256

147 Pirisi L, Creek K E, Doniger J *et al.* Continuous cell lines with altered growth and differentiation properties originate after transfection of human keratinocytes with human papillomavirus. *Carcinogenesis* 1988; **9**: 1573–1579

148 Pirisi L, Yasumoto S, Feller M *et al.* Transformation of human fibroblasts and keratinocytes with human papillomavirus type 16 DNA. *J Virol* 1987; **61**: 1061–1066

149 Gloss B, Bernard H U, Seedorf K, Klock G. The upstream regulatory region of the human papilloma virus-16 contains an E2 protein-independent enhancer which is specific for cervical carcinoma cells and regulated by glucocorticoid hormones. *EMBO J* 1987; **6**: 3735–3743

150 Mitrani-Rosenbaum S, Tsvieli R, Tur-Kaspa R. Oestrogen stimulates differential transcription of human papillomavirus type 16 in SiHa cervical carcinoma cells. *J Gen Virol* 1989; **70**: 2227–2232

151 Pater A, Bayatpour M, Pater M M. Oncogenic transformation by human papillomavirus type 16 deoxyribonucleic acid in the presence of progesterone or progestins from oral contraceptives. *Am J Obstet Gynaecol* 1990; **162**: 1099–1103

152 Syrjänen K, Syrjänen S. *Papillomavirus Infections in Human Pathology*. London: Wiley; 2000; pp 459–490

153 Morris H H B, Gatter K C, Stein H, Mason D Y. Langerhans cells in human cervical epithelium: an immunohistological study. *Br J Obstet Gynaecol* 1983; **90**: 400–411

154 Morris H H B, Gatter K C, Sykes G *et al.* Langerhans cells in human cervical epithelium: effects of wart virus infection and intraepithelial neoplasia. *Br J Obstet Gynaecol* 1983; **90**: 412–420

155 Iwasaka T, Yokoyama M, Hayashi Y, Sugimori H. Combined herpes simplex virus type 2 and human papillomavirus type 16 or 18 deoxyribonucleic acid leads to oncogenic transformation. *Am J Obstet Gynaecol* 1988; **159**: 1251–1255

156 DiPaolo J A, Jones C. The role of herpes simplex 2 and the development of HPV positive cervical carcinoma. *Papillomavirus Report* 1999; **10**: 1–7

157 Bosch F X, Schwarz E, Boukamp P *et al.* Suppression in vivo of human papillomavirus type 18 E6–E7 gene expression in nontumorigenic HeLa x fibroblast hybrid cells. *J Virol* 1990; **64**: 4743–4754

158 Matlashewski G. The cell biology of human papillomavirus transformed cells. *AntiCancer Res* 1989; **9**: 1447–1556

159 Zur Hausen H. Papillomaviruses in anogenital cancer as a model to understand the role of viruses in human cancers. *Cancer Res* 1989; **49**: 4677–4681

160 Barnes W, Delgado G, Kurman R J *et al.* Possible prognostic significance of human papillomavirus type in cervical cancer. *Gynaecol Oncol* 1988; **29**: 267–273

161 Cusick J, Sasieni P, Davies P *et al.* A systematic review of the role of human papillomavirus testing within a cervical screening programme. *Health Technology Assessment* 1999; **3**: 14

162 Cancer Research Campaign. *UK Cancer Statistics*, 2000

163 Chan S-Y, Delius H, Halpern A L, Bernard H-U. Analysis of genomic sequences of 95 papillomavirus types: uniting typing, phylogeny and taxonomy. *J Virol* 1995; **69**: 3074–3083

30 Cervical intraepithelial neoplasia and squamous cell carcinoma of the cervix

Peter A. Smith and Winifred Gray*

Introduction

It is estimated that in 1990, there were 190 000 deaths from carcinoma of the cervix world-wide. Overall, it is the sixth most common visceral cancer causing death in women, but in the developing world it is the commonest. About 78% of the mortality from this disease occurs in developing countries[1]. The epidemiology of cervical cancer shows wide geographical variation in its occurrence, as well as within local populations (Table 30.1)[2]. These differences are related to social and economic conditions, as well as religion and the influence of these factors on sexual practices.

The principal predisposing factors to the development of cervical cancer are sexual intercourse and commencement of it at an early age. The next most important epidemiological factor to early age of onset of sexual activity is the number of sexual partners, which is illustrated by the high risk of the disease in prostitutes in all parts of the world[3]. Prostitutes appear to be a reservoir of the sexually transmitted agent, now known to be certain types of human papillomavirus, which is involved in the pathogenesis of the disease. Populations, such as that of Cali, Colombia, where women traditionally are carefully shielded from sexual relations before marriage, but men customarily consort with prostitutes, have a high incidence of cervical cancer[4]. Other risk factors include cigarette smoking, the use of the oral contraceptive pill and immunosuppression. The pathogenesis of cervical cancer is discussed in detail in Chapter 29.

Squamous cell carcinoma is the commonest histological type of cervical cancer. Traditionally, adenocarcinoma of the cervix has been said to account for about 10–15% of the total of invasive carcinomas, but this figure increases if staining for mucin is routinely applied to histopathological material. It has been suggested that pure squamous cell carcinomas only account for about 70% of the total and the balance is accounted for by mixed adenosquamous or poorly-differentiated adenocarcinomas[5]. Both relative and absolute increases in incidence of adenocarcinoma of the cervix have been reported, possibly partly as a consequence of prevention of squamous cell carcinoma by screening programmes, but the changes vary considerably between different countries[6]. Adenocarcinoma of the cervix is discussed further in Chapter 32.

Clinical features of invasive squamous cell carcinoma of the cervix

Clinical invasive carcinoma usually presents with symptoms of abnormal vaginal bleeding, particularly postcoital bleeding, and vaginal discharge. After the menopause, post-menopausal bleeding may be the main presenting symptom. Advanced disease is associated with general symptoms and signs of weight loss, debility and pain. Inspection of the cervix may reveal an exophytic growth, or the cervix may be infiltrated by an endophytic or diffuse growth, in which case the condition may not be obvious to naked eye examination, until necrosis causes ulceration. Some tumours remain in the endocervical canal and are not seen. Colposcopic examination of early invasive carcinoma shows characteristic features even when the cervix has no exophytic growth[7].

Tumour spread

Squamous cell carcinoma of the cervix spreads principally by local extension to the vagina, parametrium and adjacent structures, including the ureters, bladder and rectum, but also to the pelvic lymph nodes. Involvement of lymphatics or blood vessels carries a poor prognosis. Distant

Table 30.1 Geographical variation in age standardized incidence rates for cancer of the cervix per 100 000 population

Colombia, Cali	34.4
Brazil, Belem	64.8
India, Bombay	20.2
India, Madras	38.9
Japan, Osaka	9.2
Israel, all Jews	5.3
Finland	3.6
Australia, NSW	9.2
USA, Atlanta: black	12.0
white	7.0
UK, West Midlands	13.2
UK, South Thames	9.2

Figures from the IARC, Cancer Incidence in Five Continents, vol. VII, 1997[2]

*The authors gratefully acknowledge their debt to Dr Elizabeth A Hudson, whose contribution to the previous edition of this chapter provided a substantial basis for this revised edition.

Table 30.2 The FIGO staging classification for cervical cancer (1994)

Stage	Description
0	Preinvasive carcinoma (CIN, carcinoma *in situ*)
I	Carcinoma confined to the cervix (extension to the corpus should be disregarded)
Ia	Invasive cancer identified only microscopically. All gross lesions, even with superficial invasion, are Stage Ib cancers. Measured stromal depth should not be greater than 5 mm and no wider than 7 mm*
Ia1	Measured invasion no greater than 3 mm in depth and no wider than 7 mm
Ia2	Measured depth of invasion greater than 3 mm and no greater than 5 mm, and no wider than 7 mm
Ib	Clinical lesions confined to the cervix or preclinical lesions greater than Ia
Ib1	Clinical lesions no greater than 4 cm in size
Ib2	Clinical lesions greater than 4 cm in size
II	Carcinoma extending beyond the cervix and involving the vagina (but not the lower third) and/or infiltrating the parametrium (but not reaching the pelvic side wall)
IIa	Carcinoma has involved the vagina
IIb	Carcinoma has infiltrated the parametrium
III	Carcinoma involving the lower third of the vagina and/or extending to the pelvic side wall
IIIa	Carcinoma involving the lower third of the vagina
IIIb	Carcinoma extending to the pelvic wall and/or hydronephrosis or non-functioning kidney not known to be due to other causes
IVa	Carcinoma involving the mucosa of the bladder or rectum and /or extending beyond the true pelvis
IVb	Spread to distant organs

* The depth of invasion should not be more than 5 mm from the base of the epithelium, either surface or glandular, from which it originates. Vascular space invasion, either venous or lymphatic, should not alter the staging.

metastases are less common although they are frequently found at autopsy in patients who die of the disease. Local spread of the tumour is responsible for most of the serious effects and infiltration or compression of the ureters is present in two thirds of fatal cases. The clinical staging of carcinoma of the cervix of the International Federation of Obstetrics and Gynaecology is summarized in Table 30.2[8].

Diagnosis

Diagnosis and staging are carried out by a sequence of cytology, colposcopy, histology and clinical and imaging findings. Cervical smears taken in the presence of invasive carcinoma will usually show severe dyskaryosis and may show features suggestive of the presence of invasive carcinoma (see below). The smear test is, however, less sensitive for the detection of invasive carcinomas than for preinvasive disease, termed cervical intraepithelial neoplasia (CIN)[9]. Smears taken from invasive tumours of the cervix are frequently dominated by blood cells and purulent exudate with relative exclusion of tumour cells. Moreover, the cells from invasive tumours are sometimes more difficult to interpret than those from CIN. Signs and symptoms that raise suspicion of invasive cancer are therefore an indication for referral to a specialist for

colposcopic examination and histological biopsy, even if the smear test is negative.

Histological classification

Cytological appearances reflect the histological types of invasive squamous cell carcinoma of the cervix defined by the World Health Organization[10] as follows:

> Invasive squamous carcinoma of the cervix
> Keratinizing carcinoma
> Large cell non-keratinizing carcinoma
> Small cell non-keratinizing carcinoma

This classification equates with a grading system of well-, moderately- and poorly-differentiated squamous cell carcinoma. The presence of a mixed histological type of squamous cell carcinoma may not always be evident from the cervical smear because of the limitations of the cytological sample, which is derived from the exposed surface of the tumour.

The relationship between CIN and cervical cancer

Invasive squamous carcinoma of the cervix is preceded by precancerous changes in the cervical epithelium of the transformation zone, which can be identified histologically; the precancerous changes are usually described now as cervical intraepithelial neoplasia (CIN)[11].

Evidence that CIN is a precursor of invasive squamous cell carcinoma is provided by the following:

▶ Studies of patients with CIN who did not receive treatment[12,13]
▶ Temporal relationship between CIN, microinvasive carcinoma and invasive carcinoma[14,15]
▶ CIN is found at the periphery of invasive carcinoma in histological sections
▶ Cells from CIN show morphological and cytogenetic similarity to cells from invasive cancer[16]
▶ Successful screening programmes[17] are based on the detection and eradication of CIN

These preinvasive changes represent a continuous spectrum of morphology, which has been divided arbitrarily into three stages, CIN 1, CIN 2 and CIN 3. These are equivalent in the conventional terminology respectively to mild dysplasia, moderate dysplasia, and severe dysplasia/carcinoma *in situ*.

Estimation of the duration of the preinvasive changes is based on the difference between the mean age of diagnosis of CIN 3 and the mean age of the development of invasive cancer, an interval of 10–15 years[14]. Similarly, the mean age for diagnosis of the grades of CIN is consistent with progression from CIN 1 (mild dysplasia) through CIN 2 (moderate dysplasia) to CIN 3 (severe dysplasia and carcinoma *in situ*) over a further period of around 10 years. One series reported a mean age of detection of 34.2 years for mild or slight dysplasia and 41.4 years for severe dysplasia[15].

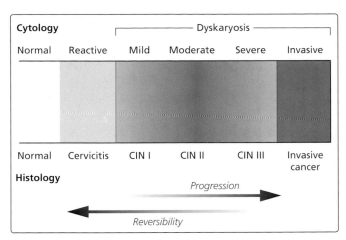

Cytology			Dyskaryosis		
Normal	Reactive	Mild	Moderate	Severe	Invasive

| Normal | Cervicitis | CIN I | CIN II | CIN III | Invasive cancer |

Histology

Progression

Reversibility

Fig. 30.1 The diagram represents the spectrum of changes in the cervical epithelium between normal, through intraepithelial neoplasia to invasive squamous cell carcinoma with arrows depicting potential for progression and reversibility.

Figures vary with the population studied and the time of the study. The incidence of carcinoma *in situ* in British Columbia peaked in the 25–29 age group in 1980[18]. In England and Wales, the modal age of diagnosis of CIN 3 appeared to have fallen to around 29–30 years by 1984[19]. It is uncertain whether this is the result of earlier diagnosis but the possibility of a cohort of women with a higher risk of the disease is important[20,21] because the cohort is likely to retain this potential throughout the lifetime of the women in the age group[22].

The similarity of the cytomorphology of CIN 3 to invasive cancer is supported by cytogenetic studies, which show similar chromosomal constitution of severe dysplasia, carcinoma *in situ* and invasive squamous cell carcinoma of the cervix[16]. There is evidence that up to one-third of cases will progress to invasive carcinoma if untreated, and other cases will persist as CIN 3[12,13] but it is uncertain whether CIN 3 regresses to less severe grades of CIN or to normal epithelium without intervention. A smaller proportion of cases of CIN 1 and CIN 2 progress to CIN 3 or invasive cancer and others persist or appear to regress to normal. The progression and regression of CIN is summarized in Figure 30.1. It has also been established that invasive carcinoma can develop from CIN 1 or CIN 2 without an intermediate stage of CIN 3[23].

Progression and regression of CIN

Follow-up studies confirm that a single punch biopsy increases significantly the proportions of CIN 1 and CIN 2 which regress to normal. Nasiell *et al.* found progression of moderate dysplasia to severe dysplasia or carcinoma *in situ*, persistence of moderate dysplasia and regression to normal of moderate dysplasia in 30%, 16% and 54% of cases respectively when 894 patients were followed up for up to 78 months[24]. Comparison of half of their patients who had biopsies taken with those who did not have biopsies showed progression in 27% and 35%, persistent moderate

dysplasia in 16% and 15% and regression in 57% and 50% (*p*<0.05). Follow-up of 555 with cytology indicating mild dysplasia showed progression to severe dysplasia, carcinoma *in situ* or invasive carcinoma (two patients) in 16%, persistence of dysplasia in 22% and regression to normal in 62% over a period of 39 months[25].

Richart and Barron required three abnormal smears before admission of women to their follow-up study in order to exclude temporary cytological changes due to repair or other benign conditions which could not reliably be distinguished from dysplasia. Biopsies were not taken during the period of the study and regression rates were very low[26].

Nasiell *et al.* noted in their follow-up of moderate dysplasia that cytology of 3.8% of their patients was normal for more than 12 months before moderate dysplasia returned, which emphasizes that patients with abnormal cytology should be followed up with continuously normal cytology for a longer period before regression can be confirmed[24].

If a normal distribution of progression rate is assumed, some cases will develop very rapidly and may outstrip even the most assiduous preventive screening (resulting in a true 'interval cancer'), whereas cases at the other end of the distribution will not progress to invasion within the woman's lifetime. At the onset of screening the excess of cases of CIN 3 should be of the order of 4:1, which would correlate adequately with the known risk of progression of CIN 3 to invasive cancer[12,13]. When data are available from a screened population, very many more cases of CIN 3 are detected than clinical cancers would be expected. Herbert and Smith report a ratio of 10:1[27].

Area of cervical epithelium with CIN

The proportion of the transformation zone affected by CIN, including crypt involvement, appears to be related to the risk of progression. The cervical smear test does not detect all CIN, particularly low-grade CIN, which involves small areas of the transformation zone[28]. The probability of detection by the cervical smear test rises with increase in the grade of CIN and increase in the area of the epithelium affected[29]. In earlier successful screening programmes, such as that in North East Scotland[30], treatment by cone biopsy or hysterectomy was only given to women whose smears indicated severe dysplasia or carcinoma *in situ* (CIN 3), from which it is deduced that many women with very small areas of CIN 3 had smears reported as only mildly abnormal and were followed up by cytology alone, and some may even have had normal smears. Progression of these undergraded abnormalities to involve larger areas of the cervix and increase in the cytological abnormality detected at a subsequent screening would prevent progression to invasive cancer in most cases.

Screening for prevention of cervical cancer
Background

Papanicolaou's observation[31] of abnormal cells exfoliated from the cervix gave rise to the use of the cervical smear test for detection of preinvasive cancer. Suitability of a disease for prevention by a screening programme is determined by high prevalence, a long detectable preclinical phase and benefit from early treatment. The screening test must have a high sensitivity, high specificity and be of low cost and low risk to the patient. Screening programmes should be preceded by a randomized controlled trial and demonstrate a reduction in morbidity and mortality.

Carcinoma of the cervix is a common disease in many unscreened populations, with a long preinvasive stage, which is treatable by surgery or ablation with a probability of success that approaches 100%. The preinvasive stage can be detected by the cervical smear test, which is simple, safe, inexpensive and generally acceptable to women. Screening programmes have now been shown to reduce morbidity and mortality from cancer of the cervix, but they were introduced before any randomized controlled trials had been carried out. The knowledge that women with carcinoma *in situ*, as it was called at the time, risked progression to invasive cancer would have made such a trial unethical. Although it was known that detected and treated cases of carcinoma *in situ* had little risk of developing invasive disease, it was not known if the cervical smear test would be sufficiently sensitive to detect a proportion of precancers, which when treated would significantly reduce mortality and morbidity.

There were serious doubts in the 1950s and 1960s about the wisdom of embarking on population screening programmes. To clarify the situation the Canadian Deputy Ministers of Health convened a task force under the chairmanship of Dr R J Walton to evaluate the effectiveness of screening programmes for preventing cervical cancer throughout the world. The result of this thorough investigation was published in 1976 and is known as the Walton Report[14]. The main conclusions of this report were that squamous cell carcinoma of the cervix does lend itself to control by cervical cytology screening and that the reduction of the disease is directly related to the proportion of the population screened. The Canadian Task Force was reconvened in 1980 to produce a second report[32]. It commented that when a certain proportion of the population at risk had been screened an increase in the frequency of screening yielded a diminishing return, and resources could be more effectively employed by increasing the number of women being screened and by improving the quality and sensitivity of screening programmes.

The favourable conclusions of the 1976 Walton Report reassured many of those who had been sceptical previously about the suitability of the cervical smear test for population screening. The report recognized the importance of the results from British Columbia, where a provincial programme was introduced in 1949. Between 1955 and 1985, the incidence of invasive carcinoma of the cervix had fallen by 78% and mortality by 72%[18].

Comprehensive population coverage of women between 25 and 60 years of age had also been obtained in the Grampian Region of North East Scotland between 1960 and 1980. In this small and then comparatively isolated community, 186 384 women were screened out of 187 000 in this age group. During this period, 584 women presented with cervical cancer, of whom 526 (90%) had no record of a cervical smear test[30]. This group of 526 was composed of women who had refused screening, some who had moved into the area after the population database had been established, and others who were found to have an invasive cancer at the time of screening, or were above the age (60 years) for inclusion in the screening programme in NE Scotland at that time[30]. These results emphasized that the woman who does not have a smear test is at a high risk of developing cervical cancer.

By 1987 Finland, Iceland and Sweden had also achieved reductions of up to 60% in the incidence of invasive cancer of the cervix[33].

Organization of a screening programme

The success of screening depends on a properly organized programme. First, the target population should be defined. The individuals must be identified and receive personal invitation and encouragement to attend for a screening test. The test must be taken reliably by a trained professional and screened and interpreted by properly regulated laboratories. Sufficient resources for investigation, treatment and follow-up of patients with abnormal screening test results must be available and quality control procedures and mechanisms for evaluation of the programme established.

Failure to screen a high enough proportion of women in the population was the main reason for the failure of the screening programme in much of the rest of the UK to emulate the early success in North East Scotland. For many years there were about 4000 registrations of, and 2000 deaths from, cancer of the cervix in England and Wales. It is probable that enough screening was taking place to keep the number of invasive cancers steady, but by 1986 an increase in incidence and mortality at the beginning of the twenty-first century was predicted[22]. In the later 1980s, a computerized national screening programme was introduced, using lists of women registered with general practitioners as the database. Over the next few years vastly increased population coverage was obtained and this now exceeds 80% of women in nearly all health districts in the UK. Deaths from cancer of the cervix in England and Wales fell from 2004 in 1986 to 1158 in 1998 and in the later 1990s were falling at a rate of about 7% per year (UK Department of Health figures). It has been estimated, based on relative risk between women screened and not screened, that there were about 1300 fewer deaths in 1997, and 8250 fewer deaths between 1988 and 1997 as a result of screening[34]. Others have suggested that this method may have significantly underestimated the effect of screening[27,35].

A screening interval of 5 years was successful in North East Scotland[30] and Finland[33]. It has been estimated that 5-yearly screening should prevent 84% of invasive cancers but that 3-yearly screening will prevent 91%. More frequent screening gains no significant further advantage[36]. It is noteworthy that screening a high proportion of the population every 5 years will prevent more disease than screening a low proportion more frequently.

All women who have ever been sexually active are at risk of developing cervical cancer and should be screened. CIN occurs in teenagers, but at least in the UK invasive carcinoma is very rare in the 20–24 year age group, and almost unknown in the under 20s. It is therefore considered that there is no justification for screening teenagers. Women who have been screened regularly with normal results up to the age of 60 have a negligible risk of developing the disease and need not have further tests[32]. Older women who have not been screened should, however, be tested at least twice. Those who avoid screening have an especially high risk of developing cervical cancer and women who have had abnormal cytology which has been treated or resolved spontaneously remain at increased risk and should be followed up with regular smear tests[13].

Technological and scientific advances in cervical screening

Increased sensitivity for the detection of preinvasive disease can be achieved by colposcopic examination[28] or by cervicography[37], but these methods result in more over-treatment of small, mostly mild, abnormalities than cervical cytology. The smear test, if properly carried out, is sufficiently sensitive for screening for prevention of cervical cancer.

A major objective is to automate the demanding, labour-intensive process of primary screening. Automated microscopic scanning of conventionally stained material, automated scanning for cell markers and measurement of chemical constituents have so far failed to replace the original method. The development of automated microscopic scanning has achieved limited success, however, and it appears likely that clear superiority of automated scanning over human screening will soon be achieved. In 1998, the Papnet ®system (Neuromedical Systems Inc., Suffern, NY) received approval from the US Food and Drug Administration (FDA) as a quality control tool. Papnet used automated screening and image analysis to display 128 'tiles' with cells analysed as the least normal on the smear, on a VDU screen. Human observation of the tiles coupled with conventional microscopy completed the examination. The NHS 'Prismatic' trial results[38] suggested that Papnet screening was, statistically, similar to human screening for all degrees of abnormality. A prospective trial in Liverpool found that, statistically, Papnet was as good as human screening for moderate and severe dyskaryosis but less sensitive for mild dyskaryosis and borderline changes (LS Turnbull and PA Smith 1999, unpublished data).

Further evaluation and consideration of its suitability as a primary screening tool within the UK cervical screening programme was brought to an abrupt halt by the liquidation of the parent company in 1999. Use of Papnet as a quality control tool only was not cost effective in the UK programme.

Also in 1998 the Autopap® system (NeoPath Inc., now TriPath Imaging Inc., Burlington, NC) received FDA approval to be used as a primary screening device so that the 25% of slides read as least abnormal could be reported as negative without human examination. A limited saving in human labour can therefore be achieved with this device, but its use has not been demonstrated to be cost effective in the setting of the UK cervical screening programme.

Alternative cell preparation systems to the conventional smear offer important advantages. The use of liquid based, thin layer preparations potentially offers better specimen sampling and quality, reduction in inadequate and borderline nuclear change reporting rates, an increase in sensitivity and specificity, and increased productivity of screening staff. Thin layer preparations are also more amenable to automated analysis than conventional smears and may become an absolute requirement for use with automated systems in the future. The potential disadvantages are increased capital, consumable materials, transport and disposal costs and the need to retrain staff to examine the new type of preparation.

Two such systems are currently in use in the USA. ThinPrep® (Cytyc Corporation, Boxborough, MA) carries FDA approval for use as an alternative to the conventional cervical smear with improved sensitivity, and the AutoCyte® (TriPath Imaging, Inc.) system carries FDA approval as an alternative with equivalence to conventional methods. The applicability of these systems within the UK cervical screening programme is currently under consideration.

The identification of certain types of human papillomavirus (HPV) as the main aetiological agent of CIN and cervical cancer raises the possibility that HPV detection and typing may have a role in screening. HPV testing has been shown to be more sensitive than cytology for CIN 2 and 3 but less specific. A recent assessment concludes that HPV testing may be of value in situations such as the management of women whose smears show borderline nuclear abnormalities or in older women, but that there is as yet no justification for widespread implementation[39].

Similarly the aetiological role of HPV raises the possibility of the clinical use of vaccines against HPV either for primary prevention, or for treatment of established HPV associated lesions. Further research and clinical trials in both these aspects are in progress.

The cervical smear test

The aim of the smear taker is to obtain a representative sample of cells from the surface of the transformation zone. The material must be spread evenly on the microscope slide and suitably preserved with fixative, so that abnormal cells can be identified by the microscopist. The smear is usually taken using a wooden or plastic spatula. Since the original Ayre spatula, a range of spatulae and brushes has been developed with the aim of improving transformation zone and/or endocervical sampling (see Fig. 28.36). Opinion is divided between those who recommend that a brush sample as well as a spatula sample is essential for every cervical screening test[40,41], and others who take a brush sample only when the external os of the cervix is so small that it will not admit the pointed tip of the spatula, or if an endocervical glandular abnormality is being investigated or followed up. Stenosis of the external os occurs principally with post-menopausal atrophy or after treatment of CIN. Submission of two slides for each sample doubles screening time, with profound resource implications for laboratories, particularly in organized screening programmes. Submission of a combined spatula and brush smear on one slide is a compromise but one or both components of such smears are likely to show air-drying artefact. A further advantage of liquid based cytology is that the material from two sampling techniques may be combined in a single preparation yielding one slide for examination.

Cytological terminology of cervical precancer

Introduction

Developments in the practice of cervical and vaginal cytology have led to changes in the terminology used. The tendency of early practitioners of cytology to work independently of histopathologists and possibly to promote cytological diagnosis as equivalent to histological diagnosis, has influenced the use of terminology in gynaecological cytology.

Papanicolaou's classification

Papanicolaou's classification[31] (Table 30.3) was used for many years and his classes I to V have been adhered to until relatively recently by some cytologists and gynaecologists. In 1953 Reagan *et al.* proposed the term dysplasia to replace atypical metaplasia and atypical hyperplasia[42] and this suggestion was approved by the First International Congress of Exfoliative Cytology[43].

World Health Organization classification

Ritton and Christopherson defined the normal and abnormal cells of cervical and vaginal smears in the World Health Organization (WHO) International Classification[10]. The abnormal cells were described in terms of the histological condition with which they correlated. The conventional histological terminology of mild, moderate and severe dysplasia and carcinoma *in situ* was used as well as atypical metaplasia. The WHO publication was widely distributed and the concise text and clear illustrations have contributed to international agreement on the application of these definitions. Grades of dysplasia, carcinoma *in situ* and invasive carcinoma have been used by a generation of cytologists to describe cervical cytology.

British Society for Clinical Cytology terminology

Dissatisfaction with the Papanicolaou classification, which was retained by some cytologists until relatively recently, led to the introduction of subdivisions, particularly of class III, but variation in the use of the classification between centres, and idiosyncratic applications resulted in deterioration of its reproducibility. There was reluctance also among some cytologists, particularly in the UK, to use histological terms to describe cell preparations.

Dyskaryosis

The British Society for Clinical Cytology's first Working Party on terminology[44] recommended the term dyskaryosis, originally coined by Papanicolaou[31] and translated from the Greek meaning 'abnormal nucleus', to describe cells from preinvasive and invasive cancer. The first Working Party classified dyskaryosis as superficial cell dyskaryosis, intermediate cell dyskaryosis and parabasal cell dyskaryosis, according to the cytoplasmic differentiation of the dyskaryotic cell and its expected histological correlation with mild, moderate and severe dysplasia and carcinoma *in situ*. Dyskaryosis or dyskaryotic proved an acceptable concept for description of abnormal cells in cervical smears but classification according to cytoplasmic differentiation using the same words used to describe normal squamous epithelial cells revealed inconsistencies. For example, parabasal cell dyskaryosis is an appropriate description of the classical or oval dyskaryotic cells with a rim of dense cytoplasm from CIN 3, but it is not a suitable description of many of the variations in appearance of cells from CIN 3 and invasive squamous cell carcinoma.

The British Society for Clinical Cytology's Working Party on terminology published a further review in 1986[45] in which dyskaryosis remained the recommended term but it was classified as mild, moderate and severe. This terminology replaces dysplasia and carcinoma *in situ* in the UK national cervical screening programme. It is used here and described in detail below (Table 30.4).

A terminology conference was held in Manchester in March 2002, at which the BSCC terminology described below was reviewed. Most importantly, the conference recommended that a change be made to a 'two-tier' reporting system of low-grade and high-grade dyskaryosis. The former category would include mild dyskaryosis and

Table 30.3	Papanicolaou's classification of cytology smear reports	
Class I	Negative	Absence of atypical or abnormal cells
Class II	Negative	Atypical cells present but without abnormal features
Class III	Suspicious	Cells with abnormal features suggestive but not conclusive for malignancy
Class IV	Positive	Cells and cell clusters fairly conclusive for malignancy
Class V	Positive	Cells and cell clusters conclusive for malignancy

Table 30.4 Terminology for reporting squamous epithelial cell abnormalities in cervical smears (BSCC, 1986[45])

Cytology	Expected histology
Mild dyskaryosis	CIN 1 (mild dysplasia)
Moderate dyskaryosis	CIN 2 (moderate dysplasia)
Severe dyskaryosis	CIN 3 (severe dysplasia/carcinoma *in situ*)
	Invasive cancer

Table 30.5 The 1991 Bethesda System for reporting cervical/vaginal cytologic diagnoses (abbreviated, after[50])

A	Statement of adequacy of the specimen:
	Satisfactory
	Satisfactory for evaluation but limited by… (specify reason)
	Unsatisfactory (specify reason)
B	General categorization of the diagnosis (optional):
	Within normal limits
	Benign cellular changes: see descriptive diagnosis
	Epithelial cell abnormality: see descriptive diagnosis
C	Descriptive diagnoses:
	Infections
	Reactive changes
	Epithelial cell abnormalities*
	Other malignant neoplasms (specify)
	Hormonal evaluation (vaginal smears only)

*Epithelial cell abnormalities:
Squamous cell
    Atypical squamous cells of undetermined significance: qualify
    Low-grade squamous intraepithelial lesion (SIL), encompassing changes of HPV and CIN 1
    High-grade squamous intraepithelial lesion (SIL), encompassing changes of CIN 2 and CIN 3
    Squamous cell carcinoma

Glandular cell
    Endometrial cells, cytologically benign, in a postmenopausal woman
    Atypical glandular cells of uncertain significance: qualify
    Endocervical adenocarcinoma
    Endometrial adenocarcinoma
    Extrauterine adenocarcinoma
    Adenocarcinoma NOS

Table reproduced with permission of *Acta Cytologica*

koilocytosis, and the latter moderate and severe dyskaryosis. The proposed changes conform very closely with the Bethesda System. Ratification of the changes proposed, and detailed guidelines for their implementation, are awaited at the time of going to press.

Cervical intraepithelial neoplasia (CIN) terminology

The disciplines of cytology and histology have converged and both cytologists and histologists have a clearer understanding of the role of cervical cytology for screening and reporting normal smears and for making a preliminary diagnosis when abnormal cells are present. The accuracy of these predictions is discussed below. Richart recommended the use of the term cervical intraepithelial neoplasia (CIN) to replace dysplasia and carcinoma *in situ*, for histological diagnosis[11]. CIN is classified into grades 1, 2 and 3, in which the artificial distinction between severe dysplasia and carcinoma *in situ* is avoided by including them both in CIN 3.

Assessment of the grade of CIN is based on the proportion of the mucosa replaced by immature crowded cells with abnormal nuclei. CIN 1 refers to a lesion in which immature cells are confined to the lowermost third of the epithelium. CIN 2 involves the middle third as well and in CIN 3 the abnormal cells extend into the upper third or even replace the entire mucosa. This terminology has been widely adopted for histological diagnosis although a more recent paper by Richart[46] supports the two categories proposed by the Bethesda Workshop described below. It is also used by some cytologists who prefer to describe cells in terms of the expected histology. The disadvantage of using histological terms for reporting cytology is the potential for misunderstanding of the report by the recipient who, untrained in pathology, may be misled into believing that the cytology is as definitive as a histological biopsy. It is well established in the literature that the cervical smear underestimates the abnormality actually present on the cervix in a significant minority of cases[47,48]. In a screening sense the abnormal smear report should be taken as indicating the least abnormality that is likely to be found on the cervix when the patient is investigated.

The Bethesda System

The *1988 Bethesda System for Reporting Cervical/Vaginal Cytologic Diagnoses* was published by a Workshop of North American experts convened by the Division of Cancer Prevention and Control of the National Cancer Institute to review existing terminology and to recommend effective methods of reporting[49]. The Workshop agreed that the Papanicolaou classification was no longer appropriate and proposed The Bethesda System, which recommends three essential components of a cervical or vaginal smear report (Table 30.5). It includes a new term, squamous intraepithelial lesion (SIL) which is divided into two grades, low-grade SIL, to include cells from HPV and CIN 1 and high-grade SIL for cells from CIN 2 and CIN 3.

The division by the Bethesda Workshop of cells from precancerous lesions of the squamous epithelium into two grades instead of three is intended to improve reproducibility of reports of abnormal cervical cytology and to relate classification to the management of the patient. High-grade SIL is an indication for excision or ablation of the abnormal tissue, whereas low-grade SIL may be followed up initially by cervical cytology alone. The Bethesda Workshop was reconvened in 1991[50] to assess the use of the Bethesda System in practice. Some minor revisions were made and these appear in Table 30.5.

A further Bethesda Workshop has been held in 2001 with proposals for further modifications, which are in draft form but are expected to be finalized in 2002. The changes that are proposed can be accessed on the Bethesda System website (http:bethesda2001.cancer.gov).

The descriptions of cytological appearances of the cells of precancerous conditions of the cervix are best understood in relation to the well defined three histological grades of cervical intraepithelial neoplasia (CIN)[11,51]. The three cytological grades of dyskaryosis defined by the British Society for Clinical Cytology, which are used in this text, relate directly to the grades of CIN. Conversion can be made to the Bethesda System or WHO terminology by reference to Table 30.6.

The cytology of CIN and invasive squamous cell carcinoma

A continuous range of abnormal nuclear morphology is seen in epithelial cells in cervical smears. The morphology reflects those abnormalities of the cervical epithelium, which involve the cells on the surface. Hence a simple basal cell hyperplasia does not produce changes at the surface of the epithelium or in the cervical smear. Lesser changes in the cells in the smear on their own are normally associated with inflammatory or reactive conditions, which are essentially benign. The more striking abnormal features described as dyskaryotic, as recommended and defined in 1986 by the Working Party of the British Society for Clinical Cytology[46], are associated with cervical intraepithelial neoplasia (CIN). If a cervical smear is correctly taken and representative of the whole of the transformation zone, an accurate correlation can be expected between the abnormal cytology and the histology when CIN is present. The factors that influence the accuracy of the cervical smear for detection of CIN are described later.

Dyskaryosis

The term dyskaryosis means literally 'abnormal nucleus'. It was used by Papanicolaou[31] and subsequently with slightly different meanings by some to describe cells from CIN 1 and CIN 2, and by others for cells from CIN 3 only. Redefined by Evans *et al.* in 1986[45], dyskaryosis or dyskaryotic describes all abnormal cells with appearances that suggest derivation from CIN and from invasive cancer of the cervix.

The morphological abnormalities seen in the nucleus of epithelial cells in cervical smears include a combination of any number of the following:

► Disproportionate nuclear enlargement
► Hyperchromasia
► Bi- and multinucleation
► Irregularity in form and outline
► Abnormal chromatin pattern, appearing as coarsening, stippling, formation of clumps or strands, and sometimes as condensation beneath the nuclear membrane producing apparent irregularities in its thickness
► Abnormalities of the number, size and form of nucleoli

The nuclear abnormalities caused by inflammation alone are usually limited to a mild degree of nuclear enlargement

and hyperchromasia. A dyskaryotic cell may show no more than a marked degree of nuclear enlargement and hyperchromasia, but the most significant and definitive feature of dyskaryosis is abnormality of the chromatin pattern (Fig. 30.2, see also Figs 30.6, 30.11). Hyperchromasia is a very common feature of dyskaryosis, (see Fig. 30.12) and easy to detect on screening examination of cervical smear slides, but it is not invariably present. Haematoxylin is not a stoichiometric stain for DNA and the intensity of staining of dyskaryotic nuclei is very variable. Some dyskaryotic nuclei are normochromatic or hypochromatic (in comparison with normal nuclei) (see Figs 30.7, 30.11, 30.14) and it is important that these less common presentations of dyskaryosis are not overlooked. Experience at least in the UK suggests that the occurrence of hypochromatic or 'pale' dyskaryosis has not received sufficient emphasis in the training of cytology medical and technical staff[52,53]. Dyskaryotic cells of these appearances are described as a significant factor leading to false negative

Table 30.6   Comparison of terminologies used for abnormal squamous epithelial cells in cervical cytology

CIN grade	WHO	BSCC	Bethesda
		Borderline	Atypia (ASCUS)
I	Mild dysplasia	Mild dyskaryosis	Low-grade SIL
II	Moderate dysplasia	Moderate dyskaryosis	High-grade SIL
III	Severe dysplasia Carcinoma *in situ*	Severe dyskaryosis	High-grade SIL
	Epidermoid carcinoma	Severe dyskaryosis ? invasive carcinoma	Squamous carcinoma

The Papanicolaou classification and other terms used in the past are not included because their equivalence is less certain. HPV infection is treated differently by the BSCC and Bethesda (see text).

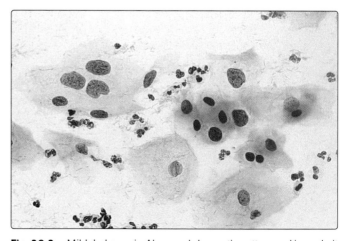

Fig. 30.2   Mild dyskaryosis. Abnormal chromatin pattern and irregularity of nuclear outline are seen in the upper part of the field as well as nuclear enlargement and hyperchromasia. The dyskaryotic cells have plentiful cytoplasm. Normal intermediate cells are present in the lower part of the field. (Papanicolaou × HP)

reporting of cervical smears[54]. Irregularity of the nuclear membrane may appear either as an irregular outline of the nucleus or irregular lines or folds across its surface. This must be distinguished from the wrinkling of the nuclear membrane in a degenerate cell as a result of inflammation. Nucleoli are not usually a conspicuous feature of dyskaryotic cells from CIN. The presence of prominent nucleoli in abnormal squamous cells in a smear suggests either widespread CIN 3 or invasive disease[55].

The difficulty in defining objective criteria for the diagnosis of dyskaryosis, the merging at the mild end of the spectrum of change with reactive or inflammatory change, and the fact that some cells from dyskaryotic populations are not always recognizable as such on an individual basis from first principles[53], are the main reasons for the necessity to use an indeterminate reporting category in practice. These changes are described as borderline nuclear changes in the BSCC terminology and will be discussed later.

Classification of dyskaryosis

Squamous cell dyskaryosis is subdivided to give a more precise indication of the severity of the abnormality. The grading depends on the nuclear cytoplasmic ratio of the cell, the cytoplasmic shape and staining quality, and the degree and diversity of nuclear abnormalities as listed above. Evaluation of these points allows subdivision into mild, moderate and severe dyskaryosis which are expected to correlate with origin from CIN 1, CIN 2 and CIN 3 respectively.

It is important that classification of dyskaryosis does not depend on the quantity and maturation of the cytoplasm alone[46] because allowance must be made for dyskaryotic cells with mature, sometimes keratinized cytoplasm, which are sometimes obtained from CIN 3 and invasive carcinoma and should be described as severely dyskaryotic (see Figs 30.51–30.53). In these circumstances the nuclear abnormalities are likely to be more pronounced in degree and diversity than usually associated with CIN 1, and the nuclear features outweigh any apparent cytoplasmic maturation. Another situation where nuclear/cytoplasmic ratio may mislead is in small parabasal cells. These sometimes have ratios more commonly associated with mild or moderate dyskaryosis but conceptually it is difficult to regard them as having arisen other than from CIN 3[53] (see Fig. 30.27).

Definitions of mild, moderate and severe dyskaryosis are made, but the changes are part of a continuous progression and absolute distinction between grades is not always possible. A smear is evaluated after careful scrutiny of all the material and rarely depends on the appearance of one cell, which may be on the borderline between accepted definitions. Normal cells usually outnumber dyskaryotic cells but the number of abnormal cells is variable. Dyskaryotic squamous cells of all grades may be seen dispersed singly or in cohesive clusters. Cell clusters, especially if large and three

dimensional, may be very difficult to interpret. Even in predominantly clustered dyskaryotic cell populations, small numbers of dispersed dyskaryotic cells are usually present. Smears with clustered dyskaryotic squamous cells with no accompanying single cells occur very rarely.

Mild dyskaryosis and CIN 1

Histology of CIN 1 (Fig. 30.3)

Despite controversy over the optimal histological classification of preinvasive lesions of the cervix there are, nevertheless, clear definitions of cervical intraepithelial neoplasia and its three-tier grading system. The case for adhering to this nomenclature has been cogently restated in recent guidelines issued by the Royal College of Pathologists and the NHSCSP[56]. CIN 1 is recognized in histological sections by increased cellularity and loss of polarity of the cells in the basal third of the epithelium due to abnormal immature cells replacing the basal and parabasal layers. Maturation appears to proceed more normally in the middle and upper thirds.

The immature cells are neoplastic and have nuclear abnormalities that relate closely to the cytological findings of dyskaryosis. These include enlargement and pleomorphism of nuclei, leading to a high nuclear cytoplasmic ratio, which is in part responsible for the appearance of cell crowding. There are also some alterations in chromatin, usually with mild hyperchromasia and stippling of the chromatin pattern. Mitoses are not infrequent, and normal and abnormal mitotic figures can be seen in the basal third of the mucosa in up to 50% of cases of CIN 1[57].

Other changes frequently seen in the upper layers include dyskeratosis due to premature keratinization of individual

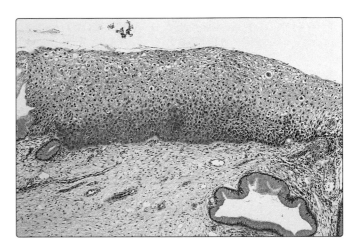

Fig. 30.3 Section of cervical squamous mucosa showing CIN 1. There is crowding of the cells in the basal third of the epithelium, so that the basal layer is no longer distinct. Nuclei in this area are enlarged and hyperchromatic and show some loss of polarity. The middle and upper layers show persistence of nuclear enlargement, but the changes are less marked and the epithelium matures normally. Koilocytes are visible towards the surface. (H&E × MP)

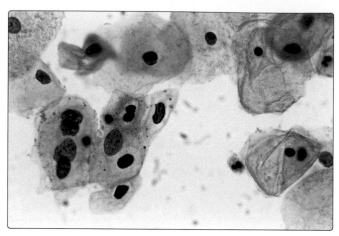

Fig. 30.4 Mild dyskaryosis. Nuclear enlargement and abnormal chromatin pattern are seen in the enlarged nuclei on the left of the field. The small abnormal pyknotic nuclei have no visible chromatin structure and amount to borderline nuclear change. The binucleated cells and cytoplasmic clearing probably indicate HPV infection but the changes do not amount to classical koilocytosis. (Papanicolaou × HP; ThinPrep ®)

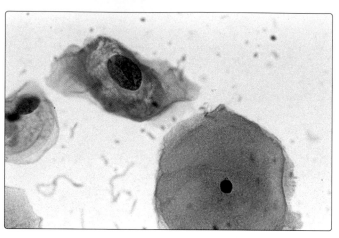

Fig. 30.5 Mild dyskaryosis and HPV infection. The cell in the upper part of the field is a koilocyte with a broad cytoplasmic perinuclear halo with condensed cytoplasm at its margin. The nucleus has a simple fold and slight coarsening of the chromatin, but is grossly enlarged, amounting to mild dyskaryosis. (Papanicolaou × HP; ThinPrep®)

squamous cells, bi- and multinucleation, pyknotic nuclei and koilocytosis, suggesting concomitant HPV infection.

It is important to note that the nuclear changes of CIN 1 persist in the mature superficial and intermediate squamous cells overlying the abnormal cells of the basal third of the epithelium. This enables recognition of lesser grades of CIN in cervical smears and allows prediction of grade of lesion based on a combination of cell maturation and degree of nuclear abnormality.

Cytological findings *(Figs 30.4–30.9)*

The morphological features of mild dyskaryosis include a combination of any of the following:

▶ Disproportionate nuclear enlargement, the nucleus usually occupying less than half the area of the cell
▶ Nuclear hyperchromasia
▶ Abnormal chromatin pattern
▶ Irregularity of the nuclear membrane
▶ Multiple abnormal nuclei
▶ Cytoplasm reduced and usually thin
▶ Cell borders usually angular

Cells sampled from an area of CIN 1 will show mild dyskaryosis. Mildly dyskaryotic cells have additional and more striking nuclear abnormalities compared with those seen in inflammatory change. The cytoplasm is usually thin, transparent and plentiful, with angular borders as seen in normal superficial and intermediate squamous cells; keratinization is sometimes seen in single cells or sheets of cells.

The nucleus is enlarged but generally occupies less than half the total area of the cell. Nuclear hyperchromasia, abnormally shaped nuclei and multiple nuclei are striking features if present but mild dyskaryosis may be represented

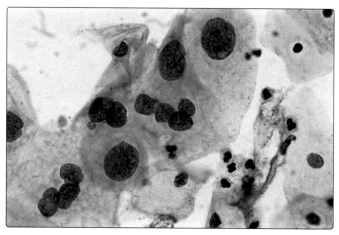

Fig. 30.6 Mild dyskaryosis. The dyskaryotic cells show varying nuclear enlargement, abnormal chromatin pattern, mild irregularities of outline and multinucleation. Normal superficial and intermediate squamous cells are seen on the right of the field. (Papanicolaou × HP. ThinPrep®)

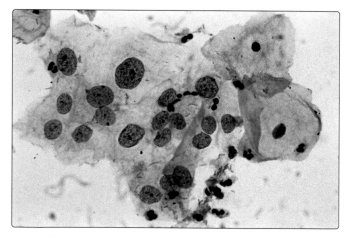

Fig. 30.7 Mild dyskaryosis. The abnormal nuclei are not hyperchromatic and are an example of 'pale' dyskaryosis. (Papanicolaou × HP; ThinPrep®)

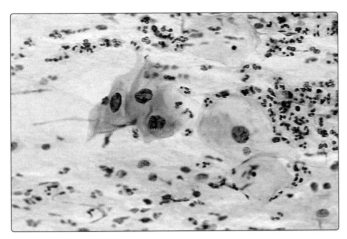

Fig. 30.8 Mild dyskaryosis with inflammatory background. The abnormal chromatin pattern clearly distinguishes the mild dyskaryosis from inflammatory nuclear change. (Papanicolaou × HP)

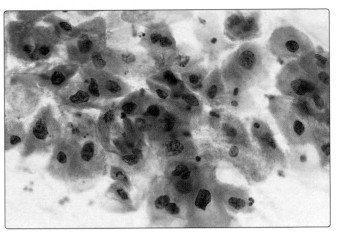

Fig. 30.9 Mild dyskaryosis. A florid example showing some binucleation and orangeophilia of keratin associated in this case with HPV infection. (Papanicolaou × HP)

by the more subtle changes of disproportionate nuclear enlargement and abnormal chromatin pattern. Nucleoli are indistinct. The abnormal nuclei associated with human papillomavirus infection cannot reliably be distinguished from dyskaryosis by light microscopy and should be evaluated according to the same criteria as dyskaryosis.

Human papillomavirus infection
(Figs 30.5, 30.9, see also Figs 30.64–30.69)

The morphological changes due to human papillomavirus (HPV) infection are summarized below. They are described more fully with infection of the female genital tract (see Chapter 28) but they must be considered further with dyskaryosis of CIN.

Cytological findings

▶ Koilocytosis
▶ Enlarged hyperchromatic nuclei
▶ Bi- and multinucleation
▶ Cytoplasmic keratinization

HPV infection may occur with or without concomitant CIN or in the same cervix as CIN but at a separate site. These distinctions can be made from a histological section of a biopsy of the cervix but cannot be made reliably from the cervical smear. The four features of HPV in the cytological specimen are koilocytosis, abnormal nuclei and multinucleation and keratinization, but not all of these characteristics are necessarily seen together. The abnormal nuclei of HPV are enlarged and usually hyperchromatic and typically have a wrinkled or collapsed appearance of the nuclear membrane. Nevertheless, the exclusion of CIN cannot be relied on from the morphology and it is advisable to manage patients whose smears show these changes according to the severity of the nuclear abnormality[58]. HPV is most commonly associated with mild dyskaryosis, but the nuclear appearance may be more comparable with

moderate dyskaryosis and suggest the presence of CIN 2. The squamous epithelial cells infected with HPV sometimes appear larger than the normal squamous epithelial cells of equivalent maturation. It is useful to take this enlargement into account if the ratio of the area of the abnormal nucleus to the area of the cell is being estimated for classification of the dyskaryosis as mild or moderate, because there is a tendency by cytologists to overestimate the degree of dyskaryosis when HPV changes are present.

Diagnostic pitfalls: mild dyskaryosis and HPV changes

Mild dyskaryosis should be distinguished from the following:

▶ Reactive/inflammatory change
▶ Navicular cells
▶ Atrophic change
▶ Keratinizing or verrucous carcinoma

Inflammatory and reactive changes involve nuclear degeneration as well as reparative or regenerative changes. Nuclear hyperchromasia and disproportionate nuclear enlargement are the principal features which are also present in mild dyskaryosis but the abnormal chromatin pattern of dyskaryosis is the most distinctive characteristic (Figs 30.2, 30.6). The spectrum of nuclear change is described as commencing with inflammation and continuing through the increasing grades of dyskaryosis, but this important diagnostic sign of abnormal chromatin pattern distinguishes mild dyskaryosis from simple reactive or inflammatory change. Severe inflammatory changes tend to affect all the cells in a smear to some extent and it is not easy to pick out particularly worrying examples because many similar cells are seen throughout the smear. Mild dyskaryosis, by contrast, will be seen in a population of cells, which is distinct from the normal and reactive squamous epithelial cells.

Nuclear degeneration leads to pyknosis and the process often includes wrinkling of the nuclear membrane at some stage. Pyknosis involves complete loss of the visible chromatin structure and it is unwise to make a diagnosis of dyskaryosis unless the diagnostic abnormal chromatin pattern is seen in some of the abnormal cells. An irregular nuclear membrane resulting from degenerative change is a sign of shrinkage of the nucleus in contrast to the folding and bulging of the nuclear membrane seen in a viable dyskaryotic cell.

Navicular cells (see Chapter 28) are boat shaped cells found in the presence of prolonged progesterone stimulation. They have eccentric nuclei and are filled with glycogen. HPV infection is epitomized cytologically and histologically by the koilocyte which typically has a wide perinuclear zone of clear cytoplasm with a clearly demarcated edge often exaggerated by a rim of condensed cytoplasm. The nucleus is usually enlarged, may be multiple and may be dyskaryotic. A navicular cell may simulate a koilocyte if it has a central nucleus surrounded by a pale area in which the granular glycogen is lightly stained. Navicular cells may have hyperchromatic nuclei but they are not enlarged or multiple. If present in a cervical smear they are usually numerous and the identity of a problem cell can easily be determined by comparison with neighbouring cells of similar appearance.

The atrophic cervical or vaginal smear (see Chapter 28) commonly shows inflammatory reaction with all its nuclear manifestations. High magnifications reveal coarser chromatin aggregation than is normal in mature squamous epithelial cells and there is often considerable nuclear enlargement. Comparison is made with the normal appearance of the nucleus in parabasal squamous cells and a distinct population of dyskaryotic cells should be identified for accurate diagnosis. If doubt persists, another smear taken immediately after completion of 7–10 days' topical application of a suitable oestrogen cream, in order to mature the epithelium, will usually resolve the difficulty.

Because of the low nuclear cytoplasmic ratios of many keratinized cells, cells from a keratinizing invasive squamous cell carcinoma may be mistaken for mild dyskaryosis if nuclear cytoplasmic ratio is relied on for assessment of dyskaryosis. When these lesions are well-differentiated, assessment of nuclear detail in terms of grading may be difficult and the appreciation of other features suggesting possible invasion such as a 'malignant diathesis' may be very important. Verrucous carcinoma (see Figs 30.62, 30.63) is a rare, but important, differential diagnosis from mild, or even moderate, dyskaryosis of CIN[59]. Typically, the smear contains a large quantity of anucleate fragments of thick keratinized cytoplasm. Nucleated cells tend to contain small hyperchromatic but pyknotic nuclei. The distinction from benign reactive hyperkeratosis or HPV infection is difficult without a description of the patient's clinical symptoms and signs.

Moderate dyskaryosis and CIN 2
Histology of CIN 2 *(Fig. 30.10)*

Histological sections from CIN 2 show replacement of normal squamous epithelium by abnormal immature cells extending into the middle third of the epithelium but, by definition, not into the uppermost third. This change imparts a crowded, disorganized appearance concentrated in the deeper layers of the epithelium, although, as with CIN 1, abnormal nuclei persist in maturing cells up to the surface. Not only do the immature cells replace more of the epithelium, but in addition they usually also show greater nuclear abnormality than is seen in CIN 1. Pleomorphism is usually marked, the chromatin pattern is coarser and irregular, and hyperchromasia is more obvious.

Abnormal mitotic figures may be quite frequent and may occur throughout the lower two thirds of the epithelium. Nucleoli remain inconspicuous.

HPV changes including koilocytosis can often be seen in the upper layers of the epithelium, affecting cells with dyskaryotic nuclei as well as less abnormal cells. The mucosa adjacent to CIN 2 frequently shows CIN 1 or HPV infection.

Cytological findings *(Figs 30.11–30.14)*

Moderate dyskaryosis is expected to correlate with CIN 2. The cytological features include any number of the following:

- ▶ Disproportionate nuclear enlargement, the nucleus usually occupying between one half and two-thirds of the total area of the cell
- ▶ Abnormal chromatin pattern, often more marked than in mild dyskaryosis
- ▶ Irregular nuclear membrane
- ▶ Nuclear hyperchromasia
- ▶ Multiple abnormal nuclei
- ▶ Cytoplasm reduced, may be thick or thin
- ▶ Cell borders may be angular or rounded

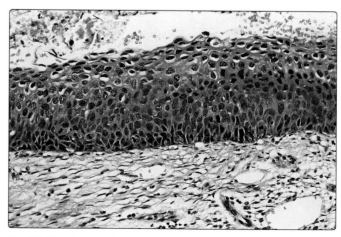

Fig. 30.10 Section of cervical squamous mucosa showing CIN 2. The squamous cells show nuclear crowding, enlargement, hyperchromasia and disorganization extending into the middle third. Above this the cells are maturing but abnormality persists to the surface. (H&E × MP)

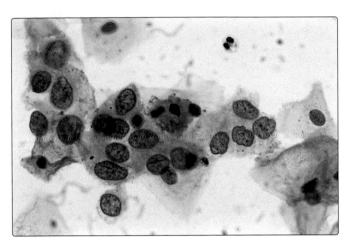

Fig. 30.11 Moderate dyskaryosis. Compare the nuclei and nuclear/cytoplasmic ratios of the dyskaryotic cells with that of the normal intermediate squamous cell on the extreme right of the field. The four dyskaryotic nuclei on its immediate left are another example of 'pale' dyskaryosis. (Papanicolaou × HP; ThinPrep®)

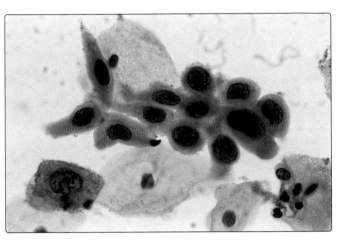

Fig. 30.13 Mild and moderate dyskaryosis. The dyskaryotic nuclei show varying hyperchromasia, abnormal chromatin pattern and sometimes irregularities of nuclear outline. Compare with the adjacent normal superficial and intermediate squamous cell nuclei. The cytoplasmic margins of two of the cells in the central group are difficult to define and their abnormality approaches severe dyskaryosis. (Papanicolaou × HP; ThinPrep®)

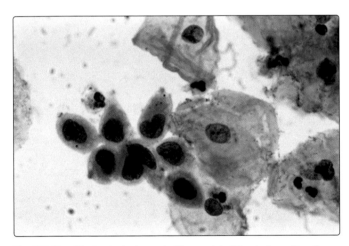

Fig. 30.12 Moderate dyskaryosis. The nuclei of the dyskaryotic cells are hyperchromatic, have irregular outlines and show complex folding. (Papanicolaou × HP; ThinPrep®)

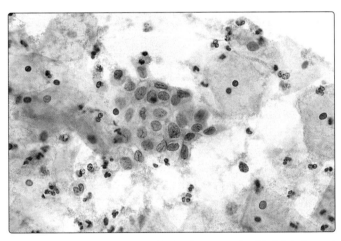

Fig. 30.14 Moderate dyskaryosis. Another example of 'pale' dyskaryosis. Irregular nuclear outlines and abnormal pattern are seen. (Papanicolaou × HP)

The abnormal nuclei in moderately dyskaryotic cells show greater disproportionate enlargement than in mildly dyskaryotic cells so that they generally occupy up to two thirds of the total area of the cell. The nuclear chromatin abnormality is usually more marked than in mild dyskaryosis. Hyperchromasia, abnormal nuclear outlines and multinucleation may be present but, as in mild dyskaryosis, disproportionate nuclear enlargement and abnormal chromatin distribution may be the only diagnostic features.

Nucleoli are not usually prominent. The quality of the cytoplasm is variable and may resemble that of superficial, intermediate or parabasal squamous cells. Moderate dyskaryosis in a smear will usually be accompanied by mild dyskaryosis as well as normal squamous cells. The proportion of the cell types can be expected to vary according to the amount and situation of the abnormal epithelium but will also depend on sampling technique.

Diagnostic pitfalls

Moderate dyskaryosis should be distinguished from the following:

▶ Immature squamous metaplasia
▶ HPV infection
▶ Endocervical cells
▶ Severe dyskaryosis

Immature squamous metaplasia (Fig. 30.15) exhibits features of both squamous and endocervical glandular epithelium. The nuclei are relatively larger than those of mature squamous cells and frequently hyperchromatic,

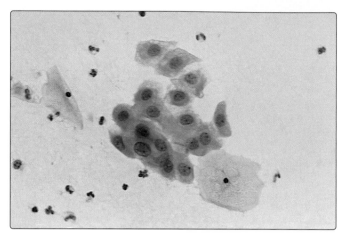

Fig. 30.15 Immature squamous metaplasia: to be distinguished from moderate dyskaryosis. The uniformity of nuclear size and texture, the abundant cytoplasm and pattern of metaplastic cells is characteristic of these normal cells. Compare with **Figs 30.11–30.14**. (Papanicolaou × HP)

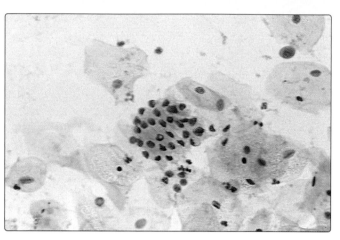

Fig. 30.16 Degenerate endocervical cells: differential diagnosis from dyskaryosis. The uniform size and distribution of the pyknotic nuclei, distinct cell borders and weak haematoxylin staining of cytoplasmic mucin identifies the central group as endocervical cells. (Papanicolaou × HP)

which may lead to misinterpretation as moderate dyskaryosis of CIN if the pattern of the squamous metaplasia and the uniformity of the cells is not recognized. Caution is necessary, however, because dyskaryosis may be present in what appear to be metaplastic cells (see Fig. 30.28). Atypical metaplasia is a term which has been applied to these appearances[10] but to avoid misunderstanding it is recommended that they should be reported as dyskaryotic and managed accordingly.

Endocervical cells (Fig. 30.16) are less likely to be confused with squamous cell dyskaryosis unless they show degenerative changes and marked hyperchromasia, in which case the nuclei are pyknotic and do not have discernible chromatin structure.

Endocervical cell cytoplasm is delicate and loss of cytoplasm is common resulting in the presence of bare endocervical cell nuclei in smears. A similar effect occurs with tubal type epithelial cells, which are being recognized more commonly in cervical smears. Bare nuclei may also originate from CIN lesions and may cause concern, but should be assessed by comparison with those of neighbouring well-preserved cells. If the bare nuclei can be assigned to a non-neoplastic cell population the problem may be resolved. (Fig. 30.17) Because degenerative changes are frequently present, dyskaryosis should not be diagnosed from the appearances of bare nuclei alone in the absence of well preserved intact dyskaryotic cells.

Enlarged, often hypochromatic nuclei with uneven chromatin distribution and anisonucleosis, often resembling reactive endocervical cell nuclei, at least at screening magnification, are sometimes seen (Fig. 30.29). Although it has been suggested that these nuclei are of atypical reserve cell origin[60], the authors consider that these cells represent severe dyskaryosis in large non-keratinizing squamous cells. When these cells are present in smears, further investigation of the patient is always warranted.

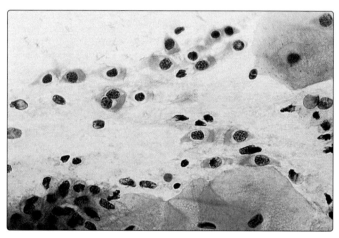

Fig. 30.17 Stripped or bare nuclei and ciliated columnar cells: differential diagnosis of dyskaryosis. The hyperchromatic nuclei with coarse but uniformly distributed chromatin may be identified within the intact columnar cells, which have terminal bars and cilia. If the bare nuclei are seen alone they may be misinterpreted as dyskaryotic. (Papanicolaou × HP)

Severe dyskaryosis in which striking nuclear abnormalities outweigh the presence of fairly abundant cytoplasm is an important differential diagnosis from moderate dyskaryosis. Keratinizing squamous cell carcinoma is a significant example, in which the dyskaryotic cells may be keratinized, with relatively abundant cytoplasm (see Figs 30.51–30.53). Occasionally, in the presence of a well-differentiated tumour, nuclei which are sufficiently well preserved to display diagnostic features, may be scarce, and diligent scrutiny of the smear is necessary.

Severe dyskaryosis and CIN 3
Histology of CIN 3 *(Fig. 30.18)*

In cases of CIN 3, the cervical squamous epithelium is replaced by immature neoplastic cells, which extend into its uppermost third and often completely replace the entire

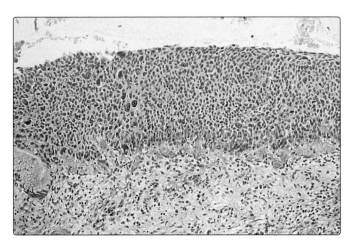

Fig. 30.18 Section of cervical squamous mucosa showing CIN 3. There is complete replacement of normal squamous cells by crowded abnormal cells with marked nuclear pleomorphism, hyperchromasia and loss of polarity. No evidence of cell maturation can be seen. Note that the basement membrane is intact. The underlying stroma shows non-specific inflammation and marked vascular engorgement. (H&E × MP)

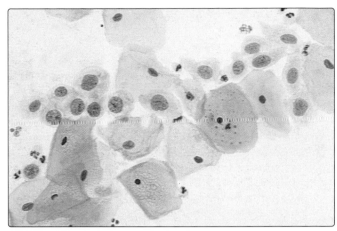

Fig. 30.19 Mild, moderate and severe dyskaryosis. A range of abnormality is seen. The small cell with scanty cytoplasm on the extreme left is severely dyskaryotic. (Papanicolaou × HP)

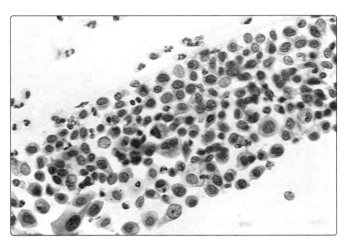

Fig. 30.20 Severe dyskaryosis. The band of cells from a case of CIN 3 includes hypochromatic nuclei and bare nuclei. Both of these may give rise to diagnostic difficulty if seen on their own. (Papanicolaou × HP)

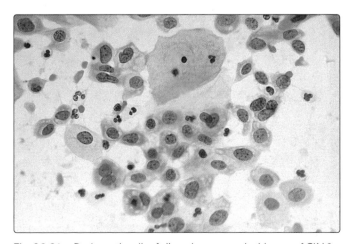

Fig. 30.21 Dyskaryotic cells of all grades are seen in this case of CIN 3. Examples of nuclei with abnormal chromatin clumping, irregular nuclear outlines and of multinucleation of dyskaryotic cells are seen. The cytoplasm of the dyskaryotic cells is of variable density. (Papanicolaou × HP)

thickness. Thus the category of CIN 3 includes both severe dysplasia and carcinoma *in situ* of previous terminology.

There is much more obvious cellular and nuclear abnormality than in lesser grades of CIN, with greater loss of polarity and crowding of cells and a tendency to vertical orientation of nuclei. The cells and their enlarged nuclei may present a monotonous appearance or can exhibit marked pleomorphism with greater cytoplasmic maturation.

This has led to subtyping of CIN 3 into small and large cell non-keratinizing types respectively. Less commonly the epithelium is replaced by large pleomorphic squamous cells with bizarre shapes and individual cell keratinization, giving the third sub-type, keratinizing CIN 3. Combinations of the different CIN 3 subtypes may be seen.

Nuclear changes include hyperchromasia, coarse granularity of chromatin pattern, irregularities of nuclear contour and mitoses. Mitoses may include obviously abnormal forms and may extend into the upper one third of the epithelium.

By definition, the basement membrane is intact in CIN 3. The abnormal epithelium extends progressively over the ectocervix or along the endocervical canal, and also into endocervical crypts. There may be a pronounced chronic inflammatory cell infiltrate in the underlying cervical stroma, representing a host response to the epithelial abnormality. There is evidence that very extensive CIN 3 lesions are associated with a greater likelihood of invasion[61]. Lesser grades of CIN and HPV changes are usually, but not invariably, present adjacent to areas of CIN 3.

Cytological findings *(Figs 30.19–30.36)*

Severely dyskaryotic cells are expected to correlate with cells from the surface of CIN 3 or invasive squamous cell carcinoma. The cytological features of severe dyskaryosis include any number of the following:

- Disproportionate nuclear enlargement with the nucleus usually occupying at least two-thirds of the total area of the cell
- Abnormal chromatin pattern
- Nuclear hyperchromasia
- Irregularity of the nuclear membrane
- Multiple abnormal nuclei
- Cytoplasm markedly reduced
- Abnormal maturation of cytoplasm, including keratinization
- Cell borders smooth or angular
- Nucleoli prominent when CIN 3 is widespread
- Bizarrely shaped cells, sometimes including fibre cells

It is clear from the description of the histological presentation that the cytological appearances of severe dyskaryosis will be variable. Similarly, the cytological abnormality may be relatively uniform in an individual case. The abnormal nuclei of severe dyskaryosis characteristically occupy almost all of the cytoplasmic area of the cell or at least two thirds of it. The narrow rim of cytoplasm surrounding the nucleus is either dense or poorly defined. The cell may be round, oval, elongated or polygonal.

Severely dyskaryotic cells occasionally have nuclear morphology more abnormal than that usually associated with CIN 1 or CIN 2, yet have plentiful cytoplasm which may be keratinized and abnormally shaped (see Figs 30.51–30.53). The diagnosis of severe dyskaryosis is confirmed by the presence of other cells, with the appearances described above, which are more frequently associated with severe dyskaryosis.

Abnormal chromatin pattern is usually the most significant nuclear abnormality in severe dyskaryosis. This may be accompanied by hyperchromasia, abnormal nuclear shape and multinucleation, or a combination of any number of these features. However, in some smears from CIN 3 the cytological abnormality is confined to an abnormal chromatin pattern in a round to oval nucleus, which fills most of the cell. Nucleoli are not usually prominent in CIN 3 unless the abnormality involves a wide area of the epithelium. Mitotic figures are infrequently observed in dispersed dyskaryotic cell populations but may sometimes be easily seen in large cohesive clusters or 'microbiopsy' fragments of dyskaryotic cells.

Although, as noted above, three cytological and histological sub-types of severe dyskaryosis and CIN 3 are recognized, they are not usually reported in routine practice, but reporting of sub-types may occasionally be useful clinically. Small cell non-keratinizing severe dyskaryosis and the corresponding CIN 3 lesion are associated with occurrence in the endocervical canal. This may explain the failure of the colposcopist to visualize a lesion diagnosed cytologically and expedite appropriate management of the patient. The histological diagnosis of keratinizing CIN 3 may adequately explain bizarre

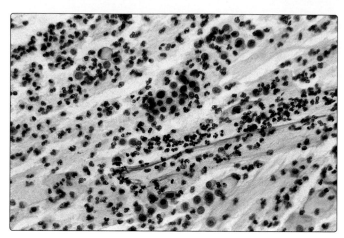

Fig. 30.22 Severe dyskaryosis in a case of small cell CIN 3. Streaks of severely dyskaryotic cells are mixed with polymorphs and may be difficult to identify. (Papanicolaou × LP)

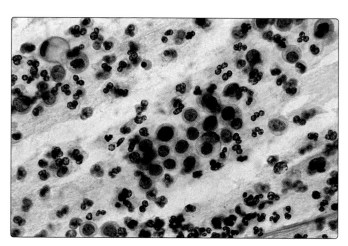

Fig. 30.23 Severe dyskaryosis in a case of small cell CIN 3. Same field as **Fig. 30.22**. There is marked hyperchromasia of a nucleus in the centre, but the abnormalities of the other nuclei are more subtle. (Papanicolaou × MP)

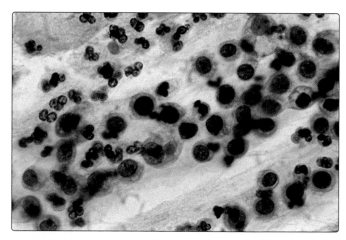

Fig. 30.24 Severe dyskaryosis in a case of small cell CIN 3. Same case as **Figs 30.22** and **30.23**. Four nuclei in the centre of the field show obvious hyperchromasia and abnormal chromatin, but other dyskaryotic nuclei in the field are much more difficult to identify as such. (Papanicolaou × HP)

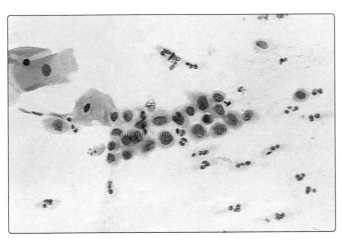

Fig. 30.25 Severe dyskaryosis. Small polychromatic cells of similar size and shape. The nuclear hyperchromasia, abnormal chromatin pattern and narrow band of cytoplasm signify severe dyskaryosis in this case of CIN 3. (Papanicolaou × HP)

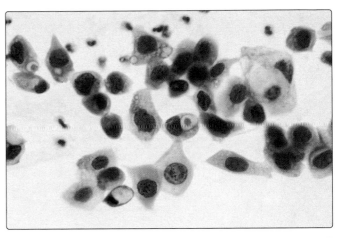

Fig. 30.28 Severe dyskaryosis. The cell pattern shows some features of immature squamous metaplasia but the nuclear chromatin, variation of nuclear size and shape and the diminished cytoplasm indicate severe dyskaryosis, in this case of CIN 3. (Papanicolaou × HP)

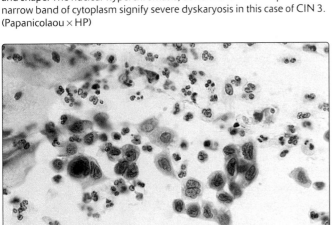

Fig. 30.26 Severe dyskaryosis. The small cells exhibit variation of size and shape as well as abnormal chromatin pattern and scanty cytoplasm. Engulfment of one dyskaryotic cell by another is seen on the left of this field from a case of CIN 3. (Papanicolaou × HP)

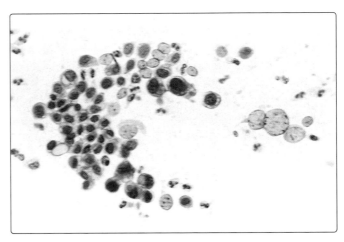

Fig. 30.29 Severe dyskaryosis. Bare, hypochromatic nuclei are associated with smaller severely dyskaryotic cells from a case of CIN 3. Bare nuclei of this type should not be mistaken for endocervical cell nuclei. (Papanicolaou × HP)

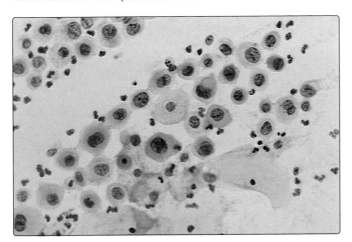

Fig. 30.27 Severe dyskaryosis from a case of CIN 3. Some of the cells have nuclear/cytoplasmic ratios more appropriate to moderate or even mild dyskaryosis. Conceptually, it is difficult to regard small parabasal cells with dense cytoplasm as having arisen from other than CIN 3. (Papanicolaou × HP)

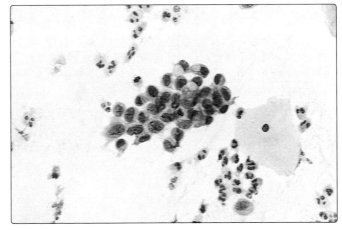

Fig. 30.30 Severe dyskaryosis. A cluster of cells from a case of CIN 3. Cytoplasmic vacuolation, which is illustrated here, may be a feature of severely dyskaryotic cells of CIN 3 or invasive squamous cell carcinoma. (Papanicolaou × HP)

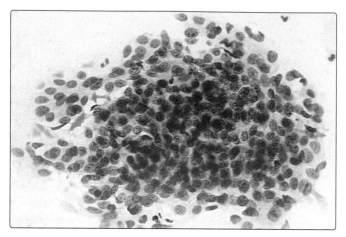

Fig. 30.31   Severe dyskaryosis. A sheet of crowded, overlapped dyskaryotic cells from a case of small cell non-keratinizing CIN 3. Sheets and clusters of abnormal cells may be more difficult to identify than dispersed dyskaryotic cells. (Papanicolaou × HP)

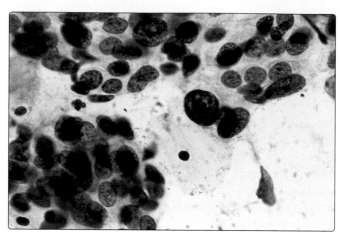

Fig. 30.34   Severe dyskaryosis, same case as **Fig. 30.33**. Abnormal chromatin clumping is confirmed and is obvious in the larger nucleus near the centre of the field. (Papanicolaou × HP)

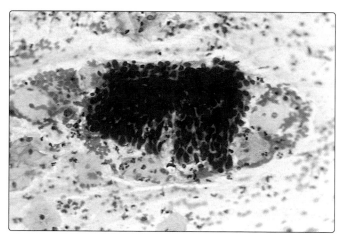

Fig. 30.32   Severe dyskaryosis. A fragment consisting of clustered severely dyskaryotic cells from a case of CIN 3. Dispersed dyskaryotic cells are usually also present, but if they are scanty, or in occasional cases entirely absent, correct identification of clustered severely dyskaryotic cells may be very difficult. (Papanicolaou × HP)

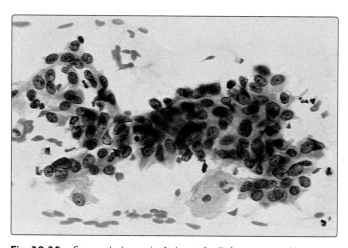

Fig. 30.35   Severe dyskaryosis. A sheet of cells from a case with widespread CIN 3. Punctate nucleoli, as seen in some of the nuclei, are not usually a feature of cells from CIN 3 unless it occupies a large proportion of the transformation zone. (Papanicolaou × HP)

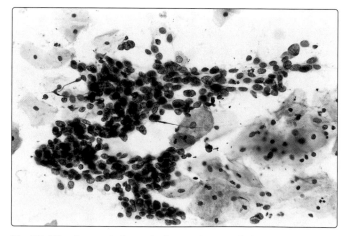

Fig. 30.33   Severe dyskaryosis. Clumped severe dyskaryosis from a case of small cell CIN 3. Compare with the endometrial cells in **Fig. 30.40**. Careful examination at high power of the detail of individual nuclei may be necessary to make the diagnosis. (Papanicolaou × LP)

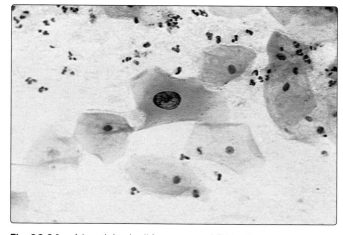

Fig. 30.36   A keratinized cell from a case of CIN 3. Seen in isolation, this cell might be interpreted as showing only mild dyskaryosis. (Papanicolaou × HP)

keratinized squamous cells in a smear reported cytologically as possibly from an invasive squamous cell carcinoma.

Diagnostic pitfalls

Severe dyskaryosis in squamous cells should be distinguished from the following:

▶ Mild and moderate dyskaryosis
▶ Histiocytes
▶ Follicular cervicitis
▶ Endometrial cells
▶ Endometrial cell exfoliation due to an IUCD
▶ HPV infection
▶ Intraepithelial and invasive adenocarcinoma

Histiocytes (Figs 30.37, 30.38) appear as single cells but less commonly in clusters especially if they are numerous, as in the late menstrual 'exodus'. Although usually small, they may vary in size. Both nucleus and cytoplasm may show degenerative changes, which occasionally may mimic small non-keratinized or keratinized dyskaryotic squamous cells very closely. If the characteristic reniform nuclei and foamy cytoplasm are not observed, distinction from a severely dyskaryotic squamous cell may usually be made by comparison with neighbouring cells which show more distinctive features[53].

Follicular (lymphocytic) cervicitis (Fig. 30.39) may result in streaks of follicular cells in a smear, often focally but sometimes dominating large areas or even the whole of a smear. The cells characteristically are dispersed, include small lymphocytes and mature plasma cells with coarse chromatin, larger follicle centre cells which may show mitotic figures, and histiocytes containing tingible bodies.

Endometrial cells (Fig. 30.40) have small hyperchromatic nuclei and scanty cytoplasm and are usually present in clusters (see Chapter 28). They are not usually difficult to distinguish from cells of CIN or invasive carcinoma but it is necessary to be aware that clustered, and sometimes single cells from small cell non-keratinizing CIN 3 or invasive carcinoma may look very similar to endometrial cells. (Fig. 30.33) The presence of characteristic biphasic endometrial cell groups is helpful to confirm endometrial exfoliation, but if there is a possibility of coexistent CIN or carcinoma, further investigation will be necessary.

Intrauterine contraceptive devices (IUCD) cause reactive changes in the endometrial epithelium at points of contact, sometimes resulting in the exfoliation of abnormal endometrial cells which appear in the cervical smear (see Chapter 28). The abnormal endometrial cells are round but enlarged, sometimes multinucleated and sometimes have visible nucleoli. The cytoplasm may be vacuolated but often forms a dense narrow rim round the nucleus, mimicking severe dyskaryosis of CIN 3. The presence of the tell-tale degenerate leucocytes and debris of endometrial material

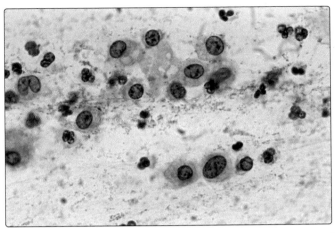

Fig. 30.37 Histiocytes. Note the coarseness of clumping of the chromatin in the nuclei of these normal cells. Failure to identify such cells as histiocytes may lead to an erroneous diagnosis of severe dyskaryosis in squamous cells. (Papanicolaou × HP)

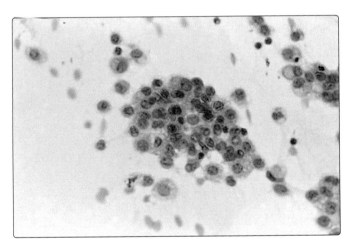

Fig. 30.38 Histiocytes: differential diagnosis of severe dyskaryosis. Reniform nuclei, nucleoli, foamy cytoplasm and size are features which aid in the identification of histiocytes. These features are seen more clearly in the single cells surrounding the cluster. (Papanicolaou × HP)

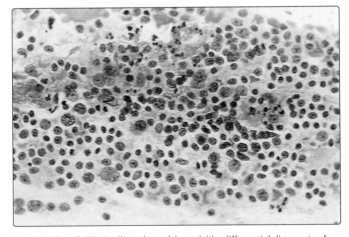

Fig. 30.39 Follicular (lymphocytic) cervicitis: differential diagnosis of severe dyskaryosis. The very coarse chromatin pattern of small lymphocytes and the presence of tingible body macrophages are important features in the correct identification of these cells. (Papanicolaou × HP)

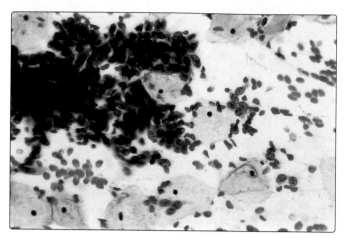

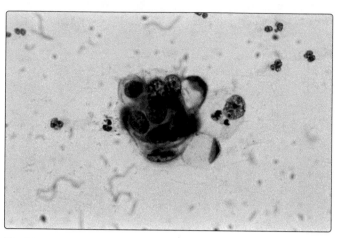

Fig. 30.40 Endometrial cells: differential diagnosis of severe dyskaryosis. Exfoliated endometrial cells tend to form 3-dimensional clusters. Distinction of such clusters from fragments of small cell CIN 3 or invasive carcinoma may require careful scrutiny of the whole smear for additional diagnostic features. Compare with **Fig. 30.33**. (Papanicolaou × LP)

Fig. 30.41 Endometrial cells in the smear of an IUCD user: differential diagnosis of severe dyskaryosis. This small three-dimensional group of endometrial cells with characteristic cytoplasmic vacuolation is easily correctly identified, but see **Fig. 30.42**. (Papanicolaou × HP)

in a streak of mucus, and the known presence of an IUCD, are helpful in arriving at the correct interpretation. (Figs 30.41, 30.42)

Human papillomavirus (HPV) infection, when represented in a smear by numerous keratinized cells, may require differentiation from keratinizing CIN 3 or invasive squamous cell carcinoma or vice versa. Careful scrutiny should reveal some severely dyskaryotic cells if CIN 3 or carcinoma is present.

Cervical adenocarcinoma, either intraepithelial or invasive, if not well-differentiated may be indistinguishable from CIN 3 or non-keratinizing squamous carcinoma in a smear. The characteristic features of rosettes, nuclear pseudostratification or palisading and feathered edges of sheets of severely dyskaryotic cells point to adenocarcinoma (see Chapter 32), but in the absence of these or distinctive squamous cell differentiation, the presence of adenocarcinoma or a mixed adenosquamous lesion may be difficult to determine. Prominent, sometimes multiple and irregular nucleoli may be present in squamous cell carcinoma or adenocarcinoma.

Adenocarcinoma cells from well-differentiated tumours of the endometrium, or less commonly, adenocarcinoma of the ovary or fallopian tube, can usually be distinguished from severe squamous dyskaryosis because of the tendency to form three-dimensional cell clusters, as well as by the presence of prominent nucleoli and cytoplasmic vacuolation. Poorly-differentiated carcinoma cells from these sites are likely to be much less numerous than severely dyskaryotic cells originating from the cervix.

Adenosquamous carcinoma of the endometrium is occasionally represented in a cervical smear (see Chapters 31, 32 and 33). A keratinizing squamous component can mislead the cytologist towards a diagnosis of cervical squamous cell carcinoma, unless the adenocarcinoma cells

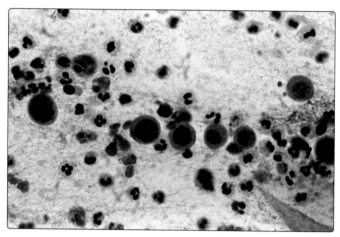

Fig. 30.42 Endometrial cells in the smear of an IUCD user, same smear as **Fig. 30.41**. The single cells with high nuclear/cytoplasmic ratios and hyper chromatic nuclei were felt probably to be degenerate endometrial cells, but that exclusion of severe squamous dyskaryosis was not possible. The patient subsequently underwent a cone biopsy and diagnostic uterine curettage; no neoplastic pathology was demonstrated in either specimen. (Papanicolaou × HP)

are represented and identified in the rounded clusters typical of endometrial origin. The dyskaryotic squamous cells will be fewer than might be expected from a cervical carcinoma.

Microinvasive and invasive squamous cell carcinoma

Histology of microinvasive and invasive squamous cell carcinoma (Fig. 30.43, see also Figs 30.46, 30.47, 30.48)

Invasive carcinoma is recognized histologically by the presence of neoplastic squamous cells which are no longer confined to the surface of the cervix or endocervical crypts by intact basement membrane, but have extended into the underlying stroma. The extent of invasion determines

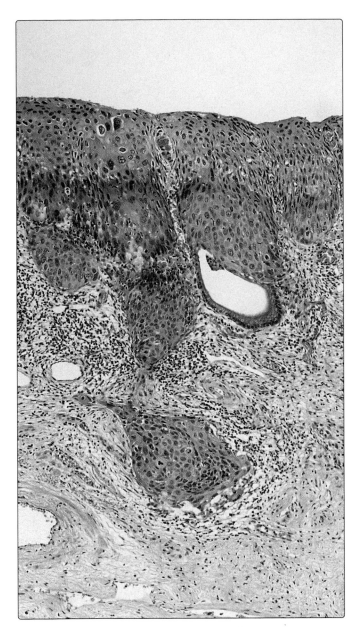

Fig. 30.43   Microinvasive carcinoma of cervix. CIN 3 is present, extending into some of the endocervical glands. Deep to this, irregular groups of squamous cells extend into the stroma to a depth of less than 3 mm. (H&E × LP) A tiny focus of microinvasion FIGO Stage Ia1 is seen extending from the basement membrane into the inflamed stroma. The invasive component shows increased cytoplasm and nesting [redifferentiation]. (H&E × MP)

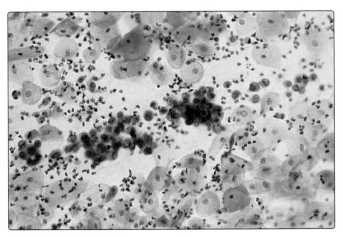

Fig. 30.44   Severe dyskaryosis from a case of early invasive squamous cell carcinoma. The smear contains many groups of severely dyskaryotic cells as well as small single keratinized cells which are seen in the background. These two features alert the cytologist to the possibility of early invasion. (Papanicolaou × MP)

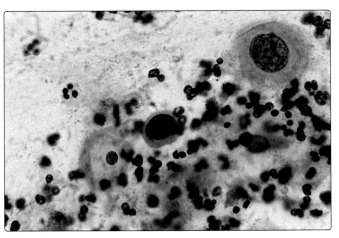

Fig. 30.45   Severe dyskaryosis in a case of invasive squamous cell carcinoma. The nucleus at the centre of the field has such coarse chromatin clumping that areas of lucency are visible. (Papanicolaou × HP)

whether the lesion is regarded as microinvasive or frankly invasive carcinoma.

The distinction is made because very early invasive (or microinvasive) carcinoma is amenable to conservative surgical treatment, that is cone biopsy, rather than a radical hysterectomy or radiotherapy, as the risk of tumour spread beyond the cervix in microinvasive disease is extremely low. Definitions of microinvasive carcinoma continue to evolve and in the latest FIGO staging[8] the term microinvasive is itself no longer used (see Table 30.2). FIGO stage Ia1 disease, i.e. with measured stromal invasion to a maximum depth of 3 mm and to a maximum width of 7 mm is generally considered that for which cone biopsy is adequate treatment.

In histological sections, microinvasive carcinoma (Fig. 30.43) usually displays extensive CIN 3 as already described, from which tongues and islands of neoplastic cells extend through the basement membrane in a spray-like pattern or later as confluent invasion.

The tumour cells frequently show greater maturation with more cytoplasmic development than those of the CIN 3 from which they have arisen, a feature reflected in their cytology (Fig 30.43). As growth proceeds beyond the stage of microinvasion, the islands of tumour cells become larger and a surrounding desmoplastic reaction may be seen, together with a variable inflammatory cell infiltrate.

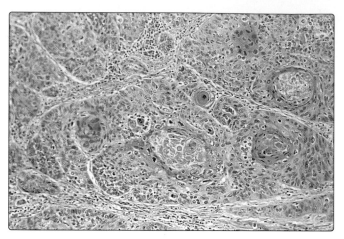

Fig. 30.46 Section of cervix with invasive well-differentiated keratinizing squamous cell carcinoma. Nests of large eosinophilic tumour cells forming keratin pearls are present. (H&E × MP)

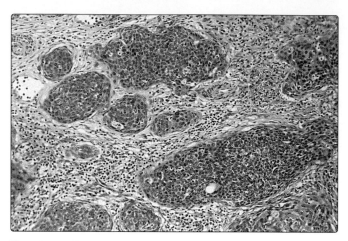

Fig. 30.48 Section of cervix showing a poorly-differentiated carcinoma composed of irregular groups of crowded abnormal epithelial cells with hyperchromatic nuclei and scattered mitoses. No differentiation can be seen but the pattern of infiltration, an origin from CIN 3 at the surface, and negative stains for mucin production indicate that this is a poorly-differentiated squamous cell carcinoma. (H&E × MP)

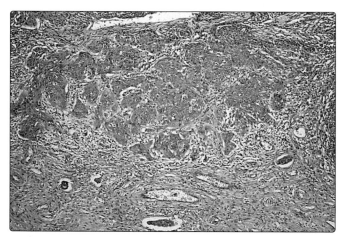

Fig. 30.47 Section of cervix with moderately-differentiated invasive squamous cell carcinoma. Multiple islands of carcinoma cells infiltrate the cervical stroma and lymphatic channels deep to the tumour contain small groups of malignant cells. (H&E × MP)

Approximately 60% of squamous cell carcinomas are moderately differentiated.

Poorly-differentiated squamous cell carcinomas (Fig. 30.48) invade as sheets, islands and single cells, often invoking a pronounced inflammatory reaction. No definite squamous features are seen and their origin may only be established with the help of special stains to exclude mucin production, or immunocytochemistry to exclude other poorly-differentiated tumour types. Identification of the pattern of keratin expression in carcinoma of the cervix by the use of monoclonal and polyclonal antibodies has proved useful in confirming the squamous nature of some of the poorly-differentiated tumours[62].

The World Health Organization has adopted a different grading system[10], following terminology proposed by Reagan and Hamonic[63], in which tumours are graded as keratinizing, large cell non-keratinizing and small cell non-keratinizing squamous cell carcinomas. These groups correlate broadly with the three grades used above, but the last group includes a number of cases, which are found to have neuroendocrine features and resemble small cell carcinoma of the bronchus. This variant is discussed further in Chapter 33.

Glandular differentiation with mucin production may be noted in isolated cells within the tumour, but this does not denote an adenosquamous carcinoma unless mucin secreting cells form more than one third of the tumour cell population[5].

Lymphatic or vascular permeation by clumps of malignant cells is increasingly likely to be found. Ultimately there is an ulcerated tumour mass, recognizable clinically as a probable carcinoma. Carcinomas are divided into well-, moderately- or poorly-differentiated grades relating to the pattern of invasion and to the cytoplasmic development in the neoplastic cells. Grading correlates broadly with prognosis for the patient and has bearing on the cytological findings.

Features indicating a well-differentiated squamous cell carcinoma (Fig. 30.46) include the presence of large islands of infiltrating tumour cells with intercellular bridges, epithelial pearl formation and obvious keratinization of the cell cytoplasm. Moderately-differentiated carcinomas (Fig. 30.47) show some evidence of a squamous origin, consisting of solid islands and smaller groups of polygonal pleomorphic cells, but keratinization and intercellular bridges are less obvious and pearl formation is not seen.

Cytological findings (Figs 30.44, 30.45, 30.49–30.61)

Microinvasive and invasive squamous cell carcinoma cannot be diagnosed reliably from a smear because the severe dyskaryosis of CIN 3 may be morphologically

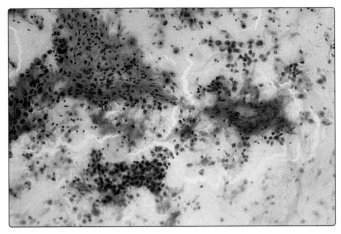

Fig. 30.49 Squamous cell carcinoma. The whole picture is abnormal. Keratinization of cytoplasm is a striking feature and severe dyskaryosis is clearly seen in the small cells, even at this magnification. (Papanicolaou × LP)

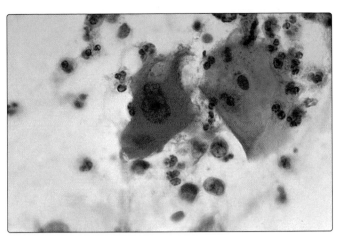

Fig. 30.52 Squamous cell carcinoma. A severely dyskaryotic squamous cell with abundant keratinized cytoplasm lies next to a normal squamous cell. (Papanicolaou × HP)

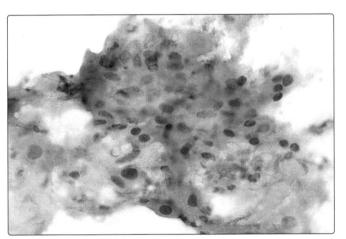

Fig. 30.50 Squamous cell carcinoma; keratinizing, well-differentiated type. Abnormal nuclear morphology is present but is less well defined in the degenerate cells. (Papanicolaou × MP)

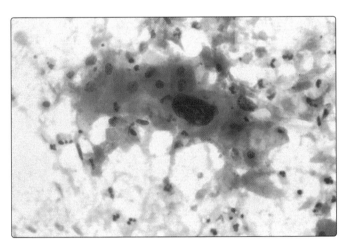

Fig. 30.53 Squamous cell carcinoma. This large keratinized cell has nuclear features amounting to severe dyskaryosis. (Papanicolaou × HP)

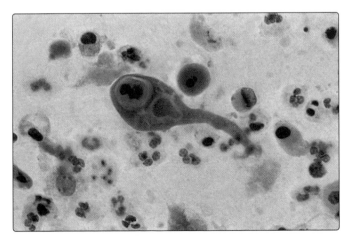

Fig. 30.51 Squamous cell carcinoma. In the centre is a bizarrely shaped keratinized dyskaryotic cell, often described as a tadpole cell. (Papanicolaou × HP)

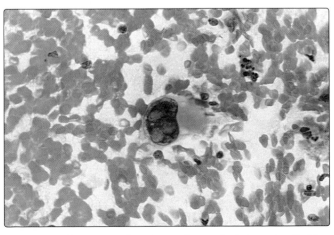

Fig. 30.54 Squamous cell carcinoma. A severely dyskaryotic cell with a degenerate nucleus. (Papanicolaou × HP)

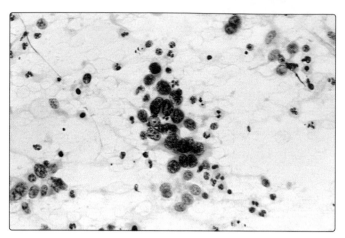

Fig. 30.55　Squamous cell carcinoma. Severe dyskaryosis of small cell type in a background of streaked exudate, debris and leucocytes. (Papanicolaou × HP)

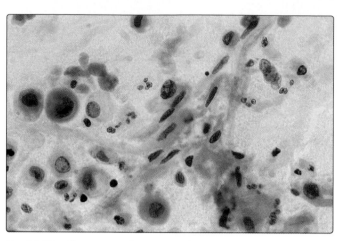

Fig. 30.58　Squamous cell carcinoma. Severe dyskaryosis with variation in size and shape of cells including elongated forms described as fibre cells. (Papanicolaou × HP)

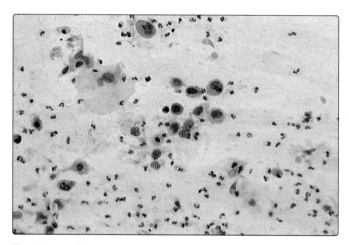

Fig. 30.56　Squamous cell carcinoma. Small severely dyskaryotic cells with scanty cytoplasm which shows keratinization in a few cells. The background 'diathesis' of leucocytes and cell debris suggests an invasive carcinoma. (Papanicolaou × HP)

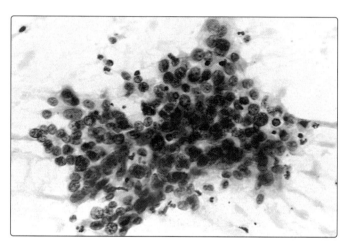

Fig. 30.59　Squamous cell carcinoma. A fragment of small cell non-keratinizing carcinoma. (Papanicolaou × HP)

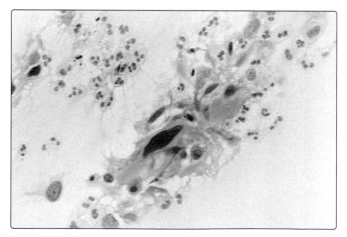

Fig. 30.57　Squamous cell carcinoma. Severe dyskaryosis with elongated nuclei. Eosinophilic and cyanophilic fragments of cytoplasm and neutrophil polymorphs in the background suggest an invasive carcinoma. (Papanicolaou × HP)

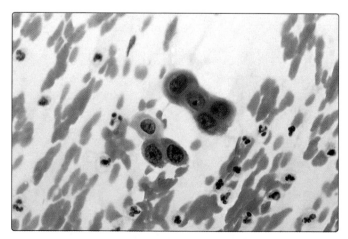

Fig. 30.60　Squamous cell carcinoma. Severe dyskaryosis from a non-keratinizing squamous cell carcinoma in which the tumour cells have prominent nucleoli and a narrow band of thick cytoplasm. (Papanicolaou × HP)

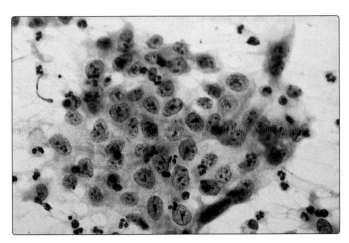

Fig. 30.61 Squamous cell carcinoma. Severe dyskaryosis from a non-keratinizing squamous cell carcinoma in which the cells have large, multiple and irregular nucleoli. (Papanicolaou × HP)

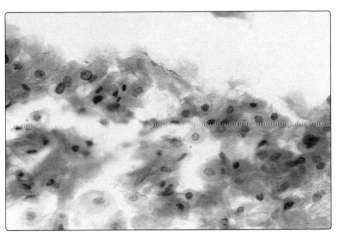

Fig. 30.62 Verrucous squamous cell carcinoma. Hyperkeratotic and keratinized cells with small degenerate nuclei dominate the cytology. Nuclear features of only mild or moderate dyskaryosis may misrepresent the malignant nature of the tumour. Awareness of the clinical appearance of the cervix should lead to early referral of the patient for biopsy. (Papanicolaou × HP)

indistinguishable from the severe dyskaryosis of invasive cancer. However, there are cytological features, which imply a strong possibility of a more advanced condition than CIN 3. These are as follows:

▶ Smears usually show very large numbers of dyskaryotic cells reflecting the widespread CIN 3 generally present with early invasion
▶ Variation in size and shape of dyskaryotic cell nuclei more than that associated with CIN 3, and often including very small cells
▶ Abnormal chromatin clumping with such coarse aggregation that areas of lucency appear between the aggregates (Fig. 30.45)
▶ Tissue fragments or 'microbiopsies' of severely dyskaryotic cells
▶ Cytoplasmic keratinization including thick anucleate fragments in keratinizing squamous cell carcinoma (Fig. 30.57)
▶ Bizarrely shaped dyskaryotic squamous cells including 'fibre' and 'tadpole cells' (Figs 30.51, 30.58)
▶ Large, sometimes irregular and multiple nucleoli especially in large cell non-keratinizing squamous cell carcinoma
▶ Smear background including fibrin, debris, leucocytes and blood described as 'tumour' or 'malignant diathesis' (Figs 30.55, 30.56). This is not sufficiently specific for diagnosis but may be an important sign drawing attention to other features

It is useful to report these features seen with severe dyskaryosis in order to convey the need for urgent investigation of the patient. That the smear test is less sensitive for invasive cancer than CIN and that false negative reports may occur have already been discussed.

Verrucous carcinoma (Figs 30.62, 30.63)

This uncommon variant of squamous cell carcinoma affects the cervix rarely. It is a slow growing exophytic tumour with a histologically well defined deep margin which extends by pushing into the neighbouring tissue. It rarely

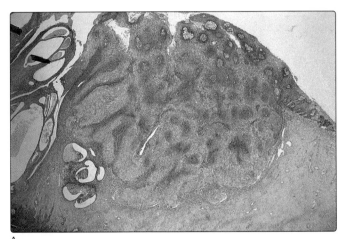

A

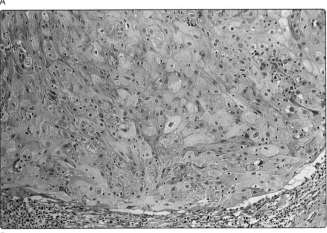

B

Fig. 30.63 (A, B) Verrucous squamous cell carcinoma. Histology shows a raised exophytic tumour mass composed of pale squamous cells with ample cytoplasm and bland nuclei. The lower border of the tumour has a pushing margin but islands of invasive carcinoma cells can be seen in the stroma. (H&E × LP and HP)

metastasizes. The cytology can be misleading because of the absence of nuclear characteristics of malignancy. The cervical smear is dominated by cells with thick, keratinized cytoplasm and small pyknotic nuclei. Ulceration of the tumour and purulent discharge may be reflected by the presence of blood and leucocytes in the smear.

The distinction from condyloma acuminatum is important and it may be the persistence or recurrence of the clinical abnormality, which eventually leads to a sufficiently large biopsy being taken to establish the correct diagnosis. Human papillomavirus has been identified in the tumour cells[59].

Borderline nuclear changes

Borderline nuclear change is the term used in the BSCC terminology[45] to categorize changes where there is genuine doubt as to whether or not they represent neoplasia. The use of a borderline or atypical category (atypical squamous cells and atypical glandular cells of undetermined significance (ASCUS and AGUS) in the Bethesda system[50] is necessary in the practice of cervical cytology because some smears cannot confidently be classified as normal or dyskaryotic. This relates to the lack of robust and objective criteria for clear distinction between reactive or inflammatory change and dyskaryosis, which form a continuum of change; the difficulty in assessing the significance of minor nuclear changes associated with human papillomavirus infection; and the difficulty of confident diagnosis of the more subtle presentations of dyskaryosis, especially if the suspect cell population is scanty.

In screening terms, the significance of the borderline category is that a proportion of women with persistent borderline nuclear change will be found to have CIN when they are investigated by colposcopy. For example, Parham *et al.*[64] found that there was a 23% excess of dyskaryosis in the repeat smear of patients after a report of borderline nuclear change compared with controls, and of those who attended for colposcopy 11% had biopsy confirmed CIN. Nevertheless, the vast majority of these women do not have CIN, and the consequence is that large numbers of women who have no risk of developing invasive cancer in the next screening interval are investigated by colposcopy. This adds substantially to the costs of screening and is a significant cause of psychosexual morbidity. This need for investigation seriously impairs the effective specificity of the cervical smear test, and probably the most serious valid criticism of cervical screening programmes is the lack of specificity of the smear test. There is a need for improvement in the screening process in this respect, and testing for human papillomavirus and its subtypes to decide which of these women with borderline nuclear changes in their cervical smears require further investigation, is a possible way forward[39]. The reporting of borderline nuclear change may be regarded as an unsatisfactory outcome of the test and, within the limits of safe reporting, its use should be minimized.

The BSCC terminology[45] stressed that this categorization should be made only after careful scrutiny of all the material on the smear, as this may reveal unequivocal abnormalities in other cells. In practice, its use is difficult to monitor because the smear test is less sensitive for minor abnormalities, the area from which the cells are originating on the cervix may be small and difficult to sample reliably, the lesion is likely to progress or regress in a short time scale, and there is no definite histological equivalent. The use of the borderline (or atypical) smear report tends to vary widely between centres and individual cytologists[65]. Concern arose in the UK about borderline reporting rates in the early 1990s and a working party was convened to examine the problem and attempt to refine the use of the term borderline nuclear change[66].

In 1995, the UK NHS cervical screening programme published targets for reporting rates[67], that for mild dyskaryosis and borderline nuclear changes being combined at $5.5 \pm 1.5\%$ of all smears (the need to combine the two categories is itself an indicator of the difficulty in consistent classification of the two groups). An appropriate target range will vary with the population being screened and the reporting system in use, but the establishment of such a range for a particular screening programme may be a valuable quality assurance tool. The Bethesda system suggests as a general guide that the rate of reporting of ASCUS should not exceed 2–3 times the rate of SIL[68].

Cytomorphology of borderline nuclear change
Changes associated with human papillomavirus (HPV) infection

The cell changes associated with HPV infection have already been described in detail in Chapter 28 and here above. Nuclear abnormality is usual, if not invariable, but the nuclear changes may fall short of mild dyskaryosis. The changes may include nuclear enlargement, minimal irregularities of outline, pyknosis, or coarsening of the chromatin pattern (Figs 30.64–30.68). Abnormal keratinization or dyskeratosis frequently accompanies HPV infection but is not specific for it. If anucleate or dyskeratotic squamous cells are present in smears they should be examined carefully but if the nuclei are entirely normal and no koilocytes are present the smears, in the absence of other significant abnormality, may be reported as negative[67]. Dyskeratotic cells with nuclear enlargement and chromatin condensation (Fig. 30.69) not amounting to mild dyskaryosis should be reported as borderline nuclear change. Whether or not koilocytes may have entirely normal nuclei is debated but current UK recommendations[67] are that all smears considered to show morphological evidence of HPV infection should be considered at least borderline. This differs significantly from the Bethesda System. In Bethesda cells showing HPV cytopathic effect are classified as LSIL, but the criteria for HPV effect are strict and demand well-defined, optically

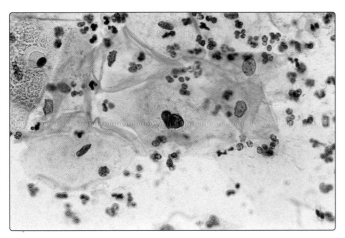

Fig. 30.64   Borderline nuclear change. In the centre is a binucleated cell with slight nuclear enlargement and hyperchromasia, but no abnormality of chromatin pattern. Compare with the adjacent normal nuclei. The change may be HPV related. (Papanicolaou × HP)

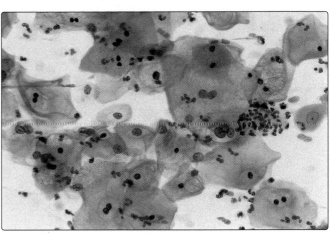

Fig. 30.66   HPV related borderline nuclear change. Koilocytosis, and nuclear changes including pyknosis, nuclear enlargement, bi- and multinucleation are seen in this field. (Papanicolaou × MP)

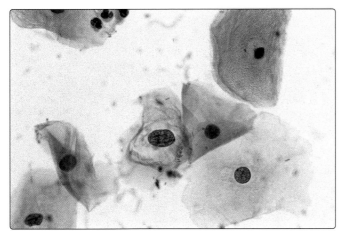

Fig. 30.65   Borderline nuclear change. The cell in the centre is a koilocyte with nuclear enlargement, longitudinal nuclear folding and slight coarsening of the chromatin pattern, but not amounting to mild dyskaryosis. Compare with the adjacent normal intermediate squamous cell nuclei. (Papanicolaou × HP; ThinPrep®)

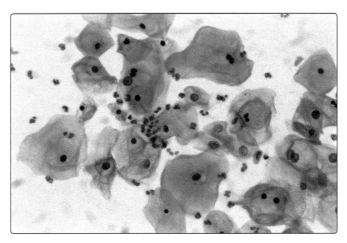

Fig. 30.67   HPV related borderline nuclear change. Koilocytosis, binucleation, nuclear pyknosis and enlargement are seen in this field. (Papanicolaou × MP)

clear perinuclear cytoplasmic vacuolation with a thickened peripheral cytoplasmic rim as well as nuclear abnormality. Cells with perinuclear cytoplasmic haloes without nuclear abnormality are considered to show a benign cellular change and are not classified as ASCUS or LSIL[69].

Changes associated with inflammation

Mild hyperchromasia and nuclear enlargement are commonly associated with inflammatory and reactive changes, but if coarsening of the chromatin pattern is present or there are degenerative or minor irregularities of nuclear outline confident distinction from dyskaryosis may not be possible. Immature metaplastic squamous cells may present particular problems as a wider range of morphological features is acceptable as normal than in mature squamous cells. Small metaplastic cells in particular

may have high nuclear/cytoplasmic ratios. Simple nuclear folds are not uncommon and degenerative changes may occur. Some metaplastic cells have intracytoplasmic vacuoles which indent the nuclear membrane leading to apparent irregularities of outline which may be deceptive especially at screening magnification. There may be bi- or multinucleation. The usual problems leading to a categorization of such cells as borderline are: hyperchromasia beyond that acceptable as reactive change; coarsening of the chromatin pattern in the absence of overt dyskaryosis; difficulty in distinguishing between simple nuclear folding, degenerative change and the irregular folding associated with dyskaryosis; minor variations in nuclear shape with smooth outlines.

Interpretation of such details may be exceptionally difficult especially in scanty populations or if the cells are

747

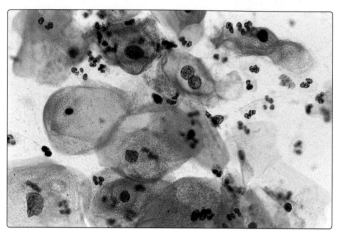

Fig. 30.68 HPV related borderline nuclear change. Koilocytosis, binucleation, nuclear enlargement and slight coarsening of the chromatin pattern, falling short of mild dyskaryosis, are seen in this field. (Papanicolaou × HP)

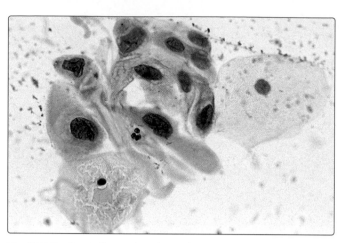

Fig. 30.70 Borderline nuclear change in metaplastic cells. The nuclei of these metaplastic cells show nuclear folding and angulation, but no convincing chromatin abnormality. (Papanicolaou × HP)

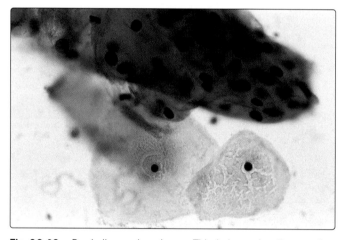

Fig. 30.69 Borderline nuclear change. This dyskeratotic cell group shows mild nuclear enlargement and anisonucleosis. Peripheral condensation of the chromatin can be seen in some of the nuclei. Compare with the adjacent normal superficial cell nuclei. Koilocytes were present elsewhere in the smear. (Papanicolaou × HP; ThinPrep®)

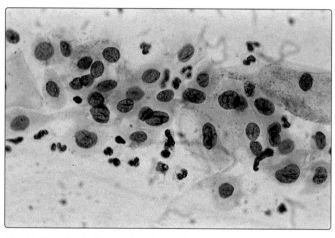

Fig. 30.71 Borderline nuclear change in metaplastic cells. These nuclei show a range of change from normality and include slightly enlarged and folded nuclei, but there is no convincing chromatin abnormality. (Papanicolaou × HP)

partly obscured by polymorphs or other smear components. (Figs 30.70, 30.71) When a confident decision cannot be reached the borderline category may have to be used.

Repair and regeneration

This type of change is described in Chapter 28. Usually it can be recognized as an entity and dismissed as insignificant. Although the cells may have large nuclei with prominent, sometimes multiple nucleoli and some granularity or coarsening of the chromatin, it remains evenly distributed. Repair cells often occur in more or less monolayered sheets and consist of cells with usually low nuclear/cytoplasmic ratios. If the cells are not monolayered, and particularly if they occur in three-dimensional clusters the nuclear detail may be difficult to observe and dismiss as insignificant. In these circumstances the borderline nuclear

change category may need to be used. Care should be taken in the assessment of apparent repair change, especially when the cells form three-dimensional clusters. Occasionally severe dyskaryosis mimics repair change, and it is important not to overlook this especially when large nucleoli are present in severely dyskaryotic nuclei, a feature likely to be associated with invasive carcinoma. Squamous dyskaryosis of more usual appearance can usually be found in the smear when this occurs.

Three-dimensional cell clusters

Three-dimensional cell clusters frequently pose problems in smear interpretation. Examination of the architecture may readily reveal the cell type as squamous, endocervical or endometrial. Abnormal cell clusters frequently have thick or 'steep' edges and disorderly cell arrangements.

Especially when crowded, it may be very difficult to discern individual nuclear detail. There may be doubt about the type of cell within the group leading to, for example, a differential diagnosis of small cell severe squamous dyskaryosis *vs* endometrial cells. Alternatively the type of cell may be in no doubt, but there is difficulty in deciding whether the nuclei are dyskaryotic or not. Careful attention to cytological detail is necessary where the cells can be clearly seen, and sometimes this is possible only if cells are breaking away at the edges of such groups. Cells in three-dimensional fragments of CIN 3 may appear deceptively orderly and occasionally clustered severely dyskaryotic cells merge with morphologically normal endocervical cells. Mitotic figures may be seen in benign or neoplastic cell groups and unless they are recognizably abnormal or particularly numerous, their observation may not be helpful in reaching a diagnosis. In abnormal three-dimensional clusters, nuclear crowding and overlap may lead to over-estimation of the degree of dyskaryosis present.

If a decision cannot be made, it may be necessary to use the borderline category but it is important that the nature of the cytological problem is transmitted in the report.

Borderline nuclear changes in endocervical cells

The range of inflammatory or reactive change in endocervical cells and their nuclei is considerable. There is overlap between the nuclear features which may be seen in extreme inflammatory change, and those which may be seen in at least some examples of cervical glandular intraepithelial neoplasia (CGIN) (see Chap. 32). Recognition of the characteristic architectural features in cell groups is very important in the diagnosis; without obvious and unequivocal endocervical cell dyskaryosis, the cytological diagnosis of CGIN should not be made in the absence of those architectural features. In the absence of overt dyskaryosis, the following features may be considered borderline nuclear change in endocervical cells[67]:

▶ Three-dimensional cell groups with disorderly cell arrangements (Figs 30.72, 30.73)
▶ Coarse grainy chromatin (Figs 30.72, 30.73)
▶ Hyperchromasia with intercellular variation in nuclear staining intensity
▶ An irregular nuclear membrane (not due to distortion by a cytoplasmic vacuole)

None of the architectural abnormalities characteristic of CGIN is absolutely specific or diagnostic and if CGIN is present examples of the abnormalities will usually be seen repeated in the abnormal cellular material. This means that if the cellular material in question is scanty in a smear confident diagnosis of CGIN may not be possible. It may be justifiable to use the borderline category in these cases (see below).

Management of women whose smears show borderline changes

Where borderline nuclear changes are apparently HPV related, or the differential diagnosis is between inflammatory change and mild dyskaryosis, repeat cytology in six months is appropriate, with referral for colposcopy after no more than three such smears in total over a period of, e.g. one year. If, however, the differential is between normality (including reactive or benign cellular changes) and severe dyskaryosis, as is sometimes the case, for example, in small metaplastic or parabasal cell populations, or in the case of three-dimensional cell groups, immediate referral for colposcopy may be warranted. It is important that the reason for the use of the borderline category and nature of the problem are transmitted in the report. In the Bethesda system, it is recommended that the categorization of a smear as showing ASCUS should be qualified to indicate whether a reactive process or SIL is favoured;

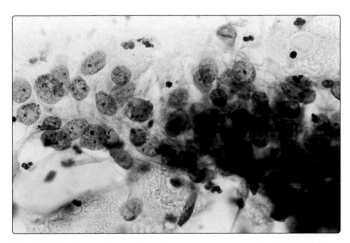

Fig. 30.72 Borderline nuclear change in endocervical cells. This cell group is three-dimensional with nuclear crowding. Where individual nuclei can be seen there is anisonucleosis and mild coarsening of the chromatin. (Papanicolaou × HP)

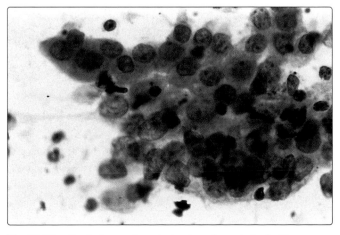

Fig. 30.73 Borderline nuclear change in endocervical cells. The endocervical cells in the upper part of the field appear normal but they merge with cells showing disorderly, crowded and enlarged nuclei with coarsening of the chromatin pattern. (Papanicolaou × HP)

communication to the clinician of the degree of concern about the cytological changes may help determine the appropriate management[69].

Borderline nuclear changes in endocervical cells, especially if used for scanty suspect endocervical cellular material for which a more definite categorization cannot be made, should be recognized as a special group. If immediate referral is not warranted, the smear should be repeated after a maximum of three months with endocervical brushings. If any doubt persists, the patient should be referred for investigation without further delay[67].

The cervical smear test in pregnancy

Dyskaryosis is seen in cervical smears from pregnant women. The cytological appearances and their origin from CIN are the same as in non-pregnant women. There is no evidence that the disease behaves differently in pregnancy, contrary to the views expressed in early papers. It was noticed that some women with abnormal smears during pregnancy, some of whom had biopsies which confirmed preinvasive disease, appeared not to have any CIN after delivery. The disappearance of lesions may be the result of removal by biopsy and resolution of residual CIN, but it is also possible that the trauma of delivery accounts for the loss of abnormal epithelium. The failure to obtain abnormal cells from a part of the transformation zone which is within the endocervical canal during the involutionary period post partum must also be considered and further smear tests should be undertaken subsequently over a period of at least two years because the abnormality tends to reappear.

Management of dyskaryosis in pregnancy

The management of women with an abnormal smear during pregnancy depends to some degree on the abnormality in the smear. Women with borderline changes or mild dyskaryosis may be followed by repeat smears but those with moderate dyskaryosis or worse should be referred for colposcopy. The cervix may be examined to exclude the presence of an invasive lesion but if CIN only is identified the patient is best managed conservatively and biopsies avoided[69]. Biopsy and treatment can be carried out postnatally.

Accuracy of cervical cytology

The preceding descriptions of dyskaryotic cells are comparable with the surface layer of cells seen in histological sections of the cervix with CIN. It is this close relationship which gives the cervical smear test its remarkable value as an indication of the condition of the whole thickness of the epithelium. In practice, however, the relationship is not perfect and merits further scrutiny.

Specificity of the cervical smear test

Severe dyskaryosis in a cervical smear which has been properly taken and interpreted, is the most accurate or specific abnormal cytological diagnosis, because the patient

is at least 90% certain to have a high-grade of CIN or invasive carcinoma. Figures taken from the earlier years of the UK cervical screening programme, when knife cone biopsies were used routinely for simultaneous diagnosis and treatment by excision, are shown in Table 30.7. These are derived from the Department of Health returns (on form SBH 140) from every National Health Service laboratory in England and Wales and include histological biopsy results for cervical smears indicating severe dysplasia or carcinoma *in situ*, for 3 out of 12 months of each year. The use of colposcopy for smaller directed biopsies may be responsible for the slight rise in false positive cytological diagnosis in 1985, because the small tissue sample restricts the search for histological confirmation of the abnormality perceived in the cervical smear. The overall accuracy of the cytological prediction of CIN 3 collected from many centres is apparent in these figures.

Since 1995, the positive predictive value of a cervical smear showing moderate dyskaryosis or worse for a histological diagnosis of CIN 2 or worse has been used as a laboratory performance indicator in the UK cervical screening programme. The target range is 65–85%[68]. In 1998-9 three-quarters of a total of 171 laboratories in England returned positive predictive values between 70% and 90%. For all laboratories the outcome for smears showing moderate dyskaryosis or worse was invasive cancer 2.7%; CIN 2, CIN3 or adenocarcinoma *in situ* 72%; and CIN 1 13%; no CIN was detected in only 13%[70]. Mild and moderate dyskaryosis in cervical smears provide a less accurate prediction of CIN 1 and CIN 2 than the prediction of CIN 3 or carcinoma with a smear report of severe dyskaryosis. Colposcopic examination and biopsy of the cervix when cytology has shown mild dyskaryosis gives a range of histology results from normal to CIN 1, CIN 2, CIN 3 and even an occasional invasive carcinoma. In 1984, Singer *et al.*[71] reported a series of 145 patients with cervical smears which predicted CIN 1. Colposcopically directed biopsies confirmed CIN 1 in 44 cases (30%), HPV infection in 16 (11%) and normal epithelium in 34 (23%), but in 32

Table 30.7 Negative cervical biopsies in women with positive cervical smears in the first three months of each year, England and Wales 1973–85

	Number of Positive* smears	Percentage biopsied	Percentage negative** histology
1973	2533	79.2	3.4
1976	3023	74.1	2.9
1979	3643	72.8	3.6
1982	5080	77.4	2.9
1985	7296	82.3	4.7

UK Department of Health Statistics (Form SBH 140)
*Positive cervical smear indicates severe dysplasia/carcinoma *in situ* (CIN 3)
**Negative histology indicates no dysplasia or carcinoma *in situ* (no CIN)

patients (22%) histology showed CIN 3, one had microinvasion and 18 patients had CIN 2. In the same series, cytological prediction of CIN 3 was confirmed histologically in 95 out of 141 cases; three had microinvasion, and another three had invasive carcinoma.

Similar results have been reported by others, including Robertson *et al.*,[72] who found a poor correlation between a single smear showing mild dyskaryosis and the biopsy result, although agreement improved with a series of smears. They followed up 1347 women who had mildly dyskaryotic smears initially. Over the first two years 625 cases (46%) regressed to normal on cytology and 140 (10%) had normal biopsies, 355 (26%) had CIN 1 or CIN 2 on biopsy and four had HPV, whereas 201 (15%) had CIN 3, four had invasive cancer and for 18 the biopsy result was not known. This evidence provides the basis for management of patients with abnormal cervical cytology. It also demonstrates the probability of making a correct or incorrect histological prediction from the cytological specimen.

Sensitivity of the cervical smear test

The accuracy of a normal (or negative) cervical smear result, if the specimen is properly taken and reliably screened and interpreted, gives good protection against the development of cervical cancer within the next three to five years, but it does not exclude the presence of small areas of usually low-grade CIN. Colposcopic examination and cervicography are more sensitive tests for CIN, but they are not practical screening procedures, because they are too sensitive and would involve too many women in largely unnecessary investigations and treatment for small, mostly low-grade CIN and HPV infections. Giles *et al.*[28] offered cervical cytology and colposcopic examination with biopsy when appropriate to 200 asymptomatic women in a general practice. The results show prevalence of CIN detected by one cervical smear as 5%, whereas by colposcopy it was 11%. The sensitivity of the cervical cytology was related to the area of cervical epithelium with CIN (Table 30.8). The availability of colposcopy has made it easier to estimate the sensitivity of the smear test. In a study comparing the cervical smear test with colposcopy and cervicography, Campion *et al.* reported a sensitivity for detection of CIN 2 and CIN 3 of 78%, and an overall sensitivity of 68%[73]. Failure of the cervical smear test to detect all CIN is largely due to the sampling method. A small area of epithelium may not be abraded by the spatula if pressure is too light or if the whole of the transformation zone is not scraped. Cells from a relatively large area of CIN 1, for example, may be present in the sample, but smaller areas of CIN 2 or CIN 3 may not be represented. A significant proportion of the cellular material sampled remains adherent to the traditional wooden spatula and is not transferred to the glass slide. Some areas of the traditionally prepared smear may be too thick for accurate microscopy. Thus even when abnormal cells are scraped from the cervix they may not be transferred

Table 30.8 Cervical cytology and colposcopic biopsy histology related to the area of abnormality in 22 cases out of 200 asymptomatic women screened by cytology and colposcopy

Area of CIN on cervix	No. of cases	Histology	Cytology
Greater than two quadrants	3	CIN 3	Severe dyskaryosis
	1	CIN 3	Mild dyskaryosis
	1	CIN 2	Moderate dyskaryosis
	1	CIN 2	Unsatisfactory smear
	1	CIN 1	Moderate dyskaryosis
	3	CIN 1	Mild dyskaryosis
Two quadrants	2	CIN 2	Normal
	2	CIN 1	Normal
One quadrant	1	CIN 2	Normal
	1	CIN 1	Mild dyskaryosis
	2	CIN 1	Normal
	4	CIN 1	Unsatisfactory

After Giles *et al.*[28], reproduced with permission, *BMJ* Publishing Group

to, or be visible on the slide. Liquid-based cytology offers a solution to these last two factors. Unfortunately, laboratory errors occur resulting in false negative test results. Some laboratory false negatives are difficult to explain, but scanty abnormal cells are difficult to detect. There is now strong evidence suggesting that fewer than about 200 dyskaryotic cells in a smear, especially if dispersed singly and not showing marked nuclear hyperchromasia, are not reliably detectable by a human screener[54,74,75].

Nevertheless, despite the above imperfections, the cervical smear is a sufficiently accurate test for a screening programme for prevention of cervical cancer, as shown in the successful screening programmes already referred to[17].

Management of the patient with abnormal cytology

It is widely agreed that the risk of progression to invasive cancer is an indication for further investigation and treatment of women who have cervical smears showing moderate or severe dyskaryosis (high-grade SIL in the Bethesda system).

The management of the much more common cytological diagnosis of mild dyskaryosis (low-grade SIL in the Bethesda system) and changes of HPV is less well defined. Until there is a reliable means of distinguishing the premalignant mild dyskaryosis from the mild dyskaryosis that will regress, many more women will be treated for CIN than would develop cervical cancer if they were not treated. The probability of approximately 30% of regression to normal after one mildly dyskaryotic smear must be balanced against the generally slightly lower probability of the presence of CIN 2 or CIN 3.

Mild dyskaryosis on more than one occasion requires colposcopic examination and biopsy of abnormal epithelium. One cervical smear test showing mild dyskaryosis or borderline changes may be followed up by cytology alone approximately six months later in an asymptomatic woman[76].

It is important to be aware of the relatively poor sensitivity of the smear test in the presence of invasive cervical cancer and to advise examination by a gynaecologist even for a mildly dyskaryotic smear if there is abnormal bleeding or discharge.

Follow-up after dyskaryosis or CIN

Patients who have had dyskaryosis either treated or untreated remain at risk of development of invasive cancer. The risk is higher than for women who have never had abnormal cervical cytology[14,77]. Close surveillance is advised for at least five years after treatment of CIN 2 or CIN 3[77]. Women who have had just one mildly dyskaryotic smear followed by three normal smear tests may return to the screening interval advised for well women[78].

Hysterectomy for women with a past or current history of CIN should be carefully carried out so that all of the abnormal epithelium is removed. If there is any suspicion that it has not all been excised, a follow-up programme of vaginal vault cytology will be required beyond the normal postoperative period of close surveillance[77]. Fawdry's review of cytology records of 1062 patients with histologically proven CIN 3 at the time of hysterectomy found that 10 of them had positive cytology in the first postoperative year and only one other patient had a recurrence after four years[79]. His findings suggest that the low detection rate after the first postoperative year does not justify annual vault smears thereafter if the CIN has been completely excised at hysterectomy.

References

1 Pisani P, Parkin D M, Bray F, Ferlay J. Estimates of the worldwide mortality from 25 cancers in 1990. *Int J Cancer* 1999; **83**: 18–29

2 Parkin D M, Whelan S J, Ferlay J et al. eds. *Cancer Incidence in Five Continents*, vol. VII. Lyon: IARC Scientific Publications, 1997; No. 143

3 Keighley E. Carcinoma of the cervix in prostitutes in a women's prison. *Br J Vener Dis* 1968; **44**: 254–255

4 Skegg D C G, Corwin P A, Paul C, Doll R. Importance of the male factor in cancer of the cervix. *Lancet* 1982; **2(8298)**: 581–583

5 Buckley C H, Fox H. Carcinoma of the cervix. In: Anthony P P, MacSween R N M eds. *Recent Advances in Histopathology* 14. Edinburgh: Churchill Livingstone, 1989; chap 4, 63–78

6 Vizcaino A P, Moreno V, Bosch F X et al. International trends in the incidence of cervical cancer: 1 Adenocarcinoma and adenosquamous cell carcinomas. *Int J Cancer* 1998; **75**: 536–545

7 Anderson M, Jordan J, Morse A, Sharp F. In: *A Text and Atlas of Integrated Colposcopy*. London: Chapman and Hall, 1992; 108–110

8 FIGO 1994. Cervical and vulva cancer: changes in FIGO definitions of staging. *Br J Obstet Gynaecol* 1996; **103**: 405–406

9 Jafari K. False negative Pap smear in uterine malignancy. *Gynecol Oncol* 1987; **6**: 76–82

10 World Health Organization. International classification of tumours, no. 8. In: Ritton G, Christopherson W M eds. *Cytology of the Female Genital Tract*. Geneva: World Health Organization, 1973

11 Richart R M. Natural history of cervical intraepithelial neoplasia. *Clin Obstet Gynecol* 1967; **10**: 748–784

12 Kinlen L J, Spriggs A I. Women with positive cervical smears but without surgical intervention. *Lancet* 1978; **2(8087)**: 463–465

13 McIndoe W A, McLean M R, Jones R W. The invasive potential of carcinoma *in situ* of the cervix. *Obstet Gynecol* 1984; **64**: 451–458

14 Walton R J. Cervical cancer screening programs. *J Can Med Assoc* 1976; **114**: 1003–1033

15 Reagan J W, Hicks D J, Scott R B. Aytpical hyperplasia of the uterine cervix. *Cancer* 1955; **8**: 42–45

16 Spriggs A I, Bowey C E, Cowdell H. Chromosomes of precancerous lesions of the cervix uteri. *Cancer* 1971; **27**: 1239–1254

17 Gustafsson L, Ponten J, Zack M, Adami H-O. International incidence rates of invasive cervical cancer after introduction of cytological screening. *Cancer Causes and Control* 1997; **8**: 755–763

18 Anderson G H, Boyes D A, Benedet J L et al. Organisation and results of the cervical cytology screening programme in British Coumbia, 1955–1985. *BMJ* 1988; **296**: 975–978

19 Cook G A, Draper G J. Trends in cervical cancer and carcinoma *in situ* in Great Britain. *Br J Cancer* 1984; **50**: 367–375

20 Wolfendale M R, King S, Usherwood M M. Abnormal cervical smears: are we in for an epidemic? *BMJ* 1983; **287**: 526–528

21 Parkin D M, Nguyen-Dinh X, Day N E. The impact of screening on the incidence of cervical cancer in England and Wales. *Br J Obstet Gynaecol* 1985; **92**: 150–157

22 Beral V, Booth M. Predictions of cervical cancer incidence and mortality in England and Wales. *Lancet* 1986; **1(8479)**: 495

23 Burghardt E. Premalignant conditions of the cervix. *Clin Obstet Gynecol* 1976; **3**: 257–294

24 Nasiell K, Nasiell M, Vaclavinklova V. Behaviour of moderate cervical dysplasia during long term follow-up. *Obstet Gynecol* 1983; **61**: 609–614

25 Nasiell K, Roger V, Nasiell M. Behaviour of mild cervical dysplasia during long term follow-up. *Obstet Gynecol* 1986; **67**: 665–669

26 Richart R M, Barron B A. A follow-up study of patients with cervical dysplasia. *Am J Obstet Gynecol* 1969; **105**: 386–393

27 Herbert A, Smith J A E. Cervical intraepithelial neoplasia grade III (CIN III) and invasive cervical carcinoma: the yawning gap revisited and the treatment of risk. *Cytopathol* 1999; **10**: 161–170

28 Giles J A, Hudson E A, Crow J et al. Colposcopic assessment of the accuracy of cervical cytology screening. *BMJ* 1988; **296**: 1099–1102

29 Jarmulowicz M R, Jenkins D, Barton S E et al. Cytologicastatus and lesion size: a further dimension in cervical intraepithelial neoplasia. *Br J Obstet Gynaecol* 1989; **96**: 1061–1066

30 McGregor J E. In: Jordan J A, Sharp F, Singer A eds. Preclinical neoplasia of the cervix. *Proceedings of the Ninth Study Group of the Royal College of Obstetricians and Gynaecologists*. London: Royal College of Obstetricians and Gynaecologists, 1982; 95–110

31 Papanicolaou G N, Traut H F. *Diagnosis of Uterine Cancer by the Vaginal Smear*. New York: Commonwealth Fund, 1943

32 Canadian Task Force. Cervical cancer screening programme: summary of the 1982 Canadian Task Force report. *J Can Med Assoc* 1982; **127**: 581

33 Läärä E, Day N E, Hakama M. Trends in mortality from cervical cancer in Nordic countries: association with organised screening programmes. *Lancet* 1987; **1**: 1247–1249

34 Sasaeni P, Adams J. Effect of screening on cervical cancer mortality in England and Wales: analysis of trends with an age period cohort model. *BMJ* 1999; **381**: 1244–1245

35 Herbert A. Effect of screening may have been underestimated (letter). *BMJ* 1997; **314**: 1277

36 IARC Working Group on Evaluation of Cervical Cancer Screening Programmes. Screening for squamous cervical cancer: duration of low risk after negative results of cervical cytology and its implication for screening policies. *BMJ* 1986; **293**: 659–664

37 Szarewski A, Cuzick J, Edwards R et al. The use of cervicography in a primary

screening service. *Br J Obstet Gynaecol* 1991; **98**: 313–317

38   Prismatic Project Management Team. Assessment of automated primary screening on Papnet of cervical smears in the Prismatic trial. *Lancet* 1999; **353**: 1381–1385

39   Cuzick J, Saseini P, Davies P et al. A systematic review of the role of human papillomavirus testing within a cervical screening programme. *Health Technology Assessment* (NHS R&D HTA Programme) 1999; vol. 3, No. 14

40   Mitchell H, Medley G. Longitudinal study of women with negative smears according to endocervical cell status. *Lancet* 1991; **337**: 265–267

41   Boon M E, Alons-van Kordelaar J J M, Rietveld-Scheffers P E M. Consequences of the introduction of combined spatula and cytobrush sampling for cervical cytology. *Acta Cytol* 1986; **30**: 264–270

42   Reagan J W, Seidemann I L, Saracusa Y. Cellular morphology of carcinoma *in situ* and dysplasia or atypical hyperplasia of uterine cervix cancer. *Cancer* 1953; **6**: 224–235

43   Wied G L. Editorial In: *Proceedings of the 1st International Congress of Exfoliative Cytology*, Vienna. Philadelphia: Appleton-Century Crofts, 1962; p 297

44   Spriggs A I, Butler E B, Evans D M D et al. Problems of cell nomenclature in cervical cytology smears. *J Clin Pathol* 1978; **31**: 1226–1227

45   Evans D M D, Hudson E A, Brown C L et al. Terminology in gynaecological cytopathology: report of the working party of the British Society for Clinical Cytology. *J Clin Pathol* 1986; **39**: 933–944

46   Richart R M. A modified terminology for cervical intraepithelial neoplasia. *Obstet Gynaecol* 1990; **75**: 131–133

47   Soutter W P, Wisdom S, Brough A K, Monaghan J M. Should patients with mild atypia in a cervical smear be referred for colposcopy? *Br J Obstet Gynaecol* 1986; **93**: 70–74

48   Walker E M, Dodgson J, Duncan I D. Does mild atypia on a cervical smear warrant further investigation? *Lancet* 1986; **ii**: 672–673

49   National Cancer Institute Workshop. The 1988 Bethesda system for reporting cervical/vaginal cytologic diagnoses. *J Am Med Assoc* 1989; **262**: 931–934

50   Bethesda Workshop. The Bethesda system for reporting cervical/vaginal cytologic diagnoses. *Acta Cytol* 1993; **37**: 115–124

51   Buckley C H, Butler E B, Fox H. Cervical intraepithelial neoplasia. *J Clin Pathol* 1982; **35**: 1–13

52   Stanbridge C M, Suleman B A, Persad R V, el-Katib S. A cervical smear review in women developing cervical carcinoma with particular reference to age, false negative cytology and the histologic type of the carcinoma. *Int J Gynecol Cancer* 1992; **2**: 92–100

53   Smith P A, Turnbull L S. Small cell and 'pale' dyskaryosis. *Cytopathol* 1997; **8**: 3–8

54   Mitchell H, Medley G. Differences between Papanicolaou smears with correct and incorrect diagnoses. *Cytopathol* 1995; **6**: 368–375

55   Vooijs G P. Benign proliferative reactions, intraepithelial neoplasia and invasive cancer of the uterine cervix. In: Bibbo M ed. *Comprehensive Cytopathology*. Philadelphia: Saunders, 1991; 153–230

56   Fox H, Buckley C H. *Histopathology Reporting in Cervical Screening*. Working Party of the Royal College of Pathologists and the NHS Cervical Screening Programme. NHSCSP Publication 1999; No. 10, 2–15

57   Jenkins D, Tay S K, Campion M J et al. Histological and immunocytochemical study of cervical intraepithelial neoplasia associated with HPV 6 and HPV 16 infections. *J Clin Pathol* 1986; **39**: 1177–1180

58   Kaufman R, Koss L G, Kurman R J et al. Editorial: statement of caution in the interpretation of papillomavirus-associated lesions of the epithelium of the uterine cervix. *Acta Cytol* 1983; **27**: 107–108

59   Powell J L, Franklin E W, Nickerson J F, Burrell M O. Verrucous carcinoma of the female genital tract. *Gynecol Oncol* 1978; **6**: 565–573

60   Beyer-Boon M E, Verdonk G W. The identification of atypical reserve cells in smears of patients with premalignant and malignant changes in the squamous and glandular epithelium of the uterine cervix. *Acta Cytol* 1978; **22**: 305–312

61   Tidbury P, Singer A, Jenkins D. CIN 3: the role of lesion size in invasion. *Br J Obstet Gynaecol* 1992; **99**: 583–586

62   Smedts F, Ramaekers F, Troyanovsky S et al. Keratin expression in cervical cancer. *Am J Pathol* 1992; **141**: 497–511

63   Reagan J W, Hamonic M J. Dysplasia of uterine cervix. *Ann NY Acad Sci* 1956; **63**: 1236–1244

64   Parham D M, Wiredu E K, Hussein K A. Significance of borderline nuclear abnormality in cervical smears. *Cytopathol* 1992; **3**: 85–91

65   Reiter, R C. Management of initial atypical cervical cytology: a randomized prospective study. *Obstet Gynecol* 1986; **68**(2): 237–240

66   Buckley C H, Herbert A, Mackenzie E F D et al. Borderline nuclear changes in cervical smears: guidelines on their recognition and management. *J Clin Pathol* 1994; **47**: 481–492

67   Herbert A, Johnson J, Patnick J et al. Achievable standards, benchmarks for reporting and criteria for evaluating cervical cytopathology. *NHS Cervical Screening Programme*, Sheffield 1995; 1st edn, p 24

68   Kurman R J, Solomon D. *The Bethesda System for reporting cervical/vaginal cytologic diagnoses*. New York: Springer-Verlag, 1994

69   Hellberg D, Axelsson O, Gad A, Nillson S. Conservative management of the abnormal smear in pregnancy. *Acta Obstet Gynecol Scand* 1987; **66**: 195–199

70   Department of Health Statistical Bulletin. 1999/32. *Cervical Screening Programme*, England: 1998–99

71   Singer A, Walker P, Tay S K, Dyson J. Impact of introduction of colposcopy to a district general hospital. *BMJ* 1984; **289**: 1049–1051

72   Robertson J H, Woodend B E, Crozier E H, Hutchinson J. Risk of cervical cancer associated with mild dyskaryosis. *BMJ* 1988; **297**: 18–21

73   Campion M J, di Paola F M, Vellios F. The value of cervicography in population screening. *J Exp Clin Cancer Res* 1990; **suppl**, FC/107

74   O'Sullivan J P, A'Hern R P, Chapman P A et al. A case control study of true positive versus false negative smears in women with cervical intraepithelial neoplasia (CIN) III. *Cytopathol* 1998; **9**: 155–161

75   Baker R W, O'Sullivan J P, Hanley J, Coleman D V. The characteristics of false negative cervical smears – implications for the UK cervical cancer screening programme. *J Clin Pathol* 1999; **52**: 358–362

76   Evans D M D, Hudson E A, Brown C L et al. Management of women with abnormal cervical smears: supplement to terminology in gynaecological cytopathology. *J Clin Pathol* 1987; **40**: 530–531

77   Duncan I D, ed. 1997. *Guidelines for Clinical Practice and Programme Management*, Sheffield: NHS Cervical Screening Programme, NHSCSP Publication 1997, 2nd edn, No. 8

78   Jones M H, Jenkins D, Cuzick J et al. Mild cervical dyskaryosis: safety of cytological surveillance. *Lancet* 1992; **339**: 1440–1443

79   Fawdry R D S. Carcinoma *in situ* of the cervix: is post hysterectomy cytology worthwhile? *Br J Obstet Gynaecol* 1984; **91**: 67–92

31 New technologies in cervical screening: an overview

Euphemia McGoogan

Introduction

Over the last 15 years, cervical screening using the cervical smear test (Pap smear) has been introduced successfully in many countries of the world, but during the same period the test has been the subject of recurrent adverse criticism in the world's press. The *Wall Street Journal* headline on 2 November 1987[1] 'Pap test misses much cervical cancer through labs' errors' is now probably the most quoted article in cervical screening. While it led to a critical appraisal of the quality of cervical screening, it unfortunately focused attention on the laboratory as the only source of 'errors'. An earlier article in *The Lancet* in 1985[2], 'Cancer of the cervix: death by incompetence', had identified lack of organization and coordination of call-recall as the cause of the failure of the screening programmes in the UK and Norway, compared with those in other Nordic countries, but this was given scant attention world-wide.

Until the 1990s, the accuracy of the cervical smear had rarely been questioned although its efficacy has never been tested in a prospective blinded trial. The general public and most health care professionals failed to recognize the fundamental limitations of the cervical smear as a screening test and expect standards that even most diagnostic tests cannot achieve[3].

Since the introduction of an organized call/recall programme in the UK in 1988, there has been a sustained increase in population coverage of women in the screening age group (20–64 years) to over 80%, with a concomitant halving of the invasive cancer rate by the mid-1990s and an accelerated decrease in mortality[4,5].

The success of the cervical screening programme in the UK so far, is due to the high population coverage and women regularly attending at an interval of between 3 and 5 years. All areas of the screening programme are now working together as a co-ordinated team. There has been an extensive 'smear taker training programme', which has improved the quality of cervical smears. Implementation of national quality standards and quality assurance not only for laboratories but also for all aspects of the programme including colposcopy and public health has further contributed to improvements in the screening programme.

Despite this, the UK's incidence and mortality from cervical cancer remains one of the highest in the European community. Data from the relatively static population in central Scotland[6], which has been well screened for three decades, suggest that a plateau may have been reached, reflecting a background mortality rate uninfluenced by more frequent cervical screens. If further reductions in the incidence and mortality of cervical cancer are to be achieved, attention must be focused on the screening test itself. Notwithstanding the effectiveness of the cervical smear in an organized screening programme, there is good evidence that the smear test is not sufficiently sensitive, specific, and consistent in reliably detecting the presence of cervical intra-epithelial neoplasia (CIN) in the cervix[7].

In the literature[8-12], the sensitivity of a single cervical smear is assessed at around 50–60%. This is perhaps not surprising since, unlike most other laboratory tests, the cervical smear methodology has remained essentially unchanged in over 60 years. The method of collecting and preparing a cervical sample has inherent limitations that, in organized screening programmes, lead to high inadequate rates and low sensitivity that can only be overcome by repeating the test at regular intervals.

The deficiencies of conventional cervical smears are due to many factors including the use of wooden samplers that are cheap and designed to collect material from the cervix, but are not flexible or designed to spread material evenly on to a glass slide. In addition to variable dexterity in collecting and preparing the sample, smear takers use a multiplicity of different fixatives in a variety of different ways. Thus there are great variations in the quality of smears sent to the laboratory: cellular distribution on the glass slide is uneven; cells may be obscured by blood or inflammatory exudate or thick streaks of other cells; total numbers of abnormal cells may be very few; fixation is variable and partial drying artefact is common, leading to poor staining and loss of microscopic detail. Not only do all of these influence the adequacy of the sample, they also limit the ability of laboratory staff to interpret the cells present in a smear correctly[13]. Sometimes the result is just too few intact cells on the slide, particularly in the presence of atrophy or cytolysis, rendering it inadequate for assessment.

It is worth noting that abnormal cells are not collected evenly on the sampling device and only a selected proportion of the cells are placed on the glass slide[14]. In fact, the amount of material transferred successfully to the glass slide ranges from around 60% at best, to less than 10% at worst and some samplers have more of a trapping effect than others[15]. Thus, depending on the sampler used, up to 90% of the material scraped from the cervix may be discarded with the sampler. Furthermore material is transferred from the sampler to the slide in a non-randomized way and therefore the cells on the glass slide are not necessarily representative of the sample removed from the cervix. The cell distribution on the glass slide is uneven[14,16,17] and abnormal cells may be present only in one small area, rather than evenly distributed across the slide. Contrary to public belief, sampling and preparation together are responsible for about two-thirds of false negative tests[10,18].

The low sensitivity of a single cervical smear is therefore mainly due to incorrect or inadequate sampling of the cervix; poor transfer of cells to the glass slide; a non-representative sample being placed on the slide; sub-optimal preparation and fixation and only to a lesser extent, the microscopic assessment in the laboratory. However all of the above affect the ability of the cytotechnologist to identify abnormal cells on the slide. Only a small proportion of all false negative tests are due to human error in microscopic assessment in the laboratory[3,19].

It is also worth noting that the false negative cervical smear may not be the biggest problem in organized cervical screening programmes. In order to decrease the false negative rate (increase sensitivity), many laboratories have increased the inadequate and false positive rates (decreased specificity). This is particularly true in a climate of litigation. Loss of specificity is particularly important in screening programmes, because false positives cause morbidity and there are social, emotional and economic costs associated with unnecessary referral of women who are essentially normal for a repeat smear or colposcopy. Some 'true positives' may also be a problem if they identify and lead to treatment of conditions such as transient human papillomavirus infection that would not progress to significant neoplastic disease. Several studies have reported spontaneous regression rates up to 60% for squamous lesions identified on cervical smears and referred for colposcopic treatment, especially where the abnormality detected on the smear was low-grade[20]. The false positive cervical smear is far more prevalent and far more costly to the health-care system and causes emotional stress for women.

The move towards new technologies is driven by the need to improve these deficiencies in the current methods of cervical screening. Improvements in diagnostic accuracy of the cervical smear need to begin in the doctor's clinic with improved techniques of specimen collection to allow better quality samples and better slide preparations. If a representative sample is not removed and sent to the laboratory, there is little that laboratory staff can do to improve the sensitivity of the test. Thus the quality of the sample sent to the laboratory, the presentation for microscopic assessment and the accuracy of the observer all need to be addressed. In addition, the world-wide shortage of trained cytologists must also be taken into consideration.

Liquid-based cytology

Over the years different methods to improve the cytological specimen have been proposed. Neugebauer *et al.*[21] in 1981 described a sedimentation velocity separation method; and Näslund[22] suggested a pulse wash method. More recently, Steven *et al.*[23] suggested chemical depolymerization of cervical mucin to help produce monolayers. However, the development of better preparations has been driven by the demands of the early automated scanning devices[24–33] which required a monolayer with as little cellular overlap as possible.

The liquid-based cytology (LBC) technique involves rinsing all the material collected on the sampling device into a preservative fluid, creating a cell suspension. This is the specimen sent to the laboratory rather than a glass slide pre-smeared with cellular material. All of the cells collected from the cervix should therefore be present in the cell suspension sent to the laboratory and the cells remain well preserved for several weeks at room temperature in the preservative fluid[14,16]. In the laboratory the cell suspension can be processed to remove excess blood and inflammatory exudate and a small representative aliquot of epithelial cells deposited in a thin layer on a glass slide. The slide preparations therefore should contain a proportional representation of all epithelial cell types in the sample deposited within a small well-demarcated area on the glass slide.

Slides from the cell suspension may be prepared manually but this is very labour intensive and it is difficult to ensure that a randomized, i.e. a representative, sample of cells is transferred on to the glass slide. There are, however, several devices now commercially available that can do this task in either a semi- or fully-automated fashion. At the time of writing, three of these devices have been approved by the United States Food and Drug Administration (FDA) as suitable for cervical screening: two ThinPrep® Processors manufactured by Cytyc Corporation (Massachusetts, USA) and AutoCyte-Prep® manufactured by TriPath Imaging Inc. (North Carolina, USA).

With the two ThinPrep® processors a plastic collection device is rinsed thoroughly into a vial containing a proprietary transport fluid (PreservCyt®). The basic component of the Cytyc ThinPrep process is a disposable plastic tube with a filter at one end. The uncapped tube with the vial of cell suspension, a labelled electronically charged glass slide and the filter are loaded into the T2000. There are three key phases to the process. Dispersion: the device inserts the tube into the vial of cell suspension, spins it round to disperse mucus and any clumps of cells that have settled at the bottom of the vial. Cell collection: a negative pressure pulse is produced in the tube, which draws the fluid through the filter, trapping a layer of cellular material. Some red cells, polymorphs and cell debris may pass through the filter pores. The flow of fluid through the filter is monitored and controlled to optimize cell collection. Cell transfer: the filter tube is then turned upside down and gently brought in contact with the electronically charged glass slide so that the cells transfer to the glass slide. The glass slide is immediately dropped into a vial of fixative.

The AutoCyte-Prep (previously known as CytoRich) uses a different process. A sample from the cervix is collected using a plastic collection device, such as Cervex®. The head of the broom is detached into a vial containing a proprietary transport fluid (CytoRich™). In the laboratory the vials are vortexed to detach the cells from the broom head. Next, the cell suspension is treated through a density gradient centrifugation process to remove red blood cells and other clinically non-significant material and to enrich the cell suspension. These pre-processing stages are only semi-automated but proprietary Cell-Shaker and Prep-Mate devices are available to facilitate the handling of multiple vials. Racks of up to 48 centrifuge tubes containing cell pellets are placed on an AutoCyte-Prep 'robot' (a Tecan device). Individual settling chambers are clamped to pre-coated glass slides and placed on the Tecan base plate. A robotic arm using disposable pipette tips delivers fluid to re-suspend the pellets and an aliquot is transferred to each settling chamber. The cells are allowed to sediment under gravity to form a thin layer on the slide. After a period of time the excess fluid, including any cells that have not stuck to the glass slide, is pipetted off and then the robotic arm delivers the Papanicolaou stain individually to each staining well. Thus each slide is stained *in situ*.

The ThinPrep device produces slides with cell deposition area of 1.9 cm in diameter containing around 100,000 cells. In contrast the AutoCyte-Prep produces a circle of deposition of 1.3 cm but, since the cells in AutoCyte-Prep are more closely associated than those of ThinPrep, this has a similar number of cells in the area of deposition.

The general appearance of a liquid-based preparation is that of an evenly distributed circular deposit of cells (Fig. 31.1). The margins of the deposit are usually well demarcated and all the cellular material is contained well within the coverslip. The cellular deposit is of uniform thickness and thus the need for frequent focus changes is reduced. Cellular preservation is enhanced and the good fixation allows more consistent staining, resulting in improved microscopic detail (Fig. 31.2). Although liquid-based preparations are flat layers of cells, they are not single cell monolayers. Some sheets of cells are retained, but the cell aggregates are smaller than in conventional smears and, even within groups, most of the nuclei can be assessed

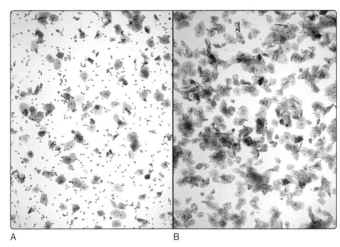

Fig. 31.1   Cellular distribution: low power. (A) ThinPrep (B) AutoCyte-Prep

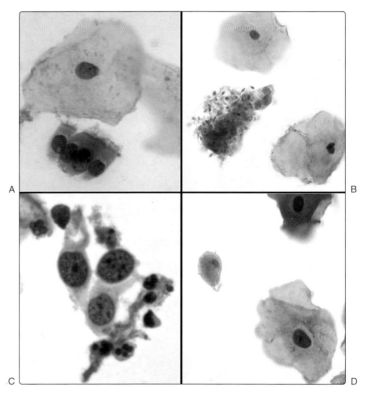

Fig. 31.2   (A,B,C,D) Examples of the good preservation: cilia on endocervical cells, sperm, nuclear chromatin detail in severe squamous dyskaryosis and flagellum on *Trichomonas vaginalis*.

microscopically (Figs 31.3, 31.4). Mucus, blood and cell debris are diminished, as are preparation artefacts such as partial air drying, air bubbles in the mountant or 'cornflake' artefact (Fig. 31.5). With a heavy neutrophil polymorph exudate the preservative fluid tends to stick the cells together to form balls, thus not obscuring epithelial cells on the slide. Background material such as menstrual or inflammatory exudate, cytolysis, microorganisms and tumour diathesis can still be identified, albeit not obscuring the epithelial cells (Figs 31.2, 31.3).

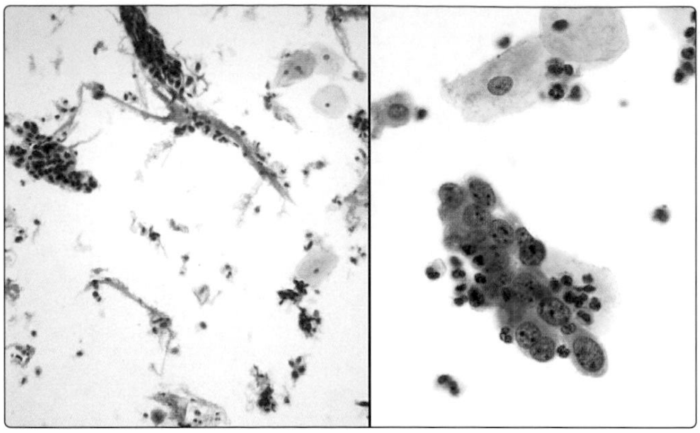

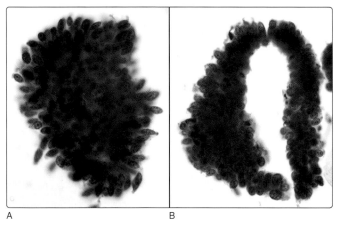

Fig. 31.3 (A,B) Non-keratinizing squamous cell carcinoma: background diathesis and nuclear chromatin detail of malignant cells.

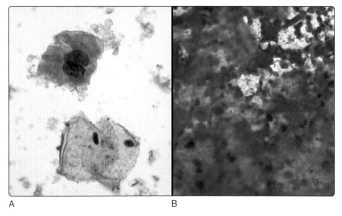

Fig. 31.4 Cervical glandular intraepithelial neoplasia: (A) Feathering at edges of clump (B) Nuclear crowding and pseudostratification.

Fig. 31.5 Split sample (A and B). Conventional smear obscured by blood: unsatisfactory. ThinPrep prepared from left over sample is satisfactory and shows dyskaryotic squamous cells.

Although there is very little available information in peer reviewed literature, the author is aware of a number of other devices currently under development which will also prepare liquid-based cytology samples. These include CYTOSCREEN with its proprietary fluid CYTeasy® and

collection device CYTOPREP® (Seroa), EasyPrep® (Labonord), CellPrint (3t), Cyto-Tek (Bayer), ThinSpin (Shandon), InPath System (Ampersand Medical Corporation) and CYPREP (Veracel, previously known as Morphometrics). While these systems offer alternative and often cheaper methods of processing cell suspensions, evidence of their ability to deliver an appropriate representative cell sample on to the glass slide consistently is not yet available in peer reviewed literature.

Whatever system is used to prepare the liquid-based cytology sample, the difference is obvious even to the naked eye (Fig. 31.1). At present, liquid-based cytology appears to offer an opportunity for improvements to cervical screening through improved collection and preparation techniques designed to provide a more representative sample on the slide, better preservation and staining and less obscuring background material. All the cellular material removed from the cervix is rinsed from the sampler into a preservative fluid so that the entire sample is sent to the laboratory preserved in an optimal state. Thus adequacy is improved, inadequate rates drop, sensitivity can be at least maintained if not improved and specificity is overall improved[19,34–36].

In the UK, with a strict 3 to 5 year screening interval, the criteria for adequacy are more stringent than those of the Bethesda Terminology and the inadequate rate is therefore higher. However, the inadequate rate has increased over the last 10 years to a level of 10%. Therefore, up to 1 in 10 women attending for routine screening must return for a repeat test simply because the first smear was unsatisfactory for interpretation. The main reasons for unsatisfactory smears are that the material is too scanty, too heavily blood-stained, is obscured by inflammatory exudate or too thickly spread. Some samples exhibit so much fixation deficiency and air-drying that the interpretation of the material on the glass slide is compromised. All of these problems could be addressed by liquid-based cytology. For countries with organized screening programmes and stringent criteria for adequacy, the improvements that could be obtained in the inadequate rate alone merit consideration of converting to liquid-based preparations.

Many studies have considered adequacy of liquid-based preparations compared to conventional smears. Unfortunately, the criteria used to define adequacy vary between the studies. Even where the Bethesda System was used, it is likely that it was interpreted in different ways since the criteria applied are either not stated or are very subjective and variable. This makes comparative evaluation difficult. Furthermore, most published studies prior to 1999 were 'split sample', rather than direct to vial. In the split sample studies, a conventional smear was prepared as normal from a single cervical scrape sample and then the liquid-based preparation was made by rinsing the residual material on the device into a vial of preservative fluid. Clearly with split samples there is a substantial 'loss' of cellular material that would otherwise be included in the

Table 31.1 Results of ThinPrep for cervical screening in a Routine Primary Screening Setting in Edinburgh, Scotland

Result	*n*	ThinPrep Health centres 2000–2001	Conv smears Health centres 1999	Overall lab conv smears 2000	UK National standard range 1995–2000	UK National standard range 2001
Inadequate	69	0.55%	10%	10%	7 ± 2%	5.8–12.9%
Negative	11 647	92.03%	82%	00%		
Borderline	333	2.63%	4%	4.5%		
Mild dyskaryoisis	349	2.76%	2.2%	2.5%	5.5 ± 1.5%	4.1–9.5%
Moderate/severe dyskaryosis/glandular neoplasia	256	2.02%	1.4%	1.7%	1.6 ± 0.4%	1.0–2.0%
Total	12 655		8670	86 700		

cell suspension for the liquid-based preparation. In this case one might expect the liquid-based preparation to be scanty and at higher risk of being considered inadequate. However, the majority of studies report that liquid-based methods had a larger proportion of samples classed as totally satisfactory (Fig. 31.5)[7,11,37–43]. According to the calculations of Payne *et al.*[11], the split sample liquid-based preparations appear to have half the unsatisfactory specimen rate of conventional smears (relative risk 0.54, 95% confidence interval 0.51 to 0.56).

Table 31.1 shows the author's experience of a significant decrease in the inadequate rate using ThinPrep direct to vial drawn from routine smears collected from a small number of Primary Care teams in Edinburgh, Scotland. These were compared with conventional smears from the same teams in the previous year and with the overall rates for the laboratory covering all smear takers in South East Scotland.

From the cytologist's point of view, the main advantages of liquid-based preparations are that the cellular material on the glass slide is evenly spread and any abnormal cells present are well preserved, making identification, evaluation and grading easier (Figs 31.4, 31.6, 31.7). Hutchinson *et al.*[14] and Bergeron[37] showed that the liquid-based preparations had greater specimen homogeneity than conventional smears and suggested that this accounted for increased diagnostic accuracy. Since a randomized aliquot of cells is placed on the glass slide, the cell population is representative of the cervical epithelium.

It is difficult to draw clear conclusions due to deficiencies in the study design of many published articles. Many studies lack verification of the diagnosis, negative results are not verified and total study numbers are small, often highly selected and carried out on populations with a high incidence of disease. Nonetheless a consistent finding is an increased detection of abnormal cells in liquid-based preparations using both ThinPrep and AutoCyte-Prep[14,17,19,38,40–72].

Table 31.2 has been extracted from the literature review of Payne *et al.*[11] and contains split sample studies published in the last 6 years where the study number was greater than 1000. Unfortunately the prevalence of significant

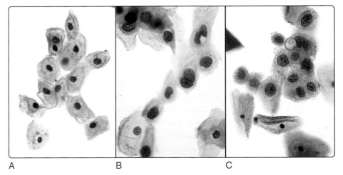

Fig. 31.6 Borderline nuclear changes in (A) Squamous cells (B) Mild squamous dyskaryosis and (C) Moderate squamous dyskaryosis.

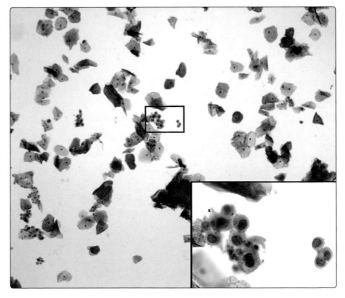

Fig. 31.7 Severe squamous dyskaryosis (inset: cells at high power).

abnormality and hence the type of population studied varies considerably, as shown in column 7. Column 5 indicates the percentage of cases where the conventional smear contained abnormal cells that were not identified in the liquid-based preparation made from the residual material on the sampling device. Column 6 shows where the residual material on the sampling device contained

Table 31.2   Summary of split sample studies with over 1000 cases since 1994

Author	Date	Country	n	Conv >Liq LSIL+	Liq >Conv LSIL+	Both are LSIL+	LBC type
Awen[4]	1994	USA	1000	0.0%	0.5%	1.3%	ThinPrep
Laverty[51]	1994	Australia	1872	2.4%	3.3%	7.5%	ThinPrep
Wilbur[115]	1994	USA	3218	0.8%	3.1%	17.0%	ThinPrep
McGoogan[56]	1996	Scotland	3091	1.0%	0.3%	3.6%	Both AutoCyte-Prep and ThinPrep
Sprenger[89]	1996	Germany	2863	2.0%	5.1%	36.2%	AutoCyte-Prep
Takahashi[95]	1997	Japan	2000	0.4%	0.3%	3.2%	AutoCyte-Prep
Bishop[13]	1997	USA	2032	1.1%	3.1%	3.1%	AutoCyte-Prep
Laverty[50]	1997	Australia	2064	3.9%	1.6%	5.0%	AutoCyte-Prep
Lee[52]	1997	USA	6747	1.9%	3.3%	6.1%	ThinPrep
Roberts[80]	1997	Australia	35 560	0.3%	0.5%	1.7%	ThinPrep
Stevens[93]	1998	Australia	1325	1.3%	0.2%	3.9%	AutoCyte-Prep
Corkill[24]	1998	USA	1583	0.8%	3.7%	1.9%	ThinPrep
Hutchinson[43]	1999	CostaRica	8636	2.5%	2.8%	2.4%	ThinPrep

abnormal cells not identified on the matched conventional smear. In almost all instances the liquid-based preparation found abnormal cells more frequently than the matched conventional smear.

The American College of Obstetricians and Gynecologists gave a Committee Opinion Statement on new screening techniques in 1998. This too concluded that, at that time, there was no large, population-based prospective study to determine whether any of these techniques (including liquid-based cytology) lower the incidence of invasive cervical cancer or improve the survival rate. They recommended that efforts to reduce the false negative rate should not detract from encouraging greater participation in the screening programme[44].

Austin and Ramzy[73] carried out a review of split sample studies in 1998. These authors concluded that liquid-based preparations showed an overall increased detection of epithelial cell abnormalities. They suggested that more recent studies using newer versions of liquid-based preparation devices appeared to be associated with enhanced detection.

Another method of comparing the outcome of liquid-based preparations and conventional cytology is a two cohort analysis. This examines two groups of women whose cervical scrape specimens have been examined by either liquid-based cytology or conventional smears. Vassilakos et al.[74] found that the high-grade abnormality detection rate increased from 0.38% to 0.68% with the use of the AutoCyte liquid-based cytology method, and Diaz-Rosario et al.[52] found a similar increase of 0.27% to 0.53% using ThinPrep. However, as with all split sample studies, these cohort studies only provide a proxy guide to improvements in sensitivity.

Broadstock[75] published a literature review for the New Zealand Health Technology Assessment in 2000. In her opinion the paucity of high quality research meant that it was not possible to reliably determine conclusions from the current evidence base that would be applicable within the New Zealand Cervical Screening Programme.

However, while acknowledging that lack of verification of diagnoses and no randomized control trials with invasive cancer or mortality as the outcome made assessment of sensitivity difficult, Payne et al. concluded for the Screening Programme in the UK 'it is likely that the liquid-based cytology technique will reduce the number of false negative test results, reduce the number of unsatisfactory specimens and may decrease the time need for examination of specimens by cytologists'[11].

More recent direct to vial published studies[37,76] offer a better evaluation of the methodology. Table 31.1 shows the results of direct to vial ThinPrep used in a routine screening situation in Edinburgh for the 18 months, January 2000–June 2001. When compared with the same primary care teams' results for conventional smears in the previous year (1999, column 3) and overall laboratory profile for conventional smears during the same time period (column 4), the LBC method showed a major reduction in inadequates from 10% to 0.6%, a reduction in the borderline from 4% to 2.6%, an overall increase in the detection of dyskaryosis from 3.6% to 4.8% and the high-grade dyskaryosis detection rate increased from 1.4% to 2.2%.

In August 2001, the USA FDA accepted Cytyc Corporation's claim that ThinPrep improves the sensitivity of the Pap test. The submitted data was from a multi-site direct to vial clinical study evaluating T2000 ThinPreps prepared prospectively and compared with a historical control cohort of conventional smears. The results showed a detection rate of 511/20,917 for the conventional smear vs 399/10,226 for the ThinPrep slides. This indicated a 59.7% ($p > 0.001$) increase in the detection of high-grade lesions by ThinPrep.

Factors other than sensitivity and adequacy must be taken into account when considering the clinical and cost effectiveness of liquid-based cytology.

Table 31.3   Primary screening times

Screener	Average time per slide (min)		
	ThinPrep	CytoRich (AutoCyte–Prep)	Conventional smear
A	2.89	2.33	5.45
B	3.06	3.18	6.32
C	4.18	3.94	8.15
Average	3.37	3.11	6.64

There is a world-wide shortage of trained cytotechnologists and cytopathologists and the situation in the UK has currently reached crisis point, with many cytotechnologist and cytopathologist vacancies remaining permanently unfilled. There is much anecdotal evidence that liquid-based preparations are very popular with cytotechnologists. Certainly the initial response is very favourable when viewing liquid-based preparations for the first time. The clarity of presentation, the improved cell preservation and lack of overlapping by other cells, blood or inflammatory exudate are much appreciated. Depositing a representative sample on a discreet small area of the glass slide allows faster and more reliable assessment by laboratory staff. The cells are in a predetermined smaller area on the slide and are mainly in one focus plane when using the ×10 screening objective. The need for continuous major adjustments in focus is therefore eliminated and this allows for significant timesaving when screening the slide. In the Edinburgh study[7] (see Table 31.3), three cytotechnologists of varying experience routinely assessed ThinPrep slides in approximately half the time taken for conventional smears. The paper work, checking the identity of the slide and writing the report take the same amount of time whether using liquid-based preparations or conventional smears but it is clear that the work output of cytotechnologists can increase significantly and up to 60% saving is reported in other studies[17,19,54]. Since the number of unnecessary early repeat smears for inadequate and borderline results will be reduced, overall laboratory workloads should decrease. Thus backlogs can be reduced and turnaround times enhanced even with depleted staffing levels.

Since only an aliquot of cell suspension is removed from the vial, there is sufficient material left to prepare multiple glass slides with an identical cell population that can be used for teaching slide libraries or for external quality assurance schemes. The residual cell suspension can be used for additional investigations such as reflex HPV testing that may further improve the sensitivity and specificity of the screening test (see Chapter 29). Improved distinction between low and high-grade lesions may be achieved on morphology alone using liquid-based cytology and thus over treatment of lesions that would regress spontaneously could be avoided. Additional investigations for sexually transmitted infections such as chlamydia and

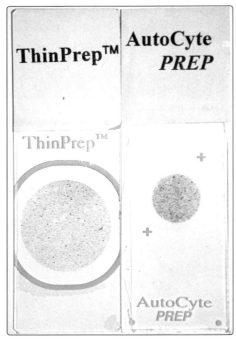

Fig. 31.8   Comparison of ThinPrep and AutoCyte-Prep slides

gonorrhoea can also be carried out on the cell suspensions as can molecular biological techniques and cytogenetic studies. This would prove invaluable should other more specific molecular tests become available in the future to identify women already harbouring or likely to progress to a high-grade lesion that requires treatment.

The nature of the evenly dispersed discreet cell deposit on the slide makes liquid-based preparations eminently suitable for immunocytochemical or immunobiological processes such as *in situ* hybridization and they are also ideal for automated scanning systems[77].

It is somewhat surprising that so much attention has been placed on the use of liquid-based cytology for cervical cytology as a screening test when it is being routinely used for non-gynaecological cytology diagnostic tests. Cytospin preparations have been used for many years for serous fluid and fine needle aspiration samples and more recently an increasing number of laboratories in the UK and North America have been using liquid-based methods for a wide variety of non-gynaecological specimens including respiratory cytology.

However, before a laboratory converts a cervical cytology service to liquid-based cytology, serious consideration must be given to some important issues. Smear takers must use a broom-style plastic sample collection device. Smear taker training in the new technology is critical in that the sampling device must be rotated five times around the full circumference of the transformation zone to collect enough material for an adequate sample. Care must be taken to transfer all the cellular material on the head of the broom or the head of the broom itself if using AutoCyte-Prep, into the vial immediately.

Material management must also be seriously considered. The delivery of supplies of preservative fluid to the clinics and storage space within those clinics must be identified. Vials of preservative fluid have a long shelf life but storage and stock control of collection fluid in such clinics is required. The transport of cell suspensions rather than dry glass slides to the laboratory must also be considered. Transport of samples to the laboratory may need different arrangements. The vials are bulkier, and thus require greater capacity in the collection vehicles.

In the laboratory, an additional resource is required to produce the new slide preparations. Conventional cervical smears arrive in the laboratory already 'prepared' and only require to be stained and coverslipped. Liquid-based cytology samples require preparation first and this has equipment, consumable and staffing resources attached to it. Extra storage space is needed for the vials prior to and following preparation; and disposal of the cell suspensions may also require additional arrangements and resources.

In addition, since the microscopic appearances of liquid-based preparations differ from conventional smears, staff must learn how to interpret these new appearances as well as recognize new 'alarms' to replace the loss of the more familiar clues in conventional smears. There is a steep learning curve and both cytotechnologists and cytopathologists must undertake significant additional training in order to achieve the same sensitivity and specificity on liquid-based preparations as for conventional smears[19,64]. Care must also be taken in the microscopic screening of liquid-based preparations. Fields of view must be overlapped more than for conventional smears; up to 30% overlap is recommended by the author. A high power lens must be used much more frequently to check clumps and single cells since the nuclear detail may indicate that these are neoplastic cells. It must be fully understood that, since only an aliquot of the sample is used for the liquid-based preparation, the total number of abnormal cells on the slide may be considerably fewer than are seen in cellular conventional smears. Great care must be taken not to miss small numbers of single severely dyskaryotic cells from a high-grade lesion.

In conventional smears there are streaks of clear areas with no cellular material, which allow the eye and brain milliseconds of 'rest' during the screening of a smear. Although liquid-based preparations are quicker to screen, the circle of deposition is completely filled by cells that must be analysed and thus the human observer needs to concentrate more intensely during the whole of the screening episode. Some cytologists have reported that, at least initially, they needed to take more frequent rest periods than for conventional smears.

To date, there is no international definition of adequacy for liquid-based cytology samples and it is inappropriate to use the criteria for conventional smears. Bethesda 2001 will attempt to provide a definition for adequacy for liquid-based preparations that may be acceptable in North America. However, in the UK reporting terminology (the dyskaryosis terminology) and criteria for adequacy are markedly different from Bethesda and a definition for use in the UK is required. This should be addressed by the Review of the British Terminology Conference being organized by the British Society for Clinical Cytology in Spring 2002 (website: clinicalcytology.co.uk), the outcome of which is discussed in Chapter 30.

Cost is a major consideration within organized screening programmes and the additional cost of consumables for laboratories is perceived as the disadvantage of liquid-based cytology. The Sheffield School of Health and Related Research (ScHARR) Report[11] estimated the marginal gross cost of consumables and relevant equipment initially associated with introducing the new technique in a typical health authority population of 500 000, and generating around 44 000 smears, at approximately £160 000 per annum. It acknowledged that this cost would decrease as liquid-based preparations reduce numbers of inadequate smears and thus reduce the need to recall women for a repeat smear. The initial capital costs of equipment and staffing efficiencies could be saved if preparation was centralized in a smaller number of processing laboratories. Prepared slides could then be distributed to peripheral laboratories for microscopic assessment. However, major savings from liquid-based cytology will be seen in primary care with fewer women returning to have repeat samples for inadequate tests and borderline results and reductions in the administration for call and recall and fail-safe follow up. There should also be savings in colposcopy clinics if fewer normal women with recurrent inadequate or borderline smears are referred for assessment. Some mechanism to transfer costs from these settings to laboratories must be identified.

The modelling studies in the ScHARR report[11] suggested that the cost effectiveness of liquid-based preparations might be in the ratio of under £10 000 per life saved (at a 5 years screening interval) and under £20 000 per life saved (at an under 3 years screening interval).

Automated scanning devices

Screening of cervical smears is a very monotonous, time consuming and taxing occupation that places great demands on trained staff who are expected to find even a few abnormal cells lying in a cell population of anywhere from 50 000 to 300 000 cells. It is recognized that the monotony of screening large numbers of smears from normal women promotes periods of lack of attention during which rare abnormal cells may be overlooked. It is therefore not surprising that major efforts have been made to automate this function of screening. The development of computerized scanning devices capable of identifying abnormal slides has raised hopes that machines could assume some of the burden of primary screening thus reducing the human effort required to perform this enormous task.

Automated primary screening devices have been promised for more than 20 years. Initial developments took place mainly in Europe but with little success until very recently when computer technology improved enough to meet the challenge. Many companies have attempted to produce an automated primary screening device and millions of dollars have been spent in the process. However, new computer software and hardware developments offer the hope that automated scanning systems may, in the near future, be available to assist with the primary assessment of liquid-based preparations.

One of the early devices was the Cytoanalyser[78], first published in 1956; almost 50 years ago! This brought attention to the fundamental problems with automation of cervical smears. It became quite evident that the similarities between benign and malignant cells were much greater than the differences. Furthermore, differentiating cells touching each other was a very complex task for machines. The TICAS system[79] was capable of more sophisticated cell analysis using not only measurements but also mathematical algorithms derived from histograms of cells. Many other attempts were made to develop systems that would be of practical value in cytology laboratories but without success until very recently[26,31,32,80–93].

The early attempts at automation, however, resulted in the development of principles, which are still applicable to all automated systems and must be taken into consideration by commercial companies developing new systems. The International Academy of Cytology (IAC) Task Force in 1997[94] recommended that the professional in charge of a clinical cytopathology laboratory continues to bear the ultimate medical responsibility for diagnostic decisions made at the facility whether automated devices are involved or not. The IAC Task Force also recommended that the introduction of automated procedures into clinical cytology should under no circumstances lead to a lowering of standards of performance. A prime objective should be to ensure that an automated procedure does not expose any patient to new risks, nor should it increase already existing inherent risks. The Task Force reaffirmed the guidelines developed by the IAC in 1984[95]. The mandatory conditions for all automated systems whether interactive or not were:

1. The system shall not be so designed or constructed as to pass as negative any sample that contains malignant tumour cells
2. The system shall not flag more 'false alarms' on normal cells than could be readily handled by visual manual review
3. The system shall not use up the entire sample nor render the sample unusable for classic microscopic review; the pathologist must be able to examine the sample after routine staining
4. The system shall yield reproducible results on repeated scannings of the same sample (within appropriate confidence limits)
5. The system shall have an internal calibration standard for quality control
6. The system shall identify the inadequate (or empty) slide

Other highly desirable features included were that the system should be able to demonstrate clearly the item that led to an 'alarm' for subsequent review by a human observer and should be able to identify dyskaryotic as well as malignant cells.

Two systems were eventually approved by the Food and Drug Administration (FDA) in the USA in the 1990s; AutoPap 300 (Neopath, Seattle, USA) and PAPNET (Neuromedical Systems Inc., New York, USA). The PAPNET system showed great promise and many laboratories throughout Europe were poised to implement this when the company went into receivership in 1999. A new company, TriPath Imaging Inc., formed from the amalgamation of AutoCyte and Neopath bought the intellectual property rights for the PAPNET system. Tripath chose not to support PAPNET as a primary scanning system and therefore AutoPap 300 remains the only FDA approved commercially available system at present.

AutoPap is a computerized image processor, which uses specially designed algorithms to recognize, analyse and classify both cells and slides and to select a proportion of slides for manual screening by a cytologist. High speed video microscopy, image analysis software and field of view computers are used to classify cell images from conventional smears. The AutoPap 300QC received FDA approval in September 1995 for use in selecting the 10% of slides for full manual rescreening mandated by CLIA 88 (Clinical Improvement Amendment Act 1988, USA). Several studies suggested that the AutoPap 300QC device could provide a five-fold improvement over a 10% random selection method in the detection of false-negative slides[96,97] However, AutoPap 300QC was not Y2K compliant and is no longer commercially available. The AutoPap Primary Screening System[12], which received FDA approval in 1998 for both primary screening and quality control, has replaced it. This system categorizes up to 25% of conventional smears into 'no further review' (i.e. within normal limits requiring no manual microscopic assessment) or 'review' (requiring full microscopic assessment). The review slides are ranked into quintiles according to the probability that they contain abnormal cells and the cytotechnologist is aware of the ranking when screening the slide. A proportion of slides fail processing by AutoPap due to physical characteristics or insufficient cellularity. There is a paucity of studies published in peer review literature and the Agency for Health Care Policy and Research review[10] suggested that further research was needed which allowed the estimation of specificity as well as sensitivity, and used a histological reference standard.

Prior to its merger into TriPath Imaging Inc., AutoCyte was marketing another automated scanning device AutoCyte-Screen, which scanned AutoCyte-Preps[98]. While this system showed great promise TriPath has only continued to market the AutoPap Primary Screener and AutoCyte-Screen is no longer available. However, TriPath Imaging Inc. is at the time of writing exhibiting a new version of their system, the AutoPap GS (Guided Screener), at Trade Exhibitions. This development of the AutoPap uses AutoCyte-Prep slides rather than convention smears and software is available to guide the cytotechnologist to the most suspicious areas on the glass slide using a motorized microscope stage. A slide gallery presented on a monitor adjacent to the microscope supports the cytotechnologist.

It must be recognized that assessing digitized cell images on a monitor is a very different mode of working for cytotechnologists and cytopathologists who are used to assessing moving 3-dimensional microscope images. Digitized images are 2-dimensional and tend to be presented in static phase. Additional training will be inevitably required.

The PAPNET system[99] analysed conventionally prepared smears with a device that used both traditional computer image technology and neural network software. The system selected and displayed up to 128 images of potentially abnormal cells for each case. Images were displayed on a monitor with 16 images per screen at low magnification with the option for viewing tiles at a higher power. When the reviewer identified abnormal cells in any images, the slide was referred for full manual screening. A multicentre trial in the UK[100] had been completed just prior to the company going into receivership.

The Cytyc Corporation is at the time of writing, showing an automated scanning system, the ThinPrep Image Processor, at Trade Exhibitions. A bench-top image processor analyses ThinPrep slides that the cytotechnologist reviews on a microscope with a motorized stage networked to the Processor. Special software takes the reviewer to the 10 most abnormal fields on the slide. No digitized images are presented on a monitor. Other companies such as Veracel (formerly Morphometrics) are also showing primary screening devices at Trade Shows, but there is as yet no data published in peer review journals.

AutoPap is in use in several laboratories in the USA and is used for quality control and occasionally primary screening. In the UK, it is unlikely that the screening programme could afford to use automated scanning devices simply for quality control. Bethesda 2001 recommends that laboratories using automated devices for primary screening or quality control should specify the name of the device and result when a case is examined by an automated device.

Since a variable proportion of slides can be archived without microscopic assessment by trained human observers, it was thought that this might offer major advantages to countries in the developing world, where invasive cancer of the cervix is a major cause of morbidity and mortality. Unfortunately, automated scanning devices are likely to be expensive, require a special environment, a stable electricity supply, appropriate technical and maintenance support and training of staff, especially if these are to be interactive. It is therefore unlikely they will provide an immediate solution for the problems of implementing cervical screening in poorer developing countries. Koss[101] in 1997 stated 'Their (automated scanning devices) use will probably lead to some savings in the cost of screening personnel but I do not envision a fully automated future in which the verdict will be rendered by machine alone. The need for trained personnel will remain but the results of screening may prove to be superior to the current systems.'

Computer assisted microscopy

In the 1990s, there was a vogue to develop computers attached to the microscope, which would support the cytotechnologist with conventional microscopy. One of the most successful was Pathfinder[76,102], manufactured by CompuCyte. The system connected sensors to the microscope stage to a computer and monitor display. This provided a map of which areas of the slide had been screened, useful when training in microscopy techniques and in ensuring the complete screening of slides by cytotechnologists. The device offered feedback to the cytologist and laboratory managers on screening techniques. Quality control data including time spent per slide, percentage coverage of the slide surface and total workload was also collected and analysed. Prior to its merger into TriPath Imaging Inc., Neopath bought CompuCyte and Pathfinder is no longer supported. Zeiss Microscopes produced a similar system called the Highly Optimized Microscope Environment (HOME) and Acumed had a system called ACcell[103]. Unfortunately these systems were costly and perceived as having only 'quality' and cytotechnologist support value and have not been commercially successful. Most are no longer being developed.

Teleconferencing and telepathology

Much of new technology is placing cytopathology and histopathology as a core imaging discipline[104]. Modern technology must be used to input into multidisciplinary networks, facilitate inclusion of images and reference literature in reports and to generate an electronically accessible patient record. Telepathology has been used for remote frozen section diagnosis in Norway for many years[105] and the AFIP and other expert institutions in the USA offer forms of telepathology consultation with specialists and expert pathologists.

Teleconferencing and telepathology are becoming increasingly important in day-to-day working in Pathology in the UK due to the shortage of consultant pathologists and the need for immediate training of more junior medical staff in pathology, particularly in cytology. These systems can be used in training and education; in the assessment of competence and proficiency testing and to allow the 'virtual' attendance at clinical meetings in buildings or hospitals at distant locations. Telepathology offers easier access to peer or expert opinion for difficult slides or for confirmation prior to expensive oncological therapy. It has the added advantage of the interactive educational value of a 'consultation' rather than a written expert opinion received if slides are sent by mail to experts at a distance with inherent time delays. It could also be used to develop standards and standardized criteria by allowing expert groups to view images simultaneously. The development of inter-centre telepathology is a high priority in countries where access to expert pathologists is difficult due to shortages of staff or geography.

Visual inspection of the cervix

In developing countries visual inspection of the cervix is being considered as the screening test. It shows variable sensitivity in the detection of invasive cancer, limited by the experience of the user, but both the sensitivity and specificity in detecting pre-invasive lesions is unsatisfactory. However, it has been promoted as a screening test in India[106]. Aided visual inspection after impregnation with 3–4% acetic acid (cervicoscopy) is being investigated as a means of detecting high-grade CIN lesions as an adjunct to the cervical smear[107]. Aided visual inspection can be further improved using a small lightweight monocular telescope called a gynoscope to visualize the acetic acid impregnated cervical tissue. But it is not clear whether this low-power magnification offers any real benefits over colposcopy and cervicoscopy.

Cervicography

Cervicography involves taking a photograph of the cervix after application of 5% acetic acid under standard conditions of illumination and focal length and then having the pictures reviewed at a later stage by an expert colposcopist for evidence of CIN or cancer[108,109]. Although first developed in 1981 and shown in initial publications to be a sensitive method of detecting cervical lesions, it has a high false positive rate and thus it has not been widely taken up as a primary screening method in countries with organized screening programmes.

Polarprobe

Polarprobe is an electronic method of cervical screening, which uses electrical and optical techniques to distinguish between malignant and non-malignant tissues *in situ*[110]. Unlike other methods of screening it does not rely on the appearance of individual cells but on the characteristics of the cervical epithelium *in situ*. The instrument is 25 cm long, with a 5 mm tip fitted with elements for optical and electrical stimulation of tissue. It relays response signals to a computer. Low voltage electrical impulses and four different wavelengths of light are applied to the surface of the cervix. Normal epithelium, CIN and invasive cancer reflect the light and the voltage in different and characteristic ways. The responses detected by the tip of the probe are relayed to the computer, which has a catalogue of pre-programmed signal patterns for each type of tissue. The probe is gently passed over the surface of the cervix and the operator is immediately informed as to whether abnormal tissue is present. The device is still in research at the time of writing until its efficacy has been fully assessed. It is designed for use in the primary care setting by either the nurse or the doctor. Its potential advantages are its potential for immediate diagnosis, high patient acceptability and objectivity. However low specificity is likely to limit its use as a primary screening tool.

Summary

The key questions facing new technologies in cervical screening are: Will it improve the false negative rate? Can this be done without a significant increase in the false positive rate? Can this be achieved in a cost effective and timely manner? The aims of automation are: to improve the quality of service by decreasing the false negative rate and increasing the recognition of significant precursors; to address the human resource issue by decreasing the work required to be carried out by each cytotechnologist and to address cost effectiveness, allowing at least cost containment for quality screening.

There are major implications for laboratories if such automated systems are introduced. The organization, physical environment and workflow and the role, skills and training of cytologists could all completely change. The increased throughput might allow more frequent screening of the population at no extra cost, decreasing the effect of sampling errors.

New health-care technologies are being marketed more frequently each year. They are usually more expensive, but possibly also more effective. Not only is there a challenge in relation to determining cost effectiveness but, more importantly, in relation to determining clinical effectiveness. It is often not clear which patients will benefit most, what is the balance between benefit and harm, what overall value for money the new technology offers, and whether it will be affordable. Without this information, there is a risk of distorted priorities, as political pressure to keep a lid on budgets creates tension between the claims of different technologies for a part of health-service funding.

References

1 Bogdanich W. Pap test misses much cervical cancer through labs' errors. *Wall Street Journal* 1987: 2 November

2 Cancer of the cervix: Death by incompetence. *Lancet* 1985; **2**: 363–364

3 Koss L G. The Papanicolaou test for cervical cancer detection: a triumph and tragedy. *J Am Med Assoc* 1989; **261**: 737–743

4 Quinn M, Babb P, Jones J, Allen E. Effect of screening on incidence and mortality from cancer of the cervix in England: evaluation based on routinely collected statistics. *BMJ* 1999; **318**: 904

5 Sasieni P, Cusick J, Farmery E. Accelerated decline in cervical cancer mortality in England and Wales. *Lancet* 1995; **346**: 1566–1567

6 van Wijngaarden W J, Duncan I D, Hussain K A. Screening for cervical neoplasia in Dundee and Angus: 10 years on. *Br J Obstet Gynaecol* 1995; **102**: 137–142

7 McGoogan E, Reith A. Would monolayers provide more representative samples and improved preparations for cervical screening? Overview and evaluation of systems available. *Acta Cytol* 1996; **40**: 107–119

8 Fahey M T, Irwig L, Macaskill P. Meta-analysis of Pap test accuracy. *Am J Epidemiol* 1995; **141**: 680–689

9 Hutchison M L, Zahniser D J, Sherman M E *et al*. Utility of liquid-based cytology for cervical carcinoma screening: results of a population-based study conducted in a region of Costa Rica with a high incidence of cervical carcinoma. *Cancer* 1999; **87**: 48–55

10 McCrory D C, Mather D B, Bastian L *et al*. Evaluation of cervical cytology. Evidence Report. *Technology Assessment* No 5. Rockville, Maryland: Agency for Health Care Policy and Research, 1999

11 Payne N, Chilcott J, McGoogan E. Liquid-based cytology in cervical screening: a rapid and systematic review. *Health Technology Assessment* 2000; **4**: No 18

12 Wilbur D C, Prey M U, Miller W M *et al*. The AutoPap system for primary screening in cervical cytology: comparing the results of a prospective, intended use study with routine manual practice. *Acta Cytol* 1998; **42**: 214–220

13 McGoogan E, Colgan T J, Ramzy I *et al*. Cell preparation methods and criteria for adequacy IAC Task Force. *Acta Cytol* 1998; **42**: 25–32

14 Hutchinson M L, Isenstein L M, Goodman A *et al*. Homogenous sampling accounts for the increased diagnostic accuracy using the ThinPrep processor. *Am J Clin Pathol* 1994; **101**: 215–219

15 Rubio C A. The false negative smear II: the trapping effect of collection instruments. *Obstet Gynaecol* 1977; **49**: 576–580

16 Laverty C R, Farnsworth A, Thurloe J K, Bowditch R C. The importance of the cell sample in cervical cytology: a controlled trial of a new sampling device. *Med J Australia* 1989; **150**: 432–436

17 Papillo J L, Lee K R, Manna E A. Clinical evaluation of the ThinPrep method for the preparation of nongynecologic material. *Acta Cytol* 1992; **36**: 651

18 Bergeron C, Debaque H, Ayivi J *et al*. Cervical smear histories of 585 women with biopsy proven carcinoma *in situ*. *Acta Cytol* 1997; **41**: 1676–1680

19 Hutchinson M L, Cassin C, Ball H. The efficacy of an automated preparation device for cervical cytology. *Am J Clin Pathol* 1991; **96**: 300–305

20 Koss L G. In: *Diagnostic Cytology and its Histopathologic Basis*. Philadelphia: Lippincott, 1992; 4th edn, pp 399–414

21 Neugebauer D, Otto K, Soost H J. Numerical analysis of cell populations in smear and monolayer preparations from the uterine cervix. I. The proportions of isolated, abnormal epithelial cells in slides from one applicator. *Anal Quant Cytol* 1981; **3**: 91–95

22 Näslund I, Auer G, Pettersson F *et al*. The pulse wash instrument. A new sampling method for uterine cervical cancer detection. *Am J Clin Oncol* 1986; **9**: 327–333

23 Steven F S, Palcic B, Sin J *et al*. A simple clinical method for the preparation of improved cervical smears-approximating to monolayers. *AntiCancer Res* 1997; **17**: 629–632

24 Bahr G F, Bibbo M, Oehme M *et al*. An automated device for the production of cell preparations suitable for automatic assessment. *Acta Cytol* 1978; **22**: 243–249

25 Barrett D L, King E B. Comparison of cellular recovery rates and morphologic details obtained using membrane filter and cytocentrifuge techniques. *Acta Cytol* 1976; **20**: 174–180

26 Carothers A, McGoogan E, Vooijs P *et al*. A collaborative trial of a semi-automatic system for slide preparation and screening in cervical cytopathology. *Anal Cell Pathol* 1994; **7**: 261–274

27 Husain O A N, Watts K C. Preparatory methods for DNA hydrolysis, cytochemistry, immunocytochemistry and ploidy analysis: Their application to routine diagnostic cytopathology. *Anal Quant Cytol Histol* 1987; **9**: 218–224

28 Oud P S, Zahniser D J, Harbers-Hendriks R *et al*. The development of a cervical smear preparation procedure for the bioPEPR image analysis system. *Anal Quant Cytomet* 1981; **3**: 73–80

29 Oud P S, Zahniser D J, Haag D J *et al*. A new disaggregation device for cytology specimens. *Cytometry* 1984; **5**: 509–514

30 Rosenthal D L, Stern E, McLatchie C *et al*. A simple method for producing a monolayer of cervical cells for digital image processing. *Anal Quant Cytomet* 1979; **1**: 84–240

31 Tanaka N, Ikeda H, Ueno T *et al*. CYBEST-CDMS: Automated cell dispersion and monolayer smearing device for CYBEST. *Anal Quant Cytomet* 1981; **3**: 96–102

32 Tucker J H, Burger G, Husain O A N *et al*. *Measuring the Accuracy of Automated Cervical Cytology Pre-Screening Systems Based on Image Analysis*. Luxembourg: Commission of the European Communities, 1988; EUR 11451 EN

33 Van Driel Kulker A N J, Ploem-Zaaijer J J, Van der Zwan M, Tanke H J. A preparation technique for exfoliated and aspirated cells allowing different staining procedures. *Anal Quant Cytomet* 1980; **2**: 243–246

34 Linder J. The coming era of cytologic automation. *Am J Clin Pathol* 1991; **96**: 293–294

35 Schumann J L. Standardization of specimen acquisition for automated pap smear screening. In: Grohs H K and Husain O A N, Igaku-Shoin eds. *Automated Cervical Cancer Screening*. New York and Tokyo 1994; **11**: 165–175

36 Wilbur D C, Cibas E S, Merritt S *et al*. ThinPrep processor clinical trials demonstrate an increased detection rate of abnormal cervical cytologic specimens. *Am J Clin Pathol* 1994; **101**: 209–214

37 Bergeron C, Bishop J, Lemarie A *et al*. Accuracy of Thin layer cytology in patients undergoing cervical cone biopsy. *Acta Cytol* 2001; **45**: 519–524

38 Guidos B J, Selvaggi S M. Use of the ThinPrep Pap test in clinical practice. *Diagn Cytopathol* 1999; **20**: 70–73

39 Roberts J M, Gurley A M, Thurloe J K *et al*. Evaluation of the ThinPrep Pap test as an adjunct to the conventional Pap smear. *Med J Australia* 1997; **167**: 466–469

40 Shield P W, Nolan G R, Phillips G E, Cummings M C. Improving cervical cytology screening in a remote, high risk population. *Med J Australia* 1999; **170**: 255–258

41 Vassilakos P, Cossali D, Albe X *et al*. Efficacy of monolayer preparations for cervical cytology: emphasis on suboptimal specimens. *Acta Cytol* 1996; **40**: 496–500

42 Weintraub J. The coming revolution in cervical cytology: a pathologist's guide for the clinician. *References en Gynecologie Obstetrique* 1999; **5**: 1–6

43 Wilbur D C, Facik M S, Rutkowski M A *et al*. Clinical trials of the CytoRich specimen-preparation device for cervical cytology. Preliminary results. *Acta Cytol* 1997; **41**: 24–29

44 ACOG Committee. Opinion on new Pap test screening techniques. *Int J Gynecol Obstet* 1998; **63**: 312–314

45 Aponte-Cipriani S, Teplitz C, Rorat E *et al*. Cervical smears prepared by an automated device versus the conventional method. A comparative analysis. *Acta Cytol* 1995; **39**: 623–630

46 Awen C, Hathway S, Eddy W *et al*. Efficacy of ThinPrep preparation of cervical smears: a 1,000-case, investigator-sponsored study. *Diagn Cytopathol* 1994; **11**: 33–36

47 Bishop J. Comparison of the CytoRich system with conventional cervical cytology.

Preliminary data on 2,032 cases from a clinical trial site. *Acta Cytol* 1997; **41**: 15–23

48 Bur M, Knowles K, Pekow P *et al.* Comparison of ThinPrep preparations with conventional cervicovaginal smears. Practical considerations. *Acta Cytol* 1995; **39**: 631–642

49 Carpenter A, Davey D D, ThinPrep Pap Test: performance and biopsy follow-up in a university hospital. *Cancer* 1999; **87**: 105–112

50 Cheuvront D A, Elston R J, Bishop J. Effect of a thin-layer preparation system on workload in a cytology laboratory. *Lab Med* 1998; **29**: 174–179

51 Corkill M, Knapp D, Hutchinson M L. Improved accuracy for cervical cytology with the ThinPrep method and the endocervical brush-spatula collection procedure. *J Low Gen Trac Dis* 1998; **2**: 12–16

52 Diaz-Rosario L A, Kabawat S E. Performance of a fluid-based, thin-layer Papanicolaou smear method in the clinical setting of an independent laboratory and an outpatient screening population in New England. *Arch Pathol Lab Med* 1999; **123**: 817–821

53 Dupree W B, Suprun H Z, Beckwith D *et al.* The promise of a new technology. The Leigh Valley Hospital's experience with liquid-based cytology. *Cancer* 1998; **84**: 202–207

54 Ferenczy A, Robitaille J, Franco E *et al.* Conventional cervical cytologic smears vs. ThinPrep smears. A paired comparison study on cervical cytology. *Acta Cytol* 1996; **40**: 1136–1142

55 Geyer J W, Hancock F, Carrico C *et al.* Preliminary evaluation of Cyto-Rich: an improved automated cytology preparation. *Diagn Cytopathol* 1993; **9**: 417–422

56 Howell L P, Davis R L, Belk T *et al.* The AutoCyte preparation system for gynecologic cytology. *Acta Cytol* 1998; **42**: 171–177

57 Hutchinson M L, Agarwal P, Denault T *et al.* A new look at cervical cytology. ThinPrep multicenter trial results. *Acta Cytol* 1992; **36**: 499–504

58 Iverson D K. Impact of training on cytotechnologists' interpretation of gynecologic thin-layer preparations. *Diagn Cytopathol* 1998; **18**: 230–235

59 Laverty C R, Thurloe J K, Redman N L, Farnsworth A. An Australian trial of ThinPrep: a new cytopreparatory technique. *Cytopathol* 1995; **6**: 140–148

60 Lee K R, Ashfaq R, Birdsong G G *et al.* Comparison of conventional Papanicolaou smears and a fluid-based, thin-layer system for cervical cancer screening. *Obstet Gynecol* 1997; **90**: 278–284

61 McGoogan E. Improved adequacy rates using ThinPrep Pap test for routine cytopathology. *Cytopathol* 1999; **10**: 2

62 Papillo J L. Current status of cytotechnology manpower: will thin layer preparations play an important role? *Diagn Cytopathol* 1994; **10**: 385–387

63 Papillo J L, Zarka M A, St John T L. Evaluation of the ThinPrep Pap test in clinical practice. A seven-month, 16,314-case experience in Northern Vermont. *Acta Cytol* 1998; **42**: 203–208

64 Spitzer M. Cervical screening adjuncts: recent advances. *Am J Obstet Gynecol* 1998; **179**: 544–556

65 Sprenger E, Schwarzmann P, Kirkpatrick M *et al.* The false negative rate in cervical cytology. Comparison of monolayers to conventional smears. *Acta Cytol* 1996; **40**: 81–89

66 Stevens M W, Nespolon W W, Milne A J, Rowland R. Evaluation of the CytoRich technique for cervical smears. *Diagn Cytopathol* 1998; **18**: 236–242

67 Takahashi M, Naito M. Application of the CytoRich monolayer preparation system for cervical cytology. A prelude to automated primary screening. *Acta Cytol* 1997; **41**: 1785–1789

68 Tezuka F, Oikawa H, Shuki H *et al.* Diagnostic efficacy and validity of the ThinPrep method in cervical cytology. *Acta Cytol* 1996; **40**: 513–518

69 Vassilakos P, Cossali D, Albe X *et al.* Efficacy of monolayer preparation for cervical cytology. Emphasis on suboptimal specimen. *Acta Cytol* 1995; **39**: 368

70 Vassilakos P, Griffin S, Megevand E *et al.* CytoRich liquid-based cervical cytologic test. Screening results in a routine cytopathology service. *Acta Cytol* 1998; **42**: 198–202

71 Vassilakos P, Saurel J, Rondez R. Direct-to-vial use of the AutoCyte PREP liquid-based preparation for cervical-vaginal specimens in three European laboratories. *Acta Cytol* 1999; **43**: 65–68

72 Wilbur D C, Dubeshter B, Angel C, Atkinson K M. Use of thin-layer preparations for gynecologic smears with emphasis on the cytomorphology of high-grade intraepithelial lesions and carcinomas. *Diagn Cytopathol* 1996; **14**: 201–211

73 Austin R M, Ramzy I. Increased detection of epithelial cell abnormalities by liquid-based gynecologic cytology preparations. A review of accumulated data. *Acta Cytol* 1998; **42**: 178–184

74 Vassilakos P, Saurel J, Rondez R. Direct-to-vial use of the AutoCyte PREP liquid-based preparation for cervical-vaginal specimens in three European laboratories. *Acta Cytol* 1999; **43**: 65–68

75 Broadstock M. Effectiveness and cost effectiveness of automated and semi-automated cervical screening devices: a systematic review of the literature. *New Zealand Health Technology Assessment (NZHTA)* 2000; **3**: No 1

76 Berger B M. Statistical Quality Assurance in Cytology. The use of the Pathfinder to continuously assess screener process control in real time. *Acta Cytol* 1996; **40**: 97–106

77 Hall S, Wu T-C, Fields A L *et al.* Suitability of ThinPrep specimens for immunocytochemistry and gene amplification by polymerase chain reaction. *Acta Cytol* **36**: 585, 1992

78 Tolles W B, Bostrom R C. Automated screening of cytological smears for cancer: the instrumentation. *Ann NY Acad Sci* 1956; **63**: 1211–1218

79 Wied G L, Bartls P H, Bahr G F, Oldfield D G. Taxonomic Intracellular Analytic System [TICAS] for cell identification. *Acta Cytol* 1968; **12**: 180–120

80 Bloss W H, Greiner W, Kringler W *et al.* Fazytan-IPS-prescreening system. In: Burger G, Ploem J S, Goerdler K eds. *Clinical Cytometry and Histometry*. London: Academic Press, 1987; pp 18–23

81 Husain O A N, Henderson M J. Observations on the use of the Quantimet Image Analysing Computer in automatic scanning for malignant cells. In: Evans D M D ed. *Cytology Automation*, Edinburgh and London: E & S Livingstone, 1970

82 Husain O A N, Allen E, Hawkins J, Taylor J B. The Quantimet Cytoscreen and the interactive approach to cancer screening. *Histochem Cytochem* 1974; **22**: 678–684

83 Jakobsen A, Kristensen P B, Poulsen H K. Flow cytometric classification of biopsy specimens from cervical inter-epithelial neoplasia. *Cytometry* 1983; **4**: 166–169

84 Millett J A, Husain O A N. Analysis of chromatin on carcinoma *in situ*. In: Pattison J R, Bitensky L, Chayen J eds. *Quantitative Cytochemistry and its Application*. London: Academic Press, 1979

85 Naujoks H, Sprenger E. Planung, Durchfuhrung und Ergebnisse einer automatisierten vaginalzytologischen. *Diagnostik Gynakologe* 1990; **23**: 322–327

86 Ploem J S, van Driel-Kulker A M J, Goyarts-Veldstra L *et al.* Image analysis Combined with Quantitative Cytochemistry – Results and Instrumental Developments for Cancer Diagnosis. *Histochemistry* 1986; **84**: 549–555

87 Stenkvist B, Bergstrom R, Brinne U *et al.* Automatic analysis of Papanicolau smears by digital image processing. *Gynecol Oncol* 1987; **27**: 1–14

88 Tanaka N, Ikeda H, Ueno T *et al.* Automated cytologic screening system (CYBEST model 4): an integrated image cytometry system. *App Optics* 1987; **26**: 3301–3307

89 Tucker J H, Husain O A N, Watts K C *et al.* Automated densitometry of cell populations in a continuous motion cell scanner. *App Optics* 1987; **26**: 3315–3324

90 Tucker J H, Stenkvist B. Whatever happened to cervical cytology automation? *Anal Cell Pathol* 1990; **2**: 259–266

91 van Driel Kulker A M J, Ploem-Zaaijer J J. Image cytometry in automated cervical screening. *Anal Cell Pathol* 1989; **1**: 63–78

92 Wheeless L L, Patten S F, Berkan T K *et al.* Multi-dimensional slit-scan prescreening system: preliminary results of a single blind clinical study. *Cytometry* 1984; **5**: 1–8

93 Zahniser D J, Oud P S, Raaijmakers M C T *et al.* Field tests results using the BioPEPR cervical smear prescreening system. *Cytometry* 1980; **1**: 200–203

94 Bartels P, Bibbo M, Hutchinson M L. Computerised screening devices: development of a policy towards automation. *Acta Cytol* 1998; **42**: 59–68

95 IAC. Specifications for automated cytodiagnostic systems proposed by the IAC. *Acta Cytol* 1984; **28**: 582

96 Patten S F, Lee J S J, Nelson A C. Neopath, Inc: Neopath AutoPap 300 automatic Pap screening system. *Acta Cytol* 1996; **40**: 45–52

97 Wilbur D C, Bonfiglio T A, Rutkowski M A *et al*. Sensitivity of the AutoPAP® 300 QC system for cervical cytologic abnormalities. *Acta Cytol* 1996; **40**: 127–132

98 Bishop J W, Kaufman R H, Taylor D A. Multicenter comparison of manual and automated screening of AutoCyte gynaecologic preparations. *Acta Cytol* 1999; **43**: 34–48

99 Mango L J. Neuromedical Systems Inc., *Acta Cytol* 1996; **40**: 53–59

100 Prismatic Project Management team. Assessment of automated primary screening on PAPNET of cervical smears in the Prismatic Trial. *Lancet* 1999; **353**: 1381–1385

101 Koss LG. Performance of cytology in screening for precursor lesions and early cancer of the uterine cervix. In: Franco E, Monsonego J eds. *New Developments in Cervical Cancer Screening and Prevention*. Oxford: Blackwell Science, 1997; 147

102 Kamentsky L A, Gershman R J, Kamentsky L D *et al*. CompuCyte Corporation Pathfinder System: Computerising the microscope to improve cytology quality assurance. *Acta Cytol* 1996; **40**: 31–36

103 Grohs D H, Gombrich P P, Domanik R A. Meeting the challenges in cervical screening: The AcCell series 2000 automated slide handling and data management system. *Acta Cytol* 1996; **40**: 26–36

104 O'Brien M J, Takahashi M, Brugal G *et al*. Digital imagery/telecytology IAC task force. *Acta Cytol* 1998; **42**: 148–164

105 Nordrum I, Eide T J. Remote frozen section service in Norway. *Arch Anat Cytol Pathol* 1995; **43**: 253–256

106 Rao S R, Revathy S, Malvi S G *et al*. Pitfalls in the visual inspection of the cervix as a method of down-staging cancer of the cervix in developing countries. *Ind J Obstet Gynaecol* 1995; **28**: 659–665

107 Van Le L, Broekhuizen S F, Janzer-Steele R *et al*. Acetic acid visualisation of the cervix to detect cervical dysplasia. *Obstet Gynaecol* 1993; **81**: 293–295

108 Stafl A. Cervicography: A new method for cervical cancer detection. *Am J Obstet Gynecol* 1981; **139**: 815–821

109 Szarewski A. Cusick J, Edwards R *et al*. The use of cervicography in a primary screening service. *Br J Obstet Gynaecol* 1991; **98**: 313–317

110 Wunderman I, Coppleson M, Skladnev V N, Reid B L. Polarprobe: A pre-cancer detection instrument. *J Gynaecol Tech* 1995; **1**: 105–109

32 Glandular neoplasms of the uterine cervix

Christine Waddell*

Introduction

Evidence is accumulating which shows that the incidence of adenocarcinoma of the cervix is rising[1-4], but following analysis of data from 60 population-based cancer registries, it appears that the trends are complex[5]. While an increase in incidence of adenocarcinoma and adenosquamous carcinoma has been shown in young women in many countries, including America, Australia and the UK, in other developed countries, including the Netherlands, Germany and New Zealand, there has been no significant change. In Finland, France and Italy there has been a fall in incidence. The increase is seen particularly in women born from 1935 onwards, with women born around 1955 being at three times greater risk than those born in 1935. Epidemiological factors for cervical adenocarcinoma are less well defined than for squamous carcinoma. As with squamous carcinoma, the increase in cervical adenocarcinoma is related to the number of sexual partners and intercourse at an early age[6]. The role of parity is unclear and the widespread use of oral contraceptives is often cited in order to explain the rising frequency[7,8]. Other factors affecting recorded incidence include changes in reporting practice, with increasing awareness of glandular lesions[9]; changes in choice of sampling devices leading to better sampling of the endocervical canal[10] and the effects of organized screening programmes leading to a relative decrease in squamous lesions[5].

It is well documented that up to 50% of endocervical adenocarcinomas are associated with cervical intraepithelial neoplasia (CIN). It is tempting to speculate that both lesions share a common pathogenesis, namely an aberrant proliferation of reserve cells, which may result in the formation of either a glandular or a squamous neoplasm. Human papillomavirus (HPV) types 16 and 18 have been demonstrated in invasive and intraepithelial endocervical tumours[11-16], supporting the concept of a common pathogenesis for at least some lesions.

Endocervical adenocarcinoma and its precursor lesions

The endocervical canal is lined by columnar epithelium, which forms a single layer over the stromal ridges, villi and crypts (see Chapter 28). With the onset of neoplasia, the single layering is disturbed, initially by the development of pseudostratification. Cytologically this appears as overlapping and crowding of nuclei in sheets of epithelial cells. Most endocervical adenocarcinomas are of endocervical type, but Müllerian epithelium has the capacity to differentiate along several pathways, with the result that some tumours have histological features that closely resemble those which usually arise in the endometrium or ovary. Müllerian epithelium also readily undergoes metaplastic change and so, for example, an adenocarcinoma of enteric type may be seen[17].

This diversity of histological pattern is reflected in the classification of endocervical tumours[18] (Table 32.1).

Table 32.1 Classification of primary cervical glandular malignancy and related tumours. (From Rollason 1998, with permission)[18]

In situ	Low-grade	
	High-grade	Endocervical
		Endometrioid
		Intestinal (goblet cell)
		Adenosquamous (including glassy cell)
		Signet ring
		Serous
		Clear cell
Invasive	Adenocarcinoma	Endocervical
		Endometrioid
		Minimal deviation (including endometrioid and clear cell variant)
		Villoglandular (including endometrioid, endocervical & intestinal types)
		Clear cell
		Serous
		Mesonephric
		Non-Müllerian mucinous (intestinal signet ring)
	Adenosquamous carcinoma (including glassy cell variant)	
	Adenoid basal carcinoma	
	Adenoid cystic carcinoma	

*The author gratefully acknowledges her debt to the late Pauline Cooper, whose contribution to the previous edition of this chapter provided a substantial basis for this revised edition.

769

High-grade cervical glandular intraepithelial neoplasia (CGIN): adenocarcinoma *in situ* (AIS)

This lesion was first described histologically in 1953, by Friedell and McKay[19]. They noted that the average age of patients with CGIN was several years younger than that of patients with invasive disease, suggesting that the *in situ* form precedes the development of invasive cancer. This concept has been supported by other studies[20-24].

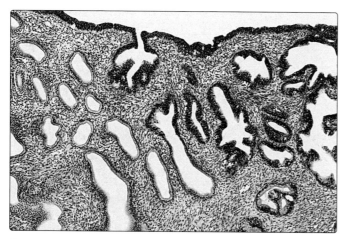

Fig. 32.1　HG-CGIN. The cervical biopsy shows the transition from normal to neoplastic glandular epithelium. (H&E × LP)

Microscopically, CGIN retains the architectural pattern of normal endocervical crypts. Usually the surface epithelium and both superficial and deep crypts are involved at or near the squamocolumnar junction. Partial crypt involvement is a frequent finding, with an abrupt transition from normal to neoplastic epithelium (Fig. 32.1)[25]. High-grade CGIN is usually a single lesion, less often multifocal and frequently extends into the endocervical canal[26-28].

Histologically, the glandular epithelium is composed of columnar cells which show an increase in nuclear size, nuclear pleomorphism, normal and abnormal mitotic activity, apoptosis and nuclear stratification. In tumours of endocervical type, the commonest form, the cells may show abundant mucin production, but often cytoplasmic mucin is diminished (Fig. 32.2). Tumours with an endometrioid or intestinal pattern[29] (Figs 32.3, 32.4) may be seen together with other histological variants, usually as focal areas within a tumour which is predominantly of endocervical type. Argyrophilic cells have also been described in association with CGIN, a finding consistent with the association between adenocarcinoma and neuroendocrine carcinoma of the cervix[30].

When high-grade CGIN is associated with an *in situ* or invasive squamous carcinoma the two cell types may be seen as adjacent lesions (Fig. 32.5). This almost certainly leads to underdiagnosis of the glandular component in lesions of mixed squamous and glandular types[31].

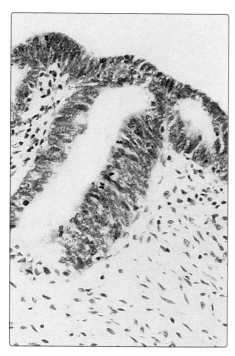

Fig. 32.2　Cervical biopsy. HG-CGIN showing a crypt lined by endocervical cells which show mucous depletion, nuclear stratification, hyperchromasia and mitotic activity. (H&E × MP)

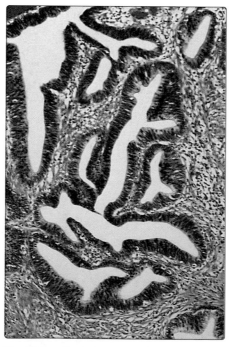

Fig. 32.3　Cervical biopsy. HG-CGIN with an endometrioid pattern. Note the total lack of mucous secretion. (H&E × LP)

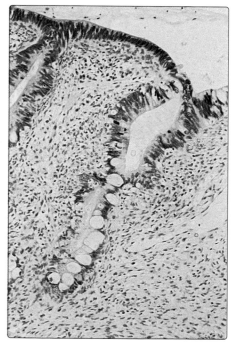

Fig. 32.4　Cervical biopsy. HG-CGIN (intestinal type). Cells in the upper part of the crypt show mucous secretion. Goblet cells are conspicuous in the deeper portion of the crypt. (H&E × LP)

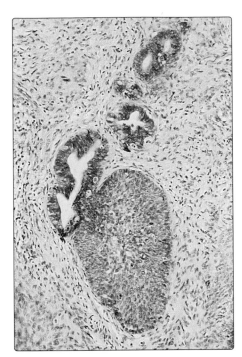

Fig. 32.5 Cervical biopsy. CGIN adjacent to an area of CIN 3. (H&E × LP)

Cytological findings

Cytological manifestations of CGIN were first published by Barter and Waters in 1970[32]. Since then further criteria have been added by a number of authors on which to base a prediction of glandular neoplasia[21,33–41]. The cytological prediction is usually made on cellular sheets and clusters and rarely on individual abnormal cells. At low power it is the disordered architecture of the cells which commands attention, whilst at higher power certain nuclear and cytoplasmic features are helpful (Fig. 32.6) (Table 32.2).

Architectural features

▶ *Exfoliation pattern*. Cohesive sheets and tissue fragments of varying size are seen in a relatively clean background. The 'honeycomb' pattern of benign epithelium is lost; the cells become crowded and their nuclei overlap. The cells often display uniformity of nuclear size within a sheet, but variation of nuclear size between sheets. Crypt openings may be seen within a sheet (Fig. 32.7).

▶ *Feathering*. Nuclei at the edge of a sheet lie at different levels due to stratification of the epithelium. The cytoplasm is usually totally or partially lost and the nuclei are somewhat attenuated. These features cause a feathered appearance at the edge of cell sheets (Fig. 32.8).

▶ *Rosettes*. A circular group of cells with peripheral nuclei where the cytoplasm is directed towards the centre (Fig. 32.9).

▶ *Pseudostratification*. Oval nuclei are seen at different levels in neighbouring cells, polarity is maintained and the cells often retain an intact brush border. This nuclear palisade is a very useful diagnostic feature at the edge of a sheet or in separate strips of epithelium (Figs 32.10, 32.11).

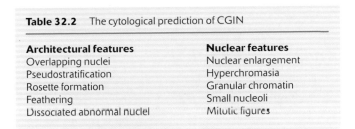

Table 32.2 The cytological prediction of CGIN

Architectural features	Nuclear features
Overlapping nuclei	Nuclear enlargement
Pseudostratification	Hyperchromasia
Rosette formation	Granular chromatin
Feathering	Small nucleoli
Dissociated abnormal nuclei	Mitotic figures

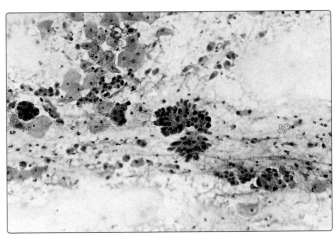

Fig. 32.6 Cervical smear. CGIN. The cervical smear contains sheets of crowded hyperchromatic endocervical cells with rosettes and feathering which may be discerned at low power. (Papanicolaou × MP)

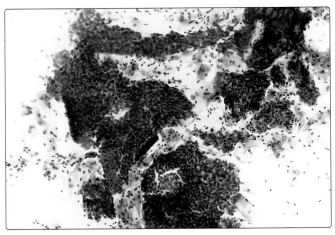

Fig. 32.7 Cervical smear. CGIN. Crowded sheet of endocervical cells with characteristic complex pattern and 'gland opening'. The nuclei are overlapping and hyperchromatic, but show only a mild variation in size within the sheet. (Papanicolaou × MP)

Nuclear features

▶ *The nuclei* within sheets of CGIN are usually larger than in benign epithelial cells and are usually oval in shape, less frequently round. The nuclear membrane is smooth and stains uniformly. The chromatin pattern is variable, but shows an even distribution and the cells often exhibit a greater degree of hyperchromasia than their benign counterparts. A range from fine to coarse granularity is seen, with moderate granularity as the most common finding, which

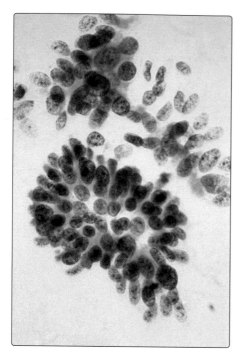

Fig. 32.8   Cervical smear. HG-CGIN. Nuclear stratification and loss of cytoplasm produces the 'feathered' appearance. (Papanicolaou × HP)

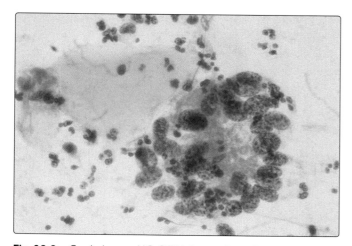

Fig. 32.9   Cervical smear. HG-CGIN. Rosette formation. Note the central location of the cytoplasm, the peripheral arrangement of the nuclei and stippled chromatin pattern. (Papanicolaou × HP)

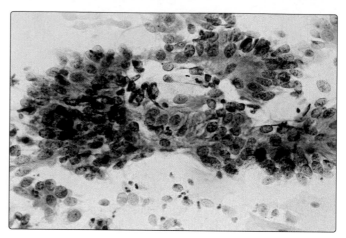

Fig. 32.10   Cervical smear. HG-CGIN. A sheet of endocervical cells shows nuclear crowding, partial rosette formation and feathering. (Papanicolaou × MP)

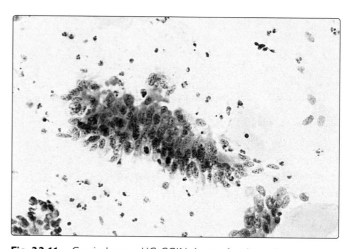

Fig. 32.11   Cervical smear. HG-CGIN. A row of endocervical cells shows nuclear stratification. (Papanicolaou × MP)

gives the nuclei a characteristic speckled salt and pepper appearance (Fig. 32.12).

▶ *Nucleoli* are not a conspicuous feature of CGIN, but when visible they are usually small and may be multiple.

▶ Very occasionally, the nuclei are of normal size or smaller. These are easy to misinterpret as benign and the diagnosis then depends on recognition of the exfoliation pattern.

▶ *Mitoses*. The frequency of mitoses varies from case to case, but their presence is a helpful diagnostic feature especially in clusters of cells with banal looking nuclei of uniform size. They are usually of normal morphology (Fig. 32.13).

▶ *Nuclear/cytoplasmic (n/c) ratio*. This is often very difficult to assess in tissue fragments. In crowded sheets there is little

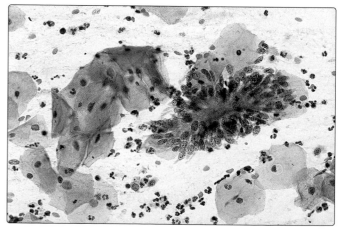

Fig. 32.12   Cervical smear. HG-CGIN. A rosette showing elongated nuclei, even chromasia, speckled chromatin, feathering and cytoplasmic tags. (Papanicolaou × HP)

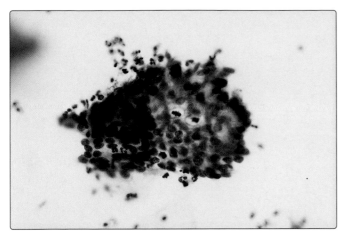

Fig. 32.13   Cervical smear. HG-CGIN. Cluster of uniform small dark cells with mitotic figures giving a clue to their neoplastic origin. (Papanicolaou × HP)

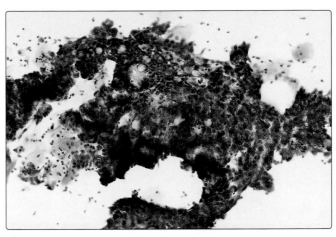

Fig. 32.14   Cervical smear. Type II CGIN. A disorganized sheet of glandular cells, with abundant cytoplasm and large vacuoles. (Papanicolaou × MP)

discernible cytoplasm. In detached strips the total cell size often exceeds that of normal endocervical cells because the cytoplasm increases concomitantly with nuclear size and so there may be no appreciable change in the n/c ratio.

Cytoplasmic features

▶ *Mucin production* in CGIN of endocervical type may be abundant, but is often diminished. The cytoplasm is usually cyanophilic, delicate, finely vacuolated and fading towards the periphery of the cell. Cytoplasmic tags[42] are often seen around the edges of cell groups and rosettes, a feature which helps in discrimination between the rosettes of CGIN and those of tuboendometrial metaplasia. Occasionally, goblet cells characteristic of enteric differentiation, are seen.

Some authors have classified high-grade CGIN into well-differentiated (Type I) and poorly- differentiated (Type II)[43–45]. Type I, the endocervical type, produces the familiar picture including rosettes and pseudostratified strips. Type II is less common, often co-exists with Type I[29], but the cytological appearances are non-specific with 'conspicuous structural disorder' and 'unequal, larger, and often clear nuclei containing large nucleoli' within cell groups[43]. In view of this, the glandular nature might not be recognized cytologically (Fig. 32.14).

Low-grade cervical glandular intraepithelial neoplasia: cervical glandular atypia

In parallel with CIN it might be anticipated that glandular epithelium would show a range of cellular abnormalities. Low-grade CGIN is not widely recognized, but histological criteria have been proposed[25,46], and cytological criteria have also been published but these are controversial[38,47–50]. The changes described represent a continuum from mild atypia to high-grade CGIN[40] the most valuable cytological feature being increase in nuclear area up to twice that of normal nuclei (Fig. 32.15). At one end of the spectrum the cytological appearances may be difficult to distinguish from inflammatory changes in endocervical cells or from atypical

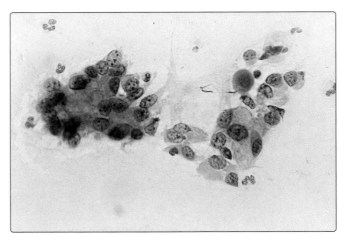

Fig. 32.15   Cervical smear. LG-CGIN. Slight overlapping in clusters of cells with delicate elongated nuclei, speckled chromatin, abundant cytoplasm and wispy cytoplasmic tags. (Papanicolaou × HP)

squamous metaplasia or reserve cell hyperplasia, but at the other, tissue repair may be so florid that it mimics adenocarcinoma (Figs 32.16–32.18)[44,51]. Reactive changes associated with HPV infection in particular may be associated with marked anisonucleosis, but the nuclei tend to be dense and hyperchromatic[50]. Sometimes on histology, enlarged or bizarre multinucleate cells seen within otherwise unremarkable endocervical glands may be due to the presence of human papillomavirus (Fig. 32.19)[46,52]. Cytologically it is the exception rather than the rule for endocervical glandular neoplasia to present with multinucleation in dyskaryotic cells[34,53].

Diagnostic accuracy

The sensitivity of cervical cytology in detecting endocervical glandular lesions is uncertain, but it is lower than for CIN. Published estimates vary between 31% and 88%[39,54]. Discrepancies may be explained by the small number of cases even in long-term or multicentre studies[21,55,56] and through changes of awareness over time leading to an

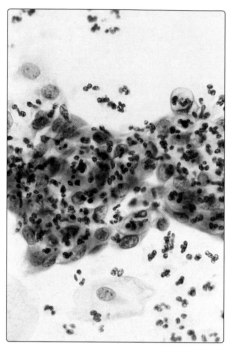

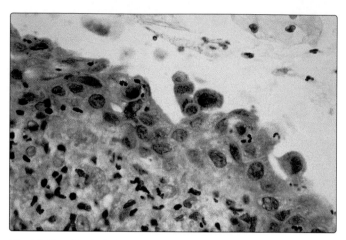

Fig. 32.18 Cervical biopsy. Inflammatory changes in endocervical cells at the tip of an endocervical polyp. (H&E × MP)

Fig. 32.16 Cervical smear. Inflammatory changes in endocervical cells which show nuclear enlargement and mucous depletion. The cell cytoplasm contains polymorphonuclear neutrophil leucocytes. (Papanicolaou × HP)

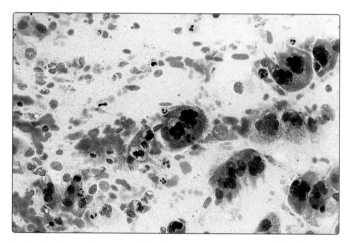

Fig. 32.19 Cervical smear. Reactive changes in endocervical cells. Multinucleate glandular cells with dense 'muddy' chromatin and abundant dense cytoplasm. Possible HPV effect. (Papanicolaou × HP)

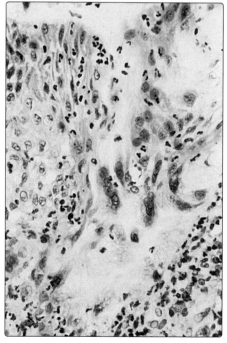

Fig. 32.17 Cervical biopsy showing an acute cervicitis. Endocervical cells show hyperchromasia, multinucleation and mucous depletion. (H&E × MP)

increase in cytological and histological recognition[9]. Sensitivity is also compromised by sampling failure. The abnormalities may be inaccessible in gland crypts beneath the transformation zone; they may be focal or high in the endocervical canal. Not infrequently, the early changes have

gone unrecognized, especially in mixed squamous and glandular lesions[20,21,26,54]. In these cases, it is the investigation of squamous or sometimes of indeterminate cytological abnormalities which lead to recognition of the glandular component[54,57].

Diagnostic pitfalls

A comprehensive account of the interpretive difficulties was published by Crum *et al.* in 1997[58]. These difficulties are reflected in the published positive predictive value (PPV) estimations of smears reported as showing glandular abnormalities. Even when the presence of high-grade glandular neoplasia is deemed highly likely, PPV estimations vary from 17 to 95.7%[59,60]. For predictions in which there is less certainty that the changes are due to glandular neoplasia, in smears reported as showing borderline nuclear abnormalities (BNA) in the UK British Society for Clinical Cytology terminology[61], PPV values as low as 2.5% are published[62]. This reflects the use of the borderline report as a holding category, comparable with the 'atypical glandular cells of uncertain significance (AGUS) favour reactive' in the Bethesda System[63]. The following may cause confusion (Table 32.3).

▶ *Inflammatory change in endocervical cells*. This is common and may be associated with cervicitis and polyps[52]. Endocervical cells are usually present in small clusters and sheets with minimal nuclear overlapping. There may be hyperchromasia and mild anisonucleosis in round or oval nuclei. Chromatin is finely stippled and may be smudged in texture[64]. Multinucleation is almost always a feature of reactive rather than neoplastic change. Nucleoli, if present, may be conspicuous and round and very occasional mitoses are seen in regenerating epithelial cells. Cytoplasm is often abundant, cyanophilic or eosinophilic and may be dense, with terminal bars and occasionally cilia[65]. The most important feature which distinguishes sheets and clusters of endocervical cells with inflammatory changes from those of CGIN is the exfoliation pattern. Nuclear stratification and feathering at the edge of sheets are features of CGIN, which are rarely present in inflammatory smears.

▶ *Severely dyskaryotic squamous cells*. Cells from gland crypts involved in CIN may pose real diagnostic problems[66]. These are often associated with the use of the more pointed samplers such as the Aylesbury spatula and endocervical brushes. However, endocervical brush samplers may produce a similar appearance in cases with no gland crypt involvement confirmed histologically[67]. Two exfoliative patterns have been recognized. Type A, described by Anderson in 1988[68], appears as rounded three-dimensional clusters of usually hyperchromatic cells arranged with central whorling and peripheral flattening of the cells within the group (Fig. 32.20). In Type B[69], the clusters show peripheral palisading and discernible pseudostratification. Occasional gland formation in the centres and fraying at the edges of these groups produce rosette look-alikes (Fig. 32.21)[58]. The streaming of elongated nuclei from the ends of crowded sheets of cells from CIN 3 may also give the impression of feathering[70]. Features in squamous dyskaryosis that help to distinguish it from endocervical dyskaryosis include smooth chromatin texture in nuclei with well-distributed chromatin or chromatin clumping and clearing in those with maldistributed chromatin. Irregular nuclear outline, anisonucleosis, variation in chromasia between adjacent nuclei within the clusters and, when present, a relative denseness of cytoplasm with an absence of peripheral cytoplasmic tags also favour squamous over endocervical dyskaryosis. By gradual assimilation of these features into reporting practice, the false positive predictions of glandular neoplasia in smears from pure squamous lesions was reduced from 43% to 24% in two consecutive eight year periods in a sixteen year audit of glandular reporting in a single centre[71].

▶ *Tubal metaplasia*. The endocervical canal and some crypts may be lined by columnar epithelium composed of ciliated, secretory and small dark intercalated cells resembling the normal lining of the fallopian tube (Fig. 32.22)[72]. Its cytological features overlap those of CGIN and adenocarcinoma[73], with the appearance of clusters of cells, which may show nuclear

Table 32.3 The cytological prediction of CGIN: Diagnostic difficulties and look-alikes

Non-neoplastic	Neoplastic
Cervicitis	Gland crypt involvement in CIN
Endocervical polyps	Type II CGIN
Tubal metaplasia	Early invasive adenocarcinoma
Endometriosis	Endometrial hyperplasia and
Microglandular hyperplasia	neoplasia
Arias-Stella reaction	Extrauterine carcinoma
Isthmic (lower uterine	
segment) sampling	

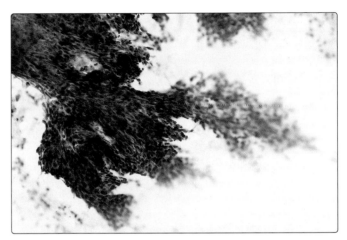

Fig. 32.20 Cervical smear. CIN 3 Type A: a three-dimensional cluster of dyskaryotic squamous cells with poor cytoplasmic differentiation peripheral streaming of nuclei mimicking feathering. (Papanicolaou × MP)

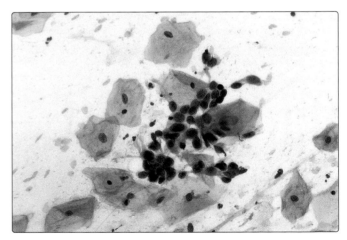

Fig. 32.21 Cervical smear. CIN 3 Type B: a rosette of dyskaryotic squamous cells but note the dense chromatin pattern and cytoplasm. (Papanicolaou × HP)

crowding, pseudostratified strips and even rosettes (Fig. 32.23). Apart from the smooth chromatin pattern of the nuclei, the most valuable feature for identification of tubal metaplasia is the denseness of cell cytoplasm, with blunted luminal edges bearing terminal bars and cilia. This is particularly useful in assessing rosettes in tubal metaplasia which are 'reversed' with dense blunt edged cytoplasm

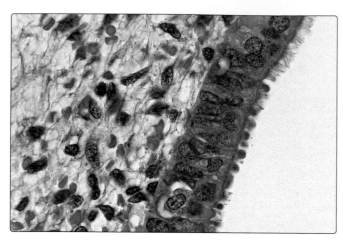

Fig. 32.22 Cervical biopsy. Tubal metaplasia in an endocervical crypt. Although the nuclei are enlarged the chromatin pattern is vesicular, there are no mitoses and ciliated cells are numerous. (H&E × OI) (see also **Fig. 32.23**)

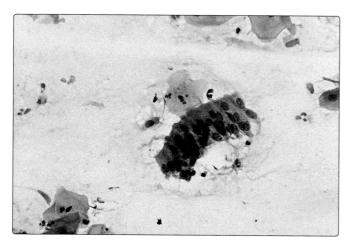

Fig. 32.23 Cervical smear. Tubal metaplasia. Columnar cells show nuclear stratification. Cilia are present along the clearly defined cell border. (Papanicolaou × HP)

clothing the outer aspect of the cell groups (Fig. 32.24). Diagnostic difficulties arise sometimes when cilia are not identified in three-dimensional and crowded groups of glandular cells[74,75]. Then, a borderline report may be justified as the possibility of coexistence of tubal metaplasia and glandular neoplasia must be borne in mind.

▶ *Endometrial cells and cervical endometriosis.* The presence of endometrial cells in cervical smears can cause confusion. This problem has been recognized in smears taken after a cone biopsy or with the endocervical brush[76,77]. The sampler may reach high into the endocervical canal and harvest cells from the lower uterine segment (LUS). These may present as blowsy poorly cohesive cuboidal cells lacking the exfoliative pattern required for a prediction of CGIN, and with the delicate vesicular nuclei consistent with endometrial origin. More striking are the large and sometimes branching fragments of crowded glandular tissue. Dense straight-sided tubular microbiopsies with peripheral palisading and associated tangles of delicate stromal cells are characteristic features particularly identifiable on low power inspection (Figs 32.25, 32.26). Capillaries may be observed running through the stromal component and mitotic figures may be evident in smears taken during the first half of the menstrual cycle[78,79]. Adenomyomatous polyps in the lower uterine segment may present cytologically as bland stromal cells in loose frayed clusters. The epithelial content is variable from few cells to tight packed clusters of crowded nuclei[80,81].

▶ *Endometriosis* is common in post-cone biopsy cervices[82] but may be seen in women with no history of previous surgery. Conflicting reports have been published of the cytological appearance of superficial cervical endometriosis. Hanau *et al.* described similarities with endocervical neoplasia including feathering and macronucleoli which may even lead to an erroneous prediction of adenocarcinoma (Fig. 32.27)[83]. Mulvaney and Surtees described changes similar to those attributed to direct LUS sampling or tubal metaplasia with an absence of feathering and pseudostratification[84]. However, the endometrioid variant of CGIN should be considered if, in the absence of endometrial stroma, extreme crowding is a feature in smears with small well preserved endometrial-type cells[85].

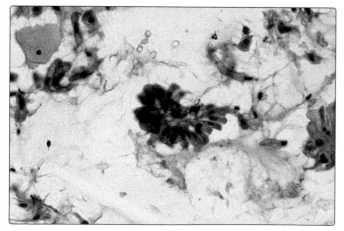

Fig. 32.24 Cervical smear. Post loop excision biopsy. An untidy rosette with centrally placed nuclei and well formed peripheral cytoplasm. Terminal bars and cilia may sometimes be observed peripherally. (Papanicolaou × HP)

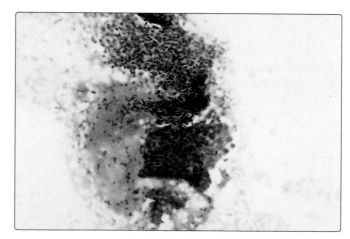

Fig. 32.25 Cervical smear. Lower uterine segment sampling. Straight-sided fragment of epithelium with nuclear crowding, mitotic figures and associated tangle of stromal cells. (Papanicolaou × MP)

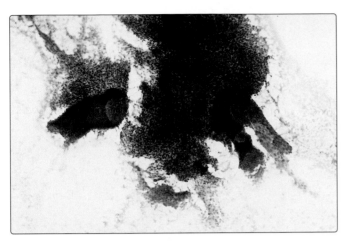

Fig. 32.26 Cervical smear. Lower uterine segment sampling. Straight-sided tubes of epithelial cells and associated stromal cells. (Papanicolaou × LP)

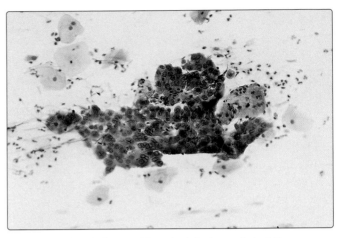

Fig. 32.28 Cervical smear. Microglandular hyperplasia. A three-dimensional fenestrated cluster of cells consisting of cuboidal and basaloid metaplastic cells. (Papanicolaou × MP)

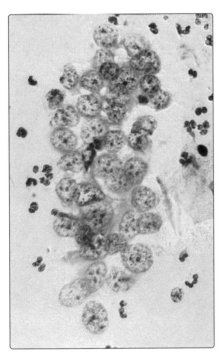

Fig. 32.27 Cervical smear. Cervical endometriosis. The cervical smear contains large groups of endometrial glandular cells. (Papanicolaou × HP)

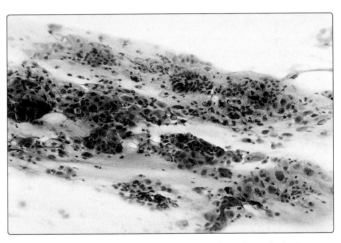

Fig. 32.29 Cervical smear. Radiation change in endocervical cells. Disorganized clusters of cells with anisonucleosis, abundant cytoplasm and minimal overlapping of nuclei. (Papanicolaou × MP)

glandular cells with finely vacuolated cytoplasm, immature metaplastic cells with dense basaloid cytoplasm and reserve cells with little or no cytoplasm (Fig. 32.28). Reactive changes resulting in anisonucleosis, nuclear enlargement and prominent nucleoli may lead to suspicion of either glandular or squamous neoplasia.

▶ *Radiation change.* Early radiation change in endocervical cells also may produce disorganized clusters of glandular cells with loss of the normal honeycomb pattern but with little overlapping of nuclei and ample cytoplasm, leading the cytologist to a non-neoplastic prediction. Nuclear enlargement with anisonucleosis is common, together with nucleolar enlargement and multinucleation (Fig. 32.29). Unlike radiation change in squamous cells, bizarre nuclear shape is unusual[91].

▶ *Mesonephric duct remnants.* The mesonephric (Wölffian) ducts in the male develop into the efferent ducts of the testis, the epididymis, vasa deferentia, seminal vesicles and ejaculatory ducts. In the female the mesonephric ducts degenerate, but remnants may persist in the broad ligament and in the lateral wall of the uterine cervix and vagina. Because the remnants are situated within cervical stroma and

▶ *Microglandular hyperplasia.* Microglandular hyperplasia of the uterine cervix may occur during pregnancy and with oral contraceptive use, but it is not confined to these groups and may be seen in postmenopausal women[86,87]. There are several studies of smears from women with histological diagnosis of microglandular hyperplasia concluding that the cytological features are nonspecific with only the most florid papillary forms causing confusion with endocervical adenocarcinoma[88], endocervical or endometrial glandular neoplasia[73], or squamous neoplasia[89]. However, Alvarez-Santín *et al.* in 1999[90] proposed cytological identification based on the histological criteria published by Greeley *et al.* in 1995[87]. These are the presence of two- and three-dimensional fenestrated sheets of a mixed population of cells consisting of cuboidal and columnar

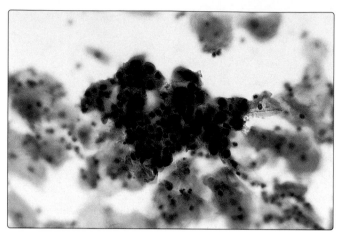

Fig. 32.30   Cervical smear. Florid mesonephric duct hyperplasia. Non-specific reactive changes in glandular cells with anisonucleosis and dense chromatin pattern. (Papanicolaou × HP)

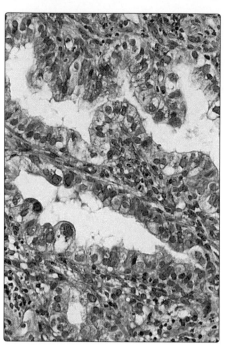

Fig. 32.31   Cervical biopsy. Arias-Stella reaction. The cells have large pleomorphic nuclei which are surrounded by abundant cytoplasm. Mitoses are absent. (H&E × MP)

rarely reach the surface cytological presentation is uncommon. In a case report, Stewart *et al.* reviewed two cervical smears from a patient with mesonephric adenocarcinoma arising in an area of diffuse mesonephric hyperplasia. They were both considered to show reactive changes only[92]. Non-specific glandular atypia was similarly encountered in a case of florid mesonephric hyperplasia (Fig. 32.30).

▶ *Arias-Stella reaction.* This is a normal phenomenon in pregnancy and may affect glandular epithelium throughout the genital tract. These changes may take place within days of fertilization[93,94]. However, the presence of large cells with ill-defined vacuolated cytoplasm, large nuclei with coarse chromatin and prominent nucleoli, accompanied by clusters of endometrial cells, is more likely to result in erroneous prediction of endometrial than endocervical neoplasia (Fig. 32.31)[95]. Moulded papillary fragments of placental tissue have also been described in post partum and post abortion smears which are open to misinterpretation as adenocarcinoma of the endocervix or of the ovary (Fig. 32.32)[96,97] (see Chapter 28).

The cytologist needs to be mindful not only of the benign mimics of glandular neoplasia but also that benign and neoplastic entities may co-exist. Masuda *et al.* have reported endometrioid adenocarcinoma arising in the lower uterine segment in a 27-year-old[98]. The presence of cilia is generally accepted as a feature of the benign epithelial cell, however, Gloor and Ruzicka recorded ciliated cells in their description of Type II CGIN[43]. Also ciliated neoplastic cells have been demonstrated by endometrial brush cytology of a histologically confirmed ciliated endometrioid adenocarcinoma of the endometrium[99]. Artefacts affecting the appearance of endocervical cells are also a potential pitfall. The cytological presentation of glandular cells is affected by the method both of cell collection and fixation. Cytobrush sampling frequently results in harvest of a surfeit of glandular cells in sheets and microbiopsies with associated difficulties in interpretation[100]. The changeover from alcohol immersion to spray fixation in many centres

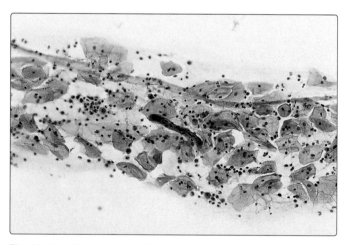

Fig. 32.32   Cervical smear. Moulded fragment of a chorionic villus in a post partum smear. (Papanicolaou × MP)

has altered cell dispersal on the slide so that feathering should be used with caution as a discriminant in prediction of CGIN[101]. Events preceding cell collection may also modify the appearance of glandular cells. Grossly attenuated endocervical cells may be observed in smears taken immediately after the application of acetic acid or Lugol's iodine used at colposcopic examination (Fig. 32.33)[102,103]. Table 32.4 summarizes useful features to take into account in the event of equivocal cytological findings.

Invasive endocervical adenocarcinoma

The majority of patients with invasive endocervical adenocarcinoma present with abnormal vaginal bleeding,

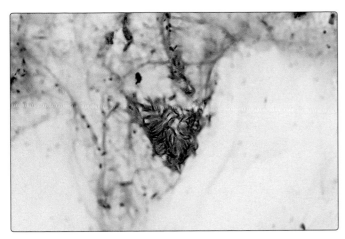

Fig. 32.33   Cervical smear. Acetic acid artefact in endocervical cells from a smear taken at colposcopy. (Papanicolaou × MP)

Table 32.4   Clues in differential diagnosis in cytological prediction of CGIN

CGIN more likely	HG-CGIN unlikely
Rosettes	Cilia
Overlapping nuclei	Anisonucleosis
Dissociated abnormal nuclei	Multinucleation
Stippled chromatin	Chromatin clumping
Round/oval nuclei	Irregular nuclear outline
Delicate cytoplasm	Dense cytoplasm
Mitotic figures	Stromal and epithelial cells

but 10–20% may be asymptomatic[104,105]. There is a wide age scatter at presentation, but most cases present in the fourth, fifth and sixth decades.

Classification

Endocervical type

Well-differentiated tumours are composed of branching glands lined by a single or stratified layer of tall columnar cells with abundant cytoplasm. Most tumours contain intracytoplasmic and intraluminal mucus (Fig. 32.34). Less-differentiated tumours are composed of poorly formed glands and display increased nuclear pleomorphism and a decrease in mucus production. Most poorly-differentiated tumours contain large pleomorphic cells, which form solid nests and sheets and a diligent search may be necessary to find any glandular differentiation. These tumours are often mistaken for squamous carcinomas. In one study up to 20–30% of tumours originally classified as squamous carcinomas were reclassified, after staining for mucins, as poorly-differentiated adenocarcinomas or as adenosquamous tumours[106].

Invasiveness

The term *microinvasive adenocarcinoma* is controversial and there is no agreed definition[25,34,53,107]. In very well-differentiated tumours, diagnosis may also be difficult as invasion occurs in the form of small glands with bland

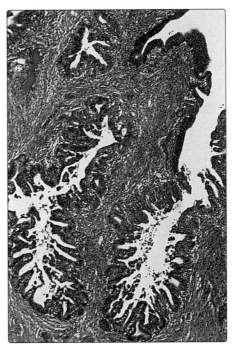

Fig. 32.34   Cervical biopsy. Well-differentiated invasive endocervical adenocarcinoma. (H&E × LP)

cytological features but extending beyond the normal crypt depth. A chronic inflammatory cell infiltrate or desmoplastic stromal reaction around the neoplastic glands are helpful diagnostic features. There is also debate about the degree of complexity of the glandular pattern which is permissible within the diagnostic spectrum of CGIN[28,29,108].

Cytological findings

Features helpful in prediction of early invasion have been identified in small retrospective studies[36,37,53,109,110]. These include:

▶ *Smear background.* This is frequently inflammatory and less often there is a recognizable tumour diathesis

▶ *Exfoliation pattern.* Very often this is indistinguishable from high-grade CGIN, but some cell groups may show super-crowding with tiny cells packed in very tight sheets. Papillary fragments may be prominent. Mulvaney[53] found high cellularity with pseudosyncytial clusters of enlarged, pleomorphic nuclei with a reduced amount of granular cytoplasm to be highly significant

▶ *Nuclear features.* The nuclei are usually hyperchromatic and often round, but variation in size and shape is common. Chromatin pattern and distribution are unhelpful as indicators of early invasion. Nucleoli are frequently present, often small and single, but occasionally large and multiple

At a later stage, the smear will show all the features of an invasive adenocarcinoma with many irregular sheets of pleomorphic cells with large nuclei, maldistribution of chromatin, prominent nucleoli[111] and frequent mitoses. The

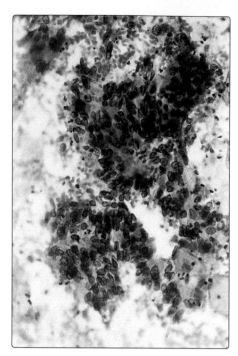

Fig. 32.35   Cervical smear. Invasive adenocarcinoma of endocervical type with large disorganized sheets of pleomorphic glandular cells. (Papanicolaou × MP)

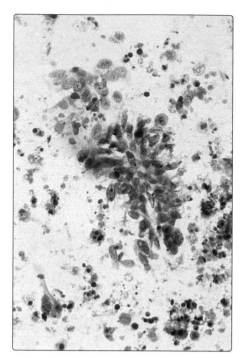

Fig. 32.37   Cervical smear. Poorly-differentiated endocervical adenocarcinoma. Malignant cells are seen in a background of cellular debris. (Papanicolaou × HP)

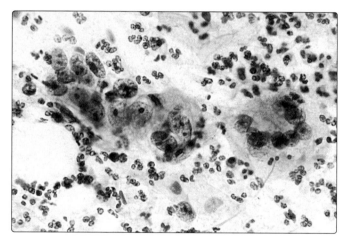

Fig. 32.36   Cervical smear. Poorly-differentiated endocervical adenocarcinoma in which the cells contain large nucleoli and show poor cytoplasmic differentiation. (Papanicolaou × HP)

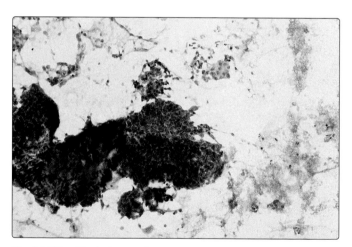

Fig. 32.38   Cervical smear. Endometrioid adenocarcinoma. Three-dimensional cluster of very small crowded cells with gland openings and mitotic figures. (Papanicolaou × MP)

cytoplasm is usually poorly defined and the cells lie in a background of blood, inflammation and necrotic cellular debris (Figs 32.35–32.37).

With tumours of endocervical type the cervical origin of the tumour may be confidently predicted from the cervical smear, but for tumours of endometrioid or other types this may not be possible[112,113].

Endometrioid adenocarcinoma

Histologically and cytologically, these tumours are identical to those arising in the endometrium and often contain areas of intraglandular squamous differentiation. The cells are small, cuboidal or columnar with eccentric nuclei and small nucleoli. The cytoplasm is scanty but dense, cyanophilic and coarsely granular (Fig. 32.38)[111]. These tumours may arise in foci of cervical endometriosis, but most are derived from reserve cells that pursue an endometrial, rather than an endocervical, pathway of differentiation. Following subtotal hysterectomy, the continuing risk of endometrioid adenocarcinoma arising in residual isthmic endometrial tissue must be borne in mind when assessing cytology from the cervical stump[114].

Minimal deviation adenocarcinoma (adenoma malignum)

This rare tumour is the most differentiated form of endocervical adenocarcinoma. Histologically, the tumour is characterized by increased complexity of crypt architecture, with large convoluted or slit-shaped glands extending deeply into the cervical stroma. The glands are usually lined by a single layer of columnar cells showing minimal cytological atypia, with basal nuclei and abundant delicate cytoplasm. There may be focal pseudostratification, an increased nucleocytoplasmic ratio and, when nuclear pleomorphism is more pronounced, large nucleoli may be seen.

Cytologically, the tumour is difficult to recognize and in many cases this is retrospective[42,115–118]. The cells are arranged in flat honeycomb sheets with focal disorganization. Typically the cells have abundant, lacy or vacuolated cytoplasm with wispy cytoplasmic tails at the periphery of the groups. Yellow-orange cytoplasmic mucin staining has been described in these cells, in contrast with the pink-green staining of normal endocervical cells[119]. Nuclei are round or oval, up to twice normal size, with fine to coarsely granular chromatin (Fig. 32.39). Occasionally nucleoli are conspicuous. The abundance of glandular material in the smear, the excessive lacy cytoplasm and occasional mitotic figures in sheets of otherwise banal uniform looking cells, are particularly helpful diagnostic features.

Villoglandular adenocarcinoma

This is an uncommon tumour with a relatively good prognosis affecting women mainly under the age of 40 years. Histologically, the diagnosis is made on recognition of papillae with normal stromal cores covered by endocervical, endometrioid or intestinal-type cells exhibiting only minor degrees of atypia[120]. It may be suspected cytologically by identifying intact papillary fronds and tight clusters of cells in cohesive three-dimensional groups with smooth borders. The nuclei are round or oval, deceptively bland with minimal pleomorphism, moderate hyperchromasia and evenly dispersed chromatin. They are relatively small, up to twice the size of intermediate squamous cell nuclei (Fig. 32.40). Apoptosis and mitotic figures may be seen[121–123].

Papillary serous adenocarcinoma

Histologically, these tumours differ from villoglandular adenocarcinoma in that the papillae are finer with delicate fibrous cores, psammoma bodies may be present and the epithelial covering shows marked cellular pleomorphism. Cytologically they are identical to serous carcinoma of the ovary (Fig. 32.41) (see Chapter 35)[120,123].

Clear cell adenocarcinoma

This form of differentiation is seen in the cervix, endometrium and ovary. In the cervix, there may be associated *in situ* foci[124]. Although vaginal and cervical clear cell carcinoma is associated with diethylstilboestrol exposure *in utero*[125], cases do occur in non-exposed women also. The tumours usually show a mixed papillary and

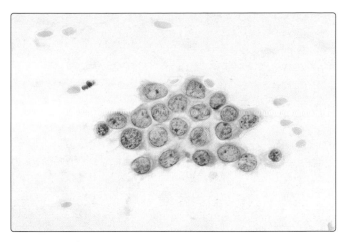

Fig. 32.39 Cervical smear. Minimal deviation adenocarcinoma. Endocervical cells retain their 'honeycomb' arrangement, but show nuclear enlargement. The cytoplasm is delicate with some fine vacuolation. (Papanicolaou × HP)

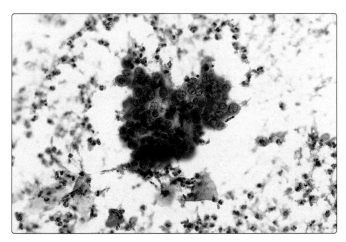

Fig. 32.40 Cervical smear. Villoglandular carcinoma. Three-dimensional cluster of crowded glandular cells with small bland oval/round nuclei. (Papanicolaou × HP)

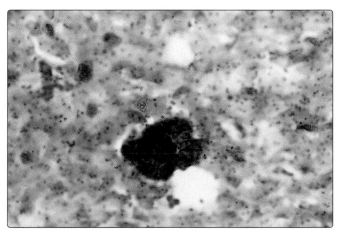

Fig. 32.41 Cervical smear. Papillary serous adenocarcinoma. Crowded cluster of small round cells surrounding a psammoma body. (Papanicolaou × MP)

tubular pattern in which the lining cells have characteristic apical or 'hob nail' nuclei and prominent nucleoli[126]. The cytoplasm contains glycogen and may be clear or eosinophilic. Cytologically, the cells appear singly or in small clusters. There is anisonucleosis. The nuclei are large, vesicular and moderately hyperchromatic, with maldistribution of the chromatin. There are usually extremely large, sometimes irregular and occasionally multiple nucleoli. When well preserved, the cytoplasm is cyanophilic or amphophilic, abundant, delicate and finely vacuolated (Fig. 32.42). Frequently cytoplasm is absent and then large pale bare nuclei are seen[111,127–129].

Enteric adenocarcinoma

These tumours probably arise from foci of intestinal metaplasia and are usually seen as part of a mixed pattern of differentiation; they rarely occur in pure form. The involved glands are lined by columnar cells with a prominent brush border and goblet cells are usually numerous. Occasionally Paneth cells and argyrophil cells may be present[130]. Cytologically, they are indistinguishable from Type II CGIN described by Gloor and Ruzicka[28,29,43].

Adenosquamous carcinoma including glassy cell carcinoma

Both squamous and glandular cervical tumours are thought to arise from undifferentiated reserve cells. Consequently it is not surprising that in some instances both patterns of differentiation are seen, either as discrete areas within the tumour (adenocarcinoma and squamous carcinoma) or with intermingling of the glandular and squamous cell components (adenosquamous carcinoma). In both of these,

there is a tendency for the glandular component to be overlooked on cytology[113,131].

Glassy cell carcinoma is an uncommon variant of adenosquamous carcinoma. Histologically it presents as sheets and nests of malignant cells with macronucleoli and marked mitotic activity. Cytologically, it appears as syncytial aggregates of large malignant cells with finely granular cytoplasm. The nuclei are round or oval with finely granular evenly distributed chromatin and large irregular nucleoli (Fig. 32.43). Dissociated malignant cells may also be seen within the tumour diathesis. It is most likely to be misinterpreted as large cell non-keratinizing squamous carcinoma[132,133].

Mesonephric, adenoid basal and adenoid cystic adenocarcinoma

These are rare tumours which are usually inaccessible to cytological sampling being either deep in the lateral wall of the cervix (mesonephric)[92] or beneath intact mucosa (adenoid basal and adenoid cystic) (Fig. 32.44).

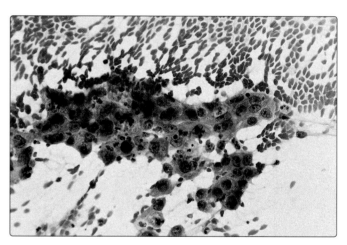

Fig. 32.43 Cervical smear. Glassy cell adenocarcinoma. Syncytial sheet of cells with round/oval nuclei and macronucleoli. (Papanicolaou × HP)

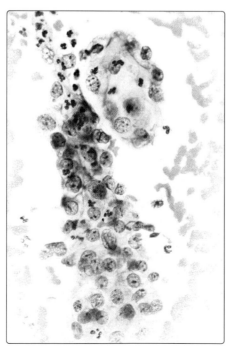

Fig. 32.42 Cervical smear. Clear cell adenocarcinoma. The cell clusters have abundant clear or finely vacuolated cytoplasm. (Papanicolaou × HP)

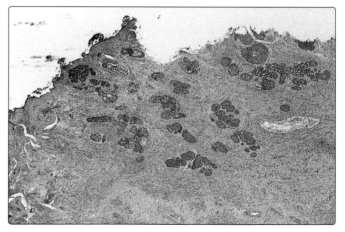

Fig. 32.44 Cervical biopsy. Adenoid basal carcinoma of the cervix. (H&E × LP)

Cytologically, adenoid basal and adenoid cystic carcinomas appear as groups and sheets of small cells with a high n/c ratio, uniform round or oval hyperchromatic nuclei and small nucleoli (Fig. 32.45). These tumours usually occur in elderly women and cytology is most likely to be misinterpreted as indicative of endometrial pathology[134–136].

Metastatic carcinoma

Malignant cells can metastasize to the cervix from tumours arising elsewhere in the genital system, notably from the ovary and endometrium, or from extragenital sites including gastrointestinal tract, breast and lung (Fig. 32.46)[137–139]. Cervical smears containing metastatic tumour cells may cause diagnostic difficulties, particularly in the absence of relevant clinical information (see Chapters 33 and 35).

Sampling

Most abnormalities of endocervical glandular epithelium occur in the transformation zone. A well-taken smear using a spatula should harvest abnormal cells and no special technique is required. However, a significant minority of false negative smears from both intraepithelial and invasive glandular lesions are associated with sampling failure[20,113]. The introduction of the more pointed spatulas such as the Aylesbury and the Cervex-Brush has gone some way towards addressing this problem, with enhancement not only of transformation zone sampling, but also with increased sampling of the more proximal endocervical canal[140,141]. Endocervical brushes extend sampling further into the canal[142] but often with the inclusion of isthmic endometrium[78]. While this has undoubtedly improved detection of glandular neoplasia especially of small foci and skip lesions, endometrial cells amongst the plethora of endocervical glandular cells and the collection of immature metaplastic and reserve cells have led to problems in interpretation with identification of minor atypias unrelated to neoplasia. The new cellular patterns thus presented greatly challenge the cytologist and during the phase of familiarization, there has been an increase in smear reports in the borderline category[62,64,69,73,75,143–146].

New techniques: thin-layer cytology and automation

New techniques including fluid-based thin-layer methods are currently under review. Preliminary trials appear favourable with the production of samples with crisp clean cell morphology[147] resulting in significant improvement in sample adequacy and a reduction in the ratio of low-grade to high-grade abnormality reports[148,149]. There has been some concern that there is reduced endocervical cell representation in thin-layer preparations, but this may be related to the use of residual material after the spread of the conventional smear in split-sample studies as this phenomenon has not been reproduced in direct-to-vial preparations[150,151].

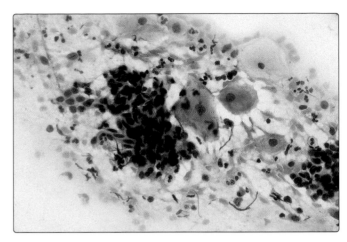

Fig. 32.45   Cervical smear. Adenoid basal carcinoma of the cervix. Clusters of small uniform cells similar to endometrial cells. (Papanicolaou × HP) (Figs 32.30, 32.44 and 32.45 courtesy of City Hospital, NHS Trust, Birmingham)

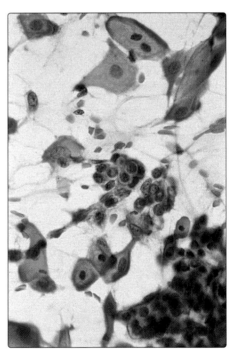

Fig. 32.46   Cervical smear. Metastatic carcinoma of the breast. Cohesive clusters of malignant cells are present in an atrophic smear. (Papanicolaou × HP)

Unfamiliarity with the cellular presentation in thin layer preparations has also been a problem. In a study of 30 paired samples from women with histologically proven high-grade CGIN, sensitivity of the conventional smears was 67% compared with 47% for the thin-layer smears. On review, 12 samples contained no diagnostic cells but four false negatives were considered to be interpretation errors owing to lack of the familiar architectural features, in particular feathering, used in identification of CGIN[152]. On finding assessment of glandular cell clusters compromised by overlapping of nuclei and absence of feathering, one group used cell block preparations from residual thin-layer cytology samples as a further aid to interpretation[153]. However, other workers have found little change in thin-layer samples in the presence of rosettes, pseudostratified strips, feathering and mitoses traditionally used for prediction of glandular neoplasia and identification of benign look-alikes[149,154]. Indeed, in one centre, changeover from conventional smear preparation to the thin-layer technique reduced their false negative rate for glandular neoplasia from 43.6% in conventional to 15.4% in thin-layer smears and reduced false positive reports associated with squamous look-alikes from 30.4% to 11.1%[155].

Alternative fixatives have also been assessed in conjunction with thin-layer methods. The use of the CytoRich Red and Yellow system, in which fixation is achieved using a buffered mixture of formaldehyde and alcohol, retains three-dimensional relationships in microbiopsies. This is usually used in preparation of Tao brush samples of the endometrium[156]. Initially, the feasibility of the use of CytoRich fixation in identification of endocervical glandular pathology was tested on hysterectomy specimens[157]. In a subsequent split-sample study, identification of glandular neoplasia based on interpretation of well presented three-dimensional microbiopsies was found to be more sensitive than reliance on feathering and other artefacts used in conventional preparations[158].

During evaluation of the now deferred Papnet neural network system, there was some evidence that the system failed to select normal endocervical components, the presence of which had been confirmed conventionally[159,160]. However, Sturgis et al. found on presentation of samples known to contain diagnostically important glandular elements, Papnet picked out 94% of the neoplastic and 98% of the benign entities. The single failure in the neoplastic group was associated with paucity of neoplastic material[161]. The use of immunocytochemical markers may improve sensitivity in cases of very well-differentiated or scanty diagnostic material. The proliferation marker MIB-1 has been used successfully in identification of cells from a well-differentiated papillary carcinoma which, although presented by Papnet, were initially misinterpreted as benign by human observers[162].

In histological preparations special techniques have been used to delineate the staining reactions of endocervical adenocarcinoma and its precursor lesions in order to distinguish them from other tumours and from benign glandular proliferations of the cervix. These are rarely applied to cytological preparations, but, with the advent of thin-layer techniques, the possibility of automation and the availability of multiple specimens from each sample, cytochemical and immunocytochemical stains as well as HPV testing[163] may be adopted as routine to identify high risk women or in addition to routine Papanicolaou staining in equivocal cases.

Silver stains of the nucleolar organizer region (AgNORs)[164–166], and MIB-1, a monoclonal antibody to the Ki-67 antigen are markers of cell proliferation[162,167]. They have been found to be useful in discrimination between benign and neoplastic endocervical cells. Similarly, MN/CA9 expression has been identified as a marker of both squamous and glandular cervical neoplasia and is particularly useful in assessment of equivocal changes in glandular cells[168].

Discrimination between different cell types is also possible using immunocytochemical and cytochemical techniques. 1C5 is a monoclonal antibody marker of endocervical, mucinous and some serous ovarian tumours but not those of endometrioid differentiation[169]. Demonstration of β-galactosidase enzyme activity by cytochemical stains indicative of endometrial epithelium may be useful in determination of the tumour subtype in cervical and endometrial adenocarcinomas[170]. LhS28, a monoclonal antibody to the basal bodies of ciliated epithelial cells, may prove useful to confirm the presence of tuboendometrial metaplasia in cases with equivocal findings on routine Papanicolaou staining[74,75,171]. The use of HK1083, which stains pyloric mucin also gives positive staining for minimal deviation adenocarcinoma[119,172]. Its use is limited, however, because of the capacity of the cervix to undergo intestinal and pyloric metaplasia[173].

Management of women with cytological prediction of glandular abnormality

Cytology may provide additional information during assessment of women presenting with signs and/or symptoms of cervical adenocarcinoma, but there are many in whom abnormal cytology is the first indication of a glandular lesion. Colposcopic appearance is non-specific in those with preinvasive or very early invasive lesions and even in those with established but occult adenocarcinoma. The lesion predicted cytologically may not be cervical at all, but may be elsewhere within the genital tract[9] or rarely, extrauterine. Good communication between clinician and cytopathologist is of utmost importance to provide optimal patient management and to ensure consideration is given to the possibility of non-cervical sources of abnormality if appropriate[174–176].

For those in whom cytology is equivocal with a differential diagnosis of a benign condition such as tubal metaplasia, cytological surveillance may be justified[60,61,63] but, because of the focal nature of CGIN and related lesions within the endocervix and the inability of cytology to discriminate between CGIN and early invasive adenocarcinoma, small diagnostic biopsies cannot be relied upon to provide representative sampling[26,34,177]. For those with persisting abnormality, or those in whom at first presentation there is a high degree of suspicion of endocervical glandular neoplasia, at one time, hysterectomy was considered to be the treatment of choice[54]. More recently, however, cone biopsy or large loop excision biopsy is regarded as the minimum on which to diagnose and, in the event of complete excision, treat CGIN[29,56,178,179]. Indeed, some advocate careful clinical and cytological surveillance even after incomplete cone biopsy of CGIN[180]. Others have reported a high risk of residual disease independent of excision margin status[181-183].

In the UK, there are no specific guidelines, separate from those for CIN, for follow-up post conservative management of CGIN other than a recommendation that endocervical sampling is undertaken[184]. From America, Johnston recommends 6-monthly smears to be undertaken indefinitely[185]. There are few long-term studies to date to test the validity of this advice. Post loop or cone biopsy smears are particularly difficult to interpret especially after management of CGIN, with the potential for the development of endometriosis, tuboendometrial metaplasia, and the likelihood of lower uterine segment sampling. Heightened awareness of the possibility of glandular neoplasia also introduces bias with an increased risk of false positive reporting of residual glandular abnormality in the presence of these benign look-alikes[60]. It is half a century since Friedell and McKay described adenocarcinoma *in situ* of the endocervix and still there are problems for clinicians and pathologists alike in recognition of this lesion and in clinical management[19].

References

1 Tasker J T, Collins J A. Adenocarcinoma of the uterine cervix. *Am J Obstet Gynecol* 1974; **118**: 344–348

2 Davis J R, Moon L B. Increased incidence of adenocarcinoma of the uterine cervix. *Obstet Gynecol* 1975; **45**: 79–83

3 Gallup D G, Abell M R. Invasive adenocarcinoma of the uterine cervix. *Obstet Gynecol* 1977; **49**: 596–603

4 Shorrock K, Johnson J, Johnson I R. Epidemiological changes in cervical carcinoma with particular reference to mucin-secreting subtypes. *Histopathol* 1990; **17**: 53–57

5 Vizcaino A P, Moreno V, Bosch F X *et al.* International trends in the incidence of cervical cancer: 1. Adenocarcinoma and adenosquamous cell carcinomas. *Int J Cancer* 1998; **75**, 536–545

6 Parazzini F, La Vecchia C. Epidemiology of adenocarcinoma of the cervix. *Gynecol Oncol* 1990; **39**: 40–46

7 Dallenbach-Hellweg G. On the origin and histological structure of adenocarcinoma of the endocervix in women under 50 years of age. *Pathol Res Pract* 1984; **179**: 38–50

8 Ursin G, Peters R K, Henderson B E *et al.* Oral contraceptive use and adenocarcinoma of the cervix. *Lancet* 1994; **344**(ii): 1390–1394

9 Jackson S R, Hollingworth T A, Anderson M C *et al.* Glandular lesions of the cervix–cytological and histological correlation. *Cytopathol* 1996, **7**, 10–16

10 Mitchell H, Medley G, Gordon L, Giles G. Cervical cytology reported as negative risk of adenocarcinoma of the cervix: no strong evidence of benefit. *Br J Cancer* 1995; **71**, 894–897

11 Tase T, Okagaki T, Clark B A *et al.* Human papilloma virus in adenocarcinoma in situ, microinvasive adenocarcinoma of the uterine cervix, and coexisting cervical squamous intraepithelial neoplasia. *Int J Gynecol Pathol* 1989; **8**: 8–17

12 Leminen A, Paavonen J, Vesterinen E *et al.* Human papillomavirus types 16 and 18 in adenocarcinoma of the uterine cervix. *Am J Clin Pathol* 1991; **95**: 647–652

13 Bjersing L, Rogo K, Evander M *et al.* HPV 18 and cervical adenocarcinomas. *AntiCancer Res* 1991; **11**: 123–128

14 Cooper K, Herrington C S, Lo E S-F *et al.* Integration of human papillomavirus virus 16 and 18 in cervical adenocarcinoma. *J Clin Pathol* 1992; **45**: 382–384

15 Duggan M A, Benoit J L, McGregor E *et al.* Adenocarcinoma in situ of the endocervix: Human papilloma determination by dot blot hybridization and polymerase chain reaction amplification. *Int J Gynecol Pathol* 1994; **13**: 143–149

16 Bosch F X, Manos M, Munos N *et al.* and the IBSCC study group. Prevalence of human papillomavirus in cervical cancer: a worldwide perspective. *J Nat Cancer Inst* 1995; **87**: 796–802

17 Trowell J E. Intestinal metaplasia with argentaffin cells in the uterine cervix. *Histopathol* 1985; **9**: 551–559

18 Rollason T P ed. Epithelial lesions of the endocervix. In: *Progress in Pathology*, vol. 4. Edinburgh: Churchill Livingstone, 1998; 179–199

19 Friedell G H, McKay D G. Adenocarcinoma in situ of the endocervix. *Cancer* 1953; **6**: 887–897

20 Boddington M M, Spriggs A I, Cowdell R H. Adenocarcinoma of the uterine cervix: cytological evidence of a long preclinical evolution. *Br J Obstet Gynaecol* 1976; **83**: 900–903

21 Bousfield L, Pacey F, Young Q *et al.* Expanded cytologic criteria for the diagnosis of adenocarcinoma in situ of the cervix and related lesions. *Acta Cytol* 1980; **24**: 283–296

22 Boon M E, Baak J P A, Kurver P J H *et al.* Adenocarcinoma in situ of the cervix: an underdiagnosed lesion. *Cancer* 1981; **48**: 768–773

23 Kurian K, Al-Nafussi A. Relation of cervical glandular intraepithelial neoplasia to microinvasive and invasive adenocarcinoma of the uterine cervix: a study of 121 cases. *J Clin Pathol* 1999; **52**: 112–117

24 Plaxe S C, Saltzstein S L. Estimation of the duration of the preclinical phase of cervical adenocarcinoma suggests that there is ample opportunity for screening. *Gynecol Oncol* 1999; **75**: 55–61

25 Fox H, Buckley C H. Working party of the Royal College of Pathologists and the NHS Cervical Screening Programme. Histopathological reporting in cervical screening. Sheffield: *NHS Cervical Screening Programme Publication* 1999; **10**: 16–36

26 Bertrand M, Lickrish G M, Colgan T J. The anatomic distribution of cervical adenocarcinoma in situ: implications for treatment. *Am J Obstet Gynecol* 1987; **157**: 21–25

27 Young R H, Clement P B, Scully R E eds. Premalignant and malignant glandular lesions of the uterine cervix. In: *Tumors and Tumorlike Lesions of the Uterine Corpus and Cervix*. New York: Churchill Livingstone 1993; 86–136

28 Jaworski R C, Pacey N F, Greenberg M L, Osborn R A. The histologic diagnosis of adenocarcinoma in situ and related lesions of the cervix uteri: adenocarcinoma in situ. *Cancer* 1988; **61**: 1171–1181

29 Östör A G, Pagano R, Davoren R A M *et al.* Adenocarcinoma in situ of the cervix. *Int J Gynecol Pathol* 1984; **3**: 179–190

30 Lee S J, Rollason T. Argyrophilic cells in cervical intraepithelial glandular neoplasia. *Int J Gynecol Pathol* 1994; **13**: 131–132

31 Keyhani-Rofagha S, Brewer J, Prokorym P. Comparative cytologic findings of in situ and invasive adenocarcinoma of the uterine cervix. *Diagn Cytopathol* 1995; **12**: 120–125

32 Barter R A, Waters E D. Cyto- and histo-morphology of cervical adenocarcinoma in situ. *Pathol* 1970; **2**: 33–40

33 Weisbrot I M, Stabinsky C, Davis A M. Adenocarcinoma in situ of the uterine cervix. *Cancer* 1972; **29**: 1179–1187

34 Qizilbash A H. In situ and microinvasive adenocarcinoma of the uterine cervix. A clinical, cytologic and histologic study of 14 cases. *Am J Clin Pathol* 1975; **64**: 155–170

35 Krumins I, Young Q, Pacey F *et al.* The cytologic diagnosis of adenocarcinoma in situ of the cervix uteri. *Acta Cytol* 1977; **21**: 320–329

36 Betsill W L, Clark A H. Early endocervical glandular neoplasia I. Histomorphology and cytomorphology. *Acta Cytol* 1986; **30**: 115–126

37 Clark A H, Betsill W L. Early endocervical glandular neoplasia II. Morphometric analysis of the cells. *Acta Cytol* 1986; **30**: 127–134

38 Lee K R, Manna E A, Jones M A. Comparative cytologic features of adenocarcinoma in situ of the uterine cervix. *Acta Cytol* 1991; **35**: 117–126

39 van Aspert-van Erp A J, van't Hof-Grootenboer A B, Brugal G, Vooijs G P. Endocervical columnar cell intraepithelial neoplasia I. Discriminating cytomorphologic criteria. *Acta Cytol* 1995; **39**: 1199–1215

40 van Aspert-van Erp A J, van't Hof-Grootenboer A B, Brugal G, Vooijs G P. Endocervical columnar cell intraepithelial neoplasia II. Grades of expression of cytomorphologic criteria. *Acta Cytol* 1995; **39**: 1216–1232

41 Biscotti C V, Gero M A, Toddy S M et al. Endocervical adenocarcinoma in situ: an analysis of cellular features. *Diagn Cytopathol* 1997; **17**: 326–332

42 Vogelsang P J, Nguyen G-K, Honoré L H. Exfoliative cytology of adenoma malignum (minimal deviation adenocarcinoma) of the uterine cervix. *Diagn Cytopathol* 1995; **13**: 146–150

43 Gloor E, Ruzicka J. Morphology of adenocarcinoma in situ of the uterine cervix: A study of 14 cases. *Cancer* 1982; **49**: 294–302

44 Ayer B, Pacey F, Greenberg M, Bousfield L. The cytologic diagnosis of adenocarcinoma in situ of the cervix uteri and related lesions I. Adenocarcinoma in situ. *Acta Cytol* 1987; **31**: 397–411

45 Tobón H, Dave H. Adenocarcinoma in situ of the cervix: Clinicopathologic observations of 11 cases. *Int J Gynecol Pathol* 1988; **7**: 139–151

46 Brown L J R, Wells M. Cervical glandular atypia associated with squamous intraepithelial neoplasia: a premalignant lesion? *J Clin Pathol* 1986; **39**: 22–28

47 Goff B A, Atanasoff P, Brown E et al. Endocervical glandular atypia in Papanicolaou smears. *Obstet Gynecol* 1992; **79**: 101–104

48 Siziopikou K P, Wang H H, Abu-Jawdeh G. Cytological features of neoplastic lesions in endocervical glands. *Diagn Cytopathol* 1997; **17**: 1–7

49 Cenci M, Mancini R, Nofroni I, Vecchione A. Endocervical atypical cells of undetermined significance I: Morphometric and cytologic characterization of cases that 'cannot rule out adenocarcinom in situ'. *Acta Cytol* 2000; **44**: 319–326

50 Cenci M, Mancini R, Nofroni I, Vecchione A. Endocervical atypical cells of undetermined significance II: Morphometric and cytologic analysis of nuclear features useful in characterizing differently correlated subgroups. *Acta Cytol* 2000; **44**: 327–331

51 Geirsson G, Woodworth F E, Patten S F, Bonfiglio T A. Epithelial repair and regeneration in the uterine cervix I. An analysis of the cells. *Acta Cytol* 1977; **21**: 371–378

52 Ghorab Z, Mahmood S, Schinella R. Endocervical reactive atypia: A histo-cytologic study. *Diagn Cytopathol* 2000; **22**: 342–346

53 Mulvaney N, Östör A. Microinvasive adenocarcinoma of the cervix: a cytohistopathologic study of 40 cases. *Diagn Cytopathol* 1997; **16**: 430–436

54 Christopherson W M, Nealon N, Gray L A. Noninvasive precursor lesions of adenocarcinoma and mixed adenosquamous carcinoma of the cervix uteri. *Cancer* 1979; **44**: 975–983

55 Nguyen G-K, Jeannot A B. Exfoliative cytology of in situ and microinvasive adenocarcinoma of the uterine cervix. *Acta Cytol* 1984; **28**: 461–467

56 Cullimore J E, Luesley D M, Rollason T P et al. A prospective study of conization of the cervix in the management of cervical intraepithelial glandular neoplasia (CIGN)–a preliminary report. *Br J Obstet Gynaecol* 1992; **99**: 314–318

57 Buscema J, Woodruff J D. Significance of neoplastic atypicalities in endocervical epithelium. *Gynecol Oncol* 1984; **17**: 356–362

58 Crum C P, Cibas E S, Lee K R, eds. Glandular precursors, adenocarcinomas, and their mimics. In: *Contemporary Issues in Surgical Pathology: Pathology of Early Cervical Neoplasia*. New York: Churchill Livingstone, 1997; 177–240

59 Novotny D B, Maygarden S J, Johnson D E, Frable W J. Tubal metaplasia. A frequent pitfall in the cytologic diagnosis of endocervical glandular dysplasia in cervical smears. *Acta Cytol* 1992; **36**: 1–10

60 Roberts J M, Thurloe J K, Bowditch R C, Laverty C R. Subdividing atypical glandular cells of undetermined significance according to the Australian modified Bethesda system: Analysis of outcomes. *Cancer (Cancer Cytopathol)* 2000; **90**: 87–95

61 Johnson J, Patnick J. Achievable standards, benchmarks for reporting, criteria for evaluating cervical cytopathology: Report of a working party set up by the Royal College of Pathologists, the British Society for Clinical Cytology and the NHS Cervical Screening Programme. Sheffield: *NHS Cervical Screening Programme Publication* 2000; **1**: 9–12

62 Lee K R, Manna E A, St John T. Atypical endocervical glandular cells: Accuracy of cytologic diagnosis. *Diagn Cytopathol* 1995; **13**: 202–208

63 Solomon D, Frable W J, Vooijs G P, Wilbur D C. ASCUS and AGUS criteria. IAC Task Force summary. *Acta Cytol* 1998; **42**: 16–24

64 Bose S, Kannan V, Kline T S. Abnormal endocervical cells. Really abnormal? Really endocervical? *Am J Clin Pathol* 1994; **101**: 708–713

65 Di'Tomasso J, I Ramzy, Mody D R. Glandular lesions of the cervix. Validity of cytologic criteria used to differentiate reactive changes, glandular intraepithelial lesions and adenocarcinoma. *Acta Cytol* 1996; **40**: 1127–1135

66 Raab S S, Isacson C, Layfield L J et al. Atypical glandular cells of undetermined significance. Cytologic criteria to separate clinically significant from benign lesions. *Am J Clin Pathol* 1995; **104**: 574–582

67 van Hoeven K H, Hanau C A, Hudock J A. The detection of endocervical gland involvement by high-grade squamous intraepithelial lesions in smears prepared from endocervical brush specimens. *Cytopathol* 1996; **7**: 310–315

68 Andersen W, Frierson H, Barber S et al. Sensitivity and specificity of endocervical curettage and the endocervical brush for the evaluation of the endocervical canal. *Am J Obstet Gynecol* 1988; **159**: 702–707

69 Selvaggi S M. Cytologic features of squamous cell carcinoma in situ involving endocervical glands in endocervical cytobrush specimens. *Acta Cytol* 1994; **38**: 687–692

70 Drijkoningen M, Meertens B, Lauweryns J. High-grade squamous intraepithelial lesion (CIN3) with extension into endocervical clefts. Difficulty of cytologic differentiation from adenocarcinoma in situ. *Acta Cytol* 1996; **40**: 889–894

71 Waddell C A. Cervical cytology: an audit of 16 years of glandular prediction in a single center. *Acta Cytol* 1998; **42**: 594

72 Ducatman B S, Wang H H, Jonasson J G et al. Tubal metaplasia: A cytologic study with comparison to other neoplastic and non-neoplastic conditions of the endocervix. *Diagn Cytopathol* 1993; **9**: 98–105

73 Selvaggi S M, Haefner H K. Microglandular endocervical hyperplasia and tubal metaplasia: pitfalls in the diagnosis of adenocarcinoma on cervical smears. *Diagn Cytopathol* 1997; **16**: 168–173

74 Hirschowitz L, Eckford S D, Phillpotts B, Midwinter A. Cytological changes associated with tubo-endometrioid metaplasia of the uterine cervix. *Cytopathol* 1994; **5**: 1–8

75 Babkowski R C, Wilbur D C, Rutkowski M A et al. The effects of endocervical canal topography, tubal metaplasia, and high canal sampling on cytologic presentation of nonneoplastic endocervical cells. *Am J Clin Pathol* 1996; **105**: 403–410

76 Pacey F, Ayer B, Greenberg M. The cytologic diagnosis of adenocarcinoma in situ of the cervix uteri and related lesions III. Pitfalls in diagnosis. *Acta Cytol* 1988; **32**: 325–329

77 Lee K R. Atypical glandular cells in cervical smears from women who have undergone cone biopsy: A potential diagnostic pitfall. *Acta Cytol* 1993; **37**: 705–709

78 de Peralta-Venturino M N, Purslow M J, Kini S R. Endometrial cells of the 'lower uterine segment' (LUS) in cervical smears obtained by endocervical brushings: A source of potential diagnostic pitfall. *Diagn Cytopathol* 1995; **12**: 263–271

79 Lee K R, Genest D R, Minter L J et al. Adenocarcinoma in situ in cervical smears with small cell (endometrioid) pattern. Distinction from cells directly sampled

from the upper endocervical canal or lower segment of the endometrium. *Am J Clin Pathol* 1998; **109**: 738–742

80 Ngadiman S, Yang G C H. Adenomyomatous lower uterine segment and endocervical polyps in cervicovaginal smears. *Acta Cytol* 1995; **39**: 643–647

81 Chhieng D C, Elgert P A, Cangiarella J F, Cohen J-M. Cytology of polypoid adenomyomas: a report of two cases. *Diagn Cytopathol* 2000; **22**: 176–180

82 Ismail S M. Cone biopsy causes cervical endometriosis and tuboendometrioid metaplasia. *Histopathol* 1991; **18**: 107–114

83 Hanau C A, Begley N, Bibbo M. Cervical endometriosis: A potential pitfall in the evaluation of glandular cells in cervical smears. *Diagn Cytopathol* 1997; **16**: 274–280

84 Mulvaney N J, Surtees V. Cervical/vaginal endometriosis with atypia: A cytohistopathologic study. *Diagn Cytopathol* 1999; **21**: 188–193

85 Lee K R. Adenocarcinoma in situ with a small cell (endometrioid) pattern in cervical smears: A test of the distinction from benign mimics using specific criteria. *Cancer (Cancer Cytopathol)* 1999; **87**: 254–258

86 Nichols T M, Fidler H K. Microglandular hyperplasia in cervical cone biopsies taken for suspicious and positive cytology. *Am J Clin Pathol* 1971; **56**: 424–429

87 Greeley C, Schroeder S, Silverberg S. Microglandular hyperplasia of the cervix: A true 'pill' lesion? *Int J Gynecol Pathol* 1995; **14**: 50–54

88 Yahr L J, Lee K R. Cytologic findings in microglandular hyperplasia of the cervix. *Diagn Cytopathol* 1991; **7**: 248–251

89 Valente P T, Schantz H D, Schultz M. Cytologic atypia associated with microglandular hyperplasia. *Diagn Cytopathol* 1994; **10**: 326–331

90 Alvarez-Santín C, Sica A, Rodríguez M C et al. Microglandular hyperplasia of the uterine cervix. Cytologic diagnosis in cervical smears. *Acta Cytol* 1999; **43**: 110–113

91 Frierson H F, Covell J L, Andersen W A. Radiation changes in endocervical cells in brush specimens. *Diagn Cytopathol* 1990; **6**: 243–247

92 Stewart C J R, Taggart C R, Brett F, Mutch A F. Mesonephric adenocarcinoma of the uterine cervix with focal endocrine cell differentiation. *Int J Gynecol Pathol* 1993; **12**: 264–269

93 Schneider V. Arias-Stella reaction of the endocervix. Frequency and location. *Acta Cytol* 1981; **25**: 224–228

94 Holmes E J, Lyle W H. How early in pregnancy does the Arias-Stella reaction occur? *Arch Pathol* 1973; **95**: 302–303

95 Shrago S S. The Arias Stella reaction. A case report of a cytologic presentation. *Acta Cytol* 1977; **21**: 310–313

96 Danos M L. Post partum cytology: Observations over a four year period. *Acta Cytol* 1968; **12**: 309–312

97 Quincey C, Persad R V, Stanbridge C M. Chorionic villi in post-partum cervical smears. *Cytopathol* 1995; **6**: 149–155

98 Masuda K, Yutani C, Akutagawa K et al. Cytopathological observations in a 27 year old female patient with endometrioid adenocarcinoma arising in the lower uterine segment of the uterus. *Diagn Cytopathol* 1999; **21**: 117–121

99 Maksem J A. Ciliated cell adenocarcinoma of the endometrium diagnosed by endometrial brush cytology and confirmed by hysterectomy: A case report detailing a highly efficient cytology collection and processing technique. *Diagn Cytopathol* 1997; **16**: 78–82

100 Schumann J L, O'Connor D M, Covell J L, Greening S E. Pap smear collection devices: technical, clinical, diagnostic, and legal considerations associated with their use. *Diagn Cytopathol* 1992; **8**: 492–503

101 Fiorella R M, Casafrancisco D, Yokota S, Kragel P J. Artifactual endocervical atypia induced by endocervical brush collection. *Diagn Cytopathol* 1994; **11**: 79–84

102 De May R M eds. The Pap smear. In: *The Art and Science of Cytopathology: Exfoliative Cytology*. Chicago: ASCP Press, 1996; 161

103 Cronjé H S, Divall P, Bam R H et al. Effects of dilute acetic acid on the cervical smear. *Acta Cytol* 1997; **41**: 1091–1094

104 Brand E, Berek J S, Hacker N F. Controversies in the management of cervical adenocarcinoma. *Obstet Gynecol* 1988; **71**: 261–269

105 Leminen A, Paavonen J, Forss M et al. Adenocarcinoma of the uterine cervix. *Cancer* 1990; **65**: 53–59

106 Buckley C H, Fox H eds. Carcinoma of the cervix. In: *Recent Advances in Histopathology*, 14. Edinburgh: Churchill Livingstone, 1989; 63–78

107 Rollason T P, Cullimore J, Bradgate M G. A suggested columnar cell morphological equivalent of squamous carcinoma in situ with early stromal invasion. *Int J Gynecol Pathol* 1989; **8**: 230–236

108 Anderson M C ed. Pathology of cervical cancer. In: *Clinics in Obstetrics and Gynaecology*, 12. London: W B Saunders, 1985; 111–115

109 Ayer B, Pacey F, Greenberg M. The cytologic diagnosis of adenocarcinoma in situ of the cervix uteri and related lesions II. Microinvasive adenocarcinoma. *Acta Cytol* 1988; **32**: 318–324

110 Kudo R, Sagae S, Hayakawa O et al. Morphology of adenocarcinoma in situ and microinvasive adenocarcinoma of the uterine cervix. A cytologic and ultrastructural study. *Acta Cytol* 1991; **35**: 109–116

111 Saigo P E, Wolinska W H, Kim W S, Hajdu S I. The role of cytology in the diagnosis and follow-up of patients with cervical adenocarcinoma. *Acta Cytol* 1985; **29**: 785–794

112 Costa M J, Kenny M B, Naib Z M. Cervicovaginal cytology in uterine adenocarcinoma and adenosquamous carcinoma. Comparison of cytologic and histologic findings. *Acta Cytol* 1991; **35**: 127–134

113 Hayes M M, Matisic J P, Chen C-J et al. Cytological aspects of uterine cervical adenocarcinoma, adenosquamous carcinoma and combined adenocarcinoma-squamous carcinoma: appraisal of diagnostic criteria for in situ versus invasive lesions. *Cytopathol* 1997; **8**: 397–408

114 Goodman H M, Niloff J M, Buttlar C A et al. Adenocarcinoma of the cervical stump. *Gynecol Oncol* 1989; **35**: 188–192

115 Kaminski P E, Norris H J. Minimal deviation carcinoma (adenoma malignum) of the cervix. *Int J Gynecol Pathol* 1983; **2**: 141–152

116 Szyfelbein W M, Young R H, Scully R E. Adenoma malignum of the cervix: cytologic findings. *Acta Cytol* 1984; **28**: 691–698

117 Granter S R, Lee K R. Cytologic findings in minimal deviation adenocarcinoma (adenoma malignum) of the cervix. A report of seven cases. *Am J Clin Pathol* 1996; **105**: 327–333

118 Hirai Y, Takeshima N, Haga A et al. A clinicocytopathologic study of adenoma malignum of the uterine cervix. *Gynecol Oncol* 1998; **70**: 219–223

119 Ishii K, Katsuyama T, Ota H et al. Cytologic and cytochemical features of adenoma malignum of the uterine cervix. *Cancer (Cancer Cytopathol)* 1999; **87**: 245–253

120 Young R H, Scully R E. Villoglandular papillary adenocarcinoma of the uterine cervix. A clinicopathologic analysis of 13 cases. *Cancer* 1989; **63**: 1173–1779

121 Ballo M S, Silverberg S G, Sidawy M. Cytologic features of well-differentiated villoglandular adenocarcinoma of the cervix. *Acta Cytol* 1996; **40**: 536–540

122 Novotny D B, Ferlisi P. Villoglandular adenocarcinoma of the cervix: cytologic presentation. *Diagn Cytopathol* 1997; **17**: 383–387

123 Chang W C, Matisic J P, Zhou C et al. Cytologic features of villoglandular adenocarcinoma of the uterine cervix: Comparison with typical endocervical adenocarcinoma with a villoglandular component and papillary serous carcinoma. *Cancer (Cancer Cytopathol)* 1999; **87**: 5–11

124 Hasumi K, Ehrmann R. Clear cell carcinoma of the uterine endocervix with an in situ component. *Cancer* 1978; **42**: 2435–2438

125 Wingfield M. The daughters of stilboestrol. Grown up now but still at risk. *BMJ* 1991; **302**: 1414–1415

126 Dickersin G R, Welch W R, Erlandson R, Robboy S J. Ultrastructure of 16 cases of clear cell adenocarcinoma of the vagina and cervix in young women. *Cancer* 1980; **45**: 1615–1624

127 Vooijs P G, Ng A B P, Wentz W B. The detection of vaginal adenosis and clear cell carcinoma. *Acta Cytol* 1973; **17**: 59

128 Taft P D, Robboy S J, Herbst A L, Scully R E. Cytology of clear cell adenocarcinoma of genital tract in young females: Review of 95 cases from the registry. *Acta Cytol* 1974; **18**: 279

129 Young Q, Pacey N F. The cytologic diagnosis of clear cell adenocarcinoma of the cervix uteri. *Acta Cytol* 1978; **22**: 3

130 Fox H, Wells M, Harris M *et al*. Enteric tumours of the lower female genital tract: a report of three cases. *Histopathol* 1988; **12**: 167–176

131 Dougherty C M, Cotten N. Mixed squamous-cell and adenocarcinoma of the cervix. *Cancer* 1964; **17**: 1132–1143

132 Pak H Y, Yokota S B, Paladugu R R, Agliozzo C M. Glassy cell carcinoma of the cervix: Cytologic and clinicopathologic analysis. *Cancer* 1983; **52**: 307–312

133 Nuñez C, Abduk-Karim F, Somrak T M. Glassy-cell carcinoma of the uterine cervix. Cytopathologic and histopathologic study of five cases. *Acta Cytol* 1985; **29**; 303–309

134 Grafton W D, Kamm R C, Cowley L H. Cytologic characteristics of adenoid cystic carcinoma of the cervix uteri. *Acta Cytol* 1976; **20**: 164–166

135 Dayton V, Henry M, Stanley M W *et al*. Adenoid cystic carcinoma of the uterine cervix. Cytologic features. *Acta Cytol* 1990; **34**: 125–128

136 Peterson L S, Neumann A A. Cytologic features of adenoid basal carcinoma of the uterine cervix. A case report. *Acta Cytol* 1995; **39**: 563–568

137 Ng A B P, Teeple D, Lindner E A, Reagan J W. The cellular manifestations of extrauterine cancer. *Acta Cytol* 1974; **18**: 108–117

138 Fiorella R M, Beckwith L G, Miller L K, Kragel P J. Metastatic signet ring carcinoma of the breast as a source of positive cervicovaginal cytology. A case report. *Acta Cytol* 1993; **37**: 948–952

139 Matsuura Y, Saito R, Kawagoe T *et al*. Cytologic analysis of primary stomach adenocarcinoma metastatic to the uterine cervix. *Acta Cytol* 1997; **41**: 291–294

140 Wolfendale M R, Howe-Guest R, Usherwood M McD, Draper G J. Controlled trial of a new cervical spatula. *BMJ* 1987; **294**: 33–35

141 Waddell C A, Rollason T P, Amarilli J M, Cullimore J, McConkey C C. The Cervex: an ectocervical brush sampler. *Cytopathol* 1990; **1**: 171–181

142 Selvaggi S M, Guidos B J. Specimen adequacy and the ThinPrep Pap test: The endocervical component. *Diagn Cytopathol* 2000; **23**: 23–26

143 Nasu I, Meurer W, Fu Y S. Endocervical glandular atypia and adenocarcinoma: A correlation of cytology and histology. *Int J Gynecol Pathol* 1993; **12**: 208–218

144 Wilbur D C. Endocervical glandular atypia: A 'new' problem for the cytologist. *Diagn Cytopathol* 1995; **13**: 463–469

145 Eddy G L, Ural S H, Strumpf K B *et al*. Incidence of atypical glandular cells of uncertain significance in cervical cytology following introduction of the Bethesda system. *Gynecol Oncol* 1997; **67**: 51–55

146 Mody D R. Agonizing over AGUS. *Cancer Cytopathol* 1999; **87**: 243–244

147 Bishop J W. Comparison of the CytoRich system with conventional cervical cytology. Preliminary data on 2,032 cases from a clinical trial site. *Acta Cytol* 1997; **41**: 15–23

148 Vassilakos P, Saurel J, Rondez R. Direct-to-vial use of the AutoCyte PREP liquid-based

preparation for cervical-vaginal specimens in three European laboratories. *Acta Cytol* 1999; **43**: 65–68

149 Bai H, Sung C J, Steinhoff M M. ThinPrep Pap test promotes detection of glandular lesions of the endocervix. *Diagn Cytopathol* 2000; **23**: 19–22

150 Roberts J M, Gurley A M, Thurloe J K *et al*. Evaluation of the ThinPrep Pap test as an adjunct to the conventional Pap smear. *MJA* 1997; **167**: 466–469

151 Corkill M, Knapp D, Martin J, Hutchinson M L. Specimen adequacy of ThinPrep sample preparations in a direct-to-vial study. *Acta Cytol* 1997; **41**: 39–44

152 Roberts J M, Thurloe J K, Bowditch R C *et al*. Comparison of ThinPrep and Pap smear in relation to prediction of adenocarcinoma in situ. *Acta Cytol* 1999; **43**: 74–80

153 Yeoh G P S, Chan K W. Cell block preparation on residual ThinPrep sample. *Diagn Cytopathol* 1999; **21**: 427–431

154 Johnson J E, Rahemtulla A. Endocervical glandular neoplasia and its mimics in ThinPrep Pap tests. A descriptive study. *Acta Cytol* 1999; **43**: 369–375

155 Ashfaq R, Gibbons D, Vela C *et al*. ThinPrep Pap test. Accuracy for glandular disease. *Acta Cytol* 1999; **43**: 81–85

156 Maksem J A, Sager F, Bender R. Endometrial collection and interpretation using the Tao brush and the CytoRich fixative system: a feasibility study. *Diagn Cytopathol* 1997; **17**: 339–346

157 Maksem J A. Endocervical cell collection using cytobrush liquid-fixation, and cytocentrifugation: a feasibility study using 455 hysterectomy specimens. *Diagn Cytopathol* 1999; **21**: 419–426

158 Johnson T, Maksem J A, Belsheim B L *et al*. Liquid-based cervical-cell collection with brushes and wooden spatulas: A comparison of 100 conventional smears from high risk women to liquid-fixed cytocentrifuge slides, demonstrating a cost-effective, alternative monolayer slide preparation method. *Diagn Cytopathol* 2000; **22**: 86–91

159 Ashfaq R, Solares B, Saboorian M H. Detection of endocervical component by Papnet system on negative cervical smears. *Diagn Cytopathol* 1996; **15**: 121–123

160 Losell K, Dejmek A. Comparison of Papnet-assisted and manual screening of cervical smears. *Diagn Cytopathol* 1999; **21**: 296–299

161 Sturgis C D, Isoe C, McNeal N E *et al*. Papnet computer-aided rescreening for detection of benign and malignant glandular elements in cervicovaginal smears: A review of 61 cases. *Diagn Cytopathol* 1998; **18**: 307–311

162 Kleinschmidt-Guy E D, van Binsbergen-Ingelse A, Boon M E. The application of MIB-1 staining to identify carcinoma cells from well differentiated adenocarcinoma of the cervix in smears screened via Papnet. *Cytopathol* 1998; **9(suppl 1)**: 38

163 Syrjänen K J, Syrjänen S M. Human papillomavirus (HPV) typing as an adjunct to cervical cancer screening. *Cytopathol* 1999; **10**: 8–15

164 Darne J F, Polacarz S V, Sheridan E *et al*. Nucleolar organiser regions in adenocarcinoma in situ and invasive adenocarinoma of the cervix. *J Clin Pathol* 1990; **43**: 657–660

165 Cardillo M R. AgNOR counts are useful in cervical smears. *Diagn Cytopathol* 1992; **8**: 208–210

166 Fiorella R M, Saran B, Kragel P J. AgNOR counts as a discriminator of lesions of the endocervix. *Acta Cytol* 1994; **38**: 527–530

167 Boon M E, Beck S, Kok L P. Semiautomatic PAPNET analysis of proliferating (MiB-1–positive) cells in cervical cytology and histology. *Diagn Cytopathol* 1995; **13**: 423–428

168 Liao S-Y, Stanbridge E J. Expression of MN/CA9 protein in Papanicolaou smears containing atypical glandular cells of undetermined significance is a diagnostic biomarker of cervical dysplasia and neoplasia. *Cancer* 2000; **88**: 1108–1121

169 Koizumi M, Uede T, Shijubo N *et al*. New monoclonal antibody, 1C5, reactive with human cervical adenocarcinoma of the uterus, with immunodiagnostic potential. *Cancer Res* 1988; **48**: 6565–6572

170 Kobilková J, Lojda Z, Dohnalová A, Havránková E. Cytologic detection of cervical and endometrial carcinoma with other genital tract involvement. *Acta Cytol* 2000; **44**: 13–17

171 Comer M T, Andrew A C, Leese H J *et al*. Application of a marker of ciliated epithelial cells to gynaecological pathology. *J Clin Pathol* 1999; **52**: 355–357

172 Utsugi K, Hirai Y, Takeshima N *et al*. Utility of the monoclonal antibody HIK1083 in the diagnosis of adenoma malignum of the uterine cervix. *Gynecol Oncol* 1999; **75**: 345–348

173 Mikamai Y, Hata S, Fujiwara K *et al*. Florid endocervical glandular hyperplasia with intestinal and pyloric gland metaplasia: worrisome benign mimic of 'adenoma malignum'. *Gynecol Oncol* 1999; **74**: 504–511

174 Cullimore J E, Luesley D M, Rollason T P *et al*. A case of glandular intraepithelial neoplasia involving the cervix and vagina. *Gynecol Oncol* 1989; **34**: 249–252

175 Leeson S C, Inglis T C M, Salman W D. A study to determine the underlying reason for abnormal glandular cytology and the formulation of a management protocol. *Cytopathol* 1997; **8**: 20–26

176 Waddell C A. Glandular abnormalities: dilemmas in cytological prediction and clinical management. *Cytopathol* 1997; **8**: 27–30

177 Cullimore J E, Rollason T P, Luesley D M *et al*. Invasive cervical cancer after laser vaporisation for cervical intraepithelial neoplasia: a 10-year experience. *J Gynecol Surg* 1990; **2**: 103–110

178 Luesley D M, Jordan J A, Woodman C B J *et al*. A retrospective review of adenocarcinoma in situ and glandular atypia of the uterine cervix. *Br J Obstet Gynaecol* 1987; **94**: 699–703

179 Laverty C R, Farnsworth A, Thurloe J, Bowditch R. The reliability of a

cytological prediction of cervical adenocarcinoma in situ. *Aust NZ J Obstet Gynaecol* 1988; **28**: 307–312

180 Hitchcock A, Johnson J, McDowell K, Johnson I R. A retrospective study into the occurrence of cervical glandular atypia in cone biopsy specimens from 1977–1978 with clinical follow-up. *Int J Gynecol Cancer* 1993; **3**: 164–168

181 Wolf J K, Levenback C, Malpica A *et al*. Adenocarcinoma in situ of the cervix: significance of cone biopsy margins. *Obstet Gynecol* 1996; **88**: 82–86

182 Denehy T R, Gregori C A, Breen J L. Endocervical curettage, cone margins, and residual adenocarcinoma in situ of the cervix. *Obstet Gynecol* 1997; **90**: 1–6

183 Azodi M, Chambers S K, Rutherford T J *et al*. Adenocarcinoma in situ of the cervix;

management and outcome. *Gynecol Oncol* 1999; **73**: 348–353

184 Anderson M C, Jordan J A, Morse A R, Sharp F eds. Management of premalignant and early malignant disease of the cervix. In: *Integrated Colposcopy*. 2nd edn. London: Chapman and Hall, 1996; 176–178

185 Johnston C. Cervical adenocarcinoma in situ: a persistent clinical dilemma. *Lancet* 1997; **350**: 1337

33 Other tumours and tumour-like conditions of the cervix

Xenia Tyler and Winifred Gray

Introduction

The preceding chapters have covered the cytopathology of the commonest types of neoplasms arising in the cervix. It is the intention in the next few pages to discuss the cytological findings in some less common tumours and tumour variants, and to review briefly the cytology of non-neoplastic conditions of the cervix that may present as a tumour clinically or microscopically.

Tumour-like conditions of the cervix

Cervical polyps

The term polyp simply refers to a protuberant mass of tissue. The tissue may be regenerative, inflammatory or neoplastic in origin; less often, it may be congenital or hamartomatous. In gynaecological practice, a cervical polyp is usually a benign polypoidal overgrowth of the endocervical tissues of the cervix, although other types of polypoidal lesion are also encountered.

Cervical polyps of endocervical origin are common, occurring in approximately 5–8% of women, most commonly multigravidas between the ages of 40–60 years. The polyps are usually single and asymptomatic, but can cause vaginal discharge or bleeding. Histologically, they are composed of endocervical tissue covered by columnar, squamous or immature metaplastic epithelium and are often inflamed (Fig. 33.1). Microglandular endocervical hyperplasia may be present focally.

Although the incidence of cervical intraepithelial neoplasia (CIN), adenocarcinoma or squamous carcinoma arising in a polyp is low (0.2–0.4%)[1], removal of cervical polyps is generally advisable. Histological examination is imperative and may reveal that the polyp is in fact an unsuspected condyloma or a neoplasm (Fig. 33.2). The presence of a polyp can interfere with the cervical smear procedure if overlying part of the transformation zone.

Cytological findings

- ▶ Smears are usually entirely normal
- ▶ Endocervical cells may show reactive features

In most instances the smear is normal, but may be of poor quality if the polyp has significantly interfered with smear taking, caused bleeding or is associated with cervicitis.

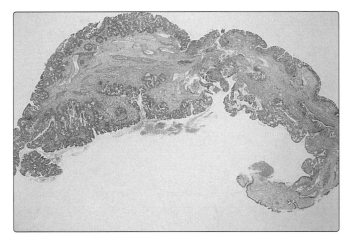

Fig. 33.1 Section of a benign endocervical polyp covered by endocervical and metaplastic epithelium. The stroma shows a light non-specific inflammatory cell infiltrate. (H&E × LP)

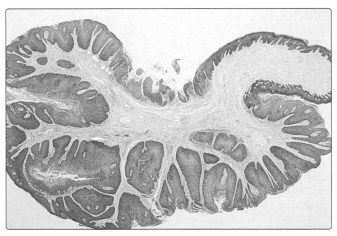

Fig. 33.2 Cervical polyp which on section shows the changes of a condyloma induced by papillomavirus infection. The covering mucosa consists of hyperplastic squamous epithelium. At this magnification maturation of the mucosa appears normal and no evidence of CIN can be seen. This example highlights the need for histological examination of all cervical lesions presenting as a polyp. (H&E × LP)

Sometimes endocervical cells from the polyp show reactive changes including marked nuclear enlargement with pleomorphism, hyperchromasia and prominent nucleoli (Fig. 33.3A,B). Occasionally polypoidal tissue fragments from the polyp appear in the smear, comprising an inner core of numerous small dark stromal cells, covered by a

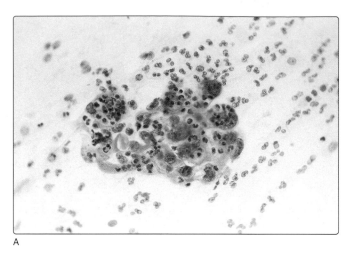 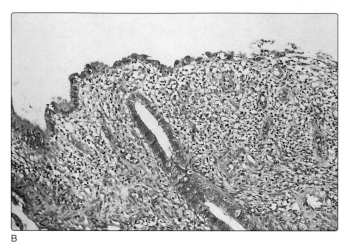

A   B

Fig. 33.3   (A) Endocervical cell cluster with reactive changes in cervical smear with a heavy inflammatory exudate. A cervical polyp was recorded in the clinical details. The smear was repeated after polypectomy and was found to be normal. The polyp showed non-specific inflammation. (Papanicolaou × HP) (B) Polypectomy specimen showed similar changes at the surface of the polyp. (H&E × MP)

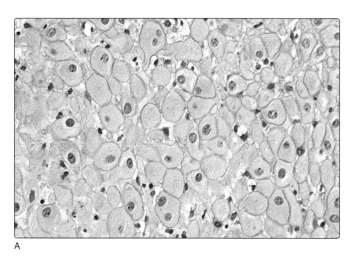 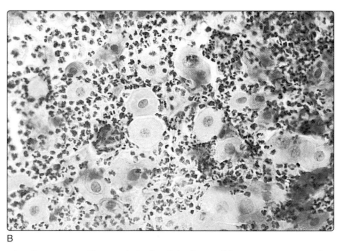

A   B

Fig. 33.4   (A) Decidual reaction in cervical stroma of a young woman at 10 weeks of pregnancy. The cervix had a clinically suspicious appearance and was biopsied to exclude a tumour. The stroma shows swollen pale cells with abundant cytoplasm, well-defined cell membranes and regular nuclei. (H&E × HP) (B) Decidual cells in a cervical smear taken from the same patient. The cells are similar to those in the biopsy, appearing swollen and pale against the background of neutrophil polymorphs. (Papanicolaou × HP) (Courtesy of Professor B Naylor, Michigan, USA)

layer of columnar cells with basal nuclei[2]. If there are interpretative problems, the smear should be repeated after removal of the polyp.

Microglandular hyperplasia, a focal clustering of small glandular elements, is sometimes seen within a polyp. Cells from these areas may have vacuolated cytoplasm and show hyperplastic features (see Fig. 33.8), but the groups lack the cell crowding and the architectural and nuclear abnormalities of endocervical dyskaryosis.

Condylomatous change, squamous or glandular precancer or invasive neoplasia within a polyp, if appropriately sampled, yields the same cytological findings as described in the preceding chapters.

Lower uterine segment polyps

This term is used to describe polyps arising at or just above the junction of endocervix with endometrium. They typically have a low gland to stroma ratio. The cytological features of two such polyps presenting in cervical smears have been described[2]. Both smears contained tissue fragments comprising small vessels running in various directions, connected by thin sheets of small ovoid cells with indistinct cytoplasm.

Decidual polyps

During pregnancy the cervical stroma frequently undergoes focal decidual change and this reaction may be so extensive as to form a polypoidal protrusion of the cervical stroma known as a decidual polyp (Fig. 33.4). The decidual change is typically subepithelial in location, often disrupting the overlying epithelium. The histological appearance may be misinterpreted as carcinoma since decidualized stromal cells have large nuclei, prominent nucleoli and abundant cytoplasm, imparting an epithelioid appearance (Fig. 33.4)[3].

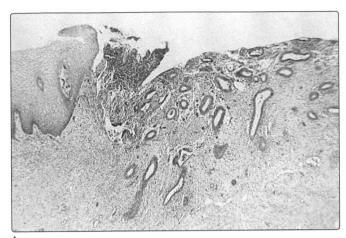

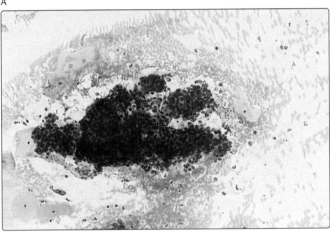

Fig. 33.5 (A) Endometriosis of cervix. The biopsy was taken from a haemorrhagic friable area at the external os in a middle-aged woman presenting with contact bleeding nine months after diathermy to a prominent nabothian follicle. Note the cellular endometrial stroma surrounding irregular glands lined by darkly stained epithelium of endometrial type. (H&E × LP) (B) Endometrial cell group composed of crowded cells with hyperchromatic nuclei in a haemorrhagic background. Cervical smear is from the patient whose biopsy is shown in (A). (Papanicolaou × MP)

Cytological findings

▶ Loose sheets of polygonal cells
▶ Abundant pale cytoplasm
▶ Large nuclei, prominent nucleoli

Decidual cells have been found in 34% of smears from women with histologically confirmed decidual change in the cervix[4]. The number of cells in a smear varies widely from less than 20 to over 3000. They tend to be arranged in loose sheets accompanied by neutrophil polymorphs. The cells are usually polygonal, more rarely having a spindled shape. Nuclei are large and usually have finely granular chromatin with prominent eosinophilic nucleoli. The cytoplasm is plentiful, transparent and delicate-looking. A history of pregnancy is helpful in avoiding confusion of decidual cells with repair cells and dyskaryotic glandular or squamous cells.

Arias–Stella change

Interpretative problems may arise during pregnancy if the endocervical glandular epithelium undergoes the type of extreme hypersecretory activity known as Arias–Stella change. This has been observed in 9% of cervices from hysterectomy specimens obtained during pregnancy[5] and is due to the action of human chorionic gonadotrophin. It can also occur in other hyperprogestational states such as gestational trophoblastic disease and with high dose progestogen therapy. Histologically, the cervix shows an exaggerated secretory pattern in the glands, associated with papillary infoldings of the epithelium, mirroring the findings in endometrium. The nuclei may be pleomorphic and hyperchromatic and the cytoplasm is vacuolated, producing a hobnail appearance at the cell surface. When superficial endocervical glands show Arias–Stella change it is possible for cells from these glands to be seen in a cervical smear.

Cytological findings

▶ Atypical glandular cells in the presence of pregnancy or other hyperprogestational state
▶ Large pleomorphic eccentric nuclei, vacuolated cytoplasm

The cytological features have been described in single case reports[6,7], and in one of these the cervical Arias-Stella reaction was associated with a cervical pregnancy. Atypical glandular cells occur singly, in syncytial clusters and cohesive sheets. They have large, hyperchromatic, pleomorphic nuclei with finely granular or smudged chromatin and one or two small nucleoli. The nuclear cytoplasmic ratio is low and the cells have abundant, frequently microvacuolated cytoplasm. A few intranuclear cytoplasmic inclusions and large, bare, hyperchromatic nuclei may also be present. Arias-Stella cells could be mistaken for malignant glandular cells if the history of pregnancy is not known.

Endometriosis

Endometriosis refers to the presence of endometrial glands and stroma outside the body of the uterus. Cervical endometriosis is considered to be uncommon unless there has been a previous operative procedure, focal endometriosis then resulting from metaplasia (Fig. 33.5A). In a study of 42 cervices from hysterectomies following conization, Ismail reported the presence of endometriosis in 43% of cases[8]. This ectopic tissue is hormonally responsive and friable and the patient may therefore present with irregular contact bleeding.

Cytological features

▶ Bloodstained smears due to contact bleeding
▶ Strips and sheets of endometrial epithelial cells

► Endometrial stromal cells in loose groups or admixed with epithelial cells

► Mitoses and mild nuclear atypia may be present

► Aspirated specimens may include degenerate red blood cells and haemosiderin laden macrophages

In smears, endometrial cells from the cervix are well preserved and are arranged in large sheets or strips showing gland openings and nuclear stratification respectively (Fig. 33.5B). The smears are often heavily blood-stained.

Endometrial cells have a high nuclear/cytoplasmic ratio, relatively hyperchromatic nuclei with irregular contours and coarse chromatin; they may have prominent nucleoli and mitoses may be found. These features, together with the exfoliation pattern described, carry the risk that the cells may be mistaken for dyskaryotic endocervical cells. The latter cells, however, typically show flat sheets of monotonous cells with crowded overlapping nuclei and the sheets have more striking architectural abnormalities (see Chapter 32). Nevertheless, diagnostic problems may arise, especially if endometriosis has developed following treatment for *in situ* glandular neoplasia of the cervix (CGIN).

Endometrial stromal cells may also be present, either in loose groups with ragged edges or admixed with the epithelial cells. Stromal cells are oval or round with rounded or reniform nuclei and scanty ill-defined cytoplasm, which is more abundant during the secretory phase of the cycle. Their presence enables the diagnosis of endometriosis to be made.

The possibility of endometriosis should also be considered when reporting fine needle aspirates from the cervix or other sites. Aspirated specimens contain endometrial epithelial and stromal cells arranged in biphasic clusters or in separate groups of one cell type. Haemosiderin laden macrophages and degenerate red blood cells are also usually present. The problem of misinterpreting mildly atypical glandular cells as adenocarcinoma in an aspirate from a caecal endometriotic mass has been reported[9].

Nabothian follicles

Nabothian follicles or mucus retention cysts are cystically dilated endocervical crypts, which develop because the opening of the gland becomes occluded by inspissated mucus or metaplastic epithelium at the orifice of the crypt. If a follicle is ruptured while taking a smear, streaks of mucoid inflammatory debris may be obtained (Fig. 33.6), associated with multinucleate cells having abundant foamy cytoplasm. While some of these cells are clearly histiocytes, others are endocervical in origin (Fig. 33.7A,B). Degenerate forms with pyknotic nuclei may be confused with dyskaryotic cells.

Microglandular endocervical hyperplasia

The term microglandular hyperplasia is applied to an alteration in endocervical glandular tissue frequently seen in pregnancy or during oral contraception and other

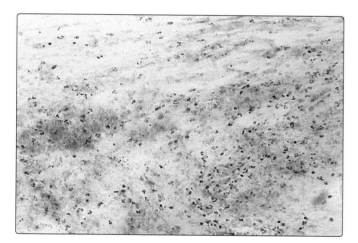

Fig. 33.6 Contents of a nabothian follicle in a cervical smear showing granular inflammatory debris mixed with thick mucoid material. (Papanicolaou × HP)

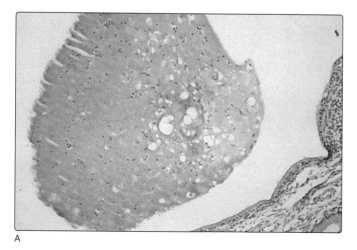

A

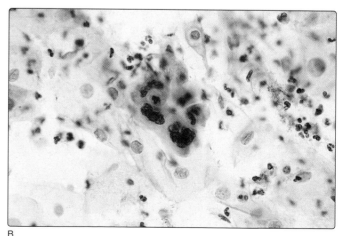

B

Fig. 33.7 (A) Section of nabothian follicle showing mucoid and inflammatory debris within the cystic gland and reactive changes in the lining epithelium. A multinucleated histiocyte can be seen within the mucoid contents. (H&E × MP) (B) Endocervical cell hyperchromasia and multinucleation in the cervical smear from this patient resembling the histological changes in the lining epithelium of the nabothian follicle. (Papanicolaou × HP)

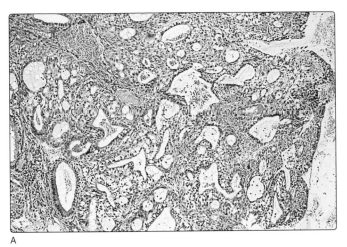

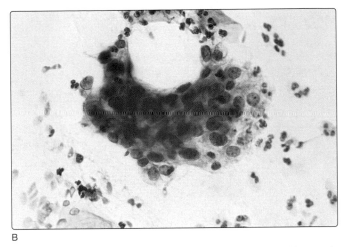

Fig. 33.8 (A) Microglandular endocervical hyperplasia in biopsy of cervix from a patient on oral contraceptive therapy. The normal gland architecture is replaced by tightly packed glands of variable size showing some secretory activity and mild nuclear pleomorphism. The findings can be mistaken for endocervical neoplasia. (H&E × MP) (B) Atypical endocervical cells found to be due to microglandular endocervical hyperplasia of cervix on biopsy. The group consists of enlarged pleomorphic endocervical cells with some loss of polarity and reactive nuclear changes. Features of endocervical dyskaryosis such as marked crowding of nuclei, feathering and architectural abnormalities are not seen. (Papanicolaou × HP) (Courtesy of Dr Al-Izzi, Welwyn Garden City, UK)

hormone therapy. It is thought to be due to progestogen stimulation and does not appear to have any premalignant potential. Typically, there are one or more small polypoidal areas arising from the endocervical canal but more extensive involvement of the endocervical epithelium also occurs.

Histologically, superficial collections or polypoidal nodules of closely packed small glands lined by flattened or cuboidal cells are seen (Fig. 33.8A). The cytoplasm of these cells may be homogeneous, finely granular and eosinophilic or vacuolated. The nuclei are generally small and uniform but may be hyperchromatic and pleomorphic with prominent nucleoli. Squamous metaplasia is frequently present and reserve cell hyperplasia may also be seen.

Atypical or florid microglandular hyperplasia can be mistaken for adenocarcinoma histologically because the glands tend to have a more solid arrangement with widespread nuclear hyperchromasia and pleomorphism. However mitoses are few and the lesion is limited to the superficial region of the endocervical canal.

Cytological findings

▶ Smears may be within normal limits
▶ Clusters of enlarged vacuolated endocervical cells may be seen
▶ Pleomorphism and nuclear changes occur in atypical hyperplasia

The changes have been described in detail by Yahr et al.[10] and Alvarez-Santin et al.[11]. The endocervical cells often appear completely normal or show benign non-specific reactive changes, namely slight enlargement of the cells and their nuclei. There may also be two- and three-dimensional clusters of moderately enlarged cells with an increased amount of cytoplasm containing vacuoles of varying size (Fig. 33.8B). These cells are sometimes ciliated; their nuclei

are enlarged with fine chromatin and small nucleoli. The cell clusters may also comprise basaloid cells with dense cytoplasm in keeping with metaplastic squamous cells and reserve cells with small round nuclei. Fenestrations and microlumina may be apparent within these clusters. In the case of florid hyperplasia, the nuclei are pleomorphic and have slightly coarse chromatin and prominent nucleoli.

Confusion with adenocarcinoma cells can be avoided by looking for a spectrum of atypical cells ranging from obviously benign endocervical cells to atypical forms. Diagnostic features of malignant glandular cells such as abnormal architecture, coarse nuclear chromatin and macronucleoli are not seen. Shidham et al.[12] report a case of grade l endometrial adenocarcinoma presenting in a smear with features simulating cervical microglandular hyperplasia. They considered the presence of single glandular cells with hyperchromatic nuclei, one to three nucleoli, easily detected mitoses, cells with karyorrhexis of nuclei and the presence of a focal watery tumour diathesis to be features suggesting neoplasia.

Malakoplakia

Malakoplakia is an uncommon chronic inflammatory condition usually involving the urinary tract but which can affect many other organs. It is thought to result from an acquired defect in macrophage function resulting in an inability to degrade ingested bacteria, particularly E. coli.

Malakoplakia of the female genital tract is rare, occurring most often in the vagina[13]. The patient is typically elderly and presents with postmenopausal bleeding. Polypoidal friable lesions may be seen in the vagina and on the cervix, simulating malignancy. Histologically, there is an infiltrate of histiocytes with abundant granular eosinophilic cytoplasm. Some of these cells contain the pathognomonic intracytoplasmic calcified laminated spherules known as

Michaelis–Gutmann bodies and microorganisms may sometimes be demonstrated.

Cytological findings

▶ Numerous plump histiocytes with large vesicular nuclei
▶ Endothelial-lined capillaries associated with histiocytes
▶ Background of mixed inflammatory cells
▶ Intracytoplasmic bacilli and Michaelis–Gutmann bodies may be seen

The cytological features have been described in cervical smears[14–17] and recently in fine needle aspiration material from a vaginal mass[18]. Both types of specimen tend to be highly cellular, the majority of cells being single histiocytes with a background of other inflammatory cells, usually neutrophil polymorphs, lymphocytes and plasma cells. The histiocytes have large vesicular nuclei with abundant granular or finely vacuolated cytoplasm.

The number of gram-negative bacilli and Michaelis–Gutmann bodies recognized within the histiocytes varies widely from case to case. Stewart and Thomas[17] describe the presence of prominent endothelium-lined capillaries associated with many of the histiocytes.

Epithelial changes simulating neoplasia

Reserve cell hyperplasia

Single reserve cells lie between the columnar endocervical cells and the basement membrane, predominantly in the proximal part of the endocervical canal. When they proliferate without maturing this is described as reserve cell hyperplasia. It is often seen in pregnant or postmenopausal women and in women using oral contraceptives, representing the earliest stage in the evolution of immature squamous metaplasia.

Histologically, there are several layers of small primitive cells beneath the columnar endocervical epithelium (Fig. 33.9). The cells have round or oval nuclei, finely granular chromatin and ill-defined cell boundaries. Atypical reserve cell hyperplasia is thought to be capable of progressing to CIN 3 or endocervical neoplasia, thus reflecting the bipotential role of the reserve cell.

Cytological findings

▶ Cells in sheets, clumps, pairs and dissociated
▶ Little or no cytoplasm
▶ Nuclei are pale or normochromatic
▶ Columnar cells may be attached
▶ Anisocytosis, nucleoli and mitoses are found in atypical hyperplasia

Hyperplastic reserve cells are typically shed in sheets and are also seen in rows with ramifications, in clumps, paired and singly. Columnar endocervical cells may be attached to these cells, arranged in a single layer (Fig. 33.10).

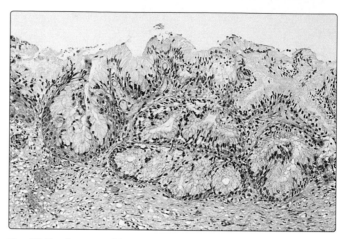

Fig. 33.9 Reserve cell hyperplasia in section of cervix. There is a multilayered row of immature cells beneath the tall columnar epithelium of the endocervical canal, showing no evidence of squamous metaplasia. (H&E × MP)

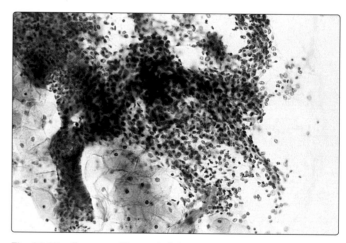

Fig. 33.10 Reserve cell hyperplasia in cervical smear. This large cellular group of endocervical origin is more crowded than normal and shows many dissociated bare nuclei at the margins. The degree of crowding was thought suggestive of endocervical dyskaryosis, but biopsy showed reserve cell hyperplasia only. (Papanicolaou × MP)

The reserve cells have oval, round or bean shaped nuclei, slightly smaller than those of endocervical cells. One end of the nucleus may be pointed and there may be a longitudinal groove. Nuclear moulding is also a recognized feature. The chromatin is finely granular and a small nucleolus may be apparent. Most nuclei are naked when the cells are dissociated, although a small amount of poorly-defined cytoplasm is occasionally present (Fig. 33.10). Sheets of reserve cells typically have a syncytial appearance because cell borders are poorly defined.

In *atypical reserve cell hyperplasia* the cells show the same exfoliation pattern, but the nuclei show anisokaryosis which may be marked. The nuclear border is prominent and the chromatin is slightly granular but evenly dispersed (Fig. 33.11A,B). The nuclei are normo- or hypochromatic rather than hyperchromatic. Nucleoli may be visible and

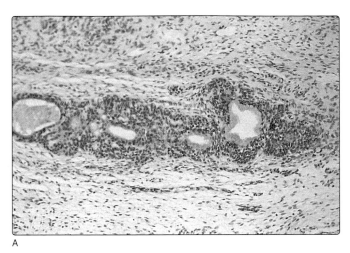

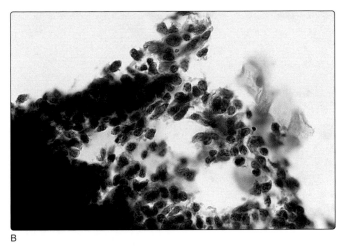

A B

Fig. 33.11 (A) Atypical reserve cell hyperplasia in cervical cone biopsy. There is a zone of multilayered reserve cells forming a cuff around most of the glands. The cells are crowded and disorganized in contrast to **Fig. 33.9**, but no mitoses are seen. (H&E × MP) (B) Atypical reserve cell hyperplasia in the cervical smear from the patient whose histology is illustrated in (A). Fragments of crowded small cells with hyperchromatic nuclei are seen, and were interpreted as severe glandular dyskaryosis. The cone biopsy showed CIN 1 in addition to the atypical reserve cell hyperplasia but no evidence of glandular intraepithelial neoplasia was found. (Papanicolaou × HP)

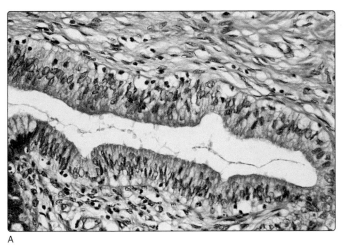

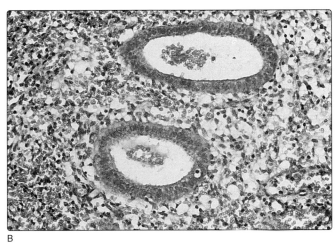

A B

Fig. 33.12 (A) Tubal metaplasia in histological section of cervix. The endocervical gland lining consists of ciliated cells with slight multilayering imparting a more disorganized appearance than is usually seen in endocervical mucosa or glands. (H&E × HP) (B) Tuboendometrioid metaplasia of cervix showing two glands lined by cells with tubal and endometrial features, set in inflamed stroma. (H&E × HP)

mitoses can be seen. Atypical reserve cells are rarely seen in negative smears, tending to be present when dyskaryotic squamous or glandular cells are also present. The higher the grade of dyskaryosis the more likely is the finding of atypical reserve cells. They can usually be distinguished from dyskaryotic cells, which have denser cytoplasm and hyperchromatic nuclei[19].

Tubal metaplasia

Tubal metaplasia refers to replacement of epithelium at mullerian derived sites, such as the endometrial cavity or endocervix, by benign epithelium resembling that of the fallopian tube. Jonasson *et al.*[20] found tubal metaplasia in 31% of cone or hysterectomy specimens, while in a more recent study Al-Nafussi and Rahilly[21] report this change in up to 70% of cervices removed for non-neoplastic

reasons and in up to 89% of cases with squamous carcinoma.

Tubal metaplasia frequently includes cells of endometrial type, producing *tubo-endometrioid metaplasia* (Fig. 33.12). Frank endometriosis, with endometrial glands and stroma present in the cervix, may also occur in the same group of patients, as already described, although a less frequent event.

These metaplastic changes tend to be multifocal, involving the upper endocervix and crypts of glands more commonly than the lower endocervix and surface epithelium. Although only infrequently seen in smears, this type of metaplasia is a recognized sequel to cone biopsy and diathermy loop treatments, having been reported in 26% of post-conization cervices[8]. It can be expected to be encountered more often in smears taken with a brush than in spatula smears.

Tubal or tubo-endometrioid metaplasia is probably a hormone-induced phenomenon. Although not thought to be preneoplastic, it is important that the cytological appearances are recognized and not misinterpreted as indicating endocervical glandular dysplasia. In a study by Novotny and co-workers[22] tubal metaplasia accounted for the smear appearances in 76% of cases in which endocervical glandular dysplasia had been suggested.

Cytological findings *(Figs 33.13A,B)*

▶ Numerous columnar cells, some ciliated and non-ciliated
▶ Large to medium-sized sheets and clusters, and single cell arrangements
▶ Nuclei larger and darker than endocervical cells
▶ Intercalary cells may be recognized

The changes have been described in detail by Ducatman *et al.*[23] and Novotny *et al.*[22]. The three cell types seen in fallopian tube epithelium should be present, namely ciliated cells, secretory non-ciliated cells and intercalary cells. Their proportion in a smear varies greatly, but ciliated columnar cells with apical terminal bars are necessary for diagnosis.

The cells are arranged in flat sheets, three-dimensional clusters, small poorly cohesive groups or they may occur singly. Cells are smaller than endocervical cells but nuclei tend to be larger and evenly spaced, although there may be overlapping of nuclei in the three-dimensional groups. They are oval, round or elongated and are usually basal in position. The chromatin is finely granular and typically slightly darker than that of endocervical cell nuclei. Nucleoli are often not visible or are small and single.

Intercalary cells, exclusive to tubal metaplasia yet not readily seen in smears, have triangular dark staining nuclei and little cytoplasm, in contrast to the other cells which have varying amounts of granular or vacuolated cytoplasm. Mitoses are rare.

Diagnostic pitfalls

The presence of aligned ciliated cells is one of the most helpful features in distinguishing tubal metaplasia from endocervical glandular dysplasia, although cilia are not often preserved in all groups in a smear. Rosettes, palisades of cells and the feathered appearance at the edge of sheets of cells typically seen in adenocarcinoma *in situ* (AIS) are rarely seen in tubal metaplasia. The nuclei are also different in AIS, since they tend to be elongated and hyperchromatic with coarsely granular chromatin and prominent nucleoli. They are invariably crowded and stratified and mitotic figures are usually present (see Fig. 33.18).

In a study of three cases of tubo-endometrioid metaplasia, Hirschowitz *et al.* describe other helpful cytological features in differentiating this change from cervical squamous or glandular intraepithelial neoplasia[24]. These include the smaller size of the cells compared with endocervical or metaplastic cells, the markedly uniform nuclear hyperchromasia and inconspicuous nucleoli, the presence of three-dimensional glandular structures and the lack of discrete squamous cell dyskaryosis.

Other differential diagnoses include cervical endometriosis, endometrial cells from the lower uterine segment, microglandular and reserve cell hyperplasia, 'reactive' endocervical cells and dyskaryotic cells from CIN 3 involving endocervical glands.

Transitional cell metaplasia

Occasionally metaplasia on the ectocervix to a transitional type of epithelium has been identified in histological

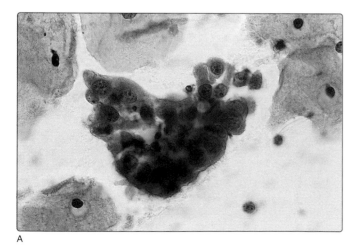
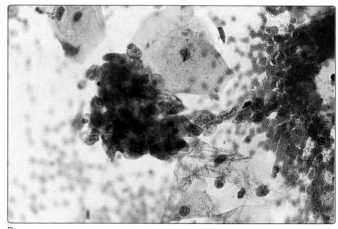

A

B

Fig. 33.13 (A) Tubal metaplasia in a group of glandular cells in a cervical smear taken as follow-up of treated CIN. There is a columnar border showing ciliated cells along the lower edge of the group. Intercalary cells cannot be identified. (Papanicolaou × HP) (B) Tuboendometrioid metaplasia in the same smear as shown (A). This group shows degenerative features with nuclear irregularities and crowding as seen in endometrial cells, although without the characteristic central core of stroma. (Papanicolaou × HP)

sections of the cervix, particularly in older post-menopausal women. The alteration is thought to represent a type of basal cell hyperplasia[25]. This change causes no symptoms and its importance appears to lie chiefly in the potential for mistaken diagnosis of a high-grade CIN lesion in hysterectomy specimens because of the lack of maturation of cells in crowded epithelium. No relationship to cervical pre-cancer or invasive disease has been established and careful examination of tissue sections reveals uniformity of nuclei, an even chromatin pattern and lack of mitotic activity, thereby excluding the possibility of neoplasia.

Recent descriptions of the cervical smear findings when cells from this type of mucosa are sampled have been published[26]. The mild nuclear changes with elongated nuclei showing longitudinal grooves and the presence of crowded cell groups can be mistaken for dyskaryosis, with the risk of over-treatment of a benign process.

Congenital transformation zone

In the normal course of events, the original squamocolumnar junction is situated at the external os from the time of its formation in utero up to the time of puberty. In conditions of altered hormonal balance during intrauterine life the upper vagina and ectocervix may fail to transform fully to mature squamous epithelium so that a residual zone of non-maturing metaplastic epithelium persists on the ectocervix, even extending on to the fornices and upper vaginal wall in some cases. This mucosa is referred to as a congenital transformation zone. The cells sampled from such an area in smear taking are indistinguishable from other partially mature squamous cells. It is nevertheless important for cytologists and histopathologists to be aware of this change since it may appear to the colposcopist as an area of CIN, leading to the risk of over-treatment of a benign process.

Leukoplakia

Leukoplakia is a clinical concept describing the presence of white patches on the mucosa of the ectocervix or in other areas of genital tract squamous epithelium. Typically, at the cervix, lesions are due to hyperkeratosis or parakeratosis of the ectocervical epithelium. The squamous mucosa may be atrophic or normal but is often hyperplastic and is covered by a thick layer of anucleate keratin (hyperkeratosis) or keratin in which pyknotic nuclei persist (parakeratosis). There is usually a well-defined granular layer beneath the layer of keratin.

These changes are often due to chronic irritation of the epithelium, for example, when there is uterine prolapse, especially procidentia (Fig. 33.14A), if a pessary is in place or with severe chronic inflammation. Sometimes, however, the underlying epithelium is abnormal, showing evidence of HPV infection, CIN or invasive squamous carcinoma. Colposcopic examination is therefore appropriate if leukoplakia is present, even in the absence of dyskaryotic squamous cells in the smear, to rule out serious underlying pathology.

Cytological findings

▶ Sheets and single anucleate mature squamous cells
▶ Keratohyaline granules in squamous cell cytoplasm
▶ Small irregular pyknotic nuclei within keratotic squames in parakeratosis

Anucleate squames are present singly or in sheets or plaques. They are of intermediate or superficial cell size and stain bright orange or yellow with the Papanicolaou stain (Fig. 33.14B). Some may contain pink or basophilic intracytoplasmic granules of keratohyaline. Parakeratotic cells are seen as smaller keratinized cells lying singly or in sheets with small slightly irregular pyknotic nuclei.

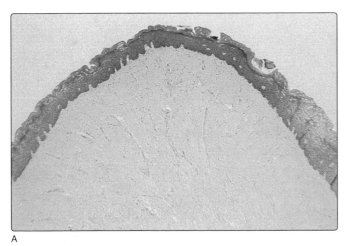

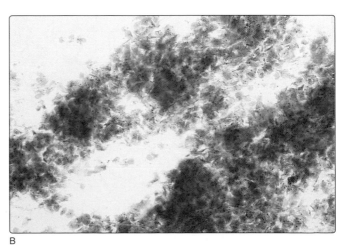

A   B

Fig. 33.14 (A) Section of cervix from a case of uterine prolapse. The squamous mucosa is thickened and covered by a dense layer of keratin. (H&E × LP) (B) Hyperkeratosis in a cervical smear from a patient with procidentia. Much of the smear consisted of deeply stained anucleate squames from the keratinized surface of the cervix. (Papanicolaou × MP)

Abnormal cells reflecting underlying pathology may also be present.

Repair and regeneration

When cervical mucosa is ulcerated or damaged re-epithelialization of denuded stroma occurs, initially by immature metaplastic epithelium, to be replaced later by mature squamous epithelium. Changes due to repair and regeneration may be seen in a smear taken after cervical biopsy, cold coagulation, laser therapy, irradiation, hysterectomy or in cases of severe cervicitis, such as in long-standing *Trichomonas vaginalis* infection[23,24]. The cells obtained can be confused with dyskaryotic squamous and glandular cells. It is therefore advisable to delay follow up smears for at least four months and preferably for six months after treatment of CIN.

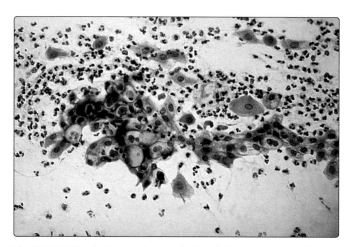

Fig. 33.15   Repair changes in metaplastic cells in a postnatal cervical smear. The cells form a ragged group with attenuated cytoplasm and have enlarged nuclei with prominent nucleoli. Note the degenerative vacuolation of the cells and the inflammatory background. (Papanicolaou × MP)

Features seen histologically include thickening of the squamous epithelium, basal cell hyperplasia and immature squamous metaplasia. The nuclei may be hyperchromatic and have prominent nucleoli but there is normal maturation of cells in the upper layers of the mucosa. Endocervical epithelium may also display similar reactive features with nuclear enlargement and hyperchromasia, loss of cytoplasmic mucus and mitotic figures. Both mucosa and underlying stroma are inflamed and there may be granulation tissue formation.

Cytological findings[27-31]

▶ Immature population of parabasals, metaplastic and reserve cells
▶ Repair cells, fibroblasts and inflammatory cells

Repair cells are thought to originate from both epithelial and stromal cells[28,30], the former showing varying degrees of differentiation towards squamous and columnar epithelium. Epithelial cells tend to occur in syncytial sheets and have enlarged oval pleomorphic nuclei containing one or more eosinophilic large nucleoli (Fig. 33.15), findings which indicate active protein synthesis in fast growing cells. Multinucleation is often seen. The chromatin pattern is usually fine and regular but may be slightly coarse and hyperchromatic. The cytoplasm is abundant and has ragged margins; there is often evidence of leukophagocytosis. Mitotic figures may be seen.

Cells thought to be fibroblasts or stromal cells tend to occur in aggregates with oval nuclei and ribbon-like extensions of poorly defined cytoplasm (Fig. 33.16). The chromatin is uniformly finely granular. Single or multiple macronucleoli are present and are occasionally irregular. Other cell types to be found include parabasal cells, metaplastic squamous cells, reserve cells which may be

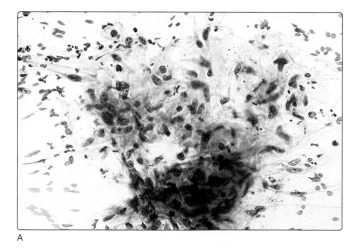

A

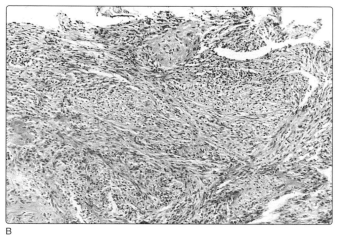

B

Fig. 33.16   (A) Repair changes in stromal cells in a cervical smear from a 79-year-old woman. The cells are elongated, with ill-defined cytoplasm and have prominent nucleoli. (Papanicolaou × HP) (B) Granulation tissue found on biopsy of cervix of patient whose smear is illustrated in (A). The fibroblasts within the newly formed tissue are similar to the stromal cells found in the smear. (H&E × MP) (Courtesy of Professor B Naylor, Michigan, USA)

atypical, neutrophil polymorphs, red blood cells and cellular debris.

Diagnostic pitfalls

Although the repair process shares some features with adenocarcinoma and large cell non-keratinizing squamous carcinoma, repair cells tend to display uniformity in numbers of chromocentres and nucleoli, an even distribution of chromatin and round smooth nuclear outlines with thin nuclear membranes; these features are not seen in malignant cells. Malignant cells occur singly as well as in groups whereas repair cells are almost invariably grouped.

A tumour diathesis may accompany carcinoma cells, while repair cells are frequently associated with neutrophil polymorphs. When the chromatin of repair cells is coarse and hyperchromatic and the macronucleoli are pleomorphic and very prominent they are said to be atypical and are difficult to distinguish from malignant cells[28,29]. A repeat smear for borderline nuclear abnormality (atypical squamous cells of undetermined significance), as discussed in Chapters 28 and 30, may be necessary, or a biopsy if there is a clinical suspicion of malignancy.

Uncommon tumours of cervix
Special types of carcinoma
Adenosquamous carcinoma

Adenosquamous carcinoma, like adenocarcinoma of the cervix, presents in slightly younger women than does squamous cell carcinoma. It is thought to have a similar prognosis to both adenocarcinoma and squamous cell carcinoma[32]. Uncommitted subcolumnar reserve cells are probably the cell type from which this neoplasm arises. Histologically, both squamous and glandular elements are combined in variable proportions (Fig. 33.17). Occasionally, a squamous carcinoma of cervix is found to have an adjoining adenocarcinoma without the intimate mingling of tissue types seen in an adenosquamous carcinoma. This is referred to as a collision tumour (Fig. 33.18). It can be that only one of the two components is invasive, the other still being an *in situ* carcinoma.

Special stains to detect mucin have shown that many tumours thought morphologically to be squamous should be classified as adenosquamous or as poorly-differentiated adenocarcinoma[33]. The glandular component may form obvious acini distinct from the squamous component or may consist of small clusters of mucus secreting cells within squamous tumour tissue, a pattern producing the picture of so-called mucoepidermoid carcinoma.

Cytological findings

▶ Severely dyskaryotic squamous and glandular cells

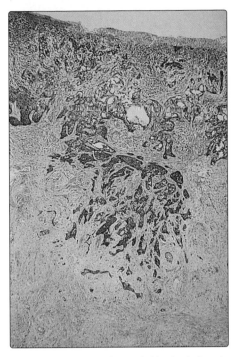

Fig. 33.17   Adenosquamous carcinoma in histological section of cervix. Solid islands of poorly-differentiated squamous carcinoma cells infiltrate deeply from the surface. Within these clumps there are areas of glandular differentiation forming acini of variable size and shape. (H&E × LP)

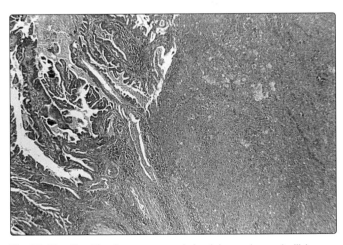

Fig. 33.18   Combined squamous and glandular carcinoma (collision tumour). This section of cervix shows a tumour mass composed of well-differentiated adenocarcinoma on the left and poorly-differentiated squamous carcinoma on the right. (H&E × MP)

▶ Poorly-differentiated tumours resemble glassy cell carcinoma
▶ Tumour diathesis.

Carcinoma cells are present and may consist of an obvious mixture of squamous and glandular cells (Fig. 33.19), or only one type of differentiation may be apparent. If both types of cell are present in the same cell cluster the possibility of a collision tumour can be excluded.

If the tumour is poorly differentiated it may be impossible to distinguish between the two types of cell and histological examination with mucin stains is required to make the

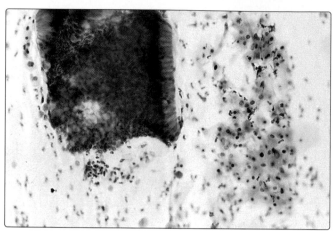

Fig. 33.19 Combined tumour. Dyskaryotic endocervical cells in large groups with obvious intestinal metaplasia visible on low magnification. A few dyskaryotic squamous cells are present below and to the right. The glandular component of this tumour was still an *in situ* lesion on histology. (Papanicolaou × LP)

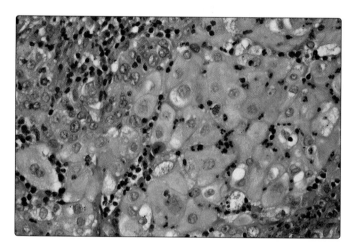

Fig. 33.20 Glassy cell carcinoma in histological section of cervix showing a compact arrangement of medium to large malignant cells with pale cytoplasm, pleomorphic nuclei, prominent nucleoli and frequent mitoses. Mucin stains showed occasional cells with mucin secretion but the majority resemble a non-keratinizing squamous carcinoma. The cytological findings in this case are shown in **Fig. 33.21**.(H&E × HP)

diagnosis. Features suggesting glassy cell carcinoma have been described in a smear taken from a poorly differentiated adenosquamous carcinoma[34].

Glassy cell carcinoma

Glassy cell carcinoma is considered to be a variant of adenosquamous carcinoma since ultrastructurally there is evidence of both glandular and squamous differentiation[35]. The prognosis is generally poor. Histologically, the tumour has an undifferentiated appearance, being composed of sheets of malignant cells with abundant finely granular cytoplasm, large vesicular nuclei and prominent nucleoli (Fig. 33.20). Mitoses tend to be numerous and the stroma is often infiltrated by lymphocytes, plasma cells and eosinophils.

Evidence of glandular and squamous differentiation may be present in the form of focal acinar formation, demonstrable intra-cytoplasmic mucin, dyskeratotic cells and an occasional keratin pearl.

Cytological findings

- ▶ Numerous large malignant cells in syncytial groups
- ▶ Large hyperchromatic nuclei, finely granular cytoplasm
- ▶ Prominent nucleoli
- ▶ Tumour diathesis

The cytological features have been described by Littman *et al.*[36] and more recently by Pak *et al.*, Nunez *et al.* and Chung *et al.*[37–39]. The tumour cells tend to be numerous and arranged in groups with a syncytial appearance or in sheets and clusters. A few single tumour cells may also be present. They are larger than severely dyskaryotic squamous cells and show marked anisokaryosis. The nuclei are large and hyperchromatic, the chromatin having a finely granular appearance. Large irregular nucleoli are often present. A moderate amount of cytoplasm is present which may have a finely granular appearance (Fig. 33.21A,B). Inflammatory cells, including eosinophils, may be conspicuous in the background and may be seen closely associated with tumour cells.

The cytological features can be confused with poorly-differentiated large cell non-keratinizing squamous carcinoma, the nuclei of which tend to have coarser chromatin and less nucleolar abnormality, and with atypical reparative cells which do not fulfil the nuclear criteria of malignancy. Misdiagnosis as a low-grade squamous abnormality can occur if the sheets of cells have bland nuclear features, leading to delay in diagnosis[40].

Adenoid cystic carcinoma

Adenoid cystic carcinoma is a rare variant of adenocarcinoma and tends to occur in post-menopausal women. It is a slowly growing, locally recurring tumour with infrequent metastases, having a similar histological appearance to adenoid cystic carcinoma of salivary glands. The cells typically demonstrate tubular, cribriform and solid growth patterns.

Cytological findings

- ▶ Groups and sheets of small uniform cells
- ▶ Hyperchromatic nuclei, indistinct nucleoli and scant cytoplasm

This tumour is rarely recognized, either because no tumour cells are present on the smear, reflecting the fact that the overlying mucosa tends to be intact, or because the tumour cells present are misinterpreted as being benign or abnormal endometrial cells[41]. The cells tend to be arranged in irregularly shaped three-dimensional groups and sheets. They may also form cords and acini, some of which contain

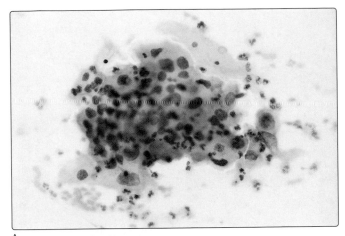

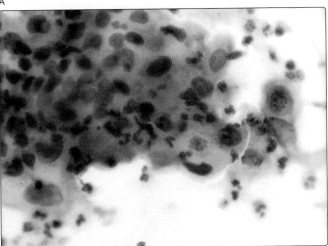

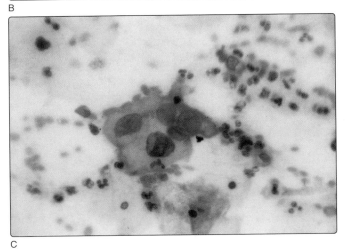

C

Fig. 33.21   (A, B, C) Medium and high power views of cells from a glassy cell carcinoma of cervix showing syncytial sheets with anisokaryosis. (Papanicolaou × MP and HP). Illustrations 33.20 and 33.21 by courtesy of Dr J Smith, Sheffield, UK, with permission of Blackwell Science, London.

globules of hyaline material. The cells are small and have small uniform hyperchromatic nuclei, occasional small nucleoli and scanty cytoplasm.

Differential diagnoses include classical endocervical adenocarcinoma, endometrial adenocarcinoma, small cell

(neuroendocrine) carcinoma, in which nuclear moulding and frequent mitoses may be seen, and severe squamous dyskaryosis, in which the cells tend to be larger and less uniform[42,43].

Adenoid cystic carcinoma frequently occurs in association with *in situ* or invasive squamous carcinoma[44,45] supporting the hypothesis that it develops from pluripotential reserve cells. Both tumour cell types may then be present in the same smear.

Neuroendocrine carcinoma

Neuroendocrine carcinoma of the cervix is rare. It is typically seen in middle aged women, causes abnormal vaginal bleeding and has a poorer prognosis than squamous or adenocarcinoma. Nearly half of these tumours show areas of squamous, glandular or adenosquamous differentiation, supporting the theory that they are derived from the pluripotential reserve cell.

The appearances range from a well-differentiated tumour (Fig. 33.22) having a trabecular or solid streaming pattern typical of a carcinoid tumour, to a small cell anaplastic carcinoma resembling oat cell carcinoma of bronchus (Fig. 33.23). Neurosecretory granules are present in the cytoplasm and are argyrophilic, staining positively with a Grimelius stain. The diagnosis can also be confirmed by immunocytochemistry, staining with Chromogranin A, synaptophysin and other neuroendocrine markers.

Cytological findings

▶ Small cells, scanty cytoplasm
▶ Round or oval nuclei with nucleoli
▶ Coarse chromatin, indistinct nucleoli, nuclear moulding if poorly-differentiated
▶ Malignant squamous and glandular cells often also present
▶ Tumour diathesis usually seen

If the tumour is well-differentiated the cells are usually in nests and have round to oval mildly pleomorphic nuclei containing small punctate reddish nucleoli and finely granular chromatin. Cytoplasm is scant and eosinophilic or basophilic, the cytoplasmic borders being ill-defined[46].

The cells of poorly-differentiated tumours tend to be ovoid and to occur singly, although papillary clusters with associated psammoma bodies have been described[47]. Nuclear moulding is typically present. The nuclei are oval and hyperchromatic with coarse or smudged chromatin and show minimal anisokaryosis. Nucleoli are indistinct. There is a thin rim of cytoplasm (Figs 33.22, 33.23).

Miles *et al.*[48] have reported the presence of large bizarre multinucleated tumour cells with prominent reddish nucleoli, finely granular chromatin and greyish blue cytoplasm in the smear from a neuroendocrine carcinoma which also contained smaller neuroendocrine-like cells and larger cells suggesting squamous and glandular

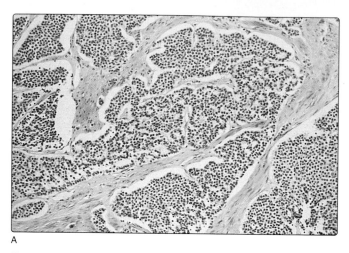

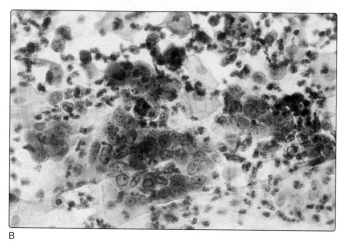

Fig. 33.22   (A) Neuroendocrine tumour of cervix of carcinoid type, composed of nests, clumps and ribbons of small regular cells set in dense fibrous stroma. (H&E × MP) (B) Neuroendocrine carcinoma cells in cervical smear showing a cohesive group of crowded cells with hyperchromatic nuclei and well-defined nucleoli. (Papanicolaou × HP) (Courtesy of Dr C Waddell and Dr M Light, Birmingham, UK)

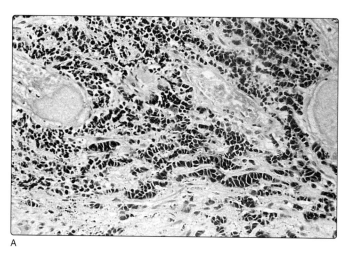

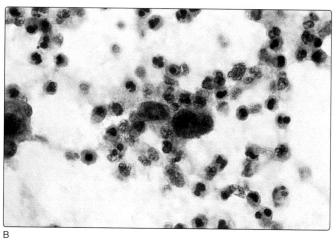

Fig. 33.23   (A) Poorly-differentiated neuroendocrine carcinoma of cervix in histological section. The tumour cells are similar to those seen in an oat cell carcinoma of bronchus, infiltrating in sheets and ribbons, with a high nuclear/cytoplasmic ratio and hyperchromatic nuclei. Nuclear moulding and pyknosis are also seen. Immunohistochemistry was in keeping with the diagnosis of neuroendocrine carcinoma. (H&E × HP) (B) Cervical smear from the same patient showed marked tumour diathesis and a few small clusters of malignant cells with little cytoplasm and coarsely granular hyperchromatic nuclei. (Papanicolaou × HP)

differentiation. The initial cytological diagnosis in this case had been adenosquamous carcinoma.

Diagnostic pitfalls

Neuroendocrine carcinoma cells can be confused with poorly-differentiated squamous carcinoma or adenocarcinoma. If the smear contains two cell populations, because a squamous or glandular component is present, confusion with an adenosquamous carcinoma can arise or the neuroendocrine component may be completely overlooked. The presence of nuclear moulding, indistinct nucleoli and scanty cytoplasm are helpful features in detecting neuroendocrine carcinoma. Metastatic small cell lung carcinoma must be considered although

metastases to the cervix are usually within the stroma and covered by intact mucosa, at least in the early stages; an appropriate history of lung tumour should be sought.

Lymphoepithelioma-like carcinoma

This tumour accounts for up to 5% of primary cervical malignancies, has a more favourable prognosis than the usual squamous cell carcinoma and tends to occur at an earlier age. Although morphologically similar to nasopharyngeal lymphoepithelioma-like carcinoma (LEC), it does not share the association with Epstein-Barr virus, nor indeed has human papillomavirus DNA been detected in the cells.

Histologically, the tumour comprises syncytial groups of anaplastic cells, intimately associated with a prominent lymphoplasmacytic infiltrate.

Cytological findings

▶ Uniform large tumour cells with indistinct borders
▶ Round or oval hyperchromatic nuclei
▶ Finely granular to flocculent cytoplasm
▶ Lymphocytes are often closely associated with tumour cells
▶ Background of blood and inflammatory cells

Reich et al.[49] and Proca et al.[50] have recently reported the cytological features in three cases of LEC. The tumour cells occur singly and in small clusters. They have a high nuclear cytoplasmic ratio. The nuclear chromatin has an irregular pattern and tends to show peripheral margination. One or more prominent nucleoli may be present. There is no evidence of dyskeratosis, keratinization or koilocytosis and no glandular features are present. Proca et al.[50] emphasize that the tumour cells can easily be overlooked in a smear containing numerous red blood cells and inflammatory cells.

LEC may be confused cytologically with squamous cell carcinoma, glassy cell carcinoma and non-Hodgkin's lymphoma, particularly of Lennert's type. The cells of a usual squamous cell carcinoma are more pleomorphic and hyperchromatic than those of a lymphoepithelioma-like carcinoma and have distinct cell borders, as do glassy cell carcinoma cells, which are also recognized by the ground-glass appearance of their cytoplasm. Immunostaining may be necessary to distinguish lymphoepithelioma-like carcinoma from lymphoma.

Mesenchymal tumours

Benign mesenchymal tumours

Approximately 8% of uterine leiomyomas (fibroids) occur in the cervix, making these the commonest benign mesenchymal neoplasms of cervix. At this site they are usually solitary. If the overlying mucosa is ulcerated benign smooth muscle cells from the lesion may be present in a smear, but their place of origin cannot be identified without appropriate clinical information. The cytological findings are described in Chapter 35.

Other benign mesenchymal tumours, namely haemangioma, neurilemmoma, lipoma, paraganglioma, and adenofibroma are uncommon and the cytological findings have not so far been documented in cervical smears.

Adenomyomatous polyps are rare. They comprise a mixture of glands and fibromuscular stroma. Their cytological features have been described by Ngadiman and Yang[2]. Numerous tissue fragments comprising bland spindle-shaped cells were present, showing tight cohesion centrally and being loosely clustered peripherally. No glandular cells were seen.

Atypical polypoid adenomyoma also occurs rarely in the cervix. The glandular component in this entity shows a variable degree of architectural and cytological atypia. Baschinsky et al. report a case in which the surface epithelium of the cervix was involved, so that atypical glandular cells were detected in the smear[51].

Malignant mesenchymal tumours

Malignant mesenchymal tumours arising as a primary neoplasm of the cervix are very rare. The most frequently encountered types are malignant mixed mesodermal (Mullerian) tumour, leiomyosarcoma and endometrial stromal sarcoma. They have similar clinical behaviour and microscopic features to their more common counterparts in the uterine corpus. Sarcoma botryoides (embryonal rhabdomyosarcoma), an aggressive rare tumour of vagina in young girls, may very occasionally develop as a primary neoplasm of the cervix.

Leiomyosarcoma

This is the commonest of the mesenchymal malignant tumours to arise in the cervix. The histological findings in a cervical leiomyosarcoma depend upon the degree of differentiation. Well-differentiated neoplasms are similar to leiomyomas apart from the higher mitotic rate, whereas poorly-differentiated tumours show cellular and nuclear pleomorphism, abnormal mitoses and loss of the characteristic interweaving pattern of the cells (Fig. 33.24A).

Cytological findings[52]

▶ Spindle cells, elongated nuclei, indefinite cytoplasm
▶ Multinucleation and tumour giant cells
▶ Pleomorphism increases with loss of differentiation

If the tumour is well-differentiated, the cells are slender and spindle shaped, with central elongated nuclei and ill-defined weakly staining cytoplasm. Cytoplasmic longitudinal microfibrils may be evident. More usually, however, the malignant cells do not display any features to indicate smooth muscle differentiation. Instead, they appear on a smear as single pleomorphic cells with variable staining of cytoplasm, anisonucleosis and frequent multinucleation. Nuclei are round or oval, hyperchromatic and often show macronucleoli.

Poorly-differentiated tumour cells may be epithelioid in appearance (Fig. 33.24B). The cells may occur in clusters, so that they can easily be misinterpreted as carcinoma cells. Their poorly defined pale staining cytoplasm is in contradistinction to that of most epithelial neoplasms of the cervix.

Malignant mixed mesenchymal tumours (MMMT)

In the majority of cases, MMMTs of cervix have arisen from the body of the uterus and, because of their aggressive behaviour, have already spread to the cervix at presentation. In a series of 202 patients with cervical involvement by this tumour only one case was shown to be a primary cervical neoplasm[53]. Most present at around the age of the menopause and the prognosis is generally poor. There is a well-established association with radiation treatment to the cervix for squamous carcinoma, usually many years previously[54].

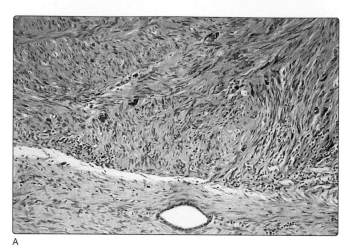

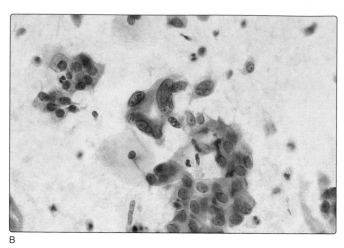

A   B

Fig. 33.24   (A) Leiomyosarcoma in histological section from a large cervical mass. The tumour occupies the upper two thirds of the illustration with a rim of cervical stroma at the lower border. There are interlacing fascicles of pleomorphic spindle-shaped malignant cells, including some tumour giant cells. (H&E × MP) (B) Leiomyosarcoma cells in cervical smear showing a central group of rather epithelioid malignant cells with ovoid or elongated nuclei and prominent nucleoli. (Papanicolaou × HP) (Courtesy of Dr J Johnson, Nottingham, UK)

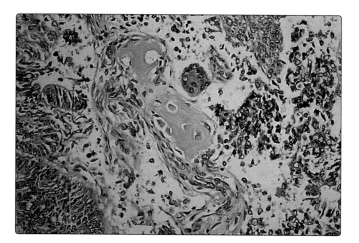

Fig. 33.25   Malignant mixed mesenchymal tumour involving cervix and uterus shown in section from hysterectomy specimen. Adenocarcinoma is seen on the left with clusters of small undifferentiated malignant cells on the right. At the centre there are some spindle cells and a focus of osteoid tissue. (H&E × HP)

The histological blend of carcinomatous and sarcomatous elements is variable but there is always a component of undifferentiated small cells and spindle cells (Fig. 33.25). Heterologous elements of rhabdomyosarcomatous, chondrosarcomatous or other type are present in about 50% of cases[55].

Cytological findings (Fig. 33.26A,B,C)

▶ Carcinomatous cells, usually adenocarcinomatous
▶ Pleomorphic and spindle-shaped sarcomatous cells
▶ Small undifferentiated cells
▶ Tumour diathesis, blood-stained smears

Most studies of smear findings are based largely on endometrial tumours, and abnormal cells are detected by

cervical cytology in only a low proportion of such cases[56,57]. Adenocarcinoma cells are the commonest epithelial abnormality to appear in cervicovaginal smears, often having a papillary arrangement[58]. Spindle-shaped malignant cells represent the sarcomatous component and these show pleomorphism and multinucleation. Heterologous elements are rare and are difficult to recognize with certainty in smears. The small undifferentiated cells of MMMTs are usually present.

The related, but less common Mullerian carcinofibroma has a better prognosis than MMMTs and occurs principally in the uterine body, but can arise in the cervix. It comprises a mixture of malignant epithelial tumour and a benign mesenchymal component, usually a fibroma. The adenocarcinoma cells in the case reported by Imai *et al.*[59] showed papillary and tubular arrangements. The spindle-shaped and ovoid cells were numerous and scattered throughout the smear. They had a thin nuclear membrane, fine chromatin and narrow, pale cytoplasm. They were larger than normal endometrial stromal cells and no mitotic activity or nuclear atypia were evident, but a tumour diathesis was present in the bloodstained smear.

Endometrial stromal sarcoma

This tumour arises primarily in the body of the uterus and although spread to the cervix can occur, cervical or vaginal smears do not usually contribute to diagnosis. The cytological findings are described in Chapter 35.

Sarcoma botryoides (embryonal rhabdomyosarcoma)

The cervix is very rarely the primary site of this aggressive tumour. It typically presents in reproductive years with vaginal discharge or a vaginal mass. The tumour develops beneath the surface epithelium and produces a polypoid mass. The cytological features of a case have been described by Matsuura *et al.*[60].

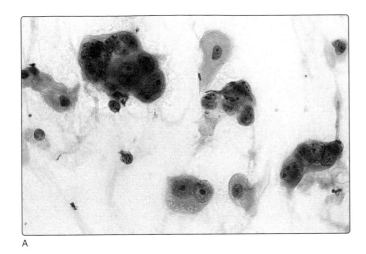

A

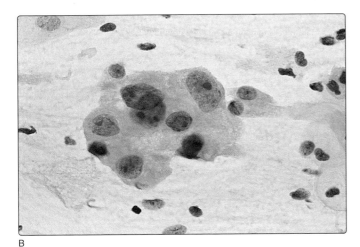

B

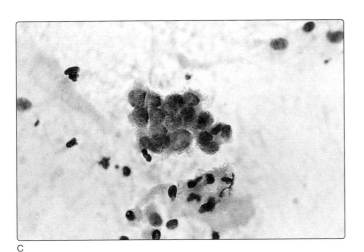

C

Fig. 33.26 (A) Cells from a malignant mixed mesenchymal tumour in a cervical smear from a woman with postmenopausal bleeding. The diversity of the malignant cell groups is obvious, with a tendency to papillary clustering suggesting adenocarcinoma at top left, while the central cluster represents the undifferentiated element seen on histology. (Papanicolaou × HP) (B) Large tumour cells from the same smear, with features of a non-keratinizing squamous cell carcinoma. (× HP) (C) Group of poorly-differentiated small cells in the same smear. No sarcomatous elements were identified. (× HP) (Courtesy of Dr Al-Izzi, Welwyn Garden City, UK)

Cytological findings

▶ Loose clusters of short spindle-shaped cells
▶ Elongated, scanty cytoplasm, with indistinct cell borders
▶ Tumour diathesis

The tumour nuclei are elongated or oval, have a variable chromatin pattern and tend to have macronucleoli. The degree of cellular atypia ranges from mild to severe. Cross striations are rarely present. Without immunostaining to demonstrate rhabdomyoblasts, distinction from a leiomyosarcoma is difficult.

Malignant melanoma

Malignant melanoma of the cervix is very rare and is usually secondary to vaginal melanoma, presenting as an ulcerated or polypoidal mass, which bleeds readily. The prognosis is poor and most patients die within two years of diagnosis. The histological features (Fig. 33.27A) are typical of melanoma at other sites, showing infiltration of tissues by epithelioid or spindle-shaped tumour cells with large pleomorphic nuclei and prominent nucleoli. Multinucleate forms are common and intracytoplasmic melanin is often present.

Cytological findings *(Fig. 33.27B,C)*

▶ Pleomorphic single cells or dissociating groups
▶ Eccentric nuclei and prominent nucleoli
▶ Intranuclear cytoplasmic inclusions
▶ Melanin may be visible
▶ Tumour diathesis

Fleming and Mein[61] report a case of primary melanoma of the cervix in which several small pigmented lesions resembling blood blisters were seen by the smear taker. The diagnosis of melanoma was suggested from the smear and confirmed on histological examination of cervical biopsies.

Although the cells can be arranged in loose groups and sheets, they typically occur singly. There is usually considerable cellular pleomorphism and the cells may be epithelioid or spindle shaped in appearance. The nuclei are pleomorphic and often eccentric. They can be hypo- or hyperchromatic, bi- or multinucleate and usually contain prominent nucleoli. The nuclear-cytoplasmic ratio is variable and nuclear moulding may be prominent[62]. Cytoplasmic inclusions, appearing as rounded intranuclear vacuoles, are a feature of some melanomas. The cytoplasm may be abundant and contain melanin pigment. Cell borders tend to be ill-defined, having a lacy appearance.

Diagnostic pitfalls

Cellular pleomorphism is usually marked but melanoma cells can be small and uniform, blending with normal

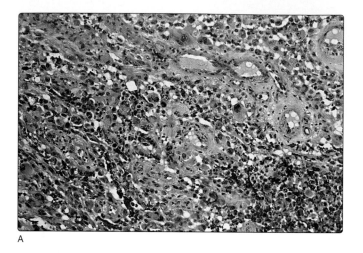

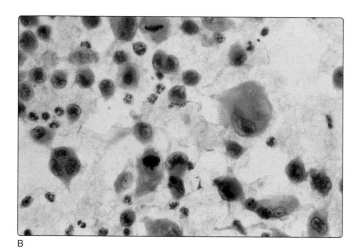

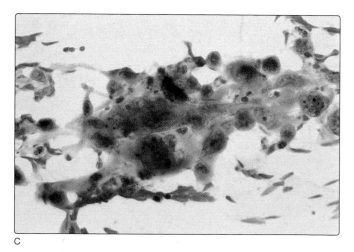

Fig. 33.27 (A) Malignant melanoma forming a polypoidal mass in the vagina, presenting with post-menopausal bleeding. There was no evidence of melanoma elsewhere. The tumour cells are mainly arranged in a ribbon-like pattern and some brown melanin pigment is visible in a few cells. (H&E × HP) (B,C) Cervical smear from the patient whose histology is illustrated in (A) showed pleomorphic malignant cells, mainly dissociated in (B), with multinucleation, prominent nucleoli and mitoses. The cells are in cohesive groups in (C), with a small amount of intracytoplasmic brown melanin pigment. (Papanicolaou × HP)

cervical cells on a smear, in which case they may be overlooked. Mudge and MacFarlane[63] report a case in which the melanoma cells were initially thought to be normal cervical cells and the intracytoplasmic brown pigment was presumed to be haemosiderin.

The differential diagnosis also includes squamous carcinoma, adenocarcinoma and sarcoma. Melanoma cells tend to be epithelioid but can be spindle shaped, in which case they may be misinterpreted as sarcomatous if the cells are exclusively of this type and no melanin is seen[64]. A Masson-Fontana silver stain to detect melanin pigment may be helpful if pigment is not apparent on a Papanicolaou-stained smear. Immunocytochemistry, using antibodies to S 100 protein or a melanoma specific marker such as HMB 45, NKI C3 or Melan A, may be helpful if sufficient material is available.

Lymphoma and leukaemia

Primary non-Hodgkin's lymphoma of the cervix is a rare but well-documented event and is usually of diffuse large B cell type[65]. Secondary involvement of the female genital tract by lymphoma or leukaemia is more commonly encountered, estimated to occur in up to 40% of cases[66]. Hodgkin's disease also may involve the cervix when advanced.

Primary non-Hodgkin's lymphoma of cervix usually presents in middle-aged or elderly patients with vaginal bleeding and a cervical tumour mass, which is then biopsied (Fig. 33.28A,B). Much less often, a cervical smear reveals abnormal cells, which may be recognized as being lymphoid.

Cytological findings (Fig. 33.28C)

▶ Blood-stained smears
▶ Dissociated abnormal lymphoid or plasma cells
▶ Tumour diathesis present

The cytological features of lymphomas have been documented by several authors[67-72], and vary with the type of lymphoma. Smears are typically normal or only show non-specific inflammation if the neoplastic cells are covered by intact mucosa. Details of the diagnostic features of the different types of lymphoma are given in Chapter 19.

Low-grade lymphomas have a relatively uniform cell population, lacking the mixed reactive features of conditions such as follicular cervicitis. High-grade tumours may be recognized by the presence of widespread pleomorphic lymphoid cells. Subtyping of lymphomas in routine cervical smears is not reliable but liquid-based preparations offer the possibility of immunostaining the abnormal cells with a panel of antibodies for phenotyping and accurate classification.

Myeloma rarely affects the female genital tract. Atypical plasma cells have been described in the smear from a woman with postmenopausal bleeding in whom the

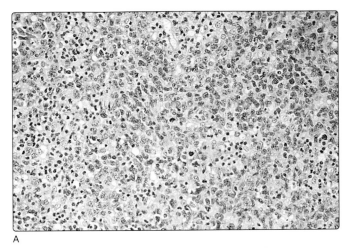

A

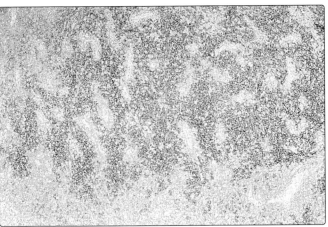

B

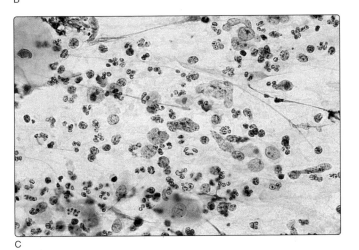

C

Fig. 33.28 (A) Non-Hodgkin's lymphoma of cervix presenting as an ulcerated tumour mass in a middle-aged woman. The H&E section shows a poorly-differentiated tumour with a scattering of small lymphoid cells throughout. (× MP) (B) Immunoalkaline phosphatase staining on the above tumour reveals strong (red) positivity for (B) cell lymphocyte marker. Other markers indicated a high-grade (B) cell non-Hodgkin's lymphoma of large cell anaplastic type. Cytokeratin staining was negative. (× MP) (C) Non-Hodgkin's lymphoma cells were found in the cervical smear from this patient, suggesting the diagnosis prior to biopsy. The malignant cells are all dissociated, mingling with the background inflammatory cells: they have little or no cytoplasm, irregular lobulated nuclear contours, coarse chromatin and prominent nucleoli. (Papanicolaou × HP)

diagnosis of myeloma had yet to be made[73]. Myeloma cells appeared as large single cells with scant or deeply basophilic cytoplasm, hyperchromatic eccentric nuclei, some of which were multinucleate and had prominent large irregular nucleoli.

Leukaemic deposits in cervical stroma can occasionally be sampled by the smear test. The appearance of the cells varies according to the type of leukaemia.

Diagnostic pitfalls

Lymphomatous cells on a smear must be distinguished from chronic inflammatory cells, small cell carcinoma, small cell cervical intraepithelial neoplasia (CIN 3), endometrial carcinoma, poorly-differentiated adenocarcinoma and sarcoma.

Reactive inflammatory cells will have a polymorphic appearance, being composed of a mixture of normal mature and immature lymphocytes, sometimes including plasma cells. A leukaemic infiltrate may be mistaken for follicular cervicitis if the appropriate history is not available. Small cell carcinoma cells tend to be irregularly shaped and pleomorphic with indistinct nucleoli. Characteristic nuclear moulding and clustering may be present. Cells of small cell severe dyskaryosis type from CIN 3 may present in sheets as well as singly and some individual cells may show evidence of keratinization.

Cells from a high-grade lymphoma may be mistaken for poorly-differentiated adenocarcinoma. Features favouring the diagnosis of lymphoma include single dissociated cells with prominent nucleoli, nipple-like projections on the nuclei, chromatin clumping at the nuclear borders and scant cytoplasm.

Metastatic tumours

Metastasis of carcinoma to the cervix is not uncommon and usually occurs in the presence of advanced metastatic disease elsewhere. The cervical mucosa tends to remain intact so that tumour cells are not often seen in smears. The most common primary sites are other areas of the genital tract, the gastrointestinal tract and breast[74]. Tumour may also involve the cervix by direct invasion from the organ primarily involved, for example, from endometrium, bladder or rectum.

Cytological findings

▶ Relative paucity of tumour cells
▶ Malignant nature of cells usually obvious
▶ Resemblance to known primary tumour
▶ Clean background

The cytological findings are variable, depending on the nature of the original tumour, the presence or absence of ulceration and the extent of cervical involvement by the

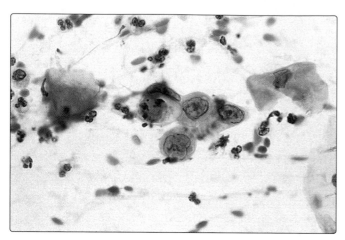

Fig. 33.29 Metastatic carcinoma cells in a cervical smear from a patient with known large bowel carcinoma. The cells are clearly malignant; the cell on the left is distended with mucin, displacing the nucleus to produce a signet ring cell. (Papanicolaou × HP)

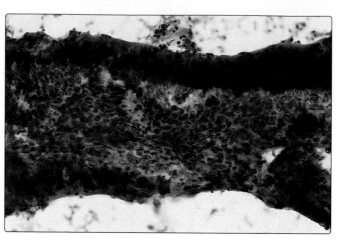

Fig. 33.30 Metastatic adenocarcinoma in a cervical smear. Large sheets of malignant tissue were present in this smear. The palisaded border of tall columnar cells at the upper edge of the sheet is unlike the usual appearances of primary cervical adenocarcinoma. This patient had had resection of a carcinoma of the rectum in the past. (Papanicolaou × MP)

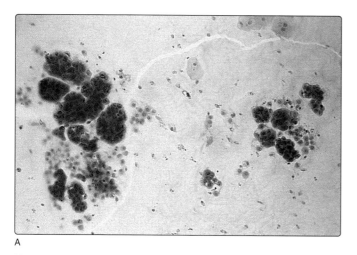

A

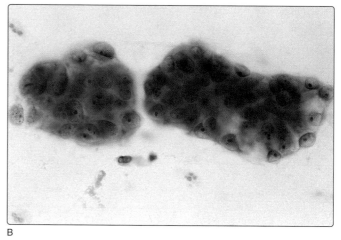

B

Fig. 33.31 Papillary clustering of adenocarcinoma cells in a cervical smear from a woman with ovarian papillary adenocarcinoma. The tumour had not spread to the cervix. (A) The abnormal cells stand out on low power against a clean background. In (B) the cells show the nuclear abnormalities of an adenocarcinoma. (Papanicolaou × HP)

metastasis. In general there are fewer abnormal cells than in smears from primary tumours of cervix. The cells are readily recognized as malignant (Fig. 33.29), but tumour typing may be difficult unless distinctive features are present. Signet ring cell formation or large sheets of tall columnar malignant cells palisaded along one edge (Fig. 33.30) may suggest an origin from the gastrointestinal tract.

While strictly not true metastases, cells exfoliated from extrauterine tumours of the fallopian tube or ovary, collected from the cervix as part of a cervical or vaginal smear, often stand out from a clear background, with little or no tumour diathesis (Fig. 33.31) as discussed in Chapters 34 and 35[75]. The cells may have a papillary pattern and psammoma bodies are sometimes noted. The appearances are striking and, if reported correctly, may lead to diagnosis of a clinically silent primary tumour.

In conclusion, awareness of the patient's history should alert one to the possibility of metastasis but it is important to remember that patients with one tumour are also more likely to develop further neoplasms. If abnormal cells are seen in a smear from a patient with a known carcinoma, the original tumour histology should be checked for comparison with the cytological findings.

References

1 Ferenczy A, Winkler B. Benign diseases of the cervix. In: Kurman R J ed. *Blaustein's Pathology of the Female Genital Tract*. New York: Springer-Verlag, 1982; 166–168

2 Ngadiman S, Yang G C H. Adenomyomatous, lower uterine segment and endocervical polyps in cervicovaginal smears. *Acta Cytol* 1995; **39**: 643–647

3 Poulsen H E, Taylor C W, Sobin L H. *Histological Typing of Female Genital Tract Tumours*. Geneva: WHO, 1975; 61–62

4 Schneider V, Barnes L A. Ectopic decidual reaction of the uterine cervix: frequency and cytologic presentation. *Acta Cytol* 1981; **25**: 616–622

5 Schneider V. Arias-Stella reaction of the endocervix: frequency and location. *Acta Cytol* 1981; **25**: 224–228

6 Mulvany N J, Khan A, Ostor A. Arias–Stella reaction associated with cervical pregnancy. Report of a case with a cytologic presentation. *Acta Cytol* 1994; **38**: 218–222

7 Yates W A, Persad R V, Stanbridge C M. The Arias–Stella reaction in the cervix: a case report with cervical cytology. *Cytopathol* 1997; **8**: 40–44

8 Ismail S M. Cone biopsy causes cervical endometriosis and tubo-endometrioid metaplasia. *Histopathol* 1991; **18**: 107–114

9 Srinivasan R, Nijhawan R, Das A, Walker R. Fine needle aspiration cytodiagnosis of endometriosis arising in scar tissue and in the caecum – case reports. *Cytopathol* 1993; **4**: 357–360

10 Yahr L J, Lee K R. Cytologic findings in microglandular hyperplasia of the cervix. *Diagn Cytopathol* 1991; **7**: 248–251

11 Alvarez-Santin C, Sica A, Rodriguez M C et al. Microglandular hyperplasia of the uterine cervix. Cytologic diagnosis in cervical smears. *Acta Cytol* 1999; **43**: 110–113

12 Shidham V B, Dayer A M, Basir Z, Kajdacsy-Balla A. Cervical cytology and immunohistochemical features in endometrial adenocarcinoma simulating microglandular hyperplasia. A case report. *Acta Cytol* 2000; **44**: 661–666

13 Chen K T K, Hendricks E J. Malakoplakia of the female genital tract. *Obstet Gynecol* 1985; **65**(suppl): 84–87

14 Wahl R W. Malakoplakia of the uterine cervix: report of two cases. *Acta Cytol* 1982; **26**: 691–694

15 Falcon-Escobedo R, Mora-Tiscareno A, Puebilitz-Peredo S. Malakoplakia of the uterine cervix. Histologic, cytologic and ultrastructural study of a case. *Acta Cytol* 1986; **30**: 281–284

16 Kapilla K, Verma K. Intracellular bacilli in vaginal smears in a case of malakoplakia of the uterine cervix. *Acta Cytol* 1989; **33**: 410–411

17 Stewart C J R, Thomas M A. Malakoplakia of the uterine cervix and endometrium. *Cytopathol* 1991; **2**: 271–275

18 Saad A J, Donovan T M, Truong L D. Malakoplakia of the vagina diagnosed by fine-needle aspiration cytology. *Diagn Cytopathol* 1993; **9**: 559–561

19 Beyer-Boon M E, Verdonk G W. The identification of atypical reserve cells in smears of patients with premalignant and malignant changes in the squamous and glandular epithelium of the uterine cervix. *Acta Cytol* 1978; **22**: 305–311

20 Jonasson J G, Wang H H, Antonioli D A, Ducatman B S. Tubal metaplasia of the uterine cervix: a prevalence study in women with gynecologic pathology. *Int J Gynecol Pathol* 1992; **11**: 89–95

21 Al-Nafussi A, Rahilly M. The prevalence of tubo-endometrial metaplasia and adenomatoid proliferation. *Histopathol* 1993; **22**: 177–179

22 Novotny D B, Maygarden S J, Johnson D E, Frable W J. Tubal metaplasia. A frequent potential pitfall in the cytologic diagnosis of endocervical glandular dysplasia on cervical smears. *Acta Cytol* 1992; **36**: 1–10

23 Ducatman B S, Wang H H, Jonasson J G et al. Tubal metaplasia: a cytologic study with comparison to other neoplastic and non-neoplastic conditions of the endocervix. *Diagn Cytopathol* 1993; **9**: 98–105

24 Hirschowitz L, Eckford S D, Phillpotts B, Midwinter A. Cytological changes associated with tubo-endometrioid metaplasia of the uterine cervix. *Cytopathol* 1994; **5**: 1–8

25 Kurman R J, Norris H J, Wilkinson E. Tumours of the cervix, vagina and vulva. In: *Atlas of Tumor Pathology*. Washington DC: AFIP, 1992; 3rd fascicle

26 Weir M M, Bell D A. Transitional cell metaplasia of the cervix: a newly described entity in cervicovaginal smears. *Diagn Cytopathol* 1998; **18**: 222–226

27 Gondos B, Smith L R, Townsend D E. Cytologic changes in cervical epithelium following cryosurgery. *Acta Cytol* 1970; **14**: 386–389

28 Gonzalez-Merlo J, Ausin J, Lejarcegui J A, Maraquez M. Regeneration of the ectocervical epithelium after its destruction by electrocauterization. *Acta Cytol* 1973; **17**: 366–371

29 Bibbo M, Keebler C M, Wied G L. The cytologic diagnosis of tissue repair in the female genital tract. *Acta Cytol* 1971; **15**: 133–137

30 Ueki M, Ueda M, Kurokawa A et al. Cytologic study of the tissue repair cells of the uterine cervix with special reference to their origin. *Acta Cytol* 1992; **36**: 310–318

31 Geirsson G, Woodworth F E, Patten S F, Bonfiglio T A. Epithelial repair and regeneration in the uterine cervix. I. An analysis of the cells. *Acta Cytol* 1977; **21**: 371–378

32 Shingleton H M, Bone H, Bradley D H, Soong S J. Adenocarcinoma of the cervix. I. Clinical evaluation and pathological features. *Am J Obstet Gynecol* 1981; **139**: 799–814

33 Buckley C H, Fox H, eds. Carcinoma of the cervix. *Recent Advances in Histopathology*. London: Churchill Livingstone, 1989; 63–64

34 Costa M J, Kenny M B, Naib Z M. Cervicovaginal cytology in uterine adenocarcinoma and adenosquamous carcinoma: comparison of cytologic and histologic findings. *Acta Cytol* 1991; **35**: 127–134

35 Ulbright T M, Gersell D J. Glassy cell carcinoma of the uterine cervix. A light and electron microscopic study of five cases. *Cancer* 1983; **51**: 2255–2263

36 Littman P, Clement P B, Henriksen B et al. Glassy cell carcinoma of the cervix. *Cancer* 1976; **37**: 2238–2246

37 Pak H Y, Yokota S B, Paladugu R R, Agliozzo C M. Glassy cell carcinoma of the cervix. Cytologic and clinicopathologic analysis. *Cancer* 1983; **52**: 307–312

38 Nunez C, Abdul-Karim F W, Somrak T M. Glassy cell carcinoma of the uterine cervix. Cytopathologic and histopathologic study of five cases. *Acta Cytol* 1985; **29**: 303–309

39 Chung J-H, Koh J-S, Lee S-S, Cho K-J. Glassy cell carcinoma of the uterine cervix. Cytologic features and expression of estrogen and progesterone receptors. *Acta Cytol* 2000; **44**: 551–556

40 Smith J H F. Cervical cytology through the looking glass. *Cytopathol* 2000; **11**: 54–56

41 Grafton W D, Kamm R C, Cowley L H. Cytologic characteristics of adenoid cystic carcinoma of the cervix uteri. *Acta Cytol* 1976; **20**: 164–166

42 Lozowski M S, Mishriki Y, Solitare G B. Cytopathologic features of adenoid cystic carcinoma of the uterine cervix. *Acta Cytol* 1983; **27**: 317–322

43 Dayton V, Henry M, Stanley M W et al. Adenoid cystic carcinoma of the uterine cervix: cytologic features. *Acta Cytol* 1990; **34**: 125–128

44 Vuong P N, Neveux Y, Schoonaert M-F et al. Adenoid Cystic (cylindromatous) carcinoma associated with squamous cell carcinoma of the cervix uteri. Cytologic presentation of a case with histologic and ultrastructural correlations. *Acta Cytol* 1996; **40**: 289–294

45 Ravinsky E, Safneck J R, Chantziuntoniou N. Cytologic features of primary adenoid cystic carcinoma of the uterine cervix. A case report. *Acta Cytol* 1996; **40**: 1304–1308

46 Hirahatake K, Hareyama H, Kure R et al. Cytologic and hormonal findings in a carcinoid tumour of the uterine cervix. *Acta Cytol* 1990; **34**: 119–124

47 Russin V, Valente P T, Hanjani P. Psammoma bodies in neuroendocrine carcinoma of the uterine cervix. *Acta Cytol* 1987; **31**: 791–795

48 Miles P A, Herrera G A, Mena H, Trujillo I. Cytologic findings in primary malignant carcinoid tumour of the cervix including immunohistochemistry and electron microscopy performed on cervical smears. *Acta Cytol* 1985; **29**: 1003–1008

49 Reich O, Pickel H, Purstner P. Exfoliative cytology of a lymphoepithelioma like carcinoma in a cervical smear. A case report. *Acta Cytol* 1999; **43**: 285–288

50 Proca D M, Hitchcock C L, Keyhani-Rofagha S. Exfoliative cytology of lymphoepithelioma like carcinoma of the uterine cervix. A report of two cases. *Acta Cytol* 2000; **44**: 410–414

51 Baschinsky D, Keyhani-Rofagha S, Hameed A. Exfoliative cytology of atypical polypoid adenomyoma. A case report. *Acta Cytol* 1999; **43**: 637–640

52 Hadju S I, Hadju E O. *Cytopathology of Sarcomas and Other Nonepithelial Tumours*. Philadelphia: W B Saunders, 1976; 183–212

53 Silverberg S G, Major F J, Blessing J A *et al.* Carcinosarcoma (malignant mixed mesodermal tumor) of the uterus. A gynecologic oncology group pathologic study of 203 cases. *Int J Gynecol Pathol* 1990; **9**: 1–19

54 Abell M R, Ramirez J A. Sarcomas and carcinosarcomas of the uterine cervix. *Cancer* 1973; **31**: 1176–1192

55 Kurman R J, Norris H J, Wilkinson E. Tumours of the cervix, vagina, and vulva. In: *Atlas of Tumour Pathology*. Washington: Armed Forces Institute of Pathology, 1992; 112

56 Barwick K W, LiVolsi V A. Malignant mixed mullerian tumors of the uterus. A clinicopathologic assessment of 34 cases. *Am J Surg Pathol* 1979; **3**: 125–135

57 Massoni E A, Hadju S I. Cytology of primary and metastatic uterine sarcomas. *Acta Cytol* 1984; **28**: 93–100

58 An-Foraker S H, Kawada C Y. Cytodiagnosis of endometrial mixed mesodermal tumor. *Acta Cytol* 1985; **29**: 137–141

59 Imai H, Kitamura H, Nananura T *et al.* Mullerian carcinofibroma of the uterus. A case report. *Acta Cytol* 1999; **43**: 667–674

60 Matsuura Y, Kashimura M, Hatanaka K *et al.* Sarcoma botryoides of the cervix. Report of a case with cytopathologic findings. *Acta Cytol* 1999; **43**: 475–480

61 Fleming H, Mein P. Primary melanoma of the cervix: a case report. *Acta Cytol* 1994; **38**: 65–69

62 Sclosshauer P W, Heller D S, Koulos J P. Malignant melanoma of the uterine cervix diagnosed on a cervical smear (letter). *Acta Cytol* 1998; **42**: 1043–1045

63 Mudge T J, MacFarlane A. Primary malignant melanoma of the cervix. *Br J Obstet Gynaecol* 1981; **88**: 1257–1259

64 Holmquist N D, Torres J. Malignant melanoma of the cervix: report of a case. *Acta Cytol* 1988; **32**: 252–256

65 Perren T, Farrant M, McCarthy K *et al.* Lymphomas of the cervix and upper vagina: a report of five cases and a review of the literature. *Gynecol Oncol* 1992; **44**: 87–95

66 Saigo P E. Unusual tumours. In: Bibbo M ed. *Comprehensive Cytopathology*. Philadelphia: W B Saunders, 1991; 307–310

67 Matsuyama T, Tsukamoto N, Kaku T *et al.* Primary malignant lymphoma of the uterine corpus and cervix: report of case with

immunocytochemical analysis. *Acta Cytol* 1989; **33**: 228–232

68 Taki I, Aozasa K, Kurokawa K. Malignant lymphoma of the uterine cervix: cytologic diagnosis of a case with immunocytochemical corroboration. *Acta Cytol* 1985; **29**: 607–611

69 Whitaker D. The role of cytology in the detection of malignant lymphoma of the uterine cervix. *Acta Cytol* 1976; **20**: 510–513

70 Krumerman M S, Chung A. Solitary reticulum cell sarcoma of the uterine cervix with initial cytodiagnosis. *Acta Cytol* 1978; **22**: 46–50

71 Al-Talib R K, Sworn M J, Ramsay A D *et al.* Primary cervical lymphoma: the role of cervical cytology. *Cytopathol* 1996; **7**: 173–177

72 Dhimes P, Alberti N, De Agustin P, Tubio J. Primary malignant lymphoma of the uterine cervix: report of a case with cytologic with immunohistochemical diagnosis. *Cytopathology* 1996; **7**: 204–210

73 Figueroa J M, Huffaker A K, Diehl E J. Malignant plasma cells in cervical smear. *Acta Cytol* 1978; **22**: 43–45

74 Way S. Carcinoma metastatic in the cervix. *Gynecol Oncol* 1980; **9**: 298–302

75 Ng A B P, Teeple D, Lindner E A, Reagan J W. The cellular manifestations of extrauterine cancer. *Acta Cytol* 1974; **18**: 108

34 Tumours of the vulva and vagina

Jane Johnson

Introduction

Vulval and vaginal smears are received in the laboratory far less frequently than diagnostic smears from the cervix. Women with vulval disease may present to dermatologists, genito-urinary physicians or gynaecologists, mainly depending upon the general practitioner's initial diagnosis but also, to some extent, upon social factors. Vulval samples tend to be dry and, because many lesions have surface keratosis, they often mainly consist of anucleate squames. Before the introduction of hormonal assays, vaginal smears were used for hormonal assessment in infertility cases but now most vaginal samples are follow-up smears from women with previously treated cervical disease which, with age and after radiotherapy, are difficult to interpret.

Vulva

Technical aspects

Smears taken from the vulva with a conventional spatula, unless from the introitus, will be dry. Improved cell preservation can be achieved by gently rubbing the area with a cotton wool swab dipped in saline and then squeezing and rolling the swab on to a glass slide to transfer the cells. Rapid fixation is paramount, followed by Papanicolaou staining. When using these smears along with colposcopic inspection of the vulva as follow-up after previous excision of vulval intraepithelial neoplasia (VIN), separate samples from the four vulval quadrants (right and left, anterior and posterior) can help to localize a recurrence. Touch preparations and brush samples may also be taken when lesions are ulcerated.

Benign tumours of the vulva

The vulva is covered with skin and benign tumours seen elsewhere are also found at this site. Naevi, pyogenic granulomata, keratoacanthomas and seborrhoeic warts are among those most often diagnosed (see Chapter 38). Vulval skin includes numerous hair follicles and sebaceous, eccrine and apocrine glands but, despite this, skin adnexal tumours are unusual. The papillary hidradenoma is the most common[1].

Papillary hidradenoma

This benign tumour is of apocrine origin; it is not seen before the apocrine glands develop at puberty. On the vulva,

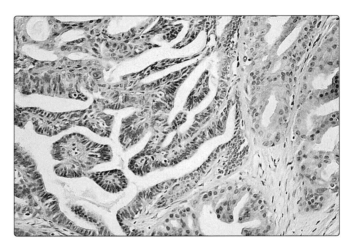

Fig. 34.1 Vulval biopsy. A papillary hidradenoma. Note the papillary structure. The cells with granular cytoplasm have undergone 'apocrine metaplasia', similar to that seen in the breast. Nuclear pleomorphism and nucleoli can be seen. (H&E × MP)

most are less than 2 cm in diameter. They are well circumscribed, mobile nodules, usually in the labia majora and although characteristically single, rare cases of women with multiple lesions have been reported[1]. Papillary hidradenomas may ulcerate and evert giving rise to a red, friable papillary mass. These lesions are most frequently diagnosed clinically, or on biopsy, but the cytological diagnosis of papillary hidradenoma of the vulva was first described in 1974 by Dupre-Froment[2] and photomicrographs published later by Schramm[3] and by Hustin et al[4].

Histologically, the lesions are composed of tubular and papillary patterns of growth. The cells seen on cytology form the outer layer of cells with, in some areas, a basal layer of smaller myoepithelial cells (Fig. 34.1).

On cytology, clumps of slightly pleomorphic glandular cells are seen with a fine, evenly distributed chromatin pattern in the nuclei. In some cells there is abundant rather granular looking cytoplasm[4].

Granular cell tumour

These rare tumours are usually solitary, well-circumscribed, subcutaneous, or submucosal nodules in the labia. Occasionally they may be bilateral[5]. They are not accessible for cytological diagnosis in vivo. They are included here because they are often associated with striking pseudocarcinomatous hyperplasia of the overlying squamous epithelium, which may lead to a misdiagnosis of VIN or squamous carcinoma. This epithelial hyperplasia may include cells with marked mitotic activity, abnormal-looking chromatin distribution and prominent nucleoli. Often the presence of an underlying granular cell tumour is the only distinguishing feature[5]. Malignant granular cell tumours have also been reported[6].

Malignant tumours of the vulva

Approximately 4% of malignant tumours in the female genital tract arise in the vulva and of these 95% are squamous cell carcinoma[7]. The remainder include basal cell carcinoma, malignant melanoma and, rarely, extramammary Paget's disease and adenocarcinoma of Bartholin's gland.

Vulval intraepithelial neoplasia (VIN)

Histologically, the characteristic features of VIN include nuclear abnormalities, decreased epithelial differentiation and increased mitotic activity. In the higher grades of VIN abnormal mitotic figures become more numerous. There is usually surface keratosis, much of which is parakeratosis with retention of pyknotic nuclear remnants. In VIN I the abnormal nuclear forms and mitotic activity are usually confined to the lower third of the epithelial thickness. In VIN II the nuclear abnormalities are usually more marked and extend to between a third and two-thirds of the thickness of the epithelium, whereas in VIN III marked nuclear abnormalities are present throughout the thickness of the epithelium with features of maturation being present in only the most superficial layer.

Until recently this disease was rarely seen before the menopause; it is, however, being diagnosed increasingly frequently in younger women, such cases being associated with human papilloma virus (HPV) infection. In one series 84% of samples of VIN III contained HPV, 96% of which were HPV 16[8]. In such cases intraepithelial neoplasia may be multicentric with lesions of the cervix, vagina, vulva and perineum including the anal canal, which may or may not present simultaneously[9].

The most common presenting feature clinically is pruritus. On gross inspection, areas of VIN may be slightly raised and reddened, or keratotic. A colposcope may be used to help outline the areas of abnormal epithelium[10]. Clinical difficulties sometimes arise in distinguishing VIN from viral warts and from squamous carcinoma.

Cytological findings

▶ Parakeratotic cells
▶ Dyskaryotic cells
▶ Anucleate squamous

Cytologically, normal anucleate squames from vulval keratinization are usually replaced by parakeratosis when

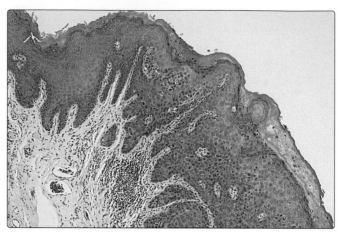

Fig. 34.2   Vulval biopsy. Vulval intraepithelial neoplasia (VIN) grade III. Note the surface parakeratosis. (H&E × MP)

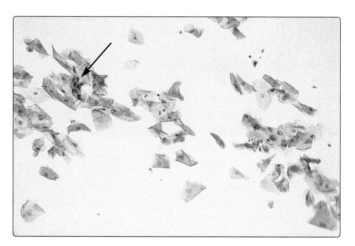

Fig. 34.3   A swab smear from the case illustrated in **Fig. 34.2**. A few parakeratotic squamous cells are present in the centre of the field. Diagnostic dyskaryotic cells with a large nuclear/cytoplasmic ratio are seen in the group at the top (arrow). (Papanicolaou × MP)

significant degrees of VIN are present (Fig. 34.2). Parakeratosis alone may be present on the slide and must always be taken seriously although it may be seen in other dermatological conditions such as psoriasis. It is helpful for the clinicians to know that if a lesion is clearly keratotic it is usually the cells beneath the white material, which rubs off, that are more likely to be diagnostic. The cells may be single or in clumps. There is an increased nuclear/cytoplasmic ratio with hyperchromatic pleomorphic nuclei (Fig. 34.3).

Squamous cell carcinoma

This tumour may affect any part of the vulva, most being more than 2 cm in diameter at presentation. Bulky, fungating masses are common, but indurated plaque-like or ulcerated lesions may also be seen. Unfortunately, lymph node metastasis occurs even in lesions showing minimal invasion and the concept of microinvasive disease is not appropriate in vulval squamous cell carcinomas[11]. The tumour is usually well to moderately differentiated and keratinizing. The rare well-differentiated exophytic variant, *verrucous carcinoma*, occurs on the vulva. Two-thirds of patients are more than 60 years of age at diagnosis with an age range of 20–90 years[7].

Cytological findings

▶ Dyskaryotic squamous cell
▶ Bizarre cell types
▶ Tumour diathesis
▶ Parakeratotic groups
▶ Anucleate squames

Cytological features are identical to those seen in squamous carcinoma of the cervix with high nuclear/cytoplasmic ratios, marked nuclear pleomorphism and fibre and tadpole forms. There may also be an inflammatory and necrotic background, the so-called 'malignant diathesis'. Parakeratotic clusters and anucleate squames may accompany the squamous carcinoma cells, having been scraped from adjacent VIN and hyperkeratotic vulval epithelium. Cells from verrucous carcinoma show minimal nuclear pleomorphism but there is usually an increased nuclear/cytoplasmic ratio and some dyskaryotic features in the nuclei. This can prove an extremely difficult diagnosis to make.

Basal cell carcinoma

This rare tumour usually involves the labia majora in postmenopausal women. The histological appearances are similar to those seen in basal cell carcinoma at other sites, including the characteristic peripheral palisading of cells (see Chapter 38)[12].

Few cases of the cytological diagnosis of basal cell carcinoma are described. The cells have scanty, poorly-defined cytoplasm. The nuclei are hyperchromatic, some having visible nucleoli. The cells are generally small and pleomorphism is not a feature.

Malignant melanoma

This is a rare tumour of the vulva. The peak incidence occurs in women aged 50–60 years but it has been reported in teenagers and in women over 80 years of age. The clitoris and labia minora are the most favoured sites. Nodular and superficial spreading types are seen and it is unusual for the woman to have noticed a pre-existing pigmented lesion[13,14]. Most present with a bleeding nodule, or with pain. As with other cutaneous melanomas, survival is related to the depth of invasion, although on the vulva, prognostic bands of greater thicknesses must be used compared with those for lesions elsewhere[15].

Cytological findings

▶ Loose clusters of pleomorphic cells
▶ Nuclei of variable size and shape
▶ Pigment often present

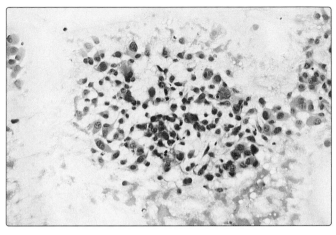

Fig. 34.4 Malignant melanoma cells in a touch preparation. A loose cluster of cells with marked pleomorphism. Brown pigment globules can be seen in some of the cells. (Papanicolaou × MP) (see **Fig. 34.5**)

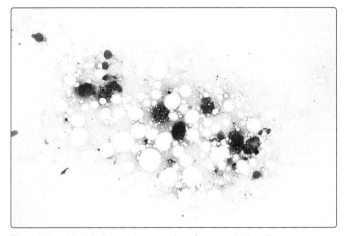

Fig. 34.5 Air-dried touch preparations from a vulval malignant melanoma. The black pigment granules are more obvious. (Giemsa × MP)

In touch preparations from ulcerated lesions, melanoma cells are usually arranged in loose clusters. The pleomorphism is remarkable with nuclei of several sizes within a cluster and round, oval and spindle-shaped forms. Pigment is present in two-thirds of cases, visible as brown granules in Papanicolaou stained smears (Fig. 34.4). The pigment is often more easily seen as black granules in the cytoplasm in Giemsa preparations (Fig. 34.5). Multinucleation is sometimes present, predominantly in amelanotic melanomas. There is no difficulty in very pleomorphic, pigmented cases, but in amelanotic melanomas S 100 immunostaining can be used as a diagnostic aid[16]. Melanoma specific antigen may also be used. This antigen is more specific, but less sensitive.

Paget's disease of the vulva

This disease occurs most often in postmenopausal white women. In one series, only one patient was below 50 years of age, the average age at diagnosis being 65 years. The

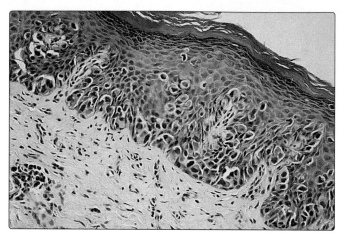

Fig. 34.6 A biopsy of Paget's disease of the vulva. The large Paget's cells are present singly and in clusters in the epidermis. (H&E × MP)

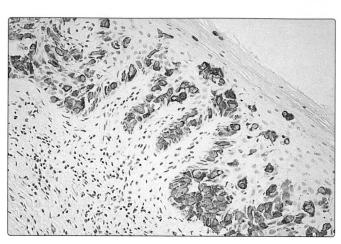

Fig. 34.7 Paget's disease of the vulva with the Paget's cells highlighted with immunoperoxidase staining. (CAM 5.2 × MP)

lesions appear as intensely itchy, reddened, excoriated areas predominantly on the labia majora. There are only occasional multifocal lesions[17].

Histologically, Paget's disease is similar wherever it occurs (Fig. 34.6), but unlike Paget's disease of the nipple of the breast, where an underlying intraduct or invasive carcinoma is the usual finding, an underlying tumour in cases of Paget's disease of the vulva is found in only 20–30%. When present, such tumours may be squamous, adeno-, or basal cell carcinomas in adjacent skin, or a tumour in the urogenital or gastrointestinal system. There may be an associated carcinoma of the breast, without evidence of Paget's disease of the nipple. Such associations are unexplained[18,19].

If left untreated, Paget's disease of the vulva spreads into the adjacent perianal skin and the top of the thigh, and rarely into the vagina and on to the cervix[20]. The clinically visible extent usually underestimates the area of histological involvement. This leads to incomplete surgical excision unless accompanied by a wide apparently disease free margin. In areas of minimal involvement of the epidermis, or where the diagnosis is in doubt, the Paget's cells can be highlighted by immunostaining with CAM 5.2 (Fig. 34.7). Mucin stains may be used, but results are variable and unreliable[21]. Rarely, Paget's cells have been seen to invade into the dermis[22].

Cytological findings

▶ Single and clustered Paget's cells
▶ Pale indistinct cytoplasm
▶ Enlarged nuclei and nucleoli

In scrapes from clinically involved areas, Paget's cells may be seen singly or in clusters. The cytoplasm is pale staining and has an indistinct outline. The nuclei are large and nucleoli are visible (Fig. 34.8). Occasionally, signet ring

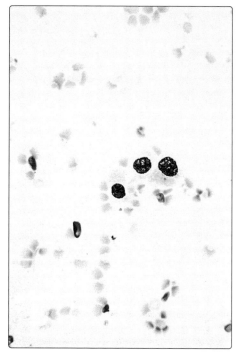

Fig. 34.8 A touch preparation from a case of Paget's disease of the vulva. Note the very scanty Paget's cells here in a small cluster. They are clearly adenocarcinoma cells with very abnormal chromatin distribution. The cytoplasm is pale staining and has an indistinct cell boundary. (Giemsa × MP)

forms are present. The cells are indistinguishable from Paget's cells in the nipple and from cells in aspirates from breast ductal carcinoma[18].

Adenocarcinoma of Bartholin's gland

These lesions are exceedingly rare. They are usually mucin-producing and have a variety of growth patterns including papillary and mucoepidermoid. If they invade to the skin surface, they can be diagnosed on cytology. They are distinguished from sweat gland carcinoma by their site.

Squamous cell carcinoma and adenoid cystic carcinomas may also arise within Bartholin's glands[23].

Vagina

Vaginal vault smears for follow-up after previously treated cervical disease are the most common vaginal smears received. The two main problem areas are interpretation of smears from the atrophic vault of an older, or oestrogen deficient, patient and the bizarre cell changes induced by radiotherapy.

Benign tumours of the vagina

In normal circumstances, there are no glandular structures in the vagina and so benign glandular tumours are not seen. There is debate over whether true benign epithelial papillomata exist other than those induced by viral infection.

Vaginal polyps

These lesions are benign connective tissue tumours with stroma similar to that seen in the loose subepithelial layer of the normal vagina. There are frequently giant fibroblasts scattered within the stroma and there may be a subepithelial condensation of fibroblasts. These polyps may represent a reactive hyperplasia of the vaginal wall rather than a true tumour[24]. Pedunculated leiomyomata and benign rhabdomyomas are also found[25,26]. All these polyps are covered with benign vaginal squamous epithelium and surface scrapes give smears in which the squamous cells are entirely normal. If the polyp has prolapsed through the introitus, however, the squamous epithelium may be keratinized on the exposed surface and anucleate squames can then be a predominant feature.

Malignant tumours of the vagina

In the female genital tract, only carcinoma of the fallopian tube is diagnosed less frequently than primary carcinoma of the vagina, which accounts for 1–2% of gynaecological malignancies. It is estimated that up to 90% of neoplasms in the vagina are secondary, many having extended on to the vagina from the cervix or, less often, the vulva. Spread from the rectum and bladder is not only possible by direct extension, but also by intravascular metastasis[27].

Vaginal intraepithelial neoplasia (VAIN)

This condition involves lack of epithelial maturation, abnormal nuclear forms and an increase in mitotic activity identical to that described in vulval intraepithelial neoplasia. It is also graded I, II and III according to the extent of replacement of the mucosa by abnormal cells. Although most often seen in association with cervical intraepithelial neoplasia (CIN), it is much less common and occurs at a later age. VAIN may be multifocal and present in women with intraepithelial neoplasia of the cervix and of the vulva, not necessarily synchronously. The diagnosis of VAIN is almost always made on cytology with confirmatory colposcopy and biopsy histology. It has been reported that, in post hysterectomy vault smears when VAIN is present, abnormal cells can be identified in 97% of the smears with an 83% sensitivity. False negatives were ascribed to obscuring inflammatory cells[28].

Histologically, intraepithelial neoplasia of the vagina is similar to that seen on the cervix, apart from lack of the underlying crypts of the cervical transformation zone. The cytological patterns seen in cells from VAIN are those seen in CIN with all the same variants (see Chapter 30).

Squamous cell carcinoma

This is primarily a tumour of older women. More than 60% of patients are aged 60 years or older[29]. Most tumours are of the large cell non-keratinizing type, but all types of squamous cell carcinoma seen in the cervix and vulva also present in the vagina. Cytological determination of site of origin cannot, therefore, be made. As with the vulva, the cytological findings are identical to those of squamous carcinoma of the cervix, which are described in Chapter 30.

Adenocarcinoma

Clear cell adenocarcinoma of the vagina has been described developing in young girls who were exposed *in utero* to diethylstilboestrol (DES). DES is a synthetic oestrogen that was prescribed to pregnant women in the UK between 1950–75, mainly to prevent miscarriage. In 1974 it was estimated that approximately 7500 women in the UK had been prescribed DES during pregnancy. Approximately one in a thousand 'DES daughters' develop clear cell adenocarcinoma[30,31] (see Chapter 28). More recently these tumours have been found in patients without a history of DES exposure, the mean age of both groups of patients being 22 years[32]. On cytology, the adenocarcinoma cells may be indistinguishable from those seen in adenocarcinoma of the endocervix or endometrium, but occasionally they have abundant clear cytoplasm[33] more typical of the cells seen from serous cystadenocarcinoma of the ovary. A metastatic deposit from such a tumour would present far more commonly than DES associated clear cell carcinoma, even in a woman of 22 years of age, and this must be borne in mind when considering the diagnosis in such cases.

In older women, adenocarcinoma cells in vaginal smears may be from other adjacent pelvic primary tumours, or from metastatic carcinomas especially of the breast, or stomach. Benign glandular cells in vault smears following hysterectomy would not be an expected finding and would give rise to concern, but they may be seen in the presence of endometriosis at the vault, in tubal prolapse (Fig. 34.9), where the fallopian tubes and ovaries had been conserved and in metaplasia in atrophic vaginal epithelium[34] or following radio/chemotherapy[35]. Other causes of benign glands in the vault include a large congenital transformation zone[36] and vaginal adenosis induced by DES exposure or Tamoxifen therapy[37].

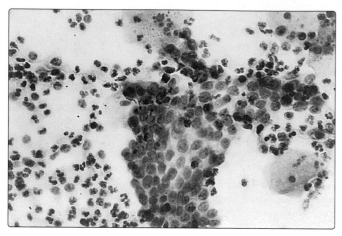

Fig. 34.9   A vault smear from a case of tubal prolapse. This is clearly a cluster of benign glandular cells, which one would not expect to see at the vault. They may, however, be seen in certain circumstances described in the text. Cells from all of these conditions may appear as in this illustration, but occasionally may look metaplastic. (Courtesy of Dr M Wolfendale, Stoke Mandeville, UK)

Malignant melanoma

This is a very rare primary tumour in the vagina. There are several cases reported in the literature, some with genuine junctional activity confirming the vagina as the primary site[38–40]. The cytological features are the same as those seen in melanoma of the vulva (Figs 34.4, 34.5).

Malignant connective tissue tumours

Embryonal rhabdomyosarcoma (sarcoma botryoides), a malignant mixed Mullerian tumour[41], and yolk sac tumours[42], both present as polypoid masses in the vagina in childhood. They are both extremely rare and highly malignant. Their diagnosis by cytological investigation is not described.

Leiomyosarcomas[43], angiosaromas[44] and other connective tissue malignancies of the vagina also appear in the literature, usually as case reports, the diagnosis having been made histologically.

References

1   Woodworth H Jr, Dockerty M B, Wilson R B, Pratt J H. Papillary hidradenoma of the vulva: a clinicopathologic study of 69 cases. *Am J Obstet Gynecol* 1971; **110**: 501–508

2   Dupre-Froment J. *Cytologie Gynecologique.* Paris: Flammarion, 1974; 41

3   Schramm G. Diagnosis of a papillary hidradenoma of the vulva by simultaneous cytology and colposcopy. *Acta Cytol* 1979; **23**: 57–60

4   Hustin J, Donnay M, Hamels J. Identification of papillary hidradenoma of the vulva by imprint cytology. *Acta Cytol* 1980; **24**: 466–467

5   Wolber R A, Talerman A, Wilkinson E J, Clement P B. Vulvar granular cell tumours with pseudocarcinomatous hyperplasia: a comparative analysis with well-differentiated squamous carcinoma. *Int J Gynecol Pathol* 1991; **10**: 59–66

6   Gamboa L G. Malignant granular cell myoblastoma. *Arch Pathol* 1955; **60**: 663–668

7   Anderson M C. Malignant tumours of the vulva. In: Anderson M C ed. *Female Reproductive System. Systemic Pathology*, vol. 6, 3rd edn. Edinburgh: Churchill Livingstone, 1991; 22

8   Buscema J, Naghashfar Z, Sawaa E et al. The predominance of human papilloma virus type 16 in vulvar neoplasia. *Obstet Gynecol* 1988; **71**: 601–606

9   Scholefield J H, Hickson W G E, Smith J H F et al. Anal intraepithelial neoplasia: part of a multifocal disease process. *Lancet* 1992; **340**: 1271–1273

10 Friedrich E G, Wilkinson E F, Fu Y S. Carcinoma *in situ* of the vulva: a continuing challenge. *Am J Obstet Gynecol* 1980; **136**: 830–843

11 Iversen T, Aalders J G, Christensen A, Kolstad P. Squamous cell carcinoma of the vulva: a review of 424 patients. *Gynecol Oncol* 1980; **9**: 271–279

12 Palladino V S, Duffy J L, Bures G L. Basal cell carcinoma of the vulva. *Cancer* 1969; **24**: 460–476

13 Podratz K C, Gaffey T A, Symmonds R E et al. Melanoma of the vulva: an update. *Gynecol Oncol* 1983; **16**: 153–168

14 Johnson T L, Kumar N B, White C D, Morley G W. Prognostic features of vulvar melanoma: a clinicopathologic analysis. *Int J Gynecol Pathol* 1986; **5**: 110–118

15 Bradgate M G, Rollason T P, McConkey C C, Powell J. Malignant melanoma of the vulva: a clinicopathological study of 50 women. *Br J Obstet Gynecol* 1990; **97**: 124–133

16 Kapila K, Kharbanda K, Verma K. Cytomorphology of metastatic melanoma – use of S100 protein in the diagnosis of amelanotic melanoma. *Cytopathol* 1991; **5**: 229–237

17 Lee S C, Roth L M, Ehrlich C, Hall J A. Extramammary Paget's disease of the vulva. A clinicopathologic study of 13 cases. *Cancer* 1977; **39**: 2540–2549

18 Russell Jones R, Spaull J, Gusterson B. The histogenesis of mammary and extramammary Paget's disease. *Histopathology* 1989; **14**: 409–416

19 Friedrich E G, Wilkinson E J, Steingraeber P H, Lewis D J. Paget's disease of the vulva and carcinoma of the breast. *Obstet Gynecol* 1975; **46**: 130–134

20 Lloyd J, Evans D J, Flanagan A M. Extension of extramammary Paget disease of the vulva to the cervix. *J Clin Pathol* 1999; **52**: 538–540

21 Alguacil-Garcia A, O'Connor R. Mucin-negative biopsy in extramammary Paget's disease. A diagnostic problem. *Histopathol* 1989; **4**: 429–431

22 Hart W R, Millman J B. Progression of intraepithelial Paget's disease of the vulva to invasive carcinoma. *Cancer* 1977; **40**: 2333–2337

23 Chamlian D L, Taylor H B. Primary carcinoma of Bartholin's gland. A report of 24 patients. *J Obstet Gynecol* 1972; **39**: 489–494

24 Al-Nafussi A I, Rebello G, Hughes D, Blessing K. Benign vaginal polyp: a histological, histochemical and immunohistochemical study of 20 polyps with comparison to normal vaginal subepithelial layer. *Histopathol* 1992; **20**: 145–150

25 Tavassoli F A, Norris H J. Smooth muscle tumours of the vagina. *Obstet Gynecol* 1979; **53**: 689–693

26 Chabrel C M, Beilby J O W. Vaginal rhabdomyoma. *Histopathol* 1980; **4**: 645–651

27 Wade-Evans T. The aetiology and pathology of cancer of the vagina. *Clin Obstet Gynecol* 1976; **3**: 229–241

28 Davila R M, Miranda M C. Vaginal intraepithelial neoplasia and the Pap smear. *Acta Cytol* 2000; **44**: 137–140

29 Benedet J L, Murphy K J, Fairey R N, Boyes D A. Primary invasive carcinoma of the vagina. *Obstet Gynecol* 1983; **62**: 715–719

30 Herbst A L, Ulfelder H, Poskanzer D C. Adenocarcinoma of the vagina. Association of maternal stilbestrol therapy with tumor appearance in young women. *N Engl J Med* 1971; **284**: 878–881

31 Vooijs G P, Ng A B P, Wentz W B. The detection of vaginal adenosis and clear cell carcinoma. *Acta Cytol* 1973; **17**: 59–64

32 Hanselaar A G J M, van Leusen N D M, de Wilde P C M, Vooijs G P. Clear cell adenocarcinoma of the vagina and cervix; a report of the central Netherlands registry with emphasis on early detection and prognosis. *Acta Cytol* 1991; **67**: 1971–1978

33 Rosati L A, Jarzynski D J. Clear cell (mesonephric) adenocarcinoma of the vagina. A case report. *Acta Cytol* 1973; **17**: 493–498

34 Sodhani P, Gupta S, Prakash S, Singh V. Columnar and metaplastic cells in vault smears: cytologic and colposcopic study. *Cytopathol* 1999; **10**: 122–126

35 Tambouret R, Pitman M B, Bell D A. Benign glandular cells in post hysterectomy vaginal smears. *Acta Cytol* 1998; **42**: 1403–1408

36 Johnson J. Commentary on the presence of glandular cells in vault smears. *Cytopathol* 1999; **10**: 131

37 Ganesan R, Ferryman S R, Waddell C A. Vaginal adenosis in a patient on Tamoxifen therapy: a case report. *Cytopathol* 1999; **10**: 127–130

38 Pomante R G. Malignant melanoma – primary in the vagina. *Gynecol Oncol* 1975; **3**: 15–20

39 Norris H J, Taylor H B. Melanomas of the vagina. *Am J Clin Pathol* 1966; **46**: 420–426

40 Chung A F, Murray J C, Flannery J T *et al.* Malignant melanoma of the vagina – report of 19 cases. *Obstet Gynecol* 1980; **55**: 720–727

41 Hilgers R D, Malakasian G D, Soule E H. Embryonal rhabdomyosarcoma (botryoid type) of the vagina. A clinicopathologic review. *Am J Obstet Gynecol* 1970; **107**: 484–502

42 Allyn D H, Silverberg S G, Salzberg A M. Endodermal sinus tumour of the vagina. Report of a case with 7-year survival and literature review of so-called 'mesonephromas'. *Cancer* 1971; **27**: 1231–1238

43 Tobon H, Murphy A I, Salazar H. Primary leiomyosarcoma of the vagina. Light and electron microscopic observations. *Cancer* 1973; **32**: 450–457

44 Pempree T, Tang C-K, Hatef A, Forster S. Angiosarcoma of the vagina; a clinicopathologic report. *Cancer* 1983; **51**: 618–622

35 Cytology of body of uterus

Paul R. McKenzie, Geoff F. Watson and Alan B. P. Ng

Introduction

The role of cytology in the screening, detection and diagnosis of diseases of the body of the uterus, fallopian tubes and ovaries is limited in comparison to the cervix. While cellular material may spontaneously exfoliate from these organs, methods to directly sample these less accessible structures are relatively more complex, time-consuming and expensive than for the cervix. The resulting preparations are also more difficult to interpret. Cytological techniques have not been routinely applied to population cancer screening programmes because of the relative difficulty of these procedures and in some cases, the low incidence of disease. They can, however be usefully applied when diseases, especially tumours, are present in these structures. The availability of other investigative techniques such as hysteroscopy and laparoscopy with capability of biopsy under direct vision, have largely supplanted cytological methods. As it does not require anaesthesia or sophisticated equipment, the value of cytological sampling is more likely to be appreciated where these other methods of investigation are not available.

There is still, however, the imperative that exfoliated cells, particularly from malignant tumours be recognized when they are present in other specimens, particularly in cervical smears, as their presence may precede clinical symptoms and lead to earlier diagnosis. This is most likely in tumours of the endometrium partly because of their frequency but also due to its close proximity to the cervix.

Normal endometrium

Histology

The uterine corpus (see Fig. 28.1) is a thick-walled muscular organ functioning as a site for foetal development. In the non-pregnant state, the uterine cavity is an elongated roughly-triangular space with the anterior and posterior walls closely apposed. The narrow endocervical canal and endocervical mucus serve as a barrier separating the sterile uterine cavity from the cervico-vaginal flora. The cavity is lined by the endometrium, which is composed of columnar glandular epithelium supported by a specialized lamina propria, the endometrial stroma.

The endometrium is a more dynamic structure than the cervix, even though it is not subjected to the effects of a microbiological flora and physical factors. The endometrium is highly sensitive to the influence of hormones, and during the reproductive years it responds to the regular cyclical changes in hormone levels, by undergoing proliferative, secretory and menstrual changes.

The endometrium consists of two layers. The deeper layer abutting the myometrium is the **basalis**, a thin layer from which the endometrium regenerates after menstruation. Above this is the **functionalis** layer, which responds to ovarian hormonal influences, undergoing rapid growth during the first half of the cycle (proliferative or follicular phase), which in the latter half of the cycle is followed by gland secretion and maturation, in preparation for implantation (secretory or luteal phase). If implantation does not occur, this is followed by menstrual shedding.

The menstrual cycle is defined as beginning at the first day of clinical menstrual bleeding. The length of the menstrual cycle varies considerably between individual women, but in a typical 28-day cycle, may be divided into the menstrual phase, days 1–4; the proliferative (follicular) phase, days 5–14; and the secretory (luteal) phase, days 15–28.

The functional layer is shed during the menstrual phase[1]. In the proliferative phase, under oestrogen stimulation, the residual endometrium regenerates and proliferates, and surface re-epithelialization marks the commencement of proliferative phase. Effete condensed stroma remaining from the previous cycle is eliminated with a cuff of surface epithelium (known as endometrial 'exodus') in the first few days (usually day 5–10). Initially, the glands of the proliferative phase are straight and narrow, and are lined by low columnar cells. In the late proliferative phase, the glands increase in size and appear tortuous with pseudostratification of the epithelium. The stromal cells are small and spindle shaped with scanty cytoplasm, and the nuclei are round to oval or reniform. Mitoses are seen in the epithelial and stromal cells. During the early secretory phase, as a result of the rise in progesterone, sub-nuclear cytoplasmic glycogen vacuoles appear and glandular mitotic activity begins to subside. This is seen in the first 4–5 days post-ovulation. During mid-secretory phase, the endometrial glands become plumper and more tortuous, the cells discharge their secretions into the gland lumen, and the stroma becomes oedematous. During the late secretory phase under the effect of progesterone, the stromal cells particularly around the spiral arteries and in the superficial endometrium, undergo a pseudodecidual reaction, characterized by an increase in cytoplasmic bulk and nucleoli may also be seen (days 9–13 post-ovulation). With the cessation of the hormonal support from the ovaries, the stroma will undergo condensation and menstrual fragmentation, while the endometrial glands show apoptosis.

Menstrual bleeding signals the end of that cycle and the commencement of the next one.

The endometrium of the lower uterine segment does not participate in these cyclical changes.

In post-menopausal women, the endometrium eventually becomes thin and atrophic. The epithelial cells become smaller, and appear low columnar or cuboidal. The stromal cells also shrink and have scanty cytoplasm.

Cytology in endometrial diagnosis

Endometrial pathology may be detected cytologically from exfoliated cells in a cervical smear or from direct sampling methods.

Endometrial cells in a cervical smear

Endometrial cells are normally detectable during the menstrual and early proliferative phases. Beyond day 10–12 of the cycle this is considered abnormal, and should be evaluated in the light of clinical details such as the presence of an intra-uterine contraceptive device, a recent pregnancy, contraceptive hormones with break-through bleeding, recent uterine instrumentation and known endometrial pathology. In post-menopausal patients, the use of hormone replacement therapy may be associated with shedding of endometrial cells. Direct abrasive sampling of endometrial tissue may also be seen in cases of previous cone biopsy, high sampling with an endocervical brush or cervical endometriosis.

Possible endometrial conditions that may cause abnormal endometrial shedding include endometritis, endometrial polyps, submucosal leiomyomas, endometrial hyperplasias and endometrial carcinoma.

Ng et al. (1974)[2] showed that the incidence of endometrial pathology detected in women with abnormal shedding of normal-appearing endometrium varied with age, such that 1 in 4 pre-menopausal women will show some endometrial pathology, rising to 1 in 2 for the post-menopausal. They found specific pathology in only about 10% of cases under 40 years of age, most being endometrial polyps; carcinoma was rare. In the 40–49 year age group, some form of endometrial pathology was found in almost 40%. In the older age groups, polyps remained a large cause, but hyperplasias and carcinomas became more frequent. Adenocarcinoma was found in 2.1% of patients in their 40s, 4.2% in their 50s and 13.2% in those over 60 years, with abnormal shedding.

In post-menopausal women, any shedding of endometrial cells seen in a cervical smear should be considered abnormal, since it is a potential indicator of endometrial pathology[3]. Studies looking at the presence of cytologically normal endometrial shedding in post-menopausal women[3] have shown that hormone replacement therapy may be responsible for many cases. In those cases examined histologically, Sarode et al.[3] found that 23% had an endometrial polyp, about 5% had hyperplasia and 5% had an endometrial carcinoma. The difference in incidence of endometrial pathology between this series and that reported by Ng et al. in 1974[2] probably relates to the greater number of benign cases resulting from current high usage of hormone replacement therapy.

Doornewaard et al. in 1993[4] found that ~6% of their post-menopausal cases with apparently normal endometrial cells present in smears proved to have carcinoma, but also noted that in cases where atypical endometrial cells were found, the incidence of carcinoma was about 48%. This is similar to findings of Van den Bosch et al.[5] who evaluated pre-curette cervical smears. Their study also addressed the converse question of the proportion of endometrial carcinomas that did not show shedding into a cervical smear. They found that two of their six carcinoma cases had negative cervical cytology.

Thus the presence of unexplained normal-appearing endometrial cells in an asymptomatic woman would still warrant investigation, particularly if there are risk factors for endometrial carcinoma. Importantly, one should not be dismissive of endometrial shedding in the post-menopausal woman purely because of the use of hormone replacement therapy, as a significant endometrial lesion may coexist.

Where abnormal or overtly malignant endometrial cells are found in the cervical smear this may expedite the diagnosis of malignancy, and the importance of their recognition cannot be overemphasized. High-grade endometrial, tubal and ovarian carcinomas, such as serous carcinoma may produce considerable cell exfoliation. However the identification of these cells in the cervical smear will not obviate the need for further histological investigation, and a cervical smear should not be regarded as an investigation of first choice for endometrial pathology.

The other important group of cervical smears containing endometrial material arises from the direct scraping of endometrium by the instrument used in obtaining the cervical specimen. This has been increasingly recognized, since the widespread use of endocervical brushes introduced to increase the yield of endocervical and transformation zone representation in smears. It is more likely to occur when the cervix is shortened after cone or loop biopsy, but enthusiastic application of the brush can yield endometrium in otherwise normal women. A similar appearance will be achieved when endometriotic lesions are present on the cervix. The smears often contain large tissue fragments with branching architecture consisting of crowded columnar cells derived from the endometrial glands, sometimes with obvious stroma attached to the outside giving a biphasic appearance to the tissue fragment. These fragments may be alarming in their resemblance to adenocarcinoma *in situ*[6,7]. It is important that their benign nature is recognized in order to avoid unnecessary ablative surgery to what may be an already damaged cervix thereby further compromising fertility.

Direct endometrial sampling *(Figs 35.1–35.4)*

The role of direct endometrial sampling is limited in diagnostic cytological practice, because of a greater reliance by clinicians on biopsy methods requiring histological processing and the interpretive problems in endometrial cytology.

Currently, the most common investigation of abnormal uterine bleeding involves ultrasound assessment, followed by hysteroscopy and curettage. The greater diagnostic accuracy of hysteroscopy with directed biopsy[8] and the expansion of medico-legal activity makes blind and minimalist procedures less acceptable to diagnostic clinicians.

Direct cytological endometrial sampling using a variety of proprietary implements which may incorporate the use of brushing, suction and high-pressure lavage have been used diagnostically as an office procedure with minimal patient discomfort and avoiding hospital admission and anaesthetic, and in experienced hands they have produced good diagnostic results[9–15].

A cytological preparation has the advantages of low cost and rapidity and there is less chance that a tiny tissue sample will be lost in processing.

However, in general, reliance on these cytological techniques should be reserved for patients in whose symptoms there is a low level of clinical suspicion. Some of the commonly used office-based endometrial samplers can collect small fragments of tissue best processed histologically. If cytological methods are used, concomitant use of a cell block preparation can bridge some of the interpretive difficulties.

These inherent interpretive problems in endometrial cytology arise from the fact that tissue fragments obtained are often large and three-dimensional rendering them opaque and difficult to study. Smearing them may distort or crush the architectural features making it difficult to discern alterations in the gland:stroma ratio or gland complexity. Cytoplasmic features (which are useful in endometrial dating) are usually better appreciated in histological sections.

Chronic endometritis, and stromal pathology generally, is difficult to interpret cytologically. Further, the interpretation of endometrial smears requires special expertise apart from general histopathological training. These problems have all limited the widespread application of direct endometrial cytology.

A series from Japan[16], looking at direct endometrial cytology sampling as a screening programme, identified amongst a cohort of 5697 patients, five test-positive carcinomas and one test-negative carcinoma, Significantly, 186 cases with positive/suspicious/non-diagnostic cytology did not have cancer. The role of endometrial cytology as a screening programme needs further evaluation and cost analysis.

Cytological appearance of normal endometrial cells

Cervical samples

Endometrial cells or tissue may be present in cervical specimens due to physiological shedding, exfoliation or due to inadvertent direct sampling, usually when an endocervical brush has been used.

As may be anticipated, endometrial cells, usually in large numbers, are frequently observed on days 1–5 of the menstrual cycle in cervical or vaginal samples, and progressively less frequently and in smaller numbers on days 6–10. Spontaneously desquamated endometrial cells are infrequently seen in normal women from samples collected during the secretory phase and when present, are usually seen in small numbers. Endometrial cells are rarely seen in cervical or vaginal samples from post-menopausal women[17,18].

Endometrial cells that are spontaneously desquamated from the endometrium and found in the cervical or vaginal secretions tend to round up like soap bubbles, obeying the law of surface tension, and as a result columnar forms are rare[17]. Menstrual shedding will appear as balled clusters, as will the physiological shedding seen in early proliferative phase ('exodus'), the difference being that in exodus, there is a cuff of epithelial cells surrounding the balled up stroma. The number of shed endometrial cells seen in cervical smears is far fewer than those seen in direct endometrial samples. They often appear no larger than inflammatory cells when screened under low power. Single endometrial cells appear round to oval, and when in aggregates they approach a cell ball pattern with moulding of the peripheral margin. The cells frequently show marked degenerative changes.

Endometrial cells may be of epithelial or stromal origin and often it is not possible to distinguish between exfoliated endometrial epithelial (Figs 35.5, 35.6) and stromal cells in a sample. Degenerative changes are frequently encountered. Apoptotic debris, a sign of degenerative change, is occasionally seen in endometrial cells. Neutrophils within the cytoplasm may be seen in degenerate endometrial cells, but this can be seen in other cell types, especially endocervical columnar and squamous metaplastic cells. Degenerate single cells and cell aggregates of endometrial cells often have an eosinophilic cast over them, a feature also seen in poorly fixed or air-dried cells. Chromatin thickening of the nuclear membrane may be seen and is an early manifestation of cell death. Pyknotic nuclei may also be present.

As endometrial stromal cells have some of the morphological features of inflammatory histiocytes, it is difficult or impossible to distinguish a single endometrial stromal cell from a true histiocyte (Figs 35.7, 35.8). Endometrial stromal cells can best be recognized when they are in aggregates or in loose clusters whereas histiocytes are usually seen singly, associated with other inflammatory cells. Superficial stromal cells appear round to oval with a scant to moderate amount of cyanophilic cytoplasm and a centrally placed round vesicular nucleus. They are slightly larger than endometrial epithelial cells (Fig. 35.7). Deep stromal cells are more comparable in size with epithelial cells. They appear oval to spindle shaped with scanty, weakly staining, cyanophilic or amphophilic cytoplasm and the oval nucleus has a more granular chromatin pattern (Fig. 35.8). A longitudinal groove in the nucleus (coffee bean nucleus) is sometimes seen. Endometrial stromal cells especially superficial stromal cells when modified by decidual change may approach the size of parabasal cells.

During the first few days of the menstrual cycle, excessive blood and degenerate material with endometrial cells are often seen in cervical or vaginal samples. The double-contoured cell masses consisting of an inner mass of stromal cells coated an outer rim of epithelial cells (Fig. 35.9) known as endometrial 'exodus' are often seen in samples obtained on days 6–10 of the menstrual cycle[17,19]. Such a smear may also contain a moderate number of stromal cells and neutrophils with a clean background.

Direct samples

Directly sampled endometrial specimens do not usually suffer from the same degenerative changes seen in exfoliated cells, but do have their own unique difficulties in interpretation.

Endometrial cells will differ in appearance depending on the stage in the cycle or the menopausal status, the perspective from which the cells are viewed, their state of preservation, and the techniques used in collection, processing and staining. For practical purposes, three cell types are recognized cytologically; endometrial epithelial cells and superficial and deep stromal cells. The predominant epithelial cell type of the endometrium consists of secretory cells, while ciliated cells and intercalated cells are less frequently seen. Low columnar cells are seen in the glands of the less active basalis layer. The endometrial stroma is composed of stromal cells, which are divided into superficial and deep stromal cells[1,17].

In a smear of normal endometrium, the cells are mostly seen in aggregates and less frequently singly. Sheets of various sizes with regular borders, small round groups and strips may be present. Gland openings may be visible in the sheets. Epithelial, stromal or both cell types may be recognized in the same aggregate. The cell and nuclear size appears uniform in the aggregates, with uniform cell polarity and distribution. Mitotic figures may be seen especially during proliferative phase. The stomas of glands are evenly distributed and uniform in size, reflecting the orderly gland architecture of proliferative phase. These become more widely separated and larger in secretory phase. The glands are lined by a single layer of regularly arranged, uniform, epithelial cells (Figs 35.1, 35.2). Occasionally blood vessels may be seen in the stroma.

Depending on the perspective from which they are viewed, epithelial endometrial cells may appear columnar, cuboidal or round to oval. The cell area is about half to two-thirds the size of a normal endocervical cell with ill-defined cell borders. The scanty cytoplasm is weakly cyanophilic, foamy or finely vacuolated. The round to oval nucleus is approximately the same size as the nucleus of a normal intermediate squamous cell and the chromatin is uniformly finely granular with one or two chromocentres. Small nucleoli are occasionally seen (Figs 35.3, 35.4). During the secretory phase, the epithelial cells initially increase in cytoplasmic volume due to the presence of cytoplasmic secretion vacuoles and the cytoplasmic border becomes more distinct. The vacuoles are located between the basement membrane and the nucleus during the early secretory phase. The cytoplasm tends to stain amphophilic or slightly eosinophilic. The nucleus remains relatively unchanged. The discharge of secretions from the cells in mid-secretory phase is followed by a reduction of cytoplasmic volume and cell size. In the late secretory phase, there is shrinkage of the nucleus with condensation of nuclear chromatin and degenerative changes.

Endometrial stromal cells and their nuclei are comparable in size with their epithelial counterparts. The cells are round to oval or slightly spindle shaped with scanty amphophilic cytoplasm. The nucleus is also round to oval, spindle shaped or reniform with a finely granular chromatin. Small nucleoli may be seen in some cells (Fig. 35.3). During the secretory phase, there is an increase in cytoplasmic volume due to glycogen accumulation and the cells appear more epithelioid especially in the late secretory phase, corresponding to decidual change. These cells may reach the size of normal parabasal cervical squamous cells. The nuclei are slightly enlarged and a nucleolus is seen in each cell. Another type of cell within the stroma is the small granular stromal granulocyte or 'K' cell. The cytoplasm of this cell contains acidophilic granules. They become more numerous in the late secretory phase.

Samples taken during the menstrual phase show degenerate or necrotic tissue fragments or cells with a background of blood, cellular debris and inflammatory cells. In the late menstrual and early proliferative phases, cell aggregates consisting of a peripheral rim of epithelial cells and a central core of stromal cells, similar to those seen in 'exodus' in cervical specimens may be present.

Specimens from atrophic endometrium in post-menopausal women usually contain fewer cells or tissue

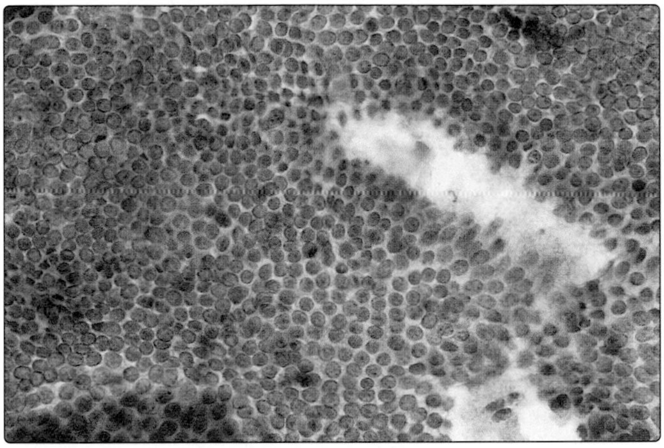

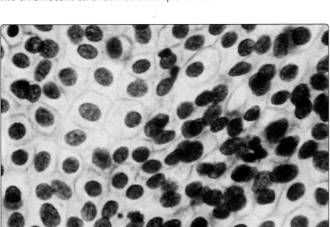

Fig. 35.1   Normal endometrial cells at proliferative phase. A sheet of regularly arranged endometrial epithelial cells with an oval glandular stoma. The cytoplasm is scanty and the nuclei are of uniform size with characteristically powdery uniformly finely granular chromatin and one or two chromocentres. Endometrial sample. (× HP)

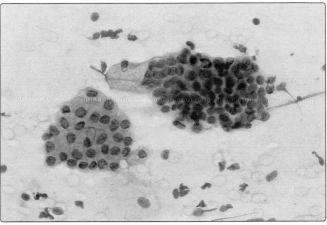

Fig. 35.4   Normal endometrial and endocervical cells. Honeycomb grouping of endocervical columnar cells (left) and endometrial epithelial cells. The endocervical cells and nuclei are larger and the eosinophilic staining cytoplasm is more abundant than the endometrial cells. Endometrial sample. (× HP)

Fig. 35.2   Normal endometrial cells at secretory phase. A sheet of larger regularly arranged endometrial epithelial cells where the cell borders are more distinctive and cytoplasmic volume is increased. Endometrial sample. (× HP)

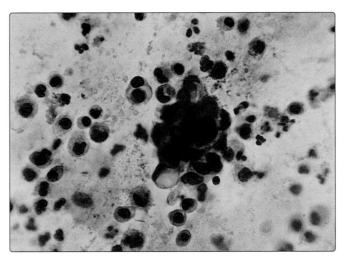

Fig. 35.5   Normal endometrial cells seen on day 4 of menstrual cycle. A tight group of epithelial cells with many single epithelial and stromal cells. The nuclei of the endometrial cells are no larger than the nucleus of the faintly appearing normal intermediate squamous cell (upper left). Endocervical sample. (× HP)

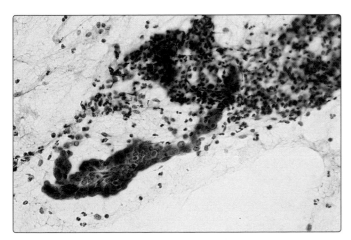

Fig. 35.3   Normal endometrial cells. Strip of epithelial cells (lower left) and a large loose aggregate of stromal cells (upper right) with single endometrial cells. Endometrial sample. (× MP)

fragments. The cells appear uniform and will not show cyclical changes or mitoses.

Endocervical cells, and less frequently squamous and metaplastic cells may be encountered in endometrial samples as contaminants.

Pathology and cytology of non-neoplastic conditions of endometrium

There are a large variety of non-neoplastic conditions that affect the endometrium and for most a specific diagnosis is not possible by cytological methods alone, as the features are not sufficiently characteristic or have not been adequately delineated. Many of the conditions however can give rise to appearances that may be misinterpreted as

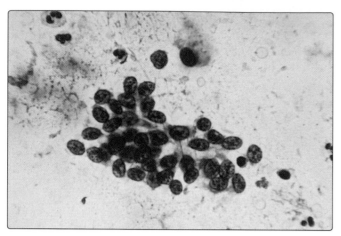

Fig. 35.6 Normal endometrial cells seen on day 5 of menstrual cycle. A loose group of epithelial cells with scanty finely vacuolated cytoplasm and uniform nuclei with finely granular chromatin. Endocervical sample. (× HP)

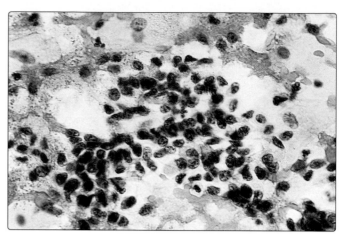

Fig. 35.8 Normal endometrial deep stromal cells. A loose aggregate of deep stromal small cells with scanty cytoplasm and oval nuclei, smaller than superficial stromal cells. The nuclei are comparable in size to nucleus of a normal intermediate squamous cell (top centre). Endocervical sample. (× HP)

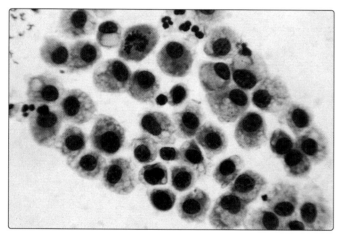

Fig. 35.7 Normal endometrial superficial stromal cells. The loose aggregate of cells is slightly larger than endometrial epithelial and deep stromal cells with relatively more cytoplasm. The nuclei are centrally or slightly eccentrically located. Note a cell in mitosis. Endocervical sample. (× HP)

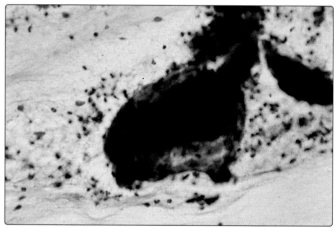

Fig. 35.9 Endometrial cells seen at exodus, day 7 of menstrual cycle. A large double contoured aggregate of endometrial cells with an outer rim of epithelial cells and centrally compact stromal cells. Endocervical sample. (× MP)

malignant, or cause endometrial shedding to be detected in a cervical smear.

Among these conditions are the various forms of metaplastic change, functional disturbances due to hormonal imbalance, changes related to oral contraceptive use, anovulation, pregnancy, endometritis, intrauterine devices and polyps[2,20,21].

Cervical and vaginal samples

As discussed, cellular changes in cervical or vaginal samples seldom reveal characteristic changes of benign endometrial lesions. However, sometimes, benign endometrial lesions cause benign or normal endometrial cells to be shed at a time they would normally not be expected to be present in cervical samples (abnormal shedding). For practical purposes, the presence of normal endometrial cells during the first half of the menstrual cycle can be attributed to

physiologic shedding, and when seen in the second half of the cycle and in the post-menopausal period, it is usually related to abnormal shedding. The number of endometrial cells due to abnormal shedding is usually few in number in the majority of cases and may be of epithelial and/or stromal origin[2].

Abnormal shedding may occur during the post-natal period as well as post-abortion and may include trophoblastic tissue (Fig. 35.10). Dysfunctional uterine bleeding, often due hormonal imbalance or conditions such as anovulatory cycling or adenomyosis can result in irregular shedding of endometrial tissue and endometrial cells are often seen in cell samples. Exogenous progesterone or contraceptive hormone may cause irregular shedding of superficial stromal or decidual cells (Fig. 35.11). Hormone replacement therapy may also be associated with abnormal shedding of benign endometrial cells.

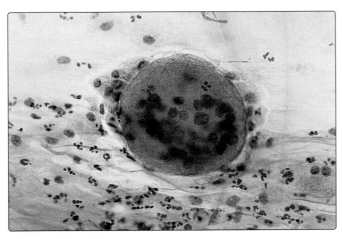

Fig. 35.10 A syncytiotrophoblast with a few attached stromal or cytotrophoblastic cells in a smear taken at the post-abortion period. Endocervical sample. (× HP)

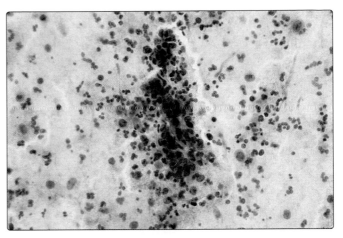

Fig. 35.12 Endometrial cells mixed with inflammatory cells in a smear from a woman using an intrauterine device, taken on day 20 of the menstrual cycle. Endocervical sample. (× HP)

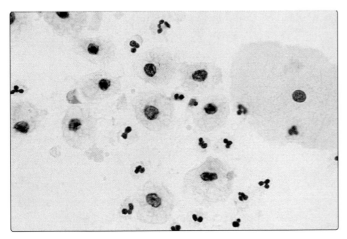

Fig. 35.11 Deciduoid cells in a smear from a patient on exogenous progesterone for dysfunctional uterine bleeding. The deciduoid cells are about the size of parabasal cells with relatively abundant foamy weakly staining cytoplasm. (×HP)

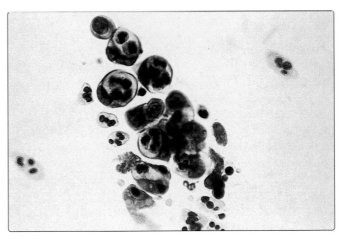

Fig. 35.13 Small groups of immature metaplastic cells of endocervical origin in a smear from a woman using an intrauterine device. Cytoplasmic vacuoles with neutrophils within them tend to push the nuclei to one side. A rim of dense staining cytoplasm confirms the metaplastic nature of the small cells. These changes can be seen in many reactive processes in the cervix and are not pathognomonic of IUD changes. Endocervical sample. (× HP)

Other causes of abnormal shedding that may show coexistent atypical change include the intrauterine devices (Figs 35.12, 35.13), recent endometrial instrumentation, endometritis, pyometra, benign endometrial polyps and submucosal leiomyomata. When endometrial cells are shed under these conditions, some of the endometrial cells may appear atypical secondary to a reactive or reparative process. These atypical cells appear slightly larger with slight nuclear enlargement, however, the relationship of the cells do not show loss of cellular or nuclear polarity and the nuclear chromatin remains uniformly granular. Nucleoli may be present in a few cells. Degenerative cytoplasmic vacuoles with or without engulfed neutrophils are also present. Benign endometrial polyps shed normal or atypical endometrial cells relatively frequently. Occasionally psammoma bodies are seen in cervical cell samples in association with benign endometrial lesions (Fig. 35.14)[22].

Most benign endometrial conditions that cause abnormal shedding of relatively normal endometrial cells occur in women during their active reproductive period. In the perimenopausal and post-menopausal period endometrial polyps and hormone replacement therapy are frequently associated with shedding of endometrial cells, though malignant causes become an important consideration.

It should be noted that in a large percentage of cases of abnormal shedding of normal-appearing endometrial cells there is no apparent cause. On the other hand, in a small percentage of cases, the presence of only normal-appearing endometrial cells in cervical samples obtained from perimenopausal or post-menopausal women is associated with pathological endometrial hyperplasia and even invasive

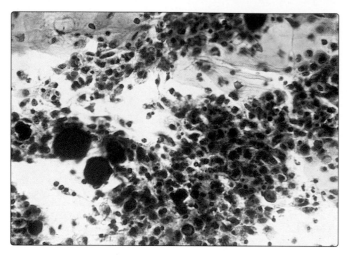

Fig. 35.14   Calcific or psammoma bodies (lower left) with a sheet of endometrial stromal cells from a patient on contraceptive hormonal therapy for 3 years. Endocervical sample. (× HP)

adenocarcinoma[2,3,23,24]. The association increases with increasing age of the patient. The endometrial cells are usually of epithelial type, a mixture of epithelial and stromal cells, or, less frequently, only endometrial stromal cells. Endometrial cells in such cell samples are usually small in number and sometimes as few as 10–15 cells per smear. These cases often do not have symptoms or abnormal vaginal bleeding. Thus, although most cases of abnormal shedding of normal-appearing endometrial cells are associated with benign endometrial conditions or have no apparent explanation, a small percentage may be associated with endometrial carcinoma and its precursors, particularly in post-menopausal women and to a lesser extent in peri-menopausal women. Evaluation of these cases by further investigation such as hysteroscopy and appropriate biopsy is warranted.

Direct endometrial samples

There are not many characteristic diagnostic cytological features in cellular samples that are associated with benign endometrial lesions except when tissue fragments are present which are then processed and evaluated as histological tissue specimens. In some cytology samples, certain cytological features may indicate specific benign endometrial lesions.

Endometrial metaplasias

Eosinophilic or oncocytic (oxyphilic) metaplasia of endometrial cells is seen on the surface epithelium and within glands[17]. The oxyphilic changes are non-specific and represent a reactive process. This change can be seen with many benign processes as well as associated with endometrial hyperplasia. Clusters of cuboidal or columnar epithelial cells with abundant granular eosinophilic cytoplasm that stains more intensely eosinophilic may be seen. The cytoplasm may contain vacuoles with neutrophils within them, a sign of degeneration. The nuclei are slightly

enlarged, round or oval, often eccentric and may contain small nucleoli. The chromatin is uniformly distributed.

Benign mucin-secreting cells of endometrial origin are also sometimes seen in cell samples as a result mucinous metaplasia[26] but distinction from endocervical cells is very difficult.

Cells derived from an area of tubal metaplastic cells with cilia will likewise be difficult to differentiate between ciliated endometrial cells or from tubal metaplasia in endocervical glands.

Endometrial squamous metaplasia may be seen in cell samples as round morules of squamous metaplastic cells, or in sheets or singly. They are also indistinguishable from squamous cells of cervical origin. Where clusters of benign squamous metaplastic cells are seen within an endometrial cell group or minute fragment of endometrial tissue a definitive interpretation of endometrial squamous metaplasia can be made. Papillary groups of benign endometrial cells will suggest papillary metaplasia, however, they are very infrequently seen.

Progesterone and pregnancy related changes

Sheets or loose aggregates of decidualized cells are seen in samples when exogenous progesterone therapy or contraceptive pill is being administered. Sometimes small narrow openings of atrophic glands widely spaced in a sheet of decidual cells are observed. This appearance correlates with the histological appearance of exaggerated decidual reaction and small inactive glands associated with progesterone therapy. In pregnancy, large multinucleated syncytiotrophoblastic cells with multiple small uniform nuclei and a moderate amount of dense cyanophilic cytoplasm may be seen in cell samples. Mononucleated cytotrophoblastic cells are less characteristic and may mimic decidualized stromal cells or epithelial cells[11,12]. Arias-Stella reaction changes are seldom recognized in cytologic specimens except when tissue fragments are present. Arias-Stella cells appear as larger atypical endometrial cells singly or among a group of normal endometrial cells. The nuclei are larger, hyperchromatic and may have irregular nuclear membranes. When present, they are few in number[26].

Inflammatory conditions

In the absence of tissue fragments, the diagnosis of acute or chronic endometritis, by cytological methods, is usually not possible as the presence of inflammatory cells in cell samples do not imply endometritis. If plasma cells are seen in the stroma of endometrial tissue fragments, chronic endometritis can be diagnosed. In suppurative inflammation or pyometra, the cell sample contains pus consisting of many neutrophils and necrotic material, and an occasional group of reactive endometrial cells may be seen. These are larger, with enlarged nuclei and small nucleoli. The overall enlargement and more prominent nucleolus may cause them to be mistaken for malignant cells. This can be a diagnostic problem as pyometra is not infrequently associated with an underlying uterine malignancy and the inflammatory exudate may mask the malignant cells. In this situation other forms of investigation would be necessary to exclude this possibility. Rarely are characteristic changes of specific infections of endometrium seen in endometrial samples such as tuberculosis, cytomegalovirus, or *herpes simplex* infection. Tuberculous endometritis may appear as a non-specific chronic endometritis and frequently lacks granulomata. The viral cytopathic changes of herpes and cytomegalovirus are similar to their appearance in other tissues. Samples from patients using an intrauterine device may also show inflammation and colonies of Actinomyces, seen as large, tangled masses of fine filamentous darkly haematoxyphilic organisms with the Papanicolaou stain (so-called 'sulphur-granules', from their macroscopic appearance as yellow flecks in actinomycotic pus).

Psammoma bodies seen free or with endometrial cells may be present[27]. They may be associated with changes of contraceptive pill effect or IUD usage[28]. Kern[29] noted the association of psammoma bodies with malignancy in four of seven cases but also noted the presence of atypical or malignant cells attached to the psammoma bodies in these cases and benign cells in the other cases. Kern concluded that when the bodies were associated with clearly benign cells a more conservative approach could be taken to investigation.

Polyps

Cell samples from women with endometrial polyps do not show characteristic changes unless tissue fragments are present to indicate the characteristic changes of a polyp as is seen in surgical specimens.

Significance of clinical information and an adequate cell sample

Based on the discussion so far, it becomes apparent that if optimal benefit is to be obtained in the detection of endometrial pathology by the cellular approach, the provision of pertinent clinical information is important. The nature of the cell sample should be indicated in the request form as it may assist in the preparation and approach to the evaluation of the cell sample. The age, the day of cycle, or menopausal status of the patient should be provided. Other important information such as presenting symptoms, the use of exogenous hormones, presence of an intrauterine device and recent intrauterine instrumentation should be included. While some of the information will not be applicable in every case, the utility of the cellular evaluation is directly related to the amount of relevant clinical information provided.

Direct endometrial sampling can provide an adequate sample for evaluation of endometrial pathology. While there are advantages in being able to do this as an out-patient procedure or in the surgery, the random nature of the specimen and the significant difficulties in interpretation when the material is prepared as a cytological smear make it less likely to be diagnostic than a hysteroscopically-directed specimen.

Endometrial hyperplasia and carcinoma

Pathogenesis of endometrial hyperplasia and carcinoma

As was mentioned earlier, the endometrium is highly sensitive to the influences of hormones. Hyperplasia of the endometrium arises in the setting of increased or uninterrupted oestrogenic stimulation and is an important factor in carcinogenesis in the endometrium. The oestrogen can be exogenous, as part of hormone replacement therapy, or endogenously produced.

The use of unopposed oestrogen in hormone replacement therapy for women with an intact uterus is now mostly of historical importance, but was previously linked to an increase in the incidence of both endometrial hyperplasia and carcinoma in the USA[30].

Tamoxifen, an anti-oestrogen drug used in breast cancer treatment and prevention, acts by competing with oestrogen for binding sites on cell oestrogen receptors and has, paradoxically, some oestrogenic effect on the endometrium in post-menopausal women. Tamoxifen has been linked to a small increase in risk for the development of endometrial carcinoma. It has been suggested that these and other patients at increased risk should be screened for the development of cancer[31-33] and that endometrial sampling may be an appropriate method.

Oestrogen is normally produced by the developing ovarian follicle, but is also produced in small amounts in the adrenal gland and by the chemical conversion of other steroid hormones in sites such as adipose tissue. It can also be secreted by oestrogen producing tumours.

Obesity is associated with raised levels of oestrone due to the conversion of the adrenal androgen to androstenedione, in the adipose tissue. It is also associated with reduced levels of sex hormone binding globulin in the serum so that there is more available free oestrogen to act on target organs such as the endometrium. In premenopausal women this can have the effect of suppressing ovulation and is an important factor in polycystic ovary disease. Other cited risk factors such as diabetes and hypertension are probably not independent of obesity.

Polycystic ovary disease occurs in young women who have bilateral ovarian enlargement with numerous follicular cysts, stromal hyperplasia and frequently hyperthecosis. These women are anovulatory or rarely ovulate and are usually infertile. Both oestrogens and androgen are raised, with a range of symptoms including menstrual abnormalities and hirsutism. They may also develop endometrial hyperplasia and about 5% may develop endometrial carcinoma, the commonest cause of that tumour in premenopausal women.

Ovarian hyperthecosis and stromal hyperplasia can occur outside the setting of polycystic disease and can be associated with the development of endometrial carcinoma. Raised oestrogen levels can also occur in ovarian tumours of the sex-cord stromal group. These include granulosa cell tumour and thecoma. Not all of these tumours secrete hormones but they are associated with a marked increase in risk of development of endometrial carcinoma.

Not all endometrial carcinomas are oestrogen related, arising in the setting of endometrial hyperplasia. Carcinoma can arise in oestrogen deprived, atrophic endometrium, usually at a later age than the group of peri-menopausal, oestrogen-related tumours. Many of these are still of endometrioid type, but are usually of higher-grade and stage. This group also includes tumours showing other types of differentiation including serous, mucinous and clear cell carcinoma and carcinomas associated with a sarcomatous component[34].

Histopathology of endometrial hyperplasia

The cytological features of hyperplasia are best understood in the light of the alterations seen on histopathological examination. High oestrogen states in premenopausal women can result in anovulatory cycling, in which there is some increase in the thickness of the endometrium and minor architectural changes to the glands with occasional elongated, branched glands, plentiful glandular and stromal mitoses and fibrin thrombi in the endometrial vessels.

A continuation of uninterrupted oestrogenic stimulation results in *simple hyperplasia* (cystic glandular hyperplasia). The glands may be branched or show cystic dilatation. Mitotic activity is pronounced but the gland-stroma ratio is not increased. The glandular epithelium is tall and regular with no nuclear atypia (Fig. 35.15). An increase in gland complexity with more elaborate branching and crowding together of gland lumina results in *complex hyperplasia without atypia* (adenomatous hyperplasia). The gland-stroma ratio is increased but the epithelium does not show atypical cytological features (Fig. 35.16).

Cytological abnormalities are present in *complex hyperplasia with atypia* (atypical hyperplasia). These usually include some loss of the polarity of nuclei and the presence of a visible nucleolus. The proportion of glands to stroma is often further increased and there may be focal areas where the glands are virtually back-to-back. Some glands may show in-folding of epithelium or gland trabeculation. Significant areas of back-to-back growth are a feature of well-differentiated carcinoma. Indeed, because of the incomplete sampling of the endometrium in curettage or other blindly obtained endometrial samples, a significant number of cases diagnosed as complex hyperplasia with atypia will prove to have carcinoma at hysterectomy.

Blind curettage and office-based endometrial sampling have diminished in their role in the investigative pathway of endometrial carcinoma and hyperplasia with the increased usage of transvaginal ultrasound and hysteroscopically-directed biopsy, but continue to have a role where dictated by necessity or surgical preference.

Cytological features of endometrial hyperplasia *(Figs 35.17–35.22)*

Cervical smears

▶ Often a normal but well oestrogenized smear
▶ Normal endometrial cells present not in keeping with menstrual cycle
▶ Normal endometrial cells present in postmenopausal smears
▶ Atypical endometrial cells in some atypical hyperplasias

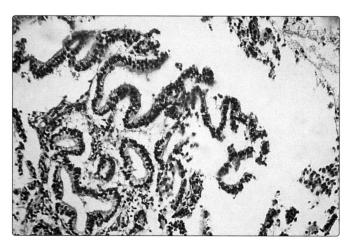

Fig. 35.15 Simple hyperplasia of endometrium. Small fragments of hyperplastic endometrium with no significant cytologic atypia. Interpretation is based on tissue morphology changes as well as evaluation of cytologic changes in the tissue fragments. Endometrial sample (Vabra technique). (H&E × LP)

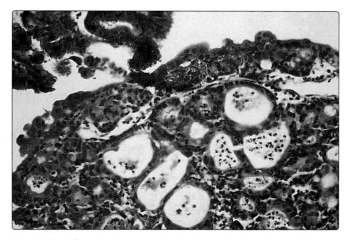

Fig. 35.16 Complex hyperplasia with atypia of endometrium. A tissue fragment showing glandular crowding with small and normal size glands with little separating stroma. The epithelial cells are larger than normal and appear less columnar with some increase in cytoplasmic volume. There is no significant change of cellular and nuclear polarity. The nuclei are also larger than normal and appear round with a vesicular nuclei and occasional micronucleoli. Endometrial sample (Vakutage procedure). (H&E × LP)

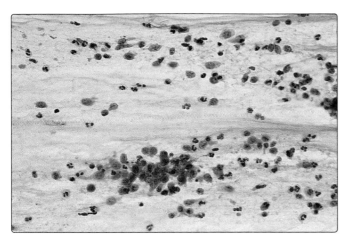

Fig. 35.17 Complex hyperplasia without atypia (adenomatous hyperplasia) of endometrium. Single and clustered of endometrial cells which appear within normal limits except for slight cellular and nuclear enlargement with no significant nuclear abnormality. Diagnosis of this type of hyperplasia in an endometrial sample smear based on cytologic changes without microfragments or tissue fragments can be difficult and often is impossible to differentiate from normal or benign endometrial conditions. Endometrial sample smear. (Papanicolaou × MP)

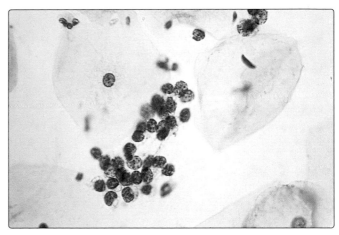

Fig. 35.19 Simple hyperplasia (cystic glandular hyperplasia) of endometrium. Endometrial cells with slightly enlarged (slightly larger than nucleus of normal intermediate squamous cell) hyperchromatic nuclei in smear taken from a 51-year-old woman, 2 years post-menopausal. Oestrogenic effect in the smear is noted. Endocervical sample. (Papanicolaou × HP)

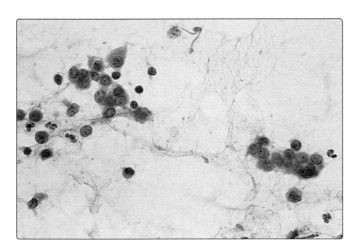

Fig. 35.18 Complex hyperplasia with atypia (atypical hyperplasia) of endometrium. When compared with **Fig. 35.17**, the endometrial epithelial cells and nuclei are larger with no significant irregular cellular polarity. Some of the oval nuclei show slight nuclear clearing and contain micronucleoli. Endocervical sample smear. (Papanicolaou × HP)

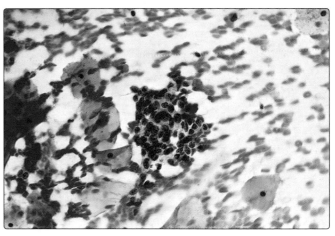

Fig. 35.20 Complex hyperplasia without atypia (adenomatous hyperplasia) of endometrium in smear from a 49-year-old woman with abnormal vaginal bleeding. The cellular changes are comparable with those seen in **Fig. 35.19** Endocervical sample. (Papanicolaou × HP)

The spontaneous exfoliation of endometrial cells, which can be detected in a cervical smear, is an inconstant feature of hyperplasia and the smear will be normal in many cases, although usually well oestrogenized. The presence of normal endometrial cells in a cervical smear can be caused by endometrial hyperplasia but is not a specific finding and can be seen in the first 10–12 days of a normal menstrual cycle and a wide range of conditions including irregular shedding, endometrial polyps, hormone replacement therapy and even carcinoma[35,36]. In a post-menopausal woman however, their presence should be a reason for further investigation, particularly in the absence of hormone replacement.

The cytological appearance of endometrial cells as seen in cervical smears was discussed previously. The cells are generally few in number and may be present as single cells about the size of a histiocyte or may be present in clusters, which may round up into cell balls. Endometrial cells should be distinguished from histiocytes, which are of no particular significance on their own[37].

The cells show degenerative features and it is difficult to distinguish glandular cells from endometrial stromal cells in this situation. The cells have round to oval nuclei and the chromatin may become condensed and pyknotic or coarse and block-like, due to cellular degeneration. Engulfment of neutrophils, also a degenerative feature, may be present.

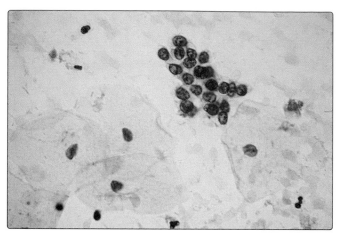

Fig. 35.21   Atypical hyperplasia of endometrium. Slight cellular and nuclear enlargement of endometrial cells with nuclear clearing in a few cells and occasional micronucleoli. Cellular relationship is not significantly altered. Note clean background and oestrogenic effect. Smear is from a 56-year-old asymptomatic woman, who is 4 years post-menopausal. Endocervical sample. (Papanicolaou × HP)

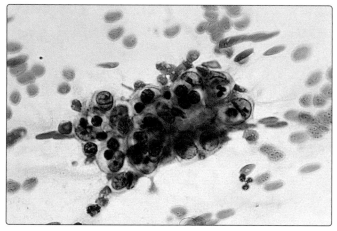

Fig. 35.22   Atypical hyperplasia of endometrium. Cellular and nuclear enlargement of endometrial cells with nuclear clearing and micronucleoli in some cells in the aggregate. Endocervical sample. (Papanicolaou × HP)

It is not possible to make a diagnosis of endometrial hyperplasia on the basis of a cervical smear containing endometrial cells. While abnormal, and in many cases, an indication for further investigation, this occurrence is not specific to a particular condition. In complex hyperplasia with atypia however, abnormal cytological features may be present but it will then not be possible to exclude a carcinoma[38–40].

Direct endometrial sampling

Although endometrial sampling has been undertaken for at least three decades, it has not attained the same degree of acceptance as cervical cytology. Diagnostic criteria and the assessment of specimen adequacy have not reached a consistent level of agreement among cytologists. While in most countries where there is a cervical cancer screening programme endometrial carcinoma is more common than

cervical carcinoma, screening programmes have not been developed for this cancer. This is partly because of the difficulty in obtaining specimens for cytology cheaply, easily and with good patient acceptance and partly because the need for screening is less as many of the cancers are low-grade and become symptomatic while still at low stage. New sampling devices continue to be developed, however, and although transvaginal ultrasound and hysteroscopic biopsy are very useful in investigation of symptomatic patients neither is likely to be an acceptable screening method.

The endometrial tissue can be obtained using either aspiration or washing, using one of a large number of proprietary devices. The resulting specimen is then smeared or, now more commonly, processed as a cell block. The difficulties associated with this type of sampling were discussed previously. Many of these devices can produce sizeable tissue fragments, which are best, processed and examined histologically. This has the advantage of displaying the architectural features of the fragments and their internal structure as well as still allowing cellular features to be visible. Further, it does not require expertise beyond histopathological training to interpret. The disadvantage is that small cell groups and single cells are difficult to evaluate and the fine structure of the nucleus is less visible than in a smear preparation. However cytological features are of lesser importance as the distinction between complex hyperplasia with atypia and carcinoma relies more on the architectural features than the cellular changes. In instances where histopathological examination is not possible or cytological examination is preferred, for example, in cases where the material does not contain visible tissue particles, the specimen can then be prepared as a wet-fixed, Papanicolaou stained smear. This would in most instances be in the nature of a screening process with later histopathological confirmation required before definitive treatment such as hysterectomy is considered.

Cytological findings

In smear preparations, the cellular material consists of single cells, small aggregates and larger tissue fragments. The diagnosis of hyperplasia is based on the evaluation of both the architectural features of the larger tissue fragments and on cellular characteristics. As hyperplastic changes in the endometrium can be patchy, there may be a mixture of normal and hyperplastic endometrium. The architectural evaluation of these tissue fragments in a smear is difficult and differentiating features between normal cyclical changes, hyperplasia and well-differentiated carcinoma are not well documented. However some features are described.

The tissue fragments consist of cell sheets of varying size, intact or partial glandular structures and strips of epithelial cells. In simple hyperplasia glandular stomas, the surface openings of the endometrial glands, are markedly enlarged but are not crowded together. In complex hyperplasia, with and without atypia these stomas are crowded closely together with variable size ranging from normal to slightly enlarged. Very closely packed glands with a back-to-back pattern would suggest the possibility of carcinoma[38].

At a cellular level the epithelial cells in simple hyperplasia and complex hyperplasia without atypia are slightly enlarged and are regularly arranged in the glands and cell aggregates. The nuclei are uniform in size and show a uniform, finely granular chromatin pattern with inconspicuous nucleoli.

In complex hyperplasia with atypia the epithelial cells are crowded around the gland structures and may be multilayered. There is nuclear enlargement and mild pleomorphism. The nuclei are round, hyperchromatic and some may show irregular chromatin distribution. Small to intermediate-sized nucleoli are present. The cytoplasm shows variable staining from cyanophilic to weakly eosinophilic. Necrosis is not a feature of hyperplasia but blood and inflammatory cells may be present[38].

Metaplasias, particularly squamous metaplasia, are commonly associated with hyperplasias, as previously mentioned.

Endometrial carcinoma

Endometrial carcinoma is the commonest malignancy of the female genital tract in countries where there is effective cervical cancer screening or a low prevalence of cancer related HPV types. About two-thirds of these cases arise in the setting of endometrial hyperplasia. The others, which are not related to hyperplasia and frequently arise in atrophic endometrium, may occur in an older age cohort. These are more often of high histological grade and include, though not exclusively, types of tumour differentiation other than endometrioid[34].

Histopathology of endometrial carcinoma

Endometrial carcinoma exhibits a range of differentiation, which parallels that of the remainder of the Mullerian system. The commonest carcinoma, endometrioid adenocarcinoma, replicates the histological features of the endometrium. Other types include serous, mucinous, clear cell and squamous carcinoma. These carcinomas frequently show mixed patterns of differentiation with two or more types present in the one tumour. Carcinomas associated with coexistent sarcomatous differentiation will be discussed in a subsequent chapter.

Endometrioid carcinoma forms the majority of low-grade carcinomas, but can also exist as a high-grade tumour. Grading is on the basis of nuclear changes and architectural differentiation. The low-grade tumours show a predominantly glandular or villo-glandular growth pattern, with regular columnar cells showing slight nuclear enlargement and a small nucleolus. Higher-grade tumours show increasing areas of solid growth with cells that are no longer recognizable as columnar, having more variable rounded pleomorphic nuclei, a prominent nucleolus and chromatin clearing. High-grade tumours may show recognizable endometrioid features only focally.

Focal squamous differentiation is a common feature in endometrioid carcinoma. Benign appearing squamous differentiation in small clusters (squamous morules) is a common feature in endometrioid carcinomas and is not of prognostic significance independent of the grade and stage of the glandular component. Overtly malignant squamous differentiation usually occurs in higher-grade tumours and has been previously termed adenosquamous carcinoma. The grade of the glandular component is usually in parallel with the squamous component and these tumours are more commonly termed endometrioid carcinoma with squamous differentiation.

Serous carcinoma resembles its more common and familiar counterpart in the ovary and coexistent ovarian and endometrial serous carcinomas are not uncommon. The tumour may have a growth pattern of papillae or may have gland-like spaces or solid areas. The spaces and papillae are lined by cells with a protuberant apical cytoplasm giving an undulating appearance to the surface. Psammoma bodies may be present. These tumours are mostly of high-grade[41,42].

Mucinous carcinoma resembles endocervical adenocarcinoma, making its distinction from that tumour difficult by cytology without knowledge of the distribution of the tumour. The tumour is mostly gland-forming or villo-glandular.

Clear cell carcinoma shows a growth pattern of loose gland-like spaces or papillae with large cells with abundant clear or pale staining cytoplasm. The nuclei tend towards the apical portion of the cytoplasm so that the apex is wider than its point of attachment, giving rise to the so-called hob-nail appearance of the cells. These tumours are also usually of high-grade and are frequently mixed with high-grade endometrioid carcinoma.

Cytological features of endometrial carcinoma *(Figs 35.23–35.36)*

Cervical smears

▶ Normal endometrial cells sometimes present
▶ Abnormal or malignant endometrial cells may be found
▶ Degenerative changes in cells
▶ Tumour diathesis present

Normal endometrial cells may be observed in the cervical smears of women with endometrial carcinoma. In a study by Sarode *et al.*[35] of 81 cases of postmenopausal women who had endometrial cells detected on routine cervical smears about 5% proved to have carcinoma on endometrial sampling and about the same number had endometrial hyperplasia. In about 42% of their cases no endometrial pathology was found.

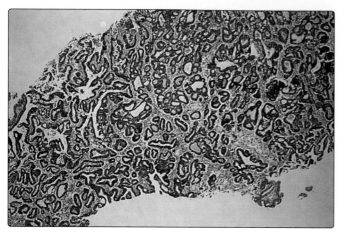

Fig. 35.23 Adenocarcinoma of endometrium in a tissue fragment. Endometrial sample (Jet-wash technique). (H&E × LP)

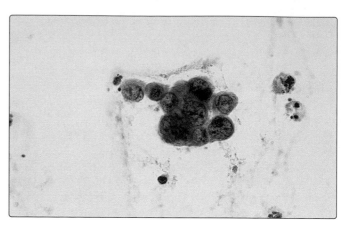

Fig. 35.26 Poorly-differentiated adenocarcinoma (grade III) of endometrium. The malignant cells and nuclei are larger than those seen in **Fig. 35.25** and the nucleoli are larger. Endometrial sample smear. (Papanicolaou × HP)

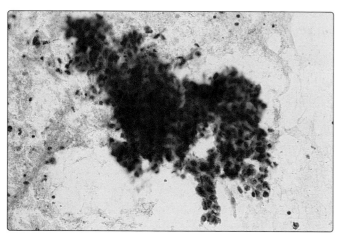

Fig. 35.24 Adenocarcinoma of endometrium. A large irregular aggregate of malignant endometrial cells with irregular arrangement of cells and nuclei and an irregular glandular stoma. Endometrial sample smear. (Papanicolaou × MP)

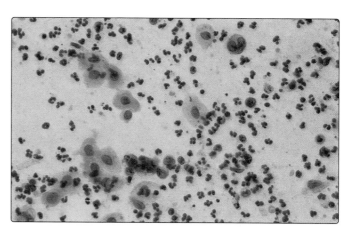

Fig. 35.27 Well-differentiated adenocarcinoma (grade I) of endometrium. Single and small group of malignant cells among inflammatory cells may be overlooked in screening. Endocervical sample. (Papanicolaou × HP)

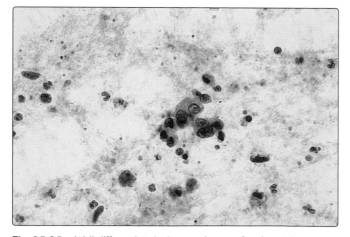

Fig. 35.25 Well-differentiated adenocarcinoma of endometrium. Malignant cells occur singly and a small aggregate with a granular watery background of a tumour diathesis. Endometrial sample smear. (Papanicolaou × HP)

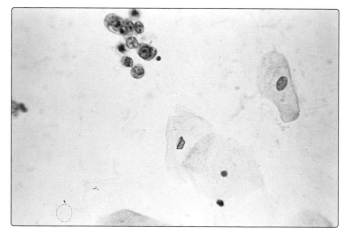

Fig. 35.28 Well-differentiated adenocarcinoma (grade I) of endometrium. Part of abnormal acinar group with loss of cellular and nuclear polarity and malignant cellular features. Endocervical sample. (Papanicolaou × HP)

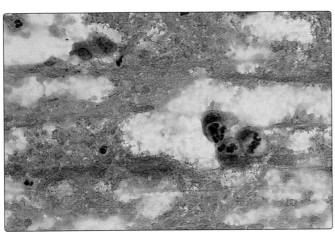

Fig. 35.29 Adenocarcinoma of endometrium. Few malignant endometrial cells with degenerative cytoplasmic vacuoles containing neutrophils in vaginal sample which may be confused for benign degenerative cells. Vaginal sample. (Papanicolaou × HP)

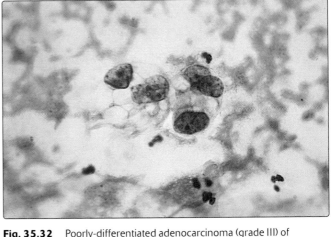

Fig. 35.32 Poorly-differentiated adenocarcinoma (grade III) of endometrium, clear cell type. The malignant cells and nuclei are relatively large with moderate amount of clear vacuolated cytoplasm. The nuclei are eccentrically located with macronucleoli. These are probably hob-nail cells modified in their passage to the cervical canal. Endocervical sample. (Papanicolaou × HP)

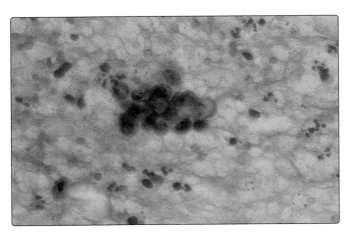

Fig. 35.30 Adenocarcinoma of endometrium. A group of malignant cells with a watery, granular background, altered blood, cellular detritus and few inflammatory cells (tumour diathesis). Endocervical sample. (Papanicolaou × HP)

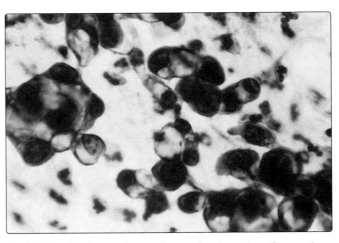

Fig. 35.33 Mucinous adenocarcinoma of endometrium. Groups of adenocarcinoma cells with slightly eosinophilic mucin in cytoplasmic vacuoles. Some cells have a signet-ring appearance. Endocervical sample. (Papanicolaou × HP)

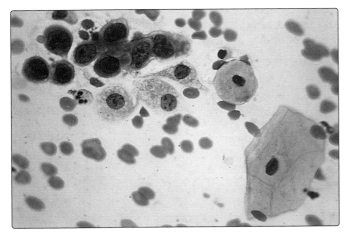

Fig. 35.31 Poorly-differentiated adenocarcinoma (grade III) of endometrium. Cellular and nuclear enlargement is present and nucleolar size is larger than well-differentiated adenocarcinoma cells. Endocervical sample. (Papanicolaou × HP)

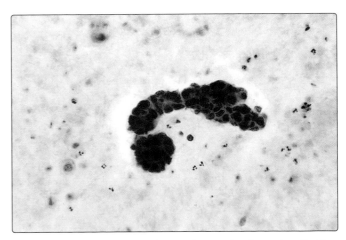

Fig. 35.34 Serous papillary adenocarcinoma of endometrium. Papillary elongated aggregate of malignant cells with fronds characteristic of papillary adenocarcinoma. Endocervical aspirate. (Papanicolaou × MP)

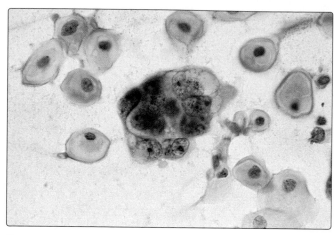

Fig. 35.35   Adenosquamous carcinoma of endometrium. A group of poorly-differentiated malignant cells representing the glandular component. Note atrophic cell pattern (see **Fig. 35.36**). Endocervical sample. (Papanicolaou × HP)

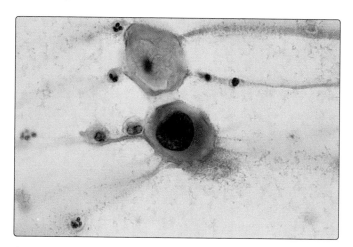

Fig. 35.36   Adenosquamous carcinoma of endometrium. A malignant squamous cell, large cell non-keratinizing type, representing the squamous component from the case in **Fig. 35.35**. Endocervical sample. (Papanicolaou × HP)

Malignant cells of endometrial origin are important to recognize in cervical smears as they may be the first indication of malignancy before symptoms become apparent, thereby leading to earlier diagnosis. Specific types of carcinoma other than endometrioid carcinoma may be difficult to distinguish in the exfoliated material present in a cervical smear. This is partly due to degenerative changes but also these higher-grade tumours may show less obvious differentiation at a cellular level. However, it is more important for future management to recognize the material as malignant and that it is likely to be from the endometrial cavity than it is to identify a specific cell type.

As a general rule, carcinomas of higher-grade and stage will be more likely to have exfoliated cells present in a cervical smear. The cells are, however, likely to be fewer in number and less conspicuous than cells from a primary cervical carcinoma. The cells of endometrial carcinoma are also larger than normal endometrial cells.

Malignant endometrial cells appear as single cells and aggregates, which can show a number of patterns ranging from tight cell balls with a smooth moulded surface to loose clusters and papillary formations. The cells may show nuclear crowding and overlapping, reflecting a loss of cell polarity. The cells show mild pleomorphism. The cytoplasm may contain vacuoles but these are frequently degenerate in nature and may be associated with engulfed material and neutrophils.

The nuclear changes vary with grade, with the higher-grade tumours showing more obvious malignant features. Nuclei are round, oval or occasionally reniform or multiple. The nuclei are mildly hyperchromatic with at least a small nucleolus. Higher-grade tumours will show chromatin clearing and a more prominent nucleolus. Tumour diathesis, containing necrotic material and old blood is likely to be more prominent in tumours of higher-grade or where there is direct involvement of the cervix. In tumours directly involving the cervix, with tumour present at the surface, the smear will also be likely to contain directly scraped, better preserved material which will be difficult to differentiate from endocervical adenocarcinoma.

Specific types of carcinoma other than endometrioid are difficult to define cytologically in exfoliated material other than usually being of high grade. Papillary serous carcinoma can sometimes be recognized by the presence of papillary groupings, psammoma bodies and cells with large, pleomorphic nuclei and abundant dense cytoplasm[43].

Endometrial sampling

▶ Abundant tumour fragments and round or hyperplastic fragments
▶ Obvious malignant features in cells of high-grade carcinomas
▶ Tumour diathesis in high-grade tumours
▶ Foam cells in low-grade tumours

Directly sampled cellular material from the endometrial cavity may include fragments of normal endometrium and hyperplastic endometrium as well as carcinoma. Much more abundant malignant material is present than in cervical smears and cell aggregates are larger. The tissue fragments present vary in size and shape, gland stomas are crowded and compressed with marked variability in size and shape. Papillary formations and solid aggregates with no visible glands may also be present.

At a cellular level the malignant cells are variable in size and shape, ranging from low columnar or cuboidal to round or oval. The cells in glands will be crowded with overlapping of nuclei or stratification. Both the cell and nucleus are relatively enlarged. The cytoplasm may be inconspicuous due to the cell crowding. The nuclei show irregularity of chromatin. Nucleoli are present but their degree of prominence varies with tumour grade. Mitoses may be prominent but are not a reliable feature of malignancy as they can be present in normal endometrium, particularly in proliferative phase. Psammoma bodies may be present. Tumour diathesis consisting of necrotic cellular debris, old blood and inflammatory cells is frequently present. Endometrial carcinoma can be associated with pyometra which may make recognition of the tumour difficult if it is obscured by inflammatory exudate, and the cells that are present may appear more pleomorphic or may be degenerate.

Features suggesting a carcinoma of low grade include more obvious gland formation with visible gland stomas, cells that are more columnar or cuboidal, small nucleoli, less prominent tumour diathesis and abundant foam cells in the background. High histological grade is suggested by less gland formation with more solid tumour fragments, larger more rounded or oval cells, prominent nucleolus and abundant tumour diathesis.

Specific types of differentiation other than endometrioid may be difficult to recognize, partly because they tend to be high-grade tumours. Squamous morules are infrequently recognized and may be confused with benign squamous metaplastic cells from the cervix, which can be present as contaminants of the endometrial sample. Overtly malignant squamous elements resemble their counterparts in the cervix. Serous carcinoma may show prominent papillary groupings and tissue fragments and psammoma bodies may be present. Clear cell carcinoma is difficult to recognize cytologically as anything other than a high-grade carcinoma but 'hobnail' cells may be recognized within glands in some cases. Mucinous carcinoma contains cytoplasmic mucin vacuoles, which may have a pale, slightly eosinophilic, staining reaction and occasionally 'signet ring' cells may be observed. The presence of mucin is more confidently distinguished from degenerative vacuoles by mucin staining in a cell-block preparation.

Problems in diagnosis (Figs 35.37–35.39)

Direct endometrial sampling is often limited by the amount of material present on the slide. The fact that the sample is taken blindly also introduces problems of representative sampling. In cervical smears the recognition of endometrial cells can be impeded by the presence of blood, tumour diathesis or inflammation. They are often few in number and as they are small and similar in size to histiocytes they may be overlooked. Reactive immature squamous metaplastic cells with degenerative vacuoles as seen in association with intrauterine device usage can show engulfment of neutrophils and resemble degenerate endometrial cells. These should, however, have the characteristic dense cytoplasm of metaplastic cells and are usually single or in sheets rather than in small clusters of cells.

Finally, there are the limits of the art and science of cytology itself, the specificity of diagnostic criteria and the ability of humans to apply them consistently. Occasionally cervical lesions could be confused with an endometrial carcinoma, particularly uncommon tumours of the cervix

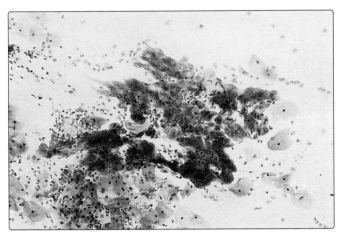

Fig. 35.37 Regenerative endocervical columnar cells. Large aggregate of endocervical columnar cells with cytoplasmic processes and relatively low nuclear/cytoplasmic ratio. The nuclei, except for nucleoli, lack malignant features. Single cells are rarely seen and there is no tumour diathesis. Endocervical sample. (Papanicolaou × MP)

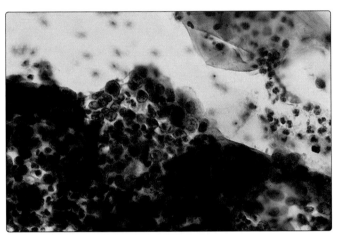

Fig. 35.38 Squamous cell carcinoma of cervix. A large syncytium of malignant squamous cells with hyperchromatic nuclei and some nucleoli. Endocervical sample. (Papanicolaou × HP)

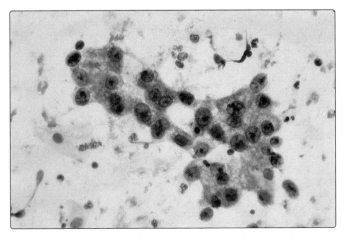

Fig. 35.39 Endocervical adenocarcinoma. Loose sheet of malignant endocervical cells with glandular stomas. The malignant cells appear columnar with characteristic slightly eosinophilic granular cytoplasm. Endocervical sample. (Papanicolaou × HP)

such as small cell carcinoma or melanoma. In these cases the cells are likely to be recognizably malignant but unless characteristic features are present it is likely that specific diagnosis would require further biopsy and even immunochemical staining. A similar problem may arise with carcinomas of extrauterine origin where recognition of specific cell type can be very difficult and further clinical work-up is necessary before final diagnosis.

Cytopathology of extrauterine and non-epithelial uterine tumours

Extrauterine cancer

Tumour cells detected in cervical smears may originate from a primary cervical tumour, a secondary tumour involving the cervix (either a metastasis or direct extension into the cervix of a tumour in a neighbouring organ) or from an extra-cervical site where exfoliated tumour cells travel via the endometrial cavity and/or the fallopian tube. The appearances of endometrial carcinoma have been discussed previously.

Non-cervical tumour cells in cervical smears are a rare finding in most laboratories[44–48]. Ng *et al.*[45] reported an incidence of 11/100 000 smears and Australian data from the New South Wales Cervical Screening Program[49] shows an incidence of 3.3/100 000 for extra-cervical cancers excluding the uterine corpus and vagina.

The occurrence of malignant cells in cervical mucus is probably a common event in patients with malignant ascites and intact fallopian tubes but most of these patients will not have cervical smears taken as it would not be likely to assist in their management[50]. The importance of the detection of these cells lies in the possibility of earlier diagnosis in asymptomatic women with ovarian, tubal or peritoneal lesions and to direct the pathway of investigation, where possible, away from unnecessary surgery.

While the features of endometrial adenocarcinoma are well described and relatively familiar, cells from these more remote sites or unusual tumour types are less familiar and are therefore less likely to be correctly interpreted. To raise the suspicion that the abnormal cells may originate outside the cervix or even the uterus can be useful in guiding clinical investigation and management. The persistence of abnormal cells in repeat smears after normal colposcopy, particularly if they are not typical of a squamous lesion, also should prompt the consideration of a more remote origin. The clinical response would usually be hysteroscopy and imaging (ultrasound or CT) to determine the presence of ovarian enlargement or free fluid in the peritoneal cavity, before cone biopsy is performed speculatively.

Cytological features (Figs 35.40–35.46)

▶ Clusters of tumour cells, usually adenocarcinomatous in type
▶ Papillary grouping may be apparent

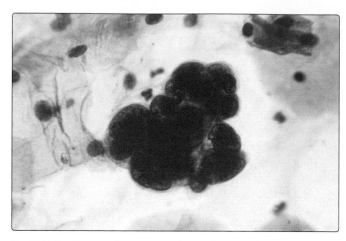

Fig. 35.40   Extrauterine adenocarcinoma. A group of poorly-differentiated papillary adenocarcinoma consistent with papillary serous adenocarcinoma. Note lack of a tumour diathesis and the background of the smear is clean. Endocervical sample. (× HP)

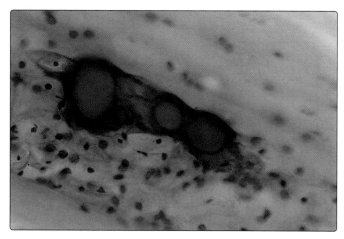

Fig. 35.41   Extrauterine adenocarcinoma. Psammoma bodies seen together with malignant cells shown in **Fig. 35.42**. Endocervical sample. (× HP)

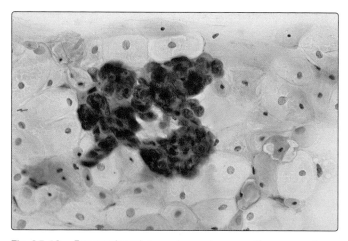

Fig. 35.42   Extrauterine adenocarcinoma. Large papillary group of malignant cells showing degenerative changes consistent with papillary serous adenocarcinoma of ovary. Note lack of tumour. Endocervical sample. (× MP)

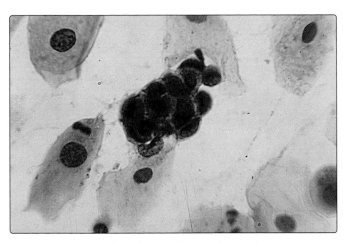

Fig. 35.43 Extrauterine adenocarcinoma, primary tubal adenocarcinoma. Group of malignant cells with many of the features of endometrial adenocarcinoma. Tumour diathesis is absent. Endocervical sample. (× HP)

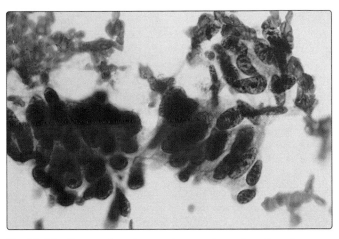

Fig. 35.45 Extrauterine adenocarcinoma, primary from the colon. Groups of malignant cells arranged in a palisade pattern with overlapping elongated nuclei characteristic of well- to moderately well-differentiated adenocarcinoma of colon. Vaginal sample.

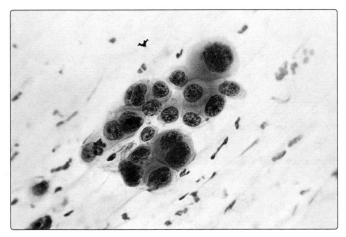

Fig. 35.44 Extrauterine adenocarcinoma, primary from the breast. Relatively large oval or polygonal malignant cells of undifferentiated adenocarcinoma similar to those seen in large cell infiltrating ductal carcinoma of breast. (× HP)

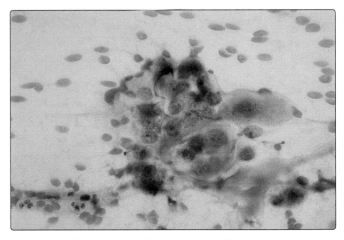

Fig. 35.46 Extrauterine malignant tumour, malignant melanoma metastatic to cervix. Few malignant cells and some with a powdery fine brown melanin pigment in their cytoplasm. Endocervical sample. (× HP)

► Psammoma bodies occasionally seen
► Absence of tumour diathesis unless tumour is directly sampled

The cytological appearances will differ depending on whether the cells are being sampled directly from a metastatic, directly spreading tumour or are derived from exfoliated cells traversing the endometrial cavity.

Tumours metastatic to the cervix may be predominantly submucosal and the material may not always be accessible to the sampling instrument. Where the tumour breaches the surface there is likely to be ulceration associated with necrosis, inflammation and haemorrhage. Similarly, if the tumour is invading the cervix from a neighbouring structure such as the rectum or bladder there is likely to be ulceration or fistula formation. Material directly scraped from such lesions is likely also to include fresh, well-preserved cells and even large tumour fragments.

A tumour diathesis (an exudate with cell debris, old blood and inflammatory cells) often reflects local ulceration and is more likely to be present in a smear where the lesion is directly sampled or is associated with bleeding, as in endometrial carcinoma. Where the cells are derived from a more distant lesion this background is diluted or less apparent. The study by Ng *et al.*[45] found 80% of cases of extrauterine cancer diagnosed on cervical smear did not have a tumour diathesis. The remaining 20% all had uterine or vaginal metastases with mucosal involvement. This has however not been shown to be a consistent finding in other studies[51]. The cells in the smear will frequently show degenerative features and may be trapped in streams of mucus.

In the case of cells traversing the uterine cavity to be deposited in the cervical mucus, this is most likely to occur where there is malignancy within the pelvic or abdominal cavities or less likely within the fallopian tube itself. The presence of ascites may assist the passage of cells and obviously this route requires patency of the fallopian tubes. In common with the causes of malignant ascites generally, the ovaries, gastrointestinal system and breast are the commonest sites of origin[51], with other sites including pancreas, pelvic/abdominal mesothelium, melanoma, lymphoma and leukaemia occurring less frequently[50]. Primary carcinoma confined to the fallopian tube, usually serous papillary carcinoma, is uncommon but may present in this way.

Of particular types of differentiation, the majority will be adenocarcinomas[45] but the cytological features are frequently not sufficiently distinctive to be reliable in predicting the site of origin and correlation with medical history and the clinical and imaging findings is essential. A pattern of predominantly papillary formations suggests the possibility of a papillary serous carcinoma. Serous papillary carcinoma of the ovary has the highest rate of positive cytology[51] reflecting a propensity for surface exfoliation. This tumour, apart from usually obvious cytological features of malignancy, may show papillary fragments, hollow spheres and in some cases psammoma bodies. However, neither the papillary architecture nor psammoma bodies are seen in this tumour exclusively. Papillae may be seen in endometrioid carcinomas and those of breast, large intestine, pancreas, thyroid and lung as well as mesothelioma. Psammoma bodies may also be seen in these tumours and, unaccompanied by malignant cells, in some benign conditions. As they are frequently serous carcinomas, fallopian tube primary carcinomas will have a similar appearance. Cell groups with tall columnar cells, often appreciated as the palisading of nuclei at the edge of the group, would suggest either large intestinal or endometrial origin. A pattern of linear cell arrangements might suggest breast or possibly gastric carcinoma. Small hyperchromatic cells with scant cytoplasm may suggest small cell carcinoma or if they are present exclusively as single dispersed cells, lymphoma should be considered.

Non-epithelial uterine lesions

Cytological material from these lesions may be encountered occasionally in both cervical smears and in direct endometrial sampling methods.

Benign mesenchymal lesions

Leiomyoma (Fig. 35.47)

These benign smooth muscle tumours (fibroids) are the commonest tumour of the female genital tract but are relatively inaccessible and are rarely sampled unless they involve the cervix or are submucosally located in the uterine corpus. The tumour does not spontaneously exfoliate cells and is not likely to be sampled unless it is ulcerated or particularly vigorous abrasion has been

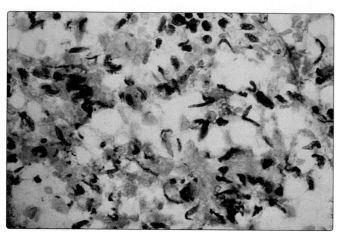

Fig. 35.47 Uterine leiomyoma, submucosal type. Elongated smooth muscles with centrally placed benign oval to elongated nuclei and eosinophilic cytoplasm. Endometrial sample smear. (× HP)

applied. The number of cells is likely to be few as these tumours are of very firm consistency. The cells appear as regular, elongated, spindle-shaped cells with an oval, vesicular nucleus and a small nucleolus. It would not be possible to distinguish these cells from smooth muscle cells of the myometrium. Pleomorphism, abundant cellularity or mitoses would be suspicious for malignancy.

Benign endometrial stromal tumours (stromal nodule)

These tumours are less common and consist of a circumscribed proliferation of the specialized endometrial stromal cells. Cytology is not useful in the diagnosis of these lesions as cells derived from these tumours are indistinguishable from those of the endometrial stroma itself and are therefore unlikely to be recognized as abnormal. Distinction from low-grade stromal sarcoma relies largely on the presence of local or vascular invasion and this cannot be assessed cytologically.

Adenomatoid tumours

These benign tumours of mesothelial origin are located in the serosa or sub-serosal myometrium and are not accessible to cytological sampling methods.

Benign papillary adenofibroma

The cytological features of this lesion have not been described and the glandular and stromal elements of the tumour would in any case be indistinguishable from their benign counterparts.

Malignant mesenchymal tumours

These tumours are much less common than endometrial carcinoma. They include malignant mixed Mullerian tumour and its variants, leiomyosarcoma, endometrial stromal sarcoma, other heterologous sarcomas and other non-epithelial tumours such as lymphoma and leukaemic infiltrates.

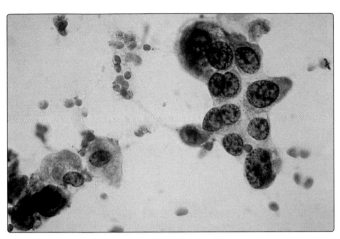

Fig. 35.48 Malignant mixed mesodermal tumour of endometrium. A group of poorly-differentiated adenocarcinoma cells (right) and few malignant cells with relatively more cytoplasm (left) probably representing sarcoma cells. (× HP)

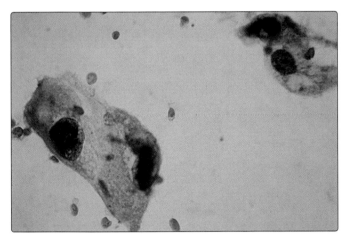

Fig. 35.49 Malignant mixed mesodermal tumour of endometrium. Large bizarre sarcoma cells consistent with malignant rhabdomyoblasts representing heterologous component. Endocervical sample. (× HP)

Malignant mixed Mullerian tumour *(Figs 35.48, 35.49)*

Mixed Mullerian tumours (mixed mesodermal tumours) express both epithelial and mesenchymal differentiation. Both components are benign in *papillary adenofibroma* (see above). When the tumour is composed of a combination of benign glands with a malignant stroma the tumour is termed an *adenosarcoma*.

The commonest tumour of this group however is the *malignant mixed Mullerian tumour*, in which both the epithelial and mesenchymal elements are malignant. These are high-grade tumours, which are commoner in elderly women, usually presenting with abnormal bleeding. As they are frequently polypoid, they may occasionally protrude through the cervical os. The epithelial component is most commonly composed of conventional endometrial adenocarcinoma, usually of high grade. Other forms of epithelial differentiation, particularly squamous, may be

present, as well as other types of Mullerian differentiation such as serous, clear cell and mucinous, either alone or in combination. The stromal component may consist of sarcoma showing differentiation native to the uterus (leiomyosarcoma or endometrial stromal sarcoma) in which case the tumour is termed homologous mixed Mullerian tumour or carcinosarcoma. When the stromal component also includes other forms of differentiation not analogous to normal uterine tissues, such as rhabdomyosarcoma or osteosarcoma, the tumour is termed heterologous.

Cellular material from these tumours may be obtained by sampling from the endometrial cavity, or less commonly may be encountered in cervical smears.

Cytological features

▶ Carcinomatous elements predominate
▶ Sarcomatous component may be overlooked
▶ Pleomorphic spindle-shaped cells
▶ Tumour diathesis is present

The cytological features of adenosarcoma have been described from imprint cytology[52]. These included aggregates and single sarcomatous cells with scanty cytoplasm and oval nuclei with coarse chromatin and conspicuous nucleoli. These were admixed with a mildly atypical glandular component in clusters.

The rate of cytological identification of malignant mixed Mullerian tumour is less than for conventional endometrial carcinoma[53–55]. Further, the carcinomatous component appears to be more frequently represented in the cytological material than the sarcomatous component, so that while the case may be recognized as malignant, the correct diagnosis may not always be possible cytologically. This is not, however, likely to be of clinical importance as the diagnosis will be amended when larger tissue biopsies or the excised lesion is examined and the treatment is not likely to be significantly altered. A finding of positive cytology in cervical smears appears to correlate with high tumour stage in malignant mixed Mullerian tumour[54]. In cervical smears the carcinomatous cells will most commonly resemble those of endometrial carcinoma, as small groups or single degenerate cells with hyperchromatic nuclei and often vacuolated cytoplasm. Directly sampled material from the uterine cavity or prolapsed tumour may contain larger fragments of tumour and a bloody diathesis, sometimes with necrosis. The sarcomatous component can be easily overlooked and is likely to consist of a scanty background population of single abnormal spindle-shaped cells with marked variation in size and shape. Bizarre, multinucleated, elongated or tadpole-shaped forms can be present. The cytoplasm can vary from lacy or fibrillary to dense and homogeneous. In many cases the sarcoma will resemble leiomyosarcoma or high-grade endometrial stromal sarcoma (see below). Specific forms of sarcomatous differentiation, particularly heterologous forms, are difficult to recognize in the sarcomatous component. Cytoplasmic cross striations are relatively rare even in histological sections of rhabdomyosarcoma so that their occurrence is very unlikely in scanty cytological samples. Osteosarcoma and chondrosarcoma are generally more cohesive and are less likely to be represented. The bizarre elongated single cells need to be distinguished from poorly-differentiated squamous carcinoma, which may also show a wide range of cell morphology but will frequently show some evidence of keratinization. Extreme examples of epithelial reparative change can result in clusters of highly atypical cells, often with a very prominent nucleolus in which a diagnosis of sarcoma may be considered. These cells usually show cell-to-cell cohesion and a spectrum of cell changes ranging through to obviously benign cells. A background of inflammation is present usually without necrosis unless there is an ulcerated inflammatory lesion on the cervix.

Leiomyosarcoma *(Fig. 35.50)*

Unlike their benign counterpart, malignant smooth muscle tumours of the uterus are uncommon. They present, usually in peri-menopausal or post-menopausal women, with abnormal bleeding, pelvic discomfort or uterine enlargement. Cytological diagnosis in these cases is very unusual, as the tumours are usually intramural and therefore inaccessible to cytological sampling. This is further complicated by the fact that histological diagnosis in low-grade tumours relies on assessment of mitotic rate and infiltration into adjacent myometrium rather than abnormalities of cellular morphology.

Rarely the tumour may be ulcerated or submucosal and can either shed cells or be abraded by a sampling device[56]. Better-differentiated tumours show slender spindle-shaped cells, larger than the normal smooth muscle cells of the myometrium with a centrally placed, slightly enlarged nucleus. The cytoplasm is poorly defined, thin or fibrillary with cyanophilic or amphophilic staining. Rounder more epithelioid cells may have a dense cytoplasm. Higher-grade tumours show general features of sarcoma with single, abnormal, often elongated or bizarre cells in which specific cellular features of smooth muscle differentiation are not recognizable.

Endometrial stromal sarcoma *(Fig. 35.51)*

Endometrial stromal sarcoma is less common than malignant mixed Mullerian tumour and leiomyosarcoma. Cytological diagnosis is possible in cervical and endometrial cytological samples when the endometrial surface or the cervix is involved directly and where tumour grade is high enough for the cells to be distinguished from normal endometrial stromal cells. The cells are round with ill-defined cell borders and scanty fine weakly cyanophilic cytoplasm. They tend to be single rather than clustered (as in normal stromal cells) and the nuclei are two to three

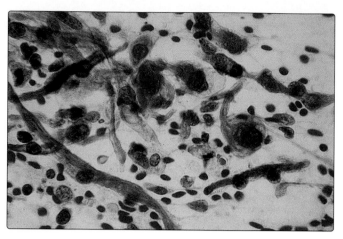

Fig. 35.50   Leiomyosarcoma of uterus. Marked spindle, caudate and oval malignant cells with variable size nuclei, some containing macronucleoli. The cytoplasm is fibrillar and stains cyanophilic. Endometrial sample. (× HP)

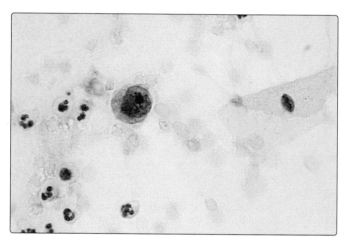

Fig. 35.51   High-grade stromal cell sarcoma of endometrium. A single malignant cell with a thin rim of cytoplasm and a large nucleus with irregular distribution of granular chromatin and a macronucleolus. Endocervical sample. (× HP)

times larger. Nucleoli are prominent in the higher-grade tumours[57,58]. Low-grade tumours require histological sampling for assessment of mitotic rate and invasion of adjacent tissue or vessels for diagnosis and cannot be distinguished by cytological appearances. A rich capillary network in tumour fragments can be a useful clue.

Lymphoma and leukaemia

Primary lymphoma of the uterus or cervix is very rare, but secondary involvement in advanced lymphoma or leukaemia is more common. Gynaecological sampling is rarely carried out on late stage patients but the potentially useful finding of abnormal lymphoid or leukaemic cells in a cervical smear could herald recurrence in otherwise well, long-term survivors. A primary diagnosis of lymphoma or leukaemia would virtually never be made on this type of cytological preparation. Recognition of these cells types is important however in distinguishing them from other types of malignancy such as small cell carcinoma and endometrial stromal sarcoma.

Cytological findings (Fig. 35.52)

The cellular appearances of non-Hodgkin's lymphoma and leukaemias depend on the cell type and in general resemble the features seen in other sites examined by similar exfoliative methods[59]. Low-grade lymphomas may differ little at a cellular level from the range of lymphoid cells present in follicular cervicitis but cervicitis will usually include plentiful plasma cells and may show tingible body macrophages with engulfed pyknotic nuclear material. Definite diagnosis would always require biopsy in low-grade lymphoma. High-grade lymphomas may show a more uniform infiltrate of larger single cells with a round to oval nucleus and coarse chromatin. Again, depending on the cell type, the nucleolus may be single and prominent or multiple. The cells are mostly single with only occasional loose aggregates. The lack of nuclear moulding and the presence of nucleoli help to distinguish them from small cell carcinoma. As most of these patients will have been previously diagnosed with lymphoma, correlation with the clinical history and comparison with any previous material may be useful in resolving diagnostic problems.

Hodgkin's lymphoma is only likely to be encountered when the disease is widespread.

Trophoblastic tumours (Figs 35.53, 35.54)

Gestational trophoblastic disease arises from the abnormal growth or neoplasia in cells derived from trophoblast that forms placental tissue.

Partial hydatidiform mole exhibits triploidy, may be associated with the presence of a fetus and has a low risk for the development of choriocarcinoma.

Complete hydatidiform mole is diploid, but has two Y-chromosomes and virtually never has an associated fetus. The placental villi develop as hollow grape-like vesicles filled with fluid. There is usually a rapid increase in uterine size and high levels of beta-human chorionic gonadotrophin (β-HCG) which may result in hyperemesis gravidarum. Diagnosis is usually made on uterine ultrasound and serum β-HCG measurement. There is an increased risk of subsequent development of choriocarcinoma.

Choriocarcinoma is a malignant tumour of placental trophoblast consisting of both cytotrophoblast and syncytiotrophoblastic elements. The tumour can present as uterine enlargement, abnormal bleeding or as a result of metastases. Metastases can be haemorrhagic and can be a cause of cerebral haemorrhage. Diagnosis is frequently made again by β-HCG measurement.

Placental site trophoblastic tumour is an uncommon tumour derived from an intermediate trophoblast, which secretes human placental lactogen (HPL).

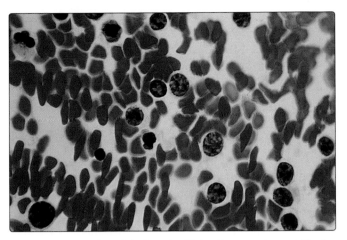

Fig. 35.52 Lymphocytic leukaemia with involvement of uterus. Single large malignant lymphoid cells with red blood cells. Endocervical sample. (× HP)

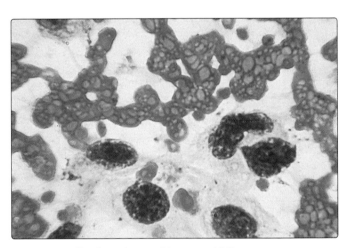

Fig. 35.53 Choriocarcinoma of the uterus. Malignant syncytiotrophoblastic and cytotrophoblastic cells are present. Endocervical sample. (× HP)

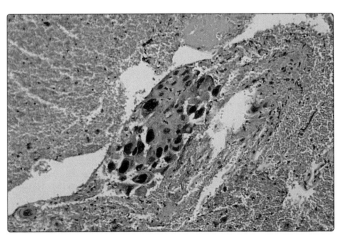

Fig. 35.54 Hydatidiform mole, complete type, of uterus. There is a small group of abnormal trophoblastic cells among blood. No molar villi seen in the sample. Endometrial sample. (× MP)

Cytology has little role to play in the routine diagnosis of these tumours, although the cytological features of trophoblastic cells have been described[60]. In the personal experience of one of the authors (ABPN) of 35 cases of confirmed choriocarcinoma with immediate pre-treatment cervical smears, only one specimen contained scanty malignant syncytiotrophoblastic cells. These were large pleomorphic cells with sharp cell borders, moderately abundant dense cytoplasm which could be eosinophilic or cyanophilic. Multiple enlarged nuclei were present but less numerous than in benign syncytiotrophoblast, usually 3–6 per cell, and located centrally.

Hydatidiform mole may also be associated with the presence of trophoblastic cells in cervical smears and occasionally placental villi are also seen. Again, diagnosis will depend more on the ultrasound and hormonal findings.

References

1 Ng A B P. *Gynecologic Pathology for Clinicians.* Miami: University of Miami Publishing, 1991; 167–209

2 Ng A B P, Reagan J W, Hawkiczek S, Wentz B W. Significance of endometrial cells in the detection of endometrial carcinoma and its precursors. *Acta Cytol* 1974; **18**: 356–361

3 Sarode V R, Rader A E, Rose P G *et al.* Significance of cytologically normal endometrial cells in cervical smears from post-menopausal women. *Acta Cytol* 2001; **45**: 153–156

4 Doornewaard H, Sie-Go D M, Woudt J M, Kooijman C D. The significance of endometrial cells in the cervical smear (abstract). *Ned Tijdschr Geneeskd* 1993; **24**: 137(17): 868–872

5 Van den Bosch T, Vandendael A, Wranz P A, Lombard C J. Cervical cytology in menopausal women at high risk for endometrial disease. *Eur J Cancer Prev* 1998; **7**(2): 149–152

6 Heaton R B, Harris T F, Larson D M, Henry M R. Glandular cells derived from direct sampling of the lower uterine segment in patients status post-cervical cone biopsy: A diagnostic dilemma. *Am J Clin Pathol* 1996; **106**: 511–516

7 Hong S R, Park J S, Kim H S. Atypical glandular cells of undetermined significance in cervical smears after conization. Cytologic features differentiating them from adenocarcinoma *in situ*. *Acta Cytol* 2001; **45**(2): 163–167

8 Cooper J M, Erickson M L. Endometrial sampling techniques in the diagnosis of abnormal uterine bleeding. *Obstet Gynecol Clin North Am* 2000; **27**(2): 235–244

9 Bibbo M. The vacutage method in the detection of endometrial cancer and its precursors. Compendium of Diagnostic Cytology. In: Wied G L, Keebler C M, Koss L G, Reagan J W eds. *Tutorials of Cytology*, Chicago IL: Publisher, 6th edn., 1990; 273–275

10 Farre J, Bernard P, Besoncon D, Siebert S. A five year experience with intrauterine washing cytology. *Acta Cytol* 1982; **26**: 623–629

11 Milan A R, Markley R L. Endometrial cytology by a new technic. *Obstet Gynecol* 1973; **42**: 469–475

12 Veneti S Z, Kyrkou K A, Kittas C N, Perdes A T. Efficacy of the Isaacs endometrial cell sampler in the cytologic detection of endometrial abnormalities. *Acta Cytol* 1984; **28**: 546–554

13 Tao L C. Direct intrauterine sampling: The IUMC endometrial sampler. *Diagn Cytopathol.* 1997; **17**: 153–159

14 Maksem J, Sager F, Bender R. Endometrial collection and interpretation using the Tao brush and the Cytorich fixative system; a feasibility study. *Diagn Cytopathol.* 1997; **17**(5): 339–346

15 Sato S, Yaegashi N, Shikano K *et al.* Endometrial cytodiagnosis with the Uterobrush and Endocyte. *Acta Cytol.* 1996; **40**(5): 907–910

16 Yoshida Y, Sato S, Okamura C *et al.* Evaluating the accuracy of uterine cancer screening with the regional cancer registration system. *Acta Cytol* 1998; **7**(2): 263–269

17 Reagan J W, Ng A B P. *The Cells of Uterine Adenocarcinoma*, 2nd edn. Basel: S. Karger, 1973

18 Vooijs G P, Van der Graaf Y, Vooijs M A. The presence of endometrial cells in cervical smears in relation to the day of the menstrual cycle and the method of contraception. *Acta Cytol* 1987; **31**: 162–166

19 Walfson W L. Histologic and cytologic correlation of endometrial wreaths. *Acta Cytol* 1983; **27**: 63–64

20 Ng A B P, Reagan J W. Normal endometrial cells and their significance in the detection of benign and malignant endometrial lesions. Compendium of Diagnostic Cytology. In: Wied G L, Keebler C M, Koss L G, Reagan J W eds. *Tutorials of Cytology*, Chicago, IL: 6th edn., 1990; 162–166

21 Schneider V. Cytology in pregancy. Compendium of Diagnostic Cytology. In: Weid G L, Keebler C M, Koss L G, Reagan J W eds. *Tutorials of Cytology*, Chicago IL: 6th edn., 1990; 51–53

22 Kern S M. Presence of psammoma bodies in Papanicolaou-stained cervicovaginal smears. *Acta Cytol* 1991; **35**: 81–88

23 Blumenfeld W, Holly E A, Mansur D L, King E B. Histiocytes and the detection of endometrial carcinoma. *Acta Cytol* 1985; **29**: 317–322

24 Cherkis R C, Patten S F Jr, Andrews T J *et al.* Significance of normal endometrial cells detected by cervical cytology. *Obstet and Gynecol* 1988; **71**: 242–249

25 Galera-Davidson H, Fernandez A, Navarro J *et al.* Mucinous metaplasia to neoplastic lesions in endometrial samples with cytohistologic correlation. *Diagn Cytopathol* 1989; **5**: 150–153

26 Shrago S S. The Arias-Stella reaction: A case report of a cytologic presentation. *Acta Cytol* 1977; **21**: 310–313

27 Fujimoto I, Masubuchi S, Miwa H *et al.* Psammoma bodies found in cervicovaginal and/or endometrial smears. *Acta Cytol* 1982; **26**: 317–322

28 Gupta P K. Intrauterine contraception devices: vaginal cytology, pathologic changes and clinical implication. *Acta Cytol* 1982; **26**: 571–613

29 Kern S B. Prevalence of psammoma bodies in Papanicolaou-stained cervicovaginal smears. *Acta Cytol* 1991; **35**(1): 81–88

30 Feeley K M, Wells M. Hormone replacement therapy and the endometrium. *J Clin Pathol* 2001; **54**(6): 435–440

31 Suh-Burgmann E J, Goodman A. Surveillance for endometrial cancer in women receiving tamoxifen. *Ann Intern Med* 1999; **131**(2): 127–135

32 Tao L C. Direct intrauterine sampling: the IUMC endometrial sampler. *Diagn Cytopathol* 1997; **17**: 153–159

33 Yoshida Y, Sato S, Okamura C *et al.* Evaluating the accuracy of uterine cancer screening with the regional cancer registration system. *Acta Cytol* 2001; **45**(2): 157–162

34 Anderson M C, Robboy S J, Russell P, Morse A. *Endometrial Carcinoma in Pathology of the Female Reproductive Tract*. London: Churchill Livingstone, 2002; 331–359

35 Sarode V, Rader A E, Rose P G *et al.* Significance of cytologically normal endometrial cells in cervical smears from postmenopausal women. *Acta Cytol* 2001; **45**(2):153–156

36 Chang A, Sandweiss L, Bose S. Cytologically benign endometrial cells in the Papanicolaou smears of postmenopausal women. *Gynecol Oncol* 2001; **80**(1):37–43

37 Tambouret R, Bell D A Centeno B A. Significance of histiocytes in cervical smears from peri/postmenopausal women. *Diagn Cytopathol* 2001; **24**(4): 271–275

38 Ng A B P, Reagan J W. Histology and cytology of normal and hyperplastic endometrium in Compendium on Diagnostic Cytology. In: Weid G ed. *Tutorials of Cytology*. Chicago IL: 8th edn., 1997; 128–142

39 Meisels A, Jolicoeur C. Criteria for the cytologic assessment of hyperplasias in endometrial samples obtained by the endopap endometrial sampler. *Acta Cytol* 1985; **29**(3): 297–340

40 Kashimura M, Baba S, Shinohara M *et al.* Cytologic findings in endometrial hyperplasia. *Acta Cytol* 1988; **32**(3): 335–340

41 Ng A B P, Reagan J W. Pathology and Cytopathology of adenocarcinoma of the uterus. Compendium on Diagnostic Cytology. In: Weid G ed. *Tutorials of Cytology*. Chicago IL: publisher, 8th edn., 1997; 157–172

42 Kuebler D L, Nikrui N. Cytologic features of endometrial papillary serous carcinoma. *Acta Cytol* 1989; **33**(1): 120–126

43 Wright C A, Leiman G, Burgess S M. The cytomorphology of papillary serous carcinoma of the endometrium in cervical smears. *Cancer* 1999; **87**(1): 12–18

44 Mallow D W, Humphrey P A, Soper J T *et al.* Metastatic lobular carcinoma of the breast diagnosed in cervicovaginal samples. A case report. *Acta Cytol* 1997; **41**: 549–555

45 Ng A B, Teeple D, Lindner E A *et al.* The cellular manifestations of extrauterine cancer. *Acta Cytol* 1974; **18**: 108–117

46 Zweizig S, Noller K, Reale F *et al.* Neoplasia associated with atypical glandular cells of undetermined significance in cervical cytology. *Gynecol Oncol* 1997; **65**: 314–318

47 Schooland M, Sterrett G F, Knowles S A *et al.* The inconclusive-possible high-grade epithelial abnormality category in Papanicolaou smear reporting. *Cancer* 1998; **84**: 208–217

48 Rahmipanah F, Reid R I. Fallopian tube carcinoma detected by ThinPrep cytology smear. *Med J Aust* 2000; **172**: 38

49 NSW Cervical Screening Program. Cytology/Histology. Cervical Cancer Screening in New South Wales. *First Annual Statistical Report* 1997. NSW: Australian Government Printing, 1999; 37–69

50 Ng A B P, Reagan J W. The diagnosis of extrauterine cancer. Compendium of Diagnostic Cytology. In: Wied G L, Keebler C M, Koss L G, Reagan J W eds. *Tutorials of Cytology*. Chicago IL: publisher, 6th edn. 1990; 204–207

51 Gupta D, Balsara G. Extrauterine malignancies: role of Pap smears in diagnosis and management. *Acta Cytol* 1999; **43**(5): 806–813

52 Takeshima N, Tabata T, Nishida H *et al.* Mullerian adenosarcoma of the uterus: report of a case with imprint cytology. *Acta Cytol* 2001, **45**(4): 613–616

53 An-Foraker S H, Kawada C. Cytodiagnosis of endometrial malignant mixed mesodermal tumour. *Acta Cytol* 1985; **29**: 137–141

54 Costa M J, Tidd C, Willis D. Cervicovaginal cytology in carcinosarcoma [malignant mixed mullerian (mesodermal) tumour] of the uterus. *Diagn Cytopathol* 1992; **8**(1): 33–40

55 Massoni E A, Hajdu S I. Cytology of primary and metastatic uterine sarcomas. *Acta Cytol* 1984; **28**: 93–100

56 Hajdu S I, Hajdu E O. *Cytopathology of Sarcomas and Other Nonepithelial Malignant Tumours*. Philadelphia: W B Saunders, 1976; 182–212

57 Becker S N, Wong J Y. Detection of endometrial stromal sarcoma in cervicovaginal smears: Report of three cases. *Acta Cytol* 1980; **25**: 272–276

58 Morimoto N, Ozawa M, Kato Y, Kuramota H. Diagnostic value of mitotic activity in endometrial stromal sarcoma: Report of two cases. *Acta Cytol* 1982; **26**: 695–698

59 Ohwada M, Suzuki M, Onagawa T *et al.* Primary malignant lymphoma of the uterine corpus diagnosed by endometrial cytology. A case report. *Acta Cytol* 2000; **44**(6): 1045–1049

60 Taki I. Cytology of hydatidiform mole, invasive mole and choriocarcinoma. Compendium of Diagnostic Cytology. In: Wied G L, Keebler C M, Koss L G, Reagan J W eds. *Tutorials of Cytology*, 6th edn. Chicago, IL: publisher, 1990; 232–235

36 Ovaries and fallopian tubes

Sanjiv Manek and Alan B. P. Ng

Ovaries

Introduction

The application of cytological techniques such as fine needle aspiration (FNA) for routine screening for ovarian lesions used to be limited, particularly for malignant neoplasms, but is now less so with the advent of accurate imaging and the introduction of key monoclonal antibodies for immunocytochemistry. When judiciously employed, fine needle aspiration of ovarian lesions can be valuable as a diagnostic or therapeutic procedure and this is reflected by the increasing number of articles in the recent literature[1–10]. As has already been described, malignant cells of ovarian origin are also occasionally identified in vaginal, cervical and endometrial samples (see Chapter 35).

Fine needle aspiration technique

Ovarian lesions can be approached through the vagina or rectum, transabdominally, during laparoscopy and at the time of laparotomy. The transvaginal route is generally favoured as the vagina can be cleansed before puncture and is the preferred route for aspirations performed in the infertility unit, in conjunction with transvaginal ultrasonography[1–4]. Transrectal aspirates are usually performed in conjunction with examination of the patient under general anaesthesia[1–3]. Ovarian cysts and solid lesions, especially those that extend into the abdomen or are associated with omental lesions, can be readily aspirated via the transabdominal route[2]. Laparoscopic visualization and aspiration can also be safely and effectively employed in the diagnosis and management of ovarian cysts[2,5]. Occasionally, ovarian cysts are found incidentally during laparotomy undertaken for other reasons. Aspiration of these cysts can provide useful diagnoses to ascertain further management.

The laboratory procedure is also crucial in determining the diagnostic potential of a given sample. The fluid can be smeared directly or cytocentrifuged depending on its viscosity. It is useful to have at least two MGG and two Papanicolaou preparations to improve the diagnostic yield as quite often, only one slide may contain the relevant cells. It is also advisable to prepare spare slides for immunocytochemistry.

Non-neoplastic cystic lesions

Prior to the cytological interpretation of ovarian needle aspirate smears, cytopathologists should be thoroughly familiar with the aspiration route and with clinical and radiographic findings[2–4]. Knowledge of the former is essential as normal cells from various sites may be inadvertently aspirated during the passage of the needle towards the ovary[1,3]. These contaminants include squamous epithelial cells from vaginal mucosa, columnar cells from rectal mucosa and mesothelial cells from the peritoneum[1,3].

The clinical and radiographic features are extremely important in order to formulate a differential diagnosis and determine if the findings are representative of the aspirated lesion.[1,11] The decision to aspirate an ovarian lesion is usually determined by the radiographic findings, especially ultrasonography[2,4,11,12]. FNA of cystic and solid lesions present different problems and opinions concerning these diagnostic and therapeutic measures are not unanimous[2,4,8,9].

Ultrasound can generally distinguish unilocular cysts from those that are multiloculated, which have thick septa or contain solid areas[2,4,12]. Unilocular cysts, especially when present in young or pregnant women, are usually benign, while multiloculated cysts could be associated with a more serious lesion. Unilocular ovarian cysts measuring less than 5 cm in diameter are usually functional and resolve spontaneously[4,11,12]. Those between 5–10 cm are more likely to be symptomatic and associated with a more significant condition, including a neoplastic process, and are more often investigated by FNA[12,13].

In the proper clinical setting, if the aspirate from one of these cysts is straw coloured or clear, most patients are managed conservatively[4,12]. A high fluid level of unconjugated oestradiol-17β (E_2) favours a functional follicular cyst rather than a neoplastic process. However, certain ovarian neoplasms such as granulosa cell tumour also produce oestrogen and the measurement may therefore be of limited significance[4,12,14]. A high CA-125 level in the fluid may indicate a neoplastic process[15]. If, however, the cyst recurs after aspiration or the aspirated fluid is haemorrhagic, removal may be necessary[4,11,14]. When necrotic material or pus is aspirated, distinction between abscess and necrotic tumour may be cytologically difficult[4].

The use of immunocytochemical techniques enables, in most cases, the distinction between functional cysts and neoplastic cysts, which are usually lined by epithelial cells[10]. Positivity of cells with the antibody to the α-subunit, and to a lesser extent to the βA-subunit, of inhibin indicates follicular cells of a functional cyst. Positivity with BerEP4 or CA-125 indicates epithelial cells and hence a neoplasm, which can include endometriotic cysts[16].

Non-neoplastic cystic lesions of the ovary include follicular and corpus luteal cysts, germinal inclusion cysts and para-ovarian and paratubal cysts. In most aspirates from benign unilocular cysts with clear fluid the specimens are usually sparsely cellular, containing lymphocytes and macrophages[3,4,12]. It is often not possible to make a definitive diagnosis or differentiate the various types of cysts on the basis of the cytological findings alone[3,4,11,12].

Follicular cysts

Specimens from follicular cysts may include numerous granulosa cells arranged singly and in tight clusters (Fig. 36.1)[17]. The cells generally have round and sometimes oval nuclei, some of which have longitudinal nuclear grooves, producing a coffee bean appearance. They have coarsely granular chromatin rendering a pepper-pot appearance and a small rim of distinct cytoplasm (Fig. 36.2)[2,12,17]. Mitotic

figures may be present[17]. The existence of ciliated bodies (detached ciliary tufts in fluids of ovarian cysts) indicate the presence of ciliated columnar epithelial cells on the wall of the cysts, which would exclude cysts of follicular origin[18].

Luteinized follicular cysts

In addition to clusters of granulosa cells, luteinized follicular cysts are characterized by the presence of large polyhedral luteinized cells with abundant granular or vacuolated cytoplasm and slight anisocytosis (Fig. 36.3)[2,12,17]. The nuclei are often eccentric and have finely granular chromatin with one or two small prominent nucleoli[10]. Such cells are commonly seen during IVF treatment when the ovary is being stimulated with hormones. There may also be anisonucleosis in these circumstances.

Corpus luteum and luteal cysts

The presence of numerous luteinized granulosa cells in a background of fresh blood, haemosiderin-laden macrophages, fibrin and fibroblasts is consistent with haemorrhage into a corpus luteum or luteal cyst (Fig. 36.4)[17].

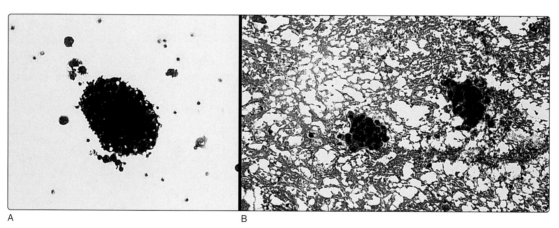

A   B

Fig. 36.1 Tightly packed clusters of follicular cells with round to oval nuclei and scanty cytoplasm. FNA of ovary. (A, MGG; B, Papanicolaou × MP)

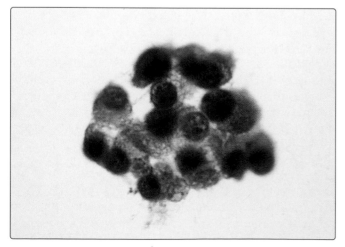

Fig. 36.2 Follicular cells with rounded nuclei containing multiple nucleoli and coarse chromatin rendering a pepper-pot appearance. FNA of ovary. (Papanicolaou × HP)

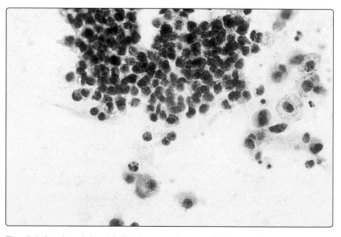

Fig. 36.3 Luteinized follicular cyst of ovary. A cluster of granulosa cells with round to oval nuclei and small rim of cytoplasm surrounded by larger luteinized granulosa cells with ample foamy cytoplasm. FNA of ovary. (Papanicolaou × MP)

The granulosa cells are often in small clusters, unlike the macrophages. Macrophages with haematoidin pigment and numerous fibroblasts suggest a regressing corpus luteum.

Luteinized follicular cysts of pregnancy

Aspirates from luteinized follicular cysts of pregnancy and the puerperium may yield cells with atypical cytological features[19]. These atypical luteinized granulosa cells exhibit an increased nuclear/cytoplasmic ratio, having enlarged nuclei with granular chromatin, chromocentres and prominent nucleoli. In some cells chromatin clearing and irregular nucleoli are present. Similar findings of cytological atypia, however, have been reported in cellular follicular cysts not associated with current or recent pregnancy[20]. Accurate clinical correlation is essential in order to minimize rendering a false positive diagnosis of malignancy.

Endometriotic cysts

Aspirates from endometriotic cysts are usually haemorrhagic and contain numerous haemosiderin-laden macrophages (Fig. 36.5)[1,3]. The presence of haemorrhage alone, recent or old, is insufficient for a diagnosis of endometriosis as many types of cysts may also show haemorrhage, including corpus luteal cysts and all forms of neoplastic cysts. In the background of degenerate blood, there is quite often cytonuclear debris including wisps of cytoplasm admixed with degenerate nuclear material, both generally of small size, but of variable shapes. Intact endometrial cells are seldom seen[3,5,17]. These cells are isolated or arranged in tight clusters. The cytoplasm is scanty and the nuclei are round or oval with finely granular chromatin (Fig. 36.6). In the absence of characteristic luteinized granulosa cells or intact endometrial cells, aspirates from haemorrhagic luteal cysts are difficult to distinguish from endometriosis[1,6,12,21,22].

Immunocytochemistry does help in distinguishing between haemorrhagic functional (corpus luteal or follicular) cysts and endometriotic cysts. Inhibin positivity indicates the former and BerEP4/CA-125 positivity, particularly in the cytoplasmic debris (Fig. 36.7) indicates the latter, although with BerEP4 positivity, it is not possible to exclude a neoplastic epithelial cell-lined cyst[16].

Occasional cases of clinically unsuspected endometriosis may be diagnosed by examining ovarian cyst fluid cytology

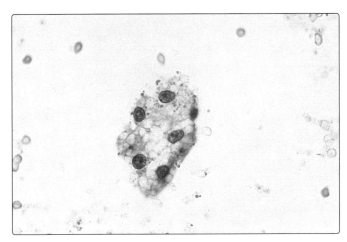

Fig. 36.4 Corpus luteum cyst of ovary. A loose cluster of luteinized granulosa cells containing round to oval nuclei with small prominent nucleoli. The cytoplasm is abundant with vacuolization. FNA of ovary. (Papanicolaou × MP)

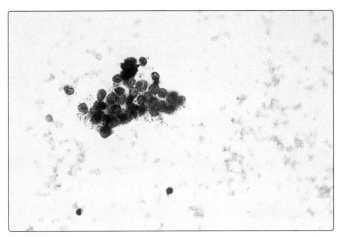

Fig. 36.6 Endometriosis of ovary. A tight cluster of small uniform endometrial cells. The background usually shows numerous haemosiderin-laden macrophages as illustrated in **Fig. 36.3**. FNA of ovary. (Papanicolaou × HP)

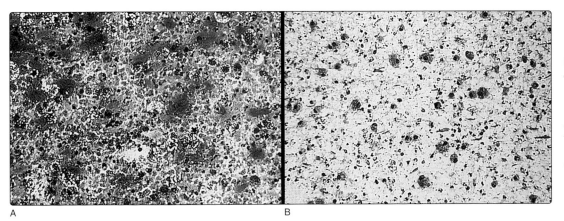

Fig. 36.5 Endometriosis of ovary. Degenerate blood in the background with haemosiderin-laden macrophages, indicative of old haemorrhage into cyst, with cytonuclear debris. Other types of cysts may also show old and recent haemorrhage. FNA of ovary. (A, MGG; B, Papanicolaou × HP)

A   B

849

as part of an *in vitro* fertilization (IVF) protocol[23]. Neither the cytomorphological features of this fluid nor the presence of endometrial cells, however, were useful in predicting IVF outcome[23].

Neoplasms

Benign ovarian tumours

Most benign epithelial tumours of ovary are cystic, filled with fluid and appear distended and tense, and are therefore seldom aspirated. In general, the finding of epithelium with or without atypia in needle aspirate smears warrants surgical intervention.

Serous cystadenomas

Aspirates from serous cystadenomas can be hypocellular and appear similar to non-neoplastic cysts[1,4,21]. They can only be diagnosed with confidence if in addition to macrophages, there are occasional single epithelial cells or aggregates of uniform cuboidal or columnar epithelial cells, sometimes papillary and lacking atypia and if these cells are ciliated (Fig. 36.8)[1,21,24].

Mucinous cystadenomas

Aspirates from mucinous cystadenomas are characterized by the presence of columnar mucin-secreting cells, arranged in honeycomb or picket-fence configurations in a mucinous background (Fig. 36.9)[1,3,24]. The cytoplasm contains either many small vacuoles or a single large vacuole displacing the nucleus to the periphery. The nuclei are homogeneous and have finely granular evenly distributed chromatin. Colonic cells contaminating transrectal aspirates can simulate the appearance of cells derived from mucinous cystadenomas[25].

Brenner tumours

Aspirates from Brenner tumours may contain both epithelial and mesenchymal cells[24]. Epithelial cells are

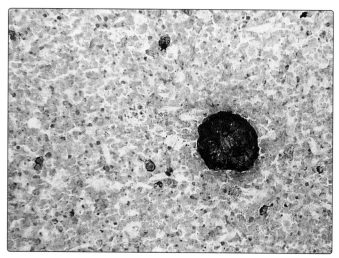

Fig. 36.7 BerEP4 positivity in cytoplasmic debris and scanty endometrioid cells in ovarian endometriosis. FNA of ovary. (× HP)

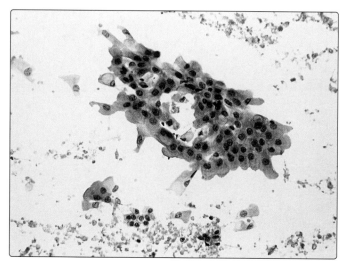

Fig. 36.9 Mucinous cystadenoma of ovary. A sheet of mucin secreting epithelial cells displaying both a honeycomb pattern and a picket-fence arrangement at the edges. FNA of ovary. (MGG × MP)

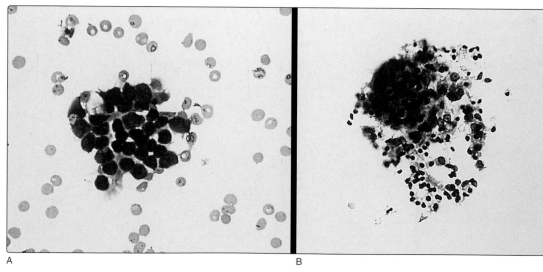

A   B

Fig. 36.8 Serous cystadenoma of ovary. A cluster of uniform cuboidal cells with round to oval nuclei and amphophilic cytoplasm, some of which are ciliated. FNA of ovary. (A, MGG; B, Papanicolaou × MP)

polygonal or cuboidal and occur singly or in sheets. The nuclei are ovoid and often have a linear groove giving them a coffee bean appearance. In some cases eosinophilic amorphous globules can be seen at the centre of the cell groups or lying free in the background. These correspond to the inspissated colloid material that is often present at the centre of epithelial islets in histological sections.

Epithelial tumours of low malignant potential (borderline tumours)

These present with greater cellularity and cytological features of malignancy (Fig. 36.10). The nuclei of the borderline tumours vary from slightly to markedly atypical and may contain nucleoli. The cells are seen singly or more frequently in groups with sheet-like or papillary configurations[24]. Serous and endometrioid tumours include columnar cells with eosinophilic cytoplasm; some of the cells are ciliated. Mucinous tumours show columnar cells with vacuoles of different sizes. Tumours with marked cellular atypia are almost invariably classified as carcinomas whereas tumours with mild atypia may be difficult to distinguish from benign cystadenomas[24]. The presence or absence of invasion cannot be determined from the aspirate smears; thus borderline malignant tumours are not cytologically distinguishable from malignant tumours[2,3,24].

Patients with a borderline (low malignant potential) mucinous neoplasm may have associated pseudomyxoma peritonei. Needle aspirate smears of pseudomyxoma peritonei are characterized by the presence of macroscopically gelatinous fluid that contains a dual population of mesothelial and fibroblastic cells in a background of fibrillary mucin. A few epithelial cells may be admixed[26].

Malignant ovarian tumours

Ovarian carcinomas are usually predominantly multicystic with a solid component and in roughly three-quarters of patients peritoneal tumour seeding is present at the time of diagnosis[1]. Aspirates may be obtained from primary, recurrent or metastatic sites and in most instances do not present a diagnostic problem[1–3,8].

The cytological diagnosis of ovarian carcinoma by FNA has a diagnostic accuracy in the range of 90–95%[25]. It is important to realize that a negative cytology result in the presence of a suspected lesion does not exclude malignancy. In these situations another aspirate or a surgical biopsy should be undertaken as the initial aspirate may have sampled a benign component of the tumour[1,8,24]. Subclassification of ovarian carcinomas on the basis of the cytological findings is possible in low and intermediate grade neoplasms; however, subtyping may be extremely difficult in high-grade tumours[2,8].

Serous cystadenocarcinomas

Serous cystadenocarcinomas (Fig. 36.11) are characterized by the presence of cuboidal to low columnar cells with moderate amounts of homogeneous basophilic cytoplasm

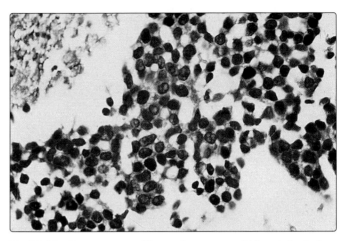

Fig. 36.10 Serous tumour of low malignant potential (borderline) of ovary. A loose cluster of cuboidal to columnar cells with irregular arrangement, nuclear hyperchromasia and an irregular chromatin pattern. FNA of ovary. (Papanicolaou × MP)

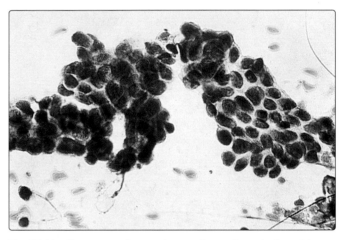

Fig. 36.11 Serous cystadenocarcinoma of ovary. Irregular branching group of malignant columnar cells with syncytial and papillary configurations. FNA of ovary. (Papanicolaou × MP)

arranged in syncytial and branching papillary groups[2,3,8,24]. The nuclei tend to be eccentric and are hyperchromatic with irregularly distributed chromatin. Nuclear pleomorphism and nucleoli are usually conspicuous. Although psammoma bodies (Fig. 36.12) are present in one third of these tumours, they are infrequently observed in aspirates[24,25].

Mucinous cystadenocarcinomas

Mucinous cystadenocarcinomas (Fig. 36.13) are characterized by the presence of numerous clusters of abnormal columnar cells surrounded by mucus. The cells can occur singly, in papillary groups, and in a picket-fence or honeycomb arrangement in low-grade tumours[1,3,8,21]. The tumour cells from low-grade lesions have abundant cytoplasm with single or multiple vacuoles. High-grade tumour cells have a high nuclear/cytoplasmic ratio and the enlarged nuclei are eccentrically placed and are often indented by the vacuoles. They have irregularly distributed chromatin material and

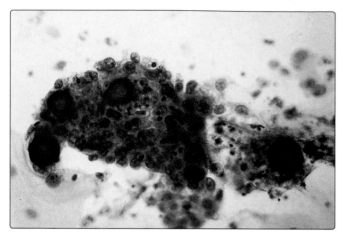

Fig. 36.12 Serous cystadenocarcinoma of ovary. Clusters of atypical cells centred around psammoma bodies. FNA of ovary. (Papanicolaou × HP)

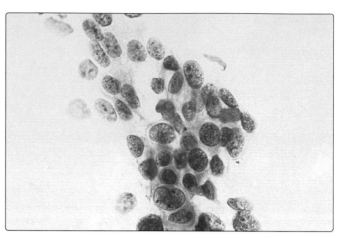

Fig. 36.14 Metastatic colonic adenocarcinoma to ovary. The cytological features are those of a mucinous adenocarcinoma and are indistinguishable from those of primary ovarian mucinous adenocarcinoma. The clinical findings were those of metastatic disease to the ovary. FNA ovary. (Papanicolaou × HP)

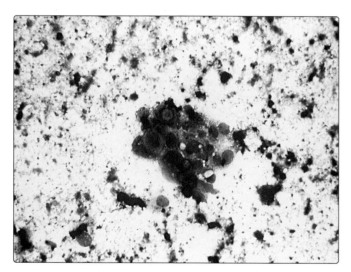

Fig. 36.13 Mucinous cystadenocarcinoma of ovary. Cytologically malignant mucin-secreting cells in a vague picket-fence arrangement. FNA of ovary. (MGG × MP)

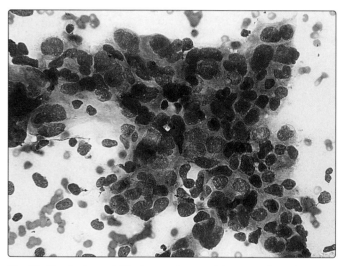

Fig. 36.15 Endometrioid adenocarcinoma of the ovary. Syncytial sheets of malignant cells with moderate amounts of granular cytoplasm and atypical nuclei. (MGG × MP)

nucleoli are seen. Metastatic mucin secreting carcinomas involving the ovary, known as Krukenberg tumours, can have the same cytological appearances as primary mucinous ovarian carcinomas (Fig. 36.14)[1]. In such cases, using a panel of antibodies, it may be possible to suggest a primary site of the tumour if the ovary itself is not considered to be the source of the malignant cells[16].

Endometrioid carcinomas

Primary carcinomas of endometrium and endometrioid carcinomas of the ovary have a similar appearance. They can be difficult to distinguish from serous carcinomas[1,3,24,25]. FNA samples from endometrioid tumours have abundant cells in syncytial groups and cell clusters with frequent acinar arrangements. Papillary groups are occasionally seen. Individual cells are cuboidal to polygonal and have small

amounts of homogeneous to finely granular cytoplasm (Fig. 36.15). Multiple small vacuoles and large single vacuoles may be present. The nuclei are round to oval, eccentric in position and have finely granular irregularly distributed chromatin with prominent nucleoli.

Clear cell carcinomas: adenosquamous carcinomas

Needle aspirates of clear cell carcinomas (Fig. 36.16) yield cells with abundant pale staining, finely granular, vacuolated cytoplasm[3,17]. Aspirates from adenosquamous carcinomas are composed of an admixture of malignant glandular cells with adenocarcinomatous features and malignant squamous cells. The glandular component usually predominates and is more easily identified than the squamous component, which is usually of the large cell non-keratinizing type.

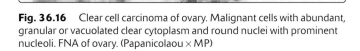

Fig. 36.16 Clear cell carcinoma of ovary. Malignant cells with abundant, granular or vacuolated clear cytoplasm and round nuclei with prominent nucleoli. FNA of ovary. (Papanicolaou × MP)

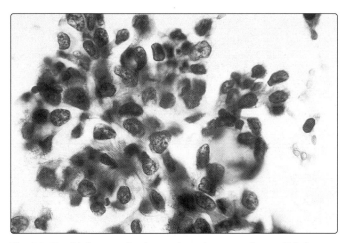

Fig. 36.17 Malignant mixed mesodermal tumour of ovary. This figure illustrates the malignant epithelial component, which is poorly-differentiated with features of adenocarcinoma. FNA of ovary. (Papanicolaou × HP)

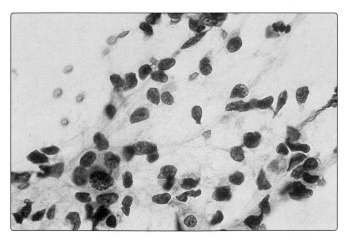

Fig. 36.18 Malignant mixed mesodermal tumour of ovary. This illustrates a malignant spindle cell mesenchymal component from the same case as **Fig. 36.17**. FNA of ovary. (Papanicolaou × HP)

Malignant mixed mesodermal tumours

Aspirates from malignant mixed mesodermal tumours (Figs 36.17, 36.18) tend to yield mostly the malignant epithelial component that appears as an adenocarcinoma. The sarcomatous component can present with isolated or small groups of spindle cells with features of malignancy, or as predominantly isolated large cells with bizarre configurations, dense cytoplasm and markedly abnormal nuclei[23]. If both epithelial and stromal elements are present an accurate diagnosis can be achieved; otherwise, the tumours are classified as adenocarcinomas or less frequently as sarcomas.

Granulosa cell tumours

Aspirates from granulosa cell tumours (Fig. 36.19) usually produce many tumour cells, which are arranged in solid, trabecular or follicular patterns[2,3,8,27]. In some tumours it is possible to observe small acinar-like structures with centrally placed amorphous, reddish violet bodies[3,23]. They correspond to the Call-Exner bodies which are characteristic of this type of tumour[3,23,28]. The cell pattern and the presence of Call-Exner bodies on aspirated cyst fluid aid in distinguishing cystic granulosa cell tumour from a follicular cyst[17]. The individual cells of granulosa cell tumour are homogeneous in appearance and have scanty cytoplasm. The nuclei are round to oval with granular evenly distributed chromatin and small nucleoli. Nuclear grooves can be seen in a number of nuclei[22,29]. The presence of cells with nuclear grooving, giving a coffee bean appearance and also, extracellular hyaline bodies may make the distinction between granulosa cell and Brenner tumour difficult although immunocytochemistry is useful in resolving this[16].

Sertoli cell tumours

Similarly, Sertoli-cell tumours, which show uniform oval nuclei with prominent nucleoli and irregularly distributed chromatin, are difficult to differentiate from granulosa cell tumour in cytological material[22].

Juvenile granulosa cell tumour

This differs cytologically from its adult counterpart by the lack of prominent grooved nuclei, absence of Call-Exner

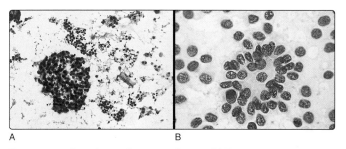

Fig. 36.19 Granulosa cell tumour of ovary. (A) Tumour cells in a cluster with a vague acinus-like arrangement. (Papanicolaou × MP) (B) Scattered nuclei show nuclear grooves. (Papanicolaou × HP) FNA of ovary.

bodies and the presence of mucin and prominent lipid vacuoles in granulosa cells[30].

Sex cord tumours with annular tubules

Cytologically, sex cord tumours with annular tubules present with relatively uniform cells that are predominantly isolated but also occur in solid, follicular and trabecular arrangements[31]. The tumour cells have a small to medium amount of pale cytoplasm. The nuclei are round to oval with evenly distributed chromatin, a small nucleolus and occasional nuclear grooving. Round or oval shaped hyaline bodies with palisading producing rosette or ring-like arrangements of the nuclei at their periphery are typically present. Again it is difficult to distinguish these tumours cytologically from granulosa cell tumours[31].

Dysgerminomas

Dysgerminomas usually have a distinctive appearance on needle aspirate samples. They are composed of numerous large poorly cohesive cells, with relatively abundant delicate pale staining cytoplasm. The nuclei are large with clumped, irregularly distributed chromatin and macronucleoli. Mitotic figures can be numerous. Mature lymphocytes and occasional multinucleated giant cells of trophoblastic origin are usually present in the background[24]. These cells are usually positive on staining immunocytochemically with placental alkaline phosphatase (PLAP).

Yolk sac tumours

The cells obtained from aspiration of yolk sac tumours are often large with voluminous cytoplasm, but small nuclei. The cytoplasm is generally clear or eosinophilic and granular. The cells are usually arranged in small flat sheets. These cells would be positive on staining immunocytochemically with alpha-fetoprotein (AFP).

Other common ovarian tumours

Fibrothecomatous tumours

Aspirations from this group of tumours contain sparse cellular material. They are composed of spindle cells, either isolated or in bundles, with scant cytoplasm and elongated nuclei in which coarsely granular, but evenly distributed chromatin is seen. In some cases, luteinized cells with more abundant, finely vacuolated cytoplasm may be present. Aspirates from these tumours can be misinterpreted as leiomyomas[24].

Benign cystic teratoma (dermoid cyst)

These tumours usually yield a viscous, oily substance, amorphous debris, numerous anucleate squames, superficial squamous cells and hair (Figs 36.20, 36.21). Other epithelial components such as respiratory and intestinal epithelium may occasionally be present. Occasionally colloid and thyroid follicular cells can be identified if there is a large component of struma ovarii. Transvaginal aspirates contaminated with vaginal squamous cells can sometimes simulate a dermoid cyst.

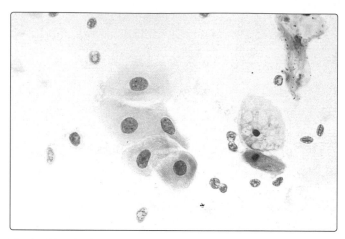

Fig. 36.20   Benign mature cystic teratoma of ovary. Mature superficial squamous cells are present. FNA of ovary. (Papanicolaou × MP)

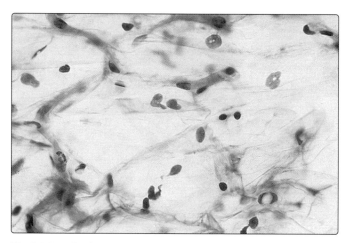

Fig. 36.21   Benign mature cystic teratoma of ovary. Mature adipose tissue. Abundant cellular and keratin debris were also present. This is from the same aspirate as shown in **Fig. 36.20**. FNA of ovary. (Papanicolaou × MP)

If hair is identified in smears and contamination can be ruled out, this is pathognomonic for teratoma[3,17,32].

Laboratory procedures in FNA cytology of ovarian cysts

The advent of immunocytochemistry has altered the potential of cytological diagnoses in ovarian cysts. In the last 5 years, there has been a surge of research into inhibin and no less in cytology[10,16]. The availability of monoclonal antibodies to the subunits of inhibin has enabled confident detection of follicular (granulosa) cells in aspirates (Figs 36.22, 36.23)[10], and when used in conjunction with epithelial markers such as BerEP4, CA-125 and cytokeratin (CK) 7 (the latter two are relatively specific for ovary), it allows the distinction between functional, non-neoplastic cysts and neoplastic epithelial cell-lined cysts which require removal[16].

In cases of metastatic carcinoma, it may be possible to determine the site of origin of the malignant cells. For example, gastrointestinal tumours are generally positive on staining with antibodies to carcinoembryonic antigen

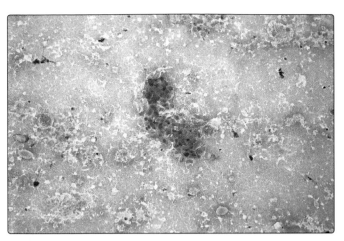

Fig. 36.22 Follicular cells from a functional cyst staining positively with α-inhibin immunocytochemistry. FNA of ovary. (Immunoalkaline phosphatase × MP)

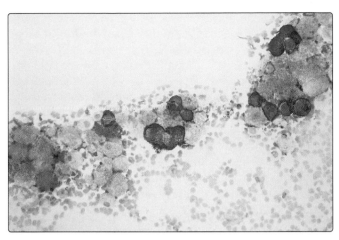

Fig. 36.24 Metastatic colonic carcinoma in the ovary. These cells stain positively with CK 20 immunocytochemistry. FNA of ovary. (Immunoalkaline phosphatase × MP)

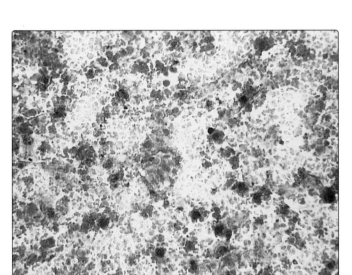

Fig. 36.23 Corpus luteal cells from an haemorrhagic cyst staining positively with α-inhibin immunocytochemistry. FNA of ovary. (× MP)

(CEA) and CK20 (Fig. 36.24). These tumours are CK7 negative[16].

In germ cell tumours, it may be possible to diagnose dysgerminomas (PLAP positive), yolk-sac tumours (AFP positive) and choriocarcinomas (β human chorionic gonadotrophin (βHCG) positive). Sex-cord/stromal tumours are usually inhibin positive[16].

Value of FNA in ovarian tumour diagnosis

In summary, under appropriate conditions fine needle aspiration cytology of the ovary is useful in the diagnosis of ovarian lesions. It is especially helpful in the diagnosis and management of benign cysts and in the diagnosis of recurrent ovarian cancer. It is also ideal in rare cases where laparoscopy cannot be performed because of poor physical condition of the patient[9,21]. However, it is difficult, if not impossible, to separate most primary ovarian carcinomas from metastatic carcinomas to the ovary solely on the basis of the cytological findings[3,24,25]. Full knowledge of the clinical and radiographic findings and the implications of the cytological diagnosis on management cannot be overemphasized.

Fallopian tubes

The application of cytological techniques for detection of fallopian tube lesions is limited. Malignant cells from the fallopian tubes are occasionally accidentally detected in endometrial, cervical or vaginal samples. Data are not available on the specific use of fine needle aspiration in detecting tubal carcinoma. The cytopathological features of tubo-ovarian abscess, cysts and endometriosis are discussed in Chapter 37.

Benign fallopian tube lesions

Occasionally aspiration of a hydrosalpinx is undertaken either in the IVF unit or at laparoscopy/laparotomy. The fluid obtained from such aspirates is generally hypocellular and comprises of macrophages, lymphoid cells and scanty epithelial cells, which are variably degenerate. A diagnosis of hydrosalpinx can only be proffered or confirmed if these epithelial cells are ciliated. In such circumstances, it may not be possible to exclude a benign serous cystadenoma of the ovary although the ovarian lesion is often more cellular.

Carcinoma of fallopian tubes

The reported incidence of primary fallopian tube cancer ranges from 0.13–1.8% of gynaecological malignancies[33,34]. Most patients are post-menopausal, with a mean age of 56 years. They present with a variety of symptoms including profuse watery discharge (hydrops tubae proliferans), vaginal bleeding and abdominal pain[33–35]. At the time of presentation, approximately three-quarters of patients have local and distant spread, often making it difficult to ascertain the primary site of origin[35].

A variety of cytological techniques can be employed, separately or in combination, in the study of fallopian tube carcinoma. Watery vaginal discharge is observed in up to 15% of patients and is potentially rich in tumour cells. Brewer and Guderian reported two patients presenting with watery discharge in whom the diagnosis of carcinoma was made in one and suspected in the other[36]. Harai et al. studied ten patients where two patients presenting with vaginal discharge had no tumour cells in cytological samples[37]. In their experience, endometrial samples showed malignant cells in six patients and this was the most effective means of detecting fallopian tube cancer. All endometrial aspirates from eight patients with fallopian tube carcinoma reported by King et al. were, however, negative[38]. Vaginal, ectocervical and endocervical samples have similarly proved to be insensitive methods for screening patients with fallopian tube carcinoma, detection rates ranging from 0–20%[39].

Cytological findings

The cytopathological features of adenocarcinoma of the fallopian tube are not distinctive or unique to the site[35]. The smears usually show a clean background and when malignant cells are present, there is a paucity of cellular material, features noted in cervicovaginal smears that contain malignant tumour cells from any other extrauterine origin (see Fig. 35.43)[37,38]. The malignant cells are most commonly glandular in origin and occur singly or in clusters. They are medium-sized, with round to oval nuclei, coarse chromatin, nucleoli and variably vacuolated cytoplasm[40]. A second population of small cells with pyknotic nuclei and scant cytoplasm has been described[40].

The neoplastic cells from fallopian tube adenocarcinoma are histopathologically and cytopathologically similar to those from ovarian, endometrial and endocervical carcinomas. In the absence of diagnostic features, the cytopathologist is more likely to suggest an origin from these more common sites than from the fallopian tube[39]. In general, fallopian tube carcinoma should be suspected when malignant cells are noted in patients with unremarkable pelvic examination and negative endometrial curettings.

Malignant tumour cells from fallopian tube adenocarcinoma may also be encountered in ascitic fluid or peritoneal washings and are similarly nondescript. Primary mixed mesodermal tumours and squamous cell carcinomas of the fallopian tube have been reported; however, the cytological features should be similar to their counterparts seen in the endometrium and cervix respectively.

References

1 Kjellren O, Angstrom T. Transvaginal and transrectal aspiration biopsy in diagnosis and classification of ovarian tumors. In: Zajicek K ed. *Aspiration Biopsy Cytology, Part II: Cytology of Infradiaphragmatic Organs.* Basel: S Karger, 1979; 80–103

2 Ganjei P, Nadji M. Aspiration cytology of ovarian neoplasms: a review. *Acta Cytol* 1984; **28**: 329–332

3 Angstrom T. Aspiration cytology of ovarian tumors. In: Wied G L, Keebler C M, Koss L G, Reagan J W eds. Compendium on diagnostic cytology. *Tutorials of Cytology*, 6th edn. Chicago, IL: 1988; 507–512

4 Buckley C H. Review article. Is needle aspiration of ovarian cysts adequate for diagnosis? *Br J Obstet Gynaecol* 1989; **96**: 1021–1023

5 Hasson H M. Laparoscopic management of ovarian cysts. *J Reproductive Med* 1990; **35**: 863–867

6 Salat-Baroux J, Merviel P, Kuttenn F. Management of ovarian cysts. *BMJ* 1996; **313**: 1098

7 Zanetta G, Lissoni A, Torri V et al. Role of puncture and aspiration in expectant management of simple ovarian cysts: a randomised study. *BMJ* 1996; **313**: 1110–1113

8 Granados R. Aspiration cytology of ovarian tumours. *Curr Opin Obstet Gynaecol* 1995; **7**: 43–48

9 Trimbos J B, Hacker N. The case against aspirating ovarian cysts. *Cancer* 1993; **72**: 828–831

10 McCluggage W G, Maxwell P, Sloan J. Immunocytochemical staining of ovarian cyst aspirates with monoclonal antibody against inhibin. *Cytopathol* 1998; **9**: 336–342

11 Khaw K T, Walker W J. Ultrasound guided fine needle aspiration of ovarian cysts: diagnosis and treatment in pregnant and non-pregnant women. *Clin Radiol* 1990; **41**: 102–108

12 De Crespigny L, Robinson H P, Davoren R A, Fortune D. The 'simple' ovarian cyst: aspirate or operate? *Br J Obstet Gynaecol* 1989; **96**: 1035–1039

13 Rodin A, Coltart T N, Chapman M G. Needle aspiration of simple ovarian cysts in pregnancy. Case reports. *Br J Obstet Gynaecol* 1989; **96**: 994–996

14 Geier G R, Strecher J R. Aspiration cytology and E₂ content in ovarian tumors. *Acta Cytol* 1981; **25**: 400–406

15 Menczer J, ben-baruch G, Moran O, Lipitz S. Cyst fluid CA-125 levels in ovarian epithelial neoplasms. *Obstet Gynecol* 1993; **81**: 25–28

16 Manek S. The role of immunohistochemistry in gynaecological diseases. *CPD Bull Cell Pathol* 1999; **1**: 162–166

17 Selvaggi S M. Cytology of non-neoplastic cysts of the ovary. *Diagn Cytopathol* 1990; **6**: 77–85

18 Rivasi F, Gasser B, Morandi P, Phillipe E. Ciliated bodies in ovarian cyst aspirates. *Acta Cytol* 1993; **37**(4): 489–493

19 Selvaggi S M. Fine needle aspiration cytology of ovarian follicle cysts with cellular atypia from reproductive-age patients. *Diagn Cytopathol* 1991; **7**: 189–192

20 Stanley M W, Horwitz C A, Frable W J. Cellular follicular cyst of the ovary. Fluid cytology mimicking malignancy. *Diagn Cytopathol* 1991; **7**: 48–52

21 Kovacic J, Rainer S, Levicnic A, Cizelj T. Cytology of benign ovarian lesions in connection with laparoscopy. In: Zajicek J ed. *Aspiration Biopsy Cytology, Part II: Cytology of Infradiaphragmatic Organs.* Basel: S Karger, 1979; 57–79

22 Ramzy I, Delaney M, Rose P. Fine needle aspiration of ovarian masses. II. Correlative cytologic and histologic study of non-neoplastic cysts and non-celomic epithelial neoplasms. *Acta Cytol* 1979; **23**: 185–193

23 Greenebaum E, Mayer J R, Stangel J J, Hughes P. Aspiration cytology of ovarian cysts in in vitro fertilization patients. *Acta Cytol* 1992; **36**(1): 11–18

24 Nunez C. Cytopathology and fine needle aspiration in ovarian tumors: its utility in diagnosis and management. In: Nogales F ed. *Current Topics in Pathology*, vol. **78**: *Ovarian Pathology*. Berlin: Springer-Verlag, 1989; 69–83

25 Kjellgren O, Angstrom T, Bergman F, Wiklund D-E. Fine needle aspiration biopsy in diagnosis and classification of ovarian carcinoma. *Cancer* 1971; **28**: 967–976

26 Leiman G, Goldberg R. Pseudomyxoma peritonei associated with ovarian mucinous tumours. Cytologic appearance in five cases. *Acta Cytol* **36**(3): 299–304

27 Bjersing L, Frankendal B, Angstrom T. Studies on a feminizing ovarian mesenchymoma (granulosa cell tumor). I. Aspiration biopsy cytology, histology and ultrastructure. *Cancer* 1973; **32**: 1360–1369

28 Ehya M, Lang W R. Cytology of granulosa cell tumor of the ovary. *Am J Clin Pathol* 1986; **85**: 402–405

29 Benda J A, Zaleski S. Fine needle aspiration cytologic features of hepatic metastasis of granulosa cell tumor of the ovary: differential diagnosis. *Acta Cytol* 1988; **32**: 527–532

30 Stamp G W, Kraus Z T. Fine needle aspiration cytology of a recurrent juvenile granulosa cell tumor. *Acta Cytol* 1988; **32**: 533–539

31 Yazdi H M. Fine needle aspiration cytology of ovarian sex cord tumor with annular tubules. *Acta Cytol* 1987; **31**: 340–344

32 Miller S J, Waddell C A, Rollason T P, Barber P. Perplexing findings in a cystic teratoma. *Cytopathol* 2001; **12**: 49–53

33 Eddy G L, Copeland L J, Gershenson D M *et al*. Fallopian tube carcinoma. *Obstet Gynecol* 1984; **64**: 546–552

34 Podratz K C, Podczaski E D, Gaffey T A *et al*. Primary carcinoma of the fallopian tube. *Am J Obstet Gynecol* 1986; **154**: 1319–1326

35 Saigo P E. Unusual tumors. In: Bibbo M ed. *Comprehensive cytopathology*. Philadelphia: WB Saunders, 1991; 299–302

36 Brewer J I, Guderian A M. Diagnosis of uterine-tube carcinoma by vaginal cytology. *Obstet Gynecol* 1956; **8**: 664–672

37 Harai Y, Chen J-T, Hama T *et al*. Clinical and cytologic aspects of primary fallopian tube carcinoma. A report of ten cases. *Acta Cytol* 1987; **31**: 834–840

38 King A, Seraj I M, Thrasher T *et al*. Fallopian tube carcinoma: a clinicopathological study of 17 cases. *Gynecol Oncol* 1989; **33**: 351–355

39 Garrett R. Extrauterine tumor cells in vaginal and cervical smears. *Obstet Gynecol* 1959; **14**: 21–27

40 Benson P A. Cytologic diagnosis in primary carcinoma of fallopian tube. Case report and review. *Acta Cytol* 1974; **18**: 429–434

37 Fine needle aspiration of benign and malignant gynaecological lesions

Geoff Watson, Paul McKenzie and Alan B P Ng

Introduction

While exfoliative cytology represents the commonest cytological screening modality for gynaecological lesions, fine needle aspiration (FNA) cytology has a diagnostic role in delineating the nature of pelvic mass lesions, some of which may be gynaecological in nature. FNA requires a clinically or radiologically defined lesion for targeted biopsy, and the usual guidance modality for intra-pelvic masses will be ultrasound or computed tomography (CT), although occasionally laparoscopic and transvaginal/transrectal approaches are also done. Transvaginal FNA is mainly used for diagnosing vaginal vault or low pelvic recurrences in patients with previous gynaecological malignancies[4]. Lymph node FNA of inguinal and supraclavicular sites is occasionally done[1-6].

The role of FNA is in obtaining a tissue diagnosis via the least invasive method, and, if supervised by the cytologist, may be used in conjunction with core tissue sampling if the FNA indicates a requirement for further tissue. In certain situations, FNA can be used to circumvent more invasive modalities of tissue diagnosis or to obviate the need for a 'second-look' laparotomy/laparoscopy, or it can be used to plan the surgery.

Although the interpretive skills are similar, the issue of immediate cytology used as an adjunct to frozen section diagnosis is beyond the scope of this chapter but it should be stated that such activity provides excellent training in FNA interpretation.

Indications

The main role of FNA in gynaecological lesions is in detecting recurrences of malignancy, mainly at intra-abdominal, vault, inguinal, pelvic and para-aortic node sites, or in acting as a staging modality for assessing spread beyond the abdominal cavity.

In primary diagnosis of pelvic lesions the main use of FNA is where the mass is not clearly gynaecological in origin or when a benign diagnosis is suspected, but requires further investigation because the patient has intercurrent pathology.

FNA has been used to determine the response to radiotherapy or chemotherapy by assessing whether a residual mass lesion contains viable tumour cells, although positron emission tomography (PET) scanning has an evolving role in this.

Core biopsies have become increasingly common as an adjunct to FNA where the aspirate is minimally yielding, where the diagnosis is unusual or if the case requires significant immunohistochemical study.

Contraindications

1. Ovarian primary neoplasms are usually not aspirated, because they are often cystic and as such carry a small risk of the FNA puncture, producing leakage of cyst content into the peritoneal cavity, upstaging the lesion. The risk of spillage from a cyst is related to the tension and thinness of the cyst wall, as well as the needle size.

   A more cogent reason for not performing FNA is that the investigation does not alter the subsequent management of surgical exploration and excision. Before undertaking any investigation on a patient it is important to address how the test is likely to influence subsequent clinical management. Furthermore the architectural patterns are very important in ovarian tumour diagnosis, and FNA can have diagnostic limitations with low-grade and borderline tumours.

2. In the presence of bowel obstruction or ileus, where the needle may traverse a distended bowel and carry the risk of bowel puncture/perforation, FNA is contra-indicated.

3. Other FNA contraindications, as at other sites, include bleeding diathesis and patient compliance.

Normal cytological findings

While it is important to be aware of what regions were traversed by the needle to sample the lesion, the use of stiletted needles by many radiologists tends to reduce the sampling to the lesion or possibly contiguous structures.

The cytologist should insist on finding out as much information about the site and size of a mass and the clinical background of the case for the purpose of assessing what questions the investigation is attempting to answer.

FNA findings in benign lesions

FNA of benign solid gynaecological lesions is an uncommon procedure, generally confined to those cases where an unusual site produces diagnostic uncertainty and the subsequent treatment plan is non-surgical. Leiomyomas in usual locations such as pedunculated

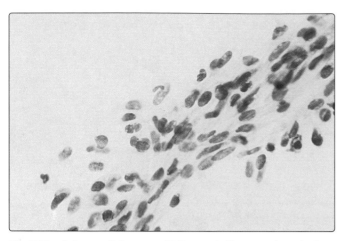

Fig. 37.1   Subserosal leiomyoma. Uniform spindle mesenchymal cells with oval and elongated nuceli. FNA of pelvic mass. (Papanicolaou × MP)

subserosal fibroids and those in broad ligament, or large degenerate fibroids growing up out of the pelvis are occasionally aspirated to exclude other lesions. The aspirates from a leiomyoma (Fig. 37.1) usually have a firm consistency and contain scant material comprising tightly clustered spindle cells or occasional single cells, sometimes with stripped nuclei: the low yield precluding certainty as to whether this is perilesional smooth muscle sampling and careful radio-pathological correlation is required. Definitive diagnosis on smooth muscle lesions often requires a core sample.

Adenomatoid tumours may enter into the differential diagnosis.

Aspiration of adnexal/ovarian cystic lesions under laparoscopic or ultrasound guidance is a more frequent procedure[7-11]. Aspirating cystic lesions is generally reserved for cases in which the imaged diagnosis favours a benign lesion, and its main role is in delineating between functional and non-functional cysts. Non-functional cysts are generally subsequently excised. As such, ovarian cyst aspiration tends to have its role in the pre-menopausal group, where there is the possibility of functional cysts needing to be excluded.

A recent paper looking at the sensitivities of aspiration cytology in adnexal cysts[7] found limitations in the sensitivity of the test (particularly for functional cysts and benign serous cysts), but a high specificity when a cell yield was achieved.

In general terms, functional cysts have a variable cellularity (often very scant) with the follicular cell morphology also varying depending on luteinization. Concomitant hormone studies (e.g. cyst fluid estradiol content >20 nmol/l)[9] may increase the diagnostic accuracy.

Non-functional cysts include epithelial cysts, endometriotic cysts and cystic neoplasms. Simple epithelial cysts contain macrophages, but usually do not exfoliate cells, resulting in their low rate of diagnosis by aspiration.

Old endometriotic cysts tend to yield mainly altered degenerate blood and haemosiderin-laden macrophages, while endometrial cells are seldom seen, and if present are degenerate.

Cystic neoplasms may be of surface epithelial or germ cell origin. Aspiration of cystic neoplasms acts to direct these cases for laparoscopic/surgical removal, and FNA is not considered part of the diagnostic work-up of these lesions.

The cytological appearances of diagnostic ovarian cyst aspiration is covered in greater detail in the preceding chapter.

Inflammatory pelvic lesions are rarely submitted to FNA, though pelvic abscesses and occasional tubo-ovarian abscesses may be initially aspirated for diagnosis prior to drainage. Cytologically these contain neutrophils, fibrin, necrotic debris and variable numbers of macrophages. Culture can be performed on aspirates.

Transvaginal fine needle aspiration has been utilized in establishing a diagnosis of actinomycotic infection of the parametrium in the absence of tubo-ovarian abscess[12].

FNA findings in malignant lesions
Squamous cell carcinoma

FNA of squamous cell carcinoma (SCC) derived from the female genital tract may be seen as a transvaginal aspirate for vault recurrence, radiological guided aspirate of pelvic nodes or percutaneous biopsy of distant metastases such as in the supraclavicular fossa. The cytological findings are similar to SCC elsewhere. The initial diagnosis on a Giemsa-based stain may be hindered by necrosis, so collecting adequate material for Papanicolaou staining (Fig. 37.2) or cell block, is important. SCC metastatic in distant sites requires close clinicopathological correlation to exclude the possibility of a second primary. No current immunochemistry is useful in resolving this issue.

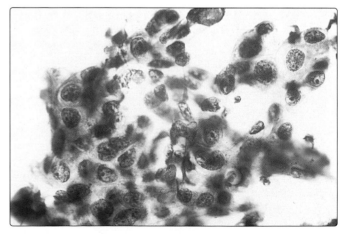

Fig. 37.2   Squamous cell carcinoma. A needle aspirate of a retroperitoneal lymph node in a patient with squamous cell carcinoma of the cervix, large cell non-keratinizing type, yielded a syncytium of malignant epithelial cells. The cells are pleomorphic with indistinct cytoplasmic borders, irregular nuclei, coarsely granular, unevenly distributed chromatin and prominent nucleoli. (Papanicolaou × HP)

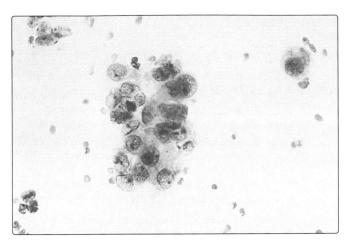

Fig. 37.3   Metastatic endometrial carcinoma. Needle aspirate of a pelvic mass in a patient previously treated for endometrial carcinoma yielded a cluster of malignant glandular cells consistent with metastatic tumour. (Papanicolaou × HP)

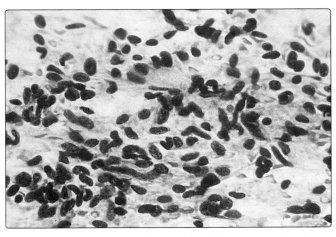

Fig. 37.4   Leiomyosarcoma. Pleomorphic and hyperchromatic malignant spindle mesenchymal cells consistent with sarcoma. FNA of pelvic mass. (Papanicolaou × MP)

Adenocarcinoma

Again, the main role of FNA is in identifying recurrences locally in the pelvis or assessing distant metastasis.

The main difficulty usually lies not in establishing malignant criteria, but determining the likely primary site. A history of a previous gynaecological adenocarcinoma (Fig. 37.3) is very helpful, but the issue of dual pathologies needs also to be considered, particularly breast and colon carcinoma. Comparison with the previous surgical material is worthwhile, but care must be taken to consider grade progression or morphological alteration resulting from intercurrent radiotherapy/chemotherapy, as well as remembering that the FNA is sampling only a tiny and often degenerate part of the tumour. The use of immunochemistry using CA125, cytokeratin 7 and 20 subsets, as well as oestrogen and progesterone receptors can be worthwhile. Inhibin and CEA also have their roles.

It is necessary to remember the limitations of cytology in sub-typing some gynaecological adenocarcinomas, particularly those which are very high grade, with which histopathology, with the added dimension of architecture, may also struggle.

Some of the clinical features of an adenocarcinoma may help lead to a diagnosis. A case, seen by one of us (GW), of a 42-year-old woman presenting with cerebellar dysfunction found to be on the basis of anti-Purkinje cell antibodies, was tracked by CT to having L1-2 para-aortic lymphadenopathy. FNA of the node identified metastatic serous carcinoma suggesting ovary as a primary site since cerebellar dysfunction is a recognized paraneoplastic phenomenon in ovarian serous carcinoma. A sub-imageable ovarian primary was then identified laparoscopically. Similarly the hypercalcaemia of ovarian small cell carcinoma can be useful.

Sometimes the radiological appearance may offer some clues to subtyping. Heavy calcification may be seen in lower-grade serous carcinomas, but also mucinous tumours and some germ cell tumours may need to be considered.

Cystic change within a tumour may be merely an indicator of central degeneration, but serous and mucinous carcinoma, mixed differentiation (e.g. adenosquamous), carcinoma arising in or overgrowing a benign lesion, and metastatic colon carcinoma should also be considered.

It is wise to think critically about each case, and not to default to diagnose all pelvic epithelial malignancy as adenocarcinoma, although statistically, most are indeed adenocarcinomas. Similarly, the apparently undifferentiated gynaecological tumour found on FNA may present problems, with minimal immunochemical reactions being obtained. It is then necessary to reconsider initial assumptions and to extend the differential to non-epithelial neoplasms, such as chloroma, Burkitt's lymphoma, granulosa cell tumour and germ cell tumour. Electron microscopy can be used on FNA material, but remember that if it is poorly differentiated by light microscopy, it is similar for the electron microscopist, and such difficult FNA cases may be better investigated surgically.

Malignant mixed mesodermal tumour (MMMT)

This tumour is characterized by an admixture of malignant epithelial and malignant stromal components[13,14]. The relative mix may vary within different areas of the tumour and FNA tends to obtain a greater amount of epithelial sampling. If the stromal component is sampled, it may be difficult to recognize the isolated small groups of spindle cells and stripped bizarre nuclei amongst the adenocarcinoma cells and they may be incorrectly dismissed as being part of the desmoplastic reaction to the tumour or degenerative changes within the carcinoma. The stromal component may include features of leiomyosarcoma (Fig. 37.4), rhabdomyosarcoma, or osteo- or chondrosarcoma. Metastasis from MMMT may have an altered proportion of the two elements. Heterologous elements may be present in MMMTs but are rarely identifiable by the cytologist.

Endometrial stromal sarcomas (ESS)

These are difficult lesions cytologically. They tend to yield fairly large amounts of cells in tightly packed aggregates with limited cytoplasm. The cell size will vary from slightly larger than normal stromal cells in low-grade ESS, to large pleomorphic cells in high-grade ESS (see Chapter 35). The key to recognizing ESS cytologically is the rich capillary vascularity within them. There are few immunochemical markers which are useful, though oestrogen and progesterone receptors are expressed in low-grade ESS, permitting distinction from a non-uterine sarcoma. High-grade ESS is usually negative for ER and PR. Desmin is typically negative distinguishing a cellular leiomyoma.

Non-gynaecological malignancy

Lesions metastatic to the pelvis from the colon, stomach and pancreas via transcoelomic seeding must be considered by both the cytopathologist and surgical pathologist reporting pelvic lesions. Aside from pancreas, CT imaging has major limitations, and the pathologist may be presented with a flawed premise from the clinicians of a primary gynaecological lesion. Serum CA125 elevation to low levels (100–200 IU/ml) may be a non-specific peritoneal reaction, but may be misinterpreted by clinicians. Carcinoembryonic antigen (CEA) in serum and on immunoperoxidase staining may be useful, although ovarian mucinous adenocarcinomas and cervical adenocarcinomas often have strong CEA staining. Cytokeratin 20 can help delineate the colonic primaries.

Breast carcinoma, particularly lobular carcinoma, may metastasize and tends to form a solid mass with cells growing in a permeative fashion. Distinction from a poorly-differentiated gastric carcinoma may be difficult. Lymphoma should also be considered in any permeative malignancy. Melanoma can metastasize anywhere, although small bowel is usually more common than gynaecological organs. Amelanotic forms and cases with a hitherto unknown primary or prolonged latency for recurrence can be missed if melanoma is not considered.

Diagnostic accuracy

The diagnostic accuracy of FNA is influenced by factors such as the size of the lesion, the accessibility of its location, the tissue consistency and operator experience for both radiologist and pathologist. The cytopathologist should ideally have access to the full clinical history of previous neoplasia, as well as radiological details of the lesion being sampled. It should be remembered that radiology, like cytology, is also an interpretive modality, so in the region of the uterus and adnexa, exact anatomical siting of a lesion may require ultrasound in addition to CT, and the pathologist should not make cytological assumptions based on a perceived site of sample.

In general, the specificity of FNA of the female genital tract has been reported as high as 85–100% and the sensitivity has ranged from 65–91%. In most studies, not only has it been possible to differentiate between benign and malignant lesions, but it was usually also possible to classify tumours accurately in histological terms. The degree of reporting accuracy will of course vary if FNA is being used mainly for staging or detecting recurrences.

A diagnostic result on FNA may obviate the need for surgical biopsy in the follow-up of patients with malignancy and can direct management for the oncologist or radiotherapist. However a negative result should be viewed judiciously, and important therapeutic decisions should not be based on a negative FNA result. Inadequate or negative aspirates in the presence of a suspected lesion should be followed by either a repeat aspirate or a surgical biopsy. The evolving use of PET scanning may help the clinician apportion an appropriate degree of suspicion on an imaged lesion; however PET may have spurious positivity in the presence of inflammation, and the test cannot replace obtaining a tissue diagnosis.

In reporting FNA cases, it is recommended that the cytopathologist's report be expressed in terms as close as possible to those used in histopathology avoiding 'positive' and 'negative' terminology.

In conclusion, FNA as a test has a defined role and is capable of high accuracy, but its indications and limitations need to be appreciated.

References

1 Ganjei P. Fine-needle aspiration cytology of the ovary (review). *Clin Lab Med* 1995; **15**(3): 705–726

2 Sevin B U, Greening S E, Nadji M et al. Fine needle aspiration cytology in gynaecologic oncology. *Acta Cytol* 1979; **23**: 277–281 and 380–388

3 Moriaty A T, Glant D, Stehman F B. The role of fine needle aspiration cytology in the management of gynaecologic malignancies. *Acta Cytol* 1986; **30**: 59–64

4 Ylagan L R, Mutch D G, Davila R M. Transvaginal fine needle aspiration biopsy. *Acta Cytol* 2001; **45**: 927–930

5 Helmkamp B F, Sevin B U, Greening S E et al. Fine needle aspiration cytology of supraclavicular lymph nodes in gynaecologic malignancies. *Gynaecol Oncol* 1981; **11**: 89–95

6 Burke T W, Heller P B, Hoskins W J et al. Evaluation of the scalene lymph nodes in primary and recurrent cervical carcinoma. *Gynaecol Oncol* 1987; **28**: 312–317

7 Martinez-Onsurbe P, Villaespesa A R, Anquela J M S, Ruiz P L V. Aspiration cytology of 147 adnexal cysts with histological correlation. *Acta Cytol* 2001; **45**: 941–947

8 Higgins R V, Matkins J F, Marroum M C. Comparison of fine-needle aspiration

cytologic findings of ovarian cysts with ovarian histologic findings. *Am J Obstet Gynecol* 1999; **180**(3): 550–553

9 Mulvany N J Aspiration cytology of ovarian cysts and cystic neoplasms. A study of 235 aspirates. *Acta Cytol* 1996; **40**(5): 911–920

10 Ganjei P, Dickinson B, Harrison T et al. Aspiration cytology of neoplastic and non-neoplastic ovarian cysts: is it accurate. *Int J Gynecol Pathol* 1996; **15**(2): 94–101

11 Wojcik E M, Selvaggi S M. Fine-needle aspiration cytology of cystic ovarian lesions. *Diagn Cytopathol* 1994; **11**: 9–14

12 Lininger J R, Frable W J. Diagnosis of pelvic actinomycosis by fine needle aspiration. A case report. *Acta Cytol* 1984; **28**: 601–604

13 Donat E E, McCutcheon J M, Alper H. Malignant mixed mullerian tumour of the ovary. Report of a case with cytodiagnosis by fine needle aspiration. *Acta Cytol* 1994; **38**(2); 231–234

14 Nguyen G-K. Cytopathologic aspects of a metastatic malignant mixed Mullerian tumour of the uterus. Report of a case with transabdominal fine needle aspiration biopsy. *Acta Cytol* 1982; **26**: 521–526

15 Nguyen G-K, Berendt R C. Aspiration of metastatic endometrial stromal sarcoma

and extragenital mixed mesodermal tumour. *Diagn Cytopathol* 1986; **2**: 256–260

16 Michael C W, Lawrence W D, Bedrossian C W. Intraoperative consultation in ovarian lesions: a comparison between cytology and frozen section. *Diagn Cytopathol* 1996; **15**(5): 387–394

Skin, soft tissues and musculoskeletal system

38 Skin

Marigold Curling and Rachel Oommen

Normal, reactive and inflammatory conditions of skin

Introduction

A relative latecomer to the field, cytodiagnosis in dermatology has not achieved as much popularity as the cytological assessment of lesions at other sites. This may be due to the reluctance of cytologists to attempt skin scrapes, which they are inexperienced at interpreting, or to the preference of dermatologists for the more traditional small biopsies, which they feel are more reliably diagnosed on histology and for which, with skin, there is such ease of access.

Skin cytology is without doubt a rapid, easy technique in experienced hands, however, and it is possible to provide valuable information in certain skin conditions. The procedure is sometimes preferable to biopsy from areas such as the face, to avoid or minimize scarring.

Anatomy of the normal skin

The skin can be divided into three main functional areas:

▶ Epidermis
▶ Dermis
▶ Skin appendages: pilosebaceous unit comprising hair follicles, sebaceous glands and arrector pili muscles; apocrine and eccrine sweat glands

Epidermis

The epidermis is derived from the primitive ectoderm and is composed of multilayered squamous cells or keratinocytes, which possess intercellular bridges, and dendritic cells, which are devoid of them, but have cytoplasmic processes extending between the squamous cells. Keratinocytes form the bulk of cells found within the epidermis. The two main dendritic cell types are melanocytes, which supply melanin pigment to the deep layers of the epidermis, and Langerhans cells, mediators of local skin immunity.

The epidermis is further divided histologically into four layers (Fig. 38.1). From the surface inwards these are:

▶ The horny layer or stratum corneum
▶ The granular layer or stratum granulosum
▶ The squamous cell layer or stratum spinosum
▶ The basal cell layer or stratum basalis

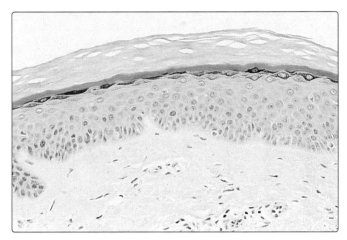

Fig. 38.1 Skin biopsy. (A) horny layer; (B) granular layer; (C) squamous cell layer; (D) basal cell layer. (H&E × HP)

The horny layer is anucleate and composed of non-homogeneous keratin, deposited in layers forming a partially waterproof covering of variable thickness over the body surface. The thin granular layer is easily identified because the cell cytoplasm contains deeply basophilic, irregular keratohyaline granules. The squamous or prickle cell layer is the most prominent and it is here that the bulk of the keratinocytes lie, their long axes parallel to the skin surface. They increase in size as they mature towards the surface.

The basal cell layer is composed of a single row of small regular columnar cells lying with their long axes perpendicular to the underlying basement membrane, which anchors them. They are germinative cells from which the outer squamous cells are derived. Melanocytes are scattered along the basal layer, conspicuous because of their clear cytoplasm and small dark nuclei. The melanin they produce is stored within the adjacent basal cells, the amount determining skin colour.

Dermis

The dermis is divided into papillary and reticular areas. The papillary dermis is superficial and interdigitates with rete pegs of the epidermis. The collagen bundles of the papillary dermis are fine and run at right angles to the surface. The reticular dermis forms the deep dermis and is characterized by thicker coarser bundles of collagen, which lie parallel to the surface and form a criss-cross network.

Skin appendages

Each pilosebaceous unit consists of a hair follicle with associated sebaceous glands. The glands are composed of several lobules of vacuolated cells rimmed by cuboidal germinative cells with large nucleoli and basophilic cytoplasm. Arrector pili muscles insert into a bulge at the lower half of the hair follicle. Various microorganisms, including *Staphylococcus epidermidis*, yeasts of Pityrosporum and the mite *Demodex folliculorum* are found lodged within the upper part of the hair follicle.

Eccrine and apocrine sweat glands are coiled glands situated in the deep dermis. Eccrine glands are found all over the body but are in high concentrations in the palms, soles, forehead and axillae. Apocrine glands are similar to eccrine glands except that the epithelial cells lining the glands are larger with abundant eosinophilic cytoplasm. Eccrine and apocrine cells are rarely seen in cytological preparations.

Technical procedures

Two methods are in common use for cytological assessment of a skin lesion: examination of a skin scrape and fine needle aspiration. For superficial lesions involving the epidermis, a skin scrape is the method of choice. Deeper lesions are best sampled by fine needle aspiration.

Direct skin scrape

The skin scrape was first used in the late 1940s in the differential diagnosis of bullous lesions by Tzanck[1]. Since then there has been a growing interest in cytodiagnosis in dermatology, confirmed by the increasing number of references in the literature[2–8]. The commonest use of a skin scrape nowadays is in the differential diagnosis of a basal cell carcinoma. Scrapes of normal skin show anucleate squames, superficial and intermediate squamous cells.

The double-ended elevator (Fig. 38.2) is a useful instrument for skin scrapes and is just sharp enough to make superficial cuts into the lesion. Scalpel blades and curettes can also be used, although there is a risk of heavier bleeding with the former. The skin is first cleansed with alcohol. Any surface crust topping the lesion should be lifted with the instrument. It is then directed towards the periphery of the lesion for sampling, as the centre is likely to be inflamed and necrotic. Cutting action may be necessary for dislodging tissue from the lesion, but this should be done as gently as possible.

With non-crusted nodular or flat lesions, it is important not to scrape the top, but to cut into it first and then to direct the blade into the cut parallel to the skin surface in order to sample the growing edge of the lesion. The minute fragment of tissue obtained should be spread on a previously labelled glass slide. The elevator used should then be sterilized by flaming and immersed in a jar containing alcohol for re-use.

Wet films enable a rapid diagnosis to be made[9–11]. The slide is first stained with a drop of 0.5% methylene blue, the addition of a coverslip spreading the stain evenly. With this method, certain features are highlighted and help to differentiate a basal cell carcinoma from a squamous cell carcinoma. In the former, there are groups of tightly packed nuclei showing palisading and more deeply staining cells around the periphery of the groups than in the centre (Fig. 38.3). Intercellular bridges are absent (Fig. 38.4A). In squamous cell carcinoma and proliferative squamous lesions, intercellular bridges can be identified (Fig. 38.4B). They are most easily demonstrated at high power with the substage diaphragm closed, the condenser lowered and the light intensity increased. It is not possible to see intercellular bridges in the permanent Papanicolaou stained smear.

Ideally, two smears should be made, one stained with methylene blue and the other fixed immediately in alcohol for Papanicolaou staining. However if only one smear is available, after looking at the methylene blue stain, which should be done immediately as the intercellular bridges fade, the smear can be fixed in ethyl alcohol, which washes

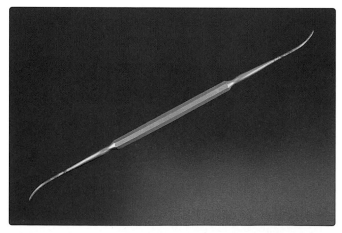

Fig. 38.2   Double-ended elevator.

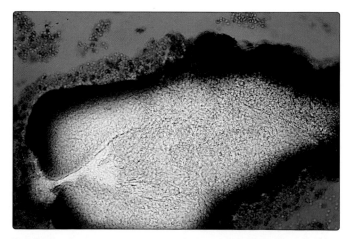

Fig. 38.3   Skin scrape: basal cell carcinoma. (Methylene blue preparation × HP)

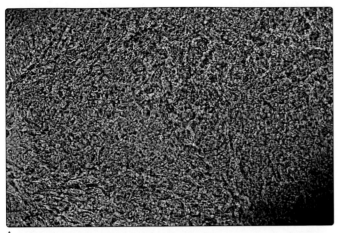

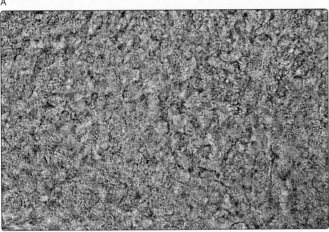

Fig. 38.4 (A) Skin scrape: intercellular bridges absent in basal cell carcinoma. (B) Intercellular bridges present in squamous cell carcinoma. (Methylene blue preparation)

off the stain and at the same time fixes the slide for permanent Papanicolaou staining.

Fine needle aspiration

The technique is similar to that employed for fine needle aspiration elsewhere in the body. Fine needle aspiration of skin nodules is usually performed to confirm secondary deposits in a patient with a known carcinoma or lymphoma and diagnosis in these cases is usually not difficult. It is advisable to have spare smears fixed in methanol if dealing with a nodule in which it is anticipated that immunostaining may be required, or to rinse the needle into tissue culture fluid for centrifuge preparations.

Bacterial lesions

It is unusual for a pustular lesion to be sampled for cytological diagnosis. Secondary bacterial infection, however, may influence the appearance of a viral or bullous lesion. Occasionally, an intradermal cystic skin lesion is found to be an abscess on aspiration.

A scraping or aspirate of pus smears easily. It is important to send a sample or swab for microbiological culture and to make extra smears for special stains for identification of Gram-positive organisms or, rarely, acid-fast bacilli and fungi, which may be accompanied by a neutrophilic infiltrate. Smears show large numbers of polymorphs, degenerate cells and debris, with varying numbers of lymphocytes and plasma cells.

Viral lesions

Although there are at least five groups of viruses that can affect the skin, there are only two that produce lesions, which can be reliably diagnosed by skin cytology. They are the herpes virus group, consisting of *Herpes simplex* and *Varicella-zoster* viruses, and the poxvirus group, of which *Molluscum contagiosum* is the common virus seen cytologically. The human papillomavirus causes skin warts, which are seldom sampled for cytology except when they occur on the vulva, and then usually in the context of investigating intraepithelial neoplasia associated with papillomavirus infection of the lower genital tract (see Chapter 28).

Usually, viruses can be seen by light microscopy only when aggregated into inclusion bodies. In the herpesvirus group they are found within the nucleus while in the poxvirus group the inclusion bodies are seen within the cytoplasm. Other cytopathic cell changes may also be found.

Herpes virus infection

Herpes virus infection of skin causes vesicle formation whether due to *Herpes simplex* or *Varicella-zoster* virus. There are clinical differences between the two infections, but in their earliest stages, both *Herpes simplex* and *Varicella-zoster* show grouped vesicles on an inflamed base, which later may become pustular and then covered by crusts. The cytological findings in both are indistinguishable[12] and viral studies are required for firm differentiation between them.

Two types of *Herpes simplex* infection occur. These are the orofacial type caused by *Herpes simplex* virus type 1 (HSV-1), and the genital type due to *Herpes simplex* virus type 2 (HSV-2). This division, based on the distribution of lesions, is not absolute, as each can infect other sites. Primary infection is always transmitted from an infected person while recurrent infection can result either from reactivation of a latent infection or a new infection.

Varicella, or chickenpox, and herpes zoster, or shingles, are caused by the same virus, *Varicella-zoster*. Around 95% of varicella infections occur as systemic infections in childhood, with a generalized rash, whereas herpes zoster occurs in adults, particularly in the elderly and the lesions are located along the course of a sensory nerve.

Cytological findings

► Multinucleate giant cells showing ground glass appearance of nuclei, nuclear moulding and margination of chromatin
► Eosinophilic intranuclear inclusion bodies

It is best to sample the lesion at an early stage, as degenerative changes and superimposed infection obscure cytological features that are essential for diagnosis.

The most characteristic finding is the presence of large multinucleated cells, thought to be caused by cell fusion, which measure between 20–30 μm in diameter (Fig. 38.5). They contain up to 30 nuclei that have a pale ground glass appearance due to accumulation of intranuclear viral particles. The nuclear chromatin is pushed to the periphery and is marginated along the nuclear membrane. There is little overlapping of the swollen nuclei, but instead there is nuclear moulding due to their crowding, which results in a cobblestone pattern. In herpes zoster the multinucleated cells contain more nuclei than in herpes simplex. In some cells large eosinophilic intranuclear inclusion bodies are seen in the centre of the pale staining nucleus. These are not to be confused with a prominent nucleolus.

Diagnostic pitfalls

Multinucleated cells accompanied by acantholytic cells are seen in pemphigus vulgaris and are a potential source of error. The nuclei, however, are unlikely to show the typical characteristics seen in herpes. Also, unlike the grouped vesicles seen clinically in herpes, pemphigus is a bullous dermatosis.

Molluscum contagiosum
Molluscum contagiosum presents as small, dome-shaped papules with umbilicated centres. In fully developed lesions, white keratinous material can be expressed from the lesion.

Cytological findings

▶ Numerous single, large, round cells with the nucleus pushed against the cell membrane
▶ The cytoplasm is eosinophilic and has a mosaic appearance

Skin scrapes show groups of squamous epithelial cells and numerous 'molluscum bodies' lying singly. The molluscum bodies consist of ballooned squamous cells with eosinophilic cytoplasm that has a mosaic appearance due to conglomeration of viral particles. The nucleus is generally pushed to the periphery where it appears as a crescent against the cytoplasmic membrane (Figs 38.6–38.8). Small, round eosinophilic bodies may be liberated from a ruptured cell. The clinical and cytological features of molluscum contagiosum are diagnostic[13].

Bullous lesions
The Tzanck test was first used in the differential diagnosis of bullous lesions. It is a rapid test used to demonstrate acantholytic epidermal cells in pemphigus and other bullous conditions characterized by dissolution of intercellular bridges. These cells are not seen in

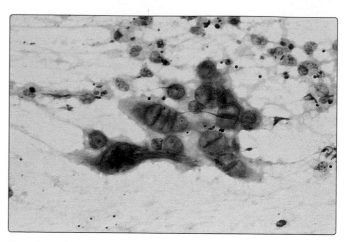

Fig. 38.5   Skin scrape: herpes infection. (Papanicolaou × HP)

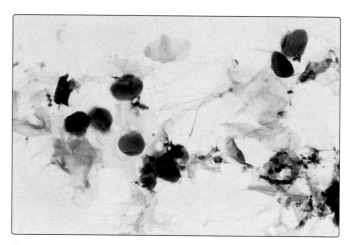

Fig. 38.6   Skin scrape: molluscum contagiosum. (Papanicolaou × HP)

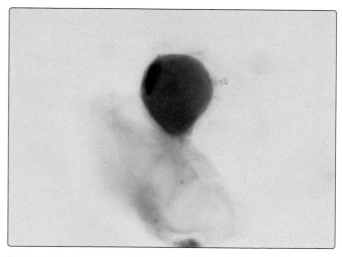

Fig. 38.7   Skin scrape: molluscum body. (Papanicolaou × OI)

subepidermal bullae of the type occurring in, for instance, bullous pemphigoid. However, the test is non-specific and cannot be used to differentiate between the various bullous diseases and other blisters associated with acantholysis

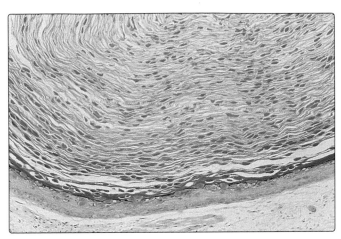

Fig. 38.8   Skin biopsy: molluscum contagiosum. (H&E × HP)

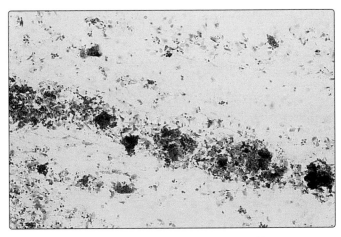

Fig. 38.9   Skin scrape: pemphigus. (Papanicolaou × HP)

secondary to cell damage, such as viral vesicles. In fact it is probably more profitable to biopsy an early bulla for histological diagnosis and to demonstrate antibody binding by immunological techniques.

Cytological findings

▶ Fluid containing acantholytic cells and inflammatory cells
▶ Rounded acantholytic cells with fuzzy cytoplasmic outlines, hyperchromatic nuclei and perinuclear haloes
▶ Multinucleated giant cells occasionally

For cytological diagnosis, a sample can either be obtained by fine needle aspiration of an early bulla or by scraping the base of a freshly opened bulla. An intraepidermal bulla contains numerous single acantholytic epidermal cells, clusters of epidermal cells and some inflammatory cells. The epidermal cells round up and the cytoplasmic outlines appear fuzzy. The nucleus is hyperchromatic and contains a large nucleolus. Mild atypia in the form of irregular chromatin pattern and nuclear enlargement is seen[14,15]. There is often a prominent perinuclear halo (Figs 38.9, 38.10). Occasionally in pemphigus, multinucleated giant cells are present which may be mistaken for herpes virus change. Pericellular and intercellular deposits of IgG have been demonstrated on immunofluorescence[16].

Subepidermal bullae contain fluid and inflammatory cells. The absence of acantholytic cells helps to differentiate them from intraepidermal bullae. The nature of the inflammatory cell component is usually not specific, consisting of variable numbers of neutrophil polymorphs and eosinophils.

Benign and malignant skin tumours

Basal cell papilloma (seborrhoeic keratosis)

This is a common benign pigmented hyperplastic and keratotic skin lesion, which occurs mainly on the trunk in adults. Scrapings consist of anucleate squames and sheets of squamous cells and basal cells. A wet film preparation

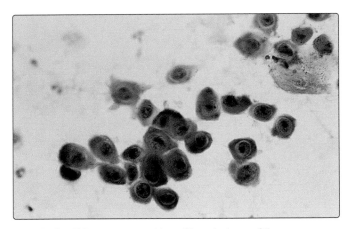

Fig. 38.10   Skin scrape: pemphigus. (Papanicolaou × OI)

will reveal intercellular bridges which is useful in excluding a basal cell carcinoma.

Keratoacanthoma

A keratoacanthoma presents as a dome-shaped lesion with a central keratin-filled crater. In its typical form, it grows rapidly for 4–6 weeks, leaving a depressed scar. Immunosuppressed patients have a high incidence of keratoacanthoma.

Scrapings consist of anucleate squames and keratinized mature squamous cells. Biopsy is always appropriate as a highly differentiated squamous cell carcinoma cannot be excluded on cytology because it is only possible to scrape the superficial part of the lesion. Skin scrapings are consequently less commonly requested now.

Solar keratosis

Solar keratosis occurs on sun-exposed skin of the face, dorsum of hand and bald portions of the scalp in men. Clinically, it occurs as erythematous, scaly areas usually less than 1 cm in diameter. Scrapings often reveal only the features of a keratotic lesion in which there is a combination of anucleate squames and keratinized mature squamous epithelial cells. Nuclear atypia if present is generally not marked.

Bowen's disease

The skin lesions of Bowen's disease (carcinoma *in situ*) are similar to those of solar keratosis except that Bowen's disease lesions tend to be larger and may occur in skin not exposed to sunlight.

Cytological findings

► A cellular smear
► Cells are arranged singly or in sheets
► Atypical squamous cells with basophilic cytoplasm
► The presence of atypical highly keratinized cells is unusual

Skin scrapings reveal atypical small cells in sheets or lying singly, similar to those seen in carcinoma *in situ* of the cervix. These cells have large hyperchromatic nuclei with little surrounding basophilic cytoplasm (Figs 38.11, 38.12). A few highly keratinized atypical cells may be present, but this is not a prominent feature and bizarre cell shapes are generally absent. If they are present a well-differentiated squamous cell carcinoma cannot be excluded by cytology.

Basal cell carcinoma

This is the most common skin tumour encountered and one which can be easily diagnosed by scrape cytology if sufficient material is obtained[17–20]. The face is the most commonly affected area because of exposure to sunlight. Basal cell carcinomas have a variable clinical appearance but common forms of presentation are as an area of central ulceration (Fig. 38.13), with pearly white rolled borders, a smooth nodule with dilated vessels coursing over the surface (Fig. 38.14), or an ill-defined flat lesion.

It should be remembered that with crusted lesions, the surface crust should be removed first so that the growing edge of the lesion can be sampled. Cystic basal cell carcinomas present as nodules and scrapes will yield clear watery fluid with tissue fragments. A fragment of tumour

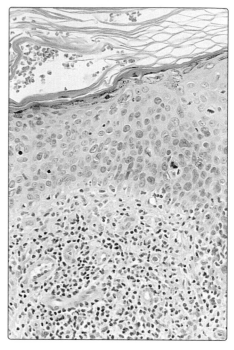

Fig. 38.12   Skin biopsy: Bowen's disease. (Papanicolaou × HP)

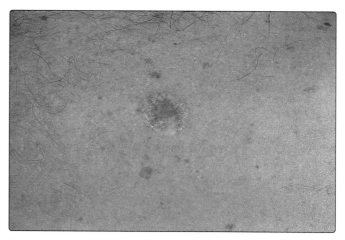

Fig. 38.13   Ulcerated basal cell carcinoma.

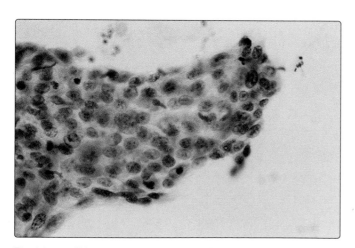

Fig. 38.11   Skin scrape: Bowen's disease. (Papanicolaou × HP)

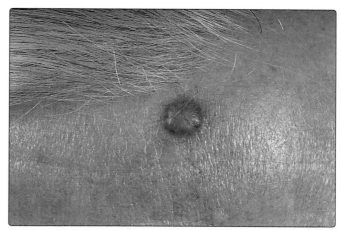

Fig. 38.14   Nodular (cystic) basal cell carcinoma.

tissue from a basal cell carcinoma has a characteristic translucent appearance when spread on the slide.

Cytological findings

▶ Cellular smear
▶ Cohesive sheets of small hyperchromatic cells with scanty cytoplasm and indistinct cell borders
▶ Peripheral palisading
▶ Absence of intercellular bridges in a wet preparation

Microscopy reveals cellular smears consisting of cohesive sheets of hyperchromatic cells showing mild nuclear pleomorphism and crowding. The nuclei are round or oval and approximately two to three times the size of red blood cells. They may contain one or two small eosinophilic nucleoli (Figs 38.15, 38.16). The nuclear chromatin is finely granular. In rapidly growing lesions, occasional mitotic figures may be seen. The cell cytoplasm is scanty and cell borders are indistinct. Peripheral palisading is commonly seen and should be looked for in groups of tumour cells forming cell balls with a smooth rounded margin (Fig. 38.17). The cell palisades may not be as striking as those

seen in H&E sections because of the three-dimensional nature of the cell groups (Fig. 38.18).

A pigmented pattern with tumour cells containing melanin and a keratotic pattern in which keratinized cell whorls are recognizable within sheets of tumour cells, are sometimes encountered. These findings reflect the histological variants of basal cell carcinoma and have no clinical significance.

Diagnostic pitfalls

Pilomatrixoma (calcifying epithelioma of Malherbe) is a differential diagnosis. Basaloid cells closely resembling cells of basal cell carcinoma are found in pilomatrixoma. Errors in diagnosis can be avoided if it is remembered that pilomatrixoma occurs in young people and is a hard subcutaneous tumour which usually occurs in the neck. FNA is required for sampling this tumour.

Metastatic small cell carcinoma may cause confusion on FNA but can usually be distinguished by the nuclear pleomorphism and moulding, and by the presence of necrosis.

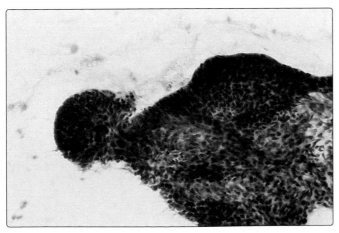

Fig. 38.15 Skin scrape: basal cell carcinoma. (Papanicolaou × LP)

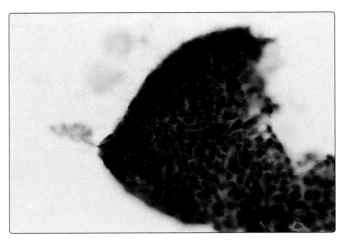

Fig. 38.17 Skin scrape: basal cell carcinoma. (Papanicolaou × HP)

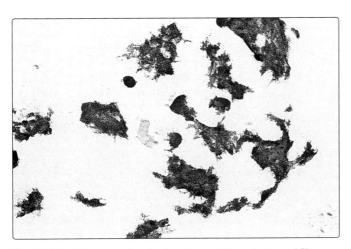

Fig. 38.16 Skin scrape: basal cell carcinoma. (Papanicolaou × MP)

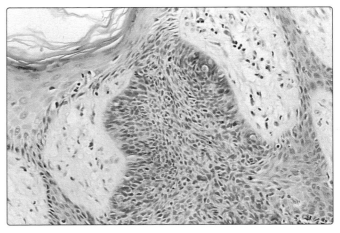

Fig. 38.18 Skin biopsy: basal cell carcinoma. (H&E × HP)

Squamous cell carcinoma

Squamous cell carcinoma presents clinically as a shallow ulcer with irregular margins or a cauliflower-like exophytic growth. Exposure to sunlight is a major factor in pathogenesis, but other factors such as immunosuppression play a major part in some cases.

Cytological findings

▶ Single cells due to loss of cohesion although solid cohesive fragments of tumour may be present in the less well-differentiated tumours
▶ Bizarre cell shapes
▶ Large irregular hyperchromatic nuclei
▶ Necrosis
▶ The presence of numerous polymorphs and sometimes eosinophils

Skin scrape smears show sheets and dissociated single atypical cells. They have moderate to abundant cytoplasm showing a variety of cell shapes and vesicular nuclei containing nucleoli (Figs 38.19, 38.20). As over 80% of squamous cell carcinomas are well-differentiated,

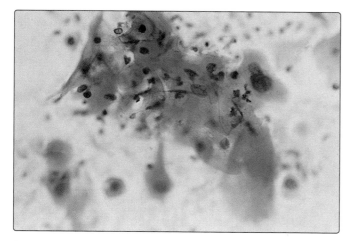

Fig. 38.19   Skin scrape: squamous cell carcinoma. (× HP)

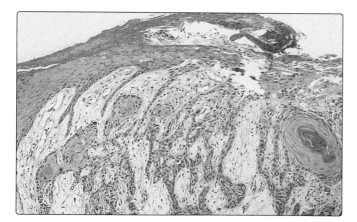

Fig. 38.20   Skin biopsy: squamous cell carcinoma. (H&E × HP)

keratinization is a common and useful feature in diagnosis, especially when Papanicolaou staining is used. Some of the cells appear highly orangeophilic. Single cell keratinization is the most reliable indicator of squamous differentiation. Inflammatory cells, particularly polymorphs, are nearly always a part of the picture.

Diagnostic pitfalls

Regenerative squamous epithelium at the edge of an ulcer will show reactive squamous cells with enlarged hyperchromatic nuclei, possibly mitotic figures and numerous polymorphs. The squamous cells are usually cohesive and nuclear atypia is not generalized or severe. Even so, it may be quite difficult to distinguish an atypical regenerative lesion from a very well-differentiated squamous cell carcinoma.

Solar keratosis and Bowen's disease have some similar features but lack the extremes of cytoplasmic and nuclear pleomorphism found in squamous carcinoma.

Naevi

These are benign tumours composed of naevus cells. They are included under the heading of melanocytic naevi, although the lesions are not always pigmented. They are divided into several types, but the junctional naevus is the most likely type to be seen by the cytopathologist. A scrape is rarely requested as these lesions do not usually resemble basal cell carcinoma, except to the very inexperienced.

Cytological findings

▶ Scanty smears
▶ Single cells predominate with few groups
▶ Melanin pigment may or may not be visible
▶ Vesicular nuclei with nucleoli

Naevi are difficult to scrape and few cells may be obtained. The naevus cells are cuboidal, or more rarely, spindle and are arranged in groups. In smears they are more commonly seen as single cells (Figs 38.21–38.23). When naevus cells are present in groups their arrangement and amount of cytoplasm is very different from the closely packed nuclei of basal cell carcinomata. The nuclei are vesicular and have nucleoli.

Although in most instances it is not possible to make a definite diagnosis, it is possible to suggest that the lesion is a naevus and to exclude basal cell carcinoma. The dysplastic naevus should not be diagnosed by cytology. Small groups of single atypical melanocytes in the epidermis may be seen in the smears and can be mistaken for malignancy. A biopsy is therefore essential to make this diagnosis. Even on histological section, the differential diagnosis between a dysplastic naevus and an early superficial spreading *in situ* melanoma may not be possible and the lesion may be reported as a borderline.

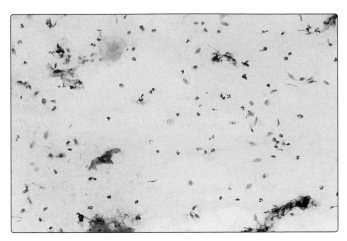

Fig. 38.21 Skin scrape: naevus. (Papanicolaou × LP)

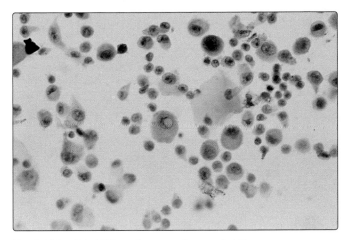

Fig. 38.24 Skin FNA: malignant melanoma. (× HP)

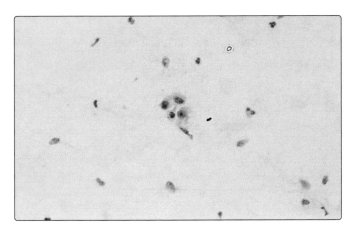

Fig. 38.22 Skin scrape: naevus. (Papanicolaou × HP)

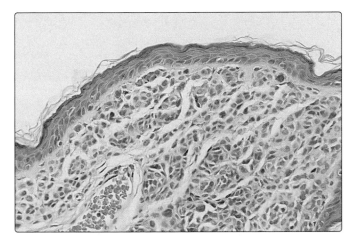

Fig. 38.23 Skin biopsy: naevus. (H&E × LP)

Malignant melanoma

Malignant tumours arising from the melanocytes of the skin are increasing in frequency in many countries. About 70% are superficial spreading melanomas, while 15% are nodular lesions. Nodular lesions infiltrate the deeper layers more rapidly. They start as raised pigmented nodules, which grow rapidly and ulcerate. Superficial spreading melanomas are usually diffusely pigmented indurated irregular lesions, which sometimes contain nodular areas.

There has been lengthy discussion concerning the method used to confirm the clinical diagnosis. Some authors suggest that incisional biopsy is contraindicated, as this may increase metastatic spread and therefore reduce survival. Reports from the USA have shown no difference in survival. No such study has been performed on scraping lesions for cytology *vs* punch biopsies as a diagnostic method. Cytology certainly is a quick and simple method of obtaining a rapid tissue diagnosis although it should be performed with care as these lesions are apt to bleed. This can be controlled by firm pressure for a few minutes.

Cytological findings

▶ Cellular smears
▶ Single cell population (aggregates of cells are rare)
▶ High nuclear/cytoplasmic ratio
▶ Binucleate and multinucleated cells are frequent
▶ Hyperchromatic nuclei with large nucleoli
▶ Cytoplasmic pigment

As with the histology of malignant melanomas, the cytological picture has a variety of forms. Some smears show single large pleomorphic undifferentiated pigmented malignant cells with moderate to abundant cytoplasm. The nuclei show great variation in size and may contain very large nucleoli with intranuclear vacuoles (Figs 38.24, 38.25). There may be pigment both within the cytoplasm and in the background. Other smears contain small spindle cells arranged in sheets or single round cells. In many cases a mixture of cell types is found. The amount of pigment varies in these tumours, some being amelanotic with no pigment[21–25].

Smears for immunocytochemical stains, such as the neural marker S 100 or the melanoma-associated antigen

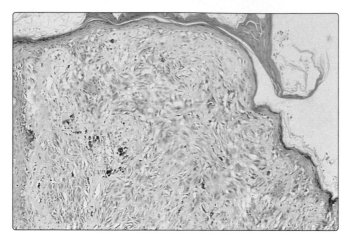

Fig. 38.25   Skin biopsy: malignant melanoma. (H&E × LP)

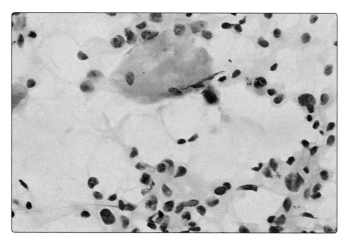

Fig. 38.26   Skin scrape: Paget's disease. (Papanicolaou × HP)

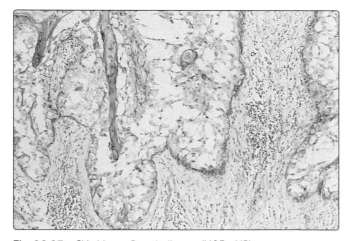

Fig. 38.27   Skin biopsy: Paget's disease. (H&E × HP)

HMB 45[26] should always be taken in cases of suspected melanoma and for the best results these should be fixed in methanol. Masson Fontana silver stain may also be helpful in identifying melanin pigment, which may be difficult to

see on the routine Papanicolaou stain, and also in differentiating melanin from haemosiderin.

Paget's disease of the nipple

Paget's disease of the nipple is characterized clinically by a crusted, eczema-like lesion, which is nearly always associated with an underlying ductal carcinoma. Occasional clear cells called Toker's clear cells are found in the epidermis of the nipple and have been shown to have the phenotype of ductal epithelial cells[27]. Paget's disease of the nipple is believed by some workers to result from malignant change in these cells in contrast to popular opinion which is that it represents spread from an underlying carcinoma. Nipple scrapings reveal dispersed malignant cells with large hyperchromatic nuclei and prominent nucleoli against a proteinaceous background (Figs 38.26, 38.27).

Eczema of the nipple is clinically very similar. However smears in eczema consist of reactive squamous epithelial cells accompanied by inflammatory cells. Bowen's disease and malignant melanoma of the nipple, though described, are very rare. The cytological appearances in these two lesions are described elsewhere.

Sebaceous gland hyperplasia and sebaceous adenoma

Sebaceous gland hyperplasia commonly arises on the face, forehead, cheeks and neck, usually in late adult life. The clinical features are very similar to those of basal cell carcinoma and these lesions may occasionally be mistaken clinically. In sebaceous adenoma the single lesions have a central duct or dimpled area surrounded by a slightly soft raised creamy area which can be mistaken for the pearly edge of a basal cell carcinoma. Sebaceous adenoma usually occurs in the same sites as hyperplasia and presents as a yellowish-white tumour.

Cytological findings

Sebaceous hyperplasia
- ▶ The lesion is usually single
- ▶ Large amount of sebaceous material
- ▶ Few sebaceous cells may be present and only rarely basaloid cells

Sebaceous adenoma
- ▶ A clinical tumour
- ▶ Sebaceous cells are present
- ▶ Basaloid cells are seen, but only up to 50% of the total cell population

The diagnosis of these lesions depends on the clinical appearance as well as the cytological findings. Scraping produces fatty sebaceous material and sometimes also groups of sebaceous cells, which appear as foamy cells with abundant cytoplasm containing fat globules (Fig. 38.28). The adenomas usually have quite a high percentage (up to 50%) of basaloid cells (Figs 38.29–38.31). These can be

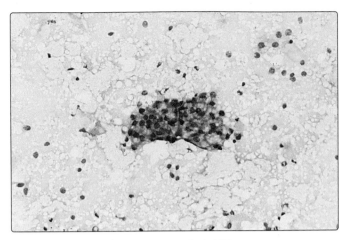

Fig. 38.28 Skin scrape: sebaceous cells. (× HP)

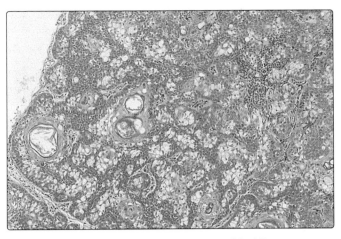

Fig. 38.31 Skin biopsy: sebaceous adenoma. (H&E × LP)

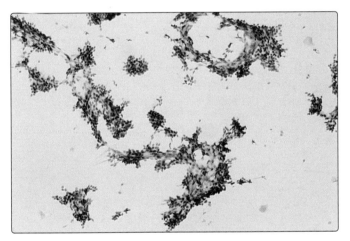

Fig. 38.29 Skin scrape: sebaceous adenoma. (× LP)

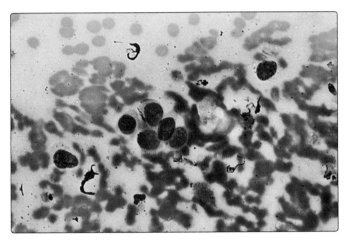

Fig. 38.32 Skin FNA: metastatic adenocarcinoma. (MGG × HP)

Hood *et al.* have described cytological features of the rare sebaceous carcinoma[28].

Other tumours

Cytological findings of skin tumours, such as pilomatrixoma[29–33], cutaneous vascular tumours[34], Merkel cell tumours[35–37], chondroid syringoma[38] and other uncommon lesions[39–40], are described by other workers.

Metastatic tumours

Although cutaneous metastases from tumours of internal organs do occur, they are uncommon. Brownstein *et al.* have shown that in women, cutaneous deposits originated from carcinoma of the breast in 69% of cases (Fig. 38.32), while in men, the commonest primary site was bronchial carcinoma.

Occasionally, skin metastases are the first sign of an internal malignancy. The location of a metastatic deposit may give a clue to the site of the primary. The so-called Sister Mary Joseph's nodule is a metastasis in the skin of the umbilicus from an intra-abdominal tumour mainly of ovary, stomach, colon or pancreas[41].

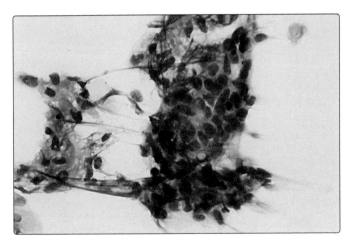

Fig. 38.30 Skin scrape: sebaceous adenoma. (× HP)

quite difficult to distinguish from a basal cell carcinoma. Rarely, the two lesions may be seen in association and the smears show groups of basal cell carcinoma and of sebaceous cells. These are now called sebaceous epithelioma: basal cell carcinoma with sebaceous differentiation.

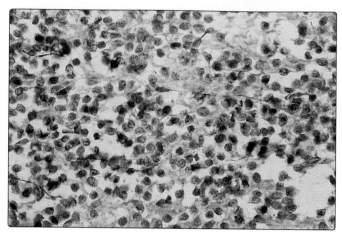

Fig. 38.33 Skin FNA: low-grade lymphoma. (× HP)

Malignant lymphomas[42] also involve the skin and must be borne in mind when assessing a smear containing poorly-differentiated cells (Fig. 38.33).

Cutaneous tumour deposits present as freely mobile lesions and are best sampled by fine needle aspiration. It is useful to prepare both air-dried and fixed smears and to prepare methanol fixed smears in reserve in case immunostaining is required for diagnosis.

Immunostaining can be useful in determining the site of origin of a metastatic tumour. Fixed direct smears can yield good results in experienced hands. Another method is to flush the remaining material in the syringe into buffered formalin from which a cell block is prepared. Sections can then be cut for immunostaining.

The choice of immunostains can sometimes be determined by the cell pattern in the smear. In tumours with a dispersed cell pattern the immunostain panel might include leucocyte common antigen for lymphoma, synaptophysin and chromogranin for neuroendocrine carcinoma, cytokeratin for carcinoma, desmin for rhabdomyosarcoma in children, S 100, HMB 45 and melan A for malignant melanoma. Smears with sheets or clusters of malignant cells are most likely to be epithelial in origin and generally cytokeratin positive. Immunostains that may help narrow the field further, include carcinoembryonic antigen gastrointestinal tract, cytokeratin 7 for ovarian tumours, cytokeratin 20 for colorectal tumours, prostate specific antigen and prostate acid phosphatase for prostatic carcinoma, thyroglobulin for thyroid carcinoma.

References

1 Tzanck A. Le cytodiagnostic immediat en dermatologie. *Ann de dermat et syph* 1948; **8**: 205–218

2 Selbach G, Keisel E. The cytological approach to skin disease. *Acta Cytol* 1962; **6**: 439–442

3 Goldman L, McCabe R M, Sawyer F. The importance of cytology technique for the dermatologist in office practice. *AMA Arch Derm* 1960; **81**: 359–368

4 Haber H. Cytodiagnosis in dermatology. *Br J Dermatol* 1954; **66**: 79–94

5 Urbach F, Burke E M, Traenkle H L. Cytodiagnosis of cutaneous malignancy. *NY State J Med* 1956; **56**(22): 3481–3485

6 Canti G. Rapid cytological diagnosis of skin lesions. In: Koss L G, Coleman D V eds. *Advances in Clinical Cytology*, vol. 2. New York: Masson Publishing, 1984

7 Mareke E, Vigneswaran N. Cytologic methods in dermatology. *Zeitschrift Fur Hautkrankheiten* 1990; **65**(2): 154–166

8 Bocking A. Cytological *vs* histological evaluation of percutaneous biopsies. *Cardiovasc Intervent Radiol* 1991; **14**(1): 5–12

9 Dudgeon L S, Barrett N R. Examination of fresh tissues by wet-film method. *Br J Surg* 1934; **22**: 4–22

10 Dudgeon L S, Patrick C V. New method for rapid microscopical diagnosis of tumours with account of 200 cases so examined. *Br J Surg* 1927; **15**: 250–261

11 Russell D S, Krayenbuhl H, Cairns H. Wet film technique in the histological diagnosis of intracranial tumours: rapid method. *J Path Bact* 1937; **45**: 501–505

12 Blank H, Burgoon C F, Baldridge G, Urbach F. Cytologic smears in diagnosis of herpes simplex, herpes zoster and varicella. *JAMA* 1951; **146**: 1410–1412

13 Oppedal B R. Molluscum contagiosum diagnosed in a cytologic smear (letter). *Acta Cytol* 1985; **29**(3): 501

14 Blank H, Burgoon C F. Abnormal cytology in epithelial cells in pemphigus vulgaris: diagnostic aid. *J Invest Dermat* 1952; **18**: 213–223

15 Coscia-Porazzi L, Maiello F M, Ruoco V, Pisani M. Cytodiagnosis of oral pemphigus vulgaris. *Acta Cytol* 1985; **29**(5): 746–749

16 Skeete M H V. Evaluation of the usefulness of immunofluorescence on Tzanck smears in pemphigus as an aid to diagnosis. *Clin Exp Dermatol* 1977; **2**(1): 57–63

17 Brown C L, Klaber M R, Robertson M G. Rapid cytological diagnosis of basal cell carcinoma of the skin. *J Clin Pathol* 1979; **32**(4): 361–367

18 Vilanova X, Pinol Aguada J, Rneda L A. The cytologic aspects of basal cell carcinoma. *J Invest Derm* 1962; **39**: 123–131

19 Malberger E, Tillinger R, Lichtig C. Diagnosis of basal cell carcinoma with aspiration cytology. *Acta Cytol* 1984; **28**(3): 301–304

20 Bocking A, Schunck K, Auffermann W. Exfoliative-cytologic diagnosis of basal cell carcinoma, with the use of DNA image cytometry as a diagnostic aid. *Acta Cytol* 1987; **3**(2): 143–149

21 Hajdu S I, Savino A. Cytologic diagnosis of malignant melanoma. *Acta Cytol* 1973; **17**: 320–327

22 Kline T S, Kannan V. Aspiration biopsy cytology and melanoma. *Am J Clin Pathol* 1982; **77**(5): 597–601

23 Svejda J, Mechl Z, Sopkova B. Cytology in the diagnosis of malignant melanoma. *Tumori* 1978; **64**(2): 229–232

24 Yamada T, Itou U, Watanabe Y, Okashi S. Cytological diagnosis of malignant melanoma. *Acta Cytol* 1972; **16**: 70–76

25 Perry M D, Gore M, Seigler H F, Johnston W W. Fine needle aspiration biopsy of metastatic melanoma: a morphologic analysis of 174 cases. *Acta Cytol* 1986; **30**(4): 385–396

26 Ordonez N G, Sneige N, Hickey R C, Brooks T E. Use of monoclonal antibody HMB-45 in the cytologic diagnosis of melanoma. *Acta Cytol* 1988; **32**(5): 684–688

27 Toker C. Clear cells of the nipple epidermis. *Cancer* 1970; **25**: 601–610

28 Hood I C, Qizilbash A H, Salama S S *et al.* Needle aspiration cytology of sebaceous carcinoma. *Acta Cytol* 1984; **28**: 305–312

29 Solanki P, Ramzy I, Durr N, Henkes D. Pilomatrixoma: cytologic features and differential diagnostic considerations. *Arch Pathol Lab Med* 1987; **111**(3): 294–297

30 Woyke S, Olszewski W, Eichelkraut A. Pilomatrixoma: a pitfall in the aspiration cytology of skin tumours. *Acta Cytol* 1982; **26**(2): 189–194

31 Kwok-Fai Ma, Man-Shan Tsui, Siu-Kwong Chan. Fine needle aspiration diagnosis of pilomatrixoma: a monomorphic population of basaloid cells with squamous differentiation not to be mistaken for carcinoma. *Acta Cytol* 1991; **35**(5): 570–574

32 Gomez-Aracil A, San Pedro C, Romero J. Fine needle aspiration cytologic findings in four cases of pilomatrixoma. *Acta Cytol* 1990; **34**(6): 842–846

33 Unger P, Watson C, Phelps R G *et al.* Fine needle aspiration cytology of pilomatrixoma. *Acta Cytol* 1990; **34**(6): 847–850

34 Perez-Guillermo M, Sola Perez J, Garcia Rojo B, Hernandez Gil A. Fine needle aspiration cytology of cutaneous vascular tumours. *Cytopathol* 1992; **3**(4): 231–244

35 Mellblom L, Akerman M, Carlen B. Aspiration cytology of neuroendocrine (Merkel-cell) carcinoma of the skin: report of a case. *Acta Cytol* 1984; **28**: 297–300

36 Szpak C A, Bossen E H, Linder J *et al.* Cytomorphology of primary small-cell (Merkel-cell) carcinoma of the skin in fine needle aspirates. *Acta Cytol* 1984; **28**: 290–296

37 Domagala W, Lubinski J, Lasota J *et al.* Neuroendocrine (Merkel-cell) carcinoma of the skin: cytology, intermediate filament typing and ultrastructure of tumour cells in fine needle aspirates. *Acta Cytol* 1987; **31**: 267–275

38 Masood S, Hardy N. Fine needle aspiration cytology of chondroid syringoma report of a case. *Acta Cytol* 1988; **32**: 428–484

39 Daskalopoulou D, Galanopoulou A, Statiropoulou P *et al.* Cytologically interesting cases of primary skin tumours and tumour-like conditions identified by fine needle aspiration biopsy. *Diagn Cytopathol* 1998; **1**: 17–27

40 Dey P, Das A, Radhika S, Nijhawan R. Cytology of primary skin tumours. *Acta Cytol* 1996, **40**(4): 708–713

41 Gupta R K, Lalhu S, McHutchison A G R, Prasad J. Fine needle aspiration of Sister Mary Joseph's nodule. *Cytopathol* 1991; **2**: 311–314

42 Binder T, Schoengen A, Bultmann B. Fine needle aspiration of the skin: diagnosis of malignant lymphoma and of cutaneous manifestations of myeloid hemoblastosis. *Hautarzt* 1988; **39**(9): 576–580

39 Normal and inflammatory conditions of soft tissue and musculoskeletal system

Måns Åkerman

Introduction

There are two main indications for fine needle aspiration (FNA) of soft tissue and bone lesions: the diagnosis of primary lesions and the investigation of lesions clinically suspicious of tumour recurrence or metastasis. The use of FNA to verify a recurrent tumour or a metastasis has never been controversial. However, the role of FNA in the initial diagnosis is still debatable, especially for soft tissue tumours although a number of articles published during recent years have indicated the value of FNA as a pre-treatment diagnostic method[1-3].

The main objections to using FNA as a pretreatment diagnostic tool for soft tissue lesions have been the inability to aspirate a sufficient number of tumour cells for diagnosis, the disadvantages of sampling material from a very limited area of large tumours and the putative unreliability of cytological diagnosis[4,5]. These objections are not surprising as the morphological diagnosis of soft tissue tumours is very often a challenge to histopathologists, as well as to cytologists. An extensive diagnostic work-up is often required, supplementing routine stains with immunohistochemistry, electron microscopy and also cytogenetic and molecular genetic methods in order to establish the histological subtype of a particular neoplasm[6,7].

At present, the main treatment for the majority of soft tissue tumours, benign or malignant, is surgical. Preoperative diagnosis is based on the combined evaluation of clinical and radiographic data, together with a surgical biopsy or core needle biopsy for histopathological diagnosis. However, the type of surgical procedure depends more on the relationship of the tumour to fasciae, blood vessels, nerves and bone, than on its histological subtype. Therefore in the majority of tumours, in which the treatment option is primary radical surgery, the most important preoperative information for the orthopaedic surgeon is whether the lesion is a true soft tissue tumour, either benign or malignant, and the histological typing of the tumour is of secondary importance. When the optimal treatment is considered to be neoadjuvant therapy (radiotherapy or chemotherapy) followed by surgery, the FNA diagnosis must equal that of a histopathological examination with regard to histotype and malignancy grade. At present this is the case with small round cell sarcomas such as rhabdomyosarcoma, neuroblastoma and Ewing´s family of tumours, but is variable in synovial sarcoma and in large, high-grade malignant intermuscular sarcoma

Using FNA instead of open biopsy, the extent of surgical excision necessary in a radical operation can be reduced. This is because with an open biopsy, seeding of tumour cells to uninvolved tissues may occur[8]; thus wider excision margins are required, with the risk of unnecessary loss of function. There are also other advantages with FNA: hospitalization is not necessary and by using rapid staining procedures a preliminary diagnosis may be rendered within 20 minutes of the aspiration. This gives the clinician the possibility of informing the patient and discussing therapy at the first visit. Core needle biopsy is an outpatient procedure, as FNA, but compared with FNA, a preliminary diagnosis is less feasible. Another advantage of FNA over core needle biopsy is the sampling of material from different parts of large tumours to diagnose tumour heterogeneity. This is an easy task with the thin needle.

With increasing experience of the use of FNA as the diagnostic method before definitive treatment, important pitfalls have been highlighted and the means to avoid them suggested[1,2].

With bone lesions, FNA may also replace open biopsy in the primary diagnosis. In this case, it is the task of the cytopathologist to distinguish benign and malignant primary bone tumours from metastatic deposits and from the range of benign reactive and inflammatory conditions of bone. Furthermore, the cytopathologist has to give a confident type-diagnosis of those primary malignant tumours of bone where neoadjuvant multidrug chemotherapy is the first treatment modality (Ewing's family of tumours and osteosarcoma). Vertebral lesions are an important example of the effectiveness of skeletal FNA. In a substantial number of cases, definitive therapy can be based with confidence on the cytological diagnosis when combined with the clinical and radiological findings, obviating the need for open biopsy[3].

In a number of soft tissue as well as bone tumour FNAs it is necessary to apply ancillary diagnostic methods on part of the aspirate in order to reach a correct diagnosis, similar to the diagnostic approach in histopathology.

Technical procedures

Soft tissue

FNA of soft tissue tumours is performed in the same way as for epithelial tumours. It is not necessary to use a local anaesthetic. A syringe holder, 10 ml syringe and 22-gauge needles (0.7 mm) are recommended. For deep-seated intramuscular or intermuscular tumours, a needle with a stylet is preferable to avoid sampling subcutaneous fat and other tissue surrounding the tumour.

All passes with the needle should go through the same site in the skin but the direction of the needle should be changed with each pass to cover different parts of the tumour. In most cases it is not necessary to make more than five passes.

As a general rule, the orthopaedic surgeon ought to decide the site of the insertion point, but if this is not possible, the vertex of the tumour is the best choice. Tattooing of the skin area at the insertion point is valuable if the surgeon wishes to include the needle tract in the surgical specimen.

Bone

Skeletal aspirations do not differ from other fine needle aspirations, but it is important to remember that it is not possible to penetrate intact cortical bone with thin needles. However, partly destroyed or eroded cortical bone can usually be penetrated quite easily with a 22-gauge needle. If the cortical bone is almost intact, an 18-gauge needle can be used, through which a 23-gauge needle may be inserted into the lesion and multiple aspirations performed. In this case, local anaesthetic must be used before aspiration.

Many malignant bone tumours have palpable soft tissue involvement and are aspirated with the aid of the palpatory findings. It is strongly recommended that aspirations of impalpable lesions are guided by the use of imaging techniques. Fluoroscopy and computerized tomographic (CT) scanning may be used. With CT scanning, it is possible to select specific small areas within the lesion for sampling.

Alcohol-fixed and air-dried smears should be prepared from soft tissue and bone lesions, staining by Papanicolaou or haematoxylin and eosin (H&E) and by May-Grünwald-Giemsa (MGG), respectively. MGG staining is superior for evaluation of cytoplasmic details and background matrix, but the findings with the different stains complement one another.

The cytological report

On the basis of clinical data and radiographic findings alone, it may be very difficult even for experienced orthopaedic surgeons and radiologists to decide whether a soft tissue tumour is benign or malignant, especially with deep-seated tumours. In these circumstances, the cytological diagnosis becomes the most important parameter in determining definitive therapy. To avoid misleading diagnoses and misinterpretation of reports, we have for many years summarized our FNA diagnoses as follows:

► Sarcoma, including highly suspicious of sarcoma
► Malignant tumour other than sarcoma
► Benign
► Non-diagnostic, including insufficient material for diagnosis and inconclusive findings

The histological type and grade of malignancy are then suggested if possible.

Soft tissue sarcomas are generally given a grading of malignancy, as this has been shown to be of prognostic importance[8]. Both three- and four-grade scales are in common usage. In either system, grade III and grades III and IV correspond to high-grade malignant tumours. In FNA material from malignant tumours it is usually possible to distinguish low-grade from high-grade sarcomas. The overall cell yield, the presence of necrosis, cellular pleomorphism, abnormalities of chromatin and nucleolar structure, and the presence of mitoses, especially if abnormal, are the most important criteria used.

With regard to soft tissue, as well as bone lesions it is very important to realize that the final diagnosis is based on a combined evaluation of clinical data, including the patient's age and the site and duration of the lesion, together with the radiographic and cytological findings. It is unwise to render a definite diagnosis on a bone lesion without knowledge of the radiographic features.

Diagnostic accuracy

The clinical usefulness of FNA depends on the ability to aspirate sufficient material for diagnostic evaluation, to diagnose true sarcomas and to separate benign tumours and other lesions from sarcomas. In general these requirements are fulfilled in soft tissue and bone.

A retrospective analysis of FNA material from the Orthopedic Oncology Group, Lund University Hospital over the last 20 years, revealed that diagnostic aspirates were obtained from 475 out of 517 soft tissue tumours (92%). These consisted of tumours of the extremities and trunk, and included 315 benign tumours and 202 sarcomas. A correct diagnosis with regard to benign vs malignant lesions was made in 447 (94%) of the 475 diagnostic aspirates[9]. The main reasons for obtaining insufficient material were the presence in sarcomas of large cystic or necrotic areas, highly vascular lesions or a collagenous background matrix. Similar accuracy figures were noted by Brosjö et al. in a retrospective study of 342 cases from the Musculoskeletal Tumour Group at the Karolinska Hospital, Stockholm[10].

At present, the criteria for cytological diagnosis have been clearly defined in a number of benign and malignant soft tissue tumours, making it possible to suggest a specific diagnosis of the tumour type (Table 39.1). In other histological types, case reports of the cytological findings have been documented but definitive diagnostic criteria are still lacking (Table 39.2).

Table 39.1   Soft tissue tumours/lesions with definitive cytological features, making diagnosis of tumour type possible*

Benign	Malignant
Nodular fasciitis	Pleomorphic sarcoma of MFH-type
Proliferative fasciitis/myositis	Leiomyosarcoma
Myositis ossificans	Liposarcoma
Lipoma	Synovial sarcoma
Neurilemmoma	Rhabdomyosarcoma
Intramuscular myxoma	Alveolar soft part sarcoma
	Clear cell sarcoma
	Ewing's family of tumours
	Neuroblastoma

* References are given in respective chapters

Table 39.2   Soft tissue tumours with cytological features reported in single cases but diagnostic criteria not yet defined*

Benign	Malignant
Desmoid fibromatosis	Haemangiopericytoma
Leiomyoma	Angiosarcoma
Rhabdomyoma	MPNST (malignant schwannoma)
Solitary fibrous tumour of soft tissue	Epithelioid sarcoma
	Extraskeletal myxoid chondrosarcoma
	Extrarenal rhabdoid tumour

* References are given in respective chapters

Table 39.3   Primary bone tumours with clearly defined cytological features enabling a specific diagnosis to be made*

Benign	Malignant
Giant cell tumour	Osteosarcoma
Osteoblastoma	Chondrosarcoma
Chondroblastoma	Ewing's family of tumours
	Chordoma

* References are given in Chapter 41

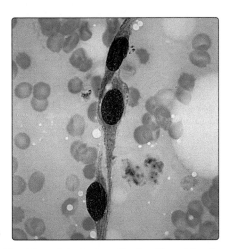

Fig. 39.1   Fibroblasts. Spindle-shaped cells with ovoid uniform nuclei and cytoplasmic processes. (MGG, × OI)

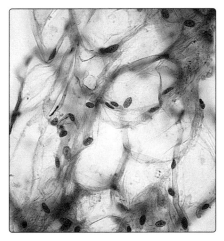

Fig. 39.2   Adipose tissue. Part of a fragment of normal adipose tissue. Large univacuolated fat cells with small regular nuclei. (H&E, × HP)

With bone tumours, the overall diagnostic accuracy is similar to that of soft tissue tumours. In a recently published retrospective evaluation of FNA of 333 bone tumours, 1980–97, from our Centre, the accuracy figures were similar; insufficient material in 6% and a correct diagnosis with regard to benign *vs* malignant lesion in 96%[3]. Kreicbergs *et al.* from the Musculoskeletal Tumour Group at the Karolinska Hospital in Stockholm reported similar figures 1996[11]. The cytological findings in FNA material have been described for all the major primary malignant bone tumours and also for a few benign primary tumours of bone (Table 39.3).

Cytological findings in normal soft tissues

Fibrous tissue

Normal fibroblasts are spindle-shaped cells with slender contours. Cytoplasmic borders may be indistinct but unipolar or bipolar processes can usually be seen. The nuclei are ovoid, rounded or elongated with regular chromatin distribution and small or absent nucleoli. Stripped nuclei are a common finding. Fibroblasts are seen either as dispersed cells or in groups or runs of loosely cohesive cells (Fig. 39.1).

Adipose tissue

Normal adipose tissue cells are found in fragments or clusters in smears showing large fat cells with abundant univacuolated cytoplasm and small dark regular nuclei. In the larger fragments a discrete network of slender capillaries may be observed. Dissociated fat cells are quite uncommon. The larger fragments resemble adipose tissue in histological sections and look like microbiopsies (Fig. 39.2).

Striated muscle

Fragments of muscle fibres are pink or amphophilic on Papanicolaou staining, eosinophilic with H&E and deep

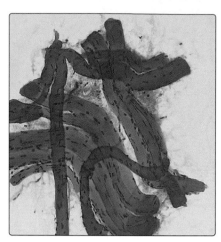

Fig. 39.3   Striated muscle. A group of striated muscle fibres. The fibres have eosinophilic faintly striated cytoplasm and small rounded dark uniform nuclei. Cross striation is not evident in this group. (H&E, × LP)

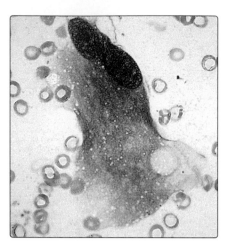

Fig. 39.4   Reactive fibroblast from a case of nodular fasciitis. A fibroblast with marked reactive changes showing binucleation, prominent nucleoli and abundant cytoplasm. (MGG × OI)

blue in MGG-stained preparations. Striation is often evident and the peripherally placed nuclei are small, rounded and dark (Fig. 39.3). Cross-striations may be observed.

Cytological findings in reactive changes

Fibroblasts

Reactive fibroblasts show wide variation in size and shape irrespective of the aetiology. The cells become fusiform, rounded or triangular, with abundant cytoplasm, which may display one or several processes or angulated cytoplasmic extensions. The nuclei vary in size and take on rounded, ovoid, spindly or irregular contours. The chromatin is often irregularly distributed and nucleoli may be prominent. Binucleated cells are common (Fig. 39.4).

Fat

Reactive adipose tissue fragments may show a myxoid background and the capillary network is often more prominent. The fragments are more cellular than normal due to a reactive increase in fibroblasts and sometimes also due to the presence of histiocytes. Between the fragments histiocytes with vacuolated or foamy cytoplasm are observed.

Striated muscle

The principal reactive changes observed in striated muscle are regenerative in origin, occurring when muscle is infiltrated by tumour tissue. Regenerating striated muscle fibres usually appear as large multinucleated cells in aspiration smears, with varying shapes including spindly, rounded and straplike forms. They are known as 'muscle giant cells'. The dense cytoplasm is deeply eosinophilic on H&E or Papanicolaou staining and dark blue on MGG. Multiple nuclei are seen, rounded or ovoid in shape, and

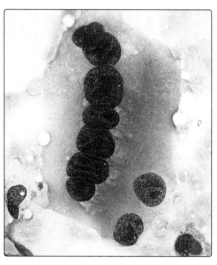

Fig. 39.5   Regenerating muscle fibre. A 'muscle giant cell' with dense blue cytoplasm and multiple rounded nuclei in a row. Note prominent nucleoli. (MGG, × OI)

often arranged in rows or eccentrically placed. Nucleoli may be large and prominent (Fig. 39.5).

Benign reactive soft tissue lesions

Clinically important examples of reactive changes in soft tissue are seen in aspirates from post-traumatic conditions, benign pseudosarcomatous lesions such as nodular fasciitis, proliferative fasciitis, proliferative myositis and myositis ossificans, and in infantile fibromatosis colli.

Nodular fasciitis

This is the commonest of the fibrous tissue tumours or tumour-like lesions, growing with great rapidity over a few weeks, but usually not reaching more than about 3 cm in diameter. Young adults are most often affected and the upper extremities are the commonest sites, although they may occur almost anywhere.

Cytological findings

▶ Cellular aspirates
▶ Cells dispersed and in closely packed sheets
▶ Myxoid background matrix
▶ Pleomorphic cells, marked anisocytosis and anisokaryosis
▶ Cells resembling ganglion cells
▶ Admixture of leucocytes and histiocytes

The cytological appearances of more than 60 examples of nodular fasciitis from the author's files reveals remarkable similarity from case to case (Åkerman, unpublished work, 1999)[12]. The most important feature is the wide variation in size and shape of the proliferating fibroblasts. Spindle-shaped cells with cytoplasmic processes and fusiform nuclei are the commonest type seen, but plump cells with ovoid, rounded, kidney-shaped or irregular nuclei are also always found.

A further typical finding is the presence of polyhedral or triangular cells with abundant cytoplasm. They have one or two rounded nuclei at the periphery near the cytoplasmic membrane, and closely resemble ganglion cells.

In spite of the pleomorphism throughout the smear, the chromatin in all of the cells is finely granular, and although their nucleoli may be very large, it is always possible to identify normal looking fibroblasts and fibroblasts with minor reactive changes mingling with the larger proliferative cells (Figs 39.6, 39.7).

Experience indicates that nodular fasciitis often decreases in size in three or four weeks[13]. We have observed 37 cases of clinically and cytologically diagnosed nodular fasciitis, which resolved and disappeared within a few weeks of FNA[14]. When the clinical findings are of a rapidly growing, tender, firm subcutaneous tumour, and the cytological appearances are typical, our policy at present is clinical observation, thereby avoiding surgical intervention.

Proliferative myositis/fasciitis

These two proliferative conditions are much rarer but are important in view of their rapid growth and pseudosarcomatous appearance histologically. They develop in adults, proliferative myositis occurring mainly on the trunk while fasciitis is more common on the extremities.

Cytological findings

▶ Proliferating fibroblasts
▶ Atypical binucleate cells with large nuclei and nucleoli
▶ Regenerating muscle fibres ('muscle giant cells')

The cytomorphology of proliferative myositis and fasciitis is less well defined than that of nodular fasciitis. Our

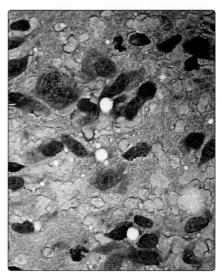

Fig. 39.6   Nodular fasciitis. A myxoid background matrix with dispersed fibroblasts displaying marked variation in shape and size. Observe the mixture of slender, almost normal-looking fibroblasts and large plump cells with abundant cytoplasm and rounded nuclei. (MGG, × LP)

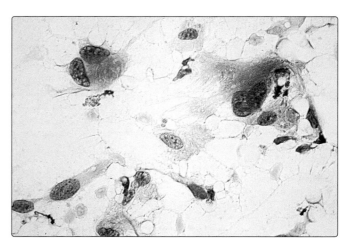

Fig. 39.7   Nodular fasciitis. Two binucleate cells, closely resembling ganglion cells, and one normal fibroblast. (H&E, × OI)

experience is similar to that of previous reports[15,16]. Smears resemble the picture of nodular fasciitis but the myxoid background matrix is seldom observed. There are usually some large rounded binucleate cells with abundant cytoplasm and enlarged round nuclei situated opposite each other very near the cytoplasmic membrane. They have prominent nucleoli (Fig. 39.8). These cells are a characteristic finding and are not seen in nodular fasciitis. In proliferative myositis, regenerating muscle fibres are also a typical feature.

Infantile fibromatosis colli

This lesion develops as a rapidly growing nodule in the sternomastoid muscle near its lower attachment, clinically resembling an enlarged firm lymph node. It usually arises in the second to fourth weeks after birth, often following a

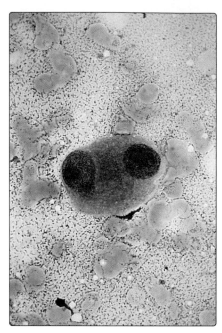

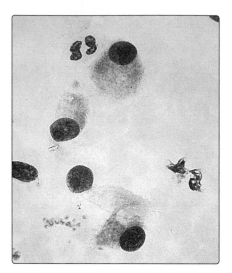

Fig. 39.9   Osteoblasts. The typical osteoblast is rounded or triangular with a round eccentrically placed nucleus and a perinuclear clear 'Hof'. (MGG, × OI)

Fig. 39.8   Proliferative myositis. A characteristic cell: large, rounded and binucleate, with abundant cytoplasm and nuclei opposite each other. (MGG, × OI)

complicated delivery, and is commoner in male infants. Histology shows proliferating fibroblasts mingled with degenerate muscle fibres, but with little pleomorphism or mitotic activity.

Cytological findings

▶ Proliferating fibroblasts
▶ Regenerating muscle fibres

The clue to diagnosis is the mixture of proliferating fibroblasts and regenerating striated muscle fibres, together with the appropriate clinical setting[17].

Normal cytological findings in aspirates from bone

The histological structure of normal bone varies with the age of the person and site of origin of the bone examined. The cytological findings reflect this variability.

Osteoblasts

Osteoblasts are most often seen as single cells but small clusters or rows are also encountered. They are uniform cells of rounded or triangular shape, with abundant cytoplasm, which contains a characteristic clear area or 'Hof' adjacent to the nucleus. The nuclei are round with a central nucleolus and are situated very close to the cytoplasmic membrane, almost protruding through it (Fig. 39.9).

Osteoclasts

Osteoclasts appear as scattered single large cells with abundant cytoplasm and multiple uniform rounded nuclei

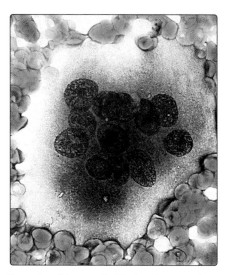

Fig. 39.10   Osteoclast. A large cell with abundant cytoplasm showing red granules on MGG and multiple uniform nuclei. (MGG, × OI)

arranged closely together. In MGG-stained smears, a characteristic cytoplasmic red granulation is seen (Fig. 39.10).

Chondrocytes

Normal chondrocytes are never seen as dissociated cells, but may be observed in lacunae in cartilaginous fragments. These are composed of a hyaline matrix, which is reddish blue to violet with MGG, or pink with H&E staining. In Papanicolaou stained preparations the matrix has a pale greyish red amphophilic fibrillary appearance.

Bone marrow cells

Bone marrow is not an uncommon finding in aspirates from ribs and vertebrae and it is important not to mistake the immature cells and megakaryocytes for malignant cells.

A mixture of erythropoietic and myelopoietic cells and megakaryocytes is characteristic. The bone marrow cells are best visualized with MGG stains.

Mesothelial cells

Occasionally, aspirates from vertebral lesions include small flat sheets of regular pavemented mesothelial cells.

Reactive changes in bone

Reactive changes in bone aspirates are seen only in osteoblasts and are found in smears from lesions such as fracture callus or proliferative periostitis[18,19]. They resemble normal osteoblasts with eccentric nuclei and a clear cytoplasmic 'Hof', but they are often larger and more variable in size and shape.

Their nuclei may also be large with prominent nucleoli (Fig. 39.11). These reactive osteoblasts are embedded in small fragments of a faintly fibrillary background matrix staining reddish violet with MGG stains. This material probably represents osteoid (Fig. 39.12).

Myositis ossificans

Myositis ossificans is a rapidly proliferating soft tissue lesion, which has been mistaken clinically as well as radiologically for a malignant tumour; a false diagnosis of osteosarcoma has also been made histologically on biopsy specimens. It is sometimes referred to as pseudomalignant myositis ossificans to stress this risk. It generally arises in the subcutaneous tissues or musculature of the extremities of young adults, forming a tender swelling which undergoes ossification in a zonal pattern after 2–3 weeks.

Cytological findings

▶ Proliferating fibroblasts
▶ Proliferating osteoblasts
▶ Osteoclastic giant cells
▶ Reactive osteoblasts also found

The characteristic feature is the mixture of proliferating fibroblasts, osteoblasts and osteoclasts. When myositis ossificans involves striated muscle, multinucleated regenerating muscle fibres are also observed. Experience indicates that a safe diagnosis of myositis ossificans may be rendered from the combined evaluation of FNA findings and radiological features. Computed tomography is especially valuable for visualizing the typical changes[20]. Experience has also shown that myositis ossificans, as with nodular fasciitis, may resolve spontaneously a number of weeks after needling[20].

Inflammatory lesions of bone

Osteomyelitis

Although much less common today in the developed world, cases of osteomyelitis are nevertheless still seen in all countries, especially in children. The metaphysis of

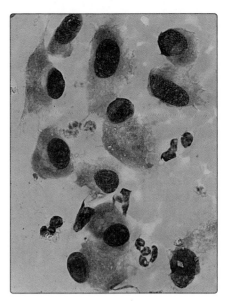

Fig. 39.11   Reactive osteoblasts. Reactive osteoblasts have the same cytological features as normal osteoblasts, including eccentric nuclei and a perinuclear 'Hof', but they vary in size and shape and anisocytosis may be marked. (MGG, × OI)

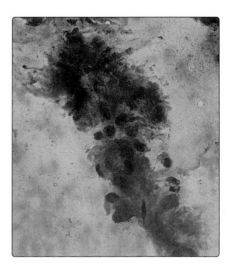

Fig. 39.12   Reactive osteoblasts. Reactive osteoblasts embedded in a reddish violet background substance which is osteoid. From a case of proliferative periostitis. (MGG, × LP)

long bones is the classical site for lesions to develop in childhood and staphylococci are the commonest infecting organism. Histologically there is an acute inflammatory reaction with necrosis of bone and regenerative changes. In cases of tuberculous osteomyelitis a more chronic inflammatory picture is seen, including giant cell granuloma formation with lymphocytes and caseation necrosis.

The radiological appearances of bacterial osteomyelitis may be difficult to differentiate from Ewing's sarcoma in children. However, the cytological findings are distinctive and when combined with microbiological culture are often diagnostic.

Cytological findings

▶ Highly cellular yields
▶ Neutrophil polymorphs
▶ Debris
▶ Histiocytes
▶ Epithelioid histiocytes in granulomatous inflammation

Aspirates are cellular and dominated by neutrophils and cellular debris, with a variable proportion of macrophages. The smears look like pus aspirated from any abscess (Fig. 39.13).

Tuberculous osteomyelitis must be suspected when clusters of epithelioid histiocytes are mixed with the neutrophils. These histiocytes are often arranged in granuloma-like clusters in FNA material. They have pale greyish blue cytoplasm with indistinct cell borders and their elongated kidney shaped nuclei are also pale staining. Small lymphocytes may also be noted (Fig. 39.14), but typical giant cells of Langhans' type as found histologically, are seldom observed and caseation necrosis is not easily recognized.

Diagnostic pitfalls in benign soft tissue and bone lesions

The most important diagnostic pitfalls are presented in Table 39.4. In general, a false diagnosis of sarcoma is attributable to the great variation in size and shape of

reactive fibroblasts and osteoblasts with their prominent nucleoli.

In doubtful cases, it is important that the final evaluation is by a combination of clinical and cytological findings. The patient's history is especially important in young people who are likely to participate in sports and athletics and have a history of trauma. The pseudosarcomatous lesions of soft tissue often grow rapidly and tenderness is not uncommon, in contradistinction to most sarcomas. Myositis ossificans has a typical appearance radiologically, especially on CT, which is a safeguard against a false positive diagnosis of malignancy.

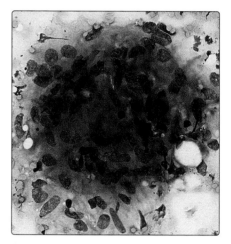

Fig. 39.14   Tuberculous osteomyelitis. A granuloma composed of epithelioid histiocytes and scattered lymphocytes. (Giemsa, × HP)

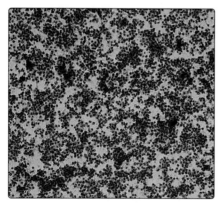

Fig. 39.13   Osteomyelitis. Pus-like smear dominated by neutrophils. (H&E, × LP).

Table 39.4   Benign soft tissue and bone lesions which may be misdiagnosed as malignant tumours in aspirate smears

Lesion	Wrong diagnosis
Nodular fasciitis	'Spindle cell' sarcoma
Proliferative fasciitis; Proliferative myositis	Pleomorphic sarcoma
Post-traumatic reaction in fibrous tissue	Pleomorphic sarcoma
Reactive changes in fat	Myxoid liposarcoma
	Well-differentiated lipoma-like liposarcoma
Regenerating muscle fibres	Multinucleated sarcoma cells
Infantile fibromatosis colli	Sarcoma with multinucleated cells
Myositis ossificans	Osteosarcoma

References

1 Åkerman M, Willén H. Critical review on the role of fine needle aspiration in soft tissue tumors. *Pathol Case Rev* 1998; **3**: 111–117

2 Åkerman M. Fine-needle aspiration cytology of soft tissue sarcoma: benefits and limitations. *Sarcoma* 1998; **2**: 155–161

3 Åkerman M, Domanski H. Fine needle aspiration (FNA) of bone tumours: with special emphasis on definitive treatment of primary malignant bone tumours based on FNA. *Curr Diagn Pathol* 1998; **5**: 82–92

4 Shiu M M, Hajdu S. Management of soft tissue sarcoma of the extremity. *Semin Oncology* 1981; **8**: 172–179

5 Hajdu S, Melamed M R. Limitations of aspiration cytology in diagnosis of primary neoplasms. *Acta Cytol* 1984; **28**: 337–345

6 Ninfo V, Chung E B, Cavazzana A O. *Tumors and Tumorlike Lesions of Soft Tissue*. New York: Churchill Livingstone, 1991

7 Rydholm A. Chromosomal aberrations in musculoskeletal tumors: clinical importance. *J Bone Joint Surg (Br)* 1996; **78**: 501–506

8 Angervall L, Kindblom L-G, Rydholm A, Stener B. The diagnosis and prognosis of soft tissue tumors. *Semin Diagn Pathol* 1986; **3**: 240–258

9 Åkerman M, Rydholm A. *Fine Needle Aspiration Cytology in 517 Primary Soft Tissue Tumors*. Abstract 2nd Combined Meeting of MSTS/EMSOS, Boston, 1992

10 Brosjö O, Bauer H C P, Kreicbergs S. Fine needle aspiration biopsy of soft tissue tumors. *Acta Orthop Scand* 1994; **65**(suppl 256): 108–109

11 Kreicbergs A, Bauer H C P, Brosjö O *et al.* Cytologic diagnosis of bone tumors. *J Bone Joint Surg (Br)* 1996; **78–B**: 258–263

12 Dahl I, Åkerman M. Nodular fasciitis: a correlative cytologic and histologic study of 13 cases. *Acta Cytol* 1981; **25**: 215–223

13 Stanley M, Skoog L, Tani E, Horwitz Ch. Spontaneous resolution of nodular fasciitis following diagnosis by fine needle aspiration. *Acta Cytol* 1991; **35**: 616–617, Abstract

14 Willén H, Åkerman M, Rydholm A. Fine needle aspiration of nodular fasciitis – no need for surgery. *Acta Orthoped Scand* 1995; **66**(suppl 265): 54–55

15 Reif R M. The cytologic picture of proliferative myositis. *Acta Cytol* 1982; **26**: 376–377

16 Lundgren L, Kindblom L-G, Willems J *et al.* Proliferative myositis and fasciitis. A light and electron microscopic, cytologic, DNA-cytometric and immunohistochemical study. *APMIS* 1992; **100**: 437–448

17 Pereira S, Tani E, Skoog L. Diagnosis of fibromatosis colli by fine needle aspiration. *Cytopathol* 1999; **1**: 25–29

18 Sanerkin N G, Jeffre G M. *Cytology of Bone Tumours*. Bristol: John Wright, 1980

19 Mirra J. Bone tumors. *Clinical, Radiologic and Pathologic Correlations*. Philadelphia: Lea & Febiger, 1989

20 Rööser B, Herrlin K, Rydholm A, Åkerman M. Pseudomalignant myositis ossificans. Clinical, radiologic and cytologic diagnosis in 5 cases. *Acta Orthop Scand* 1989; **60**: 457–460

40 Benign and malignant soft tissue tumours

Måns Åkerman

Introduction

Modern histological classification of soft tissue tumours is based on the presumptive cell of origin of the tumour. Continuous modification is needed to incorporate newly recognized tumour variants and respond to new information on cell derivation. The most recent classification is that of the World Health Organization (1993). However, after the publication of the WHO classification a number of new entities of benign as well as malignant soft tissue tumours have been described and some established entities such as malignant fibrous histiocytoma and malignant hemangiopericytoma have been questioned[1,2]. Generally, the cytological features of the vast majority of these new entities in pathology of soft tissue tumours have not yet been investigated sufficiently. Single case reports of FNA of some entities have been published. One reason for this ignorance is that most of these new types are relatively infrequent. In Table 40.1, examples of new entities of soft tissue tumours are given.

Benign soft tissue tumours are far commoner than sarcomas. It is important to note that while most tumour types have benign and malignant counterparts, almost all sarcomas arise *de novo* rather than from malignant transformation of a benign tumour. One exception is the nerve cell tumours in von Recklinghausen's disease. At times, a neurofibroma is diagnosed in one part of the tumour, while a neurofibrosarcoma is present in another area. There is usually no clear indication of any risk factors, although putative agents such as industrial carcinogens, radiation, chronic trauma and viruses are thought to be involved in the pathogenesis of certain sarcomas.

Benign tumours

The incidence of different benign soft tissue tumours is broadly reflected in the rate of referral of various tumour

Table 40.1 Examples of new entities of benign and malignant soft tissue tumours

Benign tumours	Sarcomas
Chondroid lipoma	Low-grade fibromyxoid sarcoma
Solitary fibrous tumour of soft tissues	Spindle cell liposarcoma
Mixed tumours and myoepithelioma	

types for aspiration. Lipoma is the commonest and has been recorded most frequently during the last 20 years at the Orthopaedic Oncology Group at Lund University Hospital in Sweden[3].

Neurilemmoma, intramuscular myxoma, desmoid tumour and haemangioma are encountered somewhat less often. Ganglions are frequently subjected to aspiration. Fibrous histiocytoma or dermatofibroma, the commonest superficial benign soft tissue tumour after lipoma, is aspirated quite infrequently in our experience. A number of rare tumours such as leiomyoma, rhabdomyoma, granular cell tumour, elastofibroma, ossifying fibromyxoid tumour and perineurioma are only occasionally referred for aspiration.

Benign tumours of adipose tissue
Lipoma

Usually slow growing asymptomatic tumours of adults, lipomas may be superficial or deeply placed, solitary or multiple, and vary enormously in size at presentation. Their histological structure is also variable. They are composed of mature adipose tissue, but may include other connective tissue elements and may show evidence of trauma or degeneration.

Cytological findings

► Fatty tissue fragments
► Few dissociated adipocytes
► Fragments of striated muscle or regenerating muscle fibres in inter/intramuscular lipoma

Aspirates from lipomas have virtually the same appearance as aspirates from normal adipose tissue. It is therefore important to know that the needle was really placed within the mass. If a needle with a stylet is used for deep-seated tumours, contamination with normal subcutaneous fat is avoided.

Typically, smears from lipomas consist of fragments of adipose tissue composed of large cells containing a single vacuole of fat and a small dark peripheral nucleus. Within the fragments a few capillary strands are usually observed (Fig. 40.1). Dispersed lipocytes are rather uncommon. Intramuscular lipomas often include fragments of ordinary striated muscle. When an infiltrating intramuscular lipoma is aspirated, multinucleated regenerating muscle fibres may be observed, mimicking multinucleated giant cells and hence known as 'muscle giant cells'[3].

Lipomas with chondroid metaplasia include fragments of acellular myxoid matrix stained bluish red with MGG, along with the adipose tissue fragments. Occasionally rounded chondrocytes are observed in lacunae in this matrix. Aspirates from lipomas with myxoid degeneration often yield a few drops of colourless stringy fluid. Smears show a blue or bluish red myxoid background matrix containing isolated lipocytes or small clusters of fat cells, in addition to the usual fragments of adipose tissue.

Variants of lipoma

Angiolipoma

Angiolipomas are subcutaneous and often multiple and tender on palpation. An angiolipoma should be suspected when the tumour is tender on palpation and numerous branching thin vessel fragments are seen in the fat tissue fragments.

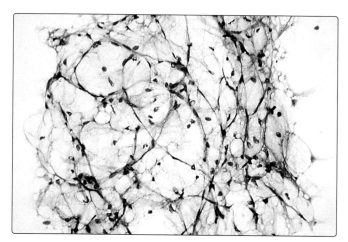

Fig. 40.1 Lipoma. Part of a fragment of adipose tissue. Large fat cells with small, dark nuclei. Thin capillary stands intersect the fragment. (MGG × MP)

Pleomorphic lipoma

Pleomorphic lipoma is a subcutaneous tumour usually found in middle-aged men in the tissues of the back of the neck. On histology, the characteristic finding is the presence of floret cells. These are multinucleated giant cells with a moderate amount of cytoplasm and multiple marginally placed hyperchromatic nuclei with indistinct chromatin[4]. The cells are easily observed in aspiration smears within and between the fatty fragments. They are large with ample cytoplasm and multiple nuclei, which in well preserved cells are overlapping and situated near the cytoplasmic membrane (Fig. 40.2A,B).

Spindle cell lipoma

Spindle cell lipoma is also a subcutaneous tumour most frequently found in the back of the neck or shoulder region in middle-aged men. The microscopic appearance in histological sections varies; lipomatous tissue is more or less replaced by bundles or fascicles of uniform spindle cells in a myxoid background matrix or associated with collagen fibres[5]. Aspirates contain a mixture of adipose tissue fragments and sheets or clusters of spindle cells with elongated, uniform nuclei and poorly demarcated cytoplasm (Fig. 40.3). A variable but important diagnostic sign is fragments of collagen fibres mixed with the other tissue constituents[6]. Runs of spindle cells may also be observed within the fragments. Due to the variable tissue pattern, aspirates from spindle cell lipomas may show a predominance of adipose tissue fragments or a predominance of spindle cell fascicles and abundant myxoid background matrix.

Hibernoma

Derived from foetal fat cells, the hibernoma is a rare slow-growing tumour not only situated in the interscapular region, on the back or chest wall (sites of normal deposits of foetal fat) but also on the extremities. Hibernomas are easily identified histologically as lobulated tumours consisting

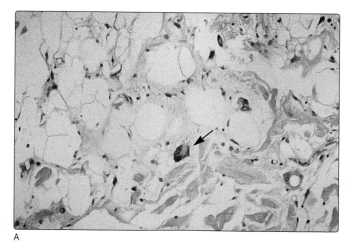

A

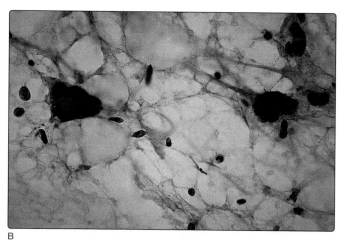

B

Fig. 40.2 (A) Histological section from a pleomorphic lipoma. One typical multinucleated floret cell (arrow). (H&E × MP) (B) Floret cells in FNA of pleomorphic lipoma. Large multinucleated cells with abundant cytoplasm and with overlapping nuclei along the cytoplasmic border. (H&E × HP)

mainly of small rounded cells with multiple cytoplasmic vacuoles or granular cytoplasm surrounding central nuclei. They are vascular tumours and contain numerous capillaries. There are few reports of the aspiration cytology of hibernoma. Typically, multivacuolated cells are found in intimate contact with capillary strands[7]. The principal cell is thus finely vacuolated with a centrally located small uniform nucleus or granulated, but ordinary large lipocytes with single vacuoles are also observed. In hibernomas, lobules of ordinary large adipose cells may predominate and the typical hibernoma cells may be in a minority. FNAs from hibernoma may thus be made up of ordinary lipoma-like fat cells.

Lipoblastoma

Lipoblastoma, a tumour of infancy involving the extremities, can be solitary or diffuse. Composed of immature fat cells histologically, with mesenchymal, myxoid and fibrotic areas, the tumour is thought to be capable of maturation to a common lipoma. The cytological findings in fine needle aspirates have only been described in single cases. Typical features were the presence of small uniform adipocytes with vacuolated cytoplasm and rounded nuclei, set in a myxoid background matrix, which also contained strands of capillaries[7].

Chondroid lipoma

Chondroid lipoma, an infrequent benign lipomatous tumour, was fully categorized in 1993[8]. Usually it is a well-defined, deep-seated tumour in the limbs, trunk or head and neck region. Histologically it is composed of an admixture of normal adipocytes, chondroblast-like cells and vacuolated, lipoblast-like cells in a myxochondroid matrix. Most neoplastic cells stain positively with S 100-protein.

We have had the opportunity to study the FNA cytology of chondroid lipoma in two cases (Fig. 40.4A,B).

Cytological findings

- ▶ More or less abundant myxoid background matrix
- ▶ Groups and clusters of ordinary fat cells
- ▶ Groups and clusters of uni- or multivacuolated, lipoblast-like cells with irregular nuclear shape, scalloped nuclei and multivacuolated cytoplasm
- ▶ Nuclei often irregular, lobulated or coffee bean-shaped
- ▶ A plexiform capillary network is not observed

The nuclei are benign-looking in spite of variation of size and shape. One important feature in the differential diagnosis from myxoid liposarcoma is the lack of a plexiform capillary network in the cell clusters.

Diagnostic pitfalls in benign adipose tissue tumours

Differentiation of these benign lipomatous lesions from various types of liposarcoma is the most serious problem.

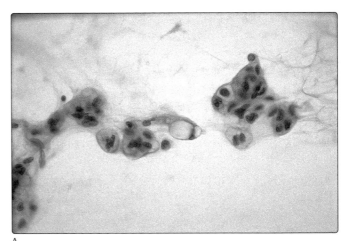

A

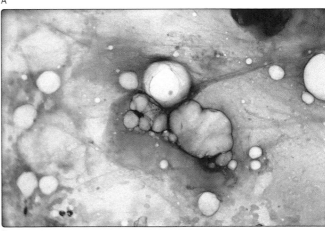

B

Fig. 40.4   (A,B) Chondroid lipoma. Group of lipoblast-cells with uni- or multivacuolated cytoplasm and irregularly shaped nuclei. (A, H&E × HP; B, MGG × HP)

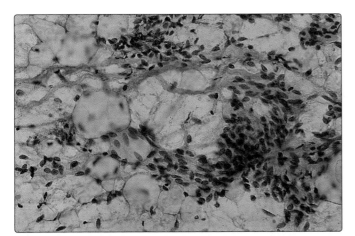

Fig. 40.3   Spindle cell lipoma. Within a fragment of adipose tissue strands and clusters of fusiform, fibroblast-like cells with ovoid or elongated nuclei are observed. (H&E × MP)

The main clue to a benign diagnosis is the absence of atypical lipoblasts. Clinical details such as age, site, size and duration of the lesion must also be taken into account.

Lipomas with chondroid metaplasia or myxoid degeneration have been mistaken for myxoid liposarcoma. The large hyperchromatic cells in pleomorphic lipoma may be misdiagnosed as sarcoma cells, suggesting a lipoma-like liposarcoma. Hibernoma can be mistaken for a well-differentiated liposarcoma because of the multivacuolated lipocytes and branching capillary strands. Regressive changes in lipoma with increased vascularity and the presence of vacuolated lipophages may also mimic liposarcoma. Chondroid lipoma is easily mistaken for liposarcoma or extraskeletal myxoid chondrosarcoma.

Nerve sheath tumours

This group of tumours, derived from the Schwann cells, which myelinate and protect all peripheral nerves, includes neurilemmoma, also known as Schwannoma, and neurofibroma, the tumour type seen classically in von Recklinghausen's disease. Granular cell tumours are also now known to be of neural origin.

Neurilemmoma

These are the commonest of the group, occurring in adults on limbs, head and neck. Encapsulated histologically, they are composed of alternating structured areas of palisaded spindle-shaped cells (Antoni A) and loose myxoid areas (Antoni B). Degenerative changes are common, earning the title of ancient neurilemmoma when large, of long duration and exhibiting the marked nuclear pleomorphism characteristic of this variant.

Cytological findings

▶ Variable cellularity
▶ Tumour tissue fragments vary in size and cellularity
▶ Cohesive cells, rarely single tumour cells
▶ Occasional palisades of cells
▶ Indistinct cytoplasm, elongated nuclei, pointed ends
▶ Moderate nuclear pleomorphism
▶ Myxoid background matrix occasionally
▶ Fragmented fibrillary background fragments

There are numerous case reports of the typical cytological features of neurilemmoma and there is also one correlative cytohistological study of 28 tumours[9]. The descriptions given correspond well with the author's experience of fine needle aspirates from over 80 neurilemmomas (M Åkerman, unpublished work, 1999).

A characteristic clinical sign is the sharp, sometimes radiating pain experienced by the patient on needling. Smears vary in cellularity, usually consisting of numerous tumour tissue fragments of different size. The fragments also vary in cellularity and have irregular borders, so that at

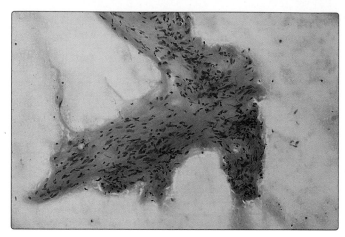

Fig. 40.5 Aspirate smear from a neurilemmoma. A tumour tissue fragment with irregular borders made up of cohesive cells with fusiform nuclei. Variable cellularity in the fragment. (H&E × LP)

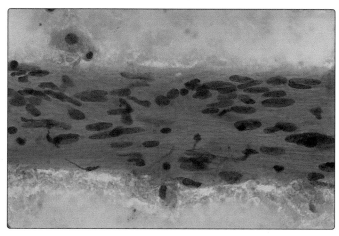

Fig. 40.6 Detail from a neurilemmoma fragment; a fibrillar background substance containing a mixture of cells with elongated nuclei with pointed ends and rounded 'lymphocyte-like' nuclei. Moderate anisokaryosis is present. (H&E × HP)

low magnification they have been compared with pieces of a jigsaw puzzle (Fig. 40.5)[9].

The cytological findings generally correspond to histological Antoni A tissue; the fragments consist of cohesive cells with very indistinct cell borders and spindle-shaped nuclei with pointed ends. Small cells with rounded 'lymphocyte-like' or ovoid nuclei are also seen. A number of the elongated nuclei are comma-shaped or have one end bent like a fishhook. Variation in nuclear size and shape is always seen and may be marked. Palisading of nuclei and Verocay body structures are sometimes observed. Dispersed cells are uncommon and mitoses are almost never seen.

Another typical feature is a fibrillary background substance in which the cells are embedded. This background is best visualized by H&E staining (Fig. 40.6). Some neurilemmomas yield a small amount of cystic fluid when aspirated. In other cases dispersed cells are embedded in a myxoid background and the tumour fragments are small with less cohesive tumour cells mingling with histiocytes. These findings correspond to Antoni B areas on histology.

Aspirates from neurofibromata may have an abundant myxoid background and dispersed cells are often more common than tumour tissue fragments. Other than this, the findings are similar to those of neurilemmomas.

Granular cell tumour

The granular cell tumour, described by Abrikosoff in 1926 and originally considered to be of myogenic origin, is now regarded as a tumour of peripheral nerve derivation[10]. Much commoner in adults than children, it is mainly situated subcutaneously but occasionally found in muscle and skin, and more rarely in internal organs. Breast and tongue are quite common sites. Histologically there is a tendency to packaging of the tumour cells. They are rounded with central nuclei and coarsely granular cytoplasm, with some smaller PAS positive cells between.

Cytological findings

► Dispersed cells and cell clusters
► Naked nuclei common
► Abundant granular cytoplasm when preserved
► Round nuclei, bland chromatin, prominent nucleoli

The cellular yield is usually good, consisting of tumour cells with abundant but fragile cytoplasm and stripped nuclei are therefore common. In preserved cells the cytoplasm is typically granular, staining eosinophilic with H&E and blue with MGG. The chromatin structure in the rounded nuclei is uniformly regular and nucleoli are quite small but prominent.

Diagnostic pitfalls in benign nerve sheath tumours

The most difficult problem lies in correctly diagnosing the so-called ancient neurilemmoma, which is easily mistaken for a sarcoma, especially leiomyosarcoma[11,12]. The large cells with pleomorphic, hyperchromatic sometimes bizarre nuclei typical of an ancient neurilemmoma are deceptively like sarcoma cells. However, careful inspection of the enlarged nuclei reveals degenerative changes, including the so called 'kern-loche', which are large intranuclear vacuoles usually present if looked for carefully (Fig. 40.7). Mitoses are not observed cytologically. A leiomyosarcoma can be excluded by immunohistochemical staining of smear or cell block with S 100-protein and anti-desmin. Ancient neurilemmoma displays strong S 100 positivity and is desmin negative.

Neurilemmoma and neurofibroma with a myxoid background matrix in smears may be misdiagnosed as a number of other soft tissue tumours exhibiting a similar background. These are listed in Table 40.2.

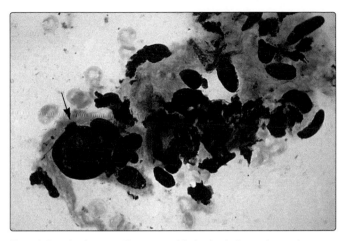

Fig. 40.7 Ancient neurilemmoma. Marked anisokaryosis, one large rounded nucleus with a typical 'kern-loche' (arrow). Faintly fibrillar background matrix. (MGG × HP)

Table 40.2 Soft tissue tumours with a myxoid background matrix. Important cytological features in the differential diagnosis

Tumour	Cytologic findings
Nodular fasciitis	Marked anisocytosis and anisokaryosis in dispersed proliferating fibroblasts. Single and binucleated cells resembling ganglion cells
Neurilemmoma	Mainly tissue fragments, dispersed cells uncommon. Fibrillary background in fragments. Nuclei with pointed ends, comma or fish-hook shaped. Nuclear palisading. Verocay body structures
Neurofibroma	Mixture of dispersed cells and cell clusters. Cell morphology as neurilemmoma
Intramuscular myxoma	Abundant myxoid background. Rather poor cellularity. Slender tumour cells with long cytoplasmic processes and elongated nuclei. Occasional vessel fragments and 'muscle-giant cells' in background
Ganglion	Abundant myxoid background. Poor cellularity. Scattered round cells with rounded nuclei
Myxofibrosarcoma	Abundant myxoid background. Tumour tissue fragments with branching vessels mixed with dispersed cells. Vessel fragments in background matrix. Cellular and nuclear atypia
Low-grade fibromyxoid sarcoma	Abundant myxoid background. Small clusters of spindle cells mixed with dispersed cells. Slight to moderate cellular atypia. Occasional vessel fragments in background matrix
Myxoid liposarcoma	Abundant myxoid background. Tumour tissue fragments with myxoid background, vacuoles and distinct branching capillary network. Lipoblasts present. Slight to moderate cellular atypia
Extraskeletal myxoid chondrosarcoma	Branching uniform cells with elongated cytoplasm and ovoid or rounded nuclei with slight atypia, or dispersed cells with sharp cellular borders and rounded nuclei with prominent nucleoli. Varying amount of myxoid background matrix. Rarely cartilage-like fragments

The richly cellular yield of granular cell tumours and large numbers of naked nuclei with prominent nucleoli seen in these lesions have been misinterpreted as malignant in smears. In fact, malignant granular cell tumour is very rare, and the key to the correct diagnosis lies in awareness of the characteristic cellular features of the benign lesion.

Fibrous and fibrohistiocytic tumours
Fibrous histiocytoma

This common tumour occurs in young adults, especially on the extremities. The lesions may be solitary or multiple, and either subcutaneous or deep. They are composed of cells resembling histiocytes and fibroblasts with a storiform pattern of growth, likened to a cartwheel. There are usually some inflammatory cells and deposits of iron within the tumour.

Cytological findings

▶ Solid cell clusters and dispersed cells
▶ Fibroblastic and histiocyte-like cells
▶ Multinucleated giant cells of Touton type
▶ Phagocytosis with haemosiderin deposits in histiocytes

The variable histological features of fibrous histiocytomas are reflected in the cytological findings in aspirate smears. A common picture is the dual presence of fibroblastic cells with ovoid or elongated nuclei and histiocytic cells, which have rounded or irregular nuclei and rather abundant cytoplasm. Giant cells of Touton type, with their characteristic peripheral circlet of nuclei, are almost always found, as are deposits of haemosiderin in the histiocytic cells. Capillary strands may be observed.

Desmoid tumour

This tumour is a type of fibromatosis affecting young adults, arising from connective tissue associated with muscle or fascia especially around the shoulder and pelvic girdle. It has a tendency to local recurrence and may behave aggressively. Histologically there are bundles of uniform elongated cells with bland nuclei and intercellular collagen or mucoid material.

Cytological findings

▶ Variable cell yield
▶ Cell clusters and dispersed cells
▶ Fragments of collagenized stroma
▶ Spindle-shaped nuclei with moderate anisokaryosis
▶ Stripped nuclei common
▶ Preserved cells show cytoplasmic processes
▶ 'Muscle giant cells' if infiltrating striated muscle

The cytological appearance of desmoid tumours has only been described in case reports[13]. The 15 cases from our files have all shown similar features in smears (M Åkerman, unpublished work 1999). The cellularity is variable and at times only a few spindle-shaped cells are aspirated. Because of the highly collagenized stroma vigorous aspirations are necessary. Desmoid tumours are very firm to palpate and a rubbery resistance is felt when needling.

A finding common to all our cases has been the presence of quite numerous fragments of collagenized stroma staining bluish grey with MGG and showing a faintly fibrillary background (Fig. 40.8). Stripped nuclei are also commonly seen. The nuclei are elongated or ovoid with finely granular chromatin and small nucleoli (Fig. 40.9). Preserved cells have well demarcated pale cytoplasm, often with unipolar or bipolar cytoplasmic processes. The cells appear in small cohesive clusters or are dissociated. Sometimes faintly outlined nuclei are seen in the stromal fragments. When infiltration of striated muscle occurs, 'muscle giant cells' are found.

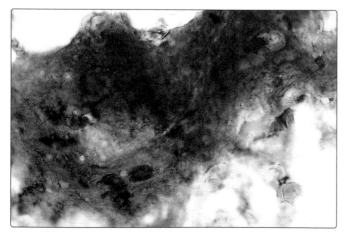

Fig. 40.8 Desmoid tumour. Part of a fragment of collagenized stroma with a faintly outlined fibrillar background material and scattered nuclei. (MGG, × HP)

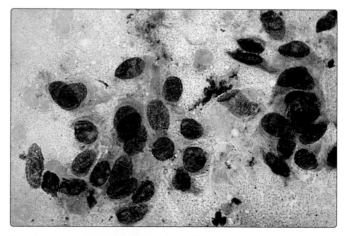

Fig. 40.9 Desmoid tumour. A cluster of loosely attached fibroblast-like cells with ovoid nuclei and pale greyish blue cytoplasm. (MGG, × OI)

Diagnostic pitfalls

Important diagnostic pitfalls arise when the cellular yield is poor and stromal fragments are lacking. Low-grade malignant fibrosarcoma and monophasic fibrous synovial sarcoma may be cytologically misdiagnosed as desmoid tumour and vice versa. Other differential diagnoses include nodular fasciitis, neurilemmoma and leiomyoma. The uniform spindle cell population, fragments of collagenized stroma, absence of a myxoid background and ganglion-like cells exclude nodular fasciitis; while tumour tissue fragments with elongated or comma-shaped nuclei in a fibrillar background are the hallmarks of neurilemmoma rather than desmoid tumour.

Soft tissue solitary fibrous tumour

Solitary fibrous tumour has been described under several names in the literature, most commonly as localized mesothelioma, fibrous mesothelioma or pleural fibroma. Tumours with the same histologic features have been described in almost every part of the body, including soft tissue. At present, the consensus is that solitary fibrous tumour is mesenchymal rather than a mesothelial lesion and the immunohistochemical profile as well as ultrastructural studies have shown that the tumour cells are predominantly fibroblastic. The essential histological features are alternating hypercellular and hypocellular sclerotic areas of bland looking short spindly or ovoid cells with poorly defined, scanty cytoplasm. Thick or thin collagen fibrils are intimately mixed with the spindle cells. The most diagnostically important feature is the CD34 positivity of the spindle cells. In some cases the cells are also CD99 positive[14].

The cytological features of soft tissue solitary fibrous tumour have been briefly described in eight cases[15]. The cytology seems to equate to that of pleural tumours[16].

Cytological findings

▶ Variably cellularity
▶ Stripped nuclei
▶ Cells in tight, at times fascicle-like clusters, or dispersed
▶ Bland chromatin structure
▶ Inconspicuous nucleoli

In aspirate smears, the soft tissue solitary fibrous tumour appears as a spindle cell tumour with bland-looking cell. Without the aid of ancillary immunocytochemistry a correct cell-type diagnosis is probably almost impossible (Fig. 40.10A,B)

Diagnostic pitfalls

The most important pitfalls are monomorphic fibrous synovial sarcoma, low-grade malignant fibrosarcoma and low-grade malignant peripheral nerve sheath tumour (MPNST). One feature, which may be useful with regard to monophasic synovial sarcoma, is the absence of mitotic figures. A clue to a correct diagnosis is CD34 positive spindle cells.

Tumours of smooth muscle

Benign smooth muscle tumours, known as leiomyomas, can be divided into visceral and extravisceral types. The latter are separated into two groups depending on whether superficial or deep-seated. Superficial leiomyomas, which are very common and often small, are thought to arise from arrector pili muscles of skin or from walls of blood vessels. In our experience they are almost never referred for FNA.

Leiomyoma of deep soft tissues

The rare leiomyomas of deep soft tissue are usually larger than their superficial counterparts and the clinical impression is that of a deep-seated, rather firm and well

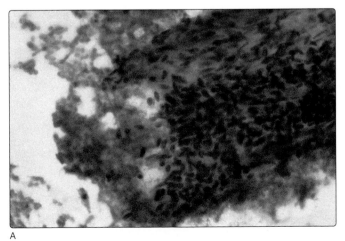
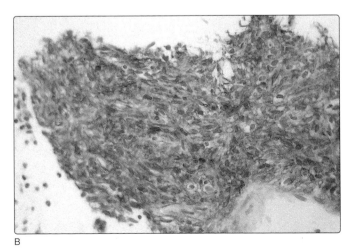

A

B

Fig. 40.10   (A,B) Solitary fibrous tumour of soft tissue. (A) A fascicle of tightly packed cells with bland looking fusiform nuclei. (H&E × MP) (B) Cell-block preparation stained with CD34. (Immunoperoxidase × MP)

circumscribed soft tissue tumour. They occur in children or adults, usually in the deep musculature of the extremities. Histologically, they are composed of interlacing bundles of eosinophilic cells with no mitotic activity and little nuclear pleomorphism, features, which they share with the superficial tumours.

Cytological findings

- ▶ Dispersed cells, clusters, a few small tissue fragments
- ▶ Naked nuclei common
- ▶ Moderate anisokaryosis
- ▶ Blunt-ended elongated or truncated nuclei
- ▶ Fragments have a bluish red background matrix (MGG)
- ▶ Abundant grey or blue cytoplasm (MGG) in dispersed cells
- ▶ Small nucleoli in dispersed cells

The author's experience of FNA of deep-seated leiomyoma is limited, being based on only five tumours. However the cytological findings in each of the aspirate smears were remarkably similar. The typical tumour cell exhibited the same nuclear characteristics as described in histological sections[10]; this included blunt-ended, 'cigar-shaped', elongated or ovoid nuclei of varying size, often truncated and sometimes containing vacuoles. The chromatin was finely granular and nucleoli were small. Naked nuclei were a common finding.

Preserved cells were arranged in clusters and also dissociated. Small fragments of tumour tissue were observed in two cases; tumour cells with indistinct cytoplasmic borders were embedded in a reddish blue background matrix. The cytoplasm in better preserved cells was light grey to blue on MGG staining. Mitoses were not observed (Fig. 40.11A,B). (Personal observation 1992).

Diagnostic pitfalls

There are two important differential diagnoses: low-grade malignant leiomyosarcoma and extra-abdominal desmoid tumour. At low power magnification, the overall pattern in smears is similar in leiomyomas and desmoid tumours: a mixture of dispersed cells and cell clusters, many stripped nuclei and stromal fragments. The clue to the diagnosis is the nuclear characteristics of smooth muscle cells, which are blunt-ended and truncated.

The diagnostic cytological criteria of the unusual epithelioid variant of leiomyoma are incomplete but their round cell pattern may easily be mistaken for an epithelial tumour.

Tumours of striated muscle

An exception to the generalization that the benign soft tissue tumours outnumber their malignant counterparts, rhabdomyoma is a rare neoplasm compared with rhabdomyosarcoma. Two main variants, adult and foetal, are distinguished, and a third similarly rare tumour, the

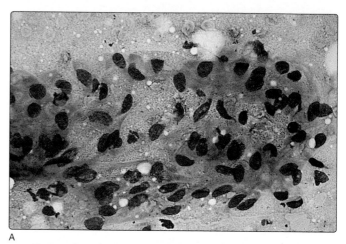

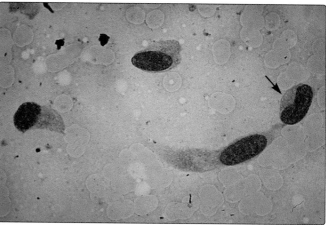

Fig. 40.11 (A) Leiomyoma. A cellular cluster of loosely attached cells which are embedded in a bluish red background substance. Pale grey or blue uni- or bipolar cytoplasm. (MGG, × HP) (B) Typical leiomyoma cells: blunt-ended, cigar-shaped nuclei. One nucleus segmented (arrow). (MGG, × OI)

genital type, develops in the vagina. Descriptions of the cytological features have been published in single case reports[17-19]. Similar findings have been described in these cases, the smears including large elongated cells resembling muscle fibres, with large nuclei and prominent nucleoli.

Tumours of blood vessels

Localized haemangiomas are extremely common, particularly in childhood. Structurally, they are difficult to distinguish from hamartomas, malformations and reactive vascular proliferations, such as pyogenic granuloma, since all of these lesions are composed of well formed blood vessels. Capillary and cavernous patterns are recognized microscopically, and there are other less common variants.

Aspiration of any type of haemangioma invariably yields copious blood. The smears are usually poor in cells, but often include cells with spindle-shaped or ovoid nuclei with a varying amount of indistinct cytoplasm. Macrophages containing haemosiderin pigment may be found. In our experience, aspirates are not characteristic and are usually non-diagnostic. However, clinical findings in the case of intramuscular haemangiomas may be highly suggestive since these are deep-seated tumours, which increase in size and become painful during exercise, yielding abundant blood on aspiration, with very few cells.

Soft tissue tumours of uncertain histogenesis
Intramuscular myxoma

The intramuscular myxoma is a benign soft tissue tumour of uncertain histogenesis which generally occurs in the middle-aged or elderly. Most common sites are the thigh, shoulder region and buttock. Because of its firm consistency and deep location the lesion is often suspicious of a sarcoma clinically.

Cytological findings

► Colourless stringy fluid on aspiration
► Abundant myxoid background
► Single vessel fragments in background matrix
► Scanty tissue fragments and dispersed cells
► Slender tumour cells, long cytoplasmic processes
► Elongated nuclei, uniform chromatin

The cytological findings on FNA have been described in ten cases[20] and we have had the opportunity of studying aspirate smears from a further 30 tumours. Characteristically, the aspirate consists of a few drops of stringy myxoid colourless fluid, not easily spread. This fluid is blue or violet on MGG and faintly eosinophilic on H&E stains.

The cellularity is generally poor. Dispersed cells mingle with a few tissue fragments of loosely attached cells in the myxoid background matrix (Fig. 40.12). The cells are usually elongated, with cytoplasmic processes which may be extremely long (Fig. 40.13). They have ovoid, elongated or sometimes rounded nuclei. Cells with rounded nuclei may have abundant triangular or polyhedral cytoplasm, blue or violet with MGG stains, and which may contain a single large vacuole or sometimes several. Binucleated cells may also be found. The chromatin texture is uniformly finely granular and nucleoli, if any, are small. A few capillary vessel strands may be observed in the background matrix as well as in the tumour fragments.

Diagnostic pitfalls

A number of benign and malignant soft tissue tumours with abundant myxoid background in smears must be considered in the differential diagnosis. Benign nerve sheath tumours, nodular fasciitis, ganglion, myxoid liposarcoma, low-grade myxofibrosarcoma, low-grade fibromyxoid sarcoma and myxoid extraskeletal chondrosarcoma are important diagnostic pitfalls (Table 40.2).

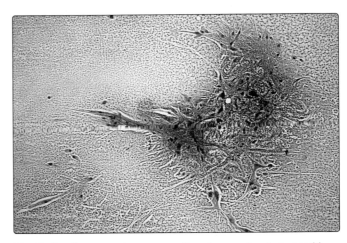

Fig. 40.12   Intramuscular myxoma. Overview: an abundant myxoid background matrix and myxoid tumour fragment containing spindle cells with bipolar cytoplasm. (MGG, × LP)

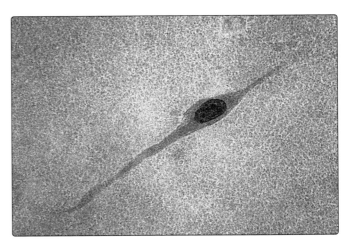

Fig. 40.13   The typical myxoma cell has very long, thin cytoplasmic processes. (H&E, × OI)

Mixed tumours and myoepitheliomas of soft tissue

Recently the possible occurrence of mixed tumours and/or myoepitheliomas in the subcutis or deep soft tissues has been studied by Kilpatrick et al.[21]. These tumours have been described predominantly in the extremities of middle-aged adults. Microscopically a mixed tumour of soft tissue resembles pleomorphic adenoma of salivary glands and chondroid syringoma. We have had the opportunity to study aspirates from two tumours and their cytomorphology was similar to that of a pleomorphic adenoma or a chondroid syringoma (Fig. 40.14)). The most important differential diagnosis in subcutaneous tumours is chondroid syringoma and in deep-seated tumours extraskeletal myxoid chondrosarcoma.

A common target for FNA is the *ganglion*, a cystic degenerative lesion arising in relation to tendon sheaths or occasionally nerve sheaths. Ganglia are not true soft tissue tumours but their clinical appearance is that of a superficial well demarcated firm soft tissue tumour on palpation. They

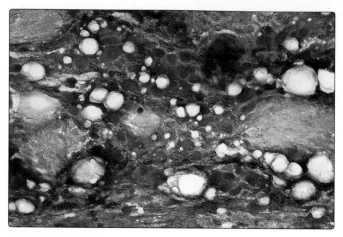

Fig. 40.14   Mixed tumour of soft tissue. In a partly fibrillar myxoid background matrix epithelial-like cells arranged in small clusters and rows. (MGG × HP)

typically yield some droplets of thick colourless myxoid stringy fluid. In smears, this material is dark blue on MGG and pale pink in H&E stains. There are scanty single cells with pale cytoplasm and small rounded or ovoid nuclei with regular chromatin texture[22]. Aspirates from ganglia are never misdiagnosed as malignant tumours but other benign tumours with a prominent myxoid background in smears must obviously be considered (Table 40.2).

Malignant tumours

There are approaching 30 different histological types of soft tissue sarcoma. Of these, malignant fibrous histiocytoma, liposarcoma and leiomyosarcoma are generally found to be the most common entities[10]. In the data-based Central Soft Tissue Sarcoma Registry of the Scandinavian Sarcoma Group (a multidisciplinary association of the Nordic Countries) 2799 soft tissue sarcomas of the extremities and trunk wall were registered 1986–August 1998. The most common sarcoma was malignant fibrous histiocytoma followed by leiomyosarcoma, liposarcoma, synovial sarcoma and malignant peripheral nerve sheath tumour.

Among adult soft tissue sarcomas of the extremities and trunk investigated by FNA from 1972–91, approximately 50% were malignant fibrous histiocytomas, while liposarcomas, leiomyosarcomas and synovial sarcomas represented 30–35% of the material. Malignant peripheral nerve sheath tumours and haemangiopericytomas were uncommon. Rare tumours, such as clear cell sarcoma, epithelioid cell sarcoma, alveolar soft part sarcoma, angiosarcoma, fibrosarcoma and extraskeletal myxoid chondrosarcoma, extraskeletal osteosarcoma and extrarenal rhabdoid tumour were only occasionally referred for FNA. The small round cell sarcomas in childhood and adolescence, which include neuroblastoma, rhabdomyosarcoma and extraskeletal neoplasms belonging to the Ewing's family of tumours, were also just occasionally aspirated.

Malignant fibrous and fibrohistiocytic tumours
Malignant fibrous histiocytoma

Recognized as a distinctive tumour of soft tissue and bone since 1963, malignant fibrous histiocytoma (MFH) was originally thought to arise from tissue histiocytes[10]. However, MFH as a specific tumour entity has been questioned during the last decade. Consensus has never been reached on the histogenesis, whether fibroblastic, dual fibroblastic/histiocytic or from primitive mesenchymal cells. Furthermore the various subtypes of MFH (storiform/pleomorphic, myxoid, giant cell, angiomatoid and inflammatory) show obvious clinical and morphologic heterogeneity. Due to these conflicting data some soft tissue pathologists have proposed that MFH, especially the storiform/pleomorphic subtype could represent the final morphological appearance of a number of poorly-differentiated sarcomas. Although this hypothesis is under debate, it has been suggested that the diagnosis of storiform/pleomorphic MFH is a diagnosis of exclusion only valid when thorough examination has failed to demonstrate any line of differentiation to prove that the tumour in question is a poorly-differentiated example of a specific histogenetic sarcoma-type. Myogenic, lipogenic and Schwann cell differentiation have been ascertained in a surprisingly high number of storiform/pleomorphic MFH on re-evaluation of various materials[23,24]. Myxoid MFH (of low-grade as well as high-grade malignancy) is regarded as a specific entity and is proposed to be diagnosed as myxofibrosarcoma, a term previously reserved for subcutaneous, predominantly low-grade, malignant myxoid MFH[25]. For a more detailed appraisal of the various subtypes of MFH reader is referred to the paper of Hollowood and Fletcher 1995[26]. In view of this new perspective on MFH, aspirates from storiform/pleomorphic MFH are classified as aspirates from pleomorphic sarcoma of MFH-type and those from myxoid MFH are classified as myxofibrosarcoma in this chapter.

The pleomorphic sarcomas of MFH type and myxofibrosarcoma are the most common and their cytomorphology has already been described in detail[27,28].

Cytological findings of pleomorphic sarcoma of MFH type

► Highly cellular yield
► Tissue fragments, cell clusters, dispersed tumour cells
► Spindle-shaped fibroblast-like cells
► Pleomorphic histiocyte-like tumour cells
► Tumour cells of indeterminate origin
► Multinucleation
► Nuclear pleomorphism, coarse chromatin, irregular nucleoli
► Mitotic figures

Smears are generally cellular, but necrosis, cystic degeneration or haemorrhage occasionally dominate the

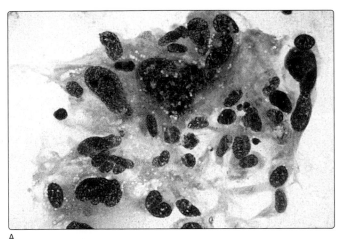

A

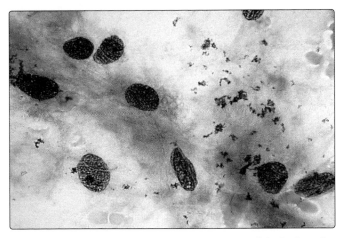

Fig. 40.16 Low-grade malignant myxofibrosarcoma. Spindle-shaped moderately atypical cells in a myxoid background matrix. (MGG, × HP)

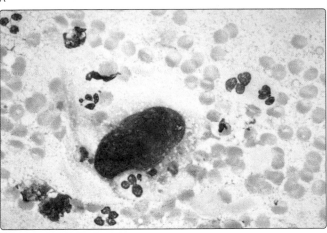

B

Fig. 40.15 (A,B) Pleomorphic sarcoma of MFH type. (A) A cluster of loosely attached pleomorphic cells with marked anisokaryosis. (MGG × HP) (B) Pleomorphic sarcoma of MFH type. A large histiocytic type cell with phagocytosis. (MGG × OI)

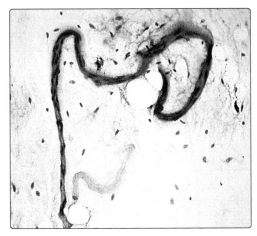

Fig. 40.17 Myxofibrosarcoma. Vessel fragment in the myxoid background. (MGG, × MP)

picture. In such cases, very few preserved sarcoma cells may be found, despite thorough screening. Dispersed cells are mixed with small clusters or tumour tissue fragments.

Marked anisocytosis and anisokaryosis are the rule in high-grade malignant tumours. However it is always possible to recognize fibroblast-like cells with fusiform or ovoid atypical nuclei and elongated cytoplasm, as well as cells resembling histiocytes with abundant cytoplasm and large eccentric rounded or irregular nuclei. The cytoplasm in the histiocyte cell types is often vacuolated or contains phagocytosed material, such as iron or lipid. Multinucleated giant cells are always found and bizarre nuclei are often seen (Fig. 40.15A,B). Normal and atypical mitoses are common.

Myxofibrosarcoma
▶ Abundant myxoid background matrix
▶ Dispersed cells and cell clusters
▶ Predominantly spindle-shaped cells with slight to moderate nuclear atypia in low-grade malignant tumours

▶ Mixture of atypical spindle cells and rounded, polyhedral pleomorphic histiocyte-like tumour cells and multinucleated cells in high-grade tumours
▶ Curved vessel fragments in the myxoid background

Myxofibrosarcomas occur in skeletal muscle, subcutaneously and in the retroperitoneum, and have a better prognosis than other variants. The subcutaneous myxofibrosarcoma has a typical histological appearance[24] with slight to moderate cellular atypia leading to a diagnosis of low-grade sarcoma. In FNA smears atypical fibroblast-like cells predominate, singly and in clusters, embedded in a myxoid background matrix, which is bright pink with MGG staining (Fig. 40.16). Scattered cells of histiocytic type are usually found with careful searching[28]. In high-grade tumours atypical, histiocyte-like cells may predominate. A profuse network of capillary vessels is a characteristic feature of the histology[25], and cytologically, vessel fragments often appear in the myxoid background (Fig. 40.17) as well as in the tissue fragments.

Aspirate smears from the 'giant cell type' contain benign osteoclast-like multinucleated giant cells in addition to the malignant pleomorphic tumour cell population[29].

Atypical fibroxanthoma

The superficial cutaneous atypical fibroxanthoma is histologically indistinguishable from pleomorphic malignant fibrous histiocytoma and is at present regarded as a cutaneous variant of this lesion. In FNA material, too, the cell pattern resembles that of storiform-pleomorphic malignant fibrous histiocytoma. The prognosis is excellent.

Fibrosarcoma

Fibrosarcoma was previously considered one of the most common types of sarcoma, but is now rarely diagnosed, as most examples can be placed in other categories by immunochemical methods or by electron microscopy[10] or cytogenetic methods. The tumour is only infrequently aspirated but when encountered, smears consist of atypical spindle-shaped cells with fusiform nuclei and elongated cytoplasm. Stripped nuclei are common. Multinucleated giant cells are not found.

Diagnostic pitfalls of pleomorphic sarcoma of MFH type

High-grade pleomorphic sarcoma of the MFH type may be difficult to distinguish from other pleomorphic sarcomas, such as pleomorphic liposarcoma, high-grade pleomorphic leiomyosarcoma and malignant peripheral nerve sheath tumour. The absence of phagocytosis and presence of atypical, often multinucleated lipoblasts favours liposarcoma and cigar-shaped, often segmented nuclei are typical of a leiomyosarcoma.

Clinically, the most important pitfall is to distinguish cells from pleomorphic sarcoma, whatever histotype, from the rare occurrence of soft tissue metastasis arising from a large cell pleomorphic carcinoma or sarcoma-like malignant melanoma or soft tissue presentation of large cell anaplastic lymphoma. Immunocytochemistry will resolve this problem conclusively if the cells stain with cytokeratin markers or with melanoma specific antibody (HMB 45 or NK1C3) in case of melanoma or with CD30, EMA and the ALK-antibody in case of anaplastic large cell lymphoma.

Intramuscular myxoma and myxoid liposarcoma may be misdiagnosed as low-grade malignant myxofibrosarcoma or vice versa (Table 40.2). Myxomas lack pleomorphic tumour cells, while the absence of lipoblasts favours a diagnosis of fibrohistiocytic tumour. Fibrosarcoma is difficult to differentiate from other predominantly spindle cell sarcomas, such as monophasic fibrous synovial sarcoma and nerve sheath tumours. Low-grade malignant fibrosarcoma may be misdiagnosed as a desmoid tumour.

Low-grade fibromyxoid sarcoma

This sarcoma was first described by Evans in 1987 and 1993[30]. Low-grade fibromyxoid sarcoma has been considered a specific entity separated from low-grade myxofibrosarcoma. Histologically, these tumours are composed of bland, uniform fibroblasts often arranged in a whorled pattern in a myxoid matrix, variably collagenous. Vascularity is low as is the mitotic activity. Immunohistochemical stains most often show nothing but vimentin-positivity. The cytology of low-grade fibromyxoid sarcoma has been described in one case report[31]. We have had the opportunity to examine FNA smears from one case. In an abundant myxoid background matrix numerous predominantly dispersed fibroblast-like cells with slight atypia were observed (Fig. 40.18A,B). The cellularity and uniformity of the tumour cells indicated a low-grade spindle cell sarcoma.

The most important differential diagnosis is low-grade myxofibrosarcoma and one important feature is the presence of curved vessel fragments in the myxoid background in myxofibrosarcoma (see Fig. 40.17).

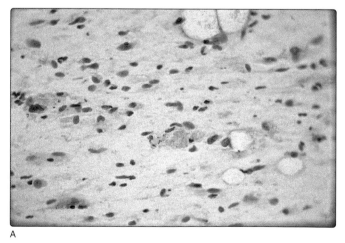
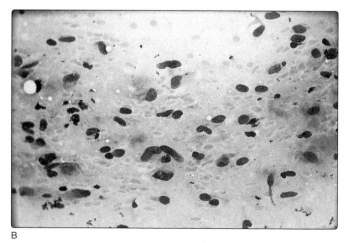

A   B

Fig. 40.18   Low-grade fibromyxoid sarcoma. (A) Dispersed fibroblast-like cells exhibiting slight to moderate atypia. (H&E × HP) (B) The tumour cells are embedded in a myxoid background matrix. (MGG × HP)

Malignant tumours of adipose tissue

Liposarcomas occur predominantly in adults and are among the largest of the soft tissue tumours at presentation. They arise from primitive mesenchymal cells rather than from mature adipose tissue, and are found most frequently in the deep tissues of the limbs and retroperitoneum.

In the WHO classification of soft tissue tumours, lipomas are divided in five different types:

1 Well-differentiated, of which there are three subtypes: lipoma-like, sclerosing and inflammatory
2 Myxoid liposarcoma, which is the commonest type, consisting of a mixture of lipoblasts and anastomosing capillaries set in a mucopolysaccharide matrix
3 Round cell liposarcoma, composed of poorly-differentiated small rounded lipoblasts with very little background matrix
4 Dedifferentiated liposarcoma
5 Pleomorphic liposarcoma, in which many giant cells are seen, sometimes containing finely dispersed lipid droplets. There are numerous mitoses

Mixed liposarcomas consist of two or more of these types in the same tumour. However, considering recently available data, especially on the specific chromosome changes in lipomatous tumours, it has been proposed that liposarcomas should be divided into three groups.

1 Well-differentiated liposarcoma (lipoma-like, sclerosing, inflammatory, spindle cell and dedifferentiated variants), featuring ring chromosomes and long marker chromosomes from Chromosome 12
2 Myxoid and round cell (poorly-differentiated myxoid) liposarcoma with reciprocal translocation t(12;16)
3 Pleomorphic liposarcoma featuring a complex karyotype

This proposed classification scheme may be of interest in FNA cytology of liposarcoma as chromosomal and molecular genetic analyses may be performed on aspirated material.

The cytological appearance of myxoid, round cell and pleomorphic liposarcomas have been described in two retrospective studies comprising 35 tumours[3,7], but the cytology of the well-differentiated type has only been documented in a few cases[7] and so far, there are no reports of the cytology of the spindle cell variant.

Cytological findings

► Cellular smears
► Tumour cells dissociated and in fragments
► Myxoid background, varying with the tumour type
► Capillary networks
► Lipoblasts and small tumour cells in variable proportions
► Atypia and pleomorphism vary with the type of liposarcoma

Experience of the FNA findings in myxoid liposarcoma reveals a characteristic picture. There is an abundant myxoid background, often rather granular in appearance, and within this, tissue fragments of variable size mingle with dispersed tumour cells. The tissue fragments also show a myxoid matrix and have a distinct network of thin branching capillaries.

Lipoblasts with single or multiple vacuoles impart a vacuolated appearance to the tumour fragments at low magnification. These lipoblasts have moderately atypical scalloped nuclei and are usually found along the capillaries. However, the most frequent tumour cells are small, with indistinct cytoplasm and rounded or ovoid slightly atypical nuclei (Fig. 40.19). Mitoses are very seldom observed. The myxoid matrix and the lipoblasts with their scalloped nuclei are best diagnosed on MGG staining.

Pure round cell liposarcomas are generally highly cellular. FNA smears are either composed predominantly of dissociated cells with many stripped nuclei, or consist of cell-rich tumour tissue fragments with closely packed overlapping cells. A myxoid background and branching capillary network are less prominent than in myxoid liposarcoma. Lipoblasts with one or several cytoplasmic vacuoles and scalloped atypical nuclei are always present (Fig. 40.20). Nuclear atypia is more pronounced than in myxoid liposarcoma and nucleoli may be large and prominent. The cytoplasm of the lipoblasts gives the fragments a vacuolated appearance. Mitotic figures are not uncommon.

The pleomorphic liposarcoma is cytologically a high-grade malignant sarcoma with marked anisocytosis and anisokaryosis. Aspiration smears resemble those of malignant fibrous histiocytoma. Markedly atypical lipoblasts with vacuolated cytoplasm, multinucleation and highly irregular scalloped nuclei are the diagnostic cells (Fig. 40.21). These cells may, however, be infrequent.

Well-differentiated liposarcomas of the lipoma-like or sclerosing subtypes are sometimes referred to as atypical lipomata, when localized to the subcutis or musculature of

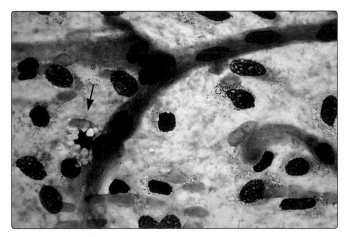

Fig. 40.19   Myxoid liposarcoma. Detail of a tumour fragment; capillary strands and one multivacuolated lipoblast (arrow). (MGG, × OI)

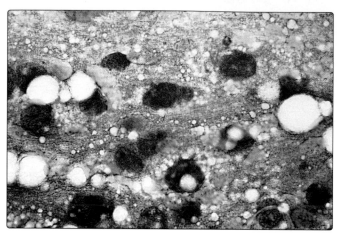

Fig. 40.20 Round cell liposarcoma. Atypical uni- and multivacuolated lipoblasts. (MGG, × OI)

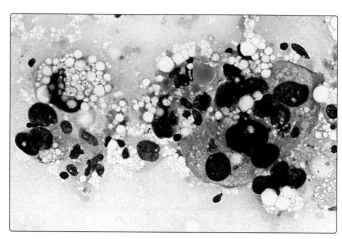

Fig. 40.21 Pleomorphic liposarcoma. Highly atypical lipoblasts some of which are multinucleated. (MGG, × OI)

Table 40.3   Important cytologic features in liposarcoma

Type	Background	Cytology
Well-differentiated	No background	Lipoma-like fragments. In and between them large atypical cells with hyperchromatic nuclei. Lipoblast-like cells
Myxoid	Granular myxoid, bluish red (MGG)	Vacuolated tissue fragments with distinct branching capillary network. Lipoblasts. Slight to moderate cellular atypia
Round cell	May be myxoid or granular or none	Numerous dissociated cells or vacuolated highly cellular tumour tissue fragments. Atypical lipoblasts present
Pleomorphic	Necrosis and cell debris may be seen	Mixture of dispersed cells and cell clusters. Marked cellular atypia. Multinucleated tumour cells. Highly atypical lipoblasts which may be multinucleated.
Spindle cell	Not evaluated	Not evaluated

the extremities. The term atypical lipoma is used because these tumours follow a benign clinical course and do not metastasize, in contrast to retroperitoneal well-differentiated liposarcomata[10]. Thus it is the anatomical site and not the cytological appearance on FNA which determines the diagnosis. The important cytological findings in smears from these tumours is the mixture of ordinary lipoma-like fragments and a varying number of atypical cells with large, irregular hyperchromatic nuclei. Some of these are lipoblastic in appearance, with cytoplasmic vacuoles and scalloped nuclei.

The dedifferentiated variant is diagnosed when aspirates from a well-differentiated liposarcoma also display cellular material from a high-grade malignant sarcoma, spindle cell type or pleomorphic. This variant is most often diagnosed in retroperitoneal liposarcoma.

A summary of the main cytological findings in the different types of liposarcoma can be seen in Table 40.3.

Diagnostic pitfalls

The most important benign tumours, which may be misdiagnosed as liposarcoma, are lipoma with regressive changes, hibernoma, chondroid lipoma and intramuscular myxoma[3,7]. The two former tumours are cytologically bland, while myxomas do not include lipoblasts.

Among sarcomas, high-grade malignant fibrous histiocytoma, myxofibrosarcoma and extraskeletal myxoid chondrosarcoma are the most frequent pitfalls. Soft tissue metastasis from a renal clear cell carcinoma has been misdiagnosed as round cell liposarcoma (personal observation). The best clue to a correct diagnosis of liposarcoma is the identification of true lipoblasts.

Malignant tumours of smooth muscle

Leiomyosarcomas occur in adults, arising most frequently within the abdomen or retroperitoneum, but also in the soft tissues of the extremities where they have a better prognosis because of their superficial position. More rarely, leiomyosarcomas are of vascular origin.

The histology of these tumours is diverse regardless of the site of origin, but the cutaneous and subcutaneous varieties are usually moderately differentiated. The tumour cells have a fascicular growth pattern and are elongated with cigar shaped nuclei. The better differentiated cells show longitudinal cytoplasmic striations. Multinucleated giant cells are a frequent finding. Epithelioid changes occur within some leiomyosarcomas, with rounded cells showing clear or vacuolated cytoplasm, and if this change is widespread, the term leiomyoblastoma is applied.

Cytological findings

▶ Very variable cell yield
▶ Cohesive clusters or large fascicular tumour fragments
▶ Few dissociated cells
▶ Blue or magenta background matrix
▶ Abundant cell cytoplasm with indistinct borders
▶ Degenerate bare nuclei
▶ Blunt ended elliptical nuclei, sometimes segmented
▶ Pleomorphism in high-grade tumours

The FNA cytology of leiomyosarcoma has been described by Dahl et al.[32] and the author's experience, based on approximately 70 tumours, is similar (M Åkerman, unpublished work, 1999). Most examples display a spindle cell population with variable pleomorphism of the tumour cells. These sarcomas are often difficult to aspirate due to resistance to the needle. The material is therefore often scanty and many cells may be damaged.

A typical smear includes tissue fragments, clusters or fascicles of cohesive tumour cells mixed with a few dispersed cells, the latter often appearing as naked nuclei. The cells in fragments and clusters are embedded in a dense matrix, which is blue or magenta on MGG staining. Cell borders are indistinct. The nuclei are cigar shaped and often appear segmented or vacuolated (Fig. 40.22A,B). Palisading of nuclei may be observed. The better preserved dispersed cells have abundant cytoplasm staining greyish blue with MGG stains. Pleomorphism is most marked in high-grade leiomyosarcomas and in these tumours multinucleated tumour giant cells can be seen. Mitotic figures are almost always present on careful screening.

Diagnostic pitfalls

Leiomyosarcomas of low-grade malignancy with only moderate cellular atypia may be misdiagnosed as leiomyoma or neurilemmoma. However, cigar shaped segmented nuclei are not a feature of neurilemmoma, and the presence of mitotic figures is consistent with leiomyosarcoma.

Among the sarcomas, malignant peripheral nerve sheath tumour may be difficult to distinguish from a leiomyosarcoma in FNA material, and high-grade leiomyosarcoma with marked cellular pleomorphism is easily mistaken for a malignant fibrous histiocytoma. Immunocytochemistry can be helpful in these cases, since leiomyosarcomas stain positively with desmin and smooth muscle actin, whereas both the nerve sheath tumours and malignant fibrous histiocytomas show no reaction.

The cytology of epithelioid leiomyosarcoma is not well defined but the epithelioid tumour cells may be mistaken for malignant cells of carcinomatous type. Immunocytochemical markers for cytokeratins are positive in carcinoma cells, whereas leiomyosarcoma cells stain with smooth muscle actin.

Malignant tumours of striated muscle

Rhabdomyosarcoma is an aggressive tumour of young adults or children, widely distributed anatomically, but found principally in the head and neck region, the genitourinary tract and retroperitoneum, and in the extremities. The classical main histological types in order of frequency are:

1 Embryonal rhabdomyosarcoma, composed of tumour tissue of variable cellularity which resembles developing muscle in the early embryo with some recognizable

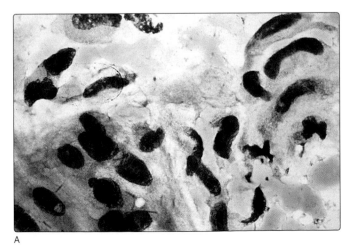
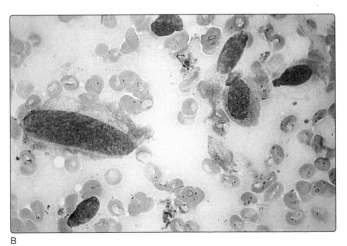

A B

Fig. 40.22 (A) Leiomyosarcoma. Part of a fascicle of elongated cells with blunt-ended nuclei. The cells are embedded in a bluish red background substance. (MGG, × OI) (B) Dispersed leiomyosarcoma cells. Although marked anisokaryosis, blunt-ended cigar shaped nuclei are present. (MGG, × OI)

racquet-shaped rhabdomyoblasts. This is the commonest type and includes the botryoid sarcoma, a lobulated oedematous tumour that protrudes into various body cavities at its site of origin, particularly in the vagina as well as the spindle cell type predominantly occurring in the peritesticular area.

2   Alveolar rhabdomyosarcoma, showing an ill-defined alveolar pattern of packaging of tumour cells which cling to the surrounding fibrous tissue septa, mimicking an adenocarcinoma. In the solid type of alveolar rhabdomyosarcoma the alveolar pattern is replaced by sheets of tumour cells.

3   Pleomorphic rhabdomyosarcoma, consisting of a mixture of rounded and pleomorphic tumour cells including bizarre rhabdomyoblasts.

The classification of rhabdomyosarcoma in children and adolescents has been debated during the last decade due to the need for an accepted and reproducible histopathological classification with a prognostic significance. In 1995, the 'International classification of rhabdomyosarcoma' was introduced[33]. This classification scheme is based on prognostically verified histopathological subgroups. As is evident from the classification, alveolar rhabdomyosarcoma belongs to the poor prognosis group. Furthermore, it was proposed that any degree of alveolar pattern or cytomorphology in a rhabdomyosarcoma would imply a bad prognostic sign[34]. This is of interest in the FNA diagnosis of rhabdomyosarcoma when the diagnosis also includes subtyping.

Cytological findings

▶ Cell rich aspirates
▶ Stripped nuclei in cytoplasmic background
▶ Predominantly dissociated cells
▶ Variable pleomorphism
▶ Myoblast like cells
▶ Cytoplasmic vacuolation
▶ Binucleated and multinucleated cells

In two reports, Seidal et al. have defined the cytological appearances of alveolar and embryonal rhabdomyosarcoma in FNA material[35,36]. The cytomorphology has also been described in a series of 15 cases by Akhtar et al.[37]. Although rhabdomyosarcoma is grouped with the so-called small round cell malignancies the overall pattern in embryonal rhabdomyosarcoma, apart from the spindle type, is predominantly pleomorphic. The alveolar rhabdomyosarcoma, however, is a true small cell malignant tumour. Dispersed cells are more common than cell clusters or fragments and the cytoplasm is fragile. Stripped nuclei in a blue-grey background of smeared cytoplasm are not uncommon. The typical cells resemble myoblasts, being triangular, strap-shaped or ribbon-like with eccentric nuclei. The cytoplasm is eosinophilic on H&E or greyish blue with

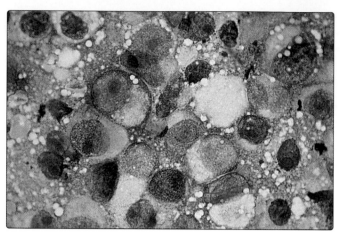

Fig. 40.23   Embryonal rhabdomyosarcoma. Variation in size and shape; many cells myoblast-like with eccentric nuclei. Note cytoplasmic background and vacuolization. (MGG, × OI)

MGG staining, which also often reveals cytoplasmic vacuolation due to dissolved glycogen. Multinucleated tumour cells are found: the nuclei are generally rounded and nucleoli may be prominent (Fig. 40.23).

Experience of the cytological diagnosis of over 30 cases has shown that definitive typing of alveolar and embryonal rhabdomyosarcoma is possible in most cases[38]. Our findings correspond with those of Atahan et al.[39]. In the alveolar type acinar structures may be observed and the predominant cell type is small to medium-sized with insignificant cytoplasm and ovoid or rounded nuclei. According to Seidal et al.[36] fragments of tumour tissue in which the cells are embedded in a myxoid background is typical of the embryonal type.

We have also had the opportunity to study a case of the spindle cell variant of embryonal rhabdomyosarcoma[40]. In a cellular aspirate the majority of cells were spindle shaped with fusiform or elongated nuclei. The nuclei had alternating pointed or blunt ends and showed moderate pleomorphism.

The pleomorphic rhabdomyosarcoma may be difficult to distinguish from other types of pleomorphic sarcomas. Highly atypical myoblast-like cells may be present in the smears.

Diagnostic pitfalls

The most important diagnostic difficulties lie in distinguishing between the different histological types of small round cell malignant tumours. These include rhabdomyosarcoma, neuroblastoma, the Ewing's family of tumours and precursor lymphoma/leukaemia (Table 40.4 and Chapter 19).

Malignant tumours of synovial tissue
Synovial sarcoma
These tumours may present in the vicinity of joints but most often occur in the extremities without any connection

Table 40.4   Important cytological findings in the differential diagnosis of small cell malignant tumours in childhood and adolescence

Tumour	Cytology
Embryonal rhabdomyosarcoma	Often marked anisocytosis and anisokaryosis. Fusiform, strap-shaped, ribbon-like, triangular or rounded myoblast-like cells. Binucleated cells. Nuclei rounded or elongated, occasionally prominent nucleoli. Predominance of fusiform cells in the spindle-cell type. Occasionally myxoid background matrix. Cytoplasmic vacuolation
Alveolar rhabdomyosarcoma	Predominantly small cell pattern. Rounded or pear-shaped primitive myoblast-like cells with eccentric nuclei. Cytoplasmic vacuolation
Neuroblastoma	Small cell pattern. Occasionally large cells resembling ganglion cells. Mixture of dispersed cells and cell clusters of loosely attached cells. Neuropil background, moulded cell clusters. Occasional rosettes. Dark rounded or irregular nuclei. In preserved cells often long thin cytoplasmic processes connecting one cell to another
PNET	Small cell pattern. Occasional rosettes. No neuropil. Bland nuclei. Cytoplasmic vacuolation and cells with small unipolar cytoplasmic processes
Classical Ewing's sarcoma	Double cell population. Large light cells with rounded nuclei and abundant thin cytoplasm with vacuoles and clear spaces. Small dark cells with scanty cytoplasm and irregular hyperchromatic nuclei. Stripped nuclei and cytoplasmic background. Bland nuclear morphology

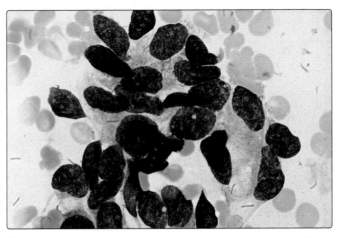

Fig. 40.24   Part of a tumour fascicle from a synovial sarcoma. Medium-sized cells with ovoid nuclei; faintly outlined gland-like structures. (MGG, × OI)

The cytology of synovial sarcoma has been described in relatively few cases. Biphasic synovial sarcoma is said to be composed of a mixture of epithelial structures and fascicles or clusters of spindle-shaped cells. In the author's experience, two distinctly different cell populations are very rarely encountered. Kindblom and Walaas have reported the FNA findings in nine synovial sarcomas[13] and in many aspects, their findings correspond to the cytological appearance in the smears from our own cases[42]. As a rule the smears are rich in cells, with a mixture of dispersed cells and different sized fragments of tightly packed cells. Tumour cells attached to ramifying capillary fragments are occasionally seen in the clusters as well as small glandular-type structures (Fig. 40.24).

In only one of our cases could a double cell population be discerned, consisting of gland-like structures surrounded by dissociated spindle cells. The most common cells were small to medium sized with scanty unipolar or bipolar cytoplasm. They had ovoid to rounded nuclei with finely granular chromatin and insignificant nucleoli (Fig. 40.25). Mitoses were not uncommon, especially in the clusters. Smears from one of the monophasic tumours were composed entirely of fusiform rather uniform cells with elongated nuclei. In yet another case the sarcoma cells were predominantly small, resembling lymphocytes, and very few spindle cells were seen. In the majority of our cases mast cells were a common finding. The cells in the poorly-differentiated variant or in aspirates from poorly-differentiated areas may be rhabdoid-like, Ewing's sarcoma cell-like or appear as highly atypical spindle cells[41]. This variant has not yet been investigated in FNA.

to joints and are also found at other sites such as trunk wall, the pharyngeal region or the abdominal wall. Young adults are most often affected, especially males; synovial sarcoma is also found in children. The long term outlook is poor due to a high incidence of late metastases, particularly in large tumours.

Histologically, synovial sarcomas are divided into biphasic tumours, monophasic fibrous, monophasic epithelial and poorly-differentiated tumours. Poorly-differentiated areas may also occur in any of the other types[41].

Cytological findings

▶ Cellular aspirates
▶ Dispersed cells and tissue fragments
▶ Stripped nuclei
▶ Branching capillaries with attached tumour cells
▶ Spindly or ovoid, bland nuclei
▶ Frequent mitoses in the tissue fragments
▶ The presence of mast cells in many aspirates

Diagnostic pitfalls

Synovial sarcoma may be very difficult to distinguish from the other spindle cell sarcomas, such as

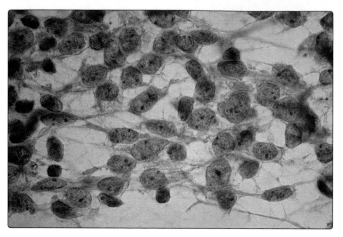

Fig. 40.25   Typical cells from a synovial sarcoma. Bland rounded or ovoid nuclei with small nucleoli. (H&E, × OI)

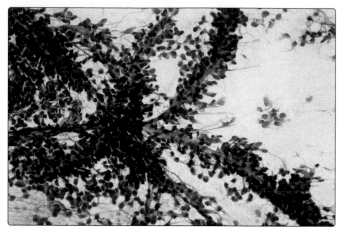

Fig. 40.26   Hemangiopericytoma. The tumour cells are attached to branching capillaries. (H&E, × MP)

haemangiopericytoma, fibrosarcoma and malignant peripheral nerve sheath tumour, especially the monophasic fibrous type. Sparsely cellular aspirates have been misdiagnosed as desmoid tumours (Table 40.4). The poorly-differentiated type may be difficult to distinguish from high-grade malignant fibrosarcoma, the Ewing's family of tumours and extrarenal rhabdoid tumour.

Cytogenetic examination of aspirated material is most probably the most effective ancillary method for achieving a correct diagnosis[43].

Malignant tumours of blood vessels

Several different types of sarcoma are known to arise from blood vessels, including angiosarcoma, Kaposi sarcoma and malignant haemangiopericytoma. Experience of FNA of malignant vascular tumours is still limited. The majority of publications have been case reports of 'malignant haemangiopericytoma'[44–47] Malignant haemangiopericytoma has for many years been considered as a pericytic tumour. However, in recent textbooks this hypothesis has been questioned and it has been proposed that malignant haemangiopericytoma of the soft tissues is a diagnosis of exclusion, only valid when other tumours with the same vascular pattern have been excluded, above all monophasic synovial sarcoma, solitary fibrous tumour and mesenchymal chondrosarcoma. Our experience, based on these new data, is limited to two tumours. The diagnosis of malignant haemangiopericytoma, according to these new data is difficult in FNA material and ancillary diagnostic methods are necessary to exclude the other tumours with 'haemangiopericytoma pattern'.

Malignant haemangiopericytoma

Cytological findings

▶ Ramifying tissue fragments and dissociated cells
▶ Thin capillary strands within the fragments
▶ Loose capillary fragments with attached tumour cells

▶ Small to medium sized spindle-shaped tumour cells
▶ Mast cells within fragments

The typical smear from a haemangiopericytoma shows a mixture of branching tissue fragments and dispersed cells. Naked nuclei are common. The fragments are composed of tightly packed cells and very often branching capillaries are seen, albeit indistinctly. Capillary fragments with attached tumour cells are occasionally observed (Fig. 40.26). The tumour cells are small to medium sized, spindle shaped, with a variable amount of cytoplasm and have rounded, ovoid or fusiform bland nuclei. Mitotic figures are rare but mast cells are often encountered. High-grade malignant tumours exhibit marked nuclear pleomorphism.

Single cases of the FNA findings in angiosarcoma have been reported[48–50]. Distinctive cytological features indicative of a vascular tumour were a mixture of rather epithelial and spindle-shaped malignant cells and also microacinar structures composed of atypical spindly cells.

Diagnostic pitfalls

It is clear from the descriptions of the cytology of synovial sarcoma and haemangiopericytoma that synovial sarcoma is the most important differential diagnosis and may be distinguishable by its biphasic cell pattern in some cases. The epithelial appearance of angiosarcoma tumour cells may suggest an epithelial tumour, a problem which can be resolved by immunocytochemistry, using cytokeratin staining to confirm an epithelial origin and endothelial markers such as factor VIII to stain the endothelial cells of an angiosarcoma.

Malignant tumours of peripheral nerves

This group of tumours includes those malignant nerve sheath tumours, which develop in patients with von Recklinghausen's disease as well as those arising spontaneously in relation to a major nerve.

Cytological findings

The cytological findings on FNA have been reported in single cases[51,52] and in short descriptions in current textbooks. Their cytology is either that of a spindle cell sarcoma (Fig. 40.27A,B) or, in some high-grade malignant tumours, that of a pleomorphic sarcoma with marked cellular and nuclear atypia and the presence of multinucleated tumour cells.

The majority of cases in our files produced cellular smears composed of a mixture of fascicles of tightly packed sarcoma cells, dispersed cells and stripped nuclei. The cells within fascicles had indistinct cytoplasm and elongated nuclei, often with pointed ends. These cells were embedded in a fibrillary background substance similar to the background in neurilemmoma aspirates. The extent of nuclear and nucleolar atypia varied considerably and a uniform appearance of the sarcoma cells with only slight atypia was not uncommon.

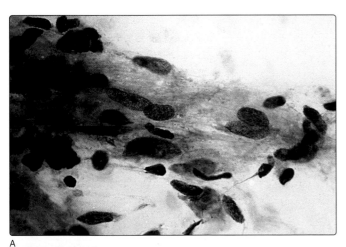

A

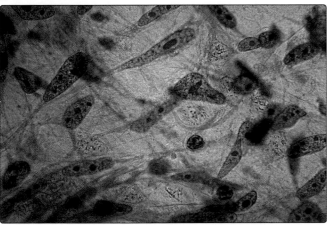

B

Fig. 40.27 (A) Malignant peripheral nerve sheath tumour. Atypical spindle cells in a fibrillary background matrix. Note the nuclei with pointed ends. (MGG, × OI) (B) Malignant peripheral nerve sheath tumour. Atypical spindle cells with fibrillar cytoplasm; nuclei have coarse chromatin and prominent nucleoli. (H&E, × OI)

Diagnostic pitfalls

With regard to benign tumours, ancient neurilemmoma is the most important diagnostic pitfall and among the sarcomas, leiomyosarcomas may be a problem. High-grade malignant pleomorphic peripheral nerve sheath tumour may be difficult to distinguish from other pleomorphic sarcomas.

Spindle cell sarcoma in FNA

One of the most difficult areas in FNA of soft tissue sarcoma is the diagnosis of various histological tumour types exhibiting a predominantly spindle cell pattern. In most cases it is possible to render a diagnosis of spindle cell sarcoma, based on the highly cellular smears with a mixture of dispersed cells and fascicles, or clusters of tightly packed cells with a variable degree of nuclear atypia. Mitoses are usually found with careful searching. However in routinely stained material it very often remains impossible to differentiate synovial sarcoma from malignant haemangiopericytoma, and malignant peripheral nerve sheath tumour from leiomyosarcoma or fibrosarcoma (Table 40.5).

Rare sarcomas of unknown or debated origin with epithelioid appearance on FNA

Alveolar soft part sarcoma

This rare sarcoma, occurring mainly in young women, is presumed to be of myogenic origin[10] and develops in the

Table 40.5 Cytological characteristics of spindle-cell sarcoma

Sarcoma	Cytology
Biphasic synovial sarcoma	Fascicles or clusters of tightly packed cells. Dispersed cells between. Cells predominantly small, fusiform with rounded or ovoid bland nuclei and small nucleoli. Occasional acinar-like structures in fragments. Rarely an obvious double cell population. Often mast cells
Monophasic synovial sarcoma	Uniform population of spindle cells. Ovoid or elongated bland nuclei.
Fibrosarcoma	Uniform population of spindle cells. In high-grade malignant tumours marked nuclear atypia
Hemangiopericytoma	Fascicles, fragments or clusters of tightly packed small to medium sized cells with ovoid or rounded nuclei. Short cytoplasmic processes. Tumour cells attached to capillary fragments. Mast cells
MPNST	Fascicles of cells with elongated nuclei and indistinct cytoplasmic borders in a fibrillar background. Variable number of dispersed cells. Slender nuclei with pointed ends and elongated cytoplasm. Variable cellular and nuclear atypia. High-grade malignant tumours markedly pleomorphic

deep soft tissues of the lower extremities or in soft tissues internally. It is aspirated infrequently and at present, the cytomorphology has only been described in detail in five cases[53,54]. Common to all descriptions was the presence of large tumour cells with abundant often granular cytoplasm, and rounded nuclei with prominent nucleoli. Binucleate or multinucleated cells were not uncommon. The cells appeared either singly or in clusters containing a capillary network.

Clear cell sarcoma

Clear cell sarcoma was first described in 1965 by Enzinger[55] and although controversial at first, it is now accepted as a clinicopathological entity considered to be of neural crest origin[10]. Another term recently proposed for the tumour is malignant melanoma of soft parts. It is prone to occur in relation to tendons and aponeuroses in young adults.

Based on the author's experience of two cases and those of Almeida et al.[56] of this relatively rare tumour, the sarcoma cells were mostly dissociated, but small clusters of loosely attached cells were also present. The cells were spindle shaped or polygonal with abundant pale cytoplasm and rounded or ovoid large nuclei. The nucleoli were prominent and the cytoplasmic borders ill-defined (Fig. 40.28).

Epithelioid sarcoma

Epithelioid sarcoma, first reported by Enzinger[57], is a peculiar tumour of unknown histogenesis developing in young adults. The sarcoma usually involves subcutaneous tissues or fascial planes and tendon sheaths of deeper soft tissues and appears as a multinodular growth, frequently showing central necrosis of nodules. An inflammatory cell infiltrate around the tumour nodules is common, as is hyalinization.

The cytological appearance of epithelioid sarcoma on FNA is only reported in single cases[58–60]. In the author's file, two cases are reported; the most important feature was the difficulty in aspirating sufficient tumour material for microscopic examination. Because of the necrosis and hyalinization, sarcoma cells were sparse and were mixed with histiocytes, lymphocytes, plasma cells and necrotic debris. The tumour cells were spindly and polygonal, with fragile abundant cytoplasm and rounded or ovoid nuclei with large nucleoli (Fig. 40.29). Small tight clusters of cells looked like cell aggregates from a large cell carcinoma, reflecting their epithelioid appearance on histology.

Diagnostic pitfalls of rare sarcomas

It is apparent from the descriptions above that these three sarcomatous entities are difficult to distinguish from each other if the final diagnosis is based only on cytological examination of routine smears. The granuloma-like appearance of epithelioid sarcoma with admixture of fibroblasts and inflammatory cells is a source of error; the

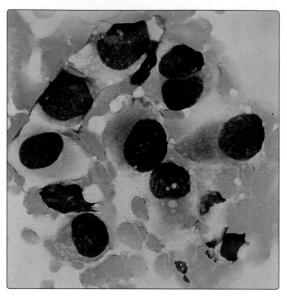

Fig. 40.28 Clear cell sarcoma. A group of cells of epithelial appearance with sharp cytoplasmic borders and rounded nuclei. (MGG, × OI)

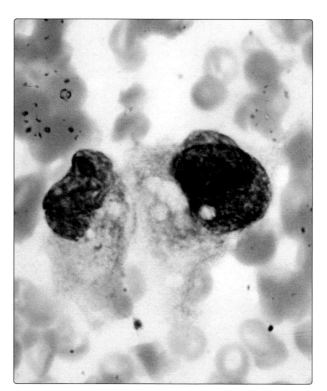

Fig. 40.29 Epithelioid sarcoma. Large cells with abundant cytoplasm and irregular nuclei with prominent nucleoli. (MGG, × OI)

malignant cells may be very infrequent and an inflammatory condition may be wrongly diagnosed.

Another diagnostic pitfall is the extent to which these sarcomatous cells resemble epithelial cells; soft tissue metastasis from large cell carcinoma is a rare, but possible diagnostic difficulty. However alveolar soft part sarcoma has a typical electron microscopic appearance, with membrane-bound crystals forming a cross-grid pattern in the cytoplasm[54], while clear cell sarcoma is usually positive for S 100 protein and HMB 45[61], and epithelioid sarcoma reacts positively with cytokeratin antibodies as well as vimentin[62].

Extrarenal rhabdoid tumour

Extrarenal rhabdoid tumours have been described as having a wide anatomical distribution in the soft tissues[63]. The age range is broad although most cases occur in children. The histological features common to all these tumours irrespective of site are rather large cells with various amounts of cytoplasm, eccentric large vesicular nuclei with prominent nucleoli and paranuclear hyaline globular inclusions. Akhtar *et al.* have published the fine needle aspiration cytology of two cases of extrarenal rhabdoid tumour[64]. We have one case in our files and our findings correspond with those of Akhtar *et al.*

Clusters of loosely attached cells were mixed with dispersed cells. The tumour cells were elongated, rounded or polygonal with vesicular nuclei exhibiting prominent nucleoli. A number of cells displayed rounded cytoplasmic inclusions. To confirm the diagnosis electron microscopic examination shows aggregates of intermediate filaments corresponding to the cytoplasmic inclusions and the tumour cells stain for vimentin and keratin, but not for desmin.

Extraskeletal myxoid chondrosarcoma

Extraskeletal myxoid chondrosarcoma (EMS) as a clinipathologic entity was first described in 1972. A comprehensive study of 117 cases has been published by Meis-Kindblom *et al.*[65]. EMS has been diagnosed in children and adults, predominantly in the middle-aged and elderly. The extremities and trunk are the sites of predilection. EMSs display an abundant myxoid matrix and are variably cellular. The tumour cells are arranged in strands and rings, and appear as small tumour balls embedded in the myxoid background or show a cribriform growth pattern. The tumour cells are variably shaped, spindly, epithelioid-like or rounded, with ovoid or spindle-shaped nuclei with finely granular chromatin and small nucleoli. Well developed hyaline cartilage is not present. There is no typical immunohistochemical profile, although 30–40% of cases have been reported to be S 100 protein positive. Electron microscopic examination has been considered useful in the diagnosis[65] as has cytogenetics. The t(9;22) translocation is typical for EMC[65].

We have examined aspirates from three cases of EMS, all harbouring the typical chromosomal abnormality on examination of the operative specimen. The cytological findings were similar in all cases (Fig. 40.30A,B,C).

Cytological findings

▶ Abundant myxoid background

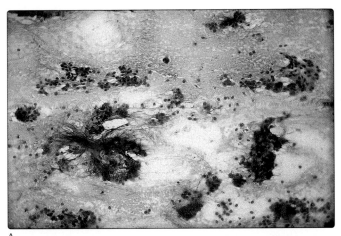

A

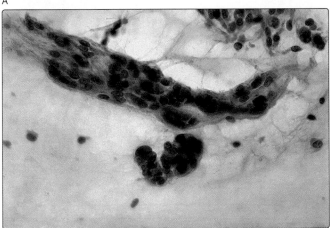

B

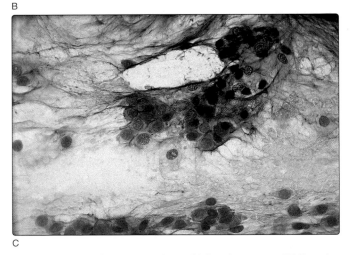

C

Fig. 40.30 (A,B,C) Extraskeletal myxoid chondrosarcoma. (A) Strands and clusters as well as dispersed cells embedded in an abundant, partly fibrillar myxoid background substance. (MGG × LP) (B) Cell-balls and clusters of rounded cells with ovoid rather bland nuclei. (H&E × HP) (C) The myxoid background is better visualized in MGG. (MGG × HP)

▶ Tumour cells arranged in cell-balls, branching strands or clusters or dispersed
▶ Rounded or spindly cells with rounded or ovoid nuclei
▶ Bland nuclear chromatin and small nucleoli

Differential diagnosis

Of all tumours exhibiting an abundant myxoid background matrix, myxoid liposarcoma, myxofibrosarcoma, low-grade fibro-myxoid sarcoma and mixed myoepithelial tumour are the most important.

Intra-abdominal desmoplastic small round cell tumour

Intra-abdominal desmoplastic small round cell tumour (DSRCT) is of uncertain histogenesis but its predilection for serosal involvement may suggest that it is a primitive mesothelial tumour. It occurs predominantly in male adolescents and young adults. The typical histopathological pattern is that of well defined nests and trabeculae of small to medium-sized tumour cells within a desmoplastic stroma[66]. The tumour cells are uniform with scanty cytoplasm and rounded or ovoid hyperchromatic nuclei. Nucleoli are small. The immunohistochemical profile indicates a multi-linear phenotype with positive staining for keratin antibodies, neuroendocrine markers, desmin and vimentin. Cytogenetic analysis has revealed a unique translocation t(11;22), however, with a gene fusion product different from that found in the Ewing's family of tumours.

The cytological features of four cases have been described by Caraway et al.[67]. Clusters of loosely attached cells that were small to medium sized with oval to rounded nuclei with finely granular chromatin and small nucleoli. The main differential diagnoses are the other tumours within the group of malignant small round cell tumours.

Neuroectodermal tumours

Neuroblastoma

This aggressive malignant tumour of infancy and childhood occurs mainly in the adrenal gland but is occasionally encountered as a soft tissue mass at sites of sympathetic nerve trunks or as metastatic tumour. Histologically, sheets of small round undifferentiated tumour cells are found, sometimes showing rosette formations around small foci of delicate neurofibrillary matrix known as neuropil. If maturation of the tumour occurs, large ganglion cells are seen.

Cytological findings

▶ Dissociated cells and clusters of loosely attached cells
▶ Rosette formations with central fibrillary material
▶ Tumour cells with small irregular nuclei and unipolar or bipolar cytoplasmic processes connecting adjacent cells
▶ Neuropil in the background of cell clusters
▶ Tumour cells arranged in indian file or in moulded clusters
▶ Occasional cells resembling ganglion cells

The cytological findings in FNA of neuroblastoma have been thoroughly described by Miller et al.[68] and Akhtar et al.[69]. In a recent re-evaluation of 19 tumours we found that the most frequent diagnostic combination of cytological features

were neuropil, moulded clusters and thin cytoplasmic processes often connecting adjacent tumour cells[70].

The smears are generally very cellular with a mixture of dispersed cells and clusters of loosely cohesive cells. In the clusters, rosettes of cells with a fibrillary centre of neuropil are observed (Fig. 40.31). At times the clusters are embedded in neuropil. Neuroblastoma cells are small to medium sized with dark irregular nuclei, a coarse chromatin structure and insignificant nucleoli. Their cytoplasm is scanty but drawn out in long thin processes connecting one cell to another (Fig. 40.32). Arrangement of cells in indian file or moulded clusters is a common finding.

Ganglion cell differentiation is sometimes seen in the form of large cells with abundant cytoplasm and eccentric nuclei with prominent nucleoli. In aspirates from primitive neuroblastoma, rosettes are not found and the tumour cells are small with scanty cytoplasm devoid of processes.

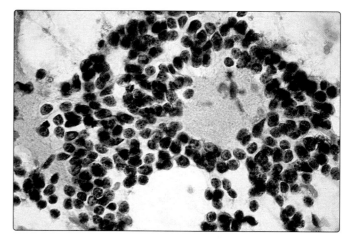

Fig. 40.31 Neuroblastoma. Rosette-like structure composed of small cells around a fibrillary centre. (H&E, × MP)

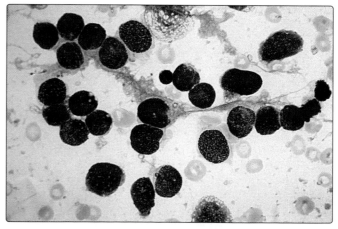

Fig. 40.32 Neuroblastoma cells have fragile fibrillar cytoplasm; the cells are often connected by thin cytoplasmic strands. (MGG, × OI)

Table 40.6   Examples of the diagnostic use of ancillary methods

Electron microscopy	Smooth muscle *vs* nerve sheath tumour
	Rhabdomyosarcoma *vs* Ewing's family of tumours
	Synovial sarcoma *vs* other spindle cell sarcoma
	Alveolar soft part sarcoma
	Pleomorphic sarcoma *vs* carcinoma, melanoma
Immunocytochemistry	Pleomorphic sarcoma *vs* carcinoma, melanoma
	Smooth muscle tumour *vs* nerve sheath tumour
	Pleomorphic sarcoma *vs* anaplastic large cell lymphoma
DNA-ploidy analysis	Pseudosarcomatous soft tissue lesion *vs* pleomorphic sarcoma (aneuploid cell population consistent with sarcoma)
Chromosomal analysis	Synovial sarcoma t(X;18)
	Alveolar rhabdomyosarcoma t(2;13)
	Ewing's family of tumours t(11;22)
	Extraskeletal myxoid chondrosarcoma t(9;22)
Molecular genetic analysis	Ewing's family of tumours *EWS/FLI1*
	Synovial sarcoma *SYT/SSX*

Primitive neuroectodermal tumour (PNET)

This round cell malignant tumour of presumed neuroectodermal origin[10] belongs to the Ewing's family of tumours. The term is at present used to include skeletal as well as extraskeletal Ewing's sarcoma, atypical Ewing's sarcoma, peripheral neuroepithelioma and the so-called Askin tumour or malignant small cell tumour of thoracopulmonary region. The rationale for lumping these neoplasms together and diagnosing them as belonging to the Ewing's family of tumours is because all share the same chromosomal abnormality t(11;22). This translocation fuses the EWS gene in chromosome 22 with the FLI1 gene in chromosome 11 and detection of the fusion protein is an important diagnostic sign in this family of tumours.

PNET is most frequent in older children and adolescents and arises predominantly in the chest wall, retroperitoneum, pelvis and the extremities. It is a rare tumour and its cytology in FNA has only been described in a few cases. Silverman *et al.*[71] have described three cases with immunocytochemical, electron microscopic and cytogenetic studies, and a further two have been documented by Gonzales-Campora *et al.*[72].

PNET is characterized in FNA material by a mixture of dispersed cells, small cell clusters and occasional rosette formations. The cells have scanty to moderate cytoplasm and rounded, oval or slightly irregular nuclei, finely granular chromatin and small but prominent nucleoli. Cytoplasmic vacuolation is a frequent finding, as are cells with small unipolar cytoplasmic processes.

Diagnostic pitfalls

The important pitfalls are the other tumours belonging to the small round cell malignancies of childhood and adolescence, Ewing's sarcoma, rhabdomyosarcoma and precursor lymphoma. Important cytological features in the differential diagnosis are listed in Table 40.4.

Ancillary methods in the diagnosis of soft tissue sarcoma

Fine needle aspirates, when cellular and technically satisfactory, provide suitable material for use of specialized techniques to assist in the diagnosis of malignant soft tissue tumours. Electron microscopy[13], immunocytochemistry[16,31,60], DNA-ploidy analysis[73,74], chromosomal analysis[75,76] and molecular genetic analysis[43,77] are some of the main adjunctive methods helpful in the differential diagnosis.

Table 40.6 gives examples of the diagnostic features of these ancillary methods.

Chromosomal analysis and molecular genetic examinations such as FISH and RT-PCR have emerged as powerful adjunctive diagnostic methods. To date the Ewing's family of tumours and synovial sarcoma are the sarcomas most frequently investigated[43,75,76]. Other candidates for these ancillary methods are myxoid and round cell liposarcoma, clear cell sarcoma, extraskeletal myxoid chondrosarcoma and alveolar rhabdomyosarcoma[77,78].

References

1 Fletcher C D M. Pleomorphic malignant fibrous histiocytoma: fact or fiction? A critical reappraisal based on 159 tumors diagnosed as pleomorphic sarcoma. *Am J Surg Pathol* 1992; **16**: 213–228

2 Fletcher C D M. Hemangiopericytoma – A dying breed? Reappraisal of an 'entity' and its variants: a hypothesis. *Curr Diagn Pathol* 1994; **1**: 19–24

3 Åkerman M, Rydholm A. Aspiration cytology of lipomatous tumors. A ten year experience at an orthopedic oncology center. *Diagn Cytopathol* 1987; **3**: 295–302

4 Shmookler B M, Enzinger F M. Pleomorphic lipoma: a benign tumor simulating liposarcoma. A clinicopathologic analysis of 48 cases. *Cancer* 1981; **47**: 126–132

5 Bolen J W, Thorning D. Spindle cell lipoma: a clinical, light – and electron microscopic study. *Am J Surg Pathol* 1981; **5**: 435–441

6 Domanski H A, Åkerman M. Fine needle aspiration cytology of spindle cell lipoma. *Acta Orthop Scand* 1998; **69**(suppl 282): 40

7 Walaas L, Kindblom L-G. Lipomatous tumors. A correlative cytologic and histologic study of 27 tumors examined by fine needle aspiration cytology. *Hum Pathol* 1985; **16**: 6–18

8 Meis J M, Enzinger F M. Chondroid lipoma: A unique tumor simulating liposarcoma and myxoid chondrosarcoma. *Am J Surg Pathol* 1993; **17**: 1103–1112

9 Dahl I, Hagmar B, Idvall I. Benign solitary neurilemoma. A correlative cytological and histological study of 28 cases. *Acta Pathol Microbiol Immunol Scand* (A) 1984; **92**: 91–101

10 Ninfo V, Chung E B, Cavazzana A O. *Tumors and Tumor-like Lesions of Soft Tissue*. New York: Churchill Livingstone, 1991

11 Ryd W, Mugel S, Ayyash K. Ancient neurilemoma. A pit-fall in the cytologic diagnosis of soft tissue tumors. *Diagn Cytopathol* 1988; **2**: 244–247

12 Dodd L, Marom E M, Dash R C et al. Fine needle aspiration cytology of 'ancient schwannoma'. *Diagn Cytopathol* 1999; **20**: 307–311

13 Kindblom L-G, Walaas L. Ultrastructural studies in the preoperative diagnosis of soft tissue tumors. *Sem Diagn Pathol* 1985; **3**: 317–344

14 Chan J K C. Solitary fibrous tumour – everywhere, and a diagnosis in vogue. *Histopathol* 1997; **31**: 568–576

15 Willen H, Carlen B, Rydholm A, Gustason P. Solitary fibrous tumor of the soft tissue. *Acta Orthop Scand* 1999; **70**(suppl 289): 31–32

16 Hoon A S Z, Hoda S, Heelan R, Zakowski M F. Solitary fibrous tumor. A cytologic-histologic study with clinical, radiologic, and immunohistochemical correlations. *Cancer* 1997; **81**(2): 116–121

17 Bondeson L, Andreasson L. Aspiration cytology of adult rhabdomyoma. *Acta Cytol* 1986; **30**: 679–682

18 Bertholf M F, Frierson H F, Feldman P S. Fine needle aspiration cytology of an adult rhabdomyoma of the head and neck. *Diagn Cytopathol* 1988; **4**: 152–155

19 Domanski H, Dawiskiba S. Adult rhabdomyoma in fine needle aspirates; A report of two cases. *Acta Cytol* 1999; **44**: 223–226

20 Åkerman M, Rydholm A. Aspiration cytology of intramuscular myxoma. A comparative clinical, cytologic and histologic study of ten cases. *Acta Cytol* 1983; **27**: 505–510

21 Kilpatrick S E, Hitchcock M G, Kraus M D et al. Mixed tumors and myoepitheliomas of soft tissues: a clinicopathologic study of 19 cases with a unifying concept. *Am J Surg Pathol* 1997; **1**: 13–22

22 Dodd L, Layfield L J. Fine-needle aspiration cytology of ganglion cysts. *Diagn Cytopathol* 1997; **15**: 377–381

23 Åkerman M. Malignant fibrous histiocytoma – the commonest soft tissue sarcoma or a nonexistent entity? *Acta Orthop Scand* 1997; **68**(suppl 273): 41–46

24 Meis-Kindblom M, Bjerkehagen B, Bohling T et al. Morphologic review of 1000 soft tissue sarcomas from the Scandinavian Sarcoma Group (SSG) Register. The peer-review committee experience. *Acta Orthoped Scan* 1999; **70**(suppl 285): 18–26

25 Angervall L, Kindblom L-G, Merck Ch. Myxofibrosarcoma. A study of 30 cases. *Acta Pathol Microbiol Scand* (A) 1977; **85**: 127–140

26 Hollowood K, Fletcher C D M. Malignant fibrous histiocytoma. Morphologic pattern or pathologic entity? *Sem Diagn Pathol* 1995; **12**: 210–220

27 Walaas L, Angervall L, Hagmar B, Säve-Söderberg J. A correlative cytologic and histologic study of malignant fibrous histiocytoma. An analysis of 40 cases examined by fine needle aspiration cytology. *Diagn Cytopathol* 1986; **2**: 46–54

28 Merck Ch, Hagmar B. Myxofibrosarcoma. A correlative cytologic and histologic study of 13 cases examined by fine needle aspiration cytology. *Acta Cytol* 1980; **22**: 137–144

29 Angervall L, Hagmar B, Kindblom L-G. Malignant giant cell tumor of soft tissue. A clinicopathologic, cytologic, ultrastructural, angiographic and microangiographic study. *Cancer* 1981; **47**: 736–747

30 Evans H L. Low-grade fibromyxoid sarcoma. A report of 12 cases. *Am J Surg Pathol* 1993; **17**: 595–600

31 Lindberg G M, Maitra A, Gokaslan S T et al. Low-grade fibromyxoid sarcoma: fine-needle aspiration cytology with histologic, cytogenetic immunohistochemical, and ultrastructural correlation. *Cancer* 1999; **87**(2): 75–82

32 Dahl I, Hagmar B, Angervall L. Leiomyosarcoma of the soft tissue. A correlative cytologic and histologic study of 11 cases. *Acta Pathol Microbiol Immunol Scand* (A) 1981; **89**: 285–291

33 Coffin C M. The new international rhabdomyosarcoma classification, its progenitors, and considerations beyond morphology. *Adv Anat Pathol* 1997; **4**: 1–16

34 Tsokos M, Webber B L, Parham D M et al. Rhabdomyosarcoma: a new classification scheme related to prognosis. *Arch Pathol Lab Med* 1992; **116**: 847–856

35 Seidal T, Mark K, Angervall L. Alveolar rhabdomyosarcoma. A cytogenetic and correlated cytological and histological study. *Acta Pathol Immunol Scand* (A) 1982; **90**: 345–354

36 Seidal T, Walaas L, Kindblom L-G, Angervall L. Cytology of embryonal rhabdomyosarcoma. A cytologic, light microscopic, electron microscopic and immunohistochemical study of seven cases. *Diagn Cytopathol* 1988; **4**: 292–300

37 Akhtar M, Ali M, Bakry M et al. Fine-needle aspiration biopsy diagnosis of rhabdomyosarcoma. Cytologic, histologic and ultrastructural correlations. *Diagn Cytopathol* 1992; **8**: 465–474

38 Åkerman M, Willen H, Carlen B. Fine needle aspiration cytology of rhabdomyosarcoma. Is a reliable type diagnosis possible to render? – a retrospective study of 23 cases. *Acta Orthop Scand* 1996; **67**(suppl 272): 55

39 Atahan S, Aksu O, Ekinci C. Cytologic diagnosis and subtyping of rhabdomyosarcoma. *Cytopathol* 1998; **9**: 389–397

40 Cavazzana A O, Schmidt D, Ninfo V et al. Spindle cell rhabdomyosarcoma. A prognostically favorable variant of rhabdomyosarcoma. *Am J Surg Pathol* 1992; **16**(3): 229–235

41 Bergh P, Meis-Kindblom J M, Gherlinzoni F et al. Synovial sarcoma: identification of low and high risk groups. *Cancer* 1999; **85**(12): 2596–25607

42 Åkerman M, Willen H, Carlen B et al. Fine needle aspiration (FNA) of synovial sarcoma – a comparative histological-cytological study of 15 cases, including immuno-histochemical, electron microscopic and cytogenetic examination and DNA-ploidy analysis. *Cytopathol* 1996; **7**: 187–200

43 Nilsson G, Ming M D, Wejde J. Reverse transcriptase polymerase chain reaction on fine needle aspirates for rapid detection of translocations in synovial sarcoma. *Acta Cytol* 1998; **42**: 1317–1324

44 Nguyen G-K, Neifer R. The cells of benign and malignant hemangiopericytomas in aspiration biopsy. *Diagn Cytopathol* 1985; **1**: 327–331

45 Kumar N, Misra K. Aspiration cytology of hemangiopericytoma: a report of two cases. *Diagn Cytopathol* 1990; **6**: 341–344

46 Jimenes-Ayala M, Diez-Nau M, Larrad A et al. Hemangiopericytoma in a male breast. Report of a case with cytologic, histologic and immunochemical studies. *Acta Cytol* 1991; **35**: 234–238

47 Nickels I, Koivuniemi A. Cytology of malignant hemangiopericytoma. *Acta Cytol* 1979; **23**: 119–125

48 Abele J, Miller Th. Cytology of well-differentiated and poorly differentiated hemangiosarcoma in fine needle aspirates. *Acta Cytol* 1982; **26**: 341–348

49 Liu K, Layfield L J. Cytomorphologic features of angiosarcoma on fine needle

aspiration biopsy. *Acta Cytol* 1999; **43**: 407–415

50 Gupta R, Naran S, Dowle C. Needle aspiration cytology and immunocytochemical study in a case of angiosarcoma of the breast. *Diagn Cytopathol* 1991; **7**: 363–365

51 Hood I, Qizilbash, Young J, Archibald S. Needle aspiration cytology of a benign and a malignant Schwannoma. *Acta Cytol* 1984; **28**: 157–163

52 Jimenez-Heffernan J A, Lopez-Ferrer P, Vicandi B *et al*. Cytologic features of malignant peripheral nerve sheath tumor. *Acta Cytol* 1999; **43**: 175–184

53 Shabb N, Fanning Ch. Dekmezian R. Fine needle aspiration cytology of alveolar soft part sarcoma. *Diagn Cytopathol* 1991; **7**: 293–298

54 Persson S, Willems J-S, Kindblom L-G, Angervall L. Alveolar soft part sarcoma. An immunohistochemical, cytologic and electronmicroscopic study and quantitative DNA analysis. *Virchows Arch A Pathol Anat Histopathol* 1988; **412**: 499–513

55 Enzinger F M, Weiss S W. *Soft Tissue Tumours*, 2nd edn. Washington DC: Mosby, 1988; 945–951

56 Almeida M M, Nunes A M, Frable W J. Malignant melanoma of soft tissue. A report of three cases with diagnosis by fine needle aspiration cytology. *Acta Cytol* 1994; **38**: 241–246

57 Enzinger F M, Weiss S W. *Soft Tissue Tumours*, 2nd edn. Washington DC: Mosby, 1988; 936–945

58 Ahmed M N, Feldman M, Seemayer T A. Cytology of epithelioid sarcoma. *Acta Cytol* 1974; **18**: 459–461

59 Goswitz J J, Kappel T, Klingaman K. Fine needle aspiration of epithelioid sarcoma. *Diagn Cytopathol* 1993; **9**: 677–681

60 Zepa P, Errico M E, Palombini L. Epithelioid sarcoma: report of two cases diagnosed by fine-needle aspiration biopsy with immunocytochemical correlation. *Diagn Cytopathol* 1999; **21**: 405–408

61 Lucas D, Nascimento A, Sim F. Clear cell sarcoma of soft tissues. Mayo Clinic experience with 35 cases. *Am J Surg Pathol* 1992; **16**(2): 1197–1204

62 Persson S, Kindblom L-G, Angervall L. Epithelioid sarcoma. An electron-microscopic and immunohistochemical study. *Appl Pathol* 1988; **6**: 1–16

63 Fanburg-Smith J C, Hengge M, Hengge U R *et al*. Extrarenal rhabdoid tumors of soft tissues: a clinicopathologic and immunohistochemical study of 18 cases. *Ann Diagn Pathol* 1998; **2**: 351–362

64 Akhtar M, Kfoury H, Haider A *et al*. Fine-needle aspiration biopsy diagnosis of extrarenal malignant rhabdoid tumor. *Diagn Cytopathol* 1994; **11**: 271–276

65 Meis-Kindblom J M, Bergh P, Gunterberg B, Kindblom L-G. Extraskeletal myxoid chrondrosarcoma. A reappraisal of its morphologic spectrum and prognostic factors based on 117 cases. *Am J Surg Pathol* 1999; **23**: 636–650

66 Ordonez N G, Adel K, El-Naggar K *et al*. Intra-abdominal desmoplastic small cell tumor: A light microscopic, immunocytochemical, ultrastructural, and flow cytometric study. *Hum Pathol* 1993; **24**: 850–865

67 Caraway N P, Fanning C V, Amato R J *et al*. Fine-needle aspiration of intra-abdominal desmoplastic small cell tumor. *Diagn Cytopathol* 1993; **9**: 465–470

68 Miller Th, Bottles K, Abele J, Beckstead H. Neuroblastoma diagnosed by fine needle aspiration biopsy. *Acta Cytol* 1985; **29**: 461–470

69 Akhtar M, Ali A, Sabbah R *et al*. Aspiration cytology of neuroblastoma. Light and electron microscopic correlations. *Cancer* 1986; **57**: 797–803

70 Åkerman M, Carlen B. Diagnosis of neuroblastoma in fine needle aspirates. *Acta Orthop Scand* 1997; **68**(suppl 274): 72

71 Silverman J F, Berns L, Tate Holbrook C *et al*. Fine needle aspiration cytology of primitive neuroectodermal tumors. A report of three cases. *Acta Cytol* 1992; **36**: 543–550

72 Gonzales-Campora R, Otal-Salaverri C, Flores P *et al*. Fine needle aspiration of peripheral neuroepithelioma of soft tissues. *Acta Cytol* 1992; **36**: 152–158

73 Åkerman M, Killander D, Rydholm A, Rööser B. Aspiration of musculoskeletal tumors for cytodiagnosis and DNA analysis. *Acta Orthop Scand* 1987; **58**: 523–528

74 Lundgren L, Kindblom L-G, Willems J *et al*. Proliferative myositis and fasciitis. A light and electron microscopic, cytologic, DNA-cytometric and immunohistochemical study. *APMIS* 1992; **100**: 437–448

75 Sreekantiaiah C, Appaji L, Hazarika D. Cytogenetic characterization of small round cell tumours using fine needle aspiration. *J Clin Pathol* 1992; **45**: 728–730

76 Åkerman M, Dreinhofer K, Rydholm A *et al*. Cytogenetic studies on fine needle aspiration samples from osteosarcoma and Ewing's sarcoma. *Diagn Cytopathol* 1996; **15**: 17–22

77 Åkerman M, Åman P, Lindholm K, Carlen B. Primary Ewing's sarcoma of bone in a 73 year old man. Diagnosis by fine needle aspiration cytology, electron microscopy, immunocytochemistry and molecular genetic analysis. *Acta Cytol* 1995; **39**: 265–266

78 Choong P, Rydholm A, Mertens F, Mandahl N. Musculoskeletal oncology. Advances in cytogenetics and molecular genetics and their clinical implications. *Acta Oncologica* 1997; **36**: 245–254

41 Benign and malignant tumours of bone

Måns Åkerman

Introduction

Definition of the cytological criteria for interpreting aspiration samples from primary bone tumours is at present largely confined to malignant neoplasms, since FNA findings in only a few benign tumours have been thoroughly documented. Nevertheless a combination of the cytological diagnosis and careful evaluation of clinical and radiographic data can be the basis of definitive treatment in a substantial number of primary bone tumours, both benign and malignant. This approach may at times replace the need for bore needle or open biopsy and histological examination. FNA will also frequently distinguish primary bone tumours from metastatic deposits.

The cytological descriptions and comments on differential diagnosis and diagnostic pitfalls given below are the culmination of recent publications and based on the author's experience of FNA in the initial diagnosis of more than 300 primary bone tumours, as well as almost 200 metastatic lesions[1,2].

Benign tumours of bone

Primary benign bone tumours with the fullest documentation of their cytology include giant cell tumours, chondroblastomas and chondromas. Others, such as osteoblastoma, chondromyxoid fibroma and the tumour-like conditions aneurysmal bone cyst, non-ossifying fibroma and osteitis fibrosa cystica have been described in relatively few cases.

Giant cell tumour (osteoclastoma)

An easy target for FNA, giant cell tumour is the primary benign bone tumour which has been most thoroughly investigated by cytology[2–4].

Giant cell tumour is most common in the second and third decades of life and the majority of cases occur in females. The epiphyses of long bones are common sites, especially on either side of the knee joint.

Histologically, the tumour is composed of stromal cells, probably neoplastic, and osteoclastic giant cells, which are probably reactive. The cortical bone is either very thin and weakened, or destroyed over the lesion and it is not difficult to aspirate with a 22-gauge needle.

Cytological findings

- ▶ Easy to needle, abundant yield
- ▶ Mixture of cell clusters and dispersed cells
- ▶ Double cell population
- ▶ Elongated mononuclear cells variable in shape
- ▶ Regular rounded or ovoid nuclei, inconspicuous nucleoli
- ▶ Large multinucleated cells of osteoclastic type
- ▶ Bi- or tri-nucleated osteoclastic cells
- ▶ Osteoclast-like cells attached to periphery of cell clusters

Typically, the smears are richly cellular, consisting of a mixture of cell clusters and dissociated cells. A double cell population is always obvious. The majority of tumour cells are elongated and mononuclear with moderate to abundant cytoplasm and sharp cytoplasmic borders. The nuclei are round or ovoid and of uniform appearance. Chromatin is regularly distributed and one or two small nucleoli are common.

The other cell type resembles an osteoclast with abundant cytoplasm and numerous uniform rounded nuclei. Fine red granules are often observed in the cytoplasm on MGG. A typical cell cluster has irregular borders along which the osteoclast-like cells are attached, the central part being composed of tightly packed mononuclear cells (Fig. 41.1A,B). Among the dispersed cells bi- or trinucleated forms may be found, suggesting a transition to the multinucleated forms.

In cell-poor aspirates the clusters are few, small or absent. The smears consist of a mixture of dispersed mononuclear and multinucleated cells. Occasionally mitoses are found in the mononuclear cells.

Chondroblastoma

As with giant cell tumours, chondroblastomas occur most often in young people, especially in the second decade, but are commoner in males, and are often painful. The most usual site is the epiphysis of the long bones, but they may also be found in small tubular and flat bones. Histologically, the tumour is composed of immature chondroblasts and giant cells, with focal calcification. Areas resembling an aneurysmal bone cyst may be present.

917

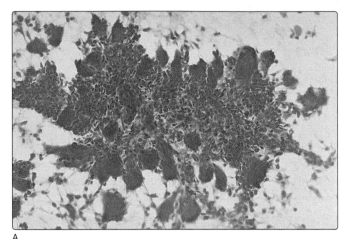

A

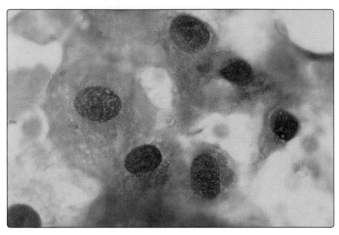

Fig. 41.2 Chondroblastoma. Chondroblast-like cells embedded in a red-blue chondroid matrix. (MGG, × OI)

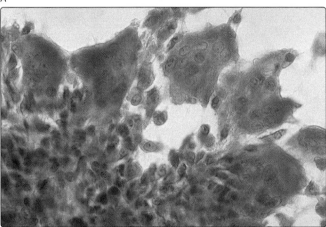

B

Fig. 41.1 Giant cell tumour. A typical cell cluster with the osteoclast-like giant cells attached to the periphery. (H&E, × LP) (**B**) Detail from (**A**). Tightly packed mononuclear cells with uniform nuclei and a peripheric row of giant cells. (H&E, × MP)

Cytological findings

► Mononuclear cells, well formed cytoplasm, round nuclei
► Multinucleated osteoclast-like cells
► Fragments of chondroid matrix

Although a rare tumour, the cytological features of 12 cases of chondroblastoma have been published[5] and there are also a few other reports[6-8]. These reports all indicate findings similar to those of the few cases in our files.

Diagnostic features in FNA smears are the mixed pattern of chondroid matrix fragments, cells of chondroblastic type and multinucleated osteoclast-like cells. According to Fanning et al.[5], the most characteristic finding is the presence of cells resembling chondroblasts. These are typically monomorphic and rounded with well-demarcated cytoplasm and round or occasionally lobulated or reniform nuclei. Nuclei are generally central and vary in size; binucleated forms are not uncommon and mitotic figures may be found.

The chondroblastic cells are either dissociated or seen in small ill-defined clusters embedded in chondroid matrix (Fig. 41.2). The chondroid matrix fragments are usually acellular and fibrillary, and stain red to reddish blue with MGG and faintly eosinophilic in H&E preparations.

Chondromyxoid fibroma

A benign cartilaginous tumour of young adults, chondromyxoid fibroma is rare, being less common than chondroblastoma. Patients are most often in the second and third decades and the tumours typically arise in the metaphyseal region of long tubular bones, especially the tibia.

Histologically, lobular masses of myxochondroid tissue are seen, surrounded by cellular areas with a mixture of spindle cells of fibroblastic type and osteoclasts.

Cytological findings

► Myxoid background matrix
► Cartilaginous fragments
► Dispersed or clustered spindle-shaped fibroblastic cells
► Osteoclastic giant cells

Only single cases of FNA cytology from chondromyxofibroma have been published[9,10] and the author's experience is limited to two cases.

Smears show fragments of cartilaginous matrix, fusiform spindle cells and osteoclastic cells embedded in a myxoid background matrix. The spindle cells vary in size and have elongated nuclei. They appear either singly or in ill-defined groups. In the cartilaginous fragments rounded chondroblast-like cells in lacunar spaces may be found. Both chondroblastic and spindle-shaped cells may show a certain polymorphism with plump nuclei and small but prominent nucleoli. Binucleated chondroblast-like cells are not uncommon (Fig. 41.3A,B,C). In our two cases the most striking finding was the presence of cartilage fragments.

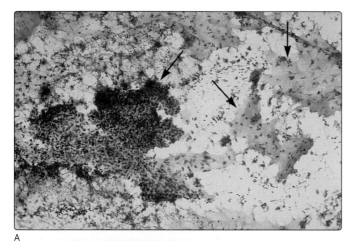

A

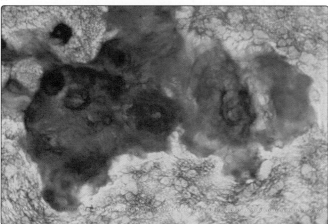

B

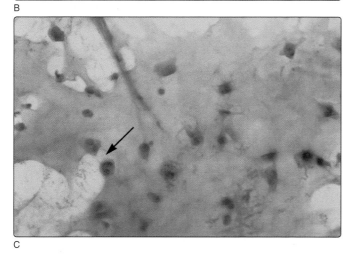

C

Fig. 41.3 Chondromyxoidfibroma. In a haemorrhagic background a cluster of spindle-shaped cells (arrow) and several fragments of cartilage (arrowhead) are evident. (H&E, × LP) (B) The cartilaginous fragments are stained red-blue in MGG and the chondroblast-like cells are only faintly visible. (MGG, × MP) (C) In wet-fixed smears the cartilaginous fragments are faintly stained and the tumour cells better visualized than with MGG. Note slight anisokaryosis and binucleated cell (arrow). (H&E, × MP)

Osteoblastoma

This benign bone-forming tumour has a definite predilection for males in the first three decades of life and

may be difficult to distinguish from osteosarcoma. The majority of cases occur in the vertebral column, long bones being next in frequency. Structurally, there are close similarities to the related tumour osteoid osteoma, with a central nidus of osteoid and vascular osteoblastic tissue, surrounded by sclerotic bone. Some cases have bizarre tumour cells but mitoses are not a prominent feature.

Cytological findings

▶ Cells of osteoblastic type, mononuclear and binucleated
▶ Clusters of spindle cells
▶ Osteoclastic cells

Only single cases of the cytology of osteoblastoma have been recorded[11] and our experience is limited to two tumours. These few cases were characterized by a mixed cell pattern. The diagnostic cells resembled osteoblasts, with eccentric rounded nuclei and a more or less distinct clear space or 'Hof' in the cytoplasm of many of the cells. Cell and nuclear size were variable and binucleated cells were observed. These osteoblast-like cells were either dispersed in the smear or arranged in small groups or rows. A blue to red or pink matrix was seen between the cells in some groups on MGG. A few clusters of tightly packed spindle cells with elongated nuclei were found in all smears and there were also scattered osteoclastic multinucleated cells.

Chondroma

Another benign tumour subjected to FNA is the chondroma. These are the most common tumours in the small bones of the hand and feet. Chondromas are evenly distributed throughout life and also occur in children. They may be single or multiple and are composed of mature hyaline cartilage interspersed with areas of degeneration.

Cytological findings

▶ Cartilaginous fragments with cells in lacunar spaces
▶ Cells with small regular nuclei
▶ Cellular pleomorphism not uncommon

It is usually not difficult to aspirate tumour tissue from chondromas. Characteristically, the smears are made up of numerous fragments of cartilage; dispersed cells are very uncommon. The fragments stain strongly violet or blue with MGG and faintly pink with H&E. Within fragments small rounded uniform cells with regular nuclei are seen in lacunar spaces. Binucleated cells are not found but the fragments may be highly cellular and exhibit cellular polymorphism, especially in chondromas of small peripheral bones.

Diagnostic pitfalls

The one cytological feature common to all the above tumours, apart from chondroma, is the presence of osteoclastic giant cells. These cells are also common in a number of tumour-like benign conditions as well as in osteosarcoma (Table 41.1).

The radiological features of aneurysmal bone cyst are similar to those seen in giant cell tumour and combinations of the two have been described. The most characteristic finding in FNA material from aneurysmal bone cyst is the very large amount of blood obtained, such that the syringe fills with blood immediately on sampling. The cellular yield is usually sparse; besides scattered osteoclastic cells, spindle-shaped fibroblastic cells and haemosiderin laden macrophages are typical findings.

Non-ossifying fibroma or metaphyseal fibrous defect is a rare lesion on FNA and only one case with thorough evaluation of the cytology has been reported[12]. The most important finding was the presence of groups or clusters of fibroblast-like spindle cells. Histiocytic cells with foamy or vacuolated cytoplasm and osteoclastic cells were also found.

Similar cytology has been described in a case of osteitis fibrosa cystica, also known as 'brown tumour' of hyperparathyroidism[13]. As well as osteoclasts, spindly mononuclear cells and macrophages were found. In the author's file, there is one case of brown tumour consisting of fragments of tightly packed spindle cells with numerous giant cells attached to the periphery, an appearance almost indistinguishable from that of a typical giant cell tumour.

The most important diagnostic pitfall is the misinterpretation of these benign lesions as malignant. There is a particular risk of giant cell tumour and osteoblastoma being mistaken for osteosarcoma, and chondromyxoid fibroma for a chondrosarcoma. Smears from osteosarcomas contain highly atypical osteoblast-like cells and multinucleated tumour cells but benign osteoclastic cells are often present in variable numbers.

Typical cases of osteoblastoma should not be mistaken for osteosarcoma but the so-called aggressive osteoblastoma[14] and those tumours containing large cells with pleomorphic hyperchromatic nuclei[15] may be, albeit rarely, misdiagnosed as osteosarcoma.

Chondromyxoid fibroma has been wrongly diagnosed as a chondrosarcoma[2,9,10]. The presence of chondroid fragments and the variation in nuclear size and shape make low-grade malignant chondrosarcoma an important diagnostic pitfall. Similarly, the cytological findings in cellular chondromas are easy to confuse with those of low-grade malignant chondrosarcoma.

When FNA smears are amply cellular and of good technical quality the combined evaluation of clinical, radiological and cytological findings may suggest a definitive diagnosis of giant cell tumour, chondroblastoma, osteoblastoma, chondromyxoid fibroma or chondroma. However, aspirates with a paucity of cells should be assessed with caution as the diagnostic cell type may be difficult to evaluate. The main criteria for the cytological diagnosis of benign bone tumours are listed in Table 41.2.

Malignant tumours of bone

Most types of primary malignant tumour of bone can be investigated effectively by FNA for diagnosis and management. In selected cases, combination of the cytological diagnosis with clinical and radiographic findings can be taken as a basis for planning definitive treatment. At other times, cytological examination is of assistance in further evaluation of the lesion.

The aggressive growth exhibited by many malignant bone tumours is often associated with destruction of cortical bone and also with local soft tissue extension of tumour

---

Table 41.1   Bone tumours/lesions exhibiting osteoclast-like giant cells in FNA

Benign
Giant cell tumour
Chondroblastoma
Chondromyxoidfibroma
Osteoblastoma
Aneurysmal bone cyst
Metaphyseal fibrous defect
Osteitis fibrosa cystica
('Brown tumour' of hyperparathyroidism)
Malignant
Osteosarcoma

Table 41.2   Main diagnostic criteria of benign bone tumours in FNA

	Age	Site	Radiology	Cytology
GCT	20–50	Epiphysis	Expansive; destructive	Double cell population of spindle cells and osteoclast-like multinucleated cells attached to the periphery of spindle cell clusters
CB	20–30	Epiphysis	Destructive; 'sharp borders'	Cartilaginous fragments; chondroblast-like cells; multinucleated osteoclast-like cells
OB	20–30	Vertebral column	Destructive; sclerotic rim	Spindle cell fragments, osteoblasts; multinucleated osteoclast-like cells
CMF	10–40	Metaphysis	Eccentric; expansive	Myxoid background substance; cartilaginous fragments with cellular polymorphism; spindle cells
CH	All ages	Small bones; hands and feet	Expansive: calcifications	Cartilaginous fragments with cells in lacunae; cellular polymorphism in variably cellular fragments

GCT, giant cell tumour; CB, chondroblastoma; OB, osteoblastoma; CMF, chondromyxoid fibroma; CH, chondroma

tissue. These factors ensure that in most cases it is easy to obtain sufficient material for cytological examination by FNA.

Osteosarcoma

The commonest of all primary malignant bone tumours, osteosarcoma has in the past been associated with a 5-year survival rate of only 20%. Recent improvements in therapy have increased this to more than 50%, but the outlook remains very poor in some of the more aggressive variants. Little is known of the pathogenesis although there are associations with pre-existing bone lesions such as Paget's disease, and with exposure to radiation or some chemotherapeutic agents.

The majority of patients are within the second and third decades of life, but osteosarcomas have been reported in children below 10 years and in middle-aged or elderly patients. There is a slight male preponderance. The metaphysis of long bones is the site of predilection, especially distal femur and proximal tibia.

Their classification can be according to site, including conventional intramedullary with cortical destruction, parosteal, periosteal and exclusively intramedullary, or by morphology, the histological findings being osteoblastic, chondroblastic, telangiectatic, fibroblastic or of small cell type. Mixed forms, especially osteoblastic/chondroblastic types, occur.

Cytological findings

▶ Mixture of cell clusters and dispersed cells
▶ Pleomorphic pattern of obviously malignant cells
▶ Relatively frequent mitoses, including atypical forms
▶ Intercellular tumour matrix of osteoid within clusters
▶ Benign osteoclastic giant cells
▶ Epithelioid tumour cells, which may be of osteoblastic type or resemble chondroblasts in osteoblastic or chondroblastic variants respectively
▶ Atypical spindle-shaped fibroblast-like cells in fibroblastic types

The FNA cytology of osteosarcoma has been thoroughly described in two articles, comprising a total of 72 tumours[11,16]. The results of these reports correspond well with the author's experience of 47 cases[2].

Intramedullary osteosarcoma

Conventional intramedullary osteosarcoma with cortical destruction is the commonest subtype histologically and on cytology, and may be osteoblastic, chondroblastic or mixed. Smears from these tumours are obviously malignant; dispersed cells are mixed with cell clusters or cohesive groups of variable size. The cell pattern is pleomorphic; in the pure osteoblastic type, the majority of tumour cells are rounded or polygonal with sharp cytoplasmic borders and eccentric nuclei. The nuclei are rounded, oval or occasionally irregular, with coarse chromatin and

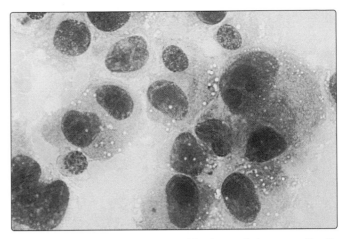

Fig. 41.4   Osteoblastic osteosarcoma. Mostly rounded tumour cells with eccentric nuclei and abundant cytoplasm. (MGG, ×HP)

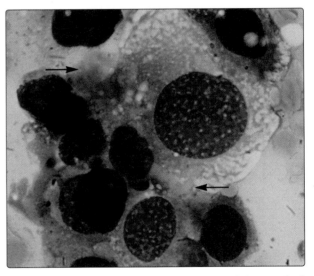

Fig. 41.5   Osteoblastic osteosarcoma. Thin intercellular strands of osteoid (arrow). (MGG, ×HP)

prominent large nucleoli. Many cells resemble osteoblasts but the clear 'Hof' is usually not visible (Fig. 41.4).

In the cell clusters and groups thin strands of a tumour matrix stained red or purple by MGG is occasionally observed between the cells (Fig. 41.5). Small clumps of similar matrix are also found in the background. This matrix, which is difficult to detect in wet-fixed smears, is considered to represent osteoid[8] and is an important diagnostic sign, especially when observed between the tumour cells in clusters or groups.

In the pure chondroblastic type, the predominant cell is mainly rounded with sharp cytoplasmic borders and a central rounded nucleus with relatively small nucleoli. In general, the cellular pleomorphism is less pronounced in the chondroblastic than in the osteoblastic type. A myxoid background and fragments of cartilaginous matrix staining blue or purple on MGG are common in chondroblastic osteosarcoma, while the thin strands of osteoid are less

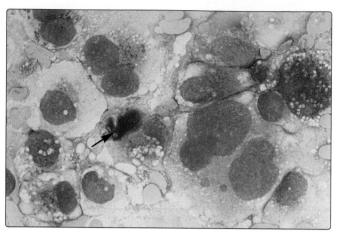

Fig. 41.6   Chondroblastic osteosarcoma. The tumour cells are embedded in a myxoid background matrix and a small fragment of purple-stained cartilage matrix is seen (arrow). (MGG, × OI)

Table 41.3   Differential diagnoses of osteosarcoma in FNA
Benign tumours/lesions
Reactive osteoblastic proliferations (pseudomalignant myositis ossificans)
Fracture callus
Aggressive osteoblastoma
Giant cell tumour
Malignant tumours
Primary pleomorphic sarcoma of bone (MFH-like)
High-grade malignant chondrosarcoma
Dedifferentiated chondrosarcoma
Metastatic anaplastic carcinoma
Anaplastic large cell lymphoma
Ewing's family of tumours (small cell OS)

MFH, Malignant fibrous histiocytoma; OS, osteosarcoma

frequent (Fig. 41.6). In the cartilage fragments, tumour cells are sometimes seen in lacunar spaces.

Both types contain multinucleated tumour cells and scattered benign osteoclastic cells are a common finding. Mitotic figures, including atypical mitoses, are seen, especially in the osteoblastic type. Aspiration smears from osteosarcoma are usually blood-stained. In the telangiectatic type, which is very haemorrhagic, the cell yield may be poor.

Fibroblastic osteosarcoma

Experience of the fibroblastic type is limited to single cases. Atypical spindle-shaped cells with fusiform nuclei predominate and cellular pleomorphism moderate.

Small cell osteosarcoma

The rare small cell osteosarcoma[17] has been only briefly described in two cases[18]. The main cytological features were a mixture of cohesive fragments and dispersed cells; the cells were small to medium sized, with round or spindle-shaped nuclei, and the overall pattern was less pleomorphic than in other types.

Parosteal osteosarcoma

FNA of the parosteal type is only documented in one case[11]. The majority of cells were atypical and spindle shaped, and resembled fibroblasts. In the author's limited experience, parosteal osteosarcomas are less suitable for FNA than other types since it is difficult to aspirate sufficient material by thin needle.

Diagnostic pitfalls

The principal differential diagnoses are listed in Table 41.3.

Reactive osteoblasts exhibit a wide range of shapes and sizes, their nuclear size is variable and nucleoli may be large and prominent. The chromatin pattern is, however, uniformly regular and their clear 'Hof' is often visible.

In pseudomalignant myositis ossificans, multinucleated tumour cells with atypical nuclei are never encountered nor are there any atypical mitoses[19].

Typical osteoblastomas are composed of spindle cell fragments, cells resembling osteoblasts with slight atypia and osteoclastic cells, producing a cell pattern different from that of a typical osteosarcoma. Predictably, the rare aggressive osteoblastoma and osteoblastoma with bizarre cells, both of which have pleomorphic hyperchromatic nuclei, do pose diagnostic problems.

Giant cell tumour has been regarded as another pitfall in diagnosis[11]. However the mononuclear cells of giant cell tumours never show the pleomorphism and nuclear atypia found in osteosarcoma.

Primary pleomorphic sarcoma of the malignant fibrous histiocytoma (MFH) type can occur in bone as well as in soft tissue, and the smear pattern may resemble that of an osteosarcoma. However, osteoblastic tumour cells are not found in the former tumour, nor are there intercellular strands of osteoid matrix. Furthermore the multinucleated giant tumour cells seen in malignant fibrous histiocytoma often show phagocytic activity. Osteosarcomatous tumour cells of either osteoblastic or chondroblastic type have an epithelioid appearance and therefore may be mistaken for carcinoma cells when seen in cohesive groups. This problem can be resolved by the use of immunocytochemical markers as described below.

The most difficult of all the differential diagnoses is between chondroblastic osteosarcoma and high-grade malignant chondrosarcoma. It may be impossible to distinguish these two malignancies by cytological examination. A similar problem arises in the diagnosis of osteosarcoma versus dedifferentiated chondrosarcoma when the aspirate contains osteosarcomatous tissue, but no fragments of well-differentiated chondrosarcoma.

The small cell variant of osteosarcoma has been considered to cause confusion with the Ewing's family primary in bone in smears[17]. However classical Ewing's tumour of bone has a very typical cell pattern in FNA material, which is quite different from that described in small cell osteosarcoma[2].

Parosteal osteosarcoma is usually less pleomorphic and of lower grade malignancy than the other types, and therefore poses other diagnostic problems. The presence of well formed cartilage and the insignificant atypia found in parosteal osteosarcoma may lead to misdiagnosis of benign chondromatous tumour.

Those osteosarcomas that are purely intramedullary often show bland-looking tumour cells that may also give diagnostic problems. However, pure intramedullary osteosarcomas are not usually subjected to FNA because of their intact cortical bone.

Ancillary techniques

Aspirated material may be used for a number of ancillary methods as aids to diagnosis. Electron microscopic examination is of value in the recognition of osteoid[2,11]. Immunocytochemical staining will help to exclude carcinomatous metastases which react with cytokeratin markers, whereas osteosarcoma cells are strongly positive when stained for alkaline phosphatase. This reaction excludes carcinoma and chondrosarcoma[2].

The role of alkaline phosphatase staining in differentiating between osteosarcoma and pleomorphic sarcoma of the MFH type is unclear. According to Magnusson et al.[20], alkaline phosphatase has been found in the spindle cells of the histiocytic tumour, while Myhre-Jensen et al.[21] claim that alkaline phosphatase is important in distinguishing malignant fibrous histiocytoma from extraskeletal osteosarcoma.

Apart from the parosteal type, the majority of osteosarcomas are aneuploid on DNA-ploidy analysis[2,22]. Unequivocal aneuploidy on DNA analysis excludes a benign osteoblastic proliferation.

Chondrosarcoma

This group of tumours has a better prognosis than osteosarcoma, and occurs in an older age group, most chondrosarcomas appearing in adults in the fourth to seventh decades. Predominant sites are the bones of the trunk and upper ends of femur and humerus, and a few are extraskeletal. Histologically, cartilage forming tumour cells permeate the local tissues, often engulfing normal or reactive bone. Thus chondrosarcomas may include bone, but it is never formed by the tumour cells themselves, in contrast to osteosarcomas, which may produce bone and cartilage.

Cytological findings

▶ Myxoid background matrix
▶ Fragments of hyaline cartilage
▶ Variable cellularity within fragments
▶ Mononuclear and binucleated tumour cells often in lacunae
▶ Large rounded individual cells and well-defined cytoplasm
▶ Nuclei rounded or irregular and lobulated

Most chondrosarcomas are easy targets for FNA. A surprisingly rich cell yield may be obtained and fragments or 'microbiopsies' of tumour tissue are found relatively commonly in smears.

The cytology of chondrosarcoma, including different histological subtypes, has been described in relatively few cases[23]. The largest series, evaluating 18 and 27 cases, respectively, has been reported by Walaas et al.[6] and the author[2].

The cytological findings depend on the grade of malignancy. Classical chondrosarcoma of low-grade malignancy yields tumour cells in fragments of variable size, cell dissociation being infrequent. The fragments are embedded in a myxoid background matrix and are of variable cellularity, with some cells lying in lacunar spaces. Matrix and fragments stain strongly reddish blue or violet on MGG, sometimes obscuring cell details, but this is not a problem with the paler pink staining on H&E (Figs 41.7, 41.8A,B). Individual tumour cells are generally large and rounded or elongated with distinct cell borders, and some are binucleate. There is slight to moderate nuclear atypia but mitoses are very rare. Well preserved cells sometimes have vacuolated or foamy cytoplasm.

Smears from high-grade chondrosarcomas are generally very cellular, showing many dissociated cells in a myxoid matrix. The number of fragments is variable but lower than in well-differentiated tumours. The fragments are also cellular and there is marked pleomorphism with nuclear atypia, enlarged nucleoli and occasional mitoses.

The histological subtypes clear cell chondrosarcoma, mesenchymal chondrosarcoma and dedifferentiated chondrosarcoma are rare and their FNA cytology has rarely been described.

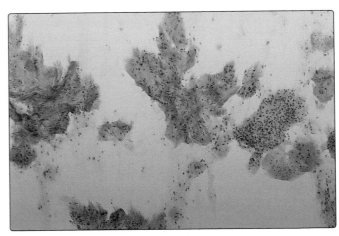

Fig. 41.7 Chondrosarcoma. Several different sized cartilaginous fragments. Note variable cellularity. (H&E, × LP)

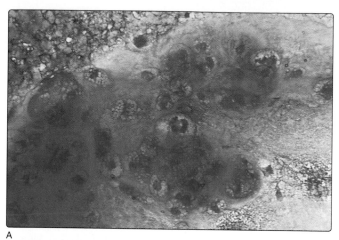

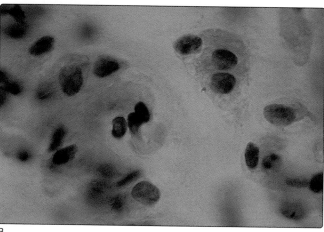

Fig. 41.8 High grade malignant chondrosarcoma. With MGG the cellular and nuclear details are difficult to assess due to the strong staining of the matrix. (MGG, × HP) (**B**) The nuclear atypia is easy to recognize in the wet-fixed smear. (H&E, × OI)

Clear cell chondrosarcoma

The only case reported[6] showed a cellular smear dominated by large tumour cells. The cells had an abundance of finely vacuolated cytoplasm with central hyperchromatic nuclei and prominent nucleoli.

Mesenchymal chondrosarcoma

The cytological features of mesenchymal chondrosarcoma in FNA smears have been reported in a few cases[6]. Small, monomorphic tumour cells in cohesive clusters have been described as a network of fibrillar matrix encircling cells and clusters. A cartilaginous matrix may be observed as giant cells of osteoclast-like type.

The extraskeletal myxoid chondrosarcoma is not related to mesenchymal chondrosarcoma of the bone[24].

Dedifferentiated chondrosarcoma

Dedifferentiated chondrosarcoma is a rare subtype, comprising about 10% of all chondrosarcoma. Histopathologically, it has the characteristics of a low-grade chondrosarcoma, which contains areas of high-grade

malignant non-chondroid sarcoma such as fibrosarcoma, osteosarcoma or malignant fibrous histiocytoma. The cytology of one case has been published, composed of a cell population similar to that of a malignant fibrous histiocytoma in addition to the cartilaginous component[25].

The single case in our file displayed a population of highly atypical spindle cells besides the low-grade chondrosarcoma component.

Diagnostic pitfalls

Chondroma may be difficult to distinguish from chondrosarcoma of low-grade malignancy on histology and the same problem is present in FNA material[2]. This is due to the presence of only insignificant atypia in low-grade chondrosarcomas and cellular pleomorphism in some chondromas.

Chondrosarcoma cells may be epithelioid and hence mistaken for carcinoma cells if only wet fixed smears are examined. This is because the characteristic background matrix and cartilaginous fragments are weakly stained unless MGG is used.

A pitfall already mentioned is the similarity between chondroblastic osteosarcoma and high-grade chondrosarcoma. Tumour bone formation is confined to osteosarcomas.

When situated in the vertebral column, chordoma is another differential diagnosis, because of the similar myxoid background matrix, but the tumour cell morphology in chordoma is different from that of chondrosarcoma.

The small cell population in mesenchymal chondrosarcoma may be misdiagnosed as a small cell tumour of other aetiology if the cartilaginous component is not represented in the smear.

Ancillary techniques

Adjunctive methods, such as electron microscopy and immunocytochemistry using S 100 protein[2,6] may help to prove the chondromatous nature of a tumour but do not assist in distinguishing between chondroma and chondrosarcoma. DNA-ploidy analysis may be helpful when the cytological findings are inconclusive with regard to benignity or malignancy. A non-diploid histogram strongly suggests a chondrosarcoma[2,26].

Chordoma

This slow growing malignant tumour arises from cells of the notochord, which are fetal remnants found in vertebral bodies and intervertebral discs. The tumour is more common in males than females and very uncommon before 30 years of age. Chordomas are found in the midline of the body, usually in the sacrococcygeal and spheno-occipital regions. They form gelatinous masses composed of large and small tumour cells arranged in ribbons or lobules set in mucinous material. Some of the cells are enormous,

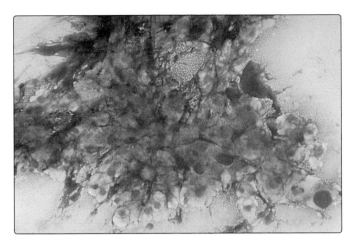

Fig. 41.9 Chordoma. The myxoid matrix encircles single cells as well as groups of tumour cells. (MGG, × LP)

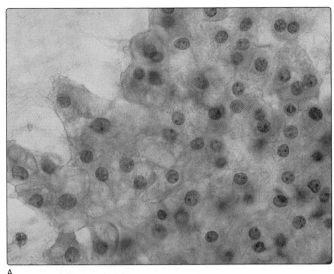

A

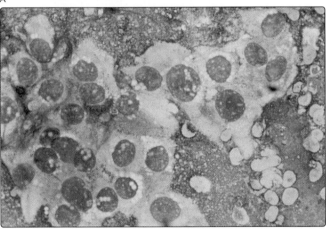

B

Fig. 41.10 Chordoma. The myxoid matrix is almost non-visible in wet-fixed smears and the cell cluster may be misinterpreted as coming from a clear cell carcinoma metastasis. (H&E, × MP) (**B**) Cytoplasm-rich tumour cells with rounded nuclei and vacuolated cytoplasm. Note the purple-stained myxoid background matrix. (MGG, × HP)

showing marked cytoplasmic vacuolation and large vesicular nuclei. They are known as physaliferous cells.

Cytological findings

- ► Abundant myxoid background
- ► Tumour cells singly or in groups
- ► Network of myxoid matrix round single cells and groups
- ► Tumour cells have abundant vacuolated cytoplasm
- ► Physaliferous cells

Because of their ability to destroy bone and invade soft tissues, chordomas are often easy to needle and the yield is usually good. The cytology of chordomas has been described in a large number of tumours[27,28]. The findings in ten neoplasms from our file are similar to other reports[2].

An abundant myxoid, often fibrillary, background matrix is the rule. Within this, dispersed tumour cells are mixed with cells in groups or cords. Characteristically, the matrix forms a network encircling these cells individually, whether isolated or in groups or cords (Fig. 41.9). The myxoid matrix is difficult to identify in wet fixed smears but easily detected in air-dried MGG-stained preparations (Fig. 41.10A,B).

The predominant tumour cell is medium sized to large, with rounded well-demarcated cytoplasm and central nucleus. The cytoplasm is often vacuolated or bubbly (Fig. 41.11). Cells may occasionally look like signet ring cells with a large cytoplasmic vacuole pushing the nucleus to the periphery, at times producing nuclear indentation. Generally some cells are very large, with abundant foamy or vacuolated cytoplasm and central prominent nuclei, corresponding to the typical physaliferous cells seen in tissue sections. Binucleated cells are found and there are also small uniformly rounded cells with scanty cytoplasm. In the so-called dedifferentiated chordoma a population of large highly atypical, mono or multinucleated cells are present besides the typical cellular pattern[29].

Diagnostic pitfalls

The main pitfalls are chondrosarcoma and metastatic clear cell carcinoma or mucus producing carcinoma. In other cases where the soft tissue component is dominant, it may be interpreted as a true soft tissue tumour if the cytopathologist is unaware of the radiographic findings. A number of myxoid soft tissue sarcomas then become important in the differential diagnosis, such as myxoid liposarcoma, myxoid MFH and myxoid extraskeletal chondrosarcoma. Immunocytochemical staining with keratin antibodies may help in the differential diagnosis between chordoma and chondrosarcoma and other myxoid sarcomas since chordoma reacts with epithelial markers. However these are not helpful with metastatic carcinoma. Carcinoembryonic antigen may be positive in some metastatic tumours.

The family of Ewing's tumours

Primary Ewing's sarcoma of bone is an aggressive tumour occurring predominantly in the first, second and third decades of life. Any bone in the skeleton may be involved but the lower extremities and the pelvic girdle account for more than 60% of cases. Histologically, it is composed of solid masses of small uniform tumour cells containing glycogen. There may be some tendency to rosette formation or an organoid pattern in the atypical variant and necrosis is often present.

Cytological findings

- Dispersed cells and cell clusters
- Cell fragility with naked nuclei and cytoplasmic background
- Double cell population
- Large vacuolated cells with bland nuclei
- Small dark cells with irregular hyperchromatic nuclei
- Abundant glycogen

Although arising centrally in bone, the rapid growth pattern of Ewing's tumour leads to early soft tissue extension, making it an easy target for needling. When aspiration is not preceded by radiological examination, the lesion may even be considered a true soft tissue tumour, clinically. The cytomorphology of Ewing's sarcoma of bone has been thoroughly evaluated[30,31]. FNA of a further 33 cases from the author's file corresponds well with these published reports[2].

Technically satisfactory cellular aspirates from Ewing's sarcoma have distinctive diagnostic cytological features. As a rule, the aspirates are highly cellular, containing a mixture of single cells and clusters of loosely attached cells. The cells are fragile so that forceful smearing results in naked deformed nuclei in a background of cytoplasmic debris.

Characteristically, there is a double cell pattern, the first being 'large light cells' with abundant poorly-defined cytoplasm containing vacuoles or clear spaces. The nuclei are rounded or ovoid with finely granular evenly distributed chromatin and small nucleoli. The second cell type consists of 'small dark cells' with scanty cytoplasm and irregularly shaped hyperchromatic nuclei. These two cell types are best observed within cell clusters in which the 'small dark cells' are interspersed between the 'large light' ones, sometimes in moulded small groups (Fig. 41.11A,B). Some nuclei in the 'large light cells' may be cleaved or lobulated. Mitotic figures are rare. In the atypical variant rosette-like structures may be observed, and the cellular and nuclear pleomorphism is more marked than in the classical type. Pear shaped cells with eccentric nuclei with evident nucleoli are present as well as cells with thin cytoplasmic extensions[32]. Peripheral neuroectodermal tumour (PNET) primary in bone exhibits the same cytological features as in soft tissue PNET (see Chapter 40)

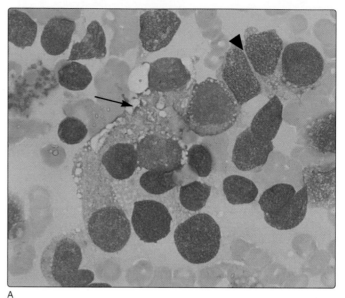

A

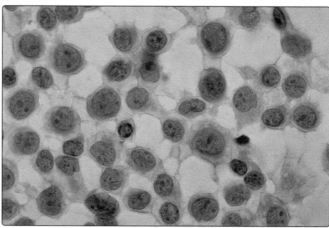

B

Fig. 41.11 Primary Ewing's sarcoma of bone. A mixture of 'large light' (arrow) and 'small, dark' (arrowhead) cells. (MGG, × OI) (**B**) The cytoplasmic details are less well evident in the wet-fixed smear but the nuclei with their finely granular chromatin and small nucleoli are well visualized. (H&E, × OI)

Diagnostic pitfalls

The major differential diagnoses are other small round cell tumours of childhood and adolescence (see Table 40.4, Chapter 40)

Ancillary techniques

Ancillary methods valuable in the differential diagnosis include electron microscopy and immunocytochemistry. Electron microscopic examination typically demonstrates abundant glycogen corresponding to the clear spaces and vacuoles seen in the cytoplasm in MGG-stained smears. No evidence of neuroepithelial or myogenic differentiation is found. Immunocytochemical staining reveals MIC[2] and vimentin positivity only, desmin and leucocyte common antigen both giving negative reactions. Cytogenetic and/or molecular genetic analyses provide a further important complementary method of investigation. The translocation t(11;22) giving rise to the EWS/FLI1 gene fusion found in family of Ewing's tumours[33,34] excludes neuroblastoma, rhabdomyosarcoma and lymphoblastic leukaemia.

Lymphohistiocytic lesions

Primary non-Hodgkin's lymphoma and Hodgkin's disease are rare in bone. The cytological features are identical to those described in FNA of lymph nodes (see Chapter 19).

Solitary plasmacytoma

Solitary plasmacytoma is a lesion that is difficult to diagnose radiologically and the findings are often misdiagnosed as metastatic carcinoma. Aspirates from plasmacytoma are often very haemorrhagic, containing a variable number of normal-looking and atypical plasma cells. Slightly atypical enlarged plasma cells may resemble osteoblasts. Poorly-differentiated plasmocytomas are composed of markedly atypical plasma cells, resembling carcinoma cells. For the most part clinical data are not helpful in diagnosis as the sedimentation rate often is within normal limits and light chain restriction is not found in the blood. In doubtful cases immunocytochemical staining is helpful.

Eosinophilic granuloma

Eosinophilic granuloma, also known as Langerhan's cell histiocytosis, is a benign lesion characterized by proliferation of histiocytic cells of Langerhan's type, with a variable number of eosinophils, neutrophils, lymphocytes and plasma cells. Most cases occur before the age of 20 and the majority of lesions are monostotic. The most frequent sites are skull, vertebrae, ribs, clavicle and scapula. Radiologically, the main differential diagnoses are osteomyelitis in the younger age group and metastasis in adults. The cytological findings on FNA have been well described in two recent publications comprising 30 cases[35,36], and the author's experience of 15 cases is in agreement with these reports[2].

Cytological findings

A richly cellular yield is common. Smears are composed of a mixed population of eosinophils, neutrophils, lymphocytes, plasma cells, osteoblasts and osteoclasts in addition to the Langerhan's histiocytes. The latter are large to medium sized cells with plentiful cytoplasm and rounded, bean or

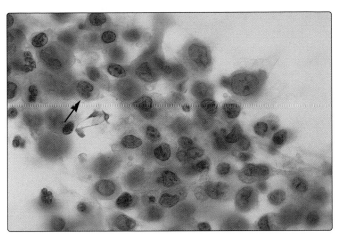

Fig. 41.12   Eosinophilic granuloma. A cluster of Langerhans' cell histiocytes. Note irregular nuclei with folded nuclear membrane. A 'coffee-bean' nucleus to the upper left is evident (arrow). (H&E, × OI)

kidney shaped nuclei. Characteristically, the nuclei are irregular and lobulated or show folded nuclear membranes (Fig. 41.12); so-called 'coffee-bean' nuclei have been reported to be especially typical. Some of these cells are binuclear or multinucleated.

In the author's opinion, osteomyelitis is the most important differential diagnosis. Electron microscopy for identification of specific Birkbeck granules, and immunocytochemistry using histiocytic markers including CDI(a) are of value in establishing a reliable diagnosis.

Metastatic tumours

In hospitals other than those specializing in the diagnosis and treatment of musculoskeletal tumours, metastatic lesions are the malignant tumours most commonly encountered in bone. Carcinomatous metastases in the skeleton are mainly derived from breast, kidney, lung, prostate, thyroid and liver. Malignant melanoma is another important primary site.

The cytological features in skeletal metastases are the same as those of the primary tumours. When the bone deposits are the first manifestation of the tumour, immunocytochemistry may help to disclose the primary site. Prostatic specific antigen for prostatic carcinoma, alpha-fetoprotein for hepatocellular carcinoma, thyroglobulin for follicular thyroid carcinoma and S 100 protein or melanoma associated antigen (HMB 45 or NK1C3) for malignant melanoma, are among the most helpful of these.

References

1   Åkerman M, Berg N O, Persson B. Fine needle aspiration biopsy in the evaluation of tumor-like lesions of bone. *Acta Orthoped Scand* 1976; **47**: 129–136

2   Åkerman M, Domanski H. Fine needle aspiration (FNA) of bone tumours: with special emphasis on the definitive

treatment of primary malignant bone tumours based on FNA. *Curr Diagn Pathol* 1998; **5**: 82–92

3   Sneige N, Ayala A, Carrasco H et al. Giant cell tumor of bone. A cytologic study of 24 cases. *Diagn Cytopathol* 1985; **1**: 111–117

4   Vetrani A, Fulciniti F, Boschi R et al. Fine needle aspiration biopsy diagnosis of giant cell tumour of bone. *Acta Cytol* 1990; **34**: 863–867

5   Fanning C V, Sneige N, Carrasco H et al. Fine needle aspiration cytology of chondroblastoma of bone. *Cancer* 1990; **65**: 1847–1863

6 Walaas L, Kindblom L-G, Gunterberg B, Bergh P. Light and electron-microscopic examination of fine needle aspiration in the preoperative diagnosis of cartilaginous tumours. *Diagn Cytopathol* 1990; **6**: 396–408

7 Pohar-Marinsek Z, Us-Krasovec M, Lamovec J. Chondroblastoma in fine needle aspirates. *Acta Cytol* 1992; **36**: 367–370

8 Kilpatrick S E, Pike E J, Geisinger K R, Ward W G. Chondroblastoma of bone: use of fine-needle aspiration biopsy and potential diagnostic pitfalls. *Diagn Cytopathol* 1997; **16**: 65–71

9 Bhatia A. Problems in the interpretation of bone tumours with fine needle aspiration (letter). *Acta Cytol* 1984; **28**: 91–92

10 Layfield L, Ferreiro J. Fine-needle aspiration cytology of chondromyxoid fibroma: a case report. *Diagn Cytopathol* 1988; **4**: 148–151

11 Walaas L, Kindblom L-G. Light and electron-microscopic examination of fine needle aspirates in the preoperative diagnosis of osteogenic tumours. A study of 21 osteosarcomas and 2 osteoblastomas. *Diagn Cytopathol* 1990; **6**: 27–38

12 Troncone G, Vetrani A, Boschi R et al. Il difetto fibroso metafisario (DFM) in biopsia aspirativa per ago sottile. *Istocitopatologia* 1988; **10**: 113–118

13 Watson C, Unger P, Kaneko M, Gabrilove J. Fine needle aspiration of osteitis fibrosa cystica. *Diagn Cytopathol* 1985; **1**: 157–160

14 Dorfman H D, Weiss S W. Borderline osteoblastic tumours Problems in the differential diagnosis of aggressive osteoblastoma and low-grade osteosarcoma. *Sem Diagn Pathol* 1984; **1**: 215–234

15 Mirra J M, Kendrick R A, Kendrick R E Pseudomalignant osteoblastoma versus arrested osteosarcoma. *Cancer* 1976; **37**: 2005–2014

16 White V A, Fanning C V, Ayala A et al. Osteosarcoma and the role of fine needle aspiration: a study of 51 cases. *Cancer* 1988; **62**: 1238–1246

17 Ayala A, Jae Y, Raymond K et al. Small cell osteosarcoma. A clinicopathologic study of 27 cases. *Cancer* 1989; **64**: 2162–2174

18 Park S H, Kim I. Small cell osteogenic sarcoma of the ribs: cytological, immunohistochemical, and ultrastructural study with literature review. *Ultrastruct Pathol* 1999; **23**: 133–140

19 Rööser B, Herrlin K, Rydholm A, Åkerman M. Pseudomalignant myositis ossificans. Clinical, radiologic, and cytologic diagnosis in 5 cases. *Acta Orthop Scand* 1989; **60**: 457–460

20 Magnusson B, Kindblom L-G, Angervall L. Enzyme histochemistry of malignant fibrous histiocytic tumours. A light and electron microscopic analysis. *Appl Pathol* 1983; **1**: 457–460

21 Myhre-Jensen O, Bendix-Hansen K. Enzyme histochemistry of soft tissue tumours. In: Fletcher C D M, McKee D H eds. *Pathobiology of Soft Tissue Tumours*. Edinburgh: Churchill Livingstone, 1990; 185–198

22 Bauer H C F, Kreicbergs A, Silfversvärd C. DNA analysis in the differential diagnosis of osteosarcoma. *Cancer* 1988; **61**: 2532–2540

23 Tunc M, Ekinici C. Chondrosarcoma diagnosed by fine needle aspiration cytology. *Acta Cytol* 1996; **40**: 283–288

24 Antonescu C, Argani P, Erlandson R et al. Skeletal and extraskeletal myxoid chondrosarcoma. A comparative clinicopathologic, ultrastructural, and molecular study. *Cancer* 1998; **83**: 1504–1521

25 Dee S, Meneses M, Ostrowski M et al. Pleomorphic ('dedifferentiated') chondrosarcoma. Report of a case initially examined by fine needle aspiration biopsy. *Acta Cytol* 1991; **35**: 467–471

26 Kreicbergs A, Söderberg G, Zetterberg A. Prognostic significance of nuclear DNA content in chondrosarcomas. *Anal Quant Cytol* 1980; **4**: 271–278

27 Finley J, Silverman J, Dabbs D et al. Chordoma, diagnosis by fine needle aspiration biopsy with histologic, immunocytochemical and ultrastructural confirmation. *Diagn Cytopathol* 1986; **2**: 330–337

28 Walaas L, Kindblom L-G. Fine needle aspiration biopsy in the preoperative diagnosis of chordoma. A study of 17 cases with application of electron microscopy, histochemical and immunohistochemical examination. *Hum Pathol* 1990; **22**: 22–28

29 Bergh P, Kindblom L-G, Gunterberg B et al. Prognostic factors in chordoma of the sacrum and mobile spine. *Cancer* 2000; **88**: 2122–2134

30 Akhtar M, Ashraf A, Sabbah R. Aspiration cytology of Ewing's sarcoma. Light and electron microscopic correlations. *Cancer* 1985; **56**: 2051–2060

31 Dahl I, Åkerman M, Angervall L. Ewing's sarcoma of bone. A correlative cytological and histological study of 14 cases. *Acta Pathol Microbiol Immuno Scand (A)* 1986; **94**: 363–369

32 Renshaw A, Perez-Atayde A, Fletcher J, Granter S. Cytology of typical and atypical Ewing's sarcoma/PNET. *Am J Clin Pathol* 1996; **106**: 620–624

33 Åkerman M, Åman P, Lindholm K, Carlén B. Primary Ewing's sarcoma of bone in a 73 year old man. Diagnosis by fine needle aspiration cytology, electron microscopy, immunocytochemistry and molecular genetic analysis. *Acta Cytol* 1995; **39**: 265–266

34 Åkerman M, Dreinhöfer K, Rydholm A et al. Cytogenetic studies of fine needle aspiration samples from osteosarcoma and Ewing's sarcoma. *Diagn Cytopathol* 1996; **15**: 17–22

35 Elsheikh T, Silverman J, Wakely P et al. Fine needle aspiration cytology of Langerhan's cell histiocytosis (eosinophilic granuloma) of bone in children. *Diagn Cytopathol* 1991; **7**: 261–266

36 Shabb N, Fanning C H, Carrasco C et al. Diagnosis of eosinophilic granuloma by fine needle aspiration with concurrent institution of therapy. *Diagn Cytopathol* 1993; **9**: 3–12

42 The cytology of synovial fluid

Anthony J. Fremont and J. Denton

Introduction

Normal synovial fluid

Joints permit bones to move relative to one another. The structure of joints is very variable, the most simple being a dense fibrous band joining two bone ends. The range of movements permitted by this mechanism is limited. By contrast, the most sophisticated joints are synovial or diarthrodial joints that allow a much greater variety of movement. In these joints, the bone ends are not directly tethered to one another: each is capped by a discrete piece of hyaline cartilage. As a consequence, the diarthrodial joint is inherently unstable, stability being imparted by a dense fibrous sheath or capsule which, rather than joining the bone ends, forms a strong flexible sleeve that surrounds the joint and envelops the peripheral segments of the two bones. This creates a cavity inside the joint which, except for the cartilage, is completely lined by a specialized form of connective tissue called synovium. The space operates under a negative pressure and contains a small amount of a viscid liquid called synovial fluid, which acts as a lubricant for the two moving articular surfaces and distributes nutrients throughout the joint.

Synovial fluid consists of a transudate of plasma from synovial blood vessels, supplemented with high molecular weight saccharide-rich molecules, notably hyaluronans, produced by one of the two main types of synovial cells: type B synoviocytes. Type A synoviocytes are phagocytes that remove debris from the synovial fluid.

Synovial fluid differs from all other body fluids in that the surface of synovium and cartilage (the tissues in immediate contact with the synovial fluid) are not covered by an intact cellular layer seated on a basement membrane, but rather an incomplete layer of cells. Thus the matrix of cartilage and synovium are in contact with the synovial fluid, allowing a relatively homogenous chemical environment to develop within the joint. Because of this unusual arrangement it is perhaps better to regard the synovial fluid as a semi-liquid, avascular hypocellular connective tissue rather than a true body fluid, such as may form in a pericardial effusion.

Synovial fluid in diseased joints

Variations in the volume and composition of synovial fluid reflect pathological processing occurring within the joint.

Because of the unusual relationship between the tissues within the joint, chemically mediated events, such as inflammation or enzyme-mediated degradation occurring within the synovium and cartilage are reflected in changes within the synovial fluid. These changes include the production of factors responsible for the accumulation of different cell types within the fluid and it is this that is the basis of understanding synovial fluid cytology.

Synovial fluid cytology

Cytoanalysis of synovial fluid differs in three important regards from that of other body fluids. First, synovial joints are very rarely affected by neoplastic processes. Second, 'cytology' of synovial fluid is better described as 'microscopy', as accurate recognition of non-cellular particulate material, such as crystals and matrix fragments, is essential to an understanding of the disease process within the joint. Third, the greatest diagnostic information comes not only from the recognition of cell types but also from their quantification[1-3].

The basic approach to synovial fluid microscopy

So that no part of the analysis is omitted, there is a sequential examination of all synovial fluid specimens arriving in the laboratory. It follows four steps:

1 Gross analysis
2 The nucleated cell count
3 The 'wet prep'
4 The cytocentrifuge preparation

Gross analysis

Because synovial fluids from inflamed joints have a tendency to clot, they should be received in the laboratory in anticoagulant. The fluid is best anticoagulated with lithium heparin. It is not possible to fix synovial fluid and the specimen therefore represents fresh tissue, and should be treated as such in every case. Even with refrigeration the optimum cytological information can only be extracted if the sample is examined within 48 hours of aspiration, and preferably as soon as possible within the first 24 hours. Upon arrival the synovial fluid should be examined macroscopically.

Macroscopic analysis involves a subjective assessment of colour, clarity and viscosity and the performance of an old established, but none the less useful, piece of bench chemistry called the 'mucin clot test'.

Colour

Synovial fluid is normally pale yellow. In haemarthroses it will be red or orange and in inflammatory arthropathies may appear cream or white. Occasionally in septic arthritis it may be coloured by bacterial chromogens.

Clarity

Normal synovial fluid is clear. As the number of particles and/or cells it contains increases so it passes through a phase of opalescence to one of being frankly opaque. Examination of the clarity therefore gives a clue to the cellularity and/or crystal content of the fluid specimen.

Viscosity

Normal synovial fluid has a thick mucoid consistency because of the complex saccharide based molecules it contains. These are fundamental to its lubricating properties. In inflammatory joint disease the viscosity of the fluid falls due to enzymatic digestion and altered synthesis of these saccharides.

Mucin clot

Mixing synovial fluid and a dilute solution of acetic acid leads to the formation of a white precipitate, produced by aggregation of proteins and hyaluronans. The nature and amount of precipitate varies from a tight dot to a fluctuant precipitate and reflects the quality and quantity of the protein/hyaluronan complex. In inflammatory joint diseases the release of digestive enzymes into the fluid leads to the breakdown of these complexes and poor clot formation. Non-inflammatory arthropathies exhibit a good mucin clot. Haemorrhage dilutes the synovial fluid and prevents good mucin clot formation.

The nucleated cell count

A sample of synovial fluid, agitated to achieve the most uniform distribution of cells, is diluted to a known concentration with normal saline containing methyl violet as a supravital stain. The diluted fluid is placed on to a haemocytometer chamber and a manual count performed of nucleated viable cells. Automated counting is possible, but because of the viscosity of some samples and the danger of producing a mucin clot within the delicate tube system of the counter through the use of standard acetic acid-based carrier media, it is more convenient to use a manual method. For convenience the nucleated cell count of synovial fluid is expressed in cells per mm³. To convert this to cell counts per ml necessitates multiplying the cell count by 1000. Normal synovial fluid contains approximately 200 cells per mm³[3-5]. In inflammatory joint disease the cell count exceeds 1000 cells per mm³ and in non-inflammatory arthropathies is usually less than 1000 cells per mm³. Cell counts in excess of 20 000 cells per mm³ are found predominantly in three clinical settings: rheumatoid arthritis, septic arthritis

and reactive arthritis: a form of arthropathy associated with infection at an extra-articular site and caused by the presence of, and reaction to, epitopes of the organism, but not the whole organism, within the joint.

The 'wet prep'

Synovial fluid often contains small particles that can be recognized with the naked eye. In making the 'wet prep' the specimen is agitated and a small aliquot containing as many of these particles as possible is aspirated into a glass pipette, then placed as a large drop on to a microscope slide. The drop is gently squeezed flat beneath a coverslip and viewed unstained with a conventional microscope. For optimal results the microscope condenser diaphragm should be nearly closed to produce diffused light in which the unstained cells and particles are more clearly seen. In addition to particulate matter including crystals and fragments of tissues from joint associated structures, such as cartilage, meniscus and ligament, the preparation is examined for one type of cell: the 'ragocyte'.

Crystals

Several classes of crystalline material are found in joints. They consist of:

▶ *Monosodium urate*. These are typically needle shaped, highly birefringent crystals usually 5–30 μm long (Fig. 42.1). They can be distinguished from other crystals in that they are negatively birefringent when viewed in polarized light with an interposed quarter wave plate. These crystals are diagnostic of gout. If found within the background of a high cell count fluid, their presence usually signifies acute gout[6], but even if the cell count is low the diagnosis is beyond doubt.

▶ *Calcium pyrophosphate dihydrate*. These crystals accumulate naturally within joints with advancing age. In elderly patients, particularly in joints containing fibrocartilage, such as the knee, they can therefore be regarded as a normal finding, a condition known as chondrocalcinosis. Sometimes the crystals are associated with a high nucleated cell count in an acute monoarthritis. This is the typical presentation and synovial fluid findings of pseudogout. Calcium pyrophosphate crystals may be found in association with otherwise characteristic features of osteoarthritis (OA). This is typical of the more common form of degenerative joint disease: hypertrophic OA[7].

▶ *Hydroxyapatite*. Crystals of hydroxyapatite within synovial fluid indicate damage either to the calcified zone of cartilage or underlying subarticular bone. Loss of cartilage sufficient to expose these structures to the synovial fluid is seen in the non-inflammatory disorder osteoarthritis and in the inflammatory rheumatoid disease. Sometimes the crystals are too small and amorphous to be seen with the conventional light microscope but staining with Alizarin red stain produces a birefringent bright red product (calcium alizarate) which is easily visualized[8-10].

▶ *Lipids*. Various lipids enter the synovial fluid from the blood in inflammatory joint disease and following haemarthrosis. Different lipids have different crystalline shapes varying from

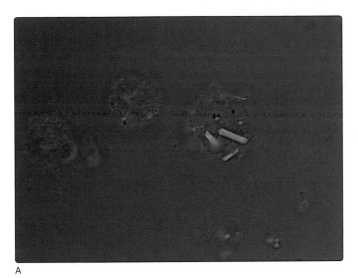
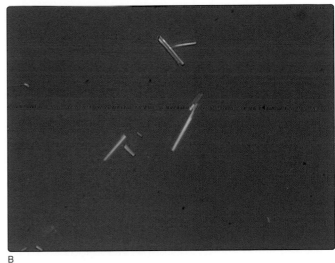

A   B

Fig. 42.1 Photomicrographs of crystals taken in polarized light with a quarter wave plate between the polarizers. (A) Intracellular crystals of calcium pyrophosphate. Note the crystals are weakly birefringent and that the crystal appears blue. Contrast this with the crystals of sodium urate in (B). These crystals appear much 'brighter'. The difference in colour is a reflection of the difference in axis of the crystal lattice. The pyrophosphate crystal is commonly described as having weak positive birefringence and the urate crystal strongly negatively birefringent.

the notched plates of cholesterol to the spherical liquid crystals of cholesterol esters[11–13].

▶ *Steroids*. Intra-articular injection of depot steroids is conventional management of certain arthropathies. Unfortunately the crystalline steroid preparation may remain within the joint for up to 10 weeks and may mislead the unwary if the characteristic appearance is not recognized[14].

▶ *Others*. Many other crystals may be found within the synovial fluid specimen but they are too numerous and rare to describe here. A more exhaustive analysis is given in Fremont and Denton[15].

Non-crystalline, non-cellular particulate material

The inside of conventional synovial joints is lined by cartilage and synovium and may be crossed by ligaments and bands of fibrocartilage. Alteration to the physical structure of any of these components by primary disease or trauma may lead to small fragments appearing free within the synovial fluid. Most common are fragments of cartilage, or following trauma, particularly to the knee, fragments of cruciate ligament and meniscal fibrocartilage[15].

Cartilage can be recognized by the silken sheen of its matrix. In osteoarthritis, the most common disorder in which fragments of cartilage are found in the joint, cartilage fragments have many of the characteristics of osteoarthritic cartilage seen in tissue sections. In particular they may show surface crimping of early fibrillation and contain clustered chondrocytes (Fig. 42.2).

Fragments of meniscal fibrocartilage can be recognized by the curved arrays of collagen fibres and flattened chondrocytes they contain. They are typically found within traumatized knee joints.

In the knee in both twisting trauma and in rheumatoid disease, small fragments of ligament may be found within synovial fluid. These fragments usually consist of long thin

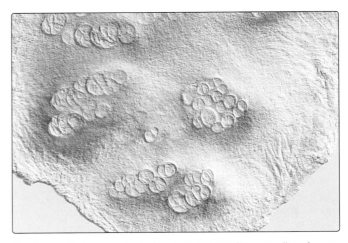

Fig. 42.2 A chondrocyte cluster within a piece of loose cartilage from a joint of a patient with osteoarthritis. (unstained × 750)

fibrils consisting of parallel collagen fibril bundles.

With the advent of prosthetic surgery, and particularly as the number of ageing prostheses increases, wear of implanted material also leads to the presence of fragments of foreign material within the joint. Many of the modern plastics, such as high density polyethylene used for articular surfaces, methyl methacrylate used as a cement, and fibres such as dacron and carbon fibre used as replacement ligaments can mimic crystals as they fragment and can cause diagnostic problems. Metal debris from metal-based prostheses can be shed or abraded and appear as tiny black particles. These may be as harbingers of imminent prosthetic failure[15,16].

Occasionally, peculiar extraneous material is found within the synovial fluid, usually introduced by a clinician. We have found structures as diverse as paper and pollen.

931

Ragocytes

Ragocytes are cells of various lineages, most often macrophages and polymorphs, which are recognized by the presence within their cytoplasm of refractile granules that vary from apple green to black (depending on the focus) when viewed with a microscope with a partially closed condenser diaphragm. The granules are larger than those of conventional neutrophil granules and can be distinguished on the basis of their size and refractility (Fig. 42.3). They are called ragocytes as they were first described as cells seen specifically in rheumatoid arthritis[17]. Extensive study of these cells shows them to contain immune complexes, including rheumatoid factors.

Ragocytes are counted and their number expressed as a proportion of all nucleated cells seen in the 'wet preparation'. In rheumatoid arthritis the proportion of ragocytes is typically greater than 70% of all nucleated cells, and, in diagnostic terms, a ragocyte count of 70–95% of all nucleated cells is typical of, and specific to, rheumatoid disease. More detailed studies have shown that ragocytes are not restricted to rheumatoid arthritis and, indeed, are a constant feature of all inflammatory arthropathies. However with the exception of septic arthritis, gout and pseudogout, ragocytes rarely account for more than 50% of all nucleated cells in the majority of the inflammatory arthropathies. A ragocyte count in excess of 95%, in the absence of crystals, is typical of septic arthritis and can be used to diagnose this condition even in the absence of detectable organisms.

The cytocentrifuge preparation

Synovial fluid cytoanalysis is best conducted on cytocentrifuge preparations stained with a modified Jenner-Giemsa stain. Optimal cytospin preparations are made by diluting the fluid down to 400 cells per mm^3 with isotonic saline. The one exception is when septic arthritis is suspected, when the greatest likelihood of identifying organisms is afforded by diluting the fluid to a concentration of 1200 cells per mm^3.

Organisms

Careful microscopic examination of synovial fluid allows microorganisms to be identified in approximately 87% of instances of clinical infective arthritis[15]. Most infective arthritis is caused by Gram-positive bacteria (Fig. 42.4).

The greatest problems in diagnosing infective arthritis are first, the recognition of Gram-negative organisms and organisms rendered Gram-negative by incomplete antibiotic therapy, and second, distinguishing contaminating organisms from those that are truly pathogenic. The latter is made more difficult because synovial fluid is a live tissue and accidental contamination of the fluid by organisms may lead to those organisms becoming intracellular, one of the features suggestive of infection.

Most bacterial infections result in a neutrophil response. However, in contrast to this infections resulting from

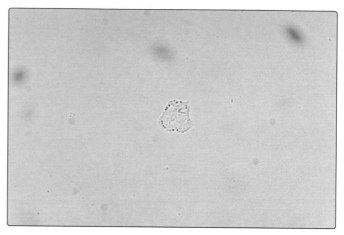

Fig. 42.3   A ragocyte viewed in 'pseudophase' optics. (unstained × 550)

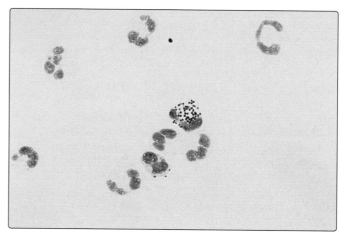

Fig. 42.4   A cytocentrifuge preparation showing Gram-positive cocci. (Gram × 750)

Mycobacterium spp, are characteristically lymphocyte rich fluids.

With an increase in the number of patients who are immunosuppressed, either as a consequence of disease, or through therapy, there is an increasing incidence of non-suppurative infective arthritis, particularly caused by mycobacteria and fungi. Although it is often possible to see organisms in these cases, close cooperation between clinician and cytopathologist is necessary to achieve the optimal detection rate.

Care must also be taken in patients who have a pre-existing arthropathy, particularly rheumatoid disease. These patients are both at a greater risk of developing a superimposed infective arthritis and of receiving treatment that may mask the presence of infection.

Cells

For reasons that are not clearly understood, primary neoplastic disease is exceptionally rare in joints. Occasionally, leukaemic cells may be found in synovial fluid, but there are only a handful of cases of other neoplastic processes involving joints. Malignant cells are therefore so rare as to be disregarded in everyday practice.

The cells that are found most frequently in synovial fluid are a reflection of the two major groups of joint diseases, namely the inflammatory arthropathies such as septic arthritis, gout, seronegative spondylarthropathies and rheumatoid disease, and the non-inflammatory arthropathies resulting from trauma or due to osteoarthritis.

In very general terms, in inflammatory arthropathies, polymorphs dominate the cytological picture and in non-inflammatory arthropathies macrophages, lymphocytes and synoviocytes are the most commonly encountered cells. Although making up the overwhelming majority of the cells within diseased joints, these four groups represent only a small proportion of the cell types that can be identified regularly within diseased joints. Most of these cell types are identifiable on morphological grounds in conventional Jenner-Giemsa stained cytocentrifuge preparations. The following are the 15 most commonly identified cells in synovial fluid.

1. *Neutrophil polymorphs*. These cells are recognized by their characteristic nuclear morphology. They are the predominant cells in inflammatory arthropathies and in intra-articular haemorrhage, the former as a consequence of specific traffic into the synovial fluid and the latter because they are the most abundant nucleated cell in blood. As a proportion of all nucleated cells, they most commonly account for between 60–80% of the cells in these conditions. In septic arthritis they frequently amount to more than 95% of the total, an observation that can be diagnostic in septic arthritis even when organisms cannot be identified.

2. *Small lymphocytes*. These are up to 12 μm in diameter with a nuclear/cytoplasmic ratio greater than 9:1. They predominate in approximately 10% of all cases of inflammatory arthritis, and in rheumatoid disease, they indicate a better long-term prognosis[18,19]. When seen in the company of LE cells they strongly suggest the diagnosis of systemic lupus erythematosus.

3. *Plasma cells*. Considering the number of plasma cells within inflamed synovium, these cells are rare in synovial fluid even in the most active inflammatory arthropathies. When seen they suggest a diagnosis of rheumatoid disease.

4. *Reider cells*. These cells are up to 15 μm in diameter with a nuclear/cytoplasmic ratio of 6:1. The nuclei are lobed, the lobes showing symmetry about a pale, attenuated, central region. This peculiar morphology is almost certainly a consequence of cytoskeletal abnormalities brought about by the cellular environment. They are seen almost exclusively in rheumatoid disease (Fig. 42.5)[15].

5. *Mott cells*. These cells resemble plasma cells, from which they are derived, except that they contain a large

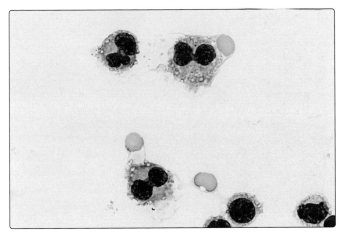

Fig. 42.5 A Reider cell; note the attenuated nucleus. (Jenner Giemsa × 350)

number of intracytoplasmic Russell bodies. They are also found almost exclusively in synovial fluid of patients with rheumatoid disease. Again, their morphology probably reflects an abnormality of intracellular structural elements, in this case the enclosing membrane of the non-secreted immunoglobulin.

6. *Monocytoid mononuclear cells*. These form one of the three morphologically distinct categories of large mononuclear cells encountered in synovial fluid. They are effectively macrophages and have all the structural characteristics of these cells. They are common in all types of arthritis and are frequently the most common cell found in non-inflammatory arthropathies, particularly in some cases of osteoarthritis and in joints in which previously implanted prostheses are breaking down. True viral arthritis, i.e. one in which the virus is present in the joint, and a rare form of acute inflammatory arthropathy of unknown cause called acute monocytic arthritis, are the only two types of inflammatory arthropathy in which macrophages predominate.

7. *Cytophagocytic mononuclear cells (CPM)*. This category refers to mononuclear cells that have phagocytosed apoptotic polymorphs (Fig. 42.6). The cells are normally seen wherever apoptosis is occurring and, as this is the usual way in which polymorphs are removed from joints, they are common. They are, however, most abundant in the seronegative spondylarthropathies[20,21]. These are a group of diseases which includes the peripheral arthritis associated with psoriasis, inflammatory bowel disease, Behçet's disease and ankylosing spondylitis. Reactive arthritis, which is an oligoarthropathy occurring in association with extra-articular infection, notably of the gastrointestinal and genito-urinary tracts[22], and the arthritis which follows vaccination and viral infection. If more than 5% of all large mononuclear cells are CPM a confident diagnosis of a seronegative spondylarthropathy can be made. The only exception to these general rules is rheumatoid disease in which apoptosis occurs in the absence of CPM formation, a

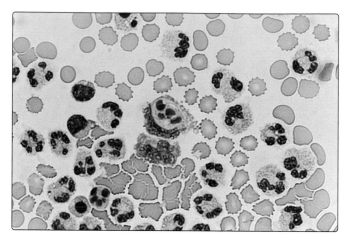

Fig. 42.6   A cytophagocytic mononuclear cell (CPM). (J-G × 350)

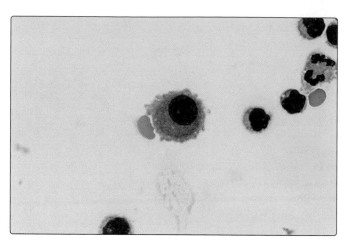

Fig. 42.7   The typical appearance of a synoviocyte. (J-G × 350)

feature of such universal occurrence that it can be used diagnostically.

8. *Synoviocytes*. These are a morphologically distinct subgroup of the large mononuclear cells, with a low nuclear/cytoplasmic ratio, round eccentrically placed nuclei and a 'pericellular frill' (Fig. 42.7). They are shed from the surface of the synovium and are found most commonly in non-inflammatory arthropathies where multinucleate forms may occur.

9. *Eosinophils*. Eosinophils are seen following intra-articular haemorrhage and arthrography, as well as in the rare parasitic infestations of joints.

10. *Mast cells*. Although mast cells can be found in most arthropathies, they are seen most commonly in inflammatory arthritis in patients with a seronegative spondylarthropathy and in non-inflammatory arthropathies associated with trauma[21].

11. *Multinucleate cells*. These may be synoviocytes or plasma cells and have no more significance than the mononuclear variants of these cells.

12. *Cells in mitosis*. Neoplastic infiltration of joints is very rare. Mitotic figures are relatively common by comparison and, no matter how bizarre they appear, are usually of little diagnostic or prognostic significance.

13. *LE cells*. Phagocytes containing a cytoplasmic inclusion of nuclear material are not uncommon and do not have the same significance in synovial fluid as they do in blood. In the presence of a fluid rich in lymphocytes, however, they are strongly suggestive of systemic lupus erythematosus.

14. *Tart cells*. These cells resemble LE cells, except that the inclusions have a distinct nuclear chromatin pattern. They predominate in rheumatoid disease.

15. *Dohle body cells*. Macrophages or polymorphs are the source of these cells, which are recognized by the presence of duck-egg blue intracytoplasmic inclusions composed of abnormal aggregates of cytoskeletal microfibrils. As in all aberrations of cell membrane and cytoskeleton, the cells are

Table 42.1	Typical synovial fluid findings in osteoarthritis
Macroscopic and wet prep findings	
Colour	: Pale yellow; sometimes haemorrhagic in acute episodes
Clarity	: Opalescent
Mucin clot	: Good
Viscosity	: High
Ragocytes (%)	: Nil
Crystals	: Often contains hydroxyapatite and, in hypertrophic OA, calcium pyrophosphate
Particles	: Coated strands; crimped cartilage; cartilage with chondrocyte clusters
Lipid	: Lipid droplets in acute episodes; lipid crystals in droplets if fluid haemorrhagic
Cytocentrifuge preparation findings	
Nucleated cells	: <1000/mm³
Polymorphs (%)	: 10 (may be higher if associated haemarthrosis)
Lymphocytes (%)	: 35
Macrophages (%)	: 30
Synoviocytes (%)	: 25
CPM (%) (of LMN)	: Nil
Mast cells	: May be up to 5%
Eosinophils	: Seen in 10–15% of cases
Other cells	: Multinucleate cells; cells (usually synoviocytes) in mitosis
Features indicating a poor prognosis	: Haemorrhage

almost invariably restricted to synovial fluid of patients with rheumatoid disease.

Clinical applications of synovial fluid microscopy

The features described above represent a short analysis of the important microscopic findings in synovial fluid. By retrospective analysis of proven cases it is possible to recognize patterns of microscopic features specific for certain arthropathies (Tables 42.1–42.8). It is also possible to take all these features and summate them into a

Table 42.2 Typical synovial fluid findings in rheumatoid disease

Macroscopic and wet prep findings

Colour	:	Pale yellow
Clarity	:	Translucent
Mucin clot	:	Variable
Viscosity	:	Variable
Ragocytes (%)	:	70
Crystals	:	Hydroxyapatite
Particles	:	Small fibrin aggregates; fragments of cartilage, ligament and meniscus
Lipid	:	Nil

Cytocentrifuge preparation findings

Nucleated cells	:	10 000/mm³
Polymorphs (%)	:	80
Lymphocytes (%)	:	15
Macrophages (%)	:	5
Synoviocytes (%)	:	0
CPM (%) (of LMN)	:	Nil (unless the patient has a non-articular infection, i.e. superimposed reactive arthritis)
Mast cells	:	Nil
Eosinophils	:	Rare
Apoptotic cells	:	Sometimes up to 100% of polymorphs
Other cells	:	Immunoblasts; Reider cells; Mott cells; DB cells; plasma cells; tart cells
Features indicating a poor prognosis	:	High nucleated cell or ragocyte count; tissue fragments

Table 42.4 Typical synovial fluid findings in systemic lupus erythematosus

Macroscopic and wet prep findings

Colour	:	Pale yellow
Clarity	:	Clear
Mucin clot	:	Fair
Viscosity	:	Low
Ragocytes (%)	:	5
Crystals	:	Nil
Particles	:	Nil
Lipid	:	Nil

Cytocentrifuge preparation findings

Nucleated cells	:	2500/mm³
Polymorphs (%)	:	10
Lymphocytes (%)	:	65 (20)*
Macrophages (%)	:	65 (20)*
Synoviocytes (%)	:	5
CPM (%) (of LMN)	:	Nil
Mast cells	:	Few
Eosinophils	:	Few
Apoptotic cells	:	Nil
Other cells	:	LE cells
Features indicating a poor prognosis	:	None known

* Typically either lymphocytes or macrophages account for approximately 65% of the cells, the other about 20%

Table 42.3 Typical synovial fluid findings in the seronegative spondylarthropathies

Macroscopic and wet prep findings

Colour	:	Pale yellow
Clarity	:	Translucent
Mucin clot	:	Fair
Viscosity	:	Intermediate
Ragocytes (%)	:	25
Crystals	:	Nil
Particles	:	Small fibrin aggregates
Lipid	:	Nil

Cytocentrifuge preparation findings

Nucleated cells	:	6000/mm³
Polymorphs (%)	:	70
Lymphocytes (%)	:	20
Macrophages (%)	:	5
Synoviocytes (%)	:	5
CPM (%) (of LMN)	:	>5
Mast cells	:	Present, sometimes >2% of all cells; CPM and mast cells
Eosinophils	:	Few
Apoptotic cells	:	Present (number proportional to CPM)
Other cells	:	LE cells
Features indicating a poor prognosis	:	None known

Table 42.5 Typical synovial fluid findings in traumatic haemarthrosis

Macroscopic and wet prep findings

Colour	:	Haemorrhagic
Clarity	:	Opaque
Mucin clot	:	Nil
Viscosity	:	Low
Ragocytes (%)	:	Nil
Crystals	:	Nil
Particles	:	Fragments of normal cartilage; pieces of bone; fragments of meniscal fibrocartilage or ligament; in cases of penetrating trauma, debris
Lipid	:	Lipid droplets which may or may not contain lipid crystals

Cytocentrifuge preparation findings

Nucleated cells	:	2000/mm³
Polymorphs (%)	:	70 (mostly blood derived)
Lymphocytes (%)	:	10
Macrophages (%)	:	15
Synoviocytes (%)	:	5
CPM (%) (of LMN)	:	Nil
Mast cells	:	<1
Eosinophils	:	May be high if there have been previous episodes of haemorrhage
Apoptotic cells	:	Nil
Other cells	:	Nil
Features indicating a poor prognosis	:	Tissue fragments, particularly bone

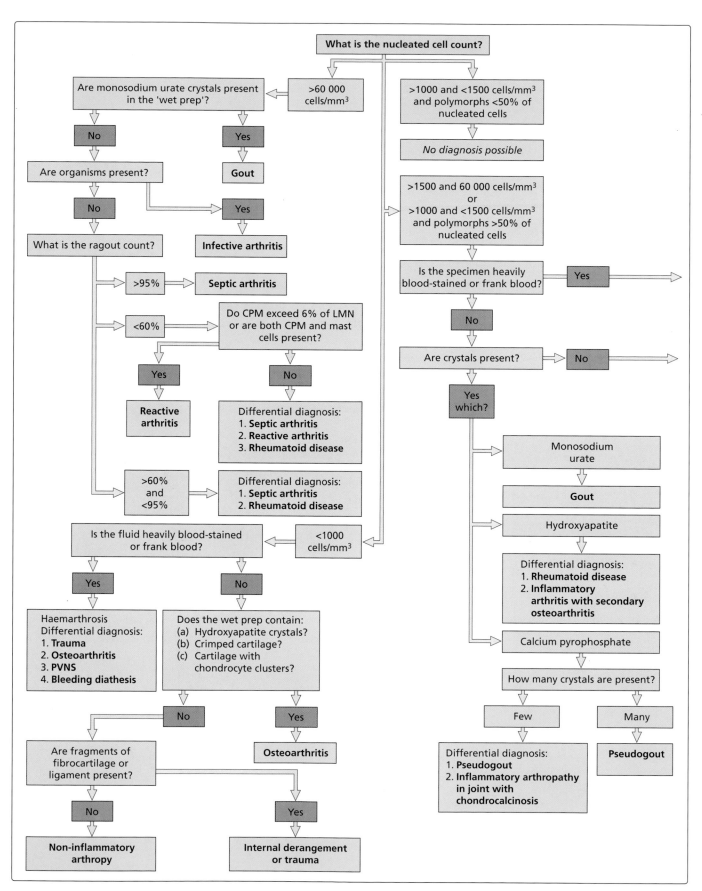

Fig. 42.8 (A) The diagnostic algorithm.

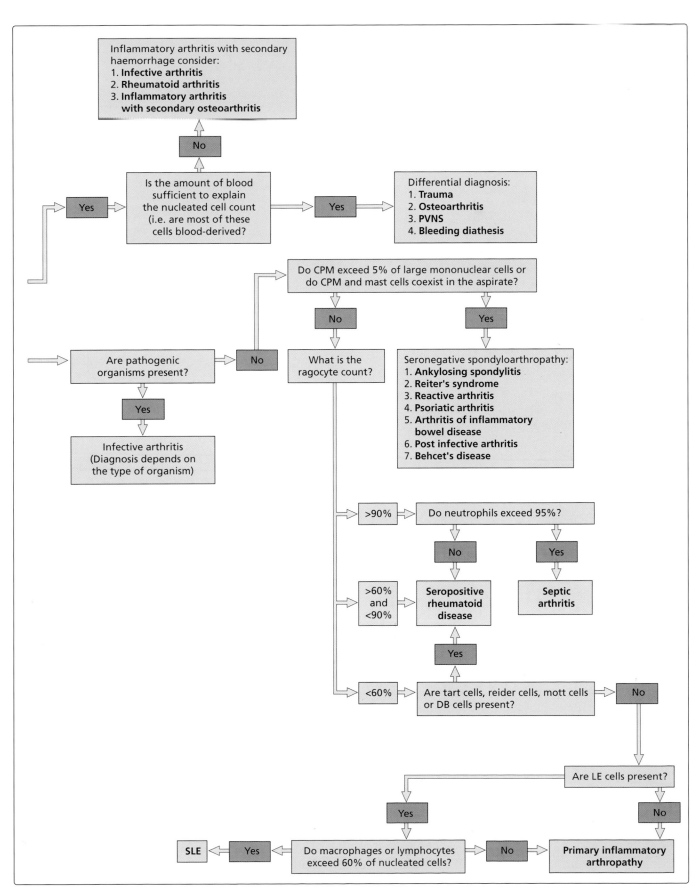

Fig. 42.8   (B) The diagnostic algorithm.

Table 42.6   Typical synovial fluid findings in septic arthritis

Macroscopic and wet prep findings

Colour	:	Brown, green or yellow
Clarity	:	Opaque
Mucin clot	:	Poor
Viscosity	:	Low
Ragocytes (%)	:	High, often >90%
Crystals	:	Nil
Particles	:	Fibrin aggregates; necrotic debris including cartilage
Lipid	:	Nil

Cytocentrifuge preparation findings

Nucleated cells	:	60 000/mm³
Polymorphs (%)	:	>95
Lymphocytes (%)	:	Nil
Macrophages (%)	:	<5
Synoviocytes (%)	:	Nil
CPM (%) (of LMN)	:	Nil
Mast cells	:	Nil
Eosinophils	:	Nil
Apoptotic cells	:	Nil
Other cells	:	Bacteria
Features indicating a poor prognosis	:	High nucleated cell count; necrotic tissue; tissue fragments

Table 42.8   Typical synovial fluid findings in gout

Macroscopic and wet prep findings

Colour	:	Pale yellow or white
Clarity	:	Opaque or opalescent
Mucin clot	:	Poor
Viscosity	:	Low
Ragocytes (%)	:	40
Crystals	:	Monosodium urate
Particles	:	Small aggregates of fibrin
Lipid	:	Nil

Cytocentrifuge preparation findings

Nucleated cells	:	20 000/mm³
Polymorphs (%)	:	>70
Lymphocytes (%)	:	Rare
Macrophages (%)	:	<20
Synoviocytes (%)	:	<10
CPM (%) (of LMN)	:	Sometimes >5
Mast cells	:	Present
Eosinophils	:	Nil
Apoptotic cells	:	Occasionally
Other cells	:	Plasma cells
Features indicating a poor prognosis	:	None known

Table 42.7   Typical synovial fluid findings in tuberculous arthritis

Macroscopic and wet prep findings

Colour	:	Pale yellow
Clarity	:	Opaque
Mucin clot	:	Fair
Viscosity	:	Low
Ragocytes (%)	:	<10
Crystals	:	Nil
Particles	:	Fibrin
Lipid	:	Nil

Cytocentrifuge preparation findings

Nucleated cells	:	15 000/mm³
Polymorphs (%)	:	30
Lymphocytes (%)	:	60
Macrophages (%)	:	10
Synoviocytes (%)	:	<1
CPM (%) (of LMN)	:	Nil
Mast cells	:	Nil
Eosinophils	:	Nil
Apoptotic cells	:	Nil
Other cells	:	Acid fast bacilli
Features indicating a poor prognosis	:	Necrotic tissue fragments

diagnostic algorithm[15,23]. This can be used to produce diagnostic and prognostic data of value in clinical practice and a practical version of value on a day-to-day basis is given in Figure 42.8.

The algorithm has been tested blind in several trials. In randomized anonymous trials conducted in ignorance of clinical data it proved possible to produce an accurate diagnosis in approximately 45% of cases[23]. In a further 25% a short differential diagnosis can be produced and in all but 4% of the remainder, it proves possible to say whether the patient has an inflammatory or non-inflammatory basis to their joint disease.

The overall diagnostic rate in synovial fluid cytoanalysis is therefore 96%, although it is true that in half of these the diagnosis is not precise. The false positive rate is almost zero and, as such, synovial fluid cytoanalysis represents the most selective and specific of all rheumatological and orthopaedic investigations. Even a relatively imprecise diagnosis may be of considerable clinical value to non-specialist physicians and general practitioners for whom referral policy to a specialist can be influenced by the inflammatory or non-inflammatory nature of the arthropathy in a given patient. For example, the specialist rheumatologist confronted with the problem of a red hot swollen joint in a patient believed to have 'burnt out' rheumatoid disease is interested in knowing whether this represents a recrudescence of the arthritis or an acute episode of osteoarthritis.

A short list of differential diagnoses may be equally important, particularly where further clinical information, unknown to the pathologist, is available to the clinician. For instance, the presence of mast cells and CPM is typical of ten or so disorders which together constitute the seronegative spondylarthropathies. However, to identify a patient as not having rheumatoid disease is both reassuring and also leads the clinician into a new line of investigation which could reveal hidden psoriatic plaques, evidence of inflammatory bowel disease or undiagnosed venereal infection.

The place of synovial fluid microscopy in diagnostic pathology

Histopathologists have very limited access to tissue from diseased joints. The articular surfaces are rarely biopsied except in end stage disease when they are removed, usually as part of joint replacement surgery. These specimens offer little of diagnostic value.

Synovium is not infrequently biopsied. Synovial biopsy is the investigation of choice in joint diseases with specific appearances, such as granulomatous inflammation and pigmented villonodular synovitis. However, most biopsies are performed for the diagnosis of one of the inflammatory or non-inflammatory arthropathies. Experienced histopathologists can have difficulty in distinguishing inflammatory from non-inflammatory arthropathies since the latter frequently have a moderate lymphocytic infiltrate in the synovium. Even if a distinction can be made it is usually impossible to be more specific because there are few microscopic differences between disorders in the same broad group.

Synovial fluid microscopy is therefore of greatest value in distinguishing inflammatory from non-inflammatory arthropathies and in defining specific disorders within these two groups. It is also important in the diagnosis of early inflammatory disease where it might be possible, on the basis of cytology, to identify a specific arthropathy before the clinical syndrome develops. In these cases accurate early diagnosis often allows the institution of specific therapy before irreversible joint damage has occurred. Finally, it permits the very rapid diagnosis of joint disease, particularly in disorders such as septic arthritis, where the prognosis is inversely related to delay in diagnosis.

Summary

The simple observations described above are based on conventionally stained and illuminated preparations. More specialized techniques are starting to be applied in the field of diagnostic synovial fluid cytoanalysis. It is to be hoped that when they are, synovial fluid microscopy may become even more selective.

By necessity this chapter has been unable to cover all aspects of synovial fluid microscopy, giving only a flavour of the important areas in the subject. For more detailed discussions, other texts are available[1,3,15,23–25].

References

1 Ropes M W, Bauer W. *Synovial Fluid Changes in Joint Diseases*. Cambridge, Massachusetts: Harvard University Press, 1953

2 Revell P A. The value of synovial fluid analysis. *Curr Topics Pathol* 1982; **71**: 1–24

3 Cohen A S, Brandt K D, Krey P R. In: Cohen A S ed. *Laboratory Diagnostic Procedures in the Rheumatic Diseases*, 2nd edn. Boston: Little, Brown, 1975

4 Currey H L F, Vernon-Roberts B. Examination of synovial fluid. *Clin Rheum Dis* 1976; **2**: 149–177

5 Wolf A W, Benson D R, Shiji H et al. Current concepts in synovial fluid analysis. *Clin Orthop* 1978; **134**: 261–265

6 Dieppe P A, Crocker P R, Corke C F et al. Synovial fluid crystals. *Quart J Med* 1979; **192**: 533–553

7 Dieppe P A, Calvert P. *Crystals and Joint Disease*. London: Chapman and Hall, 1983

8 Paul H, Reginato A J, Schumacher H R. Alizarin red-S staining as a screening test to detect calcium compounds in synovial fluid. *Arth Rheum* 1983; **26**: 191–200

9 Alwan W H, Dieppe P A, Elson C J, Bradfield J W B. Hydroxyapatite and urate crystal induced cytokine release by macrophages. *Ann Rheum Dis* 1989; **48**: 476–482

10 McCarty D J, Halverson P B, Carrera G F et al. Milwaukee shoulder: association of microspheroids containing hydroxyapatite crystals, active collagenase, and neutral protease with rotator cuff defects. II. Synovial fluid studies. *Arth Rheum* 1981; **24**: 474–483

11 Fremont A J. The role of cytological analysis of synovial fluid in diagnosis and research. *Ann Rheum Dis* 1991; **50**: 120–123

12 Riordan J W, Dieppe P A. Cholesterol crystals in shoulder synovial fluid. *Br J Rheumatol* 1987; **26**: 430–432

13 Fremont A J, Denton J. Synovial fluid findings early in traumatic arthritis. *J Rheumatol* 1988; **15**: 881–882

14 Kahn C B, Hollander J L, Schumacher H R. Corticosteroid crystals in synovial fluid. *JAMA* 1970; **211**: 807–809

15 Fremont A J, Denton J. *Atlas of Synovial Fluid Cytopathology*, vol. 18. Current histopathology. Dordrecht, Boston, London: Kluwer Academic Publishers, 1991

16 Kitridou R, Schumacher H R, Sparbaro J L, Hollander J L. Recurrent haemarthrosis after prosthetic knee arthroplasty: identification of metal particles in the synovial fluid. *Arth Rheum* 1969; **12**: 580–588

17 Rawson A J, Abelson N M, Hollander J L. Studies of the pathogenesis of rheumatoid joint inflammation. II. Intracytoplasmic particulate complexes in rheumatoid synovial fluids. *Ann Int Med* 1965; **62**: 281–284

18 Davies M J, Fremont A J. Synovial fluid cytology in rheumatoid arthritis. *Int Med for the Specialist* 1990; **11**: 121–128

19 Davies M J, Denton J, Fremont A J, Holt P J L. Comparison of serial synovial fluid cytology in rheumatoid arthritis; delineation of subgroups with prognostic implications. *Ann Rheum Dis* 1988; **47**: 559–562

20 Spriggs A I, Boddington M M, Mowat A G. Joint fluid in Reiter's disease. *Ann Rheum Dis* 1978; **37**: 557–560

21 Fremont A J, Denton J. The disease distribution of synovial fluid mast cells and cytophagocytic mononuclear cells in inflammatory arthritis. *Ann Rheum Dis* 1985; **44**: 312–315

22 Moll J M H, Haslock I, Wright V, eds. Seronegative spondarthritides. In *Copeman's Textbook of the Rheumatic Diseases*. Edinburgh: Churchill Livingstone, 1986

23 Fremont A J, Denton J, Chuck A et al. The diagnostic value of synovial fluid cytoanalysis; a reassessment. *Ann Rheum Dis* 1991; **50**: 101–107

24 Henderson B, Edwards J C W. *Synovial Lining in Health and Disease*. London: Chapman and Hall, 1987

25 Hasselbacher P. Variation in synovial fluid analysis by hospital laboratories. *Arth Rheum* 1987; **30**: 637–642

Central nervous system

43 Cerebrospinal fluid examination and direct brain preparations

Walter R. Timperley

General introduction

The cellular findings in cerebrospinal fluid were not studied until after the introduction of lumbar puncture in 1891 in Germany, where it was used as a technique for investigating cases in hydrocephalus[1]. Initially, the findings were of limited value, partly because the fluid was not concentrated by centrifugation, as it would be today, and also because the stains used did not enhance diagnostic features. Nevertheless different types of meningitis were recognized cytologically, and the lymphocytosis of neurosyphilis became a familiar finding.

Tumour cells in cerebrospinal fluid were first reported in 1904 and metastatic carcinoma cells were recognized increasingly from 1908[2]. The technique of making brain smears from cerebral tumours was developed in London by Leonard Dudgeon in the 1920s[3], but its practical use as a rapid diagnostic method for tumour diagnosis during craniotomy arose independently in Boston under Harvey Cushing in the 1930s. The procedure has been taken up by neuropathologists, often separated from mainstream exfoliative cytology, especially in Britain.

The principles of cytodiagnosis by brain smears and by examination of cerebrospinal fluid are those of cytopathology in general. This chapter covers the diagnostic applications of cytopathology in reactive, inflammatory and neoplastic disorders of the central nervous system as manifested in both of these approaches. Similar findings are obtained by fine needle aspiration of space-occupying lesions of the brain.

Anatomy of cerebrospinal fluid production and drainage

Anatomy and physiology

The cerebrospinal fluid (CSF) is enclosed in a compartment composed of the subarachnoid space and the system of ventricles within the brain. The arachnoid membrane forms the outer surface of the subarachnoid space and the pia mater, which covers and follows the surface contours of the brain and spinal cord, provides the inner surface. The outer aspect of the arachnoid membrane is separated from the dura mater lining the skull by a potential space known as the subdural space. Unlike pia mater, arachnoid mater does not extend into the sulci of the brain, thus resulting in the

formation of a continuous pathway between the two membranes, around which CSF is in constant circulation. The subarachnoid space widens in certain areas over the brain surface, forming cisterns, and extends through the foramen magnum at the base of the skull to surround the spinal cord. CSF may therefore reflect pathological processes occurring within the brain or spinal cord, or in the membranes themselves.

The spinal cord continues to the lower border of the first or upper border of the second lumbar vertebra in most cases, although it can extend as low as the upper border of the third lumbar vertebra. The arachnoid membrane, on the other hand, lines the dura mater as low as the mid-sacral vertebrae, creating a sac filled with CSF and containing the filum terminale. It is for this reason that lumbar puncture for the removal of CSF is usually carried out through the intervertebral disc space between L3 and L4. Occasionally it is removed via the cisternum magnum, or the ventricles via a burr-hole, and in infants via the fontanelle.

It is important to understand the nature of the cellular components of the various tissue layers between the skin and subarachnoid space in assessing potential contaminants that may appear in CSF samples. Squamous epithelial cells can also be introduced on to a slide from the hands of staff during slide preparation. The introduction of shunts communicating with other cavities such as the peritoneum, plasma or atrium may result in transfer of cells, including neoplastic cells, to other sites.

There is free communication of cerebrospinal fluid throughout the central nervous system via the foramina of Munro, connecting the lateral and third ventricles, the aqueduct of Sylvius, between the third and fourth ventricles, and the foramina of Magendie and Luschka which open between the fourth ventricle and the subarachnoid space.

Cerebrospinal fluid is produced mainly by the choroid plexuses, which are modified invaginations of ependyma protruding into the lumen of the lateral, third and fourth ventricles (Fig. 43.1). The luminal surface of these papillary structures is covered by specialized ependymal cells known as choroidal epithelial cells; these epithelial cells are separated from the pia layer by a highly vascular stroma.

Cerebrospinal fluid drains into the venous sinuses enclosed within the dura mater via the arachnoidal

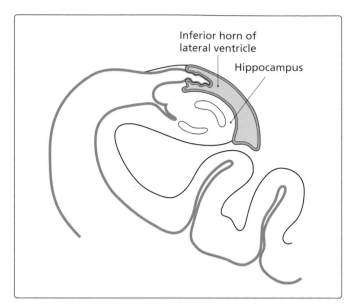

Fig. 43.1 Coronal section of temporal lobe showing choroid plexus protruding into lateral ventricle.

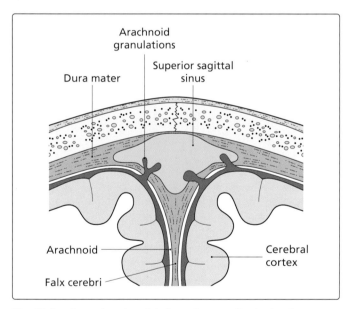

Fig. 43.2 Coronal section of skull, meninges and brain showing arachnoid granulations protruding into venous sinus.

granulations. These are derived from the arachnoidal membrane and protrude into the lumen of the sinuses, functioning as a valvular mechanism whereby CSF can pass into the blood but blood will not pass in the reverse direction (Fig. 43.2).

Indications for sampling of CSF

The main indications for sampling CSF are to investigate the possibility of infection, primary or metastatic neoplasia, leukaemia and lymphoma, and some non-neoplastic neurological problems such as haemorrhage, infarction, degenerative and demyelinating disorders. The types of cells present in CSF vary both with the disease process and

its duration. The cellular infiltrate in many cases is non-specific, but this may nevertheless be helpful in excluding neoplasia.

It is important to be aware of the relationship of the timing of the sampling to any previous surgery or invasive diagnostic and therapeutic procedure, such as a myelogram. Reactive cells can show confusing cytological abnormalities and when forming clusters they can be confused with epithelial cells. Foreign material can also be introduced during surgery and tissue fragments are sometimes seen after trauma, including epithelium from the nasal sinuses in basal skull fractures.

Most specimens of cerebrospinal fluid are derived by lumbar puncture and the amount of fluid is usually small. CSF may also be obtained by cisternal puncture, from shunt drainage, or directly from the ventricles either operatively via burr holes or by transfontanelle puncture in infants. It is essential that the pathologist is aware of relevant clinical details and that the specimen is received in the laboratory as quickly as possible and preferably no later than 30 minutes after removal.

Preparative technique

The most common methods of cell concentration in use today are cytocentrifugation and membrane filtration or a combination of both. The author's laboratory relies entirely on the cytocentrifuge technique, which results in excellent cell recovery and a wide range of stains can subsequently be used. Haematoxylin and eosin, Papanicolaou and Wright's or May-Grünwald-Giemsa stains are routinely employed. Cellular preservation is good, provided that the specimen is not centrifuged over 1000 rpm for 5 minutes and that the specimen is fresh. Individual cells vary considerably in their sensitivity to the speed of centrifugation, excessive speeds causing marked flattening, distortion and loss of cytological detail.

False negative results are common, but the chances of obtaining a positive result are increased when larger volumes of CSF are examined, with rapid processing and by taking the sample from a site of symptomatic or radiologically demonstrated disease. A positive result may be obtained from a repeat specimen if the initial result is negative[4]. Neuroimaging may establish or support the diagnosis in some cases, particularly when leptomeningeal, subependymal, dural, or cranial nerve enhancement; or superficial cerebral lesions are demonstrated. In the presence of typical clinical features neuroimaging abnormalities may be adequate to make the diagnosis of leptomeningeal involvement. This is particularly important in the case of medulloblastoma following radiotherapy, which may alter the cytological appearances of non-neoplastic cells.

The number of cells on the slide can be increased by using polylysine-coated (PLC) slides, but this only results in minor improvements in diagnostic sensitivity[5].

Fine needle aspiration samples can usually be spread directly on to slides and air-dried or wet-fixed. If large tissue fragments are included, a cell block method with histological processing is more appropriate. After expelling the aspirated material, the needle should be rinsed with tissue culture medium and prepared by cytocentrifugation. The specimen thus obtained is available for immunocytochemistry or other special stains.

Immunocytochemistry can be used for the identification of cell types (see Fig. 43.7). This is particularly helpful in identifying lymphoid cell types and in differentiating these from epithelial cells. Occasionally, marker studies are useful in detecting glial and neuroendocrine tumours and in identifying specific metastatic tumour cell types, such as melanoma or prostate, but great care should be taken in interpreting positive staining, particularly when the number of cells is small. Careful attention must be given to the method and duration of fixation and the dilution and reliability of antibodies. It is important that the pathologist knows in advance and that an adequate amount of CSF is provided. Fixation in acetone for 10 minutes is satisfactory for most antibodies, particularly monoclonal forms, but non-specific background staining can be a problem, particularly with polyclonal antibodies. In some cases, formalin fixation is preferable.

Cytological characteristics of normal CSF

Grossly, CSF is normally clear and colourless. The volume of specimen received must be documented as part of the report and a description should be given of the gross appearance, particularly whether blood-stained or xanthochromic.

Cytological findings

▶ No more than 5 cells/mm³
▶ A few lymphocytes, occasional monocytes and polymorphs
▶ Blood is frequently present from the sampling procedure
▶ Infrequently, cells from brain or membranes found
▶ Cells from surrounding tissues occasionally seen
▶ Extraneous contaminants may be present

A normal specimen should contain no more than 5 cells per mm³ or 10 per mm³ in neonates. Although cytological examination does not include an assessment of cell numbers, the pathologist will be familiar with the cellularity of concentrated specimens and will recognize when the number of cells is increased. A normal centrifuged deposit should show a few scattered lymphocytes, an occasional histiocyte of monocyte origin and one or two neutrophilic polymorphs.

Occasionally, isolated ependymal, arachnoidal (Fig. 43.3) or choroid plexus cells (Fig. 43.4) may be seen and fragments of tissue including squamous epithelium, connective tissue, muscle or intervertebral disc material may be introduced via the lumbar puncture needle. Starch particles from glove powder are easily recognized, particularly with polarized

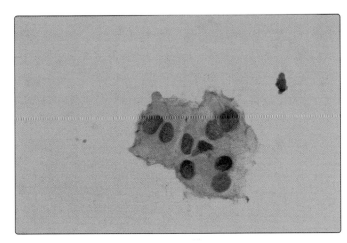

Fig. 43.3 CSF. Normal arachnoidal endothelial cells. The cells are cohesive and regular with well formed cytoplasm. (H&E × HP)

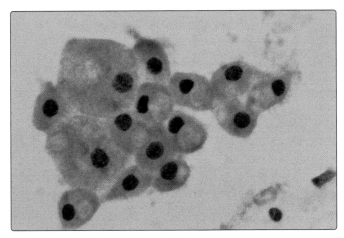

Fig. 43.4 CSF. Normal choroid plexus epithelial cells. A sheet of regular cells with small dark uniform nuclei. (H&E × HP)

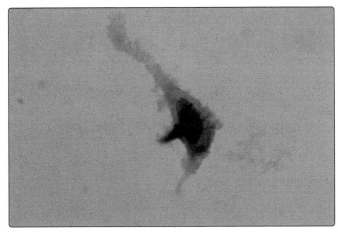

Fig. 43.5 CSF. Normal neurone following removal of CSF from lateral ventricle. Note the triangular shape, the large nucleus and prominent nucleolus. (H&E × HP)

light. During removal of ventricular fluid, fragments of meninges, grey and white matter (Figs 43.5, 43.6), ependyma or choroid plexus may be introduced. Preissig

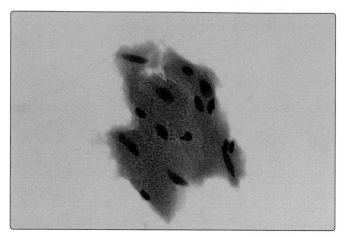

Fig. 43.6 CSF. Fragment of normal grey matter following ventricular puncture. The cells are irregularly spaced with granular cytoplasm and elongated nuclei. (H&E × HP)

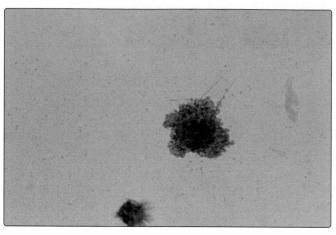

Fig. 43.7 CSF. Monocyte with bean-shaped nucleus and well developed cytoplasm showing positive reaction with CD14 antibody. (Immunoalkaline phosphatase × HP) (Courtesy of Dr D A Winfield, Sheffield, UK)

and Buhaug[6] emphasized the importance of not confusing corpora amylacea from the brain with yeasts.

CSF findings in inflammatory conditions

Many types of bacteria, fungi, viruses and parasites are capable of invading the central nervous system. This may result in infection of the meninges, causing meningitis, or direct infection of the brain parenchyma, producing encephalitis; a mixed pattern of infection can also occur. CSF may show changes in any of these conditions, but the findings are usually most intense in meningitis and are sometimes specific, providing a definitive diagnosis. If there is any possibility of infection, a specimen should be retained for culture and relevant special stains such as Gram or Ziehl-Neelsen stain.

The commonest route of infection is via the bloodstream, but direct implantation of organisms or spread from an adjacent focus of infection may occur. The peripheral nervous system also provides access for organisms to reach the central nervous system, a mechanism exploited by *Herpes simplex* virus, for example.

Different organisms are more likely to be encountered among different age groups. The meningococcus, *Neisseria meningitidis*, is commonest in adolescence, while the pneumococcus, *Streptococcus pneumoniae*, is seen at extremes of life. *Escherichia coli* is normally found only in neonates. Most bacteria cause acute pyogenic meningitis, in contrast to viral infections, which run a milder clinical course with some lymphocytosis. Tuberculous meningitis is also indolent, but the exudate is prone to undergo organization with serious complications if local structures are involved.

Cytological findings

▶ Neutrophil polymorphs present in most acute infections
▶ Mononuclear inflammatory cells supervene later
▶ Mild lymphocytosis is seen in viral infections

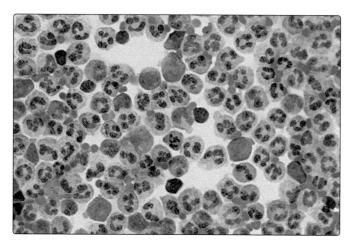

Fig. 43.8 CSF. Acute pyogenic meningitis. Reactive picture with numerous polymorphs. (Wright's × HP)

▶ Rarely, specific viral inclusions are detected
▶ Tuberculosis causes mixed inflammation with lymphocytes
▶ Eosinophils often present in parasitic infections but also appear in CSF after operative procedures involving the subarachnoid space

The cell population will vary depending on whether the inflammation is acute, subacute or chronic. Neutrophilic polymorphs are the most characteristic cell of acute inflammation and they are usually numerous (Fig. 43.8). They are the usual response to the commoner bacterial causes of meningitis. In the early stages of infection, however, there may be few and considerable experience is needed in assessing the proportion of red and white cells in a specimen contaminated with blood. As infection moves into the subacute phase, increasing numbers of histiocytes, plasma cells and lymphocytes appear (Fig. 43.9) and in the chronic stage lymphocytes predominate.

Various forms of lymphocyte may be present, including mature forms, reactive forms with prominent nucleoli and plasmacytoid cells (Fig. 43.10); mitotic figures may be seen

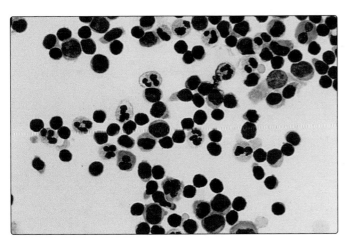

Fig. 43.9   CSF. Subacute inflammation due to tuberculous meningitis. The majority of cells are lymphocytes. (Romanowsky × HP)

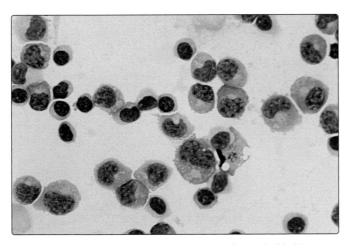

Fig. 43.10   CSF. Chronic inflammation in case of encephalitis. Numerous plasmacytoid and monocytoid cells are present and these show some variation in nuclear size and shape. Nucleoli may be prominent. (Wright's × HP)

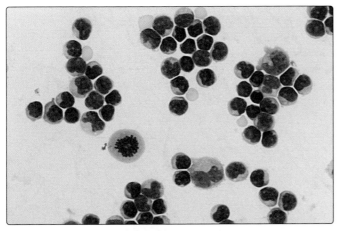

Fig. 43.11   CSF. Viral encephalitis. The cells are almost entirely lymphocytes, with a few histiocytes. Mitotic figures may be conspicuous. (Wright's × HP)

(Fig. 43.11). The cytological appearances may closely resemble those of malignant lymphocytes and mistakes are easily made; if in doubt it is best to assume a reactive cause until proved otherwise. Virus infections, tuberculosis and even multiple sclerosis, in particular, can produce a confusing picture.

Immunocytochemistry may be helpful in defining the lymphocyte types, but it is important to remember that reactive cells can also accompany lymphoma or leukaemia and that in a bloody tap leukaemic cells may be derived from the blood. A repeat specimen several days later may be advisable in these circumstances; a reactive picture will often subside whereas a neoplastic population should remain.

Immunodeficient patients are particularly vulnerable to infection and there is an increased incidence of neoplasia, including lymphoma. Infection is usually more severe and involves a wider variety of organisms including many that are not normally pathogenic or not often encountered in normal patients. Infections with fungi, such as Candida species or *Cryptococcus neoformans* are seen, as are viruses, such as *Cytomegalovirus* and *Herpes simplex,* although their characteristic inclusion bodies may not be found. *Toxoplasma gondii* is one of the protozoal infections to which these patients are susceptible.

The most common fungus found in the CSF is *Cryptococcus neoformans*; the organisms are easily missed. The yeasts vary in size up to about 15 μm in diameter and they are usually encapsulated and show evidence of budding (see Fig. 43.12A,B). The inflammatory response is not always marked and they may be difficult to find. There is often a striking histiocytic response and some of the yeasts may be intracellular. The organisms are PAS positive and the capsule stains with Alcian Blue. Indian ink preparations are particularly helpful (see Fig. 43.12C).

Very few parasites are detected within the CSF; however the presence of eosinophils should raise this possibility. Various forms of amoebae, including *Entamoeba histolytica, Naegleria fowleri,* and *Acanthamoeba culbertsoni* can produce meningitis and are detectable in the CSF[7]. The flagellated protozoan *Trypanosoma rhodesiense,* the causative agent of sleeping sickness, is readily identified in the CSF on Romanowsky stains. Other causes of eosinophilia in CSF include the presence of an intraventricular shunt.

Diagnostic pitfalls

Reactive histiocytes are easily confused with malignant cells (Fig. 43.13). Their nuclei may show considerable variation in shape and have prominent nucleoli and show some clumping of chromatin granules. Rarely, malignant histiocytes can appear in the CSF[8].

When assessing the cause of a reactive picture the possibility of invasive investigation procedures, spinal anaesthesia, cytotoxic therapy or irradiation should be considered. Both irradiation and cytotoxic drugs may

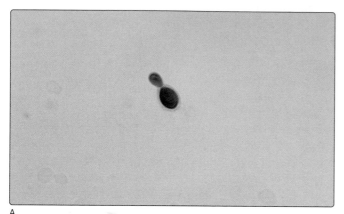

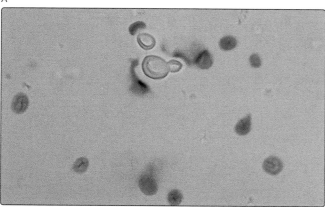

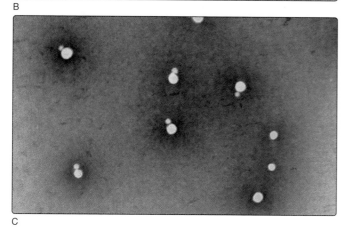

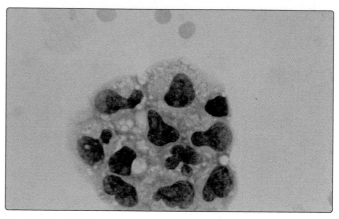

Fig. 43.13   CSF. Reactive histiocytes in tuberculous meningitis. These may clump together and are easily confused with malignant cells. The nuclei may have prominent nucleoli and show marked variation in shape. (Wright's × HP)

Fig. 43.12   CSF. (A) *Cryptococcus neoformans*. Yeast form showing evidence of budding. (PAS × HP) (B) The organisms are easily missed on routine stains. (H&E × HP) (C) Using an Indian ink method, the capsule of the organisms becomes very obvious. (Indian ink × MP) (A,B, Courtesy of Dr J C Broome, Stoke on Trent, UK. C, Courtesy of Dr D M Harris, Sheffield, UK)

produce marked cytological abnormalities that can easily be confused with neoplasia. Operative procedures and even a lumbar puncture can lead to the appearance of many eosinophils in CSF.

There is a tendency to underdiagnose infection in the early stages, particularly in the case of fungi and other unusual organisms. Familiarity with the clinical history is essential and this will also highlight the need for special stains and culture requirements. A reactive picture as seen postoperatively, following trauma or investigative

procedure, or in multiple sclerosis may suggest infection; it is better to alert the clinician to the possibility of infection and exclude it rather than take the risk of missing the diagnosis of a treatable infection.

CSF findings in neoplasia

Leukaemia

Between 1947–60 the incidence of meningeal complications in childhood leukaemia rose ten-fold[9] and in the early 1970s more than 50% of children with acute lymphoblastic leukaemia had evidence of CNS involvement[10]. Improved methods of treatment have resulted in longer survival and also in a greater chance of meningeal involvement. Clinical signs are not a reliable indication of CNS involvement. Most treatment protocols include CNS prophylactic therapy in both children and adults.

The increased incidence of neurological complications is seen in both acute lymphoblastic and nonlymphoblastic leukaemia. The most common method of spread is probably haematogenous leukaemic cells appearing first of all in the walls of arachnoidal veins from which they are released into the CSF and tissues. Infiltration may be so heavy so to result in hydrocephalus.

Staining a sample for naphthol-ASD chloroacetate esterase and myeloperoxidase may be useful in confirming the myeloid origin of neoplastic cells[11].

The CSF is rarely involved in chronic leukaemia. The cells in these cases are better differentiated and more regular in size and shape (Fig. 43.14). Leucocytosis in the CSF of patients with either chronic myeloid or chronic lymphatic leukaemia is more likely to be due to infection than to leukaemic infiltration.

Cytological findings

▶ Increased numbers of leucocytes of immature blast type
▶ Cell types are best recognized on Romanowsky stains

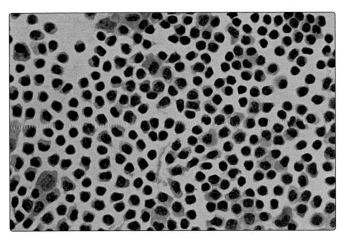

Fig. 43.14 CSF. Chronic lymphocytic leukaemia showing a monotonous pattern of well-differentiated lymphocytes. (H&E × HP)

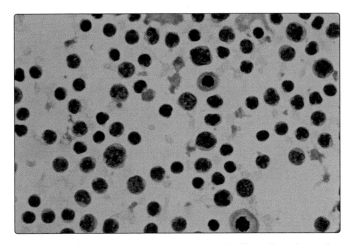

Fig. 43.15 CSF. Acute lymphoblastic leukaemia. The cells are larger than normal lymphocytes and have a higher nuclear/cytoplasmic ratio. Nuclei show some variation in size and shape and usually have visible nucleoli. Mitotic figures are seen at the centre and lower border of the field. (Wright's × HP)

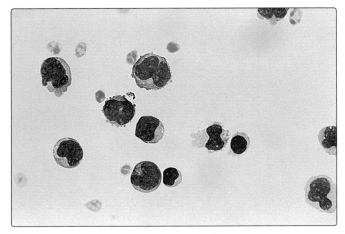

Fig. 43.16 CSF. Acute myeloid leukaemia. The cells vary in size and shape and have a high nuclear/cytoplasmic ratio. They may resemble lymphoblasts or blast cells of the myelomonocytic series. Cytoplasmic granules may be present in some cells. (Wright's × HP)

▶ Immunocytochemistry can establish monoclonality
▶ Contamination by blood may require a repeat sample
▶ Chronic leukaemic patients are more prone to infection than to leukaemic involvement of CNS

Patients receiving prophylactic therapy usually have periodic examination of the CSF. Differentiating leukaemic blast cells from normal and reactive cells requires considerable experience, especially if the cells are in small numbers. Both the cells and their nuclei are larger than those of normal lymphocytes and they have one or more prominent nucleoli (Fig. 43.15). Nuclei may be round, oval or irregular in shape and they are surrounded by variable amounts of cytoplasm. Mitotic figures are usually seen. It is important to emphasize that it is sufficient to establish whether or not blast cells are present. Immunocytochemistry may be helpful in establishing monoclonality of the abnormal cell population.

The differentiation of acute lymphocytic from acute non-lymphocytic leukaemia may be difficult, particularly on Papanicolaou stains. Leukaemic myeloblasts (Fig. 43.16) and monocytic blasts can usually be recognized in Romanowsky stained material. It is important to remember that blast cells can be introduced into the CSF by blood contamination; if in doubt the investigation should be repeated in several weeks.

Lymphoma

Neurological complications in lymphoma may be a result of compression, direct invasion, or as a result of 'remote' effects such as encephalomyelopathy, neuropathy, cerebellar degeneration, polymyositis or progressive multifocal leukoencephalopathy. There is also an increased incidence of infections such as meningitis and herpes zoster. The nervous system may also be affected by cytotoxic therapy and irradiation, and haemorrhage may complicate thrombocytopenia. Although spinal cord compression from extradural deposits is the commonest neurological complication of Hodgkin's disease, involvement of the CSF is rare in this condition. Non-Hodgkin's lymphoma involves the nervous system in approximately 5% of cases, with evidence of leptomeningeal infiltration in 3.7%[12].

Cytological examination of CSF often results in a failure to diagnose lymphomatous meningitis in patients who actually have the disease. The development of polymerase chain reaction techniques for the diagnosis of lymphoma based on the detection of clonal rearrangements of the immunoglobulin or T-cell receptor genes offers an alternative, DNA-based test for the diagnosis of lymphoma in the CSF. It sometimes provides the diagnosis when conventional cytology fails[13].

Cytological findings

▶ An excess of lymphoid cells, all dissociated
▶ Usually high-grade lymphoma with large tumour cells

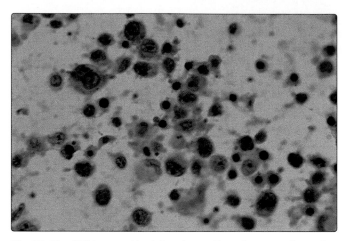

Fig. 43.17 CSF. Immunoblastic lymphoma. The cells are usually smaller than carcinoma cells and have a higher nuclear/cytoplasmic ratio. Nucleoli are prominent and may be multiple. Cell degeneration is a prominent feature. (H&E × HP)

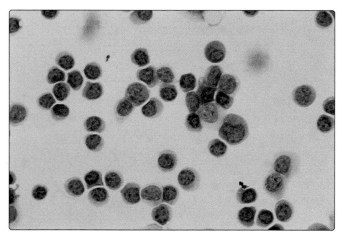

Fig. 43.18 CSF. Oat cell carcinoma. The cells have a high nuclear/cytoplasmic ratio with evenly dispersed chromatin. Some nuclei are irregular in outline. Nucleoli are not prominent. (H&E × HP)

▶ Immunocytochemical markers are helpful
▶ Infections and therapeutic complications occur

The majority of cases are poorly differentiated, or histiocytic in type. The picture can be particularly difficult to interpret (Fig. 43.17) in view of the fact that many reactive cell forms may be present and cells and their nuclei may show considerable variation in size. Larger cells may be difficult to differentiate from carcinoma cells, particularly oat cell carcinoma. Both lymphoma and carcinoma cell nuclei may contain one or more nucleoli, although in oat cell carcinoma nucleoli are inconspicuous (Fig. 43.18). Immunocytochemical markers for lymphocyte subsets and epithelial cells may be helpful. Most lymphomas are B cell in type, although T cell forms do occur; neoplastic B cells are usually monoclonal[14]. The picture is particularly difficult to assess when there is a mixture of reactive and neoplastic cells, but kappa or

lambda light chain restriction on immunocytochemical staining may be convincing.

Metastases

Many types of tumour metastasize to the nervous system and release cells into the CSF. The most common are carcinomas and melanomas, and Russell and Rubinstein[15] state that 20–40% of intracranial tumours are metastatic. The most common primary sites are lung, breast and stomach[16,17].

Evidence of meningeal involvement may be the presenting feature, particularly in the case of tumours that metastasize early, such as small cell carcinoma of the lung, adenocarcinoma of the stomach or pancreas and, in those parts of the world where it is common, choriocarcinoma[18].

Cytological findings

▶ Variable cellularity, highest in meningeal carcinomatosis
▶ Cells dispersed and in clusters
▶ Characteristic features of tumour type may be seen: oat cells – nuclear moulding; adenocarcinoma cells – mucin production; melanoma cells – rarely pigmented but have large nucleoli
▶ Immunocytochemistry is often helpful (Fig. 43.19)

The number of cells present is very variable, the largest numbers being seen in meningeal carcinomatosis. Cells may appear individually or in small groups (Figs 43.20 A,B,C); the latter is particularly useful in distinguishing undifferentiated carcinoma from lymphoma, in which the cells do not cluster. There is a tendency for cells to round up in CSF so that the cells from different types of neoplasm more closely resemble one another. The nuclei of oat cell carcinoma cells also show a marked tendency for moulding and they have inconspicuous nucleoli.

In many cases it may not be possible to determine the cell type; clinical data and the results of other investigations, particularly radiological, will usually suggest a likely origin. It is often impossible on cytological observations alone to identify the type of a primitive neuroectodermal tumour, or

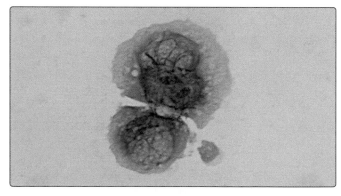

Fig. 43.19 CSF. Metastatic carcinoma cells showing positive reaction for cytokeratin, CKKI. (Immunoperoxidase × HP)

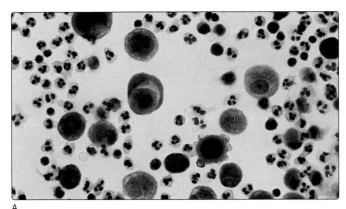

A

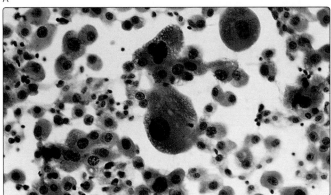

B

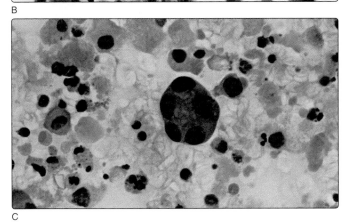

C

Fig. 43.20 CSF. (A) Malignant epithelial cells. The cells do not necessarily cluster. Nuclei are often eccentrically situated and may show marked irregularity in shape and outline. (Papanicolaou × HP) (B) Malignant epithelial cells from breast carcinoma. (H&E × HP) (C) Malignant epithelial cells from metastatic bronchial carcinoma. The cells form small clusters. Note the inflammatory and necrotic debris in the background. (H&E × HP)

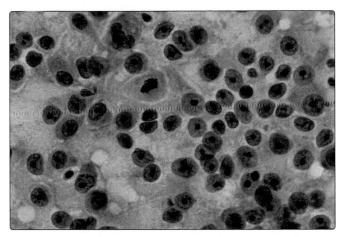

Fig. 43.21 CSF. Malignant melanoma. Macronucleoli strongly suggest melanoma. Note the absence of pigment. (H&E × HP)

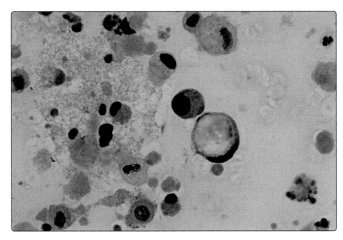

Fig. 43.22 CSF. Malignant epithelial cells from an adenocarcinoma of lung. The cells have eccentric nuclei and the cytoplasm contains vacuoles. (H&E × HP)

blast cell tumour of either CNS or systemic origin. The presence of clusters or rosettes is helpful, but these are frequently not seen.

Large undifferentiated neoplastic cells usually have an obvious abnormal chromatin pattern and prominent nucleoli. Melanoma cells may or may not contain pigment, but the presence of macronucleoli is highly suggestive (Fig. 43.21).

Cells from adenocarcinoma may also appear individually or in small groups. The nuclei are often eccentric and have malignant criteria, including irregularity of outline and

marked clumping of chromatin. The cytoplasm frequently contains vacuoles (Fig. 43.22), but they do not always contain mucin; special stains will be required to confirm that. It is not usually possible to determine the site of origin of the cells although lung is the most frequent primary site.

There is no reliable method of distinguishing carcinoma of the breast from other carcinomas (Fig. 43.23). Cells from lobular carcinoma are smaller than those of ductal origin, but the formation of morulae and chains of cells is unusual in the CSF.

A panel of immunocytochemical markers is helpful in distinguishing between metastatic carcinoma, lymphoma and primary CNS tumour when malignant cells are identified in CSF. Antibodies to cytokeratin for carcinoma cells (see Fig. 43.19), leucocyte common antigen for lymphoid cells and glial fibrillary acidic protein for tumour cells of glial origin are invaluable in this situation.

The diagnosis of metastatic melanoma can be confirmed using the melanoma specific antigen (HMB 45 or NK1C3) and the characteristic macronucleoli of the tumour cells add

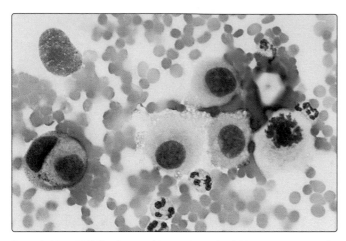

Fig. 43.23 CSF. Carcinoma of breast. Large individual tumour cells with a cell-in-cell arrangement on the left. (Romanowsky × HP)

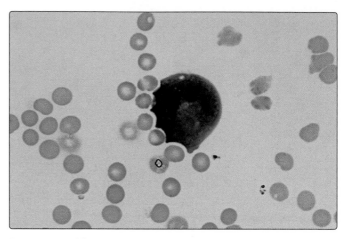

Fig. 43.24 CSF. Poorly-differentiated multinucleated glial cell from a malignant glioma showing no evidence of fibre formation and closely resembling an epithelial cell. (H&E × HP)

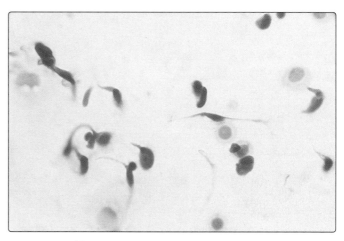

Fig. 43.25 CSF. Poorly-differentiated astrocytoma. Some of these spindle cells show evidence of fibre formation. (H&E × HP)

support to the diagnosis. Carcinoembryonic antigen is positive in some carcinoma cells but does not indicate the exact site of origin of the tumour. Where appropriate, prostate specific antigen can be used to identify cells of prostatic origin. Oat cells react with UJ13A, the neural cell adhesion molecule marker, but it is important to remember that primary neural tumours also react with this antibody. Cell morphology is important in assessing the significance of immunocytochemical stains.

Primary CNS tumours

The classification and main cytological features of these tumours are described in the section on interpretation of brain smears and fine needle aspiration samples. Primary tumours of the central nervous system commonly shed cells into cerebrospinal fluid which are recognizably malignant, but it is usually not possible to categorize the tumour type without clinical and histological correlation.

The figures vary for different neoplasms and their grade, and with the anatomical site, those occurring near the surface shedding cells more readily into either the subarachnoid space or the ventricles. There is a greater tendency for high-grade malignant neoplasms to shed cells than the more benign variants. Well-differentiated gliomas, for instance, rarely exfoliate cells into the CSF and it is extremely difficult to differentiate these from reactive astrocytes. Poorly-differentiated gliomas, on the other hand, shed cells more readily; Balhuizen *et al.*[19] quote a preoperative incidence of 13.9% for all gliomas and the percentage increases postoperatively. The author's own experience suggests a much lower incidence than this. The presence of these cells rarely creates clinical problems. In the case of medulloblastoma, on the other hand, Balhuizen *et al.* quote an incidence of 91% preoperatively, and prophylactic craniospinal irradiation is required to prevent dissemination. As with gliomas, the author's experience suggests a much lower incidence of medulloblastoma cells

in CSF. Periodic examination of the CSF is required to assess recurrence.

Cytological findings

▶ Poorly-differentiated tumours are more prone to exfoliate
▶ Glial tumour cells usually single and rounded with loss of cytoplasmic processes
▶ Glial cells difficult to distinguish from blast cells but immunocytochemistry is helpful
▶ Germ cell tumours resemble seminoma cells
▶ Choroid plexus tumours exfoliate cells readily but the cells may not be neoplastic, e.g. in hydrocephalus

It is often difficult to determine the nature of poorly-differentiated tumour cells and blast cells. Poorly-differentiated glial cells show a tendency to lose their processes and closely resemble epithelial cells (Fig. 43.24), but there may be some evidence of fibre formation (Fig. 43.25). There is also a marked tendency for the cells to

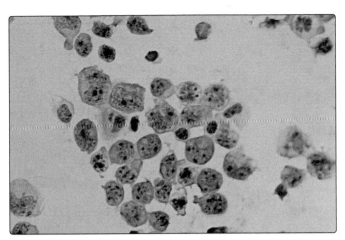

Fig. 43.26 CSF. Germ cell tumour cells. These malignant cells have fragile cytoplasm and irregular nuclear contours with prominent nucleoli. Typically, a few lymphocytes are also present. (H&E × HP)

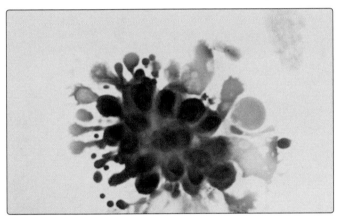

Fig. 43.27 CSF. Choroid plexus papilloma. Tumours situated near the surface readily shed cells into the CSF. (H&E × HP)

Table 43.1 Characteristic features of main abnormal cell types in CSF

Reactive pleocytosis
Atypical forms consistent with immunoblasts may be present, closely resembling leukaemic blast cells. Nuclei have smoother outlines than neoplastic cells and there is usually more cytoplasm. Mitoses may be present.

Acute leukaemia
Cells are larger and blast cell in type. Chromatin is paler. Nuclear outlines more irregular. Nucleoli may be present. Mitotic figures often plentiful.

Chronic leukaemia
Cells are smaller than those of acute leukaemia, but more variation is evident. Nucleoli are not prominent. Mitotic figures are scanty or absent. Usually monoclonal. Granulocytic precursors present when relevant.

Primitive neuroectodermal
Cells may form clusters. When present, rosettes are virtually diagnostic. Clinical history may be the only indicator.

Lymphoma
Cell type varies with degree of differentiation and nature of lymphoma. Mitoses are often plentiful. Nucleoli are usually prominent and may be multiple. Predominantly monoclonal, but beware reactive component.

Carcinoma
Cells are usually larger but some (e.g. oat cell and melanoma) may be small. Nucleoli are inconspicuous in oat cell; very much larger in melanoma. Lymphocyte markers negative. Adenocarcinoma cells are usually large and may be vacuolated. Mitoses usually present.

appear singly and the cell outlines are indistinct compared with those of metastatic carcinoma cells[20]. The cells are larger than lymphocytes and show variation in size, shape and staining properties of nuclei, but usually have poorly defined nucleoli. On cytological criteria alone it is often impossible to differentiate between blast cells of different types, including leukaemia, lymphoma, pineoblastoma and other tumours of neural crest origin. Immunocytochemistry may be helpful if sufficient sample is available as glial tumours usually react with glial fibrillary acidic protein.

Germ cell tumours sometimes shed cells into the CSF. These are indistinguishable from testicular seminoma (Fig. 43.26) and ovarian dysgerminoma; they are composed of a mixture of large spheroidal cells with vesicular nuclei and prominent nucleoli, together with lymphocytes. A variety of cell types may be found in immature teratoma[21].

Tumours of choroid plexus frequently shed groups of cells into the CSF (Fig. 43.27). It is important to realize, however, that these are not always neoplastic and it may be impossible to determine the nature of the cells on cytological criteria alone. There is an increased tendency for ependymal and choroid plexus cells to be found in the CSF in hydrocephalus. Malignant tumours of the choroid plexus usually occur in adults and these can easily be confused with adenocarcinoma.

Table 43.1 summarizes the main differences between reactive and neoplastic cells found in cerebrospinal fluid.

Miscellaneous conditions affecting CSF
Haemorrhage

The cytological picture shows similar features irrespective of the cause of the haemorrhage. In the early stages red cells are intact, but later there will be evidence of erythrophagocytosis, and macrophages containing haemosiderin pigment are seen.

The most common cause of blood in the specimen is puncture of a vessel during specimen collection. Occasionally, pathological cell types are present that will establish the cause of the haemorrhage.

Staining a specimen for iron using Perl's reagent is useful in detecting evidence of subarachnoid haemorrhage up to 15–17 weeks later. Iron-positive cells appear at 1 week, increase up to 4–6 weeks and decrease up to 15–17 weeks[22].

Infarction

The likelihood of CSF changes in the presence of cerebral infarction depends upon the extent and site of the infarct, those near the surface of the brain and extensive being more prone to evoke a reaction in the overlying meninges. In the early stages of an infarct, polymorphonuclear leucocytes are present followed by macrophages, often containing phagocytosed material. Haemorrhagic infarcts may also release blood into the CSF.

Degenerative and demyelinating diseases

Changes in the CSF in these conditions are variable, depending mainly on disease activity at the time of investigation, and CSF may even be normal on routine cytology in phases of complete remission. At other times there is a mild increase in cellularity. The cell population is non-specific and reactive in type, usually consisting of lymphocytes and histiocytes.

Histiocytic disorders

Morphologically atypical histiocytes may be found in the cerebrospinal fluid of patients with histiocytic proliferative disorders, including Letterer-Siwe disease, Hand-Schüller-Christian disease and malignant histiocytosis[23].

Diagnostic procedures in Whipple's disease usually focus on the intestine, but symptomatic involvement of the nervous system is a major threat. A high incidence of positive results (80% in patients with neurological symptoms and 70% in those without neurological symptoms) was reported by von Herbay et al.[24].

Diagnostic accuracy of CSF cytology

In general, the accuracy of tumour diagnosis from CSF examination relates directly to the extent of involvement of the leptomeninges by the disease process and is highest when frank meningeal carcinomatosis is present. There are considerable differences in success rates in different laboratories. Balhuizen et al.[19] reported a positive preoperative success rate of 15.3% of all cases of primary cerebral malignancies (13.9% of all gliomas) and in 40% of postoperative CSF samples (91% of the medulloblastomas). In all cases of single or multiple secondary cerebral tumours, positive preoperative CSF samples were found in 20%. Gondos and King[25] reported an overall detection rate of 32.2% for primary tumours and 53.3% for metastatic tumours, those occurring in lung (70%) and breast (83%) being the most frequently detected. A correct diagnosis has been recorded in two-thirds of cases with widespread meningeal infiltration by Glass et al. and false positive reports were only given in 2.6% of 117 patients coming to autopsy[26]. Diagnostic accuracy is enhanced if multiple examinations of CSF are made[27].

Lymphoma and leukaemia have been found to have a higher rate of false positive reporting than other tumours, especially chronic lymphatic leukaemia, which is easily misdiagnosed in patients known to have leukaemia and who develop viral or fungal infections with reactive lymphocytosis[28]. This problem can be overcome by the use of immunocytochemistry to identify a clonal proliferation in patients with neoplasia.

Other diagnostic problems concern the recognition of extraneous cells in CSF, either from the lumbar puncture procedure as already described, or from laboratory handling. However in experienced hands examination of CSF by cytological methods has proved to be a reliable source of readily obtainable diagnostic information.

The role of cytopathology in direct preparations of CNS origin

Although fine needle aspiration (FNA) of supratentorial space-occupying lesions of brain is undertaken with increasing frequency in some centres, direct smears of brain tumours as an intraoperative procedure is still the chief source of cytological material from the central nervous system. The experience described here is derived mainly from brain smear samples but the findings are similar in FNA specimens. Smears can be completed within a few minutes with simple equipment and facilities near to the operating theatres, allowing closer communication with relevant staff. Some form of extraction cabinet is essential.

Inflammatory lesions, such as cerebral abscess or granuloma and localized infarcts or foci of gliosis are sometimes the target for FNA and may occasionally be submitted for brain smear if presenting as a tumour clinically. Recognition of normal and reactive changes in brain is therefore necessary.

The main aim in interpretation of smears from the brain is to determine tumour cell type and to assess the rate of growth if possible. Since there may be considerable variation in the degree of differentiation within a tumour it may not always be possible to achieve the latter on a small biopsy. It is usually sufficient to classify the cell type within broad groups and ignore the subclassification. A useful classification of tumours is given in Table 43.2[29].

Rapid diagnosis is particularly important in neurosurgery. Most biopsy specimens from the CNS smear easily and this provides a useful method of determining the nature of a space-occupying lesion. The quality of cytological detail is usually excellent and better than in either frozen or paraffin-embedded sections. Even if a complete diagnosis cannot be made at the time of the operation, it is useful for the surgeon to know whether or not the relevant tissue has been sampled, avoiding the need for a second anaesthetic and invasive procedure. Many tumours of the nervous system will not be surgically removed, but accurate classification of the lesion is nevertheless essential in planning other forms of therapy, such as radiotherapy or chemotherapy.

Occasionally a sample is too tough to smear and the pathologist will need to resort to frozen section; this takes longer to complete, but is particularly useful in defining patterns, the type of lining of a cyst, lesions containing fat, and complex lesions, such as vascular malformations. It is usually apparent which approach is likely to be required at the time that the specimen is received. Occasionally a

Table 43.2   Classification of CNS tumours

A.   *Gliomas*
       Mainly astrocytic: fibrillary, protoplasmic, gemistocytic,
           pilocytic, anaplastic, glioblastoma multiforme (may contain
           a sarcoma-like component), astroblastoma, subependymal
           giant cell astrocytoma, pleomorphic xanthoastrocytoma
       Mainly oligodendroglial
       Ependymoma and subependymoma
B.   *Choroid plexus tumours*
       Papilloma
       Carcinoma
C.   *Primitive neuroectodermal tumours (PNET) and other*
           embryonic tumours
       Medulloblastoma, neuroblastoma, ependymoblastoma,
           pineoblastoma, spongioblastoma
D.   *Tumours containing neurones*
       Gangliocytoma, ganglioglioma, ganglioneuroma,
           desmoplastic infantile ganglioglioma, neuroblastoma,
           dysembryoplastic neuroepithelial tumour, central
           neurocytoma, olfactory neuroblastoma
E.   *Meningioma*
       Meningothelial, transitional, fibroblastic, psammomatous,
           angiomatous are the main types
       Atypical and malignant
       Haemangiopericytoma occurs in the meninges but has now
           been separated from the main group of meningiomas.
F.   *Nerve sheath tumours*
       Schwannoma, neurofibroma
G.   *Haemangioblastoma*
H.   *Pituitary adenoma*
I.   *Craniopharyngioma*
J.   *Dermoid and epidermoid cysts*
K.   *Lymphoma and plasma cell neoplasms*
L.   *Pineal and parapineal tumours*
       Germinoma, teratoma, pineal parenchymal tumours
M.   *Tumours invading the nervous system from a local source*
N.   *Metastatic tumours*

specimen is too tough to smear and too small for frozen section and/or paraffin embedded sections. This is particularly important in the case of spinal lesions causing pressure upon the spinal cord, when early diagnosis is essential for rapid clinical management. In these circumstances a rapid paraffin processing procedure may be useful, but it is important to realize that the quality of the result may not be as good as that of a longer procedure and that this may occasionally decrease diagnostic potential. Many of these cases, such as lymphomas may require complex immunohistochemical techniques for accurate classification and grading, but a diagnosis of lymphoma may be sufficient to enable rapid radiotherapy in order to decrease the mass effect.

It is essential when reporting a smear that the pathologist is familiar with the clinical and radiological details of the case. Knowledge of the age, sex, location and radiological appearance of the lesion will considerably reduce the differential diagnosis. It is also important that the pathologist is familiar with the normal appearance of smears from different anatomical sites and with the different pathological processes that affect those sites.

Small granular neurones from the cerebellum, for example, are easily misinterpreted as 'blast cells' and choroid plexus can superficially resemble adenocarcinoma.

The smear technique has been used for many years. Eisenhardt and Cushing[30] reported their experience using a supravital technique in 1930, but this had the disadvantage that the preparations were not permanent. Russell et al.[31] described the wet film technique that has formed the basis of current practice. The two main advantages of the smear technique are that a diagnosis can be made on a very small sample and there is excellent preservation of cytological detail. The wider use of fine needle aspiration biopsy through a burr-hole, rather than craniotomy, and the move towards thinner gauge needles with stereotactic localization has greatly reduced patient morbidity and mortality, but has also resulted in the removal of yet smaller amounts of tissue for diagnosis. This can create additional problems for the pathologist in that it becomes more difficult to assess patterns and to assess the grade of a neoplasm. The accuracy of the biopsy site becomes increasingly important if misleading information is to be avoided. The latter is particularly relevant if the neoplasm has areas of necrosis or varied radiological appearances.

Diagnostic accuracy

The smear technique provides a high degree of accuracy in experienced hands. Liwnic et al.[32] found that cytology agreed with histological assessment in 92% of their cases and this appears to be fairly representative. Marshall et al.[33] and Berkeley et al.[34] reported the results of a retrospective analysis of material in the Department of Neuropathology in Glasgow; a correct diagnosis was attained in 93.6% and in 4.6% the error was a failure to classify malignant tumour correctly and had no effect on the immediate management of the patient. It is important to emphasize, however, that unless absolutely necessary (e.g. in the case of infection) specific therapy should not be given before the diagnosis is confirmed.

Technical methods

For urgent diagnosis the pathologist has a choice of either frozen sections or smears, or a combination of these. To a certain extent, technique will be determined by the toughness and size of the specimen: some specimens are too tough to smear, although helpful and sometimes diagnostic information can often be obtained from such preparations. Frozen sections are particularly useful in assessing the architectural features of a lesion, although there is significant loss of cytological detail.

Some tissues smear more readily than others, so there is usually some variation in thickness of the smear and in the quality of fixation and staining. Interpretation involves assessment of both architectural pattern and cytological features and different parts of the preparation provide information of these two components. Architectural pattern is usually better preserved in the thicker areas and cytological detail in those areas where the cells have spread out more thinly.

Tissue sent for a smear diagnosis should not be allowed to dry out and should be placed in a closed container containing moistened gauze: the authors use a Coplin jar. Laboratory staff must be aware of the health and safety aspects of the smear technique and take appropriate precautions, including the routine use of a ventilated safety cabinet and disposable rubber gloves. The incidence of human immunodeficiency virus (HIV) will vary from laboratory to laboratory: where this risk is significant, all cases should be handled on the assumption that they are positive. Patients suffering from AIDS develop a wide variety of lesions in the CNS, including a diffuse encephalopathy, lymphoma and lesions caused by a variety of different pathogens. All biopsies from cases of dementia must be regarded as Creutzfeldt-Jacob disease until proved otherwise and instruments that are used, dealt with appropriately afterwards. Other potential dangers include tuberculosis, hepatitis, agents causing various forms of encephalitis, and agents that have so far not been identified.

Macroscopical appearances are important and will provide valuable information on the most likely part of the biopsy to contain diagnostic material. Even normal-looking tissue can, however, contain pathological abnormalities and the neurosurgeon should not take further samples until each smear has been assessed. Occasionally, paraffin embedded sections will show no further pathological tissue; the pathologist will then have to rely on the smear for diagnosis.

Sometimes there is a dilemma as to whether a tiny specimen should be smeared or retained for paraffin embedded sections and this may result in the whole of the specimen being used in the preparation of smears. These may be inconclusive and Smith and Laing[35] have described a technique whereby the original smear stained by haematoxylin and eosin can be re-used for an immunohistochemical stain. The glial fibrillary acid protein (GFAP) immunocytochemical stain may be particularly useful in confirming a glial origin.

The smear technique

Samples of tissue approximately 2 mm in diameter are placed at one end of a clean glass slide and smeared by pressing a second slide on top and sliding this towards the opposite end of the slide. Slides should always be handled at the same end in order to avoid contamination. If possible, several smears should be made from different parts of the specimen. Excessive pressure will produce crush artefact and may make interpretation impossible. The smear should be even but generally will decrease in thickness gradually from the area of the original specimen to the tail of the smear.

A variety of staining techniques may be used. We use a rapid haematoxylin and eosin (H&E) technique; some

pathologists prefer 1% aqueous Toluidine Blue for one to two minutes or methylene blue for 30 seconds, and a few use the Papanicolaou stain. Some pathologists use a combination of techniques together; the toluidine and methylene blue techniques are quicker than the H&E and can provide a little extra time for assessment. It is important that the same technique is used repeatedly by each pathologist. The following accelerated haematoxylin and eosin method is recommended:

► 1–2 mm pieces of tissue are smeared between glass slides using sufficient pressure to spread the tissue out. Excessive force will lead to disruption of the cells
► Slides are immersed in acetic alcohol fixative for 1 minute (95% alcohol and 5% glacial acetic acid)
► Slides are then rinsed in tap water and stained by rapid haematoxylin and eosin method:

a. Stain in Carazzi's haematoxylin — 1 min
b. Wash in tap water
c. Differentiate briefly in 1% acid alcohol — approximately 5×1 s dips
d. Wash in tap water
e. Blue in Scott's tap water — 30 s
f. Wash in tap water
g. Stain in 1% aqueous eosin — 1 min
h. Wash in tap water
i. Rapidly dehydrate, clear and mount in DPX

Biopsy tissue should not be fixed until after smears have been examined, since further smears may be needed and occasionally smears will be useful in the identification of cell types using other techniques, including immunocytochemistry. The pathologist has to decide at this stage whether tissue needs to be retained for other investigations such as electron microscopy, culture or marker studies.

Smears should initially be examined at low power to assess overall cellularity and decide whether or not pathological tissue is present. It is important that the whole of the smear is examined since small groups of tumour cells may be confined to a limited area and they may be present in only one of several smears. The presence of 'reactive' astrocytes, reactive capillaries, inflammatory cells, histiocytes or necrosis may imply that the biopsy was taken from near a lesion or they may represent specific pathological abnormalities.

High power examination is needed for detailed cytological assessment. Before removing the slide from the microscope stage a low power objective should be in position since wet mounting medium may be raised above the level of the edge of the cover-slip and be deposited on the lens.

Normal brain

The pathologist must be familiar with the normal appearances of the various components of the nervous system in different areas.

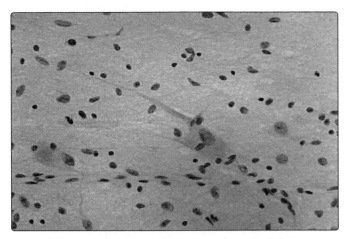

Fig. 43.28   Smear. Normal grey matter. A mixture of neurones and glial cells. (H&E × MP)

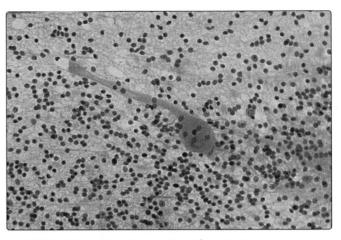

Fig. 43.30   Smear. Normal cerebellum. A large Purkinje cell is seen amongst numerous granular neurones. (H&E × MP)

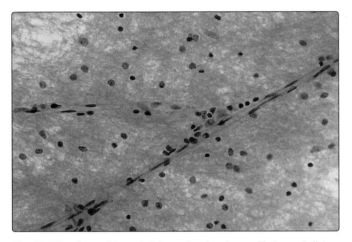

Fig. 43.29   Smear. Normal white matter showing capillaries and glial cells. (H&E × MP)

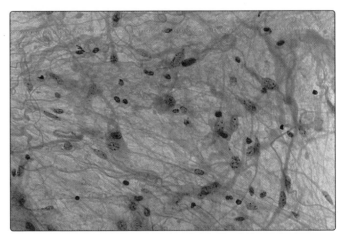

Fig. 43.31   Smear. Reactive astrocytes around the edge of a craniopharyngioma. The cells form well defined fibres. There is some variation in nuclear size and shape and they may have prominent nucleoli. Mitotic figures are often seen. (H&E × HP)

Smears from grey matter will contain a mixture of neurones, glial cells and blood vessels (Fig. 43.28), whereas smears from white matter lack neurones (Fig. 43.29). Neurones should be easily recognizable from the appearance of the nucleus and nucleolus, and from the presence of Nissl substance. The cytoplasm of normal glial cells is barely visible and it may be difficult to differentiate astrocytes from oligodendrocytes; the nuclei of oligodendrocytes tend to be more dense than those of astrocytes and the latter show a fine speckled chromatin pattern.

Smears from the cerebellum show numerous small granule cells with a few Purkinje cells scattered amongst them (Fig. 43.30) and smears from the hippocampus may contain neurones of variable size, the smaller ones having hyperchromatic nuclei. Choroid plexus, ependymal and arachnoidal endothelial cells may be encountered from time to time. Biopsies from the pituitary or pineal glands may present difficulties if the pathologist is not familiar with the normal anatomy of the area and the site of the biopsy. Choroid plexus can closely mimic adenocarcinoma.

Reactive changes

The distinction between reactive gliosis and neoplasia is difficult and sometimes impossible. Around the edge of an astrocytoma, cells often show gradual transition from reactive forms to obvious neoplastic cells. Reactive changes can be particularly marked around metastatic neoplasm, craniopharyngioma, abscess, arteriovenous malformation, infarction and following encephalitis and chronic ischaemia. If in doubt, it is safer to assume a reactive process until proved otherwise.

In a reactive area, some astrocytes usually show better defined cell borders and processes than normal astrocytes (Fig. 43.31) and gemistocytic forms are often present. Nuclei are enlarged and they often have well-defined nucleoli; an occasional mitotic figure may be seen. There may be marked proliferation of capillaries containing enlarged endothelial cells and lipid or haemosiderin-containing phagocytes may be present. The presence of perivascular cuffing with lymphocytes and plasma cells does not necessarily imply an infective process; this is sometimes seen in both primary and metastatic tumours.

Inflammatory conditions and infarction

Many types of bacteria, viruses, fungi, parasites and spirochaetes may involve the nervous system and the inflammatory response may be acute, subacute, chronic or granulomatous as in infections of the leptomeninges. Bacteria are rarely seen on a smear but sometimes fungi or parasites may be recognized, e.g. in toxoplasmosis. The presence of epithelioid cells or Langhans' giant cells should raise the possibility of tuberculosis or sarcoidosis (Fig. 43.32). Whenever the smear shows an inflammatory picture, fresh tissue should be retained for culture for bacteria, fungi and viruses. Specific viruses can sometimes be recognized by immunological techniques or electron microscopy.

The most commonly encountered inflammatory problems are abscess and encephalitis; both can mimic neoplasia clinically and radiologically. The presence of numerous polymorphs and necrotic debris should always raise the possibility of an *abscess*, but necrosis and polymorphs may also be a feature of neoplasia. The nature of the necrotic debris may be different and the presence of large numbers of 'ghost-like' remnants of cells showing variation in nuclear morphology suggests necrotic neoplasm; this can be unreliable.

Tissue from the wall of an abscess shows a mixed reactive and inflammatory picture depending on the age of the lesion and the degree of encapsulation. Reactive cells are easily confused with neoplastic cells (Fig. 43.33). The presence of collagen in the capsule may result in tissue smearing with difficulty.

The most helpful feature in encephalitis is cuffing of blood vessels by lymphocytes and plasma cells (Fig. 43.34), but this is sometimes also seen around a neoplasm, including metastatic carcinoma. The picture may be further complicated by the presence of marked reactive gliosis and

the nuclei of lymphocytes and astrocytes may be enlarged with prominent nucleoli. The most common form of encephalitis biopsied is *Herpes simplex* encephalitis, which may show a mixed population of inflammatory cells, including lymphocytes, plasma cells, polymorphs and phagocytes (Fig. 43.35).

The abnormalities seen following infarction vary with the stage of the infarct. In the early stages neurones show shrinkage of cell bodies and the cytoplasm stains deep pink with eosin, with variable degrees of loss of Nissl substance (Fig. 43.36). The nucleus becomes hyperchromatic and triangular in shape. Variable numbers of polymorphs may be present and as the infarct develops, lipid-laden phagocytes (Fig. 43.37), reactive astrocytes and proliferating capillaries appear.

Tumours of the central nervous system

The most common tumours to involve the cerebral hemispheres are astrocytomas derived from the glial tissue

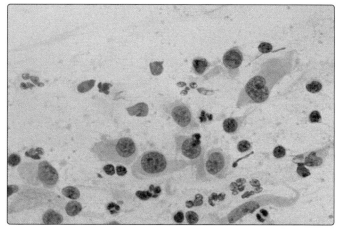

Fig. 43.33 Smear. Abscess. Reactive cells from the abscess wall may closely resemble malignant cells, with enlarged nuclei and prominent nucleoli. (H&E × HP)

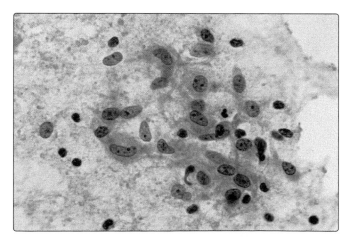

Fig. 43.32 Smear. Epithelioid histiocytes in cerebral tuberculosis. (H&E × HP)

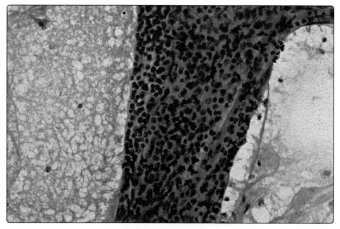

Fig. 43.34 Smear. Encephalitis. Note cuffing of vessel by lymphocytes. (H&E × MP) (Courtesy of Professor M M Esiri, Oxford, UK)

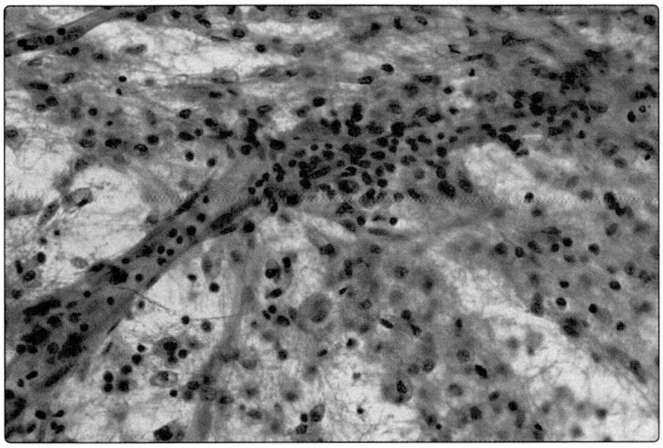

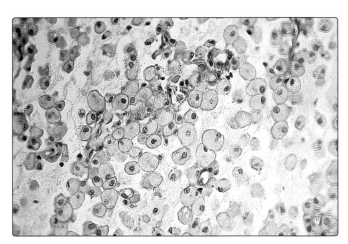

Fig. 43.35 Smear. *Herpes simplex* encephalitis with mixed population of cells including lymphocytes, plasma cells, polymorphs and phagocytes. (H&E × MP)

Fig. 43.37 Smear. Infarct containing numerous lipid-laden histiocytes. (H&E × HP)

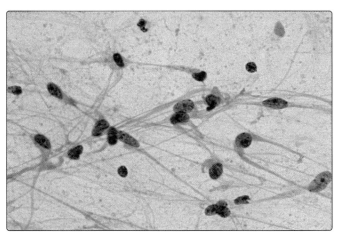

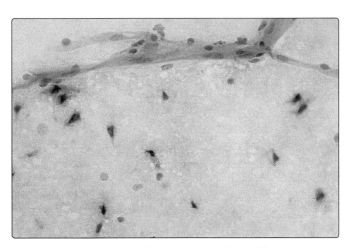

Fig. 43.36 Smear. Ischaemia. Neurones show loss of Nissl substance, eosinophilic cytoplasm and hyperchromatic shrunken nuclei. White matter stains poorly. (H&E × LP)

Fig. 43.38 Smear. Fibrillary astrocytoma grade II. Well-differentiated neoplasms show marked fibre formation. Processes often radiate towards blood vessels. Mitotic figures are difficult to find. (H&E × HP)

of the brain and metastatic tumours. In the majority of cases the tumour can be classified as one or other and an opinion given on the degree of differentiation (grade 1–4 in the case of gliomas), but it is important to remember that the biopsy sample may not represent the tumour as a whole; the neurosurgeon will need to take other factors into account in assessing further management, including radiological appearances. More detailed classification can sometimes be provided by paraffin-embedded sections and other special techniques.

In view of the enormous variety of cerebral tumours encountered in brain smears, the diagnostic cytological features will be described individually, rather than attempting an itemized summary of the findings.

Astrocytoma

Astrocytomas account for 25–30% of adult cerebral gliomas and a similar proportion of cerebellar gliomas in children. Many subtypes have been described and some

tumours contain a mixture of astrocytes and oligodendrocytes. The histological type and its biological behaviour are closely related to the age, incidence and site. These factors must be taken into account in assessing further management.

Fibrillary astrocytoma

The most common form of astrocytoma is the fibrillary astrocytoma, in which the cells form a meshwork of glial fibrils, which are often of considerable length (Fig. 43.38). The cells contain intracytoplasmic fibrils demonstrable by the phosphotungstic acid technique (PTAH). Nuclei vary a little in size, shape and chromatin content, but mitoses are rare. These tumours are not particularly cellular. There is a marked tendency for fibrillary processes to radiate towards blood vessels.

The more fibre-forming tumours smear with difficulty and the smear often shows dense clumps of cells surrounded by a peripheral rim of fibre-forming astrocytes.

959

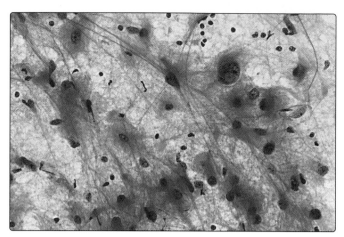

Fig. 43.39   Smear. Gemistocytic astrocytoma. These cells have abundant deeply eosinophilic cytoplasm. (H&E × HP)

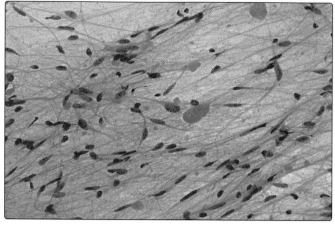

Fig. 43.40   Smear. Pilocytic astrocytoma composed of fusiform cells with long wavy processes. Rosenthal bodies are present. (H&E × HP)

Fibrillary astrocytomas usually have a poorly demarcated border and biopsies taken from the edge of such a tumour may include neurones. Focal calcification may also be present.

Protoplasmic astrocytoma

A rare form of astrocytoma, the protoplasmic astrocytoma, is composed of cells forming a fine cobweb of fibrils between which there are microcystic spaces containing eosinophilic fluid. The difference between this and the fibrillary form is usually difficult to detect on smears and from the practical point of view there is no point in trying to achieve the differentiation.

Gemistocytic astrocytoma

The gemistocytic astrocytoma is easily recognized, being composed of large cells with abundant deeply eosinophilic cytoplasm containing one or more eccentric nuclei (Fig. 43.39). This form of astrocytoma is particularly liable to differentiate to a higher grade of tumour. There is a marked tendency for blood vessels to be surrounded by lymphocytes.

Pilocytic astrocytoma

The pilocytic astrocytoma, most common in the cerebellum, is composed of fusiform cells with long wavy fine processes. They often contain elongated or globular PTAH positive bodies, known as Rosenthal fibres (Fig. 43.40). There may also be multiple foci of calcification.

Anaplastic astrocytoma

Anaplastic astrocytomas are common and any of the subtypes described above may show areas of anaplasia. These tumours are cellular and show variable degrees of dedifferentiation; the most undifferentiated cells may no longer be recognizable as astrocytic. Nuclei are often pleomorphic and bizarre and multinucleate forms are often seen; nucleoli are not usually recognizable. Mitotic figures are present and there is marked vascular proliferation, with

the formation of 'glomeruloid' buds. Parts of the tumour may be necrotic. A helpful feature in differentiating from metastatic carcinoma is the tendency of some tumour cells to remain attached to blood vessels in anaplastic astrocytomas (Fig. 43.41A–D).

Glioblastoma multiforme

This is an anaplastic form of glioma, usually astrocytic in origin, found in the cerebral hemispheres between the ages of 45 and 65 years. These tumours occasionally occur at other sites, at different ages, and in children. They contain mitotic figures, some of which may be abnormal and areas of necrosis and/or vascular hyperplasia (Fig. 43.42). The cells may have prominent nucleoli. The tumour may be very cellular and undifferentiated and contain multinucleate and bizarre cells (Fig. 43.43). The cytological features may be very diverse and may show little or no glial differentiation; differential diagnosis then includes lymphoma and metastasis. There is a tendency for the neoplastic cells to palisade around areas of necrosis. Sometimes they contain a sarcomatous component, in which case they are called gliosarcoma; the latter may smear with difficulty. The effects of irradiation therapy can produce a confusing picture with many bizarre cell types, which probably have little proliferative potential. Irradiation may also result in extensive necrosis, which can make diagnosis difficult or impossible, unless viable tissue is included. It is particularly important to realize that similar changes can be induced in lower grade neoplasms since the degree of pleomorphism can then be confused with glioblastoma multiforme (Fig. 43.44).

A rare variant known as giant cell glioblastoma has been described. This variant contains numerous large bizarre cells often with multiple nuclei with few processes.

Pleomorphic xanthoastrocytoma

This also contains pleomorphic tumour cells, many with multiple nuclei, and many of the latter contain lipid

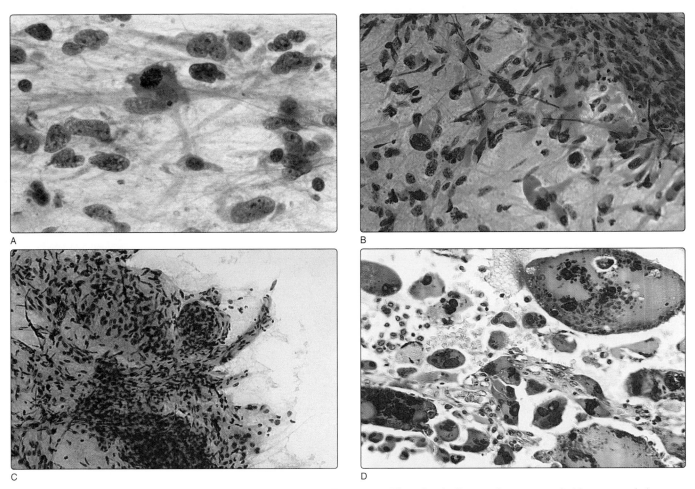

A

B

C

D

Fig. 43.41 Smear. (A) Anaplastic astrocytoma (astrocytoma grade IV). The most undifferentiated cells are no longer recognizable as astrocytic, but some fibre forming cells are usually seen. (H&E × HP) (B) Anaplastic astrocytoma showing tendency of cells to radiate towards blood vessels. (H&E × HP) (C) Anaplastic astrocytoma showing marked vascular proliferation with the formation of 'glomeruloid' structures. (H&E × HP) (D) Giant cell tumour of glial origin. The cells are large and contain one or more bizarre nuclei. It may be impossible to determine the nature of these cells. (H&E × HP)

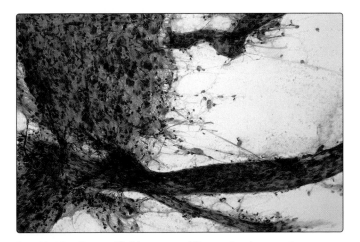

Fig. 43.42 Smear. Glioblastoma multiforme showing vascular hyperplasia. (H&E × MP)

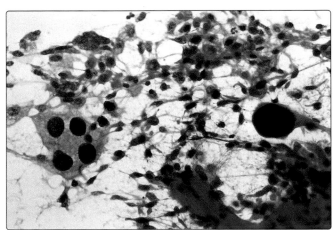

Fig. 43.43 Smear. Glioblastoma multiforme showing marked cellular pleomorphism. (H&E × HP)

vacuoles, closely resembling histiocytic neoplasms (Figs 43.45, 43.46). Mitotic figures are absent or few. Perivascular lymphocytes are often seen. Areas of necrosis, vascular proliferation and mitotic figures are usually absent.

They tend to have a better prognosis and usually behave as grade 2 neoplasms although some may grow more rapidly. They are usually associated with cysts and occur towards the surface of the brain, most commonly in the temporal or

961

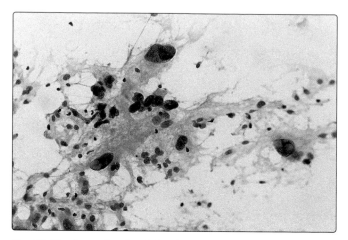

Fig. 43.44 Smear. Irradiated oligodendroglioma. Note the marked pleomorphism, which can easily be confused with glioblastoma multiforme. (H&E × MP)

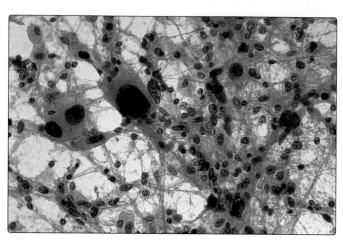

Fig. 43.46 Smear. Pleomorphic xanthoastrocytoma demonstrating pleomorphism and the presence of foamy cells. (H&E × HP)

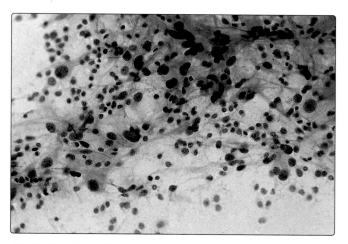

Fig. 43.45 Smear. Pleomorphic xanthoastrocytoma showing pleomorphic neoplastic cells, some with multiple nuclei, which can easily be misinterpreted as high-grade neoplasm. (H&E × MP)

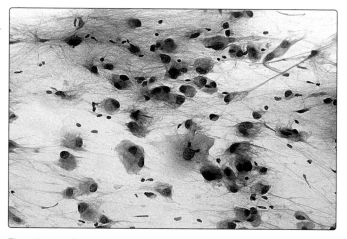

Fig. 43.47 Smear. Subependymal giant cell astrocytoma showing a mixture of large cells closely resembling neurones and fibre-forming astrocytes. (Toluidine Blue × HP)

occipital lobes. It is important that radiological appearances and age of presentation are taken into account in the assessment of this neoplasm. They tend to present in the third or fourth decade rather than later, although the patient may present with symptoms such as seizures during the first decade.

Subependymal giant cell astrocytoma

The subependymal giant cell astrocytoma typically occurs in the young as a manifestation of tuberous sclerosis. It arises from the lateral ventricle and protrudes into the lumen of the ventricle. Giant fibre-forming astrocytes and focal calcification are characteristic. The former are large cells with eccentric nuclei, abundant cytoplasm and prominent nucleoli. Morphologically, they closely resemble neurones (Fig. 43.47) but the nature of the cells is in doubt and they may stain positively or negatively for GFAP and neurofilament proteins.

Astroblastoma

Astroblastomas are usually seen in the first three decades of life in the cerebral hemispheres. They are highly malignant and there is a marked tendency for the cells to form perivascular arrangements with processes radiating towards the wall of a vessel. Cellular atypia may be present.

Polar spongioblastoma

This is a rare tumour that occurs in children and shows variable growth rate. It is of uncertain nature and shows marked palisading of nuclei, resulting in a striped pattern although this is not usually apparent on smears. The cells form fibres, which usually stain for GFAP. They may contain areas that suggest oligodendroglioma or astrocytoma and electron microscopy may show microtubules and dense-core granules, suggesting neuronal differentiation. Frozen sections are better for establishing the growth pattern (Fig. 43.48).

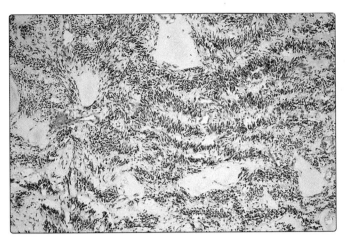

Fig. 43.48 Frozen section. Polar spongioblastoma. This neoplasm shows marked palisading of nuclei that is not usually recognizable on a smear but is easily recognized on frozen section. (H&E × MP)

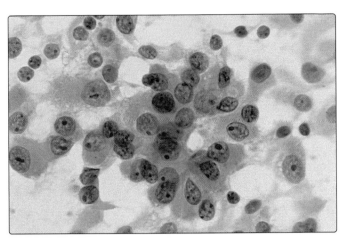

Fig. 43.50 Smear. Ependymoma. The cells resemble epithelial cells. The most helpful feature is a tendency to form rosettes. (H&E × HP)

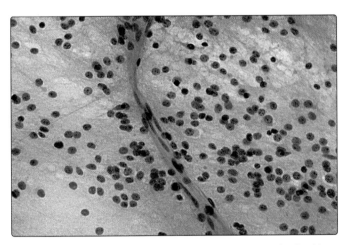

Fig. 43.49 Smear. Oligodendroglioma. Diffusely arranged cells with round or oval nuclei with a fine chromatin pattern. The cells do not show the same tendency to radiate towards blood vessels as in astrocytoma. (H&E × MP)

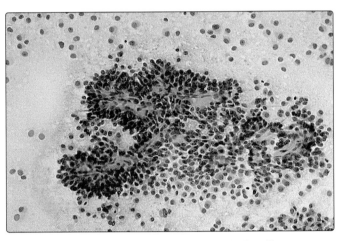

Fig. 43.51 Smear. Ependymoma showing a marked papillary pattern. (H&E × MP)

Oligodendroglioma

Oligodendrogliomas are usually situated in the cerebral hemispheres and tend to be slow growing. They are composed of diffusely arranged cells with round or oval nuclei with a fine chromatin pattern and a small nucleolus (Fig. 43.49). The nucleus is surrounded by clear cytoplasm, but this may be difficult to recognize on smears. A helpful feature is the tendency for focal calcification, which may be recognized as a gritty sensation when making the smear, and in contrast to astrocytoma, the cells show no tendency to gather around blood vessels, although the cells may produce fine short processes. The nuclei stain a little more intensely than those in astrocytomas and show a monotonously uniform pattern. Mitotic figures are rare, but dedifferentiated forms do occur. Classification of gliomas is complicated by the fact that tumours composed of a mixture of astrocytes and oligodendrocytes are often seen.

Ependymal and choroid plexus tumours

The most common site for ependymoma is the fourth ventricle, but they also arise from the ependymal lining of the lateral and third ventricles and in the spinal cord and cauda equina. They are found in children and adults.

Histologically, ependymomas exhibit several patterns. Perivascular pseudorosettes are the most frequent, but these are not easily recognized on smears. They are the result of these cells producing processes radiating towards blood vessels and they are more easily seen in frozen sections. The formation of ependymal rosettes is diagnostic (Fig. 43.50) but they can be difficult to recognize and if the 'canals' are obvious the possibility of adenocarcinoma should be considered. In smears ependymal cells have round or oval nuclei and small nucleoli. Poorly-differentiated variants also occur.

Ependymomas sometimes show a marked papillary pattern, the papillae having a connective tissue stroma covered by multiple layers of columnar epithelial cells (Fig. 43.51). This pattern closely resembles choroid plexus

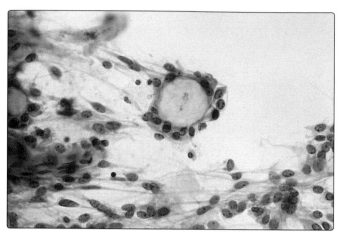

Fig. 43.52 Smear. Myxopapillary ependymoma. Ependymal cells form papillary structures around areas of hyaline collagen. (H&E × MP)

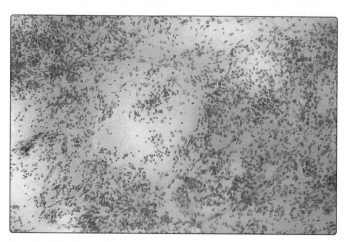

Fig. 43.53 Smear. Subependymoma. This neoplasm is most easily recognized at low power. It has an intense fibrillary background containing clusters of nuclei. (Toluidine Blue × LP)

papilloma. Calcification may be seen, particularly in supratentorial tumours. Ependymomas can closely resemble astrocytoma with a marked fibrillary component and a 'clear cell' variant closely resembles oligodendroglioma.

The *myxopapillary ependymoma* is usually found in the cauda equina region and is composed of ependymal cells with a perivascular papillary pattern around areas of hyaline collagen (Fig. 43.52). Some of the cells contain mucin, which stains positively with the PAS and Alcian blue stains, and this may also be present in the stroma.

Subependymoma

Subependymomas are usually found in the fourth ventricle and are composed of small nests of glial cells widely separated by a fine meshwork of glial fibrils. They are often asymptomatic and found incidentally at autopsy. They smear with difficulty and frozen sections may be required. They are most easily recognized at low power magnification and have an intense fibrillary background containing clusters of nuclei (Fig. 43.53). The latter resemble normal ependymal cells, being elongated or oval in shape and with a fine chromatin pattern. Mitotic figures are uncommon and difficult to find. They may show marked calcification.

Choroid plexus papilloma and carcinoma

Choroid plexus papilloma is rare and usually arises in the lateral and fourth ventricles. These tumours are seen most frequently in the first decade but can occur in adults. Smears show numerous papillae covered by cuboidal cells, which lie on a basement membrane (Fig. 43.54). They are more cellular than normal choroid plexus and have several layers of epithelial cells covering the papillae. The cells maintain cohesion in separate fragments. Nuclei are uniform in size and shape and have a fine chromatin pattern and poorly-defined nucleoli. The cells have villi and a few cilia, but these are often not recognizable without electron microscopy. The stroma is vascular and there may be dense calcification. The picture can closely resemble

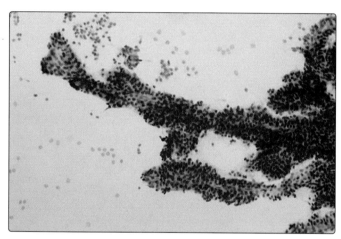

Fig. 43.54 Smear. Choroid plexus papilloma showing numerous papillae covered by cuboidal cells, which lie on a basement membrane. (H&E × LP)

adenocarcinoma. Anaplastic variants occur and these show irregularity of the papillae, mitotic figures, areas of necrosis and nuclear pleomorphism. In some cases the papillary pattern may not be present in a smear. Pigmented malignant forms also rarely occur and these have been referred to as malignant melanoma.

Primitive neuroectodermal tumours (PNET)

There is considerable confusion regarding the use of the term PNET. The World Heath Organization classification defines these tumours as 'small cell, malignant tumours of childhood with predominant location in the cerebellum and a noted capacity for divergent differentiation, including neuronal, astrocytic, ependymal, muscular and melanocytic'. They are thought to be derived from 'stem cells' showing divergent differentiation.

Some use the term to include a range of small cell neoplasms, including medulloblastoma, neuroblastoma (including olfactory neuroblastoma), ependymoblastoma, pineoblastoma and spongioblastoma, depending on site of

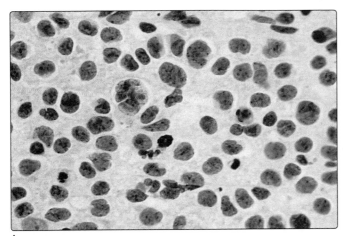

A

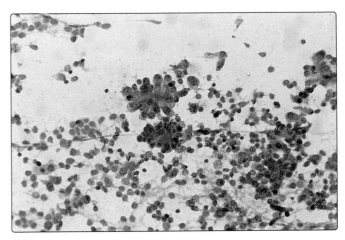

Fig. 43.56   Smear. Medulloepithelioma. The diagnostic feature is the presence of embryonic-appearing epithelium forming tubular and/or papillary structures. Primitive neuroectodermal cells often predominate. (H&E × HP).

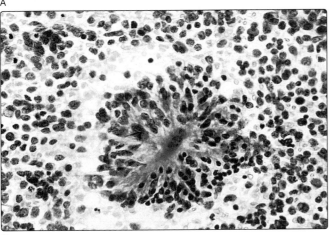

B

Fig. 43.55   Smear. (A) Primitive neuroectodermal tumour (medulloblastoma). The cells have a high nuclear/cytoplasmic ratio and the nuclei are hyperchromatic with frequent mitoses. (H&E × HP) (B) Medulloblastoma. Sometimes evidence of rosette formation is seen. These are also features of neuroblastoma and retinoblastoma. (H&E × HP)

origin. This approach should be abandoned and the term PNET should be restricted to those neoplasms fulfilling the WHO criteria. The terms medulloblastoma, pineoblastoma, ependymoblastoma and neuroblastoma should be retained for 'primitive' embryonal neoplasms composed largely of undifferentiated cells arising in specific sites.

The cells of the undifferentiated component have a high nuclear/cytoplasmic ratio and the nuclei are hyperchromatic (Fig. 43.55A). There may be considerable variation in size and shape of nuclei and in chromatin content. Nuclei may vary from oval to carrot-shaped. Mitoses are common and there may be foci of necrosis. These neoplasms may show some differentiation along a variety of cell lines. A few neoplasms have abundant reticulin and are designated 'desmoplastic' variants.

Medulloblastoma is the type most frequently encountered in smears, being the most common primary brain tumour in childhood. There is a further peak in the early 20s and a few cases occur later in life. There is a tendency for the cells to form rosettes with fine fibrils radiating towards the

centre (Fig. 43.55B). These are present in approximately 40% of cases and immunohistochemical markers may confirm neuronal (synaptophysin, neurofilament protein) or astrocytic (GFAP) differentiation.

When examining smears it is important to differentiate the small neoplastic cells from cerebellar granule cells, which have smaller nuclei of regular shape and staining properties; and granular neurones are usually associated with a few Purkinje cells.

Medulloepithelioma is a very rare variant, which consists of medullary epithelium, which retains the potential to differentiate in a variety of directions including neurones, glia, and ependyma. The epithelium rests on a basement membrane and groups of these cells can usually be recognized in a smear (Fig. 43.56). Some tumours show mesenchymal differentiation, including the formation of rhabdomyoblasts, bone and cartilage.

Pineoblastoma resembles medulloblastoma cytologically, including the presence of rosettes and they occasionally show neuronal and astrocytic differentiation. A range of tumours showing variable degrees of neuronal differentiation exist, the best differentiated being referred to as *Pineocytoma*. The rate of growth reflects the degree of differentiation.

Neuroblastoma is rare in the intracranial cavity and may also occur within the spinal cord and cauda equina. It usually occurs before the age of 2 years and may contain Homer Wright rosettes and stain for neuronal markers such as neurofilament protein and synaptophysin.

Ependymoblastoma typically occurs in children and may be congenital. It rarely occurs in adults. The neoplasm is very cellular and may form rosettes and canals but they are rarely recognizable in smears.

Neuronal tumours

Gangliocytoma and *ganglioglioma* are composed of a mixture of mature ganglion cells and glial cells (Fig. 43.57). The former consists of well-differentiated neurones within a

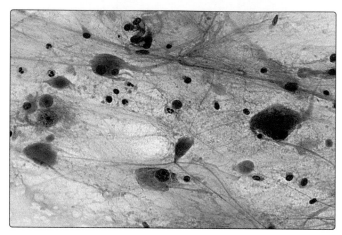

Fig. 43.57 Smear. Ganglioglioma. These neoplasms are composed of a mixture of ganglion cells and glial cells. (H&E × HP)

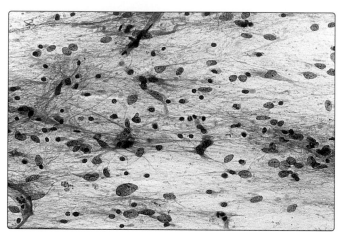

Fig. 43.58 Smear. Dysembryoplastic neuroepithelial tumour. This is composed of a mixture of neoplastic neurones, astrocytes, and oligodendrocytes. (Toluidine Blue × MP)

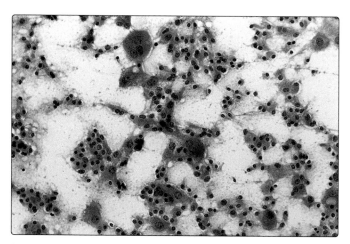

Fig. 43.59 Smear. Ganglioneuroblastoma showing a mixture of neuroblasts and well-differentiated ganglion cells. (H&E × MP)

stroma of non-neoplastic glial cells. They usually occur in children and frequently in the temporal lobe. They are slow growing and must be differentiated from glioma infiltrating neuronal tissue and from malignant gliomas containing cells with nuclei that superficially resemble those of neurones. The latter is composed of neoplastic neurones and glial cells, usually astrocytes, but sometimes oligodendrocytes. They often show cuffing of blood vessels by lymphocytes. Prognosis is usually determined by the degree of differentiation of the astrocytic component and anaplastic changes may be encountered in the glial cells.

A rare form of neoplasm called *desmoplastic infantile ganglioglioma*, containing a mixture of neurones, glial cells and fibrous stroma has been described in children below the age of 2 years. They are usually situated towards the surface of the cerebral hemispheres and smear with difficulty due to the large amount of collagen present.

Another form of neoplasm occurring within the cerebral cortex of children and young adults is the *dysembryoplastic neuroepithelial tumour*. It is composed of a mixture of neoplastic neurones, astrocytes and oligodendroglial cells and has a good prognosis. Detection of the neuronal component is essential for diagnosis. Smears show a varied picture and contain a mixture of cell types resembling astrocytes, oligodendrocytes and ganglion cells (Fig. 43.58). Mitotic figures are not seen. They closely resemble gangliocytoma or ganglioglioma.

Ganglioneuroblastoma contains a spectrum of cells varying between well-differentiated ganglion cells and neuroblasts (Fig. 43.59).

Central neurocytoma is a well circumscribed neoplasm usually found in the ventricle wall of young adults. The most common sites are in the region of the Foramen of Munro and septum pellucidum. Superficially the cells resemble oligodendroglioma but immunohistochemical stains and electron microscopy demonstrate neuronal differentiation. The cells have regular round or oval nuclei

and have fine fibrils radiating towards blood vessels (Fig. 43.60). Mitotic figures are absent or difficult to find. There may be small foci of calcification.

Meningioma

These tumours are derived from the meninges surrounding the brain and spinal cord. Most tumours arise from the arachnoidal villi concentrated in the walls of venous sinuses and their tributary veins. Approximately 50% are related to the superior sagittal sinus, but they may also occur in the spinal canal, orbit, ventricles, or skull, and they may be extra-calvarial. They most commonly occur in the middle decades of life and are more common in women.

In spite of several histological types, some characteristic features are usually recognizable. The cells generally show great cohesiveness, forming groups of arachnoidal cells with oval nuclei, which have a fine chromatin pattern and frequently show nucleoli. The most easily recognized feature is the presence of whorls (Fig. 43.61A,B). Psammoma bodies are occasionally seen. These features are not always present, particularly in the fibrous and angioblastic types.

Fibroblastic meningiomas usually smear with difficulty and form interlacing bundles of spindle-shaped cells with narrow elongated nuclei (Fig. 43.62). The cells may show some degree of whorl formation and there may even be an occasional psammoma body. It is essential that the pathologist is aware of the anatomical site and radiological features of the tumour since they closely resemble neurilemmoma and fibrillary astrocytoma. Intraventricular meningiomas are usually fibroblastic in type.

Meningiomas, particularly the *syncytial* variety, may show marked nuclear pleomorphism and a few mitotic figures. This does not indicate rapid growth but the presence of numerous mitotic figures suggests malignant change.

The *haemangioblastic, haemangiopericytic, angiomatous, microcystic, secretory, clear cell, papillary and chordoid* varieties are rare and difficult to diagnose on smears. Paraffin embedded sections are usually required to define the type. The haemangioblastic variant produces a picture similar to that of the haemangioblastoma of the cerebellum and the haemangiopericytic variant has elongated nuclei and an increased percentage of mitotic figures, reflecting their potential for aggressive behaviour.

Malignant or atypical features may be seen on the smear but the abnormalities are often patchy.

Schwannoma (neurilemmoma) and neurofibroma

Both of these tumours arise on nerve roots and are essentially tumours of Schwann cells forming the nerve sheath. They can usually be distinguished by the arrangement of the neoplastic cells; neurofibromas contain abundant collagen and nerve fibres within the tumour and are more difficult to smear than schwannomas.

The most common schwannoma biopsied is the acoustic neuroma. The tissue is usually moderately soft, but not as soft as glioma. Cells form anastomosing columns separating spaces (Fig. 43.63A). Both Antoni types A and B tissue can usually be recognized, the former consisting of interweaving bundles of spindle-shaped cells with elongated nuclei and

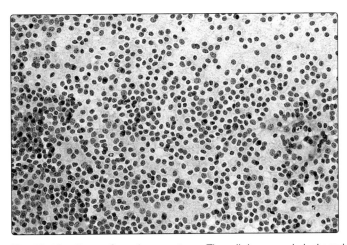

Fig. 43.60 Smear. Central neurocytoma. The cells have regularly shaped nuclei and they form fine fibrils. (H&E × MP)

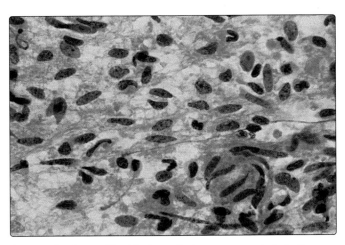

Fig. 43.62 Smear. Fibroblastic meningioma composed of spindle-shaped cells with elongated nuclei. (H&E × HP)

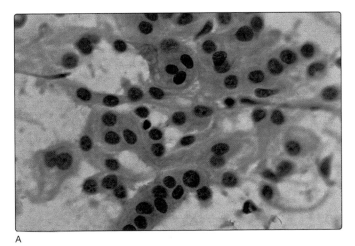

A

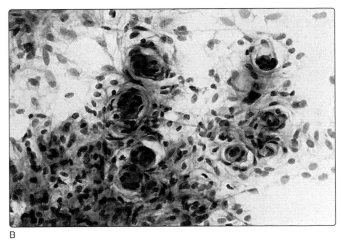

B

Fig. 43.61 Smear. (A) Meningioma showing arachnoidal endothelial cells. (H&E × HP) (B) Meningioma showing numerous whorls. (H&E × MP)

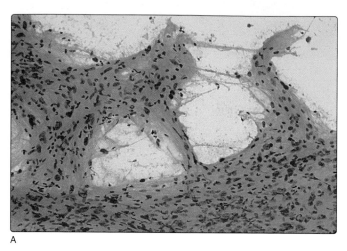

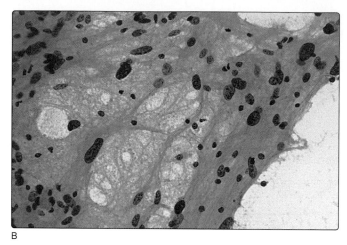

Fig. 43.63 Smear. (A) Neurilemmoma (Schwannoma) showing anastomosing columns of spindle-shaped cells separated by spaces. (H&E × MP) (B) Neurilemmoma. A mixture of cells with elongated cells and cells with abundant vacuolated cytoplasm (Antoni types A and B tissue respectively). (H&E ×

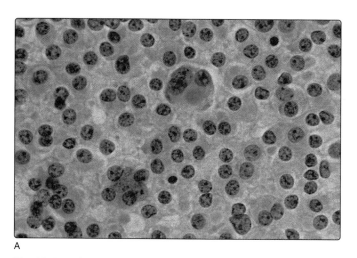

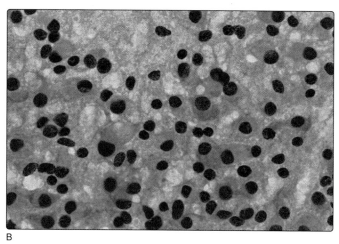

Fig. 43.64 Smear. (A) Pituitary adenoma. The nuclei are enlarged with prominent nucleoli and show some variation in size and shape. Multiple nuclei are present in some cells. In this example one cell contains a fibrous body; these are usually associated with growth hormone producing cells. Compare with normal pituitary gland in (B). (H&E × HP) (B, Courtesy of Dr P G Lynch, Preston, UK)

inconspicuous nucleoli; the latter, being larger cells with indefinite cell outlines, are less easily recognized (Fig. 43.63B). Schwannomas may show considerable nuclear pleomorphism; in the absence of mitotic figures this does not indicate rapid growth. There may be marked vascularization and evidence of recent or previous haemorrhage.

Neurofibroma is more easily recognized with frozen sections than smears. The cells are spindle shaped and form a wavy pattern within a loose stroma with clear areas and containing abundant collagen.

Pituitary gland tumours

Approximately 30% of pituitary adenomas show no clinical signs of hormonal activity. Hormonal effects usually relate to the secretion of prolactin, growth hormone and adrenocorticotrophic hormone; some tumours present with hypopituitarism. Some tumours produce more than one hormone type.

Classification depends on the immunohistochemical identification of hormones present in the tumour cells. Electron microscopy is helpful in the assessment of granule size and density. 'Fibrous bodies' may be seen in the cytoplasm of some growth hormone producing tumours. Some adenomas are oncocytomas with numerous mitochondria and few granules.

The most difficult problem for the pathologist in assessing a smear is to decide whether adenoma is present or not. It is important to realize that the normal gland may contain areas with large groups of cells of the same type that can easily be misinterpreted as adenoma on small specimens. The nuclei of adenoma cells are usually larger than normal with prominent nucleoli and show more pleomorphism (Fig. 43.64A,B). Multiple nuclei may be seen in some cells. Markedly pleomorphic forms are not uncommon (Fig. 43.65). A few tumours have regularly shaped smaller oval or round nuclei; if the site is not known

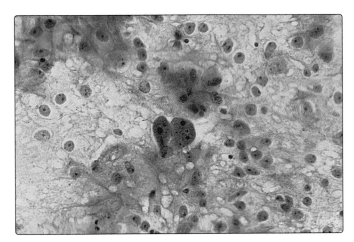

Fig. 43.65 Smear. Pituitary neoplasm showing marked nuclear pleomorphism. (H&E × HP)

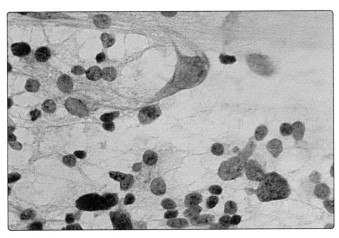

Fig. 43.66 Smear. Pineocytoma. The neoplasm is composed of a mixture of small cells with round or oval nuclei surrounded by little cytoplasm, and larger cells showing evidence of neuronal differentiation. (Toluidine Blue × HP) (Courtesy of Dr J E Bell, Edinburgh, UK)

these can easily be confused with oligodendroglioma and even with nasopharyngeal carcinoma. The cells of pituitary adenoma tend to separate individually, whereas the cells of carcinoma tend to form clusters.

Identification of the hormonal type is unreliable on smears and should be done by immunohistochemical stains on paraffin-embedded sections.

Pineal gland tumours

Tumours of the pineal cells vary in their degree of differentiation, well-differentiated tumours being known as pineocytomas and poorly-differentiated forms as pineoblastomas. Pineoblastoma tends to occur before the age of 30 and usually within the first decade; whereas pineocytoma tends to occur during or after the second decade.

Pineocytoma

Pineocytomas are composed of cells with darkly staining nuclei, which may form lobules and radiate around a central pale area containing fine argyrophilic fibrils. These are variable degrees of neuronal differentiation (Fig. 43.66). Electron microscopy shows that these cells contain dense-core vesicles. Some tumours show astrocytic differentiation. The cells of poorly-differentiated tumours have darkly staining nuclei without visible nucleoli, surrounded by small amounts of cytoplasm (Fig. 43.67).

A variety of germ cell tumours occur in the pineal region and at the base of the brain, especially within the hypothalamus. They are more common in males and usually present during the first three decades. *Germinoma* is indistinguishable from testicular seminoma and ovarian dysgerminoma. It contains a mixture of large spheroidal cells with vesicular nuclei and prominent nucleoli, and lymphocytes (Fig. 43.68). There are a variety of tumours derived from totipotential germ cells, such as *embryonal carcinoma, teratoma (mature and immature), choriocarcinoma*

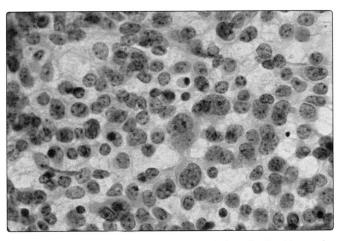

Fig. 43.67 Smear. Pineoblastoma composed of small cells with round or oval nuclei and a high nuclear/cytoplasmic ratio. In this case some cells showed positive staining with neurofilament protein indicating some neuronal differentiation. (H&E × HP)

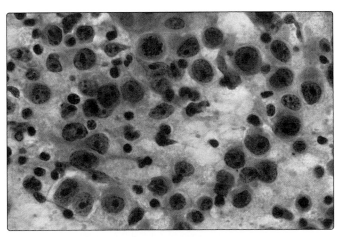

Fig. 43.68 Smear. Germinoma composed of a mixture of large spheroidal cells with vesicular nuclei and prominent nucleoli, and lymphocytes. These tumours are indistinguishable from ovarian dysgerminoma and testicular seminoma. (H&E × HP)

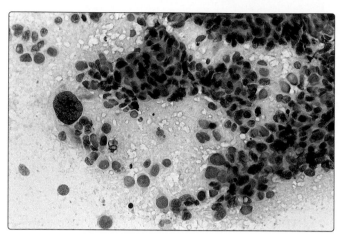

Fig. 43.69   Smear. Choriocarcinoma of pineal gland. The nuclei vary in size and shape and in staining properties. Syncytiotrophoblasts have vacuolated cytoplasm and multiple nuclei. (H&E × HP)

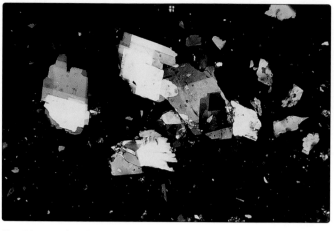

Fig. 43.71   Cyst fluid. Cholesterol crystals are easily recognized in polarized light. (× MP)

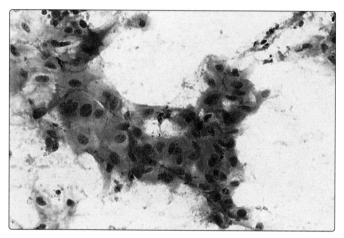

Fig. 43.70   Smear. Craniopharyngioma showing clumps of epithelial cells. (H&E × HP)

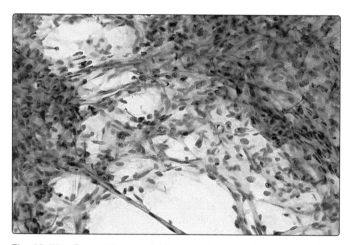

Fig. 43.72   Smear. Haemangioblastoma. Anastomosing network of blood vessels separated by cells with abundant foamy cytoplasm and small nuclei. (H&E × HP)

(Fig. 43.69), *yolk-sac carcinoma* and tumours containing mixtures of these are rare. The various types can be extremely difficult to diagnose on smears and paraffin-embedded sections are usually required. A variety of antibodies including placental alkaline phosphatase, alpha-fetoprotein, human chorionic gonadotrophin, human placental lactogen, pregnancy-specific protein and epithelial membrane antigen are useful in classification.

Craniopharyngioma and epidermoid/dermoid cysts

Smears usually show easily recognizable sheets of transitional or squamous epithelial cells (Fig. 43.70). The lesions are often cystic and cholesterol crystals and/or flakes of keratin can often be detected; polarizing filters are helpful in detecting cholesterol crystals (Fig. 43.71). These lesions may induce intense gliosis, which can easily be mistaken for astrocytoma. There may be evidence of previous haemorrhage.

Haemangioblastoma

These usually arise in the cerebellum but sometimes occur in the spinal cord. They smear with difficulty and it is not easy to recognize the vascular nature of the neoplasm. Smears usually show anastomosing trabeculae composed of blood vessels, elongated cells and occasional foamy cells (Fig. 43.72) and haemosiderin-containing histiocytes may be seen amongst them. Lipid stains (oil red-O) reveal neutral lipid droplets within the cytoplasm of the tumour cells. The lesion is usually associated with a cyst and the wall of the cyst may show intense gliosis, easily misinterpreted as astrocytoma. They tend to occur between the ages of 20 and 50 but some occur in children; the latter are more likely to be associated with the features of von Hippel-Lindau's disease. They may be multiple.

Lymphoma and leukaemia

Both lymphoma and leukaemia may involve the nervous system. The main varieties of neurological syndrome complicating lymphoma are acute or subacute spinal cord compression, cranial nerve involvement, or meningeal invasion. Both B-cell and T-cell lymphomas occur as primary tumours. There is an increasing incidence related to immunosuppression, particularly with the acquired immunodeficiency syndrome and following transplantation procedures. Health and safety issues are, therefore, very important and laboratory staff should be made aware of the HIV status in advance.

Lymphoma cells are seen particularly around blood vessels but they may invade the brain, meninges and nerve roots.

The most common form of leukaemia to involve the nervous system is *lymphoblastic leukaemia*, particularly in children treated by systemic chemotherapy. An increased incidence of neurological complications associated with longer survival is also seen in acute non-lymphoblastic leukaemia.

Smears can be difficult to interpret and distinction from undifferentiated carcinoma, 'oat cell' carcinoma, primitive neuroectodermal tumour and reactive lymphocytes in viral encephalitis or tuberculous meningitis requires considerable experience; sometimes it may not be possible. Both neoplastic and reactive smears can contain a mixture of small and large cell forms and the larger cells sometimes have irregular nuclei. Mitotic figures may be present (Fig. 43.73). Plasma cells, polymorphs and histiocytes may also be present amongst the neoplastic cell population. If in doubt a firm diagnosis should not be made and tissue should be sent for culture to exclude an infective process. 'Oat cells' appear very similar to large centrocytes and centroblasts and are easily confused if cell groups are not seen. Nucleoli are not prominent in 'oat cells' but usually are in centroblasts and immunoblasts.

Leukaemic cells may also closely resemble lymphoblastic lymphoma cells.

Lymphomatoid granulomatosis can also produce a confusing picture with a mixed population of cells including lymphocytes, plasma cells, histiocytes, and atypical lymphoid cells (Fig. 43.74). The lesion is angiocentric and necrotizing.

When appropriate material is available, immunocytochemical methods can be used to solve these problems.

Plasma cell neoplasms

The nervous system is commonly involved in myeloma and occasionally by localized plasmacytomas. The spinal vertebrae are usually infiltrated by myeloma cells and these may extend into the extradural space, producing cord compression. As a cause of cord compression, myeloma comes second to metastatic carcinoma. Vertebral collapse due to myelomatous infiltration may also result in neurological deficits.

The tissue smears easily and typical features of plasma cells with eccentric nuclei and adjacent cytoplasmic clearing

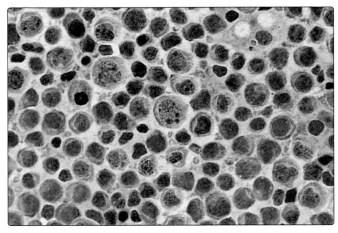

Fig. 43.73 Smear. Lymphoma. Characteristically, all of the cells are dissociated. The majority of lymphomas are B-cell in type. (H&E × HP)

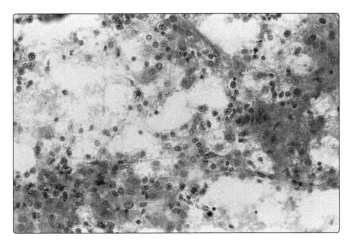

Fig. 43.74 Smear. Lymphomatoid granulomatosis showing a mixed population of cell types including lymphocytes (some of which may be atypical), plasma cells and histiocytes, which can easily be misinterpreted. (H&E × MP)

are usually easily recognized, although the degree of differentiation varies from case to case (Fig. 43.75). It can be difficult to distinguish the well-differentiated tumours from reactive plasma cells. Binucleate forms are often seen and the cells usually show prominent multiple nucleoli.

Leukaemic deposits

These predominantly occur in acute myeloid leukaemia and the cells show variable degrees of differentiation and show the relevant cytoplasmic granules. The patient is usually known to suffer from leukaemia. Great care is required in making a diagnosis since a variety of haematological cell types may be present, including megakaryocytes.

Metastatic intracranial and spinal tumours
Carcinoma

Carcinomas are the most common form of metastases in the central nervous system; bronchus, lung, breast, gastrointestinal tract, kidney and thyroid gland being the

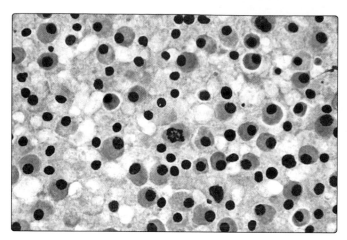

Fig. 43.75 Smear. Myeloma. The degree of differentiation varies from case to case but the plasma cell nature of the cells is usually easily recognized. (H&E × HP)

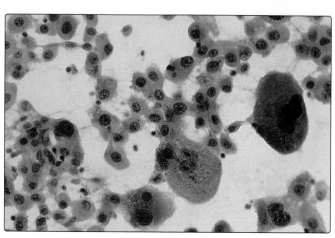

Fig. 43.77 Smear. Metastatic carcinoma from lung showing marked pleomorphism of malignant cells. It may be impossible to be certain of the origin of highly pleomorphic cells. (H&E × HP)

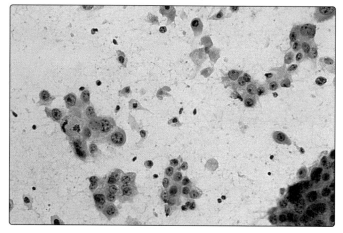

Fig. 43.76 Smear. Metastatic carcinoma showing tendency of cells to form small groups. (H&E × LP)

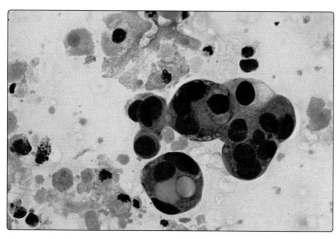

Fig. 43.78 Smear. Adenocarcinoma metastatic from lung. Cells may show an acinar pattern, but intracellular vacuoles are usually present. (H&E × HP)

commonest primary sites. Smear appearances usually reflect the tumour of origin, but architectural pattern is better recognized on frozen sections. The cells tend to stick together in small groups (Fig. 43.76) even in the more pleomorphic forms (Fig. 43.77). Adenocarcinoma may show an acinar pattern and intracellular vacuoles can usually be recognized in cells from mucin-secreting adenocarcinoma (Fig. 43.78).

The more undifferentiated *small cell carcinoma* and *oat cell carcinoma* can closely resemble anaplastic astrocytoma, malignant embryonal tumours, and lymphoma (Fig. 43.79). The most helpful feature in differentiating small cell carcinoma from anaplastic astrocytoma is the tendency of some cells in the latter to retain their relationship to blood vessels and it is unusual not to be able to find some obvious neoplastic cells from an astrocytoma showing some evidence of fibre formation. Clumps of neoplastic cells within fragments of normal or gliotic brain are almost

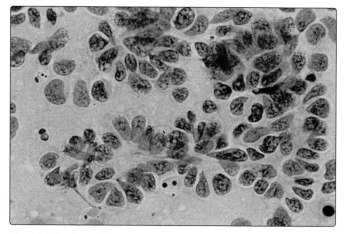

Fig. 43.79 Smear. Oat cell carcinoma. The cells have little cytoplasm and a high nuclear/cytoplasmic ratio. Nuclear chromatin is evenly dispersed and nucleoli are not prominent. There is a tendency for the cells to form small clusters; this is useful in differentiating them from lymphoid cells. (H&E × HP)

always metastatic carcinoma. Tissue removed from around the edge of metastatic carcinoma may show marked reactive gliosis, difficult to differentiate from astrocytoma and blood vessels may show marked cuffing with lymphocytes that can easily be mistaken for encephalitis.

Melanoma

Melanoma usually contains some cells containing pigment and the classical appearances with enlarged slightly eccentric nuclei and prominent angular nucleoli are usually characteristic (Fig. 43.80); even in the absence of pigment, these features will usually raise the possibility of melanoma. Some cases are heavily pigmented (Fig. 43.81)

Rarely, melanoma arises within the meninges and extends into the brain or spinal cord. These tumours vary in their degree of differentiation, the well-differentiated forms containing large amounts of pigment. Melanin may also be present in other tumours of the nervous system, including ependymoma, medulloblastoma, choroid plexus papilloma, meningioma and schwannoma.

Renal carcinoma

Renal carcinoma is often recognizable from the vacuolated cytoplasm, which is PAS positive due to glycogen but not diastase resistant. Great care is needed in the cerebellum, since the picture closely resembles haemangioblastoma (Fig. 43.82).

Local extension from regional tumours

A wide variety of tumours can extend into the CNS from adjacent structures and smears can provide a definite or highly suggestive diagnosis in many cases.

Nasopharyngeal carcinoma

Nasopharyngeal carcinoma often penetrates the base of the skull and meninges and involves nerve roots and pituitary gland. The neoplasm is usually squamous, but transitional cell and poorly-differentiated variants occur and these are easily confused with primary tumours of the pituitary gland (Fig. 43.83).

Cylindroma

Cylindromas are locally invasive tumours of sweat gland derivation, commonly arising on the scalp. They may infiltrate the base of the skull and involve cranial nerves.

Ceruminoma

Ceruminomas, which arise in the wax-secreting modified sweat glands of the ear, occasionally infiltrate into the intracranial cavity. The author has diagnosed a carcinoma of the ceruminous glands using the smear technique; the apocrine nature of the cells was easily recognizable.

Chordoma

Chordomas arise at both ends of the vertebral column; they are composed of physaliferous cells with vacuolated cytoplasm and this feature is readily recognized in smears (Fig. 43.84). Groups of cells are separated by extracellular

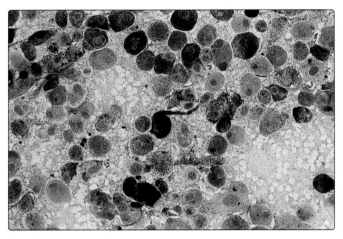

Fig. 43.81   Smear. Melanoma containing heavily pigmented cells. (H&E × HP)

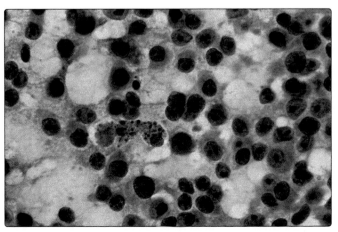

Fig. 43.80   Smear. Melanoma. The presence of macronucleoli should suggest this diagnosis. Pigment is not always present and care must be taken not to mistake haemosiderin for melanin. (H&E × HP)

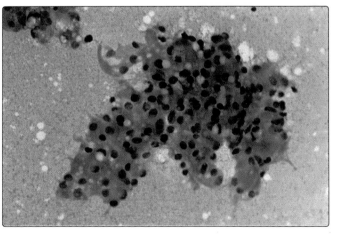

Fig. 43.82   Smear. Metastatic renal carcinoma. Cytoplasmic vacuoles are characteristic, but a similar picture can be seen in haemangioblastoma. (H&E × HP)

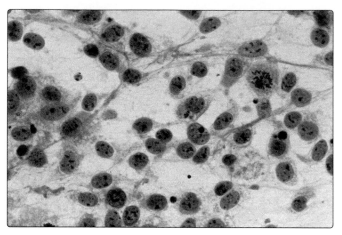

Fig. 43.83 Smear. Nasopharyngeal carcinoma. These can closely resemble pituitary gland tumours. (H&E × HP)

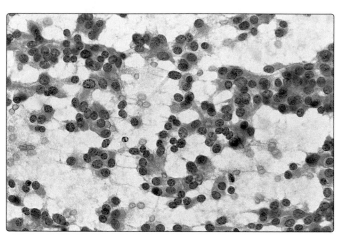

Fig. 43.85 Smear. Paraganglioma. The cells have regularly shaped nuclei, surrounded by moderate amounts of finely granular cytoplasm and they tend to form small clumps. (H&E × HP)

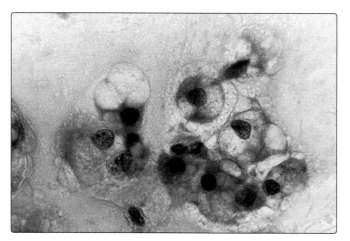

Fig. 43.84 Smear. Chordoma. The physaliferous cells with vacuolated cytoplasm are easily recognized. Chondrosarcoma can produce a similar picture. (H&E × HP)

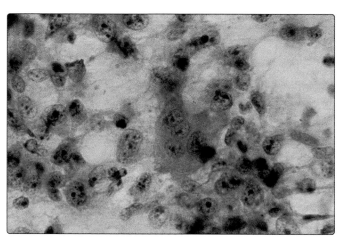

Fig. 43.86 Smear. Osteosarcoma. Tumour giant cells are usually obvious and provide a guide to the nature of the neoplasm, but the smear is not a reliable technique for diagnosing tumours of bone. (H&E × HP)

mucinous material. The connective tissue mucin is PAS positive but not diastase resistant. Mitotic figures are uncommon but pleomorphic variants occur occasionally. Chordomas may contain chondroid and chondrosarcoma produces a similar picture.

Paraganglioma

Paragangliomas derived from the glomus jugulare may extend into the posterior cranial fossa and rarely occur in the region of the cauda equina or intradural lumbo-sacral nerve roots. The cells have regularly shaped round nuclei surrounded by fine granular cytoplasm: recognition requires considerable experience and a high index of suspicion (Fig. 43.85). The cells often form small clusters. They stain positively for a variety of neuronal markers such as chromogranin, synaptophysin and somatostatin and

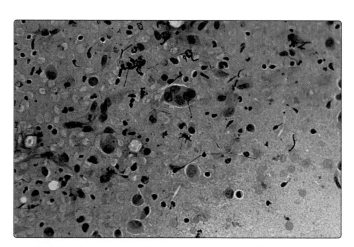

Fig. 43.87 Smear. Eosinophilic granuloma showing histiocytes and mixed inflammatory cell types. (H&E × LP) (Courtesy of Dr J M Mackenzie, Liverpool UK)

electron microscopy may demonstrate neurosecretory granules and microtubules.

Lesions of bone

Osteosarcoma is uncommon in the skull, although there is an increased incidence in Paget's disease and following radiotherapy. Osteoclasts and multinucleate giant cells are easily recognized (Fig. 43.86) and are useful in assessing the potential nature of the problem, but the smear should not be used alone as a method of diagnosing bone tumours. A variety of bone lesions may come to the attention of the neurosurgeon and they require careful assessment of sections, clinical history, site and radiological features.

Eosinophilic granuloma is a benign lesion affecting the skull in both children and adults, mainly before the age of 30. Large histiocytes and inflammatory cells, amongst which there are often some eosinophils, are easily recognized (Fig. 43.87). The histiocytes have folded and indented nuclei with small nucleoli. There is often an occasional mitotic figure and bi- or multinucleate histiocytes may be seen.

References

1 Quincke H. *Uber Hydrocephalus*. Berlin: Klin Wochenschr, 1891; **28**: 548

2 Grunze H, Spriggs Al. *History of Clinical Cytology*, 2nd edn. G-I-T Verlag: Giebeler, 1983; 81–85

3 Dudgeon L S, Barrett N R. The examination of fresh tissue by the wet-film method. *Br J Surg* 1934; **22**: 4

4 Glanz M J, Cole B F, Glanz L K *et al*. Cerebrospinal fluid cytology in patients with cancer; minimizing false-negative results. *Cancer* 1998; **82**: 733–739

5 van Oostenbrugge R J, Arends J W, Bucholtz R, Twijnsta A. Are polylysine coated slides useful? *Acta Cytol* 1997; **41**: 1510–1512

6 Preissig S H, Buhaug I. Corpora amylacea in cerebrospinal fluid: a source of diagnostic error. *Acta Cytol* 1978; **22**: 511–514

7 Fowler M, Carter R F. Acute pyogenic meningitis probably due to Acanthamoeba sp: a preliminary report. *BMJ* 1965; **2**: 740

8 Hamilton S R, Gupta P K, Marshall M E *et al*. Cerebrospinal fluid cytology in histiocytic proliferative disorders. *Acta Cytol* 1982; **26**: 22–28

9 Evans A E, Craig M. CNS involvement in children with acute leukaemia. *Cancer* 1964; **17**: 256

10 Evans A E, Gilbert E S, Zandstra R. The increasing incidence of central nervous system leukaemia in children. *Cancer* 1970; **26**: 404

11 Sindern E, Burghardt F, Voigtmann R, Malin J P. Cerebrospinal fluid cytology in granulocytic sarcoma with meningeal extension but without bone marrow involvement. *J Neurol* 1994; **241**: 320–322

12 Herman T S, Hammond N, Jones S E *et al*. Involvement of the central nervous system by non-Hodgkin's lymphoma. The Southwest Oncology Group experience. *Cancer* 1979; **43**: 390–397

13 Rhodes C H, Glantz L, Lekos A *et al*. A comparison of polymerase chain reaction examination of cerebrospinal fluid and conventional cytology in the diagnosis of lymphomatous meningitis. *Cancer* 1996; **77**: 543–548

14 Aisenberg A C, Long J C. Lymphocyte surface characteristics in malignant lymphoma. *Am J Med* 1975; **58**: 300–306

15 Russell D S, Rubinstein L J. *Pathology of Tumours of the Nervous System*, Revised by: Rubinstein L J., 5th edn. London: Arnold, 1989

16 Gonzalez-Vitale J C, Garcia-Bunuel R. Meningeal carcinomatosis. *Cancer* 1976; **37**: 2906–2911

17 Schmidt R M. Cytological investigations of the cerebrospinal fluid in secondary brain tumours. *Schweizer Arch Neurol Psychiat* 1980; **127**: 233–236

18 Wolf A L, Adcock L L, Hackiya J T, Klassen A. Choriocarcinoma with brain metastases. *Cancer* 1986; **57**: 1432

19 Balhuizen J C, Bots G T A M, Schaberg A, Bosman F T. Value of cerebrospinal fluid cytology for the diagnosis of the malignancies in the central nervous system. *J Neurosurg* 1978; **48**: 747–753

20 Naylor B. Cytological study of intracranial fluids. *Acta Cytol* 1961; **5**: 198–202

21 Kamiya M, Tateyama H, Fujiyoshi Y *et al*. Cerebrospinal fluid cytology in immature teratoma of the central nervous system. *Acta Cytol* 1991; **35**: 757–760

22 Ito U, Inaba Y. Cerebrospinal fluid after subarachnoid haemorrhage. *J Neurosurg* 1979; **51**: 352–354

23 Hamilton S R, Gupta P K, Marshall M E *et al*. Cerebrospinal fluid cytology in histiocytic proliferative disorders. *Acta Cytol* 1982; **26**: 22–28

24 von Herbay A, Ditton H J, Schuhmacher F, Maiwald M. Whipple's disease: staging and monitoring by cytology and polymerase chain reaction analysis of cerebrospinal fluid. *Gastoenterol* 1997; **113**: 434–441

25 Gondos B, King E B. Cerebrospinal fluid cytology: diagnostic accuracy and comparison of different techniques. *Acta Cytol* 1976; **20**: 542–547

26 Glass J P, Melamed M R, Chernik N L, Posner J B. Malignant cells in cerebrospinal fluid (CSF): the meaning of a positive CSF cytology. *Neurol* 1979; **29**: 1369–1375

27 Olsen M E, Chernik N L, Posner J B. Infiltration of the leptomeninges by systemic cancer: a clinical and pathological study. *Arch Neurol* 1974; **30**: 122–137

28 Borowitz M J, Bigner S H, Johnston W W. Diagnostic problems in the cytologic evaluation of cerebrospinal fluid for lymphoma and leukemia. *Acta Cytol* 1981; **25**: 665–674

29 Kernohan J W, Mabon R F, Svien H J, Adson A W. Symposium on a new and simplified classification of gliomas. *Proc Mayo Clin* 1949; **24**: 71–75

30 Eisenhardt L, Cushing H. Diagnosis of intracranial tumours by supravital technique. *Am J Pathol* 1930; **6**: 541–552

31 Russell D S, Krayenbuhl H, Cairns H. The wet film technique in the histological diagnosis of intracranial tumours; a rapid method. *J Pathol Bacteriol* 1937; **45**: 501–505

32 Liwnic B H, Masukawa T, Henderson K. Thin needle aspiration cytology of intracranial lesions: a review of 50 cases. *Acta Cytol* 1982; **26**: 779–786

33 Marshall L F, Adams H, Doyle D, Graham D I. The histological accuracy of the smear technique for neurosurgical biopsies. *J Neurosurg* 1973; **39**: 82–88

34 Berkeley B B, Adams J H, Doyle D, Graham D I, Harper C G. The smear technique in the diagnosis of neurosurgical biopsies. *NZ Med J* 1978; **87**: 12–15

35 Smith C M L, Laing R W. A useful technique for improving the diagnostic yield from single stereotactic biopsies of brain. *Neuropathol and Appl Neurobiol* 1990; **16**: 529

44

The eye

Marigold Curling*

Introduction

The eye and its adnexal tissues are amongst the least common sites in the body to be subjected to cytological investigation and even in specialist units requests for such procedures are not frequent. This creates particular problems for ophthalmologists and for cytopathologists requiring close cooperation to ensure that sampling and interpretation are both optimal. However, accessibility and the wide diversity of lesions, as well as the difficulty of tissue biopsies meant that the eye is becoming one of the most suitable organs for the practical use of diagnostic cytology in specialist hands[1].

Some of the techniques of sampling differ from those in other organs because the anatomy of the globe and its surrounding tissues pose special problems for harvesting specimens. Additional problems can arise because many pathologists, including cytologists, are unfamiliar with the range of ocular inflammatory and neoplastic conditions, which may be encountered. The paucity of references in the literature reflects these factors.

This chapter will describe the normal anatomy of the eye, the methods of sampling and the role of cytology in the investigative sequence. The pathological processes in the ocular tissues will then be discussed in relation to the cytological findings.

Anatomy of the globe and adnexa

Ocular and adnexal structures (Fig. 44.1) are predominantly derived from the surface ectoderm and neuroectoderm. The neural crest is thought to contribute most of the mesenchyme of head and neck and is a major component of the eye, true mesenchymal structures being limited to the vessels and extraocular muscles.

Skin

Cytological examination of the skin of the eyelids does not differ from that performed elsewhere, although the high level of exposure to actinic radiation confers an increased risk of development of squamous and basal cell carcinomas and malignant melanomas. This increased incidence is not confined to the pale-skinned races.

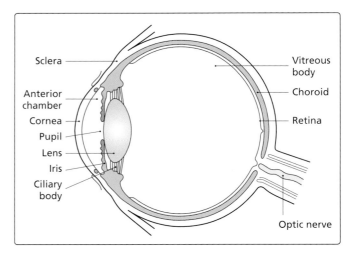

Fig. 44.1 Diagram representing principal parts of the eye.

Conjunctiva

The inner surface of the lids is lined by conjunctiva, derived from surface epithelium. The conjunctival epithelium is of non-keratinizing stratified columnar type, lubricated by goblet cells lying among the epithelial cells. The secretions of the major lacrimal serous glands and Meibomian sebaceous glands also contribute to lubrication, as do the minor glands, producing mucus and serous fluid. These glands and goblet cells all maintain hydration of the cornea and conjunctiva by producing the tear film. This surface film consists of an outer layer of lipid and an inner mucous layer, separated by an aqueous phase[2].

Lack of serous secretions in conditions such as Sjögren's disease, affecting the lacrimal glands, leads to surface drying and keratinization with squamous metaplastic transformation of the mucus producing epithelium. Loss of goblet cells is also a feature of the xerophthalmia associated with vitamin A deficiency. Impression cytology, described below, was first used on a large scale to screen for the effects of this deficiency[3].

The conjunctiva is described as palpebral when lining the lids and bulbar across the surface of the globe. The caruncle is a transformation or collision zone and as such may contain both skin and conjunctival elements.

*The authors gratefully acknowledge their debt to the late Alison McCarthy, whose contribution to the previous edition of this chapter provided a substantial basis for this revised edition.

Orbit

The bony lateral and medial orbital walls, together with the floor and roof contain the globe, lacrimal glands and fibro-fatty connective tissue. Within the cone formed by the extraocular muscles lie the optic nerve and blood supply to the eye. The orbit also contains ganglia and the branches of the cranial nerves and vessels supplying the extraocular muscles. Extension of disease processes within the sinuses can involve the orbit.

Sclera and cornea

The walls of the globe consist of the outer tough collagen and elastic tissue of the sclera, which is continuous with the clear cornea and the uvea. The uvea consists of richly vascularized pigmented choroid and more anteriorly, the ciliary body and iris. Within these structures lies the inverted erstwhile outpouching of neuroectoderm, which forms, on its inner surface, the neuroretina and on its outer surface the retinal pigment epithelium (RPE).

The sclera is relatively avascular although supplied by a network of small vessels within the episclera. The vascular choroid sustains the RPE. The limbus, which is at the junction between the sclera and the cornea, where there are no goblet cells, is the site of a circular blood supply, which maintains the clear avascular cornea. Corneal epithelial cells are replenished by epithelial stem cells at the limbus, which grow centripetally in a vortex-like fashion. The stroma and posterior epithelium, known as the corneal endothelium, are derived from the neural crest, as are the lining cells of the trabecular mesh-work in the drainage angle.

Anterior chambers, iris and ciliary body

The anterior chamber, which is accessible to paracentesis, is formed by the concave surface of the posterior cornea, which is lined by corneal endothelium, and by corneal endothelium, and by the anterior border of the iris. The iris also has three distinct layers, the anterior border and stroma deriving from the neural crest and the posterior epithelium and sphincter muscle from the neuroectoderm. These latter structures are formed from the tip of the invaginated outgrowth of the neuroectoderm; behind the iris lies the ciliary body with its muscles and ligaments, which controls movement of the lens.

Both the iris and the ciliary body have a pigmented epithelium derived from the neuroectodermal cup. The non-pigmented ciliary body epithelium is radially arranged as ciliary processes and produces aqueous humour. This maintains intraocular pressure in the anterior chambers, the aqueous flowing through the pupil and draining out through the iridocorneal angle. Accommodative movement of the lens is achieved by the ciliary muscles and suspensory ligaments.

Lens and vitreous

The lens arises from surface epithelium and consists of an anterior single layered epithelium, thick basement membrane and a collagenous nucleus of fibres.

The posterior chamber of the eye also contains about 4 ml of vitreous gel, which is usually avascular and contains very few cells, most of which produce the collagens and glycosaminoglycans which make up this translucent structure. A few macrophages may be present, but acute or chronic inflammatory cells should be regarded as abnormal.

Retina

The retina is part of the central nervous system and there is a blood-retinal barrier analogous to the blood-brain barrier. The maintenance of the photoreceptors is largely carried out by the RPE, which is itself supplied by the choriocapillaries. Waste products from phagocytosis of rod outer segments are sequestered in Bruch's basement membrane, which thickens with age. Muller cells and amacrine cells support and sustain the bipolar and ganglion cells that transmit impulses towards the brain. The axons from the ganglion cells pass in the optic nerve, surrounded by myelin sheaths proximal to the lamina cribrosa. The nerve itself is surrounded by meninges.

Choroid

The choroid contains a complex network of fenestrated vessels, which supply the outer retina and RPE with blood via the ciliary arteries. These vessels are supported in a fibrous stroma, interdigitated with dendritic melanocytes derived from the neural crest.

Sampling methods

The globe and its adnexa can be sampled in a variety of ways:

- ▶ Skin: scraping or fine needle aspiration (FNA)
- ▶ Cornea or conjunctiva: brushing, scraping, impression cytology
- ▶ The aqueous: paracentesis
- ▶ Iris and ciliary body: FNA
- ▶ The vitreous: aspiration during vitrectomy and washout
- ▶ Retina and choroid: biopsy or FNA

The orbital structures may also in some cases be accessible to FNA, bearing in mind the complexity of the anatomy and the risk of morbidity.

Open biopsy through a lateral orbitotomy may be the surgeon's preferred method of obtaining diagnostic material. Such is the case at Moorfields Eye Hospital, particularly with intraconal masses, while at St Bartholomew's Hospital, where orbital cases are rarer, FNA of intraocular masses is only performed if the mass is so posterior that it is difficult to biopsy.

Types of sampling and methods of preparation
Scraping

Lesions involving the skin, conjunctiva, and to the lesser extent, the cornea, are amenable to this form of harvesting. Scraping the cornea and conjunctiva requires local anaesthesia, but the eyelid may be scraped without. The lesions are scraped gently, removing a piece of tissue with a small platinum spatula (Swedish Dissector) or the blunt side of a scalpel blade.

If the laboratory is close to hand or the patient can attend the laboratory in person, the first slide can be stained with 0.5% methylene blue and a rapid diagnosis made. This slide can be dropped into 74% alcohol and decolourized and fixed for subsequent Papanicolaou staining.

This method should be used as the standard procedure with all basal and squamous carcinomas of the eyelid to give as rapid a preliminary report as possible so that definitive surgery and plastic reconstruction can be planned. The importance of the methylene blue stain is to identify the presence of intercellular bridges as a method of distinguishing squamous cells from basal cells. These bridges are not stained well by the Papanicolaou technique and even with methylene blue stain, the bridges fade quickly (15–20 min).

If this rapid diagnosis is not possible, the material is spread on to a number of slides and then fixed, some by air-drying, and others using a cytological fixative spray. It is important to spray from at least 12 inches away so that cells are not pushed to the edge of the slide. The slide is then stained by a conventional Papanicolaou method. If immunocytochemical analysis might be required, the slides should be fixed in methanol.

Rapid air-drying is essential and ensured by rapidly waving the slide until it is dry. These slides can be stained with Diff-Quik stain (Baxter-Dade AG), a fast fixation and staining technique requiring approximately ten dips in each component of the stain. This method compares favourably with May-Grünwald-Giemsa (MGG) and other Romanowsky staining methods and is our method of choice for the demonstration of bacteria and diagnosis of lymphomas, while the fixed Papanicolaou stained slides are superior for the diagnosis of epithelial or melanocytic lesions.

Impression cytology of the conjunctiva

Impression cytology[4] involves pressing a 2×6 mm piece of cellulose acetate Millipore (grade II) filter paper on to the surface of the conjunctiva, which need not be anaesthetized, using a pair of forceps (Fig. 44.2). The paper is gently pressed down with a glass rod if necessary. The tear film is gently mopped using a tissue before the sample is taken. After sampling, the paper is fixed in glacial acetic acid, 37% formaldehyde, absolute ethanol and distilled water. The resulting sample (Fig. 44.3) can then be stained using PAS/Papanicolaou stains and mounted in DePeX (BDH)[5]. The technique has also been used on the cornea[6]. Training in interpreting these samples is necessary and effective[7].

Conjunctival brush biopsy

This relatively underused technique was described[8] using a small cytobrush (Cytobrush-S, Medscand, Malmo, Sweden) after topical anaesthesia. A gentle brushing movement is

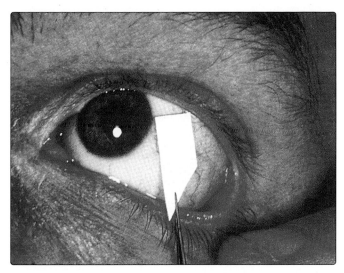

Fig. 44.2 Impression cytology of the eye. A strip of millipore paper is being applied to the unanaesthetized conjunctiva.

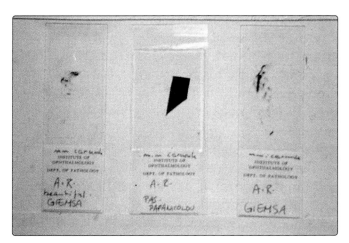

Fig. 44.3 Conventional exfoliative cytology preparations and millipore impression cytology slide.

used to dislodge cells, which are then collected, using the Millipore filter technique (SC filters, 8.0 μm pore size). The cells are collected into buffered Hank's solution, fixed using 95% ethanol and stained by the Papanicolaou method. Its protagonists argue that in contrast to impression cytology, cells of all three types, epithelial (polygonal), basal and mucus producing cells, are obtained. On the other hand, pigment-containing cells can be harvested from patients with melanotic lesions when impression cytology is used[5].

Fine needle aspiration (FNA)

Most aspirators use their own adaptation of a standard technique similar to that used at other sites. FNA has been reported as being of diagnostic use in the iris[9], retina[10] and choroid[11–16] and in the orbit[17,18]. It has also been used in the differential diagnosis of inflammatory conditions[19,20].

FNA of anterior lesions is performed at the slit lamp[9] or using ultrasound guidance[14] after retrobulbar or peribulbar anaesthesia. In the case of iris aspiration, a sterile 26 or 30 gauge needle is inserted into the anterior chamber and the lesion is 'vacuum cleaned'. In cases of suspected retinoblastoma[21], anterior chamber aspiration is no longer used in the UK due to the risk of spread along the needle track of this notoriously 'sticky' tumour. The unusual iatrogenic access to lymphatics provided by FNA may cause spread to orbit or cervical lymph nodes[22]. However anterior chamber aspirates are still performed in the USA and other countries in spite of this risk[23]. FNA is in general a very powerful and flexible investigative tool, as elsewhere in the body[24]. There are special factors in its use at differing sites in the eye.

Orbital FNA

When orbital FNA is performed, a slightly larger needle of 21–23 gauge can be used, attached to a 20 ml disposable syringe in a pistol grip (Cameco, Sweden) as described by Tijl and Koorneef[18]. This group reported 81% accuracy with histopathological control, with no false positives, but in their series of 46 cases, they reported five false negatives. They had no needle track dissemination.

Orbital FNA can usually be performed without anaesthetic. The needle is introduced through the upper or lower lid in the lateral or medial quadrants, rather than in the superior or inferior quadrants. Ultrasound guidance is occasionally necessary. Usually, the lesion has been accurately defined by palpation and computerized tomography. The most common lesions to be sampled are malignant neoplasms thought to be metastatic or extending directly into the orbit.

Choroidal FNA

Choroidal FNA[25] requires a longer needle such as a Microlance orange 0.5 × 23 using a 10 ml syringe without a holder or a short extension (Mediplus) so that the surgeon has both hands to place and manipulate the needle while the assistant controls the syringe and aspiration. With experience it is usually possible to feel when the needle is in the lesion and then to move the needle very gently within the lesion. At this stage the needle should be rotated as the cutting edge will also act by breaking up the tissue and some of the material will pass up the needle by capillary attraction alone[26,27]. Gentle aspiration is then started and the needle moved in and out of the lesion. Aspiration is maintained until material just enters the syringe, then the pressure is released and the needle extracted from the lesion. If the biopsy site is superficial, the patient can be asked to apply some pressure with a cotton wool pad to prevent bruising whilst the clinician makes the slide preparations.

The preparation is dependent on the quantity aspirated. If sufficient material is obtained, slides may be prepared by placing the specimen directly on to the slide and spreading this as in the preparation of a blood film. If only a little

material is obtained, the method of choice is to dilute with 1 ml of 3.8% sodium citrate[28] to prevent clotting and to make cytospin preparations. When possible several slides should be made to allow the use of special stains.

Intraocular tumours and FNA

The role of FNA in the diagnosis of intraocular tumours has been evaluated in several papers[12,16,29–33] since the inception by Jakobiec and colleagues in the 1970s[14,15]. Most authors are convinced of its reliability as a technique in terms of adequacy of sampling, but accept that limitations lie predominantly with the interpretation of the material. In the majority of cases, the differential diagnosis of uveal lesions in adults likely to be biopsied, lies between malignant melanoma and metastatic carcinoma[34], neither of which is likely to pose a problem to an experienced cytopathologist, but may to those who are unfamiliar with ocular work.

A much greater likelihood of misdiagnosis or missed diagnosis occurs when material from children is being reviewed. A particular problem encountered in the eye is the differential diagnosis of retinoblastoma (Fig. 44.4), and the possibility of confusion with inflammatory disease or other neoplasms, such as medulloepithelioma. This subject is further reviewed below.

The second problem encountered by some investigators is the risk of seeding along the needle track although some centres still practise this technique. The need for caution when dealing with retinoblastoma has already been mentioned and the fact that FNA should no longer be used. Some authors[35] have reported experimental data suggesting that there is a risk of seeding of melanoma cells along a track if needles greater than 25 gauge are used. The Shields, husband and wife team from Philadelphia, suggest that follow-up incisional biopsy in cases of equivocal FNA of iris

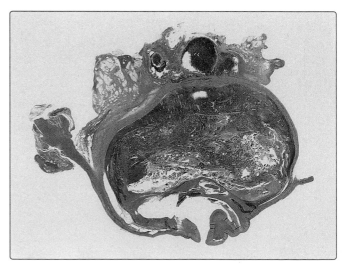

Fig. 44.4 A histological section through an enucleated eye containing retinoblastoma. (H&E × LP) (Courtesy of Dr I Cree, London, UK)

lesions should also be performed through clear cornea. They advise that biopsy-proven malignant tumours should be resected by enucleation within 24 hours of biopsy[36,37]. Others allow longer, but at most a week[16].

There is a need to exercise caution with any biopsy technique, not all of the iris or other uveal melanomas diagnosed in the Barts-Moorfields oncology service are treated by enucleation, even if FNA or open biopsy has been used, and in our experience this type of dissemination is very rare. We have not encountered an increased risk of dissemination despite using 23 gauge needles for FNA and would suggest that seeding into a scar after biopsy is commoner.

FNA has also been used for non-malignant conditions such as juvenile xanthogranuloma, epithelial down-growth and iris cysts[9,38-40]. We have recently seen a case of leiomyoma of the ciliary body, which we were able to diagnose in this way.

Diagnostic vitrectomy and vitreous aspiration

Pars plana vitrectomy has allowed aspiration biopsy of tumours within the vitreous and is especially useful in distinguishing between malignant lymphomas and uveitis[41].

The technique can also be therapeutic, clearing the visual axis of cells and debris. Aspiration of the vitreous has also been used in diagnosis of other tumours such as medulloepithelioma of the ciliary body[42,43] and can allow for the diagnosis of amyloidosis or retinal pathology such as acute retinal necrosis.

The technique of closed pars plana vitrectomy was first described by Machemer et al. in a series of papers in the early 1970s[44,45]. It has been refined to allow for removal of haemorrhage, membranes and debris from the vitreous and lens in addition to providing material for diagnosis[19,20].

The material is collected through small incisions in the pars plana, through which a light port for the fibreoptic illuminator is passed, together with a vitrectomy cutting instrument which has an integral suction component and an infusion cannula to keep the eye expanded. Methods of processing the material vary but most authors advocate the use of cytocentrifugation with or without the use of a millipore filter[20,42].

We routinely perform microbiological, cytological and histopathological examination of the washings collected within the chamber attached to the sterile outcome. After material has been collected for microbiological assessment, our preference is for immediate fixation, before cytocentrifugation, to prevent overgrowth of the contents of the chamber by exogenous bacteria or fungi, which can thrive in the highly nutritive vitreous sample. It is important to be aware that fixed vitreous has a peculiar grainy appearance, especially if MGG staining is used, and can elicit a false positive diagnosis of coccal infection.

After the addition of 10% formalin to the contents of the chamber, cytocentrifugation at 650 rpm for 5 minutes is followed by aspiration of the phase above the pellet, smearing of the aspirate and the sedimented material is collected to obtain a small block for histology. Formalin fixation allows for subsequent immunohistochemical analysis and is particularly useful when a diagnosis of intraocular lymphoma is suspected.

On rare occasions, the author has prepared specimens for electron microscopy after glutaraldehyde fixation. The most useful of these led to diagnosis of a retinoblastoma within a mass of necrotic material thought to represent an inflammatory lesion but in which the remnants of cilia-like structures pointed to the correct diagnosis.

Other authors employ a similar technique but use cytocentrifugation followed by alcohol fixation for the smears, and alcohol and formalin fixation for the histology block[27,29]. Occasionally the vitrectomy specimen may include an obvious fragment of retina. It is our practice not to proceed straight to cytocentrifugation in such a case but to attempt to process this separately, orientating it correctly[46]. Retinal membranes can also be processed from this stage[47].

Cytological diagnosis of ocular lesions

The diagnosis of lesions amenable to cytological identification will be discussed in the following pages according to the tissue of origin or their anatomical site.

Eyelids and surrounding skin
Infections

Viral disease is not usually diagnosed by cytology alone, but it is possible to identify pox virus induced *molluscum contagiosum* by eosinophilic, rounded cytoplasmic inclusions; similarly virus induced *verruca vulgaris* and the effects of the *herpes simplex viruses 1 and 2* can be diagnosed by cytological techniques, as described in Chapter 39.

Benign skin lesions

Benign cysts and tumours of the epidermis and dermis and their malignant counterparts resemble those of the skin elsewhere. *Pilomatrixoma* can be a problematic diagnosis in the lid and surrounding skin, but cytology usually shows the typical admixture of sheets of squamous cells with an inflammatory response of histiocytes and foreign body giant cells[48]. The sheets of 'shadow' or 'ghost' cells that are the most diagnostic feature for the histopathologist may not be as much in evidence in cytological preparations.

Malignant tumours
Basal cell carcinoma

Basal cell carcinomas (BCCs) are the commonest malignant lesion of the eyelid and the cytodiagnostic method of choice is by scraping the lesion as already described. Basal cell carcinomas usually occur singly, in patients who have had a long exposure to sunlight and are commoner in the lower lids. They can be multiple in patients with xeroderma pigmentosum. Because of their proximity to the eye it is particularly important that they should be diagnosed early. Although slow growing and unlikely to metastasize, they can cause considerable local destruction. Exenteration of the orbit and loss of the globe has been the necessary treatment to control the disease in neglected cases.

There are several types of BCC, with varying clinical appearances. The commonest is the ulcerative form, which appears as a nodule with an irregular raised white pearly border and an ulcerated centre, giving rise to the name 'rodent ulcer', from its supposed resemblance to rat bites (Fig. 44.5). Frequently the lesion spreads out widely in the dermis. The clinical appearance of other types may include increased pigmentation or covering by an attenuated epithelium.

The material produced by scraping appears as white or translucent, almost fatty material, which spreads easily on the slide and separates into small fragments (Fig. 44.6). This appearance is so characteristic that it is almost

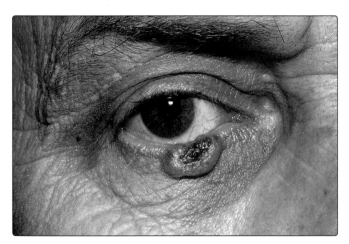

Fig. 44.5   A basal cell carcinoma of the lower eyelid showing the raised rolled edge and central ulceration. (Courtesy of Mr K Barton, London, UK)

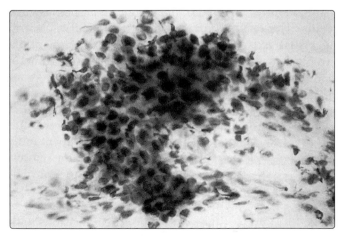

Fig. 44.6   Basal cell carcinoma of the eyelid. Scrape cytology reparation, showing characteristic easily spread clumps of cells obtained by this method. Note the crowding and hyperchromasia of the nuclei with scant cytoplasm. (scrape cytology, Papanicolaou × HP)

possible to make the diagnosis on the macroscopic appearance of the slide before staining.

Cytological findings

▶ Groups of crowded basal cells
▶ Smooth contours with peripheral palisading of basal cells
▶ Regular but hyperchromatic nuclei with granular chromatin

Examination under the microscope of the wet Papanicolaou stained slide shows that the small fragments seen macroscopically are clusters of tightly packed basal cells. These cells are usually arranged in one layer with palisading and a smoother outline. The cytological picture is very similar to that seen in the histological section.

The cells themselves show monomorphic nuclei with hyperchromatic, rather fine granular chromatin. Sometimes there are nucleoli. Mitosis is rare except in rapidly growing tumours, where there may also be a little pleomorphism, but this is not marked. In cases where marked pleomorphism is seen it is important to ensure that the lesion is not a squamous carcinoma. In the wet methylene blue stained film it is particularly easy to see the intercellular bridges and if present to make the diagnosis of squamous cell carcinoma. The bridges are rarely seen in the fixed preparations. This demonstrates the value of looking at the wet stain, although the bridges fade rapidly within 15–20 minutes even with methylene blue staining.

In the Papanicolaou permanent slides of basal cell carcinoma, the diagnostic feature is the intense hyperchromasia of the cells in their tightly packed clusters. If the first scrape only shows a few single cells, the diagnosis of BCC should not be made since single basaloid cells from a naevus can resemble cells from a basal cell carcinoma. The scrape should be repeated in the hope of obtaining a diagnostic slide showing typical clumps of cells.

Squamous carcinoma

Squamous carcinomas of the eyelid are much less common than basal carcinomas and little is known about predisposition, but like BCCs, they occur on exposed surfaces and are commoner in xeroderma pigmentosum. The clinical appearance is of an indurated ulcer with a raised irregular border. Scraping is frequently quite painless; however the lesions usually bleed easily.

Cytological findings

▶ Cell dissociation is prominent
▶ Pleomorphism of cells and nuclei
▶ Intercellular bridges are visible
▶ Well-differentiated tumours show marked keratinization

Scraping usually produces numerous single cells due to the lack of cohesion. The cytological appearances vary according to the degree of differentiation. In poorly-

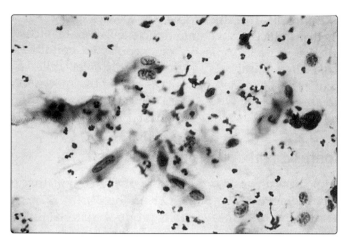

Fig. 44.7 Squamous cell carcinoma of the eyelid. High power showing keratinization and atypical cells with altered nuclear/cytoplasmic ratio. (Papanicolaou × HP)

differentiated lesions they may occasionally be mistaken for BCCs, but the larger vesicular nuclei, prominent nucleoli, pleomorphism and lack of polarity, and most importantly in rapid methylene blue stained scrapes the presence of intercellular bridges should make it easy to reach the correct diagnosis.

In well-differentiated squamous carcinoma (Fig. 44.7), the diagnosis is much easier, particularly on Papanicolaou staining. Some of the cells may be highly keratinized and the cytoplasm have an orangeophilic appearance. The cells vary in size and shape and have differing amounts of cytoplasm, but also show an increase in the nuclear/cytoplasmic ratio. Viable nuclei have malignant features, but there are often degenerate forms, with dark hyperchromatic nuclei, and anucleate necrotic 'ghost' cells are almost always present.

Scrapes from squamous cell carcinomas almost always contain large numbers of white blood cells, mainly polymorphonuclear neutrophilic leucocytes. However, it is important to remember in the differential diagnosis that inflammatory ulcers will also have large numbers of these cells. At the healing edges of an ulcer the squamous cells are often active and slightly atypical, and occasional mitotic figures may even be seen. Clinically these inflammatory lesions do not usually look malignant and they are nearly always difficult to scrape unlike squamous carcinoma and are painful on scraping.

Sebaceous carcinoma

Tumours of the sebaceous glands, whether adenomas or carcinomas are rare. Unlike basal cell carcinomas[49] they favour the upper lid. They appear to be more malignant than similar tumours elsewhere. Sebaceous gland carcinoma, which can present on the skin surface or the conjunctival surface, arises from either the Meibomian glands or the glands of Zeiss. Misdiagnoses arise by clinical and pathological confusion with blepharitis or chalazion, a

much commoner granulomatous response to the liberated fatty contents of these glands, often accompanied by an acute inflammatory response.

A secondary misdiagnosis may occur by only appreciating the basal cell-like elements, thereby underestimating the amount of radiation that may be required to treat a sebaceous carcinoma. The tumour often spreads in a pagetoid fashion within the conjunctiva, but does so less commonly within the skin, although it may show junctional tropism. The cells show varying degrees of differentiation towards sebaceous glands and the lipid within them can often be demonstrated by oil red-O staining. Spread to the orbit can occur, and may then be misdiagnosed as a primary lacrimal gland tumour[26].

Malignant melanoma

The criteria for diagnosis of malignant melanoma are similar to those in the skin elsewhere (see Chapter 39), but primary malignant melanoma involving the skin of the eyelid is a very rare tumour despite the high level of actinic radiation to which it is exposed.

Other types of increased pigmentation include harbingers of disease elsewhere. Pigmentation of the eyelid margin occurring in association with primary conjunctival melanoma is an ominous clinical sign, although not always representing extension of the tumour. Patients with oculodermal melanocytosis may have intraocular uveal, or more unusually conjunctival melanomas but rarely have skin melanomas.

Dysplastic (atypical) naevi can occur in this region and patients with the inherited, generalized form of this lesion may also have an associated risk of increased incidence of intraocular and conjunctival melanomas (J A Newton; personal communication).

Conjunctiva and cornea
Infective and inflammatory lesions

The various techniques outlined in the Introduction can be used to diagnose a range of conditions, including viral infections[50,51] allergic rhinoconjunctivitis[52], and various chronic ocular surface disorders[53] and chlamydial infections (Fig. 44.8), some dermatological diseases such as *pemphigoid* and more specific lesions such as *vernal* and *ligneous conjunctivitis* and *keratoconjunctivitis sicca*[8,54,55]. The latter, with increased squamous metaplasia and decrease in goblet cells, can occur in a range of conditions, encompassing iatrogenic removal of the lacrimal gland, ageing and connective tissue disease, as well as overlapping with deficiency induced disease[56] such as xerophthalmia[57–59] and anorexia nervosa: self-inflicted starvation[60].

Specific features of interest are the large amounts of fibrin present in the deeper part of the scrape in ligneous conjunctivitis, a disease commoner in, but not confined to, young girls. A more superficial fibrin plaque can also develop in vernal conjunctivitis but there is also an increase

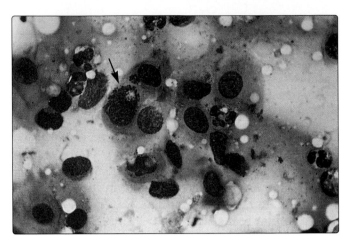

Fig. 44.8 Conjunctival scrape showing *Chlamydia trachomatis* inclusion bodies forming a dark granular cluster in the cytoplasm, partly surrounding the nucleus (arrow). (MGG × OI)

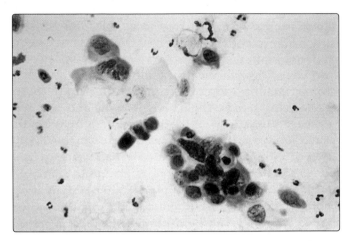

Fig. 44.9 *In situ* squamous carcinoma of the conjunctiva. Atypical squamous cells obtained by scrape cytology from anaesthetized conjunctiva. (Methylene blue × HP)

in goblet cells[61] accompanied by mast cells, basophils and eosinophils. This disease is particularly common in the Middle East and it is especially important to exclude potentially blinding TRIC chlamydial disease in these patients. Screening of MGG stained scrapes and, if relevant, monoclonal antibody staining against chlamydia is the most effective technique[29].

Conjunctival impression cytology can also be of value in thyroid associated eye disease[62]. Corneal inflammatory and infective lesions are commonly diagnosed by microbiology alone, but addition of cytology may be helpful in elucidating unusual infections, such as *actinomycosis, acanthamoebic keratitis*[63] or *blastomycosis*[64], especially when the organisms are superficial. A scrape may however, not be the most efficient way of making the diagnosis, since the acanthamoebae may have invaded much deeper than the trailing inflammatory exudate would lead one to believe. In refractory or elusive cases, a deep corneal biopsy with examination by calcofluor white or immunohistochemistry is indicated.

Keratinization of the cornea is always pathological, whether induced by vitamin deficiency[56], or climate, virus or as part of a dysplastic or neoplastic condition[65]. *Conjunctival metaplasia*, with ectopic goblet cells, can occur as part of a *choristoma*, or as part of the spectrum of disease associated with abnormalities on chromosome 11 and aniridia.

Conjunctival epithelial tumours

Cytological diagnosis of tumours of the conjunctiva includes diagnosis of premalignant *dysplastic squamous lesions*. Scrapes of these lesions produce material akin to that of intraepithelial squamous lesions elsewhere, with loss of polarity, nuclear enlargement, atypia and altered nuclear/cytoplasmic ratio (Fig. 44.9).

Infiltrating squamous carcinomas can occur at the limbus and can be diagnosed by the criteria described above as well as in the chapters on cervical cytology and skin (Chapters 30,

39). *Basal cell carcinomas* rarely, if ever, occur in the conjunctiva, although *mucoepidermoid carcinoma* may and can be diagnosed with the aid of periodic acid-Schiff staining. The presence of the normal conjunctival goblet cell population may give rise to problems of interpretation, as is also the case in conjunctival naevi, discussed below.

Occasional diagnostic problems arise with viral lesions within the conjunctiva. Human papillomavirus is present within these lesions and some evidence on incorporation of the more potentially malignant subtypes is accruing so that a long term link between subtypes and development of malignancy may be established in the near future, as has been the case with cervical neoplasia.

Conjunctival lymphomas

Lymphomas of the conjunctiva can occur within the conjunctival associated lymphoid tissue (CALT) and are similar to other mucosal associated lymphoid lesions elsewhere. Diagnosis is similar to that of other extranodal lymphomas (see Chapter 20) and below.

Conjunctival melanocytic tumours

Melanocytic primary tumours of the conjunctiva can be diagnosed by scrape cytology and impression cytology[66] as well as by histology. In *naevi*, the presence of large numbers of mucin containing goblet cells, sometimes aggregated into cysts by the proliferation of epithelium, may suggest a mucoepidermoid tumour to the unwary. These cystic downgrowths may also cause an apparent rapid increase in size in a pigmented lesion, leading to the clinical suspicion that melanoma has arisen within a naevus.

Although well described, *malignant melanoma* developing in a pre-existing naevus is an unusual sequence of events; most conjunctival melanomas either arise *de novo* or within the premalignant state known as primary *acquired melanosis with atypia*. Differentiation between this non-invasive lesion and overt malignant melanoma can be hazardous and initial

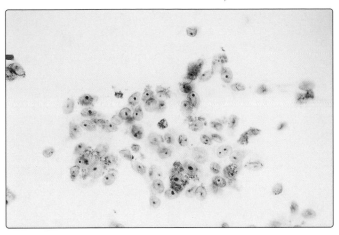

Fig. 44.10   Melanoma of the conjunctiva. Scrape cytology preparation of tumour cells. Predominantly plump spindle cells with melanin pigment. (Papanicolaou × LP)

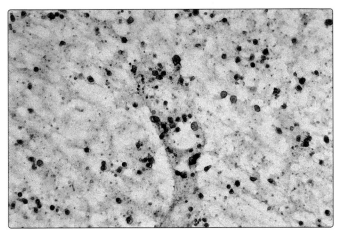

Fig. 44.12   Cytological preparation of melanoma cells, staining with immunocytochemistry HMB 45 a specific stain for melanoma. (HMB 45 × LP)

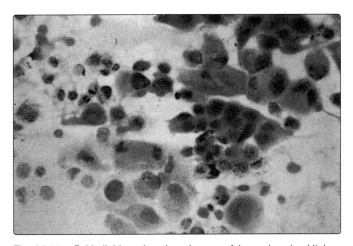

Fig. 44.11   Epithelioid amelanotic melanoma of the conjunctiva. High power view of plump epithelioid cells. A tumour such as this may require immunohistochemical confirmation using a panel of markers for melanocytic cells and negative results for cytokeratins. (Papanicolaou × HP)

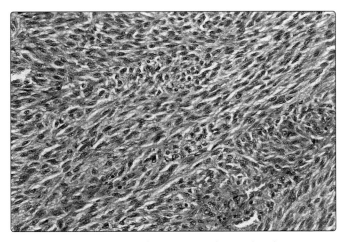

Fig. 44.13   Histopathology of a melanoma of the conjunctiva. (H&E × HP)

diagnosis is better performed using histology to delineate the lesion, although cytology may be useful in the follow-up of these patients[5].

Typically, melanoma cells are pleomorphic and tend to dissociate. They have a high nuclear/cytoplasmic ratio, rather eccentric nuclei and large prominent nucleoli. Melanin pigment is a diagnostic feature if present in the malignant cells (Fig. 44.10), but may not always be seen. *Amelanotic melanomas* occur and can be difficult to diagnose with certainty (Fig. 44.11); immunohistochemical confirmation showing positivity with a specific marker such as HMB 45 (Fig. 44.12). Figure 44.13 shows the histology of a melanoma.

Intraocular lesions

The cytological diagnosis of intraocular infections and of benign and malignant tumours arising within the eyeball is fraught with traps for the unwary. Appropriate early treatment is essential in these difficult cases if function of the eye is to be preserved. FNA sampling provides an excellent opportunity to achieve this. It is important to be aware of the diagnostic possibilities to be described, and some useful pointers to avoid misdiagnoses.

Anterior chamber infective and inflammatory lesions

Anterior chamber paracentesis has been used in the diagnosis of intraocular infections, coupled with microbiological investigations. Since the advent of HIV infection and the immunosuppression associated with the AIDS complex, previously rare intraocular infections are becoming commoner. FNA has been used to diagnose intraocular *aspergillosis* and *coccidiodomycosis*[27,29].

The acute inflammatory response engendered by bacterial and fungal infections can also be mimicked by release of lens proteins in the phacotoxic response and a more prolonged granulomatous inflammation can be seen in *phacoanaphylaxis* when both foreign body giant cells and epithelioid macrophages can be aspirated, sometimes in association with fragments of lens capsule and collagen.

Anterior chamber: tumours extending into the anterior chamber

In the past aspirates from the anterior chamber have been found to be useful in the diagnosis of retinoblastoma and other malignant tumours[10,21]. Anterior chamber aspirates in patients suspected of retinoblastoma should not be performed due to the risk of spreading the tumour. This must be stressed as the practice is still continued at some centres.

Similarly aspirates of the anterior chamber in cases of malignant melanoma may also lead to pigment-laden macrophages or even the melanoma cells becoming flushed into the anterior chamber and angle. Melanophages can usually be distinguished from hyperplastic pigment epithelial cells, derived from either the ciliary or iris pigment epithelial cells or from retinal pigment epithelium (RPE). RPE cells are typically cuboidal, with large individual melanin granules, whereas macrophages tend to have aggregates of melanin pigment present as clumps within lysosomes. Pigmented macrophages containing iron are seen in the anterior chamber and angle following intraocular haemorrhage, and are often accompanied by 'ghost' erythrocytes[10,21].

Grossniklaus's paper on iris FNA reviews the lesions that can be sampled by this technique[9], emphasizing the cytological differences between melanocytic lesions such as *aggressive iris naevi* and *melanomas* and *metastatic carcinomas*. In practice, without special stains such as S 100 and HMB 45, it can be difficult to distinguish between amelanotic melanoma and carcinoma, both at this site and in choroidal aspiration biopsies. Metastatic carcinoma, originating from the breast (Figs 44.14, 44.15), lung[13] or prostate (Fig. 44.16) is much commoner than either retinoblastoma or malignant melanoma, occurring in up to 30% of patients with disseminated carcinoma[67].

Metastatic neuroblastoma can occur within the eye and in the orbit[68] and may lead to diagnostic confusion with retinoblastomas[29]. In this case since the tumours share many markers, both being derived from primitive neuroectoderm, immunocytochemistry may not always be of use. However, cytogenetic evaluation looking for the specific chromosomal translocations common in neuroblastoma may be helpful, as is whole body imaging and search for a primary tumour. Identification of intraretinal binding protein and retinal S antigen may be of use in the identification of retinoblastoma. Flexner-Wintersteiner rosettes (Fig. 44.17) are more usually associated with retinoblastoma than neuroblastoma, but the Homer-Wright rosette is not specific. The most differentiated form, the fleurette, rarely can be aspirated. In most instances, clumps of primitive neuroectodermal cells

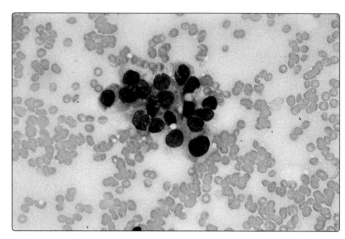

Fig. 44.14   Metastatic breast carcinoma. FNA cytological specimen obtained from a metastatic deposit in the choroid. (Giemsa × LP)

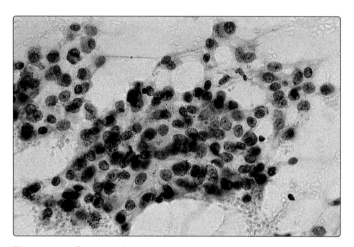

Fig. 44.15   Cytology of metastases from carcinoma of breast stained with immunocytological stains for epithelial cells Cam 5.2, which is positive. (Cam 5.2 × MP)

are the most numerous on aspiration from the anterior chamber or in vitreous taps (Figs 44.18, 44.19).

The rosette-like structures (Fig. 44.20) or primitive retinal anlages (Fig. 44.21) found in *medulloepitheliomas of the ciliary body* have occasionally proved difficult to interpret. Diagnostic confusion is less likely to occur in FNA of these ciliary body lesions if other stromal elements are aspirated as well. This is especially the case if they are heteroplastic elements such as cartilage or striated muscle[69]. Neuroretinal derivatives such as ganglion cells can also be seen (Fig. 44.22) in these ciliary body tumours, which can also have large numbers of epithelial cells derived from the non-pigmented part of the ciliary epithelium.

Melanocytic lesions of the iris include a range of variably aggressive naevi, which may grow to occlude the angle, leading to intractable glaucoma, without acquiring the potential to metastasize. Unlike true melanoma cells, the naevus cells from these lesions do not have prominent nucleoli. They may involve the iris stroma extensively as well as having plaque-like extensions across the face of the

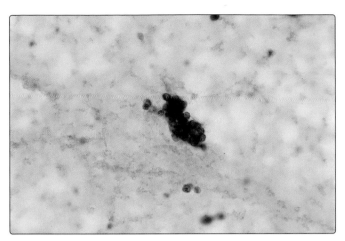

Fig. 44.16   Metastatic carcinoma. FNA of metastasis from primary prostatic adenocarcinoma stained with monoclonal antibody to prostatic specific antigen. (Immunoperoxidase × HP)

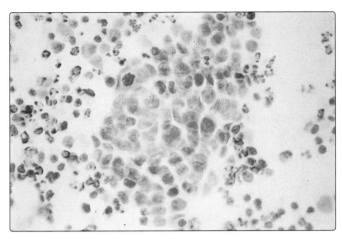

Fig. 44.19   Retinoblastoma. Undifferentiated primitive neuroectodermal cells from anterior chamber tap through clear cornea. Inflammatory cells may also be seen. (Papanicolaou × HP)

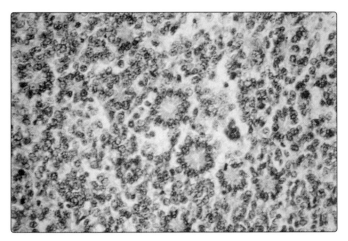

Fig. 44.17   Retinoblastoma. Histological section showing Flexner-Wintersteiner rosettes in moderately differentiated tumour. The primitive neuroectodermal cells are showing differentiation towards outer segments of photoreceptors, arranged along an external limiting membrane. (H&E × MP)

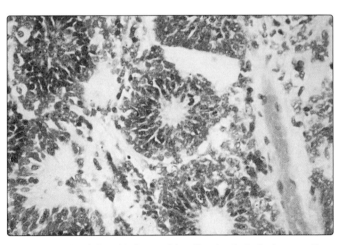

Fig. 44.20   Medulloepithelioma of the ciliary body. Retinal rosette-like structures separated by a primitive stroma. Histology section. (H&E × MP) (Courtesy of Dr A Deery, London, UK)

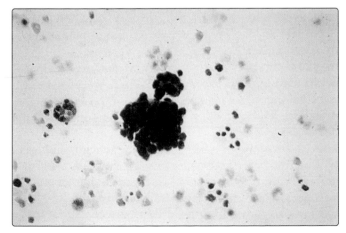

Fig. 44.18   Retinoblastoma. Cytology of vitreous aspirate showing clumps of primitive neuroectodermal cells amongst collagen strands. (H&E × LP)

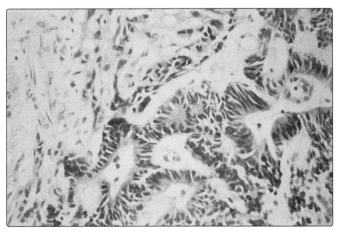

Fig. 44.21   Medulloepithelioma of the ciliary body. Histological section showing net-like areas of epithelial structures separated by stromal elements, both derived from the pluripotential cells of the outermost rim of the optic cup. (H&E × MP) (Courtesy of Dr A Deery, London, UK)

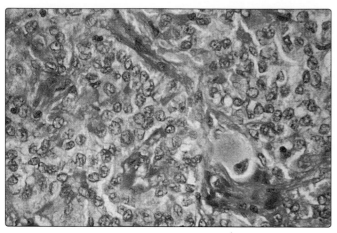

Fig. 44.22   Medulloepithelioma of the ciliary body. Retinal ganglion cells in similar tumour, presenting late in a 19-year-old girl. Most of these tumours are diagnosed in early or mid-childhood. (H&E × HP) (Courtesy of Dr A Deery, London, UK)

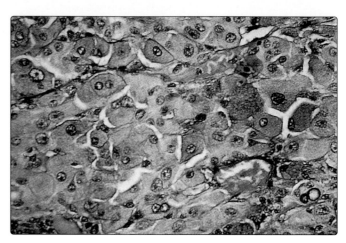

Fig. 44.24   Malignant melanoma of the choroid. Histology of high-grade epithelioid melanoma. (H&E × HP)

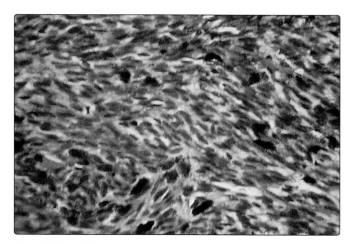

Fig. 44.23   Melanoma of the uvea. Histology showing low-grade spindle cell pigmented tumour. (H&E × MP)

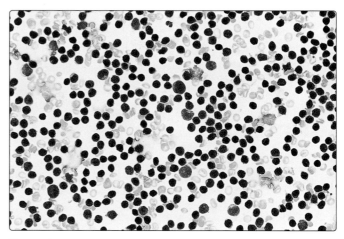

Fig. 44.25   Intraocular lymphoma. The cells here are unusually well preserved. This tumour was a B-cell lymphoma, associated with the production of a monoclonal kappa light chain. (Giemsa × MP)

iris. True melanomas, capable of metastasis, do occasionally occur within the iris and in addition, secondary involvement of the iris root from a tumour arising in the ciliary body can also occur.

FNA of *uveal, iris, choroidal* or *ciliary body melanomas*[32] may show spindle, epithelioid or mixed histological pattern[29] (Figs 44.23, 44.24). Occasionally lipoidal degeneration will lead to ballooned cells. All of these subtypes may metastasize first to the liver rather than to the lung or brain.

FNA may be used in the diagnosis of metastatic deposits[70] or to refute the diagnosis of metastasis of an adenocarcinoma and confirm the presence of a benign lesion such as a *Fuchs' adenoma*, a hyperplastic nodule arising from the non-pigmented cuboidal epithelium of the ciliary body. On aspiration, in addition to the cuboidal cells, abundant basement membrane extracellular matrix may be obtained. *Leiomyomas* arising from ectomesenchyme of

neural crest may also occur in the ciliary body but do not appear to occur within the iris (A. Garner; personal communication). Spindle cell lesions of the ciliary body are usually of melanocytic origin.

Intraocular *lymphomas* can be diagnosed by cytology (Figs 44.25–44.28), both by FNA and vitrectomy. These tumours may be preceded or accompanied by a reactive vitritis and sometimes there is involvement of the vitreous in the malignant process. This is especially true when the tumour is the large cell type of B-cell lymphoma, involving the retina and the brain. Uveal involvement can occur in these large cell lymphomas or may be concomitant with a systemic lymphoma not otherwise involving the eye. These latter lymphomas infiltrating the uvea without retinal involvement can be of any type, but commonly are of a lower grade than those seen within the retina and may disappear with low dose radiotherapy locally or as a result of systemic treatment. They may however recur if the

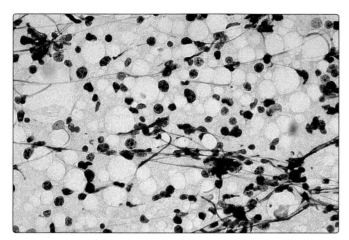

Fig. 44.26   Ocular lymphoma stained with immunocytochemical stain L26 for B lymphoid cells. (L26 × LP)

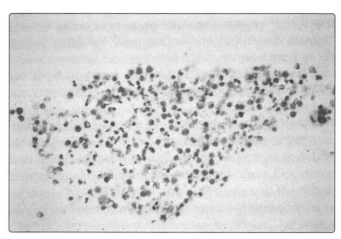

Fig. 44.28   Lymphoma showing the fragility of the cells after cytocentrifugation of material from a vitrectomy specimen. (Giemsa × LP)

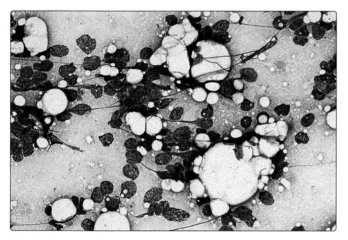

Fig. 44.27   Intraocular high-grade lymphoma. Over 90% of the lymphomas of the eye are B cell. Either MALT or centroblastic centrocytic, the remaining 10% are a mixture of the other types. (Giemsa × HP)

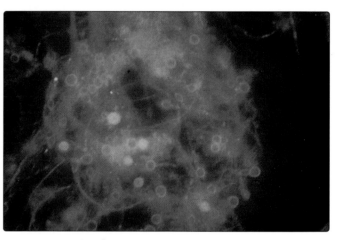

Fig. 44.29   Infective vitreitis. Calcofluor white immunofluorescent demonstration of spores and filaments of *Candida albicans* obtained by vitrectomy, with cytocentrifugation.

tumour recurs systemically or occasionally may be an isolated site of recurrence or relapse.

There has been an apparent rise in incidence of lymphomas involving the retina[71], in parallel with CNS disease, but this may reflect a greater awareness of the disease. An increase as a result of AIDS should also be expected to occur[72]. If the diagnosis of lymphoma is suspected, less rapid cytospin is advised, since the cells are fragile (Fig. 44.28) and may fragment. Light chain restriction and monoclonality can be demonstrated in some immunoblastic[73], plasmacytoid or small cell lesions. Others are lymphoblastic or undifferentiated and show restriction clearly, although their B-cell lineage can usually be demonstrated by immunocytochemistry.

Microbiological diagnosis of organisms by calcofluor white staining and subsequent immunofluorescent microscopy (Fig. 44.29) is a useful auxilliary technique in differential diagnosis of an inflammatory vitritis.

Orbital cytology

Orbital FNA, it is emphasized, requires a detailed knowledge of the anatomy, otherwise open biopsy is preferable to avoid the risk of haemorrhage and damage to the optic nerve. Nevertheless, especially when dealing with an elderly or frail patient suspected of having metastatic disease, FNA may be the technique of choice.

Some other commonly encountered orbital diagnostic problems may be very difficult to resolve. Even enthusiasts such as Kennerdell admit to problems of insufficient material or lack of distinctive cytological features in inflammatory or lymphoproliferative disease. Nevertheless, some tumours can be diagnosed with ease. These include *meningioma with psammoma bodies*[17,18] and *metastases*[74]. Rosenthal and colleagues[29] list other lesions such as *benign nerve sheath tumours* and *sarcomas* which could be aspirated and diagnosed but which in our practice would usually be approached by orbitotomy and open biopsy or excision.

Whether to use cytopathology or histopathology alone or in combination is a decision that rests entirely on the confidence in respective abilities shared between each surgeon and pathologist concerned in the management of disease at this site.

In addition to the tumours discussed below, the orbit can also be the site of *granulomatous disease* as part of a systemic disease, such as *tuberculosis* or *sarcoidosis*. *Granulomatous (Wegener's) vasculitis* can occur, either as a primary event or by extension from the nose or sinuses and a *foreign body granulomatous response* can be associated with *dermoid cysts*.

Tumours of the orbit

Primary tumours[75–79] of the orbit can arise from the adnexal glands or from the connective tissue of the orbit, which is a mixture of fat, vascular fibrous tissue, cartilage and bone. They can also arise from extraocular muscles, the peripheral nervous system and the optic nerve and its sheath. In addition there can be invasion from adjacent structures such as the sinuses and the sphenoidal ridge. Lymphoid tissue is not a normal component of the orbit in the young but lymphoid aggregates in the lacrimal gland become increasingly frequent with age. There are no lymphatics or lymph nodes behind the orbital septum.

Developmental abnormalities range from *encephaloceles* to small *dermoid cysts* and in addition, *hamartomatous lesions* of the vasculature and venous anomalies are seen. Primary *optic nerve gliomas,* especially in children, have also been regarded as hamartomatous lesions by some authors. These gliomas often produce a massive meningeal hyperplasia, which can sometimes lead to misdiagnosis of a meningioma of the optic nerve sheath. True *meningiomas* do occur in the optic nerve sheath and can also invade the orbit from the cranial cavity and the sphenoid ridge. In addition primary orbital meningioma can also arise within the bones of the orbit. It is important to differentiate these from *psammomatoid ossifying fibroma,* a benign tumour occurring predominantly in young men.

In childhood, the orbit can be the site of several of the small blue-cell tumours of childhood. These include *metastatic neuroblastoma,* invasion of the orbit by *leukaemia* and *lymphomas*[80] and *retinoblastoma.* Primary orbital tumours producing this picture also include primitive tumours classified as *embryonal sarcomas,* not arising in muscle but showing varying degrees of rhabdomyosarcomatous differentiation. These mostly occur in very young children. Extraskeletal *Ewing's tumour* can also present in the orbit. In older children, differentiation towards rhabdomyosarcoma, including the alveolar type, can be seen. *Alveolar soft-part sarcoma* can also present within the orbit as a vascularized mass.

In adults, *liposarcomas* are a source of diagnostic difficulties, often becoming myxoid, whereas in children, aggressive *lipoblastic tumours*[74] may occur. Some of the commonest orbital tumours are benign. These include *pleomorphic adenoma* of the lacrimal gland, *cavernous haemangioma* and *neurofibromas* arising with and without the other stigmata of neurofibromatosis.

Malignant tumours of the lacrimal gland include *lymphomas* and *undifferentiated carcinomas,* but *adenoid cystic carcinoma,* with its inherent propensity to invade along nerve sheaths, is a difficult tumour to treat and occurs predominantly in young patients[82].

Benign tumours
Pleomorphic adenoma

Benign mixed tumours or pleomorphic adenomas of the lacrimal gland usually present as slow growing masses. To obviate the risk of iatrogenic spread around the orbit they should not be biopsied. FNA is usually the diagnostic method of choice as there is no evidence with FNA of the increase in recurrence rate associated with incisional rather than excisional biopsy.

Smears show benign epithelial cells arranged in sheets and a transition to the myxoid stromal elements that separate them[83]. They resemble the pleomorphic adenomas of the salivary gland, described in Chapter 10, as do any of the salivary gland tumour types since all except Warthin's adenolymphoma have been described arising in the lacrimal glands. They may also present within the eyelids as masses within the palpebral lobe, or within accessory lacrimal glands of the conjunctiva, or even as choristomatous masses within the caruncle.

Other benign tumours

Other types of benign tumour arising within the orbit include *nerve sheath tumours* and *haemangiomas.* The former are often easy to diagnose by cytology but in view of the risk of haemorrhage, cavernous haemangiomas are not usually diagnosed in this way, although four cases of diagnosis by FNA have been recorded[84]. We do not advocate using this technique, and similarly feel that other cystic or vascular lesions such as haemangiopericytomas and mucoceles in this site are better diagnosed using excision biopsy and histology. This is especially the case with dermoid cysts, which should be removed in their entirety in order to preclude leakage with an extravagant foreign body reaction to the keratin and sebaceous contents.

Malignant tumours

Secondary metastatic carcinomas and other tumours are relatively common, especially in the elderly, and can be aspirated and diagnosed using immunohistochemistry if required. In addition, a number of primary malignant tumours occur within the orbit.

Malignant epithelial tumours of the lacrimal gland include adenoid cystic carcinoma and the less well-differentiated carcinoma, often presenting in older patients.

Adenoid cystic carcinomas of the lacrimal gland show clusters and single cells often forming rosette like structures, with a distinct basement membrane in the centre, which stains magenta when MGG stain is used[84], but is not demonstrated by either haematoxylin and eosin or Papanicolaou staining.

Meningiomas of the orbit may be primary within the optic nerve or extensions of disease elsewhere, as described above. Cytology shows polygonal or spindle-shaped cells[81,83], with long cytoplasmic processes. The 'empty oval' vacuolated nuclei sometimes seen in CNS histology sections are not usually as apparent on cytology and were not observed by Koss and colleagues in the two tumours they comment on. They did, however, see whorls on aspiration cytology. Psammoma bodies are not as frequent in sphenoidal ridge meningiomas within the orbit as they are within the optic nerve sheath and primary CNS tumours. In the reactive meningeal hyperplasia associated with optic nerve gliomas they are variable. Secondary

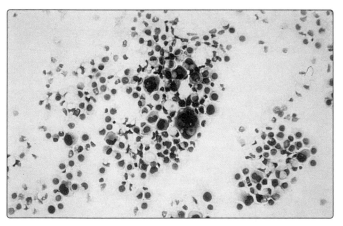

Fig. 44.30 Malignant cells in spun CSF from a case of carcinomatous meningitis due to secondary involvement of the meninges by a lobular carcinoma of the breast diagnosed and treated six years previously. The patient presented with optic nerve compression leading to loss of vision and a decompression was performed. Greenish yellow CSF was aspirated and contained these malignant cells. (Diff-Quik × HP)

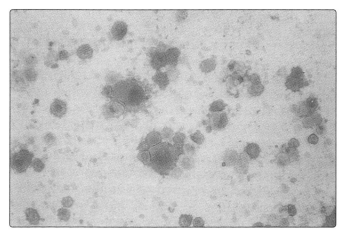

Fig. 44.31 Epithelial membrane antigen (EMA) positivity in malignant cells from the case illustrated in **Fig. 44.30**. (Immunoperoxidase × HP)

involvement of the meninges by metastatic carcinoma 'carcinomatous meningitis', can be diagnosed by aspiration cytology of the cerebrospinal fluid (CSF) from the optic nerve sheath (Figs 44.30, 44.31).

The author has no personal experience with cytological examination of *optic nerve gliomas*, but on histological grounds they fall into two categories. These are predominantly low-grade pilocytic or protoplasmic astrocytoma, producing fusiform swellings of the optic nerve in younger patients; and higher grade, more malignant tumours associated with intracranial disease in middle-aged patients. While the majority of the first group are static, almost hamartomatous lesions, there are those that are more active and will grow along the optic nerve towards the chiasma and compromise vision in the other eye.

Kennerdell reports on aspiration cytology of a malignant glioma[85]. Illustrations usually show histology rather than aspiration cytology[83] although these authors have performed over 100 orbital FNA biopsies. The rarity of optic nerve gliomas means that few authors have the opportunity to study them. Clinical and radiological evidence of increased infiltration of the optic nerve may be a much better indication of the likelihood of continued growth than cytological or histopathological criteria, despite the availability of sophisticated techniques such as nucleolar organizer region (AgNOR) counts or ubiquitin expression (A McCartney, personal observation).

In our centres the diagnosis is usually based on neuroimaging, including nuclear magnetic resonance, reinforced by histopathology if required, but as the vision may remain good, even with a large tumour, biopsy is usually only carried out on aggressive tumours. Excision is often performed for cosmetic reasons rather than to establish the diagnosis.

Lymphomas of the orbit, including *primary lymphoma of the lacrimal gland*, and those arising in association with *conjunctival lymphoma*, are similar to extranodal lymphomas elsewhere, including the thyroid, salivary gland and gut. The techniques used for the differential diagnosis of reactive lymphoid hyperplasia and lymphoma at other sites, discussed in Chapter 20, are appropriate, although T-cell lymphomas are rare, unless in continuity with skin or nasal deposits.

Most of these tumours are of B-cell lineage, and most are *well-differentiated lymphocytic, lymphoplasmacytoid*, or *centrocytic/centroblastic lymphomas* of the types associated with MALT elsewhere. Rarely, and most commonly in the orbit, a higher grade lymphoblastic tumour may occur. These may have a poorer prognosis and tend to spread to involve the abdominal lymph nodes, particularly those at the splenic axis. The diagnosis on cytology depends on the same criteria as elsewhere. A reactive T-cell component and light chain restriction can be diagnosed on immunocytochemistry. Pure *plasma cell tumours* are unusual within the orbit, unless there is widespread myeloma, although IgA producing tumours can occur within the lacrimal gland[69].

Significant amounts of reactive lymphoid tissue can also be associated with *vascular anomalies of the orbit*. These lesions, which are not malignant *per se*, probably represent regional anomalies of control of growth of vessels. They can be extremely disfiguring and show a marked tendency to recur after excision. Although many show signs of having a preponderance of venous vessels within the lesion, often with phleboliths, the number of true 'varices' is limited. Many of the vascular channels have the appearance of lymphatic vessels and are filled with clear fluid and are choristomatous within the orbit. Although there would be no practical reason for them not to be diagnosed by cytology, since they are low pressure lesions, in practice this is not usually required.

Soft tissue tumours within the orbit include small cell lesions of childhood, such as *rhabdomyosarcomas,* which can be diagnosed by aspiration[84] and six cases have been described using techniques developed for other sites[86]. The differential diagnosis of these lesions is wide. Recognition of their malignant nature may be of some help in allowing

initiation of radiotherapy or chemotherapy for these life-threatening tumours. In most instances, the auxilliary techniques of immunohistochemistry and electron microscopy will have to be used, and it is for this reason that we usually suggest open biopsy in our centres if a sarcoma is suspected.

This policy is even more important in adult malignant soft tissue tumours and those occurring later in childhood or adolescence. However, the speed of diagnosis when cytology is used successfully to diagnose other lesions such as metastatic small cell carcinomas, deposits of leukaemic or lymphoma cells or even to establish that the lesion is inflammatory, cannot be gainsaid and the position of orbital cytology seems to be assured for the future.

Conclusion

This chapter represents the author's opinion of the advantages and limitations of the techniques used in the Department over the last 18 years. In particular, the author would like to thank Mr John Hughes for his help with this chapter.

References

1 Bonshek R E. Diagnostic ophthalmic cytopathology – past, present and future. *Cytopathol* 1997; **8**: 363–365

2 McGhee C N J, Lee W R. Quantification and enzymic identification of conjunctival surface mucus. *Trans Ophthalmol Soc UK* 1985; **104**: 446–449

3 Gadomski A M, Kjolhede C L, Wittpenn J *et al.* Conjunctival impression cytology (CIC) to detect subclinical vitamin A deficiency: comparison of CIC with biochemical assessments. *Am J Nutr* 1989; **49**: 495–500

4 Divani S N, Margari C, Zikos A, Papavassilou G B. Diagnostic impression cytology: a simple technique for the diagnosis of external eye disease. *Cytopathol* 1997; **8**(6): 373–380

5 Paridaens A D A, McCartney A C E, Curling O M *et al.* Impression cytology of conjunctival melanosis and melanoma. *Br J Ophthalmol* 1992; **76**: 198–201

6 Maskin S L, Heitman K F, Lawton A W, Yee R W. Diagnostic impression for external eye disease. *Cornea* 1989; **8**: 270–273

7 Nolan G R, Hirst L W, Bancroft B J. Efficacy of a training programme designed to teach cervical smear screeners to identify ocular surface squamous neoplasia using conjunctival impression cytology. *Cytopathol*; 1997; **8**: 388–396

8 Tsubota K, Kajiwara K, Ugajin S, Hasegawa T. Conjunctival brush cytology. *Acta Cytol* 1980; **34**: 233–235

9 Grossniklaus H E. Fine-needle aspiration biopsy of the iris. *Arch Ophthalmol* 1992; **110**: 969–975

10 Char D H, Miller T R. Fine needle biopsy in retinoblastoma. *Am J Ophthalmol* 1984; **97**: 686–690

11 Char D H, Miller T R, Crawford J B. Cytopathological diagnosis of benign lesions simulating choroidal melanomas. *Am J Ophthalmol* 1991; **112**: 70–75

12 Ausburger J J, Shields J A, Folberg R *et al.* Fine needle aspiration biopsy in the diagnosis of intraocular cancer. *Ophthalmology* 1985; **92**: 39–49

13 Ausburger J J. Fine needle aspiration biopsy of suspected metastatic cancers to the posterior uvea. *Trans Am Ophthalmol Soc* 1988; **86**: 499–560

14 Jakobiec F A, Coleman D J, Chattock A, Smith M. Ultrasonically guided biopsy and cytologic diagnosis of solid intraocular tumors. *Ophthalmol* 1979; **86**: 1662–1678

15 Jakobiec F A, Chattock A. The role of cytology and needle biopsies in the diagnosis of ophthalmic tumors and simulating conditions. In: Jakobiec FA, ed. Ocular and adnexal tumors. Birmingham, AL: Aesculapius 1978; 341–358

16 Czerniak B, Woyke S, Domagala W, Krysztolik Z. Fine needle aspiration cytology of intraocular malignant melanoma. *Acta Cytol* 1981; **27**: 157–165

17 Kennerdell J S, Dekker A, Johnson B L, Dubois P J. Fine needle aspiration biopsy: its use in orbital tumors. *Arch Ophthalmol* 1979; **97**: 1315–1317

18 Tijl J W A, Koorneef L. Fine needle aspiration biopsy in orbital tumours. *Br J Ophthalmol* 1991; **75**: 491–492

19 Green W R. Diagnostic cytopathology of ocular fluid specimens. *Ophthalmol* 1984; **91**: 726–749

20 Engel H M, Green W R, Michels R G *et al.* Diagnostic vitrectomy. *Retina* 1981; **1**: 121–149

21 Das D, Das J, Chachra K L, Natarajan R. Diagnosis of retinoblastoma by fine needle aspiration and aqueous cytology. *Diagn Cytopathol* 1989; **5**: 203–206

22 Stevenson K E, Hungerford J L, Garner A. Local extraocular extension of retinoblastoma following intraocular surgery. *Br J Ophthalmol* 1989; **73**: 739–742

23 Sen S, Singha U, Kumar H *et al.* Diagnostic intraocular fine needle aspiration biopsy – an experience in three cases of retinoblastoma. *Diagn Cytopathol* 1999; **21**(5): 331–334

24 Frable W J. Needle aspiration biopsy: past, present and future. *Hum Pathol* 1989; **20**: 504–517

25 Gunduz K, Shields J A, Shields C L *et al.* Transscleral choroidal biopsy in the diagnosis of choroidal lymphoma. *Survey Ophthalmol* 1999; **43**(6): 551–555

26 Arora R, Rowar R, Bethavia S M. Fine needle aspiration of orbital and adnexal masses. *Acta Cytol* 1992; **36**: 483–491

27 Mandell D B, Levy J J, Rosenthal D L. Preparation and cytological evaluation of intraocular fluids. *Acta Cytol* 1987; **31**: 150–158

28 Kennerdell J S. Deep fine needle aspiration biopsy. In: Orsoni J G ed. *Ophthalmic Cytopathology.* Proceedings of the First Symposium on Ophthalmic Cytology, Parma, Italy 1987. Universita Degli Studi di Parma 1988; 21–23

29 Rosenthal D L, Mandell D B, Glasgow B J. Eye. In: Bibbo M ed. *Comprehensive Cytopathology.* Philadelphia: WB Saunders, 1991; 484–501

30 Scroggs M W, Johnston W W, Klintworth G K. Intraocular tumors: a cytopathologic study. *Acta Cytol* 1990; **34**: 401–408

31 Midena E, Segato T, Piermarocchi S, Boccato P. Fine needle aspiration biopsy in ophthalmology. *Surv Ophthalmol* 1985; **29**: 410–422

32 Char D H, Ljung M B, Miller T R. Intraocular fine needle biopsy: utility and accuracy. *Ophthalmol* 1987; **96**(suppl): 86

33 Eide N, Syrdalen P, Walaas L, Hagmar B. Fine needle aspiration biopsy in selecting treatment for inconclusive intraocular disease. *Acta Ophthalmol Scand* 1999; **77**: 448–452

34 Scholtz R, Green W R, Baranano E C et al. Metastatic carcinoma to the iris: diagnosis by aqueous paracentesis and response to irradiation and chemotherapy. *Ophthalmol* 1983; **90**: 1524–1527

35 Glasgow B J, Brown H H, Zaragoza A M, Foos R Y. Quantitation of seeding from fine needle aspiration of ocular melanomas. *Am J Ophthalmol* 1988; **105**: 538–546

36 Shields J A, Shields C L, eds. Melanocytic tumors of the iris stroma. In: *Intraocular Tumors: A Text and Atlas*. Philadelphia: WB Saunders, 1992; 61–83

37 Shields J A, Shields C L, Dhya H et al. Atypical retinal astrocytic hamartoma diagnosed by fine needle biopsy. *Ophthalmol* 1996; **103**(6): 949–952

38 Bruner W E, Start W J, Green W R. Presumed juvenile zanthogranuloma of the iris and ciliary body in an adult. *Arch Ophthalmol* 1982; **100**: 457–459

39 Naib Z M. Cytology of ocular lesions. *Acta Cytol* 1972; **16**: 178–185

40 Sanderson T L, Pustai W, Shelly L et al. Cytologic evaluation of ocular lesions. *Acta Cytol* 1980; **24**: 391–400

41 Fischler D F, Prayson R A. Cytologic specimens from the eye: a clinicopathologic study of 33 patients. *Diagn Cytopathol* 1997; **17**(4): 262–266

42 Engel H, de la Cruz, Jimenez-Abalahin B D et al. Cytopreparatory techniques for eye fluid specimens obtained by vitrectomy. *Acta Cytol* 1982; **26**: 551–560

43 Orellana J, Moura R A, Font R L et al. Medulloepithelioma diagnosed by ultrasound and vitreous aspirate: electron microscopic observations. *Ophthalmol* 1983; **90**: 1531–1539

44 Machemer R, Parel J M, Buettner H. A new concept for vitreous surgery, Part 1. *Am J Ophthalmol* 1972; **73**: 1–7

45 Paerl R, Machemer R, Aumayr W. A new concept for vitreous surgery part 4. *Am J Ophthalmol* 1974; **77**: 6–12

46 Schneiderman T S, Faber D W, Gross J G et al. The agar-albumin sandwich technique for processing retinal biopsy specimens. *Am J Ophthalmol* 1989; **108**: 567–571

47 Hiscott P S, Frierson I, Trombetta C J et al. Retinal and epiretinal glia: an immunohistochemical study. *Br J Ophthalmol* 1984; **68**: 698–707

48 Solanki P, Ramzy I, Durr N. Pilomatrixoma: cytologic features and differential diagnostic considerations. *Arch Pathol Lab Med* 1987; **111**: 294–297

49 Sadeghi S, Pitman M B, Weir M M. Cytologic features of metastatic sebaceous carcinoma: report of two cases with comparison to three cases of basal cell carcinoma. *Diagn Cytopathol* 1999; **21**(5): 340–345

50 Levinson R D, Hooks J J, Wang Y et al. Triple viral retinitis diagnosed by polymerase chain reaction of the vitreous biopsy in a patient with Richter syndrome. *Am J Ophthalmol* 1998; **126**(5): 732–733

51 Thiel M A, Bossart W, Bernauer W. Clinical evaluation of impression cytology in diagnosis of superficial viral infections. *Klin Monatsbl Augenheilkd* 1998; **212**(5): 388–391

52 Sapci T, Gurdal C, Onmus H et al. Diagnostic significance of impression cytology in allergic rhinoconjunctivitis. *Am J Rhinol* 1999; **13**(1): 31–35

53 Baudouin C, Brignole F, Becquet F et al. Flow cytometry in impression cytology specimens: a new method for evaluation of conjunctival inflammation. *Invest Ophthalmol Vis Sci* 1997; **38**(7): 1458–1464

54 Kobayashi T K, Tsubota K. Cytologic evaluation of dry eye by brushing procedure: value of slide preparation by ThinPrep technique. *Rinsho Byori* 1998; **46**(6): 223–228

55 Danjo Y, Watanabe H, Tisdale A S et al. Alteration of mucin in human conjunctival epithelia in dry eye. *Invest Ophthalmol Vis Sci* 1998; **39**(13): 2602–2609

56 McCullough F S, Northrop-Clewes C A, Thurnham D I. The effect of vitamin A on epithelial integrity. *Proc Nutr Soc* 1999; **58**(2): 289–293

57 Tsubota K, Fujihara T, Saito K, Takeuchi T. Conjunctival epithelium expression of HLA-DR in dry eye patients. *Ophthalmol* 1999; **213**(1): 16–19

58 Singh M, Singh G, Dwevedi K et al. Conjunctival impression cytology in xerophthalmia among rural children. *Indian J Ophthalmol* 1997; **45**(1): 26–29

59 Keenum D G, Semba R D, Wirasasmita S et al. Assessment of vitamin A status by a disc applicator for conjunctival impression cytology. *Arch Ophthalmol* 1990; **108**: 1436–1441

60 Gilbert J M, Weiss J S, Sattler A L, Koch J M. Ocular manifestations and impression cytology of anorexia nervosa. *Ophthalmol* 1990; **97**: 1001–1007

61 Butrus S I, Abelson M B. Laboratory evaluation of ocular allergy. *Ophthalmol Clin* 1988; **28**: 324–328

62 Ozkan S B, Soylev M F, Gahapoglu H et al. Evaluation of conjunctival morphology in thyroid associated eye disease by use of impression cytology. *Acta Ophthalmol Scand* 1997; 145–147

63 Karayianis S, Genack L, Lundergan M, Schumann G B. Cytological diagnosis of acanthamoebic keratitis. *Acta Cytol* 1988; **32**: 491–494

64 Desai A P, Pandit A A, Gupte P D. Cutaneous blastomycosis. Report of a case with diagnosis by fine needle aspiration cytology. *Acta Cytol* 1997; **41**: 1317–1319

65 Brown H H, Glasgow B J, Holland G N, Foos R Y. Keratinising corneal intraepithelial neoplasia. *Cornea* 1989; **8**: 220–224

66 Tseng S-H, Chen Y-T, Huang F-C, Jin Y-T. Seborrheic keratosis of conjunctiva simulating a malignant melanoma: an immunocytochemical study with impression cytology. *Ophthalmol* 1999; **1906**(8): 1516–1520

67 McCartney A C E. Intraocular metastasis. *Br J Ophthalmol* 1993; **77**: 133 (Editorial)

68 Rosenthal D L. Cytology of the central nervous system. In: Weil G L ed. *Monographs in Clinical Cytology*. Basel: S Karger 1984

69 McCartney A C E. Intraocular epithelial tumours and cysts. In: Klintworth G K and Garner A eds. *Pathobiology and Pathophysiology of Ocular Disease*. New York: Marcel Dekker, 1993

70 Martinez F, Merenda G, Bedrossian C W. Lipid-rich metastatic melanoma: diagnosis by a multimodal approach to aspiration biopsy cytology. *Diagn Cytopathol* 1990; **6**: 427–433

71 McCartney A C E, Blackwood W. Intraocular lymphomas: a rising tide? *Neuropath Appl Neurobiol* 1989; **15**: 589

72 Hofman P, Le Toureau A, Negre F et al. Primary uveal immunoblastic lymphoma in a patient with AIDS. *Br J Ophthalmol* 1992; **76**: 700–702

73 Char D H, Ljung B M, Deschenes J, Miller T R. Intraocular lymphoma; immunological and cytological analysis. *Br J Ophthalmol* 1988; **72**: 905–911

74 Logrono R, Inhorne S L, Dortzbach R K, Kurtycz D F. Leiomyosarcoma metastatic to the orbit: diagnosis by fine needle aspiration. *Diagn Cytopathol* 1997; **17**: 369–373

75 Westman-Naeser S, Naeser P. Tumours of the orbit diagnosed by fine needle biopsy. *Acta Ophthalmol* 1978; **56**: 969–976

76 Scolyer R A, Painter D M, Harper C G, Lee C S. Hepatocellular carcinoma to the orbit diagnosed by fine needle aspiration cytology. *Pathology* 1999; **31**(4): 350–353

77 Mehrotra R, Kumar S, Singh K et al. Fine needle aspiration biopsy of orbital meningioma. *Diagn Cytopathol* 1999; **21**(6): 402–404

78 Siddens J D, Fishman J R, Jackson I T et al. Primary orbital angiosarcoma: a case report. *Ophthalmic Plast Recon Surg* 1999; **15**: 454–459

79 Gupta S, Sood B, Gulati M et al. Orbital mass lesions: US-guided fine needle. *Radiol* 1999; **213**(2): 568–672

80 De Smet M D, Vancs V S, Kohler D et al. Intravitreal chemotherapy for the treatment of recurrent intraocular lymphoma. *Br J Ophthalmol* 1999; **83**: 448–451

81 Cristallini E G, Bolis G B, Ottaviano P. Fine needle aspiration biopsy of meningioma: report of a case. *Acta Cytol* 1990; **34**: 236–238

82 McCartney A C E. Tumours of the eye and adnexae. In: Fletcher C M ed. *Diagnostic Pathology of Tumours*. Edinburgh: Churchill Livingstone, 1993

83 Koss L G, Woyke S, Olszewski ??, eds.
    The orbit and the eye globe. In: *Aspiration
    Biopsy*, New York: Igaku-Shoin, 1992;
    659–678

84 Glasgow B J and Foos R Y. *Ocular
    Cytopathology*. Boston: Butterworth-
    Heinemann, 1993; 132

85 Kennerdell J S, Dubois P J, Dekker A,
    Johnson B. CT guided aspiration cytology of
    orbital optic nerve tumors. *Ophthalmol* 1980;
    97: 491–496

86 De Jong A S H, can Kessel-can Vark M, van
    Heerde P. Fine needle aspiration diagnosis of

    rhabdomyosarcoma. *Acta Cytol* 1987;
    31: 573–557

87 Zeppa P, Tranfa F, Errico ME, Troncone G,
    Fulciniti F *et al*. Fine-needle aspiration (FNA)
    biopsy of orbital masses: a critical review of
    51 cases. *Cytopathol* 1997; **8**: 366–372

Index

Page numbers in *italics* indicate figures: those in **bold** indicate tables
vs. denotes differential diagnoses, or comparisons
This index is in letter-by-letter order whereby spaces and hyphens between words are ignored in the alphabetization e.g. 'keratinization' precedes 'keratin pearls.' Terms in parentheses are also excluded from alphabetization.

To save space in the index, certain abbreviations have been used
AgNOR: silver staining nucleolar organizer regions
CGIN: cervical glandular intraepithelial neoplasia
CIN: cervical intraepithelial neoplasia
CNS: central nervous system
CSF: cerebrospinal fluid
FNA: fine needle aspiration

HCC: hepatocellular carcinoma
H&E: haematoxylin and eosin stain
MGG stain: May-Grünwald-Giemsa stain
PAS stain: periodic acid-Schiff stain
RCC: renal cell carcinoma

A

abortion, abnormal endometrial shedding 778, *778*, 826, *827*
abscess
  amoebic 380
  breast 259, *259*, 274
  CNS 958, *958*
  pancreatic 431
  perinephric 452, *452*
  pyogenic *see* pyogenic abscess
  subareolar 260
Acanthamoeba culbertsoni, in CSF in CNS inflammation 947
acanthamoebic keratitis 984
acanthosis, clear cell (glycogenic) 338
acinar cell(s) 306
  breast aspirate 248
    fibroadenoma in pregnancy 275
  sialadenosis 307, *308*
acinar cell carcinoma *see* pancreatic tumours
acinar epithelium, pancreas 429, *429*
acinar formations, in adenocarcinomas 156
acinic cell carcinoma (salivary gland) 312–313, *313*, 317
  differential diagnosis 313
  growth patterns 312–313, *313*
  sialadenosis 307, *308*
acoustic neuroma 967–968
acquired immunodeficiency syndrome (AIDS) *see* HIV infection
acquired melanosis with atypia, conjunctiva/cornea 984–985
acrosome reaction assay, sperm function tests 646
Acta Cytologica 6
actinomyces organisms
  staining 680–681
    Jones-Marres silver stain 681
  vaginal 679–682, **681**
    cytological findings *680,* 680–682
actinomycosis
  conjunctiva/cornea 984
  endometrial inflammation 829

oesophageal brush smears 334
oesophageal infection 336
pneumonia 28, *28*
pyogenic abscess 379
reactive lymphadenopathy 510
sulphur granules 259
activation markers
  kidney graft rejection 556
  liver graft rejection 557–558
active suppurative lymphadenitis, reactive lymphadenopathy 507
acute cellular rejection, kidney graft rejection 555
acute lymphoblastic leukaemia (ALL), CSF *949*
acute myeloid leukaemia (AML) *see* leukaemia, acute myeloid
acute pancreatitis *see* pancreatitis
acute respiratory distress syndrome (ARDS) 55, 89, 92
acute tubular necrosis (ATN), kidney graft rejection 555
acute vascular rejection (AVR), kidney graft rejection 555–556
Addison's disease 606, **607**
adenocarcinoid tumours 98
adenocarcinoma 76
  adenoid cystic, of cervix 782–783, *783*
  Bartholin's gland 816–817
  basal cell 311
  biliary tract *see* biliary tract adenocarcinoma
  breast *see under* breast carcinoma
  bronchioloalveolar *see* bronchioloalveolar adenocarcinoma
  bronchogenic *see* bronchogenic adenocarcinoma
  cell markers 138–139
  cervical *see under* cervical carcinoma
  clear cell, of cervix 781–782
  clumping of cells 155, *159*
  colon *see* large intestine
  differential diagnosis
    bile duct cystadenocarcinoma *vs.* 396–397
    Burkitt's lymphoma *vs.* 861

cervical malignant melanoma *vs.* 808
cervical neuroendocrine carcinoma *vs.* 804
cervical repair/regeneration *vs.* 801
chloroma *vs.* 861
chronic pancreatitis *vs.* 431
dyskaryosis (cervical) cells *vs.* 740
germ cell tumours *vs.* 861
granulosa cell tumours (ovary) *vs.* 861
low-grade CGIN *vs.* 773, *774*
mesothelial cells *vs.* 138–139, 140
mesothelioma *vs. see* mesothelioma
microglandular endocervical hyperplasia *vs.* 795
ovarian *vs.* gastrointestinal (immunocytochemistry) 194–195
ductal (endometrioid) of prostate 624–625
endocervical *see* endocervical adenocarcinoma
endometrial *see* endometrial carcinoma
extrauterine *see* extrauterine adenocarcinoma
fallopian tubes 856
gall bladder 418–419
immunocytochemistry 74, 189, 191, 861
  ascitic fluid *187, 188*
  mesothelioma *vs. see* mesothelioma
  ovarian *vs.* gastrointestinal 194–195
  pericardial fluid *186*
  pleural fluid *190*
intracytoplasmic neutral mucin 158
large intestine *see* large intestine
lung, CNS metastasis *951*
lymph node metastases 530–531, *531*
mesothelial cell hyperplasia *vs.* **155**, 159
  immunocytochemistry 188–192
morphological features of cells
  in serous fluids 155, **155**, *159,* 159–162, *160, 161*
  see also pleural fluid
mucin-negative 158
mucin staining 158, *161*
oesophagus *see* oesophagus
ovarian, mesotheliomas *vs.* 221
pancreas *see* pancreatic ductal adenocarcinoma
pelvic lesion FNA 861